医学略語コンパクト

第2版

A Collection of Medical Abbreviations, Acronyms & Symbols
2nd Edition

監修　富野 康日己

医歯薬出版株式会社

This book was originally published in Japanese
under the title of:

IGAKURYAKUGO KONPAKUTO

(A Collection of Medical Abbreviations, Acronyms & Symbols)

Editor:

TOMINO, Yasuhiko
Professor Emeritus, Juntendo University Faculty of Medicine

ISHIYAKU PUBLISHERS, INC.
7-10, Honkomagome 1 chome, Bunkyo-ku,
Tokyo 113-8612, Japan

第２版の序

本書「医学略語コンパクト」は，略語が正しく理解されなかったためにインシデントやアクシデントにつながった事例が少なくなかったことや，同じ略語であっても担当する分野によってはまったく異なった意味をもつことなどから略語の正しい理解を目指し上梓されました．初版の序には，「略語を医学系のあらゆる分野から抽出し，おのおの略語に対応する欧文とその日本語表記を記載することで，略語の意味するところを簡潔に引けるようにしたいと考えたからです．また，略語逆引き用の用語一覧を設け，逆引きを可能にした点も本書の特徴のひとつです」と述べました．

本書は，これまで医療に携わる多くの医療関連職従事者や学生に広く活用されてきたばかりか，医療事故の捜査等にかかわっている刑事や弁護士の方々にも利用されていることを知り，監修者として大変嬉しく思っています．しかし，初版の発行からすでに12年が経過しました．この間の基礎・臨床医学の進歩は目覚ましく，iPS（induced pluripotent stem cell）やAI（artificial intelligence）の発見・発明に代表されるように大きな発展を遂げています．また，臨床工学や電子工学などの分野でも新たな略語が数多く登場してきています．そのような新しい略語を収載するとともに，初版の趣旨を活かしながら内容を再検討し，ここに第2版として刊行することになりました．

本書（第2版）も医学関連分野の学生・研究者や医療スタッフの皆さんの勉学や日常診療・業務に生かしていただければ，望外の喜びです．しかし，まだまだ内容の不備な点や過不足もあろうかと思いますので，忌憚のないご意見をお寄せいただければ幸いです．

最後に，初版の作成にご協力いただきました順天堂大学医学部腎臓内科学講座の仲間たちを中心とする編集委員会スタッフに，また第2版刊行にあたり，ご尽力いただきました遠山邦男氏をはじめとする医歯薬出版の関係各位に厚く御礼申し上げます．

2018年　中秋　東京都庁を眺めつつ

富野 康日己

序

最近，日常会話のなかでも自分勝手に作ったと思われる用語や略語が氾濫し，とまどうことが少なくありません．このことは医療の現場であっても例外ではなく，よくみられる現象といえます．近年，大きな社会問題となっている医療事故のなかに，あるいは大きな事故までにはいたらないまでも「ヒヤリ・ハット」事項のなかには，記載が不十分であったり，略語が正しく理解されなかったために起こった事例も少なくないと思われます．

用語の正しい理解は，医学関係の学生のみならず，医師，歯科医師，看護師，薬剤師，臨床検査技師，放射線技師，臨床工学技士，介護福祉士など，医療に携わる多くの医療関連職従事者にとっても必須と思われます．また製薬会社の医療情報担当者（MR）にも資格試験が実施されており，医学用語や略語を学習する必要性に迫られています．

そこで今回，私が浅学非才の身をかえりみず「医学略語コンパクト」を監修した意図は，略語を医学系のあらゆる分野から抽出し，おのおの略語に対応する欧文とその日本語表記を記載することで，略語の意味するところを簡潔に引けるようにしたいと考えたからです．また，略語逆引き用の用語一覧を設け，「逆引き」を可能にした点も本書の特徴のひとつです．さらに判型も類書に比べてコンパクトにすることで，いつも手元においてすぐに確認できるようにと考えました．編集方針は後述されていますのでご一読ください．

本書を学生諸君や医療関連職従事者の皆さんの勉学や日常診療に生かしていただければ，監修者として望外の喜びです．しかし，まだまだ内容の不備な点や過不足があろうかと思われますので，忌憚のないご意見をお寄せいただければ幸いです．

最後に，本書の編集に協力していただいた順天堂大学医学部腎臓内科学講座の仲間たちと医歯薬出版の関係各位に厚く御礼申し上げます．

2006 年　盛春　神田川のほとりにて

富野 康日己

【監修者紹介】

富野（とみの） 康日己（やすひこ）

1974年　順天堂大学医学部卒業
　　　　市立札幌病院中央検査科病理部臨床修練医

1979年　東海大学医学部内科助手

1984年　同　講師

1986年　オーストラリアロイヤルアデレード病院客員研究生

1987年　アメリカミネソタ大学客員講師

1988年　順天堂大学医学部腎臓内科助教授

1994年　順天堂大学医学部腎臓内科教授

2015年　順天堂大学名誉教授
　　　　医療法人社団松和会常務理事・
　　　　アジア太平洋腎研究推進室長

主な編著書：

「尿検査のみかた，考えかた」（中外医学社）2018.

「よくわかる透析療法」（中外医学社）2011.

「メディカルスタッフのための医療禁忌なるほどブック」（中外医学社）2018.

「歯科医が押さえておきたい生活習慣病Q＆A」（デンタルダイアモンド社）2018.

「NEW エッセンシャル腎臓内科学　第2版」（医歯薬出版）2015.

他

制作スタッフ

青木（あおき）　晶子（しょうこ）

岡田（おかだ）　麻矢子（まやこ）

田中（たなか）　梨恵（りえ）

金澤（かなざわ）　哲郎（てつろう）

行方（なめかた）　誠二（せいじ）

松岡（まつおか）　優（ゆたか）

デザイン

Miyake Design

制作統括

遠山（とおやま）　邦男（くにお）

医学略語コンパクト 第1版　編集委員会

＊所属は刊行時の所属を示します

監　修

とみの　やすひこ
富野　康日己
順天堂大学医学部腎臓内科　教授

編　集

おさだ　しをり
長田　しをり
順天堂大学医学部腎臓内科　講師

ひしき　としまさ
菱木　俊匡
順天堂大学医学部腎臓内科　講師

くるす　あつし
来栖　厚
順天堂大学医学部腎臓内科　講師

すずき　ゆうすけ
鈴木　祐介
順天堂大学医学部腎臓内科　講師

しょう　いちゆう
彰　一祐
順天堂大学医学部腎臓内科　講師

はやし　かよ
林　佳代
順天堂大学医学部腎臓内科　講師

こでら　さんき
小寺　三喜
順天堂大学医学部腎臓内科

せきづか　けいこ
関塚　桂子
順天堂大学医学部腎臓内科　講師

つげ　としなお
柘植　俊直
順天堂大学医学部腎臓内科

いのうえ　さなえ
井上　早苗
順天堂大学医学部腎臓内科

かねこ　しょうご
金子　松五
順天堂大学医学部腎臓内科

しけ　としひで
四家　敏秀
順天堂大学医学部腎臓内科

かなまる　ゆたか
金丸　裕
順天堂大学医学部腎臓内科

たけだ　ゆきひこ
武田　之彦
順天堂大学医学部腎臓内科

こばた　まみ
小幡　麻美
順天堂大学医学部腎臓内科

ごうだ　ともひと
合田　朋仁
順天堂大学医学部腎臓内科

こばやし　のりよし
小林　則善
順天堂大学医学部腎臓内科

いお　ひろあき
井尾　浩章
順天堂大学医学部腎臓内科

まえだ　あつこ
前田　敦子
順天堂大学医学部腎臓内科

あさぬま　かつひこ
浅沼　克彦
順天堂大学医学部腎臓内科

しみず　あゆみ
清水　あゆみ
順天堂大学医学部腎臓内科

しいな　けんじ
椎名　健二
順天堂大学医学部腎臓内科

凡　例

編集方針

略語をアルファベット順に並べ，おのおのの略語に対応する欧文とその日本語表記を記載した．その際の表記はできるかぎり簡略化し，一略語一表記を基本的原則として対照させることで，簡潔に引け，略語の意味するところを理解できることを目指した．

医学用語，病名，症候群名などの日本語表記については，可能な限り一般的な用語を平易に表記して収載したつもりである．

全体的には，医師，歯科医師に限らず，医科ならびに歯科の学生，そのほか看護，薬学など，医療関連職従事者の方々にも，簡便・明解に利用してもらうことを第一義としている．

なお巻末には，日本語表記を50音順に並べた索引方式の用語一覧も収載し，「逆引き」を可能とすることで，よりいっそうの便宜を図っている．

ただし，収載した略語は，あらゆる分野で通用するというような普遍性を保持するものではなく，ある特定分野でのみ通用している場合もあるため，無条件で用いてよいというものではない．初出時にフルスペルを提示してから使用すべきである．

略　語

1．略語の配列は，アルファベット順に配列した．また，略語が小文字・大文字の組み合わせにより何種類もある場合における，表記の順序に優先順位はないものとした．

2．ギリシャ文字は，英語読みにした場合の頭文字で対応させたアルファベットで記載している（**表 1**）．ただし，略語や単位記号として使用されていない「文字」としてのギリシャ文字は掲載していない．また，ギリシャ文字は欧文ではなるべく英語表記のフルスペルで表示するが，日本語読みにおいては，ギリシャ文字にて表示した．

3．アルファベットに付属する記号については，シフト JIS コードに準拠し並べた．

欧　文

1．「,」で区切られた欧文が 2 種類以上あるものは，原則として用語の区切りを意味する．

2．欧文の末尾に付属している〈〉は，その欧文言語の種類を示す．また，その後につく「＝」で，英語表記があるものは，その表記を記した．言語区分は下記のとおりとする．
〈独〉＝ドイツ語，〈ラ〉＝ラテン語，〈伊〉＝イタリア語，
〈西〉＝スペイン語，〈仏〉＝フランス語，〈ギ〉＝ギリシャ語

3．イタリック表記になっているものは，ラテン語の表記と，真菌・細菌などの属名等であることを意味する．

4．多剤併用療法における抗癌剤を並列した欧文において，一般名と固有商品名が混在されている場合は，一般名を優先

表1　ギリシャ文字の欧文アルファベット対応一覧

ギリシャ文字		読み	スペル	アルファベット
大文字	小文字			
A	α	アルファ	alpha	A
B	β	ベータ，ビータ	beta	B
X	χ	カイ	chi	C
Δ	δ	デルタ	delta	D
E	ε	エプシロン，イプシロン	epsilon	E
H	η	エータ・イータ	eta	E
Γ	γ	ガンマ	gamma	G
I	ι	イオタ	iota	I
K	κ	カッパ	kappa	K
Λ	λ	ラムダ	lambda	L
M	μ	ミュー	mu	M
N	ν	ニュー	nu	N
O	o	オミクロン	omicron	O
Ω	ω	オメガ	omega	O
Φ	ϕ	ファイ	phi	P
Π	π	パイ	pi	P
Ψ	ψ	プサイ，サイ	psi	P
P	ρ	ロー	rho	R
Σ	σ	シグマ	sigma	S
T	τ	タウ	tau	T
Θ	θ	テータ，シータ	theta	T
Υ	υ	ウプシロン，ユプシロン	upsilon	U
Ξ	ξ	ザイ，グザイ	xi	X
Z	ζ	ゼータ，ジータ	zeta	Z

的に掲載することを原則とした．ただし，略語となっているアルファベットの頭文字と薬剤名の頭文字が必ずしも整合しないことがあるため，対象欧文の単語に（＝　）を付随させたうえで，商品名もしくは一般名の別名をフルスペル，もしくは略語で表記した．

日本語表記

1．「,」で区切られた語句が2種類以上あるものは，原則として用語の区切りを意味する．
2．1つの用語のなかで使われている（　）は，挿入しても意味に違いがない，または挿入・付随してもしなくても可能である語句を表す．
3．反対に〔　〕は，すぐ前の語句と言い換えが可能なものとする．言い換える語句の文字数が多い場合，または語句の区切りが不明瞭な場合は「,」で区切った並列表示を原則としている．
4．化学物質などをカタカナ読みする場合は，おおむね原則として，小社発行の「最新医学大辞典 第3版」に準拠した．
5．人名のつなぎは「・」とした．
6．末尾の《 》は，その用語の所属する分野等を表す（**表2**）．
7．末尾の〈 〉は，
〈単数〉＝その単語が単数であることを意味する．
〈複数〉＝その単語が複数であることを意味する．
〈接〉＝接頭語

表 2　分野表記略称一覧

《処》	=	処方用語
《コン》	=	コンピュータ用語
《医コン》	=	医用コンピュータ用語
《医情》	=	医用情報処理用語
《医教》	=	医用教育語
《心外》	=	心臓外科用語
《電顕》	=	電子顕微鏡用語
《画診》	=	画像診断用語
《リハ》	=	リハビリテーション用語
《超音波》	=	超音波診断用語
《脳波》	=	脳波用語
《心電》	=	心電図用語
《麻酔》	=	麻酔用語
《臨心》	=	臨床心理学用語
《統計》	=	統計学用語
《化学》	=	化学
《眼》	=	眼，眼科学
《遺伝》	=	遺伝学
《検査》	=	検査
《産婦》	=	産科・婦人科
《循環》	=	循環
《神経》	=	神経
《心理》	=	心理
《電磁》	=	電磁
《放射》	=	放射
《法医》	=	法医学用語
《ウイルス》	=	ウイルス学用語

〈元素〉＝元素に分類されることを意味する．元素については，すべての元素記号を略語として掲載しているわけではない．資料として元素表を収載（xxvii 頁）したので参照されたい．

〈単位〉＝単位に関する用語であることを意味する．

[国名]は欧文に国名が明記されていない場合の所属国を表す．

8．文末につく(属)は，真菌・細菌などの属を意味する．

9．(＝○○）は，その用語の説明，省略した表現方法など別の言い方で同じ意味を示すもの，または略語の別表記などを示す．

10．団体名等については，可能なかぎり正式名称の記載に努めたが，日本語表記の多様さから完全に把握・網羅できていない場合もある．また，収載の原則としては，なるべく医学関連を中心としたが，例外として汎用度が高いと思われる団体・機関名も載せている．

表 3　国際単位（SI）系基本単位

単位記号	SI 単位の名称	物理量
A	アンペア	電　流
cd	カンデラ	光　度
K	ケルビン	熱力学温度
kg	キログラム	質　量
m	メートル	長　さ
mol	モル	物質量
s	秒	時　間

表 4　国際単位(SI)系組立単位の例

SI 組立単位		組立て量
記　号	名　称	
A/m	アンペア毎メートル	磁場の強さ
A/m^2	アンペア毎平方メートル	電流密度
cd/m^2	カンデラ毎平方メートル	輝　度
kg/m^3	キログラム毎立方メートル	密　度
m^{-1}	毎メートル	波　数
m^2	平方メートル	面　積
m^3	立方メートル	体　積
m^3/kg	立方メートル毎キログラム	比体積
m/s	メートル毎秒	速　度
m/s^2	メートル毎平方秒	加速度
mol/m^3	モル毎立方メートル	濃度(物質の)*

* 通常，生化学ではモル濃度はモル/リットルが用いられるが，SI 単位系の正式な濃度の単位はモル/立方メートルである．モル/リットルは mol/dm^3 であり，mol/m^3 より 1,000 倍濃い

表5 固有の名称をもつ SI 組立単位

記号	欧文	名称	組立てられる量	他の SI 単位による表現	SI 基本単位による表現
Bq	becquerel	ベクレル	放射能		s^{-1}
C	coulomb	クーロン	電荷, 電気量		$s \cdot A$
F	farad	ファラド	電気容量	C/V	$m^{-2} \cdot kg^{-1} \cdot s^4 \cdot A^2$
Gy	gray	グレイ	吸収線量	J/kg	$m^2 \cdot s^{-2}$
H	henry	ヘンリー	インダクタンス	Wb/A	$m^2 \cdot kg \cdot s^{-2} \cdot A^{-2}$
Hz	hertz	ヘルツ	振動数		s^{-1}
J	joule	ジュール	エネルギー, 仕事, 熱量	N・m	$m^2 \cdot kg \cdot s^{-2}$
lm	lumen	ルーメン	光　束	cd・sr	$m^2 \cdot m^{-2} \cdot cd = cd$
lx	lux	ルクス	照　度	lm/m^2	$m^2 \cdot m^{-4} \cdot cd = m^{-2} \cdot cd$
N	newton	ニュートン	力		$m \cdot kg \cdot s^{-2}$
Pa	pascal	パスカル	圧力, 応力	N/m^2	$m^{-1} \cdot kg \cdot s^{-2}$
rad	radian	ラジアン	平面角		$m \cdot m^{-1} = 1$
S	siemens	ジーメンス	コンダクタンス	A/V	$m^{-2} \cdot kg^{-1} \cdot s^3 \cdot A^2$
sr	steradian	ステラジアン	立体角		$m^2 \cdot m^{-2} = 1$
Sv	sievert	シーベルト	線量当量	J/kg	$m^2 \cdot s^{-2}$
T	tesla	テスラ	磁束密度	Wb/m^2	$kg \cdot s^{-2} \cdot A^{-1}$
V	volt	ボルト	電圧, 電位, 起電力	W/A	$m^2 \cdot kg \cdot s^{-3} \cdot A^{-1}$
W	watt	ワット	仕事率, 放射束	J/S	$m^2 \cdot kg \cdot s^{-3}$
Wb	weber	ウェーバ	磁　束	V・s	$m^2 \cdot kg \cdot s^{-2} \cdot A^{-1}$
℃	degree centigrade, Celsius scale	セルシウス度	セルシウス温度		K
Ω	ohm	オーム	電気抵抗	V/A	$m^2 \cdot kg \cdot s^{-3} \cdot A^{-2}$

表 6　国際単位(SI)系接頭語とその記号

記号	接頭語	読み	大きさ
Y	yotta	ヨタ	10^{24}
Z	zetta	ゼタ	10^{21}
E	exa	エクサ	10^{18}
P	peta	ペタ	10^{15}
T	tera	テラ	10^{12}
G	giga	ギガ	10^{9}
M	mega	メガ	10^{6}
k	kilo	キロ	10^{3}
h	hecto	ヘクト	10^{2}
da	deca	デカ	10
d	deci	デシ	10^{-1}
c	centi	センチ	10^{-2}
m	milli	ミリ	10^{-3}
μ	micro	マイクロ	10^{-6}
n	nano	ナノ	10^{-9}
p	pico	ピコ	10^{-12}
f	femto-	フェムト	10^{-15}
a	atto-	アト	10^{-18}
z	zepto	ゼプト	10^{-21}
y	yocto	ヨクト	10^{-24}

表 7　併用が認められている単位

記　号	欧　文	名　称	SI 単位による値
B	bel	ベル**	1 B＝(1/2) ln 10 (Np)
d	day	日	1 d＝24 h＝86,400 s
h	hour	時　間	1 h＝60 min＝3,600 s
l, L	litre, liter	リットル	1 l＝1 dm^3＝$10^{-3}m^3$
min	minute	分	1 min＝60 s
Np	neper	ネーパー**	1 Np＝1
t	tonne	ト　ン	1 t＝10^3kg
°		度*	1°＝(π/180) rad
′		分	1′＝(1/60)°＝(π/10,800) rad
″		秒	1″＝(1/60)′＝(π/648,000) rad

*　1度より小さい角度の場合，分，秒を用いず十進法により表現することが勧告されている

**　ネーパーは SI 系と一貫性があるが，国際度量衡総会（CGPM）において未承認．ベルの欄において Np を括弧で囲んだのはそのためである．これらの単位を用いる時は，量を指定しておくことが必要である

表 8　CGS 単位の SI 単位系への換算

記号	欧　文	読　み	SI 単位の値
dyn	dyne	ダイン	1 dyn＝10^{-5}N
erg	erg	エルグ	1 erg＝10^{-7}J
G	gauss	ガウス	1 G＝10^{-4}T
Gal	gal	ガル	1 Gal＝1 cm/s^2＝10^{-2}m/s^2
Mx	maxwell	マクスウェル	1 Mx＝10^{-8}Wb
Oe	oersted	エルステッド	1 Oe＝(1000/4 π) A/m
P	poise〈仏〉	ポアズ	1 P＝1 dyn･s/cm^2＝0.1 Pa･s
sb	stilb	スチルブ	1 sb＝1 cd/cm^2＝10^4cd/m^2
St	stokes	ストークス	1 St＝1 cm^2/s＝$10^{-4}m^2$/s
ph	phot	フォト	1 ph (＝1 lm/cm^2)＝10^4lx

表 9　化学物質の命名に使用される数の接頭語

接頭語	数	接頭語	数
hemi-	½	heneicosa-	21
mono-	1	docosa-	22
sesqui-	1 ½	tricosa-	23
di-, bi-	2	tetracosa-	24
hemipenta-	2 ½	pentacosa-	25
tri-	3	hexacosa-	26
tetra-	4	heptacosa-	27
penta-	5	octacosa-	28
hexa-	6	nonacosa-	29
hepta-	7	triaconta-	30
octa-	8	tetraconta-	40
ennea-, nona-	9	pentaconta-	50
deca-	10	hexaconta-	60
hendeca-, undeca-	11	heptaconta-	70
dodeca-	12	octaconta-	80
trideca-	13	nonaconta-	90
tetradeca-	14	hecta-	100
pentadeca-	15	henhecta-	101
hexadeca-	16	dohecta-	102
heptadeca-	17	decahecta-	110
octadeca-	18	eicosahecta-	120
nonadeca-	19	dicta-	200
eicosa-	20		

表 10　4 桁の原子量表（12 C の相対原子量＝12）

元素記号	原子番号	原子量	元素名	
			欧　文	和　名
^{227}Ac	89	227.0	Actinium	アクチニウム
Ag	47	107.9	Silver	銀
Al	13	26.98	Aluminium	アルミニウム
^{243}Am	95	243.1	Americium	アメリシウム
Ar	18	39.95	Argon	アルゴン
As	33	74.92	Arsenic	ヒ素
^{210}At	85	210.0	Astatine	アスタチン
Au	79	197.0	Gold	金
B	5	10.81	Boron	ホウ素
Ba	56	137.3	Barium	バリウム
Be	4	9.012	Beryllium	ベリリウム
Bh	107	(272)	Bohrium	ボーリウム
Bi	83	209.0	Bismuth	ビスマス
^{247}Bk	97	247.1	Berkelium	バークリウム
Br	35	79.90	Bromine	臭素
C	6	12.01	Carbon	炭素
Ca	20	40.08	Calcium	カルシウム
Cd	48	112.4	Cadmium	カドミウム
Ce	58	140.1	Cerium	セリウム
^{252}Cf	98	252.1	Californium	カリホルニウム
Cl	17	35.45	Chlorine	塩素
^{247}Cm	96	247.1	Curium	キュリウム
Cn	112	(285)	Copernicium	コペルニシウム
Co	27	58.93	Cobalt	コバルト
Cr	24	52.00	Chromium	クロム
Cs	55	132.9	Caesium	セシウム
Cu	29	63.55	Copper	銅
Db	105	(268)	Dubnium	ドブニウム

元素記号	原子番号	原子量	元素名	
			欧　文	和　名
Ds	110	(281)	Darmstadtium	ダームスタチウム
Dy	66	162.5	Dysprosium	ジスプロシウム
Er	68	167.3	Erbium	エルビウム
^{252}Es	99	252.1	Einsteinium	アインスタイニウム
Eu	63	152.0	Europium	ユウロピウム
F	9	19.00	Fluorine	フッ素
Fe	26	55.85	Iron	鉄
Fl	114	(289)	Flerovium	フレロビウム
^{257}Fm	100	257.1	Fermium	フェルミウム
^{223}Fr	87	223.0	Francium	フランシウム
Ga	31	69.72	Gallium	ガリウム
Gd	64	157.3	Gadolinium	ガドリニウム
Ge	32	72.59**	Germanium	ゲルマニウム
H	1	1.008	Hydrogen	水素
Hs	108	(277)	Hassium	ハッシウム
He	2	4.003	Helium	ヘリウム
Hf	72	178.5	Hafnium	ハフニウム
Hg	80	200.6	Mercury	水銀
Ho	67	164.9	Holmium	ホルミウム
I	53	126.9	Iodine	ヨウ素
In	49	114.8	Indium	インジウム
Ir	77	192.2	Iridium	イリジウム
K	19	39.10	Potassium〔Kalium〕	カリウム
Kr	36	83.80	Krypton	クリプトン
La	57	138.9	Lanthanum	ランタン
Li	3	6.941*	Lithium	リチウム
^{260}Lr	103	260.1	Lawrencium	ローレンシウム
Lu	71	175.0	Lutetium	ルテチウム

元素記号	原子番号	原子量	元素名	
			欧文	和名
Lv	116	(293)	Livermorium	リバモリウム
^{256}Md	101	256.1	Mendelevium	メンデレビウム
Mg	12	24.31	Magnesium	マグネシウム
Mn	25	54.94	Manganese	マンガン
Mo	42	95.94	Molybdenum	モリブデン
Mc	115	(289)	Moscovium	モスコビウム
Mt	109	(276)	Meitnerium	マイトネリウム
N	7	14.01	Nitrogen	窒素
Na	11	22.99	Sodium〔Natrium〕	ナトリウム
Nb	41	92.91	Niobium	ニオブ
Nd	60	144.2	Neodymium	ネオジム
Ne	10	20.18	Neon	ネオン
Nh	113	(278)	Nihonium	ニホニウム
Ni	28	58.69	Nickel	ニッケル
^{259}No	102	259.1	Nobelium	ノーベリウム
^{237}Np	93	237.0	Neptunium	ネプツニウム
O	8	16.00	Oxygen	酸素
Og	118	(294)	Oganesson	オガネソン
Os	76	190.2	Osmium	オスミウム
P	15	30.97	Phosphorus	リン
^{231}Pa	91	231.0	Protactinium	プロトアクチニウム
Pb	82	207.2	Lead	鉛
Pd	46	106.4	Palladium	パラジウム
^{145}Pm	61	144.9	Promethium	プロメチウム
^{210}Po	84	210.0	Polonium	ポロニウム
Pr	59	140.9	Praseodymium	プラセオジム
Pt	78	195.1	Platinum	白金
^{239}Pu	94	239.1	Plutonium	プルトニウム

元素記号	原子番号	原子量	元素名	
			欧　文	和　名
^{226}Ra	88	226.0	Radium	ラジウム
Rb	37	85.47	Rubidium	ルビジウム
Re	75	186.2	Rhenium	レニウム
Rf	104	(267)	Rutherfordium	ラザホージウム
Rg	111	(280)	Roentgenium	レントゲニウム
Rh	47	102.9	Rhodium	ロジウム
^{222}Rn	86	222.0	Radon	ラドン
Ru	44	101.1	Ruthenium	ルテニウム
S	16	32.07	Sulfur	硫黄
Sb	51	121.8	Antimony〔Stibium〕	アンチモン
Sc	21	44.96	Scandium	スカンジウム
Se	34	78.96†	Selenium	セレン
Sg	106	(271)	Seaborgium	シーボーギウム
Si	14	28.09	Silicon	ケイ素
Sm	62	150.4	Samarium	サマリウム
Sn	50	118.7	Tin	スズ
Sr	38	87.62	Strontium	ストロンチウム
Ta	73	180.9	Tantalum	タンタル
Tb	65	158.9	Terbium	テルビウム
^{99}Tc	43	98.91	Technetium	テクネチウム
Te	52	127.6	Tellurium	テルル
Th	90	232.0	Thorium	トリウム
Ti	22	47.88**	Titanium	チタン
Tl	81	204.4	Thallium	タリウム
Tm	69	168.9	Thulium	ツリウム
Ts	117	(293)	Tennessine	テネシン
U	92	238.0	Uranium	ウラン
V	23	50.94	Vanadium	バナジウム

元素記号	原子番号	原子量	元素名	
			欧 文	和 名
W	74	183.9	Wolfram〔Tungsten〕	タングステン
Xe	54	131.3	Xenon	キセノン
Y	39	88.91	Yttrium	イットリウム
Yb	70	173.0	Ytterbium	イッテルビウム
Zn	30	65.39	Zinc	亜鉛
Zr	40	91.22	Zirconium	ジルコニウム

(注) 原子量は同位体の混合比によるので，場所によって必ずしも一定の値をとるものではない．信頼度は特に表示のない限り有効数字の 4 桁目で±1 以内であるが，* 印のついている場合は±2 以内，** のついている場合は±3 である．安定同位体がなく，特有の天然同位体組成を示さない元素は，その元素のよく知られた放射性同位体の中から一種を選んで元素記号の左肩にその質量数をつけ，その相対原子質量とともに表示してある．日本化学会・原子量小委員会（2018）による

元素の周期表

金属元素 ／ 非金属元素

原子番号
元素記号
元素名

I A	II A	III A	IV A	V A	VI A	VII A	VIII	VIII	VIII	I B	II B	III B	IV B	V B	VI B	VII B	0
1 H 水素																	2 He ヘリウム
3 Li リチウム	4 Be ベリリウム											5 B ホウ素	6 C 炭素	7 N 窒素	8 O 酸素	9 F フッ素	10 Ne ネオン
11 Na ナトリウム	12 Mg マグネシウム											13 Al アルミニウム	14 Si ケイ素	15 P リン	16 S 硫黄	17 Cl 塩素	18 Ar アルゴン
19 K カリウム	20 Ca カルシウム	21 *Sc* スカンジウム	22 *Ti* チタン	23 *V* バナジウム	24 *Cr* クロム	25 *Mn* マンガン	26 *Fe* 鉄	27 *Co* コバルト	28 *Ni* ニッケル	29 *Cu* 銅	30 *Zn* 亜鉛	31 Ga ガリウム	32 Ge ゲルマニウム	33 As ヒ素	34 Se セレン	35 Br 臭素	36 Kr クリプトン
37 Rb ルビジウム	38 Sr ストロンチウム	39 *Y* イットリウム	40 *Zr* ジルコニウム	41 *Nb* ニオブ	42 *Mo* モリブデン	43 *Tc* テクネチウム	44 *Ru* ルテニウム	45 *Rh* ロジウム	46 *Pd* パラジウム	47 *Ag* 銀	48 *Cd* カドミウム	49 In インジウム	50 Sn スズ	51 Sb アンチモン	52 Te テルル	53 I ヨウ素	54 Xe キセノン
55 Cs セシウム	56 Ba バリウム	57〜71 ランタノイド元素	72 *Hf* ハフニウム	73 *Ta* タンタル	74 *W* タングステン	75 *Re* レニウム	76 *Os* オスミウム	77 *Ir* イリジウム	78 *Pt* 白金	79 *Au* 金	80 *Hg* 水銀	81 Tl タリウム	82 Pb 鉛	83 Bi ビスマス	84 Po ポロニウム	85 At アスタチン	86 Rn ラドン
87 Fr フランシウム	88 Ra ラジウム	89〜103 アクチノイド元素	104 *Rf* ラザホージウム	105 *Db* ドブニウム	106 *Sg* シーボーギウム	107 *Bh* ボーリウム	108 *Hs* ハッシウム	109 *Mt* マイトネリウム	110 *Ds* ダームスタチウム	111 *Rg* レントゲニウム	112 *Cn* コペルニシウム	113 Nh ニホニウム	114 Fl フレロビウム	115 Mc モスコビウム	116 Lv リバモリウム	117 Ts テネシン	118 Og オガネソン

ランタノイド元素	57 *La* ランタン	58 *Ce* セリウム	59 *Pr* プラセオジム	60 *Nd* ネオジム	61 *Pm* プロメチウム	62 *Sm* サマリウム	63 *Eu* ユウロピウム	64 *Gd* ガドリニウム	65 *Tb* テルビウム	66 *Dy* ジスプロシウム	67 *Ho* ホルミウム	68 *Er* エルビウム	69 *Tm* ツリウム	70 *Yb* イッテルビウム	71 *Lu* ルテチウム
アクチノイド元素	89 *Ac* アクチニウム	90 *Th* トリウム	91 *Pa* プロトアクチニウム	92 *U* ウラン	93 *Np* ネプツニウム	94 *Pu* プルトニウム	95 *Am* アメリシウム	96 *Cm* キュリウム	97 *Bk* バークリウム	98 *Cf* カリホルニウム	99 *Es* アインスタイニウム	100 *Fm* フェルミウム	101 *Md* メンデレビウム	102 *No* ノーベリウム	103 *Lr* ローレンシウム

イタリック体は遷移金属元素，記号の上の数字は原子番号を示す．族に付した記号 A，B は，IUPAC の無機化学命名法委員会（1965 年）の取り決めによるもので従来の a，b 亜族を表わすものとは無関係である

A a

A

abnormal	異常の，不規則の
Absidia	アブシディア(属)
absolute	絶対の，無水の
absolute temperature	絶対温度
absorbance	吸光度，吸収度
Acanthocheilonema	アカントケイロネマ(属)
Acarus	コナダニ(属)
acceptor	受容器，受容体
accountable	説明できる《医教》
acetone	アセトン
acetum〈ラ〉	酢，酢剤
achievable	到達可能な《医教》
acidum〈ラ〉	酸
Acinetobacter	アシネトバクター(属)
acoustic source	音源
acromion	肩峰，かたさき
actin	アクチン
Actinobacillus	アクチノバシラス(属)
adenine	アデニン
adenoma	腺腫，アデノーマ
adenosine	アデノシン
adenylic acid	アデニル酸
admittance	アドミッタンス《電気》
adrenaline	アドレナリン
adult	成人，成人(型)の
Aedes	ヤブカ(属)
Aerobacter	アエロバクター(属)
affective domain	情意領域《医教》
age	年齢，年代
akinetic	無動の
alanine	アラニン
albumin	アルブミン
Alcaligenes	アルカリゲネス(属)
allergist	アレルギー専門医
allergy	アレルギー
alternate	交代する，交代(性)の，交互(性)の
alveolar gas	肺胞気
Amblyomma	マダニ(属)
ampere	アンペア〈単位〉
amphetamine	アンフェタミン
amphophil	両染性の，両染性細胞

ampicillin	アンピシリン
anaphylaxis	アナフィラキシー，過敏症，過敏性
Ancylostoma	鉤虫(属)
androsterone	アンドロステロン
anesthetic	麻酔の，感覚〔知覚〕脱失〔消失〕の
angiotensin	アンジオテンシン
angle	角
annus〈ラ〉＝year	年
anode	陽極
Anspannungszeit〈独〉	緊張時間
answer	答え
antagonized	拮抗された
antrectomy	(鼓室)洞摘出(術)
aorta	大動脈
aortic (valve)	大動脈(弁)，A(弁)
apnea	無呼吸
Arbeit〈独〉	労働，労務，作業
area	野，区，領域
argon	アルゴン
Ascaris	アスカリス(属)
ascending colon	上行結腸
Aspergillus	アスペルギルス(属)
assessment	事前評価，予知，アセスメント
Asterococcus	アステロコッカス(属)
asthenic	無力性
atomic weight	原子量
atria	心房〈複数〉
atrium	心房〈単数〉
atrophy	萎縮する，萎縮(症)，無栄養症
atropine	アトロピン
attack	発作
A type (blood group in ABO system)	(ABO式血液型の)A型
auricle	耳介
auscultation	聴診(法)
author	著者
axilla	腋窩，わきの下
axillary	腋窩の
axis	(円柱レンズの)軸
Azotobacter	アゾトバクター(属)
chemical activity	化学活性
deoxyadenylic acid	デオキシアデニル酸
invasion to adventitia	癌外膜浸潤

linear acceleration	直線加速
lower third (antral area)	胃下部1/3
lower third of the stomach (antral area)	胃下部1/3(区), (胃癌の)前庭部(領域), A(領域)
total activity	総合活動
a	
acute	急性の
afternoon	午後
ana〈ギ〉	各々の
audio, auditory	聴覚の
a wave	a波
a.	
absorptivity	吸収力
acceleration	加速〔促進〕度(現象)
ante	～の前に
arterial	動脈(性)の
arteriole	小動脈
atto	アト(=10^{-18})〈接〉
auris	耳
axial	軸性の, 軸面の
A0-3	
invasion to adventitia	肉眼的外膜癌浸潤程度
a0-3	
invasion to adventitia	組織学的外膜癌浸潤程度
A_1	
α_1-globulin	α_1グロブリン
A_2	
α_2-globulin	α_2グロブリン
Asian influenza virus	アジアインフルエンザウイルス
A3	
toyomycin A3	トヨマイシンA3
°A	
degree absolute	絶対温度
A-I	
angiotensin I	アンジオテンシンI
A-II	
angiotensin II	アンジオテンシンII
A-III	
angiotensin III	アンジオテンシンIII
A, a	
acid	酸(性)の
action	作用, 活動, 行為, 機能
activated	活性化
active	活動性の, 能動性の, 積極的な

activity	活性，活動度，放射能
ante〈ラ〉=before	前
anterior	前の，前方の
aqueous〈ラ〉=aqua	水の，水様の，水性の
asymmetric	非対称(性)の，左右不同の
asymmetry	非対称，左右不同
axial	軸性の，軸面の
invasion to the adventitia (pathological finding)	癌外膜浸潤の程度(病理組織所見)
total acidity	(胃液の)総酸度
A, A.	
Actinomyces	放線菌(属)，アクチノミセス(属)
Anopheles	(蚊)アノフェレス(属)
A, a, a.	
accommodation	調節，順応，適応
ampere	アンペア
anode	陽極
arteria〈ギ〉=artery	動脈
a, a.	
arterial blood	動脈血
A_2, ⅡA	
aortic second sound	第二大動脈音
AA	
absolute all	無水アルコール
absolute arrhythmia	絶対性不整脈
acetic acid	酢酸
acetoacetic acid	アセト酢酸
achievement age	学力年齢，学業成績年齢
adenocortical autoantibody	副腎皮質自己抗体
adenylic acid	アデニル酸
adjuvant arthritis	アジュバント関節炎
aggregated albumin	凝集アルブミン
agranulocytic angina	顆粒球減少性アンギナ
alcoholics anonymous	アルコール依存症者更生会，匿名断酒会
alkyl agents	アルキル化剤
allergic asthma	アレルギー性喘息
alopecia areata	円形脱毛症
aminoacetone	アミノアセトン
amino acid(s)	アミノ酸
amyloid A (protein)	アミロイドA(蛋白)
amyloid angiopathy	アミロイドアンギオパシー
aortic arch	大動脈弓
aplastic anemia	再生不良性貧血
arachidonic acid	アラキドン酸

arrythmia absoluta〈ラ〉	絶対不整脈
artificial abortion	人工流産
arylamidase	アリルアミダーゼ
Ascaris antigen	回虫抗原
ascending aorta	上行大動脈
atlantoaxial	環(椎)軸(椎)の
atomic absorption	原子吸光(分析)
Australia antigen	オーストラリア抗原
auto accident	自動車事故
axonal arborization	軸索分岐

Aa

absoluta arrhythmia〈ラ〉	絶対性不整脈

aA

azure A	アズールA

a/A

arterial-alveolar oxygen ratio	動脈・肺胞酸素分圧比

AA, aa.

ana〈ギ〉	おのおのの，おのおのを同量

Aa, AA, aa.

arteriae〈ラ〉＝arteries	動脈〈複数〉

aa, AA

aminoacyl	アミノアシル

AAA

abdominal aortic aneurysm	腹部大動脈瘤
abdominal aortic aneurysmectomy	腹部大動脈瘤切除術
acute anxiety attack	急性不安発作
amalgam	アマルガム
American Academy of Allergy	米国アレルギー学会
American Association of Anatomists	米国解剖学者協会
anti-actin antibody	抗アクチン抗体
aromatic amino acid	芳香(族)アミノ酸

AAAAI

American Academy of Allergy Asthma&Immunology	米国アレルギー喘息免疫学アカデミー

AAAD

American Asthetic Association for the Deaf	難聴者のための米国無力協会
aromatic amino acid decarboxylase	芳香(族)アミノ酸脱炭酸酵素

AAAE

amino acid-activating enzymes	アミノ酸活性化酵素

AAAIMH

American Association for the Absorption of Involuntary Mental Hospitalization	不本意な精神病院収容者解放のための米国連合

A

AAAN
American Academy of Applied Nutrition 米国応用栄養学会
AAAR
Association for Advancement of Aging Research 加齢研究進歩のための協会
AAAS
American Association for the Advancement of Science 米国科学振興協会
AAB
Association of Applied Biologists 応用生物学者協会
atrio-atrial bypass 房室・動脈バイパス
AABB
American Association of Blood Banks 米国血液バンク協会
AABD
Aid to the Aged, Blind or Disabled 高齢者・盲者・身体障害者への援助
AABEVM
Association of American Boards of Examiners in Veterinary Medicine 米国獣医学試験官協会
AABMDR
Association of American Bone Marrow Donors Registration 米国骨髄ドナー登録協会
AAbs
autoantibodies 自己抗体
AABT
Association for the Advancement of Behavior Therapy 行動治療進歩のための協会
AAC
antibiotics associated colitis 抗生物質関連大腸炎
AACC
American Association for Contamination Control 米国汚染管理協会
American Association of Clinical Chemistry 米国臨床化学協会
Association for the Aid of Crippled Children 身体障害児援助協会
AACG
acute angle-closure glaucoma 急性閉塞隅角緑内障
AACM
American Academy of Compensation Medicine 米国代償医学会
AACP
American Academy of Cerebral Palsy 米国脳性麻痺学会

American Academy of Child Psychiatry　米国小児精神医学会
American Association of Correctional Psychologists　米国矯正精神医協会

AACPR
American Association for Cleft Palate Rehabilitation　米国口蓋裂リハビリテーション協会

AACR
American Association for Cancer Research　米国癌学会

AAD
adrenalectomized alloxan diabetes　副腎摘出アロキサン糖尿病
American Academy of Dentists　米国歯科医学会
American Academy of Dermatology　米国皮膚科学会
aromatic amino(-)acid decarboxylase　芳香(族)アミノ酸脱炭酸酵素
atlanto-axial dislocation　環軸椎脱臼
atlanto-axial distance　環軸間隙

A-aDCO$_2$
alveolar-arterial carbon dioxide tension difference　肺胞気・動脈血炭酸ガス分圧較差

a-ADCO$_2$
arterial-alveolar carbon dioxide tension difference　動脈血・肺胞気炭酸ガス分圧較差

AADE
American Association of Dental Examination　米国歯科試験協会

AADM
American Academy of Dental Medicine　米国歯科医学会

AADN
American Association of Doctors Nurse　米国医師看護師協会

A(-)aDN$_2$
alveolar-arterial nitrogen tension difference　肺胞気・動脈血窒素分圧較差

a(-)ADN$_2$
arterial-alveolar nitrogen tension difference　動脈血・肺胞気窒素分圧較差

A-aDo$_2$, A-aDO$_2$
alveolar-arterial oxygen tension difference　肺胞気・動脈血酸素分圧較差

AADP
Asian American Donor Program　東洋系米国人による骨髄ドナー登録組織

A

AADPA
American Academy of Dental Practice Administration　米国歯科医業経営協会
AADS
American Association of Dental School　米国歯科大学協会
American Association of Dermatology and Syphilology　米国皮膚科学梅毒学協会
AAE
active assistive exercise　自動介助運動
acute allergic encephalitis　急性アレルギー性脳炎
annuloaortic ectasia　大動脈弁輪拡張症
AAF
acetic alcohol-formalin　酢酸アルコール・ホルマリン
ascorbic acid factor　アスコルビン酸因子
atlanto-axial fusion　環軸関節融合
2-AAF
2-acetylaminofluorene　2-アセチルアミノフルオレン
AAFB
atypical acid-fast bacilli　非定型的抗酸菌
AAFC
Agriculture and Agrifood Canada　カナダ農業農産食品省
AAFM
American Association of Feed Microscopists　米国飼料顕微鏡検者協会
AAFP
American Academy of Family Physicians　米国総合臨床〔家庭〕医学会
AAFPRS
American Association of Facial Plastic and Reconstructive Surgery　米国顔面形成再建外科協会
AAFS
American Academy of Forensic Science　米国法医学会
AAG
Asian Association of Gastroenterology　アジア消化器病学会
AAGC
American Association of Gifted Children　米国才能児協会
AAGP
American Academy of General Practice　米国医師会
AAGU
American Association of Genito-Urinary Surgeons　米国生殖泌尿器外科医協会

AAH
asymmetrical apical hypertrophy 非対称性先端肥大
atypical adenomatous hyperplasia 異型腺腫様過形成

AAHA
American Association of Hospital Accountants 米国病院計理士協会

AAHC
American Association of Hospital Consaltants 米国病院顧問協会

AAHD
American Association of History of Dentistry 米国歯科医学史協会

AAHDC
American Association of Hospital Dental Chiefs 米国病院歯科主任協会

AAHM
American Association for History of Medicine 米国医史学協会

AAHP
American Association for Hospital Planning 米国病院計画協会
American Association for Humanistic Psychology 米国人道的心理学協会
American Association of Hospital Podiatrists 米国病院足病学者協会

AAHPA
American Association of Hospital Purchasing Agents 米国病院購入代理店協会

AAHPER
American Association for Health, Psychical Education and Recreation 米国健康体育リクリエーション協会

AAHPhA
American Animal Health Pharmaceutical Association 米国動物の健康と薬物の協会

AAI
acute alveolar injury 急性肺胞障害
American Association of Immunologists 米国免疫学者協会
ankle/arm index 足首/上腕血圧指数
atlanto-axial interval 環軸間隙
atrium-atrium-inhibited pacing 心房抑制型ペーシング

AAIAN
Association for Advancement of Instruction about Alcohol and Narcotics アルコールと麻薬に関する指導進歩のための協会

A

AAIB
American Association of Instructors of Blind　米国失明者指導者協会

AAID
American Association of Industrial Dentists　米国産業歯科医協会

AAIN
American Association of Industrial Nurses　米国産業看護師協会

AAIPS
American Association of Industrial Physicians and Surgeons　米国産業内科医・外科医協会

AAIT
American Association of Inhalation Therapists　米国吸入療法士協会

AAL
anterior axillary line　前腋窩腺
arctic aeromedical laboratory　北極航空医学研究室

AAM
American Association of Microbiology　米国微生物学協会

AAMA
American Academy of Medical Administration　米国病院管理学会
American Association of Medical Assistants　米国医療補助者協会

AAMBP
Association of American Medical Book Publishers　米国医学書出版協会

AAMC
American Association of Medical Clinics　米国臨床医協会
Association of American Medical Colleges　米国医科大学協会

AAMCH
American Association for Maternal and Child Health　米国母子健康協会

AAMD
American Association on Mental Deficiency　米国精神欠陥者のための協会

AAME
acetylarginine metyl ester　アセチルアルギニンメチルエステル

AAMI
age-associated memory impairment　50歳以上の健常者に共通してみられる程度の記憶力低下

Association for Advancement of Medical Instrumentation	医療器械進歩のための協会
AAMIH	
American Association for Maternal and Infant Health	米国母親・乳児健康協会
AAMMC	
American Association of Medical Milk Commissioners	米国医療用ミルク委員会
AAMP	
American Academy of Maxillofacial Prosthetics	米国上顎顔面装具学会
AAMR	
American Academy of Mental Retardation	米国精神発達遅滞学会
AAMRL	
American Academy of Medical Record Libralians	米国病歴士学会
AAMS	
American Association of Medical Social Workers	米国医療ソーシャルワーカー協会
AAN	
acute autonomic neuropathy	急性自律神経ニューロパシー
alpha-amino acid nitrogen	αアミノ酸窒素
American Academy of Neurology	米国神経学会
American Academy of Nutrition	米国栄養学会
American Association of Neuropathologists	米国神経病理学者協会
amino-aceto-nitrile	アミノアセトニトリル
AANA	
American Association of Nurse Anesthesists	米国看護麻酔士協会
AANS	
American Association of Neurological Surgeons	米国脳神経外科医協会
AAO	
Academy of Applied Osteopathy	応用骨疾患学会
American Academy of Ophthalmology	米国眼科アカデミー
American Academy of Optometry	米国視力測定学会
American Association of Orthodontists	米国歯科矯正学会
amino-acid oxydase	アミノ酸酸化酵素
AAo	
ascending aorta	上行大動脈

A

AAOC
American Association of Ostheopathic Colleges 米国骨疾患専門医協会
AAOG
American Association of Obstetricians and Gynecologists 米国産科婦人科医協会
AAOGAS
American Association of Obstetricians, Gynecologists and Abdominal Surgeons 米国産科婦人科腹部外科医協会
AAOH
Asian Association of Occupational Health アジア労働衛生会議
AAOM
American Academy of Occupational Medicine 米国産業医学会
American Academy of Oral Medicine 米国口腔科学会
AAOME
American Association of Osteopathic Medical Examiners 米国骨疾患医学試験官協会
AAO & O
American Academy of Ophthalmology and Otolaryngology 米国眼科・耳鼻咽喉科学会
AAOP
American Academy of Oral Pathology 米国口腔病理学会
AAOPS
American Association of Oral and Plastic Surgeons 米国口腔・形成外科医協会
AAOR
American Academy of Oral Roentogenology 米国口腔放射線医学会
AAOS
American Academy of Orthopedic Surgery 米国整形外科学会
AAP
acetaminophen アセトアミノフェン
American Academy of Pediatrics 米国小児科学会
American Academy of Periodontology 米国歯周医学会
aortic annuloplasty 大動脈弁輪形成術
Association for Advancement of Psychoanalysis 心理分析進歩のための協会
Association for Advancement of Psychotherapy 心理療法進歩のための協会
Association of American Physicians 米国医師協会

Association of Applied Psychoanalysis — 応用心理分析協会

L-alanine aminopeptidase — L-アラニンアミノペプチダーゼ

AAPABIDS
anomalous arrangement of pancreatico-biliary ductal system — 膵管胆道合流異常

AAPB
American Association of Pathologists and Bacteriologists — 米国病理学者微生物学者協会

AAPC
antibiotic-associated pseudomembranous colitis — 抗生物質関連偽膜性結腸炎

AAPCC
American Association of Poison Control Centers — 米国毒物管理センター協会

American Association of Psychiatric Clinics for Children — 米国小児精神医療協会

A-aPco$_2$
alveolar-arterial carbon dioxide difference — 肺胞気・動脈血炭酸ガス分圧較差

a-APCO$_2$
arterial-alveolar carbon dioxide tension difference — 動脈血・肺胞気炭酸ガス分圧較差

AAPD
American Academy of Physiologic Dentistry — 米国生理歯科学会

AAPE
American Academy of Physical Education — 米国医学教育学会

AAPHD
American Association of Public Health Dentists — 米国公衆衛生歯科医師協会

AAPHI
Associate of Association of Public Health Inspectors — 公衆衛生監視員協会連合

AAPHP
American Association of Public Health Physicians — 米国公衆衛生医師協会

AAPMC
antibiotic-associated pseudomembranous colitis — 抗生物質関連偽膜性結腸炎

AAPMR
American Academy of Physical Medicine and Rehabilitation — 米国理学療法リハビリテーション学会

AA protein
amyloid A protein　アミロイドA蛋白

AAPS
American Association of Plastic Surgeons　米国形成外科医協会
Asian Association of Pediatric Surgeons　アジア小児外科学会
Association for Ambulatory Pediatric Services　小児科外来診療協会
Association of American Physicians and Surgeons　米国内科医外科医協会

AAPSW
Associate of Association of Psychiatric Social Workers　精神科ソーシャルワーカー協会連合

AAR
against all risks　あらゆる危険に対して
Antabus-Alkohol-Reaktion〈独〉= antabus-alchohol-reaction　抗酒剤アルコール反応
Antigen-Antikörper-Reaktion〈独〉= antigen-antibody reaction　抗原抗体反応
arousals associated with respiration　呼吸に伴う覚醒
Australia antigen radioimmunoassay　オーストラリア抗原放射免疫定量

AARC
American Association for Respiratory Care　米国呼吸ケア協会

AARD
American Academy of Restorative Dentistry　米国修復歯科学会

AARF
atlantoaxial rotatory fixation　環軸椎回旋位固定

AARIT
antigen-antibody reaction inhibition test　抗原抗体反応阻止試験

AAROM
active assistive range of motion　能動的運動補助範囲

AART
American Association for Rehabilitation Therapy　米国リハビリテーション治療協会

AAS
allgemeine Adaptation Syndrom〈独〉　汎適応症候群
anterior atlantoaxial subluxation　環軸椎前方亜脱臼
anthrax antiserum　炭疽抗血清
aortic arch syndrome　大動脈弓症候群
atlanto-axial subluxation　環軸関節不全脱臼
atomic absorption spectrophotometry　原子吸光測定

atomic absorption spectroscopy 原子吸収スペクトル測光法

AASCI
acute anterior spinal cord injury 急性前脊髄障害

AASH
American Association for Study of Headache 米国頭痛研究協会

AASND
American Association for Study of Neoplastic Diseases 米国新生物疾患研究協会

AASNS
Asian and Australarian Societry of Neurological Surgeons アジアオーストラリア脳神経外科学会

AASP
American Association for Social Psychiatry 米国社会精神医学協会

AAST
American Association for Surgery of Trauma 米国外傷外科協会

AAT
alanine aminotransferase アラニンアミノトランスフェラーゼ
asymptomatic autoimmune thyroiditis 無症候性自己免疫性甲状腺炎

AATM
American Academy of Tropical Medicine 米国熱帯医学協会

AATP
American Academy of Tuberculosis Physicians 米国結核病医協会

aa-tRNA
aminoacyl transfer RNA アミノアシル転移リボ核酸

AATS
American Association for Thoracic Surgery 米国胸部外科医協会

AAU
acute anterior uveitis 急性前ブドウ膜炎

AAV
adaptive assisted ventilation 適切な補助呼吸
adeno-associated virus アデノ関連ウイルス
adenovirus-associated virus アデノウイルス関連ウイルス

AAVB
American Association of Veterinary Bacteriology 米国獣医細菌学協会

AAVMC
Association of American Veterinary Medical Colleges 米国獣医科大学協会

A

AAVN
American Association of Veterinary Nutritionist　米国獣医栄養士協会
AAVP
American Association of Veterinary Pathologists　米国獣医病理学者協会
AAVRP
American Association of Vital Records and Public Health Statistics　米国生命記録・公衆衛生統計協会
AAWB
American Association of Workers for Blind　米国視力障害者のために働く者の協会
AB
abdominal　腹(部)の，腹(側)の
abnormal　異常の，不規則の
AB (type)　(ABO式血液型の)AB型
alcian blue　アルシアンブルー
alcian blue staining　アルシアンブルー染色
4-aninoazobenzene　4-アミノアゾベンゼン
antigen binding　抗原結合の
apex beat　心尖拍動
asbestos body　アスベスト小体
asthmatic bronchitis　喘息性気管支炎
Augenbutter〈独〉　眼脂
Ab
alabamine　アラバミン
anisotropic band　A帯
aB
azure B　アズールB
ab
about　約
A/B
acid-base (ratio)　酸・塩基(比)
AB, Ab, ab
antibodies　抗体〈複数〉
antibody　抗体〈単数〉
AB, ab
axiobuccal　軸(面)頬(面)の
AB, ab, ab.
abortion　流産
AB, A/B
aid to the blind　視力障害者への援助
ABA
abscisic acid　アブシジン酸

Agaricus bisporus agglutinin アガリクスビスポラスアグルチニン
antibacterial activity 抗細菌活性
atopic bronchial asthma アトピー型喘息
azobenzene arsonate アゾベンアルソン酸

abamp
absolute ampere 絶対アンペア

A band
anisotropic band A帯

ABAS
American Board of Abdominal Surgeons 米国腹部外科委員会

ABB
abbreviation 省略, 略字, 略語
acid-base balance 酸塩基平衡
anti bad breath 口臭防止剤

Abb.
Abbildung〈独〉 図

ABBA
American Board of Bio-Analysis 米国生物分析委員会

Abbild
Abbildungen〈独〉 図〈複数〉

abbr
abbreviated 略語にした
abbreviation 略語, 省略, 略字

ABC
acid balance control 酸バランス調節
acid-base control 酸塩基平衡
aconite, belladonna, chloroform liniment アコニット・ベラドンナ・クロロホルム塗膏
aconite, belladonna, chloroform ointment アコニット・ベラドンナ・クロロホルム軟膏
advanced breast cancer 進行した乳癌
airway, breathing and circulation 心肺蘇生のABC(気道確保・呼吸・循環)手順
alternative birth(ing) center 代替分娩センター
alum, blood, charcoal process ミョウバン・血液・木炭法
aneurysmal bone cyst 動脈瘤様骨嚢腫
antigen-binding capacity 抗原結合能
antigen-binding cell 抗原結合細胞
apnea, bradycardia, cyanosis 無呼吸, 遅脈, チアノーゼ
arousal bladder capacity 覚醒時膀胱容量
aspiration biopsy cytology 穿刺吸引細胞診
atomic biological chemical 原子生物学的化学
automatic brightness control 自動的輝度調節

avidin-biotin (peroxidase) complex — アビジン・ビオチン(ペルオキシダーゼ)複合体

axiobuccocervical — 軸面頰面頸面の

A & BC
air and bone conduction — 気導と骨導

ABCAS
automated biological cell analyzing and sorting system — 自動生体細胞分析分離装置

ABCC
Atomic Bomb Casualty Commission — 原爆障害調査委員会

ABCD
adapt, boss, creation, diplomat — 適合・上司・創造・外交

ABCDEFG
atomic, biotechnology, computer, data, electronics, fine chemical, genetic engineering — 原子物理学・生物工学・コンピュータ・情報処理・電子工学・精密化学・遺伝子操作

ABCDEFGH
airway obstruction, bleeding, critical condition, drainage of abscess, endoscopy, foreign body, golden time, honesty — 気道閉塞・出血・危急状況，膿瘍排膿・内視鏡・異物，迅速な処理・誠実な(医師の態度)

ABCM
adriamycin, bleomycin, cyclophosphamide, mitomycin C — アドリアマイシン，ブレオマイシン，シクロホスファミド，マイトマイシンC

ABC method
avidin-biotin complex method — アビシン・ビオチン結合法，ABC法

ABCP
Association of Blind Chartered Physiotherapists — 認可された重度視力障害者精神治療士協会

ABCRS
American Board of Colon and Rectal Surgery — 米国大腸直腸外科委員会

ABC syndrome
angry backfiring C-nociceptor syndrome — ABC症候群

ABCX
adriamycin, bleomycin, cisplatin, radiation therapy — アドリアマイシン，ブレオマイシン，シスプラチン，放射線療法

ABD
average body dose — (放射線の)平均身体照射量

ABD (pad)
abdominal pad 腹(部)当てガーゼ，腹部パッド

ABD, Abd, abd, abd.
abdomen 腹，腹部，腹側
abdominal 腹の，腹部の，腹側の
abduct 外転する
abduction 外転，外転運動
abductor 外転(筋)

ABD HYST, Abd Hyst
abdominal hysterectomy 腹式子宮摘出術

abdo
abdomen 腹，腹部，腹側
abdominal 腹の，腹部の，腹側の

ABDOM, Abdom, abdom
abdomen 腹，腹部，腹側
abdominal 腹の，腹部の，腹側の

ABDPH
American Board of Dental Public Health 米国歯科公衆衛生委員会

abd.poll.
abductor pollicis 母指外転(筋)

abd resp
abdominal respiration 腹式呼吸

ABDV
adriamycin, bleomycin, dacarbazine, vinblastine アドリアマイシン，ブレオマイシン，ダカルバジン，ビンブラスチン

abd XP
abdomen X-ray photography 腹部X線写真

ABE
acute bacterial endocarditis 急性細菌性心内膜炎

Abe
abequose アベコース

AB-E
astra blue-eosin アストラブルーエオジン

ABEA
American Broncho-Esophagological Association 米国気管食道科学協会

ABEM
American Board of Emergency Medicine 米国救急医療委員会

ABEPP
American Board of Examiners in Professional Psychology 米国職業心理学試験委員会

A

ABER	
auditory brain stem evoked response	聴性脳幹反応
aber	
aberrant	迷入(性)の，異所の
ABF	
antibleeding factor	抗出血因子
ABFP	
American Board of Family Practice	米国総合臨床医学認定学会
ABG	
arterial blood gas	動脈血ガス
axiobuccogingival	軸(面)頬(面)歯肉(面)の
AB gap，A-B gap	
air bone gap	気骨導聴力差，気導骨導差
ABGs	
arterial blood gases	動脈血ガス
ABHP	
earth Physics	米国健康医学委員会
ABI	
ankle brachial pressure index	足関節-上腕血圧比
atherothrombotic brain infarction	アテローム血栓性脳梗塞
a.Bic	
actual bicarbonate	実測重炭酸塩
A bile，A-bile	
gall-duct bile	胆管胆汁，A胆汁
ABIM	
American Board of Internal Medicine	米国内科学委員会
ABJS	
Association of Bone and Joint Surgeons	骨・関節外科医協会
ABL	
abetalipoproteinemia	無βリポ蛋白血症
acid-base laboratory studies〔test〕	酸塩基検査〔調査/試験〕
African Burkitt lymphoma	アフリカバーキットリンパ腫
animated biological laboratory	生命科学研究室
antigen-binding lymphocytes	抗原結合リンパ球
aquatic biological laboratory	水生生物研究室
automated biological laboratory	自動的生物研究室
axiobuccolingual	軸(面)頬(面)舌(面)の
ABLB test	
alternate binaural loudness balance test	両耳音の大きさバランス検査，ABLB検査
ABLM	
American Board of Legal Medicine	米国法医学委員会
ABLS	
atlas biomedical literature system	図表生物医学文献システム

AbLV
Abelson (leukemia) virus　エイベルソン(白血病)ウイルス

ABM
anesthesia and brain activity monitor　麻酔と脳神経活動モニター
autologous bone marrow　自家骨髄

ABMS
American Boards of Medical Specialities　米国専門医制度調整機関

ABMT
allogenic bone marrow transplantation　同種骨髄移植
autologous bone marrow transplantation　自家骨髄移植(療法)

abn
air born　空中発生の

ABN, Abn, abn
abnormal　異常の，不規則の

abnor
abnormal　異常の，不規則の
abnormality　異常，奇形

abnorm
abnormal　異常の，不規則の
abnormality　異常，奇形

ABNS
American Board of Neurological Surgery　米国神経外科委員会

ABO
ABO blood groups (A, AB, B, O)　ABO式血液型(のA, AB, B, O)
ABO blood group system　ABO式血液型
ABO blood type　ABO式血液型
abortion　流産
American Board of Ophthalmology　米国眼科学委員会
American Board of Orthodontics　米国歯科矯正委員会
American Board of Otolaryngology　米国耳鼻咽喉科学委員会
antibodies　抗体

ABOG
American Board of Obstetrics and Gynecology　米国産科婦人科学委員会

Abor, abor
abortion　流産

ABOS
American Board of Oral Surgery　米国口腔外科委員会
American Board of Orthopedic Surgery　米国整形外科委員会

A

ABP
actin-binding protein アクチン結合蛋白
adriamycin, bleomycin, prednisone アドリアマイシン,ブレオマイシン,プレドニゾン
ambulatory blood pressure 自己測定血圧
American Board of Pathology 米国病理学委員会
American Board of Pediatrics 米国小児科学委員会
American Board of Periodontology 米国歯周学委員会
American Board of Prosthodontist 米国補綴歯科学委員会
androgen-binding protein 男性ホルモン結合蛋白
arterial blood pressure 動脈血圧

ABPA
allergic bronchopulmonary aspergillosis アレルギー性気管支肺アスペルギルス症

ABPC
aminobenzylpenicillin アミノベンジルペニシリン
ampicillin アンピシリン
antibody-producig cell 抗体産生細胞

ABPD
American Board of Pediatric Dermatology 米国小児皮膚科学委員会

ABPM
allergic bronchopulmonary mycosis アレルギー性気管支肺真菌症
ambulatory blood pressure monitoring 携帯式血圧測定法, 携帯式血圧測定監視法
American Board of Preventive Medicine 米国予防医学委員会

ABPMR
American Board of Physical Medicine and Rehabilitation 米国理学療法リハビリテーション医学委員会

ABPN
American Board of Psychiatry and Neurology 米国精神医学神経学委員会

ABR
absolute bedrest 絶対安静
American Board of Radiology 米国放射線医学委員会
auditory brainstem response 聴覚脳幹反応, 聴性脳幹反応

Abr, abr
abrasions 擦過傷, 表皮剝脱

abras
abrasions 擦過傷, 表皮剝脱擦過傷

ABR test
abortus bang ring test ウシ流産菌輪テスト
agglutination test for brucellosis 波状熱の凝集反応試験

ABS
acute brain syndrome 急性脳症候群

alkyl benzenesulfonate アルキルベンゼンスルホン酸塩

aloin, belladonna, strychnine アロイン・ベラドンナ・ストリキニーネ

American Board of Surgery 米国外科学委員会

Aorten-Bogen-Syndrom〈独〉 大動脈弓症候群

at bedside ベッドサイドで

ABs

absorption 吸収

abs

absent 欠損の，無い

absolute 絶対の，無水の

@**bs.**

at bedside ベッドサイドにて，臨床にて

abs alt

absolute altitude 絶対標高

abs.feb.

absente febre〈ラ〉 無熱で，発熱がないときに，常体温

absorp

absorption 吸収

ABSP

automatic blood smear processor 全自動血液塗抹装置

AbSR

abdominal skin reflexes 腹部皮膚反射

abst

abstract 要約

abstr.

abstract 要約

abstructum〈ラ〉 抽出物《処》

abt

about 約

ABTX

alpha-bungarotoxin αブンガロトキシン

ABU

asymptomatic bacteriuria 無症候性細菌尿

ABV

actinomycin D, bleomycin, vincristine アクチノマイシンD,ブレオマイシン,ビンクリスチン

arthropod-borne virus アルボウイルス

ABVD

adriamycin, bleomycin, vinblastine, dacarbazine アドリアマイシン,ブレオマイシン,ビンブラスチン,ダカルバジン

aby

antibody 抗体

A

AC

abdominal circumference	腹囲
abdominal circumscript	腹囲
absorption coefficient	吸収係数
accelerator	促進物質
acetazolamide	アセタゾールアミド
acetylcysteine	アセチルシステイン
aconitase	アコニターゼ
aconitine	アコニチン
activated charcoal	活性炭
acute cholecystitis	急性胆嚢炎
adapted child	順応した小児
adenocarcinoma	腺癌
adenomatosis colii〈ラ〉	大腸腺腫症
adenylate cyclase	アデニレートシクラーゼ
adenyl cyclase	アデニルシクラーゼ
adrenal cortex	副腎皮質
adult castration	成人の去勢
air conditioning	換気調節
air conduction or alternative current	気導または交流
alcoholic cirrhosis	アルコール性肝硬変
anesthesia circuit	麻酔回路
angle campimetry	視角中心視野測定
anodal closure	陽極閉鎖
anterior column	前柱
anterior commissure	前交連
anticoagulant	抗凝血性の，抗凝血薬
anticomplementary	抗補体の
antiphlogistic corticoid	消炎性コルチコイド
aortic valve closure	大動脈弁閉鎖
aortocoronary	大動脈冠(状)動脈の
aperture current	細孔電流
aplastic crisis	無形成発作
applied chemistry	応用化学，工業化学
arm circumference	腕周長
Arnold-Chiari (syndrome)	アーノルド・キアリ(症候群)
arterial capillary	動脈性毛細(血)管の
ascending colon	上向結腸
asymptomatic carriers	無症候性キャリア
atopic cough	アトピー咳嗽
atranctylodes lancea varchinensis	西北蒼朮《漢方》
atriocarotid	心房頸動脈の
auditory curve	聴力曲線
axiocervical	軸位頸面の

Ac

acetate	アセテート

acetyl　アセチル
actinium　アクチニウム

aC
arabinosylcytosine　アラビノシルシトシン
azure C　アズールC

ac
antecubital　肘前の

a.c.
ad concham〈ラ〉　接耳

A-C
alveolus-capillary　肺胞・毛細管

AC, ac
acceleration　加速(度)，促進
acetylcholine　アセチルコリン
acid　酸
acute　急性の

AC, A.C.
air conduction　気導

AC, A.C., ac, a/c
alternating current　交流

AC, A.C., A-C, A/C
acromioclavicular　肩峰鎖骨の

AC, a.c.
ante cibum〈ラ〉=before a meal　食前に《処》

AC, A/C, a.c.
anterior chamber (of eye)　前(眼)房

ACA
acute cerebellar ataxia　急性小脳失調(症)
adenocarcinoma　腺癌
American College of Allergist　米国アレルギー学者専門協会
American College of Anesthetists　米国麻酔医専門協会
ammonia, copper, arsenic　アンモニア・銅・砒素
anterior cerebral artery　前大脳動脈
anterior communicating artery　前交通動脈
anticardiolipin antibody　抗カルジオリピン抗体
anticentromere antibody　抗セントロメア抗体
anticomplement activity　抗補体活性
automatic clinical analyzer　自動臨床検査分析器

7-ACA
7-amino-cephalosporinic acid　7-アミノセファロスポリン酸

AC/A
accommodative convergence/accommodation (ratio)　調節〔調整〕性輻輳対調節(比)

ac a
acetic acid　酢酸

A

ACAAI
American College of Allergy Asthma&Immunology　米国アレルギー・喘息・免疫学会
AcAc
acetoacetate　アセト酢酸，アセトアセテート
acac
acetylacetonate　アセチルアセトネート
ACAD, acad
academy　学会
Acad Med
Academy of Medicine　医学校
ACAG
acute closed angle glaucoma　急性閉塞隅角緑内障
ACAnes
American College of Anesthetists　米国麻酔医専門協会
Acanth
acanthocephaliasis　鈎頭虫症
acanthocephalous　鈎頭虫の
ACAP
American Council on Alcohol, Problems　米国アルコール問題審議会
AC/A ratio
accommodative convergence-accommodation ratio　AC/A 比(＝調整〔調節〕性輻輳対調節比)
ACAS
Asymptomatic Carotid Atherosclerosis Study　無症候性動脈硬化症研究
ACAT
acyl CoA-cholesterol acyltransferase　アシルコエンザイムAコレステロールアシルトランスフェラーゼ
ACB
antibody coated bacteria　抗体被覆細菌
AC/BC
air conduction (time)/bone conduction (time)　気導(時間)/骨導(時間)
ACBG
aorta-coronary bypass graft(ing)　大動脈・冠(状)動脈バイパス移植(術)，大動脈・冠(状)動脈吻合バイパス
A-C block
alveolar-capillary block　肺胞・毛細管ブロック，AC ブロック

ACBWS
automatic chemical biological warning system | 自動化学生物学的監視機構

A-C bypass
aorto-coronary (artery) bypass (procedure) | 大動脈・冠(状)動脈バイパス(術)

ACC
accelerin-convertin | アクセレリン・コンバルチン
acetyl coenzyme A carboxylase | アセチル補酵素〔コエンザイム〕Aカルボキシラーゼ
alveolar cell carcinoma | 肺胞細胞癌
American College of Cardiology | 米国心臓病学専門協会
anodal closure contraction | 陽極閉鎖収縮
articular chondrocalcinosis | 関節軟骨石灰症

ACC, Acc
adenoid cystic carcinoma | 腺様嚢胞(性)癌

Acc, ACC, acc
accommodation | 調節，順応，視力調節

Acc, acc
acceleration | 加速(度)，促進
accident | 事故，災害

ACCA
American College of Clinical Administrators | 米国臨床管理者専門協会

ACCCA
accessibility, comprehensiveness, coordination, continuity, accountability | 親近感・包容力・協調力・持続力・責任能力

accel
acceleration | 加速(度)，促進

AcCh, Ac Ch
acetylcholine | アセチルコリン

AcChR
acetylcholine receptor | アセチルコリン受容体

AcCHS
acetylcholinesterase | アセチルコリンエステラーゼ

accid
accident | 事故
accidental | 偶然の

ACCl
anodal closing clonus | 陽極閉鎖クローヌス

ACCM
American College of Clinic Managers | 米国臨床管理者専門協会

AcCoA, Ac CoA
acetyl coenzyme A | アセチルコエンザイムA，アセチル補酵素A

A

accom
accommodation 調節，順応
ACCP
American College of Chest Physicians 米国胸部疾患学会
American College of Clinical Pharmacy 米国臨床薬学会
ACCR
amylase creatinine clearance ratio, amylase creatinine clearance rate アミラーゼクレアチニンクリアランス比
ACCRA
Abortion and Contraception Counselling and Research Association 妊娠中絶避妊相談研究協会
ACCS
alternating covergent concomitant strabismus 交代性共同性内斜視
anterior chamber cleavage 前房分化症候群
accum
accumulated 蓄積した
accumulation 蓄積
accy
accessory 付随の，副次的な
ACD
absolute cardiac dullness 絶対心濁音界
acid citrate dextrose クエン酸ブドウ糖
actinomycin D アクチノマイシンD
alcoholic cerebellar degeneration アルコール性中毒性小脳変性
allergic contact dermatitis アレルギー性接触皮膚炎
anemia of chronic disease 慢性疾患に伴う貧血
annihilation coincidence detection 陽電子消滅γ線同時検出
anterior chest diameter 前胸部横径
axiodistocervical 軸位遠位頸面の
AC-DC, ac/dc
alternating current-direct current 交流・直流
alternating current/direct current 交流/直流
ACDK
acquired cystic disease of the kidney 後天性嚢胞性腎疾患
ACDS
acid citrate-dextrose solution クエン酸塩ブドウ糖液，ACD液
acdt
accident 事故
ACE
adrenal cortical extract 副腎皮質抽出物

adriamycin, cyclophosphamide, etoposide — アドリアマイシン,シクロホスファミド,エトポシド
alcohol-chloroform-ether (mixture) — アルコール・クロロホルム・エーテル(混合液)
angiotensin converting enzyme — アンジオテンシン変換酵素

ace, ace.
acetic — 酢酸の
acetone — アセトン

ACED
anhydrotic congenital ectodermal dyspnia — 無汗性先天性外胚葉性形成不全

ACEI
angiotensin converting enzyme inhibitor — アンジオテンシン変換酵素阻害物質〔阻害薬〕

A cell
antigen presenting cell — 抗原表示細胞

AC Em
actinium emanation — アクチニウムエマナチオン

ACEP
adriamycin, cytarabine, cyclophosphamide (=Endoxan), prednisolone — アドリアマイシン,シタラビン,シクロホスファミド(=エンドキサン),プレドニゾロン
American College of Emergency Physicians — 米国救急医療医師専門協会

ACES
N-(2-acetamido)-2-aminoethanesulfonic acid — *N*-(2-アセトアミド)-2-アミノエタンスルホン酸

acet.
acetum〈ラ〉=vinegar — 酢酸，酢

Acet, acet.
acetone — アセトン

acetab
acetabulum — 寛骨臼，脱臼

acetl
acetylene — アセチレン

ACF
Abnormal Colposcopic Findings — 異常所見
accessory clinical findings — 付随的臨床所見

ACFO
American College of Foot Orthopedists — 米国足整形外科医専門協会

ACFR
American College of Foot Roentgenologist — 米国足放射線医専門協会

ACFS
American College of Foot Surgeons 米国足の外科専門協会

ACFSA
American Correctional Food Service Association 米国改正食糧サービス協会

ACFU
agar colony-forming units 寒天コロニー形成単位

ACFUCY
actinomycin D,5-fluorouracil, cyclophosphamide アクチノマイシンD,フルオロウラシル,シクロホスファミド

ACG
American College of Gastroenterology 米国胃腸専門協会
angiocardiography 心臓(血管)造影(法)
apex cardiogram 心尖拍動図

AC-G, AcG
accelerator globulin 促進グロブリン

ACGIH
American Conference of Government Industrial Hygienists 米国産業衛生専門家会議

ACGME
Accreditation Council for Graduate Medical Education 米国医学卒後研修認定委員会

ACGPOMS
American College of General Practitioners in Osteopathic Medicine and Surgery 米国骨疾患外科医中の一般医専門協会

ACH
achalasia 弛緩不能症, 噴門痙攣
active chronic hepatitis 活動性慢性肝炎
adrenal cortical (adrenocortical) hormone 副腎皮質ホルモン
arm,chest,height 上腕囲・胸囲・身長

ACH, ACh, Ach
acetylcholine アセチルコリン

ACHA
American College of Health Association 米国健康協会専門委員会
American College of Hospital Administration 米国病院管理専門協会

AChA
anterior choroidal artery (眼の)前脈絡膜動脈

AChE
acetylcholinesterase アセチルコリンエステラーゼ

ACH index
arm girth, chest depth, hip width index　腕囲・胸の厚さ・腰幅指数

AChR
acetylcholine receptors　アセチルコリン受容体

AChRAb
acetylcholine receptor antibody　アセチルコリン受容体抗体

AChRP
acetylcholine receptor protein　アセチルコリン受容体蛋白

AC & HS
ante cibum et hora somni〈ラ〉　食前と就寝時《処》

ACI
abdominal circumference index　腹囲指標(＝肥満度指標)
acoustic comfort index　音響快適度指数
acute cerebral infarction　急性脳梗塞
acute coronary infarction　急性冠血管梗塞
acute coronary insufficiency　急性冠(状)(動脈)(機能)不全(症)
adenylate cyclase inhibitor　アデニレートシクラーゼ阻害物質〔阻害薬〕
adrenal cortical (adrenocortical) insufficiency　副腎皮質(機能)不全(症)
anticlonus index　抗痙攣指数
atomospheric pressure ionization　大気圧イオン化法

ACID
aquired cytomegalic inclusion disease　後天性巨細胞性封入体病

acid
acidosis　アシドーシス
acidulated drop　酸性化滴

acid phos
acid phosphatase　酸性ホスファターゼ

acid PO_4
acid phosphatase　酸性ホスファターゼ

acid p'tase
acid phosphatase　酸性ホスファターゼ

ACIE
affinity crossed line immunoelectrophoresis　吸着交叉〔差〕疫電気泳動法
anticomplement immunoenzymatic test　抗補体免疫酵素検査

ACIF
anticomplement immunofluorescence　抗補体免疫螢光

AC-IOL
anterior chamber intraocular lens　前房レンズ

A

ACIP

advisory committee on immunization practices	予防接種諮問委員会

ACJ

acromioclavicular joint	肩鎖関節

AC jt.

acromioclavicular joint	肩峰関節

ACK

accidentally killed	事故死の
ammonium chloride/potassium	塩化アンモニウム，カリウム

ACL

albumin, casein, lecithin	アルブミン,カゼイン,レシチン
anterior cruciate ligament	前十字靱帯

aCL

anticardiolipin	抗カルジオリピン

ACLAM

American College of Laboratory Animal Medicine	米国研究室動物専門協会

ACLE

acute cutaneous lupus erythematosus	急性皮膚エリテマトーデス

ACLM

American College of Legal Medicine	米国法医学専門協会

ACLP

Association of Contact Lens Practitioners	コンタクトレンズ取扱い者協会

ACLS

advanced cardiac life support	二次循環救命処置，二次心臓救命処置

ACM

acemetacin	アセメタシン
achromycin	アクロマイシン
aclacinomycin	アクラシノマイシン
acute cerebrospinal meningitis	急性脳脊髄膜炎
adriamycin, cyclophosphamide, methotrexate	アドリアマイシン,シクロホスファミド,メトトレキサート
alveolar capillary membrane	肺胞毛細(血)管膜

acm

albuminin-calcium-magnesium	アルブミン・カルシウム・マグネシウム

ACM-D

actinomycin D	アクチノマイシンD

ACME

Advisory Council on Medical Education	医学教育勧告審議会

angioplasty compared to medicine study　冠(状)動脈形成試験

ACMI
American Cystoscope Makers, Incorporated　米国膀胱鏡製作会社

ACMP
adriamycin, cytarabine, 6-mercaptopurine, prednisolone　アドリアマイシン,シタラビン,6-メルカプトプリン,プレドニゾロン
alveolar-capillary membrane permeability　肺胞毛細(血)管膜透過性

ACMT
American College of Medical Technologists　米国医療技士専門協会

ACMV
assist-controlled mechanical ventilation　補助・調節機械的換気

ACN
acute conditioned necrosis　急性条件下壊死
acute cortical necrosis　急性皮質壊死
American College of Neuropsychiatrists　米国神経精神科医専門協会

ACNHA
American College of Nursing Home Administrators　米国看護家庭管理専門協会

ACNM
American College of Nurse Midwives　米国看護助産術専門協会

ACNU
1-(4-amino-2-methyl-5-pyrimidinyl)-methyl-3(2-chlorethyl)-3-nitrosourea　メチルニトロソウレア
nimustine　ニムスチン

ACO
aconitase　アコニターゼ
acute coronary occlusion　急性冠(状)動脈閉塞(症)
American College of Optometry　米国視力測定士専門協会
anodal closing odor　陽極閉鎖臭
atractylodis ovota　浙江白朮《漢方》

ACOAP
adriamycin, cyclophosphamide, vincristine(=Oncovin), arabinosylcytosine, prednisone　アドリアマイシン,シクロホスファミド,ビンクリスチン(=オンコビン),アラビノシルシトシン,プレドニゾン

A

ACOG
American College of Obstetricians and Gynecologists — 米国産科婦人科医専門協会

ACOHA
American College of Osteopathic Hospital Administrators — 米国骨疾患病院管理者専門協会

ACOI
American College of Osteopathic Internists — 米国骨疾患内科医専門協会

Acom, A-com
anterior communicating artery (aneurysm) — 前交通動脈(瘤)

ACOP
adriamycin, cyclophosphamide, vincristine (=Oncovin), prednisone — アドリアマイシン，シクロホスファミド，ビンクリスチン(=オンコビン)，プレドニゾン

American College of Osteopathic Pediatricians — 米国骨疾患整形外科医専門協会

ACOPP
adriamycin, cyclophosphamide, vincristine (=Oncovin), prednisone, procarbazine — アドリアマイシン，シクロホスファミド，ビンクリスチン(=オンコビン)，プレドニゾン，プロカルバジン

ACOS
American College of Osteopathic Surgeons — 米国整骨外科医学会

ACO-S
aconitase soluble — 可溶性アコニターゼ

acous
acoustics — 音響

acous, acous.
acoustical — 聴覚の，聴音の

ACP
acid phosphatase — 酸(性)ホスファターゼ，酸性リン酸分解酵素

acyl carrier protein — アシルキャリア蛋白，アシル担体蛋白

alternative complement pathway — 補体反応副経路

alternative complement pathway — 補体別経路

American College of Pharmacists — 米国薬剤師専門協会

American College of Physicians — 米国医師学会

anodal closing picture — 陽極閉鎖図

aspirin, caffeine, phenacetin — アスピリン・カフェイン・フェナセチン

Association of Clinical Pathologists — 臨床病理学者協会

Association of Correctional Psychologists　矯正心理学者協会

ACP1
acid phosphatase 1　酸性ホスファターゼ1

ACP2
acid phosphatase 2　酸性ホスファターゼ2

ACPA
American Cleft Palate Association　米国口蓋裂協会

Ac-Pase
acid phosphatase　酸(性)ホスファターゼ

ACPC
ciclacillin　シクラシリン

AC-PC
aminocyclohexylpenicillin　アミノサイクロヘキシルペニシリン

ACPE
American Council on Pharmaceutical Education　米国調剤教育審議会

AC-PH
acid phosphatase　酸(性)ホスファターゼ

ACPM
American Congress for Preventive Medicine　米国予防医学会議

ACPMR
American Congress of Physical Medicine and Rehabilitation　米国内科学リハビリテーション学会議

ACPP
adrenocorticopolypeptide　副腎皮質ポリペプチド
American College of Preventive Physicians　米国予防医学専門協会

ACPS
acrocephalopolysyndactyly　尖頭多合指(症)

ACP-virus
adeno-conjunctival-pharyngeal virus　腺結膜咽頭ウイルス

ACQST
acquisition time　データ取り込み時間《コン》

ACR
aclarubicin　アクラルビシン
acriflavine　アクリフラビン
albumin/creatinine ratio　アルブミン/クレアチニン比
American College of Radiology　米国放射線専門協会
American College of Rheumatology　米国リウマチ学会
anti-constipation regimen　抗便秘剤

Acr
acrylic　アクリルの

A

A/C ratio
albumin/coagulin ratio　アルブミン/コアグリン比
ACR/NEMA
American College of Radiology/ National Electrical Manufactures Association　米国放射線学会/国立電機器製造協会
acro
acrophobia　高所恐怖症
ACS
acrocephalosyndactyly　尖頭合指(症)
acute confusional state　急性錯乱状態
acute confusional status　急性昏迷状態
alternating covergent strabismus　交代性内斜視
American Cancer Society　米国癌協会
American Chemical Society　米国化学協会
American College of Surgeons　米国外科学会
anodal closing sound　陽極閉鎖音
anterior coronary sinus　前冠(状)動脈洞
antireticular cytotoxic serum　抗細網性細胞傷害血清
Association of Clinical Scientists　臨床科学者協会
ACSA
adenylate cyclase stimulating　アデニレートサイクラーゼ刺激活性
ACS AO
ascending aorta　上向大動脈
ACSOA
Acoustical Society of America　米国音響協会
Ac-SPM, ACSPM
acetylspiramycin　アセチルスピラマイシン
acst
acoustic, acoustical　音響の，聴覚の
ACT
accelerated clotting〔coagulation〕 time　促進凝固時間
actin　アクチン
activated clotting〔coagulation〕 time　活性化(賦活)凝固凝血時間
activated coagulation time　活性化凝固時間
adenylate cyclase toxin　アデニレートシクラーゼ毒素
advanced coronary treatment　進歩した冠(状)動脈治療
alternative cover test　交代おおい試験
antichymotrypsin　抗キモトリプシン
anticoagulation therapy　抗凝固療法
atropine coma therapy　アトロピン昏睡療法
automatic cart transport　自動台車搬送システム
AcT
acceleration time　加速時間

act
action 作用，活動，行為
active 活動性の，能動性の
activity 活性，活動度

ACT, act
actinomycin アクチノマイシン

ACTA scanner
automatic computerised transverse axial tomographic scanner コンピュータ断層装置

ACTCM
American College of Traditional Chinese Medicine 米国東洋医学校

ACTe
anodal closing tetanus 陽極閉鎖性強直性痙攣

ACTH
adrenocorticotropic hormone 副腎皮質刺激ホルモン

ACTH-RF
adrenocorticotropic hormone releasing factor 副腎皮質刺激ホルモン放出因子

ACTH-RH
adernocorticotropic hormone-releasing hormone 副腎皮質刺激ホルモン放出ホルモン

ACTH-Z method
stimulus test of adrenal cortex 副腎皮質刺激試験，ACTH-Z法

activ
activity 活性，活動度

ACTN
alpha-actin αアクチン

ACTP
adrenocorticotropic polypeptide 副腎皮質刺激ポリペプチド

ACTS
acute cervical traumatic syndrome 急性頸部外傷症候群

actv
activate 活性化する

ACU
ambulatory care unit 救急患者収容治療室

ACUS
antithrombogenic continuous ultrafiltration system 抗血栓性持続濾過システム

ACV
acute cardiovascular (disease) 急性心血管(疾患)
acyclovir アシクロビル
atrial/carotid/ventricular 心房の・頸動脈の・心室の

ACVD
atherosclerotic cardiovascular disease アテローム硬化性心血管疾患

A

ACVP
American College of Veterinary Pathologists　米国獣医病理学者専門協会
ACW
anterior chest wall　前胸壁
anticlockwise　反時針方向
AC/W
acetone/water　アセトン/水
ACY1
aminoacylase-1　アミノアシラーゼ1
AD
academic development　大学開発
accident dispensary　調剤過誤
acute dermatomyositis　急性皮膚筋炎
addict　常用者，常習者
adjuvant disease　アジュバント病
admitting diagnosis　入院時診断
adult disease　成人病
afterdischarge　後発射
Aleutian disease　アリューシャン病
Alzheimer disease　アルツハイマー病
Anfangsdruck〈独〉　初圧
anno Domini〈ラ〉　西暦，紀元後
anodal duration　陽極持続
anterior descendence　前下行枝
antigenic determinant　抗原決定基
arginase deficiency　アルギナーゼ欠損症
arthritis deformans〈ラ〉　変形性関節炎
atlantodental　(正中)環軸の
atlanto-odontoid　環軸椎の
atopic dermatitis　アトピー性皮膚炎
atrio-dextro〈ラ〉　右(心)房(に)
autosomal dominant　常染色体(性)優性の
average deviation　平均偏差《統》
average dose　平均投与量・治療量
axis deviation　(電気)軸偏位
diphenylchlorarsine　ジフェニルクロルアルシン
drug addict　薬物嗜癖
Ad
adipocyte　脂肪細胞
admission　入院
adnexa　付属器
anisotropic disk　A帯
assay date　検査日時
ad
ad〈ラ〉=to, up to　〜まで，全量

a drug 薬剤中毒者，麻薬常用者
axiodistal 軸位遠位面の

ad.
adde，*addatur*〈ラ〉＝add 加えよ《処》

Ad2
adenovirus 2 アデノウイルス２型

AD50
anesthetic ED50 50％麻酔有効濃度

AD95
anesthetic ED95 95％麻酔有効濃度

AD，A/D
analog digital アナログ・デジタル《コン》

AD，ADH
alcohol dehydrogenase アルコールデヒドロゲナーゼ

AD，Ad，a.d.
auris dextra〈ラ〉＝right ear 右耳

Ad，AD
Adrenalin アドレナリン

A/D，A-D
analog-to-digital (converter) アナログ・デジタル(変換)

A & D，A and D
admission and discharge 入院と退院，入退院
ascending and descending 上向(性)と下向(性)の

ADA
adenosine deaminase アデノシンデアミナーゼ
American Dental Association 米国歯科協会
American Dermatological Association 米国皮膚科協会
American Diabetes Association 米国糖尿病協会
American Diabetes Association diet number 米国糖尿病協会食事番号
American with Disability Act 米国身体障害者法
anterior descending artery 前下行動脈
N-(2-acetamido) iminodiacetic acid *N*-(2-アセトアミド)イミノジ酢酸

ada
average deviation adjustment 平均偏倚調整

ADAA
American Dental Assistants Association 米国歯科助手協会

ADA diet
American Diabetes Association diet 米国糖尿病学会食

ADAM
animated dissection of anatomy for medicine エーディエーエム，アダム(＝解剖学用コンピュータソフト)

A

9-anthryldiazomethan — 9-アンスリルジアゾメタン

ADAMHA
American Drug Alcohol Mental Health Administration — 米国アルコール薬物乱用精神衛生局

adar
analog-to-digital-to-analog recording — アナログ・デジタル・アナログ記録《コン》

ADARF
Alcoholism and Drug Addiction Research Foundation — アルコール・薬物中毒研究財団

ad baln.
ad balneum〈ラ〉=to the bath — 浴槽に，浸液に

ADC
Affective Disorders Clinic — 情動疾患クリニック
albumin, dextrose, catalase — アルブミン・ブドウ糖・カタラーゼ
analog-to-digital converter — アナログ・デジタル変換器
anodal duration contraction — 陽極持続収縮
apparent diffusion coefficient — 見かけ上の拡散係数《画診》
apparent diffusion constant — 見かけ上の拡散定数《画診》
axiodistocervcal — 軸位遠位頸面の

AdC
adrenal cortex — 副腎皮質

ad-ca, Ad-Ca
adenocarcinoma — 腺癌

AD capacity
alveolar diffusing capacity — 肺胞拡散能

ad cap.amyl.
ad capsulas amylaceas〈ラ〉 — オブラートに入れて《処》

ADCC
antibody-dependent cellular cytotoxicity — 抗体依存(性)細胞性細胞毒性
antibody-dependent cell-mediated cytotoricity — 抗体依存性細胞傷害

ad chart.
ad chartam〈ラ〉 — 紙袋に入れて《処》

ad chart.cer.
ad chartam ceratam〈ラ〉 — 蠟紙に包んで《処》

ADCMC
antibody-dependent cell-mediated cytotoxicity — 抗体依存性細胞媒介性細胞傷害作用

adcom
analog-to-digital computer — アナログ・デジタル変換コンピュータ《コン》

ADCONFU
adriamycin, cyclophosphamide, vincristine (=Oncovin), 5-fluorouracil — アドリアマイシン,シクロホスファミド,ビンクリスチン(=オンコビン),フルオロウラシル

ADD
adenosine deaminase — アデノシンデアミナーゼ
atlantodental distance — 環軸歯突起間距離
attention deficit disorder — 注意(力)欠乏疾患，注意欠陥障害
average daily dose — 平均1日量

add.
addatur, *adde*〈ラ〉=add — 加えよ《処》
addition — 足し算，追加
additional — 付加の，追加の
adduct — 内転する
adductor — 内転筋

ad & d
accidental death and dismemberment — 事故死と四肢切断

add, ADD
adduction — 内転，内ひき

addar
automatic digital data acquisition and recording — 自動デジタルデータ取得と記録《コン》

ADDAS
automatic digital data assembly system — 自動デジタルデータ集合システム《コン》

addend.
addendum〈ラ〉 — 付録，追加

adder
automatic-digital data-error recorder — 自動デジタルデータ過誤記録機《コン》

ADDH
attention deficit disorder with hyperactivity — 注意欠陥多動障害

ad diag
admitting diagnosis — 明白な診断

addict
addiction — 嗜癖

addn
addition — 相加，付加，添加

addnl
additional — 追加の，付加の，補助の

add.poll
adductor pollicis — 母指内転(筋)

A

ADE
acute disseminated encephalitis 急性散在性脳炎
antibody-dependent enhancement 抗体依存増進
Ade
adenine アデニン
ade
adenoids 咽頭扁桃肥大，アデノイド
ad effect.
ad effectum〈ラ〉 効果あるまで加えよ《処》
Ade-Lec
adenotonsillectomy 咽頭扁桃〔アデノイド〕切除・口蓋扁桃摘出術
Ade-Loto
adenotonsillotomy 咽頭扁桃〔アデノイド〕切除・口蓋扁桃切除
ADEM
acute disseminated encephalomyelitis 急性散在性脳脊髄炎
ADEN
acute disseminated epidermal necrosis 急性播種性表皮壊死症
adenoca
adenocarcinoma 腺癌
Adeno-virus
adenoidal-pharyngeal-conjunctival virus アデノウイルス，咽頭・喉頭・結膜炎ウイルス
adeq
adequate 適した
ADF
acid detergent fiber 酸性デタージェント繊維
ATL-derived factor 成人T細胞性白血病誘導因子
ad.feb.
adstante febre〈ラ〉 有熱時に《処》
ADG
atrial diastolic gallop 心房拡張期駆馬音
axiodistogingival 軸位遠位歯肉面の
ad grat.acid
ad gratam aciditatem〈ラ〉 嗜好に適した酸味を加えよ《処》
ADH
Academy of Dentistry for Handicapped 障害者のための歯科学院
alcohol dehydrogenase アルコール脱水素酵素
Association of Dental Hospital 歯科病院協会
adh
adhesions 癒着，粘着
adhesive 癒着製の，粘着性の

ADH, adh
antidiuretic hormone 抗利尿ホルモン

ADHA
American Dental Hygienists Association 米国歯科衛生士協会

ADHD, AD/HD
attention deficit hyperactivity disorder 注意欠陥多動障害

adhes
adhesions 癒着，粘着
adhesive 癒着性の，粘着性の

adhib.
adhibendus〈ラ〉 投与する《処》

ad hib.
ad hibeatur〈ラ〉 飲ませる《処》
ad hibendus〈ラ〉 投薬される《処》

ADI
acceptable daily intake 1日摂取許容量
American drug index 米国最新薬剤便覧
area of interest 関心領域
atlanto-dental interval 環椎歯突起間距離
autosomal dominant ichthyosis 常染色体性優性魚鱗癬
axiodistoincisal 軸位遠位切歯面の

ADIC
adriamycin, dimethyltriazenoimidazole carboxamide アドリアマイシン，ジメチルトリアゼノイミダゾールカルボキサミド
American Dental Interfraternity Council 米国歯科学生クラブ間評議会

ad int.
ad interim〈ラ〉 中間に《処》

ADIS
anxiety disorder interview schedule 不安障害面接基準，不安障害面接試験

adj
adjacent 付近の，隣接した
adjective 形容詞，付属の
adjoining 隣接する
adjunct 付加物，付属物
adjust 調節する，順応する
adjusted 調節された，順応した，適応した
adjuvant アジュバント

ADK
adenosine kinase アデノシンキナーゼ
kanendomycin カネンドマイシン

A

ADKC
atopic dermatitis with keratoconjunctivitis　角結膜炎を伴うアトピー性皮膚炎
Adkin
adenylate kinase　アデニレイトキナーゼ
ADKM
aminodeoxy kanamycin　アミノデオキシカナマイシン
ADL
activities of daily living　日常生活動作
amplitude difference limen　(音の)強さの弁別域
automatic data link　自動データ連接
adlib., ad lib., Ad lib.
ad libitum〈ラ〉=freely, without restriction　自由に，無制限に《処》
ADL-T
activities of daily living test　日常生活動作テスト
ADM
adriamycin　アドリアマイシン(=ドキソルビシン：DOX,DXR)
musculus abductor digiti minimi　小指外転筋
AdM
adrenal medulla　副腎髄質
adm, Adm
administer　投薬，投与，管理
administration　投薬，投与，管理
adm, adm., Adm.
admission　入院
adm., ADM
administrator　管理者，理事
ADMA
American Drug Manufactures Association　米国製薬協会
ADME
absorption-distribution-metabolism-elimination　吸収・分泌・代謝・排出
ADMICS
advanced drug mixture information & consultation system　輸液情報コンサルテーションシステム
ADMIRES
automatic diagnostic maintenance information retrieval system　自動診断取得情報検索システム《医コン》
ADMIT
Coordinated Research Program on Analytical Detection Methods for Irradation Treatment of Food　食品照射の検知法に関する研究計画

ADML
acute duodenal mucosal lesion　急性十二指腸粘膜病変

admov.
admove〈ラ〉=apply, add　加える
admoveatur〈ラ〉　用いよ《処》

ADMS
assistant director of medical service　医療サービスの副支配人

ADMX
adrenal medullectomy　副腎髄質切除(術)

ADN
acide désoxyribonucléique〈仏〉　デオキシリボ核酸

ADN-B
antideoxyribonuclease-B　抗デオキシリボヌクレアーゼB

ad neut.
ad neutralizandum〈ラ〉　中和するまで《処》

ADO
axiodisto-occlusal　軸位遠位咬合面の

Ado
adenosine　アデノシン

ado
advanced development objective　客観的進歩発展

ADOAP
adriamycin, vincristine(=Oncovin), arabinosylcytosine, prednisone　アドリアマイシン,ビンクリスチン(=オンコビン),アラビノシルシトシン,プレドニゾン

Ado B12
adenosyl B12　アデノシルB12

Ado Ccl
adenosylcobalamin　アデノシルコバラミン

Ado-5′-P
adenosine-5′-monophosphate　アデノシン-5′-一リン酸

Ado-5′-P2
adenosine-5′-diphosphate　アデノシン-5′-二リン酸

Ado-5′-P3
adenosine-5′-triphosphate　アデノシン-5′-三リン酸

ADP
adenosine diphosphate　アデノシン二リン酸
adenosine-5′-diphosphate　アデノシン-5′-二リン酸
advanced pancreatitis　進行性膵炎
animal disease and parasite　動物の疾病と寄生虫
antidiuretic principle　制尿法

AdP
adductor pollicis　母指内転筋

A

ad part.dolent.
ad partes dolentes〈ラ〉=to the aching parts　疼痛部に
ADPG
adenosine-5-diphosphate-glucose　アデノシン-5-二リン酸グルコース
ADP-Glc
adenosine diphosphate glucose　ADPグルコース
ADPKD
autosomal dominant polycystic kidney disease　常染色体優性遺伝多発性嚢胞性腎疾患
adpl
average daily patient load　毎日平均患者負荷
ad pond.om.
ad pondus omnium〈ラ〉　全量まで《処》
ADP ribosylation
adenosine 5′-diphosphate ribosylation　ADPリボシル化
ad-pro
adrenaline-protalgol　アドレナリンプロタルゴール
ADQ
abductor digiti quinti　小指外転筋
adq
adequate　適した
ADR
accepted dental remedies　受容された歯科医療
adverse drug reaction　薬物有害反応，副作用
ADR，Adr
adriamycin　アドリアマイシン(=ドキソルビシン：DOX,DXR)
Adr，adr
adrenaline　アドレナリン
ADRA
Animal Disease Research Association　動物疾病研究協会
adren
adrenal　副腎の
adren，adren.
adrenaline　アドレナリン
Adrex
adrenalectomized　副腎摘出の
Adria
Adriamycin　アドリアマイシン
ADRIS
anti-dog red-cell immune serum　イヌ赤血球抗血清
ADRS
analog-to-digital data-recording system　アナログ・デジタルデータ記録システム《コン》

ADS

acid deposition system 酸性雨被害調達データベース
alternative divergent strabismus 交代性外斜視
American Dental Service 米国歯科医療サービス
anatomical dead space 解剖学的死腔
antibody deficiency syndrome 抗体欠損(性)症候群
antidiuretic substance 抗利尿物質

ADSA

American Dental Society of Anesthesiology 米国歯科麻酔協会

ad sat.

ad saturandum〈ラ〉 飽和するまで

ad satur.

ad saturandum〈ラ〉 飽和するまで

ADSC

adipose-derived stem cell 脂肪由来幹細胞

Adson's M

Adson's maneuver アドソン手技

Ad-St

Adams-Stokes syndrome アダムス・ストークス症候群

adst.feb.

adstante febre〈ラ〉＝when fever is present 発熱時に

ADT

adenosine triphosphate アデノシン三リン酸
agar-gel diffusion test 寒天ゲル拡散試験〔検査〕
alternate day therapy 隔日療法
alternate day treatment 隔日治療
any desired thing 偽薬，気休め薬，プラセボ
arm deviation test 腕偏位試験

ADTA

American Dental Trade Association 米国歯科同業組合

ADTe

anodal duration tetanus 陽極持続強直
tetanic contraction テタニー性攣縮

ad tert.vic.

ad tertium vicem〈ラ〉＝to the third time 3回まで《処》

ad ter.vic.

ad tertian vicem〈ラ〉 3回目に《処》

ADU

acute duodenal ulcer 急性十二指腸潰瘍

ad us.

ad usum〈ラ〉 習慣〔慣例〕に従って《処》

A

ad us.ext.
ad usum externum〈ラ〉=for external use　外用《処》

ad us.exter.
ad usum externum〈ラ〉=for external use　外用《処》

ad us.int.
ad usum internum〈ラ〉　内用《処》

ad us.med.
ad usum medicinalem〈ラ〉=for medicinal use　医薬用の

ad us.vet.
ad usum veterinarium〈ラ〉=for veterinary use　家畜用の，獣医用の

ADV
adenovirus　アデノウイルス
adventitia　外膜
Aleutian disease virus　アリューシャン病ウイルス

Adv
advice　助言
advisory　助言の

adv.
advanced　進行した
adverse，*adversum*〈ラ〉=against　〜に反して，〜に対して《処》，向かって，対抗して
advise　助言する

a/dv
arterio/deep venous　動脈・深部静脈(注射)

ad val.
ad valorem〈ラ〉　価値に応じて《処》

ad 2 vic.
ad duas vices〈ラ〉=at two times　2回に《処》

AD virus
adenovirus　アデノウイルス

AdVP
adriamycin, vincristine, prednisolone　アドリアマイシン，ビンクリスチン，プレドニゾロン

A5D5W
alcohol 5%, dextrose 5%, in water　5%アルコール・5%ブドウ糖水溶液

ADX
adrenalectomized　副腎摘出した
adrenalectomy　副腎切除

AE
above elbow　肘上，上腕
acrodermatitis enteropathica　腸性先端〔肢端〕皮膚炎

active exercise	自動運動
adrenal epinephrine	副腎エピネフリン
adverse event	有害事象
aftereffect	後(続)効果，後(続)作用
amyloid E (protein)	アミロイドE(蛋白)
anoxic encephalopathy	無酸素(性)脳症
anti(-)epileptic	抗てんかん作用の，抗てんかん薬
Antitoxin-Einheit〈独〉	抗毒素単位
apoenzyme	アポ酵素
arterial embolism	動脈塞栓症
artificial erection	人工(的)勃起
aryepiglottic	披裂喉頭蓋の

ae.

aetatis〈ラ〉	年齢に応じた《処》

A & E

accident and emergency	事故で緊急を要す

AEA

antierythrocyte autoantibody	抗赤血球自己抗体

AE AMP

above-elbow amputation	肘上切断

AEA solution

alcohol, ether, acetone solution	アルコール・エーテル・アセトン溶液

AEBSF

4-(2-aminoethyl)-benzenesulfonyl fluoride hydrochloride	4-(-2-アミノエチル)-ベンゼンスルホニルフルオライドヒドロクロライド

AEC

adenylate energy charge	アデニレートエネルギーチャージ
3-amino-9-ethylcarbazole	3-アミノ-9-エチルカルバゾール
at earliest convenience	可及的速やかに

AECA

anti-endothelial cell antibodies	抗血管内皮細胞抗体

AECC

aeromedical evacuation control center	航空医学避難管理センター

AECD

allergic eczematous contact dermatitis	アレルギー性湿疹性接触皮膚炎

AECM

Albert Einstein College of Medicine	アルバート・アインシュタイン医科大学

A

AED
anti(-)epileptic drug 抗てんかん薬
anti(-)epileptic drugs 抗痙攣薬
Automated External Defibrillator 自動体外式除細動器

AEDH
acute epidural hematoma 急性硬膜外血腫

AE fold
aryepiglottic fold 披裂喉頭蓋ひだ

AEG
air encephalogram 気脳造影〔撮影〕図，気脳写(像)
angio-encephalogram 脳血管造影

AEG，aeg.
aegra〈ラ〉=aeger (男性/女性)患者

AEH
alveolar epithelhyperplastic 肺胞上皮増生

AEI
annular erythema of infancy 乳児環状紅斑

AEM
analytical electron microscope 分析電子顕微鏡
analytical electron microscopy 分析電子顕微鏡検査

AEN
aseptic epiphyseal necrosis 無菌性骨端壊死

AEP
acetate-extractable ferroprotein, acetate eluted ferroprotein 酢酸抽出性フェロ蛋白
acute eosinophilic pneumonia 急性好酸球性肺炎
artificial endocrine pancreas 人工膵島
auditory evoked potential 聴覚誘発電位
averaged evoked potential 加算平均誘発電位

aEP，α-EP
alpha-endorphin αエンドルフィン

AEPL
anterior extrapleural line 前胸膜外線

aeq
age equivalent 年齢相当の

aeq.
aequales〈ラ〉=equal 等しい

AER
acoustic evoked response 聴覚誘発反応
acute exertional rhabdomyolysis 急性労作性横紋筋融解(症)
agranular endoplasmic reticulum 無顆粒小胞体
albumin excretion rate アルブミン排泄率
apical ectodermal ridge 発生学，四肢形成
auditory evoked response 聴覚誘発反応
average electroencephalic response 均等脳波反応

AERO	
aerobactor	アエロバクター
Aero, aero	
acetone-extracted serum	アセトン抽出血清
Aeromed	
aeromedicine	航空医学
AERP	
atrial effective refractory period	心房性有効不応期
AES	
acute encephalitic syndrome	急性脳炎症候群
American Epidemiological Society	米国疫学協会
American Epilepsy Society	米国てんかん協会
anterior ectosylvian gyrus	前外シルヴィウス脳回
anti-eosinophil sera	抗好酸球血清
aortic ejection sound	大動脈駆出音
atrial extrasystole	心房性期外収縮
Auger electron spectroscopy	オージェ電子分光法
AET	
aminoethyl-isothiouronium	アミノエチル・イソチウロニウム
aet.	
aetas〈ラ〉=age	年齢
aetatis〈ラ〉	年齢に応じて《処》
AEV	
avian erythroblastosis virus	トリ赤芽球症ウイルス
AF	
acid-fast (*bacilli*)	抗酸(菌)
adriamycin,5-fluorouracil	アドリアマイシン,フルオロウラシル
adult female	成人女性
afebrile	無熱(性)の
aflatoxin	アフラトキシン
after-discharge	後発射，後放電
aldehyde fuchsin	アルデヒドフクシン
amaurosis fugax	一過性黒内障
amniotic fluid	羊水
anionic ferritin	陰イオン・フェリチン
ankle flow	足関節血流量
anteflexion	前屈
antibody-forming	抗体形成(性)の，抗体産生(性)の
aortic flow	大動脈流量
apple fiber	リンゴ線維
ascitic fluid	腹水
atrial flutter	心房粗動
auranonn	アウラノフィン

A

Af
antigen frequency 抗原頻度
af
audio-frequency 可聴周波数
A-F
antifibrinogen 抗フィブリノゲン
AF, Af
atrial fibrillation 心房細動
auricular fibrillation 心房細動
AF, A-F
anterior fontanel 大泉門
AFA
alcohol-formalin-acetic acid アルコール・ホルマリン・酢酸
AFADO
Association of Food and Drug Offcials 食品・薬品公務員協会
AFASIC
Association for All Speech Impaired Children 言語障害児のための協会
AFB
acid-fast bacillus〔bacilli〕 抗酸(性)(桿)菌
aflatoxin B アフラトキシンB
American Foundation for Blind 米国視力障害者財団
aorto-femoral bypass 大動脈・大腿(動脈)バイパス
AF bypass, A-F.Bypass
axillary-femoral bypass 腋窩・大腿動脈バイパス
AFC
antibody forming cell(s) 抗体産生細胞
AFCE
acute focal cerebral edema 急性局所性脳浮腫
AFCI
acute focal cerebral ischemia 急性巣状脳虚血
American Foot Care Institute 米国足看護研究所
AFCR
American Federation for Clinical Research 米国臨床研究連合
AFD
accelerated freeze drying 加速凍結乾燥
appropriate-for-dates (infant) 相当体重(児), 適性発育(児)
AFDC
aid for dependent children 扶養小児への援助
Aid for Family & Dependent Children 米国の母子家庭生活保護制度の1つ
AFDE
American Fund for Dental Education 米国歯科教育基金

AFD infant
appropriate-for-dates infant — 相当体重児，適性発育児，AFD児（＝AGA児）

AFDOUS
Association of Food and Drug Officials of United States — 米国食品・薬品公務員協会

afeb
afebrile — 無熱（性）の

aff，aff.
afferent — 求心性の

affil
affiliated — 提携した，関連した

AFG
aflatoxin G — アフラトキシンG
amniotic fluid glucose — 羊水ブドウ糖

AFGF
acidic fibroblast growth factor — 内皮細胞増殖因子

AFI
abdominal wall fat index — 腹壁脂肪指数
amaurotic familial idiocy — 黒内障性家族性白痴
amniotic fluid index — 羊水指数
atrial〔auricular〕 fibrillation — 心房細動

AFib，A fib.
atrial〔auricular〕 fibrillation — 心房細動

AFIP
Armed Forces Institute of Pathology — 米国軍病理研究所

AFL
anti-fatty liver — 抗脂肪肝の
antifibrinolysin — 抗フィブリノリシン
artificial limb — 義肢
atrial〔auricular〕 flutter — 心房粗動

AFLP
acute fatty liver of pregnancy — 妊娠性急性脂肪肝

AFM
atomic force micoscope — 原子間力顕微鏡

AFMC
Asian Federation for Medical Chemistry — アジア医化学連合

AFO
ankle-foot orthoses — 神経疾患のリハビリテーション用短下肢装具，くるぶし奇形矯正

AFOB
American Foundation for Overseas Blind — 海外視力障害者のための米国財団

A

AFOCC
Asian Federation of Organizations for Cancer Research and Control　癌研究対策アジア連合
AFP
a diabatic fast passage　断熱高速通過
anterior faucial pillar　前口蓋弓
AFP, aFP
alpha-fetoprotein　αフェトプロテイン
AfP, AfPh
affiliate physician　提携医師，関連医師
AFPE
American Foundation for Pharmaceutical Education　米国調剤教育財団
AFPH
American Federation of Physically Handicapped　米国身体障害者連合
AFR
antifibrinolysin reaction　抗線(維素)溶(解)酵素反応
average urinary flow rate　平均尿流量率
AFRD
acute febrile respiratory disease　急性熱性呼吸器疾患
AFRI
acute febrile respiratory illness　急性熱性呼吸器疾患
AFS
adult Fanconi syndrome　成人ファンコニ症候群
AFT
aflatoxin　アフラトキシン
agglutination-flocculation test　凝集・架状検査
antifibrinolysin test　抗線維素溶解試験
Afta
Kunstafter〈独〉＝artifical anus　人工肛門
AFTM
American Foundation for Tropical Medicine　米国熱帯医学財団
AFTN
autonomous functioning thyroid nodule　自動的に作用する甲状腺小結節
AFV
amniotic fluid volume　羊水量
AFW
Association for Family Welfare　家族福祉のための協会
AFX
atypical fibroxanthoma　非定型的線維黄色腫
AG
abdominal gauge　腹囲
abdominal girth　腹囲

agarose	アガロース
aminoglycoside	アミノ配糖体
angiogram	血管造影〔撮影〕図，血管写(像)
angiography	血管造影〔撮影〕(法)，血管写
1,5-anhydro-D-glucitol	アンヒドロ・グルシトール
anion gap	アニオンギャップ
antiglobulin	抗グロブリン
antigravity	抗重力
arteriography	動脈撮影
axiogingival	軸(面)歯肉(面)の

Ag

argentum〈ラ〉＝silver	銀〈元素〉

1,5-AG

1,5-anhydroglucitol	1,5-アンヒドログルシトール

AG, Ag

antigen	抗原

AG, ag

atrial gallop (rhythm)	心房性奔馬性(リズム〔律動〕)

A-G, A/G

albumin/globulin (ratio)	アルブミン/グロブリン(比)

AGA

accelerated growth area	加速増殖野
allergic granulomatosis and angitis, allergic granulomatous angitis	アレルギー性肉芽腫性血管炎
American Gastroenterological Association	米国胃腸病協会
American Goiter Association	米国甲状腺腫協会
antiglomerular antibody	抗糸球体抗体
appropriate for gestational age	適性発育，相当体重

Ag-Ab

antigen-antibody (complex)	抗原抗体(複合体)

AGA infant

appropriate-for-gestational age infant	相当体重児，適性体重児，AGA児(＝AFD児)

AGB

antigen-antibody test	抗原抗体テスト
arteria gastrica brevis	短胃動脈

AGBAD

Alexander Graham Bell Association for Deaf	難聴者のためのアレキサンダーグラハムベル協会

AGC

automatic gain control	自動感度調節

AgCl

silver chloride	塩化銀

AGCT
antiglobulin consumption test　抗グロブリン消費検査〔試験〕

AGD
Academy of General Dentistry　一般歯科医学校
agar-gel diffusion　寒天ゲル拡散法
anogenital distance　肛門性器間距離

AGDD
agar-gel double diffusion　寒天ゲル二重拡散法

AGE
acrylamide gel　アクリルアミドゲル
acute gastroenteritis　急性胃腸炎
advanced glycation endproducts　高脂血糖症二次産物，蛋白質の最終糖化物
agarose gel electrophoresis　アガロースゲル(内)電気泳動(法)
angle of greatest extension　最大伸展角度
arterial gas embolism　動脈ガス塞栓症

AGED
arteria gastroepiploica dextra〈ラ〉　右胃大網膜動脈

AGES
arteria gastroepiploica sinistra〈ラ〉　左胃大網膜動脈

AGEs
advanced glycation end-products　グルコシル化最終産物

AGF
adrenal growth factor　副腎発育因子
angle of greatest flexion　最大屈曲角度

ag.feb.
aggrediente febre〈ラ〉　熱が上昇したときに《処》

AGG
agammaglobulinemia　無γグロブリン血症

agg
agglutinate　凝集する
agglutinated　凝集した
aggregate　凝集物
aggregated　集められた
aggregation　集合，集積

AGG, agg.
aggravated　増悪した

aggl
agglutinate　凝集する
agglutinated　凝集した
agglutination　凝集反応，凝集(作用)

Agglut, agglut, agglut.
agglutinated　凝集した
agglutination　凝集反応，凝集(作用)

aggr
aggregate 凝集する，凝集物
aggrav
aggravate 悪化させる
aggravation 悪化，増悪
aggred.feb.
aggrediente febre〈ラ〉 発熱中《処》
aggreg
aggregation 凝集，集合
AGGS
anti-gas gangrene serum 抗ガス壊疽血清
AGH
antral gastrin-cell hyperplasia 幽門洞ガストリン細胞過形成症
agit
agitated 興奮した
agitation 興奮
AGIT，agit.
agita〈ラ〉=shake 振る《処》
agit.ante sum.
agita ante sumendum〈ラ〉=shake before taking 服用前に振れ《処》
agit. a.us.
agita ante sumendum〈ラ〉=shake before taking 服用前に振れ《処》
agit.bene
agita bene〈ラ〉=shake well よく振れ《処》
agit.esu.
agitato ante sumendum〈ラ〉 使用前に振盪せよ《処》
agit.vas.
agitato vase〈ラ〉 容器を振盪せよ《処》
AGL
acute gastric lesion 急性胃病変
acute granulocytic leukemia 急性顆粒球(性)白血病
agglutination 凝集(作用)，凝集反応
aminoglutethimide アミノグルテチミド
agl
agglomerate 固める，かたまりにする
AGLMe
acetylglycyl-L-lysine methyl ester アセチルグリシル-L-リジンメチルエステル
AGM
African green monkey アフリカミドリザル
AGML
acute gastric mucosal lesion 急性胃粘膜病変
AGN
acute glomerulonephritis 急性糸球体腎炎

A

AGN，agn
agnosia 失認，認知不能(症)
$AgNO_3$
silver nitrate 硝酸銀
AgNOR
silver-stained nucleolar organizer region 銀染色仁形成体部
AGNR
anaerobic gram-negative rod 嫌気性グラム陰性桿菌
AGP
Academy of General Practice 一般医療協会
acid glycoprotein 酸性糖蛋白
AGPA
American Group Psychotherapy Association 米国集団精神医療協会
AGPT
agar-gel precipitation test 寒天ゲル沈殿試験
AgR
antigen receptor 膜免疫グロブリン
AGRF
American Geriatric Research Foundation 米国老人研究財団
agro
agrobiological 農業生物学の
agrobiologist 農業生物学者
agrobiology 農業生物学
AGS
adrenogenital syndrome 副腎性器症候群
American Geriatric Society 米国老人協会
American Gynecological Society 米国婦人科学協会
AGs
aminoglycosides アミノグリコシド，アミノ配糖体
Ags
alpha-galactosidase αガラクトシダーゼ
AGSA
arteria gastrica sinistra accesorius〈ラ〉 副左胃動脈
AGT
abnormal glucose tolerance 異常耐糖能
abnormality of glucose tolerance グルコース閾値の異常
acute generalized tuberculosis 急性全身性結核
angiotensinogen アンジオテンシノゲン
antiglobulin test 抗グロブリン検査〔試験〕
agt，agt.
agent 動因，(作用)物質〔薬/因子〕，病因

AGTH
adrenoglomerulotrop(h)ic hormone 副腎球状帯刺激ホルモン

AGTT
abnormal glucose tolerance test 異常糖負荷試験

AGV
acetic acid gentian violet 酢酸ゲンチアナバイオレット
aniline gentian violet アニリンゲンチアナバイオレット

AH
abdominal hysterectomy 腹式子宮摘出(術)
accidental hypothermia 偶発性低体温
acetohexamide アセトヘキサミド
acute hepatitis 急性肝炎
adenomatous hyperplasia 腺腫様過形成
Adie-Holmes (syndrome) アディー・ホームズ(症候群)
alcoholic hepatitis アルコール性肝炎
amenorrhea and hirsutism 無月経・多毛症
aminohippurate アミノ馬尿酸塩
anterior hypothalamus 視床下部前部
antihistamine 抗ヒスタミン剤
antihistaminic 抗ヒスタミン性の，抗ヒスタミン薬
antihyaluronidase 抗ヒアルロニダーゼ
arterial hypertension 動脈性高血圧
artificial heart 人工心臓
assisted hatching ふ化補助術
ataxic hemiparesis 失調性片麻痺
axillary hair 腋毛

Ah
ampere hour アンペア時

A & H
accident and health 事故にあったが健康である
alive and healthy 健康で生存している

AHA
acquired hemolytic anemia 後天性溶血性貧血
acute hemolytic anemia 急性溶血性貧血
American Heart Association 米国心臓協会
American Hospital Association 米国病院協会
antihemophilic A factor 抗血友病A因子
autoimmune hemolytic anemia 自己免疫性溶血性貧血

AH block
supra-Hisian block ヒス束上ブロック

AHC
Academy of Hospital Counselors 病院顧問協会
acute hemorrhagic conjunctivitis 急性出血性結膜炎
acute hemorrhagic cystitis 急性出血性膀胱炎

arteria hepatica communis〈ラ〉 総肝動脈

AHCM

apical hypertrophic cardiomyopathy 先端肥大性心筋症

AHD

acquired heart disease 後天性心疾患
acute heart disease 急性心(臓)疾患
alcoholic heart disease アルコール性心疾患
antihyaluronidase 抗ヒアルロニダーゼ
antihypertensive drug 抗高血圧薬，降圧薬
arteriolopathia hypertonica diffusa〈ラ〉 汎発性高血圧性細動脈症
arteriosclerotic heart disease 動脈硬化性心(臓)疾患
autoimmune hemolytic disease 自己免疫(性)溶血(性)疾患

AHE

acute hemorrhagic encephalomyelitis 急性出血性脳脊髄炎

AHF

acute heart failure 急性心不全
American Hospital Formulary 米国病院薬剤師会発行の病院医薬品集
American Hospital Foundation 米国病院財団
antihemolytic factor 抗溶血性因子
antihemophilic factor 抗血友病因子
antihemophilic globulin F 抗血友病グロブリンF
Argentinian hemorrhagic fever アルゼンチン出血(性)熱

AHF(-)A

antihemophilic factor A 抗血友病因子A

AHF(-)B

antihemophilic factor B 抗血友病因子B

AHFS

American Hospital Formulary Service 米国病院薬剤師会発行の病院医薬品集

AHG

aggregated human globulin 凝集ヒトグロブリン
(heat) aggregated human IgG (熱)凝固ヒト免疫グロブリンG
antihemolytic globulin 抗溶血性グロブリン
antihemophilic globulin 抗血友病グロブリン
antihemophilic globulin A 抗血友病グロブリンA
anti-human globulin 抗ヒトグロブリン

AHGG

aggregated human gamma globulin 凝集ヒトγグロブリン
anti-human gamma globulin 抗ヒトγグロブリン

AHGS

acute herpetic gingival stomatitis 急性ヘルペス性歯根口内炎

AHH

alpha-hydrazine analog of histidine ヒスチジン類似αヒドラジン
aromatic hydrocarbon hydroxylase 芳香族炭化水素水酸化酵素

AHI
acromiohumeral interval 肩峰骨頭間距離
American Health Institute 米国健康研究所

AHIL
Association of Hospital and Institution Libraries 病院・研究所図書館協会

A & H ins
accident and health insurance 事故・健康保険

AH interval
atrio-His bundle interval 心房・ヒス束時間

AHL
artificial heart lung 人工心肺

AHLE
acute hemorrhagic leukoencephalitis 急性出血性白質脳炎

AHLG
anti-human lymphocyte globulin 抗ヒトリンパ球グロブリン

AHLS
anti-human-lymphocyte serum 抗ヒトリンパ球血清

AHM
ambulatory Holter monitor 携行用ホルターモニター

AHMA
anti-heart muscle autoantibody 抗心筋自己抗体

AHMC
Association of Hospital Management Committees 病院管理委員会連合

AHN
assistant head nurse 副看護師長

AHO
Albright's hereditary osteodystrophy オルブライト遺伝性骨ジストロフィ

AHP
acute hemorrhagic pancreatitis 急性出血性膵炎
after-hyperpolarization 後過分極電位
antihyaluronidase reaction 抗ヒアルロニダーゼ反応
Assistant House Physician 家庭医助手
Association for Humanistic Psychology 人道的心理学協会

AHPR
Academy of Hospital Public Relation 病院公的関係協会

AHR
acceptable hazard rate 許容できる危険率
Association for Health Record 健康記録協会

AHS
acute hypersensitivity syndrome 急性過敏性症候群
African horse sickness アフリカウマ病
American Hearing Society 米国聴力協会

A

American Hospital Supply 米国病院供給(会社)

A.H.S.

Assistant House Surgeon 開業外科医助手

AHSB

authorized health and safety branch 公認健康安全支部

AHSC

American Hospital Supply Company 米国病院供給会社

AHT

antihyaluronidase test 抗ヒアルロニダーゼ試験
antihyaluronidase titer 抗ヒアルロニダーゼ(力)価
augmented histamine test 増強ヒスタミン試験

AHTG

anti-human thymocytic globulin 抗ヒト胸腺細胞グロブリン

AHTP

anti-human thymocytic plasma 抗ヒト胸腺細胞血漿

AHTS

anti-human thymus serum 抗ヒト胸腺血清

AHU

antihyaluronidase 抗ヒアルロニダーゼ

AHWA

Association of Hospital and Welfare Administrators 病院と福祉の管理者協会

AI

accidentally incurred 事故誘発の
acetabular index 臼蓋指数，臼蓋迫害角
acidophilic index 好酸性細胞指数
activity index 活動指数《リハ》
adoptive immunotherapy 養子免疫療法
agranular insular cortex 無顆粒島状皮質
allergy アレルギー
aluminium アルミニウム〈元素〉
anaphylatoxin inhibitor 過敏毒阻害剤
androgen index アンドロゲン指数
angiotensin I アンジオテンシンI
anxiety index 不安指数
aortic incompetence〔insufficiency〕 大動脈弁閉鎖不全(症)
apical impulse 先端衝撃
apnea index 無呼吸指数
articulation index 構音指数
artificial insemination 人工授精
artificial intelligence 人工知能
atherogenic index 動脈硬化指数
atherosclerosis index 動脈硬化指数
atrial insufficiency 心房不全
autoimmune 自己免疫の
axioincisal 軸位切歯面の

a.i.
ad interium〈ラ〉 暫定的な《処》

A & I
abstracting and indexing 抄録化と目録化
Allergy and Immunology アレルギーと免疫学

AIA
accumulation index of atherosclerosis 動脈硬化集積指数
affinity isolated antibody アフィニティ精製抗体
Allrgy Information Association アレルギー情報協会
anti-immunoglobulin antibodies 抗免疫グロブリン抗体
anti-insulin antibody 抗インスリン抗体
aspirin-induced asthma アスピリン誘発(性)喘息
Association Internationale d'Allergologic 国際アレルギー学会

AIAO
autoimmune aspermatogenic orchitis 自己免疫性精巣炎
autoimmune aspermatogenic orchitis 自己免疫性無精子症性睾丸炎

AIB
amino-isobutyric acid アミノイソ酪酸
avian infectios bronchitis 鳥類から感染する気管支炎

AIBL
angioimmunoblastic lymphadenopathy 血管免疫芽球性リンパ節症

AIBS
American Institute of Biological Science 米国生物科学研究所

AIC
Akaike's information criterion 赤池情報量基準
American Institute of Chemists 米国化学者研究所
aminoimidazole carboxamide アミノイミダゾールカルボキサミド
Association des Infermieren Canadiennes カナダ看護師協会

AICA
anterior inferior cerebellar artery 前下小脳動脈
anterior inferior communicating artery 前下交通動脈

AICAR
aminoimidazole carboxamide ribonucleotide アミノイミダゾールカルボキサミドリボ核酸

AICD
activation-induced cell death 活性化による細胞死
automatic implantable cardioverter defibrillater 埋込み型除細動器

AICE
angiotensin I converting enzyme アンジオテンシンⅠ変換酵素

A

AICF
autoimmune complement fixation 自己免疫(性)補体結合
AICT
adoptive immunochemotherapy 受動免疫化学療法
AID
acquired immunodeficiency disease 後天性免疫不全病
acute infectious disease 急性感染症
Agency for International Development 国際発展のための機関
American Instructors of the Deaf 米国難聴指導者
artificial insemination with donor('s semen) 非配偶者間人工授精
aspiration and infusion device 白内障吸引灌流装置
autoimmune disease 自己免疫疾患
automatic implantable defibrillator 埋込み型除細動器
dorsal agranular insular cortex 後無顆粒島状皮質
AIDP
acute inflammatory demyelinating polyradicuropathy 急性炎症性脱髄性多発根神経炎
AIDS
acquired immunodeficiency syndrome 後天性免疫不全症候群，エイズ
AIE
acute inclusion (body) encephalitis 急性封入体脳炎
acute infectious encephalitis 急性感染(性)脳炎
AIED
International Association of Dental Student 国際歯学生協会
AIEP
amount of insulin excretion from pancreas 膵からのインスリン分泌量
AIF
anemia-inducing factor 貧血誘発因子
anterior interbody fusion 前方固定
anti-inflammatory 抗炎症(性)の
AIFD
acute intrapartum fetal distress 急性分娩時胎児仮死
AIFM
Association Internationale des Femmes Medecins〈仏〉＝International Woman Medical Association 国際女医会
AIG
anti-immunoglobulin 抗免疫グロブリン
AIH
American Institute of Homeopathy 米国ホメオパシー研究所

artificial insemination (with) husband('s semen) 配偶者間人工授精
autoimmune hepatitis 自己免疫性肝炎
autoimmune hyperlipidemia 自己免疫性高脂血症

AIHA
American Industrial Hygiene Association 米国産業衛生協会
autoimmune hemolytic anemia 自己免疫(性)溶血性貧血

AIHC
American Industrial Health Conference 米国産業健康協議会

AIHD
acquired immune hemolytic disease 後天性免疫出血性疾患

AIIS
anterior inferior iliac spine 前下腸骨棘，下前腸骨棘

AIJ
atherogenic index of Japanese 日本人動脈硬化指数

AIL
acute infectious lymphocytosis 急性感作性リンパ球増加(症)
angioimmunoblastic lymphadenopathy 血管免疫芽球性リンパ節症

AILD
alveolar-interstitial lung disease 肺胞間質性肺疾患
angio-immunoblastic lymphadenopathy with dysproteinemia 異常蛋白血症を伴う血管リンパ芽球性リンパ節症

AIM
abnormal involuntary movement 異常不随意運動
allograft induced macrophage 同種移植による活性化マクロファージ

AIMBE
International Association of Enviromental and Biological Medicine 国際環境医学・生物学協会

AIMD
abnormal involuntary movement disorder 異常不随意運動疾患

AIMES
Association of Interns and Medical Students インターンと医学生の協会

AIMS
abnormal involuntary movement scale 異常不随意運動尺度
All-India Institute of Medical Science 全インド医科学研究所
arthritis impact measurement scales 関節炎衝撃測定尺度

A

AIN

acute interstitial nephritis, acute tubulo-interstitial nephritis	急性間質性腎炎
American Institute of Nutrition	米国栄養研究所
anti-inflammatory nonsteroidal	抗炎症(性)非ステロイド(性)の
autoimmune neutropenia	自己免疫性好中球減少症

AINSUF

aortic insufficiency	大動脈不全

AION

anterior ischemic optic neuropathy	前部虚血性視神経症

AIP

acute idiopathic pericarditis	急性特発性心膜炎
acute infectious polyneuritis	急性感染性多発神経炎
acute inflammatory polyradiculoneuropathy	急性炎症性多発根ニューロパシー
acute intermittent porphyria	急性間欠性ポルフィリン症
acute interstitial pneumonia	急性間質性肺炎
alcohol-induced pancreatitis	アルコール性膵炎
aldosterone-induced protein	アルドステロン誘発性蛋白
American Institute for Psychoanalysis	米国心理分析研究所
Association Internationale de Pediatrie〈仏〉=International Association of Pediatrics	国際小児学会
average intravascular pressure	平均血管内圧

AIPC

International Association for Prevention of Blindness	国際失明予防協会

AIPD

acute idiopathic pandysautonomia	急性特発性汎自律神経失調症
autoimmune progesterone dermatitis	自己免疫プロゲステロン皮膚炎

AIPHE

Association of Institution of Public Health Engineers	公衆衛生工学研究所協会

AIQ

antero-inferior quadrant	前下象限

AIR

5-aminoimidazole ribonucleotide	5-アミノイミダゾールリボヌクレオチド
average injection rate	平均注射率

AIRS

Aerometric Information Retrieval System	大気測定情報修正組織
Amphetamine Interview Rating Scale	アンフェタミン面接評点尺度

AIRX
American Industrial Radium and X-ray Society　米国産業ラジウムX線協会

AIS
abbreviated injury scale　簡略外傷重症度尺度
anti-insulin serum　抗インスリン血清

AISIC
autologous insoluble immune complex　自己不溶性免疫複合体

AIT
acquired immunological tolerance　獲得性免疫寛容
acute intensive treatment　急性時集中治療
amiodarone-induced thyrotoxicosis　アミオダロン誘発性甲状腺中毒症
Analytischer Intelligenztest〈独〉　分析的知能テスト
autoimmune thyroiditis　自己免疫性甲状腺炎

AITD
autoimmune thyroid disease　自己免疫性甲状腺炎

AI tip
aspiration-irrigation tip　吸引灌流チップ

AITP
autoimmune thrombocytopenic purpura　自己免疫性血小板減少性紫斑病

AITT
agrinine insulin tolerance test　アルギニンインスリン負荷試験
augmented insulin tolerance test　増強性インスリン耐性試験

AIU
absolute iodine uptake　(甲状腺)ヨウ素摂取絶対量

AIV
ventral agranular insular cortex　腹側無顆粒島状皮質

AIVPA
Association Internationale Veterinaire de Production Animale〈仏〉=International Association of Veterinair for Animal Production　国際家畜増殖獣医学協会

AIVR
accelerated idioventricular rhythm　加速性心室固有リズム

AIVV
anterior internal vertebral vein　前内側脊椎静脈

AJ
Atractylodes Japonica　北鮮白朮《漢方》

a.j.
ante jentaculum〈ラ〉=before breakfast　朝食前

A

AJ, A-J
ankle jerk(s) reflex　くるぶし反射，アキレス腱反射

AJC
American Joint Committee for Cancer Staging and End Results Reporting　癌の病期分類と予後の報告のための米国連合委員会

AK
acetate kinase　アセテートキナーゼ
actinic keratosis　光線性角化症
adenylate kinase　アデニレートキナーゼ
anomalous killer　異常キラー細胞
Antikörper〈独〉　抗体
aortic knob　大動脈球
artificial kidney　人工腎臓
astigmatic keratotomy　乱視矯正角膜切開術

AK, a.k.
above knee　膝(より)上の，大腿

AKA
above knee amputation　膝上切断術
alcoholic ketoacidosis　アルコール(性)ケトアシドーシス

AKA, a.k.a.
also known as　～としても知られている

AK amp., A/K Amp, Ak amp.
above knee amputation　膝上切断術

AKBR
arterial ketone body ratio　動脈血中ケトン体比

AKC
atopic keratoconjunctivitis　アトピー性角膜結膜炎

AKI
acute kidney injury　急性腎障害

AKM
aminodeoxykanamycin　アミノデオキシカナマイシン(＝ベカナマイシン)

AKP
above-knee prosthesis　大腿義肢
alkaline phosphatase　アルカリホスファターゼ
anterior knee pain　膝前方痛

AL
absolute latency　絶対潜時
acute leukemia　急性白血病
adaptation level　適応水準
albumin　アルブミン
anti-human lymphocytic (globulin)　抗ヒトリンパ球(グロブリン)
asset location　アセットロケーション

atractylodes lancea 古玄蒼朮《漢方》
attenuation length 減衰の長さ
axiolingual 軸(面)舌(面)の
lethal antigen 致死抗原

Al
alminium アルミニウム〈元素〉

A-L
Albert-Lembert (anastomosis) AL(吻合)(=消化管 2 層吻合)

AL, al
alignment 配列, アラインメント

a.l., AL
auris laeva〈ラ〉=left ear 左耳

ALA
American Laryngological Association 米国喉頭科学協会
aminolevulinic acid アミノレブリン酸
antilymphocyte antibody 抗リンパ球抗体

Ala
alanine アラニン

ALA, ALa, A La
axiolabial 軸(面)唇(面)の

ALA, Ala
aminolevulinic acid アミノレブリン酸

ALAD
aminolevulinic acid dehydrogenase アミノレブリン酸脱水素酵素

ALAD, ALA-D
abnormal left axis deviation 異常左軸偏位

ALAG, ALaG
axiolabiogingival 軸(面)唇(面)歯肉(面)の

ALAL, ALaL, A La L
axiolabiolingual 軸位口唇舌面の

ALANON
alcoholics anonymous 匿名アルコール中毒者《リハ》

ALAS
aminolevulinic acid synthetase アミノレブリン酸合成酵素

Alas-2
aminolevulinate acid synthase-2 アミノレブリン酸合成酵素 2

ALAT
alanine aminotransferase アラニンアミノトランスフェラーゼ
alanine transaminase アラニントランスアミナーゼ

alb.
albus〈ラ〉=white 白い

ALB, Alb, alb
albumin アルブミン

A

alb.C
albumin clearance　アルブミンクリアランス
ALB/GLOB
albumin/globulin ratio　アルブミン・グロブリン比
ALbL
acute lymphoblastic leukemia　急性リンパ芽球性白血病
ALC
allogeneic lymphocyte cytotoxicity　同種免疫リンパ球細胞傷害性
anterolateral commissure　全交連
approximate lethal concentration　近似致死濃度
avian leukosis complex　トリ白血病複合体
axiolinguocervical　軸(面)舌(面)歯頸(面)の
Alc, alc
alcohol　アルコール
ALCL
anaplastic large cell lymphoma　未分化大細胞性リンパ腫
alcoh
alcohl　アルコール
alcoholic　アルコール(性)の，飲酒家
ALD
adrenoleukodystrophy　副腎白質ジストロフィ
alcohol liver disease, alcoholic liver disease　アルコール性肝疾患
aldosterone　アルドステロン
argi(ni)nosuccinate lyase deficiency　アルギ(ニ)ノコハク酸リアーゼ欠損症
assistive listening device　補聴器補助装置
ALD, Ald
aldolase　アルドラーゼ
ALDA
aldioxa　アルジオキサ
AlDH, ALDH
aldehyde dehydrogenase　アルデヒド脱水素酵素
aldo
aldosterone　アルドステロン
ALF
acute liver failure　急性肝不全
alfacalcidol　アルファカルシドール
ALG
allergic　アレルギーの
allergical　アレルギー性
Annapolis lymphoblast globulin　アナポリスリンパ芽球グロブリン
antilymphoblastic globulin　抗リンパ芽球グロブリン
antilymphocyte globulin　抗リンパ球グロブリン
axiolinguogingival　軸(面)舌(面)歯肉(面)の

alg
algebraic 代数の，代数的な
ALG，alg.
allergy アレルギー
AL Gel
alumigel アルミゲル
ALGLYN
aluminium glycinate アミノ酪酸アルミニウム
ALGOL
algorithmic language アルゴル
algy
allergy アレルギー
ALH
anterior lobe hormone 前葉ホルモン
anterior lobe of the hypophysis 下垂体前葉
ALI
acute lung injury 急性肺障害
annual limit of intake 年摂取限度
argon laser iridotomy アルゴンレーザー虹彩切開(術)
ALIS
advanced life information system 進歩した生命情報システム
Alk，alk
alkaline アルカリ(性)の
Alk phos.，alk.phos.
alkaline phosphatase アルカリホスファターゼ
Alk PO_4
alkaline phosphatase アルカリホスファターゼ
alk.p'tase
alkaline phosphatase アルカリホスファターゼ
ALL
acute lymphoblastic leukemia 急性リンパ芽球(性)白血病
acute lymphocytic leukemia 急性リンパ性白血病
anterior longitudinal ligament 前縦靱帯
All
allose アロース
ALL，all
allergy アレルギー
allgem
allgemeine〈独〉 一般の
allogenic MLCR
allogenic mixed lymphocyte culture reaction 同種混合リンパ球培養反応
allo-THA
allo-tetrahydro-aldosterone アロテトラハイドロアルドステロン

A

allo-THC
allo-tetrahydro-corticosterone　アロテトラハイドロコルチコステロン

allo-TLAK
allogenic tumor and lymphocytes activated killer　同種培養癌細胞刺激誘導キラー細胞

ALM
acral lentiginous melanoma　肢端黒子型黒色腫

A-LM
acetylleucomycin　アセチルロイコマイシン

A-LM, ALM
acetylkitasamycin　アセチルキタサマイシン

ALME, ALMe
acetyl-L-lysine methyl ester　アセチル-L-リシンメチルエステル

ALMI
anterior lateral myocardial infarction　前外側(壁)心筋梗塞

ALN
anterior lymph node　前リンパ節

Alnsuf, A insuf.
aortic insufficiency　大動脈弁閉鎖不全(症)

ALO
apraxia of lid opening　開眼失行
average lymphocyte output　平均リンパ球排出量
axiolinguoclusal　軸位舌面咬合面の

ALOMAD
adriamycin, Leukeran, vincristine (=Oncovin), methotrexate, actinomycin D, dacarbazine　アドリアマイシン,ロイケラン,ビンクリスチン(=オンコビン),メトトレキサート,アクチノマイシンD,ダカルバジン

aloteen
alcoholic teenagers　10歳代のアルコール中毒者

ALOX
aluminium oxide　酸化アルミニウム

ALP
acute lupus pericarditis　急性狼瘡(性)心膜炎
alkaline phosphatase　アルカリホスファターゼ
(pulmonary) alveolar proteinosis　肺胞蛋白症
anterior lobe of pituitary　下垂体前葉
antilymphocyte plasma　抗リンパ球血漿
argon laser photocoagulation　アルゴンレーザー光凝固(術)

AL-Pase
alkaline phosphatase　アルカリ性リン酸分解酵素,アルカリホスファターゼ

alpha-2 M
alpha-2 macroglobulin　α_2マクログロブリン
alpha-2 PM
alpha-2 plasmin inhibitor　α_2プラスミン阻害物質〔インヒビター〕
ALPM
anterolateral papillary muscle　前側乳頭筋
AL protein
amyloid L protein　アミロイドL蛋白
ALRI
anterolateral rotatory instability　前外方回旋不安定性
ALROS
American Laryngological Rhinological and Otological Society　米国耳鼻咽喉科学会
ALS
acute lateral sclerosis　急性側索硬化症
adaptive least squares　適応最小二乗法
advanced life support　二次救命処置
afferent loop syndrome　輸入脚症候群
amyotrophic lateral sclerosis　筋萎縮性側索硬化症
angiotensin-like substance　アンジオテンシン様物質
antilymphatic serum　抗リンパ球血清
antilymphocyte serum　抗リンパ球血清
antilymphocytic serum　抗リンパ球血清
antiviral lymphocyte serum　抗ウイルスリンパ球血清
ALSD
Alzheimer-like senile dementia　アルツハイマー様老年性痴呆
ALSL
acute lymphosarcoma cell leukemia　急性リンパ肉腫細胞性白血病
ALSV
avian leukosis sarcoma virus　ニワトリリンパ肉腫ウイルス
ALT
alanine aminotransferase　アラニンアミノトランスフェラーゼ
Alt
altrose　アルトロース
ALT, alt
alternate　交代する，交互の
alternative　交代(性)の，交互の
altitude　高さ，高度
ALTB
acute laryngotracheobronchitis　急性喉頭気管気管支炎
alt.die.
alternis diebus〈ラ〉＝every other day　隔日に《処》

alt.dieb.
- *alternis diebus*〈ラ〉=every other day　隔日に《処》

ALTe
- apparent life threatening　明瞭な生命険悪状態

alt.h.
- *alternis horis*〈ラ〉=every other hour　隔時に，2時間ごとに《処》

alt.hor.
- *alternis horis*〈ラ〉=every other hour　隔時に，2時間ごとに《処》

alt.noc.
- *alterna noct*〈ラ〉=every other night　一晩おきに，隔夜に《処》
- *alternis nocta*〈ラ〉　一晩おきに，隔夜に《処》

alt.noct.
- *alterna noct*〈ラ〉=every other night　一晩おきに，隔夜に《処》

ALTS
- acute lumbar traumatic syndrome　急性腰部外傷症候群

ALUM
- aluminium adjuvant　アルミニウムアジュバント

ALV
- adeno-like virus　アデノ様ウイルス
- avian leukemia virus　トリ白血病ウイルス
- avian leukosis virus　トリ白血病ウイルス

ALV，alv，alv.
- alveolar　肺胞の，胞状の，歯槽の
- alveolus　肺胞

alv.adstrict.
- *alvo adstricto*〈ラ〉　便秘中《処》

alv.deject.
- *alvi dejectiones*〈ラ〉　腸排泄物《処》

ALVF
- acute left ventricular failure　急性左(心)室不全

ALVH
- asymmetric left ventricular hypertrophy　非均等型左(心)室肥大

alv vent，alv. vent.
- alveolar ventilation　肺胞換気(量)

Alvx，ALVX
- alveolectomy　歯槽骨切除(術)，歯槽突起切除

ALW
- arch-loop-whorl　弓状係蹄渦巻指紋《法医》

ALX
- alloxane　アロキサン

AM
- acral melanoma　末端型黒色腫
- actomyosin　アクトミオシン
- adrenal medulla　副腎髄質

adriamycin	アドリアマイシン(=ドキソルビシン)
aerospace medicine	(航空)宇宙医学
alveolar macrophage	肺胞マクロファージ
amacrine cell	アマクリン細胞
amethopterin	アメトプテリン
amperemeter	アンペア計，電流計
ampicillin	アンピシリン
amplitude modulation	振幅変調
amygdala〈ラ〉	(脳の)扁桃，扁桃核
anovular menstruation	無排卵月経
antimetabolite	代謝拮抗物質
atypical mycobacteria	非定型抗酸菌
atypical mycobacteriosis	非定型抗酸菌症
aureomycin	オーレオマイシン
aviation medicine	航空医学
axiomesial	軸(面)近心(面)の
Am	
allotype marker on human immunoglobulin A	ヒト免疫グロブリンAの異種型マーカー
amenorrhea	無月経
americium	アメリシウム
amylase	アミラーゼ
a.m.	
ante menstruationem〈ラ〉=before menstruation	月経前に
AM, Am	
American	アメリカ人，アメリカの，合衆国の
AM, am, Am	
amyl	アミル基
AM, A.M., a.m.	
ante meridiem〈ラ〉=before noon	午前中に，午前に《処》
AM, A/M	
adult male	成人男性
Am, am	
ametropia	非正視
ammeter	電流計
meter angle	メートル角
myopic astigmatism	近視性乱視
am, am.	
ametropia〈ラ〉	屈折異常
amplitude	振幅
AMA	
Aerospace Medical Association	航空医学協会
American Medical Association	米国医師会

antimitochondrial antibodies　抗ミトコンドリア抗体
anti(-)mitochondrial antibody　抗ミトコンドリア抗体
antimyocardial antibody　抗心筋抗体
antimyosin antibody　抗ミオシン抗体

ama,
as many as, as much as　〜だけ多く

AMA, a.m.a.
against medical advice　医学的助言に逆らって

AMAA
Association of Medical Advertising Agencies　医療宣伝機関協会

AMA-DE
American Medical Association Drug Evaluations　米国医師会薬品評価

AMADIB
American Medical Association Drug Information Data Base　米国医師会薬品情報データベース

AMAERF
American Medical Association Education and Research Foundation　米国医学連合教育研究財団

AMAP
as much as possible　できるだけ多く

A-mat
amorphous material　無晶形物質

AMAV
Association Mondiale des Anatomistes Veterinaires　世界獣医解剖学協会

AMAWA
American Medical Association Women's Auxiliary　米国医療婦人協力者協会

amb
ambient　周囲の
ambiguous　不明瞭な，多義の，あいまいな
ambulate　移動する

Amb, amb.
ambulance　救急車
ambulation　歩行，移動
ambulatory　外来〔通院〕の，歩行(可能)の，移動性の

AMBER
advanced multiple beam equalization radiography　新しい胸部X線撮影装置

ambig
ambiguous　不明瞭な

ambul
ambulate 移動する
ambulation 歩行，移動
ambulatory 外来(通院)の

AMC
acetylmethyl carbinol アセチルメチルカルビノール
Animal Medical Center 動物医学センター
antibody-mediated cytotoxicity 抗体媒介細胞毒性
anti-malaria campaign 抗マラリアキャンペーン
arm muscle circumference 上腕筋囲
arthrogryposis multiplex congenita 先天性多発性関節拘縮症
axiomesiocervical 軸(面)近心(面)歯頸(面)の

AMCA
7-amino-4-methylcoumarin-3-acetic acid 7-アミノ-4-メチルクマリン-3-酢酸

AMCC
Academic Medical Center Consortium 米国学術的医療センター協会

AM & CT
antibiotic medicine and clinical therapy 抗生物質と臨床療法

AMD
acid maltase deficiency 酸性マルターゼ欠損
actinomycin D アクチノマイシンD
alpha-methyl-dioxyphenylalanine αメチルジオキシフェニルアラニン
alpha-methyldopa αメチルド(ー)パ
aminosidine アミノサイジン
amiodarone アミオダロン
antimorphine dose 抗モルヒネ投与量
axiomesiodistal 軸位正中遠位の

AMDA
Airline Medical Directors Association 航空医療指導者協会
Association of Medical Doctor for Asia アジア医師連絡協議会

Am Dent
American Dental Association 米国歯科協会

Amd Evac
aeromedical evacuation 航空避難医療

AMDGF
alveolar macrophage-derived growth factor 肺胞マクロファージ由来成長因子

Amdoc
American Doctor 米国医師(組織)

AME
amebic meningoencephalitis アメーバ性髄膜脳炎

A

AMEL
Aeromedical Equipment Laboratory 航空医学装備研究室
Amer
American アメリカの，アメリカ人，合衆国の
AMF
abnormal mitotic figure 非定型的有糸核分裂像
Acquired Immunodeficiency Syndrome Medical Foundation エイズ医学基金
acute myelofibrosis 急性骨髄線維症
anterior malleolar fold 前ツチ骨ひだ
anti-müllerian factor 抗ミュラー因子
am/fm
amplitude modulation/frequency modulation 振幅変調と周波数変調の比
AMG
amygdala〈仏〉 扁挑
amyloglucosidase アミログルコシダーゼ
antimacrophage globulin 抗マクロファージグロブリン
axiomesiogingival 軸(面)近心(面)歯肉(面)の
AMH
accreditation manual for hospital 病院認定マニュアル
anti-müllerian hormone 抗ミュラー管ホルモン
automated medical history 自動既往症
Am Heart
American Heart Association 米国心臓協会
AMHT
automated multiphasic health testing 自動化検診
AMHTS
automated multiphasic health testing and services 自動健診施設
automated multiphasic health testing and services system 自動化検診システム
automated multiphasic health testing system 自動総合健診システム
AMI
acute myocardial infarction 急性心筋梗塞
acute myocardial insufficiency 急性心筋不全
amitriptyline アミトリプチリン
anterior myocardial infarction 前壁心筋梗塞
antibody-mediated immunity 抗体関与免疫
Association of Medical Illustrators 医学イラストレーター協会
axiomesioincisal 軸面近位切歯面の
AMIM
acute massive ischemic myopathy 急性かつ広範な阻血性筋壊死

AMIS
aspirin myocardial infarction study　アスピリン心筋梗塞研究
AMK
amikacin　アミカシン
AMKL
acute megakaryoblastic leukemia　急性巨核芽球性白血病
AML
acute monocytic leukemia　急性単球性白血病
acute mucosal lesion　急性粘膜病変
acute myeloblastic leukemia　急性骨髄芽球性白血病
acute myeloblastic leukemia, acute myelocytic leukemia, acute myeloid leukemia　急性骨髄性白血病
Aeromedical Laboratory　航空医学研究室
angiomyolipoma　血管筋脂肪腫
anterior malleolar ligament　前ツチ骨靱帯
anterior mitral leaflet　僧帽弁前尖
AMLR
autologous mixed lymphocyte reaction　自己混合リンパ球反応
AMLS
anti-mouse-lymphocyte serum　抗マウスリンパ球血清
AMM
agnogenic myeloid metaplasia　原因不明骨髄様化生
Association Medicale Mondiale〈仏〉= World Medical Association　世界医師会
AMM, amm
ammonia　アンモニア
AMML
acute myelomonocytic leukemia　急性骨髄単球性白血病
AMMoL
acute myelomonocytic leukemia　急性骨髄単球性白血病
ammon
ammonia　アンモニア
AMN
adrenoleukomyeloneuropathy　副腎白血球脊髄神経疾患
adrenomyeloneuropathy　副腎脊髄ニューロパシー
AMO
acute mucocutaneous ocular (syndrome)　急性粘膜皮膚眼(症候群)
axiomesioocclusal　軸位近心咬合面の
amo
amorphous　無定形の
AMOL, AMoL
acute monoblastic leukemia　急性単芽球性白血病
acute monocytic leukemia　急性単球性白血病

A

AMonoL
acute monocytic leukemia 急性単球性白血病
amor
amorphous 無定形の
amorph
amorphous 無定形の
AMP
acid mucopolysaccharide 酸性ムコ多糖類
adenosine monophosphate アデノシン一リン酸
adenosine 5′-monophosphate アデノシン5′-一リン酸
2-amino-2-methyl-1-propanol 2-アミノ-2-メチル-1-プロパノール
aminopterin アミノプテリン
amitriptyline アミトリプチリン
amphetamine アンフェタミン
ampicillin アンピシリン
astigmatism with myopia predominating 近視優勢の乱視
average mean pressure 平均中間圧
Amp
amputation 切断
amp
amperage アンペア数
ampere アンペア
amplification 増幅
amplitude 振幅
ampoule アンプル
amputate 切断する
amputated 切断した
amp.
amplus〈ラ〉=ampl 大きい，たくさんの《処》
A5MP
adenosine5′-monophosphate アデノシン5′-一リン酸
AMP，amp
ampule アンプル
amputation 切断術〔法〕
AMPAC
American Medical Political Action Committee 米国医療行政行動委員会
AMPC
amino-hydroxybenzyl penicillin アミノヒドロキシベンジルペニシリン
AMPC，AM-PC
amoxicillin アモキシシリン
AMPH
amphetamine アンフェタミン

amphotericin	アムホテリシン
amphotericin B	アムホテリシンB
amph	
amphoric	壺音性の
amph.	
amphibian, *amphibous*〈ラ〉	両生類
AMPH-B	
amphotericin B	アムホテリシンB
amphet	
amphetamine	アンフェタミン
amphetamine	
alpha-methyl-beta-phenyl-ethyl-amine	アンフェタミン
amp-hr	
ampere-hour	アンペア・時
ampl.	
amplus〈ラ〉=ampl	大きい，たくさんの《処》
AMPN	
aminopeptidase N	アミノペプチダーゼN
AMP-P-P	
adenosine triphosphate	アデノシン三リン酸
A-M PR	
Austin-Moore prosthesis	オースチン・ムーア補綴
AMPS	
acid mucopolysaccinic acid	酸性ムコ多糖類
AMP-S	
adenylosuccinic acid	アデニロコハク酸
ampt	
amputation	切断術〔法〕
amputee	(肢)切断患者
ampul.	
ampulla〈ラ〉=ampule, ampoule	アンプル
AMQ	
American Medicai Qualification	米国医師免許証
AMR	
acoustic muscle reflex	聴骨筋反射
activity metabolic rate	活性代謝率
alternating motion rate	交代運動率
average minimum requirement	平均最小必要量
AMRA	
American Medical Records Association	米国医療記録協会
AMRF	
African Medical and Research Foundation	アフリカ医学研究財団

AMRI
anteromedial rotatory instability 前内方回旋不安定性

AMS
accelerator mass spectrometry 加速器質量分析計
acute mountain sickness 急性高山病
(alpha-)amylase (α)アミラーゼ
Antikörpermangelsyndrom〈独〉 抗体欠乏症候群
antimacrophage serum 抗マクロファージ〔大食細胞〕血清
Army Medical School 陸軍軍医学校[米国]
Army Medical Service 陸軍医療サービス[米国]
atypical mole syndrome 非定型母斑症候群
auditory memory span 聴覚の記憶幅

AMS Ⅲ method
Army Medical School Ⅲ method 陸軍軍医学校Ⅲ法[米国]

AMSMH
Association of Medical Superintendents of Mental Hospital 精神病院医療管理者協会

AMT
acute miliary tuberculosis 急性粟粒結核(症)
alpha methyltyrosin αメチルチロシン
amethopterin アミトプテリン
amitriptyline アミトリプチリン
amphetamine アンフェタミン

amt, am't
amount 量

AMTIC
Ambient Monitoring Technology Information Center 環境技術情報センター

AMTR
angiomesenchymal tissue reaction 血管実質組織反応

amu
atomic mass unit 原子質量単位

AMuLV
Abelson murine leukemia virus アーベルソン白血病ウイルス

AMV
alpha mosaic virus αモザイクウイルス
assisted mechanical ventilation 補助機械的換気
Atemminutenvolumen〈独〉 毎分換気量
avian myeloblastosis virus トリ骨髄芽球性ウイルス

AMWA
American Medical Women's Association 米国女医会

AMX
amoxicillin アモキシシリン

AMY
amytal　アミタール

AMY, Amy
amylase　アミラーゼ

AMYG
amygdaloid nucleus　類扁桃核

amyl
amylase　アミラーゼ

AN
acanthosis nigricans　黒色表皮(肥厚)症
acid number　酸価
acoustic neurinoma　聴神経腫(瘍)
acute nephritis　急性腎炎
adrenergic neuron　アドレナリン作動性ニューロン
ala nasi　鼻翼，小鼻
aminonucleotide　アミノヌクレオチド
amyl nitrate　亜硝酸アミル
anomaly　異常
anorexia nervosa　神経性食思不振症
antenatal　出生前の
anterior　前方の
anxiety neurosis　不安神経症
aseptic epiphysenecrosis　無菌性骨端壊死
aseptic necrosis　無菌性壊死
Aspergillus niger　黒色アスペルギルス
associate in nursing　看護上の同僚

An
actinon　アクチノン〈元素〉
Anamnese〈独〉　病歴
anatomy　解剖(学)
aniridia　無虹彩(症)
anisometropia〈ラ〉　不同視
anodal　陽極の
anode　陽極
antrum　洞，腔，室
normal atmosphere　正常気圧

A/N
as needed　必要に応じて

a/n
acid and neutral　酸性と中性

An, AN
aneurysm　動脈瘤

ANA
acetylneuraminic acid　アセチルノイラミン酸
American Neurological Association　米国神経学協会

A

American Nurse('s) Association 米国看護師協会
anesthesia 知覚脱失〔消失〕，麻酔
anesthetic 知覚脱失〔消失〕の，麻酔の
antinuclear antibody 抗核抗体

ANAE
acid$_{\alpha}$-naphthyl acetate esterase アシドαナフチルアセテートエステラーゼ

Anaes
anesthesia 知覚脱失〔消失〕，麻酔
anesthetic 知覚脱失〔消失〕の，麻酔の

Anaesth
anesthesia 知覚脱失〔消失〕，麻酔
anesthetic 知覚脱失〔消失〕の，麻酔の

ANAG
acute narrow angle glaucoma 急性狭隅角緑内障

anal
analgesia 痛覚脱失(症)，無痛(症,法)
analgesic 鎮痛性の，鎮痛薬

ANAL., anal, anal.
analysis 分析
analyst 分析者
analytical 分析の
analyze 分析する

analog
analogous 相似している

Anal.Psychol.
analytical psychology 分析心理学

analyt
analytical 分析の

Anamn
Anamnese 既往歴

ANAS
anastomosis 吻合(術)

Anat, anat
anatomic 解剖学的な，解剖(学)の
anatomical 解剖(学)の
anatomy 解剖(学)

ANBPS
Australian national blood pressure study オーストラリア国際血圧実態調査

ANC
Alzheimer neurofibrillary change アルツハイマー神経原線維変性

ANCA
anti(-)neutrophil cytoplasmic (auto) antibody 抗好中球細胞質抗体

ANCC, AnCC
anodal closing contraction 陽極閉鎖収縮
ANCOVA
analysis of covariance 共分散分析
ANDA
abbreviated new drug application 簡易新薬申請
ANDI
acquired nephrogenic diabetes insipidus 後天性腎性尿崩症
ANDRO
androsterone アンドロステロン
AnDT
anodal duration tetanus 陽極持続強縮
ANE
angioneurotic edema 血管神経性浮腫
ANEA
antinuclear envelope antibody 抗核抗体
Anes, anes
anesthesia 知覚脱失〔消失〕, 麻酔(法)
anesthesiology 麻酔学
anesthetic 知覚脱失〔消失〕の, 麻酔の
anesth
anesthesia 知覚脱失〔消失〕, 麻酔(法)
anesthesiology 麻酔学
anesthetic 知覚消失〔脱失〕の, 麻酔薬
AnEx, an ex, an.ex., anex.
anodal excitation 陽極(性)興奮
anode excitation 陽極(性)興奮
ANF
alpha-naphthoflavone αナフトフラボン
American Nurse's Foundation 米国看護協会
antineuritic factor(s) 抗神経炎因子
antinuclear factor 抗核因子
atrial natriuretic factor 心房性ナトリウム利尿因子
avascular necrosis of femoral head 大腿骨頭無腐性壊死
ANG
Alles-oder-Nichts-Gesetz〈独〉 悉無律(=しつむりつ), 全か無(か)の法則
angiotensin アンジオテンシン
ANG I
angiotensin I アンジオテンシンI
ANG II
angiotensin II アンジオテンシンII
ANG, Ang, ang.
angiogram 血管写(像), 血管造影〔撮影〕図

A

Ang, ang.	
angle	角
angulation	(屈曲)角形成
Angio, angio	
angiogram	血管写(像), 血管造影〔撮影〕図
angiography	血管写, 血管造影〔撮影〕(法)
ang.pect	
angina pectoris	狭心症
anh	
anhydrous	無水の
ANHE	
acute necrotizing hemorrhagic encephalopathy	急性壊死性出血性脳症
anhyd	
anhydrous	無水の
ANI	
acute nerve irritation	急性神経刺激
anil	
aniline	アニリン
anim	
animal	動物
animate	生かす, 活動させる
aniso	
anisocytosis	赤血球(大小)不同(症)
Anisometr	
anisometropia	屈折(左右)不同(症), 不同視
ANIT	
alpha-naphthylisothiocyanate	αナフチルイソチオシアネート
ank	
ankle	くるぶし
ANL	
all or nothing〔none〕 law	悉無律(=しつむりつ), 全か無(か)の法則
ANLL	
acute non-lymphoblastic leukemia	急性非リンパ芽球性白血病
acute non-lymphocytic leukemia	急性非リンパ性白血病
ANM	
Anamnese	病歴
N-(1-anilinonaphthyl-4)-maleimide	N-(1-アニリノナフチル-4)-マレイミド
Ann, ann	
annals	年報, 雑誌
annual	1年の, 毎年の

Annls
annals — 年報，雑誌

annot
annotation — 注釈

ANoA
antinucleolar antibodies — 抗核小体抗体

ANOC, AnOC, AnOc
anodal opening contraction — 陽性開放収縮

anorex
anorexia nervosa〈ラ〉 — 神経性食欲不振症

ANOV
analysis of variance — 分散分析，分散解析

ANOVA
analysis of variance — 分散分析，分散解析

ANP
acute necrotizing pancreatits — 急性壊死性膵炎
A-norprogesterone — Aノルプロゲステロン
atrial natriuretic peptide — 心房性ナトリウム利尿ペプチド
atrial natriuretic polypeptide — 心房性ナトリウム利尿ポリペプチド

ANRC
Anthony Novan Research Center — アンソニーノーバン研究センター

ANRI
acute nerve root irritation — 急性神経根刺激

ANS
American Nutrition Society — 米国栄養学会
anterior nasal spine — 前鼻棘
antineutrophilic serum — 抗好中球血清
autonomic nervous system — 自律神経系

ans
answer — 答え(る)，解答

ANS, 1,8-ANS
1-anilinonaphthalene-8-sulfonic acid — 1-アニリノナフタレン-8-スルホン酸

ANSI
American National Standards Institute — 米国規格協会

ansth
anesthesia — 麻酔

AnSZ
Anodenschließungszuckung〈独〉 — 陽極閉鎖収縮

ANT
Alzheimer neurofibrillary tangle — アルツハイマー神経線維変化

2-amino-5-nitrothiazole 2-アミノ-5-ニトロチアゾール

ant
antenna アンテナ
antimycin アンチマイシン

ANT, ant
anterior 前の，前方の

Ant A
antimycin A アンチマイシンA

antag, antag.
antagonism 拮抗(作用)
antagonist 拮抗
antagonistic 拮抗する，拮抗(作用)的な

ant.ax.
anterior axillary 前腋窩

anthro
anthropologist 人類学者
anthropology 人類学

Anthrop
anthropology 人類学

anthropom.
anthropometry 人体計測(法)

anti-BM antibody
anti-basement membrane antibody 抗基底膜抗体

anti-coag
anticoagulant 抗凝血性の，抗凝固薬

anti-GBM
anti-glomerular basement membrane 抗糸球体基底膜

anti HA
anti-hepatitis A antibody 抗A型肝炎抗体

anti HBc
anti-hepatitis B core antibody 抗B型肝炎コア抗体

anti HBe
anti-hepatitis B-e antibody 抗B型肝炎e抗体

anti HBs
anti-hepatitis B surface antibody 抗B型肝炎表面抗体

anti-HGH
anti-human growth hormone 抗ヒト成長ホルモン

antitox
antitoxinum アンチトキシン，抗毒素

ant.jentac.
ante jentaculum〈ラ〉=before breakfast 朝食前に《処》

ant.long.ligs.
anterior longitudinal ligaments 前縦靱帯

Ant pit., ant.pit.
anterior pituitary　下垂体前葉
ant.prand.
ante prandium〈ラ〉＝before dinner　夕食前に《処》
ant.sup.sp.
anterior superior spine　前上棘，上前棘
Ant.sup.spine
anterior superior spine (of ilium)　(腸骨の)上前棘
ant.tib.
anterior tibial　前脛骨の
ANTU
alpha-naphthylthiourea　αナフチルチオウレア
ANUG
acute necrotizing ulcerative gingivitis　急性壊死性潰瘍性歯肉炎
anx
anxiety　不安
anxious　不安な
AO
abdominal aorta　腹部大動脈
absorption ointment　吸収軟膏
acridine orange (test)　アクリジンオレンジ(試験)
anodal opening　陽極開放
aortic ostium　大動脈口
area of operation　手術野
ascending aorta　上行大動脈
atlanto-occipital　環椎後頭骨の
atom-orbital　原子軌道
atractylodes ovota　浙江白朮《漢方》
atrioventricular valve opening　房室弁開口
axio-occlusal　軸位(面)咬合(面)の
Ao
anterior oblique　前斜
antioxidant　抗酸化剤，酸化防止剤
aorta　大動脈
aortic opening　大動脈開放
AO, Ao
aorta　大動脈
AOA
American Optometric Association　米国視力測定協会
American Orthopedic Association　米国整形外科協会
American Osteopathic Association　米国骨疾患協会
AOAC
Association of Official Analytical C　眼科分析公定法[米国]
AOAN
Asian and Oceanian Association of Neurology　アジアオセアニア神経学会

AoAW
anterior wall of the aorta 大動脈前壁
AOC
American Optical Company 米国光学会社
American Orthoptic Council 米国視力矯正審議会
anodal opening clonus 陽極開放クローヌス
anodal opening contraction 陽極開放収縮
AOCL
adsorbable organic bounded chloride 活性炭吸着塩素化合物
AOD
adult-onset diabetes 成人発症(型)糖尿病
aorta diameter, aortic diameter, aortic dimension 大動脈径
arterial occlusive disease 動脈閉塞性疾患
arteriosclerotic occlusive disease 動脈硬化性閉塞性疾患
atlanto-occipital dislocation 環椎後頭骨変位
auriculo-osteodysplasia 房室骨形成異常
AO diag
acridine-orange diagnosis アクリジンオレンジ診断
AODM
adult-onset diabetes mellitus 成人発症(型)糖尿病
AOEHI
American Organization for Education of Hearing Impaired 米国聴覚障害者教育のための組織
AOFNMB
Asian and Oceanian Federation of Nuclear Medicine and Biology アジアオセアニア核医学生物学連盟
AOG
aortography 大動脈造影法
auditory electro-oculomotogram 聴覚性電気眼球運動図
Aogen
angiotensinogen アンジオテンシノゲン
1α-OHCC
1α-hydroxycholecalciferol 1αヒドロキシコレカルシフェロール
17α-OHP, 17-α-OH-P
17α-hydroxyprogesterone 17αヒドロキシプロゲステロン
AOI
area of interest 関心領域
AOL
acro-osteolysis 先端(肢端)骨溶解(症)
amenity of life 生命の快適さ
AOM
active oxygen method 能動酸化法
acute otitis media 急性中耳炎

Master of Obstetric Art 産科学修士

AoMP

aortic mean pressure 大動脈平均圧

AON

all or none law 悉無律(=しつむりつ)，全か無(か)の法則

anterior olfactory nucleus 前嗅神経核

AOO

anodal opening odor 陽極開放時臭

AOP

acetoxy-pregnenolone アセトキシプレグネノロン

anodal opening picture 陽極開放像

aortic pressure 大動脈圧

aortic pressure pulse 大動脈圧脈波

Association of Optical Practitioners 光学者協会

Association of Osteopathic Publications 骨疾患出版協会

AOP-syndrome

adipositas-hyperthermia-oligomenorrhea-parotid-syndrome 脂肪過多・高温・過小月経・耳下腺症候群

AoPW

aortic posterior wall 大動脈後壁

AORN

American Operating Room Nurses 米国手術室看護師協会

AOrPA

American Orthopsychiatric Association 米国精神矯正学協会

AORT

Association of Operating Room Techniques 手術室技術協会

AORTF

American Organization for Rehabilitation through Training Federation 訓練によるリハビリテーションのための米国組織

aort.regurg.

aortic regurgitation 大動脈弁逆流

aort.sten

aortic stenosis 大動脈(弁)狭窄

AOS

active oxygen species 活性酸素種

American Ophthalmological Society 米国眼科学会

American Otological Society 米国耳科学会

anodal opening sound 陽極開放時音

AOSC

acute obstructive suppurative cholangitis 急性閉塞性化膿性胆管炎

A

AOSPS
American Otorhinologic Society for Plastic Surgery　形成外科のための米国耳鼻科学会

AOT
anodal opening tetanus　陽極開放強縮

AOTF
acoustico-optic tunable filter　音響光学変調フィルター

AoV，AV
aortic valve　大動脈弁

AOZ
Anodenöffnungszuckung〈独〉　陽極開放収縮

AP
Academy of Psychologists　心理学者協会
acid phosphatase　酸(性)ホスファターゼ
aclarubicin, prednisolone　アクラルビシン, プレドニゾロン
action potential　活動電位
active pepsin　活性ペプシン
acute phase　急性相，急性期
acute pneumonia　急性肺炎
acute proliferation　急性増殖
adolescent population　青年期人口
after parturition　分娩後に
alkaline phosphatase　アルカリホスファターゼ
alternative pathway　(補体系の)副経路
alum precipitate　ミョウバン沈降物
aminopeptidase　アミノペプチダーゼ
2-aminopurine　2-アミノプリン
aminopyrine　アミノピリン
angina pectoris　狭心症
ankle pressure　足関節収縮期圧
antegrade pyelography　順行性腎盂造影
anterior pituitary　下垂体前葉
anteroposterior diameter of the pelvic outlet　骨盤出口縦径
antiplasmin　抗プラスミン
antipyrine　アンチピリン
aortic pressure　大動脈圧
appendectomy　虫垂切除術
appendix　付属物，虫垂
apridine　アプリジン
apurinic acid　アプリン酸
area postrema　最後野
arithmetic progression　等差級数
arterial pressure　動脈圧
artificial pneumothorax　人工気胸(法)

associate professer 准教授
aspiration pneumonia 誤嚥性肺炎
atom-probe アトムプローブ
atrial pacing 心房調律
axiopulpal 軸(面)歯髄(面)の

ap
periodic albinoism 周期性白皮症

AP5
D-2-amino-5-phosphonovalerate D-2-アミノ-5-ホスホノ吉草酸塩

A_2P_2
aortic second sound greater than pulmonary second sound 第二大動脈音が第二肺動脈音より大

AP-2
acetylpiperadine アセチルピペラジン

a.p.
ante partum〈ラ〉 分娩前に
ante prandium〈ラ〉=before dinner 夕食前に
a priori〈ラ〉=first 最初に

A/P
ascites/plasma (ratio) 腹水/血漿(比)
assessment and plan 評価と計画

A & P
anatomy and physiology 解剖(学)と生理(学)
anterior and posterior 前後(方向)の

AP, Ap, ap
apothecary 薬剤師

AP, A-P
abdominal-perineal 腹部・会陰の
anterior posterior (view) 前後(方向)の(像)
anteroposterior 前後(方向)の

3AP, 3-AP
3-acetylpyridine 3-アセチルピリジン

A & P, A+P
auscultation and palpation 聴診と触診
auscultation and percussion 聴診と打診

APA
action potential amplitude 活動電位波高
aldosterone producing adenoma アルドステロン産生腺腫
Ambulatory Pediatric Association 外来小児科学会
American Patients Association 米国患者同盟
American Pharmaceutical Association 米国製薬協会
American Physiotherapy Association 米国理学療法協会
American Psychiatric Association 米国精神医学協会
American Psychological Association 米国心理学協会

American Psychotherapy Association 米国心理療法協会
anti-pernicious anemia (factor) 抗悪性貧血(因子)
antiplatelet antibody 抗血小板抗体
axial pressure angle 腋下加圧角

6-APA
6-aminopenicillanic acid 6-アミノペニシラン酸

APAAP
alkaline phosphatase antialkaline phosphatase (complex) アルカリホスファターゼ抗アルカリホスファターゼ(複合体)

APACHE
acute physiology (assessment) and chronic health evaluation (system) ICU患者の急性生理学的異常・慢性度による重症度評価システム，アパシェ

APAF
anti-pernicious anemia factor 抗悪性貧血因子

APAO
Asian-Pacific Academy of Ophthalmology アジア太平洋眼科学アカデミー

APAP
N-acetyl-*p*-aminophenol *N*-アセチル-*p*-アミノフェノール

APAS
annular phased array system 環状層化整列システム

APB
abductor pollicis brevis (muscle) 短母指外回転(筋)
atrial〔auricular〕 premature beat(s) 心房性期外収縮

a-PBC
asymptomatic primary biliary cirrhosis 無症候性原発性胆汁性肝硬変

APC
activated protein C 活性型プロテインC
adenoid-pharyngeal conjunctivitis アデノイド咽頭結膜炎
adenomatous polyposis coli 大腸腺腫性ポリポーシス，大腸腺腫様ポリープ
aerobic plate count 好気性菌数の測定
allophycocyanin 螢光色素蛋白
all purpose capsule 多目的カプセル
antibody producing cell 抗体産生細胞
antigen presenting cell 抗原提示細胞
antiphlogistic corticoid 消炎性コルチコイド
apneustic center 持続性吸息中枢
argon plasma coagulation アルゴンプラズマ凝固法
aspirin(=acetylsalicylic acid), phenacetin, and caffeine アスピリン(=アセチルサリチル酸)・フェナセチン・カフェイン

A

atrial〔auricular〕 premature contraction(s) — 心房性期外収縮

APCC
activated prothrombin complex concentrate — 活性プロトロンビン複合物質
aspirin, phenacetin, caffeine, with codeine — アスピリン・フェナセチン・カフェインとコデイン

APCD
adult polycystic disease — 成人型多嚢胞症

APCF
acute pharyngoconjunctival fever — 急性咽頭結膜熱

APCG
apexcardiogram — 心尖拍動図

$APCH_{50}$
alternative pathway CH_{50} — 副経路性50%溶血活性

APCI
atmospheric pressure chemical ionization — 大気圧化学イオン化法

$aPco_2$
actual pressure of carbonic acid gas — 実測炭酸ガス分圧

APCP
antibody producing cell precursor — 抗体産生前駆細胞

APCS
alcohol-induced pseudo-Cushing syndrome — アルコール誘発クッシング類似症候群

APCs
atrial premature contractions — 心房性期外収縮

APCT
alternative prism cover test — 交代プリズムおおい試験

APC tabs
aspirin, phenacetin, and caffeine tablets — アスピリン・フェナセチン・カフェイン錠(剤)

APC-virus
adenoidal-pharyngeal-conjunctivitis virus — 咽頭・喉頭・結膜炎ウイルス，アデノウイルス

APCY
allophycocyanin — 螢光色素蛋白

APD
action potential duration — 活動電位持続(時間)
acute pandysautonomia — 急性汎自律神経失調症
adult polycystic disease — 成人型多嚢胞症
amino-hydroxypropane diphosphonate — アミノヒドロキシプロパン二リン酸塩
autoimmune progesterone dermatitis — 自己免疫性プロゲステロン皮膚炎
automated peritoneal dialysis — 自動腹膜灌流

A

APD, A-PD
anterioposterior diameter　前後径

APDF
Asian Pacific Dental Federation　アジア太平洋歯学連盟

APDL
activities parallel to daily living　生活関連動作

APdS
American Pediatric Society　米国小児科学会

APDT
acellular pertussis-diphteria-tetanus　百日咳・ジフテリア・破傷風の新タイプ3種混合ワクチン
anteroposterior diameter of thorax　胸郭の前後径

APE
acute polioencephalitis　急性ポリオ脳炎
aminophylline, phenobarbital, ephedrine　アミノフィリン・フェノバルビタール・エフェドリン
anterior pituitary extract　下垂体前葉抽出物
apparent effect　明瞭な効果

APECED
autoimmune polyendocrinopathy-candidosis-ectodermal dystrophy　自己免疫多内分泌病・カンジダ症・外胚葉ジストロフィ

APECS
autoimmune polyendocrine candidiasis syndrome　自己免疫多内分泌カンジダ症候群

AP-endonuclease
apurinic/apyrimidinic endonuclease　無プリン/無ピリミジンエンドヌクレアーゼ

APF
animal protein factor　動物蛋白因子

AP-FIM
atom probe field ion microscopy　アトムプローブ電界イオン顕微鏡

AP Fistel
aortopulmonale Fistel　大動脈中隔欠損症，大動脈肺動脈窓

AP fistula
aortico-pulmonary fistula　大動脈中隔欠損症

APG
auricular plethysmograph　耳垂プレチスモグラフ

Apgar score
appearance, pulse, grimace, activity, respiration score　顔貌・心拍数・足底刺激に対する反射・筋の緊張・呼吸のスコア，アプガースコア

APH
antepartum hemorrhage　分娩前出血

anterior pituitary hormone 下垂体前葉ホルモン
apical hypertrophy 心尖部肥大

apH
actual pH 実測水素イオン濃度

APH, aph
aphasia 失語症

APHA
American Public Health Association 米国公衆衛生協会

APhA
American Pharmaceutical Association 米国製薬協会

APHB
American Printing House for Blind 米国盲人のための印刷所

APHI
Association of Public Health Inspectors 公衆衛生監視者協会

APHP
antipseudomonas human plasma 抗シュードモナスヒト血漿

API
acute panic inventory 急性パニック特性尺度
alkaline protease inhibitor アルカリ性プロテアーゼ阻害剤
ankle pressure index 足頸圧指標，足関節血圧指数
Association Phonétique Internationale〈仏〉 国際音声学協会

APIC
Association for Practitioners in Infection Control （米国）感染症防止担当協会

A-pill
abortion pill 堕胎薬

APIM
Association Professionale Internationale des Medicine〈仏〉 医学国際職業協会

APIPRS
Asian-Pacific Section of the International Confederation of Plastic and Reconstructive Surgery 国際形成外科学連合アジア太平洋部会

APIS
arteria phrenica inferior sinistra〈ラ〉 左下横隔膜動脈

APIVR
artificial pacemaker-induced ventricular rhythm 人工ペースメーカー誘導心室調律

APKD
adult polycystic kidney disease 成人多嚢胞性腎疾患

APL
abductor pollicis longus (muscle) 長母指外転（筋）

acute promyelocytic leukemia 急性前骨髄球性白血病
anterior pituitary-like (substance) 下垂体前葉類似物質
antiphospholipid 抗リン脂質抗体
α_2 plasmin inhibitor α_2プラスミン阻害物質〔インヒビター〕

apla, APLA
aplastic anemia 再生不良性貧血

ap/lat
anteroposterior and lateral 前後位と側位

APLPMR
Asian Pacific League of Physical Medicine and Rehabilitation アジア太平洋物理医学リハビリテーション連盟

APL valve
adjustable pressure limiting valve 調節式圧開放弁

APM
aminopeptidase microsomal 細胞顆粒アミノペプチダーゼ
anterior papillary muscle 前乳頭筋

APMPPE
acute posterior multifocal placoid pigment epitheliopathy 急性後部多発性板状色素上皮症

APMR
Association for Physical and Mental Rehabilitation 心身リハビリテーション協会

APN
acute pyelonephritis 急性腎盂腎炎
adult periarteritis nodosa 成人型結節性動脈周囲炎
aminopeptidase N アミノペプチダーゼN
average peak noise 平均ピーク音響

APO
adriamycin, prednisone, vincristine (= Oncovin) アドリアマイシン, プレドニゾン, ビンクリスチン (=オンコビン)
apomorphine アポモルヒネ

Apo
apolipoprotein アポリポ蛋白
apoplexy 脳卒中, 脳出血, 脳梗塞, 脳血管障害
apoprotein アポ蛋白

APO, Apo
apoplexia cerebri〈ラ〉 脳卒中

APOM
acute purulent otitis media 急性化膿性中耳炎

APORF
acute postoperative renal failure 急性術後腎不全

Apoth, apoth.
apothecary 薬剤師

A

APP
acute phase protein 急性期蛋白
adenine diphosphate アデニン二リン酸
amyloid precursor protein, amyloid protein precursor アミロイド前駆体蛋白
antiplatelet plasma 抗血小板血漿
avian pancreatic peptidase トリ膵ペプチダーゼ
avian pancreatic polypeptide トリ膵臓性ポリペプチド

App
appendectomy 虫垂切除術

app
apparatus 装置，器具
apparent 明らかな，見かけの
apparently 明らかに
appetite 食欲
appointment 予約
appropriate 適切な

APP, app, app.
appendix 付属物，虫垂

App, app
appendicitis 虫垂炎

appar
apparatus 装置，器具
apparent 明らかな，見かけの

APPC
apalcillin アパルシリン

AP-PCR
arbitrarity primed polymerase chain reaction 任意ポリメラーゼ鎖反応

Appe, appe.
appendectomy 虫垂切除
appendicitis 虫垂炎

APPG
aqueous procaine penicillin G 水溶性プロカインペニシリンG

appl
appliance 器具，器械
application 適用
applied 応用された

applan.
applanatus〈ラ〉=flattened, flat 平坦な

applic
application 適用

applicand.
applicandus〈ラ〉=to be applied 塗布せよ《処》

appoint
appointment 予約
appos
apposition 付加
appr, appr.
approximate(ly) おおよその
approx
approximation 近似
approx, approx.
approximate(ly) おおよその
A(-)P psychiatrist
analytic-psychological psychiatrist 分析心理学的精神科医
App.T
applanation tonometer 圧平眼圧計
Appt, appt.
appointment 予約
Appx
appendix 虫垂，付属物
APPY, Appy, appy
appendectomy 虫垂切除(術)
APQ
amplitude perturbation quotient (声の)振幅動揺指数
APR
abdomino-perineal resection of rectum 腹会陰式直腸切断術
acute phase reactant 急性(期)反応(性)物質
anterior pituitary reaction 下垂体前葉反応
auropalpebral reflex 耳性眼瞼反射，耳性瞬目反射
apr
annual percentage rate 年百分率
apraxia 失行(症)
aprax
apraxia 失行(症)
APRF
acute phase response factor 急性(期)反応因子
AProL, A ProL
acute promyelocytic leukemia 急性前骨髄球性白血病
APrS
American Proctologic Society 米国直腸肛門学会
APRT
adenine phosphoribosyltransferase アデニンホスホリボシルトランスフェラーゼ
APRT deficiency
adenine phosphoribosyltransferase deficiency アデニンホスホリボシルトランスフェラーゼ欠損症

A

APRV
airway pressure release ventilation 気道内圧緩和換気
aprx
approximately おおよそ
APS
adenosine phosphosulfate アデノシンリン硫酸
adenosine-5′-phosphosulfate アデノシン-5′-ホスホサルフェート
American Pediatric Society 米国小児科学会
American Proctologic Society 米国直腸肛門学会
American Psychosomatic Society 米国心身学会
antiphospholipid syndrome 抗リン脂質抗体症候群
Apgar score アプガースコア
atmosphere pressure spray 大気圧スプレー法
atrial premature systole 心房性早期収縮
automatic sensor positioning system 自動血圧計の測定センサーが動脈を探す方式
APSB
aid to potentially self-supporting blind 潜在的に自己支持のできる視力障害者への援助
APSC
Asian-Pacific Society of Cardiology アジア太平洋心臓学会
APSD
aortico-pulmonary septal defect 大動脈・肺動脈中隔欠損症
APSGN
acute poststreptococcal glomerulonephritis 急性溶連菌感染後糸球体腎炎
acute poststreptococcal leukemia 急性連鎖球菌後糸球体腎炎
APSH
Asian and Pacific Society of Hematology アジア太平洋血液学会
AP shunt
artrey-portal vein shunt 動脈門脈シャント
APSS
Association of Psychophysiological Study of Sleep 睡眠精神生理研究協会
APSSEAR
Association of Pediatric Societies of South-East Asian Region 東南アジア小児科学会
APT
abnormal prothrombin 異常プロトロンビン
alminium (aluminum) precipitated tetanus toxoid アルミニウム沈降破傷風トキソイド
alum-precipitated toxoid ミョウバン沈殿毒素

A

Antiplatelet Trialists, Collaboration 血栓性疾患における抗血小板療法の有効性を調査解析している国際的な機関

applied potential tomography エーピーティー(＝胃排出検査の1つ)

APTA

American Physical Therapy Association 米国物理療法協会

APTT

activated partial thromboplastin time 活性化部分トロンボプラスチン時間

APUD

amine precursor uptake and decarboxylase〔decarboxylation〕 アミン前駆物質摂取と脱炭酸

APUDoma

APUD producing tumor APUD系腫瘍，アプドーマ

APVD

anomalous pulmonary venous drainage 肺静脈還流異常症

APVR

Artificial pacemake ventricular rhythm 人工ペースメーカーによる心室リズム

APW

aortic pulmonary window 大動脈中隔欠損

APWA

American Public Welfare Association 米国公共福祉協会

Ap window

aortopulmonary window 大動脈中隔欠損(症)

apx

appendix 付属

AQ

accomplishment quotient 成就指数《臨心》

acoustic quantification 音響量比

aequorin エクオリン

AQ, aq, aq.

aqua〈ラ〉＝water 水

aqueous 水性の

AQ, A.Q.

achievement quotient 学力指数

aq.aerat.

aqua aerata〈ラ〉＝aerated water, soda 炭酸水

aq.aster.

aqua astricta〈ラ〉＝frozen water 氷，凍結水

aq.astr.

aqua astricta〈ラ〉＝frozen water 氷，凍結水

aq.bul.
aqua bulliens〈ラ〉=boiling water　沸騰水，熱湯

aq.bull.
aqua bulliens〈ラ〉=boiling water　沸騰水，熱湯

aq.cal.
aqua calida〈ラ〉=hot water　温水

aq.com.
aqua communis〈ラ〉=common water　通常水

aq.dest., Aq dest
aqua destillata〈ラ〉=distilled water　蒸留水

aq.ferv.
aqua fervens〈ラ〉=boiling water　沸騰水，熱湯

aq.fig.
aqua frigida〈ラ〉=cold water　冷水

aq.font.
aqua fontis〈ラ〉=city water, running water　水道水

aq.frig.
aqua frigida〈ラ〉=cold water　冷水

aql
acceptable qualifying level　許容しうる適格レベル
acceptable quality level　許容しうる品質標準
approved quality level　承認された品質標準

aq.mar.
aqua marina〈ラ〉=sea water　海水

aq.menth.pip.
aqua menthae piperitae〈ラ〉=peppermint solution　ハッカ水

aq.pluv.
aqua pluvialis〈ラ〉=rain water　雨水

aq.pur.
aqua pura〈ラ〉=pure water　純水

Aq.puri.
Aqua purificata　精製水

aq.r.
aqua regia〈ラ〉　王水

AQS
additional qualifying symptoms　追加的適格症状

aq.tep.
aqua tepida〈ラ〉=tepid water　微温湯

aqu
aqueous　水性の

AR
achievement ratio　達成比
active resistance　活発な抵抗
acrosome reaction　先体反応

airway reactivity	気道反応性
airway resistance	気道抵抗
alarm reaction	警告反応
aldose redactase	アルドース還元酵素
alkali(ne) reserve	アルカリ予備
allergic rhinitis	アレルギー性鼻炎
analytical reagent	分析用試薬
androgen receptor	アンドロゲン受容体
angle recess	隅角底
annual report	年報
anterior resection	前方切除術
aortic regurgitation	大動脈閉鎖不全症
apical-radial	先端放射性の
Argyll Robertson (pupil)	アーガイル・ロバートソン（瞳孔）
arousal reaction	覚醒反応
arousal response	覚醒反応
arsphenamine	アルスフェナミン
artificial respiration	人工呼吸
assisted respiration	補助呼吸
atrophic rhinitis	萎縮性鼻炎
attributable risk	寄与危険度
augmentation reaction	促進反応
aural reflex	音響性耳内筋反射
autoradiography	オートラジオグラフィ
autosomal recessive	常染色体劣性の
autosomal recessive inheritance	常染色体劣性遺伝

Ar

arcuate nucleus	(脳の)弓状核
aryl	アリル

ar

aromatic	芳香性の

ARA

American Rheumatic Association	米国リウマチ協会

Ara

arabinose	アラビノース

ara-A, Ara-A

adenine arabinoside	アデニンアラビノシド

Ara-AMP

adenine-arabinoside-5′-monophosphate	アデニンアラビノシド-5′-一リン酸

Ara C, Ara-C, ara-C

arabinosylcytosine	アラビノシルシトシン(＝シトシンアラビノシド)

A

ara-FC
arabinosyl-5-fluorocytidine — アラビノシル-5-フルオロシチジン

ARAS
ascending reticular activating system — 上行性網様体賦活系

ara-U, Ara-U
arabinosyluracil — アラビノシルウラシル(=ウラシルアラビノシド)

ARB
adrenergic receptor binder — アドレナリン受容体結合体
angiotensin II receptor — アンジオテンシンII受容体拮抗薬

arb
arbitrary — 任意の
arbitration — 任意

Arbo, ARBO
arthropod borne (virus) — アルボウイルス

ARC
abnormal retinal correspondence — 網膜対応異常
AIDS related complex — エイズ関連症候群
AIDSrelated condition — エイズ関連状態
American Red Cross — 米国赤十字
anomalous retinal correspondence — 網膜対応異常
antigen reactive cell(s) — 抗原反応(性)細胞
arcuate nucleus — 弓状核
Association of Rehabilitation Center — リハビリテーションセンター連合
automatic recruitment control — 自動明聴調節
average response computer — 平均加算機

ARCA
automated rapid chemistry apparatus — 自動迅速化学測定装置

ARCET
automatic recording crystal electric tonometer — 自動記録水晶電気眼圧計

Arch
archives — 記録，雑誌

ARCI
addiction research center inventory — 嗜癖研究センター特性尺度

ARCNS
American Red Cross Nursing Service — 米国赤十字看護師サービス

ARCR
Arthritis and Rheumatism Council for Research — 関節炎リウマチ研究審議会

ARCVS
Association of Royal College of Veterinary Surgeons — 獣外科医ロイヤル大学協会

A

ARD
acute respiratory disease　急性呼吸器疾患
adult respiratory disease　成人呼吸器疾患
AIDS-related disease(s)　エイズ関連疾患
allergic respiratory disease　アレルギー性呼吸器疾患
antimicrobial removal device　細菌除去装置
aortic root diameter　大動脈径
arthritis and rheumatic disease　関節炎とリウマチ性疾患
atopic respiratory disease　アトピー性呼吸器疾患

ARDMD
autosomal recessive distal muscular dystrophy　常染色体劣性遠位型筋ジストロフィ

ARDS
acute respiratory distress syndrome　急性呼吸切迫症候群
adult respiratory distress syndrome　成人型呼吸窮迫症候群
AIDS-related disease　エイズ関連疾患

ARDs
antirheumatic drugs　抗リウマチ薬

ARE
active resistive exercise　自発的抵抗運動

ARF
acute renal failure　急性腎不全
acute respiratory failure　急性呼吸不全
acute rheumatic fever　急性リウマチ熱
American Rehabilitation Foundation　米国リハビリテーション財団
Arthritis and Rheumatism Foundation　関節炎リウマチ財団

ARG
autoradiogram　オートラジオグラム
autoradiography　オートラジオグラフィ

Arg
arginine　アルギニン

arg.
argentum〈ラ〉=silver　銀

Arg-Rob
Argyll Robertson　アーガイル・ロバートソン

ARI
acute respiratory illness　急性呼吸器疾患
acute respiratory infection　急性呼吸器感染症
acute respiratory insufficiency　急性呼吸不全
acute respiratory tract infection　急性気道感染症
airway reactivity index　気道反応係数
aldose reductase inhibitor　アルドース還元酵素阻害剤

ARIA
automated radioimmunoassay　自動放射標識免疫検定

ARM
aerosol rebreathing method エアロゾル再呼吸法
allergy relief medicine アレルギー治療医学
artificial rupture of membranes 人工破水
atomic resolution microscope 原子レベル分解能顕微鏡

ARMD
age-related macular degeneration 加齢(性)黄斑変性(症)

ARMI
acute refractory myocardial ischemia 急性不応性心筋虚血

ARMS
amplification refractory mutation system 拡大難治性突然変異システム

ARMSA
Asian Regional Medical Student Association アジア医学生協会

ARN
acute retinal necrosis 急性網膜壊死

ARNMDI
Association for Research in Nervous and Mental Disease 神経精神疾患研究協会

ARO
Academic Research Organization アカデミック臨床研究機関
Association for Research in Ophthalmology 眼科学研究協会
Association of Roentogenological Organization 放射線組織連合

AROM
active range of motion 能動的運動範囲
artificial rupture of membranes 人工破水

arom
aromatic 芳香性の

ARP
absolute refractory period 絶対不応期
advanced research projects 高度研究計画
American Registry of Pathologists 米国病理学者登録
angiotensin related peptide アンジオテンシン関連ペプチド
at risk period 危険期間の
attributable risk percent 寄与危険度割合

ARPA
Advanced Research Projects Agency 高等研究計画局

ARPKD
autosomal recessive polycystic kidney disease 常染色体劣性遺伝多発性囊胞腎

A

ARPT
American Registry of Physical Therapist — 米国物理療法士登録
a-r pulse
apical-radial pulse — 橈骨先端脈
ArQ
arithmetic quotient — 算術指数
ARR
absolute risk reduction — 絶対リスク減少率
arr
arrested — 停止した
A/R ratio
albumin/creatinine ratio — アルブミン/クレアチニン比
ARRS
American Roentgen Ray Society — 米国放射線協会
ARRT
American Registry of Radiologic Technologists — 米国放射線技士登録
Arry
arrhythmia — 不整脈
ARS
alizarin red S — アリザリンレッドS
antirabies serum — 抗狂犬病血清
Ars, ars
arsphenamine — アルスフェナミン
ARSA
arylsulfatase A — アリルスルファターゼA
ARSB
arylsulfatase B — アリルスルファターゼB
ART
accredited record technician — 認定記録技士
Achilles relaxation time — アキレス腱反射弛緩相時間
Achilles tendon reflex test — アキレス腱反射検査
acoustic ray tracing — 音響線追跡
adverse reaction terminology — 副作用用語集
assisted reproductive technology — 生殖補助技術
automated reagin test — 自動感作抗体試験
art
article — 文献
articulation — 関節
ART, Art, art.
arterial — 動脈(性)の
artery — 動脈
art, art.
artifact — 人工
artificial — 人工の

arth
arthritic 関節炎の
arthritis 関節炎
arthr
arthrotomy 関節切開(術)
arthrot
arthrotomy 関節切開(術)
ARTI
acute respiratory tract illness 急性呼吸器疾患
artic
articular 関節(性)の
articulation 関節
artif
artificial 人工の
art.insem
artificial insemination 人工受精
ARTN
aureothricin オーレオスライシン
artt
articulations 関節
ARU
absolute resistance unit 絶対抵抗単位
ARV
AIDS-associated retrovirus ヒトT細胞好性ウイルスIII型
AIDS related retrovirus エイズ関連レトロウイルス
atrialized right ventricle 不整脈原性右室異型性症
ARVD
arrythmogenic right ventricular dysplasia 不整脈原性右室異形成
ary
arytenoid region 披裂部
ARZ
Achillessehnenreflexzeit〈独〉 アキレス(腱)反射時間
AS
acid-saline 酸と塩
acoustic shadow 音響陰影《超音波》
activated sleep レム(=REM)睡眠
active sarcoidosis 活動(型)サルコイドーシス
active sleep 活動睡眠
adolescent suicide 青年(期)自殺
aethoxysklerol エトキシスクレロール
alveolar sac 肺胞嚢
alveolar space 肺胞腔
ampere second アンペア秒
amyloid substance アミロイド物質
anabolic steroid 蛋白同化ステロイド

A

anal sphincter 肛門括約筋
androstanolone アンドロスタノロン
ankylosing spondyl-arthritis 強直性脊椎関節炎
ankylosing spondylitis 強直性脊椎炎
antiseptic 防腐剤
antiserum 抗血清
antisocial 反社会的な
antistreptolysin 抗ストレプトリジン
anxiety state 不安状態
aortic stenosis 大動脈弁狭窄症
aqueous solution 水溶液
aqueous suspension 水性懸濁液
artificial sweetener 人工甘味料
Astrup method アストラップ法
atherosclerosis アテローム(性動脈)硬化(症)
atrial septum 心房中隔
atriostenosis 心房弁狭窄
atropine sulfate 硫酸アトロピン

As

arsenic ヒ素〈元素〉
apnea 無呼吸
ascendance social extroversion 支配性社会的外向

as

adenosquamous carcinoma 腺平上皮癌

5-AS

5-aminosalicylic acid 5-アミノサリチル酸

AS, As, as.

astigmatism 乱視

AS, A.S., a.s.

auris sinistra〈ラ〉=left ear 左耳

AS, A-S

Adams-Stokes (syndrome) アダムス・ストークス(症候群)
arteriosclerosis 動脈硬化(症)

AS, a-s, a.s.

ampere(-)second アンペア秒

ASA

acetylsalicylic acid(=aspirin) アセチルサリチル酸(=アスピリン)
active systemic anaphylaxis 全身アナフィラキシー陽性
Adams-Stokes attack アダムス・ストークス発作
American Society of Anesthesiology 〔Anesthesiologists〕 米国麻酔学会
American Standards Association 米国標準協会
American Surgical Association 米国外科協会
aminosalicylic acid アミノサリチル酸

argi(ni)nosuccinic acid アルギ(ニ)ノコハク酸
arylsulfatase-A アリルスルファターゼA
aspirin-sensitive asthma アスピリン過敏喘息
as soon as 〜するとすぐに

AsA
ascorbic acid アスコルビン酸(=ビタミンC)

ASAIO
American Society for Artificial Internal Organs 米国人工臓器協会

ASAP, asap
as soon as possible できるだけ早く

ASAS
anterior spinal artery syndrome 前脊髄動脈症候群

ASAT
aspartate aminotransferase アスパラギン酸アミノトランスフェラーゼ

ASB
American Society of Bacteriologists 米国細菌学者協会
Arbeiter-Samariter Bund〈独〉 労働者救護団
asymptomatic bacteriuria 無症候性細菌尿

asb
apostilb アポスチルブ〈単位〉

ASBAH
Association for Spina Bifida and Hydrocephalus 脊椎分裂・水頭症協会

ASBC
American Society of Biological Chemists 米国生化学者協会

ASC
acetyl sulfanyl chloride アセチルスルファニールクロライド
alter(nat)ed states of consciousness 意識変容状態
American Society of Cytology 米国細胞学会
antibody-secreting cell(s) 抗体分泌細胞
antigen-sensitive cell(s) 抗原感受性細胞
arteria subclavia〈ラ〉 鎖骨下動脈
ascorbic acid アスコルビン酸(=ビタミンC)

AsC
asymptomatic carrier 無症候性保因者，無症候性保菌者

Asc
ascaris 回虫

asc
ascending 上行性の

A

ASC, asc, asc.
arteriosclerosis 動脈硬化(症)
arteriosclerotic 動脈硬化(性)の

ASCA
American Speech Correction Association 米国発語矯正協会

ASCAD
arteriosclerotic coronary artery disease 動脈硬化性冠(状)動脈疾患

AscAo, ASCAO
ascending aorta 上行大動脈

ASCC
American Society for Control of Cancer 米国癌制圧協会

ASCI
American Society for Clinical Investigation 米国臨床観察学会

ASCII
American standard code for information interchange 情報交換用米国標準コード

Ascit Fl
ascitic fluid 腹水

ASCN
American Society of Clinical Nutrition 米国臨床栄養学会

ASCO
American Society of Clinical Oncology 米国臨床腫瘍学会

A Scot
type-A Scottish influenza virus A型スコットランドインフルエンザウイルス

ASCP
American Society of Clinical Pathologists 米国臨床病理学会
American Society of Consulting Pharmacists 米国顧問薬剤師協会

ASCPT
American Society for Clinical Pharmacology and Therapeutics 米国臨床薬学・治療学会

ascr.
ascriptum〈ラ〉=ascribed to 〜に基づく

ASCRS
American Society of Colon and Rectal Surgeons 米国大腸直腸外科医協会

ASCs
adipose-derived stem〔stromal〕cells 脂肪幹〔間質〕細胞

ASCVD
arteriosclerotic cardiovascular disease 動脈硬化性心血管病
arteriosclerotic coronary artery disease 動脈硬化性冠(状)動脈疾患
atherosclerotic cardiovascular disease アテローム硬化性心血管疾患

ASD
accouchement sans douleur〈仏〉= childbirth without pain 無痛分娩
aldosterone secretion defect アルドステロン分泌欠損
Alzheimer senile dementia アルツハイマー(型)老人性痴呆
antistreptodornase 抗ストレプトドルナーゼ
aortic septal defect 大動脈中隔欠損
applicator skin distance 装着器皮膚間隔
argi(ni)nosuccinate synthase deficiency アルギ(ニ)ノコハク酸合成酵素欠損症
arthritis syphilitica deformans 変形性梅毒性関節炎
atrial septal defect 心房中隔欠損症
autosensitized dermatitis 自家感作性皮膚炎

ASD-I
atrial septal defect ostium primum defect 心房中隔一次孔欠損

ASD-II
atrial septal defect ostium secundum defect 心房中隔二次孔欠損

ASDA
American Sleep Disorders Association 米国睡眠障害学会

ASDC
Association of Sleep Disorders Centers 睡眠障害センター連合

ASDH
acute subdural hematoma 急性硬膜下血腫

ASDR
American Society of Dental Radiographers 米国歯科放射線写真技士協会

ASEP
American Society for Experimental Pathology 米国実験病理学会

asex
asexual 無性の

ASF
Acetobacter suboxydans factor アセトバクタースボキシダンス因子
aldosterone-stimulating factor アルドステロン刺激因子

A

American Schizophrenia Foundation 米国統合失調症財団
aniline, sulfur, formaldehyde アニリン・イオウ・ホルムアルデヒド
anterior spinal fusion 脊椎前方固定術
anterior stapedial fold 前アブミ骨ひだ

ASFV
African swine fever virus アフリカブタコレラウイルス

ASG
American Society of Genetics 米国遺伝学会

ASGBI
Association of Surgeons of Great Britain and Ireland 英国・アイルランド外科医協会

ASGE
American Society for Gastrointestinal Endoscopy 米国消化器内視鏡学会

ASH
action on smoking and health 喫煙と健康に関する活動
aldosterone-stimulating hormone アルドステロン刺激ホルモン
American Society of Hematology 米国血液病学会
ankylosing spinal hyperostosis 強直性脊椎骨化過剰
antistreptococcal hyaluronidase 抗連鎖球菌ヒアルロニダーゼ
asymmetric hypertrophy 非対称性心肥大
asymmetric septal hypertrophy 非対称性中隔肥厚

ASH, AsH, As.H
hyper(metr)opic astigmatism 遠視性乱視

A & sh, A & SH
arm and shoulder 腕と肩

ASHA
American School Health Association 米国学校保健協会
American Social Health Association 米国社会保健協会
American Social Hygiene Association 米国公衆衛生協会
American Speech and Hearing Association 米国言語聴覚協会

ASHBEAMS
American Society for Hospital-Based Emergency Air Medical Services 米国救急ヘリコプター搬送システム

ASHCVD
arteriosclerotic hypertensive cardiovascular disease 動脈硬化性高血圧性心血管疾患

ASHD
arteriosclerotic heart disease 動脈硬化性心疾患
atrial septal heart defect 心房中隔欠損

ASHE
American Society of Hospital Engineering 米国病院工学技術協会

A

ASHG
American Society of Human Genetics　米国人間遺伝学会
ASHH
American Society for Hard of Hearing　米国難聴学会
ASHI
Association for Study of Human Infertility　不妊研究会
ASHP
American Society of Hospital Pharmacists　米国病院薬剤師協会
ASHRM
American Society for Healthcare Risk Management　米国の病院で働くリスクマネージャー支援協会
ASI
active specific immunotherapy　積極的な特異的免疫療法
addiction severity index　嗜癖重症度指数
anxiety status inventory　不安状態調査票
aortic stenoinsufficiency　動脈弁狭窄兼閉鎖不全
Association Stomatologique Internationale〈仏〉=International Stomatological Association　国際口腔病学会
ASI & H
American Society of Ichthyologists and Herpetologists　米国魚鱗癬ヘルペス学者協会
ASIM
American Society of Internal Medicine　米国内科学会
ASIS
anterior superior iliac spine　前上腸骨棘
ASK
antistreptokinase　抗ストレプトキナーゼ
ASL
American sign language　米国式手話
antistreptolysin　抗ストレプトリジン
ASLE
acute systemic lupus erythematosus　急性全身性紅斑性狼瘡
ASLHA
American Speech Language and Hearing Association　米国言語聴覚学会
ASLO
antistreptolysin O　抗ストレプトリジンO
ASLOT
antistreptolysin O test　抗ストレプトリジンOテスト
ASM
airway smooth muscle　気道平滑筋

American Society for Microbiology 米国微生物学会
atrial systolic murmur 心房(性)収縮期雑音
atrio-systolic murmur 心房(性)収縮期雑音

ASM, AsM, As.M.
myopic astigmatism 近視性乱視

ASMA
Aerospace Medical Association 航空医学協会
anti-smooth muscle antibody 抗平滑筋抗体

ASMC
arterial smooth muscle cell 動脈平滑筋細胞

ASME
Association for Study of Medical Education 医学教育研究協会

ASMFS
American Society of Maxillofacial Surgeons 米国顎顔面外科医協会

ASMH
Association for Social and Moral Hygiene 社会精神衛生協会

ASMI
anteroseptal myocardial infarction 前壁中隔梗塞

ASMT
American Society of Medical Technologists 米国医療技術者協会

asmt
assessment アセスメント，事前評価

ASN
arteriosclerotic nephritis 動脈硬化性腎炎

Asn, asn
asparagine アスパラギン

ASO
allele specific oligonucleotide 対立遺伝子特異的オリゴヌクレオシド
American School of Orthodontists 米国歯牙矯正学校
antistreptolysin O 抗ストレプトリジンO
arteriosclerosis obliterans 閉塞性動脈硬化症
Association for the Study of Obesity 肥満症研究会

ASOC
acute suppurative obstructive cholangitis 急性化膿性閉塞性胆管炎

ASOM
asialoorosomucoid 脱シアル化オロソムコイド

ASOS
American Society of Oral Surgeons 米国口腔外科医協会

ASOT
antistreptococcal antibody titer 抗連鎖球菌抗体価

A

antistreptolysin O titer 抗ストレプトリジンO力価

ASP
acute suppurative parotitis 急性化膿性耳下腺炎
American Society of Parasitologists 米国寄生虫学者協会
American Society of Pharmacognostics 米国生薬学会
amnesic shellfish poisoning 記憶喪失性貝中毒
antisocial personality 反社会的人格
anti-streptococcal polysaccharide 抗ストレプトコッカルポリサッカライド
aortic systolic pressure 大動脈収縮期血圧
aspirin アスピリン
ateles species〈ラ〉 クモザル
automatic signal processor 自動信号処理器

Asp
arteria spinalis posterior 後脊髄動脈

asp
aspartate アスパラギン酸塩
aspect 外観
aspirate(d) 吸収する〔した〕
aspiration 吸引

Asp, asp.
asparaginase アスパラギナーゼ
aspartic acid アスパラギン酸

ASPAC
anisoylated plasminogen streptokinase activating complex アニソ化プラスミノーゲンストレプトキナーゼ

aspAT
aspartate aminotransferase アスパラギン酸アミノ基転移酵素

ASPC
aspoxicillin アスポキシシリン

ASPEN
American Society for Parenteral and Enteral Nutrition 米国輸液栄養学会

ASPET
American Society for Pharmacology and Experimental Therapeutics 米国薬理学実験治療学会

ASPG
anti-spleen cell globulin 抗脾(臓)細胞グロブリン

A-SPM
acetyl-spiramycin アセチルスピラマイシン

ASPRS
American Society for Plastic and Reconstructive Surgery 米国形成外科・再建外科学会

American Society of Plastic and Reconstructive Surgeons 米国形成外科・再建外科医協会

ASPVD

arteriosclerotic peripheral vascular disease 動脈硬化性末梢血管疾患

ASQ

anterosuperior quadrant 前上象限

ASR

Achilles Sehnen Reflex〈独〉 アキレス腱反射
aldosterone secretion rate アルドステロン分泌率
antistreptolysin reaction 抗ストレプトリジン反応
aortic valve stenosis and regurgitation 大動脈弁狭窄兼閉鎖不全
atrial septal resection 心房中隔切除術

ASRPP

American Society for Research in Psychomatic Problems 米国精神問題研究会

ASRT

American Society of Radiologic Technologists 米国放射線技師協会

ASS

anterior superior spine 前上棘
argi(ni)nosuccinate synthetase アルギ(ニ)ノコハク酸合成酵素

ASSA

American Society for Study of Allergy 米国アレルギー研究会

ASSArth

American Society for Study of Arthritis 米国関節炎研究会

assby

assembly 集合

ASSH

American Society for Surgery of Hand 米国手の外科学会

assim

assimilate(d) 同化する〔した〕

assist

assistance 助け
assistant 助手

Assn, assn.

association 協会

Assn Clin Biochem

Association of Clinical Biochemists 臨床生化学者協会

assoc, assoc.

associate(d) 連合する〔した〕

association	協会
assocd, assoc'd	
associated (with)	(～に)関連した
ASSS	
American Society for Study of Sterility	米国不妊研究会
Asst, asst	
assist	助ける
assistant	助手
AST	
angiotensin sensitivity test	アンジオテンシン感受性検査
anterior spinothalamic tract	前脊髄視床路
antistreptolysin test	抗ストレプトリジン検査
antistreptolysin titer	抗ストレプトリジン力価
aspartate aminotransferase	アスパラギン酸アミノトランスフェラーゼ
astrocytoma	星細胞腫
AST, Ast, ast	
astigmatism	乱視
ASTA	
antistaphylolysin	抗スタフィロリジン
Asten, A sten.	
aortic stenosis	大動脈弁狭窄(症)
Astg	
astigmatism	乱視
asth	
asthenia	無力(症)
asthma	喘息
Asth, asth.	
asthenopia〈ラ〉	眼精疲労，弱視
astig	
astigma	乱視
astigmatic	乱視の
astigmatism	乱視
astigmatizer	乱視者
astigmometer	乱視計
astigmoscope	乱視計
Astigm	
astigmatism	乱視
ASTM	
American Society for Testing and Materials	米国検査材料協会
American Society of Tropical Medicine	米国熱帯医学会
astromicin	アストロミシン

A

ASTMH
American Society of Tropical Medicine and Hygiene　米国熱帯医学衛生学会
ASTO
anti-snake venom　抗ヘビ毒
antistreptolysin O (titer)　抗ストレプトリジンO(力価)
AS TOL
as tolerated　耐性のあるような
ASTR
antistaphylolysin-reaction　抗スタフィロリジン反応
ASTZ
antistreptozyme test　抗ストレプトザイム検査
ASV
adeno-associated satellite virus　アデノ衛星ウイルス
antero-superfacial venous　前上顔面静脈の
anti-snake venom　抗蛇毒液
avian sarcoma virus　ニワトリ肉腫ウイルス
ASVIP
atrial synchronized ventricular inhibited pacemaker　心房同期型ペースメーカー
ASVR
anomalies of systemic venous return　体静脈還流異常
ASVS
arterial stimulation venous sampling　選択的カルシウム動注負荷後肝静脈採血法
Asx
asparagine　アスパラギン
aspartic acid　アスパラギン酸
asx
asymptomatic　無症候(性)の
asym
asymmetrical　非対称(性)の
asymmetry　非対称
async
asynchronous　非同時性の
ASZ
Anodenschließungszuckung〈独〉　陽極閉鎖収縮
Anspannungszeit〈独〉　緊張時間
AT
achievement test　アチーブメントテスト，学力考査
Achilles tendon　アキレス腱
acoustic tumor　聴神経腫瘍
adjunctive therapy　補助(的)療法
air temperature　気温
air trapping　エアートラッピング

aminotransferase アミノトランスフェラーゼ
aminotriazole アミノトリアゾール
amitriptyline アミトリプチリン
anaerobic threshold 無酸素性作業閾値
anaphylatoxin アナフィラトキシン
antithrombin アンチトロンビン
antitrypsin 抗トリプシン
arterial thrombosis 動脈血栓症
art therapy 芸術療法
ataxia telangiectasia〈ラ〉 運動失調毛細血管拡張病，毛細血管拡張性失調症
atmosphere 大気
atraumatic 非外傷(性)の
atrial tachycardia 心房性頻拍
atropine アトロピン
attenuated 弱毒化された
attenuation 衰弱
atypical transformation 異型移行
autogenic training 自律訓練法
autoimmune thrombocytopenia 自己免疫(性)血小板減少(症)
axillar temperature 腋窩温度
axonal terminal 軸索終末

At
astatine アスタチン〈元素〉
attic 上鼓室

AT.10
anti-tetany 10 抗テタニー剤

AT-Ⅲ
antithrombin Ⅲ アンチトロンビンⅢ

A & T
adenoidectomy and tonsillectomy アデノイド摘出兼扁桃摘出術

AT，at，at.
atom 原子

AT，A-T
ataxia telangiectasia 毛細血管拡張性運動失調(症)

aT，AT
atypical transformation zone 異型移行帯

at，at.
atomic 原子の

ATA
alimentary toxic aleukia 食物性中毒性無白症
American Thyroid Association 米国甲状腺協会
American Tinnitus Association 米国耳鳴研究会
aminotriazole アミノトリアゾール
antithyroglobulin antibody 抗サイログロブリン抗体
anti-Toxoplasma antibodies 抗トキソプラズマ抗体

A

ATA, ata
absolute atmosphere 絶対大気圧
atmosphere absolute (at sea level) 絶対大気圧

ATB
atypical tuberculosis 異型結核(症)

ATBI
athero-thrombotic brain infarction アテローム血栓性脳梗塞

ATC
activated T cell 活性化T細胞
activated thymus cells 活性化胸腺細胞

ATCase
aspartate transcarbamylase アスパルテートカルバミール転移酵素

ATD
Alzheimer-type dementia アルツハイマー型痴呆
antithyroid drugs 抗甲状腺薬
articulatio-trochanteric distance 関節面大転子間距離
asphyxiating thoracic dysplasia 窒息を伴う胸郭形成不全

ATDLG
antithoracic duct lymphoglobulin 抗胸管リンパ球グロブリン

ATE
acute toxic encephalopathy 急性中毒性脳症
adipose tissue extract 脂肪組織抽出物

ATEE
N-acetyl-L-tyrosine-ethylester *N*-アセチル-L-チロシンエチルエステル

ATEM
analytical transmission electron microscopy 分析電子顕微鏡

ATEN
atenolol アテノロール

A tetra P
adenosine tetraphosphate アデノシン四リン酸

ATF
anterior talofibular ligament 前距腓靱帯

At Fib, at.fib.
atrial fibrillation 心房細動

ATG
adenine, thymine, guanine アデニン・チミン・グアニン
anti-human thymocyte globulin 抗ヒト胸腺細胞グロブリン
anti(-)thymocyte globulin 抗胸腺細胞グロブリン
antithyroglobulin 抗サイログロブリン

ATGAM
anti(-)thymocyte gamma globulin 抗胸腺細胞ガンマグロブリン

ATH
abdominal total hysterectomy 腹式子宮全摘術

ATHC
3α-allotetrahydrocortisol　3αアロテトラヒドロコルチゾール

ATHR
aureothricin　オーレオスライシン

ATHSC, Athsc, athsc.
atherosclerosis　アテローム(性動脈)硬化(症)

ATI
air trapping index　エアートラッピング指数
anterior tympanic isthmus　前鼓室狭部
anti-tumor immunity　抗腫瘍免疫

atk
attack　発作

ATL
Achilles tendon lengthening　アキレス腱延長術
adult T cell leukemia　成人T細胞(性)白血病
adult T cell lymphoma　成人T細胞(性)リンパ腫
anterior tricuspid leaflet　三尖弁前尖
atypical lymphocytes　異型リンパ球

ATLA
adult T cell leukemia-associated antigen　成人T細胞(性)白血病(関連)抗原
ATL-virus-associated antigens　成人T細胞(性)白血病ウイルス性抗原

ATLAK
autologous tumor and lymphocytes activated killer　自己癌細胞刺激誘導キラー細胞

ATL-L
adult T cell leukemia-lymphoma　成人T細胞性白血病リンパ腫

ATLS
acute tumor lysis syndrome　急性腫瘍融解症候群
advanced trauma life support　二次外傷救命処置
advanced trauma life support course　上級外傷患者蘇生コース

ATLV
adult T cell leukemia virus　成人T細胞性白血病ウイルス

ATLV-Ⅰ,Ⅱ,Ⅲ…
adult T cell leukemia virus type Ⅰ, Ⅱ, Ⅲ…　成人T細胞性白血病ウイルスⅠ(Ⅱ,Ⅲ…)型

ATM
acute transverse myelitis　急性横断性脊髄炎
acute transverse myelopathy　急性横断性ミエロパシー

ATM, atm
atmosphere　空気, 雰囲気
atmosphere, atmospheric pressure, atmospheric　気圧

A

atmos
atmosphere 空気，雰囲気
atmospheric 空気の，雰囲気の
ATN
acute tubular necrosis 急性尿細管壊死
ATNC
atraumatic normocephalic 非外傷性正常頭部の
ATNG
angiotensinogen アンジオテンシノゲン
at.no.
atomic number 原子番号
ATNR
asymmetrical tonic neck reflex 非対称性緊張性頸反射
ATP
adenosine triphosphate アデノシン三リン酸
ambient temperature and pressure 室温と圧
atypical epithelia, atypical epithelium 異型上皮
autoimmune thrombocytopenic purpura 自己免疫性血小板減少性紫斑病
ATPA
anterior thalamoperforating arteries 前視床穿通動脈
ATPase
adenosine triphosphatase アデノシントリホスファターゼ
ATPD
ambient temperature and pressure, dry 室温，大気圧，乾燥状態
ATPS
ambient pressure 大気圧
ambient temperature 室温
saturated with water vapor 水蒸気飽和状態，飽和水蒸気
ATR
Achilles tendon reflex アキレス腱反射
aotus trivirgatus〈ラ〉 ヨザル〈オマキザル科〉
arm tonus reaction 上肢筋緊張反応
attenuated total reflection 全反射吸収，減衰全反射
atr
atrophy 萎縮
ATRA
all trans retinoic acid レチノイン酸
ATR FIB, atr.fib.
atrial fibrillation 心房細動
atrop, atrop.
atrophy 萎縮
atropine アトロピン

ATS
American Therapeutic Society　米国治療学会
American Thoracic Society　米国胸部疾患学会
anti-rat thymocyte serum　抗ラット胸腺細胞血清
antitetanic serum　抗破傷風血清
antitetanus serum　抗破傷風血清
anti-T lymphocyte serum, antithymocyte serum　抗胸腺細胞血清
anxiety tension state　不安緊張状態
arteriosclerosis　動脈硬化(症)
atherosclerosis　アテローム(性動脈)硬化(症)
autotransfusion system　自家輸血返血法

ATs
aminotransferase(s)　アミノ基転移酵素

ATT
arginine tolerated test　アルギニン負荷試験

AT type
adenine and thymine type　アデニンおよびチミン型

AtV
arteriovenous　動静脈の
atrioventricular　房室の

at vol
atomic volume　原子容量

at.wt.
atomic weight　原子量

ATx
adult thymectomized　成獣胸腺摘除
adult thymectomy　成人胸腺摘出(術)

atyp
atypical　異型の

ATZ
Austreibungszeit〈独〉　娩出時間

AU
antitoxin unit　抗毒素単位
arbitrary units　任意単位

Au
aurum〈ラ〉=gold　金〈元素〉

a.u.
ad usum〈ラ〉=according to custom　慣習に従って

AU, Au
Australia(n) antigen　オーストラリア抗原

AU, A.U., a.u.
aures unitae〈ラ〉=both ears together　両耳とも
aures utrae〈ラ〉=both ears　両耳
auris utraque〈ラ〉=each ear　片耳

A

AUA
American Urological Association — 米国泌尿器科学会
AuAg, Au-Ag
Australia(n) antigen — オーストラリア抗原
AUB
abnormal uterine bleeding — 異常子宮出血
AuBMT
autologous bone marrow transplantation — 自家骨髄移植
AUC
acute uncomplicated cystitis — 急性単純性膀胱炎
area under concentration curve — (薬物血中)濃度時間曲線下面積
area under curve — 曲線下領域
area under the plasma level-time curve — 薬物血中濃度時間曲線下面積
AUCAS
Association of University Clinical Academic Staff — 大学臨床教員協会
auct.
auctorum〈ラ〉=of authors — 著者の
AUD
arthritis of unknown diagnosis — 未確認診断の関節炎
aud
auditory — 聴覚の
AUDI
International Society of Audiology — 国際オージオロジー学会
auding
auditory hearing — 聴解，聴覚と理解
audio
audiofrequency — 可聴周波数
audiogenic — 聴覚原性の
audiogram — 聴力図，オージオグラム
audiology — 聴覚学
audiometer — 聴力計，オージオメーター
audiometry — 聴力測定
audiophone — 補聴器
audiovisual — 視聴覚
audiovisual aids — 視聴覚(教育)器具
audiol
audiology — 聴覚学
audiovis
audiovisual — 視聴覚
audiovisual aids — 視聴覚(教育)器具
auf 4×6 Stund.
4 mal (jede) 6 Stunden — 6時間ごとに4回

AUFS
absorbance unit(s), full scale　吸光度単位・フルスケール

auf 3×T
Täglich 3 mal　1日3回

auf 3×Tgl, auf 3×tgl
Täglich 3 mal　1日3回

AUG
acute ulcerative gingivitis　急性潰瘍性歯肉炎
adenine, uracil, guanine (=initiating codon)　アデニン・ウラシル・グアニン(=開始コドン)

aug.
augere〈ラ〉=to increase　増加する

Auge
Augenarzt　眼科(医)

AUHAA
Australia hepatitis-associated antigen　オーストラリア肝炎関連抗原

AUI
Alcohol Use Inventory　アルコール使用調査票

AUL
acute unclassified leukemia　急性分類不能白血病
acute undifferentiated leukemia　急性未分化白血病

AUO
amyloid of unknown origin　原因不明アミロイド

AuP
Australia antigen protein　オーストラリア抗原蛋白

AUR
American Uuiversity Radiologists　米国大学放射線科医

aur.
aures〈ラ〉=ear　耳
auricle　耳介
auricular　心房の，耳の
auris〈ラ〉=ear　片耳
aurum〈ラ〉=gold (element)　金

AUR FIB, aur.fib.
auricular fibrillation　心房細動

auric
auricle　耳介
auricular　心房の，耳の

aurist.
auristillae〈ラ〉=ear drops　点耳薬

AUS
acute urethral syndrome　急性尿道症候群

Aus
Auskratzung〈独〉　子宮内膜掻爬術
Ausraumung und Auskratzung〈独〉　掻爬除去
Uterus-ausräumung〈独〉　子宮内容除去術

A

aus.
auscultation 聴診(法)
AUSC, ausc
auscultation 聴診(法)
auscul
auscultation 聴診(法)
AuSH, AuSh
Australia serum hepatitis オーストラリア血清肝炎
Aus & Perc
auscultation and percussion 聴診(法)と打診(法)
auto
automation 自動制御装置
autop
autopsy 剖検
au tr
aural training 聴覚訓練
aux
auxiliary 補助的の
AV
adenoid vegetation 腺様増殖症，アデノイド
adriamycin, vincristine アドリアマイシン，ビンクリスチン
alveolar duct 肺胞管
angular vision 角視力
anteversion 前傾
anteverted 前傾の
aortic valve 大動脈弁
artificial ventilation 人工換気
assisted ventilation 補助換気(法)
audiovisual 視聴覚
azygos vein 奇静脈
aV
atypical vessel(s) 異型血管
av
avoirdupois 体重
avulsion 摘出
av.
acuite visuelle〈ラ〉 視力
A/V
arterial/venous 動脈・静脈の
artery-to-vein ratio 動脈/静脈比
atrial/venticular 心房・心室の
auricular/ventricular 心房・心室の
A-V
azygos vein 奇静脈

AV, Av
air velocity 空気速度
AV, Av, av.
average 平均の
AV, A-V
arteriolar-venular 動脈・静脈
arterio(-)venous 動静脈の
atrio(-)ventricular 房室の
auriculoventricular 房室の
AVA
aminovaleric acid アミノ吉草酸
antiviral antibody 抗ウイルス抗体
aortic valve area 大動脈弁領域
aortic valve atresia 大動脈弁閉鎖
arteriovenous anastomosis 動静脈吻合
audiovisual aids 視聴覚(教育)器具
AV-AF, AV/AF
anteverted/anteflexed 前傾・前屈
AVB
atrioventricular block 房室ブロック
AVC
allantoid vaginal cream ソーセージ様腟クリーム
Association of Vitamin Chemists ビタミン化学者協会
atrioventricular canal 房室間孔，房室管
audiovisual center 視聴覚(教育)センター
automatic volume control 自動音量調節
AV canal, A-V canal
atrio(-)ventricular canal 房室間孔，房室管，共通房室弁口
AV communis, A-V communis
atrio(-)ventricular(is) communis 房室間孔，共通房室弁口
AVCS
atrio(-)ventricular conduction system 房室伝導系
AVD
aortic valve deviation 大動脈弁逸脱
aortic valve disease 大動脈弁疾患
aortic valvlar disease 大動脈弁疾患
atrioventricular dissociation 房室解離
AVDA
American Venereal Disease Association 米国性病学会
AV Dis, A-V dis
atrio(-)ventricular dissociation 房室解離
$AVD\text{-}O_2$
arterio(-)venous oxygen content difference 動静脈酸素分圧較差

A

AvDP
average diastolic pressure 平均拡張期圧
avdp
avoirdupois 常用式(重量)
AVDP, avdp
asparaginase, vincristine, daunorubicin, prednisone アスパラギナーゼ,ビンクリスチン,ダウノルビシン,プレドニゾン
AVE
aortic valve echocardiogram 大動脈弁超音波心臓検査図
aver
average 平均(の)
AVF
acute ventilatory failure 急性換気不全
antiviral factor 抗ウイルス因子
arteriovenous fistula 動静脈瘻, 動静脈フィステル
aVF
augmented vector of left foot 左足増高単極肢誘導
av.fx.
avulsion fracture 裂離骨折
avg
average 平均(の)
AVH
acute viral hepatitis 急性ウイルス性肝炎
AVI
air velocity index 気速指数, 換気速度係数
AVID
audiovisual instruction department 視聴覚教育部
AVIP
adriamycin, vincristine, ifosfamide, prednisolone アドリアマイシン,ビンクリスチン,イホスファミド,プレドニゾロン
AVJ
atrioventricular junction 房室接合部
aVL
augmented vector of left arm 左手増高単極肢誘導
AVM
adriamycin, vinblastine, methotrexate アドリアマイシン,ビンブラスチン,メトトレキサート
arteriovenous malformation 動静脈奇形
atrioventricular malformation 房室奇形
AVMA
American Veterinary Medical Association 米国獣医学会
AVN, A-VN
atrio(-)ventricular node 房室結節

AVNRT
atrioventricular node reentry　房室結節リエントリー性頻拍
AVO
ampere, volt, ohm　アンペア・ボルト・オーム
aortic valve opening　大動脈弁口径
AVO_2
arteriovenous oxygen difference　動静脈酸素較差
avoir
avoirdupois　常用式(重量)
AVP
actinomycin D, vincristine, cisplatin (=Platinol)　アクチノマイシンD, ビンクリスチン, シスプラチン(=プラチノール)
adenosine vasopressin　アデノシンバソプレシン
adriamycin, vincristine, procarbazine　アドリアマイシン, ビンクリスチン, プロカルバジン
aortic valveplasty　大動脈弁形成術
aortic valvoplasty　大動脈弁形成術
arginine vasopressin　アルギニンバソプレシン
avp
antiviral protein　抗ウイルス蛋白
AVR
accelerated ventricular rhythm　促迫状心室調律
anomalous venous return　異常静脈還流
aortic valve replacement　大動脈弁置換術
atrioventricular refractory　房室無反応
average voiding rate　平均排尿比
aVR
augmented vector of right arm　右手増高単極肢誘導
AVR, A-V R
arterio(-)venous ratio　動静脈(口径)比
AVRA
Audiovisual Research Association　視聴覚研究協会
AVRP
atrioventricular refractory period　房室不応期
AVRT
atrioventricular reciprocating reentrant tachycardia　房室回帰性頻拍
AVS
Anti-vivisection Society　生体解剖反対同盟
aortic valve stenosis　大動脈弁狭窄(症)
Association for Voluntary Sterilization　随意不妊協会
AVS, A-V S
arterio(-)venous shunt　動静脈シャント, AVシャント

A

AVSD
atrioventricular septal defect 房室中隔欠損
AVSP
atrioventricular sequential pacing 房室順次ペーシング
AVSS
audiovisualsexual stimulation 視聴覚性的刺激
AVSV
aortic valve stroke volume 大動脈弁駆出量
AVT
Allen vision test アレン視覚検査
arginine vasotocin アルギニンバソトシン
audiovisual tutorial 視聴覚個別指導
Aviation Medicine Techinician 航空医学技術者
AVTA
automatic vocal transaction analyzer 自動発声処理分析器
AVTRW
Association of Veterinary Teachers and Research Workers 獣医学教官・研究者協会
AV3V
anteroventral 3rd ventricle 第三脳室腹側前方
AVZ
avascular zone 無血管帯
AW
alcohol withdrawal アルコール離脱
anal wedge 肉眼的癌肛門側断端
anterior wall 前壁
aortic window 大動脈窓
aw
anal wedge 組織学的癌肛門側断端
AW(+),(−)
anal wedge (+),(−) 幽門側断端肉眼的癌浸潤の有無
aw(+),(−)
anal wedge (+),(−) 幽門側断端組織学的癌浸潤の有無
A.W.
atomic weight 原子量
A/W
(in) according with ～に従って
A & W
alive and well 元気でいきいきした状態
aw, aw.
airways 気道
a.w.a.
as well as ～と同じく

A waves
atrial contraction waves　心房性収縮波
AWBM
alveolar wall basement membrane　肺胞壁基底膜
AWD
alive with disease　病気状態で生存
AWF
adrenal weight factor　副腎体重因子
AWI
anterior wall infarction　前壁梗塞
AWMI
anterior wall myocardial infarction　前壁心筋梗塞
AWO
airway obstruction　気道閉塞
AWP
airway pressure　気道圧
AWR
air way resistance　気道抵抗
average weighted ratio　平均加重比
AWTA
aniridia-Wilms tumor (syndrome)　無虹彩ウィルムス腫瘍(症候群)
AWU, awu
atomic weight unit　原子量単位
AX
amoxapine　アモキサピン
auxillary　補助的
ax
axial　軸性の
axon　軸索
ax.
axungia〈ラ〉　脂肪
AX, Ax, ax
axis　軸
Ax, ax
axilla　腋窩
axillary　腋窩の
AX-F
axillo-femoral bypass　腋窩・大腿バイパス
AX grad
axial gradient　軸傾度
AXL
axillary lymphoscintigraphy　腋窩リンパシンチグラフィ
AXT
alternating exotropia　交代性外斜視

A

AYA
acute yellow atrophy 急性黄色(肝)萎縮(症)
AYF
antiyeast factor 抗酵母因子
AYV
aster yellow virus アスター黄色ウイルス
AZ
Allgemeinzustand〈独〉 全身状態
azathioprine アザチオプリン
Az
Azobacter アゾバクター(属)
azote〈仏〉 窒素
AZ, A.-Z., Az
Aschheim-Zondek (pregnancy) (test) アッシュハイム・ツォンデック(妊娠)(検査)
5-Aza
5-azacytidine 5-アザシチジン
5-azaC
5-azacytidine 5-アザシチジン
5-AzCdR
5-aza-2′-deoxycytidine 5-アザ-2′-デオキシシチジン
5-AzCR
5-azacytidine 5-アザシチジン
AZG, azg.
azaguanine アザグアニン
AZL
azalomycin F アザロマイシンF
azulene アズレン
AZM
azotometry 窒素測定
AZP
azathioprine アザチオプリン
AZQ
aziridinylbenzoquinone アジリジニルベンゾキノン
AZR
alizarin red アリザリン赤
Aschheim-Zondek (pregnancy) reaction アッシュハイム・ツォンデック(妊娠)反応
AZS
automatic zero test 自動ゼロ設定
AZT
Aschheim-Zondek (pregnancy) test アッシュハイム・ツォンデック(妊娠)検査
azidodeoxythymidine アジドデオキシチミジン
azidothymidine アジドチミジン
azt(h)reonam アズトレオナム

AZTEC
amplitude-zone-time-epoch-coding　アズテック法

AzU
6-azauracil　6-アザウラシル

5-AzU
5-azauracil　5-アザウラシル

6-AzU
6-azauracil　6-アザウラシル

AZUR, AzUR
6-azauridine　6-アザウリジン

5-AzUR, 5-AZUR
5-azauridine　5-アザウリジン

6-AzUR, 6-AZUR
6-azauridine　6-アザウリジン

AZY
alizarin yellow　アリザリンイエロー

B b

B

asparagine	アスパラギン
aspartic acid	アスパラギン酸
baby	乳児
bacitracin	バシトラシン
bacterium	細菌
Bacteroides	バクテロイデス(属)
bad	悪い
Balantidium	バランチジウム(属)
barometric	気圧の
barometric pressure	大気圧
Bartonella	バルトネラ(属)
baseline	基線
Basidiobolus	バシジオボルス(属)
basophil	好塩基球
basophilic	好塩基性の
bath	入浴，沐浴
behavior	行動
behavioral	行動の
bel	ベル〈単位〉
Benoist scale	ベノア度盛
benzoate	安息香酸塩，安息香酸エステル
Bertiella	ベルチエラ(属)
beta-globulin	βグロブリン
bicuspid	小臼歯
black	黒色の，黒人の
Blastomyces	ブラストミセス(属)
blue	青色の
body	体，身体
boils at	～で煮沸する
bone	骨
bone-marrow derived	骨髄由来の
Bordetella	ボルデテラ(属)
born	生まれた，先天性の
boron	ホウ素〈元素〉
Borrelia	ボレリア(属)
Borrmann	ボルマン
bowel	腸
bradycardia	徐脈
breakfast	朝食
breathy	気息性
Brewster	ブルースター

brightness　輝度
bronchial　気管支の
bronchiole　気管支枝
brother　兄弟
Brugia　ブルギア(属)
bruit　雑音，ブリュイ
buccal　頬(側)の
bursa　関節包
bypass　バイパス，短絡
Gauss　ガウス
Gàussian units　ガウス単位《電磁》
tracheal bifurcation　気管分岐部下縁
whole blood　全血

b

barn　バーン〈単位〉
byte　バイト〈単位〉

B，b

Blut〈独〉=blood　血液

B，B.

Bacillus　バシラス，桿菌
Baumé scale　ボーメ尺度〔スケール〕
Brucella　ブルセラ(属)

B，b.

balneum〈ラ〉　沐浴
base　塩基
beta=β〈ギ〉　ベータ
bis〈ラ〉=twice，two times　2回

B-Ⅰ，BⅠ

Billroth Ⅰ (type)　ビルロートⅠ法
Magenresektion nach Billroth erste Methode〈独〉　ビルロートⅠ法

B-Ⅱ，BⅡ

Billroth Ⅱ (type)　ビルロートⅡ法
Magenresektion nach Billroth zweite Methode〈独〉　ビルロートⅡ法

BA

background activity　背景活動
balneum arenae〈ラ〉=sand bath　砂浴
basilar artery　脳底動脈
basion　基底点
betamethasone acetate　酢酸ベタメタゾン
bile acid　胆汁酸
biliary atresia　胆管閉鎖(症)
biologic activity　生物学的活性
biological assay　生物学的検定
blind approach　盲目的接近

blocking antibody	遮断抗体
blood agar	血液寒天(培地)
blood alcohol	血中アルコール
bone age	骨年齢
bovine albumin	ウシアルブミン
branchial artery (pressure)	上腕動脈(圧)
breathing apparatus	呼吸装置，呼吸器
bronchial asthma	気管支喘息
bronchoalveolar	気管支肺胞の
Brucella abortus	ブルセラアボータス
buccoaxial	頬軸位の

Ba

barium	バリウム

BA，B/A

backache	背痛，背部痛
boric acid	ホウ酸

BAA

benzoylarginine amide	ベンゾイルアルギニンアミド
bromoacetamide	ブロモアセトアミド

BAAH

body acceleration given synchronously with heartbeat	心拍動と同期した身体加速

BAB

blood agar base	血液寒天基礎培地

Bab

Babinski (reflex)	バビンスキー(反射)

BAC

bacterial antigen complex	細菌抗原複合体
bacterial artificial chromosome	大腸菌人工染色体
basal acid concentration	基礎分泌最高酸濃度
bischloroethylnitrosourea, arabinosylcytosine, cyclophosphamide	ビスクロロエチルニトロソ尿素,アラビノシルシトシン,シクロホスファミド
blood alcohol concentration	血中アルコール濃度
blood alcohol content	血中アルコール含量
bronchoalveolar cells	気管(支)肺胞細胞
bronchus alveolar cell	気管(支)肺胞細胞
buccoaxiocervical	頬軸位頸面の

Bac，Bac.

Bacillus	バシラス，桿菌

Bac.C.

bacteriological code	細菌命名規約

BACILL

bacilli〈ラ〉	桿剤

$BaCl_2$

barium chloride	塩化バリウム

B

BACO
bleomycin, adriamycin, cyclohexylchloroethylnitrosourea, vincristine (=Oncovin) — ブレオマイシン,アドリアマイシン,シクロヘキシルクロロエチルニトロソ尿素,ビンクリスチン(=オンコビン)

BACOD
bleomycin, adriamycin, cyclophosphamide, vincristine (=Oncovin), dexamethasone — ブレオマイシン,アドリアマイシン,シクロホスファミド,ビンクリスチン(=オンコビン),デキサメタゾン

BACON
bleomycin, adriamycin, cyclohexylchloroethylnitrosourea, vincristine (=Oncovin), nitrogen mustard — ブレオマイシン,アドリアマイシン,シクロヘキシルクロロエチルニトロソ尿素,ビンクリスチン(=オンコビン),ニトロゲンマスタード

BACOP
bleomycin, adriamycin, cyclophosphamide, vincristine (=Oncovin), prednisone — ブレオマイシン,アドリアマイシン,シクロホスファミド,ビンクリスチン(=オンコビン),プレドニゾン

BACT
bischloroethylnitrosourea, arabinosylcytosine, cyclophosphamide, 6-thioguanine — ビスクロロエチルニトロソ尿素,アラビノシルシトシン,シクロホスファミド,6-チオグアニン

bleomycin, adriamycin, cyclophosphamide, tamoxifen citrate — ブレオマイシン,アドリアマイシン,シクロホスファミド,クエン酸タモキシフェン

bact
bacteria — 細菌,バクテリア
bacterial — 細菌(性)の
bacteriologist — 細菌学者
bacteriology — 細菌学
bacterium — 細菌,バクテリア

BACT, Bact, bact, bact.
Bacterium — バクテリウム(属)

bact, bact.
bacteriological — 細菌学の

BACTEc
bacterial growth detector — 細菌増殖検出器

bacter
bacteriologist — 細菌学者

B

bacti
bacteriology 細菌学
BAD
branch atheromatous disease 穿通枝領域アテローム硬化性疾患
BADL
basic activity of daily living 日常生活動作
BADS
British Association of Dermatology and Syphilology 英国皮膚科・梅毒学会
BAE
bovine aortic endothelial ウシ大動脈内皮細胞
bovine aortic endothelium ウシ大動脈内皮
bronchial artery embolization 気管支動脈塞栓術
BaE
barium enema バリウム浣腸
BAEe
benzoylarginine ethyl ester ベンゾイルアルギニンエチルエステル
BaEn
barium enema バリウム浣腸
Ba enem.
barium enema バリウム浣腸
BAEP
brain stem auditory evoked potential 脳幹聴覚誘発電位
BAER
brain stem auditory evoked response 脳幹聴覚誘発反応
BAF
B cell activating factor B細胞活性化因子
B lymphocyte activating factor Bリンパ球活性化因子
BAFM
British Association of Forensic Medicine 英国法医学会
BAFS
British Association of Forensic Science 英国法医科学会
BAG
brachial angiography 上腕動脈造影法
bronchial arteriogram, bronchial arteriography 気管支動脈造影
buccoaxiogingival 頰(面)軸(面)歯肉(面)の
BAHOH
British Association of Hard of Hearing 英国難聴学会
BAI
basilar artery insufficiency 脳底動脈不全(症)

bronchial aerozol inhalation	気管支噴霧吸入
bronchial arterial infusion	気管支動脈内注入(療法)
bronchial artery infusion	気管支動脈(内)注入(療法)

BAIT

bacterial automated identification technique	菌自動同定法

BAL

blood alcohol level	血中アルコールレベル
British anti-lewisite (factor)	バル(=ジメルカプロール)
broncho-alveolar lavage	気管支(肺胞)洗浄(法)

bal

balance	平衡

BAL, bal.

balneum〈ラ〉=bath	入浴
balsamum〈ラ〉=balsam	バルサム

bal.arenae

balneum arenae〈ラ〉=sand bath	砂浴

BALF

bronchoalveolar lavage fluid	気管支(肺胞)洗浄液

BALL, B-ALL

B cell acute lymphoblastic leukemia	B細胞急性リンパ芽球性白血病

bal.mar.

balneum maris〈ラ〉=salt bath, sea-water bath	塩水浴, 海水浴

BALS

bile acid-losing syndrome	胆汁酸喪失症候群

bals.

balsamum〈ラ〉=balsam	バルサム

BALT

broncho-associated lymphatic tissue	気管支関連リンパ組織
bronchus associated lymphoid tissue	傍気管支リンパ組織

bal.vap., BAL VAP

balneum vaporis〈ラ〉, *balneum vapour*〈ラ〉=steam bath, vapor bath	蒸気浴

BAM

basilar artery migraine	脳底動脈型片頭痛
bronchoalveolar macrophage	気管支肺胞大食細胞

BAm

mean brachial artery (pressure)	平均上腕動脈(圧)

BAME

benzoylarginine methyl ester	ベンゾイルアルギニンメチルエステル

B

BAMON

bleomycin, adriamycin, methotrexate, vincristine (=Oncovin), nitrogen mustard	ブレオマイシン,アドリアマイシン,メトトレキサート,ビンクリスチン(=オンコビン),ニトロゲンマスタード

BAO

Bachelor of Art of Obstetrics	産科学士
basal acid output	基礎酸分泌量

BAOMP

behenoyl arabinofuranosylcytosinet, aclarubicin, vincristine (=Oncovin), 6-mercaptopurine, prednisolone	エノシタビン,アクラルビシン,ビンクリスチン(=オンコビン),6-メルカプトプリン,プレドニゾロン

BAP

bleomycin, adriamycin, prednisone	ブレオマイシン,アドリアマイシン,プレドニゾン
blood agar plate	血液寒天平板
brachial artery prressure	上腕動脈圧
bronchial arterial pressure	気管支動脈圧

BAPC

bacampicillin	バカンピシリン

BAPG

biauricular plethysmography	両耳垂プレチスモグラフィ

Ba Phys Med

British Association of Physical Medicine	英国内科学会

BAPS

British Association of Pediatric Surgeons	英国小児外科医協会
British Association of Plastic Surgeons	英国形成外科医協会

BAPT

British Association of Physical Training	英国体育協会

bar

barometer	気圧計，指標
barometric	気圧計の，気圧の

Barb，barb

barbiturate	バルビツレート

BARI

bypass angioplasty revascularization investigation	バイパス血管形成血行再建術調査(＝BART)

BARN

bilateral acute retinal necrosis	両側性急性網膜壊死

//bars
parallel bars　平行棒
BART
bypass angioplasty revascularization trial (investigation)　バイパス血管形成血行再建術比較試験(＝BARI)
BAR-therapy
BUdR-antimetabolite-(continuous intraarterial infusion-)radiation therapy　バー療法(＝脳腫瘍治療法の１つ)
BAS
balloon atrial septostomy　バルーン心房中隔切開術
balloon atrioseptostomy　バルーン心房中隔裂開術
benzyl analogue of serotonin　セロトニンのベンジル同族体
BAs
boric acid solution　硼酸水
B.A.S.
British Anatomical Society　英国解剖学会
bas, bas.
basilar　基底の，基部の
basophile　好塩基球
basophilic leucocyte　好塩基球
BASIC
beginner's all-purpose symbolic instruction code　ベイシック《コン》
baso
basophil(s)　好塩基球
basophile　好塩基性リンパ球
Ba swallow
barium swallow　バリウム嚥下
BAT
brain-associated T cell antigen　脳関連T細胞抗原
brain associated theta antigen　脳関連テータ抗原
brown adipose tissue　褐色細胞腫
BA top
basilar top aneurysm　脳底動脈頂点動脈瘤
batt
battery　電気，器具
BAUS
British Association of Urological Surgeons　英国泌尿器外科医協会
BAV
balloon aortic valvuloplasty　バルーン大動脈弁形成術
BAVA
Bureau of Audiovisual Aids　視聴覚(教育)器具事務局
BAVE
Bureau of Audiovisual Education　視聴覚教育部

B

BAVIP
bleomycin, adriamycin, vinblastine, imidazole carboxamide, prednisone　ブレオマイシン,アドリアマイシン,ビンブラスチン,イミダゾールカルボキサミド,プレドニゾン

BAW
broncho alveolar washing　気管支(肺胞)洗浄

BB
bed bath　全身清拭
Besnier-Boeck (syndrome)　ベスニエ・ベック(症候群)
beta blocker　β遮断薬
blood bank　血液バンク
Blutbild〈独〉　血液像
both bones　両方の骨
brachial plexus block　腕神経叢ブロック
breakthrough bleeding　破綻出血
breast biopsy　乳房生検
brush border　刷子縁
buffer base　緩衝塩基

Bb
bursae　関節包

bb
ball bearing　ボールベアリング，玉軸受け

BBA
born before arrival　病院到着前出産
4-brome-1,2-benzencarbaldehyde　4-ブロモ-1,2-ベンゼンカルバルデヒド

BB-Ag
brush border antigen　BB抗原

BBB
blood buffer base　血液緩衝塩基
bundle branch block　脚ブロック

BBB, B.B.B.
blood brain barrier　血液脳関門

BBBB
bilateral bundle branch block　両脚ブロック

BBC
bromobenzyl cyanide　ブロモベンジルシアニド

BBF
bronchial blood flow　気管支血流量

B bile, B-bile
cystic bile　胆嚢胆汁
gallbladder bile　胆嚢胆汁

BBL
barrel　バレル

BBM
Bernheim basal medium ベルンハイム基礎培地
brush border membrane 刷子縁膜
BBMV
broad bean mottle virus ソラマメ斑紋状ウイルス
brush border membrane vesicle 刷子縁膜小胞
BBN
N-butyl-*N*-butanol nitrosoamine 発癌剤
N-nitrosobutyl-4-hydroxybutylamine *N*-ニトロソブチル-4-ヒドロキシブチルアミン
BBO
bronchobronchiolitis obliterans 閉塞性気管支細気管支炎
BBOT
2,5-bis-2-(5-*t*-butylbenzoxyazolyl)-thiophene 2,5-ビス-2-(5-*t*-ブチルベンゾオキサゾリル)チオフェン

B & B pericarditis
bread and butter pericarditis パン・バター心膜炎
BBS
Besnier-Boeck-Schaumann (syndrome) ベスニエ・ベック・シャウマン(症候群)
borate buffered saline ホウ酸緩衝食塩水
BBT
basal body temperature 基礎体温
BBW
birth body weight 出生時体重
B Bx
breast biopsy 乳房生検
BC
bacitracin バシトラシン
back care 背部清拭
back-cross もどし交配
bactericidal concentration 殺菌濃度
basal cell 基底細胞
base curve 基本曲線
benign chondroblastoma 良性軟骨芽細胞腫
bicarbonate 重炭酸塩
biliary colic 胆(道)疝痛
bioclean バイオクリーン
bipolar cell 双極細胞
birth control 出生調節，産児制限
blastic crisis 急性転化
blood center 血液センター
blood count 血球算定(法)，血算
blood culture 血液培養
Blue Cross ブルークロス

bone conduction　骨導，骨伝導

bone connection　骨接合

Bowman capsule　ボーマン嚢

brachiocephalic　腕頭の

branchial carcinoma　気管支癌

breast cancer　乳癌

breathing capacity　呼吸容量

bromocriptine　ブロモクリプチン

bronchial cancer　気管支癌

bronchitis chronica〈ラ〉　慢性気管支炎

buccocervical　頬(面歯)頸(面)の

Budd-Chiari (syndrome)　バッド・キアリ(症候群)

B.C.

Bachelor of Chemistry　化学士

before Christ　西暦紀元前

b/c

because　〜なので，〜だから

B & C

biopsy and curettage　生検掻爬

BCA

brachiocephalic artery　腕頭動脈

breast cancer antigen　乳癌抗原

BCAA

branched chain amino acid　分岐鎖アミノ酸

BCAP

bischloroethylnitrosourea, cyclophosphamide, adriamycin, prednisone　ビスクロロエチルニトロソ尿素，シクロホスファミド，アドリアマイシン，プレドニゾン

B-CAVe

bleomycin, cyclohexylchloroethylnitrosourea, adriamycin, Velban　ブレオマイシン，シクロヘキシルクロロエチルニトロソ尿素，アドリアマイシン，ベルバン

BCB

brilliant cresyl blue　ブリリアントクレシルブルー

BCC

basal cell carcinoma　基底細胞癌

biliary cholesterol concentration　胆汁コレステロール濃度

birth control clinic　計画出産外来

British Cancer Campaign　英国癌征圧運動

BCCG

British Cooperative Clinical Group　英国協同臨床グループ

BCCP

biotin carboxyl carrier protein　ビオチンカルボキシル運搬蛋白質

BCD
bleomycin, cyclophosphamide, dactinomycin　ブレオマイシン，シクロホスファミド，ダクチノマイシン
border of comfortable dazzling　眩惑快不快限界域

BCDF
B cell differentiation factor　B細胞分化因子

BCDSP
Boston Collaborative-Drug Surveillance Program　ボストン合同薬監視計画

BCE
basal cell epithelioma　基底細胞上皮腫
B cell clonal excess　B細胞クローン過多

BCECT
benign childhood epilepsy with centrotemporal spike　中心側頭部に棘波をもつ良性小児てんかん

B cell
bone marrow derived cell　B細胞

BCF
bacterial culture filtrate　細菌培養炉液
basophil chemotactic factor　好塩基球化学走性因子

BCFS
breast cancer frozen section　乳癌凍結切片

BCG
Bacillus Calmette-Guérin (vaccine)　カルメット・ゲラン桿菌(ワクチン)，カルメット・ゲラン・ウシ結核菌(ワクチン)
ballistocardiogram　心弾動図，バリストカルジオグラム
ballistocardiograph　心弾動図(法)，バリストカルジオグラフ
brom-cresol-green　ブロムクレゾールグリーン，臭素クレゾールグリーン

BCG-CWS
BCG cell wall skeleton　BCG細胞壁骨格

BCGF
B cell growth factor　B細胞増殖因子

BCG test
bicolour guaiac test　二色グアヤック試験

BCH
basal cell hyperplasia　基底細胞過形成
basal cell hypoplasia　基底細胞形成不全

B.Ch.
Bachelor of Chemistry　化学士

B.Ch.D.
Baccalauleus Chirurgiae Dentium〈ラ〉=Bachelor of Dental Surgery　歯科口腔外科学士(=B.D.S.)

B.Chir
Bachelor of Chirurgery　外科学士

BChL
bacteriochlorophyll　バクテリオクロロフィル，細菌クロロフィル

BCIC
British-Control Investigation Committee　英国制御監視委員会

BCKA
branched chain keto acid　側鎖ケト酸

BCL
basic cycle length　基本周期

Bcl-2
B cell lymphoma gene2　アポトーシス阻害

B-CLL
B cell chronic lymphatic leukemia　B細胞慢性リンパ(球)性白血病

BCLS
basic cardiac life support　一次心臓救命処置

BCM
birth control medication　出産調節薬

BCME
bis chloromethyl ether　ビスクロロメチルエーテル
bis ether　ビスエーテル

BC muscle
bulbocavernous muscle　陰茎海綿体筋

BCN
basal cell nevus　基底細胞母斑

BCNS
basal cell nevus syndrome　基底細胞母斑症候群

BCNU
1,3-bis(2-chloroethyl)-1-nitrosourea　ビスクロロエチルニトロソ尿素(=カルムスチン)

BCO
bilateral carotid occlusion　両側頸動脈閉鎖
blood carbon monoxide　血液一酸化炭素

BCO_2
blood carbon dioxide　血液二酸化炭素

B comp.
B complex　(ビタミン)B複合体

BCP
birth control pill　経口避妊薬

bischloroethylnitrosourea, cyclophosphamide, prednisone — ビスクロロエチルニトロソ尿素, シクロホスファミド, プレドニゾン

bromcresol purple — ブロムクレゾール紫

BCPP

bischloroethylnitrosourea, cyclophosphamide, procarbazine, prednisolone — ビスクロロエチルニトロソ尿素, シクロホスファミド, プロカルバジン, プレドニゾロン

BCQ

breast cancer chemotherapy questionnaire — 乳癌化学療法に対するアンケート

BCR

B cell antigen receptor complex — Ig受容体α・β鎖

B cell reactivity — B細胞反応性

biological clean room — 無菌室

bulbocavernosus response — 球海綿体反応

bulbocavernous renex — 球海綿体反射

BCRD

British Council for Rehabilitation of Disabled — 英国身体障害者リハビリテーション審議会

BCRUM

British Committee on Radiation Units and Measurements — 英国放射線単位・測定委員会

BCS

battered child syndrome — 被虐待児症候群

British Cardiac Society — 英国心臓協会

Budd-Chiari syndrome — バッドキアリ症候群

B.C.S.

Bachelor of Chemical Science — 化学学士

BCSC

Blue Cross of Southern California — 南カリフォルニアブルークロス

BCSFB

blood-cerebrospinal fluid barrier — 血液・脳脊髄液関門

BCT

blood coagulation time — 血液凝固時間

breast conservation treatment — 乳房温存療法

BCTR

bovine chymotrypsin — ウシキモトリプシン

BCU

burn care unit — 熱傷集中監視室

B

BCVPP

bischloroethylnitrosourea, cyclophosphamide, vinblastine, procarbazine, prednisone	ビスクロロエチルニトロソ尿素,シクロホスファミド,ビンブラスチン,プロカルバジン,プレドニゾン
bleomycin, cyclophosphamide, vincristine, procarbazine, prednisone	ブレオマイシン,シクロホスファミド,ビンクリスチン,プロカルバジン,プレドニゾン

BCW

biological and chemical warfare	生物化学戦

BCYE

buffered charcoal-yeast extract	BCYE寒天

BD

base deficit	塩基欠乏
base of prism down	下方プリズム基底
Batten's disease	バッテン病
Baudelocque diameter	ボドロック(直)径
behavioral disorder, behavior disorder	行動異常，行動疾患
Behçet's disease	ベーチェット病
belladonna	ベラドンナ
bile duct	胆管
birth date	生年月日
Black Death	黒死(病)
Blackfan-Diamond (syndrome)	ブラックファン・ダイヤモンド(症候群)
bladder drainage	膀胱ドレナージ
Blu-lay Disk	ブルーレイディスク
Blutdruck〈独〉	血圧
brain damage	脳障害，脳損傷
brain death	脳死
bronchodilator	気管支拡張薬
buccodistal	頬(面)遠心(面)の
bundle	束

BD, Bd, bd

board	板，委員会

BD, b.d.

bis die〈ラ〉=twice a day	1日2回《処》

bd, bd.

band	帯
blind	盲目の

BDA

beclomethasone dipropionate aerosol	ジプロピオン酸ベクロメタゾンエアゾール
bile duct adenoma	胆管腺症

British Deaf Association　英国難聴者協会
British Dental Association　英国歯科医師会
British Dermatological Association　英国皮膚科学会

BDAC
Bureau of Drug Abuse Control　薬物悪用管理局

BDAE
Boston diagnostic aphasia examination　ボストン診断学的失語症検査法

BDB
bis-diazotized benzidine　ビスジアゾ化ベンチジン

BDBR
bisdiazotized benzidine reaction　タンニン酸処理血球凝集反応

BDC
biodynamic calorimeter　全身熱量計

BDDA
British Deaf and Dumb Association　英国聾唖者協会

BDE
bile duct examination　胆管検査
bile duct exploration　胆管探査

BDF
B cell differentiating factor　B細胞分化因子

BDG
bilirubin diglucuronide　ビリルビンジグルクロナイド

BDGFs
bone-derived growth factors　骨由来成長因子

BDH
British Drug Houses　英国薬局

3β-DH
3β-oxyhydro dehydrogenase　3β水酸化脱水素酵素

BDI
Beck depression inventory　ベックうつ病尺度
beclomethasone dipropionate inhaler　(気管支喘息治療の)プロピオン酸ベクロメタゾン吸入
burn depth indicator　熱傷深達度指標

BDL
below detectable limit　検出限界以下
bundle　束

BDM
birth, death, marriage　出生・死・結婚

B-DOPA
bleomycin, dacarbazine, vincristine (= Oncovin), prednisone, adriamycin　ブレオマイシン,ダカルバジン,ビンクリスチン(=オンコビン),プレドニゾン,アドリアマイシン

BDP
beclomethasone dipropionate — ジプロピオン酸ベクロメタゾン
bilateral diaphragm paralysis — 両側(性)横隔膜麻痺

BDPEC
Bureau of Disease Prevention and Environmental Control — 疾患予防・環境管理局

BDR
Bauchdeckenreflex〈独〉 — 腹壁反射

bds
beiderseitig, beiderseits〈独〉 — 両側の

B.D.S.
Bachelor of Dental Surgery — 歯科口腔外科学士(＝B.Ch.D.)

b.d.s.
bis in die sumendus〈ラ〉＝to be taken twice a day — 1日2回摂取《処》

B.D.Sc.
Bachelor of Dental Science — 歯科学士

BDT
basophile degranulation test — 好塩基球脱顆粒試験

BDUR
bromodeoxyuridine — ブロモデオキシウリジン

BDV
blood dilution value — 血液希釈値

BDW
bufferd distilled water — 緩衝蒸留水

BDZ
benzodiazepine — ベンゾジアゼパン

BE
bacillary emulsion — 細菌乳濁液
bacterial endocarditis — 細菌性心内膜炎
barium enema (method) — バリウム注腸(検査)
Barrett esophagus — バレット食道
base excess — 過剰塩基
Baumé specific gravity scale — ボーメ比重計
below elbow — 肘下, 前腕
biological electronics — 生物電子工学
biological engineering — 生物工学, 生体工具
blood volume expansion — (循環)血(液)量増加
both eyes — 両眼
bottom echo — 底エコー
brain edema — 脳浮腫
breast examination — 乳房検査
bronchiectasia — 気管支拡張症
bronchiectasis — 気管支拡張症

broncho-esophagology　気管支食道科(学)

Be

Baumé degree　ボーメ度

beryllium　ベリリウム〈元素〉

BEAC

bischloroethylnitrosourea, etoposide, arabinosylcytosine, cyclophosphamide　ビスクロロエチルニトロソ尿素, エトポシド, アラビノシルシトシン, シクロホスファミド

BEAM

bischloroethylnitrosourea, etoposide, arabinosylcytosine, melphalan　ビスクロロエチルニトロソ尿素, エトポシド, アラビノシルシトシン, メルファラン

brain electrical activity mapping　脳電位分布図(法)

BEAMP

below-elbow amputation　前腕切断

BEAR

brain stem evoked auditory response　聴性脳幹反応

BECCT

benign epilepsy of children with centrotemporal EEG foci　中心側頭部脳波焦点を伴う小児良性てんかん

BEE

basal energy expenditure　基礎エネルギー消費量

bef

before　～の前に

beg

begin　始める, 始まる

beginning　初め, 始まり, 初期

beh

behavior　行動, 態度

behaviorism　行動主義

BEI

biological exposure indices　生物学的曝露指数

butanol extractable iodine　ブタノール抽出性ヨード

Beibl

Beiblatt〈独〉　補足, 補遺, 付録

BEIS

balloon expandable intravascular stent　バルーン拡張式血管内ステント

Beitr

Beitrag〈独〉　寄稿

BEL

Beckenendlage〈独〉　骨盤位

BELD

bleomycin, Eldisine, lomustine, dacarbazine　ブレオマイシン, エルジシン, ロムスチン, ダカルバジン

B

BELIR
beta-endorphin-like immunoreactivity — βエンドルフィン様免疫反応性

bella
belladonna — ベラドンナ

BEMP
bleomycin, cyclophosphamide (= Endoxan), 6-mercaptopurine, prednisolone — ブレオマイシン，シクロホスファミド(＝エンドキサン)，6-メルカプトプリン，プレドニゾロン

BEN
benign epidemic nephropathy — 良性流行性腎症

ben.
bene〈ラ〉 — よく《処》

B-encephalitis
encephalitis japonica — 日本脳炎

benz, benz.
benzedrine — ベンゼドリン
benzene — ベンゼン
benzin (e) — ベンジン
benzoate — 安息香酸塩，安息香酸エステル

BEP
basic fetoprotein — 塩基性フェトプロテイン
bleomycin, etoposide, cisplatin (= Platinol) — ブレオマイシン，エトポシド，シスプラチン(＝プラチノール)
brain-evoked potential — 脳誘発電位

BEpA
British Epilepsy Association — 英国てんかん協会

BEPI
beta-endorphin immunoreativity — βエンドルフィン免疫反応性

BER
basal electrical rhythm — 基本電位リズム

BERA
brainstem electric response audiometry — 聴性脳幹反応
brainstem evoked response audiometry — 脳幹誘発反応聴力検査(法)

BERC
Biomedical Engineering Research Cooperation — 生物医学工学研究協同体

BES
balanced electrolyte solution — 平衡電解質溶液
Biological Engineering Society — 生物工学会

N, *N*-bis(2-hydroxyethyl)-2-aminoethanesulfonic acid — *N*, *N* ビス(2-ヒドロキシエチル)-2-アミノエタンスルホン酸

B

BESRL
Behavioral Science Research Laboratory — 行動科学研究室

BET
benign epithelial tumor — 良性上皮(性)腫瘍
blood for exchange transfusion — (新生児の)交換輸血

bet
between — ～の間に

beta GAL
β-D-galactosidase — β-D-ガラクトシダーゼ

beta2 GP1
β_2 glycoprotein 1 — β_2グリコプロテイン1

bev
beverage — 飲物，飲料

BEx
blood exchange — 交換輸血

BF
biofeedback — バイオフィードバック，生体自己制御
biological feedback — バイオフィードバック，生体自己制御
blastogenesis factor, blastogenic factor — 芽球化因子
blocking factor — 遮断因子
blood flow — 血流(量)
body fat — 体脂
body floating — 体幹絶縁
Bolivian (hemorrhagic) fever — ボリビア(出血性)熱
bouillon filtre〈仏〉 — ブイヨン濾液
breast feed — 母乳で育てる
breast feeding — 母乳を飲ませること，母乳で育てること
bronchofiberscope — 気管支鏡
bronchofiberscopy — 気管支鏡検査法
burning foot syndrome — 灼熱脚症候群
bursa of Fabricius — ファブリチウス嚢
butterfat — 乳脂肪

Bf
properdin factor B — プロペルジンB因子

bf
buffered — 緩衝された

B/F
bound and free ratio — 結合遊離比

BF, B/F, b/f
black female 黒人女性
BFB
bio(logical) feedback バイオフィードバック，生体自己制御
BFC
benign febrile convulsion 良性熱性痙攣
BFDI
bronchodilation following deep inspiration 深吸気時気管支拡張
BFE
blood flow energy 血流エネルギー
BF ERG
bright flash electroretinogram 高輝度網膜電図
bFGF
basic fibroblast growth factor 基本的線維芽成長〔増殖〕因子
BFH
benign fibrous histiocytoma 良性線維性組織球腫
BFHR
basal fetal heart rate 基礎胎児心拍数
BFI
brain function index 脳機能係数
BFO
balanced forearm orthosis バランス式前腕装具
beat-frequency oscillator 拍動性周波発振器
blood forming organs 造血臓器
BFP
balanced forearm prosthesis バランス前腕補助具
basic fetoprotein 塩基性胎児蛋白
biological false positive (reaction) 生物学的偽陽性(反応)
BFPPS
Bureau of Foods, Pesticides and Product Safety 食品・殺虫剤・生産物安全局
BFR
biological false reactor 生物学的偽反応体
blood flow rate 血流速度
bone formation rate 骨形成率
bfr
buffer 緩衝
bfR sol
buffered Ringer's solution 緩衝リンゲル液
BFS
blood fasting sugar 空腹時血糖
burning feet syndrome 灼熱足症候群
BFS, BFs
bronchofiberscope 気管支鏡

BFT
bentonite flocculation test ベントナイト綿状反応試験
bentonite inoculation test ベントナイト絮状反応試験

BFU-E
burst forming unit-erythrocyte 赤芽球バースト形成単位
burst forming unit erythroid 赤芽球コロニー群形成細胞

BG
background バックグラウンド，背景
Bender Gestalt (test) ベンダー・ゲシュタルト(検査)
bicipital groove 結節間溝
biguanide ビグアナイド剤
blood glucose 血中グルコース，血糖
bone graft 骨移植(片)
breast girth 胸囲
brilliant green ブリリアントグリーン
bronchography 気管支造影
buccogingival 頰側歯肉面の
Buerger-Grütz (syndrome) ビュルガー・グリュッツ(症候群)

bG
bluish green 青緑色

BG，B-G
Bordet-Gengou (bacillus) ボルデー・ジャング(桿菌)

BGA
blood gas analysis 動脈血ガス分析
brachial angiography 上腕動脈経由による脳血管撮影

BGABG
beta galactosidase anti-beta galactosidase BG・抗BG複合体

BGAg
blood group antigen 血液型抗原

BGC
blood group class 血液型分類

BGCA
bronchogenic carcinoma 気管支原発癌

BGDF
B cell growth and differentiation factor B細胞増殖と分化因子

BGG
bovine gamma globulin ウシガンマグロブリン

BGGT
bilirubin glucuronoside glucuronosyl transferase ビリルビングルクロノシドグルクロノシル転移酵素

B

BGH
bovine growth hormone　ウシ成長ホルモン
BGLB
brilliant green lactose broth　ブリリアントグリーン乳糖胆汁ブイヨン
BGlu
blood glucose　血中グルコース，血糖
BGM
background music　背景音楽
BG medium
Bordet-Gengou medium　ボルデ・ジャング培地
BGP
biliary glycoprotein　胆汁糖蛋白質
bone Gla protein　骨グラ蛋白質
B group
borderline group　境界群
BGS
blood group substance　血液型物質
BGSA
blood granulocyte specific activity　血液顆粒細胞特異的活動
BG subtraction
background subtraction method　バックグラウンド減算法
BGT
Bender Gestalt test　ベンダー・ゲシュタルト検査
Bender's test　ベンダー試験
Bild-Geschichten-Test〈独〉　絵画物語検査
Bgt, BGT
bungarotoxin　ブンガロトキシン
BGTT
borderline glucose tolerance test　境界(型)ブドウ糖負荷試験
BH
base hospital　基幹病院
Bernard-Horner (syndrome)　ベルナール・ホルナー症候群
Bill of Health　健康表
birth history　出生歴
borderline hypertensive　高血圧の境界(域)
breast height　乳房の高さ
breath holding　息こらえ
bronchial hyperactivity　気管支活性亢進
bronchial hyperreactivity　気管支反応性亢進
bundle of His　ヒス束
BHA
bilateral hilar adenopathy　両側(性)肺門リンパ節症
butylated hydroxyanisole　酸化抑制剤
butylhydroxy-anisole　ブチルヒドロキシアニソール

B

BH-AC
behenoyl arabinofuranosyl-cytosine ベヘノイルアラビノフルラノシルシトシン(=エノシタビン)

BH-AC DMP
behenoyl arabinofuranosylcytosine, daunorubicin, 6-mercaptopurine, prednisolone ベヘノイルアラビノフルラノシルシトシン,ダウノルビシン,6-メルカプトプリン,プレドニゾロン

B HAT
β-blocker heart attack trial βブロッカーによる心発作治験

BHb
bovine hemoglobin ウシ血色素

BH block
intraHisian block ヒス束内ブロック

BHC
benzene hexachloride 六塩化ベンゼン

BHD
bischloroethylnitrosourea, hydroxyurea, dacarbazine ビスクロロエチルニトロソ尿素,ヒドロキシ尿素,ダカルバジン

BHD-V
bischloroethylnitrosourea, hydroxyurea, dacarbazine, vincristine ビスクロロエチルニトロソ尿素,ヒドロキシ尿素,ダカルバジン,ビンクリスチン

BHF
Bolivian hemorrhagic fever ボリビア出血性熱

B-HGH
biosynthetic human growth factor 生合成ヒト成長因子

BHI
biosynthetic human insulin 生合成ヒトインスリン
brain-heart infusion 脳心臓滲出液

BHIB
beef heart infusion broth ウシ心臓滲出肉汁
brain heart infusion buffer 脳心臓滲出液緩衝液

BHI medium
brain heart infusion medium 脳心臓滲出液培地

BHK 21
baby hamster kidney 21 仔ハムスター腎細胞株21

BHL
bilateral hilar lymphadenitis 両側肺門部リンパ節腫大
bilateral hilar lymphadenopathy 両側(性)肺門リンパ節症
bilateral hilar lymphadenopathy enlargement 両側(性)肺門リンパ節腫張
biological half-time 生物学的半減期

B

BHLE
bilateral hilar lymphnode enlargement　両側(性)肺門リンパ節腫脹
bHLM
basic helix-loop-helix　インスリン転写因子
BHN
basic human need(s)　人間生活の基本的欲求
bephenium hydroxynaphthoate　ベフェニウムヒドロキシナフトエート
bridging hepatic necrosis　架橋肝壊死
Brinell hardness number　ブリネル硬度数
BHP
benign hypertrophic prostatitis　良性肥大性前立腺炎
benign hypertrophy of prostate　前立腺肥大
BHR
basal heart rate　基本心拍数
biotechnology and human research　生物工学と人間研究
borderline hypertensive rat　境界領域高血圧ラット
bronchial hyperactivity　気管支反応亢進
BH-RSV
Bryan high titer-Rous sarcoma virus　ブライアン高抗体価株・ラウス肉腫ウイルス
BHS
beta hemolytic streptococcus　β(型)溶血連鎖球菌
Bluthirnschranke〈独〉　血液脳関門
breath-holding spell　息こらえ発作
BHT
biological half-time　生物学的半減期
butylated hydroxytoluene　酪酸ヒドロキシトルエン
dibutylhydroxytoluene　ジブチルヒドロキシトルエン
BHV
bovine herpes virus　ウシヘルペスウイルス
bh/vh
body hematocrit/venous hematocrit (ratio)　身体ヘマトクリット/静脈血ヘマトクリット(比)
B.Hyg.
Bachelor of Hygiene　衛生学士
BI
bactericidal index　殺菌指数
bacteriological index　細菌学的指数
base of prism in　内方プリズム基底
basilar invagination　頭蓋内陥入
beef insulin　ウシインスリン
biischial diameter　(骨盤出口の)横径
bodily injury　身体傷害
bone injury　骨損傷

bowel impaction　腸埋伏
brain injured　脳の障害された
buffer index　緩衝指数
burn index　熱傷指数

Bi
biceps　二頭(筋)の
bismuth　ビスマス〈元素〉

BI, B.I.
Brinkman index　ブリンクマン指数

BIA
bacterial inhibition assay　細菌抑制検査
bioimmunoassay　生体免疫検定

bib.
bibe〈ラ〉　飲む

biblio
bibliography　(引用)文献，参考書

bibliother
bibliotherapeutic　読書療法の
bibliotherapist　読書療法士
bibliotherapy　読書療法

BIC
blood isotope clearance　血中アイソトープクリアランス

bic
biceps　二頭(筋)の

bicarb
bicarbonate　重炭酸塩

BICER
Baikal International Center for Ecological Research　バイカル国際生態学研究センター

bichrome
sodium bichromate　重クロム酸ナトリウム

bicv
biconcave　両凹の

bicx
biconvex　両凸の

bid., b.I.d.
bigeminy　二段脈
bis in die〈ラ〉=twice daily, twice a day　1日2回《処》

BIDS syndrome
brittle hair, impaired intelligence, decreased fertility, short stature syndrome　裂毛・知能低下・生殖能低下・短軀症候群，BIDS症候群

big D
diethyltryptamine, dimethyltryptamine, dipropyltryptamine, etc. — ジエチルトリプタミン・ジメチルトリプタミン・ジプロピルトリプタミンなどの幻覚剤

bigem.
bigeminy — 二段脈，二連脈

big H
heroin — ヘロイン

BIH
benign intracranial hypertension — 良性頭蓋内圧亢進(症)

bihor.
bihorium〈ラ〉 — 2時間《処》

BIL
brother-in-law — 義(理の)兄弟

BIL, Bil, bil.
bilateral — 両側(性)の

BIL, bil
bilirubin — ビリルビン

BIL/ALB
bilirubin-to-albumin (ratio) — ビリルビン/アルブミン(比)

bilat
bilateral — 両側(性)の

bilat SLC
bilateral short leg case — 両側短下肢例

BILAT S & O, BILAT S×O
bilateral salpingo-oophorectomy — 両側(性)卵管卵巣摘出(術)

bili
bilirubin — ビリルビン

bilirub
bilirubin — ビリルビン

b.i.n.
bis in nocte〈ラ〉, *bis in noctus*〈ラ〉= twice a night — 1夜に2回《処》

bind
binding — 結合

binocs
binoculars — 両眼

bio
biological — 生物学の
biology — 生物学

Biochem, biochem, biochem.
biochemical — 生化学の
biochemist — 生化学者
biochemistry — 生化学

biochron
biochronometry 生物時間測定
bioclean
biologically clean 生物学的に清浄な
biocon
biocontamination 生物汚染
biocyb
biocybernetics 生物サイバネティクス
biodef
biological defense 生物学的防御
biodeg
biodegradable 生物学的に退化可能な
biodes
biodestructible 生物学的に破壊可能な
biodet
biodeterioration 生物学的低下
bioeng
bioengineering 生体工学
biological engineering 生物工学
bioex
biological experiment 生物学的実験
Biol, biol
biological 生物学的
biologist 生物学者
biology 生物学
biomed
biomedical 生物医学の
biomedicine 生物医学
bionics
biology and electronics 生物学と電子工学
Biophys
biophysics 生物物理学
biophys
biophysical 生物物理学の
biophysist 生物物理学者
BIOS
biological investigation of space 空間の生物学的観察
biological satellite 生物学周辺科学
biosci
bioscience 生物科学
bioscientific 生物科学の
bioscientist 生物科学者
BIP
bacterial intravenous protein 細菌性静脈内蛋白
biological index of pollution 生物学的汚染指数
biological index of water pollution 生物学的水質汚染指数

B

bismuth iodoform paraffin ヨードホルム蒼鉛パラフィン
bleomycin, ifosfamide, cisplatin (= Platinol) ブレオマイシン,イホスファミド,シスプラチン(=プラチノール)
bronchiolitis obliterans and diffuse alveolar damage 閉塞性細気管支炎性間質性肺炎
bronchiolitis obliterans-interstitial pneumonitis 閉塞性細気管支炎・間質性肺炎

BIPAP
biphasic positive airway prerssure 二相性気道内陽圧，二相性陽圧呼吸

BiPAP
bi-level positive airway pressure 両レベル設定陽圧呼吸

BIPM
Bureau International des Poids et Mesures〈仏〉 国際度量衡局
N-{*p*-(2-benzimidazolyl)phenyl} maleimide *N*-{*p*-(2-ベンズイミダゾリル)フェニル}マレイミド

BIPP
bismuth iodoform paraffin paste ヨードホルム蒼鉛パラフィン軟膏
bismuth iodoform petrolatum paste ヨードホルム蒼鉛パラフィン泥膏

BIS
Belluevue intelligence scale ベルビュー知能検査

bis
N, *N*-methylene-bisacrylamide *N*, *N*-メチレンビスアクリルアミド，ビス

bisex
bisexual 両性の

bis in 7d.
bis in septem diebus〈ラ〉=twice a week 1週(間)に2回《処》

BISP
between ischial spines 坐骨脊柱間

BIT
between great trochanters 大転子間

bitroch
bitrochanteric 両大転子の

biw
bi-weekly 隔週の，1週おきの《処》

BJ
Bence Jones (protein) ベンスジョーンズ(蛋白)
biceps jerk 二頭筋反射
Bielschowsky-Janský (syndrome) ビールショウスキー・ヤンスキー(症候群)

BJ, B/J, B & J
bone and joint 骨と関節
BJM
bones, joints, muscles 骨・関節・筋
BJP
Bence Jones protein ベンスジョーンズ蛋白
BK
Bassen-Kornzweig (syndrome) バッセン・コルンツヴァイク(症候群)
below-knee 膝下，下腿
Blutkörperchen〈独〉 血球
bradykinin ブラジキニン
Koch bacillus コッホ桿菌
Bk
berkelium バークリウム〈元素〉
bk
back 背(中)，背部
black 黒い，黒色の，黒人
BKA
below-knee amputation 下腿切断
BK AMP
below-knee amputation 下腿切断
BKD
baked 日焼けした
bkf
breakfast 朝食
bkfst
breakfast 朝食
bkft
breakfast 朝食
BKG
Ballistokardiogramm〈独〉 心弾動図
bkg
background 背景の
BKLY
back lying 仰臥位
B-K mole
Betz-Krueger mole ベッツ・クリューガー母斑，BK母斑
bkr
beaker ビーカー
BKT
Bücherkatalogtest〈独〉 書籍目録テスト
BKTT
below-knee to toe 下腿

B

BKWP
below-knee walking plaster　下腿歩行可能ギプス

BL
Baralyme　バラライム
basal lamina　基底板
baseline　基線
basement lamina　基底層
Beinlange〈独〉　脚長，下肢長
Beschwerdenlist〈独〉　愁訴リスト
beta-lipoprotein　βリポ蛋白
black light　黒光，ブラックライト
blood loss　失血，血液喪失
Blut〈独〉＝blood　血液
body length　身長
bronchial lavage，bronchus lavage　気管支洗浄
buccolingual　頰側舌面の
Burkitt'(s) lymphoma　バーキットリンパ腫

BL，bl
bleeding　出血
Blut〈独〉＝blood　血液

Bl，bl
black　黒い，黒色の，黒人
blue　青色の，青

BLa
buccolabial　頰(面)唇(面)の

BLB
Boothby-Lovelace-Bulbulian (oxygen mask)　ブースビー・ラブレス・ブルブリアン(酸素マスク)，BLBマスク

BlB
Blutbild〈独〉　血液像

BLC，BL C，BlC
blood culture　血液培養

BLCFC
B lymphocyte colony forming cell　Bリンパ球コロニー形成細胞

BLCFU
B lymphocyte colony-forming unit　Bリンパ球コロニー形成細胞

BLCL
B-lymphoid cell line　Bリンパ球系細胞株

bl.cult
blood culture　血液培養

BLD
bacteremia of long duration　長期持続性菌血症
basal (cell) liquefactive degeneration　基底(細胞)融解変性
beryllium lung disease　ベリリウム肺疾患

Bld, bid.
Blut〈独〉=blood　血液
Bld Bnk
blood bank　血液バンク
BLE
both lower extremities　両下肢
bleed
bleeding　出血
BLEO, Bleo
bleomycin　ブレオマイシン
BLEO-MOP
bleomycin, mechlorethamine, vincristine (=Oncovin), prednisone　ブレオマイシン,メクロルエタミン,ビンクリスチン(=オンコビン),プレドニゾン
bleph
blepharoplasty　眼瞼形成(術)
BLG
beta-lactoglobulin　βラクトグロブリン
BLH
Blue-light hazard　青色光網膜傷害
BLI
bombesin-like immunoreactivity　ボンベシン様免疫反応
blk
black　黒い，黒色の，黒人
BLL
below lower limit　下限以下の
benign lymphoepithelial lesion　良性リンパ上皮病変
BLM
bleomycin　ブレオマイシン
BLN
bronchial lymph nodes　気管支リンパ節
BLOBS, bl.obs
bladder observation　膀胱観察
BLP, BLp
beta-lipoprotein　βリポ蛋白
BL PR, bl.pr
blood pressure　血圧
BLQ
both lower quadrants　両側下部1/4区
BLRA
beta-lactamase resistant antimicrobial　βラクタマーゼ抵抗性抗菌薬
BLROA
British Laryngological Rhinological and Otological Association　英国耳鼻咽喉科学会

BLS
barrels　バレル〈単位〉
basic life support　一次救命処置
blind loop syndrome　盲係蹄症候群
blood and lymphatic systems　血液・リンパ系
BlS
blood sugar　血糖
Bl Skg
Blutsenkung〈独〉　血沈
BLT
blood-clot lysis time　血餅溶解時間
blood test　血液検査
BLT, BlT
blood type　血液型
B-Lt, B-LT
B-lymphotoxin　Bリンホトキシン
bl.time
bleeding time　出血時間
BLV
biologic limit value　生物学的許容値
blood volume　血(液)量，血液容量
bovine leukemia virus　ウシ白血病ウイルス
Bl vol
blood volume　血(液)量，血液容量
bl.x
bleeding time　出血時間
B-lym
B cell leukemia-lymphoma　B細胞白血病・リンパ腫
BM
bain-marie〈仏〉　蒸し鍋
barium meal　バリウム粥
basal medium　基礎培地
basal metabolism　基礎代謝
basement membrane　基底膜
betamehtasone　ベタメタゾン
between meals　食間薬《処》
biomedical　生物医学的な
birth mark　母斑
bleomycin, mitomycin-C　ブレオマイシン，マイトマイシンC
blood monocyte　血中単球
body mass　体重
body motion　体動
bone marrow　骨髄
bowel movement　便通，排便
breast milk　母乳，人乳

buccomesial 頬側近心面の
Buttermilch〈独〉 牛(酪)乳

B.M.
Bachelor of Medicine 医学士

BM, B.M., b.m.
balneum maris〈ラ〉=sea-water bath 塩水浴, 海水浴

BM, B/M
black male 黒人男性

B_2M, β_2m
beta-2-microglobulin β_2ミクログロブリン

BMA
British Medical Association 英国医学協会

BMAP
bone marrow acid phosphatase 骨髄酸性ホスファターゼ

Bmax
maximum binding 最大結合能

BMB
British Medical Bulletin 英国医学雑誌

BM-BC
bone marrow buffy coat cell 骨髄軟膜細胞

BMC
blood mononuclear cell 血中単核球
bone marrow cell 骨髄細胞
bone mineral contents 骨内鉱質含有量

BMD
Becker muscular dystrophy ベッカー型筋ジストロフィ
beclomethasone dipropionate cream ジプロピオン酸ベクロメタゾンクリーム
bone marrow depression 骨髄抑制
bone mineral densitometry 骨塩量〔骨密度〕測定
bone mineral density 骨(塩)量, 骨密度

BMDM
bone marrow-derived macrophages 骨髄由来マクロファージ

BME
biomedical engineering 医用工学
brief maximal effort 瞬時最大努力
Eagle basal medium イーグル基礎培地

B.M.E.
Bachelor of Mechanical Engineering 工学士

B.Med.
Bachelor of Medicine 医学士

BMET
bio-medical equipment technician 臨床工学技術者

BMF
B cell maturation factor B細胞成熟因子

B

BMG
benign monoclonal gammopathy — 良性単クローン性γグロブリン血症
benign mucous membrane — 良性単クローン性免疫グロブリン血症
beta-2-microglobulin — β_2ミクログロブリン
bilirubin monoglucuronide — ビリルビンモノグルクロナイド

BMHP
1-bromo mercury 2-hydroxy propane — 臭化水銀水酸化プロパン

BMI
body mass index — 体格指数，Kaup指数

B.Mic.
Bachelor of Microbiology — 微生物学士

BMJ
British Medical Journal — 英国医学雑誌

BMK，bmk
birthmark — あざ，母斑

BML
bimastoid line — 両乳様突起間線

B-ML
B-malignant lymphoma — B細胞性悪性リンパ腫

BMLM
basement membrane-like material — 基底膜様物質

BMM
bone marrow-derived macrophages — 骨髄由来マクロファージ

BMMC
bone marrow-derived mast cell — 骨髄肥満細胞
bone marrow mononuclear cells — 骨髄単核球
breast milk mononuclear cells — 母乳単核球

BMMP
benign mucous membrane pemphigoid — 良性粘膜類天疱瘡

BMN
bone marrow necrosis — 骨髄壊死

BM-NPC
bone marrow non phagocytic cell — 骨髄非貪食細胞

B-MOPP
bleomycin, mechlorethamine, vincristine (=Oncovin), procarbazine, prednisone — ブレオマイシン，メクロルエタミン，ビンクリスチン(=オンコビン)，プロカルバジン，プレドニゾン

BMP
bischloroethylnitrosourea, methotrexate, procarbazine — ビスクロロエチルニトロソ尿素，メトトレキサート，プロカルバジン

bone marrow pressure　骨髄内圧
bone morphogenic protein　骨形成促進蛋白，骨形態発生蛋白

BMPP
benign mucous membrane pemphigus　良性粘膜天疱瘡

BMPS
British Medical Protection Society　英国予防医学会

BMR
basal metabolic rate　基礎代謝率

BMRC
British Medical Research Council　英国医学研究協議会

BMS
betamethasone　ベタメタゾン
bone mineral study　骨塩定量評価
Bureau of Medicine and Surgery　内科学・外科学事務局

BMS, B.M.S.
Bachelor of Medical Science　医学士

BMSA
British Medical Student Association　英国医学生連盟

BMT
Bachelor of Medical Technology　医療技術学士
basement membrane thickening　基底膜肥厚
benign mesenchymal tumor　良性間葉(性)腫瘍
benign mesodermal tumor　良性中胚葉性腫瘍
bone marrow transplantation　骨髄移植

BMU
basic multicellular unit　基本多細胞単位

BMV
bromegrass mosaic virus　ブロムグラスモザイクウイルス

BMZ
basement membrane zone　基底膜帯

BN
Babinski-Nageotte (syndrome)　バビンスキー・ナジェット(症候群)
Bachelor of Nursing　看護学士
brachial neuritis　上腕神経炎
branchial neuritis　鰓神経炎
bridging necrosis　架橋壊死
bucconasal　頬鼻(側)の
bulimia nervosa　神経性過食症
Bureau of Narcotics　麻薬局
nucleus basalis〈ラ〉　基底核

1-BN(2)
1-bromo-naphthol(2)　ブロモナフトール

B

B.N.
bladder neck 膀胱頸部
BNA
Basel Nomina Anatomica バーゼル解剖学用語
BNB
blood nerve barrier 血液神経関門
BNC
bladder neck contracture 膀胱頸部狭窄症
BNCT
boron neutron capture therapy ホウ素中性子捕捉療法
BND
Brand-Name Drug 先発医薬品
BNDD
Bureau of Narcotics and Dangerous Drugs 麻薬・危険薬物管理局
BNG
6-bromo-2-naphtyl-beta-galactoside 6-ブロモ-2-ナフチル-β-ガラクトシド
BNGase
6-bromo-2-naphtyl-beta-galactosidase 6-ブロモ-2-ナフチル-β-ガラクトシダーゼ
BNGF
beta nerve-growth factor β神経成長因子
BNHS
British National Health Service 英国国営医療
BNO
bladder neck obstruction 膀胱頸(部)閉塞
bowels not opened 便秘
BNP
brain natriuretic peptides 脳ナトリウム利尿ペプチド
BNPA
binasal pharyngeal airway 両側鼻腔咽頭気道
BNS
benign nephrosclerosis 良性腎硬化症
Blitz-Nick-und-Salaamkrämpfe〈独〉 瞬目・点頭・遥拝・痙攣
B.NSc.
Bachelor of Nursing Science 看護学士
BNS Krampf
Blitz-Nick-Salaam Krampf〈独〉 瞬目・点頭・遥拝・痙攣
BNT
brain neurotransmitter 脳神経伝達物質
BNU
N-butyl-*N*-nitrosourea *N*-ブチル-*N*-ニトロソ尿素
BO
base of prism out 外方プリズム基底
body odor 体臭

bohemium ボヘミウム
Bolton ボルトン
bowel obstruction 腸閉塞
bowel open 排便
bronchiolitis obliterans 閉塞性細気管支炎
bucco-occlusal 頬側咬合面の

BO_2
blood oxygen 血液酸素

BO, bo.
bowel 腸

BO, B & O
belladonna and opium ベラドンナと阿片

BOA
behavioral observation audiometry 行動反応聴覚検査
born on arrival 到着時出産〔出生〕
British Optical Association 英国眼科学会
British Orthopedic Association 英国整形外科学会
British Osteopathic Association 英国骨疾患学会

BOAI
balloon occluded arterial infusion バルーン閉塞動注法

BOAP
bleomycin, vincristine (=Oncovin), adriamycin, prednisone ブレオマイシン,ビンクリスチン(=オンコビン),アドリアマイシン,プレドニゾン

BOC
t-butoxycarbonyl *t*-ブトキシカルボニル

BOD
biochemical oxygen demand 生物化学的酸素要求量

BOD Unit
Bodansky unit ボダンスキー単位

BOF
basic oxygen furnace 基礎酸素燃焼

BOHA
balloon occluded hepatic arteriography バルーン閉鎖式肝動脈造影

BOHS
British Occupational Hygiene Society 英国産業衛生学会

11β-OHSD
11β-hydroxysteroid dehydrogenase 11βヒドロオキシステロイド脱水素酵素
11β-hydroxysteroid dehydrogenase 11βヒドロオキシステロイド脱水素酵素

boil
boiling 煮沸

B

bol
bolus〈ラ〉　大粒錠剤《処》

BOLD
bleomycin, vincristine (=Oncovin), lomustine, dacarbazine　ブレオマイシン,ビンクリスチン(=オンコビン),ロムスチン,ダカルバジン

blood oxygen level dependent　血液酸素レベル依存

bolovac
bolometric voltage and current　ボロメーター〔放射エネルギー測定装置〕の電圧と電流

BOM
bilateral otitis media　両側中耳炎

BOMA
bilateral otitis media, acute　急性両耳性中耳炎

BONP
bleomycin, vincristine (=Oncovin), Natulan, prednisolone　ブレオマイシン,ビンクリスチン(=オンコビン),ナツラン,プレドニゾロン

BOOP
bronchi(oli)tis obliterans (with) organizing pneumonia　器質化肺炎を伴う閉塞性細気管支炎

booster
booster injection or inoculation　予防接種の追加免疫

BOP
bischloroethylnitrosourea, vincristine (=Oncovin), prednisone　ビスクロロエチルニトロソ尿素,ビンクリスチン(=オンコビン),プレドニゾン

bleomycin, vincristine (=Oncovin), prednisone　ブレオマイシン,ビンクリスチン(=オンコビン),プレドニゾン

BOPAM
bleomycin, vincristine (=Oncovin), prednisone, adriamycin, methotrexate　ブレオマイシン,ビンクリスチン(=オンコビン),プレドニゾン,アドリアマイシン,メトトレキサート

BOPD
BCNU (=1,3-bis(2-chloroethyl)-1-nitrosourea), VCR=vincristine (=Oncovin), procarbazine, prednisone　カルムスチン,ビンクリスチン(=オンコビン),プロカルバジン,プレドニゾン

BOPP
bischloroethylnitrosourea, vincristine (=Oncovin), procarbazine, prednisone　ビスクロロエチルニトロソ尿素,ビンクリスチン(=オンコビン),プロカルバジン,プレドニゾン

bleomycin, vincristine(=Oncovin), procarbazine, prednisolone ブレオマイシン,ビンクリスチン(=オンコビン),プロカルバジン,プレドニゾロン

B.Opt.
Bachelor of Optometry 視力測定士

BOR
bowel open regular 便通正常
bowel open regularly 規則的に便通がある

Borr 1-4
Borrmann 1-4 ボールマン1～4型
Borrmann classification 1-4 ボールマン胃癌分類Ⅰ～Ⅳ型

BOSE
bleomycin, vincristine(=Oncovin), streptozotocin, etoposide ブレオマイシン,ビンクリスチン(=オンコビン),ストレプトゾトシン,エトポシド

bot
bottle ビン

Bot, bot.
botanical 植物学の
botany 植物

Bot.c
International Code of Botanical Nomenclature 国際植物命名規約

bov
bovine ウシの

BOW
bag of water 羊膜嚢

BP
Bachelor of Pharmacy 薬学士
Bard-Pic (syndrome) バード・ピック(症候群)
basic protein 塩基性蛋白
before present 現症以前
behavior pattern 行動パターン，行動型
Bell palsy ベル麻痺
benzopyrene ベンゾピレン
biological psychiatry 生物学的精神医学
biopterin ビオプテリン
biotic potential 生物性電位
biparietal 両頭頂部
bipolar 双極(性)の
bipolar affective disorder 双極性感情障害
bipolar lead 双極導出
birthplace 出生地
bisexual potent 両性能力

body plethysmography 体プレスチモグラフィ
bronchopleural 気管支胸膜の
buccopulpal 頰(面)(歯)髄(面)の
bullous pemphigoid 水疱性類天疱瘡
bypass バイパス，副行路，側副路

BP, bp.
bedpan 便器

BP, bp, b.p.
boiling point 沸点

BP, B.P.
blood pressure 血圧
British Pharmacopoeia 英国薬局方

bp, b.p.
base pair 塩基対

BPA
Bauhinia purpurea agglutinin バウヒニア紫斑凝集素
bovine plasma albumin ウシ血漿アルブミン
British Pediatric Association 英国小児科学会
bronchopulmonary aspergillosis 気管支肺アスペルギルス症
burst-promoting activity 赤芽球コロニー群刺激細胞

BPAA
4-biphenylacetic acid 4-ビフェニリル酢酸

BPAG
Bordetella pertussis agglutination 百日咳凝集反応

BPAS
N-benzoyl-*p*-aminosalicylic acid *N*-ベンゾイル-*p*-アミノサリチル酸

BPB
bromphenol blue ブロムフェノールブルー
P-bromophenacyl bromide 臭化パラブロモフェナシル

BPC
benzylpenicillin ベンジルペニシリン
bile phospholipid concentration 胆汁リン脂質濃度

BPC, B.P.C.
British Pharmaceutical Codex 英国調剤医薬品集

BPC-G
benzylpenicillin benzathine ベンジルペニシリン・ベンザチン

B-PCO_2
blood partial pressure of carbon dioxide 血中二酸化炭素分圧

BPD
biparietal diameter 頭蓋最大横径
blood pressure decrease(d) 血圧低下
borderline personality disoder 境界型パーソナリティ〔人格〕障害

bromperidol ブロムペリドール
broncho pulmonary dysplasia 気管支肺異形成(症)

BPE
bacterial phosphatidylethanolamine 細菌性ホスファチジルエタノールアミン
bovine pituitary extract ウシ下垂体抽出液

BPEC
bipolar electrocoagulation 双極(性)電気凝固(法)

B.Ped.
Bachelor of Pediatrics 小児科学士

BPF
bradykinin potentiating factor ブラジキニン増強因子
bronchopleural fistula 気管支胸膜瘻

BPG
benzathine penicillin G ベンザチンペニシリンG
blood pressure gauge 血圧計
bypass graft バイパス移植(片)

BPH
Bachelor of Public Health 公衆衛生学士
benign prostatic hyperplasia 良性前立腺過形成(症)
benign prostatic hypertrophy 良性前立腺肥大(症)

BPh
buccopharygeal 頬咽頭の

BPh, B.Ph.
British Pharmacopoeia 英国薬局方

BPHE
Bachelor of Physical Health Education 健康教育学士

BPheo
bacteriopheophytin バクテリオフェオフィチン

B.Phy.Thy.
Bachelor of Physical Therapy 物理療法士

BPI
bactericidal permeability increasing protein 殺菌・透過性増強蛋白
Basic Personality Inventory 基礎人格評価表
beef-pork insulin ウシ・ブタインスリン
blood pressure increased 血圧上昇

BPL
benign proliferative lesion 良性増殖性病変
benzylpenicilloyl polylysine ベンジルペニシロイルポリリジン
beta-propiolactone βプロピオラクトン
birth place 出生地
bronchopulmonary lavage 気管支肺洗浄

BP-1
early B-lineage marker　初期B細胞抗原
BPLA
beta-propiolactone　βプロピオラクトン
blood pressure, left arm　左腕の血圧
BPM
births per minute　出産/分，出生/分
breaths per minute　呼吸/分
bpm
beats per minute　心拍数
BPMC
o-sec-butylphenyl methylcarbamate　ブチルフェニルメチルカルバメイト，ビーピーエムシー
BPMF
British Postgraduate Medical Federation　英国卒後医学連盟
BPMS
blood pressure measuring system　血圧測定システム
BPMV
bean pod mottle virus　豆莢斑紋状ウイルス
BPN
brachial plexus neuropathy　腕神経叢ニューロパシー
BPO
basal pepsin output　基礎ペプシン分泌量
benzylpenicilloyl　ベンジルペニシロイル
BPO_2
benzoyl peroxide　ベンゾイルペルオキシド
BPO-HSA
benzylpenicilloyl human serum albumin　ベンジルペニシロイルヒト血清アルブミン
BPP
bovine pancreatic polypeptide　ウシ膵(臓)ポリペプチド
bradykinin-potentiating factor　ブラジキニン増強因子
BP & P
blood pressure and pulse　血圧と脈拍
BPPN
benign paroxysmal positional nystagmus　良性発作性頭位眼振
BPPV
benign paroxysmal positional vertigo　良性発作性頭位変換眩暈
BPR
bioclean patient room　無菌室
blood pressure recorder　血圧記録器
blood production rate　血液産生率
BPRA
blood pressure, right arm　右腕の血圧

BPRS
brief psychiatric rating scale | 簡易精神症状スケール
brief psychiatric rating test scale | 簡便精神医学的評価尺度

BPS
beats per second | 拍動/秒
bilateral partial salpingectomy | 両側部分卵管摘出(術)
biophysical profile score | 生物物理プロフィール評価
brain protein solvent | 脳蛋白溶剤
breaths per second | 呼吸/秒

bps
bit per second | ビット/秒

B.Ps.
Bachelor of Psychology | 心理学士

BPsS
British Psychological Society | 英国精神医学会

B.Psych.
Bachelor of Psychology | 心理学士

BPT
Bachelor of Physiotherapy | 物理療法士
biological pregnancy test | 生物学的妊娠反応
bronchial provocation test | 気管支誘発試験

BPTI
basic pancreatic trypsin inhibitor | 基本的な膵(臓)トリプシン阻害剤
bovine pancreatic trypsin inhibitor | ウシ膵臓トリプシン抑制因子

BPV
benign paroxysmal vertigo | 良性発作性眩暈
benign positional vertigo | 良性頭位変換眩暈
Bordetella pertussis vaccine | ボルデテラ百日咳ワクチン
bovine papilloma virus | ウシ乳頭腫ウイルス，ウシパピローマウイルス

Bq
becquerel | ベクレル

BQA
Bureau of Quality Assurance | 品質保証局

BQC sol
2,6-dibromoquinone-4-chlorimide solution | 2,6-ジブロモキノン-4-クロリミド溶液

BR
bacteriorhodopsin | バクテリオロドプシン
bathroom | 浴室
bedrest | ベッド上安静，床上安静
bilirubin | ビリルビン
biological response | 生物学的反応
breathing rate | 呼吸速度
breathing reserve | 換気予備量

Br	
branch	領域
breast	乳房
bridge	橋(加工)義歯，(骨)橋
British	英国(人)の，英国人
bromine	臭素
Brust〈独〉	胸部
br	
brachial	上腕の
branch	枝
breathe	呼吸する，息をする
broiled	焼けた，日焼けした
brother	兄弟
bruit	雑音，ブリュイ
BR, Br	
bronchitis	気管支炎
Brucella	ブルセラ(属)
Br, Br.	
bronchus	気管支
brown	茶色(の)，褐色(の)
br, br.	
breath	呼吸，息
BRA	
brain	脳
BrA	
bronchial artery	気管支動脈
BRAC	
basic rest activity cycle	基礎的休息活動周期
brady	
bradycardia	徐脈
BRAGS	
Bioelectrical Repair and Growth Society	生物電気修復成長学会
branch	
branchial	上腕の
BRAO	
branch retinal artery occlusion	網膜動脈枝閉塞(症)
BrAP	
brachial artery pressure	上腕動脈(血)圧
BRBA	
Brucella	ブルセラ(属)
BRBC	
bovine red blood cells	ウシ赤血球
BRBN	
blue rubber bleb nevus (syndrome)	青色ゴムまり様母斑(症候群)

BRBPR
bright red blood per rectum 直腸由来の鮮血
br.bx
breast biopsy 乳房生検
BRCA1〔2〕
breast cancer gene-1〔2〕 遺伝性乳癌遺伝子1〔2〕
BRCM
below right costal margin 右肋骨縁下(方)に
BrdU
bromodeoxyuridine ブロモデオキシウリジン
BrdUrd
bromodeoxyuridine ブロモデオキシウリジン
BRE
benign rolandic epilepsy 良性ローランドてんかん
brek
breakfast 朝食
BRF
bulbar reticular formation 延髄網様体
BRH
benign recurrent hematuria 良性再発性血尿
BRI
Biological Research Institute 生物学研究所
Biomedical Research Institute 生物医科学研究所
Brain Research Institute 脳研究所
bronchoreversibility index 気管支可逆性指数
BRIAC
behavior rating instrument of autistic children 自閉症児行動評価表
BRIC
benign recurrent intrahepatic cholestasis 良性再発性肝内胆汁うっ滞
Brit
Britain 英国
British 英国(人)の，英国人
Br.J.Surg.
British Journal of Surgery 英国外科学雑誌
Brkf，brkf
breakfast 朝食
brkt
breakfast 朝食
BRM
biological response modifier 生物反応修飾〔変換〕物質
biological response modifiers 生物学的応答調節物質
brn
brown 茶色(の)，褐色(の)

B

BRO
bronchoscopy 気管支鏡検査
bro
brother 兄弟
brom.
bromide 臭素化合物
bromidum〈ラ〉 臭化物
Bron
bronchial 気管支の
Bronch
bronchoscopic 気管支鏡の，気管支鏡的な
bronchoscopist 気管支鏡検査医
bronch
bronchitis 気管支炎
bronchogram 気管支造影図
bronchus 気管支
Bronch，bronch.
bronchoscope 気管支鏡
bronchoscopy 気管支鏡(検査)法
bronchiect
bronchiectasis 気管支拡張(症)
broncho
bronchography 気管支造影法
BRP
bathroom privileges 入浴可
bilirubin production ビリルビン産生
BRPH，Brph，brph
bronchophony 気管支声
BRR
breathing reserve ratio 換気予備比
BRS
basic Rorschach score 基礎ロールシャッハスコア
behavior rating scale 行動評価尺度
BRSF
bone resorption stimulating factor 骨吸収刺激因子
br.snds
breath sound(s) 呼吸音
Br sounds，br.sounds
breath sounds 呼吸音
BRT
Brook Reaction Test ブルック反応試験
brt
bright 明るい，鮮明な，頭のいい
brth
breath 呼吸，息

B-RTO
balloon-occluded retrograde transvenous obliteration — バルーン閉塞下逆行性経静脈的塞栓術

BrU
bromouracil — ブロモウラシル

Bruc
Brucella — ブルセラ(属)

brunch
breakfast-lunch — 朝昼兼用食，ブランチ

BRV
benign recurrent vertigo — 良性再発性眩暈症

BRVO
branch retinal vein occlusion — 網膜静脈分岐閉鎖症

BS
Bachelor of Science — 科学士
Bacillus subtilis — 枯草菌
Baehr-Schiffrin (disease) — ベーア・シフリン(病)
Behçet's syndrome — ベーチェット症候群
bismuth sulfite — 亜硫酸ビスマス培地
bispecific antibody — バイスペシフィック抗体
blepharospasm — 眼瞼痙攣
blood serum — 血清
Blue Shield — ブルーシールド
boewl sound — 腸雑音
borderline schizophrenia — 近似分裂病
both side — 両側
bowel sound — 腸雑音
Boyd-Stearns (syndrome) — ボイド・スターンズ(症候群)
bronchoscopy — 気管支鏡
Brown-Séquard (syndrome) — ブラウン・セカール(症候群)
buffered saline — 緩衝食塩水
intraoperative blood salvage — 術中出血回収
standard bicarbonate — 標準塩基

B.S.
Bárány Society — バラニー協会
British Standard — 英国標準の
Bureau of Standards — 基準局

B/S
bits per second — 1秒間のビット数

B-S
Björk-Shiley (valve) — ビジョルク・シャイリー(弁)

BS, bs
bedside — ベッドサイド

BS, B.S.
blood sugar — 血糖

BS, B.S., b.s.
breath sound(s) 呼吸音
B.S., B.Sc.
Bachelor of Science 理学士
BSA
benzene-sulfonic acid ベンゼンスルホン酸
bismuth-sulfate agar 硫酸蒼鉛寒天
Blind Service Association 盲人奉仕協会
body surface area 体表面積
bovine serum albumin ウシ血清アルブミン
burn surface area 熱傷面積
BSA nephritis
bovine serum albumin nephritis ウシ血清腎炎
BSAP
B-lineage specific transcription factor B細胞特異転写因子(=CD19)
brief short-action potential 短小活動電位
BSB
body surface burned 体表面火傷
both side band 運搬波送出両側波帯
BSBC
buffer-soluble binding component 緩衝剤溶解性物質
BSC
bedside care ベッドサイドケア，看護
Biomedical Science Corporation 生物医科学協会
BSCC
British Society for Clinical Cytology 英国臨床細胞学会
B.Sc.Dent
Bachelor of Science in Dentistry 歯科学士
B.S.Ch
Bachelor of Science in Chemistry 化学士
BSCL
basic sinus cycle length 基本洞周期長
B.Sc.Nurs.
Bachelor of Science in Nursing 看護学士
BSD
baby soft diet ベビー用軟食
bedside drainage ベッドサイドドレナージ
bsd
besonders〈独〉 とくに
B.S.Dent
Bachelor of Science in Dental Hygiene 歯科衛生士
BSDR
Behavioral Scientists in Dental Research 歯科研究行動科学協会

BSE
bovine spongiform encephalopathy　ウシ海綿状脳症
breast self-examination　乳房自己検査

BSEP
brainstem evoked potentials　脳幹誘発電位

BSER
brainstem electric response　脳幹電気反応
brainstem evoked response audiometry　脳幹(誘発)反応

BSF
back scatter factor　後方散乱係数
basal skull fracture　脳底頭蓋骨折
B cell stimulating factor　B細胞刺激因子
B-lymphocyte stimulatory factor　Bリンパ球刺激因子
busulfan　ブスルファン

BSG
branchioskeletogenital (syndrome)　鰓骨格生殖器(症候群)

B & S glands
Bartholin and Skene glands　バルトリン腺とスキーン腺

BSH
benzenesulfohydrazide　ベンゼンスルホヒドラジド
British Society of Hypnotherapeutics　英国催眠治療学会

BSHA
Bachelor of Science in Hospital Administration　病院管理学士

B.S.H.Ed.
Bachelor of Science in Health Education　健康教育学士

BSI
bound serum iron　結合血清鉄

BSIHE
British Society for International Health Education　英国国際健康教育学会

BSJ
ball and socket joint　ボールソケット関節

BSL
bedside learning　臨床学習
blood sugar level　血糖レベル

BSL1
Bandeirea simplicifolia lectin 1　バンデリアマメレクチン1

BSLB
biaural simultaneous loudness balance test　両耳同時音の大きさ平衡検査

B.S.Med.
Bachelor of Science in Medicine　医学士

B.S.Med.Rec.
Bachelor of Science in Medical Records 病歴学士

B.S.Med.Rec.Lib.
Bachelor of Science in Medical Records Librarianship 病歴学士

B.S.Med.Tech.
Bachelor of Science in Medical Technology 医療技術士

BSN
bachelor of science in nursing 看護学士
bowel sound(s) normal 正常腸音

BSNA
Bachelor of Science in Nursing Administration 看護管理学士
bowel sound(s) normal and active 腸音正常活発

B.S.Nurs.
Bachelor of Science in Nursing 看護学士

B.S.Nurs.Ed.
Bachelor of Science in Nursing Education 看護教育学士

BSO
bilateral salpingo-oophorectomy 両側(性)卵管卵巣摘出(術)

B.S.Opt.
Bachelor of Science in Optometry 視力測定学士

BSP
Bachelor of Science in Pharmacy 薬剤学士
benign spontaneous pneumothorax 良性自然気胸
brom(o)sulfophthalein ブロモスルホフタレイン
Bromsulphalein ブロムスルファレイン

BSp
bronchospasm 気管支痙攣

BSPH
Bachelor of Science in Public Health 公衆衛生学士

B.S.Phar.
Bachelor of Science in Pharmacy 薬剤学士

BSPHN
Bachelor of Science in Public Health Nursing 公衆衛生看護学士

B.S.Phys.Ther.
Bachelor of Science in Physical Therapy 物理療法学士

BSPM
body surface potential mapping 体表面電位分布図

B.Sp.Thy.
Bachelor of Speech Therapy 言語治療学士

BSR
Bachelor of Science in Rehabilitation リハビリテーション学士
basal skin resistance 基礎皮膚抵抗
blood sedimentation rate 赤血球沈降速度，赤沈
Blutkörperchensenkungsreaktion〈独〉 赤血球沈降反応，赤沈
Blutsenkungsreaktion〈独〉 赤血球沈降速度
bowel sounds regular 腸雑音正常
brainstem response 脳幹反応

BSRC
Biological Serial Record Center 生物学的連続記録センター

BSRF
brain stem reticular formation 脳幹網様体

BS-RSV
Bryan standard-Rous sarcoma virus ブライアン標準株・ラウス肉腫ウイルス

BSS
balanced salt solution 平衡食塩水
Bernard-Soulier syndrome バーナード・スーリエ症候群
black silk sutures 黒色縫合絹糸
buffer salt solution, buffered saline solution 緩衝食塩水

BSSG
Biomedical Science Support Grant 生物医科学支持基会

BSSO
British Society for Study of orthodontics 英国歯科矯正学会

BST
bacteriuria screening test 細菌尿スクリーニング
bedside teaching 臨床教育
bedside training 臨床実習
blood serologic(al) test 血液血清学的試験
bradycardia-tachycardia syndrome 徐脈頻脈症候群
brief stimulus therapy 短期刺激療法

BST1
bone marrow stroma cell antigen 骨髄基質細胞抗原

BS & T
blood, sweat and tears 血・汗・涙

BSTA
British Surgical Trades Association 英国外科医協会

BSTFA
bis-trimethylsilytrifluoroacetamide ビストリメチルシリトリフルオロアセトアミド

B.Sur.
Bachelor of Surgery 外科学士

B

BSV
basal secretion volume rate, basal secretion volume 基礎分泌量
binocular single vision 両眼単一視
BSVR
basal secretion volume (rate) 基礎分泌量
BS & W
basic sediment and water 基本的沈殿物と水
BT
balance test 平衡検査
blastocyst transfer 胚盤胞移植
balloon tube 膀胱留置カテーテル，バルーンチューブ
bathytermograph 深部(海)水温温度測定器
bedtime 就寝時刻
behavior test 行動検査
behavior tharapy 行動療法
bitemporal 両側頭部
bitrochanteric 両大転子の
bladder tumor 膀胱腫瘍
Blalock-Taussig ブラロック・タウジヒ
bleeding time 出血時間
blood transfusion 輸血
blood type 血液型
blue tetrazolium (stain) ブルーテトラゾリウム(染色)
body temperature 体温
bowel tones 腸雑音
brain tumor 脳腫瘍
breast tumor 乳房腫瘍
BTA
better than average 平均より良い
Blood Transfusion Association 輸血協会
BTB
breakthrough bleeding 破綻
brom(o)thymol blue ブロモチモールブルー
BTBA
Blood Transfusion Betterment Association 輸血改善協会
BTC
basal temperature chart 基礎体温表
BTD
benzothiadiazine ベンゾチアディアジン
BTDS
O-benzoylthiamine disulfide *O*-ベンゾイルチアミンジスルフィド

BTE
behind-the-ear hearing instrument　耳かけ式補聴器
benzilic acid 3α-tropanyl ester　ベンジル酸 3 α トロパニルエステル

BTF
blood transfusion　輸血

BTg
bovine trypsinogen　ウシトリプシノーゲン

BTH
brain tumor headache　脳腫瘍頭痛

BTHU
British Thermal Unit　イギリス熱単位

Btk
Bruton's tyrosine kinase　ブルトンチロシンキナーゼ

BTL
bilateral tubal ligation　両側(性)(卵)管結紮(法)
biologically tolerable level　生物学的許容限界
blue thermoluminescence　青色熱ルミネセンス

BTLS
basic trauma life suppport　外傷一次救命救急処置

BTM
benign tertian malaria　良性三日熱マラリア
Betäubungsmittel〈独〉　麻酔剤，麻酔薬

BTME
Babcock test of mental efficiency　バブコック知能検査

BTMP
benzoylthiamine-*o*-monophosphate　ベンゾイルサイアミン-*o*-一リン酸塩

BTP
biliary tract pain　胆道痛
body temperature and pressure　体温と血圧
brain tissue pressure　脳組織圧

BTPD
body temperature and (ambient) pressure, dry　体温と乾燥状態の大気圧

BTPS
body temperature and ambient pressure saturated with water vapor　水蒸気飽和状態の体温と大気圧

BTR
biceps tendon reflex　二頭筋腱反射
branched chain amino acid and tyrosine ratio　総分岐鎖アミノ酸とチロシンの比

BTr
bovine trypsin　ウシトリプシン

BTRC
bacitracin バシトラシン

BTS
blood transfusion service 輸血サービス
bradycardia tachycardia syndrome 徐脈頻脈症候群
Brenztraubensäure〈独〉 焦性ブドウ酸

BTSH, B-TSH
bovine thyroid-stimulating hormone ウシ甲状腺刺激ホルモン

BT shunt
Blalock-Taussig shunt ブラロック・タウジヒシャント

BTU
benzyl-thiourea ベンジル・チオウレア
British Thermal unit 英国熱量単位

BTV
blue tongue virus ブルータングウイルス

BTX
benzene, toluene, xylene ベンゼン・トルエン・キシレン
bungarotoxin ブンガロトキシン

B type
B type B型

BU
base (of prism) up 上方プリズム基底
Bauchumfang〈独〉 腹囲
benign ulcer 良性潰瘍
bilirubin unbinding 非結合ビリルビン
biological unit 生物学的単位
Bodansky units ボダンスキー単位
bromouracil ブロモウラシル
Brustumfang〈独〉 胸囲
buffo unit ガマ単位
burn unit 火傷患者収容室

Bu
butyl ブチル

BUA
blood uric acid 血中尿酸
broadband ultrasound attenuation 広帯域超音波減衰率

Bucc
buccal 頬(側)の

BUDR, BUdR
5-bromodeoxyuridine 5-ブロモデオキシウリジン
5-bromo-2′-deoxyuridine 5-ブロモ-2′-デオキシウリジン

BUE
both upper extremities 両上肢

Buginar
buginarium〈ラ〉 ブジー
BUI
brain uptake index 脳摂取指数
BUL
below upper limit 上下限
Bul
bulimia 大食症
bul
bullet (小)銃弾
bull, bull.
bulletin 公報，会報
bulliat〈ラ〉=let it boil 煮沸せよ，沸騰(させよ)《処》
BuM & S
Bureau of Medicine and Surgery 内科・外科事務局
BUN
blood urea nitrogen 血液尿素窒素
bun.br.blk.
bundle branch block 脚ブロック
BUO
bilateral ureteral occlusion 両側尿管閉塞症
bleeding of undetermined origin 未決定原因による出血
buphth.
buphthalmos 牛眼
BUQ
both upper quadrants 両側上部1/4区
Bur
buried 埋葬された，包埋された
bur
bureau 局，部
Burd
Burdick suction バーディック吸引(器)
BUS
bushel ブッシェル
busulfan ブスルファン
BUS glands
Bartholin, urethral Skene glands バルトリン・尿道・スキーン腺
BUT
precorneal tear film breakup time 角膜前涙液層破壊時間
tear breakup time 涙液層破壊時間
but.
butyrum〈ラ〉=butter バター《処》
BuTX, BuTx
bungarotoxin ブンガロトキシン

B

BV	
balloon valvuloplasty	経皮的バルーンカテーテルによる狭窄弁開大術
bethamethasone 17-valerate cream	吉草酸ベタメタゾンクリーム
billion volts	10億ボルト
binocular vision	両眼視力
biologic(al) value	生物(学)的価値
blood vessel	血管
blood volume	血液量
blue violet	ブルーバイオレット
brevium〈ラ〉	簡略
bronchovesicular	気管支肺胞の
bV	
Smooth branching vessels	樹枝状血管
b.v.	
balneum vaporis〈ラ〉=vapor bath	蒸気浴
BVA	
binocular visual acuity	両眼視視力
British Veterinary Association	英国獣医学会
BVAD	
biventricular assist device	両心補助装置
BVAP	
bischloroethylnitrosourea, vincristine, adriamycin, prednisone	ビスクロロエチルニトロソウレア,ビンクリスチン,アドリアマイシン,プレドニゾン
BVCP	
bleomycin, vincristine, cyclophosphamide, prednisolone	ブレオマイシン,ビンクリスチン,シクロホスファミド,プレドニゾロン
BVD	
bischloroethylnitrosourea, vincristine, dacarbazine	ビスクロロエチルニトロソ尿素,ビンクリスチン,ダカルバジン
BVDU	
bromovinyldeoxy uridine	ブロモビニルデオキシウリジン
BVE	
binocular visual efficiency	両眼視能
blood vessel endothelium	血管内皮
blood volume expander	(循環)血(液)量増量薬
blood volume expansion	(循環)血(液)量増加
B.Vet.Med.	
Bachelor of Veterinary Medicine	獣医学士
B.Vet.Sci.	
Bachelor of Veterinary Science	獣医学士

B.Vet.Sur.
Bachelor of Veterinary Surgery　獣医外科学士
BVG
biventriculography　両心室図
BVH
biventricular hypertrophy　両心室肥大
BVI
blood vessel invasion　血管逆転症
B vit.compl
B vitamin complex　ビタミンB複合体
BVJ
British Veterinary Journal　英国獣医学雑誌
BVL
bilateral vas ligation　両側精管結紮(法)
BVM
Bachelor of Veterinary Medicine　獣医学士
broncho-vascular marking　気管支血管模様
BVMS
Bachelor of Veterinary Medicine and Surgery　獣医内科学・外科学士
BVO
branch vein occlusion　分枝血管閉塞
BVRV
both great vessels from right ventricule　両大血管右室起始症
BVS
Bachelor of Veterinary Science　獣医学士
Bachelor of Veterinary Surgery　獣医外科学士
B.V.Sc.
Bachelor of Veterinary Science　獣医学士
B.V.Sc. & AH
Bachelor of Veterinary Science and Animal Husbandry　獣医学・牧畜学士
BVU
bromvalerylurea　ブロムワレリル尿素
BVV
bovine vaginitis virus　ウシ腟炎ウイルス
BW
biological warfare　生物学的戦争
birth weight　出生時体重
blood Wassermann　血液ワッセルマン
body water　体水分
body weight　体重
Bordet-Wassermann　ボルデー・ワッセルマン反応
Brustwirbelsäule〈独〉＝Brustwirbel　胸椎

b & w
black and white 白黒
bread and water パンと水

BWA
Brustwandableeitung〈独〉 胸部誘導《心電》

BWD
bacillary white diarrhea 細菌性白色下痢

BWG syndrome
Bland-White-Garland syndrome ブランド・ホワイト・ガーランド症候群

BWS
battered woman syndrome 被虐待婦人症候群
Brustwirbelsäule〈独〉 胸椎

BWt
birth weight 出生時体重

BX
bacitracin X バシトラシンX

Bx
biopsy 生検

BXO
balanitis xerotica obliterans 閉塞性乾燥性亀頭炎

by
brilliant yellow ブリリアントイエロー

b-y
bloody 血液の

BYE
Barile-Yaguchi-Eveland バリール・矢口・エベランド

BZ
benzene ベンゼン(寒天培地)の
benzodiazepine ベンゾジアゼピン
Beobachtungszimmer〈独〉 試験室
Blutzucker 血糖

BZ，Bz
benzoyl ベンゾイル

BZD
benziodarone ベンジオダロン
benzodiazepine derivative ベンゾジアゼピン誘導体
benzothiazide ベンゾチアジド

BzH
benzaldehyde ベンズアルデヒド

BZL
benzol ベンゾール
brotizolam ブロチゾラム

Bzl
benzyl ベンジル

BzOH
benzoic acid　安息香酸

BZQ
benzquinamide　ベンズキアミド

BZS
Bor-Zink-Salbe〈独〉　ホウ酸亜鉛華軟膏

C c

C

calculus〈ラ〉	石，結石，胆石
calorie	カロリー，大カロリー
Calymmatobacterium	カリマトバクテリウム(属)
Candida	カンジダ(属)
canine	イヌの，犬歯の
canine tooth	(永久歯の)犬歯
carat	カラット〈単位〉
carbohydrate	炭水化物，糖質
carbon	炭素〈元素〉
cardiac	心臓性の
cardia of stomach	噴門部
caries dentium〈ラ〉	う歯
carrier	保菌者，保有者
cartilago	軟骨
cast	鋳造(物)，ギプス包帯，円柱
cathodal	陰極の
Catholic	カトリック(の)
Caucasian	白人
caudal	尾側の
caudate	尾形の
cecum	盲腸
Celsius	セ氏，摂氏
centigrade	セ氏，摂氏
cerebrospinal fluid	(脳脊)髄液
certified	証明された，認定された，保証された
cervical	頸(部)の
cervical nerve	頸神経
cervical spine	頸椎
cesarean section	帝王切開(術)
chest	胸(部)
Chlamydia	クラミジア(属)
chloramphenicol	クロラムフェニコール
cholesterol	コレステロール
Chromobacterium	クロモバクテリウム(属)
cicatrization	瘢痕形成
Citrobacter	シトロバクター(属)
Cladosporium	クラドスポリウム(属)
classical	古典的
clearance	クリアランス
clearance rate	クリアランス率
clonus	クローヌス

Clostridium	クロストリジウム(属)
closure	閉鎖
clubbing	(太鼓)ばち指形成
coarse	粗大な
cocaine	コカイン
Coccidioides	コクシジオイデス(属)
cochlea	蝸牛
coefficient of facility of aqueous outflow	房水流出係数
cognitive domain	認知領域
color	色
colored	色のついた，有色(人種)の
color sense	色覚
columnar epithelium	円柱上皮
complement	補体
complete	完全な
complex	複合体，コンプレックス
compliance	コンプライアンス
component	成分
component of complement	補体成分
compositus〈ラ〉=compound	化合物
concentration	濃度
concentration of gas in blood	血中ガスの濃度を示す記号
conditioning	条件付け
condyle	顆
confirmed	確認された
congius〈ラ〉=gallon	ガロン
constant	一定，定数
consultation	立ち会い診察，他科依頼
content	内容(物)
content of a gas in blood	血中ガス含量
contraction	収縮
contracture	拘縮
control	対照
convergence	輻輳，収縮
correct	訂正する，正しい
cortex	皮質
Corynebacterium	コリネバクテリム(属)
costa〈ラ〉=rib	肋骨
costal	肋骨の
coulomb	クーロン〈単位〉
Coxiella	コクシエラ(属)
coxsackie (virus)	コクサッキー(ウイルス)
Cryptococcus	クリプトコックス(属)
cube	立方
cubical	立方の

cubitus	肘
Culex	イエカ(属)
curability	根治度
cyanosis	チアノーゼ
cycle	サイクル，周期
cylinder	円柱
cylindrical	円柱(状)の
cylindrical lens	円柱レンズ
cylindric lens	円柱レンズ
cysteine	システイン
cystine	シスチン
cytidine	シチジン
cytochrome	チトクローム
cytosine	シトシン
facility of outflow	房水流出量
heat capacity	熱容量
upper third (cardia and fundus)	胃上部
upper third of the stomach	胃上部1/3区

c

calorie	カロリー，小カロリー
canine tooth	(乳歯の)犬歯
capillary	毛細血管
cardinal	基本の
case	症例
centi-	センチ(=10^{-2})〈接〉〈単位〉
chairman	座長
cold	寒い，冷たい
contuse	つき砕いた
course	経過
current	電流
c wave	c波
molar concentration	モル濃度
speed of light	光速

c.

cornu〈ラ〉=horn	角

3C

continuity, conprehensiveness, coordination	継続性・包容力・協調性
convenience, composition, competence	便利性・親切・信頼

Ⅷ：C

factor Ⅷ coagulant activity	第Ⅷ因子凝固活性

^{11}C

carbon-11	炭素11

^{12}C

carbon-12	炭素12

^{13}C
carbon-13 炭素13

^{14}C
carbon-14 炭素14

C1-7
cervical spine segments 頸椎の分節，第１頸椎～第７頸椎

C1〔-9〕
first(-ninth) component of complement 補体第１〔～９〕成分

C_5
pentamethonium bromide 臭化ペンタメトニウム

C_6
hexamethonium bromide 臭化ヘキサメトニウム

C10
decamethonium bromide 臭化デカメトニウム

$C_{14=0}$
myristic acid ミリスチン酸

$C_{16=0}$
palmitic acid パルミチン酸

$C_{16=1}$
palmitoleic acid パルミトオレイン酸

$C_{18=0}$
stearic acid ステアリン酸

$C_{18=1}$
oleic acid オレイン酸

$C_{18=2}$
linolic acid リノール酸

$C_{18=3}$
linolenic acid リノレン酸

$C_{20=3}$
homolinolenic acid ホモリノレン酸

$C_{20=4}$
arachidonic acid アラキドン酸

C♂
Caucasian male 白人男性

C♀
Caucasian female 白人女性

c′
pulmonary endcapillary 肺胞終末毛細管

C, c
candle 燭，ろうそく
central 中心部
circulation 循環
coefficient 係数，率
contact 接触・保菌容疑者

cubic	立方(体)の
cup	杯，吸角，コップ
curie	キュリー〈単位〉
cycle(s)	周波，サイクル

C, c.

centrum〈ラ〉=one hundred	百，100
cibus〈ラ〉=meal	食事
cyclic	周期(性)の

C, c, c.

capacity	容量，能力

$\overline{C}$, $\overline{C}$, c.

cum〈ラ〉=with	～を伴う

c, c.

cibus〈ラ〉	食事《処》
circa〈ラ〉=about	約《処》
concisus〈ラ〉	細切した《処》
conque〈ラ〉	煮沸せよ《処》
cum〈ラ〉	～とともに《処》

CA

anterior commissure	前交連
bromobenzyl cyanide	ブロムベンジルシアニド
calcium antagonist	カルシウム拮抗薬
Candida albicans	カンジダ菌
caproic acid	カプロン酸
carbohydrate antigen	炭水化物抗原
carbonic anhydrase	炭酸脱水酵素
cardiac arrest	心停止
cardiac arrhythmia	不整脈
carotid artery	頸動脈
carrageenin	カラゲニン
carrying angle	肘外反角度
catecholamine	カテコールアミン
celiac artery	腹腔動脈
cellulose acetate	酢酸セルロース，セルロースアセテート
cervicoaxial	頸軸面の
chemical abstracts	化学抽出物
chemotactic activity	趨化力，走化力
cholic acid	コール酸
chorea-acanthocytosis	舞踏病・有棘赤血球症
chorioadenoma destruens〈ラ〉	破壊性絨毛腺腫
chronological age	生活年齢
citric acid	クエン酸
clonogenic assay	クローン生存率
coefficient of absorption	吸収率，吸収係数
cold agglutination	寒冷凝集反応

cold agglutinin	寒冷凝集素
colloid antigen	コロイド抗原
common antigen	共通抗原
compensation act	代償作用
compressed air	圧縮空気
compression amplification	圧縮増幅
conceptual age	在胎年齢
condyloma acuminatum〈ラ〉	尖圭コンジローマ
coronary artery	冠(状)動脈
corpora allata〈ラ〉	アラタ体
corpora amylacea	アミロイド小体，デンプン様小体
corpus albicans	白体
corpus alienum	異物
cortisone acetate	酢酸コルチゾン
Coxsackie A	コクサッキーA
cyclosporin A	シクロスポリンA
cystic artery	胆嚢動脈
cytosine arabinoside	シトシンアラビノシド
cytotoxic antibody	細胞毒性抗体

Ca

calcium	カルシウム〈元素〉
carpal	手根(骨)の

ca

candle	燭，ろうそく
circa〈ラ〉=about	約

CA15-3

carbohydrate antigen 15-3	糖鎖抗原15-3

CA19-9

carbohydrate antigen 19-9	糖鎖抗原19-9
carcinoma 19-9	カルシノーマ19-9(膵癌腫瘍マーカー)

CA50

carbohydrate antigen 50	糖鎖抗原50
carcinoma 50	カルシノーマ50(膵癌・胆嚢癌腫瘍マーカー)

CA125

carbohydrate antigen 125	糖鎖抗原125
carcinoma 125	カルシノーマ125(卵巣癌腫瘍マーカー)

Ca^{2+}

calcium ion	カルシウムイオン

C3 A

C3 activator	C 3 活性化因子

C & A

clinitest and acetest	クリニテストとアセテスト

C

C

CA, Ca
cathodal 陰極の
cathode 陰極

CA, Ca, ca
cancer 癌
carcinoma 癌

CA, C/A
Caucasian adult 白人の成人

CAA
aplastic anemia 体質性の再生不良性貧血
carbon anhydrase activity 炭酸脱水酵素活性
cardiac allograft atherosclerosis 心臓同種移植片動脈硬化(症)
carotid audiofrequency analysis 頸動脈可聴周波数分析
cerebral amyloid angiopathy 脳アミロイド血管症
chloracetaldehyde クロロ酢酸アルデヒド
coloanal anastomosis 結腸肛門吻合(術)
computer-assisted assessment コンピュータ補助による評価
constitutional aplastic anemia 体質性の再生不良性貧血
coronary artery aneurysm 冠(状)動脈瘤
crystalline amino acids 結晶性アミノ酸

CAAA
Clean Air Act Amendments 空気清浄法改正条例

CAAS
Cardiovascular Angiography Analysis System 心血管造影分析システム

CAAT
computer-assisted axial tomography コンピュータ補助体軸断層撮影(法)

CAB
captive air bubble 捕獲空気泡
catheter-associated bacteriuria カテーテル関連細菌尿
cellulose acetate butyrate 酢酸酪酸セルロース
coronary artery bypass 冠(状)動脈バイパス

CABG
coronary artery bypass graft 冠(状)動脈バイパス術

CABGS
coronary artery bypass graft surgery 冠(状)動脈バイパス術

CaBI
calcium bone index カルシウム骨指数

CABOP, CA-BOP
cyclophosphamide, adriamycin, bleomycin, vincristine(=Oncovin), prednisone シクロホスファミド,アドリアマイシン,ブレオマイシン,ビンクリスチン(=オンコビン),プレドニゾン

CABP, CaBP
calcium-binding protein カルシウム結合蛋白

CABRI
Coronary Angioplasty versus Bypass Revascularization Investigation　カブリ(＝冠血管形成術とバイパス術の血管新生比較調査)

CABS
coronary artery bypass sugery　冠(状)動脈バイパス手術

CAC
cardiac accelerator center　心(臓)促進中枢
Codex Alimentarius Commission　委員会制定栄養規則

CACC, CaCC
cathodal closing〔closure〕 contraction　陰極閉鎖(時)収縮

$CaCl_2$
calcium chloride　塩化カルシウム

Ca_{CO2}
content of carbon dioxide in arterial blood　動脈血中炭酸ガス含量

CACS
celiac axis compression syndrome　腹腔動脈圧迫症候群

CaCTe
cathodal closure tetanus　陰極閉鎖強直

CACX, CaCx
cancer of the cervix　子宮頸管癌

CAD
chorioadenoma destruens　破壊性絨毛腺腫
chronic actinic dermatitis　慢性光線性皮膚炎
cold agglutinin disease　寒冷凝集素病
collision-activated dissociation　衝突活性化分離法
compressed air disease　潜水病
computer assisted diagnois　コンピュータ診断システム
congenital abduction deficiency　先天性外転欠損
congenital alveolar dysplasia　先天性肺胞異形成
coronary artery disease　冠(状)動脈疾患
cyclophosphamide, adriamycin, dacarbazine　シクロホスファミド,アドリアマイシン,ダカルバジン
cytosine arabinoside, daunorubicin　シトシンアラビノシド,ダウノルビシン

Cad
cadaverine　カダベリン
cadmium　カドミウム
caducity　老衰

CAD, Cad
cadaver(ic)　死体(の)

CADASIL
- Cerebral Autosomal Dominant Arteriopathy with Subcortical Infarcts and Leucoencephalopathy — カダシル，家族性脳血管痴呆症

CAD/CAM
- computer-aided design/computer-aided manufacturing — コンピュータ援用設計・コンピュータ援用製造
- computer-assisted design/controlled-alignment method — コンピュータ支援設計/アラインメント制御方法

CADD
- computerized ambulatory drug delivery (system) — コンピュータ内蔵携行型薬物投与用輸液ポンプ

CADD-PCA
- computerized ambulatory drug delivery-patient controlled analgesia (system) — コンピュータ内蔵携行型鎮痛自己調節投与用輸液ポンプ

CADI
- computer-assisted diabetic instruction (system) — コンピュータ補助糖尿病指導(システム)

CADIC
- cyclophosphamide, adriamycin, dacarbazine — シクロホスファミド,アドリアマイシン,ダカルバジン

CADL
- Communicative Abilities in Daily Living — 日常コミュニケーション能力《リハ》

CADLT
- Communicative Abilities in Daily Living Test — 日常コミュニケーション能力検査《リハ》

CADS
- computer applied demented scale — コンピュータ応用簡易知能スケール

CADs
- computer-assisted diagnostics — コンピュータ支援診断学

CADTe
- cathodal duration tetanus — 陰極継続痙攣

CAE
- *ceropithecces aethiops*〈ラ〉 — サバンナモンキー
- chloroacetate esterase — クロロ酢酸エステル分解酵素
- citric acid extract — クエン酸抽出物
- coronary artery embolization — 冠(状)動脈塞栓
- cyclophosphamide, adriamycin, etoposide — シクロホスファミド,アドリアマイシン,エトポシド

CaE
- calcium excretion — カルシウム排泄

CAEBV
chronic active EB virus infection　慢性活動性EBウイルス感染症

CA EDTA
calcium disodium ethylenediaminetetraacetate　エチレンジアミン四酢酸カルシウム二ナトリウム

CaEDTA, CaEdTA
calcium disodium edetate　エデト酸カルシウム二ナトリウム

CAEP
cellulose acetate electrophoresis　セルロースアセテート電気泳動法

caerul.
caeruleus〈ラ〉=sky blue　空色の，青色の

CAF
calcium-activated factor　カルシウム依存性プロテアーゼ，カルシウム賦活因子
Caucasian adult female　白人成人女性
cell adhesion factor　細胞粘着因子
cyclophosphamide, adriamycin, 5-fluorouracil　シクロホスファミド，アドリアマイシン，フルオロウラシル

caf
caffeine　カフェイン

CAFP
cyclophosphamide, adriamycin, 5-fluorouracil, prednisone　シクロホスファミド，アドリアマイシン，フルオロウラシル，プレドニゾン

CAFVP
cyclophosphamide, adriamycin, 5-fluorouracil, vincristine, prednisone　シクロホスファミド，アドリアマイシン，フルオロウラシル，ビンクリスチン，プレドニゾン

CAG
cardioangiography　心(臓)血管造影法
carotid angiography　頸動脈撮影法
carotid arteriography　頸動脈造影法
cerebral angiography　脳血管造影法
cholangiogram　胆道造影法
chronic atrophic gastritis　慢性萎縮性胃炎
coronary angiography　冠(状)動脈造影法

ⅧCAG
factor Ⅷ coagulant antigen　第Ⅷ因子凝固抗原

Ca gluc
calcium gluconate　グルコン酸カルシウム

C

CAH
central alveolar hypoventilation 中枢性肺胞低換気
central alveolar hypoventilation syndrome 中枢性肺胞低換気症候群
chronic active hepatitis 慢性活動性肝炎
congenital adrenal hyperplasia 先天性副腎過形成
congenital adrenocortical hyperplasia 先天性副腎皮質過形成
cyanoacetic acid hydrazide シアン酢酸ヒドラジド
cyanoacetohydrazide シアノアセトヒドラジド

CAHD
coronary atherosclerotic heart disease 冠(状)動脈性心(臓)疾患

CAHF
cellulose acetate hollow fiber 酢酸セルロース空洞線維

CAH-I
carbonic anhydrase inhibitor 炭酸脱水素酵素阻害剤

CAI
capsula intema〈ラ〉 (脳の)内包
carbonic anhydrase inhibitor 炭酸脱水酵素阻害剤
comprehensive asthma inventory 総合喘息性格テスト
computer-assisted instruction コンピュータ補助学習
confused artificial insemination 混合人工授精
coronary atherosclerosis index 冠(状)動脈硬化指数
cytology activity index 細胞診活動指数

$[Ca^{2+}]_i$
cytosolic free calcium concentration 細胞内遊離カルシウム濃度

CAIR
confidential anesthesia incident reporting 秘匿式麻酔安全報告

CAL
calcium test カルシウム試験
calibration 較正
Cell-Assisted Lipotransfer 細胞付加型脂肪移植
ceriocebus albigena〈ラ〉 ブラックモンガベイ
computer-aided learning コンピュータ補助学習
coracoacromial ligament 烏口肩峰靱帯

Cal
great calorie 大カロリー(＝kcal)〈単位〉
large (kirogram) calorie 大カロリー，キロカロリー(＝kcal)〈単位〉

cal
caliber 口径
calorie カロリー〈単位〉
gram calorie グラムカロリー
small calorie 小カロリー

Ca.lact.
calcium lactieum〈ラ〉 乳酸カルシウム《処》
CAlb, C alb, Calb, C.alb
albumin clearance アルブミンクリアランス
calc
calculate 計算する，推測する
calculation 計算，推測
calcd
calculated 計算した
calcif
calcification カルシウム沈着
Cal Ct, cal.ct
calorie count カロリー計算
CALD
chronic active liver disease 慢性活動性肝(臓)障害
calef.
calefac〈ラ〉=make warm 温めよ《処》
calefactus〈ラ〉=warmed 温めた《処》
CALL
commonacute lymphocytic leukemia 急性リンパ球性白血病
CALLA
common acute lymphocytic leukemia antigen 急性リンパ球性白血病共通抗原(=CD10)
caln
calculation 計算，推測
CAM
camputer-aided myelography コンピュータ補助ミエログラフィ
Caucasian adult male 白人成人男性
cell adhesion molecule 細胞接着分子
cellulose acetate membrane (immuno) electrophoresis セルロースアセテート膜(免疫)電気泳動法
clarithromycin クラリスロマイシン
cyclophosphamide, adriamycin, methotrexate シクロホスファミド，アドリアマイシン，メトトレキサート
CaM
calmodulin カルモジュリン
Cam
amylase clearance アミラーゼクリアランス
CAMA
Civil Aerospace Medical Association 市民航空医学協会
CAMAC
computer-automated measurement and control コンピュータ自動測定・管理

C

CAMB
cyclophosphamide, adriamycin, methotrexate, bleomycin — シクロホスファミド,アドリアマイシン,メトトレキサート,ブレオマイシン

Cam/Ccr
amylase creatinine clearance ratio — アミラーゼクレアチニンクリアランス比

CAMEO
cyclophosphamide, adriamycin, methotrexate, etoposide, vincristine (=Oncovin) — シクロホスファミド,アドリアマイシン,メトトレキサート,エトポシド,ビンクリスチン(=オンコビン)

CAMF
cyclophosphamide, adriamycin, methotrexate, 5-fluorouracil — シクロホスファミド,アドリアマイシン,メトトレキサート,フルオロウラシル

CAMM
Canadian Association of Medical Microbiologists — カナダ医学微生物学会

CAMP
cyclophosphamide, adriamycin, methotrexate, procarbazine — シクロホスファミド,アドリアマイシン,メトトレキサート,プロカルバジン

cAMP
cyclic AMP(=adenosine 3′,5′-monophosphate) — サイクリックAMP,サイクリック〔環状〕アデノシン3′,5′-リン酸

CAMPAS
computer-aided multivariate pattern analysis system — コンピュータ補助多変量解析システム

CAMS
computer-aided (assisted) monitoring system — コンピュータ補助モニターシステム

CAMSI
Canadian Association of Medical Students and Interns — カナダ医学生インターン連盟

CAMU
cardiac ambulatory monitoring unit — 心臓外来モニター部門
coronary arrhythmia monitoring unit — 不整脈モニター部門

CaMV
cauliflower mosaic virus — カリフラワーモザイクウイルス

CAN
Candida — カンジダ(属)
continuous albuterol nebulization — 連続的アルブテロール噴霧療法

cord (umbilical) around neck 頸部に巻きついた臍帯

Can
cancer 癌

CA/N
child abuse and neglect 小児虐待および放置

CANAG
chronic narrow angle glaucoma 慢性狭隅角緑内障

CANAP
cochlear nucleus action potential 蝸牛核活動電位

canc
cancel(ed) 取消
cancellation 解除

CANCIRCO
Cancer International Research Cooperative 国際癌研究協同体

CANDA
computer assisted new drug application submission コンピュータ補助による新薬申請

CANP
calcium activated neutral protease カルシウム依存性中性プロテアーゼ

CANS
central auditory nervous system 中枢聴神経系

CAO
chronic airway obstruction 慢性気道閉塞
chronic airway occlusion 慢性気道閉塞
chronic arterial obstruction 慢性動脈閉塞
chronic arterial occlusion 慢性動脈閉塞
coronary artery occlusion 冠(状)動脈閉塞(症)

CaO
calcium oxide 酸化カルシウム

Cao_2
arterial oxygen content 動脈血酸素含量

CaOC
cathodal opening contraction 陰極開放収縮

CAOD
coronary artery occlusive disease 冠(状)動脈閉塞性疾患

CAOM
chronic adhesive otitis media 慢性粘着性中耳炎

ca.ox.
calcium oxalate シュウ酸カルシウム

CAP
Canadian Association of Pathologists カナダ病理学者協会
capreomycin カプレオマイシン
captopril カプトプリル
carotid arterial pulse 頸動脈波

catabolite gene activator protein 異化遺伝子活性化蛋白
cell agar plate 細胞寒天平板
cellulose acetopropionate セルロースアセトプロピオン酸
central arterial pressure (網膜)中心動脈圧
chloramphenicol クロラムフェニコール
chloroacetophenone クロロアセトフェノン
chronic alcoholic pancreatitis 慢性アルコール性膵炎
ciliary artery pressure 毛様体動脈圧
College of American Pathologists 米国病理同学院
community acquired pneumonia 共同生活で感染する肺炎
compound action potential 複合活動電位
cyclic AMP-binding protein サイクリックAMP結合蛋白
cyclophosphamide, adriamycin, cisplatin (=Platinol) シクロホスファミド,アドリアマイシン,シスプラチン(=プラチノール)
cyclophosphamide, adriamycin, prednisone シクロホスファミド,アドリアマイシン,プレドニゾン
cystine aminopeptidase シスチンアミノペプチダーゼ

Cap
capillary 毛細管
carcinoma of the prostate 前立腺癌

cap
capacity 容量，能力
caput (=head) 頭，冠，筋頭

'cap
handicapped 身体障害のある

CAP, cap, cap.
capiat〈ラ〉=let the patient take 患者に服用させよ《処》
capitatur〈ラ〉=capiat 取らせよ,服用させよ《処》

cap, cap.
capsula〈ラ〉=capsule 被膜，包，カプセル(剤)《処》

CAPA
cancer-associated polypeptide antigen 癌関連ポリペプチド抗原

cap.amyl.
capsula amylacea〈ラ〉 オブラート嚢

CAP-BOP
cyclophosphamide, adriamycin, procarbazine, bleomycin, vincristine (=Oncovin), prednisone シクロホスファミド,アドリアマイシン,プロカルバジン,ブレオマイシン,ビンクリスチン(=オンコビン),プレドニゾン

cap.chart.
capsula chartacea〈ラ〉 分包散剤《処》

CAPD
chronic ambulatory dialysis　長期外来透析
continuous ambulatory peritoneal dialysis　持続的携帯型腹膜透析
CAPE
Circadian Anti-ischemic Program in Europe　ケープ試験
cap gel.
capsula gelatinosa〈ラ〉　膠嚢《処》
cap gel el.
capsula gelatinosa elastica〈ラ〉　軟膠嚢《処》
cap gel op.
capsula gelatinosa operculate〈ラ〉　蓋付膠嚢《処》
capiend.
capiendus〈ラ〉=to be taken　服用する
cap.moll.
capsula mollis〈ラ〉=soft capsule　軟カプセル《処》
CAPP
clinical appraisal of psychosocail problem　精神社会的問題の臨床鑑定
cap quant.
capiat quantum vult〈ラ〉　欲するだけ服用せしめよ《処》
CAPS
cyclohexylaminopropanesulfonic acid　シクロヘキシルアミノプロパンスルホン酸
caps.
capsula〈ラ〉=capsule　被膜，包，カプセル(剤)《処》
capsul.
capsula〈ラ〉=capsule　被膜，包，カプセル(剤)《処》
caput med
caput medusae　メドゥサ(の)頭
CAR
Canadian Association of Radiologists　カナダ放射線医学会
chronic articular rheumatism　慢性関節リウマチ
conditioned avoidance response　条件回避反応
Car
carotid pulse wave　頸動脈波
car
carotid　頸動脈の
carb
carbonaceous　炭素質の
carbonic　炭酸の
CARB, carb
carbohydrate　炭水化物，糖質
carb, carb.
carbonate　炭酸塩

C

C

carbas.
carbasus〈ラ〉 ガーゼ
carbo
carbohydrate 炭水化物，糖質
carboloy
carbon-cobalt-tungsten alloy 炭素・コバルト・タングステン合金
carbon tet
carbon tetrachloride 四塩化炭素
card
cardiac 心臓(病)(性)の
CARD, card
cardiology 心臓(病)学
card amp
cardiovascular data analysis by machine processing 機械操作による心(蔵)血管データ分析
card.insuff
cardiac insufficiency 心不全
cardio
cardiology 心臓(病)学
cardiol
cardiologist 心臓病専門医
Cardiol, cardiol
cardiology 心臓(病)学
cardio-resp
cardiorespiratory 心(臓)呼吸(器)の
cardiov
cardiovascular 心(臓)血管の
CARDOOL
cardiology 心臓(病)学
CARES-SF
cancer rehabilitation evaluation system-short form 癌治療におけるQOL診断法
Carot
carotid pulse wave 頸動脈波
CARS
Canadian Arthritis and Rheumatism Society カナダ関節炎リウマチ学会
childhood autism rating scale 小児期自閉症評価点スケール〔尺度〕
cart
cartilage 軟骨
CAS
calcarine sulcus 鳥距溝
cardiac surgery 心臓外科
Carotid Artery Stenting 頸動脈ステント留置術

central anticholinergic syndrome	中枢性抗コリン症候群
cerebral arteriosclerosis	脳動脈硬化(症)
Chemical Abstract Service	化学抄録サービス
cold-agglutination syndrome	寒冷凝集素症候群
coloboma of iris-anal atresia syndrome	虹彩部分欠損・鎖肛症候群
Con A supernatant	コンカナバリンA加培養細胞の上清
coronary artery spasm	冠(状)動脈攣縮
crystalline ammonium sulfate	硫酸アンモニウム結晶

Cas

casualty	死傷(者)

CASA

cancer-associated serum antigen	癌関連血清抗原
computer-aided〔assisted〕 self assessment	コンピュータ補助自己評価

CASE

computer-assisted sensory examination	コンピュータ補助知覚検査

CASH

Cardiac Arrest Study Hamburg	ハンブルグ抗不整脈薬大規模試験
corticoadrenal-stimulating hormone	副腎髄質刺激ホルモン

CASHD

coronary arteriosclerotic heart disease	冠(状)動脈硬化性心疾患

CASMD

congenital atonic sclerotic muscular dystrophy	先天性無力性硬化性筋ジストロフィ

CASS

computer-assisted (simulation) surgery	コンピュータ補助によるシミュレーション外科
coronary artery surgery study	冠(状)動脈外科研究

CASSI

Chemical Abstracts Service Source Index	化学抄録サービス源索引

CAST

Canterbury Alcoholism Screening Test	カンタベリーアルコール中毒スクリーニング検査
Children of Alcoholism Screening Test	アルコール中毒児スクリーニング検査
The Cardiac Arrhythmia Suppression Trial	カスト，心臓性不整脈抑制治験

CAT

carnitine acyltransferase	カルニチンアシル転移酵素
catalase	カタラーゼ

catecholamines	カテコールアミン
cellular atypism	細胞異型度
children's appreciation test	児童絵画統覚検査
chloramphenicol acetyltransferase	クロラムフェニコールアセチル転移酵素
choline acetyltransferase	コリンアセチル基転移酵素
choline acetyltransferase test	コリンアセチル基転移酵素試験
college ability test	特殊専門能力テスト
combined approach tympanoplasty	外耳道保存鼓室形成手術
computed abdominal tomography	コンピュータ腹部断層撮影
computer-assisted tomography	コンピュータ(補助)断層撮影
computerized axial tomography	コンピュータ軸位断層法
computer of averaging transient	平均経過コンピュータ
cytarabin, adriamycin, thioguanine	シタラビン,アドリアマイシン,チオグアニン

C-A-T

collage ability test	特殊専門能力テスト

CAT, Cat, cat.

cataracta〈ラ〉=cataract	白内障

cat, cat.

catalyst	触媒
cataplasm	罨法
cataplasma〈ラ〉=a poultice	パップ(剤), 湿布《処》

CATase

chloramphenicol acetyltransferase	クロラムフェニコールアセチル転移酵素

CAT-CAM

controlled adducted trochanteric controlled alignment method	坐骨収納型大腿義足

cath

catheterize urine	カテーテル尿

CATH, Cath, Cath., cath.

catharticus〈ラ〉=cathartic	下剤, 瀉下(性)の

Cath, Cath.

catheterization	カテーテル法
cathode	陰極
Catholic	カトリック(の)

Cath., cath.

catheter	カテーテル
catheterize	カテーテルを挿入する

cathar

cathartic	下剤, 瀉下性の

CAT-MET

catecholamine and metabolites	カテコールアミンと代謝産物

CaTT
calcium tolerance test — カルシウム負荷試験

CATV
cable television — 有線テレビジョン

Cau
Caucasian — 白人

Cauc
Caucasian — 白人

Caud
caudal — 尾(側)の，尾部の

caut
cauterization — 焼灼術，焼灼法
cauterize — 焼灼する
cautiously — 注意深く，用心して

CAV
congenital absence of vagina — 先天性膣欠損
congenital adrenal virilism — 先天性副腎性男性化
croup-associated virus — クループ関連ウイルス
cyclophosphamide, adriamycin, vincristine — シクロホスファミド，アドリアマイシン，ビンクリスチン

cav
cavity — 窩，空洞，腔

CAVB
complete atrio-ventricular block — 完全房室ブロック

CAVC
common atrioventricular canal — 共通房室管孔

CAVe
cyclohexylchloroethylnitrosourea, adriamycin, vinblastine — シクロヘキシルクロロエチルニトロソ尿素，アドリアマイシン，ビンブラスチン

CAVF
completion, arithmetic problems, vocabulary, following directions — 完了・計算問題・語彙・追跡

CAVH
chronic activated virus hepatitis — 慢性活動性ウイルス肝炎
continuous arteriovenous hemofiltration — 持続動静脈血液濾過

CAVI
cardio ankle vascular index — 心臓足首血管指数

CAVHD
continuous arteriovenous hemodialysis — 持続動静脈血液透析

CAVHDF
continuous arteriovenous hemodiafiltration — 持続動静脈血液透析濾過

C

CAVP
cyclophosphamide, adriamycin, vincristine, prednisone — シクロホスファミド,アドリアマイシン,ビンクリスチン,プレドニゾン

CAV-P-VP
cyclophosphamide, adriamycin, vincristine, cisplatin(=Platinol), VP16-213(=etposide) — シクロホスファミド,アドリアマイシン,ビンクリスチン,シスプラチン(=プラチノール),エトポシド

Caw
airway conductance — 気道コンダクタンス

CAZ
ceftazidime — セフタジジム

CB
calcium blocker — カルシウム遮断薬
carbenicillin — カルベニシリン
carbonate bicarbonate buffer — 炭酸・重炭酸緩衝液
carbonated beverage — 炭酸飲料
carotid body — 頸動脈小体
catheterized bladder — カテーテル挿入状態の膀胱
ceased breathing — 呼吸停止
cell bank — 細胞バンク
cesarean birth — 帝王切開出産
chair and bed — 椅子とベッド
chemical and biological — 化学・生物学の
Chirurgiae Baccalaureus〈ラ〉 — 外科学士
chocolate blood (agar) — チョコレート血液(寒天培地)
chronic bronchiolitis — 慢性(細)気管支炎
chronic bronchitis — 慢性気管支炎
ciliary body — 毛様体
circumflex branch — 回旋枝
color blind — 色盲の
compensated base — 代償塩基
conjugated bilirubin — 結合〔抱合〕型ビリルビン
contrast bath — 対比浴, 交代浴
contrast baths — (冷温)交互〔交代〕浴
coracobrachial — 烏口上腕の
cord blood — 臍帯血
critical band — 臨界帯
cytochalasin B — サイトカラシンB

Cb
columbium — コロンビウム(=ニオブ)〈元素〉

CB-154
2-bromo-α-ergocryptin=bromocryptine — ブロモクリプチン

CBA
carcinoma-bearing animal 担癌動物
chemical biological activity 化学・生物学活性度
chronic bronchitis with asthma 喘息を伴う慢性気管支炎
competitive-binding assay 競合結合定量(法)
competitive (neuromuscular junction) blocking agent 非脱分極性筋弛緩薬
congenital biliary atresia 先天性胆道閉鎖症
cost-benefit analysis 費用対利益分析
cytochemical bioassay 細胞化学的生物検定法

CBAB
complement-binding antibody 補体結合抗体

CB agar
chocolate blood agar チョコレート血液寒天培地

CBAICP
Chemical and Biological Accident and Incident Control Plan 化学・生物学事故防止計画

CBB
carbonate bicarbonate buffer 炭酸・重炭酸緩衝液
communications in behavioral biology 行動生物学における伝達
Coomassie brilliant blue クマシーブリリアントブルー

CBC
child behavior characteristics 小児気質性格
combined blood count 複合血球計測
complete blood cell count 全血球計算

CBCN
carbenicillin カルベニシリン

CBD
carotid body denervation 頸動脈体神経遮断
closed bladder drainage 閉鎖導尿
common bile duct 総胆管
congenital biliary (duct) dilatation 先天性胆道拡張症
congenital biliary dyskinesia 先天性胆道運動障害

CBDC
chronic bullous disease of childhood 小児慢性水疱症

CBDCA
cis-diamine-1,1-cyclobutane dicarbosylate platinum シスジアミン-1,1-シクロブタンジカルボシレイトプラチナム

CBE
cardiogenic brain embolism 心原性脳塞栓症
chemical binding effect 化学結合効果
computer-based education コンピュータ支援教育

CBED
convergent beam electron diffraction 収束電子線回折法

CBER
Center of Biologic(al) Evaluation and Research — (FDAの)生物製剤評価・研究センター

CBF
cancer breaking factor — 腫瘍細胞破壊因子
capillary blood flow — 毛細(血)管血流
carcino-breaking factor — 癌破壊因子
cerebral blood flow — 脳血流量
Children's Blood Foundation — 小児血液財団
ciliary beat frequency — 線毛運動周波数
coronary blood flow — 冠血流(量)
cortical blood flow — (腎)皮質血流(量)
cutaneous blood flow — 皮膚血流(量)

CBFP
chronic biological false-positive — 慢性生物学的擬陽性の

CBG
capillary blood gas — 毛細血管内血液ガス
coronary bypass grafting — 冠(状)動脈バイパス移植(術)
corticosteroid-binding globulin — コルチコステロイド結合グロブリン
cortisol-binding globulin — コルチゾール結合グロブリン

CBH
chronic benign hepatitis — 慢性良性肝炎
cutaneous basophilic hypersensitivity — 皮膚塩基性過敏症

CBHDP
Community Based Health Developement Program — 地域共同体を基にした健康開発計画

C bile
hepatic bile — 肝内胆汁

CBL
capillary basement lamina — 毛細血管基底板
circulating blood lymphocyte — 循環血中リンパ球
cord blood lymphocyte — 臍帯血リンパ球

Cbl
cobalamin — コバラミン

CBM
capillary basement membrane — 毛細血管基底膜
chromoblastomycosis — 黒色分芽菌症

Cbm
carbamoyl — カルバモイル

CBMC
cord blood mononuclear cell(s) — 臍帯血単核細胞

CBN
chemical, bacterial, nuclear — 化学・細菌・核の
chronic benign neutropenia of childhood — 小児期慢性良性好中球減少症

CBO
cells-bound organisms　菌が付着・侵入している細胞
CBOC
completion of bed occupancy　病床看護終了
CBP
calcium binding protein　カルシウム結合蛋白(質)
cap-binding protein　キャップ結合蛋白質
carbohydrate-binding protein　炭水化物結合蛋白(質)
carotid body paraganglioma　頸動脈球傍神経節腫
chromatin binding protein　クロマチン結合蛋白(質)
cobalamin binding protein　コバラミン結合蛋白(質)
continuous blood purification　持続的血液浄化療法
corticosteroid-binding protein　コルチコステロイド結合蛋白(質)
C4-bp
C4-binding protein　C 4 結合蛋白(質)
CBPC
carboxybenzylpenicillin＝carbenicillin　カルボキシベンジルペニシリン＝カルベニシリン
CBPP
contagious bovine pleuropneumonia　ウシ肺疫
CBPPA
cyclophosphamide, bleomycin, procarbazine, prednisone, adriamycin　シクロホスファミド, ブレオマイシン, プロカルバジン, プレドニゾン, アドリアマイシン
CBPZ
cefbuperazone　セフブペラゾン
CBR
chemical, bacterial, radiological　化学・細菌・放射能の
chemical-biological-radiological　化学的生物学的放射線医学的
chronic bedrest　慢性的就床安静
complement binding reaction　補体結合反応
complete bedrest　絶対的就床安静
CBRA
chemical, bacterial, radiological agency　化学・細菌・放射能機関
CBRE
chemical, bacterial, radiological element　化学・細菌・放射能要素
CBRL
chemical, bacterial, radiological laboratories　化学・細菌・放射能研究室
CBRN
chemical, bacterial, radiological and nuclear　化学・細菌・放射能・核の

C

chemical,biological,radiological and nuclear　化学・生物・放射性物質・核

CBS
chronic bed rest　長期就床安静
chronic brain syndrome　慢性脳症候群
conjugated bile salts　抱合胆汁塩

CBSP
clearance (of) bromsulfophthalein　ブロムスルホフタレインクリアランス

CBT
cognitive behavior therapy　認識行動療法
computer based testing Web　コンピュータ利用学習支援システム

CBV
capillary blood (flow) velocity　毛細血管血流速度
catheter baloon valvuloplasty for mitral valve　バルーンカテーテル僧帽弁開大術
central blood volume　中心血液量
cerebral blood volume　脳血液量
circulating blood volume　循環血液量
collected blood volume　集積血液量
corrected blood volume　補正血液量
coxsackie B virus　コクサッキーBウイルス
cyclophosphamide, bischloroethylnitrosourea, VP16-213(=etposide)　シクロホスファミド，ビスクロロエチルニトロソ尿素，エトポシド

CBW
chemical and biological warfare　化学・生物兵器戦

CBZ
carbamazepine　カルバマゼピン
carbamazole　カルバマゾール

Cbz
carbobenzoxy (chloride)　(塩化)カルボベンゾキシ

CC
calcium cyclamate　シクラミン酸カルシウム
carcinoma colli　子宮頸癌
cardiac catheterization　心(臓)カテーテル法
cardiac cycle　心(臓)周期
carotid cavernous (fistula)　頸動脈海綿静脈洞(瘻)
case conference　ケースカンファレンス
Caucasian child　白人小児
cell culture　細胞培養
cerebral commisure　脳交連
cerebral cortex　脳皮質
Cestan-Chenais (syndrome)　セスタン・シュネ(症候群)
chemotherapeutic coefficient　化学療法係数〔指数〕

chest circumference 胸囲
chief complaint 主訴
cholecalciferol コレカルシフェロール
chondrocalcinosis 軟骨石灰化(症)
choriocarcinoma 絨毛癌
ciliated cell 線毛細胞
circulation 循環
circulatory collapse 循環虚脱
citrate cycle クエン酸回路
classical conditioning 古典的条件づけ
clindamycin クリンダマイシン
clinical clerk 病棟事務
clinical conference 症例〔臨症〕検討会
clinical course 臨床過程
Cochrane Collaboration コクラン共同計画
coefficient of correlation 相関係数
colony count コロニー数
colorectal cancer 結腸直腸癌
column chromatography カラムクロマトグラフィ
common cold 感冒
computer calculated コンピュータで計算された
congenital cardiopathy 先天性心疾患
consumption coagulopathy 消費性凝固障害
continuous current 平流・直流
contractile component 収縮要素
cord compression 脊髄圧迫
corpora cardiaca〈ラ〉 強心剤
corpus callosum 脳梁
costochondral 肋軟骨の
counter coup 反対側衝撃
cranio caudal 頭尾方向《画診》
creatinine clearance クレアチニンクリアランス
critical care 危急状態管理
critical condition 危急状態
crus cerebri 大脳脚
current complaint 現在の愁訴

Cc

cartilagines 軟骨

cc

cell count 細胞数

CC, Cc

concave 凹面の，凹形の

cc, c.c.

cubic centimeter 立方センチメートル
cum correctione〈ラ〉=with correction 矯正で

C

CCA
cebus capucinus〈ラ〉 ノドジロオマキザル
chick cell agglutination dosis ヒヨコ細胞凝集量
chimpanzee coryza agent チンパンジー(の)鼻かぜウイルス
chondrocalcinose articulaire〈仏〉 関節軟骨石灰症
choriocarcinoma 絨毛癌
circumflex coronary artery 冠(状)動脈回旋枝
common carotid artery 総頸動脈
complement cold activation 補体寒冷活性化現象
conjunctivitis catarrhalis acuta〈ラ〉 急性カタル性結膜炎

C-C-A
cytidiyl-cytidyl-adenyl シチジル・シチジル・アデニル

Cca/Ccr
calcium clearance/creatinine clearance カルシウムクリアランス/クレアチニンクリアランス(比)

CCAG
chronic closed angle glaucoma 慢性閉塞隅角緑内障

CCAM
congenital cystic adenomatoid 先天性嚢胞性腺腫様奇形

CCAT
conglutination on complement absorption test 膠着補体結合反応

CCA unit
chick cell-agglutination unit 幼若細胞凝集反応単位

CCB
calcium channel blocker カルシウム拮抗剤

CCBC
Council of Community Blood Center 共同血液センター審議会

CCBV
central circulating blood volume 中心循環血液量

CCC
cathodal closure contraction 陰極閉鎖収縮
cholangio cell carcinoma 胆管細胞癌
cholangiocelluar carcinoma 胆管細胞癌
chronic complicated cystitis 慢性複雑膀胱炎
citrated calcium carbamide クエン酸カルシウム尿素
congenital cutaneous candidiasis 先天性皮膚カンジダ症
conjunctivitis catarrhalis chronica 慢性カタル性結膜炎
countercurrent chromatography 向流クロマトグラフィ

CCCl
cathodal closure clonus 陰極閉鎖間代収縮

CCCP
carbonylcyanide-*m*-chlorophenylhydrazone　カルボニルシアニド-*m*-クロロフェニルヒドラゾン

CCCR
closed chest cardiac resuscitation　閉胸式心蘇生

CCCU
comprehensive cardiovascular care unit　全心血管管理部(室)

CCD
central core disease　中心核病
charge coupled device　電荷結合素子
color-vision deficiency　色覚異常
compact couple device　小型個体撮像素子
congenital chloride diarrhea　先天性クロール下痢症
cortical collecting duct　皮質部集合尿細管
counter current distribution　対向流分配

CCDN
Central Council for District Nursing　地域看護のための中央審議会

CCE
carbon-chloroform extract　炭酸クロロフォルム抽出物
ceratoconjunctivitis epidemica　流行性角結膜炎
clear cell carcinoma　澄明細胞癌
clubbing, cyanosis and edema　バチ状指・チアノーゼ・浮腫
counterflow centrifugal elutriation　カウンターフロー遠心分離

CCF
cancer coagulative factor　癌凝固性因子
cardiolipin complement fixation　カルジオリ〔ライ〕ピン補体結合
carotid cavernous fistula　頸動脈海綿静脈洞瘻
cephalin cholesterol flocculation (test)　セファリンコレステロール絮状〔綿状〕反応
chronic cardiac failure　慢性心不全
Common Cold Foundation　流行性感冒財団
compound comminuted fracture　複合粉砕骨折
congenital club foot　先天性内反足
congestive cardiac failure　うっ血性心不全
neutrophil-derived crystal-induced chemotactic factor　好中球由来結晶誘発走化性因子

CCFA
cycloserine-cefoxitin-fructose agar　シクロセリン・セホキシチン・果糖寒天培地

CCFE
cyclophosphamide, cisplatin, 5-fluorouracil, estramustine　シクロホスファミド, シスプラチン, フルオロウラシル, エストラムスチン

CCF test
cephalin-cholesterol flocculation test　セファリンコレステロール絮状〔綿状〕試験

CCG
cholecystogram　胆嚢造影図

CCGG
cytosine-cytosine-guanine-guanine　シトシン・シトシン・グアニン・グアニン

CCH
C-cell hyperplasia　C細胞過形成
chronic cholestatic hepatitis　慢性胆汁性肝炎

CCHD
cyanotic congenital heart disease　チアノーゼ性先天性心疾患

CCHF
Crimean-Congo hemorrhagic fever　クリミア・コンゴ出血熱

CCHS
congenital central hyperventilation syndrome　先天性中枢性過呼吸症候群

CCI
chronic coronary insufficiency　慢性冠(状動脈)不全
circuit condition inhibitor　回路条件抑制因子

CCK
cholecystokinin　コレシストキニン

CCKLI
cholecystokinin-like immunoreactivity　コレシストキニン様免疫反応性

CCK-OP
cholecystokinin octopeptide　コレシストキニン・オクトペプチド

CCK-PZ
cholecystokinin-pancreozymin　コレシストキニン・パンクレオザイミン

CCL
cefaclor　セファクロル
coracoclavicular ligament　烏口鎖骨靱帯

CCLE
chronic cutaneous lupus erythematosus　慢性皮膚エリテマトーデス

CCLF
cephalin cholesterol lecithin flocculation (test)　セファリンコレテロールレシチン絮〔綿〕状反応

CCM
cell culture medium　細胞培養培地
closed chest cardiac massage　非開胸(式)心(臓)マッサージ
congestive cardiomyopathy　うっ血型心筋症
critical care medicine　重症〔危急〕管理医学

cyclophosphamide, cyclohexylchloroethylnitrosourea, methotrexate — シクロホスファミド,シクロヘキシルクロロエチルニトロソ尿素,メトトレキサート

c.cm.
cubic centimeter — 立方センチメートル

CCMSU
clean catch midstream urine — 非汚染〔無菌的〕中間尿採取

CCMT
catechol methyltransferase — カテコールメチルトランスフェラーゼ

CCMU
critical care medicine unit — 重症〔危急〕患者管理部門

CCMV
cowpea chlorotic mottle virus — ササゲマメ萎黄病斑状ウイルス

CCN
coronary care nurse — 冠(状動脈)疾患〔不全〕看護
coronary care nursing — 冠不全〔疾患〕看護
critical care nursing — 重症〔危急〕患者看護

CCNS
cell cycle nonspecific agents — (抗癌剤の)細胞周期非特異性薬剤

CCNSC
Cancer Chemotherapy National Service Center — 国立癌化学療法サービスセンター

CCNU
chloroethyl-cyclohexyl nitrosourea — クロロエチル・シクロヘキシル・ニトロソウレア
lomustine — ロムスチン

C_{CO}
diffusing capacity for carbon monoxide — CO拡散能

CCO_2
carbon oxide content — 炭酸ガス含有量

CCOP
cyclohexylchloroethylnitrosourea, vincristine (=Oncovin), prednisone — シクロヘキシルクロロエチルニトロソ尿素,ビンクリスチン(=オンコビン),プレドニゾン

CCP
carboxyl carrier protein — カルボキシル運搬蛋白質
children's cognition of parents — 小児の両親認識
chronic calcifying pancreatitis — 慢性石灰化膵炎
chronic complicated pyelonephritis — 慢性複雑腎盂腎炎
classical complement pathway — 古典的補体反応経路

critical closing pressure 臨界閉鎖圧

CCPD

continuous circulatory peritoneal dialysis 持続的周期腹膜透析

continuous cyclic peritoneal dialysis 連続循環型腹膜透析

CCPR

cardio-cerebral pulmonary resuscitation 心肺脳蘇生法

cerebrocardiopulmonary resuscitation 心肺脳蘇生法

cerebro-cardio-pulmonary resuscitation 中枢神経心肺蘇生術，脳心肺蘇生術

CCP-SF

complement control protein superfamily 補体制御蛋白遺伝子家系

CCR

calculated constriction rate 計算収縮値

complex chemical reaction 複合化学反応

Ccr

creatinine clearance クレアチニンクリアランス

CCRS

carotid chemoreceptor stimulation 頸動脈化学受容体刺激

CCRU

Common Cold Research Unit 感冒研究組織

critical care recovery unit 集中治療回復室

CCS

Calorie Control System 熱量管理システム

case control study 症例対照研究

casualty clearing station 死傷者処理所

cell cycle specific agents 細胞回転周期特異性薬剤

cloudy cornea syndrome 混濁角膜症候群

colon clean solution 経口腸管洗浄液

contact compound scan 接触複合走査

CCSG

Children's Cancer Study Group 小児癌研究グループ

CCSI

company core safety information 企業内中核安全性情報

CCSK

clear cell sarcoma of kidney 腎澄明細胞肉腫

CCT

central condition time 中枢伝導時間

chocolate-coated tablet チョコレート被覆錠

coated compressed tablet 被覆加工圧縮錠剤

cortical collecting tubule (腎)皮質集合尿細管

cranial computed tomography 頭蓋CT検査

cyclocarbo-thiamine シクロカーボ・チアミン

cycotiamine シコチアミン

cct
circuit　回路
C & CT
chemistry and chemical technology　化学と化学技術
CCTM
color, circulation, temperature and movement　色調・循環・体温・動き
CCTP
coronary care training program　冠(状動脈)疾患管理における回復訓練プログラム
CCTV
closed circuit television　閉鎖回路テレビ
CCU
cardiac care unit　心(臓)疾患管理室
cardiovascular care unit　心血管疾患管理室
chronic complicated urinary tract infection　慢性複雑性尿路感染症
coronary care unit　冠(状動脈)疾患集中治療室
critical care unit　重症治療室
CCU psychosis
coronary care unit psychosis　CCU精神病
CCU syndrome
coronary care unit syndrome　CCU症候群
CCV
closed circuit voltage　閉回路電圧
cyclohexylchloroethylnitrosourea, cyclophosphamide, vincristine　シクロヘキシルクロロエチルニトロソ尿素,シクロホスファミド,ビンクリスチン
CCVB
cyclohexylchloroethylnitrosourea, cyclophosphamide, vincristine, bleomycin　シクロヘキシルクロロエチルニトロソウレア,シクロホスファミド,ビンクリスチン,ブレオマイシン
CCVD
chronic cerebrovascular disease　慢性脳血管疾患
CC-Virus
common cold virus　かぜウイルス，感冒ウイルス
CCVPP
cyclohexylchloroethylnitrosourea, cyclophosphamide, vincristine, procarbazine, prednisone　シクロヘキシルクロロエチルニトロソウレア,シクロホスファミド,ビンクリスチン,プロカルバジン,プレドニゾン
CCW
counterclockwise　反時計方向

C

Ccw
chest wall compliance 胸壁コンプライアンス
CCXD
computer-controlled X-ray diffractometer コンピュータ制御X線回折器
CD
cadaver donor 死体提供者
canine distemper イヌ(の)ジステンパー
carbon dioxide 二酸化炭素
cardiac disease 心(臓)疾患
cardiac dullness 心濁音界
cardiac dysrhythmia 心臓性不調律
cardiovascular disease 心血管疾患
celiac disease 小児脂肪便症
cesarean delivery 帝王切開分娩
character disoder 性格異常，性格疾患
childhood disease 小児期疾患
chorioadenoma destruens〈ラ〉 破壊性絨毛腺腫
circular dichroism 円二色性
cluster of differentiation CD分類
coefficient of digestion 消化吸収率
colidyspepsie〈ラ〉 大腸性消化不良
collagen disease 膠原病
compact disk コンパクトディスク《コン》
conjugata diagonalis〈ラ〉 骨盤入口の対角線結合径
conjugate diameter 骨盤内径
contact dermatitis 接触性皮膚炎
contagious disease 接触感染症，接触伝染病
conventional dialysis 透析従来法
convulsive disoder 痙攣性疾患
convulsive dose 痙攣を引き起こす薬量
corneal dystrophy 角膜異栄養(症)，角膜ジストロフィ
Crohn disease クローン病
curative dose 治癒(線)量
cutdown 静脈切開(術)
Cd
cadmium カドミウム〈元素〉
cord 索，帯
diodrast clearance ダイオドラスト・クリアランス
radioactive cadmium 放射性カドミウム
cd
candela カンデラ〈単位〉
carcinoid tumor カルチノイド腫瘍

CD50
half〔median〕 curative dose　治効中間投与量，50%有効量
C/D
cup/disc (ratio)　視神経乳頭陥凹比
c/d
cigarettes per day　紙巻タバコ喫煙本数/日
cigars per day　葉巻タバコ喫煙本数/日
C & D
chemist and druggist　化学者と薬学者
cytoscopy and dila(ta)tion　膀胱鏡兼拡張術
CD，Cd，cd
caudal　尾の，尾側の，尾部の
CD，C.D.
communicable disease　伝染病
CDA
Canadian Dental Association　カナダ歯科学会
cell-dependent antibody　細胞依存性抗体
cellulose diacetate　酢酸セルロース
cerebral dissecting aneurysm　解離性脳動脈瘤
chiral derivatizing agents　キラル誘導化試薬
complement-dependent antibody　補体依存抗体
congenital dyserythropoietic anemia　先天性異常造血性貧血
CDAA
chloro-diallylacetamide　クロロジアリルアセトアミド
CDAD
clostridium difficile-associated diarrhea　面倒なクロストリジウム関連の下痢
CDAI
Crohn disease activity index　クローン病の活性指標
CDAMC
complement-dependent antibody-mediated cytotoxicity　補体依存(性)抗体媒介細胞傷害
CDC
Cadaver Disposal Center　死体処理センター
calculated date of confinement　分娩予定日
cancer detection center　米国癌検知センター
capillary diffuse capacity　毛細管拡散能
carboplatin, doxorubicin, cyclophosphamide　カルボプラチン,ドキソルビシン,シクロホスファミド
cell division cycle　細胞分裂周期
Centers for Disease Control and Prevention　米国疾病管理予防センター
chenodeoxycholic acid　ケノデオキシコール酸
Communicable Disease Center　米国伝染病センター
complement-dependent cytotoxicity　補体依存(性)細胞傷害性

C

CDCA
chenodeoxycholic acid ケノデオキシコール酸
CDCC
complement-dependent cellular cytotoxicity 補体依存(性)細胞傷害性
CD-choline
cytidine diphosphate choline シチジン二リン酸コリン
CDCM
carbon-dioxide concentration module 炭酸ガス濃度単位
CDD
chemically denned diet 完全栄養
chronic degenerative disease 慢性変性疾患
CDDP
cis-diammine dichloroplatinum シスプラチン
CDE
canine distemper encephalitis イヌ(の)ジステンパー脳炎
Certified Diabetes Educator 認定糖尿病教育士
chlordiazepoxide クロルジアゼポキシド
chronic enthusiasm disorder 慢性熱中障害
CDEK
computer data entry keyboard コンピュータデータ登録キーボード
CDER
Center for Drug Evaluation and Research 米国医薬品評価研究センター
CDEUS
color doppleer endoscopic ultrasonography 超音波内視鏡下カラード(ッ)プラー法
CDF
cell division factor 細胞分裂因子
Children's Defense Fund 小児保護基金
cholinergic differentiation factor コリン作動性分化因子
chondrodystrophia fetalis 胎児軟骨形成異常(症)
ciliary dyskinesis factor 毛様体機能障害因子
cumulative distribution function 累積分布関数
cd/ft^2
candela per square foot 1平方フィートあたりの輝度
CDGF
cartilage-derived growth factor 軟骨由来増殖因子
CDGS
carbohydrate deficient glycoprotein syndrome 糖蛋白質糖鎖不全症候群
CDH
ceramide dihexoside セラミドジヘキソシド
cervical disc herniation 頸椎椎間板ヘルニア
chronic daily headache 日々起こる慢性的頭痛

chronic disease hospital 慢性疾患収容病院
congenital diaphragmatic hernia 先天性横隔膜ヘルニア
congenital dislocation of (the) hip (joint) 先天性股関節脱臼(=LCC)
congenital dysplasia of hip 先天性殿部過形成

CDI
cell-directed inhibitor 細胞指向性阻害物質
central diabetes insipidus 中枢性尿崩症
cercopithecus diana〈ラ〉 ダイアナモンキー
Children's Depression Inventory 小児うつ病目録
chronic diabetes insipidus 慢性尿崩症
clinical data interchange standard 臨床データの相互交換基準
comprehensive dissertation index 広域学位論文索引

CDILD
chronic diffuse interstitial lung disease 慢性び漫性間質性肺疾患

CD-IP
collagen disease-interstitial pneumonia 膠原病性間質性肺炎

CDK
cyclin dependent kinase サイクリン依存キナーゼ

CDKN2
cyclin-dependent kinase 2 サイクリン依存キナーゼ 2

CD40L
CD40 ligand CD40リガンド

CDLC
Canadian Dental Laboratory Conference カナダ歯科研究所協議会

CDLE
chronic discoid lupus erythematosus 慢性円板状エリテマトーデス〔紅斑性狼瘡〕

CDM
chemically defined medium 化学合成培地
choline-deficient methionine-low コリン欠乏低メチオニン

cd/m²
candela per square meter 1平方メートルあたりの輝度

cDNA
circular DNA 環状DNA
complementary deoxyribonucleic acid 相補デオキシリボ核酸
complementary DNA 相補DNA

CDP
calcium dependent protease カルシウム依存性蛋白分解酵素
chronic destructive periodontitis 慢性破壊性歯周病
continuous distending pressure 持続性陽圧呼吸
cytidine 5′-diphosphate シチジン5′-二リン酸

cytosine diphosphate シトシン二リン酸

CDP choline
cytidine 5′-diphosphate choline シチジン5′-二リン酸コリン

CDP glycerol
cytidine 5′-diphosp glycerol シチジン5′-二リン酸グリセロール

CDPK
calcium-dependent protein kinase カルシウム依存性蛋白キナーゼ

Cd-probe
cadmium-probe カドミウム試験

CDPS
common data processing system 共通データ処理組織

CDR
calcium-dependent regulatory protein カルシウム依存性調節蛋白
complementarity determining region 相補性決定領域

CdR
cadmium reaction 硫酸カドミウム反応
deoxycytidine デオキシチミジン

CDRF
Canadian Dental Research Foundation カナダ歯科研究財団

CDRH
Center for Devices and Radiological Health 医療用具放射線局[米国]

CDRI
Central Drug Research Institute 中央薬物研究所[インド]

CDS
cadmium shell カドミウムシェル
cervical dry smear 子宮頸管乾燥塗抹標本
Colistin-Dextromycin-Salbe〈独〉 コリスチン・デキストロマイシン軟膏

CDSC
Communicable Disease Surveillance Center 伝染病監視センター[米国]

CDT
carbon dioxide therapy 炭酸ガス(吸入)法
Certified Dental Technician 有資格歯科技工士
Council on Dental Therapeutics 歯科治療審議会

CDV
canine distemper virus イヌ(の)ジステンパーウイルス

cdv
cadaver 死体

CDW
chilled drinking water 冷たい飲料水

CDX
cefadroxil　セファドロキシル
Cdyn
dynamic compliance　動(的)肺コンプライアンス
CDZ
chlordiazepoxide　クロルジアゼポキシド
CDZM
cefodizime　セフォジジム
CE
California encephalitis　カリフォルニア脳炎
cardiac enlargement　心拡大
cell extract　細胞抽出物
centrilobular emphysema　小葉中心性肺気腫
chemical energy　化学エネルギー
chicken erythrocyte　ニワトリ赤血球
cholesterol ester　コレステロールエステル
chorioepithelioma　絨毛上皮癌
ciliated epithelium　線毛上皮
cleansing enema　クレンジング浣腸
clinical engineering　クリニカルエンジニアリング
columnar epithelium　円柱上皮
competitive exclusion　競争排除
conjugated estrogens　結合エストロゲン
constant error　定常誤差《統》
continuing education　継続教育
contractile element　収縮要素《心外》
contrast enhancement　造影増強効果
converting enzyme　変換酵素
counter-flow centrifugal elutriation　対向流遠心洗浄法
exfoliative material　(水晶体嚢)剥脱
Ce
celeriter〈ラ〉=quickly　早く，急いで《処》
cerium　セリウム〈元素〉
cervical esophagus　頸部食道
esophageal cancer　食道癌
CE, C-E
chloroform-ether　クロロホルムエーテル
CEA
carcinoembryonic antigen　癌胎児性抗原
carotid endarterectomy　頸動脈内膜切除〔剝離〕術
cholesterol-esterifying activity　コレステロールエステル化活性
cholinesterase　コリンエステラーゼ
cost effective(ness) analysis　費用対効果分析
crystalline egg albumin　結晶性卵アルブミン
cultured epidermal autograft　培養上皮細胞移植

C

CEA-DT
carcinoembryonic antigen doubling time　癌胎児抗原倍増時間

CEARC
Computer Education and Applied Research Center　コンピュータ教育応用研究所

CEARP
Continuing Education Approval and Recognition Program　(医師)生涯教育認定評価プログラム

CEB
calcium entry blocker　カルシウム流入ブロッカー
cotton elastic bandage　綿弾性包帯
cryogenic explosive bladder　凍結による破裂膀胱

CEBD
controlled extrahepatic biliary drainage　調節肝臓外胆汁ドレナージ

CEBV
chronic Epstein-Barr virus　慢性エプスタイン・バーウイルス

CEC
capillary electrochromatography　毛細管電気クロマトグラフィ
cephacetrile, cefacetrile　セファセトリル
ciliated epitherial cell　線毛上皮細胞
circulation extracorporale　体外循環
contractile electrical complex　収縮電位複合体

CECD
congenital endothelial corneal dystrophy　先天性角膜上皮異栄養症

CECT
contrast enhancement computed tomography　造影剤増強コンピュータ断層撮影(法)

CECT, CE-CT
contrast enhanced CT(=computed tomography)　造影CT，濃淡強調CT

CED
cefradine　セフラジン
chondroectodermal dysplasia　軟骨外胚葉性形成異常〔異形成〕
chronic enthusiasm disorder　慢性熱中障害
cultural/ethnic diversity　文化的/民族的多様性
cystoscopy-endoscopy dilation　膀胱鏡・内視鏡拡張術

CEE
central European encephalitis　中央ヨーロッパ脳炎

CEEG
computer-analyzed electroencephalography　コンピュータ分析脳波

CEev
Central European encephalitis virus　中央ヨーロッパ脳炎ウイルス
CEF
central expansion factor　中央膨張因子
chicken embryo fibroblast　ニワトリ胚線維芽細胞
CEG
cardiac electrogram　心電図
cephaloglycin　セファログリシン
chronic erosive gastritis　慢性びらん性胃炎
CEH
cholesterol ester hydrolase　コレステロールエステル水解酵素
CEI
converting enzyme inhibitor　変換酵素抑制剤
CEID
crossed electroimmunodiffusion　交叉〔差〕気免疫拡散
CEJ, cej, c.e.j.
cement-enamel junction　セメント質エナメル質境界(線)
CEL, Cel
Celsius　セ氏，摂氏
cell
cellulose　線維素，セルロース
cell nitr
cellulose nitrate　硝酸セルロース
CELO
chicken embryo lethal orphan virus　ニワトリ胎致死孤児ウイルス
Cels
Celsius　セ氏，摂氏
CELSS
Controlled Ecological Life Support System　閉鎖生態系生命維持システム
CEM
central excitatory mechanism　中枢興奮機構
conventional transmission electron microscope　通常の透過型電子顕微鏡
CE mix
chloroform ether mixture　クロロホルムエーテル混合物
CEMS
conversion electron Mossbauer spectrometry　転換電子メスバウアー分光法
CEMT-PI
cefatamet pivoxil　セファタメトピボキシル
cen, cen.
center　中心，中央，中枢
central　中心の，中央の，中枢(性)の

C

centromere 動原体

CENP-B
centromere protein B 染色体動原体蛋白

CENT, Cent, cent
centigrade 摂氏(=°C)

cent, cent.
centimeter センチメートル
centrifugal 遠心の
century 100年間，世紀

centi
centigrade 摂氏(=°C)

central CFF
central critical fusion frequency 中心臨界融合頻度

CEO
chicken embryo origin ニワトリ胎起源

CEP
cephalosporin セファロスポリン
cephapirin セファピリン
cephems セフェム系抗生物質
cerebral evoked potential 大脳誘発電位
congenital erythropoietic porphyria 先天性骨髄性ポルフィリン症
cortical evoked potential 皮質誘発電位
countercurrent electrophoresis test 対向流電気泳動法
counter electrophoresis 対向電気泳動
2-cyanoethyl-phosphate 2-シアノエチルリン酸塩
cyclophosphamide, etoposide, cisplatin (=Platinol) シクロホスファミド，エトポシド，シスプラチン(=プラチノール)

Ceph
cepharanthin セファランチン

ceph
cephalic 頭(部)の

ceph floct
cephalin floculation test セファリン絮状〔綿状〕検査

CEPR
cefapirin セファピリン

CEPs
cephalosporins セファロスポリン系抗生物質

CEPT
cyclophosphamide, 5-fluorouracil, prednisone, tamoxifen シクロホスファミド，フルオロウラシル，プレドニゾン，タモキシフェン

'cept
accept 受容
except 例外

CEQ
coenzyme Q 補酵素〔コエンザイム〕Q

CER
cefradine セフラジン
cephaloridine セファロリジン
conditioned emotional response 条件情動反応
conditioned escape response 条件回避反応
cortical evoked response 皮質(性)誘発反応

cer
cervical 頸(部)の

CER, Cer
ceramide セラミド

CERA
continuous electrical response activity 持続的電気的反応能

CERCLA
Comprehensive Environmental Response Compensation & Liability Act 総合環境対策補償責任法

cereb
cerebral (大)脳の，脳性の

CERT, Cert, cert, cert.
certificate 証明書
certified 認定された，証明された
certify 証明する

cerv, cerv.
cervical 頸(部)の
cervix 頸(部)

CES
cancer family syndrome 癌家系症候群
cat eye syndrome ネコの目症候群
central excitatory state 中枢興奮状態

CESD
cholesterol ester storage disease コレステロール蓄積症

CESEMI
computer evaluation of scanning electron microscopic image 走査電顕像のコンピュータによる評価

CET
cephalothin セファロチン
cephothin セフォチン
controlled environmental elapsed time 管理された環境での経過時間
corrected effective temperature 修正実効温度

CETB
ceftibuten セフチブテン

CETE
central European tick-borne encephalopathy 中央ヨーロッパダニ媒介脳炎

CETP
cholesterol ester transport protein コレステロールエステル転送蛋白
cholesteryl ester transfer protein コレステリルエステル転送蛋白

CEU
continuing education unit 継続教育単位

CEV
California encephalitis virus カリフォルニア脳炎ウイルス
cyclophosphamide, etoposide, vincristine シクロホスファミド,エトポシド,ビンクリスチン

CE valve
Carpentier-Edwards valve CE弁

CEW
Centrum-Erker Winkel〈独〉 大腿骨中心臼蓋角

CEX
cephalexin セファレキシン

CEZ
capillary zone electrophoresis 毛細管領域電気泳動
cefazolin セファゾリン

CF
calcium folate 葉酸カルシウム
carbolfuchsin カルボールフクシン, 石炭酸フクシン
cardiac failure 心不全
casefile 症例ファイル
cationized ferritin 陽性イオンフェリチン
cephalothin セファロチン
certainty factor 確実因子
chemotactic factor (白血球)遊走因子
chest and left leg 胸部と左足
Christmas factor クリスマス因子
cisplatin, 5-fluorouracil シスプラチン,フルオロウラシル
citrovorum factor 抗葉酸物質拮抗因子
clastogenic factor 破砕因子
climbing fiber 登上線維
clotting factor 凝固因子
colonofiberscope 大腸内視鏡
colonofiberscopy 大腸内視鏡術
colony forming コロニー形成(性)の
complement fixation 補体結合
contractile force 収縮力

cord factor コードファクター
cor floating 心臓絶縁
coronary flow 冠血流
count(ing) finger(s) 指数弁
coupling factors 共役因子
cryofiltration 冷却濾過法
cytolytic factor 細胞融解因子

Cf
californium カリフォルニウム

cf
centrifugal force 遠心力
cum formula〈ラ〉 処方を記して《処》

^{252}Cf
californium-252 カリフォルニウム252

c.f.
count(ing) finger(s) 指数弁

C/F
capillary to fiber ratio 毛細血管と線維の比率

CF, C.F.
cystic fibrosis 嚢胞性線維症

CF, C'F
complement fixing 補体結合(性)の

Cf., cf.
confer 参照

CFA
colonization factor antigen コロニー形成因子抗原
complement fixing activity 補体結合活性
complement fixing antibody 補体結合抗体
complete Freund adjuvant 完全フロイントアジュバント
conjunctivitis follicularis acuta〈ラ〉 急性濾胞性結膜炎
continuous flow adapter 連続流量調整器
continuous flow analyzer 連続流動分析器
cryptogenic fibrosing alveolitis 潜在性線維性肺胞炎

C-factor
cleverness factor 聡明因子

CFAP
Canadian Foundation for Advancement of Pharmacy 薬学進歩のためのカナダ財団

CFBS
Ca free buffered saline カルシウム不含リン酸緩衝食塩水
Canadian Federation of Biological Society カナダ生物学会連合

CFC
capillary filtration coefficient 毛細管濾過係数
chlorofluorocarbon クロロフルオロカーボン

colony forming cell コロニー形成細胞
conjunctivitis follicularis chronica 慢性濾胞性結膜炎

CFC-C
colony forming cell in culture 培養コロニー形成細胞

CFC-S
colony forming cell in spleen 脾コロニー形成細胞

CFDN
cefdinir セフジニル

CFE
colony forming efficiency assay コロニー形成試験

CFF
critical flicker fusion frequency 臨界フリッカー融合頻度
critical fusion frequency 臨界融合頻度
cystic fibrosis factor 嚢胞性線維症因子

CFFA
cystic fibrosis factor activity 嚢胞性線維症因子活性

Cf-Fe
carrier bound iron 担体結合鉄

cfg
centrifuge 遠心分離

CFI
Camberwell family interview キャンバーウェル家族評価尺度
cardiac function index 心機能指数
chemotactic factor inactivator (白血球)遊走因子不活化物質
complement fixation inhibition (test) 補体結合抑制(試験)
corticofugal inhibition 皮質遠心性抑制

CF-ICA
complement fixing cytoplasmic islet cell antibody 補体結合性膵島細胞質抗体

CFIT
colorimetric flow-injection titration 電量フローインジェクション滴定法
complement fixation inhibition test 補体結合阻止試験

CFIX
cefixime セフィキシム

C'Fix
complement fixation test 補体結合試験

CFL
cisplatin, 5-fluorouracil, leucovorin calcium シスプラチン,フルオロウラシル,ロイコボリンカルシウム

CFM
chlorofluoromethane クロロフルオロメタン

cyclophosphamide, 5-fluorouracil, citoxantrone | シクロホスファミド, フルオロウラシル, シトキサントロン

cfm, cf/m
cubic feet per minute 立法フィート/分

CFNS
chills, fever, night sweats 悪寒・発熱・寝汗

CFP
carbohydrate, fat, protein 炭水化物・脂肪・蛋白質
chronic false-positive 慢性偽陽性
cyclophosphamide, 5-fluorouracil, prednisolone シクロホスファミド, フルオロウラシル, プレドニゾロン
cystic fibrosis of the pancreatitis 膵(臓)嚢性線維症
cystic fibrosis patient 嚢胞性線維症患者
cystic fibrosis protein 嚢胞性線維症蛋白

CFPC
carfecillin カルフェシリン

CFR
complement fixation reaction 補体結合反応
constant failure rate 偶発故障率
coronary flow reserve 冠(状)動脈血流予備量

CFRP
carbon fiber reinforced plastics 炭素繊維強化プラスチック

CFS
cefsulodin セフスロジン
chronic fatigue syndrome 慢性疲労症候群
colonofiberscope 大腸内視鏡

cfs
cubic feet per second 立法フィート/秒

CFSAN
Center for Food Safety and Applied Nutrition 食品安全応用栄養センター

CFSI
cumulative fatigue symptom index 蓄積的疲労徴候調査

CFT
Ca free Tyrode solution カルシウム不含タイロード液
cardiolipin flocculation test カルジオリ〔ライ〕ピン絮状〔綿状〕テスト
cefatrizine セファトリジン
clinical full time 臨床基準時間
complement fixation test 補体結合試験〔反応〕
complement-fixing titer 補体結合(力)価

CFTM-PI
cefteram pivoxil セフテラムピボキシル

C

CFTR
cystic fibrosis transmembrane conductance regulator — 嚢胞線維症膜貫通型調節物質

CFTRI
Central Food Technological Research Institute — 中央食料技術研究所

CFU
colony forming unit — コロニー形成単位

CFU-Ba
colony forming unit-basophil — 好塩基球コロニー形成単位

CFU-BL
B-lymphocyte colony forming unit — Bリンパ球系幹細胞コロニー形成単位

CFU-C
colony forming unit in culture — 培養コロニー形成単位

CFU-E
colony forming unit erythrocyte, erythroid colony forming unit — 赤芽球コロニー形成単位

CFU-Eo, CFU-EO
colony forming unit-eosinophil — 好酸球コロニー形成単位

CFU-G
colony forming unit-granule — 好中球コロニー形成単位

CFU-GEMM
colony forming unit-granule, erythrocyte, macrophage, megakaryocyte — 好中球・赤血球・マクロファージ・巨核球コロニー形成単位

CFU-GM
colony forming unit-granulocyte macrophage — 顆粒球マクロファージコロニー形成単位

CFU-L
colony forming unit lymphoid — リンパ球コロニー形成単位

CFU-M
colony forming unit-macrophage — マクロファージコロニー形成単位

colony forming unit-megakaryocyte — 巨核球コロニー形成単位

CFU-Meg
colony forming unit-megakaryocyte — 巨核球コロニー形成単位

CFU-mix
mixed colony forming unit — 混合コロニー形成単位

CFU-ML
colony forming unit on cellulose acetate membrane — セルロースアセテート膜上のコロニー形成単位

CF unit
complement fixation unit — 補体結合単位

CFU-S
colony forming units in spleen — 脾臓コロニー形成単位

CFW
cancer-free white mouse　非癌性白ハツカネズミ

CFX
cefoxitin　セホキシチン

CG
choking gas　窒息ガス
cholesterin granuloma　コレステリン肉芽腫
chorionic gonadotropin　絨毛性性腺刺激ホルモン
chronic glomerulonephritis　慢性糸球体腎炎
cingulate gyms　帯状束回
cingulate gyrus　帯状回
colloidal gold　コロイド状金
computer graphics　コンピュータグラフィックス
control group　対照群
cryoglobulin　クリオ〔寒冷〕グロブリン
cryoglobulinemia　クリオ〔寒冷〕グロブリン血(症)
cystine guanine　シスチン・グアニン
cystography　膀胱造影撮影法

Cg
conglutinin　コングルチニン

Cg, cg, cg.
centigram　センチグラム〈単位〉

CGA
cercocebes galeritus〈ラ〉　ゴールデンモンガベイ
Compressed Gas Association　圧縮ガス協会

CGAS
children's global assessment scale　小児用包括的評価尺度

CGD
chronic granulomatous disease　慢性肉芽腫症

CGE
capillary gel electrophoresis　毛細管ゲル電気泳動

CGF
chemotaxis generating factor　化学走性産出因子

CGH
chorionic gonadotropic hormone　絨毛性ゴナドトロピン
comparative genomic hybridization　比較ゲノム交配

CGI
carbimazole　カルビマゾール
chronic granulomatous inflamation　慢性肉芽腫(性)炎(症)

CGL
chronic granulocytic leukemia　慢性顆粒球性白血病
congenital generalized lipodystrophy　先天性全身脂肪萎縮

c gl, c.gl.
correction with glasses　眼鏡で矯正

C

CGM
central grey matter 中心灰白質
concentration hemoglobinique〈仏〉 ヘモグロビン濃度
continuous glucose monitoring system 連続的血糖測定装置

cgm, cgm.
centigram センチグラム〈単位〉

cGMP
cyclic guanosine 3′,5′-monophosphate サイクリックグアノシン 3′,5′-一リン酸，環状 GMP

CGN
chronic glomerulonephritis 慢性糸球体腎炎

CGOQ
cerebral glucose oxygen quotient 脳グルコース酸比

CGP
choline glycerophosphatide コリングリセロリン脂質
chorionic growth hormone prolactin 絨毛性成長ホルモンプロラクチン

CGR
captured gamma ray 捕獲γ線

CGRP
calcitonin gene related peptide カルシトニン遺伝子関連ペプチド

CGS
cardiogenic shock 心原性ショック
catgut suture 腸線縫合

CGS, cgs, c.g.s.
centimeter gram second センチメートルグラム秒〈単位〉

CGT
chorionic gonadotropin 絨毛性性腺刺激ホルモン

CGTT
cortisol glucose tolerance test コルチゾールブドウ糖負荷試験
cortisone glucose tolerance test コルチゾンブドウ糖負荷試験

CH
case history 症例の今までの経過
chain (連)鎖
(wheel) chair (車)イス
Chédiac-Higashi (syndrome) チェディアック・東(症候群)
chiasma 交叉〔差〕，キアスマ
Chinese hamster チャイニーズハムスター
chirugia〈ラ〉=surgery 外科(学)
chloral hydrate 抱水クロラール
chronic hepatitis 慢性肝炎
chronic hypertension 慢性高血圧

Clarke-Hadfield (syndrome)	クラーク・ハッドフィールド(症候群)
clinical history	病歴
communicating hydrocephalus	交通性水頭症
congenital hypothyroidism	先天性甲状腺機能低下症
constant heavy chain domains	不変H鎖領域
continuous heparinization	持続ヘパリン化
critical hours	重症〔危急〕時間
crown-heel	頭頂踵間距離
cyclohexanol	サイクロヘキサール
H(=heavy) chain constant region	H鎖不変部
optic chiasma	視束交叉〔差〕

Ch

Charriere scale	シャリエール計測板
check	チェック
chlorpromazine	クロルプロマジン
cholesterol	コレステロール
choline	コリン
chondroitin	コンドロイチン

ch

chronic	慢性の

CH_{50}

50% hemolytic unit of complement	補体50%溶血単位

cH^{+}

hydrogen ion concentration	水素イオン濃度

C & H

coarse and harsh (breathing)	粗大かつ喘鳴性の(呼吸)
cocaine and heroin	コカインとヘロイン

CH, Ch, ch

chapter	章，話題
chest	胸(部)
chief	おもな

Ch, CH

Christchurch chromosome	クライストチャーチ染色体

Ch, ch

child	小児，児童

CHA

caprylhydroxamic acid	カプリルヒドロキサム酸
chronic hemolytic anemia	慢性溶血性貧血
cold hemagglutination test	寒冷赤血球凝集素テスト
cold hemagglutinin	寒冷赤血球凝集素(価)
common hepatic artery	総肝動脈
Community Health Association	共同健康協会
concentric hemispherical autolyzer	同心半球型分光器
congenital hypoplastic anemia	先天性形成不良性貧血
continuous heated aerosols	持続的加温エアロゾル

C

cyclohexyladenosine シクロヘキシルアデノシン
cyclohexylamine シクロヘキシルアミン

ChA, Ch-A
choline acetylase コリンアセチラーゼ

CHAC, ChAc
choline acetyltransferase コリンアセチルトランスフェラーゼ

CHAD
chronic cold hemoaggulutinin disease 慢性寒冷赤血球凝集素病
cyclophosphamide, hexamethylmelamine, adriamycin, *cis*-diamminedichloroplatinum シクロホスファミド, ヘキサメチルメラミン, アドリアマイシン, *cis*-ジアミンジクロロプラチナ

CHAI
continuous hepatic arterial infusion 肝動脈持続動注法

CHAM-OCA
cyclophosphamide, hydroxyurea, actinomycin-D, methotrexate, vincristine (=Oncovin), citrovorum factor, adriamycin シクロホスファミド, ヒドロキシ尿素, アクチノマイシンD, メトトレキサート, ビンクリスチン(=オンコビン), シトロボラム因子, アドリアマイシン

CHAP
Certified Hospital Admissions Program 公認入院計画
cyclophosphamide, hexamethylmelamine, adriamycin, cisplatin (=Platinol) シクロホスファミド, ヘキサメチルメラミン, アドリアマイシン, シスプラチン(=プラチノール)

chap
chapter 章, 話題

char
character 性質, 特徴
characteristic 特徴的な

CHARGE
coloboma, heart disease, atresiachoane, retarded growth, retarded development and/or central nervous system anomalies, genital hypoplasia and/or ear anomalies and/or deaf 網脈絡膜欠損・心疾患・後鼻孔閉鎖症・成長障害・知能発育障害(ないし中枢神経系奇形)・外性器低形成(ないし耳介奇形, ないし聾)

chart, chart.
charta〈ラ〉 薬包紙《処》
chartae〈ラ〉=(a powder in) paper 分包散剤《処》

chart bib.
charta bibula〈ラ〉 吸取紙《処》

chart cera.
charta cerata〈ラ〉 パラフィン紙《処》

chartul
chartula〈ラ〉 小型薬包紙《処》

ChAT, CHAT
choline acetyltransferase コリンアセチル転移酵素

CHB
complete heart block 完全心ブロック

CHBA
Committee on Hearing and Bioacoustics 聴覚および生物聴覚委員会
congenital Heinz body anemia 先天性ハインツ(小)体(性)貧血

Ch Bu Med
Chief on Bureau of Medicine and Surgery 内科・外科主任

CHC
cyclohexylamine carbonate 炭酸シクロヘキシルアミン

Ch-ca
choriocarcinoma 絨毛癌

CHD
Cédiak-Higashi disease チェディアック・東病
child blood disease 小児血液疾患
chronic hemodialysis 慢性的透析
common hepatic duct 総肝管
compensated heart disease 代償性心(臓)疾患
congenital heart disease 先天性心(臓)疾患
congenital hip disease 先天性股関節疾患
congenital hip dislocation 先天性股関節脱臼
congestive heart disease うっ血性心疾患
coronary heart disease 冠(状)動脈性心疾患
cyanotic heart disease チアノーゼ性心(臓)疾患
1,2-cyclohexanedione 1,2-シクロヘキサンジオン

ChD, CHD
childhood disease 小児疾患

CHDF
continuous hemodiafiltration 持続性血液濾過透析

CHDM
cyclohexane dimethanol シクロヘキサンジメタノール

CHE
chronic hepatic encephalopathy 慢性肝性脳症

ChE
cholesterol ester コレステロールエステル
cholinesterase コリンエステラーゼ

chem
chemical 化学の

chemist 化学者
chemistry 化学

Chem, chem
chemotherapy 化学療法

C

CHEMFET
chemical field effect transistor シリコン半導体を応用した電気化学センサー

CHEMICS
Combined Handling of Elucidation Methods for Interpretable ChemicalStructures 化学構造自動構造決定システム

chemo
chemotherapy 化学療法

Chemother
chemotherapy 化学療法

ChemSat
chemical shift saturation 脂肪抑制

CHEOPS
Children Hospital of Eastern Ontario Pain Scale 小児の痛みの程度を判定する指標

Ch-ep
chorioepithelioma 絨毛上皮腫

CHES
cyclohexyl-aminoethanesulfonic acid シクロヘキシルアミノエタンスルホン酸

CHESS
Community Health and Environmental Surveillance System チェス疫学調査

CHF
congenital heart failure 先天性心不全
congenital hepatic fibrosis 先天性肝線維化症
congestive heart failure うっ血性心不全
continuous hemofiltration 持続血液濾過法
cyclophosphamide, hexamethylmelamine,5-fluorouracil シクロホスファミド,ヘキサメチルメラミン,フルオロウラシル

chf
cell-associated helper factor 細胞依存ヘルパー因子

chg
change 変化
charge 費用

chg'd
changed 変化した

chg's
changes 変化〈複数〉

CHH
cartilage-hair hypoplasia 短肢性小人症
CHI
chemotherapeutic index 化学療法係数
Children's Hospice International 国際小児ホスピス
closed head injury 閉鎖性頭部外傷
creatinine height index クレアチニン身長比
chi
chimera キメラ
CHILD
congenital hemidysplasia with ichthyosiform erythroderma and limb defect (syndrome) 先天性片側性形成異常・魚鱗癬様紅皮症・肢欠損症候群
CHIME
coloboma, heart anomaly, ichthyosis, mental retardation, and ear abnormality コロボーム・心奇形・魚鱗癬・精神遅滞・聴力異常
CHINA
chronic infectious neuropathic (neurotropic) agent 慢性感染性神経障害性(神経向性)物質
CHIP
cis-dichloro-*trans*-dihydroxy-*bis* isopropylamine platinum *cis*-ジクロロ-*trans*-ジヒドロキシ-*bis*-イソプロピラミンプラチナム
comprehensive health insurance plan 包括的医療保険プラン
comprehensive hospital infections project 包括的病院感染対策
chir
chiropody 手足の治療
Chir, chir.
chirurgia〈ラ〉=Chirurgie〈独〉 外科
CHIRI
Consumer Health Information Research Institute 米国消費者健康情報調査研究所
Chiro
chiropractic 脊椎指圧療法
chiropractor 脊椎指圧療法士
chiro
chirography 証書
chirurg.
chirurgicalis〈ラ〉=surgical 外科(的)の，外科手術(上)の
Chix
chickenpox 水痘
CHL
chlorambucil クロラムブシル
chloramphenicol クロラムフェニコール

C

Chl
chlorocruorin　クロロクルオリン
chl
chloride　塩化物
Chl, chl
chloroform　クロロホルム
Chl-A
chimpanzee leukocyte antigen　チンパンジー白血球抗原
Chlb
chlorobutanol　クロロブタノール
CHLD
chronic hypoxic lung disease　慢性低酸素性肺疾患
chlor
chloroform　クロロホルム
chlorid.
chloridum〈ラ〉　塩化物
chloro
chlorophyll　葉緑素
chloroprene　クロロプレン
ChlVPP
chlorambucil, vinblastine, procarbazine, prednisone　クロラムブシル, ビンブラスチン, プロカルバジン, プレドニゾン
chm
chairman, chairwoman　座長
CHMC
Children's Hospital Medical Center　小児病院医療センター
CHMD
clinical hyaline membrane disease　臨床的ヒアリン膜疾患
CHMPP
continuous hyperthermic minor pelvic perfusion　小骨盤腔内持続温熱灌流療法
CHN
carbon, hydrogen, nitrogen　炭素・水素・窒素
central hemorrhagic necrosis　中心出血性壊死
Child Neurology　小児神経学
chng
change　変化
CHO
carbohydrate　炭水化物, 糖質
Chinese hamster ovary　チャイニーズハムスター卵巣
cholesterol　コルステロール
chorea　舞踏病
cyclophosphamide, hydroxydaunorubicin, vincristine (= Oncovin)　シクロホスファミド, ヒドロキシダウノルビシン, ビンクリスチン (=オンコビン)

Cho
choline コリン

chol
cholesterin コレステリン

CHOL, Chol, chol
cholesterol コレステロール

chole
cholecystectomy 胆嚢切除(術), 胆嚢摘出(術)
cholecystitis 胆嚢炎
cholesteatoma 真珠腫

CHOL E
cholesterol ester コレステロールエステル

cholecyst
cholecystectomy 胆嚢切除(術), 胆嚢摘出(術)

cholelith
cholelithiasis 胆石症

choles
cholesterol コレステロール

cholest
cholesterol コレステロール

CHOL EST, Chol est., chol.est.
cholesterol ester コレステロールエステル

chol-ester
cholesterin ester コレステリンエステル

CHOP
cyclophosphamide, hydroxydaunomycin, vincristine (=Oncovin), prednisone シクロホスファミド, ヒドロキシダウノマイシン, ビンクリスチン(=オンコビン), プレドニゾン

CHOP-B
cyclophosphamide, hydroxydaunorubicin, vincristine (=Oncovin), prednisone, bleomycin シクロホスファミド, ヒドロキシダウノルビシン, ビンクリスチン(=オンコビン), プレドニゾン, ブレオマイシン

CHO P F
carbohydrates, proteins, and fats 炭水化物・蛋白・脂質

CHOR
cyclophosphamide, hydroxydaunorubicin, vincristine (=Oncovin), radiation シクロホスファミド, ヒドロキシダウノルビシン, ビンクリスチン(=オンコビン), プレドニゾン, 放射線

chorio
chorioepithelioma 絨毛上皮腫

CHP
capillary hydrostatic pressure 毛細(血)管静水圧

C

charcoal hemoperfusion　活性炭血液灌流〔吸着〕
child psychiatry　小児精神医学
chromalum hematoxylin phloxinestain　クロムミョウバン・ヘマトキシリン・フロキシン
comprehensive health plan　包括的健康計画
cutaneous hepatic porphyria　皮膚肝性ポルフィリン症

CHPG
colloid hydrostatic pressure　コロイド静水圧勾配

CHPP
continuous hyperthermic peritoneal perfusion　持続温熱腹膜灌流

chpx., ch.px
chickenpox　水痘

CHQ
chlorquinol　クロルキノール

CHR
cerebrohepatorenal (syndrome)　脳肝腎(症候群)
chemotheraphy hyperthermia radiation　化学・温熱・放射線療法

CHR, Chr
Chromobacterium　クロモバクテリウム(属)

CHR, chr
chronic　慢性の

C hr, c hr, chr
candle hour　燭光時，キャンドル時間〈単位〉
curie hour　キュリー時間〈単位〉

Chrbac
Chromobacterium　クロモバクテリウム(属)

ChrBrSyn, Chr Br Syn
chronic brain syndrome　慢性脳症候群

Chr B Synd
chronic brain syndrome　慢性脳症候群

CHRD
Commission on Health Research for Development　国際保健医療研究協力委員会

CHRIS
Cancer Hazards Ranking and Information System　癌危険ランキングと情報システム

CHRM
chromomycin　クロモマイシン
chromomycin A3　クロモマイシンA 3

chRNA
chromosomal ribonucleic acid　染色体リボ核酸

chromo
chromosome　染色体

chron
chronic 慢性の

Chron, chron.
chronological 暦の

CHRS
cerebrohepatorenal syndrome 脳肝腎症候群

CHS
Chédiak-Higashi Syndrome チェディアック・東症候群
cholinesterase コリンエステラーゼ
chronic hypersensitivity 慢性過敏症
Community Health Service 共同体健康サービス
contact hypersensitivity 接触過敏症

ChS
chondroitin sulfate コンドロイチン硫酸

ch s
chondrosarcoma 軟骨肉腫

ChT
chiasma of tendon 腱交叉〔差〕

ChTg
chymotrypsinogen キモトリプシノゲン

CHTZ
chlorothiazide クロロチアジド

CHU
centrigate heat unit 集中暖房装置

CHu
Centre Hospitale-Universitaire〈仏〉 大学病院センター

CHV
cytomegalovirus サイトメガロウイルス

CHW
cold and hot water 冷温水
constant hot water 恒常温水

chw
chilled water 冷水

CHX
cycloheximide シクロヘキシミド

chylo
chylomicron カイロマイクロン

CI
cardiac index 心係数
cardiac insufficiency 心不全
cellular immunity 細胞性免疫
cerebral infarction 脳梗塞
chemical ionization 化学イオン化(法)
chemotherapeuitic index 化学療法指数
clinical impression 臨床的印象
clinical investigation 臨床研究者

clonus index クローヌス指数
coefficient of intelligence 知能係数
collapsibility index 虚脱度
colloidal iron コロイド鉄
colony inhibition コロニー阻止
color index 色素指数
Congo red index コンゴーレッド係数
Consumers International 国際消費者機構
contamination index 汚染指数
continuous infusion 持続注入
convergence insufficiency 輻輳不全
cornification index 角化係数
coronary insufficiency 冠不全
crystalline insulin 結晶インスリン
curie index キュリー単位
cytotoxic index 細胞傷害指数

Ci
curie キュリー〈単位〉

C/I
certificate of insurance 保険証書

CIA
chymotrypsin inhibitor activity キモトリプシン抑制活性
Collegium Internationale Allergologicum〈ラ〉 国際アレルギー協会
colony inhibiting activity コロニー形成阻止活性
common iliac artery 総腸骨動脈
communication inter-auriculaire 耳内連絡
congenital intestinal aganglionosis 先天性腸無神経節症

cib.
cibus〈ラ〉=food, meal 食(事)《処》

CIBD
chronic inflammatory bowel disease 慢性炎症性腸疾患

CIBHA
congenital inclusion body hemolytic anemia 先天性封入体溶血性貧血

CIC
cardiac inhibitory center 心(臓)抑制中枢
cardioinhibitor center 心(機能)抑制中枢
circulating immune complex 循環血中免疫複合体
clean intermittent catheterization 清潔間欠導尿
cloud in cell 細胞内混濁

CICA
cervical internal carotid artery 頸部内頸動脈

CICAD
Concise International Chemical Assessment Document 簡潔な国際化学物質評価証書

CICC
complement independent cellular cytotoxicity (assay) 補体非依存性細胞傷害(測定法)

CICD
Collegium Internationale Chirurgiae Digesrtivae〈ラ〉 国際消化器外科学会

CICR
Ca induced Ca release カルシウム誘発カルシウム放出

CICU
cardiac intensive care unit 心(臓)疾患集中治療部〔室〕
cardiology intensive care unit 循環器集中治療部〔室〕
coronary intensive care unit 冠(状動脈)疾患集中治療室

CID
Central Institute for Deaf 難聴中央研究所
charge injection device 電荷注入装置
chick infective dose ヒヨコ感染量
collision induced dissociation 衝突誘起の解離
combined immunodeficiency (disease) 混合性免疫不全〔疾患〕
cytomegalic inclusion disease 巨大細胞封入体病

CIDA
Comité International de Andrologia〈仏〉 アンドロロジー国際学会

CIDI
Composite International Diagnostic Interview 混成国際的診断面接

CIDO
International Classification of Disease for Oncology 国際腫瘍疾患分類

CIDP
chronic inflammatory demyelinated polyneuropathy 慢性炎症性脱髄性多発ニューロパシー
chronic inflammatory demyelinating polyradiculoneuropathy 慢性炎症性脱髄性多発神経根ニューロパシー

CIDR
chronic inflammatory demyelinated radiculopathy 慢性炎症性脱髄性神経根ニューロパシー

CIDS
Canadian Implantable Defibrillator Study カナダ移植可能細動除去器研究
cellular immunity deficiency syndrome 細胞性免疫不全症候群
cellulose ion exchanger セルロースイオン交換体
Chemical Information and Data System 化学情報およびデータシステム

CID virus
cytomegalic inclusion disease virus　巨大細胞封入体病(CID)ウイルス

CIE
commision internationale de l'eclariage〈仏〉　色度座標による国際表色系
congenital ichthyosiform erythroderma　先天性魚鱗癬様紅皮症
countercurrent immunoelectrophoresis　対向免疫電気泳動(法)
crossed immunoelectrophoresis　二次交叉〔差〕免疫電気泳動法

CIE(P)
counter immunoelectrophoresis　免疫電気向流法

CIEPS
Conseil International pour l'Education Physique et le Sport〈仏〉　国際スポーツ体育学会

CIF
cartilage inducing factor　軟骨誘導因子
clonal inhibition factor　クローン化阻止因子
cloning inhibiting factor　クローン阻止因子
colony inhibiting factor　コロニー阻止因子

CIFC
Council for Investigation of Fertility Control　受精管理調査諮問委員会

CIFD
congenital intrinsic factor deficiency　先天性内因子欠損症

CIG
cold-insoluble globulin　寒冷不溶性グロブリン

cIg
(intra) cytoplasmic immunoglobulin　細胞質(内)免疫グロブリン

cig
cigarette　紙巻タバコ

C-Ig
cellular immunoglobulin　細胞(内)免疫グロブリン

cIgM
cytoplasmic immunoglobulin M　細胞質(内)免疫グロブリンM

CIH
carbohydrate-induced hyperglycemia　炭水化物由来高血糖
chronic inactive hepatitis　慢性非活動性肝炎

CIHD
chronic ischemic cardiomyopathy　慢性虚血性心疾患

Ci-hr
curie-hour　キュリー時間〈単位〉

CIIA
common internal iliac artery　総内腸骨動脈

CIIP
chronic idiopathic intestinal pseudo-obstruction 慢性特発性腸性偽閉塞症

CIIPS
chronic idiopathic intestinal pseudo-obstruction syndrome 慢性特発性腸性偽閉塞症候群

CIJ
cholesterol index for Japan 日本人に適応されるコレステロール指数

CIM
cimetidine シメチジン
computer-integrated manufacturing コンピュータ統合生産

CIMPM
Comité International de Médecine et de Pharmacie Militaire〈仏〉 仏国際軍事医薬委員会

CI-MS
chemical ionization mass spectrometer 科学イオン化質量分析

CIMTP
Congrés International de Medecine Tropicale et de Paludisme 国際熱帯医学マラリア会議

CIN
cervical intraepithelial neoplasia 子宮頸部上皮内腫瘍
chronic idiopathic neutropenia 慢性特発性白血球減少症
chronic interstitial nephritis 慢性間質性腎炎
contrast media(-induced) nephropathy 造影剤腎症《画診》

C3 in
C3 inactivator C 3 不活性化因子

CIN, Cin, c.in.
inulin clearance イヌリンクリアランス

C1INA
C1 inactivator C 1 不活性化因子

C3INA
C3 inactivator C 3 不活性物質

CINC
cytokine-induced neutrophil chemoattractant サイトカイン依存性好中球走化性

CINDI
Countrywide Integrated Noncommunicable Disease Intervention Programme 地域を統合した非伝染病の調査計画

CINE
chemotherapy-induced nausea 化学療法誘発(性)嘔気〔嘔吐〕

C

C1 INH
C1 esterase inhibitor — C１エステラーゼインヒビター

C1INH
C1 inhibitor — C１インヒビター

cin NL
within normal limits — 正常範囲内

CINP
Collegium Internationale Neuro-Psychopharmacologicum〈ラ〉 — 国際神経精神薬理学会

CINS
chronic idiopathic neutropenia syndrome — 慢性特発性好中球減少症候群

CINX
cinoxacin — シノキサシン

CIOMS
Council for International-Organization of Medical Science — 国際医療科学組織会議

CIP
calf intestine phosphatase — 仔ウシ小腸ホスファターゼ
chronic inflammatory polyneuropathy — 慢性炎症性多発ニューロパシー
chronic interstitial pneumonia — 慢性間質性肺炎
Collége International de Podologie〈仏〉=International College of Podology — 国際脚足学会

CIPC
carindacillin=carbenicillin indanyl ester — カリンダシリン=カルベニシリンインダニルエステル

CIPD
chronic intermittent peritoneal dialysis — 慢性間欠的腹膜透析

CIPM
Comité International des Poide et Mesures〈仏〉 — 国際度量衡委員会

CIPR
Commission Internationale de Protection Contre les Radiations〈仏〉 — 放射線予防国際会議

CIR, cir
circumcised — 環状切除された
circumcision — 環状切除(術)，環切(術)

cir, cir.
circle — 円
circuit — 巡回，回路
circular — 円周状の，輪状の

circulation 循環
circulatory 循環の
circumference 周(囲)径，周長
circumferential 周(囲)径の，周長の

CiRA
Center for iPS Cell Research and Application,Kyoto University 京都大学iPS細胞研究所

CIRC
Comité Internationale de Red Cross 〈仏〉=International Committee of the Red Cross 赤十字国際委員会

CIRC, Circ, circ
circumcision 環状切除(術)，環切(術)

Circ, circ
circuit 回路，巡回
circular 円周状の，輪状の
circulate 循環する
circulating 循環している
circulation 循環
circulatory 循環の
circumcised 環状切除された
circumference 周(囲)径，周長
circumferential 周(囲)径の，周長の

circad
circadian 日周期
circadianaly 日周期で
circadic 日周期の

circum
circumference 周囲
circumflex 回旋した，弓状彎曲の

CIRM
Centro Internazionale Radio-Medico 〈西〉 スペイン国際放射線医学センター

CIRPN
chronic idiopathic relapsing polyneuropathy 慢性特発性再発性多発ニューロパシー

CI-RTP
cyclodextrin-induced room-temperature phosphorescence シクロデキストリン誘起室温リン光

CIS
carcinoma *in situ* 上皮内癌
catheter-induced spasm カテーテル誘発痙攣
cellular injury score 細胞傷害度スコア
central inhibitory state 中枢抑制状態

Centre Internationale d'Informations de Securite et d'Hygine du Travail 〈仏〉=International occupational Safety and Health Information Center — 国際職業安全衛生情報センター
chemical information system — 化学情報検索システム

CIs
confidence intervals — 信頼期間

Cis
cisplatin — シスプラチン

CISCA
cisplatin, cyclophosphamide, adriamycin — シスプラチン, シクロホスファミド, アドリアマイシン

***cis*-DDP**
cis-diammine(-)dichlor platinum — シスプラチン

cist.
cista〈ラ〉 — 小箱《処》

CIT
cold ischemic time — 冷阻血時間
conventional insulin therapy — 従来型インスリン療法

cit
cited — 引用する
citrate — クエン酸塩

Cito !
Cito!〈ラ〉 — 至急《処》

cito disp. *!*
cito dispensetur!〈ラ〉=let it be dispensed quickly — 至急調剤せよ《処》

CIV
common iliac vein — 総腸骨静脈
communication interventriculaire — 脳室内連絡
continuous intravenous infusion — 持続点滴静注

CIVD
cold induced vasodilatation — 冷却による血管拡張

C-IVH
continuous intravenous hyper-alimentation — 持続静脈高栄養法

CIVII
continuous intravenous insulin infusion — 持続インスリン点滴静注

CIX
circumflex — 回旋枝

CIXU
constant infusion excretory urogram — 持続注入排泄尿路造影図

CJ
conjunctivitis 結膜炎
CJA
callithrix jachus〈ラ〉 コモンマーモセット
CJD
Creutzfeld-Jakob disease クロイツフェルト・ヤコブ病
CJR
centric jaw relationship 中心(顎)位
CJS
Creutzfeldt-Jakob syndrome クロイツフェルト・ヤコブ症候群
CK
cholecystokinin コレシストキニン
choline kinase コリンキナーゼ
creatine kinase クレアチンキナーゼ
cyanogen chloride 塩化シアノゲン
cytokine サイトカイン
CK II
casein kinase II カゼインキナーゼII
CK, ck
check チェックする
C-K, CK
Cardiakrebs〈独〉 噴門部癌
CK-BB
creatine kinase brainband isoenzyme クレアチンキナーゼ脳由来アイソザイム
CKC
closed kinetic chain 閉鎖運動連鎖
cold-knife conization 寒冷式円錐切除(術)
CKD
chronic kidney disease 慢性腎臓病
ckd
checked チェックした
CKG
cardiokymograph 心臓キモグラフ
cardiokymography 心臓キモグラフ法
C/kg
coulomb per kilogram クーロン毎キログラム
CK-ISO
creatine kinase isoenzyme クレアチンキナーゼアイソエンザイム
CK-MB
creatine kinase myocardial band クレアチンキナーゼ心筋由来アイソザイム

CK-PZ
cholecystokinin-pancreozymin　コレシストキニン・パンクレオザイミン

CKS
classic form of Kaposi sarcoma　標準的カポジ肉腫
Continuum knee system (implant)　連続体膝システム(インプラント)

CKW, ckw
clockwise　時計回りの，右回りの

CL
capillary lumen　毛細(血)管内腔
cardiolipin　カルジオリ〔ライ〕ピン
center line　中心線
chemiluminescence　化学発光
chest and left arm　胸左腕
cholelithiasis　胆石症
cholesterol-lecithin (test)　コレステロール・レシチン(試験)
chronic leukemia　慢性白血病
clamp lamp　ランプ付鉗子
clearance　クリアランス
cleft lip　兎唇
clonidine　クロニジン
colistin　コリスチン
comfortable level　快適域値
complicated lesion　複合病変
constant light chain domains　不変L鎖領域
contact lens　コンタクトレンズ
corpus luteum〈ラ〉　黄体
critical list　臨界表
cutis laxa　弛緩性皮膚
cytotoxic lymphocyte　細胞毒性リンパ球
light chain constant region　L鎖不変部
lung compliance　肺コンプライアンス

CL(H/S)
contact lens (hard/soft)　コンタクトレンズ(ハード/ソフト)

Cl
chloride　塩化(物)
chlorine　塩素
class　組，級

cl
centiliter　センチリットル〈単位〉
clean　きれいな，汚れのない
clear　明らかな，澄んだ
close　閉じる

closed 閉ざされた，閉じた
cloudy 曇った

CL, Cl
Clostridium クロストリジウム

CL, Cl
clinic 診療所，外来

CL, cl., c.l.
corpus luteum 黄体

Cl, cl
clavicle 鎖骨
clinical 臨床的な
clonus クローヌス
closure 閉鎖

CLA
cervicolinguoaxial 歯頸(面)舌(面)軸(面)の

CLAA
clinical laboratory automation architecture 臨床検査室自動化設計概念

CLAC
check list for autistic child 精研式自閉症用行動評定表

CLAIDHA
compensating loudness by analyzing input-signal digital hearing aid デジタル信号処理技術を応用した補聴システム

C lam
cervical laminectomy 頸椎椎弓切除(術)

CLAO
Contact Lens Association of Ophthalmologists 眼科医コンタクトレンズ学会

CLAS
congenital localized absence of skin 先天性限局皮膚欠損

clas
classification 分類
classify 分類する

clasn
classification 分類

class
classification 分類

class A's
class A narcotics クラスA麻薬

class B's
class B narcotics クラスB麻薬

classif
classified 分類された

class M's
class M narcotics クラスM麻薬

C

class X's
class X narcotics　クラスX麻薬
clav, clav.
clavicle　鎖骨
CLB
chlorambucil　クロラムブシル
CLBBB
complete left bundle branch block　完全左脚ブロック
CLC
Charcot-Leyden crystal　シャルコー・ライデン結晶
colchicine　コルヒチン
CL/CP
cleft lip and cleft palate　兎唇・口唇裂
CLD
chronic liver disease　慢性肝(臓)疾患
chronic lung disease　慢性肺疾患
congenital limb deficiency　先天的四肢欠損(症)
cld
cleared　清掃された
closed　閉じた，閉ざされた
colored　有色(人種)の，着色された
CLDAS
Clinical Laboratory Data Acquisition System　臨床検査データ取得システム
CLDM
clindamycin　クリンダマイシン
cldy
cloudy　濁った
CLE
cutaneous lupus erythematosus　皮膚エリテマトーデス
CLEIA
chemiluminescent enzyme immunoassay　化学発光酵素免疫(測定)法
CLF
cardiolipin fluorescence (antibody)　カルジオリ〔ライ〕ピン螢光(抗体)
ceroid lipofuscinosis　セロイド・リポフスチン症
correction log form　症例報告書の変更・修正記録
CLH
chronic lobular hepatitis　慢性葉性肝炎
corpus luteum hormone　黄体ホルモン
CLI
corpus luteum insufficiency　黄体(機能)不全
critical limb ischemia　重症虚血肢
CLIA
chemiluminescent immunoassay　化学発光免疫測定〔分析〕法

Clinical Laboratory Improvement Act 臨床検査室改良事業

CLIF
cloning inhibition factor クローニング阻止因子

Clin
clinical 臨床の，臨床的な

CLIN, Clin, clin.
clinic 診療所，外来
clinical 臨床の，臨床的な

Clinical Dx
clinical diagnosis 臨床診断

Clin Path, Clin path.
clinical pathology 臨床病理(学)

Clin proc
clinical procedures 臨床手技

CLIP
cerebral lipidosis 脳リピドーシス
contused, lacerated, incised and punctured wounds 挫・裂・切・刺創
corticotropin-like intermediate lobe peptide コルチコトロピン様中葉ペプチド

clit
clitoral 陰核の
clitoridectomy 陰核切除
clitoris 陰核

CLL
cholesterol lowering lipid コレステロール低下脂質
chronic lymphocytic leukemia 慢性リンパ性白血病

Cl Lab
Clinical Laboratory 臨床検査室

CLLS
cells of limited life span 生命期間の限られた細胞

CLM
clindamycin クリンダマイシン

CLMA
Contact Lens Manufactures Association コンタクトレンズ製造業者協会

CLMS
Clinical Laboratory Monitoring System 臨床検査モニターシステム

CLMW
cauliflower mosaic virus カリフラワーモザイクウイルス

clnc
clearance クリアランス

CLNP
colistin nonapeptide コリスチン・ノナペプチド

C

CLO
cod liver oil タラ肝油
CLOF
clofibrate クロフィブレート
Clon
Clonorchis クロノルキス
C-L op
Caldwell-Luc operation 上顎洞根本手術
closed cDNA
closed circular DNA 閉環状DNA
Clostr
Clostridium クロストリジウム
CLP
chymotripsin-like protein キモトリプシン様蛋白
cleft lip palate 口唇口蓋裂
clinical pathology 臨床病理(学)
curvilinear profile 曲直線輪郭
Cl Pal, Cl pal., cl.pal.
cleft palete 口蓋裂
clqs.
cuilibet quantum sufficiat〈ラ〉 十分な量を随意に《処》
clr
clear 澄んだ，きれいな
CLSCL
chronic lymphosarcoma cell leukemia 慢性リンパ肉腫細胞白血病
clsg
closing 閉鎖
CLSH
corpus luteum-stimulating hormone 黄体刺激ホルモン
CLSL
chronic lymphosarcomatous leukemia 慢性リンパ肉腫性白血病
clsr
closure 閉鎖
CLT
chronic lymphocytic thyroiditis 慢性リンパ球性甲状腺炎
CLT, cl T
clotting time 凝固時間
4-CLTA
4-chlorotestosterone acetate 4-クロロテストステロン酢酸
4-CLTC
4-chlorotestosterone capronate 4-クロロテストステロンカプロン酸
cl.time
clotting time 凝固時間

4-CLTP
4-chlorotestosterone propionate　4-クロロテストステロンプロピオン酸

C & L trx
cervical and lumbar traction　頸椎・腰椎牽引

CL void
clean voided specimen　非汚染排泄検体(尿)

ClVPP
chlorambucil, vinblastine, procarbazine, prednisone　クロラムブシル,ビンブラスチン,プロカルバジン,プレドニゾン

CLX
cloxacillin　クロキサシリン

CM
capreomycin　カプレオマイシン
carboxymethyl　カルボキシメチル
cardiac muscle　心筋
cardiomyopathy　心筋症
carpal-metacarpal (joint)　中手骨手根骨(関節)
carpometacarpal　手根中手骨
causa mortis〈ラ〉=cause of death　死因
cell membrane　細胞膜
centrum medianum〈ラ〉　中心核
cervical mucous　頸管粘液
cervical mucus　(子宮)頸部粘液
chemical mediator　化学伝達物質，化学媒体
chemotactic migration　化学遊走
Chirurgicalemagister〈独〉　外科修士
chloromycetin　クロロマイセチン
chondromalacia　軟骨軟化(症)
construction management　コンストラクションマネジメント
chylomicron　カイロミクロン，乳び球
circular measure　円形メジャー
circular muscle　輪状筋
cisterna magna　大槽
clindamycin　クリンダマイシン
clinical medicine　臨床医学
cochlear microphonics　蝸牛マイクロホン作用
commercial milk　人工栄養乳製品
congenital malformation　先天(性)奇形
continuous murmur　連続性雑音
contrast media, contrast medium　造影剤
cow milk　牛乳
culture medium　培養液
cystometry　膀胱内圧測定

cytoplasmic membrane　細胞質膜

Cm

curium　キュリウム〈元素〉
maximal urea clearance　最大尿素クリアランス
maximum urea clearance　最高尿素クリアランス

cM

centimorgans　センチモルガン〈単位〉

cm^2

square centimeter　平方センチメートル〈単位〉

cm^3

cubic centimeter　立方センチメートル〈単位〉

C.M.

Chirurgiac Magister〈ラ〉=Master of Surgery　外科修士

c.m.

cras mane〈ラ〉=tomorrow morning　翌朝《処》

C & M

cocaine and morphine　コカインとモルヒネ

CM, Cm, cm

complication　合併症

CM, cm

centimeter　センチメートル〈単位〉

CM, c.m.

costal margin　肋骨縁

Cm, Cm.

maximal clearance　最大クリアランス

CMA

Canadian Medical Association　カナダ医師会
Candida metabolic antigen　カンジダ代謝性抗原
chronic metabolic acidosis　慢性代謝性アシドーシス
cleaner microanalysis　クリーナーマイクロアナリシス
compound myopic astigmatism　複性近視性遠視
cow milk allergy　牛乳アレルギー
cylindrical mirror analyzer　円筒鏡型エネルギー分光器

CMAAC

Certified Medical Assistant Administrative and Clinical　公認医療管理・臨床助手

CMAAO

Confederation of Medical Associations in Asia and Oceania　アジアオセアニア医師会連合

C_{man}

mannite clearance　マンニットクリアランス

CMAP

compound muscle action potential　複合筋活動電位

contrast myocardial appearance picture 造影剤心筋出現図

cmAq
centimeter of water 水柱センチメートル〈単位〉

CMAS
children manifest anxiety scale 児童用不安尺度

CMAX
maximal concentration 最高血中濃度

CMB
carbolic methylene blue 石炭酸メチルブルー
chloromercuribenzoate 塩化水銀安息香酸塩

CMC
carboxymethyl cellulose カルボキシメチルセルロース
carpometacarpal (joint) 手根中手骨(間)の
cell-mediated cytotoxicity 細胞媒介性細胞障害
cervical mucous crystallization 頸管粘液結晶形成
chronic mucocutaneous candidiasis 慢性粘膜皮膚カンジダ症
closed mitral commissurotomy 非直視下僧帽弁交連切開術
critical micellar concentration 臨界ミセル形成濃度
critical micelle concentration 臨界ミセル濃度
cultured mast cell マウス培養肥満細胞
1-cyclohexyl-3-(2-morpholinyl-4-ethyl)carbodiimide metho-*p*-toluenesulfonate 1-シクロヘキシル-3-(2モルホリニル-4-エチル)カルボジイミド・メト-*p*-トルエンスルホン酸塩
cyclophosphamide, methotrexate, cyclohexylchloroethylnitrosourea シクロホスファミド,メトトレキサート,シクロヘキシルクロロエチルニトロソ尿素

cmc
chronic micellar concentration 臨界ミセル(形成)濃度

CMCC
chronic mucocutaneous candidiasis 慢性皮膚粘膜カンジダ症

CM-cellulose
carboxymethylcellulose カルボキシメチルセルロース

CMC-Na
carboxymethylcellulose sodium カルボキシメチルセルロースナトリウム

CMCT
cervical mucus contact test 子宮頸管粘液接触テスト

CMD
cartilage matrix deficiency 軟骨基質不全
cefamandole セファマンドール
childhood muscular dystrophy 小児期筋ジストロフィ
congenital muscular dystrophy 先天性筋ジストロフィ
cystoid macular vein occlusion 網膜分枝静脈閉塞症

C

CME
cervical mediastinal exploration 頸部縦隔探査
cervical mucous extract 子宮頸部粘液抽出物
continuing medical education 医師生涯教育
crude marijuana extract 粗マリファナ抽出物
cystic macular edema 嚢胞様〔状〕黄斑浮腫
cystoid macular edema 嚢胞様〔状〕黄斑浮腫

CMED
cyclophosphamide, methotrexate, etoposide, dexamethasone シクロホスファミド，メトトレキサート，エトポシド，デキサメタゾン

c.medium
cocleare medium〈ラ〉＝a half spoonful スプーン半分，半さじ《処》

CMF
Ca, Mg-free カルシウム・マグネシウムを含まない
catabolite modular factor 異化代謝産物モジュール因子
chondromyxoid fibroma 軟骨粘液線維腫
chronic myelofibrosis 慢性骨髄線維形成
cortical magnification factor 皮質拡大因子
craniomandibulofacial 頭蓋下顎顔面の
cyclophosphamide, methotrexate, 5-fluorouracil シクロホスファミド，メトトレキサート，フルオロウラシル

CMFH
cyclophosphamide, methotrexate, 5-fluorouracil, hydroxyurea シクロホスファミド，メトトレキサート，フルオロウラシル，ヒドロキシ尿素

CMFP
cyclophosphamide, methotrexate, 5-fluorouracil, prednisone シクロホスファミド，メトトレキサート，フルオロウラシル，プレドニゾン

CMFPTH
cyclophosphamide, methotrexate, 5-fluorouracil, prednisone, tamoxifen, Halotestin シクロホスファミド，メトトレキサート，フルオロウラシル，プレドニゾン，タモキシフェン，ハロテスチン

CMF-TAM
cyclophosphamide, methotrexate, 5-fluorouracil, tamoxifen シクロホスファミド，メトトレキサート，フルオロウラシル，タモキシフェン

CMFV
cyclophosphamide, methotrexate, 5-fluorouracil, vincristine シクロホスファミド，メトトレキサート，フルオロウラシル，ビンクリスチン

CMFVP
cyclophosphamide, methotrexate, 5-fluorouracil, vincristine, prednisone　シクロホスファミド，メトトレキサート，フルオロウラシル，ビンクリスチン，プレドニゾン

CMG
canine myasthenia gravis　イヌの重症筋無力症
chromogranin　色素顆粒
congenital myasthenia gravis　先天性重症筋無力症
cyanmethemogloblin　シアンメトヘモグロビン
cystometrogram　膀胱内圧測定図
cystometrography　膀胱内圧測定(法)

CMGN
chronic membranous glomerulonephritis　慢性膜性糸球体腎炎

CMH
congenital malformation of heart　心臓先天(性)奇形

CMHA
Canadian Mental Health Association　カナダ精神健康協会

CMHC
Community Mental Health Center　共同体精神健康センター

cmH_2O
centimeters of water pressure　水柱センチメートル〈単位〉

CMI
carbohydrate matabolism index　炭水化物代謝指数
cell-mediated immunity　細胞媒介免疫
chronic mesenteric ischemia　慢性腸管膜虚血
colon motility index　結腸運動係数
Commonwealth Mycological Institute　連邦微生物研究所
computer managed instruction　コンピュータ管理指導
concentration minima inhibition　最小抑制濃度
Cornell Medical Index　コーネル医学指数

CMID
cytomegalic inclusion disease　巨細胞性封入体病

c.min., c/min, c/min.
cycle per minute　サイクル/分

CMIR
cell-mediated immune response　細胞媒介免疫反応

CMJ
carpometacarpal joint　手根中手骨関節

CMK
cynomolgus monkey kidney　カニクイザルの腎

CML
canthomeatal line　外眼角耳孔線
cell mediated lympholysis　細胞介在リンパ球融解〔溶解〕(反応)

chronic myeloblastic leukemia	慢性骨髄芽球性白血病
chronic myelocytic〔myelogenous/ myeloid〕leukemia	慢性骨髄性白血病
circuit micrologic	微生物回路
clinimeal	クリニミール
cutaneous malignant lymphoma	皮膚悪性リンパ腫

cml

chemical	化学の

CMM

cutaneous malignant melanoma	皮膚悪性黒色腫
cystic medial necrosis	嚢性中心壊死

cmm, c mm

cubic millimeter	立方ミリメートル〈単位〉

CMME

carcinogenesis of chloromethylmethyl ether	クロロメチルメチルエーテルの発癌性
chloromethylmethyl ether	クロロメチルメチルエーテル

CMML

chronic myelomonocytic leukemia	慢性骨髄単球性白血病

CMMoL

chronic myelomonocytic leukemia	慢性骨髄単球性白血病

CMMS

Columbia Mental Maturity Scale	コロンビア大学知能成熟度表

CMN-AA

cystic medial necrosis of ascending aorta	上行大動脈嚢性中心壊死

CMNX

cefminox	セフミノクス

CMO

cardiac minute output	分時心拍出量
cephamandole	セファマンドル
chief medical officer	医療事務主任

cmo

centimorgan	センチモルガン

C-MOPP

cyclophosphamide, mechlorethamine, vincristine(=Oncovin), procarbazine, prednisolone	シクロホスファミド, メクロルエタミン, ビンクリスチン(=オンコビン), プロカルバジン, プレドニゾロン

CMP

cardiomyopathy	心筋症
cervical mucus penetration	子宮頸管粘液貫通
chondromalacia patellae	膝蓋軟骨軟化症
competitive medical plans	競合する医療プラン
comprehensive medical plan	包括的医療プラン
cow milk protein	牛乳蛋白

cytidine monophosphate　シチジン一リン酸

2′-CMP
cytidine 2′-monophosphate　シチジン 2′-一リン酸

3′-CMP
cytidine 3′-monophosphate　シチジン 3′-一リン酸

CMPD
chronic myeloproliferative disorder　慢性骨髄増殖性疾患

cmpd
compound　化合物

CM-Pf
centromedian-parafascicular thalamotomy　中内側傍索状視床切除

CMPGN
chronic membranoproliferative glomerulonephritis　慢性膜性増殖性糸球体腎炎

cmps
centimeter per second　センチメートル/秒

cmpt
component　成分

cmptr
computer　電子計算機，コンピュータ

CMR
cerebral metabolic rate　脳代謝率
common mode rejection ratio　同相弁別比

CMRG
cerebral metabolic rate of glucose　脳ブドウ糖代謝率

CMR glu
cerebral metabolic rate of glucose　脳ブドウ糖代謝率

CMRM
courmermycin　クーマーマイシン

CMRO$_2$
cerebral oxygen metabolic rate　脳酸素消費比率，脳酸素代謝率

CMR-O$_2$
cerebral metabolic rate of oxygen　脳酸素消費量

CMRR
common mode rejection ratio　同相弁別比

CMS
cervical mucous solution　子宮頸部粘液
Christian Medical Society　キリスト教医学協会
cochlear microphonics-spiralography　蝸牛マイクロフォニックス・スパイラログラフィ
Codex Medicamentarius Scandinavicus 〈ラ〉　スカンジナビア薬局方

cm/s
centimeters per second　センチメートル/秒

C

c.m.s
cars mane sumendus〈ラ〉=to be taken tomorrow morning　翌朝服用《処》
cm/sec
centimeters per second　センチメートル/秒
CMT
catechol(amine) *O*-methyltransferase　カテコール(アミン) *O*-メチルトランスフェラーゼ
central microtubule　中心微小管
cervical mucus test　子宮頸管粘液検査
Charcot-Maire-Tooth disease　シャルコー・マリー・トゥース病
Current Medical Terminology　現代医学用語
CMTD
Charcot-Maire-Tooth disease　シャルコー・マリー・トゥース病
CMTL
computer mediated tutorial laboratory　コンピュータによる学習システム
CMU
concentration maximale of urine　最大尿濃度
CMu
chlorophenyl-dimethylurea　クロロフェニル・ジメチルウレア
CMV
canalicular membrane vesicle　小管膜小囊
cisplatin, methotrexate, vinblastine　シスプラチン,メトトレキサート,ビンブラスチン
continuous mandatory ventilation　持続的陽圧換気
continuous mechanical ventilation　持続性機械的人工呼吸
controlled mechanical ventilation　調節式機械的換気(法)
cytomegalovirus　サイトメガロウイルス
CMX
cefmenoxime　セフメノキシム
CMZ
cefmetazole　セフメタゾール
CN
cardiac neurosis　心臓神経症
certified nurse　認定看護師
casein　カゼイン
caudate nucleus　尾状核
central nerve　中枢神経
charge nurse　委託看護師
child nutrition　小児栄養
chloroacetophenone　クロロアセトフェノン
chronic nephritis　慢性腎炎

clinical nursing　臨床看護
cochlear nucleus　蝸牛核
congenital nephrosis　先天性ネフローゼ
congenital nystagmus　先天性眼振
cranial nerve　脳神経
cyanide radical, cyanogen radical　シアン基
cyanogen　シアン
cyanosis neonatorum　新生児チアノーゼ

c.n.
cras nocte〈ラ〉=tomorrow night　翌夜《処》

C/N
carbon to nitrogen (ratio)　炭素/窒素(比)

CNA
Canadian Nurses Association　カナダ看護師協会

CNAG
chronic narrow angle glaucoma　慢性狭隅角緑内障

Cnb
caffeiinum natrium benzoicum〈ラ〉　安息香酸ナトリウムカフェイン

CNB
core needle biopsy　針生検
Central Narcotics Bureau　中央麻薬捜査局〈米国〉

CN-B_{12}
cyano-B_{12}　シアノB_{12}

CNC
Canadian National TNM Committee　カナダ国家TNM分類委員会

CN-Cbl, CNCBL
cyanocobalamin　シアノコバラミン

CNCMH
Canadian National Committee for Mental Hygiene　カナダ国家精神衛生協会

CND
Commission on Narcotic Drugs　英国麻薬委員会

CNDC
chronic nonspecific diarrhea of childhood　小児期慢性非特異性下痢

CNDI
congenital nephrogenic diabetes insipidus　遺伝性腎性尿崩症

CNE
chronic nervous exhaustion　慢性神経疲労
concentric needle electrode　同心(性)針電極

C3NeF
C3 nephritic factor　C３腎炎因子

C4NeF
C4 nephritic factor　C４腎炎因子

C

CNEL
community noise equivalent level　共同音当量レベル
CNEMG
concentric needle electromyography　同心(性)針筋電図検査(法)
CNETP
continuous negative extrathoracic pressure　胸郭外持続陰圧
CNETPV
continuous negative extrathoracic pressure ventilation　胸郭外持続陰圧換気
CNF
cyclophosphamide, mitoxantrone (= Novantrone), 5-fluorouracil　シクロホスファミド, ノバントロン, フルオロウラシル
CNH
central neurogenic hyperpnea, central neurogenic hyperventilation　中枢(性)神経(原)性過呼吸
CNHD
congenital nonspherocytic hemolytic disease　先天性非球状赤血球(性)溶血(性疾患)
CNI
cebus nigrivistatus〈ラ〉　ナキガオオマキザル
chronic nerve irritation　慢性神経刺激
CNL
cardiolipin natural lecithin　カルジオリ〔ライ〕ピン自然レシチン
CNM
Center National de Malariologie　カンボジア国立マラリアセンター
certified nurse-midwife　公認助産師
congenital nonprogressive myopathy　先天性非進行性ミオパシー
CNP
chlomitrofen　クロルニトロフェン
continuous negative pressure　持続(性)陰圧
cranial nerve palsy　脳神経麻痺
CNPase
cyclic nucleotide phosphodiesterase　環状ヌクレオチドホスホジエステラーゼ
CNPV
chest negative pressure ventilation　胸郭外陰圧補助呼吸
continuous negative pressure ventilation　持続(性)陰圧換気
CNR
composite noise rating　合成音比率
CNS
central nervous system　中枢神経系
clinical nurse specialist　専門看護師

coagulase-negative *Staphylococcus* コアグラーセ陰性ブドウ球菌

c.n.s.
cras nocte sumendus〈ラ〉=to be taken tomorrow night 明晩服用せよ《処》

CNSDC
chronic non-suppurative destructive cholangitis 慢性非化膿性破壊性胆管炎

CNS depressant
central nervous system depressant 中枢神経系抑制薬

CNSHA
congenital nonspherocytic hemolytic anemia 先天性非球状赤血球(性)溶血性貧血

CN sign
central nerve sign 脳神経徴候

CNS injury
central nervous system injury 中枢神経系損傷

CNS-L
central nervous system leukemia 中枢神経系白血病

CNSLD
chronic non-specific lung disease 慢性非特異性肺疾患

CNT
can not test 検査不能

cnt
centigram センチグラム〈単位〉

CNTF
ciliary neurotrophic factor 毛様体向神経性因子，毛様体神経栄養因子

cntn
contain 含む，相当する

CNV
colistimethate,nystatin,vancomycin コリスチメテート,ニスタチン,バンコマイシン
contingent negative variation 随伴陰性変動

CNVP cell
converted non-virus producingcell 転換性非ウイルス産出細胞

CO
candidal onychomycosis カンジダ爪(甲)真菌症
carbon monoxide 一酸化炭素
cardiac output 心拍出量
castor oil ヒマシ油
centric occlusion 中心咬合
chiasma opticum〈ラ〉 視束交叉〔差〕
choline oxidase コリンオキシダーゼ
coccygeal 尾骨の
compositus〈ラ〉 合成
compound 化合物

C

conjugata vera obstetrica〈ラ〉 産科学的真結合線
corneal opacity 角膜混濁
critical organ 決定器官
crossover (genetics) 支配・交叉〔差〕(遺伝)
cyclooxygenase シクロオキシゲナーゼ

Co
cobalt コバルト〈元素〉
compliance コンプライアンス，承諾
county 州，郡
oil of croton tiglium クロトン油

co.
composition 複方《処》
compositus〈ラ〉＝a compound 合剤《処》

^{56}Co
cobalt-56 コバルト56

^{57}Co
cobalt-57 コバルト57

^{58}Co
cobalt-58 コバルト58

^{60}Co
cobalt-60 コバルト60
cobalt therapy コバルト(60)治療

CO_2
carbon dioxide 二酸化炭素

Co_2
O_2 content 酸素含(有)量

CO，Co
coenzyme 補酵素，コエンザイム

C/O，C/o，c/o
(under the) care of 〜様方

C/O，c/o
complain of 〜の病苦〔苦痛〕を訴える

COA
coagglutination 凝集反応
condition on admission 許可条件

CoA
coenzyme A 補酵素A，コエンザイムA

C.O.A.
Canadian Orthopedic Association カナダ整形外科医協会

COA，CoA
coarctation of aorta 大動脈縮窄症

CoAAc
acetyl coenzyme A アセチル補酵素A，アセチルコエンザイムA

CoA5Ac
5-acetyl-coenzyme A — 5-アセチル補酵素A, 5-アセチルコエンザイムA

COAC
coarctation of aorta complex — 大動脈縮窄複合

COAD
chronic obstructive airway disease — 慢性閉塞性気道疾患
chronic obstructive arterial disease — 慢性閉塞性動脈疾患

COAG
chronic open angle glaucoma — 慢性開放(隅)角緑内障

coag
coagulase — コアグラーゼ
coagulate — 凝塊

COAG, coag
coagulation — 凝固

coag.time
coagulation time — 凝固時間

COAP
cyclophosphamide, vincristine (=Oncovin), arabinosylcytosine, prednisone — シクロホスファミド,ビンクリスチン(=オンコビン),アラビノシルシトシン,プレドニゾン

Coarc
coarctation of the aorta — 大動脈縮窄

CoA-SPC
coenzymc A-synthetizing protein complex — 補酵素A〔コエンザイムA〕合成蛋白複合体

coax
coaxial — 同軸の

COB
chronic obstructive bronchitis — 慢性閉塞性気管支炎
cisplatin, vincristine (=Oncovin), bleomycin — シスプラチン,ビンクリスチン(=オンコビン),ブレオマイシン

cob^{I}
cob (I) alamin — ビタミンB_{12s}

cob^{II}
cob (II) alamin — ビタミンB_{12r}

COBD
chronic obstructive bronchial disease — 慢性閉塞性気管支疾患

COBE
chronic obstructive bullous emphysema — 慢性閉塞性嚢胞性肺気腫

COBH
carboxyhemoglobin — カルボキシヘモグロビン

COBOL
common business oriented language　事務用共通処理言語，コボル《コン》

COBS
chronic organic brain syndrome　慢性器質性脳症候群

COBSI
Committee on Biological Sciences Information　生物科学情報委員会

COBT
chronic obstruction of biliary tract　慢性胆道閉塞

COC
calcifying odontogenic cyst　石灰化歯牙嚢胞
cathodal opening clonus　陰極開放性クローヌス
cathodal opening contraction　陰極開放収縮
combination-type oral contraceptive　複合型経口避妊薬
human cumulus oocyte complex　ヒト累積卵母細胞複合

coc
cocaine　コカイン

COC, Coc, coc.
coccygeal　尾骨の

COCB
closed olivocochlear bundles　閉鎖オリーブ蝸牛束

cocc
coccygeal　尾骨の
coccyx　尾骨

coch.
cochlear＝*coclear*(*e*)〈ラ〉　さじ1杯《処》

coch.amp.
cochlear amplum〈ラ〉＝a tablespoonful　さじ1杯《処》

cochl.
cochlear〈ラ〉　さじ1杯《処》

cochl.duo
cochlearia duo〈ラ〉　さじ2杯《処》

cochl.infant.
cochlear infantis〈ラ〉　茶さじ1杯《処》

cochl.mag.
cochlear magnum〈ラ〉　大さじ1杯《処》

cochl.min.
cochlear minimum〈ラ〉　小さじ1杯《処》

coch.med.
coclear medium〈ラ〉＝a dessertspoonful　小さじ1杯《処》

coch.parv.
cochlear parvum〈ラ〉＝a teaspoonful　茶さじ1杯《処》

CO/CI
cardiac output/cardiac index 心拍出量/心係数
COCL, COCI
cathodal opening clonus 陰極開放性クローヌス
COCM
congestive cardiomyopathy うっ血性心筋症
CO_2 comb
carbon dioxide combining (power) 二酸化炭素結合(力)
CO_2 content
carbon oxide content (血中)炭酸ガス含量
COCP
closed olivocochlear potential 閉鎖オリーブ蝸牛電圧
Co-Cr-Mo
cobalt-chromium-molybdenum コバルト・クロム・モリブデン〔水鉛〕
Co-Cr-W-Ni
cobalt-chromium-tungsten-nickel コバルト・クロム・タングステン・ニッケル
COCs
cumulus-oocyte complexes 卵丘細胞-卵母細胞複合体
Coct, coct.
coctio〈ラ〉=boiling 煮沸, 沸騰
COD
cause of death 死因
chemical oxygen demand 化学的酸素必要量
codeine コデイン
condition on discharge 退院時健康状態
CoD
cholesterol oxidase コレステロールオキシダーゼ
CODA
Committee on Drugs and Alcohol 薬とアルコールの委員会
CODE
Committee on Donor Enlistment 提供者協力委員会
COD-MD
cerebroocular dysplasia-muscular dystrophy 脳眼形成不全・筋ジストロフィ
cod.phos.
codeine phosphate リン酸コデイン
CODSAT
Committee on Data Science and Technology 科学技術データ委員会
coef
coefficient 係数, 率
coeff
coefficient 係数, 率

C

COEPS
cortical(ly) originating extrapyramidal system　皮質錐体外路系
COF
cause of failure　失敗の原因
cementoossifying fibroma　セメント質骨化線維腫
cut-off frequency　遮断周波数
CoF
cobra factor　コブラ因子
cofactor　共因子
Co-F
coenzyme F　補酵素F，コエンザイムF
C of A
coarctation of aorta　大動脈縮窄(症)
COFS
cerebrooculofacial-skeletal (syndrome)　脳眼顔面・骨格(症候群)
COG
center of gravity　重心
clinical obstetrics and gynecology　臨床(的)産婦人科(学)
cognitive (function tests)　認識(機能試験)
COGENE
Scientific Committee on Genetic Experimentation　遺伝子実験委員会
COGME
Council on Graduate Medical Education　卒後医療教育協議会
CO-graphy
cobalt radiography　コバルトグラフ
COGTT
cortisone oral glucose tolerance test　コルチゾン経口ブドウ糖負荷試験
COH
carbohydrate　炭水化物，糖質
COHB, COHb
carboxyhemoglobin　一酸化炭素ヘモグロビン，一酸化炭素血色素
COHgB
carboxyhemoglobin　一酸化炭素ヘモグロビン，一酸化炭素血色素
COHO
Council of Health organization　健康組織審議会
COHSE
Confederation of Health Service Employees　健康奉仕雇用者同盟

COI
central obesity index 中心肥満指数
cost of illness 病気の費用
COIMS
Council for International Organization of Medical Science 医科学国際組織委員会
coke
cocaine コカイン
COL
cost of living 生活費
Col
collagen 膠原，コラーゲン
cortisol コルチゾール
col
cola 系(統)
collateral 側副の
color 色，色彩
colored 有色(人種)の，色のついた
column 柱
COL, col
colony コロニー
col, Col
colicin コリシン
col, col.
cola〈ラ〉 濾過せよ《処》
colat
colatus〈ラ〉 濾過した《処》，挫傷した
COLD
chronic obstructive lung disease 慢性閉塞性肺疾患
colet
coletur〈ラ〉 濾過せよ《処》
coletur strain 菌株
coll
collect 収集する，採集する
collection 収集
college 大学
colloidal コロイド状の，膠様の
coll.
collyrium〈ラ〉 点眼剤《処》
collat
collateral 側副の
collat.circ.
collateral circulation 副行循環，側副血行
Colles'fx.
Colles' fracture コリーズ骨折

collod.
collodium〈ラ〉 コロジオン

collun.
collunarium〈ラ〉＝a nose wash 点鼻剤，洗鼻剤《処》

Collut.
collutorium〈ラ〉＝a mouth wash 口腔洗浄剤《処》

coll vol
collective volume 集合容積

collyr.
collyrium〈ラ〉＝an eyewash 洗眼剤《処》

color.
coloretur〈ラ〉 着色せよ《処》
colorimetry 比色分析

colost
colostomy 人工肛門形成(術)，結腸フィステル形成(術)，結腸造ろう(術)

COM
chronic otitis media 慢性中耳炎
colimycin コリマイシン
computer output microfilm コンピュータ出力マイクロフィルム
cyclophosphamide, vincristine(＝Oncovin), methotrexate シクロホスファミド,ビンクリスチン(＝オンコビン),メトトレキサート
cyclophosphamide, vincristine(＝Oncovin), methylchloroethyl-cyclohexylnitrosourea シクロホスファミド,ビンクリスチン(＝オンコビン),メチルクロロエチル-シクロヘキシルニトロソ尿素

com
comminuted 粉砕された
common 共通の
communicable 伝染(性)の
complement 補体

COMA
cyclophosphamide, vincristine(＝Oncovin), methotrexate, arabinosylcytosine シクロホスファミド,ビンクリスチン(＝オンコビン),メトトレキサート,アラビノシルシトシン

COMB
cyclophosphamide, vincristine(＝Oncovin), methylchloroethyl-cyclohexylnitrosourea, bleomycin シクロホスファミド,ビンクリスチン(＝オンコビン),メチルクロロエチル-シクロヘキシルニトロソ尿素,ブレオマイシン

comb
combination 併用
combining 結合の

COMC
carboxymethylcellulose カルボキシメチルセルロース
chlamydial outer membrane complex クラミジアの外膜複合体

COMCA
cyclophosphamide, vincristine (= Oncovin), methotrexate, cytosine arabinoside シクロホスファミド,ビンクリスチン(=オンコビン),メトトレキサート,シトシンアラビノシド

COMDEV
commonwealth development 福祉発展

comf
comfortable 快適な

COML
Consumer Organization for Medicine & Law 医療人権センター，医療と法の消費者組織

COMLA
cyclophosphamide, vincristine (= Oncovin), methotrexate, leucovorin, arabinosylcytosine シクロホスファミド,ビンクリスチン(=オンコビン),メトトレキサート,ロイコボリン,アラビノシルシトシン

comm
comminuted 粉砕された
commission 委員会，委任
committee 委員会
commonwealth 福祉
communicable 伝達できる，伝染(性)の
communication 伝達，連絡

comm.cer.
commotio cerebri〈ラ〉 脳震盪

comm dis
communication disorder 伝達障害

commin
comminuted 粉砕された

commn
commission 委員会，委任
commissioner 委員，理事

commun
communicable 伝染(病)

commun.dis
communicable disease 伝染病

C

COMP
cyclophosphamide, vincristine (= Oncovin), methotrexate, prednisone — シクロホスファミド, ビンクリスチン(=オンコビン), メトトレキサート, プレドニゾン

comp
comparable — 比較に適した，類似点のある
comparative — 比較(的)の，比較上の
compare — 比較する，対照する
compensated (heart disease) — 代償性(心疾患)
compensation — 代償，補償作用
complete — 完全な
compress — 湿布，圧迫する
compressible — 圧縮性の，圧縮できる

COMP, COMP.
compound — 化合物

COMP, comp
complaint — 病訴，愁訴，主訴
complication — 合併症

Comp., comp.
compositus〈ラ〉= composition, compound — 複方，調合《処》，組成

compar
comparative — 比較の

compd
compressed — 圧縮された，圧迫された

compd, compd.
compound — 化合物

COMPD G-11
compound G-11 — ヘキサクロロフェン

compen
compensate — 代償する
compensation — 代償，補償作用
compensatory — 代償の

compet
competition — 競合

compic
complication — 合併症

compl
complains — 病苦，不平
complementary — 補足的な，補充的な
complete — 完全な
complicated — 複雑な
complied — 訴えられた

compl, compl.
complaint — 病訴，愁訴，主訴

complications 合併症

complete A-V block

complete atrio(-)ventricular block 完全房室ブロック

complete TGA

complete transposition of great arteries 完全大血管転位〔転換〕症

Complic, complic

complications 合併症

complt

complaint 病訴，愁訴，主訴

compn

composition 組成

compo

compensation 代償，補償作用
component 構成，成分
composite 混成の，合成の，合成物
composition 合成物，著作

Compound A

11-deoxyhydrocorticosterone デオキシヒドロコルチコステロン

Compound B

corticosterone コルチコステロン

Compound E

cortisone コルチゾン

Compound F

cortisol コルチゾール

Compound S

11-deoxycortisol デオキシコルチゾール

compr

compressed 圧縮された，圧迫された
compression 圧縮，加圧，与圧，圧迫(症)

compr.

comprime〈ラ〉 圧縮せよ《処》

comprn

compression 圧縮，加圧，与圧，圧迫(症)

compu

computability 計算可能
computable 計算可能の
computation 算定数値
computer 電子計算機，計算者
computerization 電子計算機処理
computerize 電子計算機で処理する

CO_2MR

cerebral oxygen metabolic reserve 脳酸素代謝予備

C

COMS
Continuous Opacity Monitoring System — 連続不透明度監視システム
COMT
catechol *O*-methyltransferase — カテコール *O*-メチルトランスフェラーゼ
COMT inhibitor
catechol-*O*-methyltransferase inhibitor — カテコール-*O*-メチル基転移酵素阻害薬
CON
certificate of need — 必要証明書
Con
condyloma — コンジローマ
con
conservative — 保存的な
control — 対照
con.
contra〈ラ〉=against — 反対の，～に対して
Con A
concanavalin A — コンカナバリンA
CO_2 narcosis
carbon dioxide narcosis — 炭酸ガスナルコーシス，二酸化炭素ナルコーシス
conc
concentrate — 濃縮物，集中する
conclusion — 結論
conc.
concentratus〈ラ〉 — 濃厚な《処》
concisus〈ラ〉 — 細かく切った《処》
c-onc
cellular oncogene — 細胞性癌遺伝子
CONC, conc, conc.
concentrated — 濃縮された
concentration — 濃度，濃縮
concd, concd.
concentrated — 濃縮された
concentr
concentrate — 濃縮物，集中する
concentrated — 濃縮された
concentration — 濃度，濃縮
concn
concentrate — 濃縮物，集中する
concentration — 濃度，濃縮
cond
condenced — 濃縮した

condenser 蓄電器，集光レンズ，コンデンサ
condition(s) 状態，容態，条件
conduction 伝導
conductivity 伝導率

cond.milk
condensed milk 練乳

condn
condition(s) 条件，状態，容態

cond.ref
conditioned reflex 条件反射

cond.resp.
conditioned response 条件反応

conduct
conductivity 伝導率

conelrad
control of electromagnetic radiation 電子磁気放射制御

conf
conference 会議
confined 拘束した
confused 錯乱した

conf.
confectio〈ラ〉 舐剤，糖剤，糖漬菓《処》

confab
confabulation 作話症

confus
confused 錯乱した

cong.
congested うっ血した，充血した
congius〈ラ〉=gallon ガロン

CONG, cong.
congenital 先天(性)の

cong, cong.
congress 会議，大会，団体

congen
congenital 先天(性)の

coniz
conization 円錐切除(術)

conj
conjunctiva 結膜

conjug.
conjugated 共同の，共役の
conjugation 接合，共同，共役，抱合

conn
connection 結合
connective 結合の

connector 結合物

connex
connection 結合

CONPADRI I
cyclophosphamide, vincristine (= Oncovin), L-phenylalanine mustard, adriamycin シクロホスファミド,ビンクリスチン(=オンコビン),L-フェニルアラニンマスタード,アドリアマイシン

CONPADRI II
cyclophosphamide, vincristine (= Oncovin), L-phenylalanine mustard, adriamycin, methotrexate シクロホスファミド,ビンクリスチン(=オンコビン),L-フェニルアラニンマスタード,アドリアマイシン,メトトレキサート

CONPADRI III
cyclophosphamide, vincristine (= Oncovin), L-phenylalanine mustard, adriamycin, methotrexate, intensified doxorubicin シクロホスファミド,ビンクリスチン(=オンコビン),L-フェニルアラニンマスタード,アドリアマイシン,メトトレキサート,強化ドキソルビシン

cons
conservative 保存的な
consonans〈ラ〉 共振
consultant 立会い医
consultation 立会診察，他科依頼
consulting 相談

cons.
conserva〈ラ〉＝keep, save 保存せよ《処》

conserv
conservative 保存(的)の

consperg.
consperge〈ラ〉 散布せよ《処》

conspers.
conspersus〈ラ〉 散布剤《処》

const
constant 定数

constit
constituent 成分
constitution 体質，素質，構造，組成
constitutional 体質(性)の，素質(性)の

consult
consultation 立会診察，他科依頼

consv
conserve 保存する

CONT，cont.
continue　持続する，継続する

cont，cont.
contact　接触
containing　含有する，内容，含量
content　内容物
continuous　持続(性)の，連続(性)の
continuously　連続的に
contra〈ラ〉=against　反対の，～に対して
control　対照
contusus〈ラ〉　臼でついて細かくした《処》

contag
contagion　(接触)感染，(接触)伝染
contagious　感染性の，伝染性の
containing　含有する，内容，含量

contd
contained　含まれた

cont'd
continued　継続された，連続した

contemp
contemporary　同年齢の，同時代の

conter
contere〈ラ〉　すりつぶす《処》

contg
containing　含有する，内容，含量

contin.
continue〈独〉　持続する〔した〕，継続する〔した〕
continuetur〈ラ〉=let it be continued　継続させよ，継続せよ《処》

contr
contract　収縮する
contracted　萎縮した，収縮した
contraction　収縮
contracture　拘縮

contra
contraction　収縮
contraindicated　禁忌の，配合禁忌の
contraindication　禁忌，配合禁忌

contralat，contralat.
contralateral　(反)対側(性)の

cont.rem.
continuetur remedia〈ラ〉　薬を続けよ《処》

contrit.
contritus〈ラ〉　砕いた《処》

contus.
contusus〈ラ〉　臼でついて細かくした《処》

C

conv
convalescence 回復期
convalescent 回復期の
conventional 普通の，通常の
convergence 輻輳，収束
convulsion 痙攣

converg
convergence 輻輳，収束

conv.strab
convergent strabismus 輻輳斜視

coop
cooperate 協力する
cooperation 協力
cooperative 協力的な

coor
coordination 共調，協調

CoOrd，coord
coordination 共調，協調

COP
capillary osmotic pressure 毛細管浸透圧
circumoral precipitin reaction 虫卵周囲沈降反応
cisplatin(=Platinol), vincristine(=Oncovin), peplomycin シスプラチン(=プラチノール), ビンクリスチン(=オンコビン), ペプレオマイシン
colloidal osmopressure コロイド浸透圧
colloid(al) osmotic prssure コロイド浸透圧
Community Options Program 共同選択企画
cyclophosphamide, vincristine(=Oncovin), prednisone シクロホスファミド, ビンクリスチン(=オンコビン), プレドニゾン

COPA
cyclophosphamide, vincristine(=Oncovin), prednisone, adriamycin シクロホスファミド, ビンクリスチン(=オンコビン), プレドニゾン, アドリアマイシン

COP-BLAM
cyclophosphamide, vincristine(=Oncovin), prednisone, bleomycin, adriamycin, Matulane シクロホスファミド, ビンクリスチン(=オンコビン), プレドニゾン, ブレオマイシン, アドリアマイシン, マツラン

COP-BLEO
cyclophosphamide, vincristine(=Oncovin), prednisone, bleomycin　シクロホスファミド,ビンクリスチン(=オンコビン),プレドニゾン,ブレオマイシン

COPBM
cyclophosphamide, vincristine(=Oncovin), prednisone, bischloroethylnitrosourea, mechlorethamine　シクロホスファミド,ビンクリスチン(=オンコビン),プレドニゾン,ビスクロロエチルニトロソ尿素,メクロルエタミン

COPC
community-oriented primary care　共同指向初期治療

COPD
chronic obstructive pulmonary disease　慢性閉塞性肺疾患

COPE
chronic obstructive pulmonary emphysema　慢性閉塞性肺気腫
Congress on Optimum Population and Environment　適正人口と環境に関する学会
Council on Population and Environment　人口と環境の審議会

COPH
Congress of Organizations of Physically Handicapped　身体障害者組織学会

COPP
cobaltprotoporphyrin　コバルトプロトポルフィリン
coprotoporphyrin　コプロトポルフィリン
cyclophosphamide, vincristine(=Oncovin), procarbazine, prednisone　シクロホスファミド,ビンクリスチン(=オンコビン),プロカルバジン,プレドニゾン

COPRO
coproporphyria　コプロポルフィリン症

COPROgen
coproporphyrinogen　コプロポルフィリノゲン

COP test
circumoval precipitation test　虫卵周囲沈降試験

CoQ
coenzyme Q(=ubiquinone)　コエンザイム〔補酵素〕Q(=ユビキノン)

coq.
coque〈ラ〉=boil　煮沸せよ《処》

coq in sa.
coque in sufficiente aqua〈ラ〉　十分な水で煮沸せよ《処》

C

coq.s.a.
coque secundum artem〈ラ〉 正しく沸騰させよ《処》
coq.sim.
coque simul〈ラ〉 一緒に沸騰させよ《処》
COR
cardiac output recorder (心)拍出量記録器
conditioned orientation reflex 条件詮索反射
corpus〈ラ〉=body 体，骨体
cortisone コルチゾン
COR(-audiometry)
conditioned orientation response audiometry 条件詮索反応聴力検査
CoR
cobalt reaction コバルト反応
coenzyme R 補酵素R，コエンザイムR
Cor
corium 真皮
COR，Cor
coronary 冠(状)の
CoR，Cor
Congo red コンゴーレッド
cor，cor.
correct 訂正する
corrected 訂正した
correction 矯正(術)
corrective 矯正の
CORA
conditioned orientation renex audiometry 条件詮索反射聴力検査
CORD
chronic obstructive respiratory disease 慢性閉塞性呼吸器疾患
CORP
ceramics ossicular replacement prosthesis セラミック製人工耳小骨
corp.
corpori〈ラ〉 身体に《処》
corr
corrected 訂正した
correspond(ing) 対応する
correspondence 対応，手紙
CORRA
Combined Overseas Rehabilitation Relief Appeal 海外協力リハビリテーション救助要請

corrected TGA
corrected transposition of great arteries — 修正大血管転位〔転換〕症

corresp
correspond(ing) — 対応する
correspondence — 対応，手紙

corros
corrosive — 腐蝕性の

CORRP
cuff-occluded rate of rise of peripheral venous pressure — カフ圧迫時末梢静脈圧上昇率

cort, cort.
cortex〈ラ〉 — 皮質
cortical — 皮質(性)の
cortisone — コルチゾン

Cor.TGA
corrected transposition of great arteries — 修正大血管転位〔転換〕症

COS
cheirooral syndrome — 唇口症候群
controlled ovarian stimulation — 調節卵巣刺激法

cos
cosine — コサイン，余弦

cosec
cosecant — コセカント

COSM
compound streptomycin — 複合ストレプトマイシン

Cosm
osmolar clearance — 浸透圧クリアランス

COSTAR, CO-STAR
computer stored ambulatory record — コンピュータに保存された救急記録

cost resp
costal respiration — 胸式呼吸

COSY
correlation spectroscopy — 相関法，相関二次元

COT
content of thought — 思考内容
continuous oxygen therapy — 持続酸素療法

cot
cotangent — コタンジェント

CO_2T
carbon dioxide therapy — 二酸化炭素療法

cotan
cotangent — コタンジェント

C

COTD
cardiac output by thermodilution 熱希釈法による心拍出量
COTE, COTe
cathodal opening tetanus 陰極開放強直
cotics
narcotics 麻薬
COV
cross-over value 交叉〔差〕価
CoV
coronavirus コロナウイルス
CoVF
cobra venom factor コブラ毒因子
COWS
Commission on World Standard 世界標準委員会
COX
cyclooxygenase シクロオキシゲナーゼ
cytochrome oxidase チトクローム酸化酵素
Cox-V
Coxsackie virus コクサッキーウイルス
CP
caloric pattern 温度パターン
canal palsy 半規管麻痺
canal paresis 半規管機能低下
candle power 燭光
capillary pressure 毛細血管圧
cardiopulmonary 心肺の
caudate putamen 尾状被殻
cell passage 細胞通過
cell proliferation 細胞増殖
cerebral infantile palsy 脳性小児麻痺
cerebral palsy 脳性麻痺
cerebral peduncle 大脳脚
cerebral poliomyelitis 脳性灰白髄炎
chemically pure 化学的純粋
chest pain 胸痛
Child Psychiatry 小児精神医学
Child Psychology 小児心理学
child psyshiatrist 小児精神(科)医
chloramphenicol クロラムフェニコール
chloroquine and primaquine クロロキンとプリマキン
chloroquine phosphate リン酸クロロキン
chloroquinidine and primaquin クロロキニジンとプリマキン
chlorpromazine クロルプロマジン
chronic pancreatitis 慢性膵炎
chronic pyelonephritis 慢性腎盂腎炎
cicatricial pemphigoid 瘢痕(性)類天疱瘡

cisplatin シスプラチン
cisternal pressure 脳槽圧
classical pathway 古典的経路
cleft palate 口蓋(破)裂, 口蓋披裂
Clinical Pathology 臨床病理(学)
clinical psychologist 臨床心理学者
clobetasol propionate プロピオン酸クロベタゾール
cochlear potential 蝸牛電位
code of practice 医師の実践要綱
cold pressor 寒冷昇圧(の)
colloidosmotic pressure コロイド浸透圧
colorectal 結腸直腸の
combination product 複合産物
compound 化合物
constant pressure 一定圧
constrictive pericarditis 収縮性心膜炎
consultant physician 顧問医
coproporphyria コプロポルフィリン症
cor pulmonale 肺性心
C peptide Cペプチド
critical parent 批判的親
critical point 臨界点
cryptomeria pollinosis スギ花粉症
cyclophosphamide シクロホスファミド
cyclophosphamide, cisplatin (= Platinol) シクロホスファミド, シスプラチン(=プラチノール)
cyclophosphamide, prednisone シクロホスファミド, プレドニゾン
cystopathic phenomenon 細胞変性現象
cytoplasmic process 細胞質作用

Cp
chickenpox 水痘
peak concentration 最高濃度
plasma drug concentration 血漿薬物濃度

cp
codeine phosphate リン酸コデイン
compressed tablet 錠剤

6-CP
6-chloropurine 6-クロロプリン

C/P
cholesterol/phospholipid (ratio) コレステロール/リン脂質比

C & P
cystoscopy and pyelography 膀胱鏡検査と腎盂造影

CP, cp, cp.
compare 比較する

C

Cp, CP
ceruloplasmin セルロプラスミン
cP, CP
chronic polyarthritis 慢性多発(性)関節炎
cP, cp.
centipoise センチポアズ(=1/100ポアズ)〈単位〉
cp, CP
creatine phosphate クレアチンリン酸
cp, cp.
compositus〈ラ〉=composition, compound 複方，調合《処》，組成
CPA
cardiopulmonary arrest 心肺停止(状態)
carotid phonoangiography 頸動脈音血管像
cerebello(-)pontine angle 小脳橋角(部)
chlorophenylalanine クロロフェニルアラニン
chronic pyrophosphate arthropathy 慢性ピロリン酸塩関節症
coeur pulmonaire aigu〈仏〉 急性肺性心
colony promoting activity コロニー推進活動
complementary package of activities 補完的活動パッケージ
costophrenic angle 肋横角
cyclophosphamide シクロホスファミド
cyproterone acetate 酢酸シプロテロン
C3PA
complement 3 proactivator 補体第3成分プロアクチベーター
C3 proactivaror C3活性化因子前駆体
CPAg
cryptomeria pollinosis antigen スギ花粉症抗原
CPAH
sodium para-aminohippurate clearance *p*-アミノ馬尿酸ナトリウムクリアランス
CPAH, CPAH, Cpah, cpah
p-aminohippuric acid clearance *p*-アミノ馬尿酸クリアランス
CPALP
carcinoplacental alkaline phosphatase 癌胎盤性アルカリホスファターゼ
CPAP
continuous positive airway pressure 持続的気道陽圧法
CPB
cardiopulmonary bypass 心肺バイパス
celiac plexus block 腹腔神経叢ブロック
cellulose porous beads 線維素性有孔ガラス玉

chronic pulmonary berylliosis　慢性ベリリウム中毒肺
competitive protein-binding　競合蛋白結合(性)の
cyclophosphamide, cisplatin (= Platinol), bischloroethylnitrosourea　シクロホスファミド, シスプラチン(=プラチノール), ビスクロロエチルニトロソ尿素

CPBA
competitive protein-binding analysis　競合蛋白結合分析
competitive protein binding assay　競合蛋白質結合放射測定法

CPBV
cardiopulmonary blood volume　心肺血(液)量

CPC
cœur pulmonaire chronique〈仏〉　慢性肺性心
centrifugal partition chromatography　遠心分離クロマトグラフィ
cerebellar Purkinje cell　小脳プルキンエ細胞
Cerebral Palsy Clinic　脳性(小児)麻痺診療所
cetylpyridinium chloride　塩化セチルピリジニウム
chronic passive congestion　慢性受動的うっ血
clinical pathological conference　臨床病理検討会
coil planet centrifuge (method)　コイルプラネット遠心(法)

CPCR
cardiopulmonary cerebral resuscitation　心肺脳蘇生術

CPD
cephalopelvic disproportion　児頭骨盤不適合
childhood polycystic disease　小児期多嚢胞病〔疾患〕
chronic peritoneal dialysis　慢性腹膜透析
citrate-phosphate-dextrose　クエン酸リン酸ブドウ糖
congenital polycystic disease　先天性多嚢胞疾患〔病〕
contact potential difference　接触電位差
contagious pustular dermatitis　接触性膿疱性皮膚炎
cyclopentadiene　シクロペンタジエン

CPD, cpd
compound　化合物

CPDD
cisplatinum diamine dichloride　二塩化ジアミンシスプラチン

cpds
compounds　化合物

CPD solution
citrate-phosphate-dextrose solution　クエン酸リン酸ブドウ糖液

CPDX-PR
cefpodoxime proxetil　セフポドキシムプロキシチル

CPE
cardiogenic pulmonary edema　心原性肺水腫
chronic pulmonary emphysema　慢性肺気腫
complex partial epilepsy　複雑部分てんかん

corona penetrating enzyme 冠貫通酵素
cytopathic effect 細胞変性効果，細胞病変作用
cytopathogenic effect 細胞変性効果，細胞病変作用

cpe
compensation 代償

CPEHS
Consumer Protection and Environment Health Service 消費者保護と環境健康サービス

CPEO
chronic progressive external ophthalmoplegia 慢性進行性外眼筋麻痺

C-peptide
connecting peptide Cペプチド

CPF
chorioid plexus fluid 脈絡叢液

CPFX
ciprofloxacin シプロフロキサシン

CPG
capillary blood gases 毛細(血)管血液ガス

CPGN
chronic proliferative glomerulonephritis 慢性増殖性糸球体腎炎

CPH
Certificate of Public Health 公衆衛生証明書
chance proteinuria/hematuria チャンス蛋白尿・血尿
chronic persistent hepatitis 慢性持続性肝炎

cph
counts per hour カウント/時
cycle per hour サイクル/時

CPHA
Canadian Public Health Association カナダ公衆衛生学会
Commission on Professional and Hospital Activities 職業的病院活動委員会

CPHER
Calculation of Patient and Hospital Education Resources 患者と病院教育の供給源の予測

CPHL
central public health laboratory 中央検査室

CPI
California psychological inventory カリフォルニア心理検査
chemical processing industries 化学製造工業
constitutional psychopathia inferior 素質的に劣性な精神病質

CPIB
ethyl chlorophenoxyisobutyrate クロロフェノキシイソ酪酸エチル

CPIZ
cefpimizole　セフピミゾール

CPK
creatine phosphokinase　クレアチンホスホキナーゼ

CPK-MB
creatine phosphokinase muscle and brain　クレアチンホスホキナーゼMBアイソザイム
creatine phosphokinase myocardial band　クレアチン・リン酸キナーゼ心筋束

CPL
cirrhotic, progressive and lymphatic forms　CPL分類(癌の型分類)
congenital pulmonary lymphangiectasis　先天性肺リンパ管拡張症

cpl
complete　完全な

C/PL
cholesterol to phospholipid (ratio)　コレステロール/リン脂質(比)

CPLD
congenital pancreatic lipase deficiency　先天性リパーゼ欠損症

CPM
capreomycin　カプレオマイシン
cefpiramide　セフピラミド
cefpiramide sodium　セフピラミドナトリウム
central pontine myelinolysis　橋中心性髄鞘融解症
chlorpheniramine maleate　マレイン酸クロルフェニラミン
chronic progressive myelopathy　慢性進行性ミエロパシー
cisplatin (=Platinol), pepleomycin, mitomycin-C　シスプラチン(=プラチノール), ペプレオマイシン, マイトマイシンC
continuous passive motion　持続他動運動
cyclohexylchloroethylnitrosourea, procarbazine, methotrexate　シクロヘキシルクロロエチルニトロソ尿素, プロカルバジン, メトトレキサート
cyclophosphamide　シクロホスファミド

cpm
counts per minute　カウント/分
cycles per minute　サイクル/分

CPMAS
cross polarization magic-angle spin　交叉〔差〕緩和マジック角度回転法

C

CPMG
Carr-Purcell-Meiboom-Gill method カール・パーセル・メイブーム・ギル法

CPMP
Committee for Proprietary Medicinal Products 薬事委員会

CPMS
chronic progressive multiple sclerosis 慢性進行性多発性硬化症

CPMV
cowpea mosaic virus ササゲマメ・モザイクウイルス

CPN
chronic polyneuropathy 慢性多発ニューロパシー
chronic pyelonephritis 慢性腎盂腎炎
C-polymodal nonreceptor C多形式非受容器

CPOF
centroposterior orbitofrontal cortex 中後眼窩前頭皮質

CPP
cerebral perfusion pressure 脳灌流圧
cerebral precocious puberty 脳性早熟
clinical pharmacy practice 臨床薬学的業務
conditioned place preference (test) 条件付け場所嗜好(試験)
cyclopentanophenanthrene シクロペンテノフェナントレン

CPPB
constant positive-pressure breathing 持続的陽圧呼吸(法)
continuous positive-pressure breathing 持続的陽圧呼吸(法)

CPPD
calcium pyrophosphate dihydrate カルシウムピロリン酸二水和物

CPPV
continuous positive pressure ventilation 持続的陽圧換気法

CPQ
Children's Personality Questionnaire 小児人格質問表

CPR
cardiopulmonary reserve 心肺予備力
cardiopulmonary resuscitation 心肺蘇生術
cardiopulmonary resuscitator 人工蘇生器
cefpirome セフピロム
cerebral cortex perfusion rate 脳皮質灌流速度
cochleo-pupillary response 蝸牛瞳孔反応
connecting peptide immunoreactivity 結合ペプチド免疫反応
cortisol production rate コルチゾール産生率
C-peptide immunoreactivity Cペプチド免疫測定値

CPRAM
controlled partial rebreathing anesthesia method　調節部分再呼吸式麻酔法
CPRD
continuous ambulatory peritoneal dialyzer　携帯型自己腹腔透析
CPRF
Cancer and Polio Research Fund　癌とポリオ研究基金
CPRG
clinical psychopharmacology reseach group　臨床精神薬理研究会
CPRM
capreomycin　カプレオマイシン
CPRS
clinical psychopathologic rating scale　臨床的精神症状評価尺度
comprehensive psychiatric rating scale　総合的精神症状評価尺度
CPS
carbamyl phosphate synthetase　カルバミルリン酸合成酵素欠損症
cholangio(-)pancreatoscope　胆膵管鏡
coagulase-positive staphylococci　コアグラーゼ陽性ブドウ球菌
complex partial seizure　複雑部分発作
contagious pustular stomatitis　伝染性膿疱性口内炎
count per second　カウント/秒
C-polysaccharide　C多糖類
cycles per second　サイクル/秒
Cps
pseudofacility　(房水流出率の)仮性C値
cps
constitutional psychopathic state　生来性精神疾患状態
cycles per second　振動数/秒
CPSD
carbamoyl phosphate synthetase deficiency　カルバモイルリン酸合成酵素欠損症
CPSE
complex partial status epilepticus　複雑部分てんかん重積発作
CPT
capacité pulmonaire totale〈仏〉　総肺活量
carnitine palmitate transferase　脂肪酸分解酵素
carnitine palmitoyltransferase　カルニチンパルミトイルトランスフェラーゼ
carotid pulse tracing　頸動脈拍動トレーシング〔記録法〕
chest physiotherapy　胸部理学療法
cholangioscopic papillotomy　胆道鏡的乳頭切開術

C

cold pressor test	寒冷昇圧検査
cold pressure test	寒冷昇圧試験
combining power test	二酸化炭素結合力テスト
concentration performance test	有効濃度試験
continuous performance test	持続的遂行能検査

CP & T

clinical pharmacology and therapeutics	臨床薬理学と治療学

CPT deficiency

carnitine palmitoyltransferase deficiency	カルニチンパルミトイル転移酵素〔トランスフェラーゼ〕欠損症

C & P trx

cervical and pelvic traction	頸椎および骨盤牽引

CPU

central processing unit	中央演算処理装置《コン》

CPUE

chest pain of unknown etiology	原因不明胸痛

CPV

circulating plasma volume	循環血漿量
cyclophosphamide, cisplatin(=Platinol), VP-16(=etoposide)	シクロホスファミド, シスプラチン(=プラチノール), エトポシド

CPVC

common pulmonary vein cavity	共通肺静脈腔

CPVD

congenital polyvalvular disease	先天性多弁膜症

CPX

cardio pulmonary exercise test	心肺運動負荷試験

CPX, C Px

complete physical examination	(完)全理学的検査

CPZ

cefoperazone	セフォペラゾン
chlorpromazine	クロルプロマジン

CQ

carbazilquinone	カルバジルキノン
carboquone	カルボコン
chloroquine	クロロキン
chloroquine-quinine	クロロキン・キニーネ

C1q

q subunit of C1 complement	補体第1成分のサブユニットの1つ

C1qBA

C1q binding assay	C1q結合測定法

CQM

chloroquine mustard	クロロキンマスタード

CR

calculation rate	計算速度
calorie restricted	カロリー制限された
cardiac rehabilitation	心臓リハビリテーション
cardiac respiration	心(臓)呼吸
cardiac resuscitation	心(臓)蘇生(術)
cathode ray	陰極線
cephalothin	セファロチン
chest and right arm	胸部と右腕
chest roentgenogram	胸部X線像
chick rectum	小児直腸
chief resident	チーフレジデント
choice reaction	選択反応
clinical record	臨床記録
clinical research	臨床研究
closed reduction	非観血的整復
clot retraction	血餅退縮，凝血退縮
coefficient of fat retention	脂肪蓄積係数
colon resection	結腸切除(術)
colon retention	大腸停滞
complement receptor	補体レセプター〔補体受容体〕
complete regression	完全制御
complete remission	完全寛解
complete response	著効
complete round	完全円
compression ratio	圧縮率
computed radiography	コンピュータ処理X線映像法
conditioned reflex	条件反射
conditioned response	条件反応
conference room	討議室
Congo red	コンゴーレッド
controlled respiration	調節呼吸(法)
corona radiata	放線冠
cough reflex	咳嗽反射
cremaster reflex	挙睾(筋)反射，精巣挙筋反射
cresol red	クレゾールレッド
critical ratio	臨界比
crown-rump (length)	頭頂・殿部(長)
cytidine	シチジン

Cr

chromium	クロム〈元素〉
crown	(歯)冠

cr

creatine	クレアチン

cr.

cras〈ラ〉＝tomorrow	明日《処》

C3-R
receptor for third component of complement　補体第3成分受容体，補体第3レセプター

CR39
Columbia resin　コロンビア樹脂

CR，Cr，cr，cr.
creatinine　クレアチニン

CR，C-R
cardiorespiratory　心(臓)呼吸(性)の，心肺の

Cr，cr
cranial　頭蓋

CRA
Canadian Rheumatism Association　カナダリウマチ学会
central retinal artery　網膜中心動脈
Chinese restaurant asthma　中華レストラン(性)喘息
clinical research associate　治験モニタリング担当者，臨床開発担当者
chronic rheumatoid arthritis　慢性関節リウマチ
colorectal adenocarcinoma　結腸直腸線癌
colorectal anastomosis　結腸直腸吻合(術)
coronary rotational atherectomy　冠(状)動脈回転式粥腫切除術

CRABP
cellular retinoic acid binding protein　細胞内レチノイン酸結合蛋白

CRACS
Canadian Red Cross Society　カナダ赤十字社

CRAD
Committee for Research into Apparatus for Disabled　身体障害者のための器具研究委員会

CRAG
cerebral radioangiography　脳血管撮影

CRAM
card random access memory　ランダムアクセス記憶装置

CRAMPS
combined rotation and multiple-pulse spectroscopy　回転と多振動の結合した分光測定

cran
cranial　頭蓋の

crani
craniotomy　開頭(術)

craniol
craniology　頭蓋学

craniom
craniometry　頭蓋計測法

CRAO
central retinal artery occlusion　網膜中心動脈閉塞(症)

crast.
crastinus〈ラ〉 明日の《処》
CRBBB
complete right bundle branch block 完全右脚ブロック
CRBC
chicken red blood cell ニワトリ赤血球
CRBP
cellular retinol-binding protein 細胞レチノール結合蛋白
Cr & Br
crown and bridge 歯冠と架工義歯
CRC
clinical research center 臨床研究センター
clinical research coordinator 臨床研究〔試験〕コーディネーター
colorectal carcinoma 大腸癌および直腸癌
concentrated red (blood) cell 濃縮赤血球
CrCl, Crcl
creatinine clearance クレアチニンクリアランス
CRD
childhood rheumatic disease 小児期リウマチ疾患
child restraint devices 小児用座席拘束装置
chorioretinal degeneration 脈絡網膜変性(症)
chronic renal disease 慢性腎疾患
chronic respiratory disease 慢性呼吸器疾患
complete reaction of degeneration 完全電気変性反応
CRE
creatinine クレアチニン
cumulative radiation effect 放射線蓄積効果
Crea
creatinine クレアチニン
creat
creatine クレアチン
creatinine クレアチニン
C region, C-region
constant region 不変部，C領域
crem
cremasteric 精巣挙筋の
crem.
cremor〈ラ〉 クリーム
cremas
cremasteric 精巣挙筋の
crep, crep.
crepitant 捻髪音の
crepitation 捻髪音
crepitus 捻髪音

C

CREST
subcutaneous calcinosis, Raynaud's phenomenon, esophageal motility anomalities, sclerodactyly, multiple teleangiectasia (symdrome) — クレスト(＝皮下石灰沈着症・レイノー症状・食道障害・手指硬化・多発性毛細血管拡張症)(症候群)

CRF
Case Report Form — 症例報告書
chronic renal failure — 慢性腎不全
chronic respiratory failure — 慢性呼吸不全
coronary risk factor — 冠(状)動脈危険因子
corticotropin releasing factor — 副腎皮質刺激ホルモン放出因子

CRH
corticotropin releasing hormone — 副腎皮質刺激ホルモン放出ホルモン

CRI
cardiac risk index — 心臓危険指数
chronic renal insufficiency — 慢性腎不全
chronic respiratory insufficiency — 慢性呼吸不全

CRIES
Crying, Requires oxygen for saturation, Increased vital sign, Expression, Sleepless — 新生児術後痛判定用スコア

CRIP
chronic relapsing inflammatory polyradiculoneuropathy — 慢性再発性炎症性多発根ニューロパシー

crip
cripple — 肢体不自由者

CRISPRi
Clustered Regularly Interspaced Short Palindromic Repeat — クリスパー(クリスパー インターフィアランス)

crit
critical — 臨界の，分離の，危篤(的)の

crit, Crit, crit.
hematocrit — ヘマトクリット

crit.temp.
critical temperature — 臨界温度

CRL
complement receptor lymphocyte — 補体レセプター〔受容(体)〕リンパ球
crown rump length — 頭殿長

CRM
carbomycin — カルボマイシン
certificated reference material — 認証標準物質
cross-reacting material — 交叉〔差〕反応(性)物質

Crm
cream　クリーム
CRM＋
cross-reacting material positive　交叉〔差〕反応(性)物質陽性
CRM－
cross-reacting material negative　交叉〔差〕反応(性)物質陰性
cr.mane
cras mane〈ラ〉　翌朝《処》
CRMD
children with retarded mental development　精神発達遅滞児
CRMN
carumonam　カルモナム
CRN
complement-requiring neutralization test　補体要求性中和抗体試験
cRNA
chromosomal ribonucleic acid　染色体リボ核酸
complementary ribonucleic acid　相補性リボ核酸
Cr ns, cr.ns.
cranial nerves　脳神経
CRO
cathode-ray oscillograph　陰極線オシロ(グラフ)
cathode-ray oscilloscope　陰極線オシロスコープ
central retinal or vein occlusion　網膜中心静脈閉塞(症)
Clinical Research Organization　臨床試験受託機関
Contract Research Organization　開発業務受託機関
CROP
compliance, rate, oxygenation and pressure　伸展性・速度・酸素化・圧
cyclophosphamide, rubidazone, vincristine (=Oncovin), prednisone　シクロホスファミド,ルビダゾン,ビンクリスチン(=オンコビン),プレドニゾン
CROS
contralateral routing of signals hearing aid　他側送信補聴器
CRP
child resistant package　小児用耐性容器
chronic relapsing pancreatitis　慢性再発性膵(臓)炎
corneoretinal potential　角膜網膜電位
coronary rehabilitation program　冠(疾患)リハビリテーションプログラム
craniopharyngioma　頭蓋咽頭腫
C-reactive protein (test)　C反応性蛋白(試験)
cross-reacting protein　交叉〔差〕反応(性)蛋白
cyclic AMP receptor protein　サイクリックAMP受容蛋白

C9RP
C9-related protein　C 9 関連蛋白
CrP, Crp
creatine phosphate　クレアチンリン酸，リン酸クレアチン
CRPA
C-reactive protein antiserum　C反応性蛋白抗血清
CRPD
chronic restrictive pulmonary disease　慢性拘束性肺疾患
CRPF
chloroquine-resistant *Plasmodium falciparum*　クロロキン耐性熱帯熱マラリア原虫
contralateral renal plasma flow　反対側腎血漿流量
CRPL
ceruloplasmin　セルロプラスミン
CRPS
complex regional pain syndrome　複雑型局部疼痛症候群
CRPV
cottontail rabbit papillomavirus　ワタウサギパピローマウイルス
CRQ
cerebral respiratory quotient　脳呼吸比
chronic respiratory disease questionnaire　慢性呼吸器疾患質問表
CRR
canal resonance response　管共鳴反応
CRRT
continuous renal replacement therapy　持続的腎置換療法
CRS
catheter-related sepsis　カテーテル関連敗血症
caudal regression syndrome　尾側退行症候群
central supply room　中央材料室
cherry red spot　サクランボ赤色斑(点)
Chinese restaurant syndrome　中華レストラン(性)症候群
colon rectal surgery　大腸直腸外科
colorectal surgery　結腸直腸外科(学)，結腸直腸手術
compliance of the respiratory system　呼吸器系の伸展性
congenital rubella syndrome　先天性風疹症候群
counter rotation system　逆ローテーションシステム
CRSA
congenital refractory sideroblastic anemia　先天性不応性鉄芽球性貧血
CRSM
cherry red spot myoclonus (syndrome)　サクランボ赤色斑(点)筋ミオクローヌス(症候群)

CrSp
craniospinal 頭蓋脊椎の
CRST
subcutaneous calcinosis, Raynaud's phenomenon, sclerodactyly, multiple teleangiectasia (syndrome) CRST(皮下石灰沈着症,レイノー症状,手指硬化,多発性毛細血管拡張症)(症候群)
crst.
crastinus〈ラ〉 明日《処》
CRT
cardiac resuscitation team 心(臓)蘇生チーム
cathode ray tube 陰極線管
chromium release test クロム放出試験〔検査〕
complex reaction time 複合〔複雑〕反応時間
cortisone-resistant thymocyte コルチゾン耐性〔抵抗性〕胸腺細胞, コルチゾン抵抗性胸腺細胞
Crt
creatinine クレアチニン
Crt, crt
hematocrit ヘマトクリット
CR-test
C-reactive protein test C反応性蛋白検査
CRTNN
creatinine クレアチニン
CRU
cardiac rehabilitation unit 心(臓)リハビリテーション部(病棟)
clinical research unit 臨床研究単位
CRV
central retinal vein 網膜中心静脈
cr.vesp.
cras vespere〈ラ〉=tomorrow evening 明日の夕方, 明晩《処》
CRVF
congestive right ventricular failure うっ血性右(心)不全
CRVO
central retinal vein occlusion 網膜中心静脈閉塞症
Cry
cryoglobulin クリオグロブリン
cryo
cryoprecipitate 寒冷沈降物
cryotherapy 寒冷療法
cryo-Ig
cryo-immunoglobulin クリオ免疫グロブリン
crys
crystal 結晶
crystalline 透明な, 結晶性の

C

cryst

crystal	結晶
crystalline	透明な，結晶性の
crystallization	結晶化
crystallized	結晶化した

crystn

crystallization	結晶化

CS

calf serum	子ウシ血清
camptomelic syndrome	彎曲肢症候群
carcinoid syndrome	カルチノイド症候群
cardiogenic shock	心原性ショック
caries susceptible	易う蝕性
carotid sheath	頸動脈鞘
carotid sinus	頸動脈洞
catgut suture	腸線による縫合
cat scratch (disease)	ネコひっかき(病)
cavernous sinus	海綿静脈洞
celiac sprue	セリアックスプルー
central service	中心サービス
central sheath	中心鞘
central supply	中央器材室
cerebrospinal (fluid)	脳脊髄(液)
cervical spine	頸椎
cervical spondylosis	頸部脊椎症
cervical stimulation	頸部刺激
cesarean section	帝王切開術
chemical sympathectomy	化学的交感神経切除(術)
chest strap	胸(包)帯
chief of staff	主任
2-chlorobenzylidene malonenitrile	クロロベンジリデンマロノニトリル
cholesterol stone	コレステロール結石
chondroitin sulfate	コンドロイチン硫酸
chorionic somatomammotropin	絨毛性ソマトマンモトロピン
chronic schizophrenia	慢性統合失調症
chronic sinusitis	慢性副鼻腔炎
cigarette smoke (solution)	タバコ煙(溶液)
cigarette smoker	紙巻タバコ喫煙者
citrate synthase	クエン酸合成酵素
climacteric syndrome	更年期症候群
clinical (laboratory) scientist	臨床(検査)科学者
clinical stage	臨床的分類
clinical state	症状
close supervision	厳重な監視
Cockayne syndrome	コケーン症候群

colistin	コリスチン
colla sinistra〈ラ〉	左手で
Collet-Sicard (syndrome)	コレ・シカール(症候群)
completed stroke	完了した拍動
completed suicide	自殺完遂
compression syndrome	圧迫症候群
concentrated strength	凝集力
concentrated strength (of solution)	(溶液の)凝集〔濃縮〕力
conditioned stimulus	条件刺激
conditioning stimulus	条件刺激
congenital syphilis	先天(性)梅毒
conjunctival secretion	結膜分泌物
conjunctiva-sclera	結膜・強膜
conscious	意識している，意識のある
consciousness	意識
consultation service	相談サービス
contact sensitivity	接触感度
continue same (treatment)	同じ(治療を)継続せよ
continuing smoker	継続的喫煙者
continuous stripping	連続的(静脈)抜去術
contract surgeon	契約外科医
control serum	対照血清
convalescence	回復期(の)
convalescent	回復期患者
convalescent status	回復状態
corneal size	角膜の大きさ
coronary sclerosis	冠(状)動脈硬化
coronary sinus	冠(状)静脈洞
coronary suture	冠状縫合
corpus striatum	線条体
corticosteroids	コルチコステロイド
crush syndrome	圧挫症候群
cryogenics	冷凍学，低温科学
current smoker	現行喫煙者
current strength	電流強度
Cursdmann-Steinert (syndrome)	カースドマン・スタイナート(症候群)
cycloserine	シクロセリン
cyclosporin	シクロスポリン
cystoscopy	膀胱鏡検査

^{129}Cs

cesium-129	セシウム129

^{131}Cs

cesium-131	セシウム131

Cs

cell surface (antigen)	細胞表面(抗原)

C

cesium　セシウム〈元素〉
citrate synthease mitochondorial　ミトコンドリアのクエン酸合成酵素

cs
center section　中心部
cholesterol sulfate　硫酸コレステロール
chromosome　染色体

c/s
cycles per second　振動数/秒，周波数/秒

C & S
conjunctiva(e) and sclera(e)　結膜と強膜
cough and sneeze　咳とくしゃみ

c-4-s
chondroitin-4-sulfate　コンドロイチン四硫酸

CS, Cs, cs
conscious　意識のある，意識している
consciousness　意識

CS, C.S., C/S, c/s
cesarean section　帝王切開(術)
cycles per second　サイクル/秒

Cs, cs
case(s)　症例

C/S, c/s, C & S, C+S
culture and sensitivity　培養と感受性

CSA
carbonylsalicylamide　カルボニルサリチルアミド
cell surface antigen　細胞表面抗原
central sleep apnea　中枢性睡眠時無呼吸
chondroitin sulfate-A　コンドロイチン硫酸A
colony stimulating activity　コロニー形成活性
compressed spectral array　圧縮分光列
continuous subcutaneous adiminstration　持続皮下注入法
cross-sectional area　横断面

CSA, CsA
cyclosporin A　シクロスポリンA

CSAVP
cerebral subarachnoid venous pressure　脳クモ膜下静脈圧

CSB
chemical stimulation of brain　脳の化学的刺激
Cheyne-Stokes breathing　チェーン・ストークス呼吸

CSBF
coronary sinus blood flow　冠状静脈洞血流量

CSC
cigarette smoke condensate　喫煙縮合物

csc
comea-sclera conjunctiva　角膜・強膜・結膜
coup sur coup〈ラ〉　(治療薬を)少量ずつ頻繁に投与せよ《処》

CSD
cat scratch disease　ネコひっかき病

CSDH
chronic subdural hematoma　慢性硬膜下血腫

CSE
combined spinal epidural block (anesthesia)　脊椎麻酔・硬膜外麻酔併用法
common standards for quantitative electrocardiography　心電図解析標準

cse
course　経過

C/sec
cesarean section　帝王切開(術)

CSEP
cortical somatosensory evoked potentials　皮質(性)体性感覚誘発電位

CSER
cortical somatosensory evoked response　皮質(性)体性感覚誘発反応

CSF
cell surface factor　細胞表面因子
cerebrospinal fluid　(脳脊)髄液
colony stimulating factor　コロニー形成活性化因子
coronary sinus flow　冠(状)静脈洞流量
cyanide-sensitive factor　シアン感受性因子

CSFP
cerebrospinal fluid pressure　(脳脊)髄液圧

CSF-WR
cerebrospinal fluid Wassermann reaction　(脳脊)髄液ワッセルマン反応

CSGUS
Clinical Society of Genitourinary Surgeon　臨床生殖泌尿器外科医協会

CSH
chronic subdual hematoma　慢性硬膜下血腫

CSHS
carotid sinus hypersensitivity syndrome　頸動脈洞過敏症候群

CsI
caesium〔cesium〕 iodide　ヨウ化セシウム

CSI
cavernous sinus infiltration　海綿静脈洞浸潤

cholesterol saturation index コレステロール飽和指数
coronary stenosis index 冠(状)動脈狭窄指数

CSICU
cardiac surgical intensive care unit 心臓外科集中治療部〔室〕

CSII
continuous subcutaneous insulin infusion (therapy) 持続皮下インスリン注入(療法)

CSIIP
continuous subcutaneous insulin infusion pump 持続皮下インスリン注入ポンプ

CSK
cytoskeleton 細胞体質

CSL
cornsteep liquor トウモロコシ湯煎液

CSM
carotid sinus massage 頸動脈洞マッサージ
cell surface modulation 細胞表面変調
cerebrospinal meningitis (脳脊)髄膜炎
cervical spondylotic myelopathy 頸椎症性脊髄症
Committee on Safety of Medicines 薬物安全委員会

CSMA/CD
carrier sense multi-access/collision detect 一斉同時通信

CSMMG
Chartered Society of Massage and Medical Gymnastics マッサージと医学体育学の認可団体

CSN
cardiac sympathetic nerve 心(臓)交感神経
carotid sinus nerve 頸動脈洞神経
crista septi nasi〈ラ〉 鼻中隔節

CSNRT
corrected sinus node recovery time 修正洞結節回復時間

CSNS
carotid sinus nerve stimulator 頸動脈洞神経刺激(装置)

CSO
cardiac second output 毎秒心拍出量
Consumer Safety Officer 消費者安全担当官

CSOM
chronic serous otitis media 慢性漿液性中耳炎
chronic suppurative otitis media 慢性化膿性中耳炎

CSP
carotid sinus pressure 頸動脈洞圧
cell surface protein 細胞表面蛋白
cerebrospinal pressure (脳脊)髄液圧
cyclosporin シクロスポリン

C sp
cervical spine 頸椎
CS-P
chondroitin sulfate-protein コンドロイチン硫酸・蛋白

C-spine
cervical spine 頸椎
CSP test
carotid sinus pressure test 頸動脈洞圧試験
CSR
carotid sinus response 頸動脈洞反射
central supply room 中央材料室
cesarean section rate 帝王切開率
Cheyne-Stokes respiration チェーン・ストークス呼吸
Clinical Science Research 臨床試験受託機関
corrected sedimentation rate 補正赤血球沈降速度
corrected survival rate 補正生存率
cortisol secretion rate コルチゾール分泌率
CS rhythm
coronary sinus rhythm 冠(状)静脈洞リズム〔調律〕
CSS
Cancer Surveillance System 癌監視システム
carotid sinus stimulation 頸動脈洞刺激
carotid sinus syndrome 頸動脈洞症候群
chewing, sucking, swallowing 咀嚼・吸入〔吸引〕・嚥下
chronic subclinical scurvy 慢性潜伏性壊血病
Churg-Strauss syndrome チャーグ・ストラウス症候群
coronary sinus stimulation 冠(状)静脈洞刺激
cranial sector scan 脳セクター〔扇形〕スキャン
CSSDC
Canadian Society for Study of Diseases in Children カナダ小児疾患研究学会
CSSP
Center for Studies of Suicide Prevention 自殺予防研究センター
CST
cavernous sinus thrombosis 海綿静脈洞血栓症
contraction stress test 子宮収縮負荷試験
convulsive shock therapy 痙攣ショック療法
static compliance 静(的)肺コンプライアンス
cSt
centistoke センチストーク〈単位〉
CS-T
cerulein-secretin test セルレイン・セクレチン試験
CSU
catheter specimen of urine カテーテル採取尿

C

CSV
crista supra ventricle　室上稜
crista supraventricularis　室上稜

CSW
commercial sex worker　商業的性労働者

CSWS
epilepsy with continuous spike waves during slow wave sleep　徐波睡眠時に持続性棘徐波を示すてんかん

CT
calcitonin　カルシトニン
calf thymus　仔ウシ胸腺
carboxyl-terminal　C末端
cardiothoracic (ratio)　心(臓)胸郭(比)
carpal tunnel　手根トンネル，手根管
celiac trunk　腹腔動脈
cellular therapy　細胞治療
cerebral thrombosis　脳血栓症
cerebral tumor　脳腫瘍
chemotaxis　化学走性
chemotherapy　化学療法
Chlamydia trachomatis　トラコーマクラミジア
chlorothiazide　クロロチアジド
cholera enterotoxin　コレラ腸毒素
cholera toxin　コレラ毒素
cholesterol total　総コレステロール血清中
chorda tympani　鼓索
chymotrypsin　キモトリプシン
circulating time　循環時間
clinical technologist　臨床検査技師
closed thoracotomy　閉鎖式開胸術
clotting time　凝固時間
coagulation time　凝固時間
coated tablet　被覆加工錠
cobra toxin　コブラ毒素
cognitive therapy　認知療法
collecting tubule　集合管
compressed tablet　圧縮錠(剤)
computed tomography　コンピュータ断層撮影(法)
computed topography　コンピュータ局所像
computerized tomography　コンピュータ断層撮影(法)
conduction time　伝導時間
congnitive therapy　認知療法
connective tissue　結合組織
contraceptive techniques　避妊技術，避妊手技
contraction time　収縮時間
Coombs test　クームス試験

corneal transplant　角膜移植(片)
coronary thrombosis　冠(状)動脈血栓
corrective therapist　矯正治療士
cover test　遮蔽試験
craniotabes　頭蓋癆(＝ろう)
cytotoxicity (test)　細胞毒性(試験)
cytotrophoblast　細胞栄養層
total lung/thorax compliance　全肺胸部コンプライアンス

ct
carat　カラット〈単位〉
chromatid　染色分体
count　計算

CT-1824
clearance test of Evans blue　エバンスブルー・クリアランス試験

C/T
cardiothoracic ratio　心胸比

CTA
Canadian Tuberculosis Association　カナダ結核病学会
cellulose triacetate　セルローストリアセテート
chemotactic activity　化学走性活性
chromotropic acid　クロモトロープ酸
computerized tomographic angiography　CT断層撮影による血管造影法
cortical taste area　皮質味領域
cor triatriatum〈ラ〉　三心房心
cyproterone acetate　酢酸シプロテロン
cystine trypticase agar medium　シスチントリプチケース寒天培地
cytotoxic assay　細胞傷害試験
lymphocytotoxic assay　リンパ球毒素検定

CTa, Cta, cta
catamenia〈ラ〉＝menstruation　月経

CTAB
cetyltrimethyl ammonium bromide　セチルトリメチル臭化アンモニウム

CTAC
cetyltrimethyl ammonium chloride　セチルトリメチル塩化アンモニウム

c.tant.
cum tanto〈ラ〉＝with the same amount of　～と同量の，～と一緒に

CTAP
CT during arterial portography　門脈造影下CT

CTAR
cardiothoracic area ratio　心胸郭面積比

C

CTC
chlortetracycline クロルテトラサイクリン
clinical therapeutic conference 症例治療検討会
concentration to control 抑制濃度
Counter Terrorism Committee テロ対策委員会
cultured T cell 培養T細胞

CTCAE
common terminology criteria for adverse events 有害事象共通用語集

CTCL
cutaneous T cell leukemialymphoma 皮膚T細胞白血病リンパ腫
cutaneous T cell lymphoma 皮膚T細胞リンパ腫

CTD
carpal tunnel decompression 手根管減圧(術)
chest tube drainage 胸管留置管排液
circulation time descending 循環時間延長
congenital thymic dysplasia 先天性胸腺異形成(症)
connective tissue disease 結合組織病〔疾患〕，膠原病
Corrective Therapy Department 矯正治療部
critical test dilution 臨界テスト希釈度
cumulative trauma disorder 蓄積外傷疾患

ctd
coated 被覆された

CT-D
computed tomography-discography CTディスコグラフィ

CTDF
cytotoxic T cell differentiation factor 細胞傷害性T細胞分化因子

CTE
calf thymus extract 仔ウシ胸腺抽出物
cultured thymic epithelium 培養胸腺上皮

CTEM
conventional transmission electron microscope 通常の透過型電子顕微鏡

C-terminal
carboxyl-terminal C末端

CTF
certificate 証明書
Colorado tick fever コロラドダニ熱
cytotoxic factor 細胞毒性因子

CTF virus
Colorado tick fever virus コロラドダニ熱ウイルス

CTG
cardiotocoergogram 胎児心拍数陣痛図
cardiotocoergograph 胎児心拍数陣痛計

CTGA
corrected transposition of great arteries　修正大血管転位
ct gr
centigram　センチグラム〈単位〉
CTH
ceramide trihexoside　セラミドトリヘキソシド
Cthio
sodium thiosulfate clearance　チオ硫酸ナトリウムクリアランス
CTI
cerebral thermal index　脳内温度増加指数
CTL
cercocebus torquatus lunulatus〈ラ〉　シロエリマンガベイ
cytotoxic T lymphocyte　細胞傷害性Tリンパ球
ctl
central　中心の
control　管理
CTLL
cutaneous T cell lymphoma　皮膚T細胞リンパ腫
CTLO
cervicothoracolumbar orthosis　頸・胸・腰椎装具
CTLSO
cervicothoracolumbosacral orthosis　頸・胸・腰仙椎装具
CTM
cardiotachometer　カルジオタコメータ
cefotiam　セホチアム
computed tomographic myelography　脊髄コンピュータ断層撮影法
connective tissue massage　結合組織マッサージ
cricothyroid membrane　輪状甲状軟骨間膜
cricothyroid muscle　輪状甲状筋
cytotoxic medium　細胞傷害試験培地
CTMC
connective tissue mast cells　結合織肥満細胞
CTM-HE
cefotiam hexetil　セホチアムヘキセチル
CTMM
computed tomographic metrizamide myelography　コンピュータ断層(撮影)メトリザマイド脊髄撮影(法)
CTNNB1
catenine beta 1　カテニンβ1
CTO
cerebral thromboangitis obliterans　脳閉塞性血栓動脈炎
cervicothoracic orthosis　頸・胸椎装具
CTox
cholera toxin　コレラ菌毒素

C

CTP
C terminal peptide　C末端ペプチド
cytidine triphosphate　シチジン三リン酸
CT-P
computed tomography-peridurography　CTペリドログラフィ
CTPP
cerebral tissue perfusion pressure　脳組織灌流圧
CTR
cardiothoracic ratio　心胸郭比，心胸郭係数
clinical trial report　治験総括報告書
ctr
center　中心，センター
CTRX
ceftriaxone　セフトリアキソン
C trx
cervical traction　頸椎牽引
CTS
Canadian Thoracic Society　カナダ胸部疾患学会
carpal tunnel syndrome　手根管症候群
computed thermography system　コンピュータサーモグラフィシステム
contralateral thresshold shift　対側閾値移動
corticosteroid　コルチコステロイド
CT scan
computerized tomographic scan　X線コンピュータ断層撮影
CTT
cefotetan　セホテタン
central tegmental tract　中心被蓋路
central transmission time　中枢伝導時間
compressed tablet triturate　圧縮錠剤粉末
computerized transaxial tomography　コンピュータ断層撮影(法)
CTU
centigrade thermal unit　摂氏温度単位
CTV
cervical and thoracic vertebrae　頸(椎)胸椎
CTW
central terminal of Wilson　ウィルソン中枢回路
CTX
cefotaxime　セホタキシム
cerebrotendinous xanthomatosis　脳腱黄色腫症
chemotaxis　化学走性
CTx
cardiac transplantation　心(臓)移植
CTX，Ctx
cyclophosphamide　シクロホスファミド

Ctx-Plat
cyclophosphamide-Platinol　シクロホスファミド・プラチノール

CTZ
ceftezole　セフテゾール
chemoreceptor trigger zone　化学受容器引金帯
chlorothiazide　クロロチアジド
chlorotriazine　クロロトリアジン

CU
cause unknown　原因不明
chymotrypsin unit　キモトリプシン単位
clinical unit　臨床単位
colitis ulcerosa〈ラ〉　潰瘍性大腸炎
contact urticaria　接触蕁麻疹
cytotoxicity unit　細胞傷害性単位

Cu
cuprum〈ラ〉＝copper　銅〈元素〉
urea clearance　尿素クリアランス

cu, cu.
cubic　立方の，立方体の

CUA
cost-utility analysis　費用対効用分析

Cua
uric acid clearance　尿酸クリアランス

CuB
copper band　カッパーバンド

CUC
chronic ulcerative colitis　慢性潰瘍性大腸炎

cu cm
cubic centimeter　立方センチメートル〈単位〉

CUD
cause undetermined　原因不明
congenital urinary tract deformities　先天性尿路変形，先天性尿路奇形

CUDAT
clinically undiagnosed active tuberculosis　臨床的診断未確定の活動性結核

cu ft, cuft
cubic foot　立方フット〔フィート〕

CUG
cystourethrogram　膀胱尿道造影〔撮影〕図

cu in
cubic inch　立方インチ〈単位〉

cult
culture　培養

C

C

cum
cumulative　蓄積の，累積の
cu m
cubic meter　立方メートル〈単位〉
cu mm
cubic millimeter　立方ミリメートル〈単位〉
cu μm
cubic micrometer　立方マイクロメートル〈単位〉
CUNSA
Canadian University Nursing Students Association　カナダ大学看護学生協会
CUPI
cholesterol uric acid phospholipid index　コレステロール尿酸リン脂質指数
CUPP
college & university partnership program　大学間教育交流プログラム
CUPS
carcinoma of unknow primary site　原発巣不明癌
cur
curative　治療の
current　電流，流動，現在の
curat.
curatio〈ラ〉　包帯
CURE
Care, Understaning, Research　看護・理解・研究
Curea
urea clearance　尿素クリアランス
CUS
catheterized urine specimen　カテーテル尿残渣
contact urticaria syndrome　接触蕁麻疹症候群
CUSA
Cavitron Ultrasonic Surgical Aspirator　超音波手術吸引装置，キューサー
CUT
chronic undifferentiated type (schizophenia)　慢性未分化型(統合失調症)
cover-uncover test　覆い・覆い取り試験
cutdown
cutdown on vein　静脈切開
CUTS
cubital tunnel syndrome　肘管症候群
cu yd
cubic yard　立方ヤード〈単位〉
CV
capacité vitale〈仏〉　肺活量

carcinoma ventriculi　胃癌
cardiac volume　心(臓)容量
cardiovascular　心(臓)血管の
cell volume　細胞体積，細胞容積
central vein　中心静脈
central venous　中心静脈の
central venous injection　中心静脈注射
cerebrovascular　脳血管(性)の
cervical vertebrae　頸椎
champ visuel〈仏〉　視野
cisplatin, Vepesid　シスプラチン，ベペシド
closing volume　閉鎖容積，クロージングボリュウム
coated vesicle　被覆小胞
coefficient of variation　変動係数
color vision　色視
concentrated volume　濃縮容積
conducting veins　伝導静脈
conduction velocity　伝導速度
conjugata vera〈ラ〉＝true conjugate　真結合線
conventional cuprophane dialyzer　在来型血液透析
conventional ventilation　従来の換気法
conversational voice　会話音声
coronary vein　胃冠(状)静脈
corpuscular volume　赤血球容積
cortical vision　皮質視覚
costovertebral　肋椎の，肋骨脊柱の
coxa vara〈ラ〉　内反股
coxsackie virus　コクサッキーウイルス
cresyl violet　クレシールバイオレット
crusus vitae〈ラ〉　生活歴
crystal violet　クリスタルバイオレット
curriculum vitae　履歴(書)
cutaneous vasculitis　皮膚血管炎
specific heat at constant volume　定容量における比熱

cv
concave　へこんだ，凹面の

4CV
four chamber view　四腔断面

C/V
coulomb per volt　クーロン/ボルト

CV，c.v.
cras vespere〈ラ〉＝tomorrow evening　明日の夕方，明晩《処》

CVA
cerebrovascular accidents　脳血管発作〔障害〕
clavulanic acid　クラブラン酸

C

costovertebral angle 脊柱角
cyclophosphamide, vincristine, adriamycin シクロホスファミド,ビンクリスチン,アドリアマイシン

C

CVA, cva
costovertebral angle 肋骨脊柱角

CVAA
Catford visual activity apparatus キャットフォード視力測定器

CVA/AMPC
clavulanic acid/amoxicillin クラブラン酸/アモキシシリン

CVAAS
cold-vapor generation atomic absorption spectrometry 水銀の還元・気化原子吸光分析

CVA-BMP
cyclophosphamide, vincristine, adriamycin, bischloroethylnitrosourea, methotrexate, procarbazine シクロホスファミド,ビンクリスチン,アドリアマイシン,ビスクロロエチルニトロソ尿素,メトトレキサート,プロカルバジン

CVAH
congenital virilizing adrenal hyperplasia 先天性男性化副腎過形成(症)

C-value
coefficient of aqueous outflow 房水流出率

CVAT
costovertebral angle tenderness 肋骨脊柱角叩打痛

CVA tend.
costovertebral angle tenderness 肋骨脊柱角叩打痛

CVA/TIPC
clavulanate/ticarcillin クラブラン/チカルシリン

CVB
cyclohexylchloroethylnitrosourea, vinblastine, bleomycin シクロヘキシルクロロエチルニトロソ尿素,ビンブラスチン,ブレオマイシン

CVC
central venous catheter 中心静脈カテーテル
constant vowel consonant 不変母音・子音

CV cath
central venous catheter 中心静脈カテーテル

CVCT
cardiovascular computed tomography 心(臓)血管コンピュータ断層撮影

CVD
cardiovascular disease 心(臓)血管疾患
cardiovascular dysfunction score 心(臓)血管機能障害スコア

cerebrovascular disease 脳血管疾患
chemical vapor deposition 化学気相成長法
clavulanic acid クラブラン酸
collagen vascular disease 膠原病
color-vision-deviant 色盲
combined valvular disease 連合弁膜症
congenital valvular disease 先天性心臓弁膜症
continuous ventricular drainage 持続脳室ドレナージ

CVD, cvd
curved 彎曲した

CVE
cerebrovaskulare Erkrankungen〈独〉 脳血管障害

CVEB
cisplatin, vinblastine, etoposide, bleomycin シスプラチン, ビンブラスチン, エトポシド, ブレオマイシン

CVF
cardiovascular failure 心(臓)血管不全
central visual field 中心視野
cervicovaginal fluid 頸(部)腟液
cobra venom factor コブラ毒因子

CVG
cerebral venography 脳静脈撮影
cerebral ventriculography 脳室造影

CVH
combined ventricular hypertrophy 両室肥大
common variable hypogammaglobulinemia 分類不能型低免疫グロブリン血症

CVHD
chronic valvular heart disease 慢性弁膜性心疾患

CVI
cerebrovascular insufficiency 脳血管不全(症)
check valve index 呼気閉塞指数

CVID
common variable immunodeficiency 原発型〔分類不能型〕免疫不全症
complete, verifiable and irreversible dismantlement 完全かつ検証可能で不可逆的な解体

C virus, C-virus
coxsackievirus コクサッキーウイルス

CVM
cardiovascular monitor 心(臓)血管モニター
Center for Veterinary Medicine 動物薬センター
cyclophosphamide, vincristine, methotrexate シクロホスファミド, ビンクリスチン, メトトレキサート

C

CVO
central vein occlusion 中心静脈閉塞(症)
conjugata vera obstetrica〈ラ〉= obstetric conjugate 産科学的真結合線

CVOD
cerebrovascular obstructive disease 脳血管閉塞性疾患
corporal veno,occlusive dysfunction 静脈性閉塞性性機能障害

CVP
central venous pressure 中心静脈圧
cyclophosphamide,vincristine, prednisone シクロホスファミド,ビンクリスチン,プレドニゾン

CVPA
cyclophosphamide,vincristine, prednisone,adriamycin シクロホスファミド,ビンクリスチン,プレドニゾン,アドリアマイシン

CVPD
cyclophosphamide,vincristine, prednisone,daunorubicin シクロホスファミド,ビンクリスチン,プレドニゾン,ダウノルビシン

CVPP
cyclophosphamide,vincristine, prednisone,procarbazine シクロホスファミド,ビンクリスチン,プレドニゾン,プロカルバジン

CVR
caloric vestibular reaction 前庭温熱刺激反応
cardiovascular renal 心(臓)血管腎性の
cardiovascular resistance 心(臓)血管抵抗
cardiovascular-respiratory (system) 心(臓)血管呼吸器(系)
cerebral vascular reactivity 脳血管反応性
cerebrovascular resistance 脳血管抵抗
coronary vascular resistance 冠血管抵抗

CVRD
cardiovascular renal disease 心(臓)血管腎疾患

CVRR
cardiovascular recovery room 心(臓)血管回復室

CVS
cardiovascular surgery 心(臓)血管外科(学)
cardiovascular system 心(臓)血管系
challenge virus standard 攻撃ウイルス基準
chorionic villus sampling 絨毛穿刺
clean voided specimen 非汚染〔無菌的〕排泄検体
closing valve sound 閉鎖時弁音

CVSMC
cultured vascular smooth muscle cell 培養血管平滑筋細胞

CV starus
cardiovascular status 心(臓)血管状態

C

CVTR
charcoal viral transport medium — チャコールウイルス移送培養液

CVVH
continuous veno-venous hemofiltration — 持続的静脈・静脈血液濾過

CW
cardiac work — 心仕事
caseworker — ケースワーカー
cell wall — 細胞壁
ceruminal water — 耳垢水
chemical warfare — 化学戦
chemical weapon — 化学兵器
chest wall — 胸壁
children's ward — 小児病棟
Christian-Weber (syndrome) — クリスチャン・ウェーバー(症候群)
continuous waves — 連続波
crutch walking — 松葉杖歩行

C/W
compare with — ～と比較せよ
consistent with — ～と一致する，～と両立する

CW，cw
clockwise — 時計回りの，右回りの

CWAP
children women aged patient — 災害弱者

CWBTS
capillary whole blood true sugar — 毛細血管全血の真性血糖

CWD
cell wall dialysis — 細胞壁透析
cell-wash dialysis — 細胞洗浄透析
continuous wave Doppler — 連続波ド(ッ)プラー法

C'wealth
common wealth — 社会福祉

CWG
constant wear garment — 生体現象記録装置システム

CWHB
citrated whole human blood — クエン酸処理ヒト全血

CWI
cardiac work index — 心仕事係数

CWL
cutaneous water loss — 皮膚水分喪失

CWOP
childbirth without pain — 無痛分娩

CWP
childbirth without pain — 無痛分娩

coal workers pneumoconiosis 石灰塵肺
cotton wool patch 綿花状白斑

CWPEA
Childbirth without Pain Education Association 無痛分娩教育協会

CWPL
Childbirth without Pain League 無痛分娩連盟

CWS
cell wall skeleton 細胞壁骨格
cold water soluble 冷水溶性の
corticosteroid withdrawal syndrome ステロイド離脱症候群

cws
clockwise 時計回りの，右回りの

CWT
cold water treatment 冷水治療

cwt
hundred weight 100ポンド

CX
cerebral cortex 大脳皮質
chest X-ray 胸部X線
circumflex coronary artery 回旋枝
cloxacillin クロキサシリン
cyclohexamide シクロヘキサミド

Cx
clearance クリアランス
complex 複合体，コンプレックス

cx
cylinder axis 軸索

CX, Cx, cx.
cervical 頸(部)の
cervix 頸(部)
convex 凸(形)の，凸面の

CXD
cefroxadine セフロキサジン
computed X-ray densitometry コンピュータによるX線濃度測定
cycloheximide シクロヘキサミド

CXM
cefuroxime セフロキシム

CXM-AX
cefuroxime-axetil セフロキシムアキセチル

CXR
chest X-ray (film) 胸部X線(フィルム)

CY
calendar year 暦年
current year 通用年

cyclophosphamide シクロホスファミド

Cy

cyanamide シアナミド

cyst 嚢胞，嚢腫

cytarabine シタラビン

cy

capacity 収容力，容積

cyanosis チアノーゼ

cyanotic チアノーゼの

cycle 周期，周波数

cyclosporin シクロスポリン

CY，Cy，cy

cyanogen シアン

CY，cy

copy コピー

CYA

cyclosporin A シクロスポリンA

CyADIC

cyclophosphamide, adriamycin, dimethyltriazenoimidazole carboxamide シクロホスファミド，アドリアマイシン，ジメチルトリアゼノイミダゾールカルボキサミド

cyan

cyanosis チアノーゼ

cyanotic チアノーゼの

cyath.

cyathus〈ラ〉 コップ1杯《処》

cyath.vin.

cyathus vinarius〈ラ〉=a wineglass ワイングラス1杯《処》

cyath.vinos.

cyathus vinosus〈ラ〉=wineglass ワイングラス1杯《処》

CYC

cyclophosphamide シクロホスファミド

cyc

cyclazocine シクラゾシン

cycle サイクル

CYC，cyc

cyclotron サイクロトロン

Cyc-IVH

cyclic intravenous hyperalimentation 周期的経静脈高カロリー輸液

CYCLO，Cyclo

cyclophosphamide シクロホスファミド

CYCLO，Cyclo，cyclo

cyclopropane シクロプロパン

CyD

cyclodextrin サイクロデキストリン

C

Cyd
cytidine シチジン
Cyd 5′-P
cytidine 5′-monophosphate シチジン 5′-一リン酸
Cyd 5′-P2
cytidine 5′-diphosphate シチジン 5′-二リン酸
Cyd 5′-P3
cytidine 5′-triphosphate シチジン 5′-三リン酸
CYE
charcoal-yeast extract チャコール・イースト抽出物
CyHOP
cyclophosphamide, Halotestin, vincristine(=Oncovin), prednisone シクロホスファミド,ハロテスチン,ビンクリスチン(=オンコビン),プレドニゾン
CyIg
cytoplasmic immunoglobulin 細胞質免疫グロブリン
cyl
cylinder 円柱
cylindrical lens 円柱レンズ
CYN
cyanide シアン化物
CYP
cyanofenphos シアノフェンホス
cytochrome P450 チトクロームP450
CYS
cystoscopy 膀胱鏡検査
Cys
cystathionine シスタチオニン
cysteine システイン
cystine シスチン
Cyst
cysteamine システアミン
Cysto, cysto.
cystogram 膀胱造影〔撮影〕図
cystoscope 膀胱鏡
cystoscopic 膀胱鏡の
cystoscopy 膀胱鏡検査
CYT
cytochrome チトクローム
Cyt
cytoplasm 細胞質
cytosine シトシン
cytol
cytological 細胞学的な
cytology 細胞学，細胞診断学

cyt.sys.
cytochrome system　チトクローム系
CY-VA-DIC
cyclophosphamide, vincristine, adriamycin, dimethyltriazenoimidazole carboxamide　シクロホスファミド,ビンクリスチン,アドリアマイシン,ジメチルトリアゼノイミダゾールカルボキサミド
CZ
carzinophilin　カルジノフィリン
cefazolin　セファゾリン
CZE
capillary zone electrophoresis　毛細管領域電気泳動法
CZI
crystalline zinc insulin　結晶(性)亜鉛インスリン
CZN
central zonal necrosis　中央帯壊死
CZON
cefuzonam　セフゾナム
CZP
capillary zone electrophoresis　毛細管領域電気泳動法
clonazepam　クロナゼパム
CZX
ceftizoxime　セフチゾキシム

D d

D

aspartic acid	アスパラギン酸
dead space	死腔
dead space gas	死腔気
degree of curve	彎曲度
dendrite	樹状突起
depression	うつ病
dermatologist	皮膚科医
dermatology	皮膚科学
descending colon	下行結腸
deuterium	ジュウテリウム，重水素
developing	現象
deviatio〈ラ〉=deviation	偏位，偏差，偏視
dextrogration	右旋性
dextrorotation	右旋性
dextrose	(右旋性)ブドウ糖
Diagnose〈独〉=diagnosis	診断
diagnostic plan	診断計画
diaphragm	横隔膜
diastole	拡張期，弛緩期
diathermy	ジアテルミー
didymium	ジジム〈元素〉
difference	差，較差
diffuse	広汎性の，び漫性の
diffusing capacity	拡散量，拡散能(力)
diffusing capacity in general	全身ガス拡散能力
diffusion coefficient	拡散係数
diffusion constant	拡散定数
dihydrouridine	ジヒドロウリジン
diopter	ジオプトリー，屈折度〈単位〉
Diphyllobothrium	裂頭条虫(属)
Diplococcus	双球菌(属)
disease	病気，疾患
dispense	投薬する，調剤せよ《処》
diverticulum	憩室
dog	犬，イヌ
dominant	優性の
donor	提供者
dorsal	背部の
dorsal vertebrae	胸椎
doublet	核共鳴時の
Dracunculus	ドラクンクルス(属)
drive	衝動，動因，欲求

drive or drive state	本能的行動またはそれを引き起こさせる状態
drug	薬
dual	二重の
ductus	管
duodenum	十二指腸
dwarf	矯小体軀(症)，小人
dwarf type colony	矮小型コロニー
factor D=C_3 proactivator convertase	活性化D因子=補体第3成分プロアクチベータ転換酵素
mean dose	平均用量，平均線量
vitamin D	ビタミンD

d

deci-	デシ(=10^{-1},1/10)〈接〉
decimus〈ラ〉	10番目の
definite	明確な，厳密な
depth	深さ
diarrhea	下痢
differentiation	分化
diurnal	昼間の，日内の
doctor	博士，医師
doubtful	疑わしい
dyne	ダイン
specific gravity	比重

D

absorbed dose	吸収量

1/d

once a day	1日1回《処》

1,25(OH)$_2$D$_3$

1,25-dihydroxycholecalciferol	1,25-ジヒドロキシコレカルシフェロール

2/d

twice a day	1日2回《処》

×2d〔3d,…〕

times two days〔three days,…〕	×2日〔3日,…〕

2,4-D

2,4-dichlorophenoxyacetic acid	2,4-ジクロロフェノキシ酢酸

4×d

four times a day	1日4回《処》

7D

seven D=①birth defect,②abnormal development,③behavioral deviations,④neurological disorder,⑤immunodeficiencies,⑥generalized debilitation,⑦premature death	7つのD=①出生欠陥 ②異常発達 ③行動偏倚 ④神経異常 ⑤免疫不全 ⑥全身無気力 ⑦早産死

24,25(OH)$_2$D$_3$
24,25-dihydroxycholecalciferol — 24,25-ジヒドロキシコレカルシフェロール

D$_1$〔D$_2$,D$_3$…〕
first〔second, third…〕 dorsal vertebra etc. — 第1〔2,3…〕胸椎など

D

D$_2$
ergocalciferol＝vitamin D$_2$ — エルゴカルシフェロール＝ビタミンD$_2$

D$_3$
cholecalciferol＝vitamin D$_3$ — コレカルシフェロール＝ビタミンD$_3$

D37
37% survival dose — 37%生存線量

D860
tolbutamide — トルブタマイド

D/3
distal third — 遠位部1/3区

/d
daily — 毎日の
per day — /日《処》

D, d
Damen〈独〉＝daughter — 娘
date — 日付，年月日
day(s) — 日
deceased — 死亡した，故人
degree — 度，学位
dextrorotatory — 右旋性(の)
divorced — 離婚した

D, d.
da〈ラ〉＝give — 与える
dead — 死
death — 死んだ，無感覚の
deciduous — 脱落(性)の，落葉の
density — 密度
detur〈ラ〉＝let it be given — 与えよ《処》
diameter — (直)径
died — 死亡した
dies〈ラ〉 — 日，命日，期間
distal — 遠位の
dorsal — 背側の，背(面)の
doses〈ラ〉＝doses — 服用量，分量，線量〈複数〉《処》
dosis〈ラ〉＝a dose — 服用量，分量，線量《処》
duration — 持続

D, d, *d*
deuteron　重陽子

DA
dark adaptation　暗順応
degenerative arthritis　変形性関節炎
delayed action　遅延作用
deoxyadenosine　デオキシアデノシン
developmental age　発達年齢
diabetic amyotrophy　糖尿病性筋萎縮症
digital-analog (conversion)　デジタル・アナログ(変換)
diphenylchlorarsine　ジフェニルクロルアルシン
dopaminergic　ド(ー)パミン作用(性)
drug addict　薬物嗜癖
ductus arteriosus　動脈管

Da
Dalton　ダルトン〈単位〉

da
day　日
deca-　デカ(＝×10)〈接〉

D.A.
Diploma in Anesthetics　麻酔資格認定書

D/A
date of accident　事故(年月)日
date of admission　入院(年月)日
digital-to-analog (ratio)　デジタル/アナログ(比)

DA, Da
direct access　直接閲覧
dopamine　ド(ー)パミン

DA, D.A.
developmental age　発育年齢

Da, da, da.
daughter　娘

DAA
dihydroxyaluminum aminoacetate　アミノ酢酸ジヒドロキシアルミニウム
dissecting aneurysm of the aorta　大動脈の解離性動脈瘤

2,4-DAA
2,4-diaminoanisole　2,4-ジアミノアニソール

DAAO
D-amino acid oxidase　D-アミノ酸酸化酵素

DAAVP
1-deamino-8-arginine vasopressin　1-デアミノ-8-アルギニンバソプレシン

DAB
days after birth　生後日数
deutsches Apothekerbuch〈独〉　ドイツ薬局方

diaminobenzene ジアミノベンゼン
diaminobenzidine ジアミノベンジジン
p-dimethylaminoazobenzene *p*-ジメチルアミノアゾベンゼン

DABA
Diplomate of American Board of Anesthesiology 米国麻酔学専門医資格者

DABCO
diazobicyclooctane ジアゾビシクロオクタン，ダブコ

DABD
Diplomate of American Board of Dermatology 米国皮膚科学専門医資格者

DABIM
Diplomate of American Board of Internal Medicine 米国内科学専門医資格者

DABNS
Diplomate of American Board of Neurological Surgery 米国神経外科学専門医資格者

DABO
Diplomate of American Board of Ophthalmology 米国眼科学専門医資格者

DABOG
Diplomate of American Board of Obst. and Gynecol. 米国産婦人科学専門医資格者

DABOS
Diplomate of American Board of Orthopedic Surgery 米国整形外科学専門医資格者

DABOt
Diplomate of American Board of Otolaryngology 米国耳鼻咽喉科学専門医資格者

DABP
Diplomate of Americann Board of Pediatrics 米国小児科学専門医資格者

DABPath
Diplomate of American Board of Pathology 米国病理学専門医資格者

DABPN
Diplomate of American Board of Psychiatry and Neurology 米国精神神経科学専門医資格者

DABR
Diplomate of American Board of Radiology 米国放射線医学専門医資格者

DABS
Diplomate of American Board of Surgery 米国外科学専門医資格者

D

DABU
Diplomate of American Board of Urology　米国泌尿器科学専門医資格者

DAC
data assistance and control　データ援助と管理
digital to analog converter　デジタル・アナログ変換器

DACA
dissecting aneurysm of the coronary artery　冠(状)動脈の解離性動脈瘤

DACCP
1,2-diamine-monocyclohexane　1,2-ジアミン-モノサイクロヘキサン(4-カルボフタレイト)プラチニウム

DACE
dexamethasone,arabinosylcytosine, carboplatin,etoposide　デキサメタゾン,アラビノシルシトシン,カルボプラチン,エトポシド

DACM
N-(7-dimethylamino-4-methylcoumarinyl) maleimide　*N*-(7-ジメチルアミノ-4-メチルクマリニル)マレイミド

dacor
data correction　データ収集

DACS
Document Archiving and Communication System　電子化診療記録統合管理

DACT
dactinomycin　ダクチノマイシン

dacty
dactylography　指紋術，指紋学
dactyloscopy　指紋検査法

dactygram
dactylogram　指紋

DAD
delayed afterdepolarization　遅延後脱分極
diffuse alveolar damage　び漫〔広汎〕性肺胞障害
dispense as directed　指示どおり調剤せよ《処》

DADA
diisopropylamine dichloroacetate　ジイソプロピルアミン・ジクロロアセテート

DADDS
N,*N*′-diacetyl-4,4′-diaminodiphenyl sulfone　*N*,*N*′-ジアセチル-4,4′-ジアミノフェニルスルホン

dAdo
deoxyadenosine　デオキシアデノシン

D

DADP
deoxyadenosine diphosphate　デオキシアデノシン二リン酸
DADPS
diamino-diphenylsulfone　ジアミノジフェニルスルホン
DAEC
diffuse adhering *Escherichia coli*　び漫〔広汎〕性粘着性大腸菌
DAF
decay accelerating factor　解離促進因子
delayed auditory feedback　遅延聴力フィードバック
DAFA
data accounting flow assessment　データ計算流動評価
DAFC
digital automatic frequency control　デジタル式自動周期調節
DAFO
dried agarose film overlay　乾燥アガロースフィルム被覆
DAF-S
stroma-derived decay-accelerating factor　基質由来腐敗加速因子
DAG
diacylglycerol　ジアシルグリセロール(=DG)，ジグリセリド
dihydroxy aluminium glutaminate　ジヒドロキシグルタミン酸アルミニウム
dodecyl diaminoethyl glycin hydrochloride　ドデシルジアミノエチル塩酸グリシン
dag
decagram　デカグラム〈単位〉
DAGT
direct antiglobulin test　直接抗グロブリン試験〔検査〕
DAH
disordered action of heart　心動作不整
DAI
death from accidental injuries　事故死
diffuse axonal injury　び漫〔広汎〕性軸索損傷
dal
decaliter　デカリットル〈単位〉
DALA, D-ALA
delta aminolevulinic acid　デルタアミノレブリン酸
DALE
Disabilities Adjusted Life Expectancy　障害調整平均余命
Drug Abuse Law Enforcemet　薬物乱用に対する法の施行
DALY
disability adjusted life years　障害調整生存年数
DAM
degraded amyloid　退化アミロイド
diacetylmonoxime　ジアセチルモノキシム

diacetylmorphine ジアセチルモルヒネ
draw a man (test) 人物画知能検査《心理》

dam
damage 傷害
decameter デカメートル〈単位〉

DAMA
discharged against medical advice 医学的助言に逆らって退院した

DAME
data acquisition and monitoring equipment データ取得監視器具

dAMP
deoxyadenosine monophosphate デオキシアデノシン一リン酸

DAN
diabetic autonomic neuropathy 糖尿病性ニューロパシー
diazoacetyl-DL-norleucine methylester ジアゾアセチル-DL-ノルロイシンメチルエステル

dand.
dandus〈ラ〉=to be given 与えよ《処》

DANS
1-dimethylaminonaphthalene-5-sulfonyl chloride 1-ジメチルアミノナフタレン-5-スルホニルクロライド

DAO
diamine oxidase ジアミン酸化酵素

DAo
descending aorta 下行大動脈

DAP
α-α'-diaminopimelic acid α-α'-ジアミノピメリン酸
deafferentation pain syndrome 求心神経遮断疼痛症候群
depolarizing afterpotential 脱分極性後電位
diabetes associated peptide 糖尿病に伴うペプチド
diaminopimelic acid ジアミノピメリン酸
1,3-diaminopropane 1,3-ジアミノプロパン
dianhydrogalactital, adriamycin, cisplatin (=Platinol) ジアンヒドロガラクチタル,アドリアマイシン,シスプラチン(=プラチノール)
diastolic aortic pressure 拡張期大動脈圧
1,4-dihydrazinophthalazine 1,4-ジヒドラジノフタラジン
dihydroxyacetone phoshate リン酸ジヒドロアセトン
dipeptidyl aminopeptidase ジペプチジルアミノペプチダーゼ
draw a person (test) 人物描写テスト，人物画テスト

DAP & E
Diploma in Applied Parasitology and Entomology 応用寄生虫学・昆虫学認定書

D

DAPI

diaminophenyl indole	ジアミノフェニルインドール

DAPR

digital automatic pattern recognition	デジタル自動類型認知

DAPT, Dapt

2,4-diamino-5-phenylthiazole	2,4-ジアミノ-5-フェニルチアゾール
direct agglutination pregnancy test	直接凝集妊娠検査

DAR

death after resuscitation	蘇生後死亡
differential absorption rate	吸収率較差
drug abuse rehabilitation	薬物乱用リハビリテーション
dual asthmatic response〔reaction〕	二相性喘息反応

DA-R

dopamine receptor	ド(ー)パミン受容体

DARC

Duffy antigen receptor for chemokine	ダフィ血液型抗原

DARE

Drug Abuse Research and Education	薬物乱用研究と教育
Drug Assistance Rehabilitation and Education	薬援助によるリハビリテーションと教育

DARES

data analysis and reduction system	データ分析・換算システム

DARF

direct antiglobulin rosette-forming	直接抗グロブリンロゼット形成の

DARP

drug abuse rehabilitation program	薬物乱用リハビリテーションプログラム

DART

development advanced rate techniques	発達率技術
diet and reinfarction trial	食事と再梗塞の実験

DAS

dextroamphetamine sulfate	硫酸デキストロアンフェタミン
dextrose aminogen solution	ブドウ糖アミノゲン液
seasonal affective disorder	季節性感情障害

DASP

double antibody solid phase method	二抗体固相法

DAT

daunorubicin, arabinosylcytosine, thioguanine	ダウノルビシン,アラビノシルシトシン,チオグアニン
delayed action tablet	遅延作用錠(剤)
dementia of the Alzheimer type	アルツハイマー型痴呆
desktop analysis tool	卓上分析器

diacetylthiamine ジアセチルチアミン
differential agglutinations test 鑑別凝集試験
differential agglutination titer 分化凝集力価
differential aptitude test 鑑別適性試験
diisoamyloxy-thiocarbanilide ジイソアミロキシ・チオカルバニリド
diphtheria antitoxin ジフテリア抗毒素
direct agglutination 直接凝集試験〔検査〕
direct antiglobulin test 直接抗グロブリン試験〔検査〕

datacom
data communications データ伝達

datacor
data correction データ修正
data corrector データ修正者

DATP
deoxyadenosine triphosphate デオキシアデノシン三リン酸

DATVP
daunorubicin, arabinosylcytosine, thioguanine, vincristine, prednisone ダウノルビシン,アラビノシルシトシン,チオグアニン,ビンクリスチン,プレドニゾン

dau
daughter 娘

DAUNO
daunorubicin ダウノルビシン

DAV
dacarbazine, amino-methyl-nitrosourea, vincristine ダカルバジン,アミノメチルニトロソウレア,ビンクリスチン
daunorubicin, arabinosylcytosine, vincristine ダウノルビシン,アラビノシルシトシン,ビンクリスチン
daunorubicin, arabinosylcytosine, VP-16(=etoposide) ダウノルビシン,アラビノシルシトシン,エトポシド
difference arterio-vein use 動静脈利用比

DAVF
dural arterio venous fistula 硬膜動静脈瘻

d-AVF
dual arteriovenous fistula 二重の動静脈瘻

DAVH
dibromodulcitol, adriamycin, vincristine, Halotestin ジブロモダルシトール,アドリアマイシン,ビンクリスチン,ハロテスチン

D

DAVP
dacarbazine, amino-methyl-nitrosourea, vincristine, peplomycin — ダカルバジン,アミノメチルニトロソウレア,ビンクリスチン,ペプロマイシン

dAVP
deamino arginine vasopressin — デアミノ・アルギニン・バソプレシン

DAVTH
dibromodulcitol, adriamycin, vincristine, tamoxifen, Halotestin — ジブロモダルシトール,アドリアマイシン,ビンクリスチン,タモキシフェン,ハロテスチン

DAW
dispense as written — 書かれたように調剤せよ《処》

DAZ
Druckanstiegzeit〈独〉 — 圧上昇時間

DB
data bank — データバンク
data base — データベース
dead body — 死体
deep breath — 深呼吸
deep burn — 皮下熱傷
dextran blue — デキストランブルー
diabetic — 糖尿病の
Diamond-Blackfan (syndrome) — ダイアモンド・ブラックファン(症候群)
direct bilirubin — 直接(型)ビリルビン
disability — 廃疾,作業不能
distobuccal — 遠心(面)頰(面)の
dry bulb — 乾球
dry-bulb temperature — 乾球温
duodenal bulb — 十二指腸球部
nucleus of diagonal band — (脳の)帯核

Db
diabetes — 糖尿病
dubnium — ドブニウム〈元素〉

D & B
dead and buried — 死亡埋葬

DB, D/B
date of birth — 生年月日

DB, DBil
direct bilirubin — 直接型ビリルビン

dB, db
decibel — デシベル〈単位〉

DBA
desbenzoyl-acemetacin — デスベンゾイルアセメタシン

dibenamine ジベナミン
dibenzanthracene ジベンズアントラセン
dolichos biflorus agglutinin フジマメ凝集素

dBA
decibel on A scale of sound levelmeter 騒音計のA特性デシベル

DBAS
1,2,5,6-dibenzanthracene endosuccinate 1,2,5,6-ジベンズアントラセンエンドサクシネイト

DBB
diagonal band of Broca ブローカ帯

DBC
dibencozide ジベンコジド
dye-binding capacity 色素結合能

DBcAMP
dibutyryl cyclic AMP(=adenosine mono-phosphate) ジブチリルサイクリックAMP(=アデノシン一リン酸)

DBCC
dimethylbenzimidazole cobamide coenzyme B_{12} 補酵素型ビタミンB_{12}

DBCLT
dilute blood clot lysis time 希釈血液塊溶解時間

DBCP
1,2-dibromo-3-chloropropane 1,2-ジブロモ-3-クロロプロパン

DB-CT
double-blind comparative test 二重盲検比較試験

DBD
definite brain damage はっきりした脳障害

DBE
dibromoethane ジブロモエタン

DBED
dibenzyl ethylenediamine ジベンジルエチレンジアミン

DBH
dopamine-beta-hydroxylase ド(ー)パミン-β-ヒドロキシラーゼ

DBI
deschlorobenzoyl-indomethacin デスクロロベンゾイルインドメタシン
development-at-birth index 出生時発育指数
diazepam binding inhibitor ジアゼパム結合阻害物質
diffuse brain injury び漫〔広汎〕性脳損傷
phenethyl biguanide フェネチルビグアナイド

D.Bi.Chem
Doctor of Biological Chemistry 生化学博士

D

D.Bi.Eng
Doctor of Biological Engineering 生物工学博士
D-Bil
direct bilirubin 直接(型)ビリルビン
D.Bi.Phy
Doctor of Biological Physics 生物物理学博士
D.Bi.Sc
Doctor of Biological Science 生物科学博士
dbl
double 2倍の，二重の
DBM
diabetic management 糖尿病管理
dibromomannitol ジブロモマンニトール
Division of Biology and Medicine 生物学・医学部
DBMA
desbenzoyl-desmethyl acemethacin デスベンゾイルデスメチルアセメタシン
N,*N*′-dibenzylmethylamine *N*,*N*′-ジベンジルメチルアミン
DBMI
desbenzoyl-desmethyl indomethacin デスベンゾイルデスメチルインドメタシン
DBMS
data base management system データベース管理システム
DBn
double blind (test) 二重盲(検)
DBO
distobucco-occlusal 遠心(面)頬側咬合面の
dreadful body odor ものすごい体臭
DBP
diastolic blood pressure 拡張期血圧
dibutyl phthalate フタル酸ジブチル
distobuccopulpal 遠心(面)頬(面)歯髄(面)の
DNA binding protein DNA結合蛋白質
vitamin D binding protein ビタミンD結合蛋白
DBPPEE
diisobutyl-phenoxypolyethoxyethanol ジイソブチルフェノキシポリエトキシエタノール
DBRN
decibel above reference noise 指示音以上の音圧
DBS
deep brain stimulation 脳深部刺激
deep stimulation 深部脳刺激
Denis Browne splint デニス・ブラウン副子
despeciated bovine serum 非特異化ウシ血清
dibromosalicyl anilide ジブロモサリチルアニリド

Division of Biological Standards 生物学標準局
dried blood spot 乾燥血液斑点

dB SPL
decibel sound pressure level デシベル音圧レベル，デシベルSPL

DBT
database lock データベースロック
double blind test 二重盲検法
dry bulb temperature 乾球温度

DBU
diaminobutyric acid ジアミノ酪酸

DBu
diglucuronide bilirubin unbinding ジグルクロニド非結合性ビリルビン

DBW
desirable body weight 理想体重

DC
decarboxylase 脱炭酸酵素
decompensated cirrhosis 非代償性肝硬変
defibrillative countershock 直流電気除細動
degenerating cell 変性細胞
dendritic cell 樹枝状細胞
dental corps 歯科医師団
deoxycholate デオキシコール酸塩
deoxycholic acid デオキシコール酸
descending colon 下行結腸
diagnostic center 診断センター
diagonal conjugate of the pelvic inlet 対角結合線(＝CD)
differentiated cell 分化細胞
diffusion chamber 拡散箱
direct Coombs (test) 直接クームス(試験)
discharged 退院した，排泄した
distocervical 遠心(面)歯頸(面)の
donor's cell 供血者血球浮遊液
dosis curativa〈ラ〉 治効量
dressing change 包帯交換
dyspepsie coli 大腸性消化不良

D & C
dilatation and curettage (頸管)拡張(子宮)掻爬(術)

DC, D.C., dc, d.c.
direct current 直流

DC, D/C, dc
discharge 放電，排泄(物)，退院

DC, D/C, D/c, Dc, dc, d/c
discontinue 中止する，中止

D

DC, D/C, d/c
decrease　減少(する)

DCA
deoxycholate-citrate agar　デオキシコール酸寒天培地
deoxycholic acid　デオキシコール酸
deoxycorticosterone acetate　酢酸デオキシコルチコステロン
desoxycorticosterone acetate　酢酸デスオキシコルチコステロン
dichloroacetate　ジクロロアセテート
dichloroacetic acid　ジクロロ酢酸
directional coronary atherectomy　直接冠(状)動脈拡張術
Drug Control Agency　薬物管理局

DCAT
Drug, Chemical and Associated Technologies Association　薬物・化学および準技術連合

DCB
dichlorobenzidine　ジクロロベンジジン

DCC
detected in colon carcinoma　大腸癌で発見された
dextran-coated charcol　デキストラン結合チャコール
dicyclohexylcarbodiimide　ジシクロヘキシルカルボジイミド
double concave　二重凹面

DCCI
dicyclohexylcarbodiimide　ジシクロヘキシルカルボジイミド

DCCMP
daunorubicin, cyclocytidine, 6-mercaptopurine, prednisolone　ダウノルビシン,シクロシチジン,6-メルカプトプリン,プレドニゾロン

DCC/N
day care center or nursery　託児所

DCCO
diffusing capacity for carbon monoxide　一酸化炭素肺拡散能

D & C color
drug and cosmetic color　薬と化粧品の色

DCCR
day creatinine clearance　1日クレアチニンクリアランス

DCCT
diabetes control and complications trial　糖尿病管理合併症試験

DCD
Dennis Test of Child Development　デニス小児発育検査〔試験〕

died as a consequence of disease 当該疾患による死亡
Diploma in Chest Disease 胸部疾患医認定書

Dc′d, dc′d
discontinued 中止した

DCDC
Department of Communicable Diseases Control 伝染性疾患管理局

DCE
desmosterol-to-cholesterol enzyme デモステロール・コレステロール変換酵素

DCEP
Diploma of Child and Educational Psychology 小児教育心理学認定書

DCET
dicethiamine ジセチアミン

DCF
deoxycoformycin デオキシコホルマイシン
direct contrifugal flotation 直接遠心浮遊法

dCf
detur cum formula〈ラ〉 処方箋とともに与えよ《処》

DCG
deoxycorticosterone glucoside デオキシコルチコステロングルコシド
Doppler cardiography ドップラーカルジオグラフィ
dynamic electrocardiography 動的心電図検査

DCH
delayed cutaneous hypersensitivity 遅延型皮膚過敏症
dicyclohexyl ジシクロヘキシル

D.Ch.
Doctor of Chirurgi 外科学博士

D.C.H.
Diploma in Child Health 小児保健資格〔免状〕

DCHN
dicyclohexylamine nitrite 亜硝酸ジサイクロヘキシルアミン

DChO
Diploma in Ophthalmic Surgery 眼外科学認定書

DCI
decarboxylase inhibitor 脱炭酸酵素阻害薬
dichloroisoprenaline ジクロロイソプレナリン
dichloroisoproterenol ジクロロイソプロテレノール
digital cone beam imaging デジタルコーンビーム映像法

DCIP
deep circumflex iliac artery 深腸骨回旋動脈
2,6-dichlorophenol-indophenol 2,6-ジクロロフェノールインドフェノール

DCK
deoxycytidine kinase デオキシシチジンキナーゼ

DCL
decarboxylase-inhibitor 脱炭酸酵素阻害薬
dicloxacillin ジクロキサシリン
diffuse cutaneous leishmaniasis 広汎〔び漫〕性皮膚リーシュマニア症
extract of malt and cod liver oil 麦芽エキス肝油

DCLS
deoxycholate, citrate, lactose, saccharose agar デオキシコレート・クエン酸・乳糖・サッカロース寒天

D.Cl.Sci
Doctor of Clinical Science 臨床科学士

DCM
diastole dilated cardiomyopathy 拡張型心筋症
dichloromethane ジクロロメタン
dichloromethotrexate ジクロロメトトレキサート
dilated cardiomyopathy 拡張型心筋症
Doctor of Comparative Medicine 比較医学士

DCMC
dichlorophenyl dimethylurea ジクロロフェニルジメチル尿素

DCML
dorsal column medial lemniscus 後索内側毛帯

DCMMC
decarbamoyl mitomycin C デカルバモイルマイトマイシンC

DCMP
daunorubicin, cyclophosphamide, 6-mercaptopurine, prednisone ダウノルビシン, シクロホスファミド, 6-メルカプトプリン, プレドニゾン
daunorubicin, cytarabine, 6-mercaptopurine, prednisolone ダウノルビシン, シタラビン, 6-メルカプトプリン, プレドニゾロン

dCMP
deoxycytidine monophosphate デオキシシチジン一リン酸

DCN
delayed cutaneous hypersensitivity 遅延(型)皮膚過敏(症)

D.C.O.G.
Diploma of the College of Obstetricians and Gynaecologists 産婦人科学卒業証書

DCP
daunorubicin, cytarabin, prednisolone ダウノルビシン, シタラビン, プレドニゾロン
dicalcium phosphate リン酸ジカルシウム

dicumyl peroxide 過酸化ジクミル

dCp

deoxycytidylic acid デオキシシチジル酸

D.C.P.

Diploma in Clinical Pathology 臨床病理資格〔免状〕

DCPA

3′,4′-dichloropropionanilide 3′,4′-ジクロロプロピオンアニリド

DCPC

dichlorodiphenylmethyl carbinol ジクロロジフェニルメチルカルビノール

DCPM

daunorubicin, cytarabin, prednisolone, 6-mercaptopurine ダウノルビシン,シタラビン,プレドニゾロン,6-メルカプトプリン

DC potential

direct current potential 直流電位

DCR

dacryocystorhinostomy 涙嚢鼻腔吻合(術)
diagnostic criteria for research 研究用診断基準
direct cortical responce 直接皮質反応

dcr

decrease 減少する
decreasing 減少

DCRV

double chambered right ventricle 右室二腔心

DCS

decompression sickness 潜函病
disease control serum 疾病対象血清
distal coronary sinus 遠位冠(状)静脈洞
dorsal column stimulator 後索刺激装置

DC shock

direct current shock 直流除細動

DCT

daunorubicin, cytarabin, thioguanine ダウノルビシン,シタラビン,チオグアニン
Department of Cancer Therapy 癌治療部門
dihydrochloro-thiazide ジヒドロクロロチアジド
direct Coombs test 直接クームス試験〔検査〕
distal convoluted tubule 遠位尿細管

DCTD

Diploma in Chest and Tuberculosis Diseases 胸部疾患結核病医認定書

DCTMA

desoxycorticosterone trimethyl-acetate トリメチル酢酸デスオキシコルチコステロン

D

D

DCTP, dCTP
deoxycytidine triphosphate デオキシシチジン三リン酸
DCTPA
desoxycorticosterone triphenylacetate トリフェニル酢酸デスオキシコルチコステロン
DCU
dichloral urea ジクロラール尿素
DCV
dacarbazine, cyclohexylchloroethylnitrosourea, vincristine ダウノルビシン,シクロヘキシルクロロエチルニトロソ尿素,ビンクリスチン
DCx
double convex 二重凸面
DD
dangerous drug 劇薬
day of delivery 分娩日
deaf and dumb 聾啞
deferred delivery, delayed delivery 遅延分娩
degenerative disease 変性疾患
delusional disorder 妄想疾患
dependent drainage 重力ドレナージ(法)
detur ad〈ラ〉 投与せよ《処》
developmental disability 発達障害
(left ventricular) diastolic dimension (左(心)室)拡張期径
differential diagnosis 鑑別診断
digestive disease 消化器病
digital display デジタルディスプレイ
disc diameter (網膜)乳頭径
discharged dead 死産
discharge diagnosis 退院時診断
dry dressing 乾燥被覆包帯
Duchenne dystrophy デュシェーヌ(型)ジストロフィ
Dupuytren disease デュピュイトラン病
fibrin degradation products D dimers フィブリン分解産物D二量体
Dd
diameter of diastolic 拡張末期径
dd
delivered 分娩の, 出産の
d.d.
detur ad〈ラ〉=let it be given to 与えよ《処》
dd, d.d.
de die〈ラ〉=daily 毎日《処》
DDA
Dangerous Drug Act 劇薬取締法

ddA
dideoxyadenosine ジデオキシアデノシン
DDAVP
deamino-8-D-arginine vasopressin (desmopressin acetate) デアミノ-8-D-アルギニンバソプレシン(＝酢酸デスモプレシン)

DDB
deep dermal burn 深部皮膚熱傷，深達性II度熱傷

DDBJ
DNA Data Bank of Japan 日本DNAデータバンク
DDC
dimethyldithiocarbamate ジメチルジチオカルバメート
direct digital control 計算機制御
ddC
dideoxycitidine ジデオキシシチジン
DDD
degenerative disk disease 変性円板疾患
dense deposit disease 高密度デポジット糸球体腎炎
Denver dialysis disease デンバー透析病
dichlorodiphenyldichloroethane ジクロロジフェニルジクロロエタン

double chambers-double, chambers-double (dual) 心房心室ユニバーサルペーシング
double double double (pacemaker) 心房心室同期型(ペースメーカー)

Dowling-Degos disease ダウリング・デゴス病
drink, drank, drunk 飲む・飲んだ・飲まれた
dual-mode, dual-pacing, dual-sensing (pacemaker) 二重モード・二腔ペーシング・二腔センシング(ペースメーカ)

DDEB
dominant dystrophic epidermolysis bullosa 優性栄養傷害性表皮水疱症
DDF
Dental Documentary Foundation 歯科文書財団
DDG
deoxy-D-glucose デオキシ-D-グルコース
dye-densitography 色素希釈法
DDH
developmental dislocation of the hip 先天性股関節脱臼
Diploma in Dental Health 歯科衛生認定書
DDI
dideoxyinosine ジデオキシイノシン

D

D

dd.in d.
de die in diem〈ラ〉=daily, from day to day 日ごとに《処》

DDL
Darm Durch Leuchtung 大腸X線検査

DDM
Diploma in Dermatological Medicine 皮膚科認定書
doctor of dental medicine 歯科医

DDO
Diploma in Dental Orthopedics 歯科矯正認定書

DDP
diamine dichloroplatinum ジアミンジクロロプラチナ

DDPH
Diploma in Dental Public Health 歯科公衆衛生認定書

DDQ
2,3-dichloro-5,6-dicyanobenzoquinone 2,3-ジクロロ-5,6-ジシアノベンゾキノン

DDR
diastolic descent rate (僧帽弁)拡張期後退速度
Diploma in Diagnostic Radiology 放射線診断認定書
vitamin D-dependent rickets ビタミンD依存性くる病

DDRIE
double-decker rocket immuno-electrophoresis 二段ロケット免疫電気泳動法

DDS
dialysis disequilibrium syndrome 透析(性)平衡異常症候群
diaminodiphenylsulfone(=dapsone) ジアミノジフェニルスルホン(=ダプソン)
digital dynamics simulator デジタル動的シミュレーター
drug delivery system 薬物輸送システム

D.D.S.
Doctor of Dental Surgery 口腔外科学博士

DDSA
dodecanyl succinic anhydride ドデカニル無水コハク酸

DDSc, D.D.Sc.
Doctor of Dental Science 歯科医学士，歯科学博士

DDSO
diaminodiphenyl-sulphone(=dapsone) ジアミノジフェニルスルホン(=ダプソン)

DDS syndrome
diamonodiphenylsulfone syndrome DDS症候群

DDST
Denver Developmental Screening Test デンバー発育スクリーニング検査〔試験〕

DDT

dichlorodiphenyltrichloroethane(=chlorophenothane)　ジクロロジフェニルトリクロロエタン(=クロロフェノタン)(=殺虫剤の一種)

dye dilution test　色素希釈法

DDVP

dimethyl-dichlorovinyl phosphate　リン酸ジメチルジクロロビニル

DDW

digestive disease week　消化器系学会の合同学術集会

double distilled water　蒸留水

DDX

differential diagnosis　鑑別診断

DE

digestive energy　消化エネルギー

dose equivalent　線量当量

Druckempfindlichkeit〈独〉　圧痛

drug evaluation　薬剤評価

drug experience　医薬品の使用経験

dyspnea on exertion　運動時呼吸困難

D & E

dilatation and evacuation　拡張と吸引

dilation and evacuation　(頸管)拡張(子宮)内容除去(術)

DE, d.e.

dosis effectiva〈ラ〉=effective dose　有効量

2DE, 2-DE

two-dimensional echocardiogram　断層心エコー図, 二次元エコー図

two-dimensional echocardiography　断層心エコー図法, 二次元エコー図法

3DE, 3-DE

three-dimensional echocardiogram　三次元エコー図

three-dimensional echocardiography　三次元エコー図法

DEA

dehydroepiandrosterone　デヒドロエピアンドロステロン

diethanolamine　ジエタノールアミン

Drug Enforcement Administration　薬物〔麻薬〕取締局

DEAE

diethylaminoethanol　ジエチルアミノエタノール

diethylaminoethanol salicylate　ジエチルアミノエタノールサリチル酸

diethylaminoethyl　ジエチルアミノエチル

D

DEAE-D
diethylaminoethyl dextran ジエチルアミノエチルデキストラン

DEAN
deputy educators against narcotics 麻薬に対する代理教育者

DeAR
delayed allergic response 遅延型アレルギー反応

DEAS
dehydroepiandrosterone デヒドロエピアンドロステロン

deaur.pil.
deaurentur pilulae〈ラ〉 丸剤に金箔せよ《処》

DEB
diepoxybutane ジエポキシブタン
diethylbutanediol ジエチルブタンジオル

deb
débridement 創面切除(術)，創傷清拭〔清浄化〕，挫滅〔壊死〕組織除去

DEBA
diethylbarbituric acid ジエチルバルビツール酸

debil.
debilitation 衰弱，虚弱
debility 衰弱した，虚弱した

deb.spis.
debita spissitudine〈ラ〉 適当な硬さの《処》

DEC
diethylcarbamazine ジエチルカルバマジン

dec
decantation 静かに注ぐ
deceased 故人，死亡した
deciduous 脱落(性)の
decimal 少数，十進法の，少数の
decompose 分解する，腐敗する
decomposed 分解した，腐敗した
decrease 減少する
decreased 減少した

dec.
decoctum〈ラ〉＝boiled (down) 煎剤《処》

dec，dec.
decimeter デシメートル〈単位〉

deca
deca- デカ(＝×10)〈接〉

decag
decagram デカグラム〈単位〉

DecAo
descending aorta 下行大動脈
DECD
disseminated eosinophilic collagen disease 播種性好酸球性膠原病
dec'd
decomposed 分解した，腐敗した
decd, dec'd
deceased 故人，死亡した
decel
deceleration 減速(度)
decim
decimeter デシメートル〈単位〉
decoct.
decoctum〈ラ〉=boiled (down) 煎剤《処》
decomp
decompensated 非代償(性)の
decompose 分解する
decomposed 分解した
decomposition 分解
decompn
decompensation 代償不全，代償障害
decr
decrease 減少する，縮小する，減少させる
decreased 減少した
DECT
dicarbethoxy-thiamine hydrochloride 塩酸ジカルベトキシサイアミン
decub.
decubitus〈ラ〉=lying down 衰弱性壊疽，床ずれ，褥瘡
DED
date of expected delivery 分娩予定日
delayed erythema dose 遅延(性)紅斑(線)量
de d.in d.
de die in diem〈ラ〉=daily, from day to day 毎日，1日ごとに《処》
dee-dee
deaf and dumb 聾唖
DEEG
depth electroencephalogram 深部脳波
depth electroencephalography 深部脳波検査(法)
DeePee
Doctor of Pharmacy 薬学士

D

DEET
N,*N*-diethyl-*m*-toluamide　*N*,*N*-ジエチル-*m*-トルアミド

def
defecate　排便する
defect　欠陥，欠落
defense　防御
defensive　防御の
deferred　延ばした，据え置きにした
deficient　不足している，不十分な，欠陥のある
deficit　欠損，欠乏，不足
define　定義を下す，限定する，明示する
definite　明確な，定数の，限定された
definition　制限，解像力，定義

DEF，def.
defecation　排便

Def，def.
deficiency　欠乏(症)，欠失，欠損

deff
dosis efficax〈ラ〉　有効量

defib
defibrillate　細動を除去する

defic
deficiency　欠乏(症)，欠損(症)
deficient　不足している，不十分な，欠損のある
deficit　欠損，欠乏，不足

def index
decayed extracted filled index　う蝕歯・要抜去歯・充填歯指数，def指数

deform
deformity　変形，奇形

DEFT
direct epifluorescent filter technique　直接落射螢光フィルター法

DEFY
drug education for youth　若者のための薬物教育

DEG
diethylene glycol　ジエチレングリコール

deg
degenerate　変性する，退化する
degeneration　変性，退化

Deg，deg.
degeneration　変性，変質，退化
degree　度，程度

degen
degeneration 変性，変質，退化
degenerative 変性の

deglut.
deglutia〈ラ〉=swallow 嚥下せよ《処》
deglutiatur〈ラ〉=let it be swallowed 嚥下させよ《処》

Deg.pig.
degeneratio pigmentosa retinae〈ラ〉 網膜色素変性症

dehyd
dehydrated 脱水した，脱水になった
dehydration 脱水(症)

DEJ
dento-enamel junction 象牙質エナメル質境界
dermoepidermal junction 表皮真皮結合部

del
deletion 欠失
delusion 妄想

del.
delinearit〈ラ〉=delineated 描いた

Del, del.
deliver 分娩させる，摘出する，導出する
delivery 分娩，出産

deld
delivered 分娩の

DELFIA
dissociation enhanced lanthanide fluoroimmunoassay デルフィアシステム

deli
delicatessen 調製食品

deliq
deliquescent 潮解の，溶解する

Delt
deltoid デルタ型の，三角形の，三角(筋)

delvd
delivered 分娩の

dely
delivery 分娩

DEM
diethyl malate ジエチルリンゴ酸

dem
demonstrate 論証する，実際にやって示す

DEM, Dem
Demerol デメロール
department of emergency medicine 救急医療部

D

Demen Prae
dementia praecox 早発(性)痴呆
demin
demineralization 鉱物質除去，無機質脱落
demogr
demographer 人口統計学者
demographic 人口統計の
demography 人口統計
DEN
dermatitis exfoliativa neonatorum 新生児剝脱性皮膚炎
den
dental 歯の，歯科の
dentist 歯科医
dentistry 歯科医学，歯科医術
DENA
diethylnitrosamine ジエチルニトロサミン
denat
denatured 変質した
Den Hyg
Dental Hygienist 歯科衛生士
D en M
Docteur en Medicine〈仏〉 医学士
denom
denominator 命名者，分母
dens
density 濃度
dent.
dentur〈ラ〉=give 与えよ《処》
Dent, dent.
dental 歯(性)の，歯科の
dentate 歯状の，鋸歯状の
dentist 歯科医
dentistry 歯科学
dentition 生歯
dent.ad.scat.
dentur ad scatulam〈ラ〉 箱に入れよ《処》
dent.tal.dos.
dentur tales doses〈ラ〉 同量投与せよ《処》
DEP
diesel exhaust particles ディーゼル排気ガス微粒子
diethylpropanediol ジエチルプロパンジオール
diisopropyl-fluorophosphate ジイソプロピルフルオロリン酸
dep.
deposit 沈積〔沈着〕物，底質
depuratus〈ラ〉=purified 精製した，純化した《処》

Dep, dep.
dependents 扶養家族，従属物
DEPA
diethylene phosphoramide ジエチレンホスホラミド
DEPC
diethyl pyrocarbonate ジエチルピロカルボネート
DEPCA
International Study Group for the Detection and Prevention 国際癌予見予防研究会
depr
depressed 意気消沈した，うつ状態の
depression 陥凹，うつ病，抑うつ
Dept, dept
department 部門，省，学部
depth EEG
depth electroencephalogram 深部脳波
DER
digital examination of rectum 直腸指診(=DRE)
dual-energy radiography 二重エネルギーX線吸収測定法
DeR
degeneration reaction 退行性反応
der
derivative chromosome 派生染色体
DER, DeR
reaction of degeneration 変性反応
deriv
derive 引き出す，由来する
deriv, deriv.
derivative of 誘導された，誘導的な，派生的な，誘導物
derived from ～に由来する，～に由来した
Derm
dermatitis 皮膚炎
derm
dermatological 皮膚科の，皮膚病学の
dermatome 皮(膚分)節
Derm, derm, derm.
dermatologist 皮膚科医
dermatology 皮膚科学
Derma
dermatology 皮膚科学
DER MX
dose efficacite respiratoire maxima 〈仏〉 最大呼吸効果投与量

D

DES
diethylstilbestrol　ジエチルスチルベストロール
diethyl sulfate　ジエチル硫酸
diffuse esophageal spasm　汎発性食道痙攣
disequilibrium syndrome　平衡異常症候群
drug eluting stents　薬剤溶出性ステント

desat
desaturated　脱飽和した
desaturation　脱飽和

desc
descendent　下行の，落下する
descending　下行(性)の
descent　下垂，下降，子孫

Desc AO
descending aorta　下行大動脈

descr
describe　記述する，描写する，表示する

desq
desquamation　落屑，剥離

dest
destroy　破壊する
destruction　破壊

dest.
destilla〈ラ〉=distil　蒸留する《処》
destillatus〈ラ〉=distilled　蒸留した《処》

destil
destilla〈ラ〉=distil　蒸留《処》

DET
diethyltryptamine　ジエチルトリプタミン

det
detrusor　利尿筋

det.
decoctum〈ラ〉　煎剤《処》
detur〈ラ〉=give　与えよ《処》

DETC
dendritic epidermal T cells　樹状上皮T細胞

determin
determination　測定，定量，決定

det.in dup.
detur in duplo〈ラ〉　2倍量を与えよ《処》

detn
detention　滞留，留置
determination　決定，定量，測定

detox
detoxi(fi)cation　解毒

detoxcen
detoxi(fi)cation center　解毒センター
d et s
detur et signatur〈ラ〉　記載して投与せよ《処》
det.time
detention time　滞留時間
D Ety
disease etiology　疾病原因
DEV
duck embryo vaccine　アヒル胚狂犬病ワクチン
dev
develop　発達させる，開発する，発育する
development　発育，発達，現象
deviation　偏差，偏位，偏視，偏移
devd
developed　発育した
devel
developed　発育した
development　発育，発達，現象
Devi
deviatio septi nasi〈ラ〉　鼻中隔彎曲症
deviatomy　鼻中隔彎曲矯正手術
Devi-Con
deviatomy-conchotomy　鼻中隔矯正術と下鼻介切除術
DEX
dexamethasone　デキサメタゾン
dex
dexterity　手先の器用さ，右利き
dextrorotatory　右旋性(の)
dex.
dextro〈ラ〉=right　右(側)の
DEXA
dual energy X-ray absorptiometry　二重エネルギーX線吸収法
dexies
dexedrine tablets　デキセドリン錠
dext.
dexter〈ラ〉=right　右(側)の
dextra〈ラ〉=right　右(側)の
dextro〈ラ〉=right　右，右側に向かって，右旋(性)の
dext, dext.
dexterity　手先の器用さ，右利き
DF
decapacitation factor　受精能獲得抑制因子
decontamination factor　汚染除去因子

D

deferoxamine デフェロキサミン
defibrillation 除細動
Dermatophagoides farinae ダニ
desferrioxamine デスフェリオキサミン
dietary fiber 食物繊維
digital fluorography デジタル透視法
discrimination factor 同相弁別比
disease factor 疾病因子
dorsiflexion 背屈
double filtration 二重膜濾過法

Df
duodenal fluid 十二指腸液

2DF
2-deoxy-L-fucose 2-デオキシ-L-フコース

DF, D/F, df, d.f.
degree of freedom 自由度

DFA
digital fluoroscopic angiography デジタル透視血管造影法
direct immunofluorescent antibody method 直接免疫螢光抗体法
direct immunofluorescent antibody test(ing) 直接免疫螢光抗体法

DFB
dinitrofluorobenzene ジニトロフルオロベンゼン
dysfunctional (uterine) bleeding 機能不全性(子宮)出血，不正(子宮)出血

DFC
distal finger crease 遠位指皺襞
dry-filled capsules 乾性調合カプセル剤

DFD
defined formula diets 限定栄養食

DFDT
difluorodiphenyl trichloroethane ジフルオロジフェニルトリクロロエタン

DFFT
dry-fat-free tissue 乾燥性脂肪遊離組織

DFI
disease free interval 非病期

DFLE
Disease free life expectancy 健康余命

DFMO
difluoromethyl-ornithine ジフルオロメチルオルニチン

DFN
difenidol ジフェニドール
distance from nose 鼻からの距離

DFO
deferoxamine デフェロキサミン
DFOM
deferoxamine デフェロキサミン
DFP
diastolic filling phase 拡張期充満
diisopropyl fluorophosphate ジイソプロピルフルオロリン酸
disease factor product 病因生成物
DF^{32}P
diisopropyl-fluorophosphate 放射標識ジイソプロピルフルオロリン酸
DFPE
double filtration plasma exchange 二重濾過血漿交換法
DFPP
double filtration plasmapheresis 二重濾過血漿分離交換法
DFR
decreasing failure rate 初期故障率
DFS
defibrination syndrome 脱線維素症候群
digital fan beam scanography デジタルファンビーム走査法
disease free survival 非病生存
duodenofiberscope 十二指腸内視鏡
DFSP
dermatofibrosarcoma 隆起性皮膚線維肉腫
DFT
defibrillation threshold 除細動閾値
diagnostic function test 診断的機能検査
dimension Fourier transform 次元フーリエ変換
discrete Fourier transform 離散フーリエ変換
DFU
dead fetus in uterus 子宮内死亡胎児
DFUF
dialysate-free ultrafiltration 無透析液限外濾過
5′-DFUR
5′-deoxy-5-fluorouridine デオキシフルオロウリジン
DFV
difludrocortisone valerate universal cream ジフルドロコルチゾン吉草酸一般クリーム
DFX
desferrioxamine デスフェリオキサミン
DG
dark ground 暗視野
dentate gyrus 歯状回
deoxyglucose デオキシグルコース
deoxyguanosine デオキシグアノシン

D

D

developmental glaucoma　発育異常緑内障
diacylglycerol　ジアシルグリセロール(＝DAG)，ジグリセリド
diglyceride　ジグリセリド
distogingival　遠心(面)歯肉(面)の
downward gaze　下方注視
Duodenalgeschwür〈独〉　十二指腸潰瘍

Dg
glyceraldehyde　グリセルアルデヒド

dG
deoxyguanylate　デオキシグアニレート

dg
decigram　デシグラム〈単位〉
diastolic gallop　拡張期奔馬律

DG，dg
diagnose　診断する
diagnosis　診断
diagnostic　診断(上)の

2DG，2-DG
2-deoxy-D-glucose　2-デオキシ-D-グルコース

D-GAP
D-glyceraldehyde-3-phosphate　D-グリセルアルデヒド三リン酸

DGAVP
desglycinamide-arginine-vasopressin　デスグリシナミド・アルギニン・バソプレシン

DGCS
density gradient centrifugation sedimentation　濃度傾斜遠心分離沈降

DGD
degree of genetic determination　遺伝決定率

DGDP
deoxyguanosine diphosphate　デオキシグアノシン二リン酸

DGE
delayed gastric emptying　胃内容排出遅延

dge
drainage　ドレナージ，排液(法)，排膿(法)

DGF
duct-growth-factor　管成長因子

DGGE
denaturant gradient gel electrophoresis　変性剤濃度勾配ゲル電気泳動法

DGI
disseminated gonococcal infection　び漫〔汎発〕性淋菌感染

DGL
diglyceride lipase　ジグリセリドリパーゼ
DG-L
deep gastric-longitudinal　深胃・縦断の
DGM
Diploma in General Medicine　一般医認定書
dgm
decigram　デシグラム〈単位〉
dGMP
deoxyguanosine monophosphate　デオキシグアノシン一リン酸
deoxyguanosine-5′-phosphate　デオキシグアノシン-5′-リン酸
DGMS
director general of medical service　医療サービス責任者
DGN
diffuse glomerulonephritis　び漫〔広汎〕性糸球体腎炎
D.G.O.
Diploma in Gynecology and Obstetrics　産婦人科資格〔免状〕
dGp
deoxyguanylic acid　デオキシグアニル酸
DGS
diabetic glomerulosclerosis　糖尿病(性)糸球体硬化(症)
Diploma in General Surgery　一般外科医認定書
DGTP, dGPT
2-deoxyguanosine-5′-triphosphate　2-デオキシグアノシン-5′-三リン酸
dgtr
daughter　娘
DGV
dextrose-gelatin-veronal (solution)　ブドウ糖ゼラチンベロナール(溶液)
DH
daily habit　日常の習慣
day hospital　デイホスピタル
dehydrocholic acid　デヒドロコール酸
dehydrogenase　デヒドロゲナーゼ，脱水素酵素
delayed hypersensitivity　遅延(型)過敏症
dental hygienist　歯科衛生士
Deparment of Health　健康局
dermatitis herpetiformis　疱疹状皮膚炎
detrusor hyperreflexia　利尿筋反射亢進
deutschehorizontal〈独〉　ドイツ平面
developmental history　発育歴
diethylaminoethyl hexestrol　コランジル

doxapram hydrochloride 塩酸ドキサプラム

dh

diuresis horaire〈ラ〉 利尿時間

DHA

dehydroacetic acid デヒドロ酢酸
dehydroascorbic acid デヒドロアスコルビン酸
dehydroxyacetone ジヒドロキシアセトン
dihydroalprenolol ジヒドロアロプレノロール
dihydroxyadenine ジヒドロキシアデニン
docosahexaenoic acid ドコサヘキサエン酸

DHAP

dihydroxyacetone phosphate リン酸ジヒドロキシアセトン

DHAS, DHA-S

dehydroepiandrosterone sulphate 硫酸デヒドロエピアンドロステロン

DHBE

dihydroxy dibutylether ジヒドロキシジブチルエーテル

DHBV

duck hepatitis B virus アヒル肝炎ウイルス

DHCA

dihydroxy coprostanic acid ジヒドロキシコプロスタン酸

DHCPB

deep hypothermic cardiopulmonary bypass 超低体温体外循環

DHD

dermatitis herpetiformis Duhring ジューリング疱疹状皮膚炎
distillate hydrosulfurization 抽出水硫化

DHE

deutsche horizontale Ebene〈独〉 ドイツ平面
dihematoporphyrin ether ジヘマトポルフィリンエーテル
dihydroergocryptine ジヒドロエルゴクリプチン
dihydroergotamine ジヒドロエルゴタミン

DHEA

dehydroepiandrosterone デヒドロエピアンドロステロン

DHEAS, DHEA-S

dihydroepiandrosterone sulfate 硫酸ジヒドロエピアンドロステロン

DHEC

dihydroergocryptine ジヒドロエルゴクリプチン

DHF

dengue hemorrhagic fever デング出血(性)熱
(7,8-)dihydrofolic acid (7,8-)ジヒドロ葉酸

DHFR
dihydrofolate reductase ジヒドロ葉酸還元酵素

DHFS
dengue hemorrhagic fever shock (syndrome) デング出血(性)熱ショック(症候群)

DHHS
Department of Health and Human Services 米国保健福祉省

DHIA
dehydroisoandrosterol デヒドロイソアンドロステロール
dehydroisoandrosterone デヒドロイソアンドロステロン

DHIC
detrusor hyperactivity with impaired contractility 排尿筋の収縮不全を伴う膀胱過活動
dihydroisocodeine ジヒドロイソコデイン

DHL
diffuse histiocytic lymphoma び漫〔広汎〕性細網肉腫

DHL agar
deoxycholate-hydrogen sulfide-lactose agar DHL寒天培地

DHMA
dehydroxymandelic acid デヒドロキシマンデル酸

DHO
deuterium hydrogen oxide 重曹
dihydroergocornine ジヒドロエルゴコルニン

DHOA
dihydroxyadenine ジヒドロキシアデニン

DHP
1,4-dihydropyridine ジヒドロピリジン
direct hemoperfusion 血液灌流

DHPG
dehydroxy-phenylglycol デヒドロキシフェニルグリコール
dihydroxy-propylmethyl guanine ジヒドロキシプロピルメチルグアニン
9-(1,3-dihydroxy-2-propoxymethyl) guanine ジヒドロキシプロポキシメチルグアニン

DHPN
dihydroxy-dipropylnitrosamine ジヒドロキシジプロピルニトロソアミン

DHPR
dihydropteridine reductase ジヒドロプテリジン還元酵素

D

DHPS
di-*p*-hydrazinophenyl sulphone　ジパラヒドラジノフェニルスルホン

DHR
delayed hypersensitivity reaction　遅延(型)過敏(症)反応

DHS
delayed hypersensitivity　遅延(型)過敏症
dextrose 5% in Hartmann solution　5％ブドウ糖ハルトマン液
Doctor of Health Science　保健科学士
dry heat sterilization　乾燥滅菌
duration of hospital stay　入院期間

DHSM
dihydrostreptomycin　ジヒドロストレプトマイシン

DHSS
Department of Health and Social Security　保健・社会保障局

DHT
dehydrotestosterone　デヒドロテストステロン
dihydroergotoxine　ジヒドロエルゴトキシン
dihydrotachysterol　ジヒドロタキステロール
dihydrotestosterone　ジヒドロテストステロン
dihydrothymine　ジヒドロチミン
dihydroxypropyltheophylline　ジヒドロキシプロピルテオフィリン
dihydroxytryptamine　ジヒドロキシトリプタミン
dissociated hypertropia　解離性上斜視
distillate hydrotreating　蒸留水処理

DHy, D.Hy.
Doctor of Hygiene　衛生学博士

DHZ
dihydralazine　ジヒドララジン

DI
daily inspection　毎日の観察
defective interfering　不完全干渉
degradation index　分解指数
dental index　臼歯列指数
dentinogenesis imperfecta　象牙質形成不全(症)
deoxyinosine　デオキシイノシン
deoxyribonucleic acid index　デオキシリボ核酸指数
depression inventory　うつ病項目表
desorption ionization　脱着電離
deterioration index　痴呆指数，悪化指数
detrusor instability　排尿筋不安定症
diabetes insipidus　尿崩症
diagnostic imaging　診断画像
diaphragmatic　横隔膜の

dichlorphenamide	ジクロルフェナミド
Diego blood group	ディエゴ血液型
differentiating intermitotics	分化的分裂間期
diphtheria	ジフテリア
disability insurance	廃疾保険
discomfort index	不快指数
dispensing information	調剤情報
distal intestine	遠位腸管
distoincisal	遠心面切端面の
dorsal interosseous	背側骨間(筋)
dorso-iliacus〈ラ〉	背腸骨筋
dose intensity	用量強度，線量強度
drip infusion	点滴
drop in	立ち寄る
drug information	医薬品情報
drug interaction	薬剤相互作用
duct injection	膵管充填
Dwyer instrumentation	ドワイヤー法
dyskaryosis index	核異常指数
dyspnea index	呼吸困難指数
dystocia index	難産指数

di

diameter	直径
diametral	直径の
didymium	ジジム

DI，D/I

date of injury	傷害(年月)日，受傷(年月)日

DIA

death in action	運動死

Dia

diabetes	糖尿病

dia

diagram	図表

Dia，dia.

diameter	直径
diathermy	ジアテルミー，透熱療法

diab

diabetes	糖尿病
diabetic	糖尿病(性)の

DIAC

diiodothyroacetic acid	ジヨードチ〔サイ〕ロ酢酸

diag

diagnose	診断する
diagnostic	診断(上)の
diagram	図

D

Diag, diag.
diagnosis 診断
diag, diag.
diagonal 対角線(の), 斜の, 斜めの
DIAL
differential absorption lidar 差分吸収ライダー
dia lw
long wave diathermy 長波透熱療法
diam, diam.
diameter 直径
DIAMOND
Danish Investigation of Arrhythmia and Mortality on Dofetilide デンマークでの抗不整脈III群薬の大規模試験
diaph
diaphragm 横隔膜
diaphyseal 骨幹の
diaphysis 骨幹
dias
diastolic 拡張〔弛緩〕期の
diast
diastole 拡張〔弛緩〕期
diastolic 拡張〔弛緩〕期の
dia sw
short wave diathermy 短波透熱療法
diath
diathermy ジアテルミー, 透熱療法
DIAZ
diazepam ジアゼパム
DIB
dead in bed (疾病でなく性行為による) ベッドでの死
diagnostic interview for borderlines 境界例の診断面接基準
DIC
differential interference contrast (microscopy) 較差干渉コントラスト(顕微鏡)
diffuse intravascular clotting 広汎性血管内凝固
disseminated intravascular coagulation (syndrome) 播種性血管内凝固(症候群)
disseminated intravascular coagulopathy 播種性血管内凝固障害
dissolved inorganic carbon 液体試料中の全炭酸
drip infusion cholangiography 点滴静注胆道撮影法
drug information center 薬剤情報センター
dic
dicentric chromosome 二動原体染色体

DICC
dynamic infusion cavernosometry and cavernosography — (陰茎海綿体の)灌流量と内圧記録
DICOM
Digital Imaging and Communication in Medicine — ダイコム(=医用画像規格)《画診》
dict
dictate — 口述する
dictated — 口述した
dictionary — 辞書，辞典
DID
dead of intercurrent disease — 偶発疾患死
dihydroxyphenylalanine(=DOPA) induced dyskinesia — ド(ー)パ誘発運動障害
double immunodiffusion — 二重免疫拡散
double isotope derivative method — 二重標識アイソトープ〔同位元素〕誘導体法
DIE
die in emergency department — 救急部での死亡
dieb.alt.
diebus alternis〈ラ〉=on alternate days — 隔日に《処》
dieb.secund.
diebus secundis〈ラ〉=every second day — 2日ごとに《処》
dieb.tert.
diebus tertiis〈ラ〉=every third day — 3日ごとに《処》
DIF
diffuse interstitial fibrosis — 広汎性間質性線維症
direct immunofluorescence — 直接免疫螢光(検査)
diff
difference — (較)差
different — 異なる
differential blood count — 鑑別血球計算
difficult — 困難な
diffrential — 鑑別の，区別の
diff.diag
differential diagnosis — 鑑別診断
DIFI
direct intrafollicular insemination — 直接卵胞内受精
DIFP
diffuse interstitial fibrosing pneumonitis — び漫〔広汎〕性間質性線維化肺炎
diisopropyl fluorophosphonate — ジイソプロピルフルオロリン酸
Dig
digoxin — ジゴキシン

D

dig.
digeratur〈ラ〉 消化させる《処》
digest 温浸せよ《処》
digestion 消化，蒸解
DIG, dig
digitalis ジギタリス
digas
digastric 二腹の
digi-com
digital computer デジタル〔電子〕計算機，デジコム
DIH
Diploma on Industrial Health 産業保健医認定書
DIHN
drug induced hypersensitivity nephropathy 薬剤過敏性腎障害
DIHPPA
diiode hydroxy phenyl pyruvic acid ジヨードヒドロキシフェニルピルビン酸
DIHS
drug-induced hypersensitivity syndrome 薬剤性過敏症症候群
DIL
daughter-in-law 義理の娘
drug-induced lupus 薬剤誘発ループス
dil
dilatation 拡張
dilate 拡張する
dilated 拡張した
diluted 希釈した
dilution 希釈
Dil, dil.
dilation 拡延，拡大，伸展
dilue 希薄
dilutus〈ラ〉=dilute 希釈せよ《処》
dilat
dilatation 拡張
dilate 拡張する
DILD
diffuse interstitial lung disease 広汎〔び漫〕性間質性肺疾患
dilne.
dilneulo〈ラ〉 早朝《処》
diluc.
diluculo〈ラ〉=at daybreak 夜明けに
dilut.
diluted 希釈した

dilution 希釈
dilutus〈ラ〉=dilute 希釈する

dim, dim.
dimension 長さ，寸法，大きさ
diminish 減少させる
diminution 減少
diminutus〈ラ〉=diminished 減少した
dosis infectiosa media〈ラ〉 50%感染量

Dim., dim.
dimidius〈ラ〉 半分の，1/2《処》

DIMD
Dorland Illustrated Medical Dictionary ドーランド図解医学辞典

DIME
Division of International Medical Education 国際医学教育局

dimin
diminished 減少した
diminution 減少

DIMS
disorders of initiating and maintaining sleep 睡眠の開始と持続障害

DIN
Deutsch Industrie-Norm〈独〉 ドイツ工業規格

D in B
dead in bed (疾病ではなく性行為による)ベッドでの死

DIND
delayed ischemic neurological deficit 遅発性虚血性神経脱落症状

D.in P.aeq.
dividetur in partes aequales〈ラ〉 等量に分割せよ《処》

diop
diopter ジオプトリー

diox
dioxygen 過酸化水素

DIP
desquamative interstitial pneumonia 落屑〔剥離〕性間質性肺炎
diffuse interstitial pneumonia び漫性間質性肺炎
diisopropylamine ジイソプロピルアミン
dipyridamole ジピリダモール
drip infusion pyelography 点滴静注腎盂撮影(法)

DIP(J)
distal interphalangeal joint 遠位指節間関節

Dip, dip
diphtheria ジフテリア

D

D

DIPA-DCA
diisopropylamine dichloroacetate　ジイソプロピルアミンジクロロアセテート

Dip.Amer.Bd.P. & N.
Diplomate of American Board of Psychiatry and Neurology　米国精神神経認定医

DI particle
defective interfering particle　不完全干渉性粒子

Dip.Bac.
Diploma in Bacteriology　細菌学認定書

Dip.BMS
Diploma in Basic Medical Science　基礎医学認定書

DIPC
diffuse interstitial pulmonary calcification　広汎性間質性肺石灰化

Dip.Card.
Diploma in Cardiology　心臓病学認定書

Dip.Ds.
Diploma in Dental Surgery　歯外科認定書

DIPF
diisopropyl phosphofluoridate　ジイソプロピルホスホフルオリデート

Dip.G. & O.
Diploma in Gynecology and Obstetrics　産婦人科認定書

diph
diphtheria　ジフテリア

Dip.HA.
Diploma in Hospital Administration　病院管理認定書

diph-tet, diph/tet
diphtheria-tetanus　ジフテリア・破傷風

diph-tox
diphtheria toxoid　ジフテリアトキソイド

diph-tox AP
diphtheria toxoid alum precipitated　ミョウバン沈殿ジフテリアトキソイド

DIPI
direct intraperitoneal insemination　腹腔内授精

Dip.MFOS
Diploma in Maxilar Face and Oral Surgery　顎顔面口腔外科認定書

Dip.Micro.
Diploma in Microbiology　微生物学認定書

Dip.Phar.
Diploma in Pharmacology　薬学認定書

Dip.Phys.Edu.
Diploma in Physical Education　医学教育認定書
Dip.P. & OT.
Diploma in Physical and Occupational Therapy　物理・職業治療認定書
dipso
dipsomaniac　発作性飲酒狂患者
dipt
diopter　ジオプトリー
Dir
director　支配人，重役，ディレクター
dir
direct　直接の
directory　指示的な
dir, dir.
directio〈ラ〉=directions　指示，命令
DIRD
drug-induce renal disease　薬剤誘発性腎疾患
dir.prop.
directione propria〈ラ〉　適当な用法に従って《処》
DIS
Diagnostic Information System　診断情報システム
diagnostic interview schedule　診断学的面接基準
digitalis-like substance　(内因性)ジギタリス様物質
Dis
discharge　退院，放電，発射
dis
disability　廃疾
discomfort　不快感
disease　疾病，疾患
dislocation　転位，脱臼
disorder　障害，疾患
dissoluble　融解性の
distance　距離
distant　遠隔の，遠位の
distribution　分配，配分
disab
disability　廃疾
disable　不可能な
disart
disarticulation　関節離断(術)
disartic
disarticulation　関節離断(術)
disc
discharge　退院(させる)，放電，排泄物
discomfort　不快感

D

DISC, disc, disc.
discontinue 中止する，中断する

disch
discharge 放電する，退院する
discharge 退院，放電，発射
discharged 放電した，退院した

disch.AMA
discharged against medical advice 医学的助言に逆らって退院した

Disco
discography 椎間板造影法

DISD
detrusor internal sphincter dyssynergia 利尿筋内尿道括約筋不〔非〕協調

DISH
diffuse idiopathic sclerosing hyperostosis び漫〔広汎〕性特発性硬化性骨増殖症
diffuse idiopathic skeletal hyperostosis び漫〔広汎〕性特発性骨増殖症
disseminated idiopathic skeletal hyperostosis 播種性特発性骨増殖症

disin
disinfectant 殺菌剤，消毒薬
disinfection 殺菌，消毒

DISL, Disl
dislocate 転位する，脱臼する
dislocated 転位した，脱臼した
dislocation 転位，脱臼

disloc
dislocate 転位する，脱臼する
dislocated 転位した，脱臼した
dislocation 転位，脱臼

dism
dismiss 解雇する
dismissed 解雇された

dis/min
disintegration per minute 毎分崩壊量

disod
disodium 二ナトリウム化合物

disord
disorder 障害，疾患

Disp., disp.
dispensare〈ラ〉=dispense 調剤せよ，投与せよ《処》
dispensarum〈ラ〉=dispensary 調剤室，診療所，薬局
Dispensetur〈ラ〉=dispense 投与する，調剤する
disposition 素因

displ
displace 置換する，置き換える
displacement 置換，移動，偏位
DISS
diameter-indexed safety system 直径指数〔係数〕安全方式
dissd
dissolved 溶解した
dissec
dissection 解剖，離断
dissem
disseminate 播種する
disseminated 播種性の，播種した，播種された
dissemination 播種
dissoc
dissociate 引き離す，分離する，解離する
dissociation 分離，解離
dist
distal 遠位の，末梢の，遠心の
distance 距離
distended 拡張性の，拡張した
distillation 蒸留
distilled 蒸留した
distinguish 識別する，区別する
distribute 分配する，割り当てる
district 地域
disturbance 障害
dist.
distilla〈ラ〉 蒸留せよ《処》
dist f
distinguished from 〜と区別した
distr
distribute 分布する，分配する
distribution 分布，分配
distrib
distribute 分布する，分配する
distribution 分布，分配
DIT
diet induced thermogenesis 食事誘発性熱源
diffuse intimal thickening び漫〔広汎〕性内膜肥厚
diiodotyrosine ジヨードチロシン
DIV
drip intravenous injection 点滴静脈注射
div, div.
divergence 発散，開散

dividetur〈ラ〉=divide | 分ける《処》
division | 分裂，分割
divorced | 離婚した

divid.
dividetur〈ラ〉=divide | 分ける《処》

div.in p.aeq.
dividetur in partes aequales〈ラ〉 | 同量に分割せよ《処》

DIVP
drip intravenous pyelography | 静脈内(急速)点滴腎盂撮影(法)

DIW
dead in water | 溺死

DJ
Dubin-Johnson (syndrome) | デュビン・ジョンソン(症候群)

DJD
degenerative joint disease | 変性性関節疾患

DJS
Dubin-Johnson syndrome | デュビン・ジョンソン症候群

DK
decay | う蝕(になる)，腐敗(する)，(放射性)崩壊(する)
degeneration of keratinocytes | ケラチノサイト変性値，DK値
Déjérine-Klumpke (syndrome) | デジェリーヌ・クルンプケ(症候群)
diabetic ketoacidosis | 糖尿病(性)ケトアシドーシス
diet kitchen | 治療食調理室
diseased kidney | 罹患腎
dry kata | 乾カタ寒暖計

dk
dark | 暗い

DKA
diabetic ketoacidosis | 糖尿病性ケトアシドーシス

DKB
aminodeoxykanamycin-B | アミノデオキシカナマイシンB
dibekacin | ジベカシン

DKC
dyskeratosis congenita | 先天性角化異常症

DKD
diabetic kidney disease | 糖尿病性腎臓病

DKCT
dog kidney tissue culture | イヌ腎(臓)組織培養

DKFZ
Deutsches Krebsforschungszentrum〈独〉　ドイツ癌研究センター

dkg
decagram　デカグラム〈単位〉

dkl
decaliter　デカリットル〈単位〉

dkm
decameter　デカメートル〈単位〉

DKP
diketopiperazine　ジケトピペラジン

DL
danger list　危険リスト
dextro-levo　右旋性・左旋性
difference limen　弁別閾値
diffuse large cell　び漫〔広汎〕性リンパ腫大細胞型
diffusing capacity of the lung　肺の拡散能
direct laryngoscopy　直接喉頭鏡検査(法)
discussion leader　討論の統率者
distolingual　遠心(面)舌(面)の
Donath-Landsteiner (antibody)　ドーナト・ラントシュタイナー(抗体)
Donath-Landsteiner phenomenon　ドーナト・ラントシュタイナー現象
dosis letalis〈ラ〉=lethal dose　致死量《処》
Durchleuchtung〈独〉　(X線)透視(法)
loading dose　負荷量
racemic　ラセミ化の

dl
deciliter　デシリットル〈単位〉
dilutus〈ラ〉　希釈した《処》

DLA, DLa
distolabial　遠心(面)唇(面)

D-L Ab
Donath-Landsteiner antibody　ドーナト・ラントシュタイナー抗体

DLAI
distolabioincisor　遠位口唇切歯の

DLBD
diffuse Lewy body disease　び漫〔広汎〕性レビー小体病

DLC
dendritic Langerhans cells　樹状上皮ランゲルハンス細胞
differential leukocyte count　白血球百分率数
double lumen catheter　二孔式カテーテル

D

DLCO
diffusing capacity of the lung for carbon monoxide — 一酸化炭素肺拡散能

dld
delivered — 分娩した，出産した

DLE
dialyzable leucocyte extract — 透析後白血球抽出物
discoid lupus erythematosus — 円板状エリテマトーデス〔紅斑性狼瘡〕
disseminated lupus erythematosus — 播種性エリテマトーデス〔紅斑性狼瘡〕

DLET
double lumen endotracheal tube — 二重管気管内チューブ

DLF
difference limen for frequency — 周波数弁別域
dorsolateral fusciculus — 背側索
dose limiting factor — 投与量規制因子

DLI
difference limen for intensity — 強さの弁別域

DLIA
Dental Laboratories Institute of America — 米国歯科検査室研究所

DLIS
digoxin-like immunoreactive substance — ジゴキシン様免疫反応物

DLLI
dulcitol lysine lactose iron — ダルシトールリジン乳糖鉄

DLM
dosis lethalis minima〈ラ〉 — 最小致死量

DLO
Diploma in Laryngology and Otology — 耳鼻咽喉科資格認定書

DLP
dislocation of the patella — 膝蓋骨脱臼
distolinguopulpal — 遠心(面)舌(面)歯髄(面)の

DLPC
dilauryl phosphatidylcholine — ジラウリルホスファチジルコリン

DLS
digitalis like substance — ジギタリス様物質

DLST
drug lymphocyte stimulation test — 薬剤リンパ球刺激試験

DLT
Donath-Landsteiner test — ドーナト・ラントシュタイナー検査
dose limiting toxicity — 投与量規制毒性

DL test
difference limen test　弁別閾検査
DLV
differential lung ventilation　分離肺換気，左右肺独立換気
double lumen ventilation　左右肺独立換気
dlvr
delivery　分娩，出産

dly
delay　遅らせる，遅延
dlyd
delayed　遅れた，遅延型の
DM
daunomycin　ダウノマイシン
data management　データマネジメント
dermal melanosis　黒皮症
dermatologist　皮膚科医
dermatology　皮膚科学
dermatomyositis　皮膚筋炎
Descemet membrane　デスメ膜
destructive mole　破壊胞状奇胎
dextromethorphan　デキストロメトルファン
diabetic mother　糖尿病の母
diastolic murmur　拡張期雑音
diffuse, mixed, small and large cell　び漫〔広汎〕性リンパ腫混合型
digastric muscle　顎二腹筋
distant metastases　遠隔転移
dopamine　ドパミン
dorsomedial　背内側の
dorsomedian (nucleus)　背内側核
double membrane　二重膜
double minutes　微小染色体
duodenal mucosa　十二指腸粘膜
membrane diffusing capacity　膜拡散能
dM
decimorgan　デシモルガン〈単位〉
dm
decimeter　デシメートル〈単位〉
D.M.
Doctor of Medicine　内科学博士
d/m
density/moisture (ratio)　密度/湿度比
DM, dm.
diabetes mellitus　糖尿病
DMA
desmethylacemetacin　デスメチルアセメタシン
dihydroxymandelic acid　ジヒドロキシマンデル酸

D

dimethyladenosine ジメチルアデノシン
dimethylamine ジメチルアミン
dimethylarginine ジメチルアルギニン
direct memory access 直接メモリ転送

DMAA
dimethylarsenic acid ジメチル砒素酸

DMAB(A)
p-dimethylaminobenzaldehyde *p*-ジメチルアミノベンズアルデヒド

DMAC
dimethylacetamide ジメチルアセトアミド

DMAE
dimethylaminoethanol ジメチルアミノエタノール

DMARDS
disease modifying antirheumatic drugs 修飾性抗リウマチ薬

DMAT
Disaster Medical Assistance Team 災害救援医療チーム

DMB
diaminobenzene ジアミノベンゼン

DMBA
desmethyl deschlorobenzoylacemetacin デスメチルデスクロロベンゾイルアセメタシン

DMBG
dimethyl biguanide ジメチルビグアニド

DMBI
desmethyl deschlorobenzoyl indomethacin デスメチルデスクロロベンゾイルインドメタシン

DMC
dactinomycin, methotrexate, cyclophosphamide ダクチノマイシン, メトトレキサート, シクロホスファミド
demeclocycline デメクロサイクリン
dichlorodiphenylmethyl carbinol ジクロロジフェニルメチルカルビノール
dimethylcarbinol ジメチルカルビノール
dimethylcysteine ジメチルシステイン

DMCT
doxycycline ドキシサイクリン(＝DOXY, DOTC)

DMCTC
demethyl chlortetracycline デメチルクロルテトラサイクリン

DMD
Duchenne muscular dystrophy デュシェーヌ(型)筋ジストロフィ

DMD, D.M.D.
dentarie medicinae doctor〈ラ〉= Doctor of Dental Medicine　歯学博士
DMDZ
desmethyldiazepam　デスメチルジアゼパム
DME
dimethyl ether　ジメチルエーテル
dimethyltubocurarine chloride　塩化ジメチルツボクラリン
Director of Medical Education　医学教育責任者
drug-metabolizing enzyme　薬物代謝酵素
D.Med.
Doctor of Medicine　医学士
D.Med.Sc.
Doctor of Medical Science　医学研究博士
DMEM
Dulbecco modified Eagle medium　ドゥルベコ変法イーグル培地
D-men
drug-enforcement officer　麻薬取締官
DMF
dimethylformamide　ジメチルホルムアミド
drug master file　ドラッグマスターファイル
DMFA
dimethylformamide　ジメチルホルムアミド
dmf index, DMF Index
decayed, missing or filled (teeth) index　DMF指数，う蝕歯・喪失歯・充填歯係数
DMFOS
Diploma in Maxillo-facial and Oral Surgery　顎顔面・口腔外科資格認定書
DMF rate
decayed missing filled rate　DMF比率
DMG
dimethylglycine　ジメチルグリシン
DMGG
dimethylguanylguanidine　ジメチルグアニルグアニジン
DMH
dimethylhydrazine　ジメチルヒドラジン
DMHS
Director of Medical and Health Service　医療保健サービス責任者
DMI
desmethyl imipramine　デスメチルイミプラミン
desmethyl indomethacin　デスメチルインドメタシン
diphragmatic myocardial infarct　横隔膜(面)心筋梗塞
direct migration inhibition　直接遊走抑制

D

DMJ
Diploma in Medical Jurist Prudence　医事法制士資格認定書
DMKA
diabetes mellitus ketoacidosis　糖尿病(性)ケトアシドーシス
DML
distal motor latency　遠位運動潜時
DMLT
Diploma in Medical Laboratory Technology　臨床検査技師資格認定書
DMN
dimethylnitrosamine　ジメチルニトロサミン
dorsal motor nucleus　背側運動核
DMNA
dimethylnitrosamine　ジメチルニトロサミン
DMO
dimethadion　ジメタジオン
dimethyloxazolidin　ジメチルオキサゾリジン
distinct medical officer　地域医療事務官
dmo
decimorgan　デシモルガン
DMP
diffuse mesangial proliferation　広汎〔び漫〕性メザンギウム増殖
dimercaprol　ジメルカプロール
dimethylphosphate　ジメチルリン酸
dimethylphthalate　ジメチルフタル酸
dura mater prosthesis　人工硬膜
dystrophia muscularis progressiva〈ラ〉　進行性筋ジストロフィ
DMPB
Diploma in Medical Pathology and Bacteriology　病理学・細菌学資格認定書
DMPC
dimethoxyphenyl-PC　メチシリン
DMPE
dimethoxyphenylethylamine　ジメトキシフェニルエチルアミン
DMPEA
dimethoxyphenylethylamine　ジメトキシフェニルエチルアミン
DMPP
dimethylphenylpiperazonium　ジメチルフェニルピペラゾニウム
DMPPC
dimethoxyphenyl penicillin　ジメトキシフェニルペニシリン
methicillin　メチシリン

DMPS
dimethyl polysiloxane ジメチルポリシオキサン
dysmyelopoietic syndrome 骨髄異形成症候群
DMR, D.M.R.
Diploma in Medical Radiology 医用放射線化学資格認定書
DMRD, D.M.R.D.
Diploma in Medical Radiological Diagnosis 医用放射線診断資格認定書

DMRE
Diploma in Medical Radiology and Electrology 医用放射線・電子学資格認定書
DMRF
dorsal medullary reticular formation 背側延髄網様体
D.M.R.T.
Diploma in Medical Radiotheraphy 医学放射線治療医免許
DMS
deoxyribonucleic acid デオキシリボ核酸
dermatomyositis 皮膚筋炎
diagnostic and statistical manual of mental disoder 精神障害の診断と統計の手引き
diffuse mesangial sclerosis 広汎〔び漫〕性メザンギウム硬化(症)
dimethylsterone ジメチルステロン
dimethyl sulfate ジメチル硫酸
dimethyl sulfonate ジメチルスルホン酸
dimethyl sulfoxide ジメチルスルホキシド
Director of Medical Service 医療サービス責任者
DMSA
2,3-dimercaptosuccinic acid ジメルカプトコハク酸
DMSO
dimethyl sulfoxide ジメチルスルホキシド
$DMSO_2$
dimethyl sulfone ジメチルスルホン
DMSS
Director of Medical and Sanitary Services 医療衛生サービス責任者
DMT
dermatophytosis 皮膚糸状菌症
dimethyl terephthalate ジメチルテレフタル酸
dimethyltryptamine ジメチルトリプタミン
DMTA
drug-mediated tumor antigen 薬物媒介性腫瘍抗原
DMTU
dimethylthiourea ジメチルチオウレア

D

DMW
Deutsche Medizinische Wochenschrift 〈独〉 ドイツ医学週刊誌
D MX
maximal dose 最大量
DN
Deiters nucleus ダイテルス核
diabetic nephropathy 糖尿病性腎症
diabetic neuropathy 糖尿病(性)神経障害〔ニューロパシー〕
dibucaine number ジブカイン数
dicrotic notch 重複切痕
dinitrocresol ジニトロクレゾール
Diploma in Nursing 看護師認定書
Diploma in Nutrition 栄養士認定書
dopaminergic neuron ド(ー)パミン作動性神経
dn
decinem デシネム〈単位〉
DN, D/N
dextrose-nitrogen (ratio) 尿中ブドウ糖/窒素(比)
DNA
deoxyribonucleic acid デオキシリボ核酸
DNA-P
deoxyribonucleic acid phosphorus デオキシリボ核酸リン
deoxyribonucleic acid polymerase デオキシリボ核酸ポリメラーゼ
DNase
deoxyribonuclease デオキシリボヌクレアーゼ
DNB
Diplomate of National Board of Medical Examiners 医師国家試験合格者
DNB, D.N.B.
dinitrobenzene ジニトロベンゼン
DNBP
dinitrobuthylphenol ジニトロブチルフェノール
DNC
4,4′-dinitrocarbanilide 4,4′-ジニトロカルバニリド
dinitrocresol ジニトロクレゾール
DNCB
dinitro-chlorobenzene ジニトロクロロベンゼン
DNCB test
dinitro-chlorobenzene test DNCB感作試験
DND
died a natural death 自然死
Division of Narcotic Drugs (米国)麻薬局

DNE
Director of Nursing Education　看護教育責任者
Doctor of Nursing Education　看護教育医師

DNFA
2,4-dinitrofluoroaniline　2,4-ジニトロフルオロアニリン

DNFB
2,4-dinitro-1-fluorobenzene　2,4-ジニトロ-1-フルオロベンゼン
1-fluoro-2,4-dinitrobenzene　1-フルオロ-2,4-ジニトロベンゼン

DNHW
Department of National Health and Welfare　国家保健福祉局

DNMP
deoxynucleoside monophosphate　デオキシヌクレオシド一リン酸

DNN
dinitronaphthol　ジニトロナフトール

DNO
district nursing officer　地区看護行政官

DNOC
3,5-dinitro-*o*-cresol　3,5-ジニトロ-*o*-クレゾール
dinitro orthocresol　ジニトロオルトクレゾール

DNP
dinitrophenol　ジニトロフェノール
2,4-dinitrophenyl　2,4-ジニトロフェニル

DNP, Dnp
deoxyribonucleoprotein　デオキシリボ核蛋白
dinitrophenol　ジニトロフェノール

DNPH
dinitrophenylhydrazine　ジニトロフェニルヒドラジン

DNP-KLH
dinitrophenyl-keyhole limpethemocyanin　ジニトロフェニル・鍵穴アオガイヘモシアニン

DNPM
dinitrophenyl morphine　ジニトロフェニルモルヒネ

DNP method
dinitrophenyl protein method　ジニトロフェニル蛋白法

DNP-S'L
1-hydroxy-5-*N*-(1-oxyl-2,2,5,5-tetramethyl-3-aminopyrrolidyl)-2,4-dinitrobenzene　1-ヒドロキシ-5-*N*-(1-オキシル-2,2,5,5-テトラメチル-3-アミノピロリジル)-2,4-ジニトロベンゼン

D

DNPT
diethyl-nitrophenyl thiophosphate ジエチル・ニトロフェニルチオリン酸

DNR
daunorubicin ダウノルビシン
did not respond 応答なし
do not resuscitate 蘇生不可〔不要〕，蘇生術適応除外

D/Nr
ratio of urinary glucose (排泄)尿中のブドウ糖と窒素との比

D-N ratio，D : N ratio
dextrose to nitrogen ratio (尿中の)ブドウ糖/窒素比

DNR-Order
do-not-resuscitate order 蘇生法を行わないという指示書

DNS
Desoxyribonukleinsäure〈独〉 デオキシリボ核酸
deviated nasal septum 偏位(性)鼻中隔
diaphragm nerve stimulation 横隔(膜)神経刺激

D/NS
dextrose in normal saline ブドウ糖生理食塩液

DNS，Dns
dansyl ダンシル

DNSA
Diploma in Nursing Administration 看護管理認定書

DNSc
Doctor of Nursing Science 看護学士

D_5NSS
5% dextrose in normal saline solution 5％ブドウ糖加生理食塩水

DNT
dermonecrotic toxin 皮膚壊死毒素
2,4-dinitrotoluene 2,4-ジニトロトルエン
do not test 検査せず

DNTP
diethyl-*p*-nitrophenyl thiophosphate ジエチルパラニトロフェニルチオホスフェイト，パラチオン

dNTP
deoxyribonucleotide triphosphate デオキシリボヌクレオチド三リン酸

DNV
dorsal nucleus of the vagus 迷走神経背側核

DO
densitéoptique〈仏〉 光学密度

Directive Organic Psychiatrics 指導的組織精神医学
dissolved oxygen 溶存酸素
Doctor of Optometry 視力検定学士

do.
dicto〈ラ〉=the same, as before, repeat 同じ
ditto 前と同じ，繰り返す

DO_2
oxygen delivery 酸素供給量

D_2O
deuterium oxide 重水

D.O.
Diploma in Ophthalmology 眼科資格〔免状〕
Doctor of Osteopathy 整骨医学博士

d/o
delivery order 出産指示

DOA
date of admission 入院日
date of arrival 到着日
dead on arrival 来院時(既)死亡
dominant optic atrophy 優性視神経萎縮
dopamine ド(ー)パミン

DOAC
Dubois oleic albumin complex デュボイスオレイン酸アルブミン複合体
direct oral anticoagulants 直接経口抗凝固薬

DOAP
daunorubicin, vincristine(=Oncovin), arabinosylcytosine, prednisone ダウノルビシン，ビンクリスチン(=オンコビン)，アラビノシルシトシン，プレドニゾン

DOB
date of birth 生年月日
dobutamine ドブタミン
doctor's order book 医師の指示簿

DOC
dead〔died〕 of other causes 他原因による死亡
deoxycorticosterone デオキシコルチコステロン
dissolved organic carbon 溶存全有機物
disturbance of consciousness 意識障害
sodium deoxycholate デオキシコール酸ナトリウム

doc
doctor 医師
document 文書，記録
documentation 文書提示，証拠文書

DOCA
deoxycorticosterone acetate — 酢酸デオキシコルチコステロン

DOCG
deoxycorticosterone glucoside — デオキシコルチコステロングルコシド
desoxycorticosterone glucoside — デスオキシコルチコステロングルコシド

DOCS
deoxycorticoids — デオキシコルチコイド〈複数〉

DOD
date of death — 死亡(年月)日
date of departure — 出発日
died of disease — 原疾患死

DOE
date of examination — 検査日
desoxyephedrine — デスオキシエフェドリン
desoxyephedrine hydrochloride — 塩酸デスオキシエフェドリン
direct observation evaluation — 直接観察評価
dyspnea on exercise — 運動時呼吸困難
dyspnea on exertion — 労作性呼吸困難

D-O-E
D-deoxyephedrine — D-デオキシエフェドリン

DOG
Deutsche Ophthalmologische Gesellschaft〈独〉 — ドイツ眼科学会

DOH
defence of honour — 護身術

DOI
date of injury — 傷害(年月)日
dead on injuries — 外傷死

DOL
distolinguo-occlusal — 遠心舌側咬合(面)の，遠心面舌面咬合面の
duration of life — 延命効果

dol.
dolor〈ラ〉=pain — 疼痛

dolent part.
dolenti parti〈ラ〉 — 患部に《処》

dolichocephs
dolichocephalics — 長頭人種

dollies
dolophine pills — ドロフィン錠

dolo
dolophine — ドロフィン

dol urg
dolore urgente〈ラ〉 疼痛時《処》
DOLV
double outlet left ventricle 両大血管左(心)室起始症
DOM
date of marriage 結婚(年月)日
2,5-dimethoxy-4-methylamphetamine ジメトキシ-メチルアンフェタミン
dimethyloxy alphamethyl phenethylamine ジメチルオキシアルファメチルフェネチラミン
dom
domestic 家庭の，国産の，家畜の
DOMA
dihydroxymandelic acid ジヒドロキシマンデル酸
DOMP
diseases of medical practice 医原病
DOMS
Diploma in Ophthalmic Medicine and Surgery 眼科認定医
DON
diazooxonorleucine ジアゾオキソノルロイシン
don.
donec〈ラ〉=until ～まで
donec alv.sol.
donec alvus soluta fuerit〈ラ〉 便通のあるまで《処》
donec dol.exulav.
donec dolor exulaverit〈ラ〉 痛みがやわらぐまで《処》
DOP
dermo-optical perception 皮膚・視覚認知
desoxypyridoxine デスオキシピリドキシン
DOPA, Dopa
dihydroxyphenylalanine ジヒドロキシフェニルアラニン，ド(ー)パ
DOPAA
dihydroxyphenyl acetic acid ジヒドロキシフェニル酢酸
DOPAmine, DOPAMINE
aminoethyl benzendiol ド(ー)パミン
3,4-dihydroxyphenylethylamine ド(ー)パミン
DOPA reaction
dihydroxyphenylalanine reaction ド(ー)パ反応
dopase
dopa oxidase ド(ー)パ酸化酵素
DOPIPC
hetacillin ヘタシリン

D

D

DOPS
diffuse obstructive pulmonary syndrome — 広汎〔び漫〕性閉塞性肺症候群
dihydroxyphenylserine — ジヒドロキシフェニルセリン

D.Opt.
Doctor of Optometry — 視力測定学士

DOP test
dioctylphthalate test — DOP試験

DOR
dental operating room — 歯科手術室

dor
dorsal — 背側の，背(面)の

DORCG
Diploma in Royal Collage of Obst. and Gynaecol — 英国産婦人科学資格〔免状〕

DORL
developmental orbital research laboratory — 発達眼窩研究室

dorsi
dorsiflexion — 背屈

dorsifl
dorsiflexion — 背屈

DOrth
Diploma in Orthodontics — 歯矯正資格認定書
Diploma in Orthopedics — 整形外科資格認定書
Diploma in Orthoptics — 視力矯正資格認定書

DORV
double outlet right ventricle — 両大血管右室起始症

DOS
day of surgery — (外科)手術日
density of states — 状態密度
digital operation system — デジタル操作システム
Doctor of Ocular Science — 眼科医
Doctor of Optometric Science — 視力測定士
doctor oriented system — ドクター中心システム

dos
dosimetry — 薬量〔線量〕測定

dos.
dosage〈ラ〉 — (適)用量，(投与)量，薬用量《処》
dosis〈ラ〉＝dose — 服用量，線量《処》

dosim
dosimetry — 薬量〔線量〕測定

DOSM
dihydrodesoxy streptomycin — ジヒドロデスオキシストレプトマイシン

dioxy streptomycin ジオキシストレプトマイシン

DOSS

dioctylsodium sulfosuccinate スルホコハク酸ジオクチルナトリウム

DOTC

deoxycycline デオキシサイクリン(=DOXY,DMCT)

6-deoxy-5-hydroxytetracycline 6-デオキシ-5-ヒドロキシテトラサイクリン

doxycycline hydrochloride 塩酸ドキシサイクリン

DOTS

directly observed treatment with short-course chemotherapy 直接監視下短期化学療法

DOW

died of wounds 創傷による死亡

DOX

doxorubicin ドキソルビシン(=アドリアマイシン)

DOXY

doxycycline ドキシサイクリン(=DMCT,DOTC)

DP

deep pulse 深在脈
degradation products 分解産物
dementia precox (praecox) 早発性痴呆
diabetes-prone 糖尿病傾向
diastolic pressure 拡張期圧
diffusion pressure 拡散圧
digestive protein 消化可能な蛋白
diphosgene ジホスゲン
diphosphate 二リン酸塩
dipropionate ジプロピオン酸塩
directional preponderance 方向優位性
directional preponderance of nystagmus 眼振方向優位性
disability pension 身障者用ペンション
discriminating power 識別力
disopyramide ジソピラミド
distal pancreatectomy 膵尾部切除術
distal phalanx 遠位指節骨
distribution point 分布点
donor's plasma 供血者の血漿
dorsals pedis (artery) 足背動脈
driving pressure (人工呼吸器の)動力圧
dynamic psychiatry 動的精神医学
polydysplasia 多発発育異常

D

D

polydystrophy 多発異栄養症
preoperative blood deposit 術前自家血保存

Dp
Dermatophagoides pteronyssinus (antigen) ヤケヒョウヒダニ(抗原)
dyspnea 呼吸困難

dp
dry pint 乾量パイント

D.P.
Doctor of Pharmacy 薬学博士

d.p.
directione propria〈ラ〉 適当な指示のもとに《処》

DPA
diphenolic acid ジフェノール酸
diphenylamine ジフェニルアミン
dipropylacetate ジプロピルアセテート
dual-photon absorptiometry 二重光子吸収法

3DPA
3-deoxypentonic acid 3-デオキシペントン酸

DPA reaction
diphenylamine reaction ジフェニルアミン反応

DPB
diffuse panbronchiolitis び漫〔広汎〕性汎細気管支炎

DPBS
Dulbecco phosphate buffered saline デュルベックリン酸塩緩衝塩

DPC
diagnosis procedure combination 診断群分類包括評価
diethyl pyrocarbonate ジエチルピロカルボネート
distal palmar crease 遠位手掌皮膚溝

dpc
dosi pedetentim crescente〈ラ〉 用量を漸増する《処》

D-Pc
D-penicillamine D-ペニシラミン

DPD
desoxypyridoxine hydrochloride 塩酸デソキシピリドキシン

DPDL
diffuse poorly differentiated lymphocytic lymphoma び漫〔広汎〕性未分化リンパ球性リンパ腫

dP/dT
differential pressure/differential time 圧力の時間微分

dp/dt
ratio of change of ventricular pressure to change in time 時間に対する心室圧の微分値

DPE
data processing equipment データ操作器具

DPF
diisopropyl fluorophosphate フッ素リン酸ジイソプロピル
DP flap
deltopectoral flap 胸三角筋部皮弁，DP皮弁，前胸壁有茎皮弁
dorsalis pedicle flap 足背動脈皮弁
DP fluid
dextrose phenol fluid ブドウ糖フェノール液
DPG
diphosphoglycerate ジホスホグリセレート
1,3-DPG
1,3-diphosphoglycerate 1,3-ジホスホグリセレート
2,3-DPG
2,3-diphosphoglycerate 2,3-ジホスホグリセレート
DPGM
diphosphoglycerate mutase ジホスホグリセレートムターゼ
DPGN
diffuse proliferative glomerulonephritis び漫〔広汎〕性増殖性糸球体腎炎
DPGP
diphosphoglycerate phosphatase ジホスホグリセレートホスファターゼ
DPH
Department of Public Health 公衆衛生局
diaphragm(atic) 横隔膜
diphenhydramine ジフェンヒドラミン
diphenylhexatriene ジフェニルヘキサトリエン
diphenylhydantoin ジフェニルヒダントイン
Diploma in Public Health 公衆衛生学資格認定書
Doctor of Public Health/Hygiene 公衆衛生学博士
D.Pharm.
Doctor of Pharmacy 薬学博士
DPHD
Diploma in Public Health Dentistry 公衆保健歯科認定書
D.Ph.Sc.
Doctor of Physical Science 医学士，医師
D.Phs.Med.
Diploma in Physical Medicine 内科認定書
DPI
dietary protein intake 食事性蛋白摂取
diphosphoinositid ジホスホイノシチド
diphtheria and pertussis immunization ジフテリア・百日咳免疫
dry powder inhaler 粉末吸入器

DPIP
dichlorphenolindophenol ジクロルフェノールインドフェノール

DPL
diagnostic peritoneal lavage 診断的腹腔洗浄法
dipalmitoyl lecithin 表面活性リン脂質
diplamitoyl lecithin ジプラミトイルレシチン

dpl.
diploma 卒業証書，学位記，賞状

DPLN
diffuse proliferative lupus nephritis び漫〔広汎〕性増殖性ループス腎炎

dplx
duplex〈ラ〉 両側の

DPM
diazo-positive metabolites ジアゾ反応陽性物質
Diploma in Psychologial Medicine 精神科専門医資格
dipyridamole ジピリダモール
dipyrromethene ジピロメテン
Doctor of Pediatric Medicine 小児科医

dpm, DPM
disintegrations per minute 毎分崩壊数

DPN
dermatosis papulosa nigra 黒色丘疹性皮膚病
diphosphopyridine nucleotide ジホスホピリジンヌクレオチド

DPNase
diphosphopyridine nucleotidase ジホスホピリジンヌクレオチダーゼ

DPNH
reduced diphosphopyridine nucleotide 還元ジホスホピリジンヌクレオチド(＝NADH)

DPO
diphenyloxazole ジフェニルオキサゾール

DPOB
date and place of birth 出生(年月)日と出生地

DPP
dipeptidyl peptidase ジペプチジルペプチダーゼ
disease prevention program 疾病予防計画
Drehpendelprüfung〈独〉 振子様回転試験

DPPC
dipalmitoyl-phosphatidilcholine ジパルミトイルホスファチジルコリン

DPPD
diphenyl-*p*-phenylenediamine ジフェニル-*p*-フェニレンジアミン

DP physician
displaced persons physician 移住医師
DPPK
dephosphophosphorylase kinase デホスホホスホリラーゼキナーゼ
DPR
diaminopropionic acid ジアミノプロピオン酸
DPRT
damped pendular rotation test 減衰振子様回転検査
DPS
deafferentation pain syndrome 求心神経遮断性疼痛症候群
delayed primary suture 遅延一次縫合
diffuse projection system 非特殊投射系
digital pencil-beam scanography デジタルペンシルビーム走査法《画診》
dps
disintegration per second 毎秒崩壊数
D.Psy.
Diploma in Psychiatry 精神科資格認定書
Diploma in Psychology 心理学資格認定書
D.Psy.Sci.
Doctor of Psychological Science 心理学博士
DPT
department 部門，科，教室
diphosphothiamine ジホスホチアミン
diphtheria, pertussis, tetanus (vaccine) ジフテリア・百日咳・破傷風(ワクチン)
dipropyltryptamine ジプロピルトリプタミン
DPTI
diastolic pressure time index 拡張期圧時間係数
DPTP
diphtheria, pertussis, tetanus, polimyelitis ジフテリア・百日咳・破傷風・ポリオ
DPTPM
diphtheria, pertussis, tetanus, poliomyelitis, measles ジフテリア・百日咳・破傷風・ポリオ・麻疹
dptr
Dioptrie〈独〉=diopter 屈折度，ジオプトリー，ディオプター〈単位〉
DPWV
diastolic posterior wall velocity 後壁拡張期後退速度
dpx
duplex〈ラ〉 両側の
DQ
deterioration quotient 崩壊指数
development(al) quotient 発育指数

differentiation quick 迅速分別染色

dq

dry quart 乾量クォート〈単位〉

DQE

detective quantum efficiency 量子検出効率

DR

Dahl salt-resistant rat ダール食塩抵抗性ラット
day room 昼間の居室
degeneration reaction 変性反応
deoxyribose デオキシリボース
desoxyribose デスオキシリボース
diabetic retinopathy 糖尿病(性)網膜症
diagnostic radiology 放射線診断学
differential rate 分化度
diffuse redness 広汎性発赤
digital radiography デジタルラジオグラフィ
dining room 食堂，食事室
D-related antigen D関連抗原
drug receptor 薬物受容体
dynamic range ダイナミックレンジ

dr

drain ドレーン，排液管
dressing 包帯(剤)

Dr.

doctor 医師

D.R.

Diploma in Radiology 放射線科専門医資格

DR，dr，dr.

dorsal root (脊髄)後根

DR，D.R.

delivery room 分娩室

dr，dr.

dram＝drachm (常用/薬用)ドラム〈単位〉

DRA

dextran reactive antibody デキストラン反応(性)抗体
dual energy radiographic absorptiometry 二重エネルギーX線吸収測定法

drain

drainage ドレナージ，排液，排膿

dr ap，dr.ap.

apothecaries dram 薬用ドラム〈単位〉
drachm apothecaries weight ドラム薬用度量衡法

DRB

daunorubicin ダウノルビシン

DRBC

dog red blood cell イヌ赤血球

D

Dr.Bi.Chem.
Doctor of Biological Chemistry 生化学博士
DRC
daunorubicin ダウノルビシン
dual retinal correspondence 網膜二重対応
DRCOG
Diploma of Royal College of Obstetricians and Gynecologists 英国産婦人科学会認定書
DRD
dopa responsive dystonia ド(ー)パ反応性筋緊張異常症
DRE
digital rectal examination 直腸指診(=DER)
DREZ
dorsal root entry zoon (脊髄)後根侵入部
DRF
Deutshe Rettungsflugwacht〈独〉 ドイツ救難飛行隊
DRG
diagnostic related group 診断関連グループ
dorsal root ganglion 後根神経節
drg
drainage ドレナージ，排液，排膿
DRG/PPS
diagnosis-related groups/prospective payment system 診断群別定額支払方式
Dr.Hy.
Doctor of Hygiene 衛生学博士
dRib
deoxyribose デオキシリボース
DRK
Deutshes Rotes Kreutz〈独〉 ドイツ赤十字
DRL
differential reinforcement of low response rate 低反応率補充誤差
drug-related lupus 薬剤関連ループス
Drm, d.r.m.
dosis reagens minima〈ラ〉 最小反応値
Dr Med, Dr.Med.
Doctor der Medizin〈独〉= *doctor medicinae*〈ラ〉 医学博士
DRNA
desoxyribose nucleic acid デスオキシリボ核酸
drng
drainage ドレナージ，排液，排膿
DRNT
diagnostic roentogenology X線診断学

D

D

DRP
dorsal root potential 後根電位
Dr.P.H.
Doctor of Public Health 公衆保健学博士
DRPLA
dentato-rubro-pallido-luysian atrophy 歯状核・赤核・淡蒼球・ルイ体萎縮症
DRQ
discomfort relief quotient 不快軽減指数
DRR
dorsal root reflex 後根反射
DRS
delirium rating scale せん(譫)妄による行動学的異常を評価する基準
drowsiness し(嗜)眠状態
DRSG, drsg
dressing 包帯，包剤
DRT
dark room test 暗室試験
dRTA
distal renal tubular acidosis 遠位尿細管アシドーシス
DRTF
differentiation-regulated transcriptional factor 遺伝網膜芽細胞腫の炎症に関する転写因子
DS
Dauerschlaf〈独〉 持続睡眠
Dauerschlafkur 持続睡眠療法
dead(-air) space 死腔
deamelin-S デアメリンS
Debré-Semelaigne (syndrome) デブレ・セミレーニュ(症候群)
deep sedative 強力鎮静薬
deep sleep 深睡眠
defined substrate 確定物質
dehydroepiandrosterone sulfate 硫酸デヒドロエピアンドロステロン
Déjérine-Sottas (syndrome) デジェリーヌ・ソッタ(症候群)
delayed sensitivity 遅延型感受性
dendritic spine 樹状突起棘
density (optical) standard 標準(光学)密度
dental surgery 歯科手術
Department of Sanitation 衛生施設局
deprivation syndrome 剥奪症候群
dermatan sulfate デルマタン硫酸
desynchronized sleep 脱同期性睡眠

Devic syndrome	デビック症候群
dextran sulfate	硫酸デキストラン
dextrose-saline	ブドウ糖-食塩水
dextrose stick	ブドウ糖(検査)スティック
diaphragm stimulation	横隔膜刺激
diastolic murmur	拡張期雑音
difference spectroscopy	差分光法
difference spectrum	差スペクトル
differential stimulus	鑑別刺激
diffuse scleroderma	広汎〔び漫〕性強皮症
digital scanography	デジタル走査撮影法
digit span	(最大拡張時の手親指小指間の)スパン
dihydrostreptomycin	ジヒドロストレプトマイシン
dilute strength	希釈力価
dioptric strength	曲光度，屈折度
Disaster Services (of Red Cross)	(赤十字の)災害時活動
discharge summary	退院要約
discrimination score	識別〔弁別〕スコア
discriminative stimulus	識別〔弁別〕刺激
disoriented	失見当(識)の
disseminated sclerosis	散在(性)硬化(症)
dissemination score	弁別能
dissolved solids	溶解固体
Doctor of Science	理学博士
donor's serum	供血者血清
Doppler ultrasound sonography	ド(ッ)プラー超音波診断法
double-stranded	二本鎖の
double strength	二倍強力
Down syndrome	ダウン症候群
drug store	薬局，薬品店
dry syrup	ドライシロップ
dumping syndrome	ダンピング症候群
duodenal sonde	十二指腸ゾンデ
duration of systole	(心)収縮(持続)時間
dual screen	デュアルスクリーン
(left ventricular) systolic dimension	(左(心)室)収縮期径

Ds

diameter in systolic	収縮末期径

D.S.

Doctor of Science	理学博士

D/S

dextrose in saline	ブドウ糖食塩液
dextrose-saline ratio	ブドウ糖・食塩比
Doerfler-Stewart (test)	デルフラー・スチュアート(試験)

D

D-5-S
dextrose 5% in saline 5%ブドウ糖食塩溶液
DS, ds
double-stranded (=DNA) 二重鎖(=DNA)
D.S., d.s.
da signa〈ラ〉=give and label 表示して与えよ，与えて書け《処》
DSA
Datura stramonium agglutinin 白花朝鮮アサガオ凝集素
destructive spondylarthropathy 破壊性脊椎症
digital substraction angiography デジタル減算処理血管造影法
digital subtraction angiography デジタル減算処理血管造影法
dsabl
disability 無能，不具
disable 無能にする
disabled 不具の，無能の
DSAK
disseminated superficial actinic keratosis 播種状表在性光線性角化症
DSAN
distantia subauriculonasalis〈ラ〉 耳下点・鼻下点間距離
DSAP
disseminated superficial actinic porokeratosis 播種性表在性光線性汗孔角化症
DSAT
digital subtraction angiotomography デジタル減算処理血管断層撮影
DSB
double side-band 両側波帯
DSBCT
donor specific buffy-coat transfusion 血縁者間軟層輸血
DSBT
donor-specific blood transfusion 血縁者間生体腎移植でのドナー血輸血
DSC
decussation of superior cerebellar (peduncles) 上小脳脚交叉
De Sanctis-Cacchione (syndrome) ドサンクティス・カッキオーネ〔症候群〕
differential scanning calorimetry 示差走査熱量測定
diffuse, small cleaved cell び漫〔広汎〕性リンパ腫小切れ込み核細胞型
digital scan converter デジタルスキャンコンバーター
disodium c(h)romoglycate クロモグリク酸二ナトリウム
Doctor of Surgical Chiropody 足の外科学博士

dobutamine stress echocardiography ドブタミン(負荷)心エコー法
Down syndrome child ダウン症児

D.Sc.
Doctor of Science 理学博士

DSCG
disodium c(h)romoglycate クロモグリク酸二ナトリウム

D.Sc.Os.
Doctor of Science of Osteopathy 整形外科医

DSCT
dorsal spinocerebellar tract 背側脊髄小脳路

DSD
depression sine depression 抑うつ感情のないうつ病
detrusor sphincter dyssynergia 排尿筋括約筋協調不全
disaster stress disorder 災害ストレス障害
dry sterile dressing 乾燥無菌包帯
dry surgical dressing 乾燥外科包帯

dsDNA
double-stranded deoxyribonucleic acid 二重鎖DNA〔デオキシリボ核酸〕

d.secund.〔tert.〕
diebus secundis〔*tertiis*〕〈ラ〉=every second〔third〕days 2日〔3日〕ごとに《処》

d.seq.
die sequente〈ラ〉=on the following day 翌日《処》

DSF
digital subtraction fluorography デジタル減算処理間接撮影

Dsg, dsg
dressing 包帯(剤)

DSHR
delayed skin hypersensitivity reaction 遅延(型)皮膚過敏反応

DSI
depression status inventory うつ状態評価尺度
direct sample insertion 試料直接導入法
direct sillicone intubation 直接シリコンチューブ挿入

DSIP
delta sleep inducing peptide デルタ睡眠誘発ペプチド

DSL
deep scattering layer 深部散乱層

dslv
dissolved 溶解した

DSM
degradable starch microsphere 塞栓療法に用いるデンプン製剤

diagnostic and statistical manual of mental disorders (米国精神医学会による)精神障害分類基準，精神疾患診断と統計マニュアル
dried skim milk 乾燥脱脂乳
drink skim milk 脱脂乳を飲む

DSMA
distal spinal muscular atrophy 遠位型脊髄性筋萎縮症

DSN
deviatio septi nasi〈ラ〉 鼻中隔彎曲症

d.s.n.
detur suo nomine〈ラ〉 内容〔薬名〕を明記せよ《処》

DSO
dermal sutures out 抜糸

DSP
decreased sensory perception 知覚の低下
delayed sleep phase 睡眠相後退
deoxyspergualin デオキシスパーガリン
dexamethasone sodium phosphate デキサメタゾンリン酸ナトリウム
diarrhetic shellfish poison 下痢性貝毒
dibasic sodium phosphate 二塩基リン酸ナトリウム
digital subtraction phlebography デジタル減算静脈造影(法)
disulfanilamide phenolphthalein ジスルファニルアミドフェノールフタレイン

D-spine
dorsal spine 胸椎

DSPS
delayed sleep pause insomnia 睡眠相遅延不眠症

DSR
Dahl salt-sensitive rat ダール食塩感受性ラット
daily secretion rate 1日分泌量
digital subtraction radioangiography デジタル減算処理血管像
digital subtraction radiography デジタル減算処理X線像
disaster stress reaction 災害ストレス反応
dynamic spatial reconstructor 動的空間再構築装置

dsRNA
double-stranded ribonucleic acid 二重鎖リボ核酸

DSRS
distal splenorenal shunt 遠位脾腎静脈吻合術

DSRU
Drug Safety Research Unit (英国)医薬品安全性研究所

DSS
dengue shock syndrome デング(熱)ショック症候群
developmental sentence scale 発達文章段階
dextrose sucrose starch agar ブドウ糖・ショ糖・デンプン寒天

dioctyl sodium sulfosuccinate　スルホコハク酸ジオクチルナトリウム
disuccinimidyl suberate　架橋剤
double simultaneous stimulation　二点同時刺激
droopy shoulder syndrome　下垂萎縮肩症候群

DSSc
Diploma in Sanitary Science　衛生学認定書

DST
daylight saving time　夏時間
Denksport Test〈独〉　謎解きテスト
dermatology and syphilology technicians　皮膚・梅毒学技士
desensitization test　脱感作テスト
dexamethasone suppression test　デキサメタゾン抑制試験
dihydrostreptomycin　ジヒドロストレプトマイシン
donor-specific blood transfusion　ドナー限定輸血
donor-specific transfusion　ドナー限定輸液

D-S test
Doerfler-Stewart test　デルフラー・スチュアート試験

dstr
distribution　分布

DSTT
delayed side tone test　緩速語音聴取検査

DSUH
direct suggestion under hypnosis　催眠状態下の直達暗示

D.Surg.
Dental Surgeon　口腔外科医
Doctor of Surgery　外科医

DSW
Doctor of Social Welfare　社会福祉学士

DT
dead time　死亡時間
delayed tanning　遅延型黒化
delirium tremens　振戦せん(=譫)妄
Dental Technician　歯科技工士
depression of transmission　伝達抑制
deviation test　かたより試験
Dicktropfenpräparat〈独〉　濃(厚層)塗抹標本
differential titer　鑑別滴定量
differential tonometry　示差眼圧測定
diphtheria and tetanus vaccine　ジフテリアと破傷風の混合ワクチン
diphtheria toxoid　ジフテリア毒素
disappearance time　消失時間
discharge tomorrow　明日退院

dispensing tablet 調剤錠
distal tubles 遠位尿細管
distance test 距離試験
double time 重複時間
doubling time (細菌・ウイルスの増殖における)2倍化時間

D

dye test 色素試験

Dt
decoctum〈ラ〉 煎剤《処》
duration tetany 強直持続時間, テタニー持続時間

dT
deoxythymidine デオキシチミジン

D/T
date of treatment 治療日
death total ratio 死亡率

D/T, d.t.
due to ～による

DTA
differential thermoanalysis 示差寒暖分析
diphtheria toxin A ジフテリア毒素A

DTAA
dissecting thoracic aortic aneurysm 解離性胸部大動脈瘤

DTAB
dodecyl trimethyl ammonium bromide 臭化ドデシルトリメチルアンモニウム

DTC
differentiated thyroid carcinoma 分化(型)甲状腺癌

DTC, d-TC
D-tubocurarine D-ツボクラリン

DTCD
Diploma in Tuberculosis and Chest Disease 結核症・胸部疾患認定書

DTD
document of definition 文書型定義

d.t.d.
detur talis dosis〈ラ〉 この量を与えよ《処》

d.t.d.no Ⅳ
da tales doses numero quattuor〈ラ〉＝ let four such doses be given 同量4個が与えられるべし《処》

dTDP
deoxythymidine diphosphate デオキシチミジン二リン酸

DTE
dithioerythritol ジチオエリトリトール

DTF
Debré-de Toni-Fanconi (syndrome) ドゥブレ・ドゥ・トニ・ファンコニ(症候群)
Dental Trader's Federation 歯科材料商連合
DTG
derivative thermogravimetry 微分熱重量測定
dermatothermogram 皮膚温記録図
DTH
delayed-type hypersensitivity 遅延(型)過敏症
dThd
deoxythymidine デオキシチミジン
DTHR
delayed type hypersensitivity reaction 遅延型過敏症反応
DTI
dipyridamol talium imaging ジピリダモール・タリウム画像
DTIC
dacarbazine ダカルバジン
dimethyl triazeno imidazole carboxamide ジメチルトリアゼノイミダゾールカルボキサミド
DTICH
delayed traumatic intracerebral hematoma 遅発性外傷性脳内血腫
D time
dream time 夢時間
DTM
Diploma in Tropical Medicine 熱帯医学認定書
Doctor of Tropical Medicine 熱帯医学士
DTMA
desoxycorticosterone trimethyl acetate デスオキシコルチコステロントリメチル酢酸塩
DTMH
Diploma of Tropical Medicine and Hygiene 熱帯医学衛生学認定書
DTMP, dTMP
deoxythymidine monophosphate デオキシチミジン一リン酸
DTN
diphtheria toxin normal ジフテリア標準毒素
drug trade news 薬品取引ニュース
DTNB
5,5′-dithiobis(2-nitrobenzoic acid) 5,5′-ジチオビス(2-ニトロ安息香酸)
d-to-a
digital-to-analog デジタル・アナログ(変換)
Dtox
dosis toxica〈ラ〉=toxic dose 中毒量

DTP
digital tingling of percussion 打診時振動
digital tingling on pressure 圧迫で指が痛みを感ずる
diphtheria, tetanus, pertussis (vaccine) ジフテリア・破傷風・百日咳（ワクチン）

DTPA
diethylenetriamine pentaacetic acid ジエチレントリアミン五酢酸

DTPS
diffuse thalamic projection び漫〔広汎〕性視床投射

DTPT
dithiopropylthiamine ジチオプロピルチアミン

DTR
deep tendon reflex 深部腱反射
Diploma in Therapeutic Radiology 放射線治療認定書

dtr.
daughter 娘
detur, *dentur*〈ラ〉=let be given 与えよ《処》

dtr.c.for.
detur cum formula 処方を記して与えよ《処》

dtr.s.n.
detur suo nomine 薬名を記して与えよ《処》

DTS
dense tubular system 高密度細管システム
dyphtheria toxin sensitivity ジフテリア毒素感受性

dt's
dementia tremors〈ラ〉 振戦痴呆

DTs, Dt's, dt's
delirium tremens 振戦せん(＝譫)妄

DTSS
Drug Therapy Screening System 薬物治療審査システム

DTT
device for transverse traction 横牽引装置
diphtheria tetanus toxoid ジフテリア破傷風毒素
dithiothreitol ジチオトレイトール

dTTP
deoxythymidine triphosphate デオキシチミジン三リン酸

DT-VAC
diphtheria-tetanus vaccine ジフテリア破傷風ワクチン

DTVM
Diploma in Tropical Veterinary Medicine 熱帯獣医認定書

DTX
detoxification 解毒
diphtheria toxin ジフテリア毒素

DTZ
diatrizoate ジアトリゾエート

DU
density unknown 濃度不明
deoxyuridine デオキシウリジン
dermal ulcer 皮膚潰瘍
diagnosis undetermined 診断未確定，診断未決定
diazouracil ジアゾウラシル
died unmarried 未婚死亡
dog unit イヌ単位
duodenal ulcer 十二指腸潰瘍

du
apothecaries drachm 薬用ドラム〈単位〉

DUA
dorsal uterine artery 背側子宮動脈

DUB
dysfunctional uterine bleeding 機能不全性子宮出血

DUC
died of unrelated cause 無関係な原因による死亡

Duco
diffusing capacity for carbon monoxide 一酸化炭素拡散能

DUD
detrusor urethral dyssynergia 利尿筋尿道(筋)不〔非〕協調

dUDP
deoxyuridine diphosphate デオキシウリジン二リン酸

DUE
drug use evaluation 薬剤使用評価

DUF
Doppler ultrasonic flowmeter ド(ッ)プラー超音波流量計

Dukes A,B,C
Dukes classification デュークス分類(=大腸・直腸癌の分類)

DUL
diffuse undifferentiated lymphoma 広汎〔び漫〕性未分化(型)リンパ腫

dulc.
dulcis〈ラ〉=sweet 甘い，おいしい

dUMP
deoxyuridine monophosphate デオキシウリジン一リン酸

DUMP，dUMP
deoxyuridine-5′-phosphate デオキシウリジン-5′-リン酸

duod
duodenal 十二指腸の
duodenum 十二指腸

dup
duplicate 複製する
duplication 重複，複製

DUR
drug utilization〔user〕 review 薬物使用調査,医薬品使用評価

dur.
durus〈ラ〉=hard 硬い

dur, dur.
durante〈ラ〉=duration, during 持続,～の間

dur.dol.
durante dolore〈ラ〉=while the pain lasts 痛みが持続する間

DUSN
diffuse unilateral subacute neuroretinitis 広汎〔び漫〕性片側(性)亜急性視神経網膜炎

DV
dependent variable 従属変数
dilute volume 希釈量
Diploma in Venerology 性病医認定書
direct vision 直接視力
distemper virus ジステンパーウイルス
divorced 離婚した
domestic violence 配偶者や恋人など親密な関係にある，またはあった者から振るわれる暴力
dorsoventral 背腹の方向
double vision 複視

dv
double vibrations 二重振動

D & V
diarrhea and vomiting 下痢と嘔吐

DVA
distance visual acuity 遠見視力

DVA test
duration of voluntary apnea test 努力性無呼吸持続試験

DVB
cis-diamminedichloroplatinum, vindesine, bleomycin シスジアミンジクロロプラチナ,ビンデシン,ブレオマイシン

DVC
dorsal vagal nucleus complex 背側迷走神経核群

DVD
digital versatile disk ディー・ブイ・ディー
dissociated vertical deviation 交代性上斜視

DV & D
Diploma in Venerology and Dermatology 性病と皮膚科認定書

DVH
Diploma in Veterinary Hygiene 獣医衛生認定書
DVI
double chambers-ventricle-inhabited 房室順次ペーシング
DVLP
daunorubicin, vincristine, L-asparaginase, prednisone ダウノルビシン,ビンクリスチン,L-アスパラギナーゼ,プレドニゾン
dvlp
develop 発育する，発達する
development 発育，発達，現象
DVM
Doctor of Veterinary Medicine 獣医学博士
DVMS
Doctor of Veterinary Medicine and Surgery 獣内科外科学博士
DVO
divisional veterinary office 地域獣医事務所
DVP
daunomycin, vincristine, predonisolone ダウノマイシン,ビンクリスチン,プレドニゾロン
daunorubicin, vincristine, prednisolone ダウノルビシン,ビンクリスチン,プレドニゾロン
DVPA
daunorubicin, vincristine, prednisone, L-asparaginase ダウノルビシン,ビンクリスチン,プレドニゾン,L-アスパラギナーゼ
DVPH
Diploma in Veterinary Public Health 獣医学公衆保健認定医
DVPL-ASP
daunorubicin, vincristine, prednisone, L-asparaginase ダウノルビシン,ビンクリスチン,プレドニゾン,L-アスパラギナーゼ
DVR
Division of Vocational Rehabilitation 職業リハビリテーション局
Doctor of Veterinary Radiology 獣放射線医学博士
double valve replacement 二弁置換
D.V.S.
Doctor of Veterinary Surgery 獣外科学博士
DVSA
digital venous subtraction angiography デジタル減算静脈血管造影(法)
DVSc
Doctor of Veterinary Science 獣医学博士
DVT
daily volume turnover 1日容量交代

deep vein thrombosis 深部静脈血栓症
deep venous thrombosis 深部静脈血栓症

DVV
diastolic ventricular volume 拡張期心室内容積

DW
dry weight 乾燥重量

D/W
δ〔delta〕-wave デルタ波
dextrose in water ブドウ糖水溶液

DW, D/W
distilled water 蒸留水

D5W, D5/W, D5W, D-5%-W, D-5/W
5% dextrose in water 5%ブドウ糖液

DWD
died with disease 病死

DWDL
diffuse well differentiated lymphocytic lymphoma 汎発性分化型リンパ球性リンパ腫

DWI
diffusion weighted image 拡散強調画像

DWSCL
dailywear soft contact lenses 常用ソフトコンタクトレンズ

dwt
denarius weight デナリウス重量
penny weight ペニー重量

DX
dextran デキストラン
dicloxacillin ジクロキサシリン

dx
difficulties 障害，困難
duplex〈ラ〉=double 2倍

DX, Dx, dx
diagnosis 診断

DXA
dual energy X-ray absorptiometry 二重エネルギーX線骨塩量測定装置

DXD, dxd
discontinued 中止した

DXI
digital X-ray imaging デジタルX線映像法

Dx Imp
diagnostic impression 診断的印象

DXM
dexamethasone デキサメタゾン

DXR
deep x ray 深部X線
delayed xenograft rejection 遅発性異種移植
doxorubicin ドキソルビシン(=アドリアマイシン)

DXRT
deep X-ray therapy 深部X線治療

Dxs
dextran sulfate デキストラン硫酸

DXT
dextrose ブドウ糖

Dy
dysprosium ジスプロシウム〈元素〉

dy
delivery 分娩，出産
dystrophia muscularis 筋層ジストロフィ

DYN
dynorphin ダイノルフィン，下垂体後葉

dyn
dynamics 力学，力動(論)
dynamometer 力量型，握力計，筋力計
dyne ダイン〈単位〉

dysen
dysentery 赤痢

dyslex
dyslexia 失読症

dysme, DYSM
dysmenorrhea 月経困難症

dysp
dyspepsia 消化不良
dyspnea 呼吸困難
dyspneic 呼吸困難の

dysto
dystopia 異所

DZ
diazepam ジアゼパム
dizygotic (twins) 二卵性(双胎)
dizziness めまい〔眩暈〕(感)

Dz
disease 疾病，疾患

d.Z
der Zeit〈独〉 時間

dz, dz.
dozen 12個，ダース

DZAPO
daunorubicin, azacytidine, arabinosylcytosine, prednisone, vincristine (=Oncovin) — ダウノルビシン,アザシチジン,アラビノシルシトシン,プレドニゾン,ビンクリスチン(=オンコビン)

DZP
diazepam — ジアゼパム

E e

E	
expired gas	呼気ガス《麻》
E	
air dose	空中線量
cortisone	コルチゾン
each	各自の，各々の，個々の
earth	接地，アース
east	東
Echinococcus	包虫(属)
Echinostoma	棘口吸虫(属)
edema	浮腫，水腫
educational plan	教育計画
effective dose	有効量，実効線量
Einheit〈独〉=unit	単位
einstein	アインシュタイン〈単位〉
einsteinium	アインスタイニウム
elastance	弾性
electric affinity	電気親和力
electric field vector	電界ベクトル
electrode potential	電極電位
electromotive force	起電力
electron	電子
embolia	塞栓症
embolic	塞栓の
embolism	塞栓症
emmetropia〈ラ〉	正眼視
enamel	エナメル質
encephalitis	脳炎
endogenous	内因性の
Endolimax	エンドリマックス(属)
Endomyces	エンドミセス(属)
endoplasm	内原形質
endotracheal	気管内の
enema	浣腸(剤)
energy	エネルギー
enflurane	エンフルレン
Entamoeba	(体内寄生性)アメーバ(属)
Enterobacter	エンテロバクター(属)
Enterobius	蟯虫(属)
Enterococcus	腸球菌
Enteromonas	エンテロモナス(属)
enzyme	酵素
eosinophilic leukocyte	好酸球

E

epicondyle	上顆
Epidermophyton	表皮菌(属)
epinephrine	エピネフリン
error	過誤，誤差
Erysipelothrix	エリジペロトリックス(属)
erythrocyte(s)	(ヒツジ)赤血球
erythroid	赤色の，紅色の，赤血球の
erythromycin	エリスロマイシン
Escherichia	エシェリキア(属)，大腸菌
esophagus	食道
esophoria	内斜位
ester	エステル
estrogen	エストロゲン
ethanol	エタノール
ether	エーテル
ethyl	エチル
exa	エクサ(＝10^{18})〈接〉
examiner	試験官
exercise	運動，練習
expected value	期待値《統》
experiment	実験
experimental	実験の
experimenter	実験者
expiration	呼息
extension	伸展，延長
external skin	肛門周囲皮膚
extinction	吸光度
extraction rate	除去率
extralymphatic	リンパ外の
eye	眼
glutamic acid	グルタミン酸
internal energy	内部エネルギー
lower intrathoracic and abdominal esophagus	胸部下部と腹部食道
redox potential	酸化還元電位
vitamin E	ビタミンE

e

ε〈ギ〉＝epsilon	エプシロン
egg transfer	卵移植
erg	エルグ〈単位〉
molar absorptivity	モル吸収係数
molar extinction coefficient	モル消衰係数

E.

Escherichia	エシェリキア(属)

3E

education, enforcement, engineering	プライバシー保守の 3 大条件：教育・法的規制・技術
effort, eating, emotion	狭心症誘発の 3 大因子：労作・食事・情動

E_0

electric affinity	電気親和力

E_1

estrone	エストロン

E_2

estradiol	エストラジオール

E_3

estriol	エストリオール

E_4

estetrol	エステトロール

E_{10}

tocoquinone-10	トコキノン10

E107

tribromoethanol	トリブロモエタノール《麻》

e^+

positron	陽電子

e^-

negative electron	陰電子

E, e

early	早期の
electric charge	電荷
electron	電子

e, e.

ex	～の外へ，～から(離れて)〈接〉

EA

early amniocentesis	初期羊水穿刺
early antigen	初期抗原
educational age	教育年齢
effort angina	労作性狭心症
egg albumin	卵アルブミン
electric affinity	電気親和性
electroacupuncture	電気鍼療法
electroanesthesia	電気麻酔
electrophysiological abnormality	電気生理学的異常
embryonic antigen	胎児抗原
enteric coated aspirin	アスピリン腸溶錠
enteroanastomosis	腸吻合術
entorhinal area	鼻内領域
enzymatic active	酵素活性〔反応性〕のある
epiandrosterone	エピアンドロステロン

epithelial antigen 上皮抗原
erythrocyte amboceptor 赤血球両受体
erythrocyte antibody complex 赤血球抗体複合体
erythrocyte-anti-erythrocyte complex 赤血球・抗赤血球複合体
erythrocyte antisera 赤血球抗血清
erythrocyte sensitized with antibody 抗体感作赤血球
ethacrynic acid エタクリン酸
Extremitätenableitung〈独〉 (四)肢誘導

Ea
abdominal esophagus 腹部食道

ea
each 各々の

EAA
essential amino acid(s) 必須アミノ酸
extrinsic allergic alveolitis 外因性アレルギー肺胞炎

EAAO
experimental allergic aspermatogenic orchitis 実験的アレルギー性精巣炎(=EAO)

EAATs
excitatory amino-acid transporter 興奮性アミノ酸輸送体

EAB
elective abortion 選択的流産

EABT
European Association of Behavior Therapy 欧州行動療法学会

EABV
effective atrial blood volume 有効動脈血(液)量

EAC
Ehrlich ascites carcinoma エールリッヒ腹水癌
electroacupuncture 電気刺針術
erythema annulare centrifugum 遠心性環状紅斑
erythrocyte amboceptor complement 赤血球両受体補体
erythrocyte (sensitized with) antibody and complement 抗体補体結合感作(ヒツジ)赤血球
erythrocyte antibody complement complex (ヒツジ)赤血球抗体補体複合体
erythrocyte-anti-erythrocyte complement complex 赤血球・抗赤血球補体複合体
external auditory canal 外耳道

EACA
epsilon aminocaproic acid εアミノカプロン酸

EACD
eczematous allergic contact dermatitis 湿疹性アレルギー性接触皮膚炎

EAD
early afterdepolarization 早期後脱分極

early afterdischarge 早期後発射
extracranial arterial disease 頭蓋外動脈疾患

ead.
eadem〈ラ〉=the same 同じ

EA-D
early-antigen diffuse type 早期抗原拡散型

EAE
evoked acoustic emission 誘発耳音響放射
experimental allergic encephalomyelitis 実験的アレルギー性脳脊髄炎

EAEC
entero-adherent *Escherichia coli* 腸管付着性大腸菌

EAE protein
experimental allergic encephalomyelitis protein EAE蛋白(=MBP)

EAF
enteropathogenic *Escherichia coli* adherent factor 腸内病原性大腸菌付着因子

EAG
electroatriogram 心房電図

EAggE
enteroaggregative *Escherichia coli* 腸管凝集性大腸菌

EAGLE
easy analysis in graphics of long-term ECG system 12誘導連続記録解析心電図装置

EAHF
eczema, asthma, hay fever (complex) 湿疹・喘息・枯草熱(の複合症状)

EAHLG
equine antihuman-lymphoblast globulin ウマ抗ヒト芽球グロブリン

EAI
ethyl amyl ketone エチルアミノケトン

EALG
equine antilymphocyte globulin ウマ抗リンパ球グロブリン

EAM
electron-beam acoustic microscopy 電子線超音波顕微鏡による観察
experimental allergic myocarditis 実験的アレルギー性心筋炎
experimental allergic myositis 実験的アレルギー性筋炎
experimental autoimmune myositis 実験的自己免疫性筋炎
external acoustic meatus 外耳道
external auditory meatus 外耳道

EAMG
experimental autoimmune myasthenia gravis 実験的自己免疫性重症筋無力症

E

EAN
experimental allergic neuritis 実験的アレルギー性神経炎
EAO
experimental allergic orchitis 実験的アレルギー性精巣炎
experimental autoimmune orchitis 実験的自己免疫精巣炎
EAP
electric acupuncture 電気鍼療法
epiallopregnanolone エピアロプレグナノロン
erythrocyte acid phosphatase 赤血球酸ホスファターゼ
etoposide, adriamycin, cisplatin (= Platinol) エトポシド,アドリアマイシン,シスプラチン(=プラチノール)
evoked action potential 誘発活動電位
eye artifact potential 眼球人工電位
EAR
earphone イヤホン
EaR, Ea.R.
Entartungsreaktion〈独〉, Elektroentartungs-reaktion〈独〉 電気変性反応
E/A ratio
enzyme/antibody ratio 酵素・抗体比
EA-RFC
EA-rosette-forming cell (ヒツジ)赤血球抗体ロゼット形成細胞
EARP
exposed group attributable risk percent 曝露群寄与危険率
EASD
European Association for the Study of Diabetes 欧州糖尿病研究協会
EAST
Emory angioplasty surgical trial エモリー血管形成術・外科的比較試験
EAT
eating attitude test 摂食態度検査
ectopic atrial tachycardia 異所性心房性頻拍
Ehrlich ascites tumor エールリッヒ腹水腫瘍
electroaerosol therapy 電気エアロゾール療法
epidermolysis acute toxia 急性毒性表皮剝脱
experimental autoimmune thymitis 実験的自己免疫性胸腺炎
experimental autoimmune thyroiditis 実験的自己免疫性甲状腺炎
EATC
Ehrlich ascites tumor cell エールリッヒ腹水腫瘍細胞
EATL
enteropathy-associated T cell lymphoma 腸症に関連したT細胞リンパ腫

EAU
experimental allergic uveitis 実験的アレルギー性ブドウ膜炎

EAV
equine abortion virus ウマ流産ウイルス

EAVM
extramedullary arteriovenous malformation 髄外動静脈奇形

EB
eastbound 東回りの
ebullition 沸騰，沸点
electroporation buffer 電気穿孔用緩衝液
elementary body 基本小体
epidermal burn 表皮熱傷(＝I度熱傷)
epidermolysis bullosa 表皮水疱症
Erlebnistypus〈独〉 体験型
esophageal body 食道体部
estradiol benzoate 安息香酸エストラジオール
ethambutol エタンブトール
ethidium bromide 臭化エチジウム
Evans blue エバンスブルー

EBA
epidermolysis bullosa acquisita〈ラ〉 後天性表皮水疱症

EBAA
Eye-bank Association of America 米国眼球銀行協会

EBAS
endogenous brain analgesia system 内在性脳内鎮痛系

EBBS
European Brain and Behavior Society 欧州脳行動学会

EBC
enuretic bladder capacity 夜尿時膀胱容量
esophageal balloon catheter 食道内バルーンカテーテル
ethylbenzyl chloride 塩化エチルベンジル

EBD
effective biological dose 有効生物学的量
endoscopic biliary drainage 内視鏡的胆汁ドレナージ
epidermolysis bullosa dystrophica 栄養障害性表皮水疱症

EBF
erythroblastosis fetalis 胎児赤芽球症

EBI
emetine bismuth iodide ヨウ化蒼鉛エメチン
ergosterol biosynthesis inhibitor エルゴステロールの選択的生合成阻害薬
estradiol-binding index エストラジオール結合指数

E

EBK
embryonic bovine kidney　ウシ胎仔腎
EBL
erythroblastic leukemia　赤芽球性白血球
estimated blood loss　推定出血量
Ebl
erythroblast　赤芽球
Ebl-p
polychromatic erythroblast　多染性赤芽球
EBM
Eagle basal medium　イーグル基本培地
electrophysiologic behavior modification　電気生理学的行動修正
evidence based medicine　科学的根拠に基づいた医学
expressed breast milk　しぼった母乳
EBNA
Epstein Barr nuclear antigen　EBウイルス核抗原
Epstein Barr virus associated nuclear antigen　EBウイルス関連特異核抗原
EBP
epidural blood patch　硬膜外血液斑
estradiol-binding protein　エストラジオール結合蛋白
EBR
electron-beam recorder　電子線記録装置
EBRT
external beam radiation therapy　外部放射線照射療法
EBS
electric brain stimulator　電気脳刺激装置
emergency bed service　救急ベッドサービス
emergency broadcast system　緊急放送システム
epidermolysis bullosa simplex　単純性表皮水疱症
EBSR
eye-bank for sight restoration　視力回復のためのアイバンク
EBUS
endobronchial ultrasound　超音波気管支鏡
EBV
effective blood volume　有効血(液)量
epirubicin, bleomycin, vinblastine　エピルビシン,ブレオマイシン,ビンブラスチン
Epstein-Barr virus　EBウイルス，エプスタインバーウイルス
EB virus
Epstein-Barr virus　EBウイルス
EC
effective concentration　有効濃度
effector cell　エフェクター細胞

Ehrlich carcinoma	エールリッヒ癌
ejection click	駆出性クリック
electrochemical	電気化学の
electrocoagulation	電子凝固術
Ellis-van Creveld (syndrome)	エリス・ファン・クレフェルト症候群
emergency capability	緊急対応能力
emetic center	嘔吐中枢
endocarditis	心内膜炎
endothelial cell	内皮細胞
enteric-coated	腸溶(錠)
enteric coating	(錠剤の)腸溶皮
enzyme code	酵素番号
Enzyme Commission	(国際生化学連合の)酵素委員会
epidermal cell	表皮細胞
epithelial cell	上皮細胞
Erb-Charcot (syndrome)	エルブ・シャルコー(症候群)
Escherichia coli	大腸菌
esophagial carcinoma	食道癌
esterified cholesterol	エステル型コレステロール
ether and chloroform	エーテルとクロロホルム
excitation-contraction	興奮・収縮
expiratory center	呼吸中枢
external carotid	外頸動脈
extracellular	細胞外の
extracranial	頭蓋外の

EC50

50% effective concentration	50%有効濃度

E/C

estriol/creatinine	エストリオール/クレアチニン(比)
estrogen-to-creatinine	エストロゲン・クレアチニン比

E-C

ether-chloroform (mixture)	エーテルクロロホルム(混合液)

ECA

enterobacterial common antigen	腸内細菌性共通抗原
eosinophil chemoatractant	好酸球走化因子
external carotid artery	外頸動脈

ECAOV

enteric cytopathogenetic avian orphan virus	腸内細胞傷害性仔トリウイルス

E-care

evening care	イブニングケア

E

ECBO
enteric cytopathogenic bovine orphan virus 腸内細胞傷害性仔ウシウイルス
ECBV
effective circulating blood volume 有効循環血液量
ECC
electrocorticogram 皮質脳波
embryonal cell carcinoma 胚細胞癌
emergency cardiac care 緊急〔救急〕心疾患治療
estimated creatinine clearance 推定クレアチニンクリアランス
excitation-contraction coupling 興奮収縮連関
external cardiac compression 胸壁外心臓圧迫法
extracorporeal circulation 体外循環
ECCC
European Congress of Clinical Chemistry 欧州臨床化学会議
ECCD
endocardial cushion defect 心内膜床欠損(症)
ECCE
extracapsular cataract extraction 水晶体囊外摘出術
EC cell
enterochromaffin cell 腸クロム親和細胞，EC細胞
ECCLS
European Committee for Clinical Laboratory Standards 欧州臨床検査標準委員会
ECCO
enteric cytopathogenetic cat orphan virus 腸内細胞性仔ネコウイルス
$ECCO_2R$
extra-corporeal carbon dioxide removal 体外人工肺炭酸ガス〔二酸化炭素〕除去装置
ECCU
emergency cardiac care unit 緊急〔救急〕心疾患治療部
ECD
electrochemical detector 電気化学検出器
electron capture detector 電子捕獲型検出器
endocardial cushion defect 心内膜床欠損(症)
endothelial corneal dystrophy 角膜内皮変性症
^{99m}Tc-ethyl cysteinate dimer テクネシウムエチルシステイン二量体
EC detector
electron capture detector 電子捕捉検出器
ECE
endothelin-converting enzyme エンドセリン変換酵素

ECF
East Coast fever 東海岸熱
effective capillary flow 有効毛細血(管)流(量)
eosinophil chemotactic factor 好酸球遊走因子
extended care facility 広範な看護施設
extracellular fluid 細胞外液

ECF-A
eosinophilic chemotactic factor of anaphylaxis アナフィラキシー好酸球遊走因子

ECF-C
eosinophilic chemotactic factor complement 補体に誘導された好酸球遊走因子

ECFE
endocardial fibroelastosis 心内膜線維弾性症

ECF-L
lymphocyte-derived eosinophil chemotactic factor リンパ球由来好酸球遊走因子

ECFMG
Educational Commission for Foreign Medical Graduates 米国外人医師卒後教育委員会
Educational Commission for Foreign Medical Graduates Examination 外国医学校卒業者試験教育委員会

ECFV
extracellular fluid volume 細胞外液量

ECG
electrocardiogram 心電図
electrocardiograph 心電計
electrocardiography 心電図(検査)法

ECGF
endotherial cell growth factor 内皮細胞増殖因子

ECH
ethylene chlorhydrin エチレンクロルヒドリン

ECHO
echocardiogram 心エコー図
echocardiography 心エコー検査
enteric cytopathogenic human orphan (virus) エコーウイルス
etoposide, cyclophosphamide, hydroxydaunomycin, vincristine(= Oncovin) エトポシド,シクロホスファミド,ヒドロキシダウノマイシン,ビンクリスチン(=オンコビン)

Echo
esterified cholesterol エステル型コレステロール

echo
echocardiogram 心エコー図
echoencephalography エコー脳写

E

echography　超音波検査
ECI
extracorporeal irradiation　体外照射
EC-IC
external carotid arteria-internal carotid arteria　外頸・内頸動脈
extracranial-intracranial　頭蓋外・頭蓋内
EC-IC bypass
extracranial-intracranial bypass　頭蓋内・(頭蓋)外バイパス術
ECJ
esophago-cardiac junction, esophago-columnar junction　食道噴門接合部
e-c junction, EC-junction
esophagocardial junction　食道噴門接合部
ECK
embryonic chicken kidney　トリ胎仔腎
ECL
electrocardiograph logarithm　心電図対数
electrogenerated chemiluminescence　電気起因性化学発光
enterochromaffin-like (type)　腸クロム親和様(型)
euglobulin clot lysis　真性グロブリン溶解
extent of cerebral lesion　大脳の損傷範囲
extracapillary lesion　毛細血管外病変
ECLA
extracorporeal lung assist　膜型人工肺と部分体外循環による体外式肺補助
eclamp
eclampsia　子癇(=しかん)
ECL cell
enterochromaffin-like cell　腸内クロマフィン様細胞
ECLE
extracapsular lens extraction　囊外レンズ摘出術
Eclec, eclec
eclectic　取捨選択の
ECLHA
extracorporeal lung and heart assist　体外式心肺補助法
ECLP
extracorporeal liver perfusion　体外式肝灌流
ECLS
extracorporeal life support　体外式生命維持装置
ECLT
euglobulin clot lysis time　真性グロブリン溶解時間
ECM
encephalo-myocarditis　脳心筋炎
erythema chronicum migrans　慢性遊走性紅斑
external cardiac massage　体外心マッサージ

extracellular matrix 細胞外マトリックス〔基質〕

EC mix

ether-chloroform mixture エーテルクロロホルム混合物

ECMO

extracorporeal membrane oxygenation 膜型人工肺体外循環

extracorporeal membrane oxygenator 膜型人工肺

ECMO virus

enterocytopathogenic monkey orphan virus 腸細胞病原性サルウイルス

EC number

enzyme code number 酵素番号

enzyme commission number 酵素番号

EcochG, ECochG

electrocochleogram 蝸電図

electrocochleograph 蝸電計

electrocochleography 蝸電図(検査)法

ECOG

Eastern Cooperative Oncology Group 東部腫瘍学共同体

ECoG

electrocorticogram 皮質脳波

ECOISD

Environmental Conservation Initiative for Sustainable Development 持続可能な開発のための環境保全イニシアティブ

E coli, E.coli

Escherichia coli 大腸菌

econ

economic 経済の

economics 経済学

ECP

eosinophil cationic protein 好酸球顆粒内蛋白

erythrocyte coproporphyrin 赤血球コプロポルフィリン

Escherichia coli derived protein 大腸菌由来蛋白

Escherichia coli polypeptides 大腸菌ポリペプチド

estradiol cyclopentyl-propionate エストラジオールシクロペンチルプロピオネート

external cardiac pressure 胸壁外心臓圧迫

external counterpulsation 胸壁外カウンターパルゼーション法

ECPOG

electro-chemical potential gradient 電気化学的電位勾配

ECPO virus

enteric cytopathogenetic porcine orphan virus 腸内細胞性仔ブタウイルス

E

ECPR
external cardiopulmonary resuscitation 胸壁外心肺蘇生
ECR
electrocardiographic response 心電図上の反応
error cause removal 誤差原因除去
ECRB
extensor carpi radialis brevis muscle 短橈側手根伸筋
eCRF
electronic Case Report Form 電子的症例報告書
ECRI
Emergency Care Research Institute 救急管理研究施設
ECRL
extensor carpi radialis longus muscle 長橈側手根伸筋
ECS
elective cosmetic surgery 選択的美容手術
electroconvulsive shock 電撃ショック
environmental control system 環境制御装置
extracapsular spread 被膜外拡散
extracellular space 細胞外液腔
ECSO virus
enteric cytopathogenetic sheep orphan virus 腸内細胞傷害性仔ヒツジウイルス
ECSP
epidermal cell surface protein 表皮細胞表面蛋白
ECST
European Carotid Surgery Trialists' Collaborative Group 欧州頸動脈外科研究者グループ
ECSWL
extracorporeal shock-wave lithotripsy 体外腎砕石術
ECT
elcatonin エルカトニン
electric convulsive therapy 電撃療法，電気痙攣療法
electroconvulsive shock therapy 電撃療法，電気痙攣療法
emission computed tomography 放射型コンピュータ断層撮影法
enteric-coated tablet 腸溶剤
extracellular tissue 細胞外組織
ect
ectopic 異所性の
EC/TC
esterified cholesterol/total cholesterol (ratio) エステル型/総コレステロール(比)
ECTD
epicardial conduction time difference 噴門上部興奮伝播時間差

ECU
environmental control unit 環境管理単位
extensor carpi ulnaris (muscle) 尺側手根伸(筋)
ECUM
extra-corporeal ultrafiltration method 限外濾過法
ECV
extracellular volume 細胞外容量
extracorporeal volume 体外循環容量
ECW
extracellular water 細胞外液
ECZ
econazole エコナゾール
ED
diodrast extraction ratio ダイオドラスト除去率
ectodermal dysplasia 上皮異形成症
ectopic depolarization 異所性脱分極
educational development 教育開発
effective dose 有効量，実効線量
Ehlers-Danlos syndrome エーラース・ダンロス症候群
Einfallsdosis〈独〉 入射線量
electrodesiccation 電気乾燥術
electrodiagnosis 電気診断
electrodialysis 電気透析
elemental diet (tube) 成分栄養(チューブ)
emergency department 救急治療部
emotional disturbance 情動障害
end-diastole 拡張期終期
Enddruck〈独〉 終圧
enteric exocrine drainage 腸管ドレナージ
enzyme deficiency 酵素欠乏症
epidural 硬膜外の
equilibrium dialysis 平衡透析
erectile dysfunction 勃起不全
erythema dose 紅斑量
ethylenediamine エチレンジアミン
extensive disease 全身進展型
extensor digitorum 指伸筋
external diameter 外径
E_d
depth dose 深部(線)量
ed
edema 水腫，浮腫
edit 編集する
edited 編集された
edition 版

editor	編集者
editorial	編集者の
educated	教育された
education	教育
educational	教育の
educator	教育者
ED_{50}	
50%effective dose	50%有効量
ED, Ed	
estradiol	エストラジオール(=E_2)
EDA	
electrodermal activity	皮膚電位
ethylenediamine	エチレンジアミン
ED-AC	
elemental diet, Azinomoto, Chiba University	成分栄養・味の素・千葉大学
EDAM	
electron dense amorphous material	高電子密度無晶性物質
EDAMS	
encephalo-duro-arterio-myo-synangiosis	脳硬膜動脈・筋血管癒合術
EDAS	
encephalo-duro-arterio-synangiosis	脳硬膜動脈血管癒合術
EDB	
extensor digitorum brevis	短指伸筋
EDC	
electronic data capture	電子データ収集(システム)
enramycin	エンラマイシン
estimated date of conception	推定受胎日
expected date of confinement	分娩予定日
extensor digitorum communis (muscle)	総指伸(筋)
1-ethyl-3-(3-dimethylaminopropyl)-carbodiimide	1-エチル-3-(3-ジメチルアミノプロピル)カルボジイミド
EDCF	
endothelium-derived constricting factor	血管内皮細胞由来収縮因子
EDCI	
energetic dynamic cardiac insufficiency	エネルギー動的心不全
EDD	
end-diastolic dimension	拡張終(末)期径
expected date of delivery	分娩予定日
EDDA	
ethynodiol diacetate	二酢酸エチノジオール

edent
edentulous 無歯の
EDF
extradural fluid 硬膜外液
EDG
electrodermogram 皮膚電気抵抗図
EDGF
eye-derived growth factor 眼由来増殖因子
EDH
epidural hematoma, extradural hematoma 硬膜外血腫
EDHF
endothelium-derived hyperpolarizing factor 血管内皮細胞由来過分極因子
EDHI
Energisch-dynamische Herzinsuffizienz〈独〉 エネルギー性力学的心不全
EDI
eosinophil derived inhibitor 好酸球由来抑制因子
EDIM virus
epizootic diarrhea of infant mouse virus 新生マウス流行性下痢症ウイルス
E-diol
estradiol エストラジオール
Edit
electric differential therapy 電気的差動治療
edit.
editorial 論説，編集者の
EDL
end-diastolic (segment) length 拡張終(末)期(部分)長
end-diastolic load 拡張終(末)期負荷
estimated date of labor 推定分娩日
extensor digitorum longus 長趾伸筋
EDLF
endogenous digitalis-like factor 内因性ジギタリス様物質
EDM
early diastolic murmur 拡張初期雑音
musculus extensor digiti minimi 小指伸筋
EDMA
ethylene glycol dimethacrylate エチレングリコールジメタクリル酸
EDMD
Emery-Dreifuss muscular dystrophy エメリー・ドレフュス(型)筋ジストロフィ
EDN
electrodesiccation 電気乾燥法

eosinophil derived neurotoxin 好酸球由来神経毒
extramucosal duodenal myotomy 粘膜外十二指腸筋切開術

EDNO
endothelium-derived nitric oxide 内皮由来一酸化窒素

EDOC
estimated date of confinement 推定出産日

EDP
electronic data processing 電子的情報処理
end-diastolic pressure 拡張終(末)期圧
epidural intracranial pressure 硬膜上頭蓋腔圧
epidural pressure 硬膜外圧

EDPS
electronic data processing system 電子データ処理システム

EDQ
musculus extensor digiti quinti 小指伸筋

EDR
effective direct radiation 有効直接照射
electrodermal response 電気皮膚反応

EDRF
endothelium-derived relaxing factor 血管内皮細胞由来弛緩因子

EDS
Ego Development Scale 自我発達スケール〔尺度〕
Ehlers-Danlos syndrome エーラース・ダンロス症候群
energy dispersive X-ray spectroscopy エネルギー分散型X線分光法
epigastric distress syndrome 心窩部(胃部)不快感症候群
excessive daytime sleepiness 過剰昼間睡眠

EDT
ethylenediamine tartrate 酒石酸エチレンジアミン

EDTA
ethylenediaminetetraacetic acid エチレンジアミン四酢酸
European Dialysis and Transplant Association 欧州透析移植学会議

EDTAC
ethylenediaminetetraacetic acid cetavlon エチレンジアミン四酢酸セタブロン

EDTG
ethylenediamine tetraglutamic acid エチレンジアミン四グルタミン酸

ED tube
elemental diet tube 成分栄養チューブ

educ
education 教育
educational 教育の

EDV
end-diastolic ventricular volume 拡張終(末)期心室容量
end-diastolic volume 拡張終(末)期容積

end dilution value 体外希釈値

EDVI
end-diastolic volume index 拡張終(末)期容積指数

ED virus
Ehrlich cell destruction virus エールリッヒ細胞破壊ウイルス

EDW
estimated dry weight 推定乾燥重量

EDWGT
emergency drinking water germicidal tablet 緊急用飲用水殺菌剤

EDWTH
end-diastolic wall thickness 拡張終(末)期(心臓)壁厚

EDX
energy dispersive X-ray spectroscopy エネルギー分散X線分光法

EDX, EDx
electrodiagnosis 電気診断

EE
electric engineer 電気技師
embryo extract 胎盤エキス
end to end (anastomosis) 端々(吻合術)
energy expenditure エネルギー消費
equine encephalitis ウマ脳炎
errors excepted 例外的誤差
errors expected 期待誤差
ethynyl estradiol エチニルエストラジオール
external ear 外耳
eye and ear 眼と耳

eE
emetische Erscheinung〈独〉 嘔吐症状

EEA
end to end anastomosis 端々吻合
end to end inverting anastomosis 消化管端・端吻合

EEC
enteropathogenic *Escherichia coli* 腸病原性大腸菌

EECD
endothelial-epithelial corneal dystrophy (角膜)内皮性・(角膜)上皮性ジストロフィ

EECG
electroencephalogram 脳波
electroencephalography 脳波検査，脳波記録

EECP
enhanced external counterpulsation 外的動脈加圧強化法

EEC syndrome
ectrodactyly, ectodermal dysplasia, cleft lip-palate syndrome 指欠損・外胚葉性形成異常・口唇口蓋裂症候群

E

EEDQ
ethoxycarbonylethoxydihydroquinoline エトキシカルボニルエトキシジヒドロキノリン

EEE
eastern equine encephalitis 東部ウマ脳炎
edema, erythema and exudate 浮腫・紅斑・滲出液
experimental enterococcal endocarditis 実験的腸球菌心内膜炎
external eye examination 外からの眼検査

EEEP
end-expiratory esophageal pressure 呼気終(末)期食道圧

EEE virus
eastern equine encephalomyelitis virus 東部ウマ脳脊髄炎ウイルス

EEG
echoencephalography エコー脳写
electroencephalogram 脳波
electroencephalograph 脳波計

EEGA
electroencephalogram analysis 脳波分析

EEG A
electroencephalography audiometry 脳波聴力検査

EEG frequency analyzer
electroencephalogram frequency analyzer 脳波周波数分析装置

EEH
elemental enteral hyperalimentation 成分経腸栄養法

EEI
expected efficacy index 有効(性)期待係数
expected efficiency index 有効性期待係数

EEJ
electroejaculation 電気(的)射精

EEL
Ecology and Epidemiology Laboratory 生態学・疫学研究室

EELS
electron energy loss spectroscopy 電子線エネルギー損失分光法

EELV
end-expiratory lung volume 呼気終(末)期肺容積

EEM
ectodermal dysplasia-ectrodactyly-macular dystrophy (syndrome) 外胚葉性形成異常(異形成)・欠指・黄斑変性(症候群)
erythema exudativum multiforme 多形滲出性紅斑

EEME
ethynylestradiol methyl ether エチニルエストラジオールメチルエーテル

EEMG
evoked electromyogram 誘発筋電図
EENETP
end-expiratory negative extrathoracic pressure 胸郭外持続陰圧
EENT, E.E.N.T.
eye, ear, nose, throat 眼・耳・鼻・咽喉
EEP
end-expiratory pressure 呼気終(末)期圧
EEPI
extraretinal eye position information 網膜外眼位情報
EEPLND
extraperitoneal endoscopic pelvic lymph node dissection 腹膜外内視鏡骨盤リンパ節切除
EER
electroencephalographic response 脳波反応
EERP
extended endocardial resection procedure 広汎心内膜切除術
EES
erythromycin ethylsuccinate エチルコハク酸エリスロマイシン
ethyl ethane sulfonate エチルエタン硫酸
expandable esophageal stent 伸張式食道ステント
EESG
evoked electrospinogram 誘発脊髄電図
EEV
encircling endocardial ventriculotomy 囲繞性心内膜側心室切開術
EF
ectopic focus 異所性焦点
edema factor 浮腫因子
ejection fraction 駆出分画，駆出率
elastic fibril 弾性原線維
electric field 電界，電場
elongation factor 伸長因子
emotional factor 情動因子
endocardial fibroelastosis 心内膜線維弾性症
endurance factor 耐久因子
equivalent focus 等価焦点
erythroblastosis fetalis 胎児赤芽球症
esophagofiberscope 食道ファイバースコープ
extended-field 広範囲照射野《放射》
extrinsic factor 外因子
EFA
enhancing factor of allergy アレルギー増強因子
essential fatty acid 必須脂肪酸

ethoxyformic anhydride エトキシ蟻酸無水物
evolving factor analysis 発展因子分析

EFAD
essential fatty acid deficiency 必須脂肪酸欠乏

EFE
endocardial fibroelastosis 心内膜線維弾性症

EFF
efficiency 効率

eff
effect 効果，作用
effective 有効な
efferent 遠心性の，輸出の
efficient 効果的な，効率のよい
effusion 滲出液

effect
effective 有効な

effer
efferent 遠心性の，輸出の

EFFU
epithelial focus-forming unit 上皮病巣形成単位

EFH
explosive follicular hyperplasia 爆発的濾胞増殖(過形成)

EFHBM
eosinophilic fibrohistiocytic (lesion of) bone marrow 骨髄の好酸性線維組織球性(部位)

EFL
effective focal length 有効焦点距離
effective half life 有効半減期
external fluid loss 体外液体喪失

EFM
electronic fetal monitoring 電気式胎児監視

EFMC
European Federation for Medicinal Chemistry 欧州医薬化学連合

EFNa
excretion of functional natrium 機能ナトリウム分泌

EFP
effective filtration pressure 有効濾過圧
etoposide, 5-fluorouracil, cisplatin (= Platinol) エトポシド，フルオロウラシル，シスプラチン(＝プラチノール)

EFPIA
European Federation of Pharmaceutical Industries Associations 欧州製薬団体連合会

EFR
effective filtration rate　有効濾過率
EFS
echo-free space　無エコー域
electric field stimulation　電場刺激
EFV
extracellular fluid volume　細胞外液量
EFW
estimated fetal weight　推定胎児体重
EG
encounter group　エンカウンターグループ
enteroglucagon　腸管グルカゴン
eosinophilic granuloma　好酸球肉芽腫
esophagogastrectomy　食道胃切除
external genitalia　外性器，外生殖器
water gauge　水ゲージ
e.g.
exempli gratia〈ラ〉　たとえば
EGA
estimated gestational age　推定在胎月齢
EGC
early gastric cancer　早期胃癌
EGD
esophagogastroduodenoscopy　食道胃十二指腸内視鏡検査
EGDF
embryonic growth and development factor　胚成長発育因子
EGF
epidermal growth factor　上皮成長因子
EGFR，EGF-R
epidermal growth factor receptor　上皮成長因子受容体〔レセプター〕
eGFR
estimate glomerular filtration rate　推定糸球体濾過量
EGG
electrogastrogram　電気胃図
electrogastrography　胃筋電図記録
electro-gravitiogram　重心図
EGH
equine growth hormone　ウマ成長ホルモン
EGJ
esophago gastric junction　食道胃接合部
EG junction
esophagogastric junction　食道胃接合部
EGM
electrogram　電位図

E

EGN
experimental glomerulonephritis 実験的糸球体腎炎
EGR
erythrocyte glutathione reductase 赤血球グルタチオン還元酵素
EGT
ethanol gelation test エタノールゲル化試験
EGTA
esophageal gastric tube airway 食道胃管エアウェイ〔気道〕
ethylene glycol-*bis* (2-aminoethyl ether) tetraacetic acid エチレングリコールビス(2-アミノエチルエーテル)四酢酸

EH
enlarged heart 拡張心
Entamoeba histolytica アメーバ原虫
enteral hyperalimentation 経腸的高カロリー栄養
epidermolytic hyperkeratosis 表皮剥離性角質増殖
essential hypertension 本態性高血圧
exercise induced hyperpnea 運動時換気量増加
E & H
environment and heredity 環境と遺伝
EHAA
Eagle-Hanks amino acid medium イーグル・ハンクスアミノ酸培地(培養液)

epidemic hepatitis associated antigen 流行性肝炎関連抗原
EHB
elevate head of bed ベッドの頭部を上げる
EHBA
extrahepatic biliary atresia 肝外胆道閉鎖症
EHBD
extrahepatic bile duct 肝外胆管
EHBF
effective hepatic blood flow 有効肝血流量
estimated hepatic blood flow 推定肝血流量
extrahepatic blood flow 肝外血流量
EHC
enterohepatic circulation 腸肝循環
enterohepatic clearance 腸肝クリアランス
Environmental Health Criterion 環境衛生規準
essential hypercholesterolemia 本態性高コレステロール血症
exophthalmos-hyperthyroid factor 眼球突出・甲状腺機能亢進症因子

EHD
epizootic hemorrhagic disease 動物流行性出血性疾患

EHDP
ethan hydroxy diphosphonate(=etidronate disodium) エタンヒドロキシ二リン酸(=エチドロン酸ナトリウム)

EHE
elastica hematoxylin eosin エラスチカヘマトキシリンエオジン

EHEC
enterohemorrhagic *Escherichia coli* 腸管出血性大腸菌

EHF
Ebola hemorrhagic fever エボラ出血熱
epidemic hemorrhagic fever 流行性出血熱

EHG
electrohysterography 子宮筋電法

EHL
effective half-life 有効半減期
electro-hydraulic lithotripsy (lithotrity) 電気水圧砕石術
essential hyperlipidemia 本態性高脂血症
extensor hallucis longus 長母指伸筋

EHO
extrahepatic obstruction 肝外閉塞

EHP
effective horsepower 有効馬力
erythrohepatic protoporphyria 骨髄肝性プロトポルフィリン症
excessive heat production 過剰熱産生
extra high potency 特別高い効率

EHPBF
effective hepatic plasma blood flow 有効肝血漿血流量

EHPF
effective hepatic plasma flow 有効肝血漿流量

EHPH
extrahepatic portal hypertension 肝外性門脈高血圧症

EHPP
erythrohepatic protoporphyria 骨髄肝性プロトポルフィリン症

EHPT
Eddy hot plate test エディ熱板試験

EHS
emergency health service 救急医療サービス
environmental health service 環境保健サービス

EHSs
extremely hazardous substances 非常に危険な物質

EHT
essential hypertension 本態性高血圧症

extra high tension 超高圧

EHV
equine herpes virus ウマヘルペスウイルス

EI
electrolyte imbalance 電解質平衡異常
electron impact ionization 電子衝撃イオン化
emesis index 悪阻指数，つわり指数
endolumbar injection 脊髄腔内注入
enzyme inhibitor 酵素抑制物質
eosinophilic index エオジン好性指数
esterase inhibitor エステル分解酵素阻止因子
excretory index 排泄指数
exercise index 運動指数

Ei
esophagus, thoracic interior 胸部下部食道
lower intrathoracic esophagus 胸部下部食道

E/I
expiration-inspiration 呼気・吸気比

EIA
early infantile autism 早期幼児自閉症
electro-immunoassay 電気免疫定量法
environmental impact assessment 環境影響評価
enzyme immunoassay 酵素免疫測定法
equine infectious anemia ウマ伝染性貧血
exercise induced asthma 運動誘発喘息
external iliac artery 外腸骨動脈

EIAB
extracranial-intracranial arterial bypass 頭蓋外・内動脈バイパス

EIAn
exercise-induced anaphylaxis 運動誘発アナフィラキシー

EIB
exercise-induced bronchoconstriction 動作誘発気管支収縮

EIC
elastase inhibitory capacity エラスターゼ抑制能
extensive intraductal component 広汎性(腺)管内要素

EID
electroimmunodiffusion 電気免疫拡散
epidural-infusion-diuretics 硬膜外・輸液併用利尿排石法

EID_{50}
50% egg-ineffective dose 半数卵感染量

EIEC
enteroinvasive *Escherichia coli* 腸管組織侵入性大腸菌

eIF
eukaryotic initiation factor 真核細胞開始因子

EI mass spectrometry
electron ionization mass spectrometry 電子衝撃イオン化法
E_{IN}
inulin extraction ratio イヌリン除去率
EIP
end-inspiratory pause 吸気後休止時間
end-inspiratory plateau 吸気末プラトー
excitatory junction potential 示指固有伸筋
extensor indicis proprius (固有)示指伸筋
EIRG
electrointraretinogram 網膜内電図
EIRN
extra incidence rate in non-vaccinated groups 非種痘群の余分発生率
EIRV
extra incidence rate in vaccinated groups 種痘群の余分発生率
EIS
endoscopic embolization injection sclerotherapy 内視鏡的硬化塞栓療法
endoscopic injection sclerotherapy 内視鏡的硬化療法
EIT
eccentric intimal thickening 限局性〔偏心性〕内膜肥厚
EITR
erythrocyte iron turnover rate 赤血球鉄交替率
EIV
external iliac vein 外腸骨静脈
EJ
elbow jerk 肘反射
Ej
ejaculation 射精
EJP
excitatory junctional potential 興奮性接合部電位
EJR
extrajunctional acetylcholine receptor 神経接合部外膜アセチルコリン受容体

ejusd.
ejusdem〈ラ〉 同様に《処》
EK
electrokardiogram 心電図
enterokinase エンテロキナーゼ
Esophagus Krebs〈独〉 食道癌
EKC
electrokinetic chromatography 動電クロマトグラフィ
epidemic keratoconjunctivitis 流行性角結膜炎

E

EKG
electrokardiograph　心電計
Elektrokardiogramm〈独〉　心電図
EKT
Elektrokrampftherapie〈独〉=electric shock therapy　電気ショック療法
ekV
electron kilovolt　電子キロボルト〈単位〉
EKY
electrokymogram　電気キモグラム
electrokymograph　電気キモグラフ
EL
Eaton-Lambert syndrome　イートン・ランバート症候群
elopement status　奔流状態
endolumbar injection　髄腔内注入
erythroleukemia　赤白血病
exercise limit　運動制限
exudate line　滲出線
El
elastase　エラスターゼ
elliptocytosis　楕円赤血球症
el
elbow　肘
EL, El, el
elixir　エリキシル(剤)
ELA
elastomer lubricating agent　エラストマー潤滑剤
endotoxin-like activity　エンドトキシン様活性
Establishment License Application　生物学的製剤製造の施設許可申請
elaeos.
elaeosaccharum〈ラ〉　油糖《処》
ELAM
endothelial leukocyte adhesion molecules　血管内皮白血球粘着物質
ELB
early labelled bilirubin　早期標識ビリルビン
elb
elbow　肘
ELBF
effective liver blood flow　有効肝血流量
ELC
ear lobe crease　耳介皺
ELCA
excimer laser coronary angioplasty　経皮的レーザー冠(状)動脈形成術

eld
eldest 最年長の，最古の
eldelcare
Plan Providing Medical Care for Elderly 老人医療計画
El Dx
electrodiagnosis 電気診断法
elec
electric 電気の
electrical 電気に関する
electricity 電気
elect
elective 選択的な
electric 電気の
elect.
electuarium〈ラ〉＝electuary なめ薬，煉薬《処》
electro
electronics 電子工学
electrol
electrolysis 電気分解
elect.surg
elective surgery 選択的外科手術
elem
element 成分
elementary 成分の
elementary 元素の，初歩の
elev
elevate 上げる，高める
elevation 隆起，挙上
elevator エレベーター
ELF
extra low frequency 極低周波
ELFMF
extremely low frequency magnetic field 極低周波磁場
ELG
endoscopic lymphangiography 内視鏡的リンパ管造影法
elig
eligible 適格な
ELISA
enzyme-linked immunosorbent assay (固相)酵素免疫測定法
elix
elixir エリキシル(剤)
ELM
epiluminescence microscopy 上発光顕微鏡
external limiting membrane 外限界膜

extravascular lung mass 血管外肺腫瘤

ELND

elective regional lymph node dissection 選択的領域リンパ節郭清

elong

elongate 延ばす

elongation 延長

ELOS

estimated length of stay 推定入院期間

extralymphatic organ site リンパ外臓器部位

ELOX

electric spark erosion 電気火花びらん

ELP

early labeled peak 早期標識ピーク

elastase-like protein エラスターゼ様蛋白

electrophoresis 電気泳動

endogenous limbic potential 内因性辺縁系電位

Estimated Learning Potential 推定学習能力，学習能力評価〔推定値〕

ELPS

excessive lateral pressure syndrome 過剰側方（外側）圧迫症候群

ELS

Eaton-Lambert syndrome イートン・ランバート症候群

electron loss spectroscopy 電子損失分光検査法

extracorporeal life support 体外式生命維持装置

extralobar sequestration 肺葉外腐骨（分離片）形成

els.

elaeosaccharum〈ラ〉 油糖《処》

ELSI

ethical, legal and social issue （移植の）倫理的・法的・社会的問題

ELSS

emergency life support system 緊急生命維持装置

ELT

euglobulin (clot) lysis time 真性グロブリン溶解時間

ELUS

endoluminal rectal ultrasonography 経内腔直腸超音波検査

ELV

erythroid leukemia virus 赤白血病ウイルス

ELVSW

effective left ventricular stroke work 有効左（心）室拍出仕事量

Elx

elixir エリキシル

E_M

mannitol extraction ratio マニトール除去率

EM
early memory 早期記憶
eczema marginatum〈ラ〉 頑癬
effective masking 実効遮蔽
ejection murmur 駆出期雑音
electro(n)-microscope 電子顕微鏡
electromicroscopy 電子顕微鏡所見
electron microscopy 電子顕微鏡検査
emergency call 緊急呼び出し
emotionally 情緒的に，情動的に
emphysema 気腫
endometriosis 子宮内膜症
ergonovine maleate マレイン酸エルゴノビン
erythema multiforme 多形紅斑
erythromycin エリスロマイシン
esophageal motility 食道運動性
estramustine エストラムスチン
extensive metabolizer 高代謝患者

Em
emulsionlayer 感光乳剤層
erythroblast mitosis 赤芽球分裂

E & M
endocrine and metabolic 内分泌代謝の
endocrine and metabolism 内分泌・代謝

E-M
Emden-Meyerhof (pathway) エムデン・マイヤーホフ(経路)

EM，Em，em
emmetropia 正視

EM，em
electromagnetic 電磁の

E/M，e/m
ratio of (electron) charge to mass 電荷/電子質量比

EMA
electronic microanalyzer 電子微量分析器
epithelial membrane antigen 上皮細胞膜抗原

EMA-CO
etoposide, methotrexate, actinomycin D, citrovorum factor エトポシド，メトトレキサート，アクチノマイシンD，シトロボラム因子
etoposide, methotrexate-leucovorin, actinomycin D, cyclophosphamide, vincristine(=Oncovin) エトポシド，メトトレキサート-ロイコボリン，アクチノマイシンD，シクロホスファミド，ビンクリスチン(=オンコビン)

E

EMAS
Employment Medical Advisory Service　医療従事者勧告サービス

EMB
ethambutol　エタンブトール
explosive mental behavior　爆発的精神行動
explosive motor behavior　爆発的運動行動

emb
embolus　塞栓
embryo　胚，胎芽，胎児

EMB, Emb, emb
embryology　胎生学，発生学

EMB agar
eosin methylene blue agar　エオジンメチレンブルー培地

EMBO
European Molecular Biology Organization　欧州分子生物学協会

EMBP
estramustine binding protein　エストラムスチン結合蛋白

embry
embryology　胎生学，発生学

embryol
embryology　胎生学，発生学

EMC
electron microscopy　電子顕微鏡検査
encephalomyocarditis　脳心筋炎
essential mixed cryoglobulinemia　本態性混合性クリオグロブリン血症

EMCT
endoscopic microwave coagulation therapy　内視鏡的超短波凝固治療

EMCV
encephalomyocarditis virus　脳心筋炎ウイルス

EMC virus
encephalomyocarditis virus　脳心筋炎ウイルス

EMD
electromechanical dissociation　電導収縮解離

EME
external mechanical efficiency　外的力学的効率

EM-E
erythromycin estolate　エリスロマイシンエストレート

EMEA
European Medicines Evaluation Agency　欧州医薬品庁

EMEP
European Monitoring and Evaluation Program　欧州監視評価計画

emer
emergency　緊急，救急

emerg
emergency　緊急，救急

emet
emeticum〈ラ〉　吐物《処》

EMF
electromagnetic field　電磁場
electromagnetic flowmeter　電磁血流計
endomyocardial fibrosis　心内膜心筋線維症
erythrocyte maturation factor　赤血球成熟因子
evaporated milk formula　練乳組成
Excerpta Medica Foundation　エクセルプタ・メディカ財団

EMG
electromyelography　脊髄電図検査
electromyogram　筋電図
electromyography　筋電図検査
exomphalos, macroglossia and gigantism (syndrome)　臍ヘルニア・巨舌・巨人(症候群)
eye movement gauge　眼球運動計

EMG syndrome
exomphalos-macroglossia-gi(g)antism syndrome　臍ヘルニア・巨舌・巨人症候群，EMG症候群

EMI
electromagnetic interference　電磁障害

EMIAT
European Myocardial Infarction Amidarone Trial　エミアト

EMIC
emergency maternity and infant care　救急産院と新生児保護

EMIT
enzyme multiplied immunoassay technique　多元酵素免疫測定法

EML
effective mandibular length　有効下顎骨長
endoscopic mechanical lithotripsy　内視鏡的機械的結石破砕術
endoscopic mechanical lithotripter　内視鏡機械的砕石バスケット鉗子

EMLA
eutectic mixture of local anaesthetics　局所麻酔薬共融物

EMMA
electron microscopy and micro-analysis　電子顕微鏡検査と微細分析

eye-movement measuring apparatus 眼球運動測定器

EMO
Epstein-Macintosh-Oxford (inhaler) エプスタイン・マッキントッシュ・オクスフォード(吸入器)
exophthalmos,myxedema circumscriptum praetibiale and osteoarthropathia hypertrophicans (syndrome) 眼球突出・限局性粘液水腫・変形関節(症候群)

EMO inhaler
Epstein-Macintosh-Oxford inhaler エプスタイン・マッキントッシュ・オクスフォード吸入器，EMO吸入器

EMOS
exophthalmus,praetibial myxedema, osteoarthropathy syndrome 眼球突出・脛骨前粘液水腫・骨関節症(ばち状指)症候群

EMO syndrome
exophthalmus,pretibial myxedema, osteoarthropathy syndrome EMO(＝眼球突出・限局性粘液水腫・変形関節)症候群

emot
emotion 情動，情緒，感情
emotional 情動の，情緒の

EMP
electromagnetic pulse 電磁パルス
Embden-Meyerhof pathway エムデン・マイヤーホフ経路
epimacular proliferation 黄斑上増殖
erythromycin propionate エリスロマイシンプロピオネート
ethmoid-maxillary plate 篩骨上顎板
ethylmethane sulfonate エチルメタンスルホン酸
external membrane protein 外膜蛋白
extramedullary plasmacytoma 骨髄外プラズマ細胞腫

emp
employee 使用人
employer 雇用者
employment 雇用

Emp.
empyema paranasalis〈ラ〉 副鼻腔蓄膿症

emp.
emplastrum〈ラ〉＝a plaster 硬膏

e.m.p.
ex modo praescripto〈ラ〉＝in the manner prescribed,as directed 処方どおりに《処》

EM pathway
Embden-Meyerhof pathway エムデン・マイヤーホフ経路

emp.ext.
emplastrum extensum〈ラ〉　展布硬膏《処》

emph
emphysema　気腫

emphys
emphysema　気腫

empl
employee　使用人
employer　雇用者
employment　雇用

EMP pathway
Embden-Meyerhof-Parnas pathway　エムデン・マイヤーホフ・パルナス経路

emp.vesic.
emplastrum vesicatorum〈ラ〉　発疱膏《処》

Empy
empyema maxillaris, empyema paranasalis　副鼻腔蓄膿症

EMQ
6-ethoxy-1,2-dihydro-2,2,4-trimethylquinoline　6-エトキシ-1,2-ジヒドロ-2,2,4-トリメチルキノリン

EMR
educable mentally retarded　教育可能な精神遅滞
electromagnetic radiation　電磁放射
electromagnetic resonance　電磁気共鳴
endoscopic mucosal resection　内視鏡的粘膜切除術
ethanol metabolic rate　エタノール代謝率
eye moving recording　眼球運動記録

E/M ratio
erythroid myeloid ratio　赤芽球糸・骨髄球糸比

EMRS
eye movement recording system　眼球運動記録装置

EMS
early morning specimen　早期検体
early morning stiffness　早朝こわばり
electrical muscle stimulation　電気的筋刺激
electromechanical systole　電気的全心収縮期
emergency medical service　救急医療
emergency medical service sysytem　救急医療システム
emergency medical system　緊急医療システム
encephalo-myosin-angiosis　脳・ミオシン・血管疾患
encephalo-myo-synangiosis　脳・筋血管癒合術
eosinophilia-myalgia syndrome　好酸球増多・筋肉痛症候群
ethylmethane sulfonate　エチルメタンスルホン酸
expandable metallic stent　管腔拡張用金属ステント

E

EMSA
Electromicroscope Society of America　米国電子顕微鏡学会
electrophoretic mobility shift assay　電気泳動度移動アッセイ

EMSS
emergency medical service system　救急医療システム

EMT
emergency medical team　救急医療チーム
emergency medical technician　救急医療技術員

EMU
early morning urine　早朝尿

EMU, emu
electromagnetic unit　電磁単位

emul
emulsion　乳濁，乳濁液

Emul.
Emulsum〈独〉　乳剤

emuls.
emulsio〈ラ〉＝an emulsion　乳濁，乳濁液

EN
electronarcosis　電気麻酔
endocardial　心内膜の
enteral nutrition　経腸栄養
erythema nodosum　結節性紅斑
ethylenediamine　エチレンジアミン

En
endothelial　内皮の

EN, en, en.
enema〈ラ〉　浣腸，注腸《処》

ENA
extractable nuclear antigen　可溶性核抗原
extractable nucleic acid　抽出可能な核酸

ENBD
endoscopic biliary drainage　内視鏡的胆管ドレナージ
endoscopic nasal biliary drainage　内視鏡的経鼻的胆道ドレナージ

encap
encapsulate　カプセルに入れる
encapsulated　カプセルに入れられた
encapsulation　カプセル化

encl
enclose　封入する
enclosed　封入された

END
exaltation of Newcastle disease virus　ニューカッスル病ウイルスの亢進

End, END
endocardium 心内膜
endo
endocardial 心内膜の
endocrine 内分泌の
endocrinology 内分泌学
endotracheal 気管内の
endocr
endocrine 内分泌の
endocrinology 内分泌学
endocrin
endocrinological 内分泌学の
endocrinologist 内分泌学者
endocrinology 内分泌学
Endocrin, endocrin.
endocrinology 内分泌学
Endoc Soc
Endocrine Society 内分泌学会
endos
endosteal 骨内の
endost
endosteal 骨内の
endo-trach
endotracheal 気管内の
ENE, E.N.E.
ethylnorepinephrine エチルノルエピネフリン
ENEM, enem
enema 浣腸
ENG
electroneurography 神経電図(検査)法
electronystagmogram 電気眼振図
electronystagmograph 電気眼振計
ENI
elective neck irradiation 選択的頸部照射
ENIAC
electronic numerical integrater and computer 電子数値積算機つきコンピュータ，エニアック
ENK
enkephalin エンケファリン
ENL
erythema nodosum leprosum 癩性結節性紅斑
enl.
enlarge 拡大する
enlarged 拡大した
enlargement 拡大

E

enlgd
enlarged — 拡大された
ENM
epidemic neuromyasthenia — 流行性神経筋無力症(＝アイスランド病)
ENMG
electroneuromusculography — 神経筋電図法
ENNG
N-ethyl-*N'*-nitro-*N*-nitrosoguanidine — エチルニトロニトロソグアニジン
Eno
enolase — エノラーゼ
ENoG
electroneurography — 電気神経検査
ENOL
enolase — エノラーゼ
eNOS
endthelial nitric oxide synthase — 内皮型酸化窒素合成酵素，内皮型NOS
ENR
extrathyroidal neck radioactivity — 甲状腺外頸部放射性活動
ENS
ethylnorsuprarenin — エチルノルスプラレニン
ENT
ear-nose-throat — 耳鼻科
Ent
enterotoxin — 腸毒素
Entlassung〈独〉 — 退院
Entom.
entomology — 昆虫学
ent-vio
entero-vioform — 腸溶被ビオホルム
ENU
N-ethyl-*N*-nitrosourea — *N*-エチル-*N*-ニトロソ尿素
enur
enuresis — 夜尿〔症〕，寝小便
env
envelope — 外皮，封筒
environ.
environment — 周囲，環境
environmental — 周囲の，環境の
ENX
endoxan — エンドキサン
enoxacin — エノキサシン
enz
enzymatic — 酵素の

enzyme 酵素，エンザイム

EO
effect of opening (of eyes) 開眼効果
eosinophilia 好酸球増加症
ethanolamine oleate オレイン酸エタノールアミン
ethylene oxide 酸化エチレン
external otitis 外耳炎
eyes open 開眼

Eo
eosinophile, eosinophilic leucocyte 好酸球，好酸性の

Eo^+
oxidation-reduction potential 酸化還元電位

EO, eo.
eosinophile 好酸球

Eo, EO
estrone エストロン(=E_1)

EOA
erosive osteoarthritis びらん性変形性関節症，びらん性骨関節炎
esophageal obturator airway 食道閉鎖式エアウェイ
examination, opinion, advice 試験・意見・忠告

EOAE
evoked oto-acoustic emissions 誘発耳音響放射

EOB
emergency observation bed 救急観察用ベッド

EO-CFC
eosinophil colony-forming cell 好酸球コロニー形成細胞

Eo-CSF
eosinophil colony stimulating factor 好酸球コロニー刺激因子

EOD, eod, e.o.d.
every other day 2日ごとに，1日おきに

EOF
electroosmotic flow 電気浸透流

E of M
error of measurement 測定誤差

EOG
electro-oculogram 眼球電図
electro-oculograph 電気眼振計
electro-oculography 電気眼球図記録法
electro-oculomotogram 電気眼球運動図
electro-olfactogram 嗅電図
ethylene oxide gas エチレンオキサイドガス

EOH
emergency operation headquarters 救急司令本部

EOJ
extrahepatic obstructive jaundice 肝外閉塞性黄疸

E

E

EOL
end of life　臨終，死
EoL
eosinophilic leukemia　好酸球性白血病
EOM
error of measurement　計測誤差
external otitis media　外因性中耳炎
extraocular movement　眼球外運動
extraocular muscle　外眼筋
exudative otitis media　滲出性中耳炎
eye ocular movement　眼球運動
EOMA
ethanolamine oleate with meglumine amidotrizoate　オレイン酸エタノールアミン・加アミドトリゾ酸メグルミン
EOMI
extraocular muscles intact　外眼筋無傷
EOP
efficiency of plating　平板効率
emergency outpatient　救急外来患者
endogenous opioido peptide　内因性モルヒネ様ペプチド
EORTC
European Organization for Research and Treatment of Cancer　癌の研究と治療のための欧州共同体
EOS
endogenous opioid system　内因性オピオイド系
European Orthodontic Society　欧州歯列矯正学会
EOS, Eos, eos.
eosinophils　好酸球
Eosins, eosins.
eosinophils　好酸球
EOT
effective oxygen transport　有効酸素運搬
EP
ectopic pregnancy　外妊
electrophoresis　電気泳動
electrophysiologic　電気生理学的な
electroprecipitin　電気沈降素
emergency physician　救急医師
endocochlear direct current potential　蝸牛内電位
endocochlear potential　蝸牛内直流電位
endogenous pyrogen　内因性発熱物質
endoperoxide　エンドペルオキシド
enteropeptidase　腸ペプチダーゼ
eosinophilic pneumonitis　好酸球浸潤肺臓炎
ependymal　上衣の

ependymoma 上衣腫
epicardial 噴門上部の，心外膜の
epinephrine エピネフリン
epithelioid 類上皮の，上皮様の
epoxide エポキシド
erythrocyte protoporphyrin 赤血球プロトポルフィリン
erythropoietic protoporphyria 造血性プロトポルフィリン症
erythropoietin エリスロポエチン
esophageal pressure 食道圧
esophoria 内斜位
estrogen-progesterone エストロゲン・プロゲステロン
ethylenediamine tetraacetic acid dependent pseudothrombocytopenia エチレンジアミン四酢酸依存性偽血小板減少症
evoked potential 誘発電位

Ep
ejection period 駆出期
endorphin エンドルフィン
entrapment point 取込み点
epidural anesthesia 硬膜外麻酔
epilepsy てんかん
estimated position 指定部位

ep
intraepithelium 粘膜上皮内

EP，ep
epithelial 上皮の
epithelium 上皮

EPA
eicosapentaenoic acid エイコサペンタエン酸
embryonic prealbumin 胎芽性プレアルブミン
Environmental Protection Agency 環境保護庁
erythrocebus patas〈ラ〉 パタスモンキー
exophthalmos producing activity 眼球突出惹起作用
extrinsic plasminogen activator 外因性プラスミノゲン賦活体

E_{PAH}
paraaminohippurate(=PAH) excretion ratio パラアミノ馬尿酸ナトリウム除去率，PAH除去率

EPALD
extraperitoneal anterolateral dissectomy 腹膜外前外側椎間板摘出術

EPAP
expiratory positive airway pressure 呼気気道陽圧，呼気陽圧呼吸

EPB
endoscopic pancreatic biopsy 内視鏡的膵生検
extensor pollicis brevis (muscle) 短母指伸筋

E

EPBF
effective pulmonary blood flow 有効肺血(流)量

EPC
end-plate current 神経終板電流
epilepsia partialis continua 持続性部分てんかん
epithelial cell(s) 上皮細胞

E_{pc}
penicillin extraction ratio ペニシリン除去率

EP cell
epithelial cell 上皮細胞

EPCG
endoscopic pancreatico-cholangiography 内視鏡的膵管胆管造影法

EPD
emotionally unstable personality disorder 情緒不安定パーソナリティ〔人格〕障害
ephedrine エフェドリン

epdm
epidemiological 疫学の
epidemiologist 疫学者
epidemiology 疫学

EPDML
epidemiological 疫学の
epidemiologist 疫学者
epidemiology 疫学

EpDRF
epithelial derived-relaxant factor 上皮由来弛緩因子
epithelium-derived relaxing factor 上皮由来弛緩因子

EPE
erythropoietin-producing enzyme エリスロポエチン産生酵素

EPEC
enteropathogenic *Escherichia coli* 腸管病原性大腸菌

EPEG
etoposide エトポシド

EPF
effective pulmonary flow 有効肺血流量
endothelial proliferating factor 内皮増殖因子
exophthalmus-producing factor 眼球突出誘発因子

EPG
eggs per gram 便1グラム中の虫卵数
electronic pantography 電気的全写法
electronic pupillograph 電気瞳孔計
electropneumogram 電気呼吸記録図
electropneumograph 電気呼吸記録計

EPH
essential pulmonary hypertension 特発性肺高血圧症

EPHA
erythroagglutinating phytohemagglutinin-agarose 赤血球凝集植物性血球凝集素
ephed
ephedrine エフェドリン
EPH-gestosis
edema, proteinuria, hypertension gestosis 浮腫・蛋白尿・高血圧妊娠中毒症
EPI
echo planar image エコープラナー像
emergency public information 救急公共情報
epithelium 上皮
epitherial 上皮の
expanded programme on immunization (WHOの)予防接種拡大計画
extrinsic pathway inhibitor 外的経路阻害物
Epi
epidural 硬膜外
epiglottis 喉頭蓋
epilepsy てんかん
Epi, EPI
epicardium 心外膜
epi, Epi, EPI
epinephrine エピネフリン
Epid
epidural anesthesia 硬膜外麻酔
epid
epidemic 流行の
Epidura
epidural hematoma 硬膜外血腫
epig
epigastric 上腹部の
epiglottic 喉頭蓋の
epiglottis 喉頭蓋
epigast
epigastrium 上腹部
Epil
epilepsy てんかん
epileptic てんかんの，てんかん患者
Epin
epinephrine エピネフリン
epineph
epinephrine エピネフリン
epiph
epiphysis 骨端，松果体

epis
episiotomy 会陰切開術
episode エピソード
episodic 挿話的な
epistaxis 鼻出血

EPISTAR
echo-planar imaging and signal target with alternating radio frequency エピスター法

E

epistom.
epistomium〈ラ〉 栓《処》

epith
epithelial 上皮の
epithelial cell 上皮細胞
epithelium 上皮

EPL
essential phospholipid 必須リン脂質
extensor pollicis longus (muscle) 長母指伸筋

EPM
esperamicin エスペラマイシン

EPMA
electron probe X-ray microanalysis 電子プローブ微細X線分析
electron probe X-ray microanalyzer 電子プローブ微細X線分析器

EPMR
endoscopic piecemeal mucosal resection 内視鏡的分割的粘膜切除術

EPNP
1,2-epoxy-3-(*p*-nitrophenoxy) propane 1,2-エポキシ-3-(*p*-ニトロフェノキシ)プロパン

EPO
eosinophil peroxidase 好酸球ペルオキシダーゼ
erythropoietin エリスロポエチン

EPo
erythropoietin エリスロポエチン

EPOR
erythropoietin receptor エリスロポエチン受容体

EPP
endplate potential 終板電位
equal pressure point 等圧点
erythropoietic porphyria 骨髄性ポルフィリン症
erythropoietic protoporphyria 赤芽球増殖性プロトポルフィリン症

EPPB
end-positive pressure breathing 終(末)期陽圧呼吸

EPR
electron paramagnetic resonance 電子常磁性共鳴

electrophrenic respiration	横隔膜電気刺激性呼吸
estradiol production rate	エストラジオール産生率
exophthalmos producing reaction	眼球突出反応

EPRA

Eastern Psychiatric Research Association	東部精神病研究会

EPR system

equipotential patient reference system	EPRシステム

EPS

elastosis perforans serpiginosa	蛇行性穿孔性弾性線維症
electrophysiologic study	電気生理学的検査
exophthalmos producing substance	眼球突出誘発因子
expressed prostatic secretion	前立腺圧出液
extrapyramidal symptomatology	錐体外路症候(学)
extrapyramidal symptoms	錐体外路症状
extrapyramidal syndrome	錐体外路症候群
extrapyramidal system	錐体外路系

EP_s

sensory evoked potentials	感覚誘発電位

ep's

epithelial cell(s)	上皮細胞

EPSE

extrapyramidal side effect	錐体外路副作用

EPSP

excitatory postsynaptic potential	興奮性シナプス後電位

EPSS

E-point septal separation	僧帽弁・心室中隔間距離

EPST

endoscopic pancreatic sphincterotomy	内視鏡的膵管口切開術

EPT

early pregnacy test	早期妊娠試験
electric pressure tracing (of esophagus)	食道電気内圧曲線
endoscopic papillotomy	内視鏡的乳頭括約筋切開術

EPTFE, E-PTFE

expanded polytetrafluoroethylene	伸縮性ポリテトラフルオロエチレン

EPTU

L-ethyl-L-phenylthiourea	L-エチル-L-フェニルチオウレア

EP-X

eosinophil protein-X	好酸球蛋白X

EPZ

extraparenchymal zone	実質外域

EQ
educational quotient 教育指数
elemental quotient 栄養指数
emergency quotient エネルギー率
emotional intelligence quotient 情動指数
Entwicklungsquotient〈独〉 発達指数
equilibrium 平衡状態

eq
equal 等しい

EQ, eq
equation 方程式

Eq, eq
equivalent 当量の，同価の

EQA
external quality assessment 外部精密査定

EQCM
electrochemical quartz crystal microbalance 電気化学石英結晶マイクロバランス

eqn
equation 方程式

eqpt
equipment 装置，装備

EQU
equivalent 当量の，同価の

equilib
equilibrium 平衡状態，釣り合い

equip
equipment 装備，装置

equiv
equivalent 当量の，同価の
equivocal 曖昧な，不確かな

ER
effectual radiation 実効輻射温
embryo replacement 胚置換
emergency room 救急治療室
emptying rate 肺内ガス混合比
endocardial resection 心内膜切除術
endoplasmic reticulum 小胞体
endoscopic resection 内視鏡的切除術
enhancement ratio 増感効果比
environmental resistance 環境上の抵抗
epigastric region 上腹部，心窩部
equivalent roentgen レントゲン当量
erythrocyte receptor 赤血球受容体
esophageal rupture 食道破裂
estradiol receptor エストラジオール受容体

estrogen receptor	エストロゲン受容体
evoked response	誘発反応
extend release	解放性伸展
external resistance	外部抵抗
external rotation	外旋
extraction ratio	除去率

Er

erbium	エルビウム〈元素〉
erosion	びらん

Er, er

erythrocyte	赤血球

ERA

electric response audiometry, evoked response audiometry	誘発反応聴力検査(法)
enthesis related arthritis	無機物挿入関連関節炎
estrogen receptor assay	エストロゲン受容体試験

ERATO

Exploratory Research for Advance Technology	創造科学技術推進事業

ERB

essential renal bleeding	本態性腎出血

ERBD

endoscopic retrograde biliary drainage	内視鏡的逆行性胆道ドレナージ

ERBF

effective renal blood flow	有効腎血流量

ERBIM

endoscopic retrograde bowel insertion method	内視鏡的逆行性大腸挿入法

ERC

ECHO virus, rhino-virus, coryzavirus	エコーウイルス・ライノウイルス・感冒ウイルス
endoscopic retrograde cholangiography	内視鏡的逆行性胆道造影法
erythropoietin responsive cell	エリスロポエチン感受性細胞

ERCC

endoscopic retrograde cholecystography	内視鏡的逆行性胆囊造影

ERCP

endoscopic retrograde cannulation of the pancreatic duct	内視鏡的逆行性膵管カニュレーション
endoscopic retrograde cholangiopancreatography	内視鏡的逆行性胆道膵管造影法

ERD

evoked response detector	誘発電位検出器

E

ERDA
elastic recoil detection analysis　弾性反跳粒子検出法
ERE
external rotation in extention　伸展時の外旋
ERF
Eye Research Foundation　眼研究財団
ERFC, E-RFC
erythrocyte rosette (=E-rosette) forming cell　赤血球ロゼット形成細胞
ERG
electroretinogram　網膜電図
electroretinography　網膜電位計測
erg
erg　エルグ〈単位〉
ERG, erg
electroretinograph　網膜電計
ERGBD
endoscopic retrograde gallbladder and bile-duct drainage　内視鏡的逆行性胆嚢胆管ドレナージ
ERIBD
endoscopic retrograde internal billiary drainage　内視鏡的逆行性内胆道ドレナージ
ER-ICA
estrogen receptor-immunocytochemical assay　エストロゲン受容体免疫細胞化学分析
ERISA
Employee Retirement Income Security Act　退職後生活扶助法
Erkrkg
Erkrankung〈独〉　疾患
ERL
emergency room laparotomy　救急室開腹
Environmental Research Laboratories　環境研究室
ERM
epiretinal membrane　網膜上膜
extended radical mastectomy　拡大根治乳房切除
ERO
evoked response olfactometry　誘発加算脳波嗅覚検査
ERP
early receptor potential　早期視細胞電位
effective refractory period　有効不応期
endoscopic retrograde pancreatography　内視鏡的逆行性膵管造影
equine rhinopneumonitis　ウマ鼻肺炎
estrogen receptor protein　エストロゲン受容体蛋白
event-related potential　事象関連電位

excess relative risk 相対危険度，過剰相対リスク

ERPF

effective renal plasma flow 有効腎血漿流量

ERR

event-related response 事象関連反応

err

erroneous 誤りの

error 過誤，誤差

ERS

endoscopic retrograde sphincterotomy 内視鏡的逆行性括約筋切断

European Respiratory Society 欧州呼吸器学会

ERSP

event-related slow-brain potential 事象関連緩徐脳電位

ERT

emergency room thoracotomy 救急室開胸

estrogen replacement therapy エストロゲン補充療法

eruct

eructation おくび，吐出物

ERV

equine rhinopneumonitis virus ウマ鼻肺炎ウイルス

expiratory reserve volume 呼気予備量

ERY

erysipelas 丹毒

ERY，Ery

Erysipelothrix エリジペロスリックス

erythrocyte 赤血球

eryth

erythema 紅斑

erythrocyte 赤血球

ES

echo sound 反響音

ejection sound 駆出音

electric stimulation 電気刺激

electroshock 電気ショック

electrosyneresis 向流電気泳動法

elopement status 奔流状態

embryonic stem cells 胚性幹細胞

Emergency Service 救急サービス

empty sella 空虚トルコ鞍

Endocrine Society 内分泌学会

endoscopic esophageal varix stiffening 内視鏡的食道静脈瘤硬化術

endoscopic papillosphincterectomy, endoscopic sphincterotomy 内視鏡的乳頭括約筋切開術，内視鏡的括約筋切開術

endotoxin specific 特異的内毒素

E

end-systole 収縮末期
end to side 端側
enema saponis〈ラ〉 石鹸浣腸
enzyme substrate 酵素基質
esophagus 食道
esophoria 内斜位
esterase エステラーゼ，エステル分解酵素
extrastriate 線条外
extrasystole 期外収縮

Es
einsteinium アインスタイニウム〈元素〉
electroshock therapy 電気痙攣治療
estriol エストリオール
eye solution 眼ぬぐい液

es
electrostatic 静電の

ESA
erythropoiesis stimulating agent 赤血球造血刺激因子製剤

ESA-4
esterase A4 エステラーゼA4

ES-Act
esterase activator エステラーゼ賦活剤

ESB
electrical stimulation of brain 脳の電気刺激

ESBS
extreme sample bias shifting 大幅なサンプル・バイアスシフト法

ESC
erythropoietin sensitive cell エリスロポ(イ)エチン感受性細胞
European Society of Cardiology 欧州心臓学会

ESCA
electronspectroscopy for chemical analysis 化学的分析のためのX線電子分光法

ESCC
epidural spinal cord compression 硬膜外性脊髄圧迫

ES cell
embryonic stem cell 胚性幹細胞，ES細胞

Esch.
Escherichia エシェリキア(属)

ESchG
Gesetz zum Schutz von Embryonen〈独〉 ドイツの生殖医療に関する基本法

ESCI
European Society for Clinical Investigation — 欧州臨床調査研究協会
ESCN
electrolyte and steroid produced cardiopathy characterized by necrosis — 壊死により電解質とステロイドが産生される心臓病
E-S coupling
excitation-secretion coupling — 興奮分泌連関
ESCP
evoked spinal cord potential — 脊髄誘発電位
ESD
emission spectrometric detector — 発光スペクトル検出器
end-systolic diameter — 収縮終(末)期径
esophagus, stomach and duodenum — 食道・胃・十二指腸
ESD, EsD
esterase D — エステラーゼD
ESEP
elbow sensory potential — 肘知覚電位
ESES
electrical status epilecticus during sleep — 睡眠時電気的てんかん重延状態
epidural spinal cord electrical stimulation — 硬膜外脊髄電気刺激法
eSET
elective single embryo transfer — 選択的単一胚移植法
ESF
erythropoiesis stimulating factor — 赤血球新生促進刺激因子
ESG
Erythrozyten Senkungsgeschwindigkeit〈独〉 — 赤血球沈降速度
ESH
European Society of Haematology — 欧州血液学会
ESI
electrospray ionization — エレクトロスプレーイオン化
ESKD
end-stage kidney disease — 末期腎不全
ESL-1
E-selectin-ligand — Eセレクチンリガンド(=シアリルルイスX)
ESM
ejection systolic murmur — 駆出性収縮期雑音
ethosuximide — エトスクシミド
ESN
estrogen stimulated neurophysine — エストロゲン刺激性ニューロフィジン

E

Eso
esophagus　食道

esoph
esophageal　食道の
esophagus　食道

ESP
effective systolic pressure　有効収縮期圧
electro-sensory panel　電気感覚計器板
end-systolic pressure　収縮終(末)期の圧
eosinophil stimulating promotor　好酸球刺激プロモーター
extra-sensory perception　第六感

esp
especially　とくに

ESPA
electrical stimulation-produced analgesia　電気的刺激による鎮痛

espec
especial　特別な
especially　とくに

ESR
electric skin resistance　皮膚電気抵抗
electron skin resonance　電気皮膚反応
electron spin resonance　電子スピン共鳴
erythrocyte sedimentation rate　赤血球沈降速度

ESRD
end-stage renal disease　終(末)期腎疾患

ESRF
end-stage renal failure　終(末)期腎不全

ESS
empty sella syndrome　空虚トルコ鞍症候群
end-systolic shoulder　収縮終(末)期期隆起
end-systolic stress　収縮終(末)期ストレス
experiment support system　実験支援組織

Ess, ess.
essentia〈ラ〉　エッセンス《処》

ESSR
European Society for Surgical Research　欧州外科的研究協会

EST
electric shock therapy, electro shock therapy　電気ショック〔痙攣/衝撃〕療法
endometrial smear test　子宮内スメアテスト
endoscopic sphincteropapillotomy　内視鏡的乳頭括約筋切開術
endoscopic sphincterotomy　内視鏡的乳頭切開術
Epidemiology and Sanitation Technician　疫学，衛生学技士

esophageal stational tone　食道静止圧

est
estimated　推定された

ESTR
estrogen receptor　エストロゲン受容体

est wt
estimated weight　推定重量

ESU
electrostatic unit　静電単位

E substance
excitor substance　刺激物質

esur.
esuriens〈ラ〉　絶食で《処》

ESV
effective stroke volume　有効1回拍出量
end-systolic volume　収縮終(末)期容量

ESVEM
Electrophysiologic Study versus Electrocardiographic Monitoring　エスベム，臨床生理学的検査vs心電図モニタリング

ESWL
electrohydraulic shock wave lithotripsy　電気水圧衝撃波砕石術
extracorporeal shock wave lithotripsy　体外衝撃波砕石術
extracorporeal shock wave lithotriptor　体外衝撃波結石破砕装置

ET
educational therapy　訓練療法
effective temperature　実効温度，有効温度
ejection time　駆出時間
elastase toxoid　エラスターゼトキソイド
electroshock thearapy　電気ショック療法
electroshock treatment　電気ショック治療
embryo transfer　胚移植
embryo transplantation　胚移植術
endothelin　エンドセリン
endotracheal incubation　経気管挿管法
enterostomal therapist　ストーマ療法士
enterostomal therapy　ストーマ療法
epithelial tumor　上皮性腫瘍
ergotamine tartrate　酒石酸エルゴタミン
esotropia　内斜視
essential thrombocythemia　本態性血小板血症
essential tremor　本態性振戦

E

Eurotransplant　ユーロトランスプラント(=欧州の移植臓器配分のための非営利団体)
exchange transfusion　交換輸血
exfoliative toxin　表皮剝脱素
expiration time　呼吸時間

Et
essential thrombocytopenia　本態性血小板減少症
ethyl　エチル基

E

et
et〈ラ〉=and　および

ET'
esotropia for near　近見時の内斜視

E/T
effector cell versus target cell　エフェクター細胞対標的細胞
effector/target ratio　エフェクターT細胞/標的細胞比

ET, Et
endotoxin　エンドトキシン
estriol　エストリオール(=E_3)

ETA
elongation of tendo Achilles　アキレス腱延長術
ethylenediaminetetraacetic acid　エチレンジアミン四酢酸

ETAA
disodium ethylenediaminetetraacetic acid　エチレンジアミン四酢酸ナトリウム

et al.
et alibi〈ラ〉=*et alii*〈ラ〉　およびその他

etc.
et cetera〈ラ〉　～のほか，～など

ET_{CO_2}
end-tidal CO_2　呼気終末二酸化炭素濃度

ETD
extralobular terminal duct　小葉外終末乳管

ETEA
5,8,11,14-eicosatetraenoic acid　5,8,11,14-エイコサテトラエン酸

ETEC
enterotoxigenic *Escherichia coli*　毒素原性大腸菌

ETEL
ethynyl estrenol　エチニルエストレノール

ETF
electron-transferring flavoprotein　電子伝達フラビン蛋白
etafenone hydrochloride　塩酸エタフェノン

ETH
ethionamide　エチオナミド

eth
ether エーテル
ethmoid 篩骨(洞)
ethmoidal 篩骨(洞)の

ETHIO
sodium thiosulfate extraction ratio チオ硫酸ナトリウム除去率

ETHO
ethylene oxide 酸化エチレン

etiol
etiology 病因

ETK
erythrocyte transketolase 赤血球トランスケトラーゼ

ETMB
endotracheal tube with movable blocker 可動性ブロッカー付き一側肺換気用気管内チューブ

ETn
early transposable element 早期転移因子

ETNT
17α-ethinyl-19-nortestosterone エチニルノルテストステロン(＝ノルエチンドロン)

ETOH, EtOH
ethyl alcohol エチルアルコール

ETOX
ethylene oxide エチレンオキシド

ETP
electron transfer particle 電子伝達粒子
electron transport particle 電子伝達粒子
eustachian tube pressure 耳管圧，エウスタキオ管圧

ETR
effective thyroid ratio 有効甲状腺率
effective thyroxin ratio 有効チロキシン比
estimated time of recovery 期待回復時間

ETS
Educational Testing Service 教育試験サービス
electrical transcranial stimulation 電気経頭蓋刺激
endoscopic transthoracic sympathectomy 腹腔鏡的交感神経遮断術
endoscopic transthoracic symphathectomy 胸腔鏡下交感神経遮断術
endotracheal suction 気管内吸引
end-to-side (anastomosis) 端側(吻合)
environmental tobacco smoke 環境タバコ煙
erythromycin topical solution エリスロマイシン局所用溶液

et seq.
et sequens〈ラ〉 ～と以下のこと
et sequens〈ラ〉, *et sequentes*〈ラ〉 およびそれに続くもの

E

ETT
- endotracheal tube 気管内チューブ
- epinephrine tolerance test エピネフリン負荷試験
- esophageal transit time 食道通過時間
- exercise treadmill test トレッドミルテスト
- extrapyramidal thyroxine 錐体外路チロキシン
- extrathyroidal thyroxine 甲状腺外チロキシン
- eye tracking test 視標追跡検査

ETTN
- ethyltrimethyloltrimethane trinitrate エチルトリメチロールトリメタン三硝酸

ETU
- emergency and trauma unit 緊急外傷収容部門
- Emergency Treatment Unit 救急治療部

ETV
- educational television 教育用テレビ
- electrothermal vaporization 電気加熱気化法

Etw
- Etwas〈独〉 ある物

etw
- etwa〈独〉 約，おおよそ
- etwas〈独〉 幾分，いくらか

EU
- Ehrlich unit エールリッヒ単位
- emergency unit 救急部
- endotoxin unit 内毒素単位
- enzyme unit 酵素単位
- esterase unit エステラーゼ単位
- experimental unit 実験単位

Eu
- European ヨーロッパ人，ヨーロッパの
- europium ユーロピウム〈元素〉

E.U.
- etiology unknown 原因不明の

EUA
- examination under anesthesia 麻酔下診察

EUCD
- emotionally unstable character disorder 情緒不安定性格疾患

EUM
- external urethral meatus 外尿道口

EUP
- extrauterine pregnancy 子宮外妊娠

EUS
- endoscopic ultrasonography 超音波内視鏡検査
- endoscopic ultrasoundscopy 超音波内視鏡検査

external urethral sphincter 外尿道括約筋

EUS emg

external urethral sphincter electromyogram 外尿道括約筋筋電図測定

eust.

eustachian 耳管の，エウスタキオ管の

eutroph.

eutrophia 栄養良好

eutrophic 栄養良好の

EUV

extreme ultraviolet 超紫外線

EV

enterovirus エンテロウイルス

epidermodysplasia verruciformis 疣贅(＝ゆうぜい)状表皮異常症，いぼ状表皮異形成

evoked response 誘発反応

excessive ventilation 過剰換気

extravascular 血管外の，脈管外の

eV

electron volt 電子ボルト

EV，ev

eversion 外転症

EVA

ethylenevinyl alcohol エチレンビニルアルコール

etoposide, vinblastine, adriamycin エトポシド，ビンブラスチン，アドリアマイシン

evac

evacuate 排泄する

eval

evaluate 評価する，検討する

evaluation 評価，検討

evap

evaporate 蒸発する

evaporated 蒸発した

evap.

evapore〈ラ〉 蒸発させよ《処》

evapn

evaporation 蒸発

EVC

expiratory vital capacity 呼気肺活量

EVE

ethyl-vinyl-ether エチルビニルエーテル

ever

eversion 回外

EV-FIA

evanescent wave fluoro-immunoassay 不安定波螢光免疫測定法

E

EVG
elastica van Gieson (staining) エラスチカ・ワンギーソン(染色)
electrovaginogram 腟電図
electroventriculogram 心室電図

evid
evidence 証拠
evident 明白な

EVL
endoscopic variceal ligation 内視鏡的食道静脈瘤結紮術

EVLW
extravascular lung water 血管外肺水分量

EVM
enviomycin エンビオマイシン
extravascular mass 血管外腫瘤

evol
evolution 進化，進展

EVP
evoked visual response 誘発視覚反応

EVR
early vertex response 早期頭頂部反応
endocardial viability ratio 心内膜活性率

EVRS
electronic video recording system ビデオ記録装置

EW
effective warmth 等価温感
Emergency Ward 救急病棟
exposure wedge 肉眼的剝離面癌露出

ew
elsewhere 他の場所に
exposure wedge 組織学的剝離面癌露出

E-W
Edinger-Westphal (nucleus) エディンガー・ヴェストファル(核)

EWB
estrogen withdrawal bleeding エストロゲン消退出血

EWHO
elbow-wrist-hand orthosis 肘・手関節・手指装具

EWL
egg-white lysozyme 卵白リゾチーム

EWPHE
European Working Party on High Blood Pressure in (the) Elderly (Trial) 高齢者高血圧欧州共同研究

EWS
Ewing sarcoma ユーイング肉腫(骨)

EWSCL
extended-wear soft contact lenses 連続装用可能なソフトコンタクトレンズ

Ex
endotoxin エンドトキシン

Ex.
extractum〈ラ〉=an extract エキス，抽出物《処》

Ex, ex
endoxan エンドキサン
exacerbate 増悪する
exacerbation 増悪
exaggerate 誇張する
examination 検査，診査
examined 検査した
examiner 試験官
example 見本
excess 過剰
excision 切除
excitation 励起波長
exercise 運動，練習
exophthalmos 眼球突出
exposure 曝露，露出
extract 抽出物
extraction 摘出，抜歯

exac
exacerbate 増悪する
exacerbation 増悪，再燃

EXAFS
extended X-ray absorption fine structure X線吸収広域微細構造，エグザフス

exag
exaggerate 誇張する
exaggeration 誇張

exam
examination 検査，診査
examine 検査する
examiner 試験官，検者

ex aq.
ex aqua〈ラ〉 水に入れて《処》

exc
excel 優る，秀でる
excellent 優れた，優秀な
excepted 除いた，除外した
excision 切除

exc.bx
excisional biopsy 切除生検

E

exch，exch.
exchange 交換(する)
excis
excise 切除する
excision 切除
excl
exclude 除去する
exclusion 除外
excr
excrete 排出する，排泄する
excretion 排出，排泄
exec，exec.
execute 実行する
executive 実行の，経営者
EXELFS
extended energy loss fine structure エネルギー損失広域微細構造，エグゼルフス
exer
exercise 運動，練習
exf
extremely fine 極めて純粋な
exh
exhibit 展示する，現す，提出する
exhibition 展示，提出
exhib.
exhibeatur〈ラ〉 与えよ《処》
Eximer Laser
excited dimer laser エキシマレーザー
exist
existing 実在する，実存する
Exit
exitus〈ラ〉 死亡
EXO
exonuclease エキソヌクレアーゼ
exopholia 外斜位
exog
exogenous 外因性の
exoph
exophthalmia 眼球突出
exos
exostosis 外骨症
exp
expansion 拡大，膨張
expected 期待されている，予想されている
expecting 予期している，予想している

expectorant 去痰の
experience 体験
experiment 実験，試験
experimental 実験の
expiratory 呼気の，呼息の
expire 呼息する
exponent 指数
expose 露出する
exposure 曝露，露出

EXP, exp.
expiration 呼気，呼息，死亡

exp, Exp, EXP
expired 期限が切れた，失効した

ex paul
e(x) paul(o)〈ラ〉 少量の《処》

expec.
expectorantem〈ラ〉=expectorant 去痰の

expect.
expectoratium〈ラ〉 去痰の，去痰薬

exper
experience 体験
experiment 実験，試験
experimental 実験の

expir
expiration 呼気，呼息
expiratory 呼気の，呼息の

expl
explain 説明する
exploration 診査
exploratory 診査の
explore 診査する

exp.lap
exploratory laparotomy 診査開腹

expn
expression 圧縮，圧搾，表現，表情

exprim.
exprime〈ラ〉 急迫する《処》

expt, expt.
expected 期待されている，予想されている
expectorant 去痰の，去痰薬
expectorate 吐き出す，喀出する
experiment 実験
experimental 実験の

exptl
experimental 実験の

E

EXT
exotoxin toxoid 菌体外毒素
Ext.
extractum〈ラ〉=an extract エキス，抽出物《処》
Ext，ext
extraction 摘出，抜歯
ext，ext.
extendere〈ラ〉=extend 伸展する，拡がる
extension 伸展，延長
extensive 広範囲の，広い
extensor 伸筋
exterior 外の，外部の
extern エクスターン，通勤医
external 外の，外界の，外部の
extracted 抽出された
extractum〈ラ〉=extract 抽出物，エキス《処》
extreme 極端な
extremities 四肢，端
extremity 端，(一)肢
ext.aud
external auditory 外耳の
ext & cc
external drug and cosmetic color 外用薬と有色化粧品
extd
extended 伸展した
extracted 抽出された
extempl
extemplo〈ラ〉 ただちに《処》
extens
extension 伸展
extensor 伸筋
ext fl
extract fluid 抽出液
ext.fd
fluid extract 流動エキス剤
ext.liq.
extractum liquidum〈ラ〉 排液
extr
extremity 端，(一)肢
Extr.
extractum〈ラ〉=an extract エキス，抽出物《処》
Extra
extrasystole 期外収縮
extr.aq.
extractum aquosum〈ラ〉 水製エキス《処》

extrav
extravasation 管外遊出，溢血
extrem
extremity 端，(一)肢
extr.fl.
extractum fluidum〈ラ〉 流動エキス《処》
ext.rot
external rotation 外旋
extub
extubate 抜管する
extubated 抜管した
extubation 抜管
EXU
excretory urogram 排泄性尿路造影
exud
exudate 滲出液
exx
examples 標本，例〈複数〉
EY
egg yolk 卵黄
EYA
egg yolk agar 卵黄寒天
EZ
Edmonston-Zagreb (vaccine) エドモンストン・ザグレブ(ワクチン)
eineiige Zwillinge〈独〉 一卵性双生児
electrical zero 電気的零点
Ez
eczema 湿疹
ez
easy 容易な

F f

F

bioavailability	生物学的活性
coupling factors	共役因子
face	顔面
facies	顔
factor	因子
failed	失敗した，不合格となった
failure	不全
fair	公平な，良さそうな
false	偽りの
family	家族
Faraday constant	ファラデー定数
fascia	筋膜
fasting (test)	空腹時(検査)
fat	脂肪
father	父親
fecal	糞(便)の
feces	糞(便)
fecus	糞便
Fellow	フェロー，研究者
female	女性，雌
feminine	女性の，雌の
fermentative	酵素の，発酵の
fermi	フェルミ
fertility (factor)	受精能(因子)
fetal	胎児の
fibrous	線維(性)の
filament	細糸
filaria	フィラリア
fine	元気な，微細な，良い
finger	指
flexed	屈曲した
flow	流量
fluid	体液，液体(の)，液性(の)
fluorine	フッ素
flux	流出
focal length	(レンズの)焦点距離
foil	箔
follicle	濾胞
fontanel(le)	泉門
foramen	孔
force	力
formula	処方，式

formulary	処方集
fornix	円蓋，脳弓
fossa	窩
Fowler phenomenon	ファラー現象
fractional concentration in dry gas phase	乾性ガス分別濃度
fracture	骨折
Francisella	フランシセラ(属)
Frau〈独〉	妻
free	自由な，遊離した
free energy	自由エネルギー
French(-size)	フレンチ(サイズ)
French number	フレンチ番号
Freon	フレオン
frequency	度数，頻度，周波数
frons	額
frontal	前頭(部)の
frontal plane	前額面
full	(食餌に)満腹した
function	機能
fundus	底
Fusarium	フザリウム(属)
fusiform	紡錘状の
Fusiformis	紡錘菌(属)
fusion	融合，固定術
Fusobacterium	フソバクテリウム(属)
gilbert	ギルバート
Helmholtz free energy	ヘルムホルツ自由エネルギー
hydrocortisone	ヒドロコルチゾン
phenylalanine	フェニルアラニン
rate of aqueous humor formation	房水産生率
rate of secretion of aqueous humor	房水産生率
variance ratio	分散比

f

fast	速い，固定した
fast〈独〉	約
feet	フィート〈複数〉
femto-	フェムト(=10^{-15})〈接〉
final target	最終目標
fission	分裂
five	5
fixed	固定した，癒着した
flat	平らな，扁平な
flexion	屈曲
focal	焦点の，病巣の
focal distance	焦点距離

focal length	焦点距離
folio	一枚
following	次の，下記の
formyl	ホルミル
friction factor	摩擦係数
from	〜から
respiratory frequency	単位時間の呼吸数

°F

degree Fahrenheit	華氏(温度)

4F

fat, forty〔fifty〕, female and fertile	太った・40代〔50代〕・女性，生殖力のある

F_1

first filial generation	雑種第一代，第一世代

F_2

second filial generation	雑種第二代，第二世代
zinc oxide eugenol cement	亜鉛華ユージノールセメント

F 710

Fourneau 710	フォルノー710

F I

factor I	凝固第I因子(＝フィブリノゲン)，第I因子

F II

factor II	凝固第II因子(＝プロトロンビン)，第II因子

F III

factor III	凝固第III因子(＝組織トロンボプラスチン)，第III因子

F IV

factor IV	凝固第IV因子(＝カルシウムイオン)，第IV因子

F V

factor V	凝固第V因子(＝不安定因子)，第V因子

F VII

factor VII	凝固第VII因子(＝安定因子)，第VII因子

F VIII

factor VIII	凝固第VIII因子，第VIII因子

F IX

factor IX	凝固第IX因子，第IX因子

F X

factor X	凝固第X因子(スチュアート因子)，第X因子

F XI

factor XI	凝固第XI因子，第XI因子

F XII
factor XII　凝固第XII因子(接触因子)，第XII因子

F XIII
factor XIII　凝固第XIII因子(フィブリン安定化因子)，第XIII因子

F′
F-prime　Fプライム

F-12
freon-12　フレオン12

F, f
farad　ファラド〈単位〉
foot　足，フット，フート
forma〈ラ〉=form, figure, shape　形，形状，形式
fraction　分数，分画
fractional　分画の

F, F., f
field of vision　視野

F, F., f, f.
fac〈ラ〉=make　つくれ《処》
fiant〈ラ〉=let them be made　つくれ《処》
fiat〈ラ〉=let it be made　つくらせよ《処》
flat〈ラ〉　つくれ《処》

F-18, ^{18}F
fluorine-18　フッ素18

FA
factory automatic　作業の自動化
false aneurysm　偽動脈瘤
familiäre Anamnese〈独〉　家族歴
Fanconi anemia　ファンコニ貧血
fatty acid　脂肪酸
femoral artery　大腿動脈
femorotibial angle　膝外側角，大腿脛骨角
fibrinolytic activity　線維素溶解活性
fibroadenoma　線維腺腫
field ambulance　野戦救急車
filterable agent　濾過剤
first aid　応急処置
first attack　最初の発作
fluorescein angiography　螢光(眼底)血管造影(法)
fluorescein-labelled antibody　フルオレ(ス)セイン標識抗体
fluorescence antibody　螢光抗体
fluorescent antibody (method)　螢光抗体(法)
fluorescent assay　螢光検定(法)，螢光定量
3-fluoro-D-alanine　3-フルオロ-D-アラニン
folic acid　葉酸

forearm	前腕
formamid(e)	ホルムアミド
fortined aqueous	強化水溶液
free acid	遊離酸
free association	自由連想
Freund adjuvant	フロイントアジュバント
Friedreich ataxia	フリードリ〔ライ〕ヒ失調症
functional activity	機能的活性
fusidic acid	フシジン酸

F

Fa

family anamnesis	家族歴

FⅡa

factorⅡa	活性化第Ⅱ因子(＝トロンビン)

FAA

acetylaminofluorene	アセチルアミノフルオレン
fatty acid acceptor	脂肪酸受容体
folic acid antagonist	葉酸拮抗物質，葉酸拮抗薬
fragmental atrial activity	断裂性心房活動
free amino acid	遊離アミノ酸
N-2-fluorenylacetamide	*N*-2-フルオレニルアセトアミド

2-FAA

N-2-fluorenylacetamide	*N*-2-フルオレニルアセトアミド

2,7-FAA

N,*N′*-2,7-fluorenyl-enebis acetamide	*N*,*N′*-2,7-フルオレニルエネビアセトアミド

FAA fixative

formalin acetic acid fixative	ホルマリン酢酸固定液

FAB

fast atom bombardment	質量分析
fast atomic beam	一次ビームとして中性原子を用いる表面分析法
French-American-British (classification)	FAB(分類)(＝白血病分類方式の１つ)
functional arm brace	上肢機能固定器

FAB, Fab

fragment antigen binding (of immunoglobulin G involved in)	(免疫グロブリンGの)抗原結合フラグメント

FABER

flexion in abduction and external rotation	股関節の屈曲・外転・外旋

FABERE

flexion, abduction, external rotation and extension (test)	股関節の屈曲・外転・外旋・伸展試験

FABF
femoral artery blood flow　大腿動脈血流量
FAB-MS
fast atom bombardment mass spectrometry　高速電子衝撃質量分析法
FABP
fatty acid-binding protein　脂肪酸結合蛋白
folic acid-binding protein　葉酸結合蛋白
FAC
familial adenomatosis colitis　家族性大腸腺腫症
fluorouracil, adriamycin, cyclophosphamide　フルオロウラシル,アドリアマイシン,シクロホスファミド

F

Fac
factor　因子，要因，要素
fac.
facere〈ラ〉=to make，to form，construct，create　つくる
facial　顔面の
FACA
Fellow of American College of Anesthetists　米国麻酔科学会員
Fellow of American College of Angiology　米国血管学会員
FACAl
Fellow of American College of Allergists　米国アレルギー学会員
FACC
Fellow of American College of Cardiology　米国心臓病学会員
FACD
Fellow of American College of Dentistry　米国歯科学会員
FACDS
Fellow of Australian College of Dental Surgeons　オーストラリア歯科医会会員
FACFO
Fellow of American College of Foot Orthopedics　米国足の整形外科学会員
FACG
Fellow of American College of Gastroenterology　米国胃腸病学会員
facil
facilitate　促進する
facilitation　促進

F

FAC-LEV
fluorouracil, adriamycin, cyclophosphamide, levamisole — フルオロウラシル,アドリアマイシン,シクロホスファミド,レバミゾール

FACMTA
Fellow of Advisory Council on Medical Training Aids — 医療訓練器具勧告委員会委員

$FACO_2$
alveolar CO_2 concentration — 肺胞気二酸化炭素〔炭酸ガス〕濃度

FACOG
Fellow of American College of Obstetricians and Gynecologists — 米国産婦人科学会員

FACP
Fellow of American College of Physicians — 米国医師会会員
ftorafur, adriamycin, cyclophosphamide, cisplatin (= Platinol) — フトラフール,アドリアマイシン,シクロホスファミド,シスプラチン(=プラチノール)

FACPM
Fellow of American College of Preventive Medicine — 米国予防医学会員

FACR
Fellow of American College of Radiology — 米国放射線科学会員

FACS
Fellow of American College of Surgeons — 米国外科医師会員
fluorescence-activated cell sorter — 螢光発色セルソーター
fluorouracil, adriamycin, cyclophosphamide, streptozo(to)cin — フルオロウラシル,アドリアマイシン,シクロホスファミド,ストレプトゾ(ト)シン

FAD
familial Alzheimer disease — 家族性アルツハイマー病
flavin adenine dinucleotide — フラビンアデニンジヌクレオチド

$FADH_2$
flavin adenine dinucleotide reduced type — フラビンアデニンジヌクレオチド還元型
reduced flavin adenine dinucleotide — 還元フラビンアデニンジヌクレオチド

FADIRE
flexion, adduction, internal rotation and extension (test) — 股関節の屈曲・内転・内旋・伸展試験

FADN
flavin adenine dinucleotide フラビンアデニンジヌクレオチド

FADO
Fellow of Association of Dispensing Opticians 眼鏡商組合員

FAE
fetal alcohol effect 胎児性アルコール効果(＝妊婦の飲酒による影響)
follicle associated epithelium 貪食能をもつ上皮

FAEC
factor analysis with equilibrium constraints 化学平衡を考慮した因子分析法

FAF
fibroblast-activating factor 線維芽細胞活性化因子

FAG
fluorescein (fundus) angiography 螢光眼底(血管)造影(法)
fluorescent fundus angiography 螢光眼底(血管)造影(法)

FAHR, Fahr
Fahrenheit 華氏〈温度〉

FAI
familial amaurotic idiocy 家族性黒内障性白痴
functional aerobic impairment 機能的好気性障害
functional assessment inventory 機能評価項目表

FAIDS
feline AIDS ネコエイズ

FAIHA
Fellow of Australian Institute of Hospital Administration オーストラリア病院管理研究所員

FAIP
Fellow of Australian Institute of Physics オーストラリア医学研究所員

FAJ
fused apophyseal joints 癒合椎間関節

FAK
focal adenosine kinase 局所的アデノシンキナーゼ

FAL
femoral arterial line 大腿動脈ライン
functional and anatomic loading 機能的・解剖学的負荷

FALP
fluoro-assisted lumbar puncture X線透視下腰椎穿刺

FALS
familial amyotrophic lateral sclerosis 家族性筋萎縮性側索硬化症

FAM
fluorouracil, adriamycin, mitomycin フルオロウラシル,アドリアマイシン,マイトマイシン

F

Fam, fam
family 家族
FAMA
Fellow of American Medical Association 米国医師会会員
fluorouracil, adriamycin, mitomycin-C, alkylating agent フルオロウラシル,アドリアマイシン,マイトマイシンC,アルキル化剤
fluorouracil, cyclophosphamide, mitomycin-C, chromomycin フルオロウラシル,シクロホスファミド,マイトマイシンC,クロモマイシン
fam.doc
family doctor 家庭医
FAMe
fluorouracil, adriamycin, methylchloroethyl-cyclohexylnitrosourea フルオロウラシル,アドリアマイシン,メチルクロロエチル-シクロヘキシルニトロソ尿素
fam.hist
family history 家族歴
Fam per.par.
familial periodic paralysis 家族性周期性四肢麻痺
Fam phys, fam phys
family physician 家庭医
FAM-S
fluorouracil, adriamycin, mitomycin-C, streptozo(to)cin フルオロウラシル,アドリアマイシン,マイトマイシンC,ストレプトゾ(ト)シン
FAMT
fluorouracil, cyclophosphamide A, mitomycin-C, Toyomycin フルオロウラシル,シクロホスファミドA,マイトマイシンC,トヨマイシン
FANA
fluorescent antinuclear antibody (test) 螢光抗核抗体(法)
necked anti-nuclear antibody 斑点状抗核抗体
FANES
furnace atomization nonthermal excitation spectrometry 黒鉛炉非熱励起分光分析
F-antigen
Forssman antigen フォルスマン抗原
FAO
Food and Agriculture Organization (国連の)食糧農業機関
FAO_2
alveolar O_2 concentration 肺胞気酸素濃度

FAP
familial adenomatous polyposis　家族性大腸腺腫症
familial amyloid polyneuropathy　家族性アミロイド多発性ニューロパシー
femoral artery pressure　大腿動脈圧
FAPA
Federation of Asian Pharmaceutical Associations　アジア製薬業連盟
FAPES
furnace atomization plasma emission spectrometry　黒鉛炉原子化プラズマ発光分析法
FAPG
fatty alcohol, propylene glycol　脂肪酸アルコール・プロピレングリコール
FAPHA
Fellow of American Public Health Association　米国公衆衛生協会員
FAPS
Fellow of American Physical Society　米国内科学会員
FAR
flight aptitude rating　飛行適性評価
far
farad　ファラド〈単位〉
faradic　感応電流の，誘導電流の
FAS
fatty acid synt(het)ase　脂肪酸合成酵素
fetal alcohol syndrome　胎児アルコール症候群
food advice service　食品助言サービス
full analysis set　最大解析対象集団
FASA
Fellow of Acoustical Society of America　米国聴覚学会員
fasc
fasciculation　線維束性攣縮
fasc, fasc.
fasciculus〈ラ〉=small bundle　束
fasci
fasciculation　線維束性攣縮
FASEB
Federation of American Society of Experimental Biology　米国実験生物学会連合
FASQ
functional assessment screening questionnaire　機能的評価選別質問
FAST
fluorescence allergosorbent test　アレルギーの特異的抗原検査

F

functional assessment staging of Alzheimer disease | アルツハイマー型痴呆の機能的評価

FAT
fast axoplasmic transport | 高速軸索原形質輸送
fluorescent antibody technique | 螢光抗体法
fluorescent antibody test | 螢光抗体検査
food awareness training | 食物認識訓練

FAVA
Federation of Asian Veternary Association | アジア獣医師会連合

FB
fasting blood sugar | 空腹時血糖
feedback | フィードバック
fiberoptic bronchoscopy | 気管支ファイバースコープ検査
film badge | フィルムバッジ
foot bath | 足浴
foreign body | 異物
free bilirubin | 遊離ビリルビン
Fusobacterium | フソバクテリウム属

F.B.
foot board | 足底板

FB, fb
fingerbreadth | 横指

FBA
fecal bile acid | (糞)便胆汁酸

F′bacterium
F-prime bacterium | Fプライム菌

F^+ bacterium
F plus bacterium | F^+菌

F^- bacterium
F minus bacterium | F^-菌

FBC
functional bladder capacity | 機能的膀胱容量

FBCOD
foreign body cornea dexter eye | 右眼角膜異物

FBCOS
foreign body cornea sinister eye | 左眼角膜異物

FBCP
Fellow of British College of Physiotherapists | 英国物理療法士会員

FBD
functional bowel disorder | 機能的腸障害〔疾患〕

FBF
forearm blood flow | 前腕血流量

Frankfurter Beschwerdefragebogen 〈独〉 フランクフルト愁訴質問リスト

FBG
fasting blood glucose 空腹時血糖値
fibrinogen 線維素原，フィブリノゲン

FBI
focal brain injury 局所性脳損傷

FBM
fetal breathing movement 胎児呼吸運動

FBN
Federal Bureau of Narcotics 麻薬連合事務局

Fbn
fibrin フィブリン

FBOA
Fellow of British Optical Association 英国眼科協会員

F body
fluorescent body 螢光小体

FBP
Federation of Podiatry Boards 足治療士連合
femoral blood pressure 大腿血圧
fibrin(ogen) breakdown products フィブリン分解産物
final boiling point 最終沸点

FBPase
fructose-1,6-bisphosphatase フルクトース-1,6-ビスホスファターゼ

FBPF
fibroblast proliferation factor 線維芽細胞増殖因子

FBPsS
Fellow of British Psychological Society 英国精神科学会会員

FBS
failed back syndrome 腰椎症候群
fasting blood sugar 空腹時血糖
fasting blood sugar level 空腹時血糖値
feedback system フィードバックシステム
fetal blood sampling 胎児採血
fetal bovine serum ウシ胎仔血清
fiber bronchoscopy ファイバー気管支鏡

FBSS
failed back surgery syndrome 腰椎手術不成功症候群

FC
false cord 仮声帯
fasciculus cuneatus 楔状束
febrile convulsion 熱性痙攣
fertilization cone 一過性卵細胞質隆起
fibrocystic 線維(性)嚢胞の

F

fibrocyte 線維細胞
finger counting 指数弁
flicker campimetry フリッカー中心視野
flucytosine フルシトシン
fluorocarbon フルオロカーボン
fold convergency 陥凹性病変に伴う皺襞集中
Foley catheter フォーリーカテーテル
formalin tricresol ホルマリントリクレゾール
free cholesterol 遊離コレステロール
frontal cortex 前頭皮質

F

Fc
fluocinonide フルオシノニド
Fragment, crystallizable 易結晶化フラグメント

fc
footcandle フートキャンドル〈単位〉

5-FC
5-fluorocytosine 5-フルオロシトシン

FⅧ:C
factor Ⅷ coagulant activity 凝固第Ⅷ因子凝固活性

F+C
flare and cells フレア(発赤拡張)細胞

F-C
femoro-crural 大腿・下腿動脈バイパス

FC, Fc
crystallizable fragment 易結晶化フラグメント

FCA
Freund complete adjuvant フロインド完全アジュバント

FCAC
fluorouracil, cyclophosphamide, adriamycin, cisplatin フルオロウラシル,シクロホスファミド,アドリアマイシン,シスプラチン

FⅧ CAG
factor Ⅷ coagulant antigen 凝固第Ⅷ因子凝固抗原

FCAP
Fellow of College of American Pathologist 米国病理学会員

FCC
follicular center cell 濾胞中心細胞

FCCP
carbonylcyanide-*p*-trifluoromethoxyphenylhydrazone カルボニルシアニド-*p*-トリフルオロメトキシフェニルヒドラゾン

FCD
fibrous cortical defect 線維性骨皮質欠損
focal cytoplasmic degradation 細胞内限局性壊死

FcεR
IgE specific Fc receptor　IgE特異的Fcレセプター
FCF
fibroblast chemotactic factor　線維芽細胞化学走性因子
FCFC
fibroblast colony-forming cells　線維芽細胞コロニー形成細胞
FCGP
Fellow of College of General Practioners　一般医学会員
FcγR
IgG specific Fc receptor　IgG特異的Fcレセプター
FCHL
familial combined hyperlipidemia　家族性混合性高脂血症
FChS
Fellow of Society of Chiropodists　手足治療士協会員
FCL
fibular collateral ligament　外側側副靱帯
fc ly
face lying　顔を伏せている
FCM
flow cytometory　フローサイトメトリー
FCMD
Fukuyama type congenital muscular dystrophy　福山型先天性筋ジストロフィ
FcμR
IgM specific Fc receptor　IgM特異的Fcレセプター
FCNA
Fellow of College of Nursing　看護学会員
FCP
final common pathway　終末一般経路
fluorouracil, cyclophosphamide, prednisone　フルオロウラシル,シクロホスファミド,プレドニゾン
FCPA
Fellow of Canadian Psychological Association　カナダ心理学協会員
FCPC
Federal Committee on Pest Control　ペスト予防連合委員会
FCPD
fibrocalculous pancreatic diabetes　線維石灰化膵性糖尿病
fc pl
facial plate　顔面板
FCPS
Fellow of College of Physicians and Surgeons　英国医師・外科医会員
FCR
flexor carpi radialis　橈側手根屈筋

flexor carpi radialis muscle	橈骨側手根屈筋
Fuji computed radiography	フジラジオグラフィ
FcR, Fc-R	
Fc(=crystallizable fragment) receptor	Fcレセプター
FCRA	
Fellow of College of Radiologist of Australia	オーストラリア放射線科学会員
FcR-AD	
Fc receptor-mediated antidody dependent enhancement	Fcレセプターによる抗体依存的増強作用(=ADCC)
fecal containment system	糞便封鎖システム
FCS	
feedback control system	フィードバックコントロールシステム
fetal calf serum	ウシ胎仔血清
fiber colonoscopy	大腸ファイバースコープ
fct	
function	機能
FCTB	
Fellow of College of Teachers of Blind	盲人教師協会会員
FCU	
flexor carpi ulnaris	尺側手根屈筋
flexor carpi ulnaris muscle	尺側手根屈筋
FCX	
frontal cortex	前頭(葉)皮質
FCZ	
fluconazole	フルコナゾール
FD	
facial dyskinesia	顔面ジスキネジア
faculty development	ファカルティ・ディベロプメント，大学教員の教育能力開発
familial dysautonomia	家族性自律神経障害
family doctor	家庭医
fan douche	扇形注入器での灌注法
fetal danger	胎児危険
field desorption	電解イオン脱離
filling defect	陰影欠損
floppy disc	フロッピーディスク
forced diuresis	強制利尿
freeze-dried	乾燥凍結
functional dyspepsia	機能性ディスペプシア
furadantin	フラダンチン

F×D
four times daily　1日4回《処》

Fd
ferredoxin　フェレドキシン
fundus　底

fd
field　視野，照射野

FD_{50}
median fatal dose　50%致死量

f/d
father and daugther　父と娘

FD，F.D.
fatal dose　致死量
focal distance　焦点距離
forceps delivery　鉗子分娩

FDA
fluorescein diacetate　フルオレ(ス)セイン二酢酸
Food and Drug Administration　米国食品医薬品局
frequency dependent attenuation　周波数依存減衰
fronto-dextra anterior　右額前位(胎児)

FDB
familial defective apolipoprotein B100　家族性異常アポB血症

FDC
fluorodecalin　フッ化デカリン
follicular dendritic cell(s)　濾胞樹状細胞

FD & C
Food, Drug and Cosmetic Act　食品・薬品・化粧品条例

FDD
Foundation Documentaire Dentaire　歯科情報管理基金

FDEIA
food-dependent exercise-induced anaphylaxis　食物依存性運動誘発アナフィラキシー

FDG
F-18-deoxyglucose　F-18-デオキシグルコース

fdg
feeding　栄養補給，給食，飼育

FDGF
fibroblast-derived growth factor　線維芽細胞由来成長因子

FDH
familial dyslipidemic hypertension　家族性脂質異常高血圧
familiar dysalbuminemic hyperthyroxinemia　家族性血漿蛋白過剰過サイロキシン血症
focal dermal hypoplasia　巣状皮膚形成不全

FDI
Federation Dentaire Internationale 〈仏〉 国際歯学連盟
first dorsal interosseous 第1背側骨間(筋)
FDIU
fetal death in utero 子宮内胎児死(亡)
FDL
flexor digitorum longus 長指屈筋
F & DL
Food and Drug Laboratory 食品・薬品研究室

FDLC
flexible double lumen catheter 軟(性)2孔式〔二重式〕カテーテル
FDLI
Food and Drug Law Institute 食品・薬品・法律研究所
FDM
fetus of diabetic mother 糖尿病の母の胎児
musculus flexor digiti minimi brevis 短小指屈筋
FD-MS
field desorption mass spectrometry フィールドデソープション質量分析法
FDNB
1-fluoro-2,4-dinitrobenzene 1-フルオロ-2,4-ジニトロベンゼン
FDP
fibrin degradation product フィブリン分解産物
fibrinogen degradation products フィブリノゲン分解物
flexor digitorum profundus (muscle) 深指屈筋
fronto-dextra posterior 右額後位〈胎位〉
fructose diphosphate フルクトース二リン酸
fructose 1,6-diphosphate フルクトース1,6-二リン酸
FDPALD
fructose diphosphate aldolase フルクトース二リン酸アルドラーゼ
FDPase
fructose 1,6-diphosphatase フルクトース1,6-ジホスファターゼ
fdp/Fdp
fibrin-fibrinogen degradation products フィブリン・フィブリノゲン分解産物
FDQB
flexor digiti quinti brevis 短小指屈筋
FDS
Fellow of Dental Surgery (英国)歯科医会会員
fiberduodenoscope 十二指腸ファイバースコープ

flexor digitorum sublimis (superficialis) 浅指屈筋
flexor digitorum superficialis muscle 浅指屈筋

FDSRCS
Fellow in Dental Surgery of Royal College of Surgeons 英国歯科医会会員

FDT
fronto-dextra posterior 右額後位〈胎位〉
fronto-dextra-transversa〈ラ〉 前頭右側横位〈胎位〉

FdUMP
5-fluoro-2′-deoxyuridine monophosphate 5-フルウロデオキシウリジンーリン酸塩

FdUrd
5-fluoro-2′-deoxyuridine 5-フルオロデオキシウリジン

FDV
first desire to void 初発尿意
Friend disease virus フレンド病ウイルス

FE
fetal echo 胎児エコー《超音波》
fetal erythroblastosis 胎児赤芽球症
focal emphysema 巣状型肺気腫
formalin and ethanol ホルマリンとエタノール
fractional excretion 分画排出

Fe
ferrum〈ラ〉=iron 鉄〈元素〉

^{59}FE
radioactive iron 放射性鉄

Fe^{2+}
ferrous 鉄の，第一鉄の

Fe^{3+}
ferric 鉄の，第二鉄の

Fe, fe
female 雌，女性

feb.
febrile 熱性の，発熱している
febris〈ラ〉=fever 熱(病)

feb.dur.
febre durante〈ラ〉=while the fever lasts 発熱が続く間

FEBS
Federation of European Biochemical Societies 欧州生化学会連合

FEC
fluorouracil, etoposide, cisplatin フルオロウラシル,エトポシド,シスプラチン

forced expiratory capacity 努力性呼気肺活量

FECF
functional extracellular fluid 機能的細胞外液

FECG
fetal electrocardiogram 胎児心電図

$FeCl_3$
ferric chloride 塩化第二鉄

FeD
iron (ferrum) deficiency 鉄欠乏

Fed
federal 連邦政府の
federation 連盟，連合

Fe def
iron (ferrum) deficiency anemia 鉄欠乏性貧血

FEDL
fat extracted dry liver 脱脂肪乾燥肝

feeb
feeble 弱い
feeblemined 精神(発達)遅滞の

FEEG
fetal electroencephalogram 胎児脳波

FEES
field emission electron spectroscopy 電界放射電子分光法

FEF
family evaluation form 家族評価書式
forced expiratory flow 最大呼気流量
frontal eye field 前頭葉眼球運動野

FEF_{25}
forced expiratory flow after 25% of vital capacity 25%努力性呼気量

FEG
field emission gun 電界放射型電子銃

FEHB
Federal Employees Health Benefit 従業員健康年金連合

FEKG
fetal electrocardiogram 胎児心電図

FEL
familial erythrophagocytic lymphohistiocytosis 家族性血球貪食リンパ組織球症
free electron laser 自由電子レーザー

Fel, fel
fellow 男の子，特別会員，特別研究員

FeLV, FelV
feline leukemia virus ネコ白血病ウイルス

FEM
field emission microscope　電界放射顕微鏡

fem
female　雌(性)の，女性(の)
feminine　女性の
femoral　大腿部の

FEM，fem.
femoris〈ラ〉=of the thigh　大腿の

fem，fem.
femur〈ラ〉　大腿(骨)

fem.ext.
femur externum〈ラ〉　大腿外側

fem.int.
femur internum〈ラ〉　大腿内側

FENa
fractional excretion of filtrated Na　尿中ナトリウム排泄
fractional excretion rate of sodium　ナトリウム分画排泄率

FeO_2
fractional concentration of oxygen in a sample of expired gas　呼気ガス内酸素濃度

FEP
free erythrocyte porphyrin　遊離赤血球ポルフィリン
free erythrocyte protoporphyrin　遊離赤血球プロトポルフィリン
front end processor　フロントエンドプロセッサ《コン》

Fepisome
fertility episome　生殖遺伝子副体

FEPP-B
vindesine, etoposide, procarbazine, prednisone, bleomycin　ビンデシン，エトポシド，プロカルバジン，プレドニゾン，ブレオマイシン

FER
ferritin　フェリチン

Fer.
ferrum〈ラ〉=iron　鉄

fer'd
fertilized　受精した，受精させた

fermentol
fermentology　酵素学

Fer.red.
ferrum reductum〈ラ〉　還元鉄《処》

fert
fertility　生殖力，多産
fertilization　受精，受胎

fertd.
fertilized 受精した，受精させた
ferv.
fervens〈ラ〉=boilling 煮沸する
FES
fat embolism syndrome 脂肪塞栓症候群
Fellow of Ethological Society 動物行動学会員
forced expiratory spirogram 努力呼気曲線
functional electrical stimulation 機能的電気刺激
functional endonasal surgery 内視鏡下副鼻腔手術
further example see より詳しくは例をみよ
FESAO
Federation of Endocrine Societies of Asia and Oceania アジアオセアニア内分泌学会連合
fest
festination 加速歩行
FeSV
feline sarcoma virus ネコ肉腫ウイルス
FET
field effect transistor 電界効果型トランジスタ
final electroconvulsive threshold 最終電気痙攣閾値
forced expiratory technique 強制呼気(呼出)法
forced expiratory time 努力性呼気時間
fet
fetus 胎児
fetal CTG
fetal cardiotocograph 胎児心拍陣痛図
fetal h.
fetal hemoglobin 胎児ヘモグロビン
$FETCO_2$
fraction of end-tidal carbon dioxide 呼気終末二酸化炭素〔炭酸ガス〕濃度
fetol
fetological 胎児学の
fetologist 胎児学者
fetology 胎児学
FEUO
for external use only 外用のみ《処》
$\%^{59}$Fe util
^{59}Fe utilization 鉄(=^{59}Fe)の赤血球利用率
FEV
forced expiratory volume 努力呼気肺活量
fev
fever 熱，発熱，熱病
feverish 熱のある，熱病の

FEV1.0
forced expiratory volume in one second　1秒量

FEV1.0%
forced expiratory volume in one second percent　1秒率

FEVR
familial exudative vitreoretinopathy　家族性滲出性硝子体網膜症

FF
fat free (diet)　無脂肪(食)
fertility factor　捻出因子，受精因子
fields of Forel　フォレル野
filtration fraction　濾過率
finger flexion　指屈曲
finger to finger　指指(試験)
fixing fluid　固定液
flat feet　扁平足
forehead nap　前頭弁
foster father　養父
Fox-Fordyce (disease)　フォックス・フォーダイス(病)
free field　自由音場
fresh frozen　新鮮凍結の

ff
following　下記の，次の

F.F
Fahrenheit　華氏(温度)〈単位〉

F & F
face-to-face　互いに向きあって

F-F
femoro-femoral (bypass)　大腿・大腿動脈(バイパス)

FF，ff
forward flexion　前屈

FFA
force field analysis　力分野の分析
free fatty acid　遊離脂肪酸

F factor
fertility factor　捻出因子，受精因子

FFAP
free fatty acid phase　遊離脂肪酸相

FFC
free from chloride　塩素遊離の

FFD
1,5-difluoro-2,4-dinitrobenzene　1,5-ジフルオロ-2,4-ジニトロベンゼン
finger floor distance　指尖床間距離

focus to film distance 焦点フィルム間距離

FFE
fecal fat excretion (糞)便脂肪排泄
free-flow electrophoresis フリーフロー電気泳動法

FFF
fat, forty and female 太った・40歳代・女性
field-flow fractionation フィールドフロー分別
flicker fusion field ちらつき視野
flicker fusion frequency フリッカー融合頻度

FFG
fasciculus gracilis 薄束

FFI
fatal familial insomnia 致死性家族性不眠症
free from infection 感染していない

FFM
fat-free mass 非脂肪組織
friction force microscope 摩擦力顕微鏡

FFP
fresh frozen plasma 新鮮凍結血漿

FFPE tissues
formalin fixed paraffin embedded tissue ホルマリン固定パラフィン包埋組織

FFPS
Fellow of Faculty of Physician and Surgeons 内科・外科会員

FFQ
finger function quotient 指運動機能指数

FFR
Fellow of Faculty of Radiologist 放射線科(分科)会員
frequency following response 周波数追跡反応

FFS
failure of fixation suppression of caloric nystagmus 温度眼振の視性抑制の欠如
fat-free solids 無脂肪固体

FFT
fast Fourier transform 高速フーリエ変換
flicker fusion threshold 閃光融合域(検査)

FFU
femur, fibula, ulna (syndrome) 大腿骨・腓骨・尺骨症候群
focus forming unit 焦点形成単位

FG
fast twitch glycolytic 迅速攣縮性解糖の
fibrinogen 線維素原，フィブリノゲン
fine grain 細顆粒
French gauge フレンチゲージ

fg
femtogram フェムトグラム(=10^{-15}g)
FGAR
formylglycinamide ribonucleotide ホルミルグリシンアミドリボ核酸
N-fromylglycinamide ribotide *N*-ホルミルグリシンアミドリボチド
FGB
fasting blood glucose 空腹時血糖
fully granulated basophil 多顆粒性好塩基球
FGC
fibrinogen gel chromatography フィブリノゲンガスクロマトグラフィ
FgDP
fibrinogen degradation product フィブリノゲン分解産物
FGF
fibroblast growth factor 線維芽細胞成長〔増殖〕因子
fresh gas flow 新鮮ガス流
fully good, fair 完全に良くかつ十分な
FGFJ
Friends of the Global Fund, Japan グローバルファンド日本委員会
FGID
functional gastrointestinal disorder 機能性胃腸障害
FGL
fasting gastrin level 空腹時ガストリンレベル
FGN
focal glomerulonephritis 巣状糸球体腎炎
fgn
foreign 他の，異なる
FGS
fiber gastroscope 胃ファイバースコープ
focal glomerulo sclerosis 巣状糸球体硬化症
focal segmental glomerular sclerosis (mouse) 巣状分節状糸球体硬化症(マウス)
formaldehydogenic steroids ホルムアルデヒド形成性ステロイド
FH
familial hypercholesterolemia 家族性高コレステロール血症
family history 家族歴
Fanconi-Hegglin (syndrome) ファンコニ・ヘグリン症候群
fetal head (胎)児頭
fibromuscular hyperplasia 線維性過形成
fimbria hippocampi〈ラ〉 (脳の)海馬采(=さい)
1-(2-tetrahydrofuryl)-5-Fu 1-(2-テトラヒドロフリル)-5-フルオロウラシル

F

fulminant hepatitis 劇症肝炎
fumarate hydratase フマル酸ヒドラターゼ

fh.
fiat haustus〈ラ〉 頓服水剤をつくれ《処》

FH_2
dihydrofolic acid ジヒドロ葉酸

F.H.
fatty tissue/hematopoietic tissue ratio 脂肪組織・造血組織比

FHA
familial hypoplastic anemia 家族性低形成貧血
filamentous hemagglutinin 線状赤血球凝集素
filterable hemolytic anaemia 濾過性溶血性貧血
Fokus-Haut-Abstand〈独〉 焦点皮膚距離，線源皮膚距離

FII-HA
FII (＝γ globulin) hemagglutination test FII (＝ガンマグロブリン)赤血球凝集試験

FHB
fetal heart beat 胎児心拍

FHBLP
familiar hypobeta-lipoproteinemia 家族性低βリポ蛋白血症

FHC
familial hypercholesterolemia 家族性高コレステロール血症

FHD
family history of diabetes 糖尿病の家族歴
Fokus-Haut-Distanz〈独〉 焦点皮膚距離，線源皮膚距離

FHF
fulminant hepatic failure 劇症肝不全

FHH
familial hypocalciuric hypercalcemia 家族性低カルシウム尿性高カルシウム血症
family history of hirsutism 多毛症の家族歴
fetal heart heard 可聴胎児心音

FHHI
familial persistent hyperinsulinemic hypoglycemia of infancy 新生児期家族性永続性高インスリンによる低血糖症

FHL
flexor hallucis longus 長母指屈筋
functional hearing loss 機能性難聴

FHLDL
familial hypercholesterolemia 家族性高コレステロール血症

FHM
familial hemiplegic migraine 家族性片麻痺性片頭痛

FHP
family history positive 家族歴あり

FHR
fetal heart rate　胎児心拍数
FHR acceleration
fetal heart rate acceleration　胎児心拍数一過性頻脈
FHR baseline
fetal heart rate baseline　胎児心拍数基線
FHR baseline variability
fetal heart rate baseline variability　胎児心拍数基線細変動
FHR deceleration
fetal heart rate deceleration　胎児心拍数一過性徐脈
FHS
fetal heart sounds　胎児心音
fetal hydantoin syndrome　胎児ヒダントイン症候群
FHT
fetal heart tone　胎児心音
FHTG
familial hypertriglyceridemia　家族性高トリグリセリド血症
F Hx, FHx
family history　家族歴
FI
Färbeindex〈独〉　色素指数
fasciculus interfascicularis　半円束
fertility index　受精指数
fibrinogen　線維素原，フィブリノゲン
fluorescence index　螢光指数
folded cell index　皺襞細胞指数
forced inspiration　強制吸気
fi
fixed internal　固定内部強化《心理》
fronto-iliacus　前頭骨・腸骨
functional inquiry　機能的追求
FIA
flow injection analysis　フローインジェクション分析
flow injection analyzer　フローインジェクション分析器
fluorescent immunoassay　螢光酵素免疫法
fluoroimmunoassay　螢光酵素免疫法
Freund incomplete adjuvant　不完全フロインドアジュバント
FIAC
fluoroiodoarabinosyl cytosine　フルオロヨードアラビノシルシトシン
FIAEM
Fédération Interntionale des Associations d,Etudiants en Médecine〈仏〉　国際医学生協会連盟

F

F

FIAT
fatty acid incorporation into adipose tissue 脂肪組織への脂肪酸転入率
FIAX
solid phase fluorescence immunoassay 固相螢光免疫測定法
FIB
fibrin フィブリン
fibroblast 線維芽細胞
fibrositis 結合組織炎
fibula 腓骨
focus ion beam 収束イオンビーム
fib
fiber 線維
fibrous 線維(性)の
Fib, fib
fibrillation 細動，線維攣縮
fibrinogen 線維素原，フィブリノゲン
fibr
fibrillation 細動，線維(性)攣縮
fibrill
fibrillation 細動，線維(性)攣縮
fibrin
fibrinogen 線維素原，フィブリノゲン
Fibro
fibroblast 線維芽細胞
FIC
fluorescein isocyanate フルオレ(ス)セインイソシアネイト
FICD
Fellow of International College of Dentists 国際歯科学会員
FICS
Fellow of International College of Surgeons 国際外科医師会員
fict.
fictilis〈ラ〉 土製の《処》
FICU
fetal intensive care unit 胎児集中治療室
FID
Federation Internationale du Diabéte〈仏〉 国際糖尿病連盟
flame ionization detector 水素炎イオン化検出器
free induction decay 自由誘導減衰

FIDE
Federation de L'Industrie Dentaire en Europe〈仏〉 欧州歯科産業連盟
FIET
forearm ischemic exercise test 前腕阻血運動試験
FIF
fibroblast interferon 線維芽細胞インターフェロン
forced inspiratory flow 努力性吸気流量
formaldehyde-induced fluorescence ホルムアルデヒド誘発螢光
FIFN
fibroblast interferon 線維芽細胞インターフェロン
FIG
figuratively 比喩的に
fig
figure 形態，図
FIGLU
formiminoglutamic acid ホルムイミノグルタミン酸
FIGO
Federation Internationale de Gynécologie ert d'Obstétrique〈仏〉 国際産科婦人科連合
International Federation of Gynecology and Obstetrics 国際産婦人科学会連合
FIH
fat-induced hyperglycemia 脂質誘発高血糖
Federation Internationale des Hopitaux〈仏〉 国際病院連盟
FIL
father-in-law 義父
fil
filament 細糸
filamentous 糸状の
filt, filt.
filter〈ラ〉 濾過《処》
filter 濾過する，濾過器
filtered 濾過した
filtra〈ラ〉=filter 濾過せよ
FIM
field ion microscopy 電解イオン顕微鏡検査
functional independence measure 機能的自立度評価法
FIME
fluorouracil, ICRF-159, methylchloroethyl-cyclohexylnitrosourea フルオロウラシル，ラゾキサン，メチルクロロエチル-シクロヘキシルニトロソ尿素
FIMLT
Fellow of Institute of Medical Laboratory Technology 医学検査技士

F

FIMP
Federation Internatinale de Médecine Physique〈仏〉 国際物理医学会
FIMPR
Federation Internationale de Médecine Physique et Réhabilitation〈仏〉 国際物理医学・リハビリテーション学会
FIMS
Federation Internationale de Médecine Sportive〈仏〉 国際体力医学連盟
FI-MS
field ionization-mass spectrometry フィールドイオン化質量分析法
FIMSA
Federation of Immunological Society of Asia-Oceania アジア太平洋免疫学会連合
FIN
fine intestinal needle 細腸管針
Final Dx
final diagnosis 最終診断
FIND
Federation of Inochi No Denwa いのちの電話連盟
friendless, isolated, needy, disabled 友人のいない・孤独な・貧しい・不具の
fines
fine particulates 細微粒子
FIO$_2$
fractional concentration of oxygen in inspired gas 吸入〔吸気〕酸素濃度
inspired oxygen fractional concentration 吸気〔吸入〕酸素分画濃度
FiO$_2$
fraction index of inspired O_2 concentration 機能的残気量
fraction of inspired oxygen 吸気酸素分圧
Fior $\dot{\bar{C}}$ Cod
Fiorinal with codeine コデイン含有フィオリナール
FIP
Federation Internationale de Pharmaceutique〈仏〉 国際薬学連盟
FIPM
Federation Internationale de Psychothérapic Médicale〈仏〉 国際精神療法医学連盟
FIPV
feline infectious peritonitis virus ネコ伝染性腹膜炎ウイルス

FIRDA
frontal intermittent rhythmic δ-activity　前頭部間欠律動的デルタ波《脳波》
FIS
fiber intestinoscope　小腸ファイバースコープ
forced inspiratory spirogram　努力性吸気曲線
FISH
fluorescence in situ hybridization　フィッシュ法
Fish conc
Fishberg concentration　フィッシュバーグ濃縮試験
Fish dill
Fishberg dilution　フィッシュバーグ希釈試験
Fiss, fiss
fissure　裂溝，披裂，亀裂
fist
fistula　フィステル，瘻孔
FiT
Facility for iPS Cell Therapy　細胞調製施設
FITC
fluorescein isothiocyanate　フルオレ(ス)セインイソチオシアネート
FIV
forced inspiratory volume　努力性吸気肺活量
FIVB
fluorouracil, imidazole, vincristine, bischloroethylnitrosourea　フルオロウラシル,イミダゾール,ビンクリスチン,ビスクロロエチルニトロソ尿素
FIVC
forced inspiratory vital capacity　努力性吸気肺活量
FJ
fruit juice　果汁
FJN
familial juvenile nephropathy　家族性若年性腎症
FJPC
familial juvenile polyposis coli　家族性若年性大腸ポリポーシス
FK
Feil-Klippel (syndrome)　フェイル・クリペル症候群
Foster Kennedy (syndrome)　フォスター・ケネディ症候群
FKG
Fremdkörpergefühl〈独〉　異物感
FKOA
funktionskieferorthopädische (= Apparatus)〈独〉　機能的顎矯正装置，アクチバトール
FL
fascia lata〈ラ〉　大腿広筋膜
fatty liver　脂肪肝

F

fetal liver　胎児肝臓
fibroblast-like　線維芽細胞様の
fibrous layer　線維層
florentium　フロレンチウム
fluorescence　螢光
fluorescent　螢光の
focal length　焦点距離
follicular, predominately large cell　濾胞性リンパ腫大細胞型
foot lambert　フート・ランベルト〈単位〉
frontal lobe　前頭葉

Fl
fluoroscopy　透視診断法

fl
flank　側腹部
flexion　屈曲
flutter　粗動
follow(ing)　次の，追跡

fl.
fluidus〈ラ〉=fluid　液体

FL, Fl
fluorescein　フルオレ(ス)セイン

FL, Fl, fl
fluid　体液，流体(の)，液性(の)

fL, fl
femtoliter　フェムトリットル(=10^{-15}リットル)〈単位〉

FLA
fluorescein-labeled antibody　螢光標識抗体
fronto-laeva-anterior〈ラ〉　前頭左側前位

f.l.a., F.L.A
fiat lege artis〈ラ〉=let be made according to the law of the art　常法に従ってつくれ《処》

FLAAS
flameless atomic absorption spectrometry　フレームを用いない原子吸光法

flac
flaccid　弛緩性の

FLAG-ida
fludarabine, arabinosylcytosine, granulocyte colony-stimulating factor, idarubicin　フルダラビン,アラビノシルシトシン,顆粒球コロニー刺激因子,イダルビシン

FLASH
fast low angle shot　高速撮影法

flat EEG
flat electroencephalogram　平坦脳波

flav.
flavus〈ラ〉=yellow 黄色の
FLC
fatty liver cell 脂肪肝細胞
fetal liver cell 胎児肝細胞
Friend leukemia cells フレンド白血病細胞
FLCZ
fluconazole 抗真菌薬
FLD
fibrotic lung disease 線維性肺疾患
fld
field 視野，放射線照射野，術野
fluid 体液，流体(の)，液性(の)
fld.ext.
fluid extract 流動エキス剤
FL & DI
Food Law and Drug Information 食品法律と薬品情報
fl dr
fluid dram ドラム液量
fld.xt.
fluid extractum〈ラ〉 流動エキス《処》
FLEP
fluorouracil, leucovorin, cisplatin (= Platinol) フルオロウラシル,ロイコボリン,シスプラチン(=プラチノール)
FLEX
Federation on Leicensing Examination 米国資格試験認定機関連合
flex
flex 屈曲させる
flexed 屈曲した
flexible 可撓(性)の
flexion 屈曲
flexor 屈筋
flex-ext inj.
flexion-extension injury 屈曲・伸展障害
fl.ext.
fluid extract 流動エキス剤
fl hd
flat head 扁平頭
FLKS
fatty liver and kidney syndrome 脂肪肝・腎症候群
FLM
fasciculus longitudinalis medialis 内側縦束
Fl.m.
Flavobacterium meningosepticum〈ラ〉 フラボバクテリア髄膜炎

floc
flocculate　架状沈殿物にする
flocculation　架状反応
floccule　架状沈殿物

flocc
flocculation　凝集，綿状反応，凝結

flor.
flores〈ラ〉=flower　花

floss
flossing　絹糸で清掃する

flox
fluorine, liquid oxygen　フッ素と液体酸素

FL OZ, fl oz, fl.oz.
fluid ounce　液量オンス〈単位〉

FLP
fern leaf pattern　シダ状模様
fern-leaf phenomenon　シダ葉現象
fronto-laeva-posterior　前頭左側後位

FLR
Kayser-Fleischer ring　カイザー・フライシャー輪

FLRX
fleroxacin　フレロキサシン

FLS
flow limiting segment　気流限界区域

FLSA
follicular lymphosarcoma　濾胞性リンパ肉腫

FLSEP
family life and sex education program　家族生活・性教育計画

FLSP
fluorescein-labeled serum protein　螢光標識血清蛋白

FLT
fetal liver transplantation　胎児肝移植
fronto-laeva-transversa　前頭左側横位

flt
filter　濾過する，濾過器

flu
influenza　インフルエンザ

fluc
fluctant　波動物
fluctating　波動
fluctation　波動，変動
fluctuate　波動する

fluid.
fluidus〈ラ〉=fluid　体液，流体(の)，液性の

fluor
fluorescent 螢光の
fluorometry 螢光測定(法)
fluoroscopy (X線)透視(検査)

fluores
fluorescence 螢光
fluorescent 螢光の

fluoro
fluoroscopy (X線)透視(検査)

FL up, fl up
follow-up 継続管理, 追跡調査

FLV
feline leukemia virus ネコ白血病ウイルス
Friend leukemia virus フレンド白血病ウイルス

flx
flexible 可撓(性)の
flexion 屈曲

FM
face mask 顔マスク
facial measurement 顔面測定
feedback mechanism フィードバック機構
fetal movement 胎動
fibrin monomer フィブリンモノマー
fibromuscular 線維筋(性)の
fibromyalgia 結合織筋痛症
flavin mononucleotide フラビンモノヌクレオチド
flowmeter 流量計
follicular, mixed small cleaved and large cell 濾胞性リンパ腫混合型
foramen magnum 大後頭孔
forensic medicine 法医学
foster mother 養母, 里親
Frauenmilch〈独〉 母乳
frequency modulation 周波数変調

Fm
fermium フェルミウム

fm
femtometer フェムトメートル(＝10^{-15}メートル)〈単位〉
form 形(状), 体形, 様式
from 〜から

F.M., f.m.
fiat mistura〈ラ〉＝let a mixture be made 混合物をつくれ, 混合せよ《処》

FMA
fluorescein mercuric acetate フルオレ(ス)セイン酢酸水銀

fluorouracil, mitomycin-C フルオロウラシル, マイトマイシンC

FMC
fluorouracil, mitomycin-C, cytarabine フルオロウラシル, マイトマイシンC, シタラビン

FM card
field medical card 負傷者カード

FMD
family medical doctor 家庭医
fibromuscular dysplasia 線維筋性異形成
foot and mouth disease 口蹄疫病

F

FMEA
failure mode effect analysis 故障モード効果分析

FMEN
familial multilple endocrine neoplasia 家族性多発性内分泌新生物

FMET
formylmethionine ホルミルメチオニン

f-Met-tRNA
formylmethionyl-tRNA ホルミルメチオニル転移リボ核酸

FMF
familial Mediterranean fever 家族性地中海熱
flow microfluorometry フロー微小螢光測定
forced midexpiratory flow 最大呼気中間流量

FMG
foreign medical graduate 外国医科大学卒業生

FMg
fractionated excretion of Mg Mg排泄の分離

FMGEMS
Foreign Medical Graduate Examination in the Medical Science 海外医学校卒業生医師試験

FMH
fat-mobilizing hormone 脂質動員ホルモン
fibromuscular hyperplasia 線維筋性過形成

FML
fluorometholone フルオロメトロン

FMLP
N-formyl-1-methionyl-1-leucyl-1-phenylalanine *N*-ホルミル-1-メチオニル-1-ロイシル-1-フェニルアラニン

FMMP
formyl methyonylmethyl phosphate ホルミルメチオニルメチルリン酸

FMN
Federation Mondiale de Neurologie 〈仏〉 世界神経学連合
flavin mononucleotide フラビンモノヌクレオチド
fmn
formation 形成
FMNH
flavin mononucleotide reduced form フラビンモノヌクレオチド還元型
FMO
flavin-containing monoxygenase フラビン含有酸素酵素
Fmoc
9-fluorenylmethoxycarbonyl 9-フルオレニルメトキシカルボニル
F mode
flexible mode 可撓性モード
fmol
femtomole フェムトモル(＝10^{-15}モル)〈単位〉
FMOX
flomoxef フロモキセフ
FMP
family medicine program 家庭医療計画
final menstrual period 月経の終了
first menstrual period 初経，初潮
formerly married person 以前結婚したことのある人
fructose monophosphate フルクトース一リン酸
FMR
Friend-Moloney-Rausher (antigen) フレンド・モロニー・ラウシャー(抗原)
fmr
former 以前の
FMR-1
fragile X mental retardation-1 (Down syndromeに伴う)脆弱X染色体による精神発達遅滞
FMRI
functional magnetic resonance imaging 機能的MRI《画診》
fmrly
formerly 以前に
FMS
fat-mobilizing substance 脂質動員物質
fluorouracil, mitomycin, streptozo(to)cin フルオロウラシル，マイトマイシン，ストレプトゾ(ト)シン

F

riboflavin 5′-monosulfate リボフラビン5′-モノサルフェート

FMSC
fibrin monomer soluble complex フィブリンモノマー溶解複合体

FMSM
Federation Mondiale sur la Santé Mentale〈仏〉 世界精神健康連合

FMT
fibrin monomer test フィブリンモノマーテスト

FMV
fluorouracil, methylchloroethyl-cyclohexylnitrosourea, vincristine フルオロウラシル, メチルクロロエチル-シクロヘキシルニトロソ尿素, ビンクリスチン

FMVD
frequent moderate variable deceleration 比較的大きい軽度減速《心電》

FMWC
Federation of Medical Women of Canada カナダ女医連合

FMX
follicular mixed small and large cell 濾胞性大小細胞混合型
full mouth radiogram 全顎X線写真
full mouth radiography 全顎X線写真撮影法

FN
facial nerve 顔面神経
false-negative 偽陰性の
fast neutron 速中性子
fibrinoid necrosis 線維素様壊死
fibronectin フィブロネクチン
fluoride number フルオライドナンバー, フッ化指数
focal necrosis 巣状壊死

fn
function 機能, 機能する

FN, F-N
finger to nose (test) 指鼻(試験)

FNA
fine needle aspiration 穿刺吸引(生検)

FNAC
fine needle aspiration cytology 穿刺吸引細胞診

FNB
fine-needle biopsy 穿刺吸引生検
Food and Nutrition Board 食品・栄養委員会

FND
functional neck dissection　機能的頸部郭清術
Fneg
false-negative　偽陰性の
FNF
femoral neck fracture　大腿(骨)頸部骨折
finger-nose-finger (test)　指鼻指(試験)
FNH
focal nodular hyperplasia　(肝)限局性結節性過形成
FNI
fifty-items neurosis index　50項目の神経症尺度
FNP
family nurse practitioner　ファミリーナースプラクティショナー
FNPS
p,*p*′-difluoro *m*,*m*′-dinitrodiphenyl sulfone　*p*,*p*′-ジフルオロ*m*,*m*′-ジニトロジフェニルスルホン
FNR
fibronectin receptor　フィブロネクチン受容体
FNS
Food and Nutrition Service　食品栄養サービス
functional neuromuscular stimulation　機能的神経筋刺激
FNST
femoral nerve stretch(ing) test　大腿神経伸展テスト
FNU
first name unknown　名前不明
FNV
Finger-Nase-Versuch〈独〉　指鼻試験
FO
fiberoptic　光ファイバーの
foramen ovale　卵円孔
ford d'œil〈仏〉　眼底
fundus oculi　眼底
ocular fundus　眼底
fo
fomentation　湿布
fo.
folio, *folium*〈ラ〉　葉《処》
f/o
female oriental　東洋人の女性
FOB
fecal occult blood　便潜血
fiberoptic bronchoscope　気管支ファイバースコープ
foot of bed　ベッドの長さ
foc
focal　焦点の，病巣の

F

focus　焦点，病巣

FOCMA
feline oncogenic cell membrane antigen　ネコに腫瘍を発生する細胞膜抗原

FOCS
fiber optic chemical sensors　ファイバーオプティク化学センサー

FOD
free of damage　傷害なし
frontooccipital diameter　前後径

F

FOG
fast twitch oxidative glycolytic　迅速攣縮性酸化解糖の
fluothane, oxygen, gas　フローセン・酸素・笑気麻酔
full on gain　最大利得

FOIA
Freedom of Information Act　情報収集自由法

fol
follow　追跡する
following　次の，下記の

fol.
folia〈ラ〉=leaves　葉〈複数〉《処》
folium〈ラ〉=a leaf　葉〈単数〉

FOM
fosfomycin　ホスホマイシン

FOMI
fluorouracil, vincristine (=Oncovin), mitomycin-C　フルオロウラシル，ビンクリスチン(=オンコビン)，マイトマイシンC

FONAR
field focusing nuclear magnetic response　地場焦点核磁気共鳴法

f.op.aq.dest.
fiat ope aquae destillatae〈ラ〉　蒸留水にてつくれ《処》

FOR
forensic pathology　法医病理学

For
foramen　孔

for
foreign　外国の

for bod
foreing body　異物

fore
before　前に，～の前に

foren
forensic medicine　法医学

form
formation 構成体
formerly 以前は
formula 処方
formal
formaldehyde ホルムアルデヒド
formalin ホルマリン
for med
forensic medicine 法医学
Forr
foramina 孔〈複数〉
fort.
fortis〈ラ〉=strong 強い，強力な
for tox
forensic toxicology 法医毒物学
FORTRAN
formula translator フォートラン《コン》
FOS
fissura orbitalis superior 上眼窩裂
fos
feet per second フィート/秒
Found, found.
foundation 基礎，支持構造，財団
FOY
gabexate mesilate メシル酸ガベキサート
FP
facial palsy 顔面神経麻痺
false-positive 偽陽性の
family physician 家庭医
family planning 家族計画
Family Practice 家庭医学，ファミリープラクティス
family practioner 家庭医
family practitioner 家庭医学開業医
fibrinopeptide フィブリノペプチド
fibrous plaque 線維斑
filter paper 濾紙
filtrating pressure 濾過圧
final pressure 終圧
fixed postmitosis 固定的分裂終了期
flat plate 扁平板
flavin phosphate リン酸フラビン
flavoprotein 黄色蛋白
flicker perimetry フリッカー周辺視野
fluorobiprofen フルオロビプロフェン
food poisoning 食中毒

freezing point 氷点，凝固点
fresh plasma 新鮮液状血漿
frontoparietal 前頭頭頂の
frozen plasma 凍結血漿
frozen preserved (egg) 凍結保存受精卵

fp
fusion point 融解点

f.p.
fiat potio〈ラ〉 一服せよ《処》
flexor pollicis 母指屈筋

F

F/P
fluorescein to protein (ratio) フルオレ(ス)セイン/蛋白(比)

FP, fp
foot-pound フートポンド〈単位〉

FP, f.p.
forearm pronated 前腕回内した

fp, f.p.
fiat pulvis〈ラ〉=let a powder be made 散剤にせよ《処》

F-1-P, F1P
fructose 1-phosphate フルクトース1-リン酸，果糖-一リン酸

F-6-P, F6P
fluctose 6-phosphate フルクトース6-リン酸，果糖6-リン酸

FPA
fibinropeptide A フィブリノペプチドA
fluorophenylalanine フルオロフェニルアラニン

FPB
fibrinopeptide B フィブリノペプチドB
flexor pollicis brevis (muscle) 短母指屈筋

FPC
familial polyposis coli 家族性大腸ポリポーシス
Family Planning Center 家族計画センター
fish protein concentrate 魚蛋白濃度

FPCG
fetal phonocardiogram 胎児心音図

FPD
fetoplacental disproportion 胎児胎盤不均衡
finger tip palmar distance 指尖手掌間距離
flat panel detector X線平面検出器《画診》
focus plate distance 線源プレート間距離

F-PEEP
fluctuating PEEP 波動変動式終末呼気陽圧呼吸法

FPG
fasting plasma glucose 空腹時血漿グルコース
focal proliferative glomerulonephritis 巣状増殖性糸球体腎炎

FPH_2
flavin phosphate, reduced 還元型フラビン・リン酸塩

F.phy.S.
Fellow of Physical Society 医学会員

FPI
Freiburger Persönlichkeitsinventar〈独〉 フライブルグ人格特性尺度

FPIA
fluorescence polarization immunoassay 螢光偏光免疫(学)検定

f.pil.
fiant pilula〈ラ〉=let a pill be made 丸剤をつくれ〈単数〉《処》
fiant pilulae〈ラ〉=let pills be made 丸剤をつくれ〈複数〉《処》

FPK
fructose 6-phosphate-kinase フルクトース 6-リン酸キナーゼ

FPL
fasting plasma lipid 空腹時血漿脂質
flexor pollicis longus (muscle) 長母指屈筋
forced preferential looking 強制選択視
functional profile length 機能的尿道長

FPLN
focal proliferative lupus nephritis 巣状増殖型ループス腎炎

FPM
filter paper microscopic 濾紙顕微鏡試験

fpm
foot per minute フート/分

FPO
freezing point osmometer 氷点浸透圧計

FPP
family planning program 家族計画
finger print pattern 指紋型
free portal pressure 自由門脈圧

FPPH
familial primary pulmonary hypertension 家族性原発性肺高血圧

FPR
foot-pad reaction (マウスやモルモットの)足蹠反応

F protein
fibrous protein 線維性蛋白質
fusion protein 融合蛋白質，融合蛋白

FPS
feet per second フィート/秒
Fellow of Pharmaceutical Society 薬学会員

fps
frames per second フレーム/秒

FPS, fps
foot-pound-second フートポンド/秒

FPU
fetoplacental unit 胎児胎盤系

FPV
feline panleukopenia virus ネコ汎白血球減少症ウイルス
fowl plague virus 家禽ペストウイルス
fowl pox virus トリポックスウイルス

FPVB
femoral-popliteal vein bypass 大腿-膝窩静脈バイパス

FPZ
fluphenazine フルフェナジン

FPZ-D
fluphenazine decanoate デカン酸フルフェナジン

FQRS
filtered QRS 心室遅延電位の陽性基準であるフィルター処理後のQRS

FR
failure rate (contraception) (避妊)失敗率
fasciculus retroflexus〈ラ〉 反屈束
father 父親
Favre-Racouchot (disease) ファーブル・ラクショ(病)
Federal Register 米国政府発行の公文書
feedback regulation フィードバック制御
fibrinogen related フィブリノゲン関連(性)の
filtration rate 濾過率
Fisher-Race (notation) フィッシャー・レース(表記法)
fixed ratio 一定率
flocculation reaction 綿状反応
flow rate (尿)流量率
fluid restriction 水分制限
fluid retention 水分貯留
formatio reticularis〈ラ〉 網様体
formatio reticularis〈ラ〉=reticular formation 網様体
framework region of immunoglobulin V region V領域のなかの(変化が少ない)骨組み
free radical 遊離基
free radical フリーラジカル

frequent relapses　頻回再発
Friend (virus)　フレンド(ウイルス)
full range　最大域
functional residual (capacity)　機能的残気量

Fr
fracture　骨折
francium　フランシウム〈元素〉
Franklin　フランクリン〈単位〉
French　フランス式(カテーテルサイズ)

fR
flache Riesenzellen〈独〉　扁平巨細胞

F & R
force and rhythm　力と調律

FR, Fr
French (scale)　フレンチ(スケール)

FR, fR
frequency of respiration　呼吸頻度, 呼吸数

fr, fr.
from　〜から

FRA
fibrinogen-related antigen　フィブリノゲン関連抗原
fluorescent rabies antibody　螢光狂犬病抗体

fra
fragile site　脆弱部

FRAC
Food Research and Action Center　食品研究活動センター

frac
fracture　骨折

Fract, fract
fraction　割合, 分画
fracture　骨折

fract.dos.
fracta dosi〈ラ〉=in a divided dose　分服で《処》

frag
fragile　脆い, 壊れやすい
fragility　脆弱性
fragment　フラグメント, 断片, 破片

F Ⅷ R AG, FⅧ R : AG
factor Ⅷ related antigen　凝固第Ⅷ因子関連抗原

frag. test
fragility test　脆弱性試験

FRAME
Fund for Replacement of Animals in Medical Research　医学研究用動物補充基金

FRAT
free radical assay capacity フリーラジカル検出法
FRC
frozen red cells 凍結赤血球
functional residual capacity 機能的残気量
FRCGP
Fellow of Royal College of General Practioners 英国一般医学会員
FRCOG
Fellow of Royal College of Obst. and Gynecol. 英国産婦人科医師会員
F
FRCP
Fellow of Royal College of Physicians 英国内科学会会員
FRCS
Fellow of Royal College of Surgeons 英国外科学会会員
FRD
fumarate reductase フマル酸還元酵素
frem
fremitus vocalis〈ラ〉 音声振盪
freq
frequency 度数，頻度，周波数
frequent しばしば起こる
FRF
follicle stimulating hormone releasing factor 卵胞刺激ホルモン放出因子
FRFPS
Fellow of Royal Faculty of Physicians and Surgeons 英国内科・外科学会員
FRH
follicle-stimulating hormone-releasing hormone 卵胞刺激ホルモン放出ホルモン
fric
friction 摩擦
frict
friction 摩擦
FRIED test
Friedman test フリードマン妊娠試験法
frig.
frigidus〈ラ〉=cold 寒冷の，冷たい《処》
FRIPHH
Fellow of Royal Institute of Public Health and Hygiene 英国公衆保健衛生院会員
FRJM
full range of joint movement 関節運動の最大域

FRM
fradiomycin フラジオマイシン
frmn
formation 形成(物)
frmr
former 以前の
FROI
fixed region of interest method 固定関心領域法
FROM
full range of motion 最大可動域
full range of movement 運動の最大域
FRP
fiber reinforced plastics ガラス線維補強プラスチック
functional refractory period 機能的不応期
Fr.R
Friedman reaction フリードマン反応
FR r, Fr r, fr.r.
friction rub 摩擦音
FRS
face pain rating scale 痛みの程度の５段階評価
first rank symptoms １級症状
furosemide フロセミド
FRT
fixation reflex test 固視反射テスト
frt
fruit 果物
Fru
fructose 果糖
frust.
frustillatim〈ラ〉 少量に《処》
FⅧ RWA, FⅧ R：WA
factor Ⅷ related von Willebrand activity 凝固第Ⅷ因子フォンウィルブラント因子活性
FⅧ R：WF
factor Ⅷ related von Willebrand factor 凝固第Ⅷ因子フォンウィルブラント因子
FS
facial sinus 顔面神経洞
facial spasm 顔面痙攣
factor of safety 安全因子
Fanconi syndrome ファンコニ症候群
fatty streak 脂肪線条
Felty syndrome フェルティ症候群
fetoscope 胎児鏡
fibromyalgia syndrome 線維筋痛症候群
fibrous synovium 線維性滑膜

field stimulation	視野刺激
fine structure	微細構造
fingerstick	指穿刺
fire setter	刺激誘発者《心理》
first sensation of fullness	初発膀胱充満感
Fisher syndrome	フィッシャー症候群
fistular symptom	瘻孔症状
flexible sigmoidoscopy	軟性S状結腸鏡
food service	食事サービス
foramen spinosum〈ラ〉	棘孔
foream supination	前腕回外
forearm supinated	前腕回外した
(human) foreskin (cells)	(ヒト)包皮(細胞)
for skin	皮膚用の
Fourier series	フーリエ級数
fractional shortening	駆出短縮
fracture, simple	単純骨折，閉鎖骨折
fracture site	骨折部位
fragile site	脆弱部，染色体不安定部
Freeman-Sheldon (syndrome)	フリーマン-シェルドン(症候群)
fresh serum	新鮮血清
Friesinger score	フリージンガースコア
full and soft	十分で軟らかな(食事)
full scale (in IQ)	IQの満点
full strength	最大強度
functional shortening	機能的短縮
function study	機能検査
semissem〈ラ〉	半分を《処》

f/s

first stage	第1期

FS, f.s.

frozen section	凍結切片

FSA

fetal sulfoglycoprotein antigen	胎児硫酸グリコ蛋白抗原
fiat secundum artem〈ラ〉	常法によりつくれ《処》
Fundus-Symphysen Abstand〈独〉	子宮底・結合間距離

FSAR

fiat secundum artem regulas〈ラ〉	技術の法則に従いつくれ《処》

FSB

fetal scalp blood	胎児頭皮血液

FSBC

Société Française de Biologie Clinique〈仏〉	フランス臨床生物学会

FSC

fat-storing cell	脂肪貯蔵細胞

follicular, predominantly small cleaved cell　濾胞性リンパ腫小切れ込み核細胞型

FSD

focus sample distance　(X線写真の)焦点フィルム間距離

focus-skin distance　線源皮膚間距離

focus-surface distance　線源表面間距離

Fourier self-deconvolution　フーリエ変換を利用したデコンボリューション

fundus-symphysis distance　子宮底結合間距離

fusidic acid　フシジン酸

FSE

fast spin echo　高速スピンエコー法

feline spongiform encephalopathy　ネコ海綿状脳症

FSF

fibrin stabilizing factor　フィブリン安定化因子

FSG

fasting serum glucose　空腹時血糖

finger sphygmogram　指尖脈波曲線

focal sclerosing glomerulonephritis　巣状硬化性糸球体腎炎

FSGN

focal sclerosing glomerulonephritis　巣状硬化性糸球体腎炎

FSGS

focal segmental glomerulosclerosis　巣状分節状糸球体硬化症

FSH

facioscapulohumeral　顔面肩甲上腕の

facioscapulohumeral muscular dystrophy　顔面・肩甲・上腕型筋ジストロフィ

follicle-stimulating hormone　卵胞刺激ホルモン

FSHD

facioscapulohumeral dystrophy　顔面肩甲上腕型筋ジストロフィ

FSHRBI

follicle stimulating hormone receptor binding inhibitor　卵胞刺激ホルモンレセプター結合抑制因子

FSH-RF

follicle stimulating hormone-releasing factor　卵胞刺激ホルモン放出因子

FSH-RFH

follicle stimulating hormone releasing factor hormone　卵胞刺激ホルモン放出因子ホルモン

FSH-RH

follicle stimulating hormone-releasing hormone　卵胞刺激ホルモン放出ホルモン

FSIS

Food Safety and Inspection Service　米国食品安全検査局

FSK
frequency shift keying 周波数偏移キーイング
FSL
fasting serum level 空腹時血清レベル
FSM
film/screen method X線直接撮影法
flying-spot microscope フライングスポット顕微鏡
furosemide フロセミド
FSMB
Federation of State Medical Boards of the United States 米国医学教育委員会

FSMD
facioscapulo humeral muscular dystrophy 顔面肩甲上腕型筋ジストロフィ
FSP
familial spastic paraplegia 家族性痙性対麻痺
fibrin/fibrinogen-split products フィブリン・フィブリノゲン分解産物
FSR
fractional synthetic rate 分別合成比
fusiform skin revision 紡錘状皮膚再建
FSS
Fear Survey Schedule 恐怖調査スケジュール
focal segmental sclerosis 巣状硬化性変化
French steel sonde フランス製鋼ゾンデ
FST
foam stability test 泡沫安定試験
FSV
feline fibrosarcoma virus ネコ線維肉腫ウイルス
FT
dihydroxymethyl furatrizine ジヒドロキシメチルフラトリジン
falloposcopic tuboplasty 卵管鏡下卵管形成
false transmitter 偽性伝達物質
family therapy 家族療法
fast twitch 急速単収縮
fatigue test 疲労試検
faucial tonsil 口蓋扁桃
fetal thymus 胎児胸腺
fetal tonsil 胎児扁桃
fibrous tissue 線維組織
finger tapping 指によるタッピング
fingertip 指先
follow through 追求
formal training 正式な訓練
formol toxoid ホルマリン類毒素

Fourier transform フーリエ変換
free thyroxine 遊離チ〔サイ〕ロキシン
full term 満期
functional test 機能試験

Ft
ferritin フェリチン

ft.
fac〈ラ〉=make つくる《処》
fiant〈ラ〉=let them be made (それらを)つくれ《処》
fiat〈ラ〉=let it be made (それを)つくれ《処》

ft^2
square foot 平方フート

ft^3
cubic foot 立法フート

F3T
trifluoro thymidine トリフルオロチミジン

FT207
futraful フトラフール

Ft, ft
feet フィート(=footの複数形)
foot 足, フット, フート〈単数〉

FT_3, fT_3
free T_3(=thyronine-3) 遊離T_3, 遊離トリヨードチ〔サイ〕ロニン3

FT_4, fT_4
free T_4(=thyronine-4) 遊離T_4, 遊離チ〔サイ〕ロニン4

FTA
fault tree analysis 故障木解析法
femoral-tibial angle 膝外側角
femorotibial angle 大腿脛骨角
fluorescent titer antibody 螢光抗体価
fluorescent treponema antibody test 螢光トレポネーマ抗体試験

FTA-AB
fluorescent treponemal antibody absorption 螢光トレポネーマ抗体吸収

FTA-ABS
fluorescent treponema antibody absorption (test) 螢光トレポネーマ抗体吸収(試験)

FTAT
fluorescent treponemal antibody test 梅毒螢光トレポネーマ抗体試験

FTB
fingertip blood 指先血液

FTBA
fasting total bile acid 空腹時総胆汁酸

F

FTBD
full term born dead　満期死産

FTC
fast time constant　定着時定数

ft-c
foot candle　フィート燭光

ft.catapl.
fiat cataplasma〈ラ〉=let a poultice be made　パップ剤をつくれ《処》

ft.cataplasm.
fiat cataplasma〈ラ〉　パップ剤をつくれ《処》

ft.cerat.
fiat ceratum〈ラ〉=let a cerate be made　ろう膏〔膏薬〕をつくれ《処》

ft.chart.vi
fiant chartulae vi〈ラ〉=let six powders be made　6包の散剤をつくれ《処》

ft.collyr.
fiat collyrium〈ラ〉=let an eyewash be made　点眼液をつくれ《処》

F3TDR
trifluorothymidine　トリフルオロチミジン

FTE
fetal tobacco effects　不全型胎児タバコ症候群
full time equivalent　満期と同等の

ft.emuls.
fiat emulsio〈ラ〉=let an emulsion be made　乳剤をつくれ《処》

ft.enem.
fiat enema〈ラ〉=let an enema be made　浣腸剤をつくれ《処》

F-test
estrogen feedback test　エストロゲンフィードバック検査

FTF
finger to finger test　指指試験

FTFTN
finger-to-finger-to-nose test　指指鼻試験

FTG
full-thickness graft　全層皮膚移植片，全層植皮

ft.garg.
fiat gargarisma〈ラ〉=let a gargle be made　うがいさせる《処》

ft.haust.
fiat haustus〈ラ〉　頓服水剤をつくれ《処》

FTI
free thyroxine index　遊離チ〔サイ〕ロキシン指数

FT$_3$I
free triiodothyronine index　遊離トリヨードチ〔サイ〕ロニン指数

FT$_4$I
free thyroxine index　遊離チ〔サイ〕ロキシン指数

FT$_3$ index
free thyroxine index　遊離チ〔サイ〕ロキシン指数

FT$_4$ index
free triiodothyronine index　遊離トリヨードチ〔サイ〕ロニン指数

ft.infus.
fiat infusum〈ラ〉=let an infusion be made　浸剤をつくれ《処》

ft.injec.
fiat injectio〈ラ〉=let an injection be made　注射剤をつくれ《処》

FTIR
Fourier transform infrared spectrometer　フーリエ変換赤外分光器
functional terminal innervation ratio　機能性終末神経支配比

FTKA
failed to keep appointment　予約を守れなかった

FTL, ft-L
foot lambert　フィート輝度〈単位〉, フートランベルト

f.tl.a.
fiat lege artis〈ラ〉　常法によりつくれ《処》

FTLB
full term living birth　満期出産

ft lb, ft-lb, FT-Lb
foot pound　フート・ポンド〈単位〉

ft.linim.
fiat linimentum〈ラ〉=let a liniment be made　塗布剤をつくれ《処》

ft.m.
fiat mistura〈ラ〉　水剤をつくれ《処》

ft.mas.
fiat massa〈ラ〉=let a mass be made　塊をつくれ《処》

ft.mas.div.in pil.
fiat massa dividenda in pilulae〈ラ〉　混合して錠剤とせよ《処》

ft.mist.
fiat mistura〈ラ〉=let a mixture be made　混合物をつくれ《処》

F

FTMS
Fourier transform mass spectrometer　フーリエ変換質量分析計

FTN
finger to nose (test)　指鼻試験

FTND
full term normal delivery　満期正常産

FTNS
functional transcutaneous nerve stimulation　機能的経皮的神経刺激

FTNSD
full term, normal, spontaneous delivery　満期正常自然分娩

FTNVD
full term normal vaginal delivery　満期正常経膣分娩

FTOC
fetal thymus organ culture　胎児胸腺臓器培養

F to N test
finger to nose test　指鼻試験

FTPA
perfluorotripropylamine　ペルフルオロトリプロピルアミン

ft.pil.
fiat pilula, *fiant pilulae*〈ラ〉　丸剤をつくれ《処》

ft.pil.XXIV
fiant pilulae XXIV〈ラ〉= let 24 pills be made　24個の丸剤をつくれ《処》

ft.pulv.
fiat pulvis〈ラ〉= let a powder be made　散剤をつくれ《処》

FTR
functional test report　機能検査報告
functional test request　機能検査依頼

FTS
fetal tobacco syndrome　胎児性タバコ症候群
fingertips　指先〈複数〉
serum thymic factor　血清胸腺因子

ft.s.a.
fiat secundum artem〈ラ〉　常法によりつくれ《処》

FTSG
full-thickness skin graft　全層植皮

ft.sol.
fiat solutio〈ラ〉= let a solution be made　溶液をつくれ《処》

ft.solut.
fiat solutio〈ラ〉=let a solution be made　溶液をつくれ《処》

ft.suppos.
fiat suppositorium〈ラ〉=let a suppository be made　坐剤をつくらせる《処》

FTT
fat tolerance test　脂肪負荷試験
Fever Therapy Technician　熱治療技士
field transfusion team　戦場輸血班
fructose tolerance test　果糖負荷試験

ft.troch.
fiant trochisci〈ラ〉=let lozenges be made　トローチ剤をつくれ《処》

ft.ung.
fiat unguentum〈ラ〉　軟膏をつくれ《処》
fiat unguentum〈ラ〉=let an ointment be made　塗布させる

FU
fecal urobilinogen　便ウロビリノゲン
feces urobilinogen　糞便中ウロビリノゲン
Finsen unit　フィンゼン単位
fluorescence unit　螢光単位
fluorouracil　フルオロウラシル
fundus　底

5-FU
5-fluorouracil　フルオロウラシル

FU, F/U, f/u
follow-up　継続管理，追跡調査

FUB
functional uterine bleeding　機能性子宮出血

Fuc
fucose　フコース

FUCA
α-L-fucosidase　α-L-フコシダーゼ

FUdR
5-fluorouridine　5-フルオロウリジン

5-FUDR
5-fluoro-2′-deoxyuridine　5-フルオロ-2′-デオキシウリジン

FUDR, FUdR
5-fluoro-2′-deoxy-β-uridine　5-フルオロ-2′-デオキシ-βウリジン

fulg
fulguration　高周波療法

F

F

FUM
fumarase フマラーゼ
fumarate フマレート
fumigate 薫蒸する，薫煙する
fumigation 薫蒸，薫煙
FUMIR
fluorouracil, mitomycin-C, radiation フルオロウラシル，マイトマイシンC，放射線照射
FUMP
fluorouridine monophosphate フルオロウリジン一リン酸
funct
function 機能，機能する
functional 機能性の
fund
fundamental 基礎の
fungi
fungicide 殺真菌剤
FUO
fever of undetermined origin 原因不明熱
fever of unknown origin 不明熱
FUP
fusion point 融合点
FUR
5-fluorouridine 5-フルオロウリジン
FUra
fluorouracil フルオロウラシル
FURAM
Futrafur, adriamycin, mitomycin-C フトラフール，アドリアマイシン，マイトマイシンC
FUS
first-use syndrome ファーストユース症候群
fus
fusion 融合，癒合，固定術
FUT
fibrinogen uptake test フィブリノゲン摂取試験
fut
future 未来
FUTP
fluorouridine triphosphate フルオロウリジン三リン酸
FV
femoral vein 大腿静脈
flow volume 流量
formaldehyde vapors ホルムアルデヒド蒸気
Friend virus フレンドウイルス
fruit and vegetable 果物と野菜

Fv-4
Friend virus susceptibility-4 gene　フレンドウイルス感受性遺伝子 4

FVA
Friend virus anemia　フレンドウイルス貧血

f.va.
fiat venaesectio〈ラ〉　瀉血せよ《処》

FVC
false vocal cord　偽声帯
filled voiding flow rate　膀胱充満時排尿速度
flow-volume curve　フローボリューム曲線
forced vital capacity　努力性肺活量

FVCA
forced vital capacity analysis　努力性肺活量分析

FVD
fibrovascular tissue on disk　椎間板線維血管組織

FVE
fibrovascular tissue elsewhere　他の線維血管組織
forced volume, expiratory　努力性呼気量

FVFR
filled voiding flow rate　膀胱充満時排尿速度

FVH
focal vascular headache　巣状血管性頭痛
fulminant viral hepatitis　劇症ウイルス性肝炎

FVL
femoral vein ligation　大腿静脈結紮術
flexible video laparoscope　軟性ビデオ腹腔鏡
force, velocity, length　力・速度・長さ

FVM
familial visceral myopathy　家族性内臓筋障害

FVOP
finger venous opening pressure　指静脈開存圧

FVP
Friend virus polycythemia　フレンドウイルス赤血球増加症

FVPRA
Fruit and Vegetable Preservation Research Association　果物野菜貯蔵研究協会

FVR
feline viral rhinotracheitis　ネコのウイルス性鼻気管支炎
forearm vascular resistance　前腕血管抵抗

FVS
fetal varicella syndrome　胎児水痘症症候群

FW
Falconer-Weddell (syndrome)　ファルコナー・ウェッデル（症候群）

Felix-Weil (reaction) フェリックス・ヴァイル(反応)
Friderichsen-Waterhouse (syndrome) フリーデリックセン・ウォーターハウス(症候群)

F & W
feeding and watering 栄養と補水

fw, f.w.
fresh water 新鮮水

FWB
full weight bearing 全荷重

FWD
forward 前進の
fresh water damage 新鮮水傷害

FWHF
Federation of World Health Foundations 世界健康財団連合

FWHM
full-width at half maximum 半値全幅

FWM
Folin-Wu method フォリン・ウー法

FWR
Felix-Weil reaction フェリックス・ヴァイル反応
Folin-Wu reaction フォリン・ウー反応

FX
fluoroscopy (X線)透視(検査)
fornix 円蓋, 脳弓
frozen section 凍結切片

Fx
fractional urine 分別尿

fx
friction 摩擦, 摩擦法

FX, Fx, fx
fracture 骨折

fxd
fixed 固定された, 癒着した

Fx-dis.fx-dis
fracture-dislocation 脱臼骨折

fxg
fixing 固定, 癒着

FXR
fracture 骨折

FXS
fragile X syndrome 脆弱X症候群

FY
blood factor 〔ダ(ッ)フィの〕血液型因子
fiscal year 会計年度

FYA
Duffy A positive　ダ(ッ)フィA+(血液型)
FYAN
Duffy A negative　ダ(ッ)フィA−(血液型)
FYB
Duffy B positive　ダ(ッ)フィB+(血液型)
FYBN
Duffy B negative　ダ(ッ)フィB−(血液型)
FYI
for your information　あなたの情報の参考に
FYIG
for your information and guidance　あなたの情報と案内の参考に
FYP
first year program　初年度計画
FZ
Fingerzahlen〈独〉　指数弁
focal zone　病巣部，病変部
frozen section　凍結切片
furazolidone　フラゾリドン
FZRC
frozen section red (blood) cell　凍結切片赤血球

G g

G

acceleration of gravity	重力加速度
deoxyguanylic acid	デオキシグアニル酸
Gaffky scale	ガフキー号数
gamma-globulin	γグロブリン
ganglion	神経節，結節腫，ガングリオン
gas	ガス
Gasterophilus	ウマバエ
gastrin	ガストリン
gauge	計器，尺度
gauss	ガウス〈単位〉
Gemella	双子菌
general learning ability	一般学習能力
germinoma	胚細胞腫
Giardia	ジアルジア(属)
Giga	ギガ(＝10^9)〈接〉
gingiva	歯肉
gingivitis	歯肉炎
globulin	グロブリン
glomerulus	糸球体(腎の)
Glossina	ツェツェバエ
glycine	グリシン
glycogen	グリコーゲン
glyoxylic acid	グリオキサル酸
Gnathostoma	顎口虫
goat	ヤギ
gold inlay	金のインレー
gonidial	胞子の
gonidial type colony	胞子型コロニー
gonidium	胞子
good	良い，良好な
Gordioidea	ハリガネムシ類
grading	悪性腫瘍の異型度
granule	顆粒
gravitation	遠心力
gravitational unit	重量単位
Greek	ギリシャ語の
gross	グロス〈単位〉
guanidine	グアニジン
guanine	グアニン
guanosine	グアノシン
guanylic acid	グアニル酸

gurgle　腹鳴，グル音
gynae　女の，雌の
immunoglobulin G　免疫グロブリンG
ventricular gradient　心室グラディエント

g
gram(me)　グラム〈単位〉
great　偉大な，多くの
green　緑(の)，グリーン(の)
grey　灰色，灰色の
specific gravity　比重

G1
Grid 1　入力端子1

G2
Grid 2　入力端子2

G_4
dichlorophene　ジクロロフェン

G_6
hexachlorophene　ヘキサクロロフェン

g%
gram percent　グラムパーセント
grams per milliliter　グラム/ミリリットル

G+
gram positive　グラム陽性の

G，G
Gibbs free energy　ギブズ自由エネルギー

G，g
conductance　コンダクタンス
gallop　奔馬調律
gap　裂
gender　性
gingival　歯肉の
glucose　グルコース，ブドウ糖
grain　穀草
gravity　重力〈単位〉
group　群

G，g.
gravida〈ラ〉=pregnant woman　妊婦

G，g，g.
gauche〈仏〉　左の

GA
gastric analysis　胃液検査
general anesthesia　全身麻酔
general appearance　全身症状
general average　全体平均
gestational age　在胎月齢
gibberellic acid　ギベレル酸

gingivo-axial	歯軸の
glucuronic acid	グルクロン酸
glutaraldehyde	グルタールアルデヒド
glycated albumin	糖化アルブミン
glycyrrhetinic acid	グリシレチン酸
Golgi apparatus	ゴルジ装置
gramicidin A	グラミシジンA
granuloma annulare	環状肉芽腫
guajaretic acid	グアヤレチン酸
guessed average	推定平均値

Ga

gallium	ガリウム〈元素〉
granulocyte agglutination	顆粒球凝集

ga.

gauge	ゲージ〈単位〉

^{67}Ga

gallium-67	ガリウム67

GA, G/A

gingivoaxial	歯肉軸の

GAA

guanidinoacetic acid	グアニジノ酢酸

GABA

gamma-aminobutyric acid	γアミノ酪酸

GABA-T

gamma-aminobutyric acid transaminase	γアミノ酪酸トランスアミナーゼ

GABHS

group A beta-hemolytic streptococcus	A群β溶血性連鎖球菌

GABOB

gamma-amino-beta-hydroxybutyric acid	γアミノ-β-ヒドロキシ酪酸

G-actin

globular actin	球状アクチン

GAD

(general) acyl-CoA dehydrogenase	アシル基脱水素酵素
glutamic acid decarboxylase	グルタミン酸デカルボキシラーゼ

GADH

gastric alcohol dehydrogenase	胃アルコールデヒドロゲナーゼ

GADS

gonococcal arthritis/dermatitis syndrome	淋菌性関節炎・皮膚炎症候群

GAE

granulomatous amebic encephalitis	アメーバ性肉芽腫性脳炎

GAF
giant axon formation 巨大軸索形成
gaffer & gammer
grandfather and grandmother 祖父と祖母
GAG
Global Advisory Group on Expended Programme on Immunization 世界予防接種助言者会議
glycosaminoglycan グリコサミノグリカン
glyoxal-bis-guanyl hydrazone グリオキザルビスグアニルヒドラゾン
group specific antigen 群特異性抗原
^{67}Ga-gallium citrate
gallium-67-gallium citrate ガリウム67・クエン酸ガリウム
GAHS
galactorrhea-amenorrhea hyperprolactinemia syndrome 乳汁分泌・無月経・高プロラクチン血症症候群
GAL
galactosidase ガラクトシダーゼ
galactosyl ガラクトシル
galanin ガラニン
gallus adeno-like virus ガルスアデノ様ウイルス
gal
Galileo ガリレオ
girl 少女
Gal, gal.
galactose ガラクトース
gal, gal.
gallon ガロン〈単位〉
Gal-Act
galactase activator ガラクターゼ活性物質
GALK
galactokinase ガラクトキナーゼ
gal/min
gallons per minute ガロン/分
GalN
galactosamine ガラクトサミン
GalNAc
N-acetylgalactosamine *N*-アセチルガラクトサミン
$GalNH_2$
galactosamine ガラクトサミン
gal-1-P
galactose-1-phosphate ガラクトース-1-リン酸
GALS
gut-associated lymphoid system 消化管リンパ装置

G

GALT
galactose-1-phosphate uridyltransferase　ガラクトース-1-リン酸ウリジルトランスフェラーゼ
gut-associated lymphoid tissue　消化管関連リンパ系組織

GalTT, GAL TT
galactose tolerance test　ガラクトース負荷試験

GalU
galacturonic acid　ガラクツロン酸

GalUA
galacturonic acid　ガラクツロン酸

GALV
Gibbon ape leukemia virus　テナガザル白血病ウイルス

GaLV
Gibbon ape lymphosarcoma virus　テナガザルリンパ肉腫ウイルス

galv.
galvanism　ガルバーニ現象

Galv, galv
galvanic　ガルバーニ電流の，直流電流の
galvanized　電気メッキした

GAM agar
Gifu anaerobic medium agar　GAM寒天

GAMG
goat anti-mouse immunoglobulin G　ヤギ抗マウス免疫グロブリンG

GAMIN
Guilford-Martin personality inventory for factors　ギルフォード・マーチン人格目録

GAN
giant axonal neuropathy　巨大軸索ニューロパシー

GANC
ganciclovir　ガンシクロビル

G and D
growth and development　成長と発育

gang
ganglion　神経節，結節腫，ガングリオン
ganglionic　神経節の

gangl
ganglion　神経節，結節腫，ガングリオン
ganglionic　神経節の

gangr
gangrene　壊疽

GANS
granulomatous angitis of the nervous system 神経系肉芽腫性血管炎
GAP
Gardner Analysis of Personality Survey ガードナー人格調査分析
glutamin transpeptidase activating protein グルタミントランスペプチダーゼ活性蛋白
glyceraldehyde phosphate リン酸グリセルアルデヒド
growth associated protein 成長関連蛋白
GAPD
glyceraldehyde phosphate dehydrogenase リン酸グリセルアルデヒド脱水素酵素
GAPDH
glyceraldehyde-3-phosphate dehydrogenase グリセルアルデヒド-3-リン酸デヒドロゲナーゼ
GAPS
phosphoribosyl glycinamide synthetase ホスホリボシルグリシンアミド合成酵素
G/A quotient
globulin-albumin quotient グロブリン/アルブミン係数
GAR
genitoanorectal syndrome 陰部肛門直腸症候群
glyceraldehyde reductase グリセルアルデヒド還元酵素
glycinamide ribonucleotide グリシンアミドリボヌクレオチド
goat anti-rabbit gamma globulin ヤギ抗ウサギγグロブリン
GARD
gamma atomic radiation detector γ線検出器
GARG, garg.
gargarisma〈ラ〉=a gargle うがい剤
GARGG
goat antirabbit gamma globulin ヤギ抗ウサギγグロブリン
GAS
gastroenterology 胃腸病学
gatric acid secretion 胃酸分泌
general adaptation syndrome 汎適応症候群
generalized arteriosclerosis 全身性動脈硬化症
Global assessment scale グローバル診断法
group A streptococcus A群連鎖球菌
gast
gastric (muscle) 胃の
gastrocnemius 腓腹筋
Gastric ul
gastric ulcer 胃潰瘍

G

gastro
gastrotomy 胃切開術
Gastroc, gastroc
gastrocnemius muscle 腓腹筋
gastroenterol
gastroenterology 胃腸病学
GAT
gelatin agglutination test ゼラチン凝集試験
gerontological apperception test 老人用統覚検査
group adjustment therapy グループ適応療法
L-glutamic acid-L-alanine-L-tyrosine polymer L-グルタミン酸-L-アラニン-L-チロシンポリマー(合成抗原)

G

GATT
gastric tumor associated antigen 胃腫瘍関連抗原
GAVI
Global Alliance for Vaccine and Immunization ワクチンと予防接種のための世界同盟
Gaw
airway conductance 気道コンダクタンス
GB
gallbladder 胆嚢
gallbladder examination 胆嚢造影検査
gnotobioto 動物飼育条件
goof butts 大麻
Gougerot-Blum (syndrome) グジュロ・ブラン(症候群)
Guillain-Barré (syndrome) ギラン・バレー(症候群)
Gb
blood gravity 全血の比重
gilbert ギルバート
specific gravity of blood 血液比重
GB, G.B.
gallbladder 胆嚢
globule blanc〈仏〉 白血球
GBA
ganglionic-blocking agent 神経節遮断薬
guanidinobutyric acid グアニジノ酪酸
G-band
Giemsaband (ギムザ染色の)Gバンド
GBD
gallbladder disease 胆嚢疾患
granulomatous bowel disease 肉芽腫性腸疾患
GB exam
gallbladder examination 胆嚢造影検査
GBF
gastric blood flow 胃血流量

GBG

glycine-rich beta-glycoprotein	グリシンリッチβグリコプロテイン
gonadal steroid-binding globulin	性ステロイド結合グロブリン

GBH

graphite-benzalkonium-heparin	黒鉛・ベンザルコニウム・ヘパリン

GBI

globulin-bound insulin	グロブリン結合インスリン

GBK

Gallenblasen Karzinom〈独〉	胆嚢癌

GBM

glomerular basement membrane	糸球体基底膜

GBMF

glioblastoma multiforme	多形性膠芽腫

GBP

glucocorticoid binding protein	グルココルチコイド結合蛋白

GBPS

gallbladder pigment stones	胆嚢色素結石

GBq

gigabequerel	ギガベケレル

GBR

glutathione bicarbonate Ringer solution	グルタチオン重炭酸加リンゲル液

GBS

gallbladder series	胆嚢系
gastric bypass surgery	胃バイパス手術
group B streptococcal infection	B群連鎖球菌感染症
group B streptococcus	B群連鎖球菌

GBS, G-BS

Guillain-Barré syndrome	ギラン・バレー症候群

GC

galactocerebroside	ガラクトセレブレシド
ganglion cells	神経節細胞
gas chromatography	ガスクロマトグラフィ
gastric cancer	胃癌
gastrocamera	胃カメラ
gel chromatography	ゲルクロマトグラフィ
general condition	全身状態
germinal center	胚中心
glucocorticoid	グルココルチコイド
glycocholic acid	グリココール酸
goblet cell	杯細胞
Golgi cell	ゴルジ細胞
Golgi complex	ゴルジ体
gonococcal	淋菌の

gonococcus 淋菌
good condition 良い状態
granular casts 顆粒円柱
granular cell 顆粒細胞
granulomatous colitis 肉芽腫性大腸炎
granulosa cell 顆粒膜細胞
group specific component 群特別成分
guanidino compounds グアニジノ化合物
guanylate cyclase グアニル酸シクラーゼ

Gc
gigacycle ギガサイクル

GC, Gc
gonorrhea 淋疾, 淋病

GC, gc
gonococcal 淋菌の
gonococcus 淋菌

GCA
gastric cancer antigen 胃癌抗原
giant cell arteritis 巨細胞動脈炎

Gca, gca
gonorrhea 淋疾, 淋病

GC agar
gonococcus agar GC寒天培地

g cal, g-cal
gram-calorie グラムカロリー〈単位〉

GCB
germinal center B cells 胚中心Bリンパ球

GCBA
glucose cysteine blood agar ブドウ糖・システイン血液寒天

GCC
germinal center cell 胚中心細胞

GC/C/IRMS
gas chromatography/combustion/isotope ratio mass spectrometry ガスクロマトグラフィ・燃焼炉・同位体質量分析システム

GC content
guanine-cytosine content グアニン・シトシン含有量

GCDC
glycochenodeoxycholic acid グリコケノデオキシコール酸

GCE
general certificate of education 教育の一般認可

GC-ECD
gas chromatography with electron capture detection ガスクロマトグラフィ気道電子捕獲検出法

G cell, G-cell
gastrin secretory cell　ガストリン分泌細胞
GCF
greatest common factor　最大公約数
GCFT
gonococcal complement-fixation test　淋菌補体結合試験
GCI
glucose comsumption index　グルコース消費指数
GCIIS
glucose controlled insulin infusion system　グルコースコントロールインスリン注入システム
GCM
glioma conditioned medium　神経膠腫条件下培養基
greatest common measure　最大公約数
g-cm
gram-centimeter　グラムセンチメートル
GCMF
gas chromatography mass fragmentography　ガスクロマトグラフィ質量分離図
GCMS
gas chromatography mass spectrometry　ガスクロマトグラフィ質量分析システム
GCMS-CPU
gas chromatography mass spectrometry computer　ガスクロマトグラフィ質量分析コンピュータ
GCN
greatest common numerator　最大公約数
GCP
gastritis cystica polyposa　ポリープ状嚢胞性胃炎
good clinical practice　優良臨床試験基準
GCR
glucocorticoid receptor　糖質コルチコイド受容体
group conformity rating　集団合致等級分類
GCRC
General Clinical Research Centers　一般臨床研究センター
GCS
general clinical service　一般臨床サービス
Glasgow coma scale　グラスゴーコーマスケール
glucocorticosteroid　グルココルチコステロイド
GCSA
Gross cell surface antigen　グロス細胞表面抗原
G-CSF
granulocyte colony-stimulating factor　顆粒球コロニー刺激因子
GCSN
ganglionic cervical sympathetic nerve　頸部交感神経筋

G

G

G-C syndrome
Gianotti-Crosti syndrome　ジャノッティ・クロスティ症候群

GCT
gate control theory　ゲートコントロール説
giant cell tumor　巨細胞腫
granular cell tumor　顆粒細胞腫

GC type
guanine cytosine type　グアニン・シトシン型

GCU
gonococcal urethritis　淋菌性尿道炎
growing care unit　成長監視ユニット

GCV
ganciclovir　ガンシクロビル

GCVF
great cardiac vein flow　大心臓静脈血流量

GCW
glomerular capillary wall　糸球体毛細血管壁

GCY
gastroscopy　胃鏡検査

GD
gastric devascularization　胃周囲の血行遮断
gastroduodenal　胃十二指腸の
gel diffusion　ゲル拡散
gestation day　受精日
gonadal dysgenesis　性器発育異常，性器発育不全
good delivery　安産
grand daughter　孫娘
Graves disease　グレーヴス病
gravimetric density　比重

Gd
gadolinium　ガドリニウム〈元素〉

gd
good　良い，良好な

GD, G/D
growth and development　成長と発育

GDA
gastroduodenal artery　胃十二指腸動脈

GDC
giant dopamine-containing cell　巨大ド(ー)パミン含有細胞
glycodeoxycholic acid　グリコデオキシコール酸

Gd-DTPA
gadopentetic acid　ガドペンテト酸

GDGF
glioma-derived growth factor　神経膠腫由来成長因子

GDH
glucose dehydrogenase ブドウ糖脱水素酵素
glutamate dehydrogenase グルタメートデヒドロゲナーゼ
glutamic acid dehydrogenase グルタミン酸脱水素酵素
glycerol dehydrogenase グリセロール脱水素酵素
glycerophosphate dehydrogenase グリセロホスフェートデヒドロゲナーゼ
gonadotropic hormone 性腺刺激ホルモン
growth and development hormone 成長ホルモン
growth and differentiation hormone 成長と分化ホルモン

GDL
glow-discharge lump グロー放電ランプ

GDM
gestational diabetes mellitus 妊娠糖尿病

GDMO
General Duty Medical Officer 一般的義務のある医療事務官

GDMS
glow discharge mass spectrometry グロー放電質量分析法

Gdn
guanidine グアニジン

gdn
guardian 保護者

GDO
group of difficult organism 取扱いが難しい菌群

GDOS
glow discharge optical emission spectrometry 赤外吸収,放電発光陰極光

GDP
gel diffusion precipitation ゲル内沈降反応
Good Dispensing Practice 医療機関における医薬品管理規範
guanosine 5′-diphosphate グアノシン(5′-)二リン酸

G6DP
glucose-6-phosphate dehydrogenase グルコース六リン酸脱水素酵素

GDP-D-mannose
guanosine diphosphate-D-mannose グアノシン二リン酸-D-マンノース

GDPM
guanosine diphosphate mannose グアノシン二リン酸マンノース

GDR
granulocyte disappearance rate 顆粒球消失率

G

GDRT 1/2
granulocyte disappearance rate time 1/2 顆粒球半減時間
GDS
geriatric depression scale 老人性うつ病尺度〔スケール〕
group D streptococcus D群連鎖球菌
GDU
gastroduodenal ulcer 胃十二指腸潰瘍
GE
Gänsslen-Erb syndrome ゲンスレン・エルプ症候群
gastric emptying 胃内容排出
gastroemotional 胃情動の
gastroenteritis 胃腸炎
gastroenterology 胃腸病学
gastroenterostomy 胃腸吻合術
gastroesophageal 胃食道の
gastrointestinal endoscopy 胃腸内視鏡検査
gel electrophoresis ゲル電気泳動
generalized epilepsy 全般てんかん
gentamicin ゲンタマイシン
glandular epithelium 腺上皮
glycerin enema グリセリン浣腸
gradient echo 傾斜磁場エコー
Ge
germanium ゲルマニウム〈元素〉
G/E
granuloid/erythroid (ratio) 顆粒球系/赤芽球系(比)
G : E
granulocyte : erythroblast 顆粒球：赤芽球比
g.e., g-e
gravity eliminated 重力除去した
GEA
gastroepiploic artery 胃大網動脈
geb
geboren〈独〉 生まれた
gebunden〈独〉 結合した
GEC
glomerular epithelial cell 糸球体上皮細胞
ged
gedampft〈独〉 混濁した
GEE
glycine ethyl ester グリシンエチルエステル
GEF
glossoepiglottic fold 舌喉頭蓋ひだ
glycosylation enhancing factor グリコレーション増強因子
gonadotropin enhancing factor 性腺刺激ホルモン増強因子

G

GEH
glycerol ester hydrolase　グリセロールエステルヒドロラーゼ

gel
gelatin　ゼラチン
gelatinous　ゼラチンの

gel.quav.
gelatina quavis〈ラ〉　ゼリーに混入して《処》

gem
geminal　ジェムの，一対の

gem-
geminate　対の，二重の〈接〉

GEMM-CFU
granulocyte, erythroid, megakaryocyte and macrophage colony forming units　顆粒球・赤血球・巨核球・大食細胞コロニー形成単位

GEMS
Global Environmental Monitoring System　地球環境モニタリング計画

GEMs
genetically engineered microorganisms　遺伝子組換え微生物

GEMSA
guanidinoethyl-mercapto acetate　グアニジノエチル・メルカプト酢酸

GEN, gen
gender　性
general　一般の，全体の
generation　出産，世代
genetics　遺伝学
genital　生殖(器)の，性器の
genitalia　性器，生殖器
genus〈ラ〉＝kind　属，種類

genet
genetic　遺伝の
genetics　遺伝学

gen.et sp.nov.
genus et species nova〈ラ〉＝new genus and species　新しい属と種

Gen Hosp
general hospital　総合病院

genit
genitalia　性器，生殖器

gen'l
general　一般の，全体の

G

gen.nov.
genus novum〈ラ〉=new genus　新属
gen prac
general practice　一般医療
gen.proc
general procedure　一般手技
gen pub
general public　公衆
geohy
geohygiene　地球衛生学
geom
geometric　幾何学の

GEP
gastroenteropancreatic　胃腸膵の
gastro-entero-pancreatic-endocrine system　胃腸膵臓内分泌系
GEPG
gastroesophageal pressure gradient　胃食道圧勾配
GER
gastric emptying rate　胃内容物排出速度
gastroesophageal reflux　胃食道逆流
granular endoplasmic reticulum　粗面小胞体
Ger
German　ドイツ語，ドイツ人
Ger，ger
geriatrics　老年医学，老年病学
GERD
gastroesophageal reflux disease　胃食道逆流疾患
geriat
geriatrics　老年医学，老年病学
GERL
Golgi-associated endoplasmic reticulum lysosomes　ゴルジ関連小胞体リソソーム
germi
germicide　殺菌剤
Gerontol
gerontologist　老年病学者
gerontology　老年医学，老年病学
GERSO
Groupement European de Recherche Scientifique eu Stomaco-Odontologie〈仏〉=European Group for Scientific Research on Stomato-Odontology　欧州口腔病学研究会
GES
glucose electrolyte solution　ブドウ糖電解質溶液

Group Environment Scale グループ環境スケール

GEST

gestation 妊娠

gestational 妊娠の

GET

gastric emptying time 胃内容排出時間

GEU

gestation, extra-uterine 子宮外妊娠

GeV

giga elecron volt ギガ電子ボルト

GEX

gas exchange ガス交換

GF

gastric fistula 胃フィステル

gastric fluid 胃液

gel filtration ゲル濾過

germ free 無菌(の)

glomerular filtration 糸球体濾過

gluten-free 無グルテンの

grandfather 祖父

growth factor 増殖因子

growth failure 成長不全

growth fraction 増殖分屑

Gf

gene frequency 遺伝子頻度

G-F

globular-fibrous 球状・線維状の

GFA, GfA

germ-free animal 無菌動物

GFAAS

graphite furnace atomic absorption spectrometry 黒鉛炉原子吸光法

G factor

general factor 一般因子

GFAP

glial fibrillary acidic protein グリア線維酸性蛋白

GFATM

Global Fund to Fight AIDS, Tuberculosis and Malaria 世界エイズ・結核・マラリア対策基金

GFB

gastrofiberscope 胃ファイバースコープ

GFCI

ground fault circuit interrupter 漏電遮断機

GFD

gluten-free diet 無グルテン食

G

GFH
glucose-free Hanks' solution　無ブドウ糖ハンクス溶液
GFI
glucagon-free insulin　無グルカゴンインスリン
GFL
giant follicular lymphoma　巨大濾胞リンパ腫
G forces, G-forces
acceleration forces　加速力
GFP
gamma-fetoprotein　γフェトプロテイン
GFR
glomerular filtration rate　糸球体濾過量

GFS
gastrofiberscope　胃ファイバースコープ
gastrofiberscopy　胃内視鏡法
GFT
gel filtration technique　ゲル拡散法
green-fluorescent-protein　緑色螢光蛋白質
GFX
glucose, fructose, xylitol　グルコース・フルクトース・キシリトール混合液
GG
gamma globulin　γグロブリン
Geburtsgewicht〈独〉　出生時体重
genioglossus　オトガイ舌筋
glyceryl guaiacolate　グリセリルグアヤコール塩
glycylglycine　グリシルグリシン
granuloma gangraenescens〈ラ〉　壊疽性肉芽腫
GGA
general gonadotropic activity　一般性腺刺激活性
GGB
gasserian ganglion block　半月神経節ブロック
GGCS
gamma-glutamyl-cysteine synthetase　γグルタミルシステイン合成酵素
GGD
great granddaughter　(女の)曽孫
GGE
generalized glandular enlargement　全身性腺腫脹
gradient gel electrophoresis　勾配ゲル電気泳動
GGF
glial growth factor　グリア成長因子
GGG
glycine-rich gamma-glycoprotein　グリシンリッチγグリコプロテイン(血清蛋白成分)

GGK
Gallengangkrebs〈独〉 胆管癌
Ggl
ganglion 神経節〈単数〉，結節腫，ガングリオン
Ggll
ganglia 神経節〈複数〉
GGM
glucose-galactose malabsorption グルコース・ガラクトース吸収不全
GGO
gorilla gorilla〈ラ〉 ゴリラ
GGPNA
gamma-glutamyl-*p*-nitroanilide γグルタミル-*p*-ニトロアニリド
GGS
great grandson 曽孫(男)
GGT
gamma-glutamyltransferase γグルタミルトランスフェラーゼ
GGTP
gamma-glutamyl transpeptidase γグルタミルトランスペプチダーゼ
GGTT
glucocorticoid glucose tolerance test 糖質コルチコイド併用糖負荷テスト
GGtt
glucose glucagon tributamide tolerance グルコース・グルカゴン・トリブトアミド負荷試験
GGVB
glucose gelatin veronal buffer グルコースゼラチンベローナル緩衝液
GH
Gehörhalluzination〈独〉 幻聴
general hospital 総合病院，一般病院
genetic hypertension 遺伝性高血圧
geniohyoid オトガイ舌骨
glenohumeral 肩甲骨関節窩・上腕の
growth hormone 成長ホルモン
G+H
Gibbs and Helmholtz equation ギブズ・ヘルムホルツ方程式
GHAA
Group Health Association of America 米国グループ保健協会
GHB
gamma-hydroxybutyrate γヒドロキシ酪酸

gamma hydroxybutyric acid γヒドロキシ酪酸
glycohemoglobin グリコヘモグロビン

G-HB
glycosylated hemoglobin グリコシル化ヘモグロビン

GHBP
growth hormone binding protein 成長ホルモン結合蛋白

GHD
growth hormone deficiency 成長ホルモン欠乏症

4G×6H×10D
four grains times six hours times ten days 4グレン×6時間×10日

GHF
glomerular hyperfiltration 糸球体濾過亢進

GHIH
growth hormone inhibiting hormone 成長ホルモン分泌抑制ホルモン

GHK
Goldman-Hodgkin-Katz equation ゴールドマン・ホジキン・キャッツ方程式

GHND
growth hormone neurosecretory dysfunction 成長ホルモン調節神経分泌系異常

GH-NSD
human growth hormone neurosecretory dysfunction 成長ホルモン神経分泌異常症

GHQ
General Health Questionnaire 一般健康質問票

GHR
genetically hypertensive rat 遺伝性高血圧ラット
granulomatous hypersensitivity 肉芽腫性過敏反応

GHRF
growth hormone releasing factor 成長ホルモン放出因子

GHRH
growth hormone releasing hormone 成長ホルモン放出ホルモン

GHRIF
growth hormone release-inhibiting factor 成長ホルモン放出抑制因子

GHRP
growth hormone releasng peptide 成長ホルモン放出ペプチド

GHT
glomerular hypertension 糸球体高血圧

GHZ
geniculate herpes zoster 膝神経節帯状疱疹

GHz
gigahertz ギガヘルツ《単位》

GI
gastrointestinal　胃腸の
gastrointestinal tract　胃腸管
gingival index　歯肉指数
glomerular index　糸球体指数
glucagon and insulin (therapy)　グルカゴン・インスリン(療法)
glucagon immunoreactivity　グルカゴン免疫反応性
glycemic index　血糖上昇係数
glycogen index　グリコーゲン指数
granuloma inguinale〈ラ〉　鼠径部肉芽腫
growth inhibiting　成長抑制の

Gi
gips　ギプス
good impression　良い印象

gi
gill　ジル〈単位〉

GI, G.I.
globin insulin　グロビンインスリン

GIA
gastrointestinal anastomosis　胃腸吻合術
gastrointestinal apparatus　胃腸装置

GIBF
gastrointestinal bacterial flora　胃腸内細菌叢

GIC
glycyrrhizin iron colloid　グリシリジン鉄コロイド

GICA
gastrointestinal cancer　消化器癌
gastrointestinal cancer antigen　消化器癌抗原
gastrointestinal carcinoma antigen　消化器癌抗原

GICU
general intensive care unit　一般集中治療室

GIF
gastrointestinal fiberscope　消化管内視鏡
gastro-intestinal fiberscopy　上部消化管内視鏡
glycosylation inhibiting factor　グリコシレーション阻害因子
glycyrrhizin iron colloid　グリチルリジン鉄コロイド
gonadotropin-inhibitory factor　性腺刺激ホルモン抑制因子
graphics interchange format　画像交換フォーマット，ジフ《コン》
growth hormone inhibiting factor　成長ホルモン分泌抑制因子
somatostatin　ソマトスタチン

GIFT
gamete intrafallopian transfer　配偶子卵管内移植法
gamete intrafallopian tube transfar　性細胞輸卵管内注入法
granulocyte immunofluorescence　顆粒球免疫螢光検査

G

granulocyte immunofluorescene test 顆粒球抗体検出螢光(法)

GIH
gastrointestinal hemorrhage 消化管出血，胃腸出血
gastrointestinal hormone 消化管ホルモン
growth hormone release inhibiting hormone 成長ホルモン放出抑制ホルモン

GII
gastrointestinal infection 消化管感染
Global Issue Initiative on Population and AIDS 人口・エイズに関する地球規模問題イニシアティブ

GIK
glucose, insulin, kalium solution グルコース・インスリン・カリウム溶液
glucose-insulin-kalium (therapy) ブドウ糖・インスリン・カリウム(療法)
glucose, insulin, kalium chloride グルコース・インスリン・塩化カリウム

GIL
graft infiltrating lymphocytes 移植片浸潤性リンパ球
granulocyte inhibitory lymphocyte 顆粒球抑制リンパ球(＝LGL様細胞)

GIM
gonadotropin-inhibitory material 性腺刺激ホルモン抑制物質

GIMT
gastrointestinal mesenchymal tumor 間葉系腫瘍

GIN
glutamine グルタミン

GINA
global initiative for asthma 喘息のためのガイド

ging.
gingiva〈ラ〉＝gum 歯肉

GIO
general instructional object 一般教育目標

g-ion
gram-ion グラムイオン

GIP
gastric inhibitory peptide 胃抑制ペプチド
gastric inhibitory polypeptide 胃機能抑制ポリペプチド
giant cell interstitial pneumonia 巨細胞性間質性肺炎
glucose-dependent insulinotropic peptide ブドウ糖依存向インスリンペプチド
glucose-dependent insulin-releasing peptide ブドウ糖依存インスリン放出ペプチド
Good Import Practices 輸入医薬品の品質管理基準

GIR
global improvement rating　全般改善評点
glucose infusion rate　グルコース注入率

GIS
gas in stomach　胃内ガス
gastrointestinal series　胃腸造影図
gastrointestinal symptom　胃腸症状
gastrointestinal system　胃腸系，消化器系

GIST
gastrointestinal stromal tumor　消化管間葉系腫瘍

GIT
gastrointestinal tract　消化管
gastrointestinal tumor　消化器腫瘍
gatrointestinal tract　胃腸管
glutathione-insulin transhydrogenase　グルタチオン・インスリントランスヒドロゲナーゼ

GI tract
gastrointestinal tract　消化管

GITS
gastrointestinal therapeutic system　胃腸管治療システム

GITT
gastrointestinal transit time　胃腸通過時間
glucose-insulin tolerance test　ブドウ糖インスリン負荷試験

Giv
gigaelectron volts　ギガ電子ボルト

GJ
gap junctions　ギャップジャンクション，細隙結合
gastrojejunostomy　胃空腸吻合術

GJP
generalized juvenile periodontitis　広汎型若年性歯周炎

GK
galactokinase　ガラクトキナーゼ
Ganzkörper〈独〉　全身
Gingiva Krebs〈独〉　歯肉癌
glucokinase　ブドウ糖酵素
glycerol kinase　グリセロールキナーゼ

Gk
Greek　ギリシャ語，ギリシャ人

GL
Giardia lamblia　ランブリア鞭毛虫
Glaukomflecken of Vogt　フォーグトの緑内障斑
glycyrrhizin　グリシリジン
granular layer　顆粒層
greatest length　最大身長
group leader　グループリーダー

L-glutamic acid グルタミン酸

Gl
glucinium グルシニウム(＝ベリリウム)
glycolyl グリコリル

gl
glyceryl グリセリン基

GL, Gl, gl, gl.
glandula〈ラ〉＝gland 腺
glandular 腺の

Gl, gl
gill ジル〈単位〉，えら

G/L, g/l
grams per liter グラム/リットル

GLA
alpha-galactosidase αガラクトシダーゼ
giant left atrium 巨大左房
gingivolinguoaxial 歯肉舌面軸の
glucagon activity グルカゴン活性

Gla
gamma-carboxyglutamic acid γカルボキシグルタミン酸

glac
glacial 氷の

GLAD
gold-labeled antigen detection technique 金標識抗原検出法

gland.
glandula〈ラ〉＝gland 腺
glandular 腺の

GLAT
glutamic acid, lysine, alanine and tyrosine グルタミン酸・リジン・アラニン・チロシン

glau
glaucoma 緑内障

glauc
glaucoma 緑内障

GLB1
beta-galactosidase-1 βガラクトシダーゼ 1

GLB2
beta-galactosidase-2 βガラクトシダーゼ 2

GLC
gas-liquid chromatography ガス液体クロマトグラフィ

Glc
D-glucose D-グルコース(＝右旋性ブドウ糖)

glc
glycerin グリセリン(＝グリセロール)

GLC, Glc
glaucoma 緑内障

GlcA
gluconic acid グルコン酸

GlcN
glucosamine グルコサミン

GlcNAc
N-acetylglucosamine *N*-アセチルグルコサミン

GlcU
glucuronic acid グルクロン酸

GlcUA, Glc-UA
glucronic acid グルクロン酸

GLD
globoid cell leukodystrophy 遺伝性白質変性症
globoid leukodystrophy グロボイド白質ジストロフィ
glutamate dehydrogenase グルタミン酸デヒドロゲナーゼ

GLDH
glutamate dehydrogenase グルタミン酸脱水素酵素

GL enzyme
glycosaminoglycanlyase グリコサミノグリカン分解酵素

GLH
germinal layer hemorrhage 胚芽層出血

GLI
glicentin グリセンチン
glucagon-like immunoreactivity グルカゴン様免疫反応物質

Gll
glandulae 腺

Gln
glutamine グルタミン
glutaminyl グルタミニル

GLO
glycoxalase グリコキサラーゼ

Glob
globular 球状の，小球状の
globulin グロブリン

glob
globule 丸薬

GLOC
gravity-induced loss of consciousness 重力で引き起される意識喪失

G-LOC
loss of consciousness by G-force 急激なGによる失神

glos.dev
glossal deviation 舌偏位

GLP
glycolipoprotein 糖リポ蛋白

good laboratory practice 医薬品安全試験基準

GLP-1
glucagon-like peptide-1 グルカゴン様ペプチド

GLPD
granular lymphocyte-proliferative disorders 顆粒リンパ球増多症

GLT
glutamine, lysine, tyrosine グルタミン・リジン・チロシン

GlTN
glomerulo-tubulo-nephritis 糸球体細尿管腎炎

Glu
glucose ブドウ糖，グルコース
glutamic acid グルタミン酸
glutamine グルタミン
glutamyl グルタミル

glu
glutamate グルタミン酸塩，グルタミン酸エステル

GLU, glu.
glucose グルコース，ブドウ糖

GluA
glucuronic acid グルクロン酸

gluc
glucose グルコース，ブドウ糖

gluc.tol
glucose tolerance ブドウ糖負荷

glucur
glucuronide グルクロニド

glu.ox.
glucose oxidase グルコースオキシダーゼ

Glu-1-p
glucose-1-phosphate グルコース-1-リン酸

GLUT
glucose transporter グルコース輸送担体

Glut
gluteal 殿部の

glu.tol
glucose tolerance ブドウ糖負荷

GLV
Gross leukemia virus グロス白血病ウイルス

glv
galvanic 直流電気の

Glx
glutamic acid グルタミン酸
glutamine グルタミン

Gly
glycine グリシン
glycocoll (in peptiden) (ペプチド中の)グリココル
glycyl グリシル
gly
glycerite グリセライト
glycerol グリセロール
glyc
glyceride グリセリド
glycerin グリセリン
glyc.
glyceritum〈ラ〉=glycerite グリセライト
Glycerol-3-P
glycerol-3-phosphate グリセロール三リン酸
glyco
glycogen グリコーゲン
GM
gastric motility 胃の運動性
gastric mucosa 胃粘膜
Geiger-Müller counter ガイガー・ミュラー計数管
general medical 一般医学の
general medicine 一般医学
genetic manipulation 遺伝子操作
gentamicin ゲンタミシン，ゲンタマイシン
geometric mean 幾何平均
grand mal 大発作
grandmother 祖母
granulocyte-macrophage 顆粒球・大食細胞
immunoglobulin types 免疫グロブリン型
monosialoganglioside モノシアロガングリオシド
Gm
callotype marker on human immunoglobulin G ヒト免疫グロブリンGの異種型マーカー
gamma ガンマ，γ
granulocyte mitosis 顆粒球染色体分裂像
Gm＋
gram-positive グラム陽性の
Gm－
gram-negative グラム陰性の
g/m
gallons per minute ガロン/分
g-m
gram-meter グラムメートル
Gm, gm
gramma〈ラ〉=gram(me) (重量の)グラム

G

Gm%, gm%
gram(me) per hundred milliliters グラム/100ml
GMA
glycol methacrylate グリコールメタアクリレート
glycol methacrylic acid メタクリン酸グリコール
gross motor activity 粗大運動活性
GMB
gastric mucosal barrier 胃粘膜バリア
GMBF
gastric mucosal blood flow 胃粘膜血流量
GMC
general medical clinic 一般医学クリニック
General Medical Council 総医学評議会
gm cal
gram calorie グラムカロリー
gm/cc
grams per cubic centimeter グラム/cc〈単位〉
GMCD
grand mal convulsive disorder 大発作痙攣疾患
GM-CFC
granulocyte-macrophage colony forming cells 顆粒球・大食細胞コロニー形成細胞
GM-CFU
granulocyte-macrophage colony-forming unit 顆粒球・大食細胞コロニー形成ユニット
GM counter
Geiger-Müller counter ガイガー・ミュラー計数管
GM-CSF
granulocyte-macrophage colony stimulating factor 顆粒球・大食細胞コロニー刺激因子
GME
graduate medical education 卒後医学教育
GMEPP
giant miniature end-plate potential 巨大微少終板電位
GMF
glial maturation factor グリア成熟因子
GMFT
Graffe de Moelle-France Transplant〈仏〉 フランス国立骨髄ドナーバンク
GMH
Gaumenmandelhypertrophie〈独〉 口蓋扁桃肥大
GMK
green monkey kidney cells アフリカ・ミドリザル腎細胞
GML
gut mucosal lymphocyte 腸粘膜リンパ球

gm/l
gram(me) per liter グラム/リットル
gm-m
gram(me)-meter グラムメートル
g-mol
gram(me)-molecule グラムモル
GMP
glucose monophosphate グルコース一リン酸
Good Manufacturing Practice 医薬品の製造と品質管理に関する規準
guanosine 5′-phosphate グアノシン5′-リン酸
GM-P
G-myeloma proteins G骨髄腫蛋白
GmRH
gonadotropin releasing hormone ゴナドトロピン放出ホルモン
GMS
general medical service 一般医療
glycerine monostearate グリセリン一ステアリン酸エステル
Gomori methenamine-silver stain ゴモリメテナミン銀染色
GM & S
general medical and surgical 一般内科外科の
general medicine and surgery 一般内科外科学
GMSA
gel mobility shift assay 電気泳動分析
GM seizzure
grand mal seizure 大発作
GMT
geometric mean titer 幾何平均値
GMT, G.M.T.
Greenwich mean time グリニッジ標準時
GM tube
Geiger-Müller tube ガイガー・ミュラー管
GMV
gram molecular volume グラム分子容量
GMW
gram molecular weight グラム分子重量
GN
Gandy-Nanta disease ガンディー・ナンタ病
gaseous nitrogen 気体窒素
gaze nystagmus 注視眼振
glomerulonephritis 糸球体腎炎
glucagon グルカゴン
gram-negative グラム陰性の
guanethidine グアネチジン

Gn
gonadotropin ゴナドトロピン
GN, G/N
glucose/nitrogen (ratio) グルコース(=ブドウ糖)/窒素比
GNB
gram-negative bacillus グラム陰性桿菌
gram-negative bacterium グラム陰性菌
GNBM
gram-negative bacillary meningitis グラム陰性桿菌性髄膜炎
GN broth
gram-negative broth グラム陰性ブロス

GNC
general nursing care 一般看護ケア
General Nursing Council 一般看護審議会
gram-negative coccus グラム陰性球菌
GND
gram-negative diplococcus グラム陰性双球菌
gnd
ground 接地線
GNF-GNR
glucose nonfermentative gram-negative rods ブドウ糖非発酵グラム陰性桿菌
GNP
gross national product 国民総生産
GNR
gram-negative rod グラム陰性桿菌
G/N r
glucose-to-nitrogen ratio グルコース/窒素比
GnRBI
gonadotropin receptor binding inhibitor ゴナドトロピンレセプター結合抑制因子
GnRF
gonadotropin releasing factor 性腺刺激ホルモン出因子
GnRH
gonadotropin releasing hormone 性腺刺激ホルモン放出ホルモン
GnRH agonist therapy
gonadotropin releasing hormone agonist therapy 偽閉経療法
gnrl
general 一般の
Gns
Graduate Nurse 看護学校卒業生
G/NS
glucose in normal saline グルコース/生理食塩水

GNT
giant negative T 巨大陰性T波
GO
galactose oxidase ガラクトースオキシダーゼ
gas oxygen 気体酸素
gonorrhea 淋疾，淋病
GΩ
gigaohm ギガオーム（$=10^9\Omega$）
Go
Golgi ゴルジ
go
gore （傷からの）流血，凝血

GO_2
gaseous oxygen 気体酸素
GO，g.o.
glucose oxidase グルコースオキシダーゼ，ブドウ糖酸化酵素
GOC
genu corporis callosi〈ラ〉 脳梁膝
GOD
glucose oxidase ブドウ糖酸化酵素
GOD/POD
glucose oxidase-peroxidase method グルコースオキシダーゼ/ペルオキシダーゼ法
GOE
gas, oxygen, ether 笑気ガス・酸素・エーテル
gas-oxygen-ether anesthesia 笑気エーテル麻酔
gas (nitrous oxide)-oxygen-Ethrane (anesthesia) 亜酸化窒素・酸素・エンフルラン麻酔
GOF
gas-oxygen-fluothane anesthesia 笑気フローセン麻酔
gas (nitrous oxide)-oxygen-halothane (anesthesia) 亜酸化窒素・酸素・ハロタン麻酔
GOI
gas (nitrous oxide)-oxygen-isoflurane (anesthesia) 亜酸化窒素・酸素・イソフルレン麻酔
GOK
god only knows 診断不可能
GOL
glabello-opisthion line 眉間・オピスチン線
GOLD
generalized obstructive lung disease 全般閉塞性肺疾患
GOLDSOL
colloidal gold curve solution コロイド金曲線溶液
GON
gonococcal ophthalmia neonatorum 淋菌性新生児眼炎

G

Gonio
gonioscopy ゴニオスコピー
GONLA
gas (nitrous oxide)-oxygen-NLA(= neuoleptansthesia) (anesthesia) 亜酸化窒素・酸素・神経遮断麻酔併用法
gono
gonococcal 淋菌性の
gonococcus 淋菌
Gono, gono
gonorrhea 淋疾，淋病
GO_3OS
Global Ozone Observing System 地球オゾン観測組織
GOP
gas-oxygen-penthrance 笑気ペントレン麻酔
gas (nitrous oxide)-oxygen-Penthrane (anesthesia) 亜酸化窒素・酸素・ペントレン麻酔法
GOR
gastroesophageal reflux 胃食道逆流
general operating room 一般手術室
GOS
galactose oxidase-Schiff (reaction) ガラクトース・オキシダーゼ・シッフ反応
gas (nitrous oxide)-oxygen-sevoflurane (anesthesia) 亜酸化窒素・酸素・セボフルレン麻酔法
Glasgow outcome scale グラスゴー転帰尺度〔スケール〕
GOT
glutamic oxaloacetic transaminase グルタミン酸オキサロ酢酸トランスアミナーゼ
goals of treatment 治療目標
GOTS
great occipital trigeminus syndrome 大後頭三叉〔差〕神経症候群
Gov
governmental 政府の
govt
government 政府
GOX
gaseous oxygenium 気体酸素
GP
D-glycerophosphate D-グリセロリン酸
gastric polyp 胃ポリープ
gastroplasty 胃形成術
general paralysis 全身性麻痺
general paresis 全身性麻痺
general physician 家庭医
general practice 一般診療(所)

general practitioner	一般開業医
general purpose collimator	汎用コリメーター
geometric progression	幾何級数，等比級数
ginseng powder	高麗人参
globus pallidus	淡蒼球
glomerular pressure	糸球体圧
glucose production	グルコース産生
glutathione peroxidase	グルタチオンペルオキシダーゼ
glycoprotein	糖蛋白
Goldmann perimeter	ゴールドマン視野計
Goodpasture syndrome	グッドパスチャー症候群
gram-positive	グラム陽性の
grasping power	握力
guinea pig	モルモット，テンジクネズミ
gutta-percha	ガッタパーチャ
phosphoglycomutase	リン酸グリコムターゼ
speciific gravity of plasma	血漿比重

G1P

glucose-1-phosphate　グルコース-1-リン酸

G3P

glucose-3-phosphate　ブドウ糖-3-リン酸

G6P

glucose-6-phosphate　グルコース-6-リン酸

G-1,6-P

glucose-1,6-diphosphate　グルコース-1,6-二リン酸

GP, gp

group　群，基

G3P, G-3-P

glyceraldehyde-3-phosphate　グリセルアルデヒド-3-リン酸

GPA

Global Programme on AIDS　(WHO)世界エイズ対策計画

granulomatosis with polyangiitis　多発血管炎性肉芽腫症

guinea pig albumin　モルモットアルブミン

GPAIS

guinea pig anti-insulin serum　モルモット抗インスリン血清

G6Pase

glucose-6-phosphatase　グルコース-6-ホスファターゼ

GPB

glossopharyngeal breathing　舌咽呼吸

gram-positive bacillus　グラム陽性桿菌

GPBP

guinea pig myelin basic protein　モルモットミエリン塩基性蛋白

G

GPBS
glucose containing phosphate buffered saline　ブドウ糖含有リン酸緩衝食塩水

GPC
gastric parietal cell　胃壁在細胞
gel-permeation chromatography　ゲル浸透性クロマトグラフィ
general purpose computer　汎用コンピュータ
giant papillary conjunctivitis　巨大乳頭結膜炎
glycerophosphorylcholine　グリセロホスホリルコリン
gram-positive coccus　グラム陽性球菌
guinea-pig complement　モルモット補体

GPD
glucose-6-phosphate dehydrogenase　グルコース-6-リン酸デヒドロゲナーゼ

G-3-PD
glyceraldehyde-3-phosphate dehydrogenase　グリセルアルデヒド-3-リン酸脱水素酵素

G6PD, G-6PD, G-6-PD
glucose-6-phosphate dehydrogenase　グルコース-6-リン酸脱水素酵素

G6PDH
glucose-6-phosphate dehydrogenase　グルコース-6-リン酸脱水素酵素

GPE
guinea-pig embryo　モルモット胚

GPF
glial promoting factor　グリア促進因子
glomerular plasma flow　糸球体血漿流量
gram-positive fibers　グラム陽性線維
granulocytosis-promoting factor　顆粒球増多促進因子

GPGG
guinea pig gamma globulin　モルモットγグロブリン

GPHN
giant pigmented hairy nevus　巨大色素有毛母斑

GPHV
guinea pig herpes virus　モルモットヘルペスウイルス

GPI
general paralysis of insane　精神病の全身麻痺
glucose phosphate isomerase　グルコースリン酸イソメラーゼ
guinea pig ileum　モルモット回腸

GPIB
general purpose interface bus　計測システム標準インターフェイス

GPID
glucose-phosphate isomerase deficiency — グルコースリン酸イソメラーゼ欠乏症
GPIMH
guinea pig intestinal mucosal homogenate — モルモット腸粘膜ホモジネート
GPIT
Generic Pharmaceutical Industry Association — ジェネリック製薬工業協会
GPK
guinea pig kidney antigen — モルモット腎抗原
GPKA
guinea pig kidney absorption test — モルモット腎吸収試験
GPLA
guinea pig leukocyte antigen — モルモット白血球抗原
GPLV
guinea pig leukemia virus — モルモット白血病ウイルス
Gply
gingivoplasty — 歯肉形成
GPM
general preventure medicine — 一般予防医学
Gpm
globus pallidus〈ラ〉 — 淡蒼球
phosphoglucomutase — リン酸グルコムターゼ
GPMSP
Good Post-Marketing Surveillance Practice — 新医薬品再審査申請のための市販後調査実施に関する基準
GPN
glossopharyngeal neuralgia — 舌咽神経痛
GPO
glycerin-1-phosphate-oxydase — グリセリン-1-リン酸酸化酵素
GPP
Good Pharmacy Practice — 薬局業務基準
Good Promotional Practice — 医薬品情報基準
GPRBC
guinea-pig red blood cell — モルモット赤血球
GPS
Goodpasture syndrome — グッドパスチャー症候群
guinea pig serum — モルモット血清
guinea pig spleen — モルモット脾
GPSP
Good Postmarketing Surveilance Practice — 医薬品の製造販売後の調査および試験の実施に関する基準

GPT
glutamic-pyruvic transaminase　グルタミン酸ピルビン酸トランスアミナーゼ
guinea pig trachea　モルモット気管

GP TH, GpTh, Gp Th
group therapy　グループ療法，集団治療

GPTSM
guinea pig tracheal smooth muscle　モルモット気管平滑筋

GPU
gunea-pig unit　モルモット単位

GPX
glutathione peroxidase　グルタチオンペルオキシダーゼ

GPX1
glutathione peroxidase 1　グルタチオンペルオキシダーゼ1

GR
gamma ray　ガンマ線，γ線
gastric resection　胃切除術
generalized rash　全身発疹
general research　一般研究
globule rouge〈仏〉　赤血球
glucocorticoid receptor　糖質コルチコイドレセプター
glucose response　グルコース反応
glutathione reductase　グルタチオン還元酵素
glycyrrhizin　グリチルリチン
good recovery　回復良好
granulocyte　顆粒球
Griess-Romijin agent　グリース・ロミジン試薬
growth retardation　発育遅延

Gr
gravid　妊娠の，妊娠した

gr
grade　グレード
graft　移植(片)
grain　グレーン
gravity　重力

gr.
gravida〈ラ〉=pregnant woman　妊婦

gr+
gram-positive bacteria　グラム陽性菌

gr−
gram-negative bacteria　グラム陰性菌

GR, gr
gamma roentgen　γレントゲン

GRA
gonadotropin-releasing agent 性腺刺激ホルモン放出ホルモン

grad
gradient 勾配，傾き
graduated 目盛りをつけた

grad.
gradatim〈ラ〉=gradually 徐々に《処》

'gram
radiogram X線写真

gran
granular 顆粒の
granulation 顆粒化

GRAS
generally recognized as safe 安全認定食品添加物

grav.
gravid 妊娠中の
gravity 重力

grav.1
primigravida〈ラ〉 初妊婦

Grav, grav.
gravida〈ラ〉=gravida 妊婦

gravid.
gravida〈ラ〉=gravida 妊婦

grav.Ṫ
primigravida〈ラ〉 初妊婦

grav.Ṫ/Ab.Ṫ
gravida 1, *aborta* 1〈ラ〉 妊娠1回・流産1回

GRBAS
grade, rough, brethy, asthenic, strained 程度・粗造性・気息性・無力性・努力性

GRD
beta-glucuronidase βグルクロニダーゼ
gramicidin dubious グラミシジン

grd
ground 接地

GRE
glucocorticoid responsive element グルココルチコイド感応部位
gradient-echo グラディエントエコー

GRF
gonadotropic releasing factor 性腺刺激ホルモン放出因子
griseofulvin グリセオフルビン
growth hormone releasing factor 成長ホルモン放出因子

growth hormone releasing factor neuron　成長ホルモン放出因子ニューロン

GR-FR
grandfather　祖父

GRG
glycine-rich glycoprotein　グリシン過多糖蛋白(質)

GRH
gonadotropin-releasing hormone　性腺刺激ホルモン放出ホルモン
growth hormone releasing hormone　成長ホルモン放出ホルモン

GRID
gay-related immunodeficiency disease　ゲイ関連免疫不全疾患

G

GRIF
growth hormone releasing-inhibiting factor　成長ホルモン放出抑制因子

GR-J
gramicidin-J　グラミシジンJ

GRL
granular layer　顆粒層

grm
gram　グラム

GRMN-J
gramicidin-J　グラミシジンJ

GR-MO
grandmother　祖母

grmp
grosso modo pulverisatum〈ラ〉　粗大粉末にせよ《処》

GRN
granules　顆粒

grn
green　緑(の)，グリーン(の)

GRO
growth regulatory gene　成長調節遺伝子

gros.
grossus〈ラ〉＝coarse　粗い

GRP
gastrin releasing hormone　ガストリン放出ホルモン
gastrin releasing peptide　ガストリン放出ペプチド

GrP
gram-positive　グラム陽性の

grp
group　群

Gr_1 P_0 AB_1
one pregnancy, no births, one abortion　妊娠１回・出産０回・流産１回

GRR
gross reproduction rate　総再生産率
GRS
β-glucuronidase　βグルクロニダーゼ
GRT
gesture recognition test　身振り認知テスト
GRTP
guanosine triphosphate　グアノシン三リン酸
GrTr
graphite treatment　黒鉛療法
grwt
gross weight　総重量
GS
gallstone　胆石
Gardner syndrome　ガードナー症候群
gastrocnemius soleus　腓腹筋，ヒラメ筋
Gaumenspalte〈独〉　口蓋裂
general surgeon　一般外科医
general surgery　一般外科学
gestational sac　胎嚢
gestational stage　妊娠期
Gilbert syndrome　ジルベール症候群
ginseng saponin　ニンジンサポニン
glomerular sclerosis　糸球体硬化
glucagon secretion　グルカゴン分泌
glutamine synthetase　グルタミン合成酵素
goat serum　ヤギ血清
Goldenhar syndrome　ゴルドナール症候群
Goodpasture syndrome　グッドパスチャー症候群
Gram stain　グラム染色(法)
grandson　孫息子
granulocystein substance　顆粒球様システイン物質
granulocyte substance　顆粒球物質
Grönblad-Strandberg syndrome　グレンブラッド・ストランベリー症候群
Guérin-Stern (syndrome)　ゲラン・スターン(症候群)
Gs
gauss　ガウス〈単位〉
G/S
glucose and saline　ブドウ糖と生食水
g/s
gallons per second　ガロン/秒
GS, gs
group specific　群特異的な
GSA
general somatic afferent　一般体性求心性

G

general somatic afferent nerve 一般体性求心神経
Gross virus antigen グロスウイルス抗原
group-specific antigen 群特異的抗原
guanidinosuccinic acid グアニジノコハク酸

GS-ANA
granulocyte specific antinuclear antibody 顆粒球特異抗核抗原

GSANF
granulocyte specific antinuclear factor 顆粒球特異抗核因子

GSAS
glutamate-γ-semialdehyde synthetase グルタメートγセミアルデヒド合成酵素

GSBG
gonadal steroid-binding globulin 性腺ステロイド結合グロブリン

GSC
gas solid chromatography ガス固体クロマトグラフィ

G-SC
guanosine-coupled spleen cell グアノシン結合脾臓細胞

g scale
(force of) gravity scale 重力スケール〔尺度〕

GSCC
German Society for Clinical Chemistry ドイツ臨床化学会

GSCN
giant serotonin-containing neuron 巨大セロトニン含有ニューロン

GSD
genetically significant dose 遺伝的有意線量
glutathione synthetase deficiency グルタチオン合成酵素欠乏症
glycogen storage disease 糖原病

GSE
general somatic efferent nerve 一般体性遠心神経
geometric standard error 幾何標準誤差
gluten-sensitive enteropathy グルテン感受性過敏腸障害

GSH
γ-glutamylcysteinylglycine γグルタミルシステイニルグリシン
glomerular stimulating hormone 糸球体刺激ホルモン
glucocorticoid suppressible hyperaldosteronism グルココルチコイド奏効性アルドステロン症
glutathione グルタチオン
reduced glutathione 還元型グルタチオン

GSH-P
glutathione peroxidase　グルタチオンペルオキシダーゼ

GSHPx
glutathione peroxidase　グルタチオンペルキオシダーゼ

GSHV
ground squirrel hepatitis virus　リス肝炎ウイルス

GSLs
glycosphingolipids　糖質スフィンゴ脂質

GSN
giant serotonin neuron　巨大セロトニンニューロン

GSP
galvanic skin potential　電気皮膚電位
good supplying practice　優良医薬品供給基準

GSR
galvanic skin reflex　皮膚電気反射
galvanic skin response (audiometry)　皮膚電気反射(聴力検査)
generalized Shwartzman reaction　全身シュワルツマン反応
global severity rating　概括重症度
glutathion reductase　グルタチオン還元酵素

GSS
Gerstmann-Straussler Scheinker syndrome　ゲルストマン・シュトロイスラー・シャインカー症候群

GSSG
oxidized glutathione　酸化型グルタチオン

GSSG-R
glutathione reductase　グルタチオン還元酵素

GST
glutathione-S-transferase　グルタチオン-S-変換酵素
gold salt therapy　金塩療法
gold sodium thiomalate　金チオリンゴ酸ナトリウム

GST-P
glutathione-S-transferase placental form　グルタチオン-S-変換酵素胎盤型

GSW
gunshot wound　射創，銃創

GSWA
gunshot wound to the abdomen　腹部射創，腹部銃創

GT
gait training　歩行訓練
galanthamine　ガランサミン
gastric tube　胃チューブ
gastrocamera　胃カメラ
gastrostomy　胃造瘻術，胃瘻造設術
generation time　発生時間

G

gene targetting 遺伝子ターゲット
genetic therapy 遺伝子治療
globe thermometer グローブ寒暖計
glove temperature 黒球温
glucose therapy ブドウ糖療法
glucose transport ブドウ糖輸送量
glutamyl transpeptidase グルタミルトランスペプチダーゼ
granulation time 顆粒形成時間
greater trochanter 大転子
greater tuberosity 大結節
great toe 足の拇指
group therapy グループ療法，集団治療

gt.
gutta〈ラ〉＝drop 滴

GT1〔2,3…〕
glycogenosis type 1〔2,3…〕 1〔2,3…〕型糖原病

GT-41
myleran ミ〔マイ〕レラン

g/t
granulation tissue 肉芽組織

G & T
gowns and towels ガウンとタオル

GTB
glomerulotubular balance 糸球体尿細管調節

GTC
glucose tolerance curve 耐糖曲線

GTCS
generalized tonic-clonic seizure 全身性強直性間代性発作

GTE
glucose/tris/EDTA グルコース・トリス・EDTA

G-test
gonadotropin stimulation test ゴナドトロピン刺激検査

GTF
gastrocamera with fiberscope ファイバースコープ付胃カメラ
gastroduodenal fiberscope 上部消化管内視鏡
glucose tolerance factor ブドウ糖耐性因子

GTG
gut-type glucagon 腸管型グルカゴン

GTH
gestational transient hyperthyroidism 妊娠時一過性甲状腺機能亢進症
gonadotrophic hormone 性腺刺激ホルモン

GTN
gestational trophoblastic neoplasia　妊娠性絨毛性腫瘍
glomerulotubulonephritis　糸球体尿細管腎炎
glyceryl trinitrate　三硝酸グリセリン

GTO
Golgi tendon organ　ゴルジ腱紡錘

GTP
glutamyl transpeptidase　グルタミルトランスペプチダーゼ
gonadotropin　性腺刺激ホルモン
green tea polyphenolic fraction　グリーンティーポリフェノフラクション
guanosine 5′-triphosphate　グアノシン(5′-)三リン酸

GTR
granulocyte turnover rate　顆粒球交替率
guided tissue regeneration　組織再生誘導法

GTS
glucose transport system　ブドウ糖輸送系

GTT
gelatin-tellurite-taurocholate　ゼラチン・亜テルル酸塩・タウロコール酸塩
glucose tolerance test　ブドウ糖負荷試験

gtt.
guttae〈ラ〉=drops　滴

gtts.
guttae〈ラ〉=drops　滴
guttas〈ラ〉　滴を《処》

GU
gastric ulcer　胃潰瘍
genito-urinary　生殖・泌尿器(の)
glucose uptake　ブドウ糖摂取
glycogenic unit　グリコゲン合成単位
gonococcal urethritis　淋菌性尿道炎
gravitational ulcer　沈下性潰瘍

Gu
concentration of glucose in urine　尿中ブドウ糖濃度

GU, G-U
genitourinary　尿生殖器の

Gua
guanine　グアニン

GUI
graphical user interface　回使用中間面

guid.
guidance　誘導

GUK
guanylate kinase　グアニル酸キナーゼ

GUO, Guo
guanosine　グアノシン

GUR
global utility rating　全般有効度

GUS
genitourinary system　生殖泌尿器系

GUSB
β-glucuronidase　βグルクロニダーゼ

GUSTO
global utilization of streptokinase and tissue plasminogen activator for occluded coronary arteries　tPA・SK比較大規模治験(＝いわゆるガスト治験)

gutt.
gutturi〈ラ〉＝to the throat　喉に

guttat.
guttatim〈ラ〉＝drop by drop　一滴ずつ

gutt.quibusd.
guttis quibusdam〈ラ〉　数滴ずつ《処》

GV
germinal vesicle　卵核胞
gastric volume　胃容量
gentian violet　ゲンチアナ紫
Gross virus　グロスウイルス
guidance value　ガイダンスバリュー

GVA
general visceral afferent　一般内臓求心性
general visceral afferent nerve　一般内臓求心神経

GVB
gelatin veronal buffer　ゼラチンベロナール緩衝液

GVE
general visceral efferent　一般内臓遠心性
general visceral efferent nerve　一般内臓遠心神経

GVF
good visual fields　視野良好

GVG
gamma-vinyl-GABA　γビニルGABA

GVH
graft versus host reaction　移植片対宿主反応

GVH, GvH
graft versus host　移植片対宿主

GVHD
graft versus host disease　移植片対宿主疾患

GVHR
graft versus host reaction　移植片対宿主反応

GVL
graft versus leukemia　移植片対白血病細胞反応

GVN
gentamicin, vancomycin, nystatin ゲンタミ〔マイ〕シン・バンコマイシン・ナイスタチン

GVP
good vigilance practice 医薬品・医薬部外品・化粧品・医療機器の製造販売後安全管理の基準

Gvty
gingivectomy 歯肉切除

GW
Gaze Wechsel〈独〉 ガーゼ交換
gigawatt ギガワット
glycerin in water グリセリン水
group work グループ仕事

G/W
glucose in water ブドウ糖液

G & W
glycerin and water グリセリンと水

GWE
glycerin and water enema グリセリンと水浣腸

GWG
generalized Wegener's granulomatosis 全身性ウェゲナー肉芽腫症

GX
flagella 鞭毛
glycine xylide グリシンキシリッド

GXT
graded exercise test 段階的運動テスト

Gy
gray グレイ〈単位〉

GYN, Gyn, gyn
gynecologic 婦人科学の
gynecological 婦人科学の
gynecologist 婦人科医
gynecology 婦人科学

GYV
green yellow vegetable 黄緑野菜

H h

H

Haemaphysalis	チマダニ(属)
Haemophilus	ヘモフィルス(属)
halothane	ハロタン，ハロセン
Harn〈独〉	尿
Hartnup (disease)	ハートナップ(病)
haustus〈ラ〉=a draught, a drink	(水剤の)一服量《処》
heart	心臓
heart disease	心疾患
heavy	重い
hemagglutination	(赤)血球凝集(反応)
hemisphere	半球
Hemophilus	ヘモフィルス(属)
henry	ヘンリー〈単位〉
hepar	肝臓
heparin	ヘパリン
hepatic metastasis	癌肝転移
hernia	ヘルニア，脱出
heroin	ヘロイン
Heterophyes	異形吸虫(属)
hip	股関節部
hippocampus〈ラ〉	(脳の)海馬
histidine	ヒスチジン
Histoplasma	ヒストプラズマ(属)
Holzknecht space	ホルツクネヒト腔
Holzknecht unit	ホルツクネヒト単位
homosexual	同性愛(者)の
horizontal	水平の
horizontal plane	水平面
hormone	ホルモン
horse	ウマ
hospital	病院
hot	熱い
Hounsfield unit	ハウンスフィールド単位
H-type substance	H型物質
human response	ヒト反応
humoral factor	液性因子
hundred	100
husband	夫
hydrogen	水素
hydrolysis	加水分解
hygiene	衛生(学)
Hymenolepis	膜様条虫(属)

hyoscine	ヒオスシン
hyperemia	充血
hypermetropia〈ラ〉	遠視
hyperopia	遠視
hyperopic	遠視の
hyperphoria	上斜位
hyperplasia	過形成，増殖
hypodermic	皮下の，皮下注射(器)
hypodermic injection	皮下注射
hypothalamus	視床下部
intermittent hypertropia	間欠性上斜視
Planck constant	プランク定数
h	
hard	固い
hardness	堅固，困難
hecto	ヘクト(＝10^2)〈接〉
herba〈ラ〉	葉
humidity	湿度
viscosity	粘稠度，粘性，粘着性
h.	
haustus〈ラ〉	水薬の１服量《処》
^1H	
hydrogen(＝protium)	水素１(＝プロチウム)
^2H	
hydrogen-2(＝deuterium)	水素２，重水素(＝ジューテリウム)
^3H	
hydrogen-3(＝tritium)	水素３，三重水素(＝トリチウム)
H_3	
procaine hydrochloride	塩酸プロカイン
H^+	
hydrogen ion	水素イオン
H-2	
histocompatibility complex	マウス主要組織適合遺伝子複合体
H'	
hyperphoria for near	近見時の上斜位
[H^+]	
hydrogen ion concentration	水素イオン濃度(＝(H^+))
H, h	
height	身長
hight	高さ
hora, *horae*〈ラ〉＝hour	時,時間
human	ヒト

HA

habitus asthenicus〈ラ〉	無力性体質
hallux abductus	外反母趾
halothane anesthesia	ハロタ〔セ〕ン麻酔
H antigen	H抗原
headache	頭痛
hearing aid	補聴器
heat aggregated	熱凝固
height age	身長年齢
hemadsorption	血液吸着
hemagglutinating activity	赤血球凝集活性
hemagglutinating antibody	赤血球凝集抗体
hemagglutination test	赤血球凝集試験
hemagglutinin	赤血球凝集素
hemolytic anemia	溶血性貧血
hepatic adenoma	肝腺腫
hepatic artery	肝動脈
hepatitis A	A型肝炎
hepatitis A antibody	A型肝炎抗体
hepatitis associated (virus)	肝炎関連(ウイルス)
herpangina	ヘルパンギーナ，水疱性口峡炎
heterophil antibody	好異種抗体
high anxiety	高度不安
hippuric acid	馬尿酸
histamine	ヒスタミン
histocompatibility antigen	組織適合抗原
homogentisic acid	ホモゲンチジン酸
Horton arteritis	ホートン動脈炎
hospital admission	入院
hospital automation	病院自動化
hyaluronic acid	ヒアルロン酸
hydroxyapatite	ヒドロキシアパタイト
hyperalimentation	高栄養輸液
hyperandrogenism	アンドロゲン(分泌)過剰症，高アンドロゲン症
hypermetropic astigmatism	遠視性乱視
hypersensitivity alveolitis	過敏性肺胞炎
hypersensitivity angitis	過敏性血管炎
hypothalamic amenorrhea	視床下部性無月経
symbol for “an acid”	酸を示す記号

Ha

hahnium	ハーニウム(＝ドブニウム)
Harn〈独〉	尿
Hartmann number	ハルトマン数

H/A
head-to-abdomen (ratio) 頭部・腹部(比)

HAA
hearing aid amplifier 補聴器増幅器
hemolytic anemia antigen 溶血性貧血抗原
hemolyticanemia antigen 溶血性貧血抗原
hepatitis associated antigen 肝炎関連抗原
hospital activity analysis 病院活動分析

HA Ag, HA-Ag
hepatitis A antigen A型肝炎抗原

HAB
HTL associated bronchitis HTL関連呼吸器障害
human and animal binding ヒトと動物の結束
human T cell leukemia virus type I associated bronchopneumonopathy ヒトT細胞白血病ウイルスI型関連気管支肺病変
human T lymphotropic virus type I associated bronchopneumonopathy ヒトTリンパ球向性ウイルスI型関連気管支肺病変

HABA
HTLV-I associated bronchiolo-alveolar disorder HTLV-I関連細気管支肺胞異常症
human T lymphotropic virus associated bronchovesicular abnormality ヒトTリンパ球向性ウイルス関連気管支・肺胞異常症

HABCA
4′-hydroxy-azobenzene carboxylic acid 4′-ヒドロキシアゾベンゼンカルボン酸, ハブカ

HABF
hepatic artery blood flow 肝動脈血流

HAb/HAd
horizontal abduction/adduction 水平外転/内転

habit
habitat 居住環境, 生息場所

habt.
habeatur〈ラ〉 患者に持たせよ《処》

HAC
hexamethylmelamine, adriamycin, cyclophosphamide ヘキサメチルメラミン, アドリアマイシン, シクロホスファミド
hyperactive children 多動児

HACCP
Hazard Analysis Critical Control Point Inspection System 食品の危害分析・重要管理点監視方式

HACE
hepatic artery chemoembolization 肝動脈の化学的塞栓形成(法)
high-altitude cerebral edema 高所脳浮腫

HAChT
high affinity choline transport 高親和性コリン輸送
HACR
hereditary adenomatosis of colon and rectum 結腸と直腸の遺伝性腺腫症
HACS
hyperactive child syndrome 過活動児童〔小児〕症候群
HAD
hemadsorption 赤血球吸着現象
hexamethylmelamine, adriamycin, *cis*-diamminedichloroplatinum ヘキサメチルメラミン,アドリアマイシン,*cis*-ジアミンジクロロプラチナム
hospital administration 病院管理
hospital administrator 病院管理者
human adjuvant disease ヒトアジュバント病
hypophysectomized alloxan diabetic 下垂体切除性アロキサン糖尿病(患者)
L'Hospitalisation a Domicile〈仏〉 在宅入院制度
HAD, HAd
hemadsorption (赤)血球吸着(現象)
HADH
hydroxyacyl-CoA dehydrogenase ヒドロキシアシル・コエンザイムAデヒドロゲナーゼ
HAE
health appraisal examination 健康評価検査
hearing aid evaluation 補聴器評価
hepatic artery embolization 肝動脈塞栓形成法
hepatic artery embolization 肝動脈塞栓形成(法)
hereditary angioedema 遺伝性血管浮腫
hereditary angioneurotic edema 遺伝性血管運動神経症性浮腫
HAEC
Hirschsprung-associated enterocolitis ヒルシュスプルング関連腸炎
haem
haemolysis 溶血(現象)
haematol
haematologist 血液学者
haematology 血液学
haemorrh
haemorrhage 出血
HAF
hepatic arterial flow 肝動脈(血)流量
HaF
Hageman factor ハーゲマン因子
HAFP
human alpha-fetoprotein ヒトαフェトプロテイン

HAG
heat-aggregated globulin　熱凝集グロブリン
HAGG
hyperimmune antivariola gamma globulin　高度免疫抗痘瘡γグロブリン，過免疫抗天然痘γグロブリン
HAGL
humeral avulsion of the glenohumeral ligament　関節上腕靱帯の上腕骨剝離
HAHTG
horse antihuman-thymus globulin　ウマ抗ヒト胸腺グロブリン
HAI
hemagglutination inhibition (titer)　赤血球凝集抑制(滴定濃度)
hemagglutinin inhibition　赤血球凝集素抑制
histology activity index　組織活動性指標
HAIA
Hearing Aid Industry Association　補聴器製作会社協会
H & A Ins
Health and Accident Insurance　健康・事故保険
HAIR
hemagglutination inhibition reaction　赤血球凝集抑制反応
HAIR-AN
hyperandrogenism, insulin resistance, and acanthosis nigricans (syndrome)　アンドロゲン過剰症・インスリン抵抗性・黒色表皮腫(症候群)
HAIT
hemagglutination inhibition test　赤血球凝集抑制試験
HAL
haloperidol　ハロペリドール
halothane　ハロタ〔セ〕ン
hypoplastic acute leukemia　再生不良性急性白血病
Hal
halogen　ハロゲン
hallu
hallucinant　幻覚剤
hallucinate　幻覚を起こさせる
hallucination　幻覚
hallucinogen　幻覚剤
hallucinogenic　幻覚を生ずる
halluc
hallucination　幻覚
HALP
hyperalphalipoproteinemia　高アルファリポ蛋白血症
HALV
hamster leukemia virus　ハムスター白血病ウイルス

HAM
hearing aid microphone 補聴器マイクロフォン
hexamethylmelamine, adriamycin, melphalan ヘキサメチルメラミン,アドリアマイシン,メルファラン
human alveolar macrophage ヒト肺胞マクロファージ
human T cell leukemia virus type I associated myelopathy ヒトT細胞白血病ウイルスI型関連脊髄症
human T cell lymphoma associated virus myelopathy ヒトT細胞白血病ウイルス脊髄症
human T lymphotropic virus type I associated myelopathy ヒトTリンパ球向性ウイルスI型関連脊髄症
hypoparathyroidism-Addison-Monilia (syndrome) 副甲状腺機能低下症・アジソン病・モニリア症〔カンジダ症〕(症候群)

HAMA
Hamilton Anxiety (Scale) ハミルトン不安(尺度)
human antimouse antibody ヒト抗マウス抗体
human antimurine antibody 外来抗体に対する異型抗体

HAMD
Hamilton Depression (Scale) ハミルトンうつ病(尺度)

HAMS
hypoparathyroidism-Addison-Monilia syndrome 副甲状腺機能低下・アジソン・モニリア症〔カンジダ症〕(症候群), HAM症候群

Hams
hamstrings 膝窩腱, 膝屈曲筋

HaMSV
Harvey murine sarcoma virus ハーヴェーマウス肉腫ウイルス

HAN
heroin-associated nephropathy ヘロイン性腎症
hyperplastic alveolar nodule 過形成胞状結節

HANA
hemagglutinin neuraminidase 赤血球凝集素ノイラミニダーゼ

H and D, H & D
Hunter and Driffield (curve) ハンター・ドリフィールド(曲線)《画診》

H and E, H & E
hemorrhage and exudate 出血と滲出液
heredity and environment 遺伝と環境

H and E staining
hematoxylin and eosin (staining) ヘマトキシリン・エオジン(染色法)

H and N
head and neck 頭頸部
HANE
hereditary angioneurotic edama ハネ，遺伝性血管(運動)神経性浮腫
HANES
Health and Nutrition Examination Survey 国民健康栄養状態調査
HANP
human atrial natriuretic peptide ヒト心房性ナトリウム利尿ペプチド
hANP
human atrial natriuretic hormone ヒト心房性ナトリウム利尿ホルモン
H antigens
antigens localized in flagella of motile bacteria(=flagellar antigen, Hauch antigens) 細菌鞭毛限局抗原，H抗原
HAP
hereditary ataxic polyneuritis 遺伝性失調性多発性神経炎
heredopathia atactica polyneuritiformis 遺伝性多発神経炎性失調(症)
hospital-acquired pneumonia 院内(感染性)肺炎
humoral antibody production 体液性抗体産生
hydroxyapatite 水酸化リン灰石，ヒドロキシアパタイト
HAPA
hemagglutinating antipenicillin antibody 赤血球凝集性抗ペニシリン抗体
HAPC
high-amplitude contraction 高振幅性収縮
hospital-acquired penetration contact 院内侵入接触
HAPD
home-automated peritoneal dialysis 在宅自動化腹膜透析
HAPE
high-altitude pulmonary edema 高所肺水腫
high-altitude pulmonary oedema 高所肺水腫
HAPO
high-altitude pulmonary oedema 高所肺水腫
HAPs
hazardous air pollutants 大気中の有害化学物質
HAQ
Health Assessment Questionnaire 健康評価のための質問
4-HAQO
4-hydroxyaminoquinoline-L-oxide 4-ヒドロキシアミノキノリンL-オキサイド

HAR
hemagglutination reaction 赤血球凝集反応
high-altitude retinopathy 高高度網膜障害
high anterior resection 高位前方切除術
hyperacute rejection 超急性拒絶反応

Har
homoarginine ホモアルギニン

HARD
hydrocephalus, agyria, retinal dysplasia 水頭症・無脳回(症)・網膜形成異常〔異形成〕

HARH
high-altitude retinal hemorrage 高高度網膜出血

harm
harmonic 調和

H

HARPPS
heat, absence of use, redness, pain, pus, swelling 熱・(患部)不使用・発赤・疼痛・膿・腫脹(などの感染症状)

HARS
Hamilton Anxiety Rating Scale ハミルトン不安評点尺度

HAS
Hirnarteriosklerose〈独〉 脳動脈硬化症
hyperalimentation solution 高栄養溶液
hypertensive arteriosclerosis 高血圧性動脈硬化症

HASCHD
hypertensive arteriosclerotic heart disease 高血圧性動脈硬化性心疾患

HASCVD
hypertensive arteriosclerotic cardiovascular disease 高血圧性動脈硬化性心血管疾患

HASHD
hypertensive arteriosclerotic heart disease 高血圧性動脈硬化性心疾患

H & ASHD
hypertension and arteriosclerotic heart disease 高血圧と動脈硬化性心疾患

HAT
Halstead Aphasia Test ハルステッド失語検査
head, arms, trunk 頭・腕・体幹部
hemagglutination titer 赤血球凝集価
heparin-associated thrombocytopenia ヘパリン関連血小板減少(症)
high antigenic tumor 高抗原腫瘍
hospital arrival time 病院到着時間

HA test
hemadsorption test 赤血球吸着反応試験

HATG
horse antihuman-thymocyte globulin ウマ抗ヒト胸腺細胞グロブリン

HAT medium
hypoxanthine-aminopterin-thymidine medium ヒポキサンチン・アミノプテリン・チミジン培地, HAT培養液

HATT
heparin-associated thrombocytopenia and thrombosis ヘパリン関連血小板減少(症)と血栓症

HAU
hemagglutinating unit 赤血球凝集単位

haust.
haustus〈ラ〉=a draught, a drink (頓服水剤の)一服量《処》

HAV
hallux abducto valgus 外反〔外転〕母趾
hemadsorption virus 赤血球吸着ウイルス
hepatitis A virus A型肝炎ウイルス

HAVD
hypertensive cardiovascular disease 高血圧性心血管疾患

HA virus
hemadsorption virus 赤血球吸着ウイルス, パラインフルエンザウイルス

HAVS
hand arm vibration syndrome 手腕振動症候群

HAWIE
Hamburg-Wechsler-Intelligenz-test für Erwachsene〈独〉 ハンブルグ式成人用ウェクスラー知能テスト

HAWIK
Hamburg-Wechsler-Intelligenz test für Kinder〈独〉 ハンブルグ式児童用ウェクスラー知能テスト

haz
hazard 危険
hazardous 危険な

HB
habenula〈ラ〉 手綱
hair bath 洗髪
Handbewegung〈独〉 手動弁
Hassall bodies ハッサル小体
heart block 心ブロック
Heinz body ハインツ小体
hepatitis B B型肝炎
His bundle ヒス束
Hutchinson-Boeck (disease) ハッチンソン・ベック(病)
hybridoma bank ハイブリドーマバンク

H

hydrocortisone butyrate cream ブチル酸ヒドロコルチゾン・クリーム
hyoid body 舌骨体

Hb
hemoglobin ヘモグロビン，血色素
herbarium 植物標本室

hb
herba〈ラ〉 葉《処》

HB1°〔2°,3°〕
first〔second/third〕-degree heart block 第1～3度心(臓)ブロック

HB A
hemoglobin alpha chain 血色素α鎖

Hb A
hemoglobin A ヘモグロビンA
hemoglobin adult 成人型ヘモグロビン

Hb A_1
hemoglobin A_1 ヘモグロビンA_1

Hb A_2
hemoglobin A_2 ヘモグロビンA_2

HB Ab
hepatitis B antibody B型肝炎抗体

HBABA
2-(4′-hydroxybenzene)-azobenzoic acid 2-4′-ヒドロキシベンゼン・アゾ安息香酸

Hb A_{1c}
hemoglobin A_{1c} ヘモグロビンA_{1c}

HB Ag
hepatitis B antigen B型肝炎抗原

H band
heller band H帯

HB antigen
hepatitis virus B antigen B型肝炎抗原

Hb A-S
hemoglobin A and hemoglobin S ヘモグロビンAとヘモグロビンS

HBB
hemoglobin beta chain 血色素β鎖

Hb Bart
Bart hemoglobin バート型ヘモグロビン

HbBC
hemoglobin-binding capacity 血色素結合能

HB/BW
hold breakfast for blood work 血液検査のため朝食延食

HBC
hydrodynamically balanced capsule 水力学的平衡カプセル

H

Hb C	
hemoglobin C	ヘモグロビンC
HBc, HBC	
hepatitis B core (antigen)	B型肝炎コア(抗原)
HBcAb	
hepatitis B core antibody	B型肝炎コア抗体
HBcAg	
hepatitis B core antigen	B型肝炎コア抗原
HBCO, HbCO	
carbon monoxide hemoglobin	一酸化炭素ヘモグロビン
HBD	
α-hydroxy butyrate dehydrogenase	α水酸化酪酸脱水素酵素
β-hydroxy butyrate dehydrogenase	β水酸化酪酸脱水素酵素
hemoglobin delta chain	血色素δ鎖
hypophosphatemic bone disease	低リン酸血(症)性骨疾患
HbD	
hemoglobin D	ヘモグロビンD
HBDH	
α-hydroxybutyrate dehydrogenase	α-水酸化酪酸脱水素酵素
HBDT	
human basophil degranulation test	ヒト好塩基球脱顆粒試験
HBE	
hemoglobin epsilon chain	血色素ε鎖
His bundle electrogram	ヒス束電位図
Hb E	
hemoglobin E	ヘモグロビンE
HBe Ag, HBe-Ag	
hepatitis B envelope antigen	HBe抗原
HBF	
hand blood flow	手血流量
hemispheric blood flow	半球血流量
hepatic blood flow	肝血流量
hypothalamic blood flow	視床下部血流量
HbF	
fetal hemoglobin	胎児性ヘモグロビン
hemoglobin F	ヘモグロビンF
hemoglobin fetal	胎児ヘモグロビン
HBg	
hepatitis B antigen	B型肝炎抗原
HBG1	
hemoglobin gamma chain A	血色素γ鎖A
HBG2	
hemoglobin gamma chain G	血色素γ鎖G
HBGF	
heparin binding growth factor	ヘパリン結合性成長因子

HBGF-1
heparin binding growth factor-1 — ヘパリン結合増殖因子 1

HBGM
home blood glucose monitoring — 家庭血糖モニター

Hb H
hemoglobin H — ヘモグロビンH

Hb-HP
hemoglobin-haptoglobin (complex) — ヘモグロビン・ハプトグロビン(複合体)

HBI
half body irradiation — 半身照射

HBID
hereditary benign intraepithelial dyskeratosis — 遺伝性良性上皮内異角化症

H

HBIG, HBIg
hepatitis B immunoglobulin — B型肝炎免疫グロブリン

HBISG
hepatitis B immunoserum globulin — B型肝炎血清免疫グロブリン

HBK
habekacin — ハベカシン

Hb Kansas
mutant hemoglobin with a low affinity for oxygen — 酸素低親和性突然変異ヘモグロビン

HBL
hepatoblastoma — 肝芽細胞腫

HBLA
human B lymphocyte antigen — ヒトBリンパ球抗原

Hb Lepore
hemoglobin Lepore — ヘモグロビンレポア

HbM
hemoglobin M — ヘモグロビンM

HBO
hyperbaric oxygenation — 高圧酸素治療
hyperbaric oxygen therapy — 高圧酸素療法

HBO, HbO
oxygenated hemoglobin — 酸化ヘモグロビン

HBOC
human breast and ovarian cancer — ヒトの乳癌と卵巣癌

HBP
hepatic-binding protein — 肝結合蛋白
high blood pressure — 高血圧
hydrocortisone butylate propionate — 酪酸プロピオン酸ヒドロコルチゾン

Hb P
hemoglobin P — ヘモグロビンP
primitive hemoglobin — 胎児ヘモグロビン

HBr
hydrobromic acid　臭化水素酸

Hb R
methemoglobin reductase　メトヘモグロビン還元酵素

HBS
HEPES buffered saline　HEPES緩衝食塩水
hydrodynamically balanced system　水力学的平衡系
hyperkinetic behavior syndrome　多動行動症候群

Hb S
hemoglobin S(=sickle cell hemoglobin)　ヘモグロビンS，鎌状赤血球ヘモグロビン

HBs，HBS
hepatitis B surface　B型肝炎表面

HBSA
human B cell specific antigen　ヒトB細胞特異抗原

HBsAb
hepatitis B surface antibody　B型肝炎s抗体，HBs抗体

HBsAg，HBs-Ag
hepatitis B surface antigen　B型肝炎s抗体，HBs抗原

HbSC
hemoglobin SC(=sickle cell hemoglobin C)　ヘモグロビンSC，鎌状赤血球ヘモグロビンC

HbSC disease
hemoglobin SC disease　ヘモグロビンSC病

HbS disease
hemoglobin S disease　ヘモグロビンS病

HBSS
Hanks balanced salt solution　ハンクス平衡食塩水

HbSS
hemoglobin SS　ヘモグロビンSのホモ接合型

HBT
human breast tumor　ヒト乳腺腫瘍

HBV
hepatitis B virus　B型肝炎ウイルス

HBW
high birth weight　高出生時体重

H/BW
heart-to-body weight (ratio)　心(臓)/体重(比)
height-to-body weight (ratio)　身長/体重(比)

HBZ
hemoglobin zeta chain　血色素ζ鎖

HC
hair cell　有毛細胞
Hassall corpuscles　(甲状腺)ハッサル小体
head circumference　頭囲
head compression　頭部圧迫

health center	保健所
heart cycle	心サイクル
heavy chain	H鎖，重鎖
heavy chain of myosin	ミオシンH鎖
hemoglobin concentration	血色素濃度
hemorrhage, cerebral	脳出血
hemorrhagic colitis	出血性大腸炎
heparin cofactor	ヘパリン補因子
hepatic catalase	肝カタラーゼ
hepatitis C	C型肝炎
hepatocellular cancer	肝細胞癌
hereditary coproporphyria	遺伝性コプロポルフィリン症
hexachlorethane	ヘキサクロルエタン
high calorie	高カロリー
hippocampus	海馬
histochemistry	組織化学
home care	家庭治療
homocystinuria	ホモシスチン尿〔症〕
Huntington chorea	ハンチントン舞踏病
hyaline casts	硝子円柱
hyaline cell	硝子細胞
hydranencephaly	水無脳症
hydraulic concussion	水力振盪症
hydrocarbon	炭化水素
hydrocortisone	ヒドロコルチゾン
hydrocortisone acetate	酢酸ヒドロコルチゾン
hydroxycorticoid	ヒドロキシコルチコイド
hydroxycorticosterone acetate	酢酸ヒドロキシコルチコステロン
hypercholesterolemia	高コレステロール血症
hyperplastic cell	過形成細胞
hypertrophic cardiomyopathy	肥大型心筋症

HCII

heparin cofactor II	ヘパリンコファクターII

HC-3

hemicholinium-3	ヘミコリニウム3

H & C

heroin and cocaine	ヘロインとコカイン

h & c, H & C

hot and cold (water)	熱(い〔温かい〕水)と冷(たい水)

HCA

hepatocellular adenoma	肝細胞腺腫
hydrocortisone acetate	酢酸ヒドロコルチゾン

H

H-CAP
hexamethylmelamine, cyclophosphamide, adriamycin, cisplatin (=Platinol) ヘキサメチルメラミン,シクロホスファミド,アドリアマイシン,シスプラチン(=プラチノール)

hcap, HCAP
handicap(ped) 障害(のある), ハンディキャップ(のある)

HCAT
human cell agglutination test ヒト血球凝集試験

HCC
hepatitis contagiosa canis (virus) イヌ伝染性肝炎(ウイルス)
hepatocellular carcinoma 肝細胞癌
hepatoma carcinoma cell 肝癌細胞
hexachlorocyclohexane ヘキサクロロシクロヘキサン
history of chief complaint 主訴の病歴
hydroxycholecalciferol ヒドロキシコレカルシフェロール(=ビタミンD)

25-HCC
25-hydroxycholecalciferol 25-ヒドロキシコレカルシフェロール

HCD
heavy chain disease H鎖病
hepatocerebral disease 肝脳疾患
high carbohydrate diet 高炭水化物食, 高糖質食
homologous canine distemper antiserum 同種属イヌジステンパー抗血清
hypertensive cardiac disease 高血圧性心疾患

HCE
hypoglossal carotid entrapment 舌下頸動脈絞扼

HCF
hereditary capillary fragility 遺伝性毛細血管脆弱症
host cell factor ホスト細胞因子
hypocaloric carbohydrate feeding 低カロリー炭水化物栄養補給

HCFA
Health Care Financing Administration 保健医療資金局

HCFI
histopathologic contractility failure index 病理組織学的収縮不全度

hCFSH
human chorionic follicle-stimulating hormone ヒト絨毛性卵胞刺激ホルモン

HCFU
1-hexylcarbamoyl-5-fluorouracil 1-ヘキシルカルバモイル-5-フルオロウラシル, カルモフール

hCG
human chorionic gonadotropin　ヒト絨毛性性腺刺激ホルモン
HCGF
hemopoietic cell growth factor　造血性細胞増殖因子
HCGN
hypocomplementemic glomerulonephritis　低補体血症性糸球体腎炎
HCG test，hCG test
human chorionic gonadotropin test　ゴナドトロピン負荷試験，hCG試験
HCH
1,2,3,4,5,6-hexachlorocyclohexane　1,2,3,4,5,6-ヘキサクロロシクロヘキサン
hygroscopic condenser humidifier　吸湿性コンデンサー湿度調節器

H

HCH，Hch
hemochromatosis　ヘモクロマトーシス
H chain
heavy chain　H鎖，重鎖
HCHWA
hereditary cerebral hemorrhage with amyloidosis　アミロイド症に伴う脳出血
HCHWA-D
hereditary cerebral hemorrhage with amyloidosis of Dutch type　オランダ型アミロイド(沈着)症を伴う(遺伝性)脳出血
HCI
homologous chromatid interchanges　相同染色分体間交換
HCIA
Health Care Improvement Act　(米国)保健質的改善法
HCL
hairy cell leukemia　ヘアリーセル白血病，毛様細胞性白血病
hard contact lens　ハードコンタクトレンズ
hydrochloric acid　塩酸，塩化水素酸
hydrogen chloride　塩化水素
HCLF
high carbohydrate,low fiber (diet)　高炭水化物低線維(食)
HCM
heart-cell conditioned medium　心臓細胞条件下培地
host-controlled modification　宿主依存性変異
hypertrophic cardiomyopathy　肥大型心筋症
HCMM
hereditary cutaneous malignant melanoma　遺伝性皮膚悪性黒色腫
HCMV
human cytomegalovirus　ヒトサイトメガロウイルス

HCN
hereditary chronic nephritis　遺伝性慢性腎炎
hydrocyanic acid　シアン化水素酸，青酸
hydrogen cyanide　シアン化水素

HCNS
Health Care Network System　保健ネットワーク組織

HCO
hylotates concolor〈ラ〉　クロテナガザル

HCO_3^-
sodium bicarbonate　重炭酸イオン，炭酸水素イオン

HCP
hepatic coproporphyria　肝性コプロポルフィリン症
hereditary coporphyria　遺伝性コポルフィリン症
hereditary coproporphyria　遺伝性コプロポルフィリン症
hexachlorophene　ヘキサクロロフェン

hcp，HCP
handicap(ped)　障害(のある)，ハンディキャップ(のある)

HCR
hemin-controlled repressor　ヘミン調節性レプレッサー
host cell reactivation　宿主回復
hysterical conversion reaction　ヒステリー性変換反応

hcrit
hematocrit　ヘマトクリット

HCS
Hajdu-Cheney syndrome　ハジュ・チェネー症候群
health care support　保健医療サポート
hematocystic spot　血嚢胞点
holocarboxylase synthetase　ホロカルボキシラーゼ合成酵素
hourglass contraction of stomach　胃砂時計状収縮
human chrionic somatomammotropin　ヒト胎盤性乳腺刺激ホルモン
human chorionic somatotropin　ヒト絨毛性ソマトトロピン
human cord serum　ヒト臍帯血清
hydroxycorticosteroid　ヒドロキシコルチコステロイド

HCS，hCS，hcs
human chorionic somatomammotropin(=human placental lactogen)　ヒト絨毛性ソマトマンモトロピン(=ヒト胎盤性ラクトゲン)

HCSD
Health Care Studies Division　保健医療研究部

HCSM, hCSM

human chorionic somatomammotropin (=human placental lactogen)	ヒト絨毛性ソマトマンモトロピン(=ヒト胎盤性ラクトゲン)

HCSS

hypersensitive carotid sinus syndrome	過敏性頸動脈洞症候群

HCT

Health Check Test	健康チェック検査
heart-circulation training	心(臓)循環訓練
histamine challenge test	ヒスタミンチャレンジ試験, 攻撃誘導試験
historic control trial	病歴対照試験
homocytotrophic	同種細胞親和性の
hydrochlorothiazide	ヒドロクロロチアジド
hydrocortisone	ヒドロコルチゾン
hydroxycortisone	ヒドロキシコルチゾン

Hct

hematocrit (value)	ヘマトクリット(値)

hCT

human calcitonin	ヒトカルシトニン
human chorionic thyrotropin	絨毛性甲状腺刺激ホルモン

HCTA

homocytotropic antibody	同種細胞向抗体

HCTD

hepatic computed tomography density	肝コンピュータ断層撮影吸収度
high cholesterol and tocopherol deficient	高コレステロールおよびトコフェロール欠乏(症)

HC telephone

handicapped telephone	身体障害者用電話

HCTU

home cervical traction unit	在宅頸椎牽引ユニット

HCTZ, Hctz

hydrochlorothiazide	ヒドロクロロチアジド

HCU

high care unit	高度集中治療室
homocystinuria	ホモシスチン尿(症)
hyperplasia cystica uteri	子宮嚢胞過形成

HCV

hepatitis C virus	C型肝炎ウイルス
home care ventilation	在宅人工呼吸
host-controlled variation	宿主依存性変異
human coronary virus	ヒト冠状ウイルス

HCVD

hypertensive cardiovascular disease	高血圧性心血管疾患

H

HCVR
hypercapnic ventilatory response　高炭酸ガス換気反応

HCVS
human coronavirus sensitivity　ヒトコロナウイルス感受性

HCW
health care workers　保健従事者

HCY
haemocyanin　ヘモシアニン

Hcy
homocysteine　ホモシステイン

H-Cys
cysteine reductase　シスチン還元酵素

HD
central system of hemodialysis　多人数用透析液供給装置
Haab-Dimmer (syndrome)　ハーブ・ディンマー(症候群)
Hajna-Damon (broth)　ハジナ・デーモン(肉汁)
haloperidol decanoate　デカン酸ハロペリドール
Hanganutziu-Deicher　ハンガヌチウ・ダイヘル
Hansen disease　ハンセン病
hard disk　ハードディスク
head down　頭部低下，頭低位
hearing distance　聴取距離
heart disease　心(臓)疾患，心臓病
helium dilution　ヘリウム希釈
Heller-Dor (procedure)　ヘラー・ドール(手技)
heloma durum〈ラ〉=hard corn　硬鶏眼
hemidiaphragm　片側横隔膜
hemodialysis　血液透析
hemolytic disease　溶血性疾患
hepatitis D　D型肝炎
herniated disc　椎間板ヘルニア
high density　高密度
high dosage　多量
high dose　大量
hip disarticulation　股関節離断(術)
Hirschsprung disease　ヒルシュスプルング病
Hodgkin disease　ホジキン病
hormone dependent　ホルモン依存性の
hospital day　入院期間
house dust　ハウスダスト
Huntington disease　ハンチントン(舞踏)病
hydatid disease　包虫症
preoperative isovolumic hemodilution　術前血液希釈

hd
half desmosome　半デスモゾーム
head　頭

6-HD
6-hydroxydopamine 6-ヒドロキシド(ー)パミン

HD_{50}
50% hemolyzing dose of complement 補体の50%溶血量

h.d.
hora decubitus〈ラ〉=at bedtime 就寝時に

HDBH
α-hydroxybutyrate dehydrogenase αヒドロキシブチレートデヒドロゲナーゼ

HDC
hemodialysis chronica〈ラ〉 慢性血液透析
histidine decarboxylase ヒスチジンデカルボキシラーゼ
human diploid cell ヒト二倍体細胞

H

HDCA
hyodeoxycholic acid ヒオデオキシコール酸

HDCS
human diploid cell strain (system) ヒト二倍体細胞株(系)

HDF
hemodiafiltration 血液濾過透析(法)
host defensive factor 宿主防御因子

HDFL
human development and family life ヒトの発育と家庭生活

HDFP
hypertension detection and follow-up program 高血圧検出・追跡プログラム

HDG
high-dose group 高用量群, 高線量群
hypotonic duodenography 低緊張性十二指腸造影

HDGF
hypothalamus-derived growth factor ウシ視床下部由来成長因子

HDH
heart disease history 心疾患歴
Hostility and Direction of Hostility 敵意と敵意傾向

HDHQ
Hostility and Direction of Hostility Questionaire 敵意と敵意傾向のための質問票

HDI
Health and Development Initiative 保健と開発に関するイニシアティブ
hemorrhagic disease of infants 乳児出血性疾患
hexamethylene-diisocyanate ヘキサメチレン・ジイソシアネート
host defense index 生体防衛指数
human development index 人間開発指数

H disease
Hartnup disease　ハートナップ病
HDIT
home drug infusion therapy　在宅薬剤注入療法
HDL
high density lipoprotein　高比重リポ蛋白
HDL cholesterol
high density lipoprotein cholesterol　HDLコレステロール，高比重リポ蛋白コレステロール
HDL determination
high density lipoprotein determination　高比重リポ蛋白の測定
HDLP
high density lipoprotein　高比重リポ蛋白
HDLS
hereditary diffuse leukoencephalopathy with spheroids　遺伝性び漫性白質脳症
HDLW
hearing distance, watch at left ear　時計音による左耳聴能距離
HDM
hexadimethrine　ヘキサジメスリン
house dust mite　ハウスダストダニ
HDMP
high-dose methylprednisolone　大量メチルプレドニゾロン
HDMTX
high-dosc methotrexate　大量メトトレキサート
HDN
hemolytic disease of newborn　新生児溶血性疾患
hemorrhagic disease of newborn　新生児出血性疾患
human diabetic neuropathy　ヒト糖尿病性神経障害
hDNA
deoxyribonucleic acid, histone　デオキシリボ核酸・ヒストン
HDP
hexose diphosphate　ヘキソース二リン酸
high density polyethylene　高比重ポリエチレン
hold-down pressure　血圧センサー固定圧
HDPA
Hospital Discharge Planners Association　退院後計画協会
HDPAA
heparin-dependent platelet-associated antibody　ヘパリン依存性(血)小板関連抗体
HDRV
human diploid rabies vaccine　ヒト二倍体狂犬病ワクチン

HDRW
hearing distance, watch at right ear　時計音による右耳聴能距離
HDS
Hamilton depression scale　ハミルトンうつ病評価尺度
herniated disc syndrome　ヘルニア板症候群
hospital discharge survey　退院調査
HDS-R
Revised Hasegawa dementia scale　改訂長谷川式簡易知能評価スケール

HDU
head-drop-unit　落差単位
hemodialysis unit　血液透析室
HDV
hepatitis D virus　D型肝炎ウイルス

HDZ
hydralazine　ヒドララジン
HE
height of eye　眼の高さ
hemagglutinating encepholamyelitis　赤血球凝集性脳脊髄炎
hematoxylin eosin stain　ヘマトキシリンエオジン染色
hemoglobin electrophoresis　血色素電気泳動
hepatic encephalopathy　肝性脳症
hepatitis E　E型肝炎
hereditary elliptocytosis　遺伝性楕円赤血球症
high explosive　高度爆発性の
human engineering　人間工学
human enteric　ヒトの腸の
hyperbaric enema　高圧浣腸
hypophysectomy　下垂体切除術
hypothalamic extract　視床下部抽出物
He
helium　ヘリウム〈元素〉
H & E
heredity and environment　遺伝と環境
he, he.
head　頭(部)
HEA
hexone-extracted acetone　ヘキソン抽出アセトン
human erythrocyte antigen　ヒト赤血球抗原
human erythrocyte test　ヒト赤血球試験
HEADSS
home life, education level, activities, drug use, sexual activity, suicide ideation/attempts　(青年期病歴上の)家庭生活・教育水準・活動・薬物使用・性的行動・自殺観念/企図

HEAL
Human Exposure Assessment Locations　人体曝露評価計画

HEAR
hospital emergency administrative ratio　病院救急管理率

HEAT
human erythrocyte agglutination test　ヒト赤血球凝集試験

HEB
hematoencephalic barrier　血液脳関門

hebdom
hebdomada〈ラ〉　(生後) 1 週間

HEC
hamster embryo cell　ハムスター胚細胞
high endothelial cells　高血管内皮細胞
Hospital Ethics Committee　病院倫理委員会
human endothelial cell　ヒト内皮細胞
hydroxyergocalciferol　ヒドロキシエルゴカルシフェロール
hydroxyethyl cellulose　ヒドロキシエチルセルロース

HE classification
Heath-Edward classification　ヘス・エドワード分類

HED
Hauteinheitsdosis〈独〉　皮膚単位量
Hauterythemdose〈独〉　皮膚紅斑(線)量

HEDH
hypohidrotic ectodermal dysplasia with hypothyroidism　甲状腺(機能)低下(症)に伴う無汗性外胚芽形成異常症

HEEA
home elemental enteral alimentation　在宅経腸栄養法

HEEH
home elemental enteral hyperalimentation　在宅経腸栄養法
Home enteral elemental hyperalimentation　在宅成分栄養法

HEENT
head, eyes, ears, nose, and throat　頭・目・耳・鼻・咽喉

HEF
hamster embryo fibroblast　ハムスター胚線維芽細胞
human embryo fibroblast　ヒト胎児線維芽細胞

HEG
hemorrhagic erosive gastritis　出血性びらん性胃炎

hEGF
human epidermal growth factor　ヒト表皮性成長因子

HEH
home enteral hyperalimentation　家庭〔在宅〕用経腸高カロリー輸液
2-hydroxy ethyl hydrazine　2-ヒドロオキシ・エチルヒドラジン

HEI
homogeneous enzyme immunoassay　均一酵素免疫測定法

HE inj.
hyperextension injury　過伸展損傷

HEIR
high-energy ionizing radiation　高エネルギーイオン化放射能

HEIS
high-energy ion scattering　高エネルギーイオン散乱
high-energy ion scattering spectroscopy　高速イオン散乱分光法

HEK
human embryo kidney (cell)　ヒト胚腎(細胞)

HEL
hen egg-white lysozyme　ニワトリ卵白リゾチーム
human embryonic lung　ヒト胚肺
human erythroleukemia　ヒト赤白血病

HELF
human embryonic lung fibroblasts　ヒト胚肺線維芽細胞

HELLP
hemolysis-elevated liver (enzyme)-low platelet (syndrome)　溶血・肝酵素上昇・血小板減少(症候群), ヘルプ(症候群)

HELP
heat escape lessening posture　熱放出緩和姿勢
heparin-(induced) extracorporeal LDL precipitation　ヘパリン誘発体外LDL沈殿法
heparin-induced extracorporeal low-density lipoprotein precipitation　ヘパリン誘発体外低比重リポ蛋白沈殿法, LDL沈殿法
Heroin Emergency Life Project　ヘロイン緊急救命プロジェクト

hel rec
health record　健康記録

Hem
hematology　血液(病)学

hem
hematuria　血尿
hemoglobin　ヘモグロビン
hemorrhage　出血
hemorrhoid　痔(核)

Hem, hem.
hemolysis　溶血

hemolytic 溶血性の

HEMA

hydroxyethyl methacrylate 水酸化エチルメタクリレイト

hydroxyethyl methylcellulose ヒドロキシエチルメチルセルロース

hemat

hematocrit ヘマトクリット

HEMAT, hemat.

hematology 血液(病)学

hematem

hematemesis 吐血

Hematol, hematol.

hematologist 血液学者, 血液病専門医

hematology 血液(病)学

Hemi

hemisphere 半球

hemi

hemiparalysis 片麻痺, 半側麻痺

hemiplegia 片麻痺, 半側麻痺

Hemo

hemorrhoid 痔(核)

hemo

hemoglobin ヘモグロビン, 血色素

hemophilia 血友病

hemocyt

hemocytometer 血球計, 血球計算板

hemop

hemoptysis 喀血

hemorr

hemorrhage 出血

hemorrhagic 出血性の

hemorrh

hemorrhage 出血

HEMPAS

hereditary erythrocytic multinuclearity with positive acidified serum test 酸性血清試験陽性の遺伝性赤血球多核

HEMT

high electron mobility transistor 高電子移動度トランジスター

HEN

home enteral nutrition 在宅経管栄養法

HEOD

1,2,3,4,10,10-hexachloro-6,7-epoxy-1,4,4α,5,6,7,8,8α-octahydro-endo-1,4-exo-5,8-dimethanonaphthalene ディルドリン

HEP	
hemolysis end point	溶血終了点
hepatic	肝(性)の
hepatoerythropoietic porphyria	肝赤血球産生性ポルフィリン症
high egg passage (virus)	高度鶏卵継代(ウイルス)
high-energy phosphate	高エネルギーリン酸塩
human epithelial cells	ヒト上皮細胞
hep, HEP	
hepatitis	肝炎
HEPA filter	
high efficiency particulate air filter	高性能微粒子フィルター
Hep/Clav	
hepatoclavicular	肝鎖骨の
HEPES	
N-2-hydroxyethylpiperazine-*N*′-2-ethanesulfonic acid	*N*-2-ヒドロキシ〔水酸化〕エチルピペラジン-*N*′-2′-エタンスルホン酸
HEPM	
human embryonic palatal mesenchymal cell	ヒト胎児の二次口蓋の間葉組織から樹立された細胞
HEPPS	
N-2-hydroxyethylpiperazine-*N*′-2-propanesulfonic acid	*N*-2-ヒドロキシ〔水酸化〕エチルピラペジン-*N*′-2-プロパンスルホン酸
HER	
hemodynamic erectile response	血行動態拡張反応
hemorrhagic encephalopathy virus of rat	ラット出血性脳症ウイルス
her.	
hernia	ヘルニア，脱出
herb	
herba〈ラ〉	草《処》
herb.recent.	
herbarium recentium〈ラ〉＝of fresh herbs	新鮮薬草の
hered	
hereditary	遺伝性の
heredity	遺伝
hern	
hernia	ヘルニア，脱出
herniation	ヘルニア
HES	
hematoxylin-eosin stain	ヘマトキシリン・エオジン染色
hydroxyethyl starch	ヒドロキシエチルデンプン

hypereosinophilic syndrome	好酸球増多症候群
hES	
human embryonic skin	ヒト胚皮膚
human embryonic spleen	ヒト胚脾臓
HET	
helium equilibration time	ヘリウム平衡時間
heterozygous	異形接合の，ヘテロ接合の
HETE	
hydroxyeicosatetraenoic acid	ヒドロキシエイコサテトラエン酸
12-L-hydroxy-5,8,10,14-epicosatetraenoic acid	12-L-ヒドロキシ-5,8,10,14-エピコトラエン酸
5-HETE	
5-hydroxy-eicosatetraenoic acid	5-ヒドロキシ-エイコサテトラエン酸
heterog	
heterogenous	異種発生の
HETP	
height equivalent to a theoretical plate	理論的な高さ
hexaethyl tetraphosphate	四リン酸ヘキサエチル
HEV	
health and environment	健康と環境
hemagglutination encephalomyelitis virus	赤血球凝集脳脊髄炎ウイルス
hepatitis E virus	E型肝炎ウイルス
hepato-encephalomyelitis virus	肝脳脊髄炎ウイルス
high endothelial venules	高内皮細静脈
human enteric virus	ヒトエンテロウイルス
HEV light	
high-energy visible light	高エネルギー可視光線
HEW	
health, education and welfare	健康, 教育, 福祉
Hex	
hexose	六炭糖
hex	
hexagon	六角
hexagonal	六角の
hexa	
hexamethylene tetramine	メセナミン
HEXA, Hex A	
hexosaminidase A	ヘキソサミニダーゼA

Hexa-CAF
hexamethylmelamine, cyclophosphamide, amphotericin, B, 5-fluorouracil — ヘキサメチルメラミン,シクロホスファミド,アンホテリシンB,フルオロウラシル

HEXB, Hex B
hexosaminidase B — ヘキソサミニダーゼB

HF
Hageman factor — ハーゲマン因子
hard feces — 硬便
hay fever — 枯草熱
head flat — 頭部水平
head of fetus — 胎児頭部
heart failure — 心不全
helper factor — ヘルパー因子
hemofiltration — 血液濾過
hemorrhagic factor — 出血因子
hemorrhagic fever — 出血熱
hepatocyte function — 肝細胞機能
Herzfrequenz〈独〉 — 心拍数
high fat (diet) — 高脂肪(食)
high-flux dialyzer — 高流量血液透析
high frequency — 高頻度, 高周波数
Hooker Forbes method — フッカー・フォーブス法
human fibroblasts — ヒト線維芽細胞

Hf
hafnium — ハフニウム〈元素〉
haplotype frequency — ハプロタイプ頻度

HF, hf.
half — 半分の

HFA
hydroxy fatty acid — 水酸化肪脂酸

H_4FA
L(-)-5,6,7,8-tetrahydrofolic acid — L(-)-5,6,7,8-テトラヒドロ葉酸

HFAS
hereditary flat adenoma syndrome — 遺伝性アデノーマ〔扁平腺腫〕症候群

HFC
hard filled capsules — 固く充填されたカプセル
high-frequency current — 高周波電流

HFCWC
high-frequency chest wall compression — 高頻度胸壁圧迫法

HFD
hemorrhagic fever of deer — シカ出血(性)熱

high fiber diet 高線維食
high forceps delivery 高位鉗子分娩

HFD infant
heavy-for-dates infant 過大体重児

HFEC
human foreskin epithelial cell ヒト包皮上皮細胞

HFF
high-frequency fatigue 高周波数型疲労

HFF, hFF
human foreskin fibroblast ヒト包皮線維芽細胞

HFG
hand-foot-genital (syndrome) 手・足・性器(症候群)

HFH
hemifacial hyperplasia 片側〔半側〕顔面の過形成

hFH
heterozygous familial hypercholesterolemia ヘテロ接合性家族性高コレステロール血(症)

HFI
hereditary fructose intolerance 遺伝性果糖不耐症
hyperostosis frontalis interna〈ラ〉 内前頭骨過形成

HFI, hFI
human fibroblast interferon ヒト線維芽細胞インターフェロン
human freedom index 人間自由度指標

HFIF, hFIF
human fibroblast interferon ヒト線維芽細胞インターフェロン

HF inj
hyperflexion injury 過屈曲損傷

HFJV
high-frequency jet ventilation 高頻度ジェット換気〔呼吸〕(法)

HFK
hollow fiber kidney 中空型人工腎臓

HFL, hFL
human fetal lung ヒト胎児肺

HFM
hemifacial microsomia 片側〔半側〕顔面小人症

HFMD
hand foot and mouth disease 手足口病

HFO
high-frequency oscillation 高頻度振動

HFOV
high-frequency oscillatory ventilation 高頻度振動換気法〔呼吸法〕

HFP
hypofibrinogenic plasma 低フィブリノゲン血漿

H

HFPPV	
high-frequency positive pressure ventilation	高頻度陽圧呼吸〔換気〕
HFR	
high-frequency range	高周波域
Hfr	
high-frequency of recombination	高頻度(染色体)組換え(株)
HFRS	
hemorrhagic fever with renal syndrome	腎症候性出血熱
HFS	
habitual facial spasmus	習慣性顔面痙攣
hemifacial spasm	片側〔半側〕顔面痙攣
hydrocele funiculi spermatica	精索水瘤
HFSH, hFSH	
human follicle stimulating hormone	ヒト卵胞刺激ホルモン
HFT	
hemofiltration therapy	血液濾過療法
Hft	
high-frequency transduction	高頻度(形質)導入
HFU	
hand-foot-uterus (syndrome)	手足子宮(症候群)
HFUPR	
hourly fetal urine production rate	胎児時間尿産生率
HFV	
high-frequency ventilation	高頻度(人工)換気〔呼吸〕法
HG	
handgrip	握手，握力
head girth	頭囲
hepatogram	肝機能検査図表
herpes genitalis	陰部ヘルペス〔疱疹〕
herpes gestationis〈ラ〉	妊娠(性)疱疹，妊娠(性)ヘルペス
Herter-Gee (syndrome)	ハーター・ジー(症候群)
Heschl gyri	ヘッシュル回
histaglobin	ヒスタグロビン
Hutchinson-Gilford (syndrome)	ハッチンソン・ギルフォード症候群
hybrid granulocyte	ハイブリッド顆粒球
hypoglycemia	低血糖(症)
Hg	
hemoglobin	ヘモグロビン，血色素
hydrargyrum〈ラ〉＝mercury	水銀〈元素〉，水銀柱
hg	
hectogram	ヘクトグラム(＝100g)

H

HG, hG
human gonadotrop(h)in　ヒト性腺刺激ホルモン
human growth factor　ヒト成長〔生長〕因子

HGA
homogentisic acid　ホモゲンチシン酸

HGAAS
hydrogenation atomic absorption spectrometry　水素発生原子吸光分析

HGB, Hgb, hGB, hgb.
hemoglobin　ヘモグロビン，血色素

Hgb & Hct
hemoglobin and hematocrit　ヘモグロビン〔血色素〕とヘマトクリット

HGC
hypoglycemic coma　低血糖性昏睡

HGD
high-grade dysplasia　高度形成異常(症)

HGE
human granulocytic ehrlichiosis　ヒト顆粒球性エールリヒア症

H-G effect
hydrocarbon-glycol effect　炭化水素グリコール効果

HGF
heparin-binding growth factor　ヘパリン結合成長因子
hepatocyte growth factor　肝細胞増殖因子
hybridoma growth factor　ハイブリドーマ成長因子(＝IL-6)
hyperglycemic glycogenolytic factor　過血糖性糖原分解因子

HgF
fetal hemoglobin　胎児ヘモグロビン

HG factor
herpes gestationis factor　妊娠性疱疹因子

HGG
herpetic geniculate ganglionitis　ヘルペス性膝神経節炎
hippurylglycyl glycine　馬尿酸グリシルグリシン
Hopalemus griseus griseus〈ラ〉　ハイイロキツネザル

HGG, hGG
human gamma globulin　ヒトガンマグロブリン

hGH
human growth hormone　ヒト成長ホルモン

HGL
hepatic glyceride lipase　肝由来グリセリドリパーゼ

HGM
hog gastric mucin　ブタ胃ムチン

HGMF
hydrophobic grid membrane filter　メンブランフィルター法

H

HGN
membranous glomerulonephritis 膜性糸球体腎炎

HGO
hepatic glucose output 肝ブドウ糖排出量

HGO, hGO
human glucose output ヒトブドウ糖排出量

HGP
hepatic glucose production 肝ブドウ糖産生
hyperglobulinemia purpura 高グロブリン血(性)紫斑病, グロブリン過剰血紫斑病

HGPRT
hypoxanthine(-guanine) phosphoribosyltransferase ヒポキサンチン(グアニン)ホスホリボシルトランスフェラーゼ

HGPS
Hutchinson-Gilford progeria syndrome ハッチンソン・ギルフォード早老症候群

HGRF, hGRF
human growth hormone releasing factor ヒト成長ホルモン刺激因子

HGS
hysterosalpingography 子宮卵管造影法

HGSIL
high-grade squamous intraepithelial lesion 高度落屑性上皮内病変

Hgt
height 高さ, 身長

HGV
hepatitis G virus G型肝炎ウイルス

HH
halothane hepatitis ハロタ〔セ〕ン肝炎
hard of hearing 難聴
Head-Holms (syndrome) ヘッド・ホームズ(症候群)
hematogonadotropic hypogonadism 低ゴナドトロピン性性(腺)機能低下〔不全〕症
hemodialysis-induced hypoxemia 血液透析誘発性低酸素血症
Henderson and Haggard (inhaler) ヘンダーソン・ハッガード(吸入器)
hereditary-hyperglycemic 遺伝性過血糖症
hiatal hernia 裂孔ヘルニア
home help(er) 在宅介助(者), 在宅介護
homonymous hemianopia 同名半盲
Hunter-Hurler (syndrome) ハンター・フルラー(症候群)
hydroxyhexamide ヒドロキシヘキサミド
hypergastrinemic hyperchlorhydria 高ガストリン血症性過塩酸症
hyperhidrosis 発汗過多(症), 多汗(症)

hyporeninemic hypoaldosteronism　低レニン血症性低アルドステロン血症

Hh

hedgehog　ハリネズミ

hh

heavy hydrogen　重水素

h/h

hard of hearing　難聴

H & H

hemoglobin and hematocrit　ヘモグロビンとヘマトクリット

HHA

hereditary hemolytic anemia　遺伝性溶血性貧血

hypothalamic hypophyseal adrenal　視床下部・下垂体・副腎の

HHAA

hypothalamic hypophyseal adrenal axis　視床下部・下垂体・副腎軸

HHB

un-ionized hemoglobin　イオン化されない血色素

HHb

reduced hemoglobin　還元ヘモグロビン

HHB, HHb

hypohemoglobinemia　低ヘモグロビン血症

HHC

home health care　家庭内健康管理

HHCS

high-altitude hypertrophic cardiomyopathy syndrome　肥大型心筋症症候群，高山〔高所〕病

HHD

high heparin dose　高ヘパリン量

hogshead　ホッグズヘッド

hypertensive heart disease　高血圧性心疾患

HHE

hemiconvulsions-hemiplegia-epilepsy (syndrome)　片側痙攣・片麻痺・てんかん（症候群）

HHED

hereditary hidrotic ectodermal defect　遺伝性有汗性外胚葉形成異常症

HHG

hypertrophic hypersecretory gastropathy　過形成性過分泌性胃疾患

hHG

human hypophyseal gonadotropin　ヒト下垂性性腺刺激ホルモン

H

H

HHH
hyperornithinemia, hyperammonemia and homocitrullinemia (syndrome) 高オルニチン血症・高アンモニア血症・ホモシトリン血症(症候群)

HHHO
hypotonia, hypomentia, hypogonadism and obesity (syndrome) 筋緊張低下・精神障害・性機能不全〔低下〕・肥満(症候群)

HHI
Henderson-Heggard inhaler ヘンダーソン・ヘッガード吸入器

HHIE
Hearing Handicap Inventory for Elderly 老人の聴力障害度調査[米国]

HHL
hippuryl-L-histidyl-L-leucine 馬尿酸-L-ヒスチジル-L-ロイシン

Hypophysenhinterlappen〈独〉 下垂体後葉

HHLL
histocytoid hemangioma-like lesion 組織細胞様血管腫様病変

HHM
hemohydrometry (液体)比重測定(法)

humoral hypercalcemia of malignancy 悪性(体液性)高カルシウム血症

hyalohyphomycosis 無色糸菌症

H+Hm, H-Hm
compound hypermetropic astigmatism 複性遠視性乱視

HHN
hyperosmolar hyperglycemic nonketotic (syndrome) 高浸透圧性高血糖性非ケトン性(症候群)

HHNK
hyperglycemic hyperosmolar nonketotic (coma) 高血糖性高浸透圧性非ケトン性(昏睡)

HHNKS
hyperglycemic hyperosmolar nonketotic syndrome 高血糖性高浸透圧性非ケトン性症候群

HHO
hypotonia-hypomentia-obesity (syndrome) 筋緊張低下・精神障害・肥満(症候群)(＝H_2O症候群)

HHPC
hyperoxic-hypercapnic 高酸素(症)・高炭酸ガス(症)の

HHRH
hereditary hypophosphatemic rickets with hypercalciuria 遺伝性低リン血症性くる病

HHS

Department of Health and Human Service	保健福祉省
hereditary hemolytic syndrome	遺伝性溶血性症候群
hyperkinetic heart syndrome	運動過多性心臓症候群，心運動亢進症

HHT

hereditary hemorrhagic telangiectasia	遺伝性出血〔溶血〕性毛細(血)管拡張症
hydroxyheptadecatrienoic acid	ヒドロキシ・ヘプタデカトリエノン酸

HHTA

hypothalamo-hypophyseal-thyroidal axis	視床下部・下垂体・甲状腺軸

HHV1〔2,3…7〕

human herpes virus 1〔2,3…7〕	ヒトヘルペスウイルス 1〔2,3… 7〕型

HI

Harrington instrumentation	(側彎症に対する)ハリントン法
head injury	頭部外傷
hearing impaired	聴力障害された
heart infusion	心(臓)滲出液
heat inactivated	熱不活化された
hemagglutination inhibition	血球凝集抑制反応
hepatic insufficiency	肝(機能)不全
hormone independent	ホルモン非依存性
hormone insensitive	ホルモン非感受性の
hospital insurance	病院保険
humidity index	湿度指数
humoral immunity	体液性免疫
hydriodic acid	ヨウ化水素酸
hydroxyindole	ヒドロキシインドール
hyperglycemic index	高血糖指数
hypoglycemic index	低血糖指数
hypothermic ischemia	低体温性虚血

HI, Hi

histidine	ヒスチジン

HIA

hemagglutination inhibition antibody	(赤)血球凝集抑制抗体
hemagglutination inhibitory antibody	(赤)血球凝集抑制抗体
Hospital Industries Association	病院産業協会

HIAA

Health Insurance Association of America	米国健康保険協会

5-HIAA
5-hydroxyindoleacetic acid — 5-ヒドロキシインドール酢酸

HIB
Haemophilus influenzae type B — インフルエンザ菌B型
hemolytic immune body — 溶血性免疫体

HIC
hydrophobic interaction chromatography — 疎水性クロマトグラフィ

H-ICDA
International Classification of Disease, Adopted Code for Hospitals — 病院用の国際疾患分類

H

HICH
hypertensive intracerebral hemorrhage — 高血圧性脳(内)出血

Hi CHO
high carbohydrate (diet) — 高炭水化物(食)，高糖質(食)

HiCN
cyanmethemoglobin — シアンメトヘモグロビン

HID
hallucination, illusions and delusions — 幻覚・錯覚・妄想
headache, insomnia, depression (syndrome) — 頭痛・不眠・うつ(症候群)
herniated intervertebral disc — 椎間板ヘルニア
hyperkinetic impulse disorder — 運動過剰(症)の衝動障害

HIDA
dimethyl iminodiacetic acid — ジメチル・イミノジ酢酸

HID-AB stain
high iron diamine-alcian blue stain — 高鉄ダイアミン・アルシアンブルー染色

HIDH
heat-stable lactic dehydrogenase — 耐熱性乳酸脱水素酵素

HIE
human intestinal epithelial (cell) — ヒト腸上皮(細胞)
hyperimmunoglobulin E — 高免疫グロブリンE
hypoxic ischemic encephalopathy — 低酸素性・虚血性脳障害

HIES
hyperimmunoglobulinemia E syndrome — 高IgE症候群

HIF
Health Information Foundation — 保健情報財団
higher intellectual function — 高次精神〔知能〕機能
histoplasma tissue inhibitory factor — ヒストプラズマ組織抑制因子

HIFBS
heat-inactivated f(o)etal bovine serum　熱不活化ウシ胎仔血清

HIFC
hog intrinsic factor concentrate　ブタ内因子濃縮物
human intrinsic factor concentrate　ヒト内因子濃縮

HIFCS
heat-inactivated f(o)etal calf serum　熱不活化ウシ胎仔血清

HiFi
high fidelity　高性能の再現性

hiflex
high flexibility　高可撓性

HIFU
high intensity focused ultrasound　超音波

HIg
human immunoglobulin　ヒト免疫グロブリン

HIGMI
hyper-IgM immunodeficiency syndrome　高IgM型免疫不全(症候群)

HIH
Heidenhain-iron-hematoxylin　ハイデンハイム・鉄・ヘマトキシリン

HII
Health Insurance Institute　健康保険研究所
hemagglutination inhibition immunoassay　(赤)血球凝集抑制免疫定量(法)

HIIC
heated intraoperative intraperitoneal chemotherapy　術中腹腔内化学療法

HIL
hypoxic-ischemic lesion　低酸素性・虚血性損傷

HILA
high impulsiveness, low anxiety　強い衝動・軽度の不安

HILIC
hydrophilic interaction chromatography　親水性相互作用クロマトグラフィ

HIM
hematopoietic inductive microenvironment　赤血球産生微小環境
hepatitis-infectious mononucleosis　肝炎・伝染性単核症
hexose phosphate isomerase　リン酸六炭糖イソメラーゼ
host induced modification　宿主依存性変異

HIMA
Health Industry Manufactures Association　保健産業製造業者協会

H

HIMAC
Heavy Ion Medical Accelerator in Chiba　重粒子線癌治療装置
HIMP
high-dose intravenous methylprednisolone　大量静脈内メチルプレドニゾロン投与
HIMSS
Healthcare Information and Management Systems Society　医療情報管理システム協会
HIMT
hemagglutination inhibition morphine test　(赤)血球凝集抑制モルヒネ試験
Hind II〔III〕
restriction endonuclease from *Haemophilus influenzae* Rd II〔III〕　インフルエンザ菌由来の制限エンドヌクレアーゼ, ヒンズ・ツー〔スリー〕

H inf
hypodermoclysis infusion　皮下注入
HINI
hypoxic-ischemic neuronal injury　低酸性・虚血性ニューロン損傷
H & Ins
health and accident insurance　健康と損害保険
Hint
Hinton　ヒントン(梅毒検査)
Hint test
Hinton test　ヒントン試験
HIO
hele-in-one technique　ホールインワン技法
hypoiodism　低ヨード症
hypoiodite　次亜ヨウ素酸塩
HIO_3
iodic acid　ヨウ素酸
HIOMT
hydroxyindole-*O*-methyltransferase　ヒドロキシインドール-*O*-メチル転移酵素
HIOS
high index of suspicion　高い疑惑指数
HIP
Health Insurance Plan　健康保険計画
Help for Incontinent People　失禁患者援助協会
hippocampus〈ラ〉　海馬
homograft incus prosthesis　同種移植人工キヌタ骨
hospital insurance program　病気保険プログラム
humoral immunocompetence profile　体液(性)免疫能プロフィール
hydrostatic indifference point　流体静力学的中性点

HIPC
Health Insurance Purchasing Copperative グループ医療保険
hormone independent prostate cancer ホルモン非依存性前立腺癌(腫)

HIPE
hospital inpatient enquiry 病院入院患者調査

HiPIP
high-potential iron protein 高能力鉄蛋白

HIPO
hemihypertrophy, intestinal web, preauricular skin tag and congenital corneal opacity (syndrome) 片側〔半側〕肥大・腸ウェブ・耳介前方糸状線維腫・先天性角膜混濁(症候群)

HIPP
hippocampus〈ラ〉 海馬
Hippocrates ヒポクラテス

HiPro
high protein (diet) 高蛋白(食)

Hi Prot
high protein (diet) 高蛋白(食)

HIR
head injury routine 頭部外傷処理手順
high irradiance response 高照射応答
histological incorporation ratio 組織学的骨置換率

HIRB
Health Insurance Registration Board 健康保険登録委員会

HIRF
histamine inhibitory releasing factor ヒスタミン抑制放出因子

HIS
Hanover Intensive Score ハノーバー集中(治療)スコア
health information system 健康情報システム
Health Interview Survey 健康状態観察調査
hospital information systems 病院情報システム
hyperimmune serum 高免疫血清

His
histidyl ヒスチジル

His, HIS
histidine ヒスチジン

HISG
human immune serum globulin ヒト免疫血清グロブリン

HISS
human immune status survey ヒト免疫状態調査

Hist.
histologist 組織学者
histology 組織学

H

Hist, hist
- histamine　ヒスタミン
- histidine　ヒスチジン
- histidinemia　ヒスチジン血症
- history　病歴

histo
- histoplasmosis　ヒストプラズマ症

Histol
- histologist　組織学者
- histology　組織学

HIT
- health indication test　健康適応検査
- hemagglutination inhibition test　赤血球凝集抑制試験
- heparin induced thrombocytopenia　ヘパリン誘発〔誘因〕性血小板減少症
- histamine inhalation test　ヒスタミン吸入試験
- histamine ion transfer　ヒスタミン・イオン転換
- Holtzman inkblot technique　ホルツマンインクブロット手法
- home infusion therapy　在宅輸液療法
- hypertrophic infiltrative tendinitis　肥大性浸潤性腱炎
- hypertrophied inferior turbinate　肥大下鼻甲介
- hysteroscopic insemination into tube　子宮鏡下卵管内精子注入法，卵管内受精

HITB
- *Hemophilus influenzae* type B　インフルエンザ菌B型

HITES
- hydrocortisone, insulin, transferrin, estradiol, selenium　ヒドロコルチゾン・インスリン・トランスフェリン・エストラジオール・セレン

HI test
- hemagglutination inhibition test　赤血球凝集抑制試験

HITT
- hematoma irrigation with trephination therapy　極小開頭血腫洗浄除去法
- heparin-induced thrombocytopenia with thrombosis　血栓症に伴うヘパリン誘困性血小板減少症

HITTS
- heparin-induced thrombosis-thrombocytopenia syndrome　ヘパリン誘因性血栓症・血小板減少症候群

HIU
- head injury unit　頭部外傷ユニット
- hyperplasia interstitialis uteri　子宮間質過形成

HIV
- human immunodeficiency virus　ヒト免疫不全ウイルス

HIV-AB	
human immunodeficiency virus antibody	ヒト免疫不全ウイルス抗体，HIV抗体
HIVAN	
HIV-associated nephropathy	HIV関連腎症
HIVAT	
home intravenous antibiotic therapy	在宅静脈抗生物質療法
HIVD	
herniated interverterbral disc	椎間板ヘルニア
HIVH	
home intravenous hyperalimentation	在宅静脈内高カロリー栄養法
HIVIG	
anti-HIV immune serum globulin	抗HIV免疫血清グロブリン
HIV immunoglobulin	HIV免疫グロブリン
HIV infection	
human immunodeficiency virus infection	ヒト免疫不全ウイルス感染症，HIV感染症
HIV-P	
human immunodeficiency virus-associated periodontitis	ヒト免疫不全ウイルス関連歯周炎
HIV-SGD	
HIV-associated salivary gland disease	HIV関連唾液腺病
HJ	
Howell-Jolly (bodies)	ハウエル・ジョリー(小体)
HJB	
Howell-Jolly bodies	ハウエル・ジョリー小体
HJR	
hepatojugular reflux	肝頸静脈逆流
HK	
Hall-Kaster	ホール・カスター
Hauptklage〈独〉	主訴
heat killed	熱殺菌された
hexokinase	ヘキソキナーゼ
Hoffa-Kastert (syndrome)	ホッファー・カスタート(症候群)
human kidney (cells)	ヒト腎(細胞)
HK1	
hexokinase-1	ヘキソキナーゼ1
H-K	
hand to knee	手膝(試験)
HK, H-K	
heel to knee (test)	踵膝(試験)
HKAFO	
hip-knee-ankle-foot-orthosis	骨盤帯付き長下肢装具

HKAO
hip-knee-ankle-orthosis　股・膝・足関節装具

HKC
human kidney cells　ヒト腎細胞

HKH-syndrome
hyperkinetic heart syndrome　過運動性心症候群，心運動亢進症

HKLM
heat-killed *Listeria monocytogenes*　熱殺菌リステリア菌

HKO
hip-knee orthosis (splint)　股関節・膝装具(副子)

HK Raum
Holzknechtscher Raum〈独〉　ホルツクネヒト腔

HKS
heel-knee-shin (test)　踵・膝・脛(試験)
herpes keratitis simplex　単純ヘルペス角膜炎
hyperkinesis syndrome　多動症候群

HK virus
Hong-Kong type of influenza virus　香港型インフルエンザウイルス

HL
hairline　毛のはえぎわ
half life　半減期
hallux limitus　可動制限母趾
harelip　兎唇
Harnleiter〈独〉　尿管
hearing level　聴力レベル
hearing loss　聴力損失
heat labile　熱不耐性
hemolysin　溶血素
hemolysis　溶血
hepatic lipase　肝性リパーゼ
Hickman line　ヒックマンライン
histiocytic lymphoma　細網肉腫・組織球性リンパ腫
histocompatibility locus　組織適合遺伝子座
Hodgkin lymphoma　ホジキンリンパ腫
human leukocyte　ヒト白血球
human lymphocyte　ヒトリンパ球
hydrophil/lipophil (number)　親水性/親油性(数)
hyperlipidemia　高脂血症
hyperlipoproteinemia　高リポ蛋白血症
hypertrichosis lanuginosa　うぶ毛性多毛症
hypoplastic leukemia　低形成性白血病

hl
hectoliter　ヘクトリットル(＝100l)

H/L
high/low amplitude electromyogram (ratio) 筋電図の高低振幅比
hydrophil/lipophil (ratio) 親水性/親油性(比)

H & L
heart and lungs 心臓と肺

HL, Hl, H/L
latent hypermetropia 潜在〔潜伏〕性遠視

HL, h.l.
hearing loss 聴力損失・難聴

HLA
heart, lungs and abdomen 心臓・肺・腹
histocompatibility locus antigen 組織適合抗原
homologous leukocytic antibodies 同種白血球抗体
human leukocyte antigen ヒト白血球抗原
human lymphocyte antibody ヒトリンパ球抗体
human lymphocyte antigen ヒトリンパ球抗原
hylobates lar〈ラ〉 シロテナガザル
hypoplastic left atrium 左(心)房形成不全

HLAA
human leukocyte antigen A ヒト白血球抗原A

HLA antigen
human leukocyte antigen ヒト白血球抗原

HLAB
human leukocyte antigen B ヒト白血球抗原B
human lymphocyte antigen B ヒトリンパ球抗原B

HLAC
human lymphocyte antigen C ヒトリンパ球抗原C

HLAD
human leukocyte antigen D ヒト白血球抗原D
human lymphocyte antigen D ヒトリンパ球抗原D

HLAL
human leukocyte antigen L ヒト白血球抗原L

HLALD
horse liver alcohol dehydrogenase ウマ肝アルコール脱水素酵素

HLB
hydrophil-lipophil balance 親水性・親油性バランス

HLBI
human lymphoblastoid interferon ヒトリンパ芽球(性)インターフェロン

HLC
Hospital Library Council 病院図書館審議会

HLD
half lethal dose 50%致死量
hepatolenticular degeneration 肝レンズ核変性(症)
herniated lumbar disc 腰部椎間板ヘルニア

hypersensitivity lung disease 過敏性肺疾患
von Hipple-Lindau disease フォンヒッペル・リンダウ病

HLD, HL-D
haloperidol decanoate デカン酸ハロペリドール

HLDA
human leukocyte differentiation antigen ヒト白血球分化抗原

HLDH
heat-stable lactic dehydrogenase 耐熱性乳酸デビドロゲナーゼ〔脱水素酵素〕

HLE
human leukocyte elastase ヒト白血球エラスターゼ

HLF
heat-labile factor 熱不安定因子
human lung field ヒト肺野

HLG
hypertrophic lymphocytic gastritis 肥厚性リンパ球(性)胃炎

hlg
halogen ハロゲン

HLGF
hemolymphopoietic growth factor 血液リンパ生成成長因子

HLH
helix-loop-helix ヘリックス・ループ・ヘリックス(のDNA結合モチーフ)
hemophagocytic lymphohistiocytosis 血球貪食細胞性リンパ組織球増多(症)

hLH
human luteinizing hormone ヒト黄体化ホルモン

HLHS
hypoplastic left heart syndrome 左(心)室低形成症候群

HLI
hemolysis inhibition 溶血(反応)抑制
human leukocyte interferon ヒト白血球インターフェロン
human lymphocyte interferon ヒトリンパ球インターフェロン

HLK
heart, liver, kidney 心臓・肝臓・腎臓

HLLT
high reactive level laser treatment 高反応レベルレーザー治療

HLN
hilar lymph node 肺門リンパ節
human Lesch-Nyhan (cell) ヒトレッシュ・ナイハン(細胞)
hyperplastic liver nodule 増殖性肝(臓)小結節

H

HL number
hydrophil-lipophil number 親水性・親油性数
H & L OK
heart and lungs normal 心臓と肺正常
HLP
haloperidol ハロペリドール
hepatic lipoperoxidation 肝脂質超酸化反応
hyperkeratosis lenticularis perstans 恒久性レンズ形角質増加症
hyperlipoproteinemia 高リポ蛋白血症
HLR
heart-lung ratio 心肺係数
heart lung resuscitation 心肺蘇生(法)
HLS
Hippel-Lindau syndrome ヒッペル・リンダウ症候群
hypertonic lactated Ringer solution 高張乳酸加リンゲル液
hyperttonic lactated saline solution 高張乳酸加食塩液
HLT
heat labile toxin 易熱性毒素
hlth.
health 健康，保健
H-L Tx
heart-lung transplantation 心肺(同時)移植
HLV
herpes-like virus ヘルペス様ウイルス
hypoplastic left ventricle 左室低形成
HLVS
hypoplastic left ventricular syndrome 左室低形成症候群
HM
hand movements, hand motion 手動弁
health maintenance 健康維持
heart murmur 心雑音
Heine-Medin (disease) ハイネ・メイディーン(病)
heloma molle〈ラ〉=soft corn 軟鶏眼
hemifacial microsomia 片側〔半側〕顔面小人症
hemiplegic migraine 片麻痺性片頭痛
hepatic metabolism 肝代謝
Holter monitoring ホルターモニター
homosexual male 男性同性愛者
human milk 母乳
hydatidiform mole 胞状奇胎
hm
hectometer ヘクトメートル(=100m)
hydroxymethyl ヒドロキシメチル
H.m.
manifest hypermetropia 顕性遠視

H

HMA
hemorrhages and microaneurysm　出血・微細動脈瘤
HMB
homatropine methylbromide　メチル臭化ホマトロピン
HMBA
hexamethylenebisacetamide　ヘキサメチレンビスアセトアミド
HMC
hand-mirror cell　手鏡細胞
heroin, morphine, cocaine　ヘロイン・モルヒネ・コカイン
hydroxylmethyl cellulose　ヒドロキシルメチルセルロース
5-hydroxymethyl cytosine　ヒドロキシメチルシトシン
hypertelorism-microtia-clefting (syndrome)　隔離症・小耳症・裂(症候群)
3-HMC
3-hydroxymethyl-β-carboline　3-ヒドロキシメチル-β-カルボリン
HMCCMP
human mammary carcinoma cell membrane proteinase　ヒト乳癌細胞膜プロテイナーゼ
HMCE
hereditary multiple cartilaginous exostosis　遺伝性多発性軟骨性外骨症
HMC hypodermic tablets
hyoscine, morphine, cactus hypodermic tablets　ヒヨスチン・モルヒネ・カクタス・皮下注射剤
5hmCyt
5-hydroxymethyl cytosine　5-ヒドロキシメチルシトシン
HMD
hyaline membrane disease　肺胞硝子膜症
2-hydroxymethylene-17α-methyldihydrotestosterone　2-ヒドロキシメチレン-17αメチルジヒドロテストステロン
5hmdCyd
5-hydroxymethyl deoxycytidine　5-ヒドロキシメチルデオキシシチジン
hMDGF
human macrophage derived growth factor　ヒトマクロファージ増殖因子
5hmdUrd
5-deoxymethyl deoxyuridine　5-ヒドロキシメチルデオキシウリジン
HME
heat & moisture exchanger　熱湿交換器

HMF
hydroxymethylfurfural　ヒドロキシメチルフルフラル

HMG
high mobility group　高運動性群
hydroxymethylglutaryl　ヒドロキシメチルグルタリル

hMG
human menopausal gonadotropin　ヒト閉経期尿性性腺刺激ホルモン

HMG-CoA
β-hydroxy-β-methylglutaryl-cocarboxylase A　βヒドロキシ-βメチルグルタリル・コカルボキシラーゼA
hepatic hydroxymethyl-glutaryl coenzyme A　肝ヒドロキシメチルグルタリルコエンザイムA
3-hydroxy-3-methylglutaryl coenzyme A　3-ヒドロキシ-3-メチルグルタリルコエンザイムA

HMG-CoA reductase
hydroxymethylglutaryl coenzyme A reductase　ヒドロキシメチルグルタリルコエンザイムA還元酵素

hMG-hCG
human menopausal gonadotropin-human chorionic gonadotropin　ヒト閉経期ゴナドトロピン・ヒト絨毛性ゴナドトロピン

HMG-HCG therapy
human menopausal gonadotropin-human chorionic gonadotropin therapy　HMG・HCG療法

HMG test
human menopausal gonadotropin test　ゴナドトロピン負荷試験, HMG試験

HMI
healed myocardial infarction　治癒した心筋梗塞

HMK
high molecule kininogen　高分子キニノゲン

HML
human milk lysozyme　人乳リゾチーム
Hypophysenmittellappen〈独〉　下垂体中葉

HMM
heavy meromyosin　重メロミオシン
hexamethylmelamine　ヘキサメチルメラミン

HMMA
4-hydroxy-3-methoxymandelic acid　4-ヒドロキシ-3-メトキシマンデル酸

HMO
Health Maintenance Organization　保健維持機構
heart minute output　毎分心拍出量

HMP
hemolysis maximum point 最大溶血点
hexamethylphosphoramide ヘキサメチルホスホラミド
hexose monophosphate pathway ヘキソース一リン酸経路
human menopausal ヒト閉経期の

HMPA
hexamethylphosphoramide ヘキサメチルホスホラミド

HMPAO
^{99m}Tc-hexamethyl-propyleneamine oxime テクネチウム・ヘキサメチル・プロピレナミン・オキシム

HMPS
hexose monophosphate shunt ヘキソース一リン酸経路，HMP側路

HMPT
hexamethylphosphoric triamide ヘキサメチルリン酸トリアミド

HMR
histiocytic medullary reticulosis 髄索性組織球性細網症

H-mRNA
H-chain messenger ribonucleic acid H鎖伝令リボ核酸

hMRP
human multidrug resistance associated protein ヒト多剤耐性蛋白

HMRS
Howmedica Modular Resection System ホウメディカ基準切除

HMRTE
human milk reverse transcriptase enzyme ヒト乳逆転写酵素

HMS
Harvard Medical School ハーバード医科大学
hexose monophosphate shunt ヘキソース一リン酸経路
high molecular weight renin substance 高分子レニン抽出物
hour, minute, second 時・分・秒
hyaline membrane syndrome ヒアリン膜症候群
hydroxymesterone ヒドロキシメステロン
hyperactive malarial splenomegaly 過反応性マラリア性脾腫
hypermobility syndrome 過剰運動性症候群

HMSAS
hypertrophic muscular subaortic stenosis 肥大性〔肥厚性〕筋性大動脈弁下部狭窄(症)

HMSN
hereditary motor sensory neuropathy 遺伝性運動知覚〔運動感覚性〕ニューロパシー

HMT
hematocrit ヘマトクリット
hexamethylenetetramine ヘキサメチレンテトラミン
histamine methyltransferase ヒスタミンメチルトランスフェラーゼ
4-hydroxy-17α-methyltestosterone 4-ヒドロキシ-17α-メチルテストステロン

hMT
human molar thyrotropin ヒトモル甲状腺刺激ホルモン

HMU
5-hydroxymethyl uracil ヒドロキシメチル・ウラシル

5hmUra
5-hydroxymethyl uracil 5-ヒドロキシメチルウラシル

HMV
heart minute volume 分時心拍出量
heart minute volume index 分時心拍出量指数
Herzminutenvolumen〈独〉 毎分心拍出量
home mechanical ventilation 在宅人工換気療法
human melanoma cell line ヒト黒色腫細胞系

HMVECs
human dermal microvascular endothelial cells ヒト皮膚血管内皮細胞

HMW
high molecular weight 高分子量

HMWC
high molecular weight component 高分子量成分

HMW kininogen
high molecular weight kininogen 高分子キニノゲン

HN
Hansfield number ハンスフィールド値
head nurse 看護師長
Heller-Nelson (syndrome) ヘラー・ネルソン(症候群)
hemagglutinin neuraminidase 赤血球凝集素ノイラミニダーゼ
hematemesis neonatorum 新生児吐血
hemorrhage of newborn 新生児出血
hereditary nephritis 遺伝性腎炎
high nitrogen 高窒素
hilar node 肺門部リンパ節
histamine-containing neuron ヒスタミン含有ニューロン
home nursing 在宅看護
human nutrition ヒト栄養
hyperplastic nodule(s) 過形成節
hypertensive nephrosclerosis 高血圧性腎硬化(症)
hypertrophic neuropathy 肥厚性〔肥大性〕ニューロパシー

H

h.n.
hoc nocte〈ラ〉=tonight 今夜
H & N
head and neck 頭(部)と頸(部)
HN2, HN_2
nitrogen mustard(=mechlorethamine) ニトロゲンマスタード(=メクロルエタミン)
HNA
heparin neutralizing activity ヘパリン中和活性
HNAC
Heymann nephritis antigenic complex ハイマン腎炎抗原複合体
HNB
human neuroblastoma ヒト神経芽(細胞)腫
hydroxynitrobenzylbromide ヒドロキシニトロベンジルブロミド
HNB-DMSH
dimethyl(-2-hydroxy-5-nitrobenzyl) sulfonium halide ハロゲン化ジメチル(-2-ヒドロキシ-5-ニトロベンジル)スルホニウム
HNC
head and neck cancer 頭(部)頸部癌(腫)
human neutrophil collagenase ヒト好中球コラゲナーゼ
hypernephroma cell 副腎腫細胞
hyperosmolar nonketotic coma 高浸透圧性非ケトン性昏睡
hyperoxic normocapnic 高酸素(症)・炭酸(ガス)正常状態の
hypothalamic-neurohypophyseal complex 視床下部・神経下垂体複合体
HNCM
hypertrophic nonobstructive cardiomyopathy 非閉塞性肥大型心筋症
HNE
human neutrophil elastase ヒト好中球エラスターゼ
4-hydroxy-2-nonenale 4-ヒドロキシ-2-ノネナール
HNK
human natural killer cell(s) ヒトNK細胞
HNKC
hyperosmolar nonketotic coma 高浸透圧性非ケトン性昏睡
HNKDC
hyperosmolar nonketotic diabetic coma 高浸透圧性非ケトン性糖尿病昏睡
HNKDS
hyperosmolar nonketotic diabetic state 高浸透圧性非ケトン性糖尿病状態

HNL
heparin-novo-lente　ヘパリン・ノボ・レンテ
HNLN
hospitalization no longer necessary　もはや入院の必要なし
H & N mot.
head and neck motion　頭頸部運動
HNN
hemorrhagic nephrosonephritis　出血性ネフローゼ腎炎
HNO
Hals Nasen und ohren-heilkunde〈独〉　耳鼻咽喉科
HNOH
Hals-Nasen-Ohren-Heilkunde〈独〉　耳鼻咽喉科学
HNP
hereditary nephritic protein　遺伝性腎炎蛋白
herniated nucleus pulposus　頸椎椎間板ヘルニア，髄核ヘルニア
human neurophysin　ヒトニューロフィシン
HNPCC
hereditary non-polyposis colorectal cancer　遺伝性非ポリープ性結腸直腸癌
hnRNA, HnRNA
heterogenous nuclear RNA(=ribonucleic acid)　不均一核リボ核酸，ヘテロ(ジナス)核リボ核酸
hnRNP
heterogeneous nuclear ribonucleoprotein　ヘテロ(ジナス)核リボ核蛋白
HNS
head and neck surgery　頭頸部外科
head, neck and shaft　頭部・頸部・骨幹部
hypophyseal-neurohypophyseal system　視床下部神経下垂体系
hypothalamus-neurohypophyseal system　視床下部神経下垂体系
HNSHA
hereditary nonspherocytic hemolytic anemia　遺伝性非球状赤血球性溶血性貧血
HNTD
highest nontoxic dose　最大非中毒量
HNTLA
Hiskey-Nebraska Test of Learning Aptitude　ヒスキー・ネブラスカ学習適性検査
HNV
has not voided　無効になっていない，排尿していない
HO
heterotopic ossification　異所性骨化

H

high oxygen 高酸素
Holt-Oram (syndrome) ホールト・オーラム(症候群)
house officer 研修医
hydrophilic ointment 親水軟膏
hyperbaric oxygen 高圧酸素
hypertrophic osteoarthropathy 肥大性骨関節症

Ho
holmium ホルミウム〈元素〉

ho
hydroxy ヒドロキシの

H_2O
hypotonia-hypomentia-obesity (syndrome) 筋緊張低下・精神障害・肥満(症候群)(＝HHO症候群)
water 水

H_2O_2
hydrogen peroxide 過酸化水素

H/O, h/o
history of ～の病歴

HOA
hip osteoarthritis 股関節骨関節炎
hypertrophic osteoarthritis 肥大性骨関節炎，過形成関節症

HOADH
β-hydroxyacyl CoA dehydrogenase βヒドロキシアシルCoAデヒドロゲナーゼ

HOAP-BLEO
hydroxydaunomycin, vincristine (＝Oncovin), arabinosylcytosine, prednisone, bleomycin ヒドロキシダウノマイシン，ビンクリスチン(＝オンコビン)，アラビノシルシトシン，プレドニゾン，ブレオマイシン

HoaTTG
horse anti-tetanus toxoid globulin ウマ抗破傷風トキソイドグロブリン

HOB
head of bed ベッド頭部

HOB up SOB, HOB UP SOB
head of bed up for shortness of breath 呼吸困難のためベッド頭部を上げる

HOC
heavy organic chemical 重有機化合物
human ovarian cancer ヒト卵巣癌
hydroxycorticoid ヒドロキシコルチコイド

HOCA
high osmolar contrast agent 高浸透性造影剤

HOCM
high osmolar contrast medium　高浸透性造影剤
hypertrophic obstructive cardiomyopathy　肥大型閉塞性心筋症

hoc vesp.
hoc vespere〈ラ〉=this evening　今晩《処》

HOD
hereditary opalescent dentin　遺伝性オパール様〔乳白色〕象牙質
hospital day　入院期日
hyperbaric oxygen drenching　高圧酸素療法

HOF
hepatic outflow　肝流出
human oviduct fluid　ヒト卵管液

Hoff
Hoffmann (reflex)　ホフマン(反射)

H of F
height of fundus　子宮底の高さ，基底部高

Hoff refl
Hoffmann reflex　ホフマン反射

Hoff resp
Hoffmann response　ホフマン反応

H of sp
hybrid of species　雑種

HOG
halothane, oxygen and gas 〔nitrous oxide〕　ハロタ〔セ〕ン・酸素・ガス〔亜酸化窒素〕

HOGA
hyperornithinemia with gyrate atrophy　脳回転状萎縮に伴う高オルニチン血症

HOH
hard of hearing　難聴

HOI
hospital onset of infection　院内感染
hypoiodous acid　次亜ヨウ素酸

Holg
horse immunoglobulin　ウマ免疫グロブリン

HOM
hexamethylmelamine, vincristine (=Oncovin), methotrexate　ヘキサメチルメラミン, ビンクリスチン(=オンコビン), メトトレキサート

homatrop
homatropine　ホマトロピン，ホムアトロピン

H

HOME
Home-Oriented Maternity Experience　在宅出産経験
human omental microvascular endothelial　ヒト大網小動脈由来内皮細胞
Homeo
homeopathy　ホメオパシー，同毒療法の
homo
homeopathic　ホメオパシーの，同毒療法の
homeopathy　ホメオパシー，同毒療法
Homo, homo.
homosexaul　男性同性愛の，男性同性愛者
homolat
homolateral　同側の
H
HON
δhydroxy-γ-oxo-L-norvaline　δヒドロキシ-γ-オキソ-L-ノルバリン
HONK
hyperosmolar non-ketotic coma　高浸透圧性非ケトン性昏睡
HOOD
hereditary osteo-onychodysplasia　遺伝性骨爪異形成症
HOODS
hereditary onychoosteodysplasia syndrome　遺伝性爪甲・骨異形成(症候群)
HOP
high oxygen pressure　高酸素圧
hydroxydaunomycin, vincristine(=Oncovin), prednisone　ヒドロキシダウノマイシン，ビンクリスチン(=オンコビン),プレドニゾン
HOPA
calcium hopantenate　ホパテン酸カルシウム
HOPD
hospital outpatient department　病院外来部
HOPE
health opportunity people everywhere　どこでも健康な機会に恵まれた人々
health-oriented physical education　健康志向の体育
HOPG
highly oriented pyrolytic graphite　高配向熱分解黒鉛
HOPI
history of present illness　現症
HOPP
hepatic occluded portal pressure　肝閉塞門脈圧
HOQNO
N-heptylhydroquinoline-*N*-oxide　*N*-ヘプチルヒドロキノリン-*N*-オキシド

hor
horizontal — 水平(の), 水平面
hor.decu.
hora decubitus〈ラ〉=at bedtime — 就寝時に《処》
hor.decub.
hora decubitus〈ラ〉=at bedtime — 就寝〔就眠〕時に
hor.interm.
horis intermedius〈ラ〉, *hora intermedia*〈ラ〉=at the intermediate hour — 中間時に《処》
horiz
horizontal — 水平の
hor.som.
hora somni〈ラ〉=at the hour of sleep, at bedtime — 就寝時に《処》
hor.1 spat.
horae unius spatio〈ラ〉=one hour's time — 1時間
hor.un.spatio
horae unitus spatio〈ラ〉 — 時間の終りに《処》
horae unius spatio〈ラ〉=one hour's time — 1時間
HOS
Holt-Oram syndrome — ホールト・オーラム症候群
human osteosarcoma — ヒト骨肉腫
HoS
horse serum — ウマ血清
hosp
hospitalization — 入院
hospitalize — 入院させる
Hosp, hosp.
hospital — 病院
hosp ins
hospital insurance — 病院保険
HOST
hypo-osmotic shock treatment — 低浸透圧ショック治療
HOT
home oxygen therapy — 在宅酸素療法
human old tuberculin — ヒト旧ツベルクリン
hyperbaric oxygen therapy — 高圧酸素療法
HOTC
heterozygous ornithine transcarbamoylase — ヘテロ接合性オルニチントランスカルバモイラーゼ
hot labo
hot laboratory — 危険な実験作業室

HOTS

hypercalcemia-osteolysis-T cell syndrome	高カルシウム血症・骨溶解・T細胞症候群

HOW

hypothermia oxygen warmer	低体温(症)用酸素加温器

Ho : YAG

holmium : yttrium-aluminum-garnet	ホルミウム・イットリウム・アルミニウム・ガーネット

HP

Haemophilus pleuropneumoniae	ヘモフィルス(属)胸膜肺炎
handicapped person	身体障害者
Harding-Passey (melanoma)	ハーディング・パッセー(黒色腫)
hard palate	硬口蓋
Harnpack〈独〉	排尿パック
Harvard pump	ハーバードポンプ
heat production	熱産生
Helicobacter pylori	ヘリコバクターピロリ
hemiparesis	片側〔半側〕不全麻痺，不全片麻痺
hemipelvectomy	片側骨盤切除術，片側下肢切除術
hemodynamic profile	血液力学側面図
hemoglobinopathy	血色素異常症
hemoperfusion	血液灌流
heparin	ヘパリン
hepatomegaly	肝腫大
hereditary pancreatitis	遺伝性膵(臓)炎
heterophagosome	ヘテロファゴゾーム
highly purified	高純度の
high potency	高能力
high power	高性能
high pressure	高圧
high protein	高蛋白
history of present illness	現病歴
hormone product	ホルモン産生量
horsepower	馬力
house physician	病院住込医師
human pituitary	ヒト下垂体の
hydrocollator pack	吸水薬罨法
hydrophobic protein	疎水性蛋白
hydrostatic pressure	静水圧
hyperparathyroidism	副甲状腺機能亢進症
hyperphoria	上斜位
hypersensitive pneumonitis	過敏性肺臓炎
hypersensitivity pneumonitis	過敏性肺臓炎

hypertension and proteinuria 高血圧と蛋白尿
hypertension plus proteinuria 高血圧プラス蛋白尿
hypoparathyroidism 副甲状腺機能低下症
hypopharynx 下咽頭，咽頭喉頭部

Hp
hematoporphyrin ヘマトポルフィリン
hemiplegia 片麻痺

H/P
hemoglobin plasma ratio ヘモグロビン血漿比

H & P
history and physical examination 病歴と理学所見

H-P
Hilgenreiner-Perkins ヒルゲンライナー・パーキンス

HP，Hp
haptoglobin ハプトグロビン

HP，H→P
heel-to-patella 踵・膝蓋骨

HP，H.P.
hot pack 温パック，ホットパック

HP，H & P
Hodgen and Pearson (suspension traction) ホジェン・ピアーソン(懸吊牽引)

HPA
alpha haptoglobin αハプトグロビン
hemagglutination penicillin antibody 赤血球凝集性ペニシリン抗体
Hospital Physics Association 病院医薬協会
human platelet antigen ヒト血小板抗原
hypersomnia with periodic apnea 周期性無呼吸を伴う傾眠症
hypothalamic-pituitary-adrenal (axis) 視床下部・下垂体・副腎(軸)
hypothalamic-pituitary-adrenocortical 視床下部・下垂体・副腎皮質の
hypothalamic-pituitary-adrenocortical system 視床下部・下垂体・副腎皮質系

hPa
hectpascal ヘクトパスカル(＝mb)〈単位〉

HPAA
hydroperoxyarachidonic acid ヒドロペルオキシアラキドン酸
hydroxyphenylacetic acid ヒドロキシフェニル酢酸

HPAC
high performance affinity chromatography 高速親和性クロマトグラフィ

HPAT
home parenteral antibiotic therapy 在宅抗生物質注射療法
HPB
hypersomnia with periodic breathing 周期性呼吸を伴う傾眠症
HPBC
hyperpolarizing bipolar cell 過分極双極細胞
HPBF
hepatotropic portal blood factor 肝親和性門脈血因子
HPBL
human peripheral blood leukocyte ヒト末梢血白血球
HPC
hemangiopericytoma 血管周囲細胞腫，血管外皮細胞腫
hematopoietic precursor cell(s) 血液前駆細胞
hippocampal pyramidal cell(s) 海馬錐体細胞
history of present condition 現病歴
hydroxyphenyl-cinchoninic acid ヒドロキシフェニル・シンコニン酸
hydroxypropyl cellulose ヒドロキシプロピルセルロース
hydroxypropyl methylcellulose ヒドロキシプロピルメチルセルロース
hypopharyngeal carcinoma 下咽頭癌
HPCA
human plasma cell antigen ヒト形質細胞抗原
HPCC
high performance computing & communications 高性能情報処理通信
HPCD
hemostatic puncture closure device 止血穿刺閉鎖器具
HPCE
high performance capillary electrophoresis 高性能毛細管電気流動
HPCHA
hereditary high red cell membrane phosphatidyl choline hemolytic anemia 遺伝性高赤血球膜ホスファチジルコリン(＝レシチン)溶血性貧血
HPCM
human placental conditioned medium ヒト胎盤調整培地
human placental culture medium ヒト胎盤培養基
HPD
hemopoietic dysplasia 造血異形成
hereditary progressive dystonia 遺伝性進行性ジストニア
high protein diet 高蛋白食
home peritoneal dialysis 在宅腹膜透析

HpD
hematoporphyrin derivative　ヘマトポルフィリン誘導体
HP-D
Hough-Powell digitizer　ヒュー・パウエルのデジタル表示装置
hPDGF
human platelet derived growth factor　ヒト血小板由来成長因子
HPE
hepatic portoenterostomy　肛門部空腸吻合(術)
high permeability edema　高透過性浮腫
history and physical examination　病歴と理学的検査
hydrostatic pulmonary edema　静水性肺水腫
HPEASA
Health Professions Educational Assistance Act　保健関連職教員援助法
HPETE
hydroperoxy-eicosa-tetraenoic acid　ヒドロペルオキシ・エイコサ・テトラエノイン酸
HPF
hepatic plasma flow　肝血漿流量
high-pass filter　高周波通過フィルター
hyperplastic foci　過形成点
hypocaloric protein feeding　低カロリー蛋白食
Hp-F
heparinized fresh whole blood　ヘパリン加新鮮血液
HPF, hpf
high-power field　強拡大視野
/HPF, /hpf
per high-power field　強拡大の一視野(あたり)
HPFA
high-performance frontal analysis　高速先端分析法
HPFH
hereditary persistence of fetal hemoglobin　遺伝性高胎児ヘモグロビン症
hPFSH
human pituitary follicle stimulating hormone　ヒト下垂体卵胞刺激ホルモン
HPG
hypothalamic-pituitary-gonadal　視床下部・下垂体・性腺の
hPG
human pituitary gonadotropin　ヒト下垂体性腺刺激ホルモン
HPGF
hematopoietic growth factor　造血増殖因子
hybridoma plasma cell growth factor　ハイブリドーマプラズマ細胞増殖因子

hpGRF
human pancreatic growth hormone releasing factor　ヒト膵成長ホルモン放出因子

HPH
halothane-percent-hour　ハロタ〔セ〕ン・%・時

Hp-Hb complex
haptoglobin-hemoglobin complex　ハプトグロビン・ヘモグロビン複合体

HPI
hepatic perfusion index　肝灌流指数
Heston Personality Inventory　ヘストン人格調査表
history of present illness　現病歴

HPIC
high performance ion chromatography　高性能イオンクロマトグラフィ

HPL
Helix pomatia lectin　カタツムリレクチン
human parotid lysozyme　ヒト耳下腺リゾチーム
human peripheral lymphocyte　ヒト末梢血リンパ球
human placental lactogen　ヒト胎盤性ラクトゲン

HPL, hPL
human placental lactogen　ヒト胎盤性ラクトゲン

hPL
human prolactin　ヒトプロラクチン

HPLA
hydroxyphenyllactic acid　ヒドロキシフェニル乳酸

HPLAC
high pressure liquid affinity chromatography　高圧液体親和性クロマトグラフィ

HPLC
high performance liquid chromatography　高性能液体クロマトグラフィ

HPM
Harding-Passey melanoma　ハーディング・パッセイ黒色腫
hemiplegic migraine　片麻痺性片(側)頭痛
high performance membrane　高性能膜

HPMC
human peripheral mononuclear cell　ヒト末梢血単核細胞

HPMV
high pressure mechanical ventilation　高圧機械呼吸

HPN
home parenteral nutrition　在宅中心静脈栄養(法)

HPN, hpn.
hypertension　高血圧(症)

HPNME	
human peripheral nerve myelin extract	ヒト末梢神経ミエリン抽出物
HPNS	
high pressure nervous syndrome	高圧神経症候群
HPO	
high pressure oxygen (therapy)	高圧酸素(療法)
Hospital Physicians Organization	病院医師組織
hypertrophic pulmonary osteoarthritis	肥大性肺性骨関節炎
hypertrophic pulmonary osteoarthropathy	肥大性肺性骨関節症
Hpo-T	
hypotension	低血圧
HPP	
hereditary pyropoikilocytosis	遺伝性熱変性奇形赤血球
histaminopexic power	ヒスタミン固定力
history of presenting problems	現病歴
hPP	
human pancreatic polypeptide	ヒト膵ポリペプチド
2HPP	
two hours postprandial (blood sugar)	食後2時間の(血糖値)
HPPA	
hydroxyphenylpyruvic acid	ヒドロキシフェニルピルビン酸
HPPH	
hydroxyphenyl-phenylhydantoin	ヒドロキシフェニル・フェニルヒダントイン
HPPO	
high partial pressure of oxygen	高酸素分圧
hydroxyphenylpyruvate oxidase	ヒドロキシフェニルピルビン酸酸化酵素
hPPSH	
human pituitary follicle stimulating hormone	ヒト下垂体卵胞刺激ホルモン
HPR	
(4-)hydroxyproline	ヒドロキシプロリン
hPr	
human prolactin	ヒトプロラクチン，ヒト黄体刺激ホルモン
HPRF	
high pulse repetition frequency	高頻度繰り返し周波数
hPRL	
human prolactin	ヒトプロラクチン，ヒト黄体刺激ホルモン

H

HPRT

hypoxanthine phosphoribosyl transferase	ヒポキサンチンホスホリボシルトランスフェラーゼ

HPS

Hantavirus pulmonary syndrome	ハンタウイルス肺症候群
Health Physical Society	保健体育協会
hematoxylin, phloxine, saffron	ヘマトキシリン・フロキシン・サフロン
hemophagocytic syndrome	血球貪食症候群
Henoch-Schönlein purpura	ヘノッホ・シェーンライン紫斑病
hereditary pyloric stenosis	遺伝性幽門狭窄
Hermansky-Pudlak syndrome	ヘルマンスキー・パドラック症候群
high protein supplement	高蛋白補給
His Purkinje system	ヒス・プルキンエ系
human platelet suspension	ヒト血小板懸濁液
hypertrophic pyloric stenosis	肥厚性幽門狭窄(症)
hypothalamic pituitary system	視床下部下垂体系
hypothalamic pubertal syndrome	青春期視床下部症候群

HPSA

hepato-portal subtraction angiography	肝門脈サブトラクション血管造影法

HPSEC

high performance size-exclusion chromatography	高性能サイズ除外クロマトグラフィ

HPSN

hereditary pressure-sensitive neuropathy	遺伝性圧脆弱性神経疾患

HPT

hepaplastin test	ヘパプラスチン試験
hepatic pulse tracing	肝拍動図
histamine provocation test	ヒスタミン誘発試験
hot plate test	熱板試験
hyperparathyroidism	副甲状腺機能亢進症，上皮小体(機能)亢進症
hypothalamic-pituitary-thyroid	視床下部・下垂体・甲状腺の

Hpt

haptoglobin	ハプトグロビン

hPT

human placental thyrotropin	ヒト胎盤(性)甲状腺刺激ホルモン

HPTH

hyperparathyroid hormone	上皮小体(機能)亢進性ホルモン，副甲状腺機能亢進性ホルモン

hyperparathyroidism	上皮小体(機能)亢進(症)，副甲状腺機能亢進症
HPTIN	
human pancreatic trypsin inhibitor	ヒト膵トリプシン抑制因子
HPTLC	
high performance thin layer chromatography	高性能薄層クロマトグラフィ
HPTM	
home prothrombin time monitoring	在宅プロトロンビン時間モニタリング
hptn	
hypertension	高血圧
HPU	
heater probe unit	加熱プローブユニット
HPV	
Haemophilus pertussis vaccine	百日咳(菌)ワクチン
hepatic portal vein	肝門脈
high pressure ventilation	高圧換気
human papilloma viral infection	ヒト乳頭腫ウイルス感染
human papilloma virus	ヒト乳頭腫ウイルス
human parrot virus	ヒトオウム病ウイルス
human parvovirus	ヒトパルボウイルス
hypoxic pulmonary vasoconstriction	低酸素性肺血管攣縮
HPVD	
hypertensive pulmonary vascular disease	高血圧性肺血管疾患
HPVG	
hepatic portal venous gas	肝門脈ガス
HPVV	
human papilloma virus vaccine	HPVワクチン，子宮頸癌ワクチン
HPX	
hypophysectomized	下垂体摘出術を受けた
partial hepatectomy	部分的肝切除
Hpx	
hemopexin	ヘモペキシン，凝血酵素
HPZ	
high pressure zone	高圧帯
HQC	
hydroxyquinoline citrate	クエン酸ヒドロキシキノリン
HR	
Halstead-Reitan (battery)	ハルステッド・ライタン(検査)
Hamman-Rich (syndrome)	ハマン・リッチ(症候群)
heart rate	心拍数
hemorrhagic retinopathy	出血性網膜症

heterosexual relations (scale) 異性関係(尺度)
high resolution 高溶解性
high resolution collimator 高分解能コリメーター〔視準器〕
high resolving 高分解能の
histamine receptor ヒスタミン受容体
homing receptor ホーミング受容体
hormone responsive ホルモン反応性の
hospital record 入院記録
hospital recruit 病院補充
hospital report 病院報告
Howship-Romberg (syndrome) ハウシップ・ロンベルグ(症候群)
hyperimmune reaction 超免疫反応
hypoxic responder 低酸素(症)性応答

Hr
Harn〈独〉 尿

hr
hour 時間

H2R
histamine$_2$ receptor ヒスタミン2受容体

H & R
hysterectomy and radiation 子宮摘出術と放射線照射

HRA
health risk appraisal 健康危険度評価
high right atrium 高右心耳
histamine releasing activity ヒスタミン放出活性
hospital resources administration 病院供給源管理

HRB
histamin release (from) basophils 塩基球からのヒスタミン放出

HRBC
horse red blood cell(s) ウマ赤血球
human red blood cell(s) ヒト赤血球

HRC
horse red cell(s) ウマ赤血球

HRCT
high resolution CT 高分解能CT

HRCV
human respiratory coronavirus ヒト呼吸器コロナウイルス

HRD
human retroviral disease ヒトレトロウイルス性疾患

hrd
hard 固い，困難な

HRE
high resolution electrocardiogram 高解像度心電図
high resolution electrocardiography 高解像度心電図検査法

hormone-receptor enzyme　ホルモン受容体酵素

HREC
hepatic reticuloendothelial cell　肝細網内皮細胞

H reflex
Hoffmann reflex　ホフマン反射

HREH
high renin essential hypertension　高レニン本態性高血圧(症)

HREM
high resolution electron microscope　高解像度電子顕微鏡
high resolution electron-microscopy　高分解能電子顕微鏡法

H response
Hoffmann response　ホフマン反応

HRF
heart reactive factor　心臓反応因子
histamine releasing factor　ヒスタミン遊離因子
homologous restriction factor　均一制限因子

HRG
Health Research Group　健康資源管理局
histidine-rich glycoprotein　ヒスチジンリッチグリコプロテイン

HRH
hypothalamic releasing hormone　視床下部放出ホルモン

HRHS
hypoplastic right heart syndrome　右心発育不全〔低形成〕症候群

HRI
Harrington rod instrumentation　ハリントンロッド装具
hemin-regulated inhibitor　ヘミン調節性インヒビター

HRIG，HRIg
human rabies immune globulin　ヒト狂犬病免疫グロブリン

HRLA
human reovirus-like agent　レオウイルス様因子(＝ロタウイルス)

HRLM
high resolution light microscopy　高分解能光学顕微鏡検査

hRNA
heterogeneous ribonucleic acid　ヘテロリボ核酸

HRNB
Halstead-Reitan Neuropsychological Battery　ハルステッド・ライタン神経心理学的検査

HRP
high-risk pregnancy　高度危険妊娠，ハイリスク妊娠
horseradish peroxidase　西洋ワサビペルオキシダーゼ

HRPD
Hamburg Rating Scale for Psychiatric Disorders　ハンブルグ精神障害評価尺度

HRPO	
horseradish peroxidase	西洋ワサビペルオキシダーゼ
hypodermic (injection)	皮下(注射)
HRQOL	
health related quality of life	健康に関連した生活の質
HRR	
Hardy, Rand & Ritter pseudoisochromatic plates	ハーディー・ランド・リッター色覚異常検査表
heart rate range	心拍数範囲
HRR plates	
Hardy, Rand & Rittler plates	ハーディー・ランド・リッター色覚異常検査表
HRS	
Hamilton Rating Scale	ハミルトン評点尺度
Haw River syndrome	ホー川症候群
hepatorenal syndrome	肝腎症候群
hormone receptor site	ホルモン受容体部位
humeroradial synostosis	上腕骨橈骨(骨)癒合症
hrs	
hours	時間
HRSA	
histamine rabbit serum albumin conjugate	ヒスタミンウサギ血清アルブミン接合
HRSD	
Hamilton Rating Scale for Depression	ハミルトンうつ病評価尺度
HRT	
heart rate	心拍数
histamine release test	ヒスタミン遊離試験
hormone replacement therapy	ホルモン補充療法
hydrolysis related transport	水解輸送
HRTEM	
high resolution transmission electron microscopy	高解像度〔高分解能〕透過型電子顕微鏡
HRV	
heart rate variability	心拍変動
human rotavirus	ヒトロタウイルス
HRVL	
human reovirus-like	ヒトレオウイルス様の
HRX	
human trithorax	急性骨髄性白血病での遺伝子
HS	
Hallervorden-Spatz (syndrome)	ハレルフォルデン・シュパッツ(症候群)
hamstring	膝腱，膝屈曲筋
Hartman solution	ハートマン液

healthy subject	健常者
heart sound	心音
heat seal	熱接着包装
heat stable	熱安定性の
heavy smoker	ヘビースモーカー
Hegglin syndrome	ヘグリン症候群
heme synthtase	ヘム〔血色素〕合成酵素，ヘムシンターゼ
Henoch-Schönlein (syndrome)	ヘノッホ・シェーンライン(症候群)
heparin sulfate	硫酸ヘパリン
hereditary spherocytosis	遺伝性球状赤血球症
herpes simplex	単純疱疹，単純ヘルペス
hidradenitis suppurativa	汗腺膿瘍，化膿性汗腺炎
high sensitivity collimator	高感度コリメーター
Höhensonne〈独〉	人工太陽灯
hopelessness scale	絶望スケール
hopeless scale	悲観的尺度
Horner syndrome	ホルナー〔ホルネル〕症候群
horse serum	ウマ血清
hospital stay	入院
hours of sleep	睡眠時間
house surgeon	院内外科医
human serum	ヒト血清
Hurler syndrome	フルラー〔ハーラー〕症候群
hypereosinophilic syndrome	好酸球増多症候群
hypcrsensitivity	過敏性，過敏症
hypertonic saline	高浸透圧食塩水
hypertrophic scar	肥厚性瘢痕

Hs

hair shampoo	洗髪
hypochondriasis	心気症，ヒポコンドリー(症)

H→S

heel-to-shin (test)	踵脛(検査)

H/S

helper/suppressor (ratio)	ヘルパー/サプレッサー(比)

H & S

hemorrhage and shock	出血とショック
hysterectomy and sterilization	子宮摘出と不妊術

HS, h.s.

hora somni〈ラ〉=hour of sleep, at bedtime	就寝時(に)《処》

HSA

Health Service Administration	保健サービス管理
hemi-spherical analyzer	同心半球型エネルギー分析器
homo sapiens〈ラ〉	ヒト

horse serum albumin	ウマ血清アルブミン
human salt-poor albumin	ヒト乏塩アルブミン
human serum albumin	ヒト血清アルブミン
hypersomnia-sleep apnea (syndrome)	睡眠過剰・睡眠時無呼吸(症候群)
hypothalamic secretory factor	視床下部分泌因子
HSAA	
Health Science Advancement Award	保健科学推進補助金
HSAN	
hereditary sensory and autonomic neuropathy	遺伝性知覚性自律神経性ニューロパシー
HSAP	
heat stable alkaline phosphatase	耐熱性アルカリホスファターゼ
HSAPDT	
heat stable acellular pertussis-diphteria-tetanus	耐熱性無細胞性の百日咳・ジフテリア・テタヌス・ワクチン
HSAS	
hypertrophic subaortic stenosis	肥大〔肥厚〕性大動脈弁下部狭窄(症)
HSBG	
heel-stick blood gas	かかと穿刺血液ガス
HSC	
Hand-Schüller-Christian (disease)	ハンド・シューラー・クリスチャン病
Health and Safety Code	保健安全法
hearing speech clinic	聾唖クリニック
hematopoietic stem cell	造血幹細胞
HSCCC	
high-speed countercurrent chromatography	高速向流クロマトグラフィ
HSCL	
Hopkins Symptom Checklist	ホプキンズ症状チェックリスト
HSCR	
Hirschsprung disease	ヒルシュスプルング病，先天性巨大結腸症
HSD	
Hallervorden-Spatz disease	ハラボーデン・シュパッツ病
heavy snorer disease	重症いびき症候群
hydroxysteroid dehydrogenase	水酸化ステロイド脱水素酵素
HSDA	
high single dose alternate day	1日おきに単回大量投与せよ《処》

HSE
hemorrhagic shock and encephalopathy　出血性ショック脳症
herpes simplex encephalitis　単純ヘルペス脳炎
hypertonic saline-epinephrine　高張食塩エピネフリン
HSES
hemorrhagic shock-encephalopathy syndrome　出血性ショック脳症症候群
HSF
hepatocyte stimulating factor　肝細胞刺激因子
histamine-induced suppressor factor　ヒスタミン誘発性抑制因子
histamine-sensitizing factor　ヒスタミン増感因子
HSG
Health and Safety Guide　健康と安全のガイド
herpes simplex genitalis　陰部単純ヘルペス
hysterosalpingography　子宮卵管造影法
hSGF
human skeletal growth factor　ヒト骨格成長因子
HSGP
human sialoglycoprotein　ヒト唾液糖蛋白
HSI
heat stress index　熱ストレス指数
HSK
herpes simplex keratitis　単純ヘルペス角膜炎
hskpg.
housekeeping　家事，清掃
HSL
herpes simplex labialis　口唇単純ヘルペス
hormone-sensitive lipase　ホルモン感受性リパーゼ
HSLC
high-speed liquid chromatography　高速液体クロマトグラフィ
HSM
hepatosplenomegaly　肝脾腫大
holosystolic murmur　汎収縮期雑音，全収縮期雑音
HSMNⅢ
hereditary sensory motor neuropathy, typeⅢ　遺伝性感覚運動(性)ニューロパシーⅢ型
HSN
Hansen-Street nail　ハンセン・ストリート釘
hereditary sensory neuropathy　遺伝性感覚性ニューロパシー
herpes simplex neonatorum　新生児単純ヘルペス
h.som.
hora somni〈ラ〉=hour of sleep, at bedtime　就寝時(に)《処》
HSP
heat shock protein　熱ショック蛋白

H

hemolysis starting point	溶血開始点
Henoch-Schönlein purpura	ヘノッホ・シェーンライン紫斑病
human serum prealbumin	ヒト血清プレアルブミン
human serum protein	ヒト血清蛋白
hypersensitivity pneumonitis panel	過敏性肺(臓)炎パネル
hysterosalpingography	子宮卵管造影(法)

HSPG
heparan sulfate proteoglycan　ヘパラン硫酸プロテオグリカン

HSPM
hippocampal synaptic plasma membrane　海馬シナプス血漿膜

HSPN
Henoch-Schönlein purpura nephritis　ヘノッホ・シェーンライン紫斑病性腎炎

HSPQ
High School Personality Questionnaire　高校生人格質問表

HSR
homogeneously staining region　染色体均質染色領域

HSRA
high-speed rotational atherectomy　高速回転式粥腫切除術

HSRD
hypertension secondary to renal disease　腎疾患に続発する高血圧(症)

HSRS
Health-Sickness Rating Scale　健康疾病評点尺度

HSS

Hallermann-Streiff syndrome	ハレルマン・ストレフ症候群
Hallervorden-Spatz syndrome	ハラーフォルデン・シュパッツ症候群
Henoch-Schönlein syndrome	ヘノッホ・シェーンライン症候群
high speed scan	高速走査法
hyperstimulation syndrome	刺激(作用)過多症候群
hypertrophic subaortic stenosis	肥大〔肥厚〕性大動脈弁下部狭窄(症)

HSSCC
hereditary site-specific colon cancer　遺伝性部位特異的結腸癌

HSSP
Health Sector Support Project　保健医療分野支援プロジェクト

HST
horseshoe tear　馬蹄形裂孔

Hst
hereditary stomatocytosis　遺伝性口唇状赤血球症
HSTF
human serum thymus factor　ヒト血清胸腺因子
HSTK
herpes simplex-thymidine kinase gene　単純性ヘルペスチミジンキナーゼ遺伝子
H-subst
histamine-like substance　ヒスタミン様物質
HSV
herpes simplex virus　単純ヘルペスウイルス
hyperviscosity syndrome　高粘(稠)度症候群
HSVE
herpes simplex virus encephalitis　単純ヘルペスウイルス脳炎
HSVtk
herpes simplex virus thymidine kinase　単純ヘルペスウイルスチミジンキナーゼ
H_T
equivalent dose　等価線量
HT
half time　半減期
hammer toe　槌状趾
Hand Test　ハンド検査
Hashimoto thyroiditis　橋本甲状腺炎
hearing test　聴力検査
hearing threshold　聴覚閾値
heart　心臓
heart transplant　心臓移植
heat treated　温熱で治療〔処理〕した
heat treatment　温熱療法
hemagglutination titer　赤血球凝集価
high temperature　高温
home treatment　在宅治療
hospital treatment　病院治療
Huhner test　ヒューナー試験
human thrombin　ヒトトロンビン
hydrocortisone test　ヒドロコルチゾン試験
hydrotherapy　水治療法
hydroxytryptamine　ヒドロキシトリプタミン(＝セロトニン)
hypertension　高血圧
hyperthermia　高温熱
hyperthyroidism　甲状腺機能亢進症
hypertropia　上斜視
hypoxanthine, thymidine　ヒポキサンチン・チミジン
total hyper(metr)opia　全遠視

H

Ht
height 高さ，身長
hematocrit ヘマトクリット
hematocrit value ヘマトクリット値
heterozygote 異形接合体，ヘテロ接合体

Ht.
haustus〈ラ〉＝a draught，a drink （水剤の）一服量《処》

3-HT
3-hydroxytyramine 3-ヒドロキシチラミン（ドパミン）

5-HT
5-hydroxytriptamine（＝serotonin） 5-ヒドロキシトリプタミン（＝セロトニン）

HT'
hypertropia for near 近見時の上斜視

h.t.
hoc tempore〈ラ〉 この時点で《処》

H & T
hospitalization and treatment 入院と治療
hospitalize and treat 入院と治療

HT，Ht
hypothalamus 視床下部

HT，h.t.
heart tone 心音
high tension 高緊張，高圧
hypodermic tablet 皮下用錠剤

Ht，ht
heat （加）熱，発情

HTA
heterophil transplantation antigen 異好性移植抗原
human thymocyte antigen ヒト胸腺細胞抗原
hydroxytryptamine ヒドロキシトリプタミン（＝セロトニン）
5-hydroxytryptamine 5-ヒドロキシトリプタミン（＝セロトニン）
hypertension artérielle〈仏〉 高血圧症

HTACS
human thyroid adenyl cyclase stimulator ヒト甲状腺アデニルシクラーゼ刺激物質

HTAT
human tetanus antitoxin ヒト破傷風抗毒素

HTB
hot tub bath 温浴
house tube（feeding） 在宅経管（栄養）

HTC
heated tracheostomy collar 加熱気管切開カラー

hepatoma cell(s) 肝癌細胞
hepatoma tissue culture 肝癌組織培養
homozygous typing cell ホモ接合型タイピング細胞
hypertensive crisis 高血圧(性)クリーゼ

HTCA
human tumor colony assay ヒト腫瘍コロニー効力検定

HT cell
helper T cell ヘルパーT細胞

HTCVD
hypertensive cardiovascular disease 高血圧性心血管疾患

HTD
hospital for tropical disease 熱帯病(のための)病院
human therapeutic dose ヒト治療量

^{3}H-TdR
tritiated thymidine トリチウム化チミジン

HTF
heterothyrotropic factor 異種甲状腺刺激因子
house tube feeding 在宅経管栄養

HTG
hypertriglyceridemia 高トリグリセリド血症

HTGL
hepato-triglyceride lipase 肝(性)トリグリセリドリパーゼ

Hth
hypothalamus 視床下部

HTHD
hypertensive heart disease 高血圧性心疾患

H_2-Thy
5,6-dihydrothymine 5,6-ジヒドロチミン

HThyL
human thymus-leukemia associated antigen ヒト胸腺白血病関連抗原

HTI
hemisphere thrombotic infarction 半球血栓性梗塞

HTIG
homologous tetanus immune globulin 同種破傷風免疫グロブリン

hTIg
human tetanus immunoglobulin ヒト破傷風免疫グロブリン

HTK
heel-to-knee (test) 踵膝(検査)

HTL
hearing threshold level 聴力レベル
hemodialysis-induced transient leukopenia 血液透析誘発性一過性白血球減少症
histo(logic) technologist (病理)組織技士
human T cell leukemia ヒトT細胞白血病

H

human T cell lymphoma ヒトT細胞リンパ腫
human thymic leukemia ヒト胸腺白血病

HTLA
human thymic leukemia ヒト胸腺白血病
human T lymphocyte antigen ヒトTリンパ球抗原

HTLV
human T cell leukemia virus ヒトT細胞白血病ウイルス
human T lymphotropic virus ヒトTリンパ球向性ウイルス

HTLV-Ⅰ〔Ⅱ,Ⅲ〕
human T cell leukemia virus type Ⅰ〔Ⅱ/Ⅲ〕 ヒトT細胞白血病ウイルスⅠ〔Ⅱ/Ⅲ〕型
human T lymphotropic virus type Ⅰ〔Ⅱ/Ⅲ〕 ヒトTリンパ球向性ウイルスⅠ〔Ⅱ/Ⅲ〕型

HTLV-MA
human T cell leukemia virus associated membrane antigen ヒトT細胞白血病ウイルス関連膜抗原
human T cell lymphotropic virus associated membrane antigen ヒトTリンパ球向性ウイルス関連膜抗原

HTM
haemophilus test medium ヘモフィルス属の感受性検査用培地
high-threshold mechanoreceptor 高閾値機械受容器

HTML
Hypertext Markup Language ハイパーテキスト記述言語

HTN
hypertension 高血圧
hypertensive 高血圧性の
hypertensive nephropathy 高血圧性腎症

HTO
high tibial osteotomy 高位脛骨骨切り術
hospital transfer order 病院搬送指示

HTP
house-tree-person (test) 家・樹木・人物描画試験，HTPテスト
hydroxytryptophan ヒドロキシトリプトファン（＝セロトニン前駆体）
hypothromboplastinemia 低トロンボプラスチン血症

5-HTP
5-hydroxytryptophan 5-ヒドロキシトリプトファン（＝セロトニン前駆体）

HTPF
heat-treated plasma fraction 熱処理血漿分画

HTPN
home total parenteral nutrition 在宅における高カロリー輸液

HTS
head traumatic syndrome 頭部外傷症候群

heel-to-shin (test) 踵脛(検査)
hemangioma-thrombocytopenia syndrome 血管腫・血小板減少症候群

hTS
human T cell specific antigen ヒトT細胞特異抗原
human thyroid-stimulating (hormone) ヒト甲状腺刺激ホルモン
human thyroid stimulator ヒト甲状腺刺激因子

hTSAb
human thyroid stimulating antibody ヒト甲状腺刺激抗体

HTSCA
human tumor stem cell assay ヒト腫瘍幹細胞効力検定

hTSH
human thyroid stimulating hormone ヒト甲状腺刺激ホルモン

HTST
high temperature short time (pasteurization) 高温短時間(殺菌)法

HTV
herpes type virus ヘルペス型ウイルス

HTVD
hypertensive vascular disease 高血圧性血管疾患

HTVT
heating and ventilation 加熱と換気

HTW
high temperature water 高温水

HTX
heart transplantation 心臓移植
hemothorax 血胸

HU
heat unit X線管熱容量
hemagglutinating unit 赤血球凝集単位
hemagglutinin unit 赤血球凝集素単位
hemolytic unit 溶血単位
Hounsfield unit ハウンスフィールド単位
hydroxyurea ヒドロキシ尿素
hyperemia unit 充血単位

Hu
human ヒトの

HUC
hypouricemia 低尿酸血症

HUCVG
human umbilical cord vein graft ヒト臍帯静脈移植片

HUD
head-up display ヘッドアップディスプレイ

HuE
human erythrocyte ヒト赤血球

HUGA
human genome analyzer　自動DNA分析装置
HUI
headache unit index　頭痛単位係数
HUIFM
human leukocyte interferon milieu　ヒト白血球インターフェロン環境
HuIFN
human interferon　ヒトインターフェロン
HUK
human urinary kallikrein　ヒト尿カリクレイン
HUM
heat〔hot packs〕, ultrasound and massage　熱〔温湿布〕・超音波・マッサージ
hematourimetry　血尿測定
home uterine monitoring　在宅子宮モニタリング
hum.
humerus　上腕骨
human CMV
human cytomegalovirus　ヒトサイトメガロウイルス
humer
humerus〈ラ〉　上腕骨
HUMI
Harris-Kronner uterine manipulator injector　ハリス・クローネ子宮マニピュレーター注射器
humi
humidity　湿度
hun
hundred　100
hund
hundred　100
H unit
Holzknecht unit　ホルツクネヒト単位
hunth
hundred thousand　10万
HUR
hydroxyurea　ヒドロキシ尿素
HuRBC
human red blood cell　ヒト赤血球
HUS
hemolytic uremic syndrome　溶血性尿毒症症候群
hyaluronidase unit for semen　精液ヒアルロニダーゼ単位
hyaluronidase unit for serum　血清ヒアルロニダーゼ単位
HuSA
human serum albumin　ヒト血清アルブミン

H

husb, husb.
husband　夫
HUTHAS
human thymus antiserum　ヒト胸腺抗血清
HUV
human umbilical vein　ヒト臍静脈
HUVECs
human umbilical vein endothelial (cells)　ヒト臍帯静脈内皮細胞
HV
hallux valgus　外反母趾，母趾外反症
Hancock valve　H弁
health visitor　保健師
heart volume　心容積
hepatic vein　肝静脈
hepatic venous　肝静脈の
herpes virus　ヘルペスウイルス
high velocity　高速度
high voltage　高電圧，高電位
home visit　家庭訪問
hospital visit　受診
hydroa vacciniforme〈ラ〉　種痘様水疱症
hypersensitive vasculitis　過敏性血管炎
hyperventilation　過呼吸，過換気，換気亢進
Hysterie〈独〉=hysteria　ヒステリー
hv
heavy　重い
h.v.
hoc vespere〈ラ〉=this evening　今晩，今夕《処》
H & V
hemigastrectomy and vagotomy　胃半切除・迷走神経切断(術)
HVA
hallux valgus angle　外反母趾角
Health Visitor's Association　保健師協会
homovanillic acid　ホモバニリン酸
HVAC
heating, ventilating and air conditioning　加熱・換気・空調
HV block
infra hisian block　ヒス束下ブロック
HV & C
heating, ventilating and cooling　加熱・換気・冷却
HVD
hypertensive vascular disease　高血圧性血管疾患
hypertrophie ventriculaire droite〈仏〉　右心室肥大
hypoxic ventilatory drive　低酸素換気刺激

HVDO
hypovitaminosis D osteopathy　ビタミンD不足骨障害
HVDRR
hypophosphatemic vitamin D resistant rickets　低リン酸血症性ビタミンD抵抗性くる病
HVE
hepatic vascular exclusion　肝血管遮断
hepatic venous effluence　肝静脈流出
high voltage electrophoresis　高電圧電気泳動
high volume evacuator　高容量吸引〔吸収〕器
HVEM
high voltage electron microscope　超高電圧電子顕微鏡
HVF
hepatocyte volume fraction　肝細胞容積分画

HVFP
hepatic vein free pressure　肝静脈自由圧
HVG
hematoxylin and van Gieson (stain)　ヘマトキシリンとヴァンギーソン(染色)
host-versus-graft (disease)　宿主対移植片(疾患)
hypertrophie ventriculaire gauche〈仏〉　左(心)室肥大
HVGR
host-versus-graft reaction　宿主対移植片反応
HVH
herpesvirus hominis　ヒトヘルペスウイルス
HV-HR-TEM
high-voltage high-resolution transmission electron microscope　超高圧高分解能透過型電子顕微鏡
HVID
horizontal visible iris diameter　水平可視光彩径
HV interval
His ventricular interval　ヒス心室時間
HVJ
hemagglutinating virus of Japan　日本血球凝集ウイルス，センダイウイルス
HVL
Hypophysenvorderlappen〈独〉　下垂体前葉
hvl
half value layer　半価層
HVLP
high volume, low pressure　高容量・低圧
HVLT
high-velocity lead therapy　高速鉛療法
HVM
hybrid vesicular model　ハイブリッド血管モデル
hypothalamic ventromedial (nucleus)　視床下部腹内側(核)

HVOO
hepatic venous outflow obstruction 肝静脈流出遮断
HVPE
high-voltage paper electrophoresis 高電圧濾紙電気泳動法
HVPG
hepatic venous pressure gradient 肝静脈圧勾配
HVR
hyper-variable region 超可変領域
hyperviscosity retinopathy 血液粘性亢進網膜症
Hypophysenvorderlappenreaktion〈独〉 下垂体前葉反応
hypoxic ventilatory response 低酸素換気反応
HVS
herpesvirus saimiri ヘルペスウイルスサイミリ
herpesvirus sensitivity ヘルペスウイルス感受性
high voltage slow wave 高振幅徐波
hyperventilation syndrome 過換気症候群
HVT
half value thickness 半価層
HVTEM
high-voltage transmission electron microscopy 高電圧透過型電子顕微鏡
HV time
His-ventricle time ヒス心室時間
HVUS
hypocomplementemic vasculitis-urticarial syndrome 低補体血症性血管炎・蕁麻疹様症候群
hvy
heavy 重い
HW
Halswirbel〈独〉 頸椎
hand wash 手浴
Hayem-Widal (syndrome) エヤン・ヴィダル(症候群)
healing well 治癒良好
hemisphere width 半球幅
hot water 湯
H/W
husband and wife 夫と妻
HW, h.w.
housewife 主婦
HWD
Halbwertdose〈独〉 半数致死線量
HWHM
half width at half maximum 半値半幅
HWP
Hutchinson-Weber-Peutz (syndrome) ハッチンソン・ウェーバー・ポイツ(症候群)

H

HWS
Halbwertschicht〈独〉 半価層
Halswirbelsäule〈独〉 頸椎
hot water soluble 温湯に可溶な
HWT
histamine wheal test ヒスタミン丘斑試験
HX
histocytosis X 原因不明性組織球増殖症，ヒストサイトーシスX
hypophysectomized 下垂体摘出術を受けた
hypoxanthine ヒポキサンチン
Hx
hemopexin ヘモペキシン
hexokinase ヘキソキナーゼ
history 病歴
HXIS
hard X-ray imaging spectrometer 硬X線画像分析〔分光〕計
HXM
hexamethylmelamine ヘキサメチルメラミン
HXR
hypoxanthine riboside ヒポキサンチンリボシド
Hxs
hexose 六炭糖，ヘキソース
HXV
herpes simplex virus 単純ヘルペスウイルス
HY
hypophysis 下垂体
Hy
history 病歴
hypothenar 小指球(の)
HY, Hy
hype(rmet)ropia 遠視
hyperopic 遠視の
Hy, hy
Hysterie〈独〉=hysteria ヒステリー
H-Y antigen
histocompatibility-Y antigen H-Y抗原，組織適合性Y抗原
hyb
hybrid 雑種
HYD
hydralazine ヒドララジン
hydroxyurea ヒドロキシ尿素
Hyd
hydrocortisone ヒドロコルチゾン
hydrosalpinx 卵管留水症

hydrostatics 流体静力学

hyd

hydrate 含水化合物

Hyd.

hydration 水化，水分補給

hydrostatic 流体静力学の，静水の

Hydr，Hydr.

hydraulic 水力の，水力学的な

Hydrarg，Hydrarg.

hydrargyrum〈ラ〉 水銀

Hydro

hydrotherapy 水治療法〔学〕

Hydrochl

hydrochloride 塩化水素酸の

Hydrox

hydroxyline ヒドロキシリン

Hyg，hyg

hygiene 衛生(学)

hygienic 衛生的な，衛生学の

hygienist 保健師，衛生士，衛生技師

HYL，Hyl

hydroxylysine ヒドロキシリジン

HYLO

hyaline ヒアリンの，硝子質の

Hyp

hyper-resonance 共鳴過度

hyp

hypalgesia 痛覚鈍麻

hypochondria 沈うつ

hypophysis 下垂体

hypopnysectomy 下垂体切除(術)

hypothesis 仮説

hypothetical 仮説の

HYP，Hyp

hydroxyproline ヒドロキシプロリン

hypnosis 催眠(状)

HYP，Hyp，hyp.

hypertrophy 肥大，肥厚

Hyp，hyp

hypothalamus 視床下部

hype

hypodermic 皮下の

hyper A

hyperactive 活動亢進の

hyperact.

hyperactive 活動亢進の

hyperal	
hyperalimentation	過剰栄養，高栄養
hyper-IgE	
hyperimmunoglobulinemia E	高IgE血症
hyperpara	
hyperparathyroidism	副甲状腺機能亢進(症)
hypersens	
hypersensitive	過敏の
hyper T & A	
hypertrophy of tonsils and adenoids	扁桃の過形成およびアデノイド
hyperten	
hypertension	高血圧
hypertens	
hypertensive	高血圧性の
hypervent	
hyperventilation	過換気，過呼吸
hypes	
hypesthesia	感覚鈍麻，感覚減退
hypho, hypno.	
hypnotic	催眠薬，催眠術の
hypnotism	催眠術，催眠法
hypn	
hypertension	高血圧(症)
hypno	
hypnosis	催眠(状態)
hypnot	
hypnotism	催眠術，催眠法
hypnotist	催眠術者
hypo	
hypochondria	沈うつ
hypochondriac	心気症の患者
hypochondriacal	心気症の
hypochromia	血色素減少症，低色素血症
hypodermic (injection)	皮下の，皮下注射
hypodermically	皮下に
sodium thiosulfate	チオ硫酸ナトリウム
hypo A	
hypoactive	活動低下の
hypoact	
hypoactive	活動低下の
HYPOTH	
hypothalamus	視床下部
hypoth	
hypothesis	仮説

HYPP
hypersegmented neutrophil 過分葉好中球
HypRF
hypothalamic releasing factor 視床下部放出因子
Hypro
hydroxyproline ヒドロキシプロリン
hys.
hysterectomy 子宮摘出術
HYS，hys.
hysteria ヒステリー
hysterical ヒステリーの
HYST，hyst.
hysterectomy 子宮摘出術
hystero
hystero-salpingography 子宮卵管造影法
Hyv
hydroxyisovaleric acid ヒドロキシイソバレリン酸
HZ
herpes zoster 帯状ヘルペス
Hz
hertz ヘルツ〈単位〉
HZ，Hz
Harnzucker〈独〉 尿糖
HZO
herpes zoster ophthalmicus 眼部帯状ヘルペス
HZV
herpes zoster virus 帯状ヘルペスウイルス

I i

I	
ileum	回腸
implantation	着床
incisivus〈ラ〉	切開する
inclusion	封入体
inconsistent	不一致の
incus	キヌタ骨
independent	独立した
index	係数，指数
indicated	適応のある，示した
induction	誘発，誘導，導入，感応
inhalation	吸息，吸入
inhibition	抑制，阻止，阻害
inhibitor	抑制因子
inosine	イノシン
inspiration	吸気，吸息
inspired (gas)	吸気
insulin	インスリン
intake	摂取
intensity	超音波の強度
intensity of magnetism	磁気力，磁気強度
intermediate	中間の
intermediate inactivator	中間的不活性物
internal medicine	内科(学)
internist	内科医
Iodamoeba	ヨードアメーバ
iodine	ヨウ素〈元素〉
ionic strength	イオン強度
isoflurane	イソフルレン
isoleucine	イソロイシン
isotope	同位体，同位元素
Ixodes	マダニ
luminous intensity	光度
i	
inactive	不活性
inseparable	非分割性の
iota	イオタ
iso-	イソ〈接〉，同類の，同種の
isochromosome	同腕染色体
^{123}I	
iodine-123	ヨウ素123
^{125}I	
iodine-125	ヨウ素125

radioactive infarct particle 放射性塞栓粒子

^{131}I

iodine-131 ヨウ素131
radioactive iodine 放射性ヨウ素

I, i

incisor (乳歯の)切歯
insoluble 不溶性の

IA

image amplifier 螢光像増倍管
immune adherence 免疫粘着(反応)
immunoadsorbent 免疫吸着
immunoassay 免疫測定法
immunobiologic activity 免疫生物(学的)活性
impedance angle インピーダンス角
indolamine インドールアミン
indolic acid インドール酸
infected area 感染部位
inferior angle 下角
informed assent インフォームドアセント
infra-audible 可聴閾値下
Intelligenzalter〈独〉 精神年齢
interaural atenuation 両耳間移行減衰
internal auditory 内耳の

Ia

immune (region)-associated antigen 免疫関連抗原

IA, i.a.

intraalveolar 肺胞内の
intraaortic 大動脈内の
intraarterial 動脈内の
intraarticular 関節(腔)内の
intraatrial 心房内の
intraauricular 耳介内の，心房内の

IAA

ileo-anal anastomosis 回腸肛門吻合(術)
indoleacetic acid インドール酢酸
insulin autoantibody 抗インスリン自己抗体
International Association of Allergology 国際アレルギー学会
interruption of aortic arch 大動脈弓離断(症)
iodoacetamid ヨードアセトアミド(=モノヨードアセトアミド)
iodoacetic acid(=MIA) ヨード酢酸(=モノヨード酢酸)

^{131}I-AA

iodine-131 aggregated albumin ヨウ素131標識凝集アルブミン

I

Ia-A
I-region associated antigen　I領域関連抗原
Ia antigen
I region associated antigen　Ia抗原，I領域遺伝子関連抗原
IAAP
International Association of Applied Psychology　国際応用心理学会
IAAR
imidazoleacetic (acid) ribonucleotide　イミダゾール酢酸リボヌクレオチド
IAASM
International Academy of Aviation and Space Medicine　国際航空宇宙医学アカデミー
IAATM
International Association for Accident and Traffic Medicine　国際交通災害医学会

IAB
intraabdominal　腹腔内の
intraaorta balloon　大動脈内バルーン
IABA
intraaortic balloon assistance　大動脈内バルーン補助
IABC
intraaortic balloon counterpulsation　大動脈内バルーンカウンターパルセイション
IABCP
intraaortic balloon counterpulsation　大動脈内バルーンカウンターパルセイション
IABP
intraaortic balloon pump　大動脈内バルーンポンプ
intraaortic balloon pumping　大動脈内バルーンパンピング法
IAC
ineffective airway clearance　無効気道クリアランス
internal auditory canal　内耳道
International Academy of Cytology　国際細胞学会
intraarterial chemotherapy　動脈内化学療法,化学療法動注法
IACAPAP
International Association for Child and Adolescent Psychiatry and Allied Professions　国際児童青年精神医学会
IACB
intraaortic counterpulsation balloon　大動脈内カウンターパルセイションバルーン

IAC-CPR
interposed abdominal compressions-cardio-pulmonary resuscitation　介在腹部圧迫・心肺蘇生

IACD
implantable automatic cardioverter-defibril-lator　植込み型自動心臓除細動器
intraatrial conduction defect　心房内伝導障害

IACG
intermittent angle closure glaucoma　間欠性閉塞隅角緑内障

IACP
intraaortic counterpulsation　大動脈内カウンターパルセイション

IACPS
International Academy of Chest Physicians and Surgeons　国際胸部内科医外科医アカデミー

IACRLRD
International Association for Comparative Research on Leukemia and Related Disease　国際比較白血病および関連疾患学会

IAD
inactivating dose　不活化量
inhibiting antibiotic dose　(細菌発育)阻止抗生物質量
internal absorbed dose　内部吸収量
intractable atopic dermatitis　難治性アトピー性皮膚炎

IADH
inappropriate antidiuretic hormone　抗利尿ホルモン分泌異常

IADHS
inappropriate antidiuretic hormone syndrome　抗利尿ホルモン分泌異常症候群

IADL
instrumental activity of daily living　手段的日常生活動作

IADMFR
International Association of Dento-Maxillo-facial Radiology　国際歯顎顔面放射線学会

^{131}I-adosterol
iodine-131 adosterol　ヨウ素131アドステロール

IADR
International Association of Dental Research　国際歯科研究学会

IADS
International Association of Dental Students　国際歯学生協会

IADSA
intraarterial digital subtraction angiography　動脈内デジタル減算血管造影法，経動脈DSA

I

I

IAE
intraatrial electrocardiogram 動脈内心電図
IAEA
International Atomic Energy Agency 国際原子力機関
IAFI
infantile amaurotic familial idiocy 乳幼児黒内障性家族性精神遅滞
IAFS
International Association for Forensic Sciences 国際法科学協会
IAFT
International Association of Forensic Toxicologist 国際法毒物学協会
IAG
International Association of Gerontology 国際老年病学会
IAGP
International Association of Group Psychotherapy 国際集団精神療法学会
IAGT
indirect antiglobulin test 間接抗グロブリン試験
IAH
idiopathic adrenal hyperplasia 特発性副腎過形成
IAHA
idiopathic autoimmune hemolytic anemia 特発性自己免疫(性)溶血性貧血
immune adherence hemagglutination 免疫粘着(赤)血球凝集(反応)
IAHD
idiopathic acquired hemolytic disease 特発性後天(性)溶血性疾患
International Association of Hydatid Disease 国際胞虫症学会
IAHIA
immune adherence immunosorbent assay 免疫付着(粘着)免疫吸着検定
IAHM
International Academy of the History of Medicine 国際医史学アカデミー
IAHS
infection-associated hemophagocytic syndrome 感染症に伴う血球貪食症候群
International Association for Hospital Security 国際病院安全管理協会
IAI
intraabdominal infection 腹腔内感染

IAIA
immune adherence immunosorbent assay 免疫付着〔粘着〕免疫吸着検定
IALM
International Academy of Legal Medicine 国際法医学会
IALP
International Association of Logopedics and Phoniatrics 国際音声言語医学会
IAM
Institute of Aviation Medicine 航空医学研究所
internal accoustic meatus 内耳道
internal auditory meatus 内耳道
iodoacetamide ヨードアセトアミド
IAMB
International Association of Microbiologists 国際微生物学者連合
IAMBE
International Association for Medicine and Biology of Environment 国際環境医学生物学協会
IAMC
Institute for Advancement of Medical Communication 医学報道進歩のための研究所
IAMLT
International Association of Medical Laboratory Technologists 国際臨床検査技師協会
International Association of Microbiological Societies 国際微生物学会協会
IAMM
International Association of Medical Museum 国際医学博物館協会
IAN
idiopathic aseptic nerosis 特発性無菌壊死
indole-3-acetonitrile インドール-3-アセトニトリル
IANC
International Anatomical Nomenclature Committee 国際解剖学用語委員会
IAO
immediately after onset 発症直後(に)
intermittent aortic occlusion 間欠性大動脈閉塞症
IAOMS
International Association of Oral and Maxillofacial Surgeons 国際口腔顎顔面外科学会

IAOS
International Association of Oral Surgeons　国際口腔外科学会
IAP
immunosupprresive acidic protein　免疫抑制酸性蛋白
inosinic acid pyrophosphorylase　イノシン酸ピロホスホリラーゼ
intermittent acute porphyria　間欠性急性ポルフィリン症
International Academy of Pathology　国際病理学会
intraabdominal pressure　腹腔内圧
islet-activating protein　膵島活性化蛋白
IAPB
International Agency for the Prevention of Blindness　国際失明予防学会
IAPD
International Association of Pediatric Dentistry　国際小児歯科学会
IAPG
interatrial pressure gradient　動脈間圧勾配
IAPP
insulinoma, islet amyloid polypeptide　膵島腺腫アミロイドポリペプチド
IAR
immediate allergic response　即時型アレルギー(反応)
immediate asthmatic response　即時型喘息反応
inhibitory anal reflex　抑制肛内反射
iodine-azide reaction　ヨウ素・アジ化合物反応
IARC
International Agency for Research on Cancer　国際癌研究機構
IARF
ischemic acute renal failure　虚血性急性腎不全
IARR
indirect antiglobulin rosetting reaction　間接抗グロブリンロゼット形成反応
IARSA
idiopathic acquired refractory sideroblastic anemia　特発性後天性不応性鉄芽球性貧血
IART
intraarterial reentrant tachycardia　動脈内リエントリー性頻拍
i arter.
intraarterial　動脈内の
IAS
idiopathic ankylosing spondylitis　特発性強直性脊椎炎
immunosuppressive acidic substance　免疫抑制(性)酸性物質
inactivated serum　不活性化血清

interatrial septum	心房中隔
internal anal sphincter	内肛門括約筋
International AIDS(=Aquired Immunodeficiency Syndrome) Society	国際エイズ学会

IASA

interatrial septal aneurysm	心房中隔瘤

IASCT

International Association for the Sensitization of Cancer Treatment	国際癌治療増感研究協会

IASD

interatrial septal defect	心房中隔欠損(症)

IASH

isolated asymmetric septal hypertrophy	単独非対称中隔肥大

IASL

International Association for the Study of the Liver	国際肝臓研究協会

IASLC

International Association for the Study of Lung Cancer	国際肺癌学会

IASP

International Association for the Study of Pain	国際疼痛学会

IASSID

International Association for the Scientific Study of Intellectual Disabilities	国際知的障害研究協会

IASSMD

International Association for Scientific Study of Mental Deficiency	国際精神遅滞研究協会

IAT

immunoabsorption therapy	免疫吸着療法
immunoaugmentative therapy	免疫増強療法
indirect antiglobulin test	間接抗グロブリン試験
inside air temperature	室内気温
instillation abortion time	(薬剤)点滴注入流産時間
invasive activity test	侵襲性活性検査
iodine azide test	ヨウ素アジ化合物試験

IAU

International Association of Universities	国際大学協会
International Astronomical Union	国際天文学連合

IAV

intermittent assisted ventilation	間欠的補助換気

IAVM
- intramedullary arteriovenous malformation　髄内動静脈奇形

IB
- Ibrahim-Beck (disease)　イブラヒム・ベック(病)
- idiopathic blepharospasm　特発性眼瞼痙攣
- ileal bypass　回腸バイパス
- immune balance　免疫バランス
- immune body　免疫体
- immunoblotting　イムノブロッティング
- inclusion body　封入(小)体
- index of body build　体型指数
- indirect bilirubin　間接ビリルビン
- infectious bronchitis　感染性気管支炎
- investigator's brochure　治験薬概要書
- Institute of Biology　(英国)生物学研究所
- instruction book　指導書
- intestinal Behçet　腸管ベーチェット病
- isolation bed　隔離ベッド

ib.
- *ibidem*〈ラ〉=in the same place　同じ場所〔個所〕で

i.b.
- im besonderen〈独〉　特に

I-B
- interbody　椎体間の

IBA
- index bone area　骨皮質指数
- isobutyric acid　イソ酪酸

I band
- isotropic band　等方帯, I帯

IBAT
- intravascular bronchoalveolar tumor　血管内気管支肺胞腫瘍

IBB
- intestinal brush border　腸刷子縁

IBBB
- intrablood-brain barrier　内血液・脳関門

IBBBB
- incomplete bilateral bundle branch block　不完全両脚ブロック

IBC
- Institutional Biosafety Committee　施設内生命安全委員会
- iodine-binding capacity　ヨード結合能
- iron-binding capacity　鉄結合能
- isobutyl cyanoacrylate　イソブチルシアノアクリレート

IBCA
isobutyl cyanoacrylate イソブチルシアノアクリレート

IBCSG
International Breast Cancer Study Group 国際乳癌研究グループ

IBD
idiopathic inflammatory bowel disease 特発性炎症性腸疾患
infectious bowel disease 感染性腸疾患
inflammatory bowel disease 炎症性腸疾患
irritable bowel disease 過敏性腸疾患
ischemic bowel disease 虚血性腸疾患

IBE
International Bureau for Epilepsy 国際てんかん協会
International Bureau of Education (ユネスコ)国際教育局

IB-EP
immunoreactive beta endomorphin 免疫反応(性)ベータエンドルフィン

IBES
International Bronchoesophagological Society 国際気管食道科学会

IBF
immature brown fat (cell) 未成熟茶色脂肪(細胞)
immunoglobulin-binding factor 免疫グロブリン結合因子

IBG
iliac bone graft 腸骨移植片
insoluble bone gelatin 不溶性骨ゼラチン
iron-binding globulin 鉄結合グロブリン

IBI
intermittent bladder irrigation 間欠的膀胱洗浄
ischemic brain infarction 虚血性脳梗塞

ibid.
ibidem〈ラ〉=in the same place 同じ場所〔個所〕で

I-Bil
indirect bilirubin 間接ビリルビン

IBK
infectious bovine keratoconjunctivitis ウシの感染性角結膜炎

IBL
immunoblastic lymphadenopathy 免疫芽球性リンパ節症

IBL-T
immunoblastic lymphadenopathy-like T cell lymphoma IBL様T細胞リンパ腫

IBM
inclusion body myositis 封入体筋炎
intact bridge tympanomastoidectomy 橋保存鼓室乳突削開術

IBMTR
International Bone Marrow Transplant Registry — 国際骨髄移植登録

IBMX
3-isobutyl-1-methylxanthine — 3-イソブチル-1-メチルキサンチン

ibo
ibotenic acid — イボテン酸

IBOW
intact bag of waters — 無傷羊膜

IBP
idiopathic bacterial peritoritis — 特発性細菌性腹膜炎
initial boiling point — 初期沸点
International Biological Program — 国際生物学事業計画
intraaortic balloon pump — 大動脈内バルーンポンプ
iron-binding protein — 鉄結合蛋白

I

IBPMS
indirect blood pressure measuring system — 間接的血圧測定システム

IBQ
illness behavior questionnaire — 疾病行動質問票

IBR
immediate breast reconstruction — 即時乳房再建
Infant Behavior Record — 乳児行動記録
infectious bovine rhinotracheitis — 感染性ウシ鼻・気管炎

IBRO
International Brain Research Organization — 国際脳研究機構

IBRS
Inpatient Behavior Rating Scale — 入院患者行動評価スケール〔尺度〕

IBRV
infective bovine rhinotracheitis virus — 感染性ウシ鼻・気管炎ウイルス

IBS
immunoblastic sarcoma — 免疫芽球性肉腫
indirect bilirubin syndrome — 濃縮性胆汁症候群
inflammatory bowel syndrome — 炎症性腸症候群
irritable bowel syndrome — 過敏性(大)腸症候群
isobaric solution — 等比重液

IBSA
immunoreactive bovine serum albumin — 免疫反応性ウシ血清アルブミン

IBSN
infantile bilateral striated necrosis — 乳児両側線条体壊死

IBT

ink blot test (=Rorschach test)	インクブロット試験(=ロールシャッハテスト)
isatin-beta-thiosemicarbazone	イサチンβチオセミカルバゾン

IBTR

ipsilateral breast tumor recurrence	同側乳腺腫瘍再発

IBU

ibuprofen	イブプロフェン

IBV

infectious bronchitis vaccine	伝染性気管支炎ワクチン
infectious bronchitis virus	伝染性気管支ウイルス

IBW

ideal body weight	理想的体重

IC

icteric	黄疸(性)の
immune complex	免疫複合体
immune cytotoxicity	免疫細胞毒性
immunocytochemistry	免疫細胞化学
inclusion conjunctivitis	封入体性結膜炎
indigocarmine	インジゴカルミン
indirect calorimetry	間接熱量測定
individual counseling	個人カウンセリング
inferior colliculus	下丘
information content	情報内容
informed consent	インフォームドコンセント，説明と同意
inhibiting concentration	抑制〔阻止〕濃度
inorganic carbon	無機炭素
inspiratory capacity	最大吸気量
inspiratory center	吸気中枢
integrated circuit	集積回路
intensive care	集中治療
intercostal	肋間の
intercostal margin	肋間縁
intermittent catheterization	間欠カテーテル法
intermittent claudication	間欠性跛行
internal capsule	内包
internal carotid artery	内頸動脈
internal cholecystectomy	内視鏡下胆嚢切除(術)
interstitial cell	間(質)細胞
intracardiac	心臓内の
intracarotid	頸動脈内の
intracellular (concentration)	細胞内の(濃度)
intracerebral	(大)脳内の
intracisternal	槽内の

intracranial 頭蓋内の
intrahepatic cholestasis 肝内胆汁うっ滞
intrapleural catheter 胸膜内カテーテル
ion change イオン交換
irritable colon 過敏(性)結腸
ischemic colitis 虚血性大腸炎
islet cell (of pancreas) (膵)島細胞
isotope cisternography RI脳槽撮影
isovolumetric contraction 等容性収縮
suspect frank invasive carcinoma, infiltrating cancer 浸潤癌

IC_{50}
concentration that inhibits 50% 50%抑制濃度

i.c.
inter cibos〈ラ〉=between meals 食間(に)《処》

I-3-C
indole-3-carbinol インドール-3-カルビノール

IC, ic
intracutaneous 皮内(の)
intracutaneous injection 皮内注射

ICA
ileocolic artery 回腸結腸動脈
immunocytochemical assay 免疫細胞化学的測定法
Infertility Center of America 米国代理母斡旋センター
internal carotid artery 内頸動脈
International College of Angiology 国際脈管学会
International Conference on AIDS(=Aquired Immunodeficiency Syndrome) 国際エイズ会議
intracranial aneurysm 頭蓋内動脈瘤
islet cell antibody 膵島細胞抗体

ICAA
International Council on Alcohol and Addictions 国際アルコール・薬物依存協会

ICAAC
Interscience Conference on Antimicrobial Agents and Chemotherapy 抗生物質と化学療法の学際的学会

ICAb
islet cell antibody 膵島細胞抗体

ICADTS
International Council on Alcohol, Drugs and Traffic Safety アルコール・薬物・交通安全国際委員会

ICAF
internal carotid artery flow 内頸動脈流

ICAM
intercellular adhesion molecule 細胞間接着分子
ICAO
internal carotid artery occlusion 内頸動脈閉塞(症)
i card
intracardial 心臓内の
ICAS
intermediate coronary artery syndrome 中間冠(状)動脈症候群
International Congress on Analytical Sciences 国際分析科学会議
icav
intracavity 腔内
ICB
Institute of Comparative Biology 比較生物学研究所
intracranial bleeding 頭蓋内出血
ICBG
iliac crest bone graft 腸骨稜骨移植(片)
ICBM
International Council of Botanic Medicine 国際薬草学協議会
ICBP
intercellular binding protein(s) 細胞間結合蛋白
intestinal calcium-binding protein 腸カルシウム結合蛋白
intracellular binding protein(s) 細胞内結合蛋白
ICBPC
indanyl CBPC(= carboxybenzylpenicillin)(= carindacillin) インダニルカルベニシリン(=カリンダシリン)
ICBT
intercostobronchial trunk 肋間気管(状動脈)幹
ICC
immunocompetent cell 免疫(学的)適格細胞
immunocytochemistry 免疫細胞化学
Indian childhood cirrhosis インディアン小児肝硬変
infection control committee 感染対策委員会
intensive coronary care 冠(状)動脈疾患集中治療
interchromosomal crossing-over 染色体(間)交叉〔差〕
intermittent clean catheterization 間欠清潔カテーテル挿入
International Congress Chemotherapy 国際化学療法学会
interstitial cell of Cajal カハール(間質)細胞
ischemic cell change 虚血性細胞変化
islet cell carcinoma 膵島細胞癌
ICCA
islet cell cytoplasmic antibody 膵ランゲルハンス島細胞質抗体

ICCB
International Congress on Cell Biology — 国際細胞生物学会議

ICCC
International Conference on Coordination Chemistry — 錯体化学国際会議

ICCE
intracapsular cataract extraction — 水晶体嚢内摘出術，嚢内白内障摘出(術)

ICCM
idiopathic congestive cardiomyopathy — 特発性うっ血性心筋症

ICCU
intensive coronary care unit — 冠(状)動脈疾患集中治療部門
intermediate coronary care unit — 中間冠(状動脈)疾患治療部門

ICD
I(=inclusion) cell disease — Ｉ(＝封入体)細胞病
immune complex disease — 免疫複合体病
implantable cardioverter defibrillator — 植込み型除細動器
instantaneous cardiac death — 瞬時心臓死
intercanthal distance — 眼角間距離
International Classification of Disease — 国際疾病分類
International College of Dentists — 国際歯科医師会
International Congress on Dermatology — 国際皮膚科学会議
International League of Dermatological Societies — 国際皮膚科学会連盟
intrauterine contraceptive device — 子宮内避妊器具
ischemic coronary disease — 虚血性冠(状動脈)疾患
isocitrate dehydrogenase — イソクエン酸脱水素酵素

ICDA
International Classification of Diseases, Adapted for Use in United States — 米国で使用される国際疾病分類

ICD-ATP
implantable cardioverter-defibrillator/atrial tachycardia pacing — 植込み型心臓除細動器・心房頻脈ペーシング

ICDC
implantable cardioverter/defibrillator catheter — 植込み型心臓除細動器・除細動器カテーテル

ICDCD
International Classification of Diseases and Causes of Death — 国際疾病および死因分類

ICDH
isocitrate dehydrogenase — イソクエン酸脱水素酵素

ICDID
International Classification of Diseases, Injuries and Causes of Death — 国際疾病・傷害および死因統計分類

ICDO
International Classification of Diseases for Oncology — 国際腫瘍疾病分類

ICDRG
International Contact Dermatitis Research Group — 国際接触皮膚炎研究グループ

ICE
ichthyosis-cheek-eyebrow (syndrome) — 魚鱗癬・頬・眉(症候群)
ifosfamide, carboplatin, etoposide — イホスファミド,カルボプラチン,エトポシド
interleukin-1β converting enzyme — インターロイキン1β変換酵素
iridocorneal endothelial (syndrome) — 虹彩角膜内皮(症候群)

I cell
inclusion cell — I〔封入体〕細胞

I cell disease
inclusion cell disease — I〔封入体〕細胞病

ICE syndrome
iridocorneal endothelial syndrome — ICE(=虹彩角膜内皮)症候群

ICEUS
intracaval endovascular ultrasonography — 大動脈内血管内超音波検査(法)

ICF
informed consent form — 同意説明文書
intensive care facility — 集中治療施設
intercellular fluorescence — 細胞間螢光
intermediate care facility — 中間ケア施設
International Cardiology Federation — 国際心臓連盟
intracellular fluid — 細胞内液
intravascular coagulation and fibrinolysis (syndrome) — 血管内凝固・線溶(症候群)

ICFA
incomplete Freund adjuvant — 不完全フロイントアジュバント
induced complement-fixing antigen — 誘発補体結合抗原

ICFV
intracellular fluid volume — 細胞内液量

IC fx
intracapsular fracture — 関節包内骨折

ICG
indocyanine green — インドシアニングリーン

I

International Congress of Genetics 国際遺伝学会議
isotope cisternography 同位元素脳槽造影(法)

ICGN
immune complex glomerulonephritis 免疫複合体糸球体腎炎

ICH
idiopathic cardiac hypertrophy 特発性心(筋)肥大
idiopathic cortical hyperostosis 特発性皮質性骨化過剰症
immunocompromised host 免疫妥協宿主
immunoreactive growth hormone 免疫反応性成長ホルモン
intracerebral hematoma 脳内血腫
intracerebral hemorrhage 脳内出血
intracerebral hypertension 脳内圧亢進(症)
intracranial hemorrhage 頭蓋内出血
intracranial hypertension 頭蓋内圧亢進
International Conference on Harmonization of Technical Requirements for Registration of Pharmaceuticals for Human Use 日米EU医薬品規制調和国際会議

ICHD
Intersociety Commission for Heart Disease Resources 心疾患資料連絡協議会
ischemic coronary heart disease 虚血性冠(状動脈)心疾患

ICHPER-SD
International Council on Health, Physical Education, Recreation, Sports and Dance 国際保健・体育・リクリエイションスポーツ・ダンス協議会

ICHPPC
International Classification of Health Problems in Primary Care プライマリケアにおける保健問題の国際分類

ICI
initial chest irradiation 初期胸部照射
International Commission on Illumination System of Color-representation 国際色彩照明方式委員会
intracardiac injection 心臓内注射，心注

ICIA
International Center of Information on Antibiotics 国際抗生物質学情報センター

ICIDH
International Classification of Impairments, Disabilities and Handicaps (WHOの)国際障害分類

ICIT
intensive conventional insulin therapy 強化インスリン療法

ICJ
ileocecal junction 回盲接合部

ICL
idiopathic CD4 T cell lymphocytopenia　特発性CD4T細胞リンパ球減少症
intracorneal lens　角膜内レンズ
intracorporeal laser lithotripsy　体内レーザー砕石術
iris-clip lens　虹彩クリップレンズ

ICLA
International Committee on Laboratory Animals　国際実験動物委員会

ICLAS
International Council for Laboratory Animal Science　国際実験動物科学会議

ICLCO
International Contact Lens Council of Ophthalmology　国際眼科コンタクトレンズ会議

ICLE
intracapsular lens extraction　嚢内レンズ摘出術

ICM
idiopathic cardiomegaly　特発性心拡大
idiopathic cardiomyopathy　特発性心筋症
inner cell mass　内細胞塊
International Confederation of Midwives　国際助産師連盟
intracostal margin　肋間(辺)縁
intracytoplasmic membrane　細胞質内膜
isolated cardiovascular malformation　単独心血管奇形

ICMA
idiopathic chronic megaloblastic anemia　原発性慢性巨赤芽球性貧血

ICMJE
International Committee of Medical Journal Editors　医学雑誌編集者国際委員会

ICML
International Congress on Medical Librarianship　国際医学図書司書会議

ICMMP
International Committee of Military Medicine and Pharmacy　国際軍事医薬委員会

ICMR
inhibitor of chemical mediator release　化学伝達物質遊離抑制薬

IC muscle
ischiocavernous muscle　坐骨海綿体筋

ICN
infection control nurse　感染管理看護師
intensive care neonatal　新生児集中治療

intensive care nursery 集中治療看護部
intermediate care nursery 中間治療保育室
International Council of Nurses 国際看護師協会

ICNC
intracerebellar nuclear cell 小脳内核細胞

ICO
idiopathic cyclic oedema 特発性周期性浮腫
impedance cardiac output インピーダンス心拍出量
International Congress of Otolaryngology 国際耳鼻咽喉科学会議

i coch
intracochlear 蝸牛内の

ICOH
International Commission on Occupational Health 国際労働衛生学会

ICOI
International College of Oral Implantologists 国際口腔インプラント学士会
International Congress of Oral Implantologists 口腔インプラント国際会議

ICONS
isotopes of carbon, oxygen, nitrogen and sulfur 炭素・酸素・窒素・硫黄のアイソトープ

ICP
incubation period 潜伏期
inductively coupled plasma 誘導結合プラズマ
infectious cell protein 感染細胞蛋白
inflammatory cloacogenic polyp 炎症性総排出腔性ポリープ
International Council of Psychologists 国際心理学者協会
intracavernous pressure 陰茎海綿体(血)圧
intracranial pressure 頭蓋内圧
intracranial pressure recording 頭蓋内圧測定装置
isometric contraction period 等尺性収縮期

ICPA
International Commission for Prevention of Alcoholism and Drug Dependency 国際アルコール中毒防止委員会

ICP-AES
inductively coupled plasma atomic emission spectrometry 誘導結合プラズマ発光分析

ICPC
internal carotid posterior communicating (aneurysm) 内頸動脈後交通動脈(瘤)
internal carotid posterior communicating (artery) 内頸動脈・後交通動脈分岐部

International Classification of Primary Care　プライマリケア国際分類
intracranial pressure catheter　頭蓋内圧カテーテル

ICPD
International Commission for Prevention and Therapy of Depression　国際うつ病予防治療委員会

ICPE
International Conference on Pharmacoepidemiology　国際薬剤疫学学会

ICPFR
International Committee on Physical Fitness Research　国際体力研究委員会

ICPM
incisors, canines, premolars, molars　切歯・犬歯・小臼歯・大臼歯
International College of Psychosomatic Medicine　国際心身医学会

ICPMM
incisors, canines, premolars and molars　切歯・犬歯・小臼歯・大臼歯

ICP-MS
inductively coupled plasma mass spectrometry　誘導結合プラズマ質量分析法

ICPP
intubated continuous positive-pressure　挿管連続陽圧

ICPR
International Commission for Stage Grouping on Cancer and Presentation of Results　癌の病期分類と結果報告のための国際委員会

ICR
industrial clean room　無塵室
Institute of Cancer Research　癌研究所
International Congress of Radiology　国際放射線医学会議
International Consensus Report on Diagnosis and Management of Asthma　喘息の診断と治療の国際報告
intracardiac catheter recording　心(臓)内カテーテル記録(法)
intracavitary radium　腔内ラジウム(療法)
intracranial reinforcement　頭蓋内増強
ion cyclotron resonance　イオンサイクロトロン共鳴

icr
increase　増す，増加する

ICRC
International Committee of Red Cross　赤十字国際委員会

I

I

ICRDB	
International Cancer Research Data Bank	国際癌研究データバンク
ICRE	
International Commission on Radiological Education and Information	国際放射線学教育・情報委員会
ICRF	
Imperial Cancer Research Fund	(英国)帝国癌研究基金
I-CRF	
immunoreactive corticotropin-releasing factor	免疫反応性副腎皮質刺激ホルモン放出因子
ICRO	
International Cell Research Organization	(ユネスコ)国際細胞研究機構
ICRP	
International Commission on Radiological Protection	国際放射線防護委員会
ICRU	
International Commission on Radiation Units and Measurements	国際放射線単位測定委員会
ICS	
immotile cilia syndrome	線毛不動症候群
impulse conducting system	(心臓)刺激伝導系
intercellular cement substance	細胞間結合物質
intercellular space	細胞間腔
intercostal space	肋間腔
intermediate coronary syndrome	中間冠(状動脈)症候群
International College of Surgeons	国際外科学会
International Continence Society	国際禁欲学会
intracranial stimulation	頭蓋内刺激
irritable colon syndrome	過敏性大腸症候群
ICSA	
islet cell surface antibody	膵島細胞膜抗体
ICSB	
International Committee on Systematic Bacteriology	国際系統細菌学委員会
ICSC	
idiopathic central serous chorioretinopathy	特発性中心性漿液性脈絡網膜症
International Chemical Safety Cards	国際化学物質安全性カード
ICSD	
International Classification of Sleep Disorders	睡眠障害国際分類

ICSH
- International Committee for Standardization Hematology　国際血液学標準化委員会
- interstitial cell-stimulating hormone　間質細胞刺激ホルモン

ICSI
- intracytoplasmic sperm injection　卵(母)細胞質内精子注入法

ICSP
- International Committee on Systematic of Prokaryotes　原核生物系統学に関する国際委員会

ICSS
- intracranial self-stimulation　頭蓋内自己刺激

ICSU
- International Council for Science　国際学術連合
- International Council of Scientific Union　国際学術連合

ICSW
- International Council on Social Welfare　国際社会福祉協議会

ICT
- intracardiac thrombus　心内血栓
- intraoral cariogenicity test　口腔内う蝕原性検査

ict.
- *icterus*〈ラ〉　黄疸

iCT, ICT
- icteric　黄疸(性)の
- immunoglobulin consumption test　免疫グロブリン消費試験
- immunoreactive calcitonin　免疫反応性カルシトニン
- indigo carmine test　インジゴカルミンテスト
- indirect Coombs test　間接クームス試験
- induction chemotherapy　術前化学療法
- infection control team　感染対策チーム
- inflammation of connective tissue　結合組織炎
- insulin coma therapy　インスリン昏睡治療
- insulin convulsive therapy　インスリン痙攣療法
- intensified conventional insulin therapy　インスリン頻回注射療法
- intensive conventional therapy　集中的通常療法
- intermittent cervical traction　間欠的頸部牽引
- interstitial cell tumor　間質細胞腫瘍
- intracoronary thrombolysis　冠(状)動脈内血栓溶解療法
- intracranial tumor　頭蓋内腫瘍
- intracutaneous test　皮内反応
- isovolumic contraction time　等容収縮期

ict.ind
- icteric index　黄疸指数

ICTMM
International Congress on Tropical Medicine and Malaria　国際熱帯医学マラリア会議
ICTS
idiopathic carpal tunnel syndrome　特発性手根管症候群
ICTV
International Committee for Taxonomy of Viruses　国際ウイルス命名委員会
ICTX
intermittent cervical traction　間欠的頸椎牽引
ICU
immunologic contact urticaria　免疫接触性蕁麻疹
intensive care unit　集中治療部〔室〕
ICU psychosis
intensive care unit psychosis　ICU精神病
ICUS
intracoronary ultrasound　冠(状)動脈内超音波(検査)
ICU syndrome
intensive care unit syndrome　ICU症候群
i cut
intracutaneous　皮内の
ICV
internal cerebral vein　内大脳静脈
International Congress of Virology　国際ウイルス学会議
intracellular volume　細胞内容量
icv, ICV
into cerebral ventricles　脳室(内)へ
intracerebroventricular　脳室内の
ICVH
ischemic cerebrovascular headache　虚血性脳血管性頭痛
ICVS
International Cardiovascular Society　国際心臓血管学会
ICW
Institute of Child Welfare　小児福祉研究所
intensive care ward　集中治療棟
intracellular water　細胞内水分量
ICX
immune complex　免疫複合体
ICXA
intermediate circumflex artery　中間彎曲動脈
ID
diabetic index　糖尿病係数
identification　同定，識別，身分証明
immunodeficiency　免疫不全
immunoglobulin deficiency　免疫グロブリン欠損(症)
inclusion disease　封入体病〔疾患〕

infant death　乳児死亡
infectious disease　感染症
infective dose　感染量
inhibitory dose　抑制量
initial diagnosis　初回診断
initial dose　初回量
Initialdruck〈独〉　初圧
injected dose　注射量
inner diameter　内径
insertion/deletion　挿入・欠失
inside diameter　内径
insufficient data　不十分データ
intermediate dose　中間量
internal diameter　内部径
interstitial disease　間質(性)疾患
intraduodenal　十二指腸内の
intrinsicoid deflection　近接様効果

Id
idiotype　イディオタイプ
immunodiffusion　免疫拡散法

id.
idem〈ラ〉=the same　同じく，不変

i.d.
in diem〈ラ〉=during the day　日中，その日のうちに《処》

I & D
incision and drainage　切開排膿

ID, id, i.d.
intradermal　皮(膚)内の

ID50, ID_{50}
half inhibitory dose　50%阻害用量
median infective dose　50%感染量

IDA
idarubicin　イダルビシン
idiopathic destructive arthritis　特発性破壊性関節炎
iminodiacetic acid　イミノ二酢酸
infraduodenal angle　下十二指腸角
insulin-degrading activity　インスリン分解活性
iron deficiency anemia　鉄欠乏性貧血

IDAA
International Doctors in Alcoholics Anonymous　アルコール中毒者更生国際医師団

id.ac
idem ac〈ラ〉=the same as　～と同じ

IDAMIS
Integrated Dose Abuse Management Informational Systems　薬剤用量・乱用管理情報統合システム

IDAT
indirect antiglobulin test 間接抗グロブリン試験
IDAV
immunodeficiency-associated virus 免疫不全関連ウイルス
IDBR
indirect bilirubin 間接ビリルビン
IDBS
infantile diffuse brain sclerosis 乳児広汎〔び漫〕性脳硬化症
IDC
idiopathic dilated cardiomyopathy 特発性拡張型心筋症
infiltrating ductal carcinoma 浸潤性腺管癌
interdigitating dendritic cell(s) 相互連結樹状細胞
intraductal carcinoma (腺)管内癌
invasive ductal carcinoma 侵襲性腺管癌
IDCF
immunodiffusion complement fixation 免疫拡散補体結合
I-D curve
intensity-duration curve 強さ・持続曲線
IDD
insulin-dependent diabetes インスリン依存性糖尿病
IDDM
insulin-dependent diabetes mellitus インスリン依存性糖尿病
IDDT
immuno-double diffusion test 二重免疫拡散法
IDE
immunodominant epitope 免疫優位エピトープ
interdigitated array electrode くし型電極
iden
identification 同定，識別
identify 同定する，識別する
i derm
intradermal 皮(膚)内の
IDF
insoluble dietary fiber 非水溶性食物繊維
International Diabetes Federation 国際糖尿病連合
IDFC
immature dead female child 死亡未熟女児
IDG
interdental groove 歯間溝
intermediate-dose group 中間量群
IDH
isocitrate dehydrogenase イソクエン酸脱水素酵素
IDI
induction-delivery interval 誘発分娩感覚
interdischarge interval 発射間間隔

interpersonal dependency inventory 対人依存特性尺度

IDI, IdI
interdentale inferius 下部歯間の

idiopathic RPGN
idiopathic rapidly progressive glomerulonephritis 特発性急速進行性糸球体腎炎

I disk
isotropic disk 等方帯，I帯

IDK
internal derangement of knee (joint) 膝(関節)内障
internal derangement of the knee 膝内障

IDL
Index to Dental Literature 歯科文献索引
intensity difference limen 強さの弁別域
intermediate density lipoprotein 中間比重リポ蛋白

IDL test
intensity difference limen test 音の強さの弁別検査

IDM
idiopathic disease of the myocardium 特発性心筋疾患
immune defense mechanism 免疫防御機構
indirect method 間接法
infant of diabetic mother 糖尿病母体の出生児

IDMC
immature dead male child 死亡未熟男児
Independent Data Monitoring Committee 独立データ監視委員会

ID-MS
isotope dilution mass spectrometry 同位元素希釈質量分光法

I-DNA
informational DNA 情報DNA

Ido
idose イドース

idon.vehic.
idoneo vehiculo〈ラ〉 適当な基剤に入れて《処》

Ido U
iduronic acid イズロン酸

Ido UA
iduronic acid イズロン酸

IDP
immunodiffusion procedure 免疫拡散手技
inosine diphosphate イノシン二リン酸
inosine 5′-diphosphate イノシン5′-二リン酸
intervertebral disc protrusion 椎間板ヘルニア
intraductal proliferation 管内増殖

I

IDPH
idiopathic pulmonary hemosiderosis　特発性肺血鉄症，特発性肺ヘモジデリン沈着症

IDPN
intradialytic parenteral nutrition　透析中非経口栄養法

IDR
idarubicin　イダルビシン
idiosyncratic drug reaction　特異体質薬剤反応
Institute for Dream Research　夢研究所
intradermal reaction　皮内反応

IDS
immunity deficiency state　免疫欠乏状態
immunodeficiency syndrome　免疫不全症候群
infectious disease service　感染症部門
inhibitor of DNA synthesis　DNA合成抑制因子，DNA合成阻害薬
institutional difference study　死亡率の相違性の研究
intraduodenal stimulation　十二指腸内刺激
Investigative Dermatological Society　研究皮膚科学会

IdS
interdentale superius　上部歯間の

IDT
immunodiffusion test　免疫拡散法
intradermal test　皮内テスト
isodensitracer　等濃度トレーサー

IDU
idoxuridine　イドクスウリジン
injecting drug user　注射薬物乱用者
5-iodo-2′-deoxyuridine　ヨードデオキシウリジン

IDUR
idoxuridine　イドクスウリジン

IDUS
intraductal ultrasonograhy　膵管内超音波検査(法)，経胆管的胆道超音波検査(法)

IDV
intermittent demand ventilation　間欠的強制換気

IDVC
indwelling venous catheter　留置静脈カテーテル

IDX
index to central literature　中央雑誌索引
intelligent diagnostic X ray　早くわかるX線診断システム

IE
Immunität Einheit〈独〉　免疫単位
immunoelectrophoresis　免疫電気泳動(法)
impedance epigastrography　インピーダンス胃電図
infectious〔infective〕 endocarditis　感染性心内膜炎

initial echo	初発エコー
inner ear	内耳
Insulineinheit〈独〉	インスリン単位
internal ear	内耳
internal elastica	内部弾性線維
internationale Einheit〈独〉	国際単位
in-the-in hearing instrument	耳孔挿入式補聴器
intraepithelial	上皮内の，上皮細胞間の

I/E

inspiration time/expiration time ratio	吸気相/呼気相時間比
inspiratory-expiratory ratio	吸気相・呼気相比

I & E

internal and external	内と外(の)

ie, i.e.

id est〈ラ〉=that is	すなわち

IEA

immediate early antigen	即時早期抗原
immuno-electrophoretic analysis	免疫電気泳動法
inferior epigastric artery	下腹壁動脈
International Epidemiological Association	国際流行疫学協会
International Ergonomics Association	国際人間工学会
intravascular erythrocyte aggregation	血管内赤血球凝集

IEBD

intraesophageal balloon distention	食道内バルーン拡張

IEC

Independent Ethics Committee	独立倫理委員会
injection electrode catheter	注射電極カテーテル
International Electrotechnical Commission	国際電気標準委員会
intraepithelial carcinoma	上皮内癌
ion exchange chromatography	イオン交換クロマトグラフィ

IE Ca cx

intraepithelial carcinoma of cervix	子宮頸上皮内癌

IED

individual effective dose	個別有効量
inherited epidermal dysplasia	遺伝性表皮形成異常

IEE

inner enamel epithelium	内エナメル上皮

IEF

International Eye Foundation	国際眼財団
isoelectric focusing	等電点電気泳動

IEL

internal elastic lamina	内部弾性板
intraepithelial leukocyte	上皮内白血球
intraepithelial lymphocyte	上皮内リンパ球

I

IEM
immunoelectron microscopy 免疫電子顕微鏡法
inborn error of metabolism 先天性代謝異常
IEMG
integrated electromyogram 積算筋電図
IEMS
Institute of Experimental Medicine and Surgery 実験医学・外科学研究所
IEP
immunoelectrophoresis 免疫電気泳動法
Institute of Experimental Psychology 実験心理学研究所
isoelectric point 等電点
I/E ratio
inspiratory/expiratory time ratio 吸気/呼気時間比
IES
immunoelectrophoresis 免疫電気浸透法
IETS
inelastic electron tunneling spectroscopy 非弾性電子トンネリング分光法
IEU
idiopathic esophageal ulcer 特発性食道潰瘍
IEX
ion exchange イオン交換
IF
idiopathic fibroplasia 特発性線維増殖症
immersion foot 浸水足
immunofluorescence 免疫蛍光抗体法
infrared 赤外(線)の，赤外部の
inhibiting factor 阻止因子，抑制因子
initiation factor 開始因子
interferon インターフェロン
intermediate filament 中間糸状体，中間フィラメント
intermediate frequency 中間頻度，中間周波数
internal fixation 内固定
interstitial fluid 間質液
intimal flap 剝離内膜
intracellular fluid 細胞内液
intrinsic factor 内(因性)因子
involved field 併発部
IFA
idiopathic fibrosing alveolitis 特発性線維化肺胞炎
immunofluorescence assay 免疫蛍光測定法
immunofluorescent antibody 免疫蛍光抗体
incomplete Freund adjuvant 不完全フロインドアジュバント

indirect fluorescent antibody 間接螢光抗体
intrinsic factor antibody 内因子抗体

IFA, IF-A
inflammatory factor for anaphylaxis アナフィラキシーの炎症(性)因子

IFAA
International Federation of Association of Anatomists 国際解剖学連合

IFAD
International Fund for Agricultural Development 国連の国際農業開発基金

IFAT
indirect fluorescent antibody test 間接螢光抗体検査

IFC
intermittent flow centrifugation 間欠流遠心法

IFCB
International Federation for Cell Biology 国際細胞生物連合

IFCC
International Federation of Clinical Chemistry 国際臨床化学連合

IFCL
intermittent flow centrifugation leukapheresis 間欠流遠心白血球アフェレーシス

IFE
immunofixation electrophoresis 免疫固定電気泳動法

Ifex
ifosfamide イホスファミド

IFF
inner fracture face 内骨折面

IFFS
International Federation of Fertility Societies 国際不妊学会連合

IFG
inferior frontal gyrus 下前頭回

IFHPSM
International Federation for Hygiene, Preventive Medicine and Social Medicine 国際衛生学・予防医学・社会医学連盟

IFI
intrafollicular insemination 卵胞内受精

IFL
immunofluorescence 免疫螢光検査(法), 螢光抗体法

IFLrA
recombinant human leukocyte interferon A 組換え型ヒト白血球インターフェロンA

IFM
internal fetal monitoring 胎児子宮内モニター
intrafusal muscle 錐内線維筋

IFMBE
International Federation for Medical and Biological Engineering 国際医用生体工学連合

IFME
International Federation of Medical Electronics 国際医用電子工学連合

IFMP
International Federation for Medical Psychotherapy 国際精神療法医学連盟

IFMSA
International Federation of Medical Students' Associations 国際医学生協会連盟

IFN
immunoreactive fibronectin 免疫反応性フィブロネクチン
interferon インターフェロン

if nec
if necessary 必要ならば

IFOBT
immunological fecal occult blood test 免疫便潜血検査

IFORS
International Federation of Operational Research Societies 国際手術研究会連合

IFOS
ifosfamide イホスファミド
International Federation of Ophthalmological Societies 国際眼科学会連盟
International Federation of Oto-Rhino-Laryngological Societies 国際耳鼻咽喉科学会連合

IFP
inflammatory fibroid polyp 炎症性類線維ポリープ
intermediate filament protein 中間フィラメント蛋白
International Federation for Psychotherapy 国際精神療法医学連盟

IFPM
International Federation of Physical Medicine 国際物理療法学連盟

IFPMA
International Federation of Pharmaceutical Manufactures & Association 国際製薬団体連合会

IFPMR
International Federation of Physical Medicine and Rehabilitation 国際物理療法学リハビリテーション学会連盟
IFPW
International Federation of Pharmaceutical Wholesalers 国際医薬品卸連盟
IFR
increasing failure rate 摩耗故障率
infrared 赤外(線)の
inspiratory flow rate 吸気流量率(速度)
IFRA
indirect fluorescent rabies antibody (test) 間接螢光狂犬病抗体(検査)
IFS
International Foundation for Science 国際科学財団
interstitial fluid space 細胞間質液腔
IFSC
International Federation of Surgical Colleges 国際外科学連盟
IFSEM
International Federation of Societies for Electron Microscopy 国際電子顕微鏡学会
IFSH
International Federation of Societies of Microscopy 国際顕微鏡学会
IFT
immunofluorcscence technique 免疫螢光法
immunofluorescence test 免疫螢光検査
IFTT
intravenous fat tolerance test 経静脈性脂肪負荷テスト
IFU
inclusion forming unit 封入形成単位
interferon unit インターフェロン単位
IFV
interstitial fluid volume 細胞間質液量
intracellular fluid volume 細胞内液量
IFX
ifosfamide イホスファミド
IG
icterogen 黄疸発生物
iG
immunoreactive human gastrin 免疫反応性ヒトガストリン
I-G
insulin-glucagon インスリン・グルカゴン
Ig, IG
immunoglobulin 免疫グロブリン

I

ig, IG
intragastric　胃内の
intragastrically　胃内に

IGA
infantile genetic agranulocytosis　乳児遺伝性無顆粒球症

IgA
immunoglobulin A　免疫グロブリンA

IgA GN
IgA glomerulonephritis　IgA腎症

IgA-SC
immunoglobulin A secreting cell　免疫グロブリンA分泌細胞

IGBP
International Geosphere-Biosphere Programme　地球圏・生物圏国際協同計画

IGD
idiopathic growth hormone deficiency　特発性成長ホルモン欠損症
interglobal distance　眼球間距離
isolated gonadotropin deficiency　単独ゴナドトロピン欠損症

IgD
immunoglobulin D　免疫グロブリンD

IgE
immunoglobulin E　免疫グロブリンE

IGF
insulin-like growth factor　インスリン様成長因子
International Genetics Federation　国際遺伝学連合

IgF
immunoglobulin F　免疫グロブリンF

IGFBP
insulin-like growth factor binding protein　インスリン様成長因子結合蛋白

IgG
immunoglobulin G　免疫グロブリンG

IgG-R
immunoglobulin G receptor　IgGレセプター

IgG RF
immunoglobulin G rheumatoid factor　免疫グロブリンGリウマチ因子

IgG-SC
immunoglobulin G secreting cell　IgG分泌細胞

IgGSF
immunoglobulin gene super family　免疫グロブリン遺伝子スーパーファミリー

IgG S-T S
short-term sensitizing IgG antibody　短期感作IgG抗体

IGH
idiopathic growth hormone　自然成長ホルモン

immunoreactive growth hormone 免疫反応性成長ホルモン

IgH
immunoglobulin heavy chain 免疫グロブリンH鎖

IGHD
inherited growth hormone deficiency 家族性成長ホルモン欠損症
isolated growth hormone deficiency 単独成長ホルモン欠損症

IGIM
immunoglobulin, intramuscular 筋肉内免疫グロブリン

IGIV
immunoglobulin, intravenous 静脈内免疫グロブリン

IgL
immunoglobulin light chain 免疫グロブリンL鎖

IgM
immunoglobulin M 免疫グロブリンM

IgM-anti HA
IgM class anti hepatitis A antibody IgM-抗A型肝炎抗体

IgM-anti HBc
IgM class anti hepatitis B core antibody IgM-抗B型肝炎コア抗体

IgM RF
immunoglobulin M rheumatoid factor 免疫グロブリンMリウマチ因子

IgM-SC
immunoglobulin M secreting cell 免疫グロブリンM分泌細胞

IGN
inferior gluteal nerve 下殿神経

IGP
intestinal glycoprotein 腸糖蛋白

IgQ
immunoglobulin quantitation 免疫グロブリン定量

IGR
immediate generalized reaction 即時全身反応
immunogenic region 免疫抗原認識部位

I group
indeterminate group 非定型群

IGS
inappropriate gonadotropin secretion 不適切性ホルモン分泌
intramural glomerulosclerosis 壁内糸球体硬化症

IgSC
immunoglobulin-secreting cell 免疫グロブリン分泌細胞

IGSS
immuno-gold-silver staining (method) 免疫性金銀染色(法)

IGT
impaired glucose tolerance 耐糖能障害

I

IGTT
intravenous glucose tolerance test 静脈内ブドウ糖負荷試験

IGU
International Geographical Union 国際地理学連合

IGV
idiopathic genu valgum 特発性外反膝
intrathoracic gas volume 胸腔内気体量

IH
immediate (type) hypersensitivity 即時(型)過敏症
incomplete healing 不完全治癒
indirect hemagglutination 間接赤血球凝集(反応)
infantile hydrocephalus 乳児水頭症
infectious hepatitis 感染〔伝染〕性肝炎
inguinal hernia 鼠径ヘルニア
inhibiting hormone 抑制ホルモン
in hospital (病)院内
intermittent heparinization 間欠性ヘパリン化
intracerebral hematoma 脳内血腫
intracranial hematoma 頭蓋内血腫
iron hematoxylin 鉄ヘマトキシリン

IHA
idiopathic hyperaldosteronism 特発性高アルドステロン症
immune hemolytic anemia 免疫性溶血性貧血
implantable hearing aid 植込み型補聴器
indirect hemagglutinating antibody 間接赤血球凝集抗体
infusion hepatic angiography 〔arteriography〕 (造影剤)注入肝動脈血管造影
intrahepatic atresia 肝内胆道閉鎖

IHAS
idiopathic hypertrophic aortic stenosis 特発性肥大性大動脈狭窄(症)

IHB
incomplete heart block 不完全心(臓)ブロック

IHBD
intrahepatic bile〔biliary〕 duct 肝内胆管

IHBT
incompatible hemolytic blood transfusion 不適合溶血性輸血

IHBTD
incompatible hemolytic blood transfusion disease 不適合溶血性輸血病

IHC
idiopathic hemochromatosis 特発性ヘモクロマトーシス
idiopathic hypercalciuria 特発性高カルシウム尿症
immunohistochemistry 免疫組織化学
induced hypertension chemotheray 血圧昇圧癌化学療法

intrahepatic cholestasis | 肝内胆汁うっ滞

IHC-F(r)
immunohistochemistry for frozen sections | 凍結切片用免疫組織化学

IHD
Institute of Human Development | 人間発達研究所
International Health Division | 国際保健局
ischemic heart disease | 虚血性心疾患

iHEA
International Health Economics Association | 国際医療経済学会

IHES
idiopathic hypereosinophilic syndrome | 特発性好酸球増多症候群

IHF
Industrial Hygiene Foundation | 産業衛生財団
International Hospital Federation | 国際病院連盟

IHG
ichthyosis hystrix gravior | 重症ヤマアラシ状魚鱗癬

IHGH
iodinated human growth hormone | 放射性ヨウ素標識成長ホルモン

IHGS
intrahepatic gallstone | 肝内結石

IHH
idiopathic hypogonadotropic hypogonadism | 特発性低ゴナドトロピン性性機能低下〔不全〕症
idiopathic hypothalamic hypogonadism | 特発性視床下部性性機能低下〔不全〕(症)
infectious human hepatitis | 感染性ヒト肝炎

IHHS
idiopathic hyperkinetic heart syndrome | 特発性心運動亢進症

IHI
impact of hypertension information | 高血圧情報インパクト

IHL
International Homeopathic League | 国際同種療法協会
intrahepatic lymphocyte | 肝内リンパ球

IHMS
sodium isonicotinic acid hydrazic methanesulfonate | イソニコチン酸ヒドラジド，メタンスルホン酸ナトリウム

IHO
idiopathic hypertrophic osteoarthropathy | 特発性肥大性骨関節症

idiopathic orthostatic hypotension 特発性起立性低血圧

IHP
idiopathic hypoparathyroidism 特発性副甲状腺機能低下症
idiopathic hypopituitarism 特発性下垂体機能低下症

IHPC
intrahepatic cholestasis 肝内胆汁うっ滞

IHPH
intrahepatic portal hypertension 肝内門脈高血圧

IHR
immediate hypersensitive reaction 即時型過敏反応
International Health Regulation 国際保健規則(WHO)
intrahepatic resistance 肝内抵抗
intrinsic heart rate 固有心拍数

IHRIM
Institute of Health Record Information and Management 健康記録情報医療管理協会

I

IHS
idiopathic hypereosinophilic syndrome 特発性好酸球増多症候群
independent hemopathic syndrome 独立血液疾患症候群
International Haematophilia Society 国際血友病学会
International Headache Society 国際頭痛学会
International Hearing Society 国際聴覚学会

IHSA
iodinated human serum albumin 放射性ヨウ素標識ヒト血清アルブミン

^{123}I-HSA
iodine-123 human serum albumin 放射性ヨウ素123標識ヒト血清アルブミン

^{131}I-HSA
iodine-131 human serum albumin 放射性ヨウ素131標識ヒト血清アルブミン

IHSC
immunoreactive human skin collagenase 免疫反応性ヒト皮膚コラゲナーゼ

IHSS
idiopathic hypertrophic subaortic stenosis 特発性肥大性大動脈弁下狭窄症

IHT
insulin hypoglycemia test インスリン低血糖試験
intarvenous histamine test 静注ヒスタミン試験

IHTT
interhemispheric transfer time 半球間伝達時間

IHW
inner heel wedge 内側踵くさび

II
icteric index　黄疸指数
image intensifier　イメージ増倍管
insulinogenic index　インスリン分泌指数

IIA
internal iliac artery　内腸骨動脈

IIC
ion interaction chromatography　イオン干渉クロマトグラフィ

IICA
intracranial internal carotid artery　頭蓋内内頸動脈

IICP
increased intracranial pressure　頭蓋内圧亢進

IID
insulin-independent diabetes　インスリン非依存性糖尿病

IIDM
insulin-independent diabetes mellitus　インスリン非依存性糖尿病

IIDR
image intensifier digital radiography　螢光倍増音信号デジタル化診断用X線装置
International institute for Dream Research　国際夢研究所

IIE
idiopathic ineffective erythropoiesis　特発性無効赤血球産生

IIF
immune interferon　免疫インターフェロン
indirect immunofluorescence　間接免疫螢光法

IIFT
intraoperative intraarterial fibrinolytic therapy　術中動脈内フィブリン溶解療法

IIH
idiopathic infantile hypercalcemia　特発性乳児高カルシウム血症
iodine-induced hyperthyroidism　ヨウ素誘発性甲状腺機能亢進症

IIHCEHV
International Institute of Health Care, Ethics and Human Values　健康管理・倫理・人間の価値に関する国際研究機関

IIIC
International Intraocular Implant Club　国際眼内レンズ学会

IIIVC
intrahepatic interruption of inferior vena cava　肝内下大静脈遮断(操作)

[^{123}I]IMP
iodoamphetamine　ヨードアンフェタミン

IINB
iliohypogastric nerve block　腸骨下腹神経ブロック

ilioinguinal nerve block 腸骨鼠径神経ブロック

IIP

idiopathic interstitial pneumonia 特発性間質性肺炎

idiopathic intestinal pseudo-obstruction 特発性腸偽閉塞(症)

indirect immunoperoxidase 間接免疫ペルオキシダーゼ

IIPF

idiopathic interstitial pulmonary fibrosis 特発性間質性肺線維症

IIR

investigator initiated research〔study〕〔trial〕 研究者主導研究

ion interaction reagent イオン干渉試薬，イオン相互作用試薬

IIS

intensive immunosuppression 集中免疫抑制

I

IIT

intensive insulin therapy 強化インスリン療法

I-IVH

intermittent intravenous hyperalimentation 周期的経静脈高カロリー輸液

IIVP

intensified IVP 強化経静脈性腎盂造影法

IJ

intrajejunal 空腸内の

IJ, I-J

internal jugular (vein) 内頸(静脈)

iJ, i.J.

im Jahre〈独〉 ～年に

IJD

inflammatory joint disease 炎症性関節疾患

IJP

inhibitory junction(al) potential 抑制性接合部電位

internal jugular pressure 内頸静脈圧

IJPAC

International Journal of Polymer Analysis and Characterization 高分子化学国際誌

IJSB

International Journal of Systematic Bacteriology 国際細菌命名規約

IJV

internal jugular vein 内頸静脈

IK

interstitial keratitis 間質性角膜炎

IK, I.K.

Immunkörper〈独〉＝immune bodies 免疫体

I_2KL
iodo-iodokalium Lugol solution　ルゴール液，複合ヨードグリセリン

IKR
Interkostalraum〈独〉　肋間腔

IL
ileum　回腸
iliolumbar　腰腸の
independent laboratory　独立検査室，独立研究所
independent living　自立生活《リハ》
inside layer　内層
inside left　内左
inside length　内側の長さ
intensity level　(音の)強さのレベル
interleukin　インターロイキン
intestinal lymphocyte　腸リンパ球
intralumbar　腰椎内の

Il
illinium　イリニウム

il
illustrate　図示する，図解する
illustrated　図示された，図解された
illustrator　作図家，イラストレーター
intralesional　病変内の

IL, Il, il
illustration　図，図解

ILA
insulin-like activity　インスリン様活性
International Leprosy Association　国際ハンセン病学会

ILa
incisolabial　切端唇側壁の

ILAE
International League Against Epilepsy　国際抗てんかん連盟

ILAR
International League Association for Rheumatology　国際リウマチ連盟

ILAS
insulin-like activity substance　インスリン様活性物質

ILBBB
incomplete left bundle branch block　不完全左脚ブロック

ILC
ichthyosis linearis circumflex　回旋性線状魚鱗癬
infiltrating lobular carcinoma　浸潤性小葉癌
intermediolateral column　中間外側路

ILCP
interstitial laser coagulation prostatectomy　前立腺生体組織内深部レーザー凝固術
ILD
induced labyrinthine deviation　誘発迷路性偏倚
interaural latency difference　両耳間潜時差
interstitial lung disease　間質性肺疾患
ischemic leg disease　虚血性脚疾患
ischemic limb disease　虚血性四肢疾患
isolated lactase deficiency　単独ラクターゼ欠損症
ILDL
intermediate low density lipoprotein　中間型低比重リポ蛋白
ILDPA
International Institute of Dental Practice Administration　国際歯科医療管理協会
ILE, Ile
isoleucine　イソロイシン
isoleucyl　イソロイシル
i lesion
intralesional　病変内の
ILEU, Ileu, ileu
isoleucine　イソロイシン
ILFC
immature living female child　生存未熟女児
ILGF
insulin-like growth factor　インスリン様成長因子
ill
illusion　錯覚
illustration　図，図解
illic.lag.obturat.
illico lagena obturatur〈ラ〉=let the bottle be closed at once　ただちにビンを閉め(させ)よ
illus
illustrated　図解した
illustration　図，図解
ILM
insulin-like material　インスリン様物質
internal limiting membrane　内境界膜
ILO
International Labor Organization　国際労働機関
ILo
iodine lotion　ヨウ素入り溶液
ILP
inadequate luteal phase　(妊娠)不適黄体期
interstitial laser photocoagulation　間質レーザー光凝固
interstitial lymphocytic pneumonia　間質性リンパ性肺炎

ILR
individual life time risk　個人生涯リスク

ILS
idiopathic lymphadenopathy syndrome　特発性リンパ節疾患症候群
increase in life span　生命延長，生存期間の延長
infrared liver scanner　赤外線肝スキャナー
interferon-like substance　インターフェロン様物質
intralobular sequestration　肺葉内肺分画症
intraluminal stapler　管腔内ホチキス

ILSMH
International League of Societies of Persons with Mental Handicap　国際知的障害者育成会連盟

ILSS
integrated life support system　統合生命維持システム
intraluminal somatostatin　管腔内ソマトスタチン

ILUS
intraluminal ultrasound　管腔内超音波

ILV
induced leukemia virus　誘発白血病ウイルス

ILVD
ischaemic left ventricular dysfunction　虚血性心左(心)室機能不全

ILVEN
inflammatory linear verrucous epidermal nevus　炎症性線状疣状表皮母斑

IM
idiopathic myelofibrosis　特発性骨髄線維症
immunosuppression method　免疫抑制法
impulse modulation　衝撃変動
infectious mononucleosis　伝染性単核球症
innocent murmur　無害性雑音
inspiratory muscle　吸気筋
insuffisance mitrale〈仏〉　僧帽弁閉鎖不全(症)
intermediate modulation　中間変動
intermediate position　中間位
intermodulation distortion　相互意識のひずみ《心理》
internal malleolus　内顆，うちくるぶし
internal medicine　内科(学)
intramedullary　髄内の
invasive mole　破壊性奇胎

Im
middle intrathoracic esophagus　胸部中部食道

im
immature　未熟な，未分化の

IM, im, I.m.
intramuscular (injection)　筋肉内(注射)

IM, I.M.
Index Medicus　インデックスメディクス，医学文献集

IMA
inferior mesenteric aorta (artery)　下腸間膜動脈
internal mammary artery　内乳(房)動脈
intestinal mucous antigen　腸粘液抗原

IMAA
iodinated macroaggregated albumin　ヨウ素標識大凝集アルブミン

^{131}I-MAA
iodine-131 macroaggregate albumin　ヨウ素131標識大凝集アルブミン

IMAB
internal mammary artery bypass　内乳(房)動脈バイパス(術)

IMAC
ifosfamide, mesna uroprotection, adriamycin, cisplatin　イホスファミド,メスナによる尿道保護,アドリアマイシン,シスプラチン

IMAG
internal mammary artery graft　内乳(房)動脈移植

IMAI
internal mammary artery implant　内乳(房)動脈移植

IMAO
inhibiteur de la mono-amine-oxydase〈仏〉　モノアミン酸化酵素抑制薬

IMB
intermenstrual bleeding　月経期外出血

IMBC
indirect maximal breathing capacity　間接最大呼吸量

IMBRF
International Medical Benefit/Risk Foundation　医薬品の便益性とリスクを科学的に評価解析することを目的とした国際財団

IMC
interdigestive migrating complex　消化管間移動複合
interdigestive migrating motor complex　空腹期の消化管強収縮運動
intestinal (mucosal) mast cell　腸(粘膜)肥満細胞

IMCD
inner medullary collecting duct　髄質内層集合管

IMCI
integrated management of childhood illuness　小児疾患包括的管理

IMD
idiopathic myocardial disease　原発性心筋症
immunizing dose　免疫量

immunologically mediated disease 免疫関与疾患
inherited metabolic disorder 遺伝性代謝障害
intermediate-dose methotrexate 中等量メトトレキサート

IMDD
idiopathic midline destructive disease 特発性中心線(部分)破壊病

IMF
idiopathic myelofibrosis 特発性骨髄線維症
ifosfamide, mesna uroprotection, methotrexate, 5-fluorouracil イホスファミド・メスナによる尿道保護・メトトレキサート・フルオロウラシル
intermaxillary fixation 顎間固定
International Myeloma Foundation 国際骨髄腫基金

IMFP
inelastic mean free path 非弾性平均自由行程

IMG
idiopathic monoclonal gammopathy 特発性モノクローナル免疫グロブリン異常症
inferior mesentric ganglion 下腸間膜神経節
internal mammary graft 内乳(房)動脈移植片
internal medicine group 内科グループ

IMGG
intramuscular gamma globulin 筋肉内ガンマグロブリン

IMH
idiopathic myocardial hypertrophy 特発性心筋肥大
indirect microhemagglutination 間接ミクロ血球凝集

IMI
imipramine イミプラミン
impending myocardial infarction 切迫心筋梗塞(症)
indirect membrane immunofluorescence 間接膜免疫螢光(検査)
inferior myocardial infarction 下壁心筋梗塞(症)
intermeal interval 食間間隔，食事間隔
intramuscular injection 筋注，筋肉内注射

IMIA
International Medical Informatics Association 国際医療情報学会

^{131}I-MIBG
iodine-131 metaiodobenzylguanidine ヨウ素131メタヨウ化ベンジルグアニジン

IMIC
International Medical Information Center 国際医学情報センター

IMIG
intramuscular immunoglobulin 筋肉内免疫グロブリン

IMIP
imipramine イミプラミン

imit
imitation 模倣
imitative 模倣の
IML
internal mammary lymphoscintigraphy 内乳房リンパシンチグラフィ
IMLC
incomplete mitral leaflet closure 僧帽弁閉鎖不全
IMLNS
idiopathic minimal lesion nephrotic syndrome 特発性微小病変型ネフローゼ症候群
immat
immature 未熟の
immed
immediately ただちに
immob
immobile 不動の
immobi
immobilize 固定する，不動にする
Immun, immun, immun.
immune 免疫(性)の
immunity 免疫
immunization 免疫(法,処置)
immunize 免疫化する
immunology 免疫学
Immunol, immunol
immunology 免疫学
IMN
internal mammary (lymph) node 内乳房リンパ節
intramedullary nailing 髄内釘固定法
IMP
idiopathic myeloid proliferation 特発性骨髄増殖
idiopathic myocardiopathy 特発性心筋症
^{123}I-isopropyl amphetamine イソプロピルアンフェタミン
imipramine イミプラミン
impotence 性的不能(症)，陰萎，インポテンス
incomplete male pseudohermaphroditism 不完全男性偽半陰陽
inosine monophosphate イノシンモノリン酸，イノシン一リン酸，イノシン酸
interface message processor インターフェイス・メッセージ・プロセッサ
intramembranous particle 膜内粒子
iodoamphetamine ヨードアンフェタミン

Imp, imp
impacted 埋伏した，楔合した，嵌入した
imperfect 不完全な
important 重要な
impression 印象，圧痕，陥凹
improve 改善する
improved 改善した
improvement 改善

IMPA
incisal mandibular plane angle 切歯下顎面角

impair
impaired 障害された
impairment 欠陥，障害

imperf
imperfect 不完全な
imperforate 閉鎖した，無孔の，無開口の

impet-efferv
impetu effervescentiae〈ラ〉 沸騰時に《処》

IMPL
impulse 衝動，インパルス

IMPO
immunoperoxidase 免疫ペルオキシダーゼ

Impo
Impotenz〈独〉 性的不能(症)，陰萎，インポテンス

imposs
impossible 不可能な

impr
impression 圧痕，陥凹，印象
improve 改善する
improved 改善した
improvement 改善

imprans
impransus 断食の《処》

impreg
impregnate 受胎させる，受精させる

IMPRV
improvement 改善

IMPS
inpatient multidimensional psychiatric scale 入院患者用多次元的精神症状評価尺度〔スケール〕

impt
important 大切な

impvt
improvement 改善

Impx
impaction (歯牙)埋伏(症)，嵌入，衝撃

IMR
individual medical record 個人の病歴
infant mortality rate 乳児死亡率
infectious mononucleosis receptor 伝染性単核症受容体
International Medical Research 国際医学研究

IMS
industrial methylated spirit 工業用加メチルエタノール
international metric system 国際メートル法

IMSS
in-flight medical support system 航空機内医療サポートシステム

IMT
indomethacin インドメタシン
induced muscular tension 誘発筋緊張
inspiratory muscle training 吸気筋訓練
intima-media thickness 内膜・中膜の壁厚

IMU，ImU
international milliunit 国際ミリ単位

IMV
ifosfamide, methotrexate, vincristine イホスファミド，メトトレキサート，ビンクリスチン
inferior mesenteric vein 下腸間膜静脈
intermittent mandatory ventilation 間欠的強制換気(法)

imv
improve 改良する，活用する

IMVP
idiopathic mitral valve prolapse 特発性僧帽弁逸脱症

IMVP-16
ifosfamide, mesna uroprotection, methotrexate, etoposide イホスファミド・メスナによる尿道保護・メトトレキサート・エトポシド

IMVS
Institute of Medical and Veterinary Science 医学・獣医学研究所

IN
icterus neonatorum 新生児黄疸
impetigo neonatorum 新生児膿痂疹
incidence 出生率，出現率，発生率
incompatibility number 不適合数
infantile nephrotic (syndrome) 乳児ネフローゼ(症候群)
infantile nephrotic (syndrome) 乳児ネフローゼ(症候群)
interneuron 介在ニューロン
interstitial nephritis 間質性腎炎
intranasal 鼻内の，鼻腔内の

I

In
index　示指，人差し指，指数
indium　インジウム〈元素〉
inion　外後頭隆起点《頭蓋計測》
inulin　イヌリン

in
inch　インチ〈単数〉〈単位〉
inches　インチ〈複数〉〈単位〉

in^3
cubic inches　立方インチ

in, In
insulin　インスリン

INA
infectious nucleic acid　感染性核酸
inferior nasal artery　下鼻動脈

INAA
instrumental neutron activation analysis　機器中性子放射化分析法

inac
inactive　不活性の，非活動性の

INAD
infantile neuroaxonal dystrophy　小児神経軸索萎縮(症)，小児神経軸索ジストロフィ

INAH
isonicotinic acid hydrazide　イソニコチン酸ヒドラジド，アイナー

in aq.
in aqua〈ラ〉　水に入れて《処》

in aq.bull.
in aqua bulliente〈ラ〉　沸湯で《処》

inaud
inaudible　聴こえない

INB
ischemic necrosis of bone　骨虚血性壊死，虚血性骨壊死

INC
interstitial nucleus of Cajal　カハール間質核

Inc
including　〜を含んだ

INC, Inc, Inc., inc.
incorporated　会社

INC, inc, inc.
incision　切開(術)
incisional　切開の
incomplete　不完全な
inconclusive　決定的ではない
incontinent　失禁の

increase 増加(する)，増大(する)
increased 増加した，増大した
increment 増強，増分

inc, inc.
incisus〈ラ〉 切った《処》
inconclusive 完成していない
incorporated 結合した，合併した

Inc Ab
incomplete abortion 不全流産

INCB
International Narcotics Control Board 国際麻薬統制委員会

IncB
inclusion body 封入(小)体

INCD
infantile nuclear cerebral degeneration 乳児核大脳変性(症)

I

incd
incident 起こりがちな

incdt
incident 起こりがちな

incid
incidence 出現率
incident 起こりがちな
incidental 付帯的な

incid.
incide〈ラ〉=cut 切開する，切る

incl
include 含む
including ～を含んだ
inclusive ～を含めて

incln
inclusion 封入，包括

incoher
incoherent 非連続性の，思考(散乱)した

incompat
incompatible 不適合な，配合禁忌の

incompl
incomplete 不完全な

incont
incontinence 失禁，失調(症)
incontinent 失禁の

INCR, Incr, incr.
increase 増加(する)，増大(する)
increasing 増大している
increment 増強，増分，変化量

incur, incur.
incurable　不治の

IND
indomethacin　インドメタシン
industrial　産業の
investigational new drug　治験(新)薬
investigation new drug　新薬調査，治験薬申請
notice of claimed investigational exemption for new drug　研究用新薬届

in d.
in die〈ラ〉=in a day　1日に《処》
in dies〈ラ〉=daily　日々，毎日《処》

ind, ind.
independent　独立した
index　示指，人差し指，指数
indicate　示す
indicating　示している
indication　適応(症)，適用
indigo　インジゴ
indirect　間接的な，間接の
induction　誘発，誘導

indef
indefinite　不定の，無期限の

indeq
inadequate　不適当な

indic
indicated　適応がある，示された
indication　適応(症)，適用，指示，指標

indig
indigestion　消化障害，消化不良

indiv, INDIV
individual　個々の，個人の

Ind.Med.
Index Medicus　指数〔係数〕・メディクス，医学文献集

Ind-Med
industrial medicine　産業医学

indo, INDO
indomethacin　インドメタシン

indocin
indomethacin　インドメタシン

indo.vehic.
idoneo vehiculo〈ラ〉=in a suitable vehicle　適当な賦形剤に

ind.th.
individual therapy　個人療法

^{111}In-DTPA
indium-111 diethylene triamine pentaacetic acid — インジウム111ジエチレントリアミン五酢酸

induc
inductance — インダクタンス係数
induction — 誘導

induct
induction — 誘発

indur
induration — 硬化，硬結

indust
industrial — 産業の
industry — 産業

INE
infantile necrotizing encephalomyelopathy — 乳児壊死性脳脊髄症

I

INEOA
International Narcotic Enforcement Officers Association — 国際麻薬取締官協会

in extrem.
in extremis〈ラ〉=in the last — 最後に，臨終に

INF
infiltration — 浸潤，浸潤度
infundibulum — 漏斗
interferon — インターフェロン

inf.
infunde〈ラ〉 — 注ぐ《処》
infusum〈ラ〉=an infusion — 浸剤

INF, Inf, inf
infusion — 温浸法，注入，浸剤

INF, inf
inferior — 下(方)の
infirmary — 小病院，診療所

INF, inf, inf.
infancy — 新生児期
infant — 乳幼児
infantile — 乳幼児の
infect — 感染する
infected — 感染した
infection — 感染，伝染
infectious — 感染の，感染性

inf, inf.
infarct — 梗塞
infarction — 梗塞(症)
in fine〈ラ〉=finally, at the end — 結局は，最後に
inflammatory changes — 炎症

information 情報

infarct

infarction 梗塞(症)

infec.dis

infectious disease 感染症

infect

infection 感染，伝染

infectious 感染の

infer

inferior 下(方)の

INFH

idiopathic necrosis of the femoral head 特発性大腿骨頭壊死

ischemic necrosis of femoral head 大腿骨頭虚血性壊死

infl

inflammation 炎症

influence 影響(力)

influx 流入

inflam

inflammation 炎症

inflammatory 炎症性の

inflamm

inflammation 炎症

inflammatory 炎症性の

infl proc

inflammatory process 炎症過程

influ

influence 影響，影響を及ぼす

influential 影響を与える

INFM

infectious mononucleosis 感染性単核球症

Inf.MI

inferior myocardial infarction 下壁心筋梗塞

inf mono

infectious mononucleosis 感染性単核球症

info

information 情報，通知，資料

infor

information 情報，通知，資料

INFOTERRA

International Environmental Information System 国際環境情報源照合システム

Inf.PS

infundibular pulmonary stenosis 漏斗部肺動脈狭窄

infra

infrared 赤外(線)の

I

inf.turb
inferior turbinate 下鼻甲介

Ing., ing
inguinal 鼠径(部)の

ingest
ingestion (経口)摂取，食物摂取

InGP
indolglycerophosphate インドールグリセロリン酸塩

INH
isonicotinoylhydrazine(=isoniazid) イソニコチン酸ヒドラジド(=イソニアジド)

INH, inh
inhalation 吸入(法)

inhal
inhalation 吸入(法)

I

inher
inherent 固有の，先天的な

inhib
inhibit(ing) 抑制する，阻止する
inhibition 抑制，阻止
inhibitor 抑制因子，抑制薬
inhibitory 抑制の，阻害の

INI
Industrial Nurse Institute 産業看護研究所
International Nursing Index 国際看護索引
intranuclear inclusion body 核内封入体

INIS
International Nuclear Information System 国際原子力情報システム

inj
inject 注射する
injure 傷害する
injured 損傷された
injury 損傷，傷害，外傷

Inj, inj, Inj.
injection 注射，注射剤

inject
injection 注射，注射剤

inj.enem.
injiciatur enema〈ラ〉=let an enema be injected 浣腸(剤を注入)せよ《処》

INK
injury not known 未知外傷

inl
initial 最初の，初期の
inlay インレー

in.lb., in-lb
inch-pound　インチ・ポンド
INLH
intestinal nodular lymphoid hyperplasia　腸管結節性リンパ過形成
in litt.
in litteris〈ラ〉　書面で《処》
in loc.cit.
in loco citato〈ラ〉=in the place cited　引用した場所に
in loc frig
in loco frigido〈ラ〉　冷所に《処》
INMS
isoniazid-methasulfonate　イソニアジド・メタスルホン酸
INN
infectious nephronephritis　炎症性ネフローゼ腎炎
international nonproprietary name　国際一般名，非商標名
innerv
innervated　神経支配された
innervation　神経支配
innom
innominate　無名の
INO
internuclear ophthalmoplegia　核間眼筋麻痺
Ino
inosine　イノシン
inositol　イノシトール
inosyl　イノシル
INOC, inoc
inoculate　接種する
inoc, inoc.
inoculated　接種した
inoculation　接種(法)
INOP
internodal ophthalmoplegia　結節間眼筋麻痺
inop
inoperable　手術できない
Ino-5′-P
inosine 5′-(mono)phosphate　イノシン5′-(モノ〔一〕)リン酸
Ino-5′-P2
inosine 5′-diphosphate　イノシン5′-ジ〔二〕リン酸
Ino-5′-P3
inosine 5′-triphosphate　イノシン5′-トリ〔三〕リン酸
inor
inorganic　無機の，無生物の

I

inorg
inorganic 無機の，無生物の
iNOS
inducible nitric oxide synthase 誘導型一酸化窒素合成酵素，誘導型NOS
IN.OUT
intake/output 水分出納
in-out
input-output 入力・出力
in.oz.
inch ounce インチ・オンス
INP
idiopathic neutropenia 特発性好中球減少症
intracellular negative potential 細胞間陰性電位
INPB
intermittent negative pressure assisted ventilation 間欠的陰圧補助的換気
intermittent negative pressure breathing 間欠的陰圧呼吸法
INPC
o-isopropyl *N*-phenyl carbamate *o*-イソプロピル*N*-フェニルカルバメート
INPEA
N-isopropyl-*p*-nitrophenylethanolamine *N*-イソプロピル-*p*-ニトロフェニルエタノールアミン
INPRCNS
information processing in central nervous system 中枢神経系の情報伝達
in prep
in preparation 準備中
in pro
in proportion 比例して，〜に応じて
in pulm.
in pulmento〈ラ〉 粥に混ぜて《処》
INPV
intermittent negative pressure ventilation 間欠的陰圧換気
INQ
inferior nasal quadrant 下鼻側(部)1/4区
INR
international normalized ratio 国際標準値〔比〕
INREM
internal roentgen equivalent, man 人体内レントゲン当量
INS
idiopathic nephrotic syndrome 特発性ネフローゼ症候群
information network system 情報ネットワークシステム

ion neutralization spectroscopy イオン中和分光

ins
inches インチ〈複数〉
insertion 挿入，停止，装着

INS, Ins
insurance 保険

INS, ins
insulin インスリン

in scat
in scatula 箱に入れて《処》

insid
insidious 潜行性の

in situ
in natural〔normal〕 position 原位置に

insol
insoluble 不溶(解)性の

InsP
inositol-phosphate イノシトールリン酸

insp
inspect 視診する，監査する

Insp, insp
inspiration 吸気
inspiratory 吸気の

insp, insp.
inspection 視診，監査

INSPEC
inspection 視診，監査
inspector 監査役

Inspir, inspir
inspiration 吸気
inspiratory 吸気の

INSS
International Neuroblastoma Staging System 国際神経芽細胞腫病期分類
International Staging System 国際病期分類

Inst, inst
institute 研究所
institution 制度，公共団体
institutional 制度(上)の
instructions 指図，通達
instrument 機械，器具

instab
instability 不安定(性)

instill
instillation 点滴注入，滴注

Instn
institution 制度，公共団体

Instr
instruction 教育
instructor 教官

insuf, insuf.
insufficient 不十分な
insufflatio〈ラ〉=an insufflation 吸入，通気

insuff
insufficiency (機能)不全(症)

INT
iodo-nitro-tetrazolium ヨード・ニトロ・テトラゾリウム

Int
intimate 親密な

INT, Int
intern インターン，医学研修生
internist 内科医

INT, Int, int
intermittent 間欠性の

int, int.
intact 障害されていない，完全な
interest 興味，利子
interesting 興味深い
interior 内の，内部
internal 内(の)，内部(の)
intersection 交叉〔差〕
interval 間隔，中間(期)
intestinal 腸(管)の

int.cib.
inter cibos〈ラ〉=between meal 食間に

intcl
intercostal 肋間の

INTEG
integument 外皮

intell
intelligence 知能，知性
intelligent 知能の高い，教養のある

intens
intensive 集中的な

inter.
interetur〈ラ〉 反復すべし《処》
intermediate 中間の

INTERASMA
International Association of Asthmology 国際喘息協会

intercond
intercondylar　顆間の

intermed
intermediate　介在する，中間物

intest
intestin　内部，腸
intestinal　腸の

intl
international　国際の

Int.Med.
internal medicine　内科(学)

int.noct.
inter noctem〈ラ〉=during the night　夜間に

intox
intoxicant　麻薬
intoxicate　中毒させる
intoxication　中毒

INTREX
information transfer experiment　情報伝達実験

intvw
interview　面接，面接する

in ut
in utero　子宮内で

inv
inversion　逆位，転位，反転

invagi
invagination　腸重積症

in vas.claus.
in vaso clauso〈ラ〉　ふたのある容器に入れて《処》

invest
investigation　調査，研究

in vit.
in vitro〈ラ〉　試験管内で

in viv.
in vivo〈ラ〉　生体内で

invol
involuntary　不随意の，無意識の

Inzi
Inzision〈独〉　切開

IO
inferior oblique muscle　下斜筋
inferior olive　下オリーブ核
intraocular　眼球内の

I & O
intake and output　摂取(量)と排出(量)

I/O, I & O
input/output 入力/出力
input/output port コンピュータの入出力ポート
IOAT
International Organization Against Trachoma 国際トラコーマ予防機構
IOC
initial operational capability 初期手術可能性
in our clinic われわれの臨床で
intraoperative cholangiogram 術中胆管造影図
IOCG
intraoperative cholangiogram 術中胆管造影図
IOCV
International organization of Citrus Virologists 国際柑橘類ウイルス学者機構
IOD
injured on duty 仕事中に受傷した
integrated optical density 積分視覚濃度《コン》
interorbital distance 眼窩間距離
iodid.
iodidum〈ラ〉 ヨウ化物《処》
IOFB
intraocular foreign body 眼球内異物
IOFNA
intraoperative fine-needle aspiration 術中微小針吸引術
IOH
idiopathic orthostatic hypotension 特発性起立性低血圧(症)
IOHS
idiopathic orthostatic hypotension syndrome 特発性起立性低血圧症候群
IOI
intraosseous infusion 骨内注入(輸液)
IOL
intraocular lens 眼内レンズ
IOLI
intraocular lens implantation 眼内レンズ移植
IOM
Institute of Medicine 医学研究所
intraocular muscle 眼内筋
IOML
infraorbitomeatal line 眼窩下縁外耳孔線
ION
ischemic optic neuropathy 虚血性視神経疾患
IONIS
indirect optic nerve injury syndrome 間接視神経損傷症候群

IOP
input-output processor 入力・出力操作
intraocular pressure 眼(内)圧
IOPAB
International Organization for Pure and Applied Biophysics 国際純粋・応用生物物理学機構
IOR
intraoperative radiation 術中放射線照射
intraoperative radiotherapy 術中照射療法
I or I
illness or injuries 疾患あるいは損傷
IORT
intraoperative irradiation therapy 術中照射療法
intraoperative radiation therapy 術中放射線療法
IOS
intraoperative sonography 術中超音波検査
IOT
intraocular tension 眼(内)圧
intraocular transfer 眼内移動
ipsilateral optic tectum 同側視蓋
IoT
Internet of Things モノのインターネット
IOU
intensive (therapy) observation unit 集中観察室，集中治療室
international opacity unit 国際混濁単位
IOVP
interesophageal variceal pressure 食道静脈瘤圧
iow
in other word 他の言葉で言えば
IP
icterus praecox 早発黄疸
identified patient 依存病者
imaging plate イメージ板
immunoblastic plasma 免疫芽球プラズマ〔血漿〕
immunoperoxidase 免疫ペルオキシダーゼ
inactivated pepsin 不活性化ペプシン
incisoproximal 切歯近位の
incisopulpal 切歯髄の
incontinentia pigmenti 色素失調(症)
incubation period 潜伏期
induction period 誘発月経〔生理〕
industrial population 産業人口
infection prevention 感染予防
infusion pump インフュージョンポンプ，輸液注入器
infusion (intravenous) pyelography 静脈性腎盂造影(法)

initial pressure	初(期)圧
inorganic phosphate	無機リン酸
inorganic phosphorous	無機リン酸
inosine phosphorylase	イノシンホスホリラーゼ
inositol phosphate	イノシトールリン酸
instantaneous pressure	瞬時圧
intenstinal pseudoobstruction	腸管仮性閉塞症
International Pharmacopoeia	国際薬局方
internus paresis	内筋麻痺
interpeduncular (nucleus)	脚間(核)
interphalangeal	指節間(関節)
interstitial pneumonitis	間質性肺炎
intracellular proteolysis	細胞内蛋白分解
intraperitoneal (injection)	腹腔内(注射)
intravenous pyelography	静脈性腎盂造影
investigational product	治験薬管理
iris process	虹彩突起
isoproterenol	イソプロテレノール
iso-tachophoresis	細管式等速電気泳動法
L' Institut Pasteur	パスツール研究所

IP3

inositol thiphosphate	イノシトール三リン酸

Ip

immunophagocytosis	免疫食作用

I/P

iris and pupil	虹彩と瞳孔

I & P

indexed and paged	索引とページを示した

IP, ip, i.p.

intraperitoneal	腹腔内の，経腹膜的
intraperitoneally	腹腔内に，経腹膜的に

ip, I.p.

isoelectric point	等電点

IPA

ifosfamide, cisplatin (=Platinol), adriamycin	イホスファミド,シスプラチン(=プラチノール),アドリアマイシン
imidazole pyruvic acid	イミダゾール焦性ブドウ酸
including particular average	特殊平均を含む
International Pediatric Association	国際小児科学会
International Phonetic Association	国際音声協会
International Psychoanalytical Association	国際精神分析学会
International Psychogeriatrics Association	国際老年精神医学会
isopropyl-arterenol	イソプロピルアルテレノール

I

IPAA
ileal pouch anal anastomosis 回腸(嚢)肛門吻合術
IPABPC
isopropyliden-aminobenzylpenicillin イソプロピリデンアミノベンジルペニシリン(=ヘタシリンカリウム)
IPAO
insulin-induced peak acid output インスリン誘発最大酸分泌
IPAP
inspiratory positive airway pressure 吸気陽性気道圧
IPAS
Izumo Prehospital Apoplexy Scale 出雲急性期脳卒中病院前診断チェックリスト
IPB
infrapopliteal bypass 膝窩下バイパス(術)
IPC
intraductal papillary carcinoma (腺)管内乳頭状癌
intraperitoneal chemotherapy 腹腔内化学療法
IPCC
Intergovernmental Panel on Climate Change 気候変動に関する政府間パネル
International Pigment Cell Conference 国際色素細胞会議
IPCD
infantile polycystic disease 幼児型多嚢胞症
IPCS
International Programme on Chemical Safety 国際化学物質安全性計画
intrauterine progesterone contraceptive system 子宮内プロゲステロン避妊システム
IPD
idiopathic Parkinson disease 特発性パーキンソン病
idiopathic protracted diarrhea 特発性長期下痢(症)
immediate pigment darkening 即時型色素黒化
increase in pupillary diameter 瞳孔直径の増加
intermittent peritoneal dialysis 間欠的腹膜透析(法)
intermittent pigment darkening 間欠性色素黒化
interpupillary distance 瞳孔間距離
IPDA
inferior pancreatico-duodenal artery 下膵十二指腸動脈
IPE
initial psychiatric development 初期精神的発達
injury pulmonary edema 外傷性肺浮腫
interstitial pulmonary emphysema 間質性肺気腫

I

IPEH	
intravascular papillary endothelial hyperplasia	血管内乳頭状内皮過形成
IPF	
idiopathic pulmonary fibrosis	特発性肺線維症
infection-potentiating factor	感染増強因子
insulin promoter factor	インスリン転写因子
interstitial pulmonary fibrosis	間質性肺線維症
IPFC	
indirect plaque-forming cell(s)	間接プラーク形成細胞
IPFD	
intrapartum fetal distress	分娩時胎児仮死
IPG	
impedance phlebograph	インピーダンス静脈波計
impedance plethysmography	インピーダンスプレチスモグラフィ
iPGE	
immunoreactive prostaglandin E	免疫反応性プロスタグランジンE
IPH	
idiopathic portal hypertension	特発性門脈圧亢進症
idiopathic pulmonary hemosiderosis	特発性肺ヘモジデリン沈着症
inflammatory papillary hyperplasia	炎症性乳頭状過形成(症)
interphalangeal	指骨間の
intraparenchymal hemorrhage	(臓器)実質内出血
IPHP	
intraperitoneal hyperthermic perfusion	腹腔内温熱灌流療法
IPHR	
inverted polypoid hamartoma of rectum	内反ポリープ状直腸過誤腫
IPJ	
interphalangeal joint	指節間関節
IPK	
interphalangeal keratosis	指節間角化症
intractable plantar keratosis	難治性足底角化症
IPKD	
infantile polycystic kindney disease	乳児多嚢胞腎病
IPL	
idiopathic plasmacytic lymphadenopathy	特発性プラズマ細胞リンパ節腫脹
IPM	
Impulsiv-Petit-mal〈独〉	無動小発作
intrauterine pressure monitor	子宮内圧モニター
isopropyl myristate	ミリスチン酸イソプロピル

IPM/CS
imipenem/cilastatin sodium イミペネム/シラスタチンナトリウム

IPN
infantile periarteritis nodosa 乳児型結節性動脈周囲炎
infantile polyarteritis nodosa 乳児型結節性多発動脈炎

IPn
interstitial pneumonitis 間質性肺臓炎

IPNA
isopropyl-noradrenaline(=isoproterenol) イソプロピルノルアドレナリン(=イソプロテレノール)

IPNP
intraductal papillary neoplasm of the pancreas (膵)管内乳頭状膵癌

IPNPB
intermittent positive-negative pressure breathing 間欠的陽陰圧呼吸

IPNPV
intermittent positive-negative pressure ventilation 間欠的陽陰圧換気法

IPO
intrahepatic portal vein obstruction 肝内門脈閉塞症

IPOS
International Psycho-oncology Society 国際精神腫瘍学会

IPP
idiopathic precocious puberty 体質性早熟
intermittent positive pressure 間欠的陽圧
intrapleural pressure 胸(膜)腔内圧
isopropyl palmitate パルミチン酸イソプロピル

IPPA
inspection, palpation, percussion, auscultation 視診・触診・打診・聴診

IPPB
intermittent positive pressure breathing 間欠的陽圧呼吸

IPPF
immediate postsurgical prosthetic fitting 術直後人工装具装着
International Planned Parenthood Federation 国際家族計画連盟

IPPNW
International Physicians for Prevention of Nuclear War 国際反核医師の会

IPPO
intermittent positive pressure (inflation) with oxygen　間欠的陽圧(吹入)酸素療法

IPPR
intermittent positive pressure respiration　間欠的陽圧呼吸

IPPV
intermittent positive pressure ventilation　間欠的陽圧人工換気(法)

IPR
isoproterenol　イソプロテレノール

IPRS
International Confederation for Plastic and Reconstruction Surgery　国際形成外科学連合

IPS
idiopathic postprandial syndrome　特発性食事後症候群
impulse per second　インパルス/秒
information, production and systems　情報・生産・システム
infundibular pulmonary stenosis　漏斗状肺動脈弁狭窄(症)
International Planetarium Society　国際プラネタリウム協会
International Presentation Society　国際プレゼンテーション協会
intraparietal sulcus　頭頂間溝
intraperitoneal shock　腹腔内ショック
Inter Press Service　インタープレスサービス，国際報道機関
intrusion prevention system　侵入防止システム
ischiopubic synchondrosis　坐骨恥骨軟骨結合
isoprinosine　イソプリノシン

IPs
inositol phosphates　イノシトールリン酸

iPS
induced pluripotent stem cells　人工多能性幹細胞

ips
inches per second　毎秒インチ

IPSB
intrapartum stillbirth　分娩時死産

IPSF
International Pharmacy Students Federation　国際薬学生連盟

IPSID
immunoproliferative small intestinal disease　免疫増殖性小腸疾患

IPSP
inhibitory postsynaptic potential　抑制性シナプス後電位

IPSS
international pilot study of schizophrenia　分裂病国際試験研究
International Prostate Symptom Score　国際前立腺症状スコア

IPT
immunoperoxidase technique　免疫ペルオキシダーゼ法
indexed, paged and titled　索引・ページ・表題のついた
interpersonal psychotherapy　対人関係精神療法

IPTD
2-(*p*-aminobenzensulfamido-)5-isopropylthiadiazole　2-(パラアミノベンゼンスルファミド-)5-イソプロピルチアジアゾール

iPTH
immunoreactive parathyroid hormone　免疫反応性上皮小体ホルモン

IPTR
International Pancreas Transplant Registry　国際膵移植登録

IPV
immunoreactive polymyelitis vaccine　免疫反応性多発脊髄炎ワクチン
inactivated poliomyelitis vaccine　不活性化ポリオワクチン
inactivated poliovirus vaccine　不活化ポリオ(ウイルス)ワクチン
infectious pustular (vulvo) vaginitis　感染性膿疱性(外陰)腟炎

IPVC
interpolated premature ventricular contraction　間入性早期期外収縮

IPVD
index of pulmonary vascular disease　肺動脈疾患の重症度指数

^{131}I-PVP
iodine-131 polyvinylpyrrolidone　ヨウ素131ポリビニルピロリドン

^{131}I-PVP test
iodine-131 polyvinylpyrrolidone test　ヨウ素131ポリビニルピロリドン試験，ゴルドン試験

IPVS
International Pig Veterinary Society　国際養豚獣医学協会

IPZ
insulin/protamine-zinc　インスリン・プロタミン亜鉛
intraparenchymal zone　実質内域

IQ
intelligence quotient　知能指数

i.q.
idem quod〈ラ〉=the same as　～と同じ

IQC
internal quality control　内部精度管理
i.q.e.d.
id quod erat demonstrundum〈ラ〉　証明されたように
IQ & S
iron, quinicine and strychnine　鉄・キニシン・ストリキニン
IR
immunologic response　免疫(学的)反応
infantile Refsum disease　小児レフサム病
inferior rectus (muscle)　下直筋
information retrieval　情報検索
infrared (rays)　赤外線の
infrared absorption spectrometry　赤外線吸収分光計測
inner rotation　内旋
inspectors report　調査者の報告
inspiratory reserve　吸気予備(量)
inspiratory resistance　吸気抵抗
insulation resistance　絶縁抵抗
insulin receptor　インスリンレセプター
insulin requirement　インスリン必要量
insulin resistance　インスリン抵抗性
insulin response　インスリン応答
intrarachidian　脊髄内の
inversion recovery　反転回復法
investigation record　観察記録
iridectomy　虹彩切除
Ir
immune response　免疫応答
internal resistance　内部抵抗
iridium　イリジウム
isovolumetric relaxation　等容性弛緩
^{192}Ir
iridium-192　イリジウム192
IR, I.r.
intrarectal　直腸内の
IRA
ileo-rectal anastomosis　回腸直腸吻合術
immunoradioassay　免疫放射標識定量法，ラジオ免疫法
immunoregulatory alpha globulin　免疫調節(性)αグロブリン
inferior mesenteric artery　下腸間膜動脈
infrared A　短波長赤外線
intravenous regional analgesia　静脈内局所麻酔
IRAS
infrared reflection absorption spectroscopy　赤外線金属反射吸収スペクトル法

I

IRB
infrared B 中波長赤外線
Institutional Review Board 研究所の治験審査委員会

^{131}I-RB
iodine-131 rose bengal ヨウ素131ローズベンガル

IRBBB
incomplete right bundle branch block 不完全右脚ブロック

IRBC
infected red blood cell 感染赤血球

IRBC，iRBC
immature red blood cell 未熟赤血球

IRBP
intraretinal binding protein 網膜間結合蛋白

IRC
indirect radionuclide cystography 間接放射性核種膀胱造影(法)
infrared C 長波長赤外線
infrared coagulator 赤外線凝固薬
infrared photocoagulation 赤外線光凝固
intensive respiratory care 集中呼吸管理

IRCA
intravascular red cell aggregation 血管内赤血球凝集

IRCU
intensive respiratory care unit 集中呼吸管理治療部

IRD
idiopathic respiratory disease 特発性呼吸器疾患
immune renal disease 免疫性腎疾患
infantile Refsum syndrome 乳児レフスム症候群
ischemic renal disease 虚血性腎症

IRDA
intermittent rhythmic delta activity 間欠性律動性δ波

IRDM
insulin-resistant diabetes mellitus インスリン抵抗性糖尿病

IRDNI
idiopathic respiratory distress of newborn infant 特発性新生児呼吸窮迫障害

IRDS
idiopathic respiratory distress syndrome 特発性呼吸窮迫症候群
infantile respiratory distress syndrome 新生児呼吸窮迫症候群

IRE
immunoreactive elastase 免疫反応性エラスターゼ
insulin responsive element インスリン反応性要素
internal rotation in extension 伸展時における内旋

IRF
idiopathic retroperitoneal fibrosis 特発性腹膜後線維症

interferon regulatory factor　インターフェロン制御因子
internal rotation in flexion　屈曲時における内旋

IRG
immunoreactive gastrin　免疫反応性ガストリン
immunoreactive glucagon　免疫反応性グルカゴン
immunoreactive glucose　免疫反応性グルコース

Ir gene
immune response gene　免疫応答遺伝子

IRGH
immunoreactive growth hormone　免疫反応性成長ホルモン

IRGI
immunoreactive glucagon　免疫反応性グルカゴン

IRH
intraretinal hemorrhage　網膜内出血

IRhCG
immunoreactive human chorionic gonadotropin　免疫反応性ヒト絨毛性ゴナドトロピン

IRHCS
immunoradioassayable human chorionic somatomammotropin　ラジオイムノアッセイヒト絨毛性体乳腺成長ホルモン

IRhCS
immunoreactive human chorionic somatomammotropin　免疫反応性ヒト絨毛性体乳腺成長ホルモン

IRhGH
immunoreactive human growth hormone　免疫反応性ヒト成長ホルモン

IRhPL
immunoreactive human placental lactogen　免疫反応性ヒト胎盤性ラクトゲン

IRI
immunoreactive insulin　免疫反応性インスリン

IRIA
indirect radioimmunoassay　間接放射免疫標識定量法

IRM
immunoreactive motilin　免疫反応性モチリン
innate releasing mechanism　先天放出機構

IRMA
immunoradiometric assay　免疫放射定量法
International Rehabilitation Medicine Association　国際リハビリテーション医学会
intraretinal microangiopathy　網膜内微小血管症
intraretinal microvascular abnormalities　網膜内微小血管異常

iRNA
immune ribonuclear acid　免疫リボ核酸
informational ribonucleic acid　情報伝達リボ核酸

IRP
idiopathic recurrent pancreatitis 特発性再発性膵炎
immunoreactive plasma 免疫反応性血漿
immunoreactive proinsulin 免疫反応性プロインスリン
immunoreactive prolactin 免疫反応性プロラクチン
International Reference Preparation 国際標準品
interstitial radiation pneumonitis 間質性放射線肺炎

IRPGN
idiopathic rapidly progressive glomerulonephritis 特発性急速進行性糸球体腎炎

IRP-HMG
International Reference Preparation for Human Menopausal Gonadotropin ヒト閉経期ゴナドトロピンに関する国際文献機関

IRPTC
International Register of Potentially Toxic Chemicals 国際有害化学物質登録制度

IRPTH
immunoreactive parathyroid hormone 免疫反応性上皮小体ホルモン

IRR
intrarenal reflux 腎内逆流

IR ray
infrared ray (radiation) 赤外線(照射)

irreg
irregular 不規則

IRRG, irrg
irrigation 洗浄，灌注

irrig
irrigation 洗浄，灌注

IRS
immune response system 免疫反応系
immunoreactive somatostatin 免疫反応性ソマトスタチン
insulin receptor substrate インスリン受容体基質
Intergroup Rhabdomyosarcoma Study 国際横紋筋腫研究会
International Rhinologic Society 国際鼻科学会
International Rorschach Society 国際ロールシャッハ協会
intravenous regional sympathe(te)ctomy 静脈内局所交感神経遮断

IRSA
idiopathic refractory sideroblastic anemia 特発性不応性鉄芽球性貧血

IRT
immunological reactive tryosinogen 免疫反応性トリオシノゲン
immunoreactive trypsin 免疫反応性トリプシン
initial response time 効果発現時間
isometric relaxation time 等容拡張時間

IRU
International Radium Unit　国際ラジウム単位
International Rat Unit　国際ラット単位

IRV
inspiratory reserve volume　予備吸気量
inversed ratio ventilation　逆比率換気

IS
idiopathic scoliosis　特発性側弯症
ilial segment　回腸分節
immune serum　免疫血清
immune suppressor　免疫サプレッサー
immuno suppression　免疫抑制
incentive spirometer　インセンティブスパイロメータ
incentive spirometry　インセンティブスパイロメトリー
incudostapedial　キヌタ・アブミ骨関節
indoxyl sulfate　インドキシル硫酸
infrahyoid strap　舌骨下筋
initial axonal segment　軸索起始部
initial segment　初節
insertion sequence　挿入配列
insulin secretion　インスリン分泌
intercellular space　細胞間腔
intercostal space　肋間腔
internal standard material　中部標準物質
interventricular septum　心室中隔厚
intracardial shunt　心腔内シャント
Irvine syndrome　アービン症候群
ischemic score　虚血スコア
musculus infraspinatus　棘下筋
subcutaneous injection　皮下注射

is
islet　小島，島

ISA
ileosigmoid anastomosis　回腸S状結腸吻合
International Strabismological Association　国際斜視学会
intrinsic sympathomimetic activity　内因性交感神経刺激作用
iodinated serum albumin　ヨウ素標識血清アルブミン

ISAC
image save and carry　画像の保存と運送

ISADH
inappropriate secretion of antidiuretic hormone　抗利尿ホルモン不適合分泌

ISB
International Society of Biometeorology　国際生物気象学会

ISBI
International Society for Burn Injuries　国際熱傷学会
international standard book numbering　国際標準図書番号体系

ISC
immunoglobulin-secreting cell　免疫グロブリン分泌細胞
Inter-American Society of Cardiology　米大陸心臓学会
International Society of Cardiology　国際心臓病学会，国際循環器(外科)学会
International Society of Chemotherapy　国際化学療法学会
International Society of Criminology　国際犯罪学会
interstitial cell　間質細胞
irreversible sickle cell　不可逆性鎌状赤血球
irreversibly sickled cell　不可逆性鎌状赤血球

IsC
islands of Calleja　カレハ嗅覚小島

IS & C
image save and carry　画像ファイリングシステム

ISCD
International Statistical Classification of Disease　国際疾病分類

ISCEV
International Society for Clinical Electrophysiology of Vision　国際臨床視覚電気生理学会

ISCF
interstitial cell fluid　間質細胞液

ISCOMS
immunostimulating complexes　免疫刺激複合体

ISCP
International Society of Clinical Pathology　国際臨床病理学会

ISD
immunosuppressive drug　免疫抑制薬
inhibited sexual desire　性欲阻害
initial sleep disturbance　初期睡眠障害
interatrial septal defect　心房中隔欠損
interventricular septal defect　心室中隔欠損
intrinsic sphincter deficiency　固有括約筋欠損(症)
intrinsic sphincter dysfunction　固有括約筋機能不全(障害)

I

ISDB
indirect self-destructive behavior 間接自傷〔自損〕行為
ISDN
isosorbide dinitrate (二)硝酸イソソルビド
ISE
inhibited sexual excitement 抑制された性的興奮
inhibitor sensitive esterase 抑制物質感受性エステラーゼ
ion-selective electrode イオン選択電極
ISEK
International Society of Electrophysiological Kinesiology 国際電気生理筋運動学会
ISF
interstitial fluid 間質液
ISFET
ion sensitive field effect transistor イオン感受領域効果トランジスタ
ISG
immune serum globulin 免疫血清グロブリン
Is gene
immune suppression gene 免疫抑制遺伝子
ISGEO
International Society of Geographical Ophthalmology 国際地理眼科学会
ISG-IID
International Study Group on Diabetes Treatment with Implantable Insulin Delivery Devices 移植可能なインスリン放出装置で糖尿病を治療する国際研究グループ
ISH
icteric serum hepatitis 黄疸性血清肝炎
in situ hybridization *in situ* ハイブリダイゼーション法
International Society of Hematology 国際血液学会
International Society of Hypertension 国際高血圧学会
intrasellar subarachinoidal herniation トルコ鞍内クモ膜下腔嵌入
isolated systolic hypertension 孤立性収縮期高血圧(症)
ISHLT
International Society for Heart & Lung Transplantation 国際心肺移植学会
ISHR
International Society for Heart Research 国際心臓研究学会
ISI
infarct size index 梗塞サイズ指標
initial slope index 初期勾配指数
injury severity index 外傷重症度係数

insulin sensitivity index　インスリン感受性指数
international sensitivity index　国際感度指数
International Statistical Institute　国際統計協会

ISIM
International Society of Internal Medicine　国際内科学会

ISIS
image-selected in vivo spectroscopy　生体内画像選択分光器
international study of infant survival　国際乳児生存研究

ISKDC
International Study of Kidney Disease in Children　国際小児腎研究

ISL
International Society of Lymphology　国際リンパ学会

ISLIS
International Society of Life Information Science　国際生命情報科学会

isl of Lang
islands of Langerhans　ランゲルハンス島

ISM
industrial, scientific, medical wavelength　産業・科学・医学の波長

ISMC
International Symposium on Macrocyclic Chemistry　大環状化合物国際シンポジウム

ISMED
International Society on Metabolic Eye Disease　国際代謝異常眼疾患学会

ISMH
International Society of Medical Hydrology and Climatology　国際温泉気候学会

ISMN
isosorbide 5-mononitrate　イソソルビド 5-モノニトレート

ISMRM
International Society of Magnetic Resonance in Medicine　国際磁気共鳴医学会

ISMUS
morphinismus　モルヒネ中毒

ISN
International Society for Neurochemistry　国際神経化学会
International Society of Nephrology　国際腎臓学会
International Society of Neuropathology　国際神経病理学会

I

ISNAE
International Society for Normal and Abnormal Ethnopsychology　国際民族心理学会
ISNR
International Society of Neurovegetative Research　国際自律神経研究会
ISNY socket
Irlandic-Swedenish-New York socket　アイルランド・スウェーデン・ニューヨーク型ソケット
ISO
International Organization for Standardization　国際標準化機構
isoproterenol　イソプロテレノール
iso
isotropic　等方向性の
isoamy
isoamylase　イソアミラーゼ
ISOBM
International Society for Oncodevelopmental Biology and Medicine　国際癌胎児性蛋白質学会
isobu
isobutyl　イソブチル基
isochr
isochronal　等時性の
isoln
isolation　分離
isom
isomeric　異性の
isot
isotropic　等方向性の
ISP
distance between iliac spines　腸骨棘突起間距離
immunoreactive substance P　免疫反応物質P
Index of Social Progress　社会進歩指標
Interamerican Society of Psychology　全米心理学会
interstitial pneumonia　間質性肺炎
intrasplenic pressure　脾内圧
isepamicin　イセパミシン
isoprenaline　イソプレナリン
isp
intraspinal　脊髄内の
ISPE
International Society for Pharmacoepidemiology　国際薬剤疫学学会

ISPN
International Society for Pediatric Neurosurgery　国際小児脳神経外科学会
ISPNE
International Society for Psychoneuroendocrinology　国際精神神経内分泌学会
ISPO
International Society for Prosthetics and Orthotics　国際補綴矯正学会
International Society of Pediatric Ophthalmology　国際小児眼科学会
ISPOG
International Society of Psychosomatic Obstetrics and Gynecology　国際女性心身医学会産科婦人科学会
ISPRM
International Society of Physical and Rehabilitation Medicine　国際リハビリテーション医学会
ISQUA
International Society for Quality in Health Care　国際ヘルスケア質向上協会
ISR
Institute for Sex Research　性科学研究所
International Society of Radiology　国際放射線学会
inter scapular region　肩甲間部
ISRD
International Society for Rehabilitation of the Disabled　国際身体障害者リハビリテーション学会
ISRE
IFN stimulated response element　インターフェロン刺激反応因子
ISRP
internal surface reversed phase　内面逆相
ISRRT
International Society of Radiographers and Radiological Technologists　国際放射線技士学会
ISS
injury severity score　外傷重症度スコア
ion scattering spectroscopy　イオン散乱分光法
ion surface scattering　イオン表面散乱
irritable stomach syndrome　過敏性胃症候群
iss.
unum cum semisse〈ラ〉　1個半

I

ISSA
International Social Security Association — 国際社会保障協会

ISSBD
International Society for the Study of Behavioural Development — 国際行動発達学会

ISSDCR
International Society for the Study of Diseases of the Colon and Rectum — 国際結腸・直腸病学会

ISSLS
International for the Study of Lumber Spine Society — 国際腰椎学会

ISSN
international standard serial number — 国際標準逐次刊行物番号

IS spike
initial segment spike — ISスパイク

I

ISSVD
International Society for Study of Vulvovaginal Disease — 国際外陰部疾患学会

IST
injection sclerotherapy — 注入硬化療法
insulin secretion test — インスリン分泌試験
insulin shock therapy — インスリンショック療法
International Society on Toxinology — 国際毒物学会
isometric systolic tension — 等尺性収縮張力

ISTC
International Science and Technology Center — 国際科学技術センター

ISTD
Institute for Study and Treatment of Delinquency — 非行の研究と治療研究所

ISTH
International Society on Thrombosis and Haemostasis — 国際血栓止血学会

I-sub
inhibitor substance — 抑制物質

ISUCRS
International Society of University Colon and Rectal Surgeons — 国際大学結腸・直腸外科医学会

ISVN
International System of Virus Nomenclature — 国際ウイルス命名法

ISVR
Institute of Sound and Vibration Research — 音響・振動研究所

ISW
interstitial water 間質液
ISWT
Incremental Shuttle Warking Test 漸増シャトルウォーキングテスト
isy
intrasynovial 滑液包内の
IT
immediate tanning 即時型黒化
immunity test 免疫検査
immunologic test 免疫学的検査
immunotherapy 免疫療法
industrial therapy 産業医学
information technology 情報技術
inhalation test 吸入試験
inhalation therapy 吸入療法
insulin treatment インスリン治療
intensive therapy 集中治療
intention tremor 企図振戦
interstitial tissue 間質組織，結合組織
intertuberous 結節間の
intestinal type 腸型
intradermal test 皮内試験
intrathecal 脊髄腔内
intrathecal injection 髄腔内注射
intrathoracic 胸腔内
intratracheal 気管内
intratrachcal tube 気管内チューブ
isometric transition 核異性体転位
i.t.
intrathymic 胸腺内
I/T
intensity/duration 強度/持続時間比
ITA
inferior temporal artery 下側頭動脈
internal thoracic artery 内胸動脈
intratubal adhesion 管内癒着
itaconic acid イタコン酸
ital
italicize イタリック体で印刷する
italics イタリック体
ITCAN
inspect and correct as necessary 点検し,必要なら修正する
ITCG
intratracheal pnemocardiogram pressure 気管内心拍動波

ITCVD
ischemic thrombotic cerebrovascular disease　虚血性血栓性脳血管疾患
ITD
idiopathic torsion dystonia　特発性捻転ジストニー
intralobuar terminal duct　小葉内終末管
ITE
intrapulmonary interstitial emphysema　肺間質性気腫
iter.
iteretur〈ラ〉　反復せよ《処》
ITES
insulin, transferrin, ethanolamine, selenium　インスリン・トランスフェリン・エタノラミン・セレニウム

I

ITF
interferon　インターフェロン
ITFS
iliotibial tract friction syndrome　腸脛靱帯摩擦症候群
incomplete testicular feminization syndrome　不完全精巣性女性化症候群
ITG
isometric contraction time　等尺性収縮時間
ITGP
immunotactoid glomerulopathy　免疫接触性糸球体症
ITH
immediate type hypersensitivity　即時型過敏症
ITh
intrathecal　髄腔内の
ITI
inter α-trypsin inhibitor　インターαトリプシンインヒビター
International Team Implantologists　国際インプラント研究者チーム
intertrial interval　試行間間隔
intratubal insemination　卵管内授精
Itk
IL-2 induced T cell tyrosine kinase　インターロイキン2誘導T細胞チロシンキナーゼ
ITLC
instant thin-layer chromatography　瞬時薄層クロマトグラフィ
ITMA
International Traffic Medicine Association　国際交通医学会
ITN
intratracheal narcosis　気管内麻痺

ITOU
intensive therapy observation unit 集中観察治療部門

ITP
idiopathic thrombocytopenic purpura 特発性血小板減少性紫斑病
inosine 5′-triphosphate イノシン5′-三リン酸
islet-cell tumor of the pancreas 膵島細胞腫瘍
isotachophoresis 等速(度)電気泳動

ITPA
Illinois test of psycholinguistic abilities イリノイ言語学習能力診断検査

ITPV
intratracheal pulmonary ventilation 経気管肺換気法

ITR
International Islet Transplant Registry 国際膵島移植登録

$^{125}IT_3RSU$
iodine-125 triiodothyronine resin sponge uptake ヨウ素125トリヨードチ〔サイ〕ロニンレジン摂取率

$^{131}IT_3RSU$
iodine-131 triiodothyronine resin sponge uptake ヨウ素131トリヨードチ〔サイ〕ロニンレジン摂取率

ITS
International Thermal Scale 国際熱尺度〔スケール〕

ITSHD
isolated thyroid stimulating hormone deficiency 単独甲状腺刺激ホルモン欠乏(症)

ITT
insulin tolerance test インスリン耐性試験
internal tibial torsion 脛骨内捻

ITU
intensive therapy unit 集中治療部門

ITV
industrial television 工業用テレビ

ITX
intertriginous xanthoma 間擦性黄色腫

IU
immunizing unit 免疫単位
international unit 国際単位
intrauterine 子宮内

Iu
upper intrathoracic esophagus 胸部上部食道

iu
infectious unit 感染単位

IUA
International Union of Angiography 国際脈管学連合
intrauterine adhesion 子宮内付着

IUAC
International Union Against Cancer 世界対癌連合
IUAPPA
International Union of Air Pollution Prevention Environment Protection Association 国際大気汚染防止団体連合会
IUAT
International Union Against Tuberculosis 国際結核予防連合
IUATLD
International Union Against Tuberculosis and Lung Disease 国際結核肺疾患予防連合
IUB
International Union of Biochemistry 国際生化学連合
IUBMB
International Union of Biochemistry and Molecular Biology 国際生化学・分子生物学連合
IUBS
International Union of Biological Sciences 国際生物科学連合
IUC
idiopathic ulcerative colitis 特発性潰瘍性大腸炎
intraurethral catheter 尿道内カテーテル
IUCD
intrauterine contraceptive device 子宮内避妊器具
IUD
intrauterine death 子宮内死亡
intrauterine device 子宮内器具
intrauterine diaphragm 子宮内隔膜
IUFB
intrauterine foreign body 子宮内異物
IUFD
intrauterine fetal death 子宮内胎児死亡
intrauterine fetal distress 子宮内胎児仮死
IUFGR
intrauterine fetal growth retardation 子宮内胎児発育遅延
IUFT
intrauterine fetal transfusion 子宮内胎児輸血
IUG
infusion urogram 注入尿路造影像
intrauterine gas 子宮内ガス
intrauterine gestation 子宮内妊娠
intrauterine growth 子宮内胎児発育
IUGR
intrauterine growth rate 子宮内成長率
intrauterine growth restriction 子宮内発育遅延児

IUHE
International Union for Health Education　国際保健教育連合

IUIS
International Union of Immunological Societies　国際免疫学会連合

IUM
internal urethral meatus　内尿道口
intrauterine membrane　子宮内膜

IUMS
International Union of Microbiological Societies　国際微生物学会連合

IUNS
International Union of Nutritional Sciences　国際栄養科学連合

IUP
International Union of Phlebology　国際静脈学会
intrauterine pregnancy　子宮内妊娠
intrauterine pressure　子宮内圧

IUPAC
International Union of Pure and Applied Chemistry　国際純正・応用化学連合

IUPAP
International Union of Pure and Applied Physics　国際純粋・応用物理学連合

IUPD
intrauterine pregnancy delivered　子宮内妊娠分娩

IUPHAR
International Union of basic and clinical pharmacology　国際薬理学連合

IUPM
International Union for Protecting Public Mortality　公共死亡率防御国際連合

IUPS
International Union of Physiological Sciences　国際生理科学連合

IUSSP
International Union for the Scientific Study of Population　国際人口科学研究連合

IUT
intrauterine transfusion　子宮内輸血

IUTAM
International Union of Theoretical and Applied Mechanics　国際理論・応用力学連合

IUTOX
International Union of Toxicology　国際毒物学連合

IUVDT
- International Union Against the Venereal Disease and the Treponematosis　国際性病予防連合

IV
- *ichthyosis vulgaris*〈ラ〉　尋常性魚鱗癬
- initial velocity　初速
- interventricular　(心)室間の
- intervertebral　脊椎間の
- intravariceal injection　静脈瘤内注入法
- intravascular　血管内，脈管内
- intravenous　静脈内の
- intravenous injection　静脈内注射

iv
- inverted　逆転した，転位した

IV，i.v.
- *in vitro*〈ラ〉=in a glass (test tube)　試験管内で，非生体内で
- *in vivo*〈ラ〉=in the alive (body)　生体内で

IVA
- intraoperative vascular angiography　術中血管造影(法)

IVAAP
- International Veterinary Association for Animal Production　国際家畜増殖獣医学協会

i vac
- in vacuum　真空内の，真空で

IVBAT
- intravascular bronchioalveolar tumor　血管内気管支肺胞上皮腫瘍

IVC
- inferior vena cava　下大静脈
- inspiratory vital capacity　吸気肺活量
- intravascular coagulation　血管内凝固
- intravenous cholangiography　経静脈性胆道造影(法)
- intravenous cholecystography　経静脈性胆嚢撮影法

IVCC
- intravascular consumption coagulopathy　血管内消費性凝固障害

IVCD
- intraventricular conduction defect　心室内伝導障害
- intraventricular conduction delay　心室内伝導遅延

IVCG
- inferior venacavography　脳室内出血

IVCS
- intrapelvic venous congestion syndrome　骨盤内静脈うっ血症候群

IVCT
- intravenous coronary thrombolysis　全身静脈内血栓溶解療法

IVCY
intravenous cyclophosphamide　経静脈内シクロホスファミド(療法)

IVD
intravenous drip infusion　点滴静(脈内)注(射)

IVDSA
intravenous digital subtraction angiography, intravenous DSA　経静脈性デジタルサブトラクション血管造影, 経静脈DSA

IVDU
intravenous drug use　静(脈)注(射)薬物乱用(者)

IVECG
intravenous electrocardiography　静脈内心電図

IVF
interventricular foramen　心室間孔
intravascular fluid　血管内液
intravenous fluid　経静脈輸液
in vitro fertilization　体外受精
in vivo fertilization　体内受精

IVFB
intravascular foreign body　血管内異物

IVF & ER
in vitro fertilization & embryo replacement　体外受精と胚移植

IVF-ET
in vitro fertilization - embryo transplantation　体外受精と胚移植(法)

IVGTT
intravenous glucose tolerance test　静脈内ブドウ糖負荷試験

IVH
intravenous hyperalimentation　経中心静脈栄養(=高カロリー輸液)
intraventricular hematoma　脳室内血腫
intraventricular hemorrhage　脳室内出血

IVI
intravariceal injection　静脈瘤内注入

IVIG
intravenous immunoglobulin　静注用免疫グロブリン製剤

IVIM
intravoxel incoherent motion　IVIM法(=MRI撮影法の1つ)

IVJC
intervertebral joint complex　椎間関節複合

IVL
intravenous leiomyomatosis　静脈内平滑筋腫

I

IVM
in vitro matulation　体外成熟
involuntary movement　不随意運動
IVM-IVF
in vitro matulation, *in vitro* fertilization and embryo-transfer　体外成熟-体外受精-胚移植法
IVN
intravenous nutrition　経静脈栄養
IVP
intravenous pyelography　経静脈性腎盂造影法
intraventricular pressure　脳室内圧
IVPB
intravenous piggyback　静脈用ピギーバック
IVPF
isovolumic pressure-flow　等容圧流量
IVR
interventional radiology　インターベンショナルラジオロジー
intravaginal ring　腟内リング
IV route
intravenous route　静脈路確保
IVRT
isovolumic relaxation time　等量減張期
IVS
inferior vena cava　下大静脈
intervening sequence　介在配列(＝イントロン)
interventricular septum　心室中隔
intervillous space　絨毛間隙
intraventricular septum　心室中隔
irritable voiding syndrome　過敏性排尿症候群
IVSA
interventricular septum anterior　心室中隔前部
IVSD
interventricular septal defect　心室中隔欠損
IVSE
interventricular septal excursion　心室中隔振幅
IVST
interventricular septal thickness　心室中隔厚
IVT
intravenous transfusion　静脈内輸液
IVU
intravenous urography　(経)静脈性尿路造影〔撮影〕法
IVUS
intravascular ultrasound　血管内超音波

IVV
influenza virus vaccine | インフルエンザウイルスワクチン

IW
insensible water | 不感蒸泄水分

IYDP
International Year of Disabled Persons | 国際身体障害者年

IZS
insulin zinc suspension | 亜鉛化インスリン懸濁液

J j

J
electric current density　電流密度
esophagogastric junction　食道胃接合部
J blood factor　ジェー血液因子
Jewish　ユダヤ人(の)
joint　関節，結合(部)
joule (equivalent)　ジュール〈単位〉
journal　雑誌
juvenile　若年性(の)，小児
juxtapulmonary-capillary (receptor)　傍肺毛細血管(受容体)

j
jaundice　黄疸

J
flux (density)　磁束(密度)

J, j
juice　汁，液

J1-J3
Jaeger test type number 1-3　イエーガー視力表

JA
juvenile arthritis　若年性関節炎
juvenile atrophy　若年性萎縮症
juxtaarticular　関節近傍の

JAC
Journal of Applied Chemicals　応用化学雑誌

J-acid
2-amino-5-naphthol-7-sulfonic acid　ジェー酸

Jahrb
Jahrbuch〈独〉　年報

Jahrg
Jahrgang〈独〉　(雑誌の)巻

JAI
juvenile amaurotic idiocy　若年性黒内障(性)精神遅滞

JAIH
Japan Association of Industrial Health　日本産業衛生学会

Jak-1
Janus kinase 1　ヤーヌスキナーゼ1

JALMA
Japan Leprosy Mission for Asia　(日本)アジア救ライ協会

JALT
Japanese antiarrhythmic long-term trial　不整脈治療に関する調査

JAMA
The Journal of the American Medical Association 米国医師会雑誌
JAMEI
Japan Association of Medical Equipment Industries 日本医用器械工業会
JAMG
juvenile autoimmune myasthenia gravis 若年性自己免疫性重症筋無力症
JAMI
Japan Association for Medical Information 日本医療情報学会
JAMS
Japan Association of Mineralogical Sciences 日本鉱物科学会
Japanese Association of Medical Sciences 日本医学会
JAN
Japanese Accepted Names 日本医薬品一般名称
JAPIC
Japan Pharmaceutical Information Center 日本医薬情報センター
JAS
Japanese Agricultural Standard 日本農林規格
Jenkins Activity Survey ジェンキンス活動調査
Job Attitude Scale 職業態度〔意識〕尺度
JASA
Journal of Acoustical Society of America 米国聴覚学会誌
JASCT
Japanese Association of Sex Counselors and Therapists 日本セックスカウンセラー・セラピスト協会(現,日本性科学学会)
JAST
Japan Association for the Surgery of Trauma 日本外傷学会
JATA
Japanese Trial on Efficacy of Antihypertensive Treatment in Elderly 日本老人高血圧治療効果試験
jaund, jaund.
jaundice 黄疸
JAXA
Japan Aerospace Exploration Agency 宇宙航空研究開発機構
JBE
Japanese B encephalitis B型日本脳炎

Jber
Jahresbericht〈独〉 年報
JBF
Jochbeinfraktur〈独〉 頬骨骨折
JC
Jakob-Creutzfeldt (syndrome) ヤコブ・クロイツフェルト(症候群)
joint contracture 関節拘縮
junctional complex 複合連絡
J/C
joule per coulomb ジュール/クーロン
jc, jc.
juice 汁，液
JCA
juvenile chronic arthritis 若年性慢性関節炎
JCAH
Joint Commission of Accreditation of Hospital 病院認定連合委員会

JCAHO
Joint Commission on Accreditation of Healthcare Organization 米国医療機能評価機関
JCAR
Joint Commission of Applied Radioactivity 応用放射線学連合委員会
JCCLS
Japanese Committee for Clinical Laboratory Standard 日本臨床検査標準委員会
JCF
juvenile calcaneal fracture 若年性踵骨骨折
J chain
joining chain J鎖
JCML
juvenile chronic myelocytic leukemia 若年性慢性骨髄性白血病
JCP
juvenile chronic polyarthritis 若年性慢性多発(性)関節炎
JCPE
Japan Chemistry Program Exchange 日本化学プログラム交換機関
JCPTGP
Joint Committee on Postgraduate Training for General Practice 一般医卒後修練連合機関
JCR
Journal Citation Report 雑誌引用報告
JCRB
Japanese Cancer Research Resources Bank 日本癌研究資源バンク

JCS
Japan Coma Scale　日本昏睡スケール，意識障害分類(＝3-3-9度方式)

JCT
juxtaglomerular cell tumor　傍糸球体細胞腫瘍

jct
junction　連結，接合部

JCV
Jamestown Canyon virus　ジェームズタウンキャニオンウイルス

JD
Janet disease　ジャネー病
jaundice　黄疸
jejunal diverticulitis　空腸憩室炎
jugulodigastric (node)　頸静脈二腹筋(リンパ節)
juvenile-onset diabetes millitus　若年(発症)型〔性〕糖尿病

JDDST
Japanese Edition Denver Development Screening Test　日本版デンバー式発達スクリーニング検査

JDDW
Japan Digestive Disease Week　日本消化器病週間

JDM
juvenile-onset diabetes mellitus　若年(発症)型〔性〕糖尿病

JDMS
juvenile dermatomyositis　若年性皮膚筋炎

JDMS/PM
juvenile dermato/polymyositis　若年性皮膚筋炎/多発(性)筋炎

JDOS
joint density of states　結合状態密度

JE
Japanese encephalitis　日本脳炎
junctional escape　結節性補充収縮

JEA
Japan Ergonomics Association　日本人間工学会

JEB
junctional epidermolysis bullosa　接合(部)型表皮水疱症
junctional escape beat　結節性補充収縮

JECFA
Joint Expert Committee on Food Additives　食品添加物に関する合同専門家委員会

JEJ, Jej, jej
jejunum　空腸

JELIS
Japan Eicosapentaenoic Acid Lipid Intervention Study　日本エイコサ・ペンタエン酸検証研究

jentac.
jentaculum〈ラ〉 朝食

JET
junctional ectopic tachycardia 接合部異所性頻拍

JEV
Japanese encephalitis virus 日本脳炎ウイルス

JF
jugular foramen 頸静脈孔

JFAA
Japan Food Additives Association 日本食品添加物協会

JFC
jugular foramen syndrome 頸静脈孔症候群

JFS
jugular foramen syndrome 頸静脈孔症候群

JG
juxtaglomerular 傍糸球体の，糸球体近接の

JGA
juxtaglomerular apparatus 傍糸球体装置

J

JGC
juxtaglomerular cell (count) 糸球体近接細胞(数)，傍糸球体細胞(数)

j-g complex
juxtaglomerular complex 傍糸球体複合体

JGCT
juvenile granulosa cell tumor 若年性顆粒膜細胞腫瘍
juxtaglomerular cell tumor 傍糸球体細胞腫瘍

JGI
jejunogastric intussusception 空腸胃重積(症)
juxtaglomerular granulation index 傍糸球体肉芽(顆粒)形成指数
juxtaglomerular index 傍糸球体指数

JGOFS
Joint Global Ocean Flux Study 合同全地球海洋潮流研究

JGP
juvenile general paralysis 若年性全身(完全)麻痺

JGSP
Japanese Good Supplying Practice 医薬品の供給および品質管理に関する日本の基準

JH
juvenile hormone 若年性ホルモン

JHH
John Hopkins Hospital ジョン・ホプキンス病院

JHMI
John Hopkins Medical Institute ジョン・ホプキンス医学研究所

JHR
Jarisch-Herxheimer reaction　ヤーリッシュ・ヘルクスハイマー反応

JHS
Japan hematological standard　日本血液検査器械検定協会規格

JHUSHPH
John Hopkins University School of Hygiene and Public Health　ジョン・ホプキンス大学衛生学公衆衛生学科

JHUSM
John Hopkins University School of Medical　ジョン・ホプキンス大学医学部

JI
jejunoileal　空(腸)回腸の
jejunoileostomy　空回腸吻合(術)

JIB
jejunoileal bypass　空(腸)回腸バイパス(術)

JICA
Japan International Cooperation Agency　日本国際協力事業団

JICST
Japan Information Center of Science and Technology　日本科学技術情報センター

JIMA
Japan Internet Medical Association　日本インターネット医療協会

JIMTEF
Japan International Medical Technology Foundation　日本国際医療技術交流財団

JIP
Japan Institute of Pharasemeillance　日本医薬監視研究所

JIRA
Japan Medical Imaging and Radiological Systems Industries Association　日本画像医療システム工業会，ジラ

JIS
Japanese Industrial Standards　日本工業規格
juvenile idiopathic scoliosis　若年性特発(性)(脊椎)側彎(症)

JISA
Japan Industrial Safety Association　日本産業安全協会

JIT
just in time　適時

JJ
jaw jerk　下顎反射
jejunojejunostomy　空腸空腸吻合(術)

JJC
Japan Joint Committee for Cancer Staging and End Results Reporting 癌の病期分類と結果報告のための日本委員会
JJPEN
Japanese Journal of Parenteral and Enteral Nutrition 日本輸液栄養雑誌
JJTOM
Japan Journal of Traumatology and Occupational Medicine 日本災害・産業医学会雑誌
JKD
Junius-Kuhnt disease ジューニアス・クーント病
JKST
Johnson-Kennye Screening Test ジョンソン・ケニースクリーニングテスト

JL
Jadassohn-Lewandowski (syndrome) ヤーダッソーン・レーヴァンドウスキー(症候群)

Jaffe-Lichtenstein (syndrome) ヤッフェ・リヒテンシュタイン(症候群)

Judkins left ジャドキンス左(冠(状)動脈用カテーテル)

JLMA
Japan Leprosy Mission for Asia (日本)アジア救ライ協会
JLP
juvenile laryngeal papilloma 若年性喉頭乳頭腫
juvenile laryngeal papilloma (tosis) 若年性喉頭乳頭腫(症)
JM
josamycin ジョサマイシン
JMA
Japan Medical Association 日本医学会
JMAP
Japanese version of Miller Assessment for Preschoolers 日本版ミラー幼児発達スクリーニング検査，Jマップ
JMC
Jefferson Medical College ジェファーソン医科大学
JME
juvenile myoclonic epilepsy 若年ミオクロニーてんかん
JMG
juxtamedullary glomerulus 傍髄質糸球体
JMH
John Milton Hagen (antibody) ジョーンミルトンハーゲン(抗体)

J-MIC
Japan multicenter investigation for cardiovascular drugs 心筋梗塞の再閉塞予防に関する研究システム

JMR
Jones-Mote reactivity ジョーンズ・モート(型)反応
JMTDR
Japan Medical Team for Disaster Relief 国際緊急援助隊医療チーム
JNA
Japanese Nursing Association 日本看護協会
Jena Nomina Anatomica〈ラ〉 エーナ解剖学名
JNC
The joint national committee on detection, evaluation and treatment of high blood pressure 高血圧の診断と治療に関する米国合同委員会
JND
just noticeable difference 識別閾(値)
Juvenile Narcotics Division 青少年麻薬取締局
JNPAF
juvenile nasopharyngeal angiofibroma 若年性鼻咽頭血管線維腫
jnt
joint 関節, 結合
JOA
Japan Orthopedic Association 日本整形外科学会
JOCS
Japan Overseas Christian Medical Cooperative Service 日本キリスト教海外医療協力会
JOD
juvenile-onset type diabetes (mellitus) 若年型〔性〕糖尿病
JODM
juvenile-onset (type) diabetes millitus 若年性〔型〕糖尿病
JOHAC
Japan Overseas Health Administration Center 日本海外健康管理センター
JOIS
Japan Information Center of Science and Technology online Information System 日本科学技術情報センターオンライン文献検索システム
JOMF
Japan Overseas Medical Fund 日本財団法人海外邦人医療基金
JOR
jaw-opening reflex 下顎開反射
Jour, jour
journal 雑誌

J

JP
Jackson-Pratt (drain) ジャクソン・プラット(ドレーン)
Japanese Pharmacopoeia 日本薬局方
juvenile parkinsonism 若年性パーキンソニズム
juvenile periodontitis 若年性歯周炎

JPB
junctional premature beat (contraction) 房室(接合部)性期外収縮

JPBC
junctional premature beat contraction 房室接合部性期外収縮

JPC
junctional premature contraction 房室接合部性期外収縮

JPD
juvenile plantar dermatosis 若年性足底皮膚症

JPDQ
Japanese Edition Prescreening Development Questionnaire 日本版前選別発達質問

JPEG
joint photographic experts group 写真専門家連合

JPI
Jackson Personality Inventory ジャクソン人格調査表

JPMA
Japan Pharmaceuticals Manufactures Association 日本製薬工業協会

JPS
joint position sense 関節位置覚
junctional premature systole 結合部早期収縮

JR
Jolly reaction ヨリー反応
Judkins right ジャドキンス右(冠(状)動脈用カテーテル)

jr
junior ジュニア，年下の

JRA
juvenile rheumatoid arthritis 若年性関節リウマチ

JRC
The Japanese Red Cross Society 日本赤十字社

JRCPM
Japanese Raven Coloured Progressive Matrices 日本版レーヴン色彩マトリックス(検査)《臨心》

JRIA
Japan Radioisotope Association 日本ラジオアイソトープ協会

jrl
journal 雑誌

jrnl	
journal	雑誌
JRS	
Japan Radiological Society	日本医学放射線学会
JS	
Job syndrome	ヨブ症候群
Junkmam-Schoeller	ユンクマン・シューラー(単位)
JSA	
Japan Society of Anesthesiology	日本麻酔学会
JSC	
Japan Science Council	日本学術会議
JSCA	
Japanese Committee for Standardization of Alpha-fetoprotein	アルファフェトプロテインの標準化日本委員会
JSCC	
Japanese Society of Clinical Chemistry	日本臨床化学会
Standard Commodity Classification for Japan	日本標準商品分類
JSCP	
Japan Society of Clinical Pathology	日本臨床病理学会
JSD	
Japanese Stroke Databank	日本脳卒中データバンク
JSI	
Jansky Screening Index	ヤンスキースクリーニング指数
JSICM	
Japan Society of Intensive Care Medicine	日本集中治療医学会
JSS	
Japan Stroke Scale	日本脳卒中スケール
JSSRS	
Japan Standard Stroke Registry Study	日本脳卒中協会データバンク部門
JST	
Japanese skin type	日本人皮膚型
Japan Special Team	日本特別チーム
JSU	
Junkman-Schoeller unit	ユンクマン・シェーラー単位
JSV	
Jerry-Slough virus	ジェリー・スロウウイルス
JT	
junctional tachycardia	接合部(性)頻拍(症)

JT，jt
joint　関節，連結
jt.asp
joint aspiration　関節吸引
JTF
jejunostomy tube feeding　空腸経管栄養
JTP
jugular tympanic paraganglioma　頸静脈鼓室傍神経節腫
JTPS
juvenile tropical pancreatitis syndrome　若年性熱帯膵(臓)炎症候群
jug
jugular　頸(静脈)，頸の
jug.comp.
jugular compression (test)　頸静脈圧迫(試験)
JUH
Johaniter-Unfall-Hilfe　ヨハネ協会救急救援助隊
junct
junction　連結，結合
juscul.
jusculum〈ラ〉　肉汁《処》
juv，juv.
juvenile　若年(性)の
juve
juvenile　若年(性)の
juve para
juvenile paralysis　若年性進行麻痺
JUXT，juxt
juxta〈ラ〉　近い，傍らの
JV
jugular pressure　頸静脈圧
jugular pulse　頸静脈波
jugular vein　頸静脈
jugular venous　頸静脈の
JVC
Japan Volunteer Center　日本ボランティアセンター
jugular venous catheter　頸静脈カテーテル
JVD
jugular venous distention　頸静脈怒張
JVIS
Jackson Vocational Interest Survey　ジャクソン職業興味調査
JVP
jugular vein〔venous〕 pulse　頸静脈波
jugular venous pressure　頸静脈圧
JXG
juvenile xanthogranuloma　若年性黄色肉芽腫

J

K k

K

absolute zero	絶対零度
capsular antigen	莢膜抗原
coefficient of heat transfer	熱伝達の係数
coefficient of ocular rigidity	眼硬化係数
coefficient of scleral rigidity	強膜硬性係数
dissociation constant	解離定数
electron capture	電子捕獲
electrostatic capacity	静電容量
equilibrium constant	平衡定数
ionization constant	イオン定数
kalium	カリウム〈元素〉
kallikrein inhibiting unit	カリクレイン抑制単位
kalyx〈ギ〉＝calyx，calix	腎杯
kanamycin	カナマイシン
kappa＝$\varkappa$〈ギ〉	カッパ
Kell blood system	ケル血液型
Kell factor	ケル因子
kelvin	ケルビン〈単位〉
keratin	ケラチン
keratometer	角膜(曲率)計
keratosis	角化上皮
kerma(＝kinetic energy release in material)	ケルマ〈単位〉，カーマ
ketotifen	ケトチフェン
kidney	腎臓
killer (cell)	キラー(細胞)
kilopermeability coefficient	キロ透過性係数
kinetic energy	運動エネルギー
Klebsiella	クレブシエラ(属)
knee	膝
Küntscher (nail)	キュンチャー(針)
lysine	リジン
potassium	カリウム〈元素〉
symbol for dissociation constant	定数・常数を示す記号

k

Boltzmann constant	ボルツマン定数
constant	定数
Kell-negative	ケル陰性
Kell-positjve	ケル陽性
kilo(-)	キロ(＝10^3)〈接〉〈単位〉
magnetic susceptibility	磁化率
rate constants	速度定数

K

reaction rate constant 反応速度定数

17-K

17-ketosteroid(s) 17-ケトステロイド

K_1

vitamin K_1 (=phylloquinone) ビタミンK_1，フィロキノン

K_2

vitamin K_2 (=menaquinone) ビタミンK_2，メナキノン

K_3

vitamin K_3 (=menadione) ビタミンK_3，メナジオン

K，K.

kathode 陰極

KA

alkaline phosphatase アルカリホスファターゼ

keratoacanthoma 角化棘細胞腫

ketoacidosis ケトアシドーシス

King-Armstrong (unit) キング・アームストロング単位〈単位〉

Korean antigen 韓国抗原

künstlicher Abort〈独〉 人工妊娠中絶

kynurenic acid キヌレン酸

K

Ka

kallikrein カリクレイン

kathode 陰極

ketoadipic acid ケトアジピン酸

kA

kiloampere キロアンペア〈単位〉

k/a

ketogenic to antiketogenic ケトン対抗ケトン

KA，Ka，ka

kathodal 陰極の

kathode 陰極

K_a，K_a

acid ionization 〔dissociation〕 constant 酸のイオン化〔解離〕定数

K/A，K：A

ketogenic/antiketogenic (ratio) ケトン/抗ケトン(比)

KAAD

kerosene, alcohol, acetic acid dioxane ケローセン・アルコール・酢酸ジオキサン

K-ABC

Kaufman Assessment Battery for Children カウフマン心理・教育アセスメントバッテリー《臨心》

KAF

kinase-activating factor キナーゼ活性化因子

KAFO

knee-ankle-foot orthosis 膝・踝・足装具

KAL
Kallmann (syndrome)　カルマン(症候群)

Kal
kalium　カリウム〈元素〉

KAO
knee-ankle orthosis　膝・踵装具

KAP
knowledge, attitude, practice　知識・態度・実技

KAS
Katz adjustment scales　カッツ適応スケール

KASH
knowledge, abilities, skills and habits　知識・能力・技術および習慣

KAST
Kindergarten Auditory Screening Test　幼稚園児聴力スクリーニングテスト
Kurihama alcoholism screening test　久里浜式アルコール症選別検査

KAT
kanamycin acetyltransferase　カナマイシンアセチルトランスフェラーゼ

kat
katal　カタール〈単位〉

KAU
King-Armstrong unit　キング・アームストロング単位

KA unit
King-Armstrong unit　キング・アームストロング単位

KB
Kashin-Bek (disease)　カシン・ベック病
ketobutyric acid　ケト酪酸
ketone bodies　ケトン体
kilobytes　キロバイト〈複数〉
Klüver Barerra staining　クリューバー・バレラ染色
knuckle-bender (splint)　ナックル・ベンダー(副子)
Koagulationsband〈独〉　凝固帯
Künstliche Befruchtung〈独〉　人工受精

kb
kilobase　キロ塩基, キロベース〈単位〉

K-B
Kleihauer-Betke (test)　クライハウエル・ベトケ(試験)

K_b, K_b
base ionization constant　塩基イオン定数

KBgT
kappa-bungaro-toxin　カッパ・ブンガロ毒素
KBM
Kondylen Bettung Münster (socket)　KBMソケット
Kondylombelastungsprothese Münster〈独〉　ミュンスター式顆部下腿義足
KBM Prothese
Kondylen Bettung Münster Prothese〈独〉　KBM下腿義足
kbp
kilobase pair　キロ塩基対，1000塩基対
kBq
kilobecquerel　キロベクレル
KBR
Komplementbindungsreaktion〈独〉　補体結合反応
KBr
potassium bromide　臭化カリウム
KBS
Klüver-Bucy syndrome　クリューバー・ビューシー症候群
kbs
kilobase pair　キロ塩基対，キロベース対
KC
kathodal closing　陰極閉鎖
keratoconjunctivitis　角結膜炎
keratoconus　円錐角膜
keratoma climacterium　更年期角化腫
knuckle cracking　指関節のひび
Kupffer cell　クプファー細胞
Kc
catalytic constant　触媒定数
kc
kilocycle　キロサイクル〈単位〉
kcal
kilocalorie　キロカロリー〈単位〉
Kcat
catalytic constant　触媒定数
KCC
kathodal〔cathodal〕 closing contraction　陰極閉鎖収縮
Kulchitzky cell carcinoma　クルチッキー細胞癌(腫)
KCCT
kaolin-cephalin clotting time　カオリン・セファリン凝固時間
K cell
killer cell　キラー細胞

KCG
kinetocardiogram キネトカルジオグラム
kinetocardiogram 心運動図
kCi
kilocurie キロキュリー〈単位〉
KCL
keratoconus line 円錐角膜線
KCl
potassium chloride 塩化カリウム
KC method
Kingsbury-Clark method キングスベリー・クラーク法
KCNS
potassium thiocyanate チオシアン酸カリウム
KCP
knee-chest posture 膝胸位
kcps, kc.p.s.
kilocycles per second キロサイクル/秒
KCS
keratoconjunctivitis sicca 乾(燥)性角結膜炎
kc/s
kilocycles per second キロサイクル/秒〈単位〉
KCT
kaolin clotting time カオリン凝固時間
kathodal〔cathodal〕 closing tetanus 陰極閉鎖強直
KCTe
kathodal〔cathodal〕 closing tetanus 陰極閉鎖強直
KCZ
ketoconazole ケトコナゾール
KD
kathodal〔cathodal〕 duration 陰極持続
Kawasaki disease 川崎病
kidney donor 腎臓提供者
knee disarticulation 膝関節離断(術)
knitted Dacron ニットダクロン
K_d
dissociation constant 解離定数
Kd
distribution coefficient 分布係数
partition coefficient 分配係数
kd
killed 殺された
kilodalton キロダルトン〈単位〉
KDA
known drug allergies〔allergy〕 既知薬剤アレルギー
KDM
kanendomycin カネンドマイシン

K

KDO
2-keto-3-deoxy-octonate　2-ケト-3-デオキシオクトネート

KDS
Kaufman Development Scale　カウフマン発育尺度〔スケール〕
Kocher-Debre-Semelaigne (syndrome)　コッヘル・デブレ・セメレーニュ(症候群)

KDSM
keratinizing desquamative squamous metaplasia　角質化落屑性扁平化生

KDSS
Kurtzke Disability Status Scale　クルツケ身体障害スケール

KDT
kathodal〔cathodal〕 duration tetanus　陰極持続強縮

KDTe
cathodal〔kathodal〕 duration tetanus　陰極持続強直

KE
Kaninchen-einheit〈独〉　家兎単位
Kendall compound E　ケンダル化合物E(＝コルチゾン)
kinetic energy　運動エネルギー
klinische Einheit〈独〉　臨床単位

Ke
exchangeable body potassium　交換性カリウム

KEG
keto-enol granule　ケトエノール顆粒

KEMAR
kemales electronic manikin for acoustic research　ノールズ研究用音響的人体模型

KEP
Kelman phacoemulsification　ケルマン法

K_{eq}
equilibrium constant　平衡定数

Kera
keratitis　角膜炎

kerma
kinetic energy release in material　ケルマ

keto
ketogenic　ケトンの
keton　ケトン
ketonemia　ケトン体血症
ketonurea　ケトン尿
ketose　ケトース
ketosis　ケトン体血症
17-ketosteroid(s)　17-ケトステロイド

K

ketol
keton alcohol　ケトン・アルコール(結合物)
keV, kev
kilo-electronvolt, kiloelectron volt (s)　キロ電子ボルト
KF
Klippel-Feil (syndrome)　クリペル・フェーユ(症候群)
KFD
Kinetic Family Drawing　動的〔動態〕家族描画法《臨心》
Kyasanur Forest disease　キャサヌール森林熱
Kyasanur forest disease　キャサヌール森林病
KFR
Kayser-Fleischer ring　カイゼル・フライシャー輪
KFS
Klippel-Feil syndrome　クリペル・フェーユ症候群
KG
α-ketoglutaric acid　α-ケトグルタル酸
Körpergewicht〈独〉　体重
kG
kilogauss　キロガウス
kg
kilogram　キログラム〈単位〉
KG-1
Koeffler Golde-1　ケフラーゴールド1
KGC
keflin, gentamicin, carbenicillin　ケフリン,ゲンタマイシン,カルベニシリン
kg cal
kilogram-calorie　キログラム・カロリー
KGF
keratinocyte growth factor　角質細胞増殖因子
KGHT
kidney Goldblatt hypertension　ゴールドブラット高血圧(症)腎
KGL
kalium gluconate　グルコン酸カリウム
KGM
ketoglutaramate　ケトグルタラメート
kg・m
kilogram(me)-meter　キログラム・メートル〈単位〉
Kgn
kininogen　キニノゲン
kgps
kilogram(me) per second　キログラム/秒
KGS
ketogenic steroid(s)　ケトン生成ステロイド

17-KGS
17-ketogenic steroid(s) 17-ケトン生成ステロイド
kg/s
kilogram(me) per second キログラム/秒〈単位〉
KH
ketotic hyperglycinemia ケトーシス型高グリシン血症
Kohlenhydrat〈独〉 炭水化物，糖質
Krebs-Henseleit (cycle) クレブス・ヘンゼライト(サイクル)
KHb
potassium hemoglobinate ヘモグロビン酸カリウム
KHD
kinky hair disease 縮れ毛病
KHF
killer-helper factor キラー・ヘルパー因子
Korean hemorrhagic fever 朝鮮出血熱
KHM
keratoderma hereditaria mutilans 断指趾型先天性掌蹠角化症
KHS
kinky hair syndrome 縮れ毛症候群
Krebs-Henseleit solution クレブス・ヘンゼライト溶液
KHT
Kindesherztöne〈独〉 胎児心音〈複数〉
kHz
kilohertz キロヘルツ〈単位〉
KI
karyopyknotic index 核濃縮指数
Kaup-Davenport index カウプ・ダベンポート指数
kernikterus 核黄疸
Kupperman index クッパーマン指数
potassium iodine ヨウ化カリウム
K_I
inhibition constant 抑制定数
inhibitor constant 阻害物質定数
KIA
killed in action 作戦中死亡
Kligler iron agar (medium) クリグラー鉄寒天(培地)
KICB
killed intracellular bacteria 死滅細胞内細菌
KICU
kidney intensive care unit 腎疾患集中治療室
KID
keratitis-ichthyosis-deafness (syndrome) 角膜炎・魚鱗癬・難聴症候群

K

KIDS
Kent Infant Development Scale　ケント乳児発育尺度〔スケール〕
Kinder Infant Development Scale　乳幼児発達スケール，キッズ《臨心》

kilo
kilogram(me)　キログラム
kilometer　キロメートル

KIP
Klinische Intelligenzprüfung〈独〉　臨床知能検査

KIT
Kahn Intelligence Tests　カーン知能検査

KIU
kallikrein inhibiting unit　カリクレイン抑制単位

KIV
ketoisovaleric acid　ケトイソ吉草酸

KJ
kilojoule　キロジュール〈単位〉

KJ，kj
knee jerk　膝蓋腱反射

KK
kallikrein　カリクレイン
Kollimkarzinom〈独〉　子宮体部癌

KK，Kk
knee kick　膝蓋腱反射

KKe
Kranke〈独〉　患者

KKK
Kehlkopfkrebs〈独〉　喉頭癌

KKKK
kallikrein, kinin, kininogen, kininase　カリクレイン・キニン・キニノゲン・キニナーゼ

K. KL
Kinderklinik〈独〉　小児科

KK system
kallikrein-kinin system　カリクレイン・キニン系

KL
killed and living　不活性・活性(ワクチン)
Kleine-Levin (syndrome)　クライン・レビン症候群
Knochenleitung〈独〉　骨(伝)導
Kopflage〈独〉　頭位
Körperlänge〈独〉　身長

kl
kiloliter　キロリットル〈単位〉

KL bac
Klebs-Löffler bacillus　クレブス・レフラー桿菌

Kleb(s)
Klebsiella クレブシエラ(属)
klepto
kleptomania 病的盗癖
KLH
keyhole limpet hemocyanin キーホールリンペット〔鍵穴付着〕ヘモシアニン
KLS
kidneys, liver, and spleen 腎(臓)・肝(臓)・脾臓
Kreuzbein lipomatous syndrome クロイツバイン脂肪腫症候群
KM
kanamycin カナマイシン
K-immunoglobulin (light chain) *K*-免疫グロブリン(軽鎖)
kitasamycin キタサマイシン
Kraepelin-Morel (disease) クレペリン・モレル(病)
Kuhmilch〈独〉 牛乳
K_m
Michaelis-Menten (dissociation) constant ミカエリス・メンテン(解離)定数
km
kilometer キロメートル
Km, K_m
Michaelis constant ミカエリス定数
Michaelis-Menten dissociation constant ミカエリス・メンテン解離定数
kMc
kilomegacycle キロメガサイクル
kMcps
kilomegacycles per second キロメガサイクル/秒
KMEF
keratin, myosin, epidermin, fibrin ケラチン・ミオシン・エピデルミン・フィブリン
$KMnO_4$
potassium permanganate 過マンガン酸カリウム
kmps
kilometer per second キロメートル/秒
KMS
kwashiorkor-marasmus syndrome クワシオルコル・マラスムス症候群
km/s
kilometer per second キロメートル/秒
KMTB
alpha-keto-gamma-methylthio butyric acid α-ケト-γ-メチルチオ酪酸
KMV
killed measles vaccine (virus) 死滅麻疹ワクチン(ウイルス)

K

kN
kilonewton キロニュートン
KN, Kn, kn
knee 膝
K nail
Küntscher nail キュンチャー釘
KNF model
Koshland-Némethy-Filmer model コシュランド・ネメシー・フィルマーモデル
KNO
keep needle open (注射)針をオープンに保て《処》
knork
knife and fork ナイフとフォーク
KNRK
Kirsten sarcoma virus in normal rat kidney (cell) 正常ラット腎(細胞)におけるキリステン肉腫ウイルス
KO
killed organism 死滅(微)生物
knee orthosis 膝関節装具
Ko
catalytic precipitates 触媒定数
KO, K/O
keep on(=continue) 継続せよ《処》
keep open 開けたままにせよ《処》
knocked out ノックアウトした〔された〕
KO, K/o
keep on 続ける
KOC
cathodal〔kathodal〕 opening contraction 陰極開放拘縮
kathodal opening concentration 陰極開放濃度
KOH
potassium hydroxide 水酸化カリウム
KOT
Knowledge of Occupations Test 職業知識テスト
KOZ
Kathodenöffnungszuckung〈独〉 陰極開放収縮
KP
Kaufmann-Peterson (base) カウフマン・ピーターソン(塩基)
keratic precipitate 角膜後面〔裏面〕沈着物
keratitis parenchymatosa 実質性角膜炎
keratitis punctata〈ラ〉 点状角膜炎
keratotic patch 角化症パッチ
kidney protein 腎(臓)蛋白

K

kidney punch　腎(臓)パンチ
killed parenteral (vaccine)　非経口不活化(ワクチン)

kp
kilopond〈独〉　キロポンド〈単位〉

K-P
Kaiser-Permanente (diet)　カイザー・パーマネント(治療食)

kPa
kilopascal　キロパスカル

KPAB
potassium *p*-aminobenzoate　パラアミノ安息香酸カリウム

KPB
ketophenylbutazone　ケトフェニルブタゾン

KPE
Kelman phacoemulsification　ケルマン超音波白内障破砕吸引術

KPI
karyopyknotic index　核濃縮指数

KPR
Kuder Preference Record　クーダー選好記録

KPR-V
Kuder Preference Record-Vocational　クーダー職業選好記録

KPS
Karnofsky performance status scale　カルノフスキー行動〔活動〕評価スケール
keratitis punctata superficialis　表層点状角膜炎

KPT
kidney punch test　腎(臓)パンチ検査
Kuder Performance Test　クーダー動作性検査

KPTI
Kunitz pancreatic trypsin inhibitor　クニッツ膵臓トリプシンインヒビター

K-PTT
kaolin activated partial thromboplastin time　カオリン加部分トロンボプラスチン時間

KR
Kopper Reppart (medium)　コッパー・レパート(培地)

Kr
krypton　クリプトン〈元素〉

kR
kiloroentgen　キロレントゲン〈単位〉

^{81m}Kr
krypton-81m　クリプトン81m

KRA
Klinefelter-Reifenstein-Albright (syndrome) クラインフェルター・ライフェンスタイン・オルブライト(症候群)

KRBB
Krebs-Ringer bicarbonate buffer クレブス・リンゲル重炭酸塩緩衝剤

KRH
Krebs Ringer HEPES クレブス・リンゲルヘペス

Krkh
Krankheit〈独〉 疾患

KRP
Kolmer (test with) Reiter protein (antigen) ライター蛋白(抗原)を用いるコルマー(法)
Kolmer test with Reiter protein ライター蛋白を用いるコルマー法
Krebs Ringer phosphate buffer クレブス・リンゲルリン酸緩衝液

KRPS
Krebs Ringer phosphate (buffer solution) クレブス・リンゲルリン酸(緩衝溶液)

KRRS
kinetic resonance Raman spectroscopy 運動共鳴ラーマン分光法

KS
Kallmann syndrome カルマン症候群
Kaposi sarcoma カポジ肉種
Kartagener syndrome カルタゲナー症候群
Kawasaki syndrome 川崎病
keratan sulfate ケラタン硫酸
ketosteroid ケトステロイド
Klinefelter syndrome クラインフェルター症候群
Kochleffel syndrome コクレフェル症候群
kombinierte Sinusitis〈独〉 併合性副鼻腔炎
Kopfschmerz〈独〉 叩打痛
Korsakoff syndrome コルサコフ症候群
Kugel-Stoloff (syndrome) クーゲル・ストロフ(症候群)
Kveim-Siltzbach (test) クヴェーム・シルツバッハ(試験)

Ks
substrate constant 基質定数

ks
kilosecond キロ秒

17-KS
17-ketosteroid(s) 17-ケトステロイド

K

KSA
knowledge, skills and abilities　知識・技能および能力

KSbS
Klinische Selbsturteilungs-Skalen〈独〉　臨床的自己評価尺度

KSD
keratitis superficialis diffusa〈ラ〉　び漫〔広汎〕性表層角膜炎

KSHV
Kaposi sarcoma-associated herpesvirus　カポジ肉腫関連ヘルペスウイルス

KSM
kasugamycin　カスガマイシン

KS/OI
Kaposi sarcoma and opportunistic infections　カポジ肉腫と日和見感染

KSP
Karolinska Scale of Personality　カロリンスカ人格尺度
keratitis superficialis punctata　表在性点状角膜炎
kidney-specific protein　腎(臓)特異(的)蛋白

KSS
Kearns-Sayre-Shy (syndrome)　キーンズ・セイアー・シャイ(症候群)
Kearns-Sayre syndrome　キーンズ・セイアー症候群

K

KST
cathodal-closing tetanus　陰極閉鎖強直

KSZ
Kathodenschließungszuckung〈独〉　陰極閉鎖攣縮

KT
kidney transplant　腎移植(片)
kidney transplantation　腎(臓)移植(術)
kidney treatment　腎(臓)治療
kinesiotherapy　運動療法
Körpertemperatur〈独〉　体温
Kuder test　クーダーテスト

KT_{50}
median knock-down time　KT50，50%落下横転時間

KTI
kallikrein-trypsin inhibitor　カリクレイン・トリプシン阻害因子

KTP
potassium-titanyl-phosphate　カリウム・チタン・リン酸

KTPP
keratoderma tylodes palmaris progressiva　進行性指掌角化症

KTSA
Kahn test of symbol arrangement　カーン・シンボルテスト(＝作業式投影法)

KT syndrome	
Klippel-Trenaunay syndrome	クリッペル・テレノー症候群
KTVS	
Keystone Telebinocular Visual Survey	キーストン双眼鏡視覚調査
KTWS	
Klippel-Trenaunay-Weber syndrome	クリッペル・テレノー・ウェーバー症候群
KU	
kallikrein unit	カリクレイン単位
Karmen unit	カーメン単位
Kopfumfang〈独〉	頭囲
KUB	
kidney(s),ureter,bladder	腎(臓)・尿管・膀胱
KUS	
kidneys,ureters and spleen	腎(臓)・尿管および脾臓
KV	
kanamycin-vancomycin	カナマイシン・バンコマイシン
killed vaccine	死滅〔死菌〕ワクチン
kVA	
kilovolt-ampere	キロボルト・アンペア〈単位〉
KVE	
Kaposi varicelliform eruption	カポジ水痘様疹
KVLBA	
kanamycin-vancomycin laked blood agar	カナマイシン・バンコマイシン入り血液寒天培地
KVO	
keep vein open	静脈確保(せよ)
KVOC D5W	
keep vein open cum dextrose 5%	5%ブドウ糖液による静脈確保(せよ)
kVp	
kilovolt peak	管電圧波高値
KW	
Keith-Wagener	キース・ワグナー
kidney weight	腎(臓)重量
Kimmelstiel-Wilson (syndrome)	キンメルスティール・ウィルソン(症候群)
Koch-Weeks bacillus	コッホ・ウィークス菌
Kugelberg-Welander (disease)	クーゲルベルク・ヴェランデル(病)
kW	
kilowatt	キロワット〈単位〉

KWB
Keith-Wagener-Barker — キース・ワグナー・バーカー(本態性高血圧症)

KW classification
Keith-Wagener classification — キース・ワグナー分類，KW分類

kWh
kilowatt hour — キロワット時

kW-hr
kilowatt hour — キロワット時

K wire
Kirschner wire — キルシュナー針金〔鋼線〕

kymo
kymography — X線動態撮影

kyph
kyphosis — (脊柱)後彎(症)

KZ
Kaplan-Zuelzer (syndrome) — カプラン・ズルジャー(症候群)

KZ-Neurose
Konzentrationslagerneurose〈独〉 — 強制収容所神経症

KZS
Konzentrationslager Syndrom〈独〉 — 強制収容所症候群

L l

L

Lactobacillus	乳酸桿菌(属)
lambert	ランベルト〈単位〉
latent (heat)	潜(熱)
lateral	側方の
lateral (nucleus)	外側核
latex	ラテックス
Latin	ラテン語(の)
lecithin	レシチン
left eye	左眼
Legionella	レジオネラ(属)
Leishmania	リーシュマニア(属)
lens	水晶体
lepra	ハンセン(らい)病
Leptospira	レプトスピラ(属)
Leptotrichia	レプトトリキア(属)
leucine	ロイシン
Leuconostoc	ロイコノストック(属)
leukocyte=leucocyte	白血球
lewisite	ルイサイト
liber〈ラ〉	本
licenced to practice	開業免許
lidocaine	リドカイン
ligament(um)	靱帯
ligand	リガンド
light sense	光覚
lilac	ライラック(色)，藤紫色
lime	石灰，ライム
limen	限
limes zero	無毒界
lincomycin	リンコマイシン
lingual	舌(側)の
liquor	液(体)
Listeria	リステリア(属)
little finger	小指
liver	肝(臓)
lues〈ラ〉	梅毒
lumbar	腰(部)の，腰椎の
lumbar spine	腰椎
lung	肺
lymph	リンパ
lymphocyte	リンパ球
lymphogranuloma	リンパ肉芽腫

lysosome リソソーム，水解小体
roman numeral 50 (ローマ数字の)50

l
levo 左，左方向，レボ
line 線
links〈独〉 左
locus〈ラ〉 場所，位置，染色体の座
long 長い

0-L
0-low titer ゼロ低価

L I〔L II，L III〕
stage of lues I〔II，III〕 第I〔II，III〕期梅毒

L/3
lower third (of leg bone) (足骨の)下1/3

L+
limes tod，limes death 限界死

l，L
left 左(の)
length 長さ
lethal 致死の，致命的な
libra〈ラ〉=pound ポンド
licenced〔licensed〕 免許を受けた
light 光
liter リットル〈単位〉
living 生きている
longitudinal (section) 縦の(断面)，縦軸の
low 低い
lower より低い
lowest 最低の
lumen 管腔

LA
lactic acid 乳酸
lactic acidosis 乳酸アシドーシス
laminin ラミニン
language age 言語年齢
laparoscopic appendectomy 腹腔鏡下虫垂切除術
large amount 大量(の)
laser ablation レーザー気化法
latex agglutination ラテックス凝集反応
Latin American ラテンアメリカ人
left and above 左上(象限)
left angle 左角
left arm 左腕，左上肢
left atrial (pressure) 左(心)房の(圧)
left atrium 左(心)室房
left auricle 左(心)室耳，左耳介

leucine aminopeptidase	ロイシンアミノペプチダーゼ
leukemia antigen	白血球抗原
leukoagglutinating	白血球凝集
leukocyte adhesion	白血球接着
Lightwood-Albright (syndrome)	ライトウッド・オールブライト(症候群)
linear accelerator	リニアアクセルレータ(＝LINAC)
linolenic acid	リノール酸
Little area	リトル野
local anesthesia	局所麻酔(法)
long-acting (drug)	長時間作用(性)の(薬)
Ludwig angina	ルードウィッヒのアンギナ
lumbar artery	腰動脈
lupus anticoagulant	ループス抗凝固物質
lymphocyte antibody	リンパ球性抗体

La

labial	口唇の
lanthanum	ランタン〈元素〉

L/A

lysine/arginine ratio	リジン/アルギニン比

L & A

light and accommodation	対光調節
living and acting	生きており活動している

L.A., l.a.

lege artis〈ラ〉＝by the law of the art	常法に従って《処》

LAA

left acromion anterior (position)	第一横位第一分類(＝LScA)〈胎位〉
left atrial abnormality	左(心)房異常
left atrial appendage	左(心)室耳
leukemia-associated antigen	白血病関連抗原
leukocyte ascorbic acid	白血球アスコルビン酸

LA : A, La : A

left atrial to aortic (ratio)	左(心)房大動脈(比)

LAAL

lower anterior axillary line	低位前腋窩線

LAAM

levo-alpha acetyl-methadol	左旋性アルファ・アセチル・メタドール

LAANAM

Latin American Association of National Academies of Medicine	ラテンアメリカ医学アカデミー協会

LAAO

L-amino acid oxidase	L-アミノ酸酸化酵素

L

lab
lab ferment 凝乳酵素
LAB, Lab, lab
laboratory 実験室，検査室
LABA
Laboratory Animal Breeders Association 実験動物飼育者協会
laser-assisted balloon angioplasty レーザー補助下バルーン血管形成術
LABBB
left anterior bundle branch block 左脚ブロック
LABC
lymphadenosis benigna cutis 皮膚リンパ球腫
lab.proc.
laboratory procedure 検査室手技，検査室操作
LABV
left atrial ball valve 左(心)房ボール〔球〕(状)弁
LABVT
left atrial ball valve thrombus 左(心)房(球状)弁血栓
LAC
left atrial contraction 左(心)房収縮
long-arm cast 長上肢ギプス包帯
lung adenocarcinoma cell 肺腺癌細胞
lac
laceration 裂傷
lactate 乳酸塩，乳酸エステル
lactation 乳汁分泌，授乳(期)
LAC, LaC
labiocervical 唇側歯頸の
Lac-B
Lactobacillus bifidus〈ラ〉 ビフィズス菌
LACI
lipoprotein associated coagulation inhibitor リポ蛋白結合凝固阻害物質
lacr
lacrimal 涙の，涙液の
lact
lactate 乳酸塩，乳酸エステル
lactating 授乳している
lactation 授乳(期)，乳汁分泌
lactic acid 乳酸
lacZ
β-galactosidase gene *lacZ*遺伝子，(大腸菌の)βガラクトシダーゼ遺伝子

L

LAD

lactic acid dehydrogenase	乳酸脱水素酵素，乳酸デヒドロゲナーゼ
late after discharge	後期後発射
left anterior descendence	左冠(状)動脈前下行枝
left anterior descending artery	左冠(状)動脈前下行枝
left atrial dimension	左(心)房径
left axis deviation	左軸偏位《心電》
leukocyte adhesion deficiency	白血球接着不全(症)
lipoamide dehydrogenase	リポアミドデヒドロゲナーゼ，リポアミド脱水素酵素
lymphocyte-activating determinant	リンパ球活性化(抗原)決定基

LADCA

left anterior descending coronary artery	左冠(状)動脈前下行枝

LADD

lacrimoauriculodentodigital (syndrome)	涙・耳介・歯・指(症候群)

LADH

lactic acid dehydrogenase	乳酸脱水素酵素，乳酸デヒドロゲナーゼ
liver alcohol dehydrogenase	肝アルコール脱水素酵素，肝アルコールデヒドロゲナーゼ

LADME

liberation-absorption-distribution-metabolism-elimination	薬物の放出・吸収・分布・代謝・排泄

LADPG

laparoscopically assisted distal partial gastrectomy	腹腔鏡下遠位胃部分切除(術)

LAE

left atrial enlargement	左(心)房拡大
lysergic acid ethylamide	リゼルグ酸エチルアミド

LAEC

locally advanced esophageal cancer	局在性進行食道癌

LAEDV

left atrial end-diastolic volume	左(心)房拡張終(末)期容積

LAEI

left atrial emptying index	左(心)房排出指数

LAeq

equivalent continuous A-weighted sound pressure level	等価騒音レベル(＝Leq)

LAER

late auditory-evoked response	遅発聴覚誘発反応

LAESV

left atrial end-systolic volume	左(心)房収縮終(末)期容積

laev.
laevus〈ラ〉　左(の)

LAF
laminar air flow　層空気流
Latin American female　ラテンアメリカ(人)女性
leukocyte-activating factor　白血球活性化因子
lymphocyte-activating factor　リンパ球活性化因子

LAF-3
leukocyte antigen factor-3　白血球抗原因子 3

LAFB
left anterior fascicular block　左脚前枝ブロック

LAFR
laminar air flow room　層空気流室

LAG
lymphangiogram　リンパ管撮影図，リンパ管造影像
lymphangiography　リンパ管造影〔撮影〕法

lag.
lagena〈ラ〉　ツボ，ビン，フラスコ《処》

LAG, LaG
labiogingival　唇側歯肉の

L-α-GP
L-α-glycerophosphate　L-α-グリセロリン酸

LAH
left anterior hemiblock　左脚前枝ヘミブロック
left atrial hypertrophy　左(心)房肥大

LAHB
left anterior hemiblock　左脚前枝ヘミブロック

LAHV
leukocyte-associated herpesvirus　白血球結合型ヘルペスウイルス

LAI
latex (particle) agglutination inhibition　ラテックス(粒子)凝集抑制
leukocyte adherence inhibition (assay)　白血球粘着阻止(試験)

LAI, LaI
labioincisal　唇切縁の

LAIF
leukocyte adherence inhibition factor　白血球吸着抑制因子

LAIR
latex agglutination inhibition reaction　ラテックス凝集阻止反応

LAIT
latex agglutination inhibition test　ラテックス凝集抑制試験〔検査〕

LAK
lectin activated killer cell　レクチン活性化キラー細胞
lymphokine-activated killer (cell)　リンホカイン活性(化)キラー(細胞)

LAL
limulus amebocyte lysate　リムルス・アメーバ様細胞溶解質

L-Ala
L-alanine　L-アラニン

LALI
lymphocyte antibody lymphocytolytic interaction　リンパ球抗体リンパ球溶解相互作用

LAM
lactation amenorrhea method　授乳期無月経法
Latin American male　ラテンアメリカ(人)男性
left atrial myxoma　左(心)房粘液腫
leukocyte adhesion molecule　白血球接着分子
lymphangioleimyomatosis　リンパ管平滑筋腫症

LA_m
mean left atrial pressure　平均左(心)室房圧

LAM, Lam, lam
laminectomy　椎弓切除(術), ラミネクトミー

LAMA
laser-assisted microanastomosis　レーザー補助下微小吻合(術)

LA-MAX
maximal left atrial (dimension)　最大左(心)室房

LAMB syndrome
lentigines, atrial myxoma, mucocutaneous myxomas, blue nevi syndrome　ラム症候群, 黒子・心房粘液腫・粘膜皮膚の粘液腫・青色母斑症候群

lami
laminotomy　椎弓切開(術)

LAMMA
laser microprobe mass analyzer　レーザー微小プローブ質量分析器

LAMP
limbic system membrane-associated protein　辺縁組織膜関連蛋白

LAMP-1
lysosome associated membrane glycoprotein-1　リソソーム関連膜糖蛋白

LAN
local area network　構内情報通信網《コン》
long-acting neuroleptic　長時間作用(性)神経弛緩薬

LANC
long arm navicular cast 長上肢舟状骨ギプス包帯
LANSI
Laser Association of Neurological Surgeon International 国際神経外科医レーザー連合
LANV
left atrial neovascularization 左(心)房血管新生
LAO
left anterior oblique (position) 第二斜位(の)，左前斜位(の)
left atrial overloading 左(心)房過負荷
LAP
left acromion posterior (position) 第一横位第二分類(＝LScP)〈胎位〉
left arterial pressure 左動脈圧
left atrial pressure 左(心)房圧
leucine aminopeptidase ロイシンアミノペプチダーゼ
leukocyte alkaline phosphatase 白血球アルカリホスファターゼ
low atmospheric pressure 低(大)気圧
lyophilized anterior pituitary 凍結乾燥下下垂体前葉(組織)
LAP, lap
laparoscopy 腹腔鏡検査(法)
LAP, lap, lap.
laparotomy 開腹(術)
LAPA
latex agglutination photometric assay ラテックス凝集比濁法
leukocyte alkaline phosphatase activity 白血球アルカリホスファターゼ活性
Lapa-Chole
laparoscopic cholecystectomy 腹腔鏡下胆嚢摘出術
laparo
laparoscopy 腹腔鏡検査
LAPC
lenampicillin レナンピシリン
lapcholy
laparoscopic cholecystectomy 腹腔鏡下胆嚢摘出術
LAPF
low-affinity platelet factor 低親和性血小板因子
lapid.
lapideum〈ラ〉 石のような，硬い
LAPMS
long arm posterior-molded splint 上上肢後面形成シーネ(副子)

L

LAPOCA
L-asparaginase, prednisone, vincristine (=Oncovin), cytarabine, adriamycin — L-アスパラギナーゼ,プレドニゾン,ビンクリスチン(=オンコビン),シタラビン,アドリアマイシン

LAPS
light-addressable potentiometric sensor — 並列型光活性電位センサー

LAP stain
leukocyte alkaline phosphatase stain — 白血球アルカリホスファターゼ染色(法)

LAPW
left atrial posterior wall — 左(心)房後壁

LAR
late allergic response — 遅発型アレルギー反応
late asthmatic response — 遅発型喘息反応
late-phase allergic reaction — 後期アレルギー反応
latex agglutination reaction — ラテックス凝集反応
low anterior resection — 低位前方切除術

lar
left arm reclining — 左側臥位

LAR, lar
laryngology — 喉頭(科)学
larynx — 喉頭

LARC
leukocyte automatic recognition computer — 白血球自動測定器

large FCC
large follicular center cell — 大型濾胞中心細胞

larng
laryngological — 喉頭(科)学の
laryngologist — 喉頭(科)医
laryngology — 喉頭(科)学

laryn
laryngeal — 喉頭の
laryngitis — 喉頭炎
laryngoscopy — 喉頭鏡検査(法)

Laryng
laryngology — 喉頭(科)学

Laryngol
laryngologist — 喉頭(科)医
laryngology — 喉頭(科)学

LAS
laboratory automation system — 局所適応症候群
laparoscopically assisted surgery — 補助的腹腔鏡下外科手術
lateral amyotrophic sclerosis — 筋萎縮性側索硬化症

laxative abuse syndrome 緩下薬乱用症候群
left anterior-superior 左前上の
linear alkylbenzene sulfonate 直鎖型アルキルベンゼンスルホン酸塩(＝linear ABS)
local adaptation syndrome 局所適応症候群
long arm splint 長腕副子
lower abdominal surgery 下腹部手術
lymphadenopathy syndrome リンパ節疾患症候群

LASA
left anterior spinal artery 左前脊椎動脈

LASE
laser-assisted spinal endoscopy レーザー補助下脊椎内視鏡検査(法)

LASEC
left atrial spontaneous echo contrast 左(心)房自然エコーコントラスト

LASER, laser
light amplification by stimulated emission of radiation レーザー，励起誘導放射による光増幅

LASFB
left anterior-superior fascicular block 左前上束ブロック

LASH
left anterior-superior hemiblock 左前上ヘミブロック

LASK
laser *in situ* keratomileusis レーザー角膜内切削形成(術)，レーシック手術

L-ASP
L-asparaginase L-アスパラギナーゼ

LASS
labile aggregation stimulatory substance 不安定凝固刺激物質

LAST
left anterior small thoracotomy 左前小開胸
leukocyte-antigen sensitivity testing 白血球抗原感受性テスト
long-acting thyroid stimulator 持続性甲状腺刺激物質

LAT
lactic acidosis threshold 乳酸アシドーシス閾値
latent 潜伏(性)の
latex agglutination test ラテックス凝集試験
left anterior temporal 左側頭前部
left anterior thigh 左大腿前面
left anterior triangle 左前三角
left atrial thrombus 左(心)房血栓
low antigenic tumor 低抗原腫瘍

lat, lat.
lateral 外側の，側方の，横向きの

L

latitude　緯度
latus〈ラ〉　広い

lat admov
lateri admoveatum〈ラ〉　その側に貼付せよ《処》

lat.bend.
lateral bending　側屈

lat.dol.
lateri dolenti〈ラ〉　疼痛側に

Latero
laterotorsio cruris〈ラ〉　下腿外方捻転

lat.men.
lateral meniscectomy　外側半月(板)切除(術)

LATP
left atrial transmural pressure　左(心)房経壁圧

lat.Rin.
lactated Ringer　乳酸加リンゲル(液)

LATS
long-acting thyroid-stimulating (hormone)　持続性甲状腺刺激(ホルモン)
long-acting thyroid stimulator　持続性甲状腺刺激物質
long-acting transmural stimulator　持続性貫壁性刺激物質

LATS-P
long-acting thyroid stimulator protector　持続性甲状腺刺激物質保護体

LATu
lobuloalveolar tumor　小葉肺胞腫瘍

LAUP
laser assisted uvulopatoplasty　レーザーによる口蓋垂軟口蓋形成術

LAV
left atrial volume　左(心)室房容積
lymphadenopathy-associated virus　リンパ節症関連ウイルス(＝HIV)
lymphocyte-associated virus　リンパ球関連ウイルス

LAVC
left atrial volume change　左(心)室房容積変化

LAVH
laparoscopic vaginal hysterectomy　腹腔鏡下膣式子宮摘出術

LAW
left atrial wall　左(心)房壁

Lax, lax
laxative　緩下薬
laxity　下痢，弛緩

LB
laboratory (data)　検査(室)(データ)
Lactobacillus bulgaricus　ブルガリア乳酸菌(属)

large bowel　大腸
lateral band　側索
lateral bending　側屈(の)
Lederer-Brill (syndrome)　レデラー・ブリル(症候群)
left bundle　左脚
left buttock　左殿部
leiomyoblastoma　平滑筋芽腫
lipid body　脂肪体
live birth　生児出産，生産
liver biopsy　肝生検
loose body　遊離体
low back (pain)　腰部(症)，下背部(痛)
lung biopsy　肺生検

Lb

leghemoglobin　レグヘモグロビン

lb, lb.

libra〈ラ〉=pound　ポンド〈単位〉

L & B, LB

left and below　左下(象限)，左下部

LBA

laser balloon angioplasty　レーザーバルーン血管形成(術)

left brow anterior (position)　第一額位(=LFA)〈胎位〉
lima bean agglutinin　リマ豆〔アオイ豆〕アグルチニン

lb ap.

libra apothecary〈ラ〉　薬用式ポンド

lb av.

libra avoirdupois〈ラ〉　常用式ポンド

LBB

left bundle branch　左脚
low back bending　下背部屈曲，腰部屈曲

LBBB

left bundle branch block　左脚ブロック

LBC

lidocaine blood concentration　リドカイン血中濃度
lymphadenosis benigna cutis　皮膚良性リンパ節症

LBCD

left border (of) cardiac dullness　心濁音界左縁

LBCF

laboratory branch complement fixation (test)　実験室ブランチ補体結合(試験)

LBD

laparotomic biliary drainage　開腹下肝外胆管ドレナージ
Lewy body dementia　レヴィ(小)体痴呆

LBE
long below-elbow (cast) 長肘下(ギプス包帯)

LBF
Lactobacillus bulgaricus factor ブルガリア乳酸菌因子，LB因子
limb blood flow 四肢血液量
liver blood flow 肝血流量

lb-ft
pound-feet ポンドフィート

LBH
length, breadth, height 長さ・幅・高さ

LBI
low serum-bound iron 低血清結合鉄

LBL
labeled lymphoblast 標識リンパ芽球
Lawrence Berkeley Laboratory ローレンス・バークレー研究所
lymphoblastic lymphoma リンパ芽球性リンパ腫

LBM
lean body mass 除脂肪体重
lens basement membrane 水晶体基底膜
lumbrical muscle (指の)虫様筋
lung basement membrane 肺基底膜

LBNP
lower body negative pressure 下半身陰圧

LBO
large bowel obstruction 大腸閉塞

LBP
left brow posterior (position) 第二額位(＝LFP)〈胎位〉
lipopolysaccharide binding protein リポポリサッカライド結合蛋白(＝LPS結合蛋白)
low back pain 腰痛(症)，下背部痛
low blood pressure 低血圧

LBPP
lower body positive pressure 下半身陽圧負荷

LBRF
louse-borne relapsing fever シラミ媒介回帰熱

LBS
long spike bursts 腸平骨筋の推進性運動
low back syndrome 腰部(下背部)症候群

lbs.
librae〈ラ〉 ポンド〈複数〉

LBSA
lipid-bound sialic acid 脂肪結合シアル酸(＝シアリン酸)

LBT

left brow transverse (position)	第一額位(＝LFT)〈胎位〉
low back tenderness	腰部(下背部)圧痛
lupus band test	ループス帯試験
lymphoblast transformation	リンパ芽球化変換

LBTI

lima bean tripsin inhibitor	リマ豆〔アオイ豆〕トリプシン抑制物質

LBV

lung blood volume	肺血液量

LBW

low birth weight	出生時低体重，低出生体重

LBWD

low birth weight dwarfism	低体重出生矮小症

LBWI

low-birth-weight infant	出生時低体重児，低出生体重児

LBWR

lung-body weight ratio	肺体重比

LC

Laënnec cirrhosis	ラエネック肝硬変
Langerhans cell	ランゲルハンス細胞
laparoscopic cholecystectomy	腹腔鏡下胆嚢摘出(術)
large chromophore	大発色団
laryngitis chronica〈ラ〉	慢性喉頭炎
least concentration	最低濃度
left central	左中心部
lethal concentration	致死濃度
leukemia cell	白血病細胞
leukocyte common antigen	白血球共通抗原
light chain	L鎖，軽鎖
light coagulation	光凝固
light cone	光錐
lining cell	管壁細胞
liquid chromatography	液(体)クロマトグラフィ
lithocholic (acid)	リトコール(酸)
liver cirrhosis	肝硬変(症)
liver clinic	肝臓クリニック
locus ceruleus	青斑核
long-chain	長鎖
longus capitus〈ラ〉	頭長筋
low calorie	低カロリー
low carbohydrate	低炭水化物
lues congenita〈ラ〉	先天性梅毒
luminary brightness increment campimetry	明度識別中心視野測定

lung cancer 肺癌
lung cell 肺細胞
lymph capillary リンパ毛細管
lymphocyte count リンパ球数
lymphocytotoxin リンパ球毒素
lymphoma culture リンパ腫培養

Lc
lumichrome ルミクロム

LC_{50}
median lethal concentration 50%致死濃度

l.c.
loco citato〈ラ〉 指定の場所に《処》

%LC
percent labeled cell 標識細胞百分率

LCA
Leber congenital amaurosis レーバー先天性黒内障
left carotid artery 左頸動脈
left circumflex artery 左回旋動脈
left colic artery 左結腸動脈
left coronary artery 左冠(状)動脈
Lemur catta〈ラ〉 ワオキツネザル
lipemia clearing factor 脂血症浄化因子
lymphocyte chemoattractant activity リンパ球化学誘導物質活性
lymphocytotoxic antibody リンパ球毒性抗体

LCAL
large cell anaplastic lymphoma 未分化大細胞リンパ腫

L-CAM
liver cell adhesion molecule 肝細胞接着分子

LCAS
lipoprotein and coronary atherosclerosis study リポ蛋白と冠(状)動脈硬化に関する研究

LCAT
lecithin-cholesterol acyltransferase レシチン・コレステロール・アシルトランスフェラーゼ，エルキャット

LCAT deficiency
lecithin-cholesterol-acyltransferase deficiency エルキャット〔LCAT〕欠損症

LCB
left costal border 左肋骨縁
lymphomatosis cutis benigna 良性皮膚リンパ腫症

LCBF
local cerebral blood flow 局所(大)脳血流(量)

LCC
left common carotid 左総頸(動脈)
left coronary cusp 左冠尖

luxatio coxae congenita 先天性股関節脱臼

LCCA
late cerebellar cortical atrophy 晩発性小脳皮質萎縮症
left common carotid artery 左総頸動脈

LCCD
late cortical cerebellar degeneration 晩発性皮質性小脳変性症

LCCS
low cervical cesarean section 子宮下部帝王切開(術)

LCCSCT
large cell calcifying Sertoli cell tumor 大細胞石灰化セルトリ細胞腫

LCD
light chain disease L鎖病，軽鎖病
liver cell dysplasia 肝細胞形成異常

LCDD
light chain deposition disease L鎖沈着病，軽鎖沈着病

LCE
laparoscopic cholecystectomy 腹腔鏡下胆嚢摘出術
left carotid endarterectomy 左頸動脈(血管)内膜切除(術)

L cell
Langerhans cell ランゲルハンス細胞

LCF
leukocyte chemotactic factor 白血球遊走因子
lipemia clearing factor 脂肪血症清浄化因子
lymphocyte chemotactic factor リンパ球走化因子
lymphocyte culture fluid リンパ球培養液

LCFA
long-chain fatty acid 長鎖脂肪酸

LCFAO
long-chain fatty acid oxidation 長鎖脂肪酸酸化

LCFU，L-CFU
leukocyte colony-forming unit 白血球コロニー形成ユニット

LCG
Langerhans cell granule ランゲルハンス細胞顆粒

LCGU
local cerebral glucose utilization 局所脳ブドウ糖消費量

LCH
Langerhans cell histiocytosis ランゲルハンス細胞組織球症

LCh
Licentiate in Chirurgy 外科有資格者

L-chain
light chain (disease) L鎖(病)，軽鎖(病)

LCI
light chain I 軽鎖 I

LCIS
lobular carcinoma *in situ* 小葉上皮内癌

LCL
lateral collateral ligament 外側側副靱帯
Levinthal-Coles-Lillie (body) レビンサール・コールズ・リリー(小体)
lower control limit 下方管理限界
lymphoblastoid cell line リンパ芽球様細胞株
lymphocytic choriomeningitis (virus) リンパ球性脈絡髄膜炎(ウイルス)
lymphocytic leukemia リンパ(球)性白血病
lymphocytic lymphosarcoma リンパ球性リンパ肉腫

LCM
latent cardiomyopathy 潜在(性)心筋障害
least common multiple 最小公倍数
left costal margin 左肋骨縁
lincomycin リンコマイシン
lymphocytic choriomeningitis リンパ球性脈絡髄膜炎

LCME
Liaison Committee for Medical Education 医学教育連絡委員会

LCMRG
local cerebral metabolic rate for glucose 局所脳ブドウ糖代謝率

LCMV
lymphocytic choriomeningitis virus リンパ球性脈絡髄膜炎ウイルス

LCN
left caudate nucleus 左尾状核

LCO(S)
low cardiac output (syndrome) 低心拍出量(症候群)

LCP
Legg-Calvé-Perthes (disease) レッグ・カルベ・ペルテス(病)
leukocytephoresis 白血球伝達
lymphocytophoresis リンパ球伝達

LCPD
Legg-Calvé-Perthes disease レッグ・カルベ・ペルテス病

LCP & SA
Licentiate of College of Physicians and Surgeons of America 米国内科外科学有資格者

LCR
late cutaneous reaction 遅発皮膚反応
leurocristine ロイロクリスチン
liquide céphalo-rachidien〈仏〉 (脳脊)髄液

LCS
left coronary sinus 左冠(状)静脈洞
liquor cerebrospinalis (脳脊)髄液

L

LCSG
left cardiac sympathetic ganglionectomy — 左(心)室交感神経節切除(術)

LCT
least concentration time — 最低濃縮時間
liver cell tumor — 肝細胞腫瘍
locoregional cancer treatment — 癌の局所療法
long-chain triglyceride — 長鎖中性脂肪
lymphocyte cytotoxicity test — リンパ球細胞傷害試験
lymphocyte toxin — リンパ球毒素
lymphocytotoxicity test — リンパ球毒性試験

LCTA
lymphocytotoxic antibody — リンパ球毒性抗体

LCTCS
low cervical transverse cesarean section — 低位(子宮)頸部横帝王切開

LC therapy
ligation and cryotherapy — 結紮凍結療法

LCV
leukocytoclastic vasculitis — 白血球破壊(破砕)性血管炎

LCX
left (coronary artery) circumflex branch — 左(冠(状)動脈)回旋枝

LD
lactate dehydrogenase — 乳酸脱水素酵素，乳酸デヒドロゲナーゼ
large ducts — 中心乳管
laser desorption — レーザー脱離
L-dopa — L-ド(—)パ(=レボドパ)
learning disability — 学習(能力)障害
left deltoid — 左三角(筋)
Legionnaires disease — 在郷軍人病，レジオネラ症
Leishmania donovani — リーシュマニア・ドノヴァン
lethal dose — 致死量
leukocyte dialysate — 白血球透析物
levodopa — レボドパ(=L-ド(—)パ)
light difference — 光差，明度差閾値
limited disease — 限局疾患
limiting dilution — 限外希釈
linguodistal — 舌側遠心の
lipodystrophy — リポジストロフィ
liver disease — 肝(臓)疾患
loading dose — 負荷量
lobular disorganization — 小葉組織崩壊
longitudinal diameter — 縦(直)径
longitudinal diameter of heart — 心臓縦(直)径

low density 低比重，低密度
low dose 少量
Luftdusche〈独〉 耳管通気
lymphocyte-defined (antigen) リンパ球識別混合培養(抗原)
lymphocyte depleted リンパ球欠乏

LD_{50}
median lethal dose 50%致死量，半数致死量

LD_{100}
lethal dose 100 100%致死量

LD，Ld
laboratory data 検査(室)データ

LD，L/D
light/dark (ratio) 明/暗(比)

LD，L-D
Leishman-Donovan (bodies) リーシュマン・ドノバン(小体)

L & D，L+D
labor and delivery 陣痛と出産

LDA
left-dorso-anterior 左背前位
limiting dilution assay 限外希釈法
low density area 低吸収域，低濃度域
lymphocyte-dependent antibody リンパ球依存抗体

LD antigen
lymphocyte defined antigen LD抗原

LDAR
latex direct agglutination reaction ラテックス直接凝集反応

L-D bodies
Leishman-Donovan bodies リーシュマン・ドノバン(小)体

LDC
lymphoid dendritic cell リンパ球様樹状細胞

LDCC
lectin dependent cellular cytotoxicity レクチン依存性細胞傷害

LDCF
lymphocyte derived chemotactic factor リンパ球由来白血球遊走因子

LDCT
late distal cortical tubule 後半遠位皮質尿細管

LDD
laser disk decompression レーザー椎間板減圧術
light-dark discrimination 明暗識別

LDDS
local drug delivery system 地域薬剤搬送システム

LDER
lateral-view dual-energy radiography 側方二倍線量X線撮影(法)

LDF
laser Doppler flowmetry　レーザード(ッ)プラー流量計測(法)

LDG
low-dose group　少量群

LDH
lactate dehydrogenase　乳酸脱水素酵素
low-dose heparin　少量ヘパリン
lumbar disc herniation　腰椎椎間板ヘルニア

LDI
low-density lipoprotein distribution index　低比重リポ蛋白分布指数

LDIH
left direct inguinal hernia　左直接鼠径ヘルニア

LDL
loudness discomfort level　音量不快レベル
low-density lipoprotein　低比重リポ蛋白
low-density lymphocyte　低比重リンパ球

LDL-cholesterol
low-density lipoprotein-cholesterol　LDLコレステロール

L-DLE
localized disseminated lupus erythematosus　限局性播種性エリテマトーデス

L

LDMC
latissimus dorsi-myocutaneous flap　広背筋皮弁
lectin dependent macrophage-mediated cytotoxicity　レクチン介在によるマクロファージの殺腫瘍細胞作用

LDMS
laser desorption mass spectrometry　レーザー脱離質量分析法

L_{dn}
day-night sound level　昼夜騒音レベル

L-DOPA, L-dopa, l-dapa, L-dapa
levodopa (=3,4-dihydroxy-L-phenylalanine)　L-ド(ー)パ, レボドパ

LDP
left-dorso-posterior　左背後位〈胎位〉
lumbodorsal pain　腰背部痛

LDPE
low-density polyethylene　低密度ポリエチレン

LDR
labor-delivery-recovery　分娩・出産・回復

L/D ratio
length to diameter ratio　長さ/直径比

LDRP
labor-delivery-recovery-postpartum　陣痛・分娩・回復・(出)産後

L.D.S.
Licentiate in Dental Surgery　口腔外科免許医
L.D.Sc.
Licentiate in Dental Science　歯科学免許医
LDT
lateral dorsal tegmental nucleus　側後天蓋核
LDV
lactic dehydrogenase virus　乳酸脱水素酵素ウイルス
laser Doppler velocimeter　レーザード(ッ)プラー流速計
laser Doppler velocimetry　レーザード(ッ)プラー流速計測法
LDX
long distance xerography　長距離ゼログラフィ
LE
lactulose enema　ラクツロース浣腸
left ear　左耳
left eye　左眼
lens extraction　水晶体(核)摘出(術)
leukocyte elastase　白血球エラスターゼ
leukocyte esterase　白血球エステラーゼ
leukoegresin　好中球遊走因子
leukoencephalitis　白質脳炎
live embryo　生存胚
Long-Evans rat　ロング・エバンスラット
lupus erythematosus (cell)　エリテマトーデス(細胞)
lysosomal enzyme　リソソーム酵素
Le
Leonard　レオナルド〈単位〉
Lewis number　ルイス数
LE, L/E
lower extremity　下肢
LEA
lower extremity amputation　下肢切断(術)
lumbar epidural anesthesia　腰部硬膜外麻酔
LEAFS
laser-excited atomic fluorescence spectrometry　レーザー励起原子螢光分析
lec
tonsillectomy　扁桃摘出手術
LECAM-1
leukocyte-endothelial cell adhesion molecule-1　白血球内皮細胞接着分子1
LE cell
lupus erythematosus cell　LE細胞，エリテマトーデス細胞

L

LECP
low-energy charged particle 低エネルギー荷電粒子
lect, Lect
lecture 講義，講師
LED
light-emitting diode 発光ダイオード
lowest effective dose 最小有効量
lupus erythematosus disseminatus 播種性エリテマトーデス，播種性紅斑性狼瘡
LEED
low-energy electron diffraction 低速電子線回折
LEEM
low-energy electron microscope 低エネルギー電子顕微鏡
LEEP
left end-expiratory pressure 左側呼気終末圧
loop electrical excision procedure ループ電気メス切除法
loop electrocautery excision procedure ループ電気メス焼灼切除法
loop electrosurgical excision procedure ループ電気メス外科切除法
LEF
lupus erythematosus factor エリテマトーデス因子，LE因子
LE factor
lupus erythematosus factor エリテマトーデス因子，LE因子
leg
legal 法律(上)の，合法の，法律に関する
legally 法律的に，合法的に
legislation 立法，法律(の)
legislative 立法，法律(の)
LEI
laparoscopic ethanol injection 腹腔鏡下エタノール注入療法
LEIS
laser-enhanced ionization spectroscopy レーザー誘起イオン化分光法
low-energy ion scattering 低エネルギーイオン散乱分光法
LeIF
leukocyte interferon 白血球インターフェロン
LE/LP
lupus erythematosus/lichen planus エリテマトーデス/扁平苔癬
LEM
lateral eye movement 側方眼球運動
leukocyte endogenous mediator 白血球内因性メディエータ

light electron microscope 光学電子顕微鏡

LEMS

Lambert-Eaton myasthenic syndrome ランバート・イートン筋無力症候群

LEMSIP

Laboratory for Experimental Medicine and Surgery in Primates 霊長動物実験内科・外科研究室

lenit.

leniter〈ラ〉 穏やかに，優しく

LEOPARD syndrome

lentigines, electrocardiographic abnormalities, occular hypertelorism, pulmonary stenosis, abnormalities of genitalia, retardation of growth, deafness syndrome 黒子症・心電図異常・眼間隔開離・肺動脈狭窄・性器奇形・発育遅滞・難聴症候群，レオパード症候群

LEP

lipoprotein electrophoresis リポ蛋白電気泳動(法)

low egg passage 軽度鶏卵継代

lower esophageal (pressure) 下部食道(圧)

LEPD

low-energy positron diffraction 低速陽電子線回折

LEPRA

Leprosy Relief Association ハンセン病救助協会

LE prep

lupus erythematosus preparation LE標本，エリテマトーデス標本

Lept

Leptospira レプトスピラ(属)

LEPTOS

leptospirosis agglutinin レプトスピラ症凝集素

Leq

equivalent continuous sound pressure level 等価騒音レベル(＝LAeq)

LER

lysosomal enzyme release リソソーム酵素放出

LES

Lambert-Eaton syndrome ランバート・イートン症候群

laser endoscope レーザー内視鏡

local excitatory state 局所的興奮状態

lower esophageal segment 食道下部

lower esophageal sphincter 下部食道括約筋

lupus erythematosus, systemic 全身性エリテマトーデス，全身性紅斑性狼瘡(＝SLE)

Les

lesbianism レスビアニズム

L

les
lesion 外傷(部位)，損傷(部位)
LESP
lower esophageal sphincter pressure 下部食道括約筋圧
LET
linear energy transfer 線エネルギー付与
LETD
lowest effective toxic dose 最小有効中毒量
LE test
lupus erythematosus test LE試験，エリテマトーデス試験
LETS protein
large external transformation-sensitive protein 高分子性外在性変質感受性蛋白，レッツ蛋白
LEU
leucovorin ロイコボリン
LEU，Leu
leucine ロイシン
leu-CAM
leukocyte cell adhesion molecule 白血球接着分子
Leu-EK
leucine-enkephalin ロイシン・エンケファリン
L
leuko
leukocytes 白血球
lev，lev.
levis〈ラ〉 軽い
levorotatory 左旋性の
Levine1-6
Levine grades of cardiac murmur(1-6) レバイン心雑音強度分類1～6
levit.
leviter〈ラ〉 軽く
L ext.，l/ext
lower extremity 下肢，脚
LF
labile factor 不安定因子
laryngofiberscope 喉頭ファイバースコープ
laryngofissure 喉頭切開(術)
Lassa fever ラッサ熱
latex fixation ラテックス吸着
lavage fluid 洗浄液
left foot 左足
left forearm 左前腕
left frontal 左前頭部
low fat (diet) 低脂肪(食)

Lf
limit flocculation untis 架〔線〕状反応単位
limit of flocculation 架〔線〕出限界
lumiflavin ルミフラビン

lf
loss of function 機能喪失

LF, lf
low frequency 低周波数，低頻度

LFA
learned food aversions 特定食物の嫌悪
left femoral artery 左大腿動脈
left forearm 左前腕
left fronto anterior (position) 第一額位(=LBA)〈胎位〉
leukotactic factor activity 白血球走性因子活性
low friction arthroplasty 低摩擦関節形成術
lymphocyte function associated antigen リンパ球機能関連抗原
lymphocyte〔leukocyte〕 function-associated antigen リンパ球〔白血球〕関連抗原

LFA-1
leukocyte factor antigen-1 白血球因子抗原 1
lymphocyte function antigen-1 リンパ球機能抗原 1

LFC
left frontal craniotomy 左前頭(部)開頭(術)
low fat and cholesterol 低脂肪・(低)コレステロール(食)

LFCS
low flap cesarean section 低皮切位帝王切開

LFD
lactose-free diet 無乳糖食
least fatal dose 最小致死量
low fat diet 低脂肪食
low fiber diet 低繊維食

LFD infant
large for dates infant 過大体重児，LFD児

LFEA
low frequency electrical acupuncture (treatment) 低周波置鍼〔針〕(療法)

LFF
Lemeur fulvus fulvus〈ラ〉 ブラウンキツネザル
low frequency fatigue 低周波数型疲労

L-F f.
Laki-Lorand factor レーキ・ローランド因子(=第XIII因子)

LFG infant
light for gestational age infant 過小体重児，LFG児

L

LFH
left femoral hernia 左大腿ヘルニア
LFLX
lomefloxacin ロメフロキサシン
LFM
laser force microscope レーザー力顕微鏡
LFMF
low frequency medium frequency 低周波中周波
LFN
lactoferrin ラクトフェリン
L form
Lister form リスター型
LFP
left fronto posterior (position) 第一額位(=LBP)〈胎位〉
LFp
left frontal pole 左前頭極
LFR
lymphoid follicular reticulosis リンパ球濾胞性細網症
L fraction
labile fraction 膜電位の不安定分屑
LFS
lateral facet syndrome 椎間関節症候群
Li-Fraumeni syndrome リー・フラウメニ症候群
LFT
latex fixation test ラテックス吸着試験
latex flocculation test ラテックス凝集試験
left fronto transverse (position) 第一額位(=LBT)〈胎位〉
liver function test 肝機能検査
low frequency transduction 低頻度(形質)導入
LFV
Lassa-fever virus ラッサ熱ウイルス
low frequency ventilation 低頻度換気
L fx
linear fracture 線状骨折
LG
lactoglobulin ラクトグロブリン
laryngectomy 喉頭切除(術)
left gastric 左胃動脈
left gluteal 左殿(部)の
left gluteus 左殿(筋)
leucyl-glycine ロイシルグリシン
limb-girdle muscular dystrophy 肢帯(型)筋ジストロフィ
linguogingival 舌側歯肉の
liver graft 肝移植片
lymph gland リンパ節
lymphocytic gastritis リンパ球性胃炎

Lg X
lymphogranulomatosis X — リンパ肉芽腫症 X

LG, Lg
Lactobacillus gasseri — ラクトバチルス・ガッセリ(菌)(属)

Lg, lg.
large — 大きい
leg — 脚
long — 長い

LGA
left gastric artery — 左胃動脈

LGA infant
large for gestational age infant — 過大体重児，LGA児

LGB
Landry Guillain Barré (syndrome) — ランドリー・ギラン・バレー(症候群)
lateral geniculate body — 外側膝状体

LGBS
Landry Guillain Barré syndrome — ランドリー・ギラン・バレー(症候群)

LGBT
Lesbian-Gay-Bisexual-Transgender — エル・ジー・ビィー・ティー，性的少数者

L

LGC
lateral gain control — 側方捕獲制御
liquid gas container — 可搬性超低温液化ガス容器

LGD
low-grade dysplasia — 低度異形成

LGE
Langat encephalitis — ランガット脳炎

Lge, lge
large — 大きい

LGH
lactogenic hormone — 乳腺刺激ホルモン

LGIF
lymphocyte growth inhibitory factor — リンパ球増殖阻害因子

LGL
large granular leukocyte — 大顆粒白血球
large granular lymphocyte — 大顆粒リンパ球
lobular glomerulonephritis — 分葉性糸球体腎炎
low grade lymphoma — 軽度リンパ腫
Lown-Ganong-Levine (syndrome) — ローン・ガノン・レバイン(症候群)

LGL syndrome
Lown-Ganong-Levine syndrome — LGL症候群，ローン・ガノン・レバイン症候群

LGMD
limb-girdle muscular dystrophy　肢帯(型)筋ジストロフィ，肢帯(型)筋異栄養(症)

LGN
lateral geniculate nucleus　外側膝状核
lobular glomerulonephritis　分葉性糸球体腎炎

LGP
laser gonioplasty　レーザー隅角形成術

Lgp
lymphocyte glycoprotein　リンパ球糖蛋白

LGS
Lennox-Gastaut syndrome　レノックス・ガストー症候群

LGSIL
low-grade squamous intraepithelial lesion　軽度扁平上皮内病変

LGT
Langat encephalitis　ランガット脳炎
late generalized tuberculosis　晩期全身(性)結核

Lgt, lgt.
ligamentum〈ラ〉=ligament　靱帯〈単数〉

lgts
ligaments　靱帯〈複数〉

L

LGV
large granular vesicle　大顆粒小胞
left gastric vein　左胃静脈
left gastric venocaval shunt　左胃静脈下大静脈吻合術
lymphogranuloma venereum　性病性リンパ肉芽腫

LGV conjunctivitis
lymphogranuloma venereum conjunctivitis　性病性リンパ肉芽腫性結膜炎

LH
lateral hypothalamus　外側視床下部
left hemisphere　左半球
left hepatic　左肝動脈
left hyperphoria　左上斜位
left hypertropia　左上斜視
limulus hemocyanin　カサガイヘモシアニン
Linke Hand〈独〉=left hand　左手
loop of Henle　ヘンレ(の)わな，係蹄
lower half　下半(分)
lues hereditaria　遺伝性梅毒
luteinizing hormone　黄体化ホルモン，黄体形成ホルモン
luteotrop(h)ic hormone　黄体刺激ホルモン

LH_2
liquid hydrogen　液体水素

L/H
lymphocytic/histiocytic (cell) リンパ球系/組織球系(細胞)
LHA
lateral hypothalamic area 側視床下部領域
left hepatic artery 左肝動脈
LHBV
left heart blood volume 左(心)室血液量
LHC
Langerhans cell histiocytosis ランゲルハンス細胞組織球増殖(症)
left heart catheterization 左(心)室カテーテル法
left hypochondrium 左季肋部，左下肋部
LHD
luetic heart disease 梅毒性心疾患
LHe
liquid helium 液体ヘリウム
LHF
left(-sided) heart failure 左(心)室不全
LH/FSH-RF
luteinizing hormone/follicle-stimulating hormone-releasing factor 黄体化〔黄体形成〕ホルモン・卵胞刺激ホルモン放出因子
LHI
Ligue Homéopathique Internationale 〈仏〉 国際同種療法協会
LHL
left hepatic lobe 肝左葉
LHON
Leber hereditary optic neuropathy レーバー遺伝性視神経萎縮症
LHPA
limbic-hypothalamus-pituitary-adrenal axis 辺縁系・視床下部・下垂体・副腎系
LHPC
lipomatous hemangiopericytoma 脂肪腫性血管周囲〔血管外皮〕細胞腫
LHR
leukocyte histamine release (test) 白血球ヒスタミン放出(試験)
Lyon hypertensive rat リヨン高血圧ラット
l hr
lumen hour ルーメン時
LHRF
luteinizing hormone-releasing factor 黄体形成〔黄体化〕ホルモン放出因子
luteotropic hormone-releasing factor 黄体刺激ホルモン放出因子

L

LHRH
luteinizing hormone-releasing hormone　黄体形成〔黄体化〕ホルモン放出ホルモン

LHS
left heart strain　左(心)室負荷

LHs
left-hand side　左手側，左側

LHT
left hypertropia　左眼斜視
left hypertropia　左眼遠視

L-5-HTP
L-5-hydroxytryptophan　L-5-ヒドロキシトリプトファン

LHV
left hepatic vein　左肝静脈

LI
labeling index　標識指数
lactose intolerance　乳糖不耐症
lamellar ichthyosis　層状〔葉状〕魚鱗癬
large intestine　大腸
laser iridotomy　レーザー虹彩切開術
Leptospira interrogans serovar *icterohaemorrhagiae*　黄疸出血性レストスピラ
lithiasis index　結石生成指数
lymphocytic index　リンパ球指数

Li
links〈独〉　左の
lithium　リチウム〈元素〉

L & I
liver and iron　肝(臓)と鉄

LIA
laser immunoassay　レーザー免疫測定法
leukemia-associated inhibitory activity　白血球関連抑制活性
leukemia cell-derived inhibitory activity　白血病細胞由来抑制活性
lysine-iron agar　リジン鉄寒天(培地)

LIAH
lymphocyte-induced angiogenesis factor　リンパ球由来血管新生因子

lib.
liber〈ラ〉　本
libra〈ラ〉　ポンド〈単位〉

lib cat
library catalogue　図書館目録

L

LiBr
lithium bromide 臭化リチウム
LIC
left internal carotid 左内頸(動脈)
localized intravascular coagulation 局所的血管内凝固
LICA
left internal carotid artery 左内頸動脈
LICC
lectin-induced cell-mediated cytotoxicity レクチン誘導細胞介在細胞傷害
lectin-induced cellular cytotoxicity レクチン誘導細胞傷害
LICD
lower intestinal Crohn disease 下部消化管クローン病
LICM
left intercostal margin 左肋間縁
Lic Med
Licenciate of Medicine 開業有資格者
Li_2CO_3
lithium carbonate 炭酸リチウム
LICS
left intercostal space 左肋間腔
LID
late-onset immunoglobulin deficiency 遅発性免疫グロブリン欠乏(症)
lymphocytic infiltrative disease リンパ球浸潤(性)疾患
LID-AB
low iron diamine-alcian blue 低鉄ジアミノアルシアンブルー
LIDO
lidocaine リドカイン
lidoc
lidocaine リドカイン
LIF
laser-induced fluorescence レーザー誘発螢光
lateral incudal fold 側キヌタ骨ひだ
left iliac fossa 左腸骨窩
left index finger 左示指
leukemia inhibitory factor 白血病阻止因子
leukocyte infiltration factor 白血球浸潤因子
leukocyte inhibitory factor 白血球抑制〔阻止〕因子
leukocyte interferon 白血球由来インターフェロン
leukocyte migration inhibitory factor 白血球遊走阻止因子
leukocytosis-inducing factor 白血球増多誘発因子
LIFT
lymphocyte immunofluorescence test リンパ球免疫螢光試験

Lig, lig, lig.
ligament 靱帯，ひだ〈単数〉
ligamentum〈ラ〉 靱帯，ひだ
ligate 結紮する
ligation 結紮
ligature 結紮，結び，結紮糸，結紮法
lignum〈ラ〉 木材

ligg, ligg.
ligamenta〈ラ〉=ligament 靱帯，ひだ〈単数〉
ligaments 靱帯，ひだ〈複数〉
ligature 結紮，結び，結紮糸，結紮法

ligs
ligaments 靱帯，ひだ〈複数〉

LIH
left inguinal hernia 左鼠径ヘルニア

LII
Leisure Interest Inventory 余暇〔レジャー〕興味調査表《心理》

LILA
liposome immune lysis assay リポソーム免疫溶解試験

LIM
limes〈ラ〉 限界，境界
lysine indole motility medium リジン・インドール運動性培地

lim
limit 限界，範囲，制限する
limitation 限界，制限

lin, lin.
linear 線(状)の，直線の，線形の
linimentum〈ラ〉=liniment 塗布剤，リニメント(剤)，擦剤

linac, LINAC
linear accelerator 直線加速器，リニアック

linct
linctus〈ラ〉 舐汁《処》

ling
lingual 舌の，舌側の
lingular 小舌の

linim
liniment 塗布剤，リニメント(剤)，擦剤

Linn
linnaean リンネ式の
Linnaeus リンネ

LInstPhys
Licentiate of Institute of Physics 医学研究所有資格者

LIO
left inferior oblique (muscle) 左下斜(筋)
Li_2O
lithium oxide 酸化リチウム
LiOH
lithium hydroxide 水酸化リチウム
LIP
lithium-induced polydipsia リチウム誘発多飲(症)
lymphoid interstitial pneumonia リンパ球性間質性肺炎
Lip
lipoate(=lipoic acid) リポ酸(塩)
LIPA
lysosomal acid lipase A リソソーム酸リパーゼA
LIPB
lysosomal acid lipase B リソソーム酸リパーゼB
LIQ
lower inner quadrant 下内(部)1/4区
LIQ, Liq, liq.
liquor〈ラ〉=a liquid, a solution 液体(の), 液状(の)
LIR
left iliac region 左腸骨部
left inferior rectus 左下直(筋)
LIRBM
liver, iron, red bone marrow 肝・鉄・赤色骨髄
LIS
laboratory information system 臨床検査室情報システム
left intercostal space 左肋間腔
locked-in syndrome 閉込め症候群
LISL
laser-induced intracorporeal shock wave lithotripsy レーザー誘発体内衝撃波砕石術
LISS
low ionic-strength solution 低イオン強度溶液
LIT
leukocyte migration inhibition test 白血球遊走阻止検査
lit, lit.
liter リットル〈単位〉
literal 文字どおりの, 厳密な
literally 文字どおりに, 全く
literature 文献
little 小さい
LITA
left internal thoracic artery 左内胸動脈
litho
lithotripsy 砕石術

L

LIV
left innominate vein 左無名静脈
liver 肝(臓)
living 生きている

LIV-BP
leucine, isoleucine, valine-binding protein ロイシン・イソロイシン・バリン結合蛋白

LIVC
left inferior vena cava 左下大静脈

LIVEN
linear inflammatory verrucous epidermal nevus 線状炎症性イボ状表皮性母斑

LIXIscope
low intensity X-ray imaging scope 低強度X線顕微鏡

LJ
Larsen-Johansson (syndrome) ラーセン・ヨハンセン(症候群)

Lj
Lebensjahr〈独〉 年齢

LJM
limited joint mobility 関節可動性制限

LJP
localized juvenile periodontitis 限局型若年性歯周炎

LK
lamellar keratoplasty 表層角膜移植術
Landry-Kussmaul (syndrome) ランドリー・クスマウル(症候群)
left kidney 左腎(臓)
Lichtkegel〈独〉 光錐
Lichtkoagulation〈独〉 光凝固
locus kieselbachii〈ラ〉 キーセルバッハ部位
Löhr-Kindberg (syndrome) レール・キントベルク(症候群)
Lungenkrebs〈独〉 肺癌
lymphokine リンホカイン

LK^+
low potassium ion 低カリウムイオン

Lkc
leukocyte 白血球

LKM
liver-kidney microsomal 肝腎ミクロソームの
liver-kidney microsome 肝腎ミクロソーム

LKMAb
anti liver-kidney microsome antibody 抗肝腎ミクロソーム抗体

L

LKS
Landau-Kleffner syndrome ランドー・クレッフナー症候群
liver, kidney, spleen 肝・腎・脾
LKSB
liver, kidney, spleen, bladder 肝・腎・脾・膀胱
LKS non.pal.
liver, kidney, spleen not palpable 肝・腎・脾触知不能
LL
language laboratory 語学研究所
large lymphocyte 大リンパ球
lateral lemniscus 外側毛帯
left lateral 左外側の
left leg 左脚
left lower 左下の
left lung 下肺
lepromatous leprosy ライ腫(型)ハンセン(病)
Lewandowsky-Lutz (syndrome) レワンドウスキー・ルッツ(症候群)
lines 線〈複数〉
lipoprotein lipase リポ蛋白リパーゼ
long leg 長脚
loudness level 音量レベル
lower lid 下眼瞼
lower limit 下限
lower lobe 下葉
lues latens 潜伏梅毒
Luftleitung〈独〉 気導，空気伝導
lymphoblastic lymphoma リンパ芽球性リンパ腫
lymphocytic leukemia リンパ性白血病
lymphocytic lymphoma リンパ球性リンパ腫
lymphoid leukemia リンパ性白血病
Lyon low blood pressure strain リヨン低血圧系統
lysolecithin リゾレシチン
L1-L5, L_{1-5}
lumbar spine segments (腰神経の)第１～第５腰椎
L lam
lumbar laminectomy 腰椎椎弓切除(術)
LLB
left lateral border 左外(側)縁
long leg brace 長下肢装具《リハ》
lower lobe bronchus 下葉気管支
lung liver border 肺肝境界
LLBCD
left lower border of cardiac dullness 心濁音界左下縁

L

LLC
laparoscopic laser cholecystectomy　腹腔鏡下レーザー胆嚢摘出術
liquid-liquid chromatography　液相・液相クロマトグラフィ
lymphocytic leukemia, chronic　慢性リンパ球性白血病

LL cast
long leg cast　長脚ギプス包帯

LLCC
long leg cylinder cast　長脚円柱(状)ギプス包帯

LLD
left lateral decubitus　左側臥位
leg length discrepancy　脚長差
liquid liquid distribution　液体液体分布
long-lasting depolarization　長(時間)持続(性)脱分極

LLD factor
lactobacillus lactis donor factor　乳汁中の乳酸桿菌ドナー因子

LLE
left lower extremity　左下肢

LLF
Laki-Lorand factor　レーキ・ローランド因子
left lateral femoral　左外側大腿の

LLG
Lungenlebergrenze〈独〉　肺肝境界

LLL
left liver lobe　肝(臓)左葉
left lower leg　左下腿
left lower lid　左下眼瞼
left lower limb　左下肢
left lower lobe (of lung)　(肺の)左下葉
left lower lung　左下(肺)(野)
localized *Leishmania* lymphadenitis　局所リンパ管炎リーシュマニア(症)

LLL brace
left long leg brace　左長脚装具

LLLE
lower lid, left eye　下眼瞼・左眼(＝LLOS)

LLLI
La Loche Leaque International〈西〉　国際母乳連盟

LLLL
left lower lung lobe　左下(肺)葉

LLLNR
left lower lobe, no rales　左(肺)下葉ラ音なし

LLLSB
lower left limits of sternal border　胸骨下部左縁

LLLT
low reactive level laser therapy　低反応レベルレーザー治療

LLN
lower limit of normal 正常下限
LLOD
lower lid, oculus dexter 下眼瞼・右眼(＝LLRE)
LLOS
lower lid, oculus sinister 下眼瞼・左眼(＝LLLE)
LLP
long-lasting potentiation 長(時間)持続(性)増強作用
LLQ
left lower quadrant 左下腹部
LLR
late local reaction 遷延性局所反応
left lateral rectus 左外直(筋)《眼》
left lumbar region 左腰部
LLRA
low lateral right atrium 下側右心房
LLRE
lower lid, right eye 下眼瞼・右眼
LLS
lazy leukocyte syndrome なまけもの白血球症候群
long leg splint 長下肢装具《リハ》
LLSB
left limits of sternal border 胸骨下部左縁
left lower scapular border 左下肩甲骨縁
left lower sternal border 左下胸骨縁
LLT
left lateral thigh 左外側大腿
lysolecithin リソレシチン
LLV
lymphatic leukemia virus リンパ性白血病ウイルス
LLV-F
lymphatic leukemia virus, Friend (virus associated) リンパ性白血病ウイルス・(ウイルス関連)フレンド
LLVP
left lateral ventricular pre-excitation 左外側心室早期興奮
LLW
low-level waste 低レベル廃棄物
LLWC
long leg walking cast 長脚歩行ギプス帯
LLX
left lower extremity 左下肢
LM
lactose malabsorption 乳糖吸収不全
laminin ラミニン
laryngeal mask ラリンゲアルマスク
laryngeal muscle 喉頭筋

lateral malleolus 外果，外くるぶし
lateral medial 外内側
left median 左正中(の)
legal medicine 法医学
lemniscus medialis 内側毛帯
leucomycin(=kitasamycin) ロイコマイシン(=キタサマイシン)
Licentiate in Midwifery 助産師有資格者
light microscope, light microscopy 光(学)顕(微鏡)
lincomycin リンコマイシン
lipid microspheres 脂肪微粒子
lipid mobilizing 脂質動員
liquid membrane 液体膜，液状膜
Listeria monocytogenes リステリア・モノサイトゲネス
littermate 同腹子
longitudinal muscle 縦走筋
Looser-Milkman (syndrome) ルーザー・ミルクマン(症候群)
lower motor (neuron) 下位運動(ニューロン)

Lm
lambert ランバート〈単位〉
Lebensmonat〈独〉 月齢

lm
lumen ルーメン〈単位〉

L/M
liter per minute リットル/分

%LM
percent labeled mitosis 標識分裂細胞百分率

LMA
left mentum anterior (position) 第二顔位〈胎位〉
Lemur macaco〈ラ〉 クロキツネザル
limbic midbrain area 辺縁系中脳部
liver membrane antibody 肝細胞膜抗体
liver membrane antigen 肝細胞膜抗原
liver membrane autoantibody 肝細胞膜自己抗体

LMAF
leukocyte migration activating factor 白血球遊走促進因子

LMB
Laurence-Moon-Biedl (syndrome) ローレンス・ムーン・ビードル(症候群)
leiomyoblastoma 平滑筋芽腫

LMBB
Laurence-Moon-Bardet-Biedl (syndrome) ローレンス・ムーン・バルデー・ビードル(症候群)

LMBS
Laurence-Moon-Biedl syndrome ローレンス・ムーン・ビードル症候群

LMC
laparoscopic microwave coagulation 腹腔鏡下マイクロ波凝固療法
large motile cell 大運動細胞
left main coronary artery 左冠(状)動脈主幹部
left middle cerebral 左中大脳
lymphocyte-mediated cytolysis リンパ球媒介細胞溶解
lymphocyte-mediated cytotoxicity リンパ球媒介細胞毒性
lymphomyeloid complex リンパ骨髄系複合体

LMCA
left main coronary artery 左冠(状)動脈主幹部
left middle cerebral artery 左中大脳動脈

LMCAD
left main coronary artery disease 冠(状)動脈左主幹部疾患

LMCAT
left middle cerebral artery thrombosis 左中大脳動脈血栓症

LMCL
left midclavicular line 左鎖骨中央線

LMD
local medical doctor 地域医師，地区医師
low molecular (weight) dextran 低分子(量)デキストラン

LMDF
lupus miliaris disseminatus faciei 顔面播種状粟粒性狼瘡

LMDX
low molecular (weight) dextran 低分子(量)デキストラン

LME
Lafora myoclonic epilepsy ラフォラ型ミオクローヌスてんかん
left mediolateral episiotomy 左中外側会陰切開(術)
leukocyte migration enhancement 白血球遊走増強

LMEL
Leonard Memorial for Eradication of Leprosy ハンセン病撲滅レオナルド記念館

LMF
lateral malleolar fold 外果ひだ
left middle finger 左中指
Leukeran, methotrexate, 5-fluorouracil ロイケラン・メトトレキサート・フルオロウラシル
leukocyte mitogenic factor 白血球有糸核分裂因子
lipid mobilizing factor 脂質動員因子

LMG
lethal midline granuloma 致死性正中(部)肉芽腫

LMH
lipid mobilizing hormone 脂質動員ホルモン
low molecular weight heparin 低分子ヘパリン
LMI
leukocyte migration inhibition 白血球遊走抑制
LMIF
leukocyte migration inhibition factor 白血球遊走抑制因子
L/min
liters per minute リットル/分
L/min/m²
liters per minute per square meter リットル/分/平方メートル
LMIR
leukocyte migration inhibition reaction 白血球遊走抑制反応
LMIT
leukocyte migration inhibition test 白血球遊走抑制試験
LML
left mediolateral 左中外側の
lower midline 下部正中
LMLE
left mediolateral episiotomy 左中・側会陰切開(術)
LMM
lactobacillus maintenance medium 乳酸桿菌維持培地
lentigo maligna melanoma 悪性黒子黒色腫
light meromyosin 軽メロミオシン
LMN
lower motor neuron 下位運動ニューロン
LMNL
lower motor neuron lesion 下位運動ニューロン病変
LMO
Lemur mongoz〈ラ〉 マングースキツネザル
LMOX
latamoxef ラタモキセフ
moxalactam モキサラクタム
LMP
last menstrual period 最終月経期
left mento posterior 左頤後位
left mentum posterior (position) 第二顔位(オトガイ部後方)〈胎位〉
liver membrane protein 肝細胞膜抗原
lumbar puncture 腰椎穿刺
LMR
left medial rectus 左内直(筋)《眼》
linguomandibular reflex 舌下顎反射

L

LMS
laryngo-microsurgery ラリンゴマイクロサージェリー
lateral medullary syndrome 外側延髄症候群
leiomyosarcoma 平滑筋肉腫
levamisole レバミゾール
L.M.S.
Licentiate in Medicine and Surgery 内科および外科有資格者
LMT
left main trunk 左冠(状)動脈主幹部
left mentum transverse (position) 第二顔位〈胎位〉
left middle temporal 左側頭中部
leukocyte migration technique 白血球遊走技術
leukocyte migration test 白血球遊走試験
LMT(H)
luteomammotropic hormone 黄体乳腺刺激ホルモン
lmtd.
limited 狭い，有限(会社)，制限された
L-3-MTO
L-3-methoxy-4-hydroxyphenylalanine L-3-メトキシ-4-ヒドロキシフェニルアラニン
LMV
larva migrans visceralis 内臓幼虫移行症
lateral mesencephalic vein 側中脳静脈
LMW
low molecular weight 低分子量
LMWD
low molecular weight dextran 低分子量デキストラン
LMWK
low molecular weight kininogen 低分子量キニノゲン
LN
laser nephelometry レーザーネフェロメトリー
later (onset) nephrotic (syndrome) 遅発性ネフローゼ(症候群)
lipoid nephrosis リポイド〔変性〕ネフローゼ
lupus nephritis ループス腎炎
lymph node リンパ節
Lyon normotensive strain リヨン正常血圧系統
L_n
equivalent input noise level 等価入力雑音レベル
ln
logarithm, natural 自然対数
LN_2
liquid nitrogen 液体窒素
LNAA
large neutral amino acid 大(型)中性アミノ酸

LNC
lymph node cell リンパ節細胞
LND
left radical neck dissection 根治的左頸部郭清(術)
Lesch-Nyhan disease レッシュ・ナイハン病
LNF
laparoscopic Nissen fundoplication 腹腔鏡下ニッセン胃底皺襞形成(術)
LNG
liquefied natural gas 液化天然ガス
LNKS
low natural killer syndrome 低ナチュラルキラー症候群
LNL
lower normal limit 正常下限
LNM
lymph node metastasis リンパ節転移
LNMP
last normal menstrual period 最終正常月経
LNP
liponucleoprotein リポ核蛋白
L_{np}
noise pollution level 騒音汚染レベル
LNPF
lymph node permeability factor リンパ節透過(性)因子
LNS
Lesch-Nyhan syndrome レッシュ・ナイハン症候群
LNT
lymph node T cell リンパ節T細胞
LNU
last name unknown 姓不明
LO
left occiput 左後頭位〈胎位〉
love object 愛の対象
low 低い
lo, LO
left occipital 左後頭部
local 局所の
LOA
Leber optic atrophy レーバー視神経萎縮(症)
left occiput anterior (position) 第一頭位第一分類〈胎位〉
LOAEL
low, observed adverse effect level 最小毒性量
lobo
lobotomy 白質切截，ロボトミー
LOC
laxative of choice 選択すべき緩下剤

level of consciousness 意識レベル
loss of consciousness 意識消失

loc
local 局所の
localized 限局性の

LoCa
low calcium 低カルシウム

lo.cal
low calorie (diet) 低カロリー(食)

lo.calc
low calcium (diet) 低カルシウム(食)

loc.cit.
loco citato〈ラ〉 引用した場所に

loc.dol.
loco dolenti〈ラ〉 有痛部に《処》

Lo CHO
low carbohydrates 低炭水化物

lo.chol
low cholesterol 低コレステロール

locn
location 位置

loc.tens.
locum tenens〈ラ〉 一時的な位置

LOD
lactate oxidase 乳酸酸化酵素
laparoscopic ovarian drilling 腹腔鏡下多囊胞卵巣多孔術
loss on drying 乾燥減量

lo-d
low density 低濃度，低密度，低比重

LOF
low outlet forceps 低位出口鉗子

lo.fat
low fat 低脂肪

LOFD
low outlet forceps delivery 低位出口鉗子分娩

log
logarithm 対数

LOH
local osteolytic hypercalcemia 局所性骨溶性高カルシウム血症
loop of Henle ヘンレのわな〔係蹄〕
loss of heterozygosity 初期の癌での染色体のロス

LOHF
late onset hepatic failure 遅発性肝不全

LOI
level of incompetence 機能不全レベル

L

LOIH
left oblique inguinal hernia 左斜位鼠径ヘルニア
LoK
low kalium 低カリウム
LoKa
low kalium 低カリウム
LOM
left otitis media 左中耳炎
limitation of motion 運動制限
loss of movement 運動喪失
LOMAC
leucovorin, vincristine (=Oncovin), methotrexate, adriamycin, cyclophosphamide ロイコボリン，ビンクリスチン(=オンコビン)，メトトレキサート，アドリアマイシン，シクロホスファミド
LOMSA
left otitis media, suppurative, acute 左中耳炎・化膿性・急性
LOMSC
left otitis media, suppurative, chronic 左中耳炎・化膿性・慢性
LOMSCh
left otitis media, suppurative, chronic 左中耳炎・化膿性・慢性
LoNa
low natrium〔sodium〕 低ナトリウム
long
longitude 経度
longitudinal 縦の
long.
longus〈ラ〉 長い
LOP
laparoscopic orchiopexy 腹腔鏡下精巣〔睾丸〕固定(術)
left oblique projection 第二斜位
left occiput posterior (position) 第一頭位第二分類〈胎位〉
lymphomatoid papulosis リンパ腫様丘疹症
lymphomatous polyposis リンパ腫ポリープ症
LOPS
length of patient stay 患者入院(滞在)期間
LOQ
lower outer quadrant 下外部1/4区
LOR
lorazepam ロラゼパム
lord
lordosis (脊柱)前彎(症)
lordotic (脊柱)前彎(症)の
LOS
length of stay 滞在期間
low cardiac output syndrome 低心拍出量症候群

lo.salt
low salt 低塩(分)
LOT
lateral olfactory tract 側嗅神経路
left occiput transverse (position) 第一頭位第二分類〈胎位〉
lot.
lotio〈ラ〉 ローション(剤), 洗浄剤, 洗浄液
loto
tonsillotomy 扁桃切除術
LOWBI
low-birth-weight infant 低出生体重児, 出生時低体重児
LOX
lipoxygenase リポキシゲナーゼ
lox
liquid oxygen 液体酸素
LP
labile peptide 不安定ペプチド
labile protein 不安定蛋白
laboratory procedure 実験的方法
lactoperoxidase ラクトペルオキシダーゼ
lamina propria 固有層
latency period 潜伏期(間), 潜(刺激)期
latent period 潜伏期
late potentials 遅延電位
(nucleus) lateralis posterior (視床)後外側(核)
latex particle ラテックス粒子
left parietal 左頭頂部
leukocytic pyrogen 白血球性発熱物質
levator palati 口蓋挙(筋)
levomepromazine レボメプロマジン
lichen planus 扁平苔癬
ligamentum patellae 膝蓋靱帯
light perception 光覚, 光認知
linear programming 線形計画法
lipiodol リピオドール
lipoprotein リポ蛋白
litter patient 担架患者
liver perfusate 肝灌流液
low point 低点
low power 低拡大(顕微鏡)
low pressure 低圧
low protein 低蛋白
lumbar puncture 腰椎穿刺

L

luminary brightness increment perimetry　明度識別周辺視野測定
lung parenchyma　肺実質
lymphocyte predominant　リンパ球優位の
lymphoproliferation　リンパ球増殖

Lp(a)
lipoprotein(a)　リポ蛋白(a)

L/P
lactate/pyruvate (ratio)　乳酸/ピルビン酸(比)
liver to plasma (concentration ratio)　肝/血漿(濃度比)
lymphocyte/polymorph (ratio)　リンパ球/多形核球(比)
lymph-plasma (ratio)　リンパ/血漿(比)

L-P
left parietal　左頭頂部

LPA
latex particle agglutination　ラテックス粒子凝集(反応)
left pulmonary artery　左肺動脈
Limulus polyphemus agglutinin　カブトガニレクチン
lysophosphatidic acid　リゾホスファチジン酸

L-PAM
L-phenylalanine mustard　フェニルアラニンマスタード

L

LPAT
latex particle agglutination test　ラテックス粒子凝集テスト

LPB
lipoprotein B　リポ蛋白B

LPC
laser photocoagulation　レーザー光凝固術
late positive component　後期陽性成分
lysophosphatidyl choline　リゾホスファチジルコリン

LPCA
leukocyte procoagulant activity　白血球凝血促進活性
long posterior ciliary artery　長後毛様動脈

LPCVD
low pressure chemical vapor deposition　低圧化学的気相成長法

LPD
leiomyomatosis peritonealis disseminata　播種性腹膜平滑筋腫症
lipiodol　リピオドール
lipiodolization　リピオドール注入塞栓術
low potassium dextran　低カリウムデキストラン
low-protein diet　低蛋白食
luteal phase defect　黄体期欠損
lymphoproliferative disorder　リンパ球増殖疾患

LPDA
left posterior descending artery　左後方下行動脈

LPDS
lipoprotein deficient serum　リポ蛋白欠乏血清
LPE
lipoprotein electrophoresis　リポ蛋白電気泳動(法)
liquid phase epitaxy　液相エピタキシ
lysophosphatidyl ethanolamine　リゾホスファチジルエタノールアミン
LPerc
light perception　光覚
LPF
leukocytosis promoting factor　白血球増多因子
leukopenia factor　白血球減少因子
lipopolysaccharide factor　リポ多糖因子
lymphocytosis promoting factor　リンパ球増多因子
LPF, lpf, l.p.f.
low-power field　(顕微鏡の)低拡大野
LPFB
left posterior fascicular block　左後束ブロック
LPG
linear (gradient) polyacrylamide gel　線形濃度勾配アクリルアミドゲル
liquefied petroleum gas　液化石油ガス，LPガス
LPH
left posterior hemiblock　左脚後枝ヘミブロック
lipotropic hormone　リポトロピン
low perfusion hyperemia　低灌流充血
LPHD
lymphocyte predominance Hodgkin disease　リンパ球優勢型ホジキン病
LPI
laser peripheral iridectomy　レーザー周辺虹彩切除(術)
left posterior-inferior　左後下の
long process of incus　キヌタ骨長突起
lysinuric protein intolerance　リジン蛋白不耐症
LPIA
latex photometric immunoassay　ラテックス光学的免疫測定法
LPICA
left posterior internal carotid artery　左後内頸動脈
LPIFB
left posterior-inferior fascicular block　左後下束ブロック
LPL
lamina propria lymphocyte　固有層リンパ球
lichen planus-like lesion　扁平苔癬様病変
lipoprotein lipase　リポ蛋白リパーゼ
low-percentage leukemia　低パーセント白血病

L

LPLA
lipoprotein lipase activity　リポ蛋白リパーゼ活性
LPLK
lichen planus-like keratosis　扁平苔癬様角化症
LPLND
laparoscopic pelvic lymph node dissection　腹腔鏡下骨盤リンパ節郭清(術)
LPM
lateral pterygoid muscle　外側翼突筋
liver plasma membrane　肝臓(原)形質膜
localized pretibial myxedema　限局性脛骨前粘液水腫
lymphoproliferative malignancy　リンパ増殖性悪性病変
LPM, lpm
liters per minute　リットル/分
LPN
licenced practical nurse　准看護師
LPO
left posterior oblique (position)　左後斜位，前後方向第一斜位
light perception only　光覚のみ
lipid peroxide　過酸化脂質
LPOF
lateroposterior orbitofrontal cortex　側後眼窩前頭皮質

L

LpOH
lysopine dehydrogenase　リソピン脱水素酵素，リソピンデヒドロゲナーゼ
LPP
lateral pterygoid processus　外側翼状突起
lipopeptide　リポペプチド
liver phosphorylase phosphatase　肝ホスホリラーゼホスファターゼ
lymphocyte plasmapheresis　リンパ球プラズマ伝達
LPPH
late postpartum hemorrhage　遅発性分娩後出血
LPR
lactate-pyruvate ratio　乳酸塩・ピルビン酸塩比
late phase reaction　遅延型反応
late phase response　後期反応
lymphocyte proliferative response　リンパ球増殖反応
L/P ratio
lactate-pyruvate ratio　乳酸塩・ピルビン酸塩比
LPRC
leukocyte-poor red cell　白血球除去赤血球
LProj
light projection　光投射
LPS
laparoscope　腹腔鏡

levator palpebrae superioris (muscle) 上眼瞼挙(筋)
lipase リパーゼ
lipopolysaccharide リポ多糖類
lipopolysaccharidosis リポ多糖体症
lyophilized pig skin 乾燥凍結ブタ真皮
lyophilized porcine skin 凍結乾燥豚皮

lps
liter per second リットル/秒

LP shunt
lumbar arachnoid peritoneal shunt 腰椎クモ膜下腔腹腔シャント術
lumboperitoneal shunt 腰椎腹腔シャント術

LPSR
lipopolysaccharide receptor リポ多糖類受容体

LPT
left posterior temporal 左側頭後部
licensed physical therapy 認可された物理療法
lipotate リポテート

LPV
left portal vein 左門脈
left pulmonary vein 左肺静脈
lymphopathia venereum 性病性リンパ(節)疾患
lymphotropic papovavirus リンパ栄養パポバウイルス

LPVP
left posterior ventricular pre-excitation 左後心室早期興奮

LPW
lateral pharyngeal wall 外側咽頭壁

lpw
lumens per watt ルーメン/ワット

LpX, LPX
lipoprotein X リポ蛋白X

LPZ, LPz
levomepromazine レボメプロマジン

LQ
last quarter 最後の1/4
lowest quadrant (quartile) 最下部1/4区

LQTS
long Q-T syndrome QT延長症候群

LR
laboratory report 検査室報告
labor room 分娩室，陣痛室
lactated Ringer (solution) 乳酸加リンゲル(液)
large reticulocyte 大(型)網(状)赤血球
latency relaxation 潜伏時弛緩
lateral rectus (muscle) 外直(筋)

L

left rotation 左回転
light reaction 光反応
light reflex 対光反射

Lr
lawrencium ローレンシウム〈元素〉

lr
lower 下の

L→R
left to right 左→右

L/R
left to right (ratio) 左右(比)

l/r
lower right 右下

L & R
left and right 左と右

L<R
left less than right 左<右

L>R
left greater than right 左>右

lR, LR
letzte Regel〈独〉 最終月経

LRA
left radial artery 左橈骨動脈
left renal artery 左腎動脈
low right atrium 低位右(心)房

LRB
lisamine rhodamine B リサミンローダミンB

LRC
lack of retinal correspondence 網膜対応欠如
Lipid Research Center 脂質研究センター
living renal donor 生体腎移植ドナー

LRC-CPPT
Lipid Research Center-Coronary Primary Prevention Trial 脂質研究センター冠(状)動脈一次予防試験

LRCP
Licentiate in Royal College of Physicians 英国医師会員有資格者

LRCS
Licentiate in Royal College of Surgeons 英国外科医師会員有資格者

LRD
living-related donor 移植素材生体提供者
low residue diet 合成低残渣食

LRE
leukemic reticuloendotheliosis 白血病性(細)網内(皮)症
lymphoreticuloendothelial リンパ(細)網内(皮)の

LREH
low renin essential hypertension 低レニン本態性高血圧(症)
LRF
latex, resorcinol, formaldehyde ラテックス・レゾルシノール・ホルムアルデヒド
left rectus femoris 左大腿直(筋)
liver residue factor 肝臓残留因子
luteinizing hormone releasing factor 黄体形成〔黄体化〕ホルモン放出因子
LRFPS
Licentiate in Royal Faculty of Physicians and Surgeons 英国内科医・外科医分科会員有資格者
LRH
luteinizing hormone-releasing hormone 黄体形成〔黄体化〕ホルモン放出ホルモン
LRI
lower respiratory illness 下気道疾患
lymphocyte reactivity index リンパ球反応性指数
LRM
left radical mastectomy 根治的左乳房切断(術)
LRMP
last regular menstrual period 最終規則的月経
LRNA
low renin, normal aldosterone 低レニン・正常アルドステロン
LRND
left radical neck dissection 根治的左頸部郭清(術)
LRP
LDL related protein 低比重リポ蛋白関連蛋白
lichen ruber planus 扁平紅色苔癬
LRQ
lower right quadrant 下右(部)1/4区
LRR
labyrinthine righting reflex 迷路立ち直り反射
lower reduced rate 低減率
LRS
lactated Ringer solution 乳酸加リンゲル液
laparoscopic reproductive surgery 腹腔鏡下生殖手術
lateral recess stenosis 外側陥凹狭窄(症)
lateral recess syndrome 外側陥凹症候群
lumboradicular syndrome 腰(神経)根症候群
LRSF
lactating rat serum factor 授乳ラット血清因子
liver regenerating serum factor 肝再生血清因子
LR-SH
left-right shunt 左右シャント

L

L-R shunt
left to right shunt　左右シャント

LRSS
late respiratory systemic syndrome　遅発型呼吸性全身症候群

LR system
lymphoreticular system　リンパ網内系

LRT
leucine response test　ロイシン反応試験
lower respiratory tract　下気道

LRTI
lower respiratory tract illness　下気道疾患

LRV
left renal vein　左腎静脈

LRZ
lorazepam　ロラゼパム

LS
learning strategies　学習計画
left sacrum　左仙骨
left side　左側
legally separated　法(律)的に別居した
leiomyosarcoma　平滑筋肉腫
length of stay　滞在期間
Letterer-Siwe (disease)　レッテラー・シーベ(病)
Libman-Sacks (disease)　リブマン・サックス(病)
library searching　図書検索
Lichtsinn〈独〉=light sense　光(感)覚
light sleep　軽睡眠
liminal sensitivity　閾値の知覚度
lipid synthesis　脂質合成
low sodium　低ナトリウム
lumber spine　腰椎
lumbosacral　腰仙の
lymphocyte score　末梢血リンパ球数
lymphosarcoma　リンパ肉腫

L5-S1
lumbar fifth vertebra to sacral first vertebra　第五腰椎・第一仙椎

l.s.
Lichtsinn〈独〉=light sense, light perception　光覚弁

L/S
lecithin/sphingomyelin (ratio)　レシチン/スフィンゴミエリン(比)

L-S
lumbo-sacral　腰仙骨の

L & S, L+S
liver and spleen | 肝(臓)と脾(臓)

LSA
left sacrum anterior (position) | 第一骨盤位第一分類〈胎位〉
left subclavicular artery | 左鎖骨下動脈
leukocyte specific activity | 白血球特異(的)活性
lichen sclerosus et atrophicans〈ラ〉 | 硬化性萎縮性苔癬
liver specific antigen | 肝特異抗原
lymphosarcoma | リンパ肉腫

LS antigen
heat-liabile and heat-stable antigen | 易熱・熱安定抗原

LSA/RCS
lymphosarcoma-reticulum cell sarcoma | リンパ肉腫/細網肉腫

LSB
left scapular border | 左肩甲骨縁
left sternal border | 胸骨左縁

LS BPS
laparoscopic bilateral partial salpingectomy | 腹腔鏡下両側卵管部分切除(術)

LSC
left sided colon (cancer) | 左側結腸(癌)
lichen simplex chronicus | 慢性単純苔癬
liquid scintillation counter | 液体シンチレーションカウンター
liquid-solid chromatography | 液相・固相クロマトグラフィ

l.s.c.
loco supra citato〈ラ〉 | 前に引用された位置に

LSCA
left subclavian artery | 左鎖骨下動脈

LScA
left scapula anterior (position) | 第一横位第一分類(=LAA)〈胎位〉

LSCL
lymphosarcoma cell leukemia | リンパ肉腫細胞(性)白血病

LScP
left scapula posterior (position) | 第一横位第二分類(=LAP)〈胎位〉

LSCS
lumbar spinal canal stenosis | 腰部脊柱管狭窄症

LSCV
left subclavian vein | 左鎖骨下静脈

LSD
least significant difference | 最小有意差
leukemia significant dose | 白血病有意線量
low salt diet | 低塩(分)食

low sodium diet　低ナトリウム食
Lysergsäurediäthylamid〈独〉＝lysergic acid diethylamide　リセルグ酸ジエチルアミド

LSD 25
lysergic acid diethylamine tartrate　酒石酸リゼルグ酸ジエチラミン

LSECS
Life Support and Environmental Control System　生活支持と環境管理組織

l sect
longitudinal section　縦切

LSEP
left somatosensory evoked potential　左体性感覚誘発電位

LSF
line spread function　線像強度分布
long acting sulfonamide　持続性サルファ剤
long spacing fibril　長周期原線維
lymphocyte-stimulating factor　リンパ球刺激因子

LSFA
life supporting first aid　一次救命処置

LSG
Lymphoma Study Group　(悪性)リンパ腫研究グループ

Lsg
Lösung〈独〉　(溶)液

LSH
lutein-stimulating hormone　黄体刺激ホルモン
lymphocyte-stimulating hormone (factor)　リンパ球刺激ホルモン(因子)

LSI
large scale integrated circuit　大規模集積回路
Life Satisfaction Index　生活満足指数
light scattering index　光散乱指数

LSIO
lumbosacroiliac orthosis　腰椎・仙腸装具

LSK
liver, spleen, kidney　肝・脾・腎

LSKM
liver-spleen-kidney megalia　肝・脾・腎巨大症

LSL
left sacrolateral　左仙骨側方
lymphosarcoma (cell) leukemia　リンパ肉腫(細胞性)白血病

LSLB
left short-leg brace　左短脚固定器

LSM
late diastolic murmur　拡張終期雑音
late systolic murmur　収縮後期雑音

lipid storage myopathy 脂質蓄積型ミオパシー
lymphocyte separation medium リンパ球分離液
lysergic acid morphine リゼルグ酸モルヒネ

LSMOC
life science medical operation computer 生命科学医学情報コンピュータ《医コン》

LSN
lateral septal nucleus 側中隔核
left substantia nigra 左黒質
left sympathetic nerve 左交感神経

LSO
left salpingo-oophorectomy 左卵管卵巣摘出(術)
left superior oblique 左上斜(筋)
left superior olive 左上オリーブ(核)
lumbosacral orthosis 腰・仙椎装具

LSP
left-sacro-posterior 左仙骨部後位
left sacrum posterior (position) 第一骨盤位第二分類〈胎位〉
liver specific membrane lipoprotein 肝特異的膜リポ蛋白

LSp, L sp.
life span 寿命

L sp., L-sp
lumbar spine 腰椎

LSR
left supeiror rectus 左上直(筋)

LSRA
low septal right atrium 下中隔右心房

L/S ratio
lecithin/sphingomyelin ratio レシチン・スフィンゴミエリン比, L/S比

LSS
life saving service 生命救助サービス
life saving station 生命救助本部
Life Span Study 寿命研究
life support system 生命維持装置
lumbar spinal stenosis 腰部脊柱管狭窄症

LST
lateral sinus thrombophlebitis 外側静脈洞血栓症静脈炎
lateral spinothalamic tract 外側脊髄視床路
lateral spreading tumor 側方発育型腫瘍
left-sacro-transverse 左仙骨部横位
left sacrum transverse (position) 第一骨盤位第二分類〈胎位〉
lymphocyte stimulation test リンパ球刺激試験

LSTC
laparoscopic tubal cautery 腹腔鏡下卵管焼灼
laparoscopic tubal coagulation 腹腔鏡下卵管凝固

LSTL
laparoscopic tubal ligation 腹腔鏡的卵管結紮(法)
LST tract
lateral spinothalamic tract 外側脊髄視床路
LSU
lactose, saccharose, urea agar medium 乳糖・サッカロース・尿素寒天培地
LSV
lateral sacral vein 外側仙骨静脈
left subclavian vein 左鎖骨下静脈
LSVC
left superior vena cava 左上大静脈
LSWA
large-amplitude, slow-wave activity 大〔高〕振幅徐波活動
LT
heat-labile enterotoxin 熱不安定腸毒素
left thigh 左大腿
length of tendon 膝蓋靭帯の長さ
lethal time 致死時間
leukotriene ロイコトリエン
Levin tube レヴィン管
levothyroxine レボチロキシン
lingual tonsil 舌扁桃
long term 長期(間)
long tube 長い管
low temperature 低温
low tension 低張力
lues test 梅毒検査
lymphocyte transformation リンパ球転換
lymphocyte transitional リンパ球移行の
lymphocytic thyroiditis リンパ球性甲状腺炎
lymphocytotoxin リンパ球毒素
lymphotoxin リンホトキシン
LT50
50% lethal time 50%致死時間
LT_{50}
mean lethal temperature 半数〔50%〕致死温度
L-T
left temporal 左側頭部
Lt, lt., lt
left 左方の
light 光
LTA
laryngeal tracheal anesthesia 喉頭気管麻酔
leisure-time activity 余暇活動

L

lipoate transacetylase リポエートトランスアセチラーゼ
local tracheal anesthesia 局所気管麻酔(法)
lymphocyte-transforming activity リンパ球転換活性

LTA_4
leukotriene A_4 ロイコトリエンA_4

LTAF
local tissue advancement flap 局部組織前位縫合皮弁

LTAS
lead tetra-acetate Schiff 四酢酸鉛シッフ

LTB
laparoscopic tubal banding 腹腔鏡下卵管バンド結紮
laryngotracheal bronchitis 喉頭気管気管支炎
laryngotracheobronchitis 喉頭気管気管支炎

LTB_4
leukotriene B_4 ロイトコリエンB_4

LTBMC
long-term bone marrow culture 長期骨髄培養

LTC
large transformed cell 大(型)転換細胞
lidocaine tissue concentration リドカイン組織(中)濃度
long-term care 長期ケア，長期療養
lysed tumor cell 溶解腫瘍細胞

LTC_4
leukotriene C_4 ロイトコリエンC_4

LTCBDE
laparoscopic transcystic common bile duct exploration 腹腔鏡下経胆嚢総胆管診査

LTCF
long-term care facility 長期ケア施設

LTD
Laron-type dwarfism ラロン型小人症
long-term depression 長期抑圧(脳)
long-term disability 長期廃疾

ltd.
limited 制限された，有限(会社)，狭い

LTD_4
leukotriene D_4 ロイトコリエンD_4

LTE
laryngotracheoesophageal 喉頭気管食道の
local thermodynamic equilibrium 局所的熱平衡

LTE_4
leukotriene E_4 ロイトコリエンE_4

LTEC
long-term electrocardiogram 長期記録心電図

L

LTF
lipotrop(h)ic factor 脂肪親和性因子，脂(肪)向性因子
lymphocyte-transforming factor リンパ球転換因子

LTF_4
leukotriene F_4 ロイトコリエンF_4

LTG
low tension glaucoma 低眼圧緑内障

LTGA
left transposition of great artery 左大血管転位症

LTH
lactogenic hormone 乳腺刺激ホルモン
local tumor hyperthermia 局所腫瘍温熱(療法)
luteotropic hormone 黄体刺激ホルモン

LTHIF
luteotropic hormone inhibitory factor 黄体刺激ホルモン抑制因子

L-threo DOPS
L-threo-dihydroxy-phenyl-serine L-スレオ-ジヒドロキシフェニルセリン

LTK
laser thermal keratoplasty レーザー熱角膜移植(術)

ltk
leukocyte tyrosine kinase 白血球チロシンキナーゼ

LTL
laparoscopic tubal ligation 腹腔鏡下卵管結紮

lt.lat
left lateral 左外側の

LTM
long-term memory 長期記憶

LTNP
long-term non-progressor (HIVの)長期非進行者

LTNS
long-term non-seroconverter (HIV抗体の)長期非変換者

LTO
laparoscopic total occlusion 腹腔鏡下完全閉鎖(術)

LTOF
low temperature optical facility 低温視覚施設

LTOT
long-term oxygen therapy 長期酸素療法

LTP
laser trabeculoplasty レーザー線維柱帯形成術
leukocyte thromboplastin 白血球トロンボプラスチン
lipid transfer protein 脂質転送蛋白
lipid transport protein 脂質輸送蛋白
long-term potentiation 長時間相乗作用
L-tryptophan L-トリプトファン

luteotropin　黄体刺激ホルモン

LTPP

lipothiamide pyrophosphate　リポチアミドピロリン酸

LTR

long terminal repeat　長鎖末端反復
lymphocyte transfer reaction　リンパ球転換反応

L-Trp

L-tryptophan　L-トリプトファン

LTS

lactose　乳糖
laparoscopic tubal sterilization　腹腔鏡下卵管不妊手術
long-term storage　長期貯蔵
long-term surviving　長期生存の
long tract sign　長経路(遮断)徴候

LTs

leukotrienes　ロイコトリエン〈複数〉

LTT

lactose tolerance test　乳糖負荷試験
leucine tolerance test　ロイシン負荷試験
lymphoblastic transformation test　リンパ芽球化転換試験，リンパ球幼若転換試験
lymphocyte transformation test　リンパ球転換試験

LTV

long-term variability　ロングタームバリアビリティ
Lucké tumor virus　リュッケ腫瘍ウイルス

lt.vent.BBB

left ventricular bundle branch block　左(心)室脚ブロック

LTW

Leydig cell tumor of Wistar rats　ウィスターラット(の)ライディヒ細胞腫瘍

LTX

lophotoxin　ロホトキシン
lung transplantation　肺移植

LU

left upper　左上の
Leibesumfang〈独〉　腹囲
lytic unit　細胞溶解単位

Lu

lutetium　ルテチウム〈元素〉
Lutheran blood group (system)　リュテラン血液型

lu.

lues〈ラ〉　梅毒

L & U

lower and upper　下方と上方の，下位と上位の

LU, Lu

lung　肺

LUA
left upper arm　左上腕
Luc
luciferase　ルシフェラーゼ
lucp.
luce prima〈ラ〉　朝早く，夜明けに《処》
luc.prim.
luce prima〈ラ〉　朝早く，夜明けに《処》
LUE
left upper extremity　左上肢
LUF
lower useful frequency　低有用周波数
luteinzet unruptured follicle (syndrome)　黄体化未破裂卵胞(症候群)
LUFS
luteinzet unruptured follicle syndrome　黄体化未破裂卵胞症候群
LUHF
lowest usable high frequency　最低有用高周波
LUL
left upper (eye) lid　左上眼瞼
left upper limb　左上肢
left upper lobe　左(肺)上葉
left upper lobectomy　左(肺)上葉切除術
left upper lung　左上肺(野)，左(肺)上葉
lum
lumbago　腰痛
lumen　管腔
Lumb, lumb
lumbar　腰(部)の，腰椎の
Lumbal
Lumbalpunktion〈独〉　腰椎穿刺
LUO
left ureteral orifice　左尿管口
LUOB
left upper outer buttock　左上外殿部
LUOQ
left upper outer quadrant　左上外(部)1/4区
LUQ
left upper quadrant　左上(部)1/4区
LUS
laparoscopic ultrasonography　腹腔鏡下超音波法
LUSB
left upper scapular border　左上肩甲骨縁
left upper sternal border　左上胸骨縁

L

lut.
luteum〈ラ〉 黄色の
LUTT
lower urinary tract tumor 下部尿路腫瘍
LUV
large unilamellar vesicles 大型単層状小胞
LV
laryngeal vestibule 喉頭前庭
lateral ventricle 側脳室
left ventricle 左(心)室
leucovorin ロイコボリン
leukemia virus 白血病ウイルス
live vaccine 生ワクチン
low volume 低体積，低容量〔容積〕
lumbar vertebra 腰椎
lung volume 肺容積
L-8-V
lysine-8-vasopressin リジン-8-バソプレシン
LV, L.V.
left vision 左眼視力
Lv, lv
leave 去る，休暇
LVA
left ventricular aneurysm 左(心)室動脈瘤
left ventricular aneurysmectomy 左(心)室動脈瘤切除(術)
left vertebral artery 左椎骨動脈
L vaccine
living vaccine 活性ワクチン
LVAD
left ventricular assist device 左(心)室補助循環装置
L-VAM
leuprolide acetate, vinblastine, adriamycin, mitomycin C 酢酸ロイプロリド，ビンブラスチン，アドリアマイシン，マイトマイシンC
LVAW
left ventricular anterior wall 左(心)室前壁
LVBP
left ventricle bypass pump 左(心)室バイパスポンプ
LVC
laser vision correction レーザー視力矯正
LVCS
low vertical cesarean section 下位垂直帝王切開(術)
LVD
left ventricular dimension 左(心)室径
left ventricular dysfunction 左(心)室機能不全

LV$_D$, LVd
left ventricular (end-)diastolic (pressure) 左(心)室拡張(終(末))期(圧)

LVDd
left ventricular end-diastolic dimension 左(心)室拡張終(末)期径

LVDI
left ventricular dimension 左(心)室径

LVDM
lividomycin リビドマイシン

LVDP
left ventricular diastolic pressure 左(心)室拡張期圧

LVDs
left ventricular end-systolic dimension 左(心)室収縮終(末)期径

LVDV
left ventricular diastolic volume 左(心)室拡張期容積

LVE
left ventricular ejection 左(心)室駆出
left ventricular enlargement 左(心)室拡大

LVED
left ventricular end-diastolic 左(心)室拡張終(末)期の

LVEDa
left ventricular end-diastolic area 左(心)室拡張終(末)期領域

LVEDC
left ventricular end-diastolic circumference 左(心)室拡張終(末)期周径

LVEDD
left ventricular end-diastolic diameter 左(心)室拡張終(末)期径
left ventricular end-diastolic dimension 左(心)室拡張終(末)期径

LVEDP
left ventricular end-diastolic pressure 左(心)室拡張終(末)期圧

LVEDV
left ventricular end-diastolic volume 左(心)室拡張終(末)期容積

LVEF
left ventricular ejection fraction 左(心)室駆出率

LVEndo
left ventricular endocardial (half) 左(心)室心内膜(半分)

LVEP
left ventricular end-diastolic pressure 左(心)室拡張終(末)期圧

LVER
liver fraction elevated 肝(臓)分画上昇

LVESa
left ventricular end-systolic area 左(心)室収縮終(末)期領域

LVESD
left ventricular end-systolic diameter 左(心)室収縮終(末)期径
LVESV
left ventricular end-systolic volume 左(心)室収縮終(末)期容積
LVESVI
left ventricular end-systolic volume index 左(心)室収縮終(末)期容積指数
LVET
left ventricular ejection time 左(心)室駆出時間
LVETI
left ventricular ejection time index 左(心)室駆出時間指数
LVF
left ventricular failure 左(心)室不全
left ventricular function 左(心)室機能
left visual field 左視野
low voltage fast (wave) 低電圧速(波)
low voltage foci 低電圧焦点
LVFB
left ventricular fascicular block 左(心)室束枝ブロック
LVF-EEG
low voltage fast electroencephalogram 低電位速波脳波
LVFP
left ventricular filling pressure 左(心)室充満圧
LVFX
levofloxacin レボフロキサシン
LVG
left ventriculography 左(心)室造影
lymphogranuloma venereum 性病性リンパ肉芽腫
LVH
large vessel hematocrit 大(血)管ヘマトクリット
left ventricular hypertrophy 左(心)室肥大
LVI
left ventricular insufficiency 左(心)室(機能)不全(症)
left ventricular ischemia 左(心)室虚血
low viscosity index 低粘稠度係数
LVID(ed)
left ventricular internal diameter (end-diastole) 左(心)室内径(拡張終(末)期)
LVID(es)
left ventricular internal diameter (end-systole) 左(心)室内径(収縮終(末)期)
LVID, LVIDD
left ventricular internal diastolic (diameter) 左(心)室拡張期内(径)

L

LVID, LVIDd
left ventricular internal dimension (diastole) 左(心)室(拡張期)内径
LVIDP
left ventricular initial diastolic pressure 左(心)室初期拡張期圧
LVIDs
left ventricular internal dimension end-systole 左(心)室収縮終(末)期径
LVIV
left ventricular infarct volume 左(心)室梗塞容積
LVL
left vastus lateralis (muscle) 外側広(筋)
LVLG
left ventrolateral gluteal 左腹側側方殿部
LVM
left ventricular mass 左(心)室心筋重量
levamisole レバミゾール
Lvmas, LV mass
left ventricular mass 左(心)室体積
LVMF
left ventricular minute flow 左(心)室分時流量
LVMM
left ventricular muscle mass 左(心)室心筋重量
LVN
lateral ventricular nerve 側脳室神経
lateral vestibular nucleus 前庭神経核の外側核
LVO, LVOA
left ventricular overactivity 左(心)室過活動
LVOT
left ventricular outflow tract 左(心)室流出路
LVOTD
left ventricular outflow tract dimension 左(心)室流出路径
LVP
large volume paracentesis 大容量穿刺(術)
large volume parenteral (infusion) 大量非経口投与(注射)
left ventricular pressure 左(心)室圧
levator veil palatini 口蓋帆挙(筋)
lysine vasopressin リジンバソプレシン
LVPEP
left ventricular pre-ejection period 左(心)室前駆出期
LVPFR
left ventricular peak filling rate 左(心)室ピーク充満率
LVPSP
left ventricular peak systolic pressure 左(心)室ピーク収縮期圧

LVPW
left ventricular posterior wall (thickness) 左(心)室後壁(厚)
LVPWT
left ventricular posterior wall thickness 左(心)室後壁厚
LVR
leucovorin ロイコボリン
limb vascular resistance 四肢血管抵抗
lung volume reduction 肺容量減少
L_1〔L_2〕VR
first〔second〕 lumbar ventral (nerve) root 第1〔2〕腰椎腹側(神経)根
LVRS
lung volume reduction surgery 肺容量減少(手)術
LVS
lateral venous sinus 外側静脈洞
left ventricular strain 左(心)室緊張
low voltage slow wave 低電圧徐波
LVs
(mean) left ventricular systolic (pressure) 平均左(心)室収縮期(圧)
LVSEMI
left ventricular subendocardial myocardial ischemia 左(心)室心内膜下心筋虚血
LVSI
left ventricular systolic index 左(心)室収縮期指数
lymphvascular involvement リンパ血管併発
LVSO
left ventricular systolic output 左(心)室収縮期駆出
LVSP
left ventricular systolic pressure 左(心)室収縮期圧
LVSPI
left ventricular stroke power index 左(心)室拍出力指数
LVST
lateral vestibulospinal tract 外側前庭脊髄路
LVSV
left ventricular stroke volume 左(心)室駆出量
LVSW
left ventricular septal wall 左(心)室中隔壁
left ventricular stroke work 左(心)室(拍出)仕事量
LVSWI
left ventricular stroke work index 左(心)室1回仕事係数
LVT
left ventricular tension 左(心)室圧力
lysine vasotonin リジン血管緊張物質

LVT_1
left ventricular fast filling time　左(心)室急速充満時間

LVV
left ventricular volume　左(心)室容積
LeVeen valve　リビーン〔レヴィーン〕弁
live varicella vaccine　水痘生ワクチン

LVW
lateral vaginal wall　外側腟壁
lateral ventricular width　側脳室幅
left ventricular wall　左(心)室壁
left ventricular work　左(心)室拍出仕事量

LVW/HW
lateral ventricular width to hemispheric width　側脳室幅/大脳半球幅比

LVWI
left ventricular work index　左(心)室仕事量係数〔指数〕

LVWM, LVWMA
left ventricular wall motion (abnormality)　左(心)室壁運動(異常)

LVWMI
left ventricular wall motion index　左(心)室壁運動指数

L

LVWT
left ventricular wall thickness　左(心)室壁厚

LW
lacerating wound　裂創
lateral wall　側壁
Lee-White　リー・ホワイト
left (ear)/warm (stimulus)　左(耳)・温(刺激)
Lendenwirbel〈独〉　腰椎
Léri-Weill (syndrome)　レリー・ワイル(症候群)
line width factor　線幅因子
lower left　左下象限
lung width　肺幅

Lw
lawrencium　ローレンシウム

lW
lichte Weite〈独〉　内径

L & W
living and well　生存しており健康である

LWBS
left without being seen　診察〔検査〕されずに帰った

LWC
leave without consent　無断欠勤

LWCT
Lee-White clotting time　リー・ホワイト凝固時間

LWD
living with disease 疾病と共存して生きる
LWK
large white kidney 大白色腎
LWP
large whirlpool 大渦巻き
lateral wall pressure 側壁圧
LWS
Lendenwirbelsäule〈独〉 腰椎
LWS cone pigment
long wave sensitive cone pigment, erythrolabe 赤錐体色素
L_x
static population 定常人口
l_x
number surviving 生存数
lx
lux ルクス〈単位〉
Lx, LX
latex ラテックス
lipoxin リポキシン
local irradiation 局所照射
luxation 脱臼
lx, lx.
larynx 喉頭
lower extremity 下肢
LXT
left exotropia 左外斜視
ly 0-3
lymph invasion 病理組織学的リンパ管侵襲の有無と1～3の程度
LY, ly, ly.
langley ラングレイ
last year 昨年
lying 臥位の
lymphatic invasion リンパ管浸潤度
lymphocyte リンパ球
lymphoma リンパ腫
lyophilization 凍結乾燥(法)
Lyb
lymphocyte b リンパ球b抗原
LYDMA
lymphocyte-detected membrane antigen リンパ球検出膜抗原
LYG
lymphomatoid granulomatosis リンパ腫様肉芽腫

LYM
lymph リンパ

lym
lymphocyte リンパ球(性の)

lymph
lymphocyte リンパ球(性の)

LYMPH%
percentage of lymphocytes リンパ球の割合

lymphos
lymphocytes リンパ球〈複数〉

lymphs
lymphocytes リンパ球〈複数〉

LYN
lymph nodes リンパ節

LyNeF
lytic nephritic factor 溶解性腎炎因子

lyo
lyophilized 凍結乾燥した

Lyp
lymphosarcoma リンパ肉腫

Lys
Lysholmsche Blende〈独〉=Lysholm grid リスホルム格子

LYS, Lys
lysine リジン, リシン
lysosome リソソーム

LySLK
lymphoma syndrome leukemia リンパ腫症候群

Lyt
lymphocyte t リンパ球t抗原
series of mouse T lymphocyte surface antigen マウスTリンパ球表面抗原系列

LYTES, lytes
electrolyte 電解質

Lyx
lyxose リキソース

LZM, Lzm, lzm
lysozyme リゾチーム

LZT
lead, zirconium, titanium 鉛・ジルコニウム・チタン

M m

M

macera〈ラ〉＝macerate	浸漬せよ《処》
Mach	マッハ〈単位〉
macroglobulin	マクログロブリン
maintenance	維持，維持量
malignant	悪性の
mammillary body	乳頭体
Manie〈独〉＝mania	躁病
manual	用手の，徒手の
matching coefficient	共有度係数
matrix	気質，母質，マトリックス
maximal	最大の
maximum	最大，最高
mean	平均
measurable	測定できる《医教》
meatus	道
medial	内側の
mediator	メディエーター，媒介物質，両受体
medical	医学の，医療の，医用の
medicine	医学，薬(物)，薬剤，内科学
mega(-)	巨大な，メガ(＝10^6)〈接〉
meningioma	髄膜腫
mesial	近心の
metabolite	代謝産物
metal	金属
metanephrine	メタネフリン
metastasis	転移
methionine	メチオニン
methotrexate	メトトレキサート
Micrococcus	ミクロコッカス(属)
microgloburin	ミクログロブリン
Microsporum	小胞子菌(属)
middle finger	中指
middle third (bulk of corpus)	胃中部
middle third of the stomach	胃中部1/3区
mitochondria	ミトコンドリア
mitosis	有糸分裂
mitotic phase	有糸核分裂期
mode	モード
mol	モル
molar	大臼歯，臼歯
mole	奇胎

molecular weight	分子量
Monday	月曜日
monkey	サル
monocyte	単核球
mosaic	モザイク
mother	母(親)
motile	(自発)運動能力のある
Mucor	ムコール(属)，ケカビ(属)
mucous	粘膜
mucus	粘液
multipara	経産婦
muscle	筋肉
Mycobacterium	マイコバクテリウム(属)
Mycoplasma	マイコプラズマ(属)
myopia	近視
myopic	近視(性)の
myosin	ミオシン
organ metastasis	臓器転移

m

limited mucosa	粘膜内
main	おもな
meliorated	回復した
meta	メタ〈接〉
milli	ミリ(＝10^{-3})〈接〉
minute	分
mixed infection	混合感染
molality	重量モル濃度〈単位〉
mucosa	(光顕でみられる)粘膜内癌
murmur	心雑音
muscle layer	筋層の

m.

mane〈ラ〉	朝に《処》
manipulus〈ラ〉	ひと握り(の量)
minimum	最小，最低

3M

meningitis, measles, mumps	脳膜炎・風疹・流行性耳下腺炎

M_0

no metastasis	(癌の)転移なし

M_{0-1}

organ metastasis	(癌の)臓器転移の有無程度

M_1

metastasis present	(癌の)転移あり
mitral first sound	心尖部第一音

M_1,M_2,M_3

slight, marked and absolute dullness	弱い・著しい・絶対的濁音

M

M_2
- dose per square meter of body surface　体表 $1\ m^2$ あたりの量
- mitral second sound　心尖部第二音

m^2
- square meter　平方メートル〈単位〉

m^3
- cubic meter　立方メートル〈単位〉

MÅ
- milliangstrom　ミリオングストローム〈単位〉

M, m
- male　男性，雄
- married　既婚の，結婚した
- masculine　男性(の)，雄性(の)
- mass　質量，集団，大量
- massage　マッサージ
- mature　成熟した
- median　中央値《統》，中間
- medium　媒質，培地
- memory　記憶
- meter　メートル〈単位〉
- milli-　ミリ($=10^{-3}$)〈接〉
- minim　ミニム〈単位〉
- month　月
- morphine　モルヒネ
- murmur　雑音

M, m.
- *membrana*〈ラ〉=membrane　膜
- *mentum*〈ラ〉　頤(おとがい)
- *meridas*〈ラ〉=noon　正午，昼
- *mille*〈ラ〉　千
- *mitte*〈ラ〉　送れ《処》
- *morbus*〈ラ〉　疾病，疾患
- Morgen〈独〉=morning　朝
- *mors*〈ラ〉　死亡
- *mortuus*〈ラ〉　死亡している
- *muscula*〈ラ〉　筋肉〈複数〉
- *mutitas*〈ラ〉　啞(=おし)，無言(症)，濁音

M, m, m.
- *misce*〈ラ〉=mix　混ぜよ，混和する，混ぜる《処》
- *mistura*〈ラ〉=mixture　混合物，混和物《処》

M2, M-2
- vincristine, carmustine, cyclophosphamide, melphalan, prednisone　ビンクリスチン，カルムスチン，シクロホスファミド，メルファラン，プレドニゾン

m/3, M/3
middle third 中1/3

MA
macrophage activation マクロファージ活性化
malabsorption (syndrome) 吸収不良(症候群)
malonaldehyde マロンアルデヒド
manderic acid マンデル酸
Martin-Albright (syndrome) マーティン・オルブライト(症候群)
masseter 咬筋
maternal aunt 母方のおば
mean arterial (blood pressure) 平均動脈血圧
meconium antigen 胎便抗原
megaloblastic anemia 巨赤芽球性貧血
membrane antigen 膜抗原
menstrual age 月経年齢
mental age 精神年齢
mentor anterior 頤前方位
meta-adrenaline メタアドレナリン
Mexican American メキシコ系アメリカ人
microaneurysm 微細動脈瘤，小動脈瘤
Miller-Abbott (tube) ミラー・アボット(管)
mitochondrial antibody ミトコンドリア抗体
mitral atresia 僧帽弁口閉鎖症
monoamine モノアミン
monoclonal antibody モノクローナル抗体
Morax-Axenfeld diplococcus モラー・アクセンフェルト菌
motor aphasia 運動失語
muscle activity 筋(肉)活動
myelinated axon 有髄軸索

Ma
Mach number マッハ数
masurium マスリウム〈元素〉

M/A
mood and/or affect 気分および/または感情

MA, ma
meter angle メートル角

MA, mA, ma.
milliampere ミリアンペア〈単位〉

MAA
macroaggregated albumin 大凝集アルブミン
medical assistance for aged 高齢者のための医療介助
melanoma-associated antigen 黒色腫関連抗原
mercaptoalkylamine メルカプトアルキルアミン
methacrylic acid メタアクリル酸
methyl arsonic acid メチルアルソン酸

M

monoarticular arthritis	単関節(性)関節炎
Maanes	
Master of Anesthesiology	麻酔学士
MAAS	
Multicentre Anti-Atheroma Study	マース(＝アテローマ疾患に対する高脂血症治療薬の効果を調査した大規模臨床試験)
MAB	
Man and Biosphere Plan	人間と生物環境計画
4-methylaminoazobenzene	4-メチルアミノアゾベンゼン
mAb	
monoclonal antibody	モノクローナル抗体
MABOP	
mechlorethamine, adriamycin, bleomycin, vincristine (＝Oncovin), prednisone	メクロレタミン,アドリアマイシン,ブレオマイシン,ビンクリスチン(＝オンコビン),プレドニゾン
MABP	
mean arterial blood pressure	平均動脈圧
MAC	
malignancy associated changes	悪性(腫瘍)関連変化
maximal acid concentration	最高酸素濃度
maximum acid concentration	最大〔最高〕酸濃度
membrane attack complex	膜侵襲複合体
methotrexate, actinomycin D, chlorambucil	メトトレキサート,アクチノマイシンD,クロラムブシル
minimal antibiotic concentration	最小抗生物質濃度
minimum allowance concentration	最小許容濃度
minimum alveolar (anesthetic) concentration	最小肺胞(麻酔)濃度
minimum anesthetic concentration	最小麻酔濃度
monkey cell adapting component	サルの細胞適合因子
Mycobacterium avium complex	トリマイコバクテリウム複合体
Mac	
macula	黄斑, 斑(紋)
mac.	
macera〈ラ〉＝macerate	冷浸せよ《処》
maceration	冷浸(法), 浸軟
MAC, MAC III	
methotrexate, actinomycin D, cyclophosphamide	メトトレキサート,アクチノマイシンD,シクロホスファミド

M

MAC, M.A.C
maximum allowable (acceptable) concentration — 最大許容濃度

MACC
methotrexate, adriamycin, cyclophosphamide, cyclohexylchloroethylnitrosourea — メトトレキサート,アドリアマイシン,シクロホスファミド,シクロヘキシルクロロエチルニトロソ尿素

methotrexate, arabinosylcytosine, cyclophosphamide, cyclohexylchloroethylnitrosourea — メトトレキサート,アラビノシルシトシン,シクロホスファミド,シクロヘキシルクロロエチルニトロソ尿素

m.accur.
misce accuratissme〈ラ〉 — 非常に正確に混和せよ《処》

mAChR
muscarinic acetylcholine receptor — ムスカリン様アセチルコリン受容体

MACOB
methotrexate, adriamycin, cyclophosphamide, vincristine (=Oncovin), bleomycin — メトトレキサート,アドリアマイシン,シクロホスファミド,ビンクリスチン(=オンコビン),ブレオマイシン

MACOP-B
methotrexate-leucovorine, adriamycin, cyclophosphamide, vincristine (=Oncovin), prednisone, bleomycin — メトトレキサート-ロイコボリン,アドリアマイシン,シクロホスファミド,ビンクリスチン(=オンコビン),プレドニゾン,ブレオマイシン

M

mac.per.
macera per horas decem〈ラ〉 — 10時間冷浸せよ《処》

macro
macroscopic — 肉眼(的)の

macrocephs
macrocephalics — 大頭の

MAD
major affective disorder — 大感情障害
maximum allowable dose — 最大許容線量
mean absolute deviation — 平均絶対偏差《統》
methyl-androstenediol — メチルアンドロステンジオール
minimum average dosis — 最小有効量

MADDOC
mechlorethamine, adriamycin, dacarbazine, *cis*-diamminedichloroplatinum, vincristine (=Oncovin), cyclophosphamide — メクロルエタミン,アドリアマイシン,ダカルバジン,シスジアミンジクロロプラチナム,ビンクリスチン(=オンコビン),シクロホスファミド

MADI
maximum acceptable daily intake — 最大1日摂取許容量

MADR
minimum adult daily requirement — 成人毎日必要最小量

MADS
Montgomery and Asberg depression scale — モンゴメリ・アスベルグうつ病係数

MADs
mind-altering drugs — 精神変換薬
mothers against drugs — 薬に反対する母親

MAE
mean absolute error — 平均絶対誤差《統》
medical air evacuation — 医学的空気排除
methenolone enanthate — メテノロンエナンテート

MAF
macrophage activating factor — マクロファージ活性化因子
macrophage-agglutinating factor — マクロファージ凝集因子
methotrexate, adriamycin, Futraful — メトトレキサート,アドリアマイシン,フトラフール
minimum audible field — 最小聴域
mouse amniotic fluid — マウス羊水

MAG
menadione-linked α-glycerophosphate dehydrogenase — メナジオン結合α-グリセロリン酸脱水素酵素
myelin-associated glycoprotein — 髄鞘(=ミエリン)関連糖蛋白

Mag, mag
magnesium — マグネシウム〈元素〉
magnet — 磁気
magnetic — 磁気の
magnification — 拡大
magnify — 拡大する
magnus〈ラ〉 — 大きい

Mag.cit
magnesium citrate — クエン酸マグネシウム

MAGE
mean amplitude of glycemic excursion — 平均グリセリン変動域

MAGE-1
melanoma antigen gene-1 — メラノーマ抗原遺伝子1

M

MAggF
macrophage aggultination factor　マクロファージ凝集反応因子

magn.
magnus〈ラ〉　大きい

magnif
magnification　拡大

Mag.sul
magnesia sulfuricum　硫酸マグネシウム

Mag.ust
magnesia usta　マグネシア

MAH
malignancy-associated hypercalcemia　悪性腫瘍に伴う高カルシウム血症

MAHA
microangiopathic hemolytic anemia　微小血管障害性溶血性貧血

MAHH
malignancy-associated humoral hypercalcemia　悪性腫瘍関連体液性高カルシウム血症

MAID
mesna, adriamycin, ifosfamide, dacarbazine　メスナ,アドリアマイシン,イホスファミド,ダカルバジン

mesna, adriamycin, interleukin-3, dacarbazine　メスナ,アドリアマイシン,インターロイキン-3,ダカルバジン

MAIDS
murine acquired immunodeficiency syndrome　ネズミ後天性免疫不全症候群

maj
major　大きい
majority　大多数，過半数

Major
major tranquilizer　抗精神病薬

MAKA
major karyotypic abnormalities　おもな核の異常

MAL
malfunction　機能不全
midaxillary line　腋窩中線

mal.
malanando〈ラ〉　発疱で，水疱形式で
malanandria〈ラ〉　水疱，疱疹，発疱剤
malignant　悪性の

malad
maladjusted　適応障害の

MALDI
matrix assisted laser destruction　マトリックス支援レーザー破壊

MalE
Escherichia coli maltose binding protein　大腸菌マルトース結合蛋白

malig
malignancy　悪性(腫瘍)
malignant　悪性の

MALIMET
Master List of Medical Indexing Terms　医学基礎用語集

malprac
malpractice　不正療法
malpractioner　不正療法医

MALT
mucosal associated lymphoid tissue　粘膜関連リンパ組織
mucous membrane associated lymphoid tissue　粘膜系リンパ組織
Münchner Alkoholismustest〈独〉　ミュンヘンアルコール症テスト

malt
malted milk shake　麦芽ミルクセーキ

MAM
methylazomethanol　メチルアゾメタノール

M+Am
compound myopic astigmatism　複合近視合併性乱視

mam, mAm, MAM, MaM
milliampere minute　ミリアンペア分〈単位〉

mammal
mammalogy　哺乳動物学

MAMMO
mammography　乳房撮影(法)

MAN
N-methyl-*N*-amyl nitrosamine　*N*-メチル-*N*-アミルニトロサミン

Man
manipulation　操作，手技，処置

man
manipulate　操作する
manual　小冊子，手引き

man.
mane〈ラ〉　朝(に)《処》
manipulus〈ラ〉　ひと握り《処》

Man, MAN
mannose　マンノース

M

mand
mandible 下顎骨
mandibular 下顎骨の
manif
manifest 顕性の
manifestation (症状)発現
manifest
manifestation (症状)発現
manip.
manipulus〈ラ〉 ひと握り《処》
MANIP, manip
manipulation 操作，手技，処置
ManN
mannosamine マンノサミン
ManNAc
N-acetylmannosamine *N*-アセチルマンノサミン
MANOVA
multivariate analysis of variance 分散多変量解析
MAN-6-P
mannose-6-phosphate マンノース-6-リン酸
man.pr.
mane primo〈ラ〉 朝いちばんで《処》
man.prim.
mane primo〈ラ〉 朝いちばんで《処》

M

manu
manufacture 製造(する)，製品
manuf
manufacture 製造(する)，製品
MAO
maximal acid output 最高酸分泌量
mesenteric vascular occlusion 腸管膜血管閉塞症
monoamine oxidase モノアミン酸化酵素
MAOA
monoamine oxidase A モノアミン酸化酵素A
MAOB
monoamine oxidase B モノアミン酸化酵素B
MAOI
monoamine oxidase inhibitor モノアミン酸化酵素阻害薬
MAP
magnesium ammonium phosphate stone リン酸マグネシウムアンモニウム結石
malignant atrophic papulosis 悪性萎縮性丘疹症
mandibular advancing positioner 下顎挙出器具
mannitol-adenine-phosphate マンニトールアデニンホスフェート，赤血球MAP
mean airway pressure 平均気道内圧

mean aortic pressure 平均大動脈(血)圧
mean arterial pressure 平均動脈(血)圧
medical air post 医学航空便
Medical Audit Program 医療監査計画
methamphetamine メトアンフェタミン
microlithiasis alveolarum pulmonum 肺胞微石症
microtubule associated protein 微小管結合蛋白
minimum audible pressure 最小可聴音圧
mitogen activated protein マイトゲン活性化蛋白
mitomycin C, adriamycin, cisplatin(=Platinol) マイトマイシンC,アドリアマイシン,シスプラチン(=プラチノール)
mitral annuloplasty 僧帽弁形成術
monophasic action potential 単相性活動電位
mouse antibody production (test) マウス抗体産生(試験)
muscle action potential 筋(肉)活動電位

MAPK
mitogen activated protein kinase マイトゲン活性化蛋白キナーゼ

MAPM
macroprolactinoma プロラクチン産生下垂体腫瘍

MAPO
metepa methaphoxide マポ(=水溶性アルキル化剤の1つ)

MAPS
make a picture story 絵画創作(=性格テストの1つ)

MAPs
microtubule associated protein 微小管付属蛋白質

MAR
marasmus 消耗症, 衰弱
margin 縁, マージン
marrow 骨髄
maximal aggregation ratio 最大凝集比
medication administration record 薬剤投与記録
minimal angle resolution 最小角分解能
mixed agglutination reaction 混合凝集反応
mixed antiglobulin reaction 混合抗グロブリン反応
multifocal atrial rhythm 多源性心房性調律
multiple antibiotic resistance 多剤抗生物質抵抗型

marg
margin 縁
marginal (辺)縁の

marr
marriage 結婚

M

MARS	
Monitored Atheroscleosis Regression Study	動脈硬化回復の監視研究
mouse antirat serum	マウス抗ラット血清
marsup	
marsupialization	造袋(術)
MAS	
malabsorption syndrome	吸収不良症候群
(Taylor) manifest anxiety scale	(テイラー)不安尺度(検査), 顕在性不安(検査)《臨心》
massive aspiration syndrome	大量吸引症候群
Maternal Attitude Scale	母親態度スケール(尺度)
meconium aspiration syndrome	胎便吸引〔嚥下〕症候群
meiosis-activating sterol	減数分裂活性化ステロール
milk alkali syndrome	ミルクアルカリ症候群
mobile arm support	可動性腕支持用具
Morgagni-Adams-Stokes (syndrome)	モルガニー・アダムス・ストークス(症候群)
motion analysis system	運動分析システム
MAs	
myopic astigmatism	近視複合乱視
mas.	
masculine	男性(の), 雄性(の)
massa〈ラ〉	質量, 集団, 大量, 塊《処》
mas, mAS, MAS	
milliampere second	ミリアンペア秒〈単位〉
masc	
masculine	男性(の), 雄性(の)
MASER	
microwave amplifier by stimulated emission of radiation	放射線被刺激放出による微小波増幅器
MASH	
medical aid for sick hippies	病気ヒッピーのための医療援助
mas.pil.	
massa pilularum〈ラ〉	丸剤塊《処》
mass, mass.	
massa〈ラ〉	質量, 集団, 大量, 塊《処》
massage	マッサージ, 按摩
massive	大量の, 塊状の, 大きい
MAST	
military anti-shock trouser	軍用ショック治療ズボン, (抗)ショックパンツ
multiple antigen simultaneos test	同時多項目アレルゲン特異的IgE抗体検査

M

mAST
mitochondrial aspartate aminotransferase　ミトコンドリアアスパラギン酸アミノトランスフェラーゼ

mast
mastectomy　乳房切断(術)，乳房切除(術)
mastoid　乳頭様の，乳(様)突(起)の

MAT
manual arts therapy　手芸療法
mature　成熟した，成熟する
maturity　成熟
mean absorption time　平均吸収時間
medication administration team　薬剤投与チーム
moderate antigenic tumor　中抗原腫瘍
Motivation Analysis Test　動機分析検査
motor age test　運動年齢テスト
multifocal atrial tachycardia　多源性心房頻拍
multiple agent (chemo) therapy　多剤(化学)療法
multiple (multifocal) artrial tachycardia　多源性心房頻拍

Mat
maternity　母性，妊娠，産(科病)院

mat
material　材料，物質

mat.gf
maternal grandfather　母方の祖父

mat.gm
maternal grandmother　母方の祖母

math, math
mathematical　数学(上)の，数学的な
mathematics　数学

matr.
matrimonium〈ラ〉　結婚

MA tube
Miller-Abbott tube　ミラー・アボット管

matut.
matutinus〈ラ〉　朝に《処》

MAU
Meyenburg-Altherr-Uehlinger (syndrome)　マイエンブルク・アルテル・ユーリンガー(症候群)

MAV
multiple antigen vaccine　多抗原ワクチン

MAVR
mitral and aortic valve replacement　僧帽弁大動脈弁置換(術)

Max
maximum　最大，最高

max, max., Max
maxillaries 上顎骨

max, max., Max	
maxilla	上顎骨
maxillary	上顎(骨)の
maximal	最大の，最高の
maximum	最大，最高
MaxEP	
maximum esophageal pressure	最大食道圧
MB	
buccal margin	頬縁
macrobiotic	長寿の
Mallory body	マロリー(小)体
mamillary body	乳頭体
Marsh-Bender factor	マーシュ・ベンダー因子
maximum breathing	最大換気〔呼吸〕
medulloblastoma	髄芽腫
megabyte	メガバイト〈単位〉
mesiobuccal	近心頬側の
methyl bromide	臭化メチル
methylene blue	メチレンブルー
microbiological (assay)	微生物学的(検定)
Milwaukee brace	ミルウォーキーブレース
multibacillary	多菌型
muscle balance	筋(肉)バランス
Mycobacterium bovis	ウシ型マイコバクテリア
Mb	
mandible body	下顎(骨)体
muscle hemoglobin	筋肉ヘモグロビン
myoglobin	ミオグロビン
mb	
millibar	ミリバール〈単位〉
M.B.	
Medicinae Baccalaureus〈ラ〉= Bachelor of Medicine	医学士
mb, m.b.	
misce bene〈ラ〉	よく混和せよ《処》
MBA	
megadolicho basilar artery	メガドリコ脳底動脈
Melitensis brucella antigen	マルタ熱抗原
methylbenzyl alcohol	メチルベンジルアルコール
monobromoacetic acid	モノブロモ酢酸
M-BACOD	
methotrexate, bleomycin, adriamycin, cyclophosphamide, vincristine (= Oncovin), dexamethasone	メトトレキサート，ブレオマイシン，アドリアマイシン，シクロホスファミド，ビンクリスチン(=オンコビン)，デキサメタゾン

m-BACOD
moderate-dose methotrexate, bleomycin, adriamycin, cyclophosphamide, vincristine (= Oncovin), dexamethasone — 通常投与メトトレキサート,ブレオマイシン,アドリアマイシン,シクロホスファミド,ビンクリスチン(=オンコビン),デキサメタゾン

M-BACOS
methotrexate, bleomycin, adriamycin, cyclophosphamide, vincristine (= Oncovin), Solu-Medrol — メトトレキサート,ブレオマイシン,アドリアマイシン,シクロホスファミド,ビンクリスチン(=オンコビン),ソル・メドロール

M band
monoclonal band — モノクローナルバンド

MBAR
myocardial beta-adrenergic receptor — 心筋βアドレナリン作用性受容体

mbar
millibar — ミリバール〈単位〉

MBAS
benzoylated 4,4′-diaminostilbene-2,2′-disulfonic acid — ベンゾイル化4,4′-ジアミノスチルベン-2,2′-ジスルホン酸
methylene blue active substance — メチレンブルー活性物質

MBC
male breast cancer — 男性乳癌
maximum bladder capacity — 最大膀胱容量
maximum breathing capacity — 最大換気量
metastatic breast cancer — 転移性乳癌
methotrexate, bleomycin, cisplatin — メトトレキサート,ブレオマイシン,シスプラチン
methylbenzyl chloride — 塩化メチルベンゾール
methylene blue complex — メチレンブルー複合体
minimal bactericidal concentration — 最小殺菌濃度
minute breathing capacity — 分時換気量

MBD
Marchiafava-Bignami disease — マルチアファバ・ビグナミ病
methotrexate, bleomycin, diamminedichloroplatinum — メトトレキサート,ブレオマイシン,ジアミンジクロロプラチン
methylene blue dye — メチレンブルー色素
minimal brain damage — 微細脳機能障害
minimal brain dysfunction syndrome — 微細脳機能障害症候群

MBE
medical and biological electronics — 医学・生物学的電子工学
medical and biological engineering — 医用生体工学

MBeA
methylbenzylamine メチルベンジルアミン
MBF
mesenteric blood flow 腸間膜血流
muscle blood flow 筋(肉)血流量
myocardial blood flow 心筋血流量
MBG
mean bood glucose 平均血糖
MBH
medial basal hypothalamus 内側基底視床下部
mediobasal hypothalamic 内側基底視床下部の
MBI
may be issued 発刊予定
methylene blue instillation メチレンブルー点滴注入
M.Bi.Chem
Master of Biological Chemistry 生化学士
M.Bi.Eng
Master of Biological Engineering 生物工学士
M.Bi.Phy
Master of Biological Physics 生物物理学士
M.Bi.S
Master of Biological Science 生物科学士
MBK
methyl butyl ketone メチルブチルケトン
MBL
mechanical basket lithotripsy (胆石の)機械式砕石法
menstrual blood loss 月経量
minimal bactericidal level 最小殺菌レベル
monocytoid B-lymphocytes 単クローンBリンパ球
Mbl
myeloblast 骨髄芽球
MBLA
mouse bone marrow lymphocyte antigen マウス骨髄リンパ球抗原
MBN
methylbenzyl-nitrosoamine メチルベンジルニトロソアミン
MBO
mesiobucco-occlusal 近心頰側咬合の
MbO_2
oxymyoglobin オキシミオグロビン
MBP
major basic protein 主要塩基性蛋白
maltose binding protein マルトース結合蛋白
mannose binding protein マンノース結合蛋白
mean blood pressure 平均血圧

Melitensis bovine and porcine antigen　マルタ熱菌のウシおよびブタ株から製造した抗原
mesiobuccopulpal　近心頬側歯髄の
miscellaneous bioactive peptides　種々の生理活性ペプチド
mucoprotein binding polysaccharide　ムコ蛋白結合多糖体
myelin basic protein　ミエリン塩基性蛋白

MBRT
methylene blue reduction time　メチレンブルー還元時間

MBS
Martin-Bell syndrome　マーティン・ベル症候群

MBSA
methylated bovine serum albumin　メチル化ウシ血清アルブミン

MBSC
medial basal part of suprachiasmatic area　上交叉〔差〕域内基礎部分

MBT
mean body temperature　平均体温
2-mercaptobenzothiazole　2-メルカプトベンゾチアゾール
methylthymol blue　メチルチモールブルー
mild barbiturate therapy　緩和バルビツレート療法
mixed bacterial toxin　混合細菌毒素

MBTI
Myers-Briggs type indicator　マイヤー・ブリックス(型)性格検査《臨心》

MBV
mitral balloon valvotomy　僧帽弁バルーン切開(術)

MBVP
maximum bladder voluntary pressure　最高膀胱随意圧

MBW
maternal birth weight　妊婦自身の出生時体重

MC
masking curve　遮蔽曲線
mast cell　肥満細胞
maximum concentration　最大濃度
medical corps　衛生部隊
medicochirurgical　内・外科学の
medullary carcinoma　髄様癌
medullary cavity　骨髄腔
melanoma cell　メラノーマ細胞
meningeal carcinomatosis　髄膜癌腫症
mesangial cell　メサンギウム細胞
mesiocervical　近心歯頸の
metacarpal　中手(骨)の
methylcellulose　メチルセルロース
methylcholanthrene　メチルコラントレン

microcephaly	小頭(蓋)症
microcirculation	微小循環
midcarpal	中手根の
midline central	正中中心部
minimal change group	微小変化群
mitomycin C	マイトマイシンC
mitral closure sound	僧帽弁閉鎖音
mitral commissurotomy	僧帽弁交連切開(術)
mixed cellularity	混合細胞型
mixed cryoglobulinemia	混合寒冷グロブリン血(症)
molluscum contagiosum〈ラ〉	伝染性軟属腫
monkey cell	サル細胞
monocrotaline	モノクロタリン
mononuclear cell	単核細胞
mucolipidosis	ムコリピドーシス
mycillin	マイシリン
mycocutaneous flap	筋皮弁
myocarditis	心筋炎

Mc

mitral valve closure	僧帽弁閉鎖

mC

millicoulomb	ミリクーロン〈単位〉

3-MC

3-methylcholanthrene	3-メチルコラントレン

MC, Mc, mc

megacurie	メガキュリー〈単位〉
megacycle	メガサイクル〈単位〉

MC, M-C

mineral corticoid	鉱質コルチコイド

mc, mc.

millicurie	ミリキュリー〈単位〉

M & C, M+C

morphine and cocaine	モルヒネとコカイン

MCA

major coronary artery	主冠(状)動脈
mechanical circulatory assistance	機能的循環補助
Medicines Control Agency	医薬品庁
megestrol, cyclophosphamide, adriamycin	メゲストロール, シクロホスファミド, アドリアマイシン
methylcholanthrene	メチルコラントレン
middle cerebral artery	中大脳動脈
middle colic artery	中結腸動脈
monochloroacetic acid	モノクロロ酢酸
monoclonal antiboby	モノクローナル抗体
multiple congenital abnormality	多発性先天(性)異常

multiple congenital anomaly | 多発性先天(性)奇形
muricholic acid | ムリコール酸

mca
mucous membrane carcinoma | 粘膜層癌

McAb
anti-thyroid microsomal antibody | 抗甲状腺ミクロソーム抗体
thyroid microsomal antibody | 甲状腺ミクロソーム抗体

MCAb，MCAB
monoclonal antibody | モノクローナル抗体

MCAC
metal chelate affinity chromatography | 金属キレート親和性クロマトグラフィ

MCAR
mixed cell agglutination reaction | 混合細胞凝集反応

MCAS
middle cerebral artery syndrome | 中大脳動脈症候群

MCAT
mean corpuscular average thickness | 赤血球の平均の厚さ
Medical College Admission Test | 医科大学入学試験
middle cerebral artery thrombosis | 中大脳動脈血栓症

m.caute
misce caute〈ラ〉 | 注意深く混和せよ《処》

MCB
membranous cytoplasmic body | 膜性細胞質内封入体

McB
McBurney point | マクバーニー(圧痛)点

MCBN
muscle capillary basement membrane | 筋(肉)毛細(血)管基底膜

MCBNT
muscle capillary basement membrane thickening | 筋(肉)毛細(血)管基底膜肥厚

MCBP
melphalan, cyclophosphamide, bischloroethylnitrosourea, prednisone | メルファラン,シクロホスファミド,ビスクロロエチルニトロソ尿素,プレドニゾン

McB pt
McBurney point | マクバーニー(圧痛)点

MCBR
minimum concentration of bilirubin | ビリルビン最小濃度

MCC
maximal cell concentration | 最大細胞濃度
mean corpuscular constants | 平均赤血球恒数
mean corpuscular hemoglobin concentration | 平均赤血球血色素濃度
metastatic cord compression | 転移性脊髄圧迫

M

methylcrotonyl CoA carboxylase	メチルクロトニル補酵素Aカルボキシラーゼ
minimum cytocidal concentration	最小殺菌濃度
mucocutaneous candidiasis	粘膜皮膚カンジダ症

MCCNU

methyl-chloroethyl-cyclohexylnitrosourea (＝semustine)	メチルクロロエチルシクロヘキシルニトロソ尿素(＝セムスチン)

MC-CPA

mast cell carboxypeptidase A	肥満細胞カルボキシペプチダーゼA

MCCU

mobile coronary care unit	移動式冠(状動脈)疾患管理部門

MCD

mean cell diameter	平均細胞直径
mean corpuscular diameter	平均赤血球直径
median control death	平均対照群死
medullary cystic disease	腎髄質嚢胞症
metabolic coronary dilation	代謝性冠(状動脈)拡張
millicuries destroyed	崩壊ミリキュリー
minimal cerebral dysfunction	微小(大)脳機能不全
muscle carnitine deficiency	筋(肉)カルニチン欠乏(症)

MCDI

Minnesota Child Development Inventory	ミネソタ小児発達〔発育〕調査表

MCDP

mast cell degranulating peptide	肥満細胞脱顆粒ペプチド

MCE

multicystic encephalopathy	多嚢胞性脳症
multiple cartilaginous exostosis	多発性軟骨性外骨腫

MCES

multiple cholesterol emboli syndrome	多発性コレステロール塞栓症候群

MCF

macrophage chemotactic factor	マクロファージ化学走化性因子
medium corpuscular fragility	培地赤血球脆弱性
melanocyte contracting factor	メラニン細胞凝集因子
microsomal fraction complement fixation test	ミクロソーム分画補体結合反応
mink cell focus-inducing virus	ミンク細胞病巣誘導ウイルス
mononuclear cell factor	単核球(細胞)因子
mycoplasma fraction complement fixation test	マイコプラズマによる補体結合反応
myocardial contractile force	心筋収縮力

MCFA
medium-chain fatty acid　中鎖脂肪酸

MCG
magnetocardiogram　心磁図
mechanocardiogram　心動図
mechanocardiography　心機図
membrane coating granule　膜被覆顆粒
micturition cytography　排尿時膀胱造影法

mcg
microgram　マイクログラム〈単位〉

MCGF
mast cell growth factor　肥満細胞成長因子

mcgm
microgram　マイクログラム〈単位〉

MCGN
mesangiocapillary glomerulonephritis　メサンギウム毛細管性糸球体腎炎

MCG-S
simple mechanocardiography　簡易心機図法

MCH
maternal and child health　母子保健，母子衛生
mean cell hemoglobin　平均赤血球ヘモグロビン量
mean corpuscular hemoglobin　平均赤血球血色素量
3-methylcyclohexanone　3-メチルシクロヘキサノン
muscle contraction headache　筋収縮性頭痛

M.Ch.
Magister Chirugiae〈ラ〉　外科博士

mch, mc h, mc-h, mc.h.
millicurie hour　ミリキュリー時間〈単位〉

MCHA
microsome hemagglutination test　ミクロソーム感作血球凝集反応

MCHC
mean cell hemoglobin concentration　平均赤血球ヘモグロビン濃度
mean corpuscular hemoglobin concentration　平均赤血球血色素濃度

M.Ch.D.
Magister Chirugiae Dentalis〈ラ〉= Master of Dental Surgery　歯科外科博士，口腔外科学修士

MCHg
mean corpuscular hemoglobin　平均赤血球ヘモグロビン量

MCHgb
mean corpuscular hemoglobin　平均赤血球ヘモグロビン量

M.Ch.Orth.
Master of Orthopedic Surgery　整形外科学修士

MCHP
maternal and child health program　母子健康計画
mchr, mc-hr
millicurie(-)hour　ミリキュリー時間〈単位〉
MCHS
maternal and child health service　母子健康サービス
MChS
Member of Chiropodialis Society　足治療科協会員
MCI
mean cardiac index　平均心係数
metacarpal index　中手骨の骨皮質幅測定
methicillin　メチシリン
myocardial infarction　心筋梗塞
MCi
megacurie　メガキュリー〈単位〉
mCi
millicurie　ミリキュリー〈単位〉
mCi-hr
millicurie hour　ミリキュリー時間〈単位〉
MCINS
minimal change idiopathic nephrotic syndrome　特発性微小変化ネフローゼ症候群
MCIPC
methyl chlorophenyl isoxazolyl penicillin(＝cloxacillin natrium)　メチルクロロフェニルイソキサゾールペニシリン(＝クロキサシリン)
MCK
muscle creatine kinase　筋肉クレアチンキナーゼ
MCK, MCKD
multicystic kindey (disease)　多嚢胞性腎(病)
MCL
mantle cell lymphoma　外套細胞リンパ腫
medial collateral ligament　内側側副靱帯
midclavian line　鎖骨中線
midclavicular line　鎖骨中線
midcostal line　肋骨中線
most comfortable loudness (level)　快適大きさ曲線
mucocutaneous leishmaniasis　粘膜皮膚リーシュマニア症
MCLA
mucocutaneous lymph node arthritis　粘膜皮膚リンパ節関節炎
M.Clin.Psychol
Master of Clinical Psychology　臨床心理学士
MCLO
Medical Construction Liaison Office　医療相談連絡事務所

M

MCLS
(acute febrile) mucocutaneous lymph node syndrome　(急性熱性)皮膚粘膜リンパ節症候群
M.Cl.Sc
Master of Clinical Science　臨床科学士
MCM
mast cell medium　肥満細胞用培養液
Monte Carlo method　モンテカルロ法
MCMV
mouse cytomegalovirus　マウスサイトメガロウイルス
murine cytomegalovirus　ネズミサイトメガロウイルス
MCN
minimal change nephropathy　微小変化腎障害
MC-N
mixed cell nodular (lymphoma)　混合細胞結節性(リンパ腫)
MCNS
minimal change nephrotic syndrome　微小変化ネフローゼ症候群
MCNU
methyl-6-chloroethyl nitrosourea　メチル-6-クロロエチルニトロソウレア
M colony
mucoid colony　ムコイドコロニー
M component
monoclonal component　単クローン成分
MCOS
mucocutaneous ocular syndrome　粘膜皮膚眼症候群
mcoul
millicoulomb　ミリクーロン〈単位〉
MCP
maximal closure pressure　最大閉鎖圧
melphalan, cyclophosphamide, prednisone　メルファラン, シクロホスファミド, プレドニゾン
metacarpophalangeal　中手指節関節の
methyl-accepting chemotaxis protein　メチル基受容化学走性蛋白
metoclopramide　メトクロプラミド
mitotic-control protein　有糸分裂制御蛋白
monocyte chemotactic protein　単球遊走性蛋白
Mcp
McBurney point　マクバーニー(圧痛)点
MCP-1
macrophage chemoattractant protein-1　マクロファージ化学誘導蛋白1
MCPH
metacarpophalangeal　中手指節関節の
MCPJ
metacarpophalangeal joint　中手指節関節

M

MCPS
Member of College of Physicians and Surgeons 米国内科外科学会員

Mcps, mc p s, mcps, Mc.p.s.
megacycles per second メガサイクル/秒〈単位〉

MCPT-1
mast cell protease-1 肥満細胞プロテアーゼ1

MCP-test
mucin-clot-prevention-test ムチン・血餅・予防試験

MCQ
multiple choice question 多肢選択問題

MCR
Matsubara cutireaction 松原皮内反応
mean clearance rate 平均除去率
metabolic clearance rate 代謝クリアランス率
micronomicin ミクロノマイシン
mother-child relationship 母子関係

MCRCC
multilocular cystic renal cell carcinoma 多房性嚢胞状腎癌

MCS
malignant carcinoid syndrome 悪性カルチノイド症候群
mesocaval shunt 腸間膜静脈下大静脈シャント(術)
methylcholanthrene(-induced) sarcoma メチルコラントレン(誘発)肉腫
moisture control system 湿度制御システム
myocardial contractile state 心筋収縮状態

mc/s
megacycles per second メガサイクル/秒〈単位〉

M-CSF
macrophage colony-stimulating factor マクロファージコロニー刺激因子
megakaryocyte colony stimulating factor 巨核球コロニー形成刺激因子
monocyte colony stimulating factor 単球コロニー刺激因子

MCSP
Member of Charactered Society of Physiotherapy 物理療法協会員

MCSR
mean circumferential shortening rate 平均的内周短縮率

MCSS
multiple chemical sensitivity syndrome 化学物質頻回曝露感度症候群

MCT
mean cell threshold 平均細胞閾値

M

mean circulation time 平均循環時間
mean corpuscular thickness 平均赤血球厚径
medium chain triglyceride 中鎖脂肪
medium chain triglyceride milk 中鎖脂肪酸ミルク《処》
medullary carcinoma of thyroid 甲状腺髄様癌
medullary collecting tubule 髄質集合尿細管
microcrystalline cellulose triacetate 小結晶セルロース三酢酸塩
middle chain triacylglycerol 中鎖トリアシルグリセロール
minimum contact technology 最小接触技術
multiple compressed tablet 多重圧縮錠剤

MCTC
metrizamide computed tomography cisternography メトリザミドコンピュータ断層撮影大槽造影法

MCTD
mixed connective tissue disease 混合結合組織病

MCTF
mononuclear cell tissue factor 単核細胞組織因子

MCT oil
medium-chain triglyceride oil 中鎖トリグリセリド油

MCU
millicurie ミリキュリー〈単位〉
minimal care unit 軽症病棟

mcU
microunit マイクロ単位〈単位〉

MCUG
micturating urogram 排尿時尿路造影図
micturition cystourethrography 排尿時膀胱尿道造影法

MCV
mean cell volume 平均赤血球容積
mean corpuscular volume 平均赤血球容積
molluscum contagiosum virus 伝染性軟属腫ウイルス
motor nerve conduction velocity 運動神経伝導速度

MCx
motor cortex 運動皮質

MCZ
miconazole ミコナゾール

MD
macula densa 密集斑
magnesium deficiency マグネシウム欠乏(症)
magnetic disk 磁気ディスク
maintenance dose 維持量
major depression 大うつ病
malate dehydrogenase リンゴ酸脱水素酵素
malic acid dehydrogenase リンゴ酸脱水素酵素
manic depressive 躁うつ(病)の，躁うつ病患者
Marburg disease マールブルグ病

maternal deprivation	母性(愛)妨害
maximal dosis	最大投与量
maximum dose	極量，最大量
mean deviation	平均偏差《統》
Meckel diverticulum	メッケル憩室，臍(＝さい)腸間膜憩室
(nucleus) medialis dorsalis	(視床下部)背側内側(核)
mediastinal disease	縦隔疾患
medical department	診療科
medical discharge	医学的排泄物
medicine and duty	医療と義務
mediodorsal	正中背側の，内背側の
mediodorsal thalamic nucleus	中背側視床核
Ménétrier disease	メネトリエ病
Ménière disease	メニエール病
mental deficiency	精神遅滞
mentally deficient	精神遅滞の
mesiodistal	近(心)遠心の
microdensitometry	骨量測定法
Middlebrook-Dubos test	ミドルブルック・デュボス試験
mild dysplasia	軽度異形成
Minamata disease	水俣病
(bone) mineral density	骨塩量
minimum dosage	最小量
minimum dose	最小量
minute difference	分差
mitral disease	僧帽弁疾患
moderate dysplasia	中等度異形成
molecular rotation	モル旋光度
monocular deprivation	単眼妨害
movement disorder	運動疾患
multiple deficiency	多重欠損症，多重欠乏症
muscular dystrophy	筋ジストロフィ，筋異栄養(症)
myeloproliferative disease	骨髄増殖性疾患
myocardial damage	心筋傷害
myocardial disease	心筋疾患
myodiopter	筋曲光率
myotonic dystrophy	筋緊張性ジストロフィ

Md

mendelevium	メンデレビウム
Müllerian duct	ミュラー管

m.d.

mano dextra〈ラ〉	右手
more dicto〈ラ〉＝as directed	指示のとおり《処》

MD, M.D.
Medicinae Doctor〈ラ〉＝Medical Doctor　医学(博)士

md, md.
median　正中の，中央値《統》
more dicto〈ラ〉＝as directed　指示のとおり《処》

MDA
malondialdehyde　マロンジアルデヒド
mento-dextra anterior〈ラ〉　右頤前位
3,4-methylenedioxyamphetamine　3,4-メチレンジオキシアンフェタミン
motor discriminative acuity　運動識別精度
Muscular Dystrophy Association　筋ジストロフィ協会

MDC
maximal diffusing capacity　最大拡散能力
4-methyl-7-diethylaminocoumarin　4-メチル-7-ジエチルアミノクマリン
metoprolol dilated cardiomyopathy　メトプロロール拡張型心筋症
minimum detectable concentration　最小検出可能濃度

MDCM
mildly dilated congestive cardiomyopathy　軽度拡張型うっ血性心筋症

MDD
major depressive disorder　定型うつ病
mean daily dose　平均1日量

MDDA
Minnesota Differential Diagnosis of Aphasia　ミネソタ失語鑑別診断

MDE
Modern Drug Encyclopedia　最新医薬全集

MDF
macrophage differential factor　マクロファージ分化因子
macrophage disappearance factor　マクロファージ消失因子
myocardial depressant factor　心筋抑制因子

MDG
Magen-und-Duodenalgeschwür〈独〉　胃・十二指腸潰瘍
Medical Director General　医学総管理者

MDGF
macrophage derived growth factor　マクロファージ由来成長因子

MDH
malate dehydrogenase (malic acid dehydrogenase)　リンゴ酸脱水素酵素
minimum deviation hepatoma　最小偏倚ヘパトーマ

MDH1
soluble malate dehydrogenase　可溶性リンゴ酸脱水素酵素

MDH2
mitochondrial malate dehydrogenase　ミトコンドリア性リンゴ酸脱水素酵素

MDHM
mitochondrial malate dehydrogenase　ミトコンドリア性リンゴ酸脱水素酵素

MDHS
soluble malate dehydrogenase　可溶性リンゴ酸脱水素酵素

MDHV
Marek disease herpesvirus　マレク病ヘルペスウイルス

MDI
diphenylmethane diisocyanate　ジフェニルメタンジイソシアネート
manisch-depressives Irresein〈独〉= manic depressive insanity　躁うつ病
medical date index　健康調査表
mental deterioration index　精神変調指数
metered dose inhaler　定量噴霧式吸入器
methodological drug interferences　測定方法論的薬剤干渉
methylene diisocyanate　メチレンジイソシアネート
methylenediphenyldiisocyanate　メチレンジフェニルジイソシアネート

m.dict.
modo dictum〈ラ〉　口授どおりに《処》
more dicto〈ラ〉　指示した方法で《処》

MDIPC
methyl dichlorophenyl isoxazolylpenicillin　メチルジクロルフェニルイソキサゾリルペニシリン(=ジクロキサシリン)

MDL
median lethal dose　半致死量
method detection limit　測定最小限界

MDL, M.D.L
Magen Durchleuchtung〈独〉　胃X線透視撮影

MDLO
metoclopramide, dexamethasone, lorazepam, ondansetron　メトクロプラミド,デキサメタゾン,ロラゼパム,オンダンセトロン

MDM
medical decision marking　医学判断学
mid-diastolic murmur　拡張中期雑音
midecamycin　ミデカマイシン

MDMH
monomethylol dimethylhydantoin　モノメチロールジメチルヒダントイン

mdn
median 正中の，中央値《統計》
MDNB
mean daily nitrogen balance 平均１日窒素平衡
mdnt
midnight 深夜
MDOPA
methyldopa メチルド(ー)パ
MDP
manic-depressive psychosis 躁うつ病
mento-dextra posterior〈ラ〉 頤右後位
methylene diphosphate メチレン二リン酸
methylene diphosphonate メチレン二ホスホン酸
muramyldipeptide ムラミルジペプチド
N-acetyl-muramyl-L-alanyl-D-isoglutamate *N*-アセチル-ムラミル-L-アラニル-D-イソグルタメート
MDPI
maximum daily permissible intake 最大１日許容摂取量
MDQ
minimum detectable quantity 最小検出可能量
MDR
macrophage disappearance reaction マクロファージ消失反応
medical device reporting regulation 医療機器事故報告制度
minimum daily requirement 最小１日必要量
multidrug resistantce 多剤耐性(癌化学療法の１つ)
multiple drug resistance 多剤耐性(癌化学療法)
MDRP
multidrug-resistant *Pseudomonas aeruginosa* 多剤耐性緑膿菌
MDR-TB
multidrug-resistant *Mycobacterium tuberculosis* 多剤耐性結核菌
MDS
Master of Dental Surgery 口腔外科学修士
medical data system 医療データシステム
medical dental service 歯科医療サービス
medical dextran sulfate 医用硫酸デキストラン
microvascular defence system 微小循環による防御機構
minimum data set 最小記録一式《医情》
multidimensional scaling 多次元尺度法
multiple deficiency syndrome 多重欠損症候群
myelodysplastic syndrome 骨髄異形成症候群
M.D.S., m.d.s.
misce da signa, *misceatur detur signetur*〈ラ〉 混和し使用法を記入して与えよ《処》

M.D.Sc
Master of Dental Science　歯科学士
MDSDM
multidose streptozo(to)cin-induced diabetes mellitus　ストレプトゾ(ト)シンの頻回投与による真性糖尿病
MDSO
mentally disordered sex offender　精神異常(性)性(的)攻撃者
MDT
mast cell degeneration test　肥満細胞変性試験
mean dissolution time　平均溶解時間
mento-dextra transverse〈ラ〉　右頤横位
mirror drawing test　鏡映描写法
multidisciplinary treatment　集学的治療
multidrug therapy　多剤併用療法
MDTR
mean diameter-thickness ratio　平均直径/厚さ比
m.d.u.
more dicto utendus〈ラ〉=to be used as directed　指示のとおり用いられるべし《処》
MDUO
myocardial disease of unknown origin　原因不明心筋疾患
MDV
Marek disease virus　マレク病ウイルス
maximum desire to viod　最大尿意
mucosal disease virus　粘膜病ウイルス
MDY
month, date, year　月・日・年
ME
Mache-Einheit〈独〉　マッヘ単位
macula edema　浮腫斑
malic enzyme　リンゴ酵素
manic episode　躁(病)エピソード
Mauseinheit〈独〉　マウス単位
maximum effect　最大効果
maximum effort　最大努力
measles encephalitis　麻疹脳炎
median eminence (of hypothalamus)　(視床下部)内側隆起，正中隆起
medical education　医学教育
medical electronics　医用電子機器
medical engineering　医用電子工学
medical examination　医学試験
medical examiner　診査医，監察医
mefenamic acid　メフェナム酸
meningoencephalitis　髄膜脳炎

M

metabolizable energy	代謝可能エネルギー
metamyelocyte	後骨髄球
metencephalon	後脳，小脳
methazolamide	メタゾールアミド
methenolone enanthate	メテノロンエナンテート
micellar electrokinetic capillar chromatography	ミセル電動毛細管クロマトグラフィ
microelectronics	微細電子工学
middle ear	中耳
midline echo	中央エコー《超音波》
milligram equivalent	ミリグラム等量〈単位〉
mixing efficiency	混合効率
most excellent	最も優秀な
mouse epithelial (cell)	マウス上皮(細胞)
muscle examination	筋肉検査
myoclonus epilepsy	ミオクローヌスてんかん
myoepithelial (cell)	筋上皮(細胞)

Me

aceton	アセトン
methyl	メチル
methyl alcohol	メチルアルコール

2ME

2-mercaptoethanol	2-メルカプトエタノール

8-ME

8-mercaptoguanosine	8-メルカプトグアノシン

ME_{50}

50 percent maximal effect	50%最大効果

ME-

methyl-	メチル

M & E

music effects	音楽効果

M/E, M : E

myeloid-erythroid (ratio)	骨髄(顆粒球)系/赤芽球系細胞(比)

MEA

Medical Exhibitors Association	医科展示者協会
mercaptoethylamine	メルカプトエチルアミン
monoethanolamine	モノエタノールアミン
multiple endocrine adenomas	多発性内分泌性腺腫
multiple endocrine adenomatosis	多発性内分泌腺腫症

meas

measure	測定(する)
measured	測定した
measurement	測定
measuring	測定する

MEB	
methylene blue	メチレンブルー
MeB_{12}	
methylcobalamin	メチルコバラミン
ME & BE	
medical electronics and biologic electronics	医用電子工学と生物電子工学
MEC	
middle ear canals	中耳管
minimum effective concentration	最小有効濃度
mec	
meconium	胎便
3-MECA	
3-methylcholanthrene	3-メチルコラントレン
mecano	
mechanotherapy	機械的療法
Mec Asp	
meconium aspiration	胎便吸引
MeCbl	
methylcobalamin	メチルコバラミン
Me-CCNU	
methyl lomustine	メチルロムスチン
MECG	
mixed essential cryoglobulinemia	混合本態性寒冷グロブリン血症
mech	
mechanical	機械的な，力学的な
mechanism	機構，機序
Mechano, mechano	
mechanotherapy	機械(的)療法
MeCP	
methylchloroethyl-cyclohexylnitrosourea, cyclophosphamide, prednisone	メチルクロロエチル-シクロヘキシルニトロソ尿素，シクロホスファミド，プレドニゾン
MECY	
methotrexate, cyclophosphamide	メトトレキサート，シクロホスファミド
MeCyt	
methylcytosine	メチルシトシン
MED	
mean erythrocyte diameter	平均赤血球径
minimal effective dose	最小有効量
minimal erythema dose	最小紅斑量
minimum effective dose	最小有効量
multiple epiphyseal dysplasia	多発性骨端異形成症

M

Med
mediastinum 縦隔
MED, Med, med.
median 正中の，中央値《統》
medical 医学の，薬の
medicine 薬剤，医学，内科学
med, med.
medial 内側の
medicamentum〈ラ〉＝medication 薬剤，薬(物)，投薬
medicinal 医薬の，医薬品
medium 培地，媒質
medius〈ラ〉 中位の《処》
MEDAC
multiple endocrine deficiency, Addison disease and candidiasis (syndrome) 多発性内分泌欠乏症・アジソン病・カンジダ症(症候群)
multiple endocrine deficiency autoimmune candidiasis 多内分泌欠乏性自己免疫性糸状菌症
MedC
Medical Corporation 医療法人
MedCAP
Medical Civil Action Program 医療市民行動計画
MED-DENT
Medical Dental Division 医学歯学部門
MEDDRA
Medical Dictionary for Drug Regulatory Affairs 医薬品規制用語集
medevac
medical evacuation 医学的排泄
medex
medical expert 医療専門家
MEDIA
Manufactures Educational Drug Information Association 薬製造教育情報協会
medic
medical doctor 医師
medical student 医学生
medicaid
medical aid 医療援助，医療補助者
medicare
medical care 医療介護
MEDICATES
medical computer-aided training system 医学生教育システム
MEDICO
Medical International Corporation 医学国際協会

MEDINFO
Medical Information — 医療情報
Medio
mediotorsio cmris〈ラ〉 — 下腿内方捻転
MEDIS
Medical Information System — 医療情報システム
MEDIS-DC
Medical Information System Developing Center — 医療情報システム開発センター
medix
medical students — 医学生
med juris
medical jurisprudence — 医療法律学
med lab
medical laboratory — 医学研究室
MEDLARS
Medical Literature Analysis and Retrieval System — (米国)医学関連文献分析検索システム
MEDLARS on-Line
Medical Literature Analysis and Retrieval System on-line — オンライン医学関連文献分析システム
MEDLINE
MEDLARS On-line — オンライン医学関連文献分析システム，メドライン

M

med.men
medial meniscectomy — 内側半月(板)切除(術)
medial meniscus — 内側半月
MEDPRO
Medical Education Program — 医学教育プログラム
med ray
medullary ray — 髄線
med ray par
medullary ray parenchyma — 髄線実質
MEDRC
medical reserve corps — 医療予備隊
MEDRESCO
Medical Research Council — 医学研究協議会
MEDS
microsurgical extraction of ductal sperm — 精管摘出マイクロサージェリー〔顕微(鏡)手術〕
myocardial energy deficiency state — 心筋エネルギー欠乏状態
meds, MEDS
medications — 薬(物)，薬剤，投薬
medicines — 薬物，薬剤，医学
MEDSAC
Medical Service Activity — 医療奉仕活動

Med.Sc.D.
Doctor of Medical Science 医科学士
Med Sch
medical school 医科大学，医学部
Med Surg
medicine and surgery 内科学と外科学
Med Tech
medical technician 臨床検査技師
medical technology 臨床検査法
Med Tech，med.tech.
medical technology 医療技術
MEE
methylethyl ether メチルエチルエーテル
middle ear effusion 中耳滲出液
MEEI
Massachusetts Eye and Ear Infirmary マサチューセッツ眼科耳鼻咽喉科病院
MEF
maximal expiratory flow 最大呼気流量
middle ear fluid 中耳液
midexpiratory flow 中間呼気流量
migration enhancement factor 遊走増強因子
mouse embryo fibroblasts マウス胚線維芽細胞
MEF_{50}
mean maximum expiratory flow 平均最大呼気流量
MEFA
methylchloroethyl-cyclohexylnitrosourea, 5-fluorouracil, adriamycin メチルクロロエチル-シクロヘキシルニトロソ尿素, フルオロウラシル, アドリアマイシン
$MeFH_4$
methyltetrahydrofolate メチルテトラヒドロ葉酸
MEFR
maximal expiratory flow rate 最大呼気速度
MEFV
maximal expiratory flow-volume curve 最大呼気フローボリウム曲線
MEG
magnetoencephalogram 脳磁図
magnetoencephalograph 脳磁気図計
magnetoencephalography 脳磁気図検査法
mono-ethylene glycol モノエチレングリコール
multifocal eosinophilic granuloma 多病巣性好酸球性肉芽腫
meg
megaloblastic 巨(大)赤芽球(性)の

M

MEG, meg
megacycle　メガサイクル
megakaryocyte　(骨髄)巨核球

megamouse
one million mice　百万マウス

Meg-CSF
megakaryocyte colony stimulating factor　巨核球コロニー刺激因子

MEGD
minimal euthyroid Graves disease　最小甲状腺機能正常型グレーブス病

mEGF
mouse epidermal growth factor　マウス表皮成長因子

MEGX
monoethylglycinexylidide　モノエチルグリシンキシリジド

MEH
melanocyte expanding hormone　メラニン細胞刺激ホルモン

MEIS
medium energy ion scattering spectroscopy　中速イオン散乱分光法

MEK
methyl ethyl ketone　メチルエチルケトン

M

MEKC
micellar electrokinetic chromatography　ミセル電動クロマトグラフィ

MEKS
Mediterranean Kaposi sarcoma　地中海カポジ肉腫

MEL
melanoma antigen　メラノーマ抗原
mouse erythroleukemia　マウス赤白血病
murine erythroleukemia　ネズミ赤白血病

Mel
melarsoprol　メラルソプロール

mel
melanoma　黒色腫
melena〈英〉＝Meläna〈独〉＝melæna〈仏〉　メレナ

MELA
mitochondrial encephalomyopathy　ミトコンドリア脳筋症

MELAS
mitochondrial myopathy, encephalopathy, lactic acidosis, stroke-like episodes　乳酸血症・卒中発作を伴うミトコンドリア脳筋症，メラス

MELC
murine erythroleukemia cell　ネズミ赤白血病細胞

MELDOS
melioidosis 類鼻疽
MELI
metenkephalin-like immunoreactivity メトエンケファリン様免疫反応性
MEM
maximum entropy method 最大エントロピー法
minimum essential medium 最少必須培地
mem
member 会員，手足，メンバー
memb
membrane 膜
MEMIC
Medical Microbiology Interdisciplinary Commission 医学微生物学学際委員会
MEMO
Medical Equipment Management Office 医療装備管理事務所
memo
memorandum 覚え書き
MEMR
multiple exostoses-mental retardation (syndrome) 多発性外骨(腫)症・精神遅滞(症候群)
MEN
multiple endocrine neoplasia 多発性内分泌腺腫瘍症
multiple endocrine neoplasm 多発性内分泌腺腫瘍
Men
meningioma 髄膜腫
men
meningeal (脳脊)髄膜の
meninges 髄膜
meningitis 髄膜炎
menses 月経
menstruation 月経
mening
meningeal (脳脊)髄膜の
meninges 髄膜
meningitis 髄膜炎
meno
menopausal 更年期の
menopause 更年期，更年期障害
menorrhea 月経，帯下
menst
menstrual 月経の
menstruate 月経がある

menstru	
menstrual	月経の
menstruate	月経がある
menstruation	月経
mensur	
mensuration	計量
ment	
mental	精神(的)の，頤(＝オトガイ)の
mentation	精神機能作用
MEO	
malignant external otitis	悪性外耳炎
MeOH	
methyl alcohol	メチルアルコール
MEOS	
microsomal ethanol oxidizing system	マイクロソームエタノール酸化系
MEP	
Malaria Eradication Programme	マラリア根絶計画
maximal expiratory pressure	最大呼気圧
mean effective pressure	平均効果圧
mitomycin C, etoposide, cisplatin(＝Platinol)	マイトマイシンC, エトポシド, シスプラチン(＝プラチノール)
monoethyl phosphoric acid	モノエチルリン酸
moth-eaten phenomenon	虫くい現象
motor end plate	運動終板
multimodality evoked potential	多元的誘発電位
MEP, mep	
meperidine	メペリジン
MEPA	
Movement Education Program Assessment	ムーブメント教育プログラムアセスメント
MEPP	
miniature endplate potential	微小終板電位
MePr	
methylprednisolone	メチルプレドニゾロン
MEq, mEq, meq	
milli(gram) equivalent	ミリグラム当量〈単位〉
mEq/l	
milli(gram) equivalents per liter	ミリグラム当量/リットル
MER	
mean ejection rate	平均駆出率
methanol extraction residue	メタノール抽出残渣

M

MERB
met-enkephalin receptor biding — メトエンケファリン受容体結合性の

MERDI
Medical Equipment Research and Development Laboratory — 医療設備研究と開発研究所

MERI
Medical Relief International — 国際医療救援

MERS
Middle East Respiratory Syudrome — 中東呼吸器症候群

MERS-CoV
Middle Coronavirus — MERSコロナウイルス，マーズコロナウイルス

MES
2-(*N*-morpholino) ethanesulfonic acid — 2-(*N*-モルホリノ)エタンスルホン酸
maintenance electrolyte solution — 維持電解質溶液
maximal electroshock (seizure) — 最大電気ショック(性発作)
maximal eye speed — 最大眼球速度
middle extro-Sylvian gyms — 中外シルビウス脳回

Mes
mesencephalic — 中脳の
mesencephalon — 中脳

MESA
microscopic epididymal sperm aspiration — 顕微鏡下精巣上体精子吸引法

Mesc
mescaline — メスカリン

MeSH
Medical Subject Headings — 医学事項索引用見出し，メッシュ

MesPGN
mesangial proliferative glomerulonephritis — メサンギウム増殖性糸球体腎炎

MET
metabolic equivalent — 代謝当量
minimal electroshock threshold — 電撃痙攣閾値

Met
metronidazole — メトロニダゾール

met
metabolism — 代謝
metabolites — 代謝産物
metal — 金属
metastatic — 転移(性)の

MET, met
metabolic — 代謝の

metastasis 転移

Met, MET, met
methionine メチオニン

met, met.
metallic 金属(性)の

meta
metatarsal 中足(骨)の

metab
metabolic 代謝の
metabolism 代謝
metabolites 代謝産物

metaph
metaphysis 骨幹端

metas
metastasis 転移
metastasize 転移する
metastatic 転移(性)の

met-EK
methionine-enkephalin メチオニン・エンケファリン

M et f.pil.
misce et fiant pilulae〈ラ〉 混和し丸剤とせよ《処》

M et f.pulv.
misce et fiat pulvis〈ラ〉 混和し散剤とせよ《処》

METH
methicillin メチシリン

Meth
methedrine メセドリン

meth
method 方法, 様式
methyl メチル

metHb
methemoglobin メトヘモグロビン

metho
methodology 方法論
methyl alcohol メチルアルコール

methyl-GAG
methylglyoxyl-bis-guanylhydrazone メチルグリオキシルビスグアニルヒドラゾン

metMb
metmyoglobin メトミオグロビン

m.et n.
mane et nocte〈ラ〉 朝と夜《処》

Metr
metreurynter メトロイリンテル
metreuryse メトロイリーゼ

METS
metabolic equivalents　代謝当量

Mets
metabolic equivalents of activity　安静時の消費エネルギー
metastasis　転移

m.et sig.
misce et signa〈ラ〉　混和し用法を記せ《処》

METT
maximum exercise tolerance test　最大運動負荷試験法

Met-tRNA
methionine-transfer RNA　メチオニン転移リボ核酸

m.et v.
mane et vespere〈ラ〉=morning and evening　朝と夕方《処》

MEUC
minimum effective urinary concentration　最小有効尿濃度

MEV
maximal exercise ventilatioin　最大運動換気
methotrexate, cyclophosphamide(=Endoxan), vincristine　メトトレキサート, シクロホスファミド(=エンドキサン), ビンクリスチン
murine erythroblastosis virus　ネズミ赤芽球症ウイルス

Mev
mega volt　メガボルト〈単位〉

MeV, MEV, mev
megaelectron volt　メガ電子ボルト〈単位〉

MEVAP
melphalan, cyclophosphamide(=Endoxan), vincristine, 1-(4-amino-2-methyl-5-pyrimidinyl)-methyl-3(2-chlorethyl)-3-nitrosourea, prednisone　メルファラン, シクロホスファミド(=エンドキサン), ビンクリスチン, メチルニトロソウレア, プレドニゾン

MEVP
melphalan, cyclophosphamide(=Endoxan), vincristine, prednisone　メルファラン, シクロホスファミド(=エンドキサン), ビンクリスチン, プレドニゾン
methotrexate, cyclophosphamide(=Endoxan), vincristine, prednisone　メトトレキサート, シクロホスファミド(=エンドキサン), ビンクリスチン, プレドニゾン

MEWDS
multiple evanescent white dot syndrome　多発性一過性白色斑点症候群

MF
- main feed — 主栄養
- meat free — 肉の入っていない
- medium frequency — 中(間)周波数，中(間)頻度
- megafarad — メガファラド〈単位〉
- melamine-formaldehyde — メラミンホルムアルデヒド
- microfibrile — 細線維
- microfilament — 細糸
- microfiltration — ミクロフィルトレーション
- microscopic factor — 顕微鏡因子
- midline frontal — 正中前頭部
- Miller Fisher (syndrome) — ミラー・フィッシャー(症候群)
- millipore filter — ミリポアフィルター
- mitochondrial fragments — ミトコンドリア分画
- mitogenic factor — 分裂促進因子
- mitomycin C,5-fluorouracil — マイトマイシンC,フルオロウラシル
- mitotic figure — 有糸(核)分裂像
- modifying factor — 修正係数
- mossy fiber — 苔状線維
- mucosal fluid — 粘(膜)液
- multifactorial — 多因子(性)の
- multiplying factor — 倍率
- mutation frequency — 突然変異(発生)率
- mycosis fungoides — 菌状息肉症
- myelin figure — ミエリン形態
- myelofibrosis — 骨髄線維症
- myocardial fibrosis — 心筋線維症
- myofibrillar — 筋原線維の

M & F
- mother and father — 母親と父親

Mf, mf
- microfilaria — 糸状虫仔虫，フィラリア仔虫

mF, mf
- millifarad — ミリファラド〈単位〉

m.f., M.f.
- *misce fiant*〈ラ〉 — 混和して作れ《処》
- *misce fiat*〈ラ〉 — 混和して作れ《処》

M/F, M : F
- male to female (ratio) — 男性/女性(比)

MFA
- *macaca fascicularis*〈ラ〉 — カニクイザル
- microplate fluorescent antibody method — マイクロプレート螢光抗体法
- monofluoroacetamide — モノフルオロアセトアミド

M

multiple factor analysis 多因子解析

MFAT
multifocal atrial tachycardia 多焦点性心房頻拍

MFB
medial forebrain bundle 内側前脳束
metallic foreign body 金属性異物

MFC
middle finger crease 中位指皺襞
mitomycin C,5-fluorouracil, cytarabin マイトマイシンC,フルオロウラシル,シタラビン

MFD
mandibulofacial dysostosis (下)顎顔面骨形成不全(症)
midforceps delivery 中位鉗子分娩
milk-free diet ミルクの入っていない食事, 無牛乳食
minimum fatal dose 最小致死量
mono-rhythmic frontal delta activity 単一律動性前頭部Δ〔デルタ〕波
multiple fraction per day 多分割照射

mfd
manufactured 製造された

MFG
modified fluid heat-degraded gelatin 熱加変性ゼラチン

MFGM
milk fat globule membrane (牛)乳脂肪球皮膜

MFH
malignant fibrous histiocytoma 悪性線維性組織球腫

MFI
mean fluorescence intensity 平均螢光強度

MFIPC
methyl flucrochlorophenyl isoxazolyl penicillin メチルクロロフェニルイソキサゾリルペニシリン(=フルクロキサシリン)

M flac, M.flac., m.flac.
membrana flaccida〈ラ〉 (鼓膜)弛緩部, シュラップネル膜

MFM
magnetic force microscope 磁力顕微鏡
microfluorometry 微小螢光測定(法)
millipore filter method ミリポアフィルター法

m.f.mass.pil.
misce fiat massa pilularum〈ラ〉 混和し丸剤塊とせよ《処》

M.f.mist.
misce fiat mistura〈ラ〉 混和し水剤とせよ《処》

M.f.mixt.
misce fiat mixtura〈ラ〉 混和し水剤とせよ《処》

MFO
mixed function oxidase 混合機能酸化酵素
MFP
mean circulatory filling pressure 循環系平均充満圧
monofluorophosphate モノフルオロホスフェート
MFPE
membrane filter plasma exchange 膜濾過法血漿交換
m.f.pil.
misce fiant pilulae〈ラ〉 混和し丸剤とせよ《処》
M.f.pulv.XII
misce fiat pulvis No.XII〈ラ〉 混和し散剤12包とせよ《処》
m.f.pulv., M.f.pulv.
misce fiat pulvis〈ラ〉 混和し散剤とせよ《処》
M.f.pulv.D.t.d.XII
misce fiat pulvis Da tales doses No. XII〈ラ〉 混和し散剤１包とし同量12包とせよ《処》
MFR
maximum flow rate 最大流量率
maximum urinary flow rate 最大尿流量率
mean flow rate 平均流量率
mucus flow rate 粘液流量率
mfr
manufacture 製品
manufacturer 製造(業)者，製作者
MFRS
microvascular flow regulating system 微小循環領域の血流を調節する機構
MFS
Miller-Fisher syndrome ミラー・フィッシャー症候群
m.f.sol.
misce fiat solutio〈ラ〉 混和し水剤とせよ《処》
MF solution
merthiolate-formaldehyde solution メルチオレイトホルムアルデヒド溶液
MF/SS
mycosis fungoides/Sézary syndrome 菌状息肉症/セザリー症候群
mfst
manifest 明らかな
MFT
motor function test 運動機能テスト
mucous membrane function test 粘膜機能検査
multifocal atrial tachycardia 多焦点性心房頻拍
muscle function test 筋機能検査
m.ft., M.ft.
misce fiant〈ラ〉 混合物をつくれ，混和してつくれ《処》

misce fiat〈ラ〉 | 混合物をつくれ，混和してつくれ《処》

MFTE
mitomycin C, 5-fluorouracil (= Endoxan), Toyomycin, cyclophosphamide | マイトマイシンC, フルオロウラシル, トヨマイシン, シクロホスファミド(=エンドキサン)

m.ft.l.a., M.ft.l.a.
misce fiat lege artis〈ラ〉 | 混和し常法に従ってつくれ《処》

M.ft.pulv.
misce fiat pulvis〈ラ〉 | 混和し散剤とせよ《処》

MFU
medical follow-up | 医学的経過観察

m.f.ung., M.f.ung.
misce fist unguentum〈ラ〉 | 混和し軟膏をつくれ《処》

MG
macroglobulin | マクログロブリン
Magengeschwür〈独〉 | 胃潰瘍
Marcus Gunn (pupil) | マーカス・ガン(瞳孔)
margin | 辺縁
May-Grunward | メイ・グリュンワルド(染色)
medial gastrocnemius | 内側腓腹(筋)
membranous glomerulonephritis | 膜性糸球体腎炎
menopausal gonadotrop(h)in | 閉経期ゴナドトロピン
methylglucoside | メチルグルコシド
methylglyoxal | メチルグリオキサル
methylguanidine | メチルグアニジン
Meulengracht icteric index | モレイングラハト黄疸指数
Meulengracht unit | モレイングラハト(黄疸)指数
Michaelis-Gutmann (body) | ミハエリス・グートマン(小体)
Millard-Gubler (syndrome) | ミヤール・ギュブレ(症候群)
minigastrin | ミニガストリン
monoacyl glycerol | モノアシルグリセロール
monoclonal gammopathy | 単クローン性免疫グロブリン血症
monoglyceride | モノグリセリド
Motoaki Guilford Personality test | 本明・ギルフォード性格検査《臨心》
mucous granule | 粘液顆粒
muscle group | 筋群
myasthenia gravis | 重症筋無力症
myoglobin | ミオグロビン

Mg
magnesium | マグネシウム〈元素〉

Molekulargewicht〈独〉 分子量

mg
marginal 辺縁の
milligram ミリグラム〈単位〉
mittelgroβ〈独〉 中等大の，中ぐらいの大きさの

mγ
milligamma ミリガンマ

mg%
milligrams percent ミリグラムパーセント〈単位〉

MGA
medical gas analyzer 医用ガス分析器
melengestrol acetate 酢酸メレンゲストロール

Mg-A
myeloma globulin A 骨髄腫グロブリンA

MGB
medial geniculate body 内側膝状体

MGBG
methylglyoxal-bis-guanylhydrase メチルグリオキサルビスグアミルヒドラーゼ
methylglyoxal-bis-guanylhydrazone メチルグリオキサルビスグアニルヒドラゾン

MGBH
methylglyoxal-bis-guanylhydrazone メチルグリオキサルビスグアニルヒドラゾン

M-G body
Michaelis-Gutmann body ミハエリス・グートマン小体

MGC
minimum growth-inhibiting concentration 最小発育阻止濃度
multinucleated giant cell(s) 多核巨大細胞

$MgCl_2$
magnesium chloride 塩化マグネシウム

MGD
meibomian gland dysfunction マイボーム腺障害
mixed gonadal dysgenesis 混合性器発育異常

mg/d
million gallons per day ミリオンガロン/日

MGE
movable genetic element トランスポゾン，可動遺伝要素

mgeh
milligram-element-hour 毎時ミリグラム要素

mg-el
milligram-element ミリグラム要素

MGF
macrophage growth factor 大食細胞成長因子
maternal grandfather 母方の祖父
mother's grandfather 母方の祖父
MGG
May-Grünwald-Giemsa (stain) メイ・グリュンワルト・ギムザ(染色)
mouse gamma globulin マウスγグロブリン
Mg-G
myeloma globulin G 骨髄腫グロブリンG
MGH
Massachusetts General Hospital マサチューセッツ総合病院
monoglyceride hydrolase モノグリセリド加水分解酵素
MGH, mgh, mg h
milligram-hour ミリグラム時〈単位〉
mg/hr
milligram per hour ミリグラム/時〈単位〉
mg-hr
milligram-hour ミリグラム時〈単位〉
Mgk
megakaryocyte 巨核球
mg/kg
milligrams per kilogram ミリグラム/キログラム
M.gl
multiple myeloma globulin 多発性骨髄腫グロブリン
MGM
maternal grandmother 母方の祖母
mother's grandmother 母方の祖母
mgm
milligram ミリグラム〈単位〉
mgmt
management 管理，経営
MGN
medial geniculate nucleus 内側膝状体(核)
membrane glomerulonephritis 膜性糸球体腎炎
mgn
micrograin マイクログレイン
MgO
magnesium oxide 酸化マグネシウム
M-GOT
mitochondrial glutamic-oxaloacetic transaminase ミトコンドリアGOT
MGP
bone matrix Gla protein 骨マトリックス・グラ蛋白
marginal granulocyte pool 顆粒球の辺縁部プール
membranous glomerulopathy 膜性糸球体症

methyl-green pyronin	メチルグリーンピロニン
mucin glycoprotein	ムチン糖蛋白
mucous glycoprotein	粘液糖蛋白

mgr

manager	管理人，マネージャー

MGS

meter gram second	メートル・グラム・秒

MGSA

melanoma growth-stimulating activity	メラノーマ成長刺激活性

$MgSO_4$

magnesium sulfate	硫酸マグネシウム

mgt

management	管理，経営

mgtis

meningitis	髄膜炎

MGUS

monoclonal gammopathy of undetermined significance	原因不明の単クローン性免疫グロブリン症

MGW

macroglobulinemia Waldenström	ワルデンストレームマクログロブリン血症
magnesium sulfate, glycerin, water (enema)	硫酸マグネシウム・グリセリン・水(浣腸)

M

MH

malignant histiocytosis	悪性組織球増殖(症)
malignant hyperpyrexia	悪性高熱(症)，悪性高体温(症)
malignant hyperthermia	悪性高熱(症)，悪性高体温(症)
mammotrophic hormone	乳腺刺激ホルモン(＝プロラクチン)
marital history	結婚歴
medial habenula	中手綱部
medial hypothalamus	内側視床下部
medical history	病歴
melanophore hormone	メラニン細胞ホルモン
menstrual history	月経歴
mental health	精神衛生
methylhistidine	メチルヒスチジン
military history	軍歴
Minister of Health, Labour and Welfare	厚生労働大臣
mixed hamartoma	混合性過誤腫
moist heat	湿熱
mouse hepatoma	マウス肝癌

murine hepatitis ネズミ肝炎

mH, mh

millihenry ミリヘンリー〈単位〉

MHA

major histocompatibility antigen 主要組織適合抗原
May-Hegglin anomaly メイ・ヘグリン異常
Mental Health Administration 精神衛生管理
Mental Health Association 精神衛生協会
methemalbumin メトヘムアルブミン
microangiopathic hemolytic anemia 細血管障害性溶血性貧血
microsome hemagglutination test ミクロソーム赤血球凝集テスト〔試験〕
middle hepatic artery 中肝動脈
mixed hemadsorption 混合赤血球吸着試験

MHB

maximum hospital benefit 最大病院利益

MHb

methemoglobin(=metHb) メトヘモグロビン
myohemoglobin(=myoHb) ミオヘモグロビン

MHbCN

cyan-methemoglobin シアンメトヘモグロビン

MHC

major histocompatibility complex 主要組織遺伝子複合体
mental health center 精神保健センター
mental health clinic 精神健康クリニック

mhcp

mean horizontal candle power 平均水平燭光

MHD

magnetohydrodynamics 磁気流体力学
maintenance hemodialysis 維持血液透析
mean hemolytic dose 平均溶血量
Metahydrin メタヒドリン
minimal hemagglutinating dose 最小赤血球凝集量

MHD, M.H.D.

minimal hemolytic dose 最小溶血量

MHK

minimal hemoconcentration 最小阻止濃度

MHLW

Ministry of Health, Labour and Welfare 厚生労働省

MHMA

3-methoxy-4-hydroxymandelic acid 3-メトキシ-4-ヒドロキシマンデル酸

MHN

morbus hemolyticus neonatomm〈ラ〉= morbus haemolyticus neonatorum 新生児溶血性疾患

M

MHO
microsomal heme oxygenase — ミクロソームヘムオキシゲナーゼ

MHP
maternal health program — 母親健康プログラム
mercurie-2-hydroxypropane — 水銀-2-水酸化プロパン

MHPA
mild hyperphenylalaninemia — 軽度高フェニルアラニン血(症)

MHPG
3-methoxy-4-hydroxyphenylglycol — 3-メトキシ-4-ヒドロキシフェニルグリコール

MHR
major histocompatibility region — 主要組織適合部位
maximum heart rate — 最大心拍数
methemoglobin reductase — メトヘモグロビン還元酵素
Milan hypertensive rat — ミラノ高血圧ラット

MHS
major histocompatibility system — 主要組織適合抗原系
malignant hyperthermia susceptible (patient) — 偽悪性高熱症(患者)
malignant hyperthermia suspected — 悪性高熱症の疑い(がある)
medical history sheet — 病歴用紙
multiphasic health screening — 多相スクリーニング

M

MHT
malignant hypertension — 悪性高血圧

MHTS
multiphasic health testing services — 多相的健康診断システム

MHV
magnetic heart vector — 磁気心臓ベクトル
middle hepatic vein — 中肝臓静脈
mouse hepatitis virus — マウス肝炎ウイルス

M Hx
medical history — 病歴

M.Hyg.
Master of Hygiene — 衛生学修士

MHz
megahertz — メガヘルツ〈単位〉

MI
massa intermedia — 中間質
maturation index — 成熟指数
mechanical inflammation — 機械的炎症
medical inspection — (医学的)視診
Medicus Index — 医学文献索引
melanophore index — メラニン(保有)細胞指数
membrane intact — 処女膜

menopausal index	更年期指数
menstruation induction	月経誘発
mental illness	精神病
mentally impaired	精神障害の
mentally institution	精神病院
mercaptoimidazole	メルカプトイミダゾール
mesioincisal	近心面切端の
metabolic index	代謝指数
middle initial	中間の初期
migration index	遊走指数
migration inhibition	遊走抑制〔阻止〕
M index	M指数
mitotic index	分裂指数
mitral incompetence	僧帽弁機能不全
mitral insufficiency	僧帽弁逆流症
mononucleosis infectiosa	伝染性単核細胞症，感染性単核細胞症
morphological index	菌形指数
motility index	運動指数
myocardial infarction	心筋梗塞

Mi

mitomycin	マイトマイシン

mi

minor	小さい
minute	分〈単位〉
mitral	僧帽の

MIA

microsatellite instability assay	マイクロサテライトインスタビリティアッセイ
monoiodoacetic acid	モノヨード酢酸

MIAA

microaggregated albumin	微小凝集アルブミン
monoiodoacetic acid	モノヨード酢酸

MIBG

metaiodobenzylguanidine	*m*-ヨードベンジルグアニジン

MIBI

^{99m}Tc-methoxy isobutyl isonitrile	^{99m}Tc-メトキシイソブチルイソニトリル

MIBK

methylisobutyl ketone	メチルイソブチルケトン

MIC

maternal and infant care	母親乳児ケア
maximum inspiratory capacity	最大吸気量
minimum inhibitory concentration	最小発育阻止濃度

MiC
minocycline ミノサイクリン
Mic
microaneurysm 微細動脈瘤
microscopic findings in centrifuged urinary sediment 尿遠心分離沈渣の顕微鏡所見
MIC, mic
microscopic 顕微鏡的な，顕微鏡の
microscopy 顕微鏡検査法
MICA
monoclonal islet cell autoantibody 単クローン抗膵島細胞自己抗体
mic.pan.
mica panis〈ラ〉 パン屑《処》
micr
microscope 顕微鏡
microscopy 顕微鏡検査法
micro
microscopic 顕微鏡的な，顕微鏡の
microscopy 顕微鏡検査法
microbiol., Microbiol
microbiological 微生物学(的)の
microbiology 微生物学
microcephs
microcephalics 小頭人種
microcryst
microcrystalline 微晶質の，微晶性の
microt
microtome ミクロトーム
MICS
minimally invasive cardiac surgery 低侵襲心臓外科手術
MID
minimal infecting dose 最小感染量
minimal inhibiting dose 最小発育阻止量
multi-infarct dementia 多発性脳梗塞性痴呆
mid
middle 中央の
MIDCAB
minimally invasing direct coronary artery bypass 低侵襲冠(状)動脈バイパス手術
middle/3
middle third 中(部)1/3(区)
MIEMSS
Maryland Institute for Emergency Medical Services System メリーランド救急医療サービス研究所

MIF
macrophage inhibitory factor　マクロファージ抑制因子
macrophage migration inhibitory factor　マクロファージ遊走阻止因子
melanocyte inhibitory factor　メラニン細胞抑制因子
melanocyte-stimulation hormone release inhibiting factor　メラニン細胞刺激ホルモン放出抑制因子
membrane immunofluorescence test　膜蛍光抗体法
merthiolate iodine formaldehyde (stain)　メチルチオレートヨードホルムアルデヒド(染色)
microimmunofluorescence test　微量免疫蛍光検査法
migration inhibitory factor　遊走阻止因子
mixed immunofluorescence　混合免疫蛍光検査法
mouse interferon　マウスインターフェロン
müllerian-inhibiting foctor　ミュラー管阻害〔抑制〕因子

MIFA
mitomycin C,5-fluorouracil, adriamycin　マイトマイシンC,フルオロウラシル,アドリアマイシン

MIFR
maximum inspiratory flow rate　最大吸気流量率

MIG
mumps immunoglobulin　流行性耳下腺炎免疫グロブリン

MIg
malaria immunoglobulin　マラリア免疫グロブリン
measles immunoglobulin　麻疹免疫グロブリン
membrane immunoglobulin　膜免疫グロブリン

MIH
melanocyte inhibitory hormone　メラノサイト抑制ホルモン
minor histocompatibility loci　副組織適合性遺伝子座
MSH-inhibitory hormone　MSH抑制ホルモン

MIHPPA
3,5-monoiodo-4-hydroxyl-phenylpyruvic acid　3,5-モノヨード-4-ヒドロキシルフェニルピルビン酸

MIIA
medical information and intelligence agency　医療情報代理業

MIIT
multiple insulin injection therapy　インスリン頻回注射療法

mike
microphone　マイクロホン

MIL
medical information line　電話健康相談

mil
military　軍の

mil, mil.
milliliter　ミリリットル〈単位〉

mil, ml
mile　マイル〈単位〉

MILIS
Multicenter Investigation of the Limitation of Infarct Size Study　ミリス・スタディ(＝心理的ストレスと冠動脈疾患との強い関連性を示した大規模試験)

millihg
millimeters of mercury (pressure)　ミリメートル水銀柱(圧)

millisec
millisecond　ミリ秒〈単位〉

mil.TB
miliary tuberculosis　粟粒結核(症)

MIN
medial interlaminar nucleus　内側層間核

min
mineral　無機質，鉱質
minor　小の，小さい

/min
per minute　毎分，１分間に

MIN, min.
minim　最小
minimal　最小の
minimum〈ラ〉　最小
minute　分〈単位〉

MINA
monoisonitrosoacetone　モノイソニトロソアセトン

MINE
mesna uroprotection, ifosfamide, mitoxantrone, etoposide　メスナによる尿道保護,イホスファミド,ミトキサントロン,エトポシド

MINET
Medical Information Network　医療情報ネットワーク

MINIA
monkey intranuclear inclusion　サル核内封入体因子

mini-VAB
vinblastine, actinomycin D, bleomycin　ビンブラスチン,アクチノマイシンD,ブレオマイシン

MINO
minocycline　ミノサイクリン

Minor
minor tranquilizer　抗不安薬

M.Int.Med.
Master of Internal Medicine　内科学士

min wt
minimum weight 最小重量
MIO, M.I.O.
minimal identifiable odor 最小識別臭気
MIP
macrophage inflammatory protein マクロファージ由来炎症性蛋白
maximal inspiratory pressure 最大吸気圧
mean incubation period 平均潜伏期
mean inspiratory pressure 平均吸気圧
mean intravascular pressure 平均血管内圧
microwave-induced plasma マイクロ波誘導プラズマ
minimal pancreatitis 軽度膵炎
MIPI
mean interpotential interval 平均放電間隔
MIPM
microprolactinoma 微小プロラクチノーマ
MIP-MS
microwave-induced plasma mass spectrometer マイクロ波プラズマ微量元素質量分析装置
MIPS
million instructions per second 百万命令毎秒，ミプス
MIR
main immunogenic region 主要免疫原性部位
myocardial ischemia with subsequent reperfusion 再灌流を伴う心筋虚血
mir
mirror 鏡
MIRD
medical internal radiation dose 医療内部被曝線量
medium internal radiation dose 中間内部放射線量
MIRU
myocardial infarction research unit 心筋梗塞研究部門
MIS
management information system 治療情報システム
maturation-inducing substance 卵成熟誘起因子
medical information service 医学情報サービス
medical information system 医学情報システム
minimally invasive surgery 最小侵襲手術
motor index score 運動指標得点
müllerian inhibiting substance ミュラー管抑制物質
Mis Astig
mixed astigmatism 混合乱視，雑性乱視
Misc
miscellany 備考，雑録

misc
miscarriage 流産
miscellaneos 雑多な，その他の

mis.et sig.
misce et signa〈ラ〉 混合しラベルに記入せよ《処》

MISS
Medical Interview Satisfaction Scale 満足度面接調査

MIST
medical information service via telephone 電話による医学情報サービス
minimally invasive surgical technique 低侵襲手術法

mist
mistura〈ラ〉＝mixture 混合物，合剤《処》

MIT
macrophage migration inhibition test マクロファージ遊走阻止試験
Male Impotence Test 男性インポテンス検査
metabolism inhibition test 代謝抑制検査
minimally invasive therapy 最小侵襲治療法
miracidial immobilization test 幼仔虫運動停止試験
monoiodotyrosine モノヨードチロシン
multiple injection therapy 頻回注射療法
multiple insulin infusion therapy インスリン頻回注射療法

mit.
mitis〈ラ〉 温和な《処》
mitochondria ミトコンドリア

mit insuf
mitral insufficiency 僧帽弁不全

mitt, mitt.
mitte〈ラ〉 送れ，行かせる，放す《処》

mitt.sang.
mitte sanguinem〈ラ〉 採血せよ《処》

mitt.tal.
mitte tales〈ラ〉 同量を送れ《処》

mitt.tal.vi
mitte tales vi〈ラ〉 同量 6 個を送れ《処》

mIU
milli-international unit ミリ国際単位

mix.
mixture〈ラ〉 混合，混合物《処》

mixt.
mixtura〈ラ〉 混合物《処》

MJ
marijuana マリファナ
megajoule メガジュール〈単位〉

MJA
mechanical joint apparatus 機械的関節装置

M

MJAD
Machado-Joseph Azorean disease　マチャド・ジョセフ・アゾレア病
MJD
Machado-Joseph disease　マチャド・ジョセフ病
MK
Magen Krebs〈独〉　胃癌
menaquinone　メナキノン
midkine　ミドカイン
monkey kidney　サル腎(臓)
monokine　モノカイン
Mounier-Kuhn (syndrome)　モニエール・クーン(症候群)
myokinase　ミオキナーゼ
MK-6
menaquinone-6　メナキノン 6
MKB
megakaryoblast　巨核芽球
MKC
monkey kidney cell　サル腎(臓)細胞
MK-CSF
megakaryocyte colony stimulating factor　巨核球コロニー刺激因子
mkd
marked　印を付けた，高度の
MKDGF
megakaryocyte-derived growth factor　巨核球由来成長因子
mkdly
markedly　高度に
MKG
mandibular kinediography　下顎運動路軌跡記録装置
MKG, mkg
meter kilogram　メートルキログラム
MKH
Menke kinky hair　メンキー縮れ毛
MKHS
Menke kinky hair syndrome　メンキー縮れ毛症候群
MKM
mikamycin　ミカマイシン
MK-POT
megakaryocyte potentiator　巨核球増幅因子活性
MKR
Meinicke Klarungsreaktion〈独〉　マイニッケ清澄反応
mkr
mikroskopisch〈独〉　顕微鏡の

MKS, M.K.S., mks
meter kilogram second　毎秒メートルキログラム

MKSA
meter, kilogram, second, ampere　メートル・キログラム・秒・アンペア

MKSAP
Medical Knowledge Self Assessment Program　米国の生涯教育用の教本と問題集シリーズ

MKTC
monkey kidney tissue culture　サル腎(臓)組織培養

ML
lingual margin　舌縁
macula lutea　網膜黄斑
malignant lymphoma　悪性リンパ腫
Mamillarlinie〈独〉　乳頭線
mean level　平均レベル
medial lateral　内外側
medial lemniscus　内側毛帯
meningeal leukemia　髄膜白血病
metachromatic leucodystrophy　異染性白質異常症
meter lens　メートルレンズ
middle lobe　中肺葉
midline　正中の
molecular layer　分子層
motor latency　運動潜時
mucolipidosis　ムコリピドーシス
muscular layer　筋層
Mycobacterium leprae　ライ菌
myeloid leukemia　骨髄性白血病

mL
millilambert　ミリランベルト〈単位〉

mL, ml, ml.
milliliter　ミリリットル〈単位〉

M/L
mother-in-law　義理の母

m/l
middle left　中央部の左

ML, M.L.
Licentiate in Medicine　医師免許証所有者

ML, m.l.
midline　中央(線)，中心(線)

M : L, M/L
monocyte-lymphocyte (ratio)　単球/リンパ球比

MLA
Medical Library Association　医学図書館協会
mento-laeva-anterior　左頤前位

monocytic leukemia, acute　急性骨髄単球性白血病
mucosa lymphocyte antigen　粘膜リンパ球抗原
multilanguage aphasia　多言語失語症

mLAD
modified left anterior oblique　修正左前斜位

MLAP
mean left atrial pressure　平均左(心)房圧

MLBP
mechanical low back pain　機械的腰痛(症)

MLBT
monoaural loudness balance test　単耳大きさ平衡テスト

MLC
minimal lethal concentration　最小致死濃度
mixed leucocyte culture　混合白血球培養
mixed lymphocyte concentration　混合リンパ球濃度
mixed lymphocyte culture　混合リンパ球培養
morphine-like compound　モルヒネ様化合物
myelomonocytic leukemia, chronic　慢性骨髄単球性白血病
myosin light chain　ミオシン軽鎖

MLCB
mannitol lysine crystal violet brilliant green (medium)　マンニトール・リジン結晶バイオレット・ブリリアントグリーン(培地)

MLCK
myosin light-chain kinase　ミオシン軽鎖キナーゼ

MLCN
multilocular cystic nephroma　多房性腎嚢胞

MLCR
mixed lymphocyte culture reaction　リンパ球混合培養反応

MLD
masking level difference　遮蔽レベル較差
metachromatic leukodystrophy　異染性脳白質変性症
minimal lethal dose　最小致死量

MLD_{50}
median lethal dose　50%致死量

MLF
medial longitudinal fasciculus　内側縦束
morphine-like factor　モルヒネ様因子

MLFS
medial longitudinal fasciculus syndrome　内側縦束症候群

MLG
myelography　脊髄造影

MLGN
minimal lesion glomerulonephritis　最小病変糸球体腎炎

ML-H
hystiocytic malignant lymphoma 組織球性悪性リンパ腫
MLI
mixed lymphocyte interaction 混合リンパ球相互作用
M line
M band M線，M帯
MLL
lymphoblastic malignant lymphoma リンパ芽球性悪性リンパ腫
ml/min/m²
milliliters per minute per square meter ミリリットル/分/平方メートル
MLN
membranous lupus erythematous nephritis 膜型ループス腎炎
membranous lupus nephropathy 慢性ループス腎症
mesangial proliferative lupus nephritis 脈管膜増殖性ループス腎炎
mesenteric lymph node 腸内膜リンパ節
MLNS
minimal lesion nephrotic syndrome 微小変化型ネフローゼ症候群
mucocutaneous lymph node syndrome 粘膜皮膚リンパ節症候群
MLO
medio lateral oblique 内外側斜位
MLP
mento-laeva posterior〈ラ〉 左頤後位
microsomal lipoprotein ミクロソームリポ蛋白
multiple lymphomatous polyposis 多発性リンパ腫性ポリポーシス
ML-PDL
poorly differenciated lymphocytic malignant lymphoma 低分化リンパ球性悪性リンパ腫
MLR
middle latency response 中潜時反応
mixed leucocyte reaction 混合白血球反応
mixed lymphocyte reaction 混合リンパ球反応
multiple linear regression analysis 重回帰分析《統》
MLS
median longitudinal section 正中縦断(面)
medium life span 平均的生存期間
middle lobe syndrome (肺)中葉症候群
mouse leukemia virus マウス白血病ウイルス
mucolipidosis ムコリピドーシス
subacute myelomonocytic leukemia 亜急性骨髄単球性白血病
MLs
macrolides マクロライド類

MLSB
migrating long spike bursts 腸平滑筋推進運動
MLT
median lethal time 50%致死時間
mento-laeva transverse〈ラ〉 左頤横位
MLTC
mixed lymphocyte tumor cell 混合リンパ球腫瘍細胞
tetracycline methylene lysine テトラサイクリンメチレンリジン
MLTR
mixed lymphocyte tumor cell reaction 混合リンパ球腫瘍細胞反応
MLV
Moloney leukemia virus モロニー白血病ウイルス
mouse leukemia virus マウス白血病ウイルス
multilaminar vesicle 多層性小胞
murine leukemia virus ネズミ白血病ウイルス
MLVM
murine leukemia virus Moloney モロニー・ネズミ白血病
MLVR
murine leukemia virus Rauscher ラウシャー・ネズミ白血病
MLX
miloxacin ミロキサシン
MM
macromolecule 高分子
Magenmittel〈独〉 胃健剤
malignant melanoma 悪性黒色腫
Marshall-Marchetti (procedure) マーシャル・マーケッティ(手技)
masseter muscle 咬筋
megamitochondria メガ〔巨大〕ミトコンドリア
melanoma metastasis 黒色腫転移
meningococcal meningitis 髄膜菌性(脳脊)髄膜炎
Menschenmilch〈独〉 人乳，母乳
metastatic melanoma 転移性黒色腫
methadone maintenance メサドン維持(療法)
middle molecule 中分子
morbidity, mortality 罹病率・死亡率
mucous membrane 粘膜
multiple myeloma 多発性骨髄腫
myeloid metaplasia 骨髄(様)化生
mM
millimol ミリモル〈単位〉
millimolar ミリモルの
mm
methylmalonyl メチルマロニル

M

millimeter — ミリメートル〈単位〉
mittelmäßig〈独〉 — 中位の，中等の
motus manus — 手動弁
(to) muscularis mucosae — 粘膜筋板(まで)

mμ
millimicron — ミリミクロン〈単位〉

mm²
cubic millimeter — 立法ミリメートル〈単位〉

mm³
square millimeter — 平方ミリメートル〈単位〉

m.m.
motus manus〈ラ〉 — 手動弁

M & M
milk and molasses — ミルクと糖蜜
morbidity and mortality — 罹患率と死亡率

M-M
Michaelis-Menten — ミハエリス・メンテン

MM, mm
medial malleolus — 内果，内くるぶし
muscles — 筋，筋肉

MMA
methyl malonic acid — メチルマロン酸
methylmetacrylate — メチルメタクリル酸
middle meningeal artery — 中硬膜動脈

MMAD
mass median aerodynamic diameter — エアロゾル粒子の平均粒子径

MMC
Maternal Mortality Committee — 妊産婦死亡調査委員会
Medical Micro-Computer Club — 医用マイクロコンピュータクラブ
mitomycin C — マイトマイシンC
mucosal mast cell — 粘膜肥満細胞

mμc
millimicrocurie — ミリマイクロキュリー〈単位〉

MMCoA
methylmalonyl coenzyme A — メチルマロニルコエンザイムA

MMCP
mouse mast cell protease — マウス肥満細胞プロテアーゼ

MMD
myotonic muscular dystrophy — 筋緊張性ジストロフィ

MME
M-mode echocardiography — Mモード心エコー検査
mouse mammary epithelium — マウス乳房上皮

M.Med
Master of Medicine — 医学士

MMEF
maximum mid-expiratory flow　最大中間呼気流量
MMF
maximal mid-expiratory flow　最大中間呼気流量
mean maximum flow　平均最大流量
MMFR
maximal midexpiratory flow rate　最大中間呼気流速
MMG
mean maternal glucose　平均母体グルコース
mammography　マンモグラフィ(ー)
mμg.
millimicrogram　ミリマイクログラム〈単位〉
MMH
monomethylhydrazine　モノメチルヒドラジン
mmHg
millimeter of mercury　ミリメートル水銀柱圧〈単位〉
mmH$_2$O
millimeters of water　ミリメートル水柱圧〈単位〉
MMI
methimazole　メチマゾール
methylmercaptoimidazole　メチルメルカプトイミダゾール
M.Mic
Master of Microbiology　微生物学士
MMK
Mammakrebs〈独〉　乳癌
MML
myelomonocytic leukemia　骨髄(性)単球(性)白血病
mM/L, mM/l
millimoles per liter　ミリモル/リットル〈単位〉
MMLV
Moloney murine leukemia virus　モロニーネズミ白血病ウイルス
MMM
methylmalonyl-coenzyme A mutase　メチルマロニル・コエンザイム〔Co〕Aムターゼ
myelosclerosis with myeloid metaplasia　骨髄性化生を伴う骨髄硬化症
MMMF
man-made mineral fiber　人工鉱物繊維
MMMS
Merck molecular modeling system　メルク分子モデルシステム
MMMT
malignant mixed mesodermal tumor　悪性中胚葉混合腫瘍
malignant mixed müllerian tumor　悪性ミュラー管混合腫瘍

M

MMN
morbus maculosus neonatorum　新生児紫斑病
multiple mucosal neuroma　多発性粘膜神経腫

MMNC
marrow mononuclear cell　骨髄単核細胞

MMoL
myelomonoblastic leukemia　骨髄単芽球白血病

mmol
millimole　ミリモル〈単位〉

mmole
millimole　ミリモル〈単位〉

MMP
matrix metalloproteinase　マトリックスメタロプロテイナーゼ

4MMPD
4-methoxy-meta-phenylenediamine　4-メトキシ-メタ-フェニレンジアミン

MMPG
Medical Management Planning Group　医療管理計画グループ

MMPI
Minnesota Multiphasic Personality Inventory　ミネソタ多面的人格目録検査

MMPNC
Medical Material Program for Nuclear Causalities　放射線事故母体医療プログラム

mmpp, mm.p.p.
millimeters partial pressure　ミリメートル分圧

MMPs
matrix degrading metalloproteinase　基質分解メタロプロテイナーゼ

MMQ
Mauseley medical questionnaire　モーズレイ健康調査表

MMR
masseter muscle rigidity　咬筋硬直
measles mumps rubella (vaccine)　3種(=麻疹・おたふくかぜ・風疹)混合ワクチン
myocardial metabolic rate　心筋代謝率

MMS
metabolic monitoring system　代謝監視機構
methyl methanesulfonate　メチルメタンスルホン酸
middle molecular substance　中分子物質
mixed mesodermal sarcoma　中胚葉混合肉腫
myeloma morphology score　骨髄腫形態得点

MMSC
methylmethionine sulfonium chloride　メチルメチオニンスルホニウムクロリド

MMSE
mini-mental state examination 知能状態小検査
mm/sec
millimeters per second ミリメートル/秒〈単位〉
MMST
mini-mental state test 簡易知能テスト
MMst, mm st, mmst.
muscle strength 筋力
mm str
muscle strength 筋力
MMT
l-methyl-5-mercapto-1,2,3,4-tetrazole 1-メチル-5-メルカプト-1,2,3,4-テトラゾール
malignant mesenchymal tumor 悪性間葉性腫瘍
Mann muscle test マン筋力テスト
manual muscle test 徒手筋力検査
mouse mammary tumor マウス乳房腫瘍
mmt
monomethoxytrityl モノメトキシトリチル
MMTN
myelinated mechanothermal nociceptor 有髄性機械温熱受容器
MMTP
Methadone Maintenance Treatment Program メサドン維持治療プログラム
MMTV
mouse mammary tumor virus マウス乳房腫瘍ウイルス
MMU
Macaca mulatta〈ラ〉 アカゲザル
MMuLv
Moloney murine leukemia virus モロニーネズミ白血病ウイルス
MMV
mandatory minute ventilation 必須瞬間換気量
MMWR
morbidity and mortaliiy weekly report 疾病率と死亡率の週報
MMY
Mental Measurements Yearbook 精神測定年鑑
MN
malignant nephrosclerosis 悪性腎硬化症
mass neuropediatrics 発達スクリーニングテスト
melena neonatorum 新生児メレナ
membranous nephropathy 膜性腎症
mesenteric node 腸間膜節
metanephrine メタネフリン

MN blood type — MN式血液型
mononuclear — 単核(性)の
multinodular — 多結節性の
myoneural — 神経筋の，筋神経の

Mn
manganese — マンガン〈元素〉

mN
millinormal — ミリ規定(溶液)の

M.N.
Master of Nursing — 看護学士

M & N
morning and night — 朝と夜

MN, M/N, mn
midnight — 真夜中

MNA
maximum noise area — 最大雑音区
N′-methylnicotinamide — *N′*-メチルニコチンアミド

MNAP
mixed nerve action potential — 混合神経活動電位

MNB
murine neuroblastoma — ネズミ神経芽(細胞)腫

MNC
mononuclear cell — 単核細胞

M

MNCV
maximum nerve conduction velocity — 最大神経伝達速度
mixed nerve conduction velocity — 混合神経伝達速度
motor nerve conduction velocity — 運動神経伝導速度

MND
minimal necrotizing dose — 最小壊死量
modified neck dissection — 修飾頸部郭清術
motor neuron disease — 運動ニューロン疾患

MNG
N-methyl-*N′*-nitroso-*N*-nitroguanidine — *N*-メチル-*N′*-ニトロソ-*N*-ニトログアニジン

mng
managing — 管理
morning — 朝

MNGF
motor neuron growth factor — 運動神経成長因子

MNI
Montreal Neurological Institute — モントリオール神経学研究所

MNI virus
Mumps, Newcastle disease, Influenzavirus — 流行性耳下腺炎・ニューカッスル病・インフルエンザウイルス

MNJ
myeloneural junction 神経筋接合部，筋神経接合部
MNL
mononuclear leukocyte 単核性白血球
MNM
mononeuritis multiplex 散在性単神経炎
MNMS
myo-nephropathic metabolic syndrome 筋腎代謝症候群
MNP
mononuclear phagocyte 単核性(貪)食細胞
MNRU
Medical Neuropsychiatric Research Unit 医学神経精神病研究部門
MNS
Milan normotensive strain ミラノ正常血圧ラット
MNSF
monoclonal nonspecific suppressor factor モノクローナル非特異的抑制因子
MnSOD
manganous superoxide dismutase マンガンスーパーオキシドジスムターゼ
MNU
methyl nitrosourea メチルニトロソ尿素
MO
manually operated 手動の
medical officer 医療事務員
method of operation 手術法
micro-Ouchterlony method マイクロオクタロニー法
mineral oil ミネラル油
minute output 分時拍出量
mitral opening sound 僧帽弁開放音
molecular orbital 分子軌道
morbidly obese 病的肥満の
MΩ
megohm メガオーム〈単位〉
Mo
mitral valve opening 僧帽弁開放
mode モード
Moloney (strain) モロニー(株)
molybdenum モリブデン〈元素〉
mono 単一
monocyte 単球
mo
Morgan unit モルガン単位

M

^{99}Mo
molybdenum-99 モリブデン99

MO_2
myocardial oxygen (consumption) 心筋酸素(消費)

mo′
more もっと
morning 朝

m/o
male oriental 男で東洋人

MO, mo
month 月

MOA
mechanism of action 作用機序

MoA
monocyte specific antigen 単球特異抗原

MOAB
(murine) monoclonal antibody (ネズミ)モノクローナル抗体

MOAb
monoclonal antibody モノクローナル抗体

MOAD
methotrexate, vincristine (=Oncovin), L-asparaginase, dexamethasone メトトレキサート,ビンクリスチン(=オンコビン),L-アスパラギナーゼ,デキサメタゾン

M

MOB
mechlorethamine, vincristine (=Oncovin), bleomycin メクロレタミン,ビンクリスチン(=オンコビン),ブレオマイシン
4-methoxy-2-hydroxybenzophenone 4-メトキシ-2-ヒドロキシベンゾフェノン
multiple operated back 多数回手術腰部

mob
mobile 移動性の，可動性の
mobility 移動度，可動性
mobilization 動員，可動化，関節受動(術)

mobil
mobility 移動度，可動性

MOB-PT
mitomycin C, vincristine (=Oncovin), bleomycin, cisplatin (=Platinol) マイトマイシンC,ビンクリスチン(=オンコビン),ブレオマイシン,シスプラチン(=プラチノール)

MOC
maximum oxgen consumption 最大酸素消費量
multiple ocular coloboma 多発性眼コロボーマ
myocardial oxygen consumption 心筋酸素消費量

MOCA
methotrexate, vincristine (= Oncovin), cyclophosphamide, adriamycin　メトトレキサート，ビンクリスチン(=オンコビン)，シクロホスファミド，アドリアマイシン

MOCM
monocyte conditioned medium　単球コンディション培養液

MOCVD
metal organic chemical vapor deposition　有機金属熱分解気層エピタキシャル成長

MOD
magnetic optical disc　光磁気ディスク《コン》
maturity onset type diabetes　成人型糖尿病
medical officer of the day　日直医
mesial-occlusal distal　遠位正中咬合の

MOD, mod
moderate　中等度の，穏やかな

mod, mod.
moderately　中等度に
modicus〈ラ〉　中等大に
modification　変法
modified　修正した
modify　変える
modulation　調節

MODB
mesial occlusal distal buccal　遠位頬側正中咬合の

MODD
mean of daily difference　日差血糖変動幅

MODEM
modulator and demodulator　変復調装置

MOD/IRAN
modification, inspection and repair as necessary　必要に応じて変え・観察し・修理する

MODM
maturity-onset diabetes mellitus　成人発症型糖尿病

mod praesc, mod.praesc
modo praescripto〈ラ〉　指示どおりに，処方した方法で《処》

MODS
multiple organ dysfunction syndrome　多臓器機能障害症候群

mods
modifiers　修正する人

MODY
maturity-onset diabetes of youth　若年性成人発症型糖尿病，タタソール症候群

M

MOE
Ministry of Education　教育省，文部省[米国]
MOF
methotrexate, vincristine (= Oncovin), 5-fluorouracil　メトトレキサート，ビンクリスチン(=オンコビン)，フルオロウラシル
methoxyflurane　メトキシフルラン
multiple organ failure　多臓器不全
MOG
Master of Obstetrics and Gynecology　産婦人科学士
myel-oligodendrocyte glycoprotein　ミエリンオリゴデンドロサイトグリコプロテイン
MOH
Medical Officer of Health　公衆衛生技官，検疫官
MOI
maximum oxygen intake　最大酸素摂取量
moi, MOI
multiplicity of infection　感染多重度
MOJAC
mood, orientation, judgement, affect, content　気分・見当識・判断・情動・内容
MOL
molecular layer　分子層
MoL
monocytic leukemia　単球性白血病
mol
mole　モル〈単位〉
molecular　分子の
molecule　分子
molc
molar concentration　モル濃度
Mole
Blasenmole〈独〉　胞状奇胎
mole
molecular　分子の
molecule　分子
moll.
mollis〈ラ〉　軟らかい，軟性の
mol/l
molecules per liter　モル/リットル
mol.wgt
molecular weight　分子量
MOL WT, Mol wt, mol wt, mol.wt.
molecular weight　分子量

M

moly
molybdenum モリブデン
MOM
milk of magnesia マグネシウム乳(剤), 酸化マグネシウム(懸濁液)
miokamycin ミオカマイシン
mucoid otitis media ムコイド中耳炎
mom
middle of month 中旬
MOMA
methoxyhydroxymandelic acid メトキシヒドロキシマンデル酸
3-methoxy-4-hydroxymandelic acid 3-メトキシ-4-ヒドロキシマンデル酸(=バニリルマンデル酸)
MOMP
mechlorethamine, vincristine (= Oncovin), methotrexate, prednisone メクロルエタミン, ビンクリスチン(オンコビン), メトトレキサート, プレドニゾン
monoclonal marrow plasmacytosis 骨髄単クローン形質細胞増加症
MOMS
multiple organ malrotation syndrome 多臓器異常回転症候群
MoMSV
Moloney murine sarcoma virus モロニーマウス肉腫ウイルス
Mo-MuLV
Moloney murine leukemia virus モロニーマウス白血病ウイルス
mon
monocyte 単球, 単核細胞
month(s) 月
MON, Mon
Monday 月曜日
Mongo
mongolism 蒙古症, ダウン症
Mono
(infectious) mononucleosis (伝染性)単核細胞(症), (伝染性)単球増加(症)
mono
monocular 単眼の
monocyte 単球, 単核細胞
monophonic 単旋律の
monotype 単一形
monobas
monobasic 一塩基の
Monos
monocytes 単球, 単核細胞

M

monot
monotonus 単調な
monotony 単音
monotype 単型
monotypic 単型の

montrg
monitoring 監視

MOP
medical outpatient 外来患者
methotrexate, vincristine (=Oncovin), prednisone メトトレキサート, ビンクリスチン(=オンコビン), プレドニゾン
moderate pancreatitis 中等度膵炎
multiple operated back 何回も手術を受けた腰
myeloperoxidase ミエロペルオキシダーゼ

5-MOP
5-methoxypsoralen 5-メトキシソラレン

MOP-BAP
mechlorethamine, vincristine (=Oncovin), prednisone, bleomycin, adriamycin, procarbazine メクロルエタミン, ビンクリスチン(=オンコビン), プレドニゾン, ブレオマイシン, アドリアマイシン, プロカルバジン

MOPP
mechlorethamine, vincristine (=Oncovin), procarbazine, prednisone メクロルエタミン, ビンクリスチン(=オンコビン), プロカルバジン, プレドニゾン

MOPP/ABV
mechlorethamine, vincristine (=Oncovin), procarbazine, prednisone, adriamycin, bleomycin, vinblastine メクロルエタミン, ビンクリスチン(=オンコビン), プロカルバジン, プレドニゾン, アドリアマイシン, ブレオマイシン, ビンブラスチン

MOPS
3-(*N*-morpholino) propanesulfonic acid 3-(*N*-モルホリノ)プロパンスルホン酸

M.Opt
Master of Optometry 視力測定学士

MOPV
monovalent oral poliovirus vaccine 一価経口ポリオウイルスワクチン

MOR
morphine モルヒネ

mor
mortality　死亡率
MORA
mandibular orthopaedic repositioning appliance　下顎(骨)整形外科整復器具
mor.dict.
more dicto〈ラ〉　指示した方法で《処》
morph
morphine　モルヒネ
morphological　形態学的な
morphology　形態学
morph.hydr
morphine hydrochloride　塩酸モルヒネ
mor.sol.
more solito〈ラ〉　通常の方法で《処》
mort
mortal　死の，臨終の，人間の
mortality　人類，死亡数，死亡率
mortal
mortality　人類，死亡数，死亡率
MOS
metal oxide semiconductor　金属・酸化シリコン半導体
mitral opening snap　僧帽弁開放音
myelofibrosis osteosclerosis　骨髄線維症(性)骨硬化(症)
mOs
milliosmolar　ミリ重量モル浸透圧の
milliosmole　ミリオスモル〈単位〉
mos
month(s)　月
mosaic　モザイク
MOsm，mOsm，mosm
milliosmolar　ミリ容積モル浸透圧の，ミリオスモルの
m osmole
milliosmole　ミリオスモル〈単位〉
MOT
mini-object test　ミニ対象試験《検査》
mouse ovarian tumor　マウス卵巣腫瘍
Mot V
motor nucleus of the trigeminal V(＝fifth)　三叉〔差〕神経(＝第V脳神経)運動核
MOVC
membraneous obstruction of vena cava　大静脈膜性閉塞(症)
MOX
moxalactam　モキサラクタム

M

MOY
myoglobin　ミオグロビン

MP
macrophage　マクロファージ
matrix protein　基質蛋白
medial plantar　内側足底
medical payment　医療(費)支払い
medium pressure　平均圧
medroxyprogesterone　メドロキシプロゲステロン
melphalan, prednisone　メルファラン, プレドニゾン
membrane potential　膜電位
menstrual period　月経期
mentum posterior　頤後位の
mercaptopurine　メルカプトプリン
mesenteric panniculitis　腸間膜組織炎
metacarpophalangeal　中手指節関節の
metacarpophalangeal joint　中手指節関節
metatarsophalangeal　中足指節の
methylprednisolone　メチルプレドニゾロン
middle phalanx　中指(趾)節骨
midline parietal　正中頭頂部
mitogenic protein　有糸核分裂蛋白
modulator protein　修飾物質蛋白
monoclonal protein　M蛋白
monopolar lead　単極誘導
motion picture　映画
motor potential　運動電位
mucopolysaccharide　ムコ多糖(体)
mucoprotein　ムコ蛋白
multiparous　経産婦の
muscle potential　筋電位
mycoplasma　マイコプラズマ
mycoplasmal pneumonia　マイコプラズマ肺炎

Mϕ
macrophage　マクロファージ

mp
melting point　融点
multipolar　多極性(神経細胞)
(to) muscularis propria　固有筋層(まで)

6-MP
6-mercaptopurine　6-メルカプトプリン

m.p.
mane primo〈ラ〉　朝早く《処》
massa pilularum〈ラ〉　丸剤塊《処》

MP, m.p.
modo praescripto〈ラ〉　処方した方法で《処》

M

MPA
- main pulmonary artery 主肺動脈
- maximal pepsin activity 最高ペプシン活性
- medroxyprogesterone acetate 酢酸メドロキシプロゲステロン塩
- methylprednisolone acetate 酢酸メチルプレドニゾロン
- mycophenolic acid ミコフェノール酸

MPa
- megapascal メガパスカル

MPACS
- manual picture achieving and communication system デジタル画像伝送システム操作

mPAP, MPAP
- mean pulmonary arterial pressure 平均肺動脈圧

MPB
- male pattern baldness 男性型はげ
- meprobamate メプロバメート

MPC
- maximal permissible concentration 最大許容濃度
- mean plasma concentration 平均血漿濃度
- mecillinam メシリナム
- meperidine, promethazine, chlorpromazine メペリジン・プロメタジン・クロルプロマジン
- middle palmar crease 中位手掌皮膚溝
- minimal mycoplasmacidal concentration 最小マイコプラズマ殺菌濃度
- minimum protozoacidal concentration 最小殺原虫濃度
- mucopurulent cervicitis 粘液膿性子宮頸(管)炎
- murine plasmacytoma ネズミ形質細胞腫

MPCN
- microscopically positive, culturally negative 顕微鏡(的)陽性・培養(的)陰性

MPCUR
- maximal permissible concentration of unidentified radionuclides 未確認放射性核種の最大許容濃度

MPD
- minimal papular dose 最小丘疹量
- minimal phototoxic dose 最小光毒量
- multiple personality disorder 多重人格障害
- muscle phosphorylase deficiency 筋ホスホリラーゼ欠損症
- myeloproliferative disorder 骨髄増殖性疾患
- myofascial pain dysfunction 筋・筋膜疼痛症候群

M.Pd
- Master of Pedagology 足学士

MPD, M.P.D.
maximal permissible dose 最大許容(線)量
MPDS
mandibular pain dysfunction syndrome 下顎骨疼痛症候群
myofascial pain dysfunction syndrome 筋・筋膜疼痛症候群
MPE
malignant pleyral effusion 悪性胸水
maximum permissible exposure 最大露光許容量
MPED
minimal phototoxic erythema dose 最小光毒(性)紅斑(線)量
monopolar electrocoagulation 単極電気凝固
MPEH
methylphenylethylhydantoin メチルフェニルエチルヒダントイン
M period
mitotic period 有糸分裂期間〔周期〕
MPF
maturation promoting factor 卵成熟促進因子
multipurpose food 多目的食品
MPG
magnetopneumography 肺磁図
MPGF
male pronucleus growth factor 雄性前核成長因子
MPGN
membranoproliferative glomerulonephritis 膜(性)増殖性糸球体腎炎
mesangioproliferative glomerulonephritis メサンギウム増殖性糸球体腎炎
MPGN-I
membranoproliferative glomerulonephritis type I 膜性増殖性糸球体腎炎I型
MPGN-II
membranoproliferative glomerulonephritis type II 膜性増殖性糸球体腎炎II型
MPH
male pseudohermaphroditism 男性偽半陰陽
Master of Public Health 公衆衛生学修士
methylphenidate メチルフェニデート
mph
miles per hour マイル/時〈単位〉
MPHA
mixed passive haemagglutination 混合受身凝集法
MPHD
multiple pituitary hormone deficiency 多種下垂体ホルモン欠損症

M

MPHE
Master of Public Health Engineering 公衆衛生工学士
M.Ph.Ed.
Master of Public Health Education 公衆衛生教育学士
M.Phr.
Master of Pharmacy 薬学士
MPHTM
Master of Public Health and Tropical Medicine 公衆衛生・熱帯医学士
MPI
mannose phosphate isomerase マンノースリン酸イソメラーゼ
Maudsley personality inventory モーズレイ性格〔人格〕検査
maximal permitted intake 最大許容摂取量
maximal point of impulse 最大衝動点
minimum pass index 最低合格指数
multiphasic personality inventory 多相性格表
myocardial perfusion imaging 心筋灌流画像
M-pill
menstruation pill 月経丸薬
MPIPC
methylphenylisoxazolylpenicillin メチルフェニルイソキサゾリルペニシリン
oxacillin オキサシリン
MPJ
metacarpophalangeal joint 中手指節関節
metatarsophalangeal joint 中足指節関節
MPL
maximum permissible level 最大許容レベル
melphalan メルファラン
minimum pass level 最低合格水準
MPM
malignant papillary mesothelioma 悪性乳頭状中皮腫
malignant pleural mesothelioma 悪性胸膜中皮腫
multiple primary malignancy 多発性原発性悪性腫瘍
multiple prophylactic management 多併用予防処置
MPN
mesangial proliferative glomerulonephritis メサンギウム性増殖性糸球体腎炎
most probable number 最高確率数値
MPn
mycoplasma pneumonia マイコプラズマ肺炎
MPNST
malignant peripheral nerve sheath tumor 悪性末梢神経鞘腫瘍

M

MPO
maximal pepsin output 最高ペプシン分泌量
medial preoptic area 内側二対体前部
myeloperoxidase ミエロペルオキシダーゼ

MPOD
myeloperoxidase deficiency ミエロペルオキシダーゼ欠乏(症)

MPP
massive periretinal proliferation 高度網膜周囲増殖
maximum perfusion pressure 最大灌流圧
medial pterygoid process 内側翼状突起
mycoplasma pneumonia マイコプラズマ肺炎

MPPCF
million particles per cubic foot 100万粒子/立方フィート〔フート〕

MPPT
methylprednisolone pulse therapy メチルプレドニゾロンパルス療法

MPPV
malignant persistent positional vertigo 悪性持続性頭位眩暈症

MPQ
McGill pain questionnaire マギル痛み性状評価法

MPR
marrow production rate 骨髄産生率
massive preretinal retraction 高度網膜周囲退縮
maximum pulse rate 最大心拍数
multi-planer reconstruction 多断面再構成

6-MPR
6-mercaptopurine ribonucleoside 6-メルカプトプリンリボヌクレオシド

MP-RAGE
magnitude preparation-rapid acqusition gradient echo 高速撮影グラディエントエコー

M protein
monoclonal protein M蛋白
myeloma protein ミエローマ蛋白

MPS
meiosis preventing substance 減数分裂抑制物質
Member of Pharmaceutical Society 製薬協会員
mononuclear phagocyte system 単核性食細胞系
Montreal platelet syndrome モントリオール血小板症候群
movement produced stimuli 運動産生刺激
mucopolysaccharide ムコ多糖類
mucopolysaccharidosis ムコ多糖体症
mucoprotease 粘性蛋白質分解酵素

myeloma progression score 骨髄腫促進得点
myocardial perfusion scintigraphy 心筋灌流シンチグラフィ
myofascial pain syndrome 筋・筋膜疼痛症候群

M.Ps
Master of Psychology 心理学士

MPSW
Master of Psychiatric Social Work 精神科社会学士

MPT
maximum phonation time 最長発声時間
melting point 融点
mixed parotid gland tumor 耳下腺混合腫瘍

mpt
midpoint 中心点，中間点

MPTP
1-methyl-4-phenyl-1,2,3,6-tetrahydropyridine 1-メチル-4-フェニル-1,2,3,6-テトラヒドロピリジン

MPU
Medical Practioners Unit 医療実施者単位
Medical Practitioners Union 開業医連合[英国]
microprocessor unit 超小型演算処理装置

MPV
mean platelet volume 平均血小板体積

mpx，MPX
multiplex 多様な

MQ
maturation quotient 成熟指数
memory quotient 記憶指数

MQRO
Medical Quality Review Organization 医療質的査定機構

MR
Maddox rod マッドクス桿(状)体
Magenresektion〈独〉 胃切除術
magnetic resonance 磁気共鳴
maintenance and repair 維持，修復
mandibular reflex 下顎(骨)反射
mannose-resistant マンノース抵抗性〔耐性〕の
may repeat 繰り返してもよい
measles-rubella 麻疹・風疹
medial rectus muscle 内直筋
median raphe 中央縫合
medical rehabilitation 医学的リハビリテーション
medical representative 医療情報担当者
medicine reaction 薬物反応
Melkersson-Rosenthal (syndrome) メルカーソン・ローゼンタール(症候群)

M

mentally retardate	精神(発達)遅滞児
mentally retarded	精神(発達)遅滞の
mental retardation	精神(発達)遅滞
mesencephalic raphe	中脳縫合
metabolic rate	代謝率
methemoglobin reductase	メトヘモグロビン還元酵素
methyl red	メチルレッド
microelise autoreader	比色定量計
microradiogram	マイクロラジオグラム
microradiography	マイクロラジオグラフィ，超粒子放射線撮影(法)
milk ring (test)	ミルクリング(検査)
miscellaneous report	その他の報告
mitral reflux	僧帽弁逆流
mitral regurgitation	僧帽弁閉鎖不全症
mobile operation room	移動手術室
modulation rate	修飾率，転形〔変調〕率
monthly report	月報
mortality rate	死亡率
mortality ratio	死亡率比
multicentric reticulohistiocytosis	多中心性細網組織球症
multiplication rate	増加率，増殖率
multiplicity reactivation	複数感染再活性化
muscle receptor	筋受容体
muscle relaxant	筋弛緩薬
myotactic reflex	筋伸展反射

Mr

mandible ramus	下顎骨枝
molecular (weight) ratio	分子(量)比

mR

milliroentgen	ミリレントゲン〈単位〉

M.R.×1

may repeat one time	1回繰り返してもよい

m/r

middle right	中央部の右

M & R

measure and record	測定と記録

MRA

magnetic resonance angiography	磁気共鳴血管造影法
malignant rheumatoid arthritis	悪性関節リウマチ
Medical Record Administrator	医学記録管理者，診療記録管理者
melody, rhythm, accent	メロディー・リズム・アクセント
middle rectal artery	中直腸動脈
mitral regurgitant area	僧帽弁逆流面積

MRACP
Member of Royal Australian College of Physicians　オーストラリア医師会員

mrad
millirad　ミリラド〈単位〉

M.Rad
Master of Radiology　放射線学修士

MRAN
medicine resident admit note　内科レジデント入院記録

MRAP
maximal resting anal pressure　最大安静時肛門圧
mean right atrial pressure　平均右(心)房圧

MRAS
main renal artery stenosis　主腎動脈狭窄(症)

MRBC
maternal red blood corpuscle　母赤血球
monkey red blood (receptor)　サル赤血球(受容体)
mouse red blood cell　マウス赤血球

MRBF
mean renal blood flow　平均腎血流量

MRC
magnetic resonance cholangiography　磁気共鳴胆道撮影(法)
Medical Research Center　医学研究センター
Medical Research Corps　医学研究団体
Medical Research Council　医学研究審議会
Medical Reserve Corps　予備軍医団
medullary respiratory chemoceptor　延髄呼吸化学受容器
methyl-rosaniline chloride　塩化メチルロザニリン

MRCC
metastatic renal cell carcinoma　転移性腎細胞癌

MRCLS
mean red cell life span　平均赤血球寿命

MRCNS
methicillin-resistant coagulase-negative Staphylococci　メチシリン耐性コアグラーゼ陰性ブドウ球菌

MRCOG
Member of Royal College of Obstetricians and Gynecologists　王立産婦人科学会会員

MRCP
Member of Royal College of Physicians　王立内科学会会員

MRCPE
Member of Royal College of Physicians of Edinburgh　王立エディンバラ医師会員［英国］

MRCS
Member of Royal College of Surgeons 王立外科学会会員[英国]

MR-CT
magnetic resonance computed tomography 磁気共鳴断層撮影法
magnetic resonance computerized tomography 磁気共鳴コンピュータ画像診断法

MRCU
Medical Research Council Unit 医学研究委員会単位

MRC-UK
Medical Research Council of United Kingdom 英国医学研究委員会

MRCVS
Member of Royal College of Veterinary Surgeons 英国外科獣医師会員

MRD
Medical Record Department 医療記録部門，病歴課
Microbiological Research Department 微生物学研究科
minimal reacting dose 最小反応量
minimal renal disease 微小腎疾患
minimal residual disease 微小残存病変

mrd
millirutherford ミリラザーフォード〈単位〉

M

MRDM
malnutritional related diabetes mellitus 栄養不良関連糖尿病

MRE
manual resistive exercise 徒手抵抗運動
maximal respiratory effectiveness 最大換気有効率
metal responsive element 金属感応成分
Microbiological Research Establishment 微生物学研究施設

MR-E
methemoglobin reductase メトヘモグロビン還元酵素

MREM
milliroentgen equivalent mean ミリレントゲン当量

mrem
millirem ミリレム〈単位〉

MREP
milliroentgen equivalent physical 物理学的ミリレントゲン当量

MRF
medical record file 医事記録ファイル
medical record form 医事記録用紙
melanocyte-releasing factor メラニン細胞放出因子

melanocyte-stimulating hormone-releasing factor メラニン細胞刺激ホルモン放出因子
mesencephalic reticular formation 中脳網様体
midbrain reticular formation 中脳網様体
mitral regurgitant flow 僧帽弁逆流量
moderate renal failure 中等度腎不全
monoclonal rheumatoid factor モノクローナルリウマチ因子
müllerian regression factor ミュラー(管)退行因子

MRFC
mouse rosette-forming cells マウスロゼット形成細胞

MRFIT
Multiple Risk Factor Intervention Trial 多種因子介入的研究(=高血圧治療に関する大規模試験)

mrg
margin 辺縁
marginal 辺縁の

MRH
melanocyte stimulating hormone releasing hormone メラニン細胞刺激ホルモン放出ホルモン

MRHA
mannose-resistant hemagglutination マンノース抵抗性(赤)血球凝集(反応)

mrhm
milliroentgen per hour at one meter ミリレントゲン/時/メートル

mr/hr
milliroentgen per hour ミリレントゲン/時

MRI
magnetic resonance imaging 磁気共鳴映像法
Mental Research Institute 精神研究施設
mitral regurgitation index 僧帽弁逆流指数
moderate renal insufficiency 中等度腎不全

M.R.I.
Medical Record Librarian 医学文献司書

MRIF
medium resolution infrared 平均分解赤外線
melanocyte-stimulating hormone release-inhibiting factor メラニン細胞刺激ホルモン放出抑制因子

MRIH
melanocyte stimulating hormone release-inhibiting hormone メラニン細胞刺激ホルモン放出抑制ホルモン

M & R I & O
measure and record intake and output 摂取量と排泄量を測定・記録(せよ)

MRIS
Medical Research Information System | 医学研究情報システム

MRK
Mayer-Rokitansky-Küster (syndrome) | MRK症候群

mrkr
marker | 印，マーカー

MRL
medical record library | 病歴室
medical records librarian | 病歴士，病歴保管者

MRM
magnetic resonance mammography | 磁気共鳴マンモグラフィ
measles, rubella, mumps | 麻疹・風疹・流行性耳下腺炎
modified radical mastectomy | 非定型的乳房切除術

MRN
macroregenerative nodule | 大再生結節
malignant renal neoplasm | 悪性腎新生物

mRNA
messenger ribonucleic acid | 情報伝達リボ核酸，メッセンジャーRNA

MRP
mean resting potential | 平均静止電位
migration inhibitory factor-related protein | 遊走阻止因子関連蛋白

MRR
marrow release rate | 骨髄放出率
maximal relaxation rate | 最大弛緩率
medical research reactor | 医療研究用加速器

MRS
magnetic resonance spectroscopy | (核)磁気スペクトロスコピー
Melkersson-Rosenthal syndrome | メルカーソン・ローゼンタール症候群
methicillin-resistant *Staphylococcus aureus* | メチシリン耐性黄色ブドウ球菌

MRSA
methicillin resistant *Staphylococcus aureus* | メチシリン耐性黄色ブドウ球菌

MRSE
methicillin-resistant *Staphylococcus epidermidis* | メチシリン耐性表皮ブドウ球菌

MRSH
Member of Royal Society of Health | 王立健康協会員［英国］

MRSI
magnetic resonance spectroscopic imaging | 磁気共鳴分光画像(法)

M

MRSM

Member of Royal Society of Medicine	王立医学会員[英国]

MRT

magnetic resonance tomogrphy	磁気共鳴断層撮影法
mean radiant temperature	平均輻射温度
mean residence time	平均滞留時間
median reaction time	50%反応時間
median recognition threshold	50%認識閾値
medical records technology	医療記録技術
milk-ring test	ミルクリング検査《検査》
muscle response test	筋反応検査〔試験〕

MR test

milk ring test	ミルクリング検査〔試験〕

MRU

minimal reproductive units	最小繁殖単位

MRUS

maximum rate of urea synthesis	最大尿素合成率

MRV

minute respiratory volume	毎分呼吸量
mixed respiratory vaccine	混合呼吸器ワクチン

MRVP

mean right ventricular pressure	平均右(心)室圧

MR-VP

methyl red and Voges-Proskauer broth	メチルレッド・フォーゲス・プロスカウエル反応用ブイヨン

MS

main stream	主流煙
manuscript	論文
margin of safety	安全域
Marie-Strümpell (disease)	マリー・シュトリュンペル(病)
mass spectrometry	質量分析法
mass spectrum	質量分析
maxillary sinus	上顎洞
maximum stress	最大刺激
mechanical stimulation	機械的刺激
medial sacral artery	正中仙骨動脈
mediastinal shift	縦隔移動
Medical Specialist Corps	専門医団体
medical student	医学生
medical survey	医学的調査
Ménière syndrome	メニエール症候群
mental status	精神状態
meso	中(間部), メゾ型

M

metabolic syndrome	メタボリックシンドローム
methionine-sulfoximine	メチオニン・スルホキシミン
microscope slide	顕微鏡スライド
Mikulicz syndrome	ミクリッツ症候群
mitral sound	僧帽雑音
mitral stenosis	僧帽弁狭窄症
modal sensitivity	様相感受性
mol solution	モル液
mongolian spot	蒙古斑
morning stiffness	朝のこわばり
morphine sulfate	硫酸モルヒネ
motion sensitivity	運動感受性
multiple sclerosis	多発性硬化症
muscle strength	筋力
musculoskeletal	骨格筋の

Ms

manuscript	原稿
murmurs	雑音
muscles	筋，筋肉

ms

millisecond	ミリ秒
miscellaneous	その他

MS Ⅲ

fourth-year medical student	第 4 学年医学生

M

MS Ⅳ

third-year medical student	第 3 学年医学生

M.S.

Master of Surgery	外科学修士

m.s.

mano sistra〈ラ〉	左手
more solito〈ラ〉=in the usual manner	常法で《処》

M/S

meters per second	メートル/秒〈単位〉

M & S

Medicine and Surgery	内科と外科

MSA

major serologic antigen	主(要)血清学的抗原
male specific antigen	男性〔雄〕特異的抗原
medical short appointment	診療短時間予約
membrane-stabilizing action	膜安定化作用
membrane-stabilizing activity	膜安定化活性
membranous septal aneurysm	膜性中隔動脈瘤
mouse serum albumin	マウス血清アルブミン
multiple system atrophy	多系統萎縮症
multiplication-stimulating activity	増殖刺激活性体
muscle sympathetic nerve activity	筋の交感神経の活動

MSAA
multiple sclerosis-associated agent　多発性硬化症関連因子
MS-Ag
membrane soluble antigen　膜可溶化抗原
mSAP, MSAP
mean systemic arterial pressure　平均全身動脈圧
MSB
Martius-Scarlet-blue　マチス・スカーレットブルー
MSBLA
mouse-specific B lymphocyte antigen　マウス特異的Bリンパ球抗原
MSBOS
maximum surgical blood order schedule　最大手術血液準備量
MSBP
Münchhausen syndrome by proxy　代理ミュンヒハウゼン症候群
MSC
Medical Service Corps　医療奉仕団
mesenchymal stromal cells　間葉系間質細胞
mid-systolic click　収縮中期クリック
MSCA
McCarthy Scales of Children's Abilities　マッカーシー小児能力尺度
MSCLC
mouse stem cell-like cell　マウス幹細胞様細胞
M.Sc.Ost
Master of Science in Osteopathy　骨疾患研究学士
mscp
mean spherical candle power　平均球面燭光
MSD
Master of Scientific Diagnostics　科学的診断学士
mean survival days　平均生存日数
Medical Science Doctor　医学士
multiple sulfatase deficiency　多種スルファターゼ欠損症
MSDA
monorhythmic sinusoidal δ-activity　単調洞性デルタ波
M.S.Dent
Master of Science of Dentistry　歯科学士
M.S.Derm
Master of Science in Dermatology　皮膚科学士
MSDI
Martin S-D (suicide-depression) Inventory　マーティン自殺うつ病調査票
MSDOS, MS-DOS
Microsoft Disk Operating System　マイクロソフト社のOS《コン》

MSDS
material safety data sheets　化学物質安全性データシート

MSE
Meerschweinchen Einheit〈独〉　モルモット単位
mental status examination　精神状態検査

mse
mean square error　平均二乗誤差《統》

msec
millisecond　ミリ秒〈単位〉

MSEG
mean systolic ejection gradient　収縮期平均駆出勾配

MSEL
myasthenic syndrome of Eaton-Lambert　イートン・ランバートの筋無力症症候群

m.seq.
mane sequenti〈ラ〉　翌朝《処》

MSER
mean systolic ejection rate　平均収縮期駆出速度
Mental Status Examination Record　精神状態検査記録

MSES
medical school environmental stress　医学校環境ストレス

MSF
macrophage-spreading factor　マクロファージ拡散因子
mean systolic force　平均駆出力
Médecins Sans Frontières〈仏〉　国境なき医師団
Mediterranean spotted fever　地中海斑点熱
melanocyte-stimulating factor　メラニン細胞刺激因子
methanesulfonyl fluoride　メタンスルホニルフルオリド
migration-stimulating factor　遊走刺激因子
muscle shock factor　筋ショック因子

MSFA
maximum shunt flow area　最大シャント血流面積

MSFAI
maximum shunt flow area index　最大シャント血流面積係数

MSG
monosodium glutamate〈ラ〉　グルタミン酸ナトリウム

MSH
Master of Science in Hygiene　衛生学士
melanocyte stimulating hormone　メラニン細胞刺激ホルモン
melanophore stimulating hormone　メラニン細胞刺激ホルモン

MSHA
mannose-sensitive hemagglutination　マンノース感受性(赤)血球凝集(反応)
Master of Science in Hospital Administration　病院管理学士

MSHRF
melancocyte-stimulating hormone-releasing factor　メラニン細胞刺激ホルモン放出因子
MSH-RIF
melanocyte-stimulating hormone release-inhibiting factor　メラニン細胞刺激ホルモン放出抑制因子
MSHSC
multiple self-healing squamous carcinoma　多発性自己癒合性扁平上皮癌
MSI
magnetic source imaging　磁気画像(診断)法
medium scale integrated circuit　中規模集積回路
microbial safety index　微生物学的安全指数
mitral stenoinsufficiency　僧帽弁狭窄閉鎖不全(症)
mitral stenosis index　僧帽弁狭窄指数
MSIS
micromolecular substance having both irritating and sensitizing properties　刺激性および感作原性低分子物質
MSK
medullary sponge kidney　髄質性海綿腎
MSKCC
Memorial Sloan-Kettering Cancer Center　スローン・ケタリング記念癌センター
MSL
midsternal line　胸骨中線
mittelere Sprachstimmlage〈独〉　中間会話声域
multiple symmetric lipomatosis　多発性対称性脂肪腫症
MSLA
mouse-specific lymphocyte antigen　マウス特異的リンパ球抗原
MSLR
mixed skin (cell) leukocyte reaction　混合性皮膚(細胞)白血球反応
MSLT
multiple sleep latency test　睡眠潜時反復検査
M.S.Med
Master of Medical Science　医学士
MSN
main sensory nucleus　主知覚核
Master of Science in Nursing Major　看護学修士
medial septal nucleus　内側中隔核
M.S.N
Master of Science in Nursing　看護学士
M.S.N.Ed
Master of Science in Nursing Education　看護教育学士

M

MSO
Managed Service Organization　経営サービス組織
MSOF
multiple systemic organ failure　系統的多臓器失調
M.S.Opthal
Master of Opthalmological Surgery　眼外科学士
M.S.Ortho
Master of Orthopedic Surgery　整形外科学士
MSP
multiple signal processer　複合信号処理器
Münchausen syndrome by proxy　代理ミュンヒハウゼン症候群
Msp
muscle spasm　筋痙攣
M.S.P
Master of Science in Pharmacy　薬学士
MSpC
Medical Specialist Corps　専門医団体
MSPD
matrix solid-phase dispersion　マトリックス固相分散(法)《統》
MSPE, M.S.P.E.
Master of Science in Physical Education　医学教育学士
MSPGN
mesangial proliferative glomerulonephritis　メサンギウム増殖性糸球体腎炎
MSPH
Master of Science in Public Health　公衆衛生学士
MSPHE
Master of Science in Public Health Education　公衆衛生教育学士
Master of Science in Public Health Engineering　公衆衛生工学士
MSQ
Mental Status Questionnaire　精神状態質問表
Minnesota Satisfaction Questionnaire　ミネソタ満足度質問表《心理》
MSR
mitral stenosis and regurgitation　僧帽弁狭窄閉鎖不全(症)
monosynaptic reflex　単シナプス反射
M.S.Rd
Master of Science in Radiology　放射線科学士
MSRM
mucoid, smooth, rough mutation　粘液・均一性・粗糙変異
MSRPP
multidimensional scale for rating psychiatric patients　多面人格尺度

MS-RTP
micelle-stabilized room-temperature phosphorescence　ミセル安定化室温リン光
MSS
Marinesco-Sjögren syndrome　マリネスコ・シェーグレン症候群
Marshall-Smith syndrome　マーシャル・スミス症候群
massage　マッサージ
mass storage system　大容量記憶装置
Minnesota Satisfactoriness Scales　ミネソタ満足度尺度
minor surgery suite　小手術服
motion sickness susceptibility　動揺病感受性
mucus-stimulating substance　粘液刺激物質
multiple sclerosis susceptibility　多発性硬化症感受性
muscular subaortic stenosis　筋性大動脈弁下部狭窄(症)
Mss, MSS
manuscript　論文
MSSA
methicillin-sensitive *Staphylococcus aureus*　メチシリン感受性黄色ブドウ球菌
M.S.Sc
Master of Sanitary Science　衛生学士
MS Scale
manic-state rating scale　躁状態評価尺度
MSSG
multiple sclerosis susceptibility gene　多発性硬化症感受性遺伝子
MSSPPD
Modified subtotal stomach -presserving pancreaticoduodenectomy　改良型亜全胃温存膵頭十二指腸切除術
MSSVD
Medical Society for Study of Veneral Disease　性病研究医学協会
MST
maximal stimulation test　最大刺激検査
mean survival time　平均生存期間
mean swell time　平均腫脹時間
median survival time　50%生存時間
mst
measurement　測定
MStF
migration stimulation factor　遊走刺激因子
MSTh
mesotherium　メゾトリウム〈元素〉
MSTI
multiple soft tissue injuries　多発性軟部組織損傷

M stim
muscle stimulation 筋(肉)刺激
M str
muscle strength 筋力
MSU
maple syrup urine メープルシロップ尿
midstream specimen of urine 中間尿検体
midstream urine specimen 中間尿試料
monosodium urate 尿酸塩
MSUD
maple syrup urine disease メープルシロップ尿病
MSV
maximal secretion volume 最高胃液分泌量
maximum spatial vector 空間最大ベクトル
Moloney sarcoma virus モロニー肉腫ウイルス
mouse sarcoma virus マウス肉腫ウイルス
murine sarcoma virus ネズミ肉腫ウイルス
MSVC
maximum sustained ventilatory capacity 最大持続換気量
MSVM
murine sarcoma virus Moloney モロニーネズミ肉腫ウイルス
MSW
medical social worker 医療ソーシャルワーカー
multiple stab wounds 多刺創
MSWD
married, single, widowed, divorced 既婚・未婚・寡婦・離婚
married, single, widowed, divorced 結婚している・独身の・やもめの・離婚した

MT
empty からっぽ
Magentube〈独〉 胃チューブ
magnetic tape 磁気テープ
malaria therapy マラリア療法
malignant teratoma 悪性奇形腫
mamillothalamic tract 乳頭体視床路
mammary tumor 乳房腫瘍
manual traction 用手牽引
mean transit time computer 平均循環時間測定装置
medial thalamus 内側視床，視床内側部
medical technician 臨床検査技師
medical technologist 臨床検査技師
medical treatment 医療
membrana tympani〈ラ〉 鼓膜
mesangial thickening メサンギウム肥厚
metallothionein メタロチオネイン

metatarsal 中足(骨)の
methoxytryptamine メトキシトリプタミン
methyltyrosine メチルチロシン
microtome ミ〔マイ〕クロトーム
microtubule 微小管
Milieutherapie〈独〉 環境療法，作業療法
minimum threshold 最小閾値
minor tremor 微細振動
mitotic time 有糸分裂時間
Muir–Torre (syndrome) ミュア・トール(症候群)
Mundtherapie〈独〉 ムンテラ
muscles and tendons 筋(肉)と腱
muscle test 筋(肉)検査
music therapy 音楽療法

mt.
mitte〈ラ〉 送れ《処》

3-MT
3-methoxytyramine 3-メトキシチラミン

MT-6
mercaptomerin メルカプトメリン

M & T
Monilia and *Trichomonas* モニリア(＝カンジダ)とトリコモナス

M-T
macroglobulin-trypsin (complex) マクログロブリン・トリプシン(複合体)

mt, MT
mitochondria ミトコンドリア

MTA
anaplastic malignant teratoma 未分化悪性奇形腫
mammary tumor agent 乳房腫瘍因子
medical technology assessment 医療における技術評価
metatarsus adductus 内転中足(症)

MTAD
membrana tympana auris dextre〈ラ〉 右耳鼓膜

MTAg
mite antigen ダニ抗原

MTAI
Minnesota Teacher Attitude Inventory ミネソタ教師態度調査票《心理》

MTAS
membrana tympana auris sinistrae〈ラ〉 左耳鼓膜

MTASCP
Medical Technologist of American Society of Chemical Pathologists 米国化学病理学者協会の医学技術者

MTAU
membrana tympana auris unitae〈ラ〉 両耳鼓膜
MTB
Mycobacterium tuberculosis 結核菌，ヒト(型)結核菌
MTBA
maximum total bile acids 最高総胆汁酸
MT bar
metatarsal bar 中足骨バー
MTBF
mean time between failure 平均故障時間
MTBFL
meantime between function loss 機能喪失平均時間
MTBM
meantime between maintenance 維持平均時間
MTC
maximum tolerated concentration 最大許容濃度
maximum toxic concentration 最大中毒濃度
Medical Training Center 医学訓練センター
medullary thyroid carcinoma 甲状腺髄様癌
methacycline メタサイクリン
microwave tissue coagulation マイクロ波による組織凝血
mitomycin C マイトマイシンC
multilocular thymic cyst 多房性胸腺嚢胞
MTD
maximal tolerated dose 最大耐用量
metastatic trophoblastic disease 転移性栄養膜疾患
minimum toxic dose 最小中毒
Monroe tidal drainage モンロー還流排液法
multiple tic disorder 多発性チック疾患
mtd, m.t.d.
mitte tales doses〈ラ〉 同量を送れ《処》
MTDDA
Minnesota Test for the Differential Diagnosis of Aphasia ミネソタ失語鑑別診断検査〔試験〕
mtDNA
mitochondria deoxyribonucleic acid ミトコンドリアデオキシリボ核酸
MTDT
methylthiadiazole thiol メチルチアジアゾールチオール
MTE
medical toxic environment 医学的中毒性環境
MTF
modulation transfer function 空間周波数特性
MTFase
methyltransferase メチル基転移酵素

MTg
mouse thyroglobulin マウスチ〔サイ〕ログロブリン
MTH
mammotropic hormone 乳腺刺激ホルモン
mithramycin ミトラマイシン
mth
month(s) 月
M-Thy
mature thymocyte 成熟胸腺細胞
MTI
mammary tumor inciter 乳癌刺激物
minimum time interval 最小時間間隔
moving target indicator 移動標的指示薬
6-MTI
6-methylthioinosine 6-メチルチオイノシン
MTJ
midtarsal joint 横足根関節
MTL
minimum toxicity line 最小レベルの毒性ライン
mtl
material 材料
monatlich〈独〉 毎月
MTLP
metabolic toxemia of late pregnancy 晩期妊娠代謝性中毒症
MTM
minor tooth movement マイナー・トゥース・ムーブメント
mithramycin ミトラマイシン
mt mRNA
mitochondrial messenger RNA ミトコンドリアメッセンジャーRNA
mtn
motion 運動，行動，動き
MTO C
mitomycin C マイトマイシンC
MTP
maximum tolerated pressure 最大耐性
meet to professor 教授面接
metatarsophalangeal 中足指節の
metatarsophalangeal joint 中足指節関節
microtubule protein 微小管蛋白
muramyl tripeptide ムラミルペプチド
MTQ
metolquizolone メトルキゾロン

M

MTR
Meinicke Trübungsreaktion〈独〉= Meinicke turbidity reaction　マイニッケ混濁反応
MTR-0
no masses, tenderness or rebound　腫瘤・圧痛・反跳圧痛なし
mt rRNA
mitochondrial ribosomal RNA　ミトコンドリアリボソーム RNA
MTS
medial tibial syndrome　内側脛骨症候群
mesial temporal sclerosis　近心側頭硬化症
microtubular structure　細管状構造体
microtubular system　微小管
modified Tyrode solution　改良タイロード液
MTSS
medial tibial stress syndrome　内側脛骨ストレス症候群
MTST
maximal treadmill stress test　最大トレッドミルストレス検査
MTT
3-(4,5-dimethylthiazol)-2,5-diphenyl-tetrazolium bromide　ジメチルチアゾールジフェニルテトラゾリウム臭酸塩
malignant trophoblastic teratoma　悪性栄養膜奇形腫
maximal treadmill testing　最大トレッドミル検査
mean tidal time　平均呼吸時間
mean transit time　脳平均通過時間
mt tRNA
mitochondrial transfer RNA　ミトコンドリア転移RNA
MTU
Medical Therapy Unit　医学治療ユニット
methylthiouracil　メチルチオウラシル
M tuberc., M.tuberc
Mycobacterium tuberculosis　ヒト(型)結核菌
MTV
metatarsus varus　内反中足(症)
Mtv, MTV
mammary tumor virus　乳腺腫瘍ウイルス
MTX
methotrexate　メトトレキサート
MTZ
metronidazole　メトロニダゾール
MU
Mache unit　マッヘ単位
maternal uncle　母方の叔父
motor unit　運動単位
mouse unit　マウス単位

mU
milliunit ミリ単位
mu
micron ミクロン
0-mu
anucleolate mutation 無核突然変異
4-MU
4-methylumbelliferone 4-メチルウンベリフェロン
MUA
middle uterine artery 中子宮動脈
multiple unit activity 多様活動性
M.u.A., m.u.a
morgen und abend〈独〉 朝と夕方《処》
MUAP
motor nunit action potential 運動単位活動電位
MUC
maximum urinary concentration 最大尿(中)濃度
mucilago〈ラ〉 漿剤, 粘滑薬
mucosal ulcerative colitis 粘膜性潰瘍性大腸炎
muc
mucinous adenocarcinoma 粘液性腺癌
mucoid ムコイド(の), (類)粘液(状の)
mucous 粘液(性)の
mucus 粘液
muco-pur
mucopurulent 粘液(化)膿(性)の
MUD
minimal urticarial dose 最小蕁麻疹量
morphologically unexplained death 形態的死因不明死
MUE
motor unit estimated 推定運動単位
MUF
maximum usable frequency 最大使用可能周波数
mul.inj
multiple injuries 多発性外傷〔損傷〕
mult
multiple 多発(性)の
multiplication 増殖, 掛け算
multip., Multip
multipara 経産婦
multiparous 経産婦の
multivits
multivitamins 混合ビタミン
MuLV, MULV
murine (complex) leukemia virus ネズミ(複合)白血病ウイルス

MUMPS
Massachusetts General Hospital Utility Multi-Programming System　マンプス(=マサチューセッツ総合病院式医療コンピュータ言語)

MuMTV
murine mammary tumor virus　ネズミ乳腺腫瘍ウイルス

MUO
myocardiopathy of unknown origin　未知の原因による心筋症

MUP
maximal urethral pressure　最大尿道圧
motor unit potential　運動単位電位

MUPK
medizinische Universität Poliklinik〈独〉　医科大学の外来診療

Mur
muramic acid　ムラミン酸

mur
muriaticus〈ラ〉　塩酸の《処》

MurNAc
N-acethylmuramate　*N*-アセチルムラミン酸
N-acetylmuramic acid　*N*-アセチルムラミン酸

MuS
musculo-skeletal　筋骨格の

M

musc
muscle　筋，筋肉
muscular　筋(性)の

musc.ligt
musculoligamentous　筋，靱帯の

mus-lig
musculoligamentous　筋，靱帯の

MUST
self-contained and transportable medical unit　自己内蔵・運搬可能な医療器械

mustrgen
mustard nitrogen　ニトロゲンマスタード

mut
mutilated　断節された
mutilation　断節

MUU
mouse uterine unit　マウス子宮単位

MUW
mouse uterine weight　マウス子宮重量

MUWU
mouse uterine weight unit　マウス子宮重量単位

mux
multiplex　複合の，多様な

MV
main venule 主細静脈
mean variation 平均的変化
measles virus 麻疹ウイルス
meat and vegetable 肉と野菜
mechanical ventilation 機械的肺換気法
megavolt メガボルト〈単位〉
meningovascular 髄膜脈管の，髄膜血管の
microvesicle 微小嚢胞《電顕》
microvibration 微細振動
microvilli 微小絨毛
minute ventilation 毎分換気量
minute volume 分時量
mitral valve 僧帽弁，M弁
mitral valvuloplasty 僧帽弁開大術
mixed venous 混合静脈の
monochromatic vision 単色視
multivesicular 多小胞(性)の，多小水疱(性)の

Mv
mendelevium メンデレビウム〈元素〉

M.V.
medicus veterinarius〈ラ〉 獣医

mV，MV
millivolt ミリボルト〈単位〉

MVA
mechanical ventilatory assistance 機械的換気補助
mevalonic acid メバロン酸
mitral valve area 僧帽弁弁口面積
motor vehicle accident 自動車事故，交通事故

MVAC，M-VAC
methotrexate, vinblastine, adriamycin, cisplatin メトトレキサート，ビンブラスチン，アドリアマイシン，シスプラチン

MVB
multivesicular body 多小胞体，多小水疱体

MVC
maximal voluntary contraction 最大随意(的)収縮

mVCF
mean velocity of circumferential 円周平均速度

MVD
Marburg virus disease マールブルグウイルス病
microvascular decompression 微小血管減圧術
mitral valve disease 僧帽弁疾患
mouse vas deferens マウス精管

M

MVDDR
diastolic descent rate of the mitral valve＝mitral valve diastolic descent rate　僧帽弁(拡張期)後退速度

MVE
mitral valve excursion　僧帽弁可動域
Murray Valley encephalitis　マリー・バレー脳炎

MvEC
human microvascular endothelial cell　ヒト微小血管内皮細胞

MVG
mitral valve gradient　僧帽弁口圧勾配
myodil ventriculography　マイオジール脳室撮影

MV gard
mitral valve gradient　僧帽弁口圧勾配

MVH
massive variceal hemorrhage　大量静脈瘤出血
massive vitreous hemorrhage　大量硝子体出血
methotrexate, VP-16, hexamethylonelamine　メトトレキサート，エトポシド，ヘキサメチロネラミン
murine viral hepatitis　マウス肝炎

MVI
multi-vitamin infusion　複合ビタミン輸液

MVII
Minnesota Vocational Interest Inventory　ミネソタ職業興味調査票

M

MVM
microvillose membrane　微小絨毛膜

MVMT
movement　運動

MVN
medial vestibular nucleus　前庭神経核の内側核

MVO
maximum venous oxygen saturation　最大静脈酸素飽和
mitral valve orifice　僧帽弁口

mVO_2
minute venous oxygen consumption　分時静脈血酸素消費量

MVO_2，$M\dot{V}O_2$
maximal venous oxygen consumption　最大静脈血酸素消費量
mean venous oxygen content　平均静脈血酸素量
myocardial oxygen (volume) consumption　心筋酸素消費量

MVOA
mitral valve orifice area　僧帽弁口野(部)

MVOS
mixed venous oxygen saturation　混合静脈酸素飽和

MVP
maximum voluntary pressure 最高随意圧
microvascular pressure 微小血管圧
mitomycin, vinblastine, cisplatin (= Platinol) マイトマイシン,ビンブラスチン,シスプラチン(=プラチノール)
mitral valve prolapse (syndrome) 僧帽弁逸脱症候群

MVPP
mechlorethamine, vinblastine, procarbazine, prednisone メクロルエタミン,ビンブラスチン,プロカルバジン,プレドニゾン
6-mercaptopurine, vinblastine, procarbazine, prednisolone 6-メルカプトプリン,ビンブラスチン,プロカルバジン,プレドニゾロン
mustine, vinblastine, procarbazine, prednisone ムスチン,ビンブラスチン,プロカルバジン,プレドニゾン

MVPS
mitral valve prolapse syndrome 僧帽弁逸脱症候群

MVR
massive vitreous retraction 高度硝子体牽引
maximum voiding rate 最高排尿速度
microvascular research 微小血管研究
mitral valve replacement 僧帽弁置換術
mitral valve ring 僧帽弁輪
multiple valve replacement 多(数)弁置換(術)

MVRI
mixed vaccine respiratory infections 呼吸器感染に対する多種ワクチン

MVS
mitral valve stenosis 僧帽弁狭窄症

MV-SV
mitral valve-semilunar valve 僧帽弁・半月弁

mvt
movement 運動

MVV
maximum voluntary ventilation 分時最大呼吸量

MVV1
maximal ventilatory volume 最大換気量

MVVPP
mechlorethamine, vincristine, vinblastine, procarbazine, prednisone メクロルエタミン,ビンクリスチン,ビンブラスチン,プロカルバジン,プレドニゾン

MW
Mallory-Weiss (syndrome) マロリー・ワイス(症候群)

mean weight 平均重量
medical waste 医療用廃棄物
microwave マイクロ波
midwife 助産師
molecular weight 分子量

mW
milliwatt ミリワット〈単位〉

M-W
men and women 男性と女性

mW, M.W
Meterwinkel〈独〉 メートル角

m wave
Müller cell activity ミュラー細胞活動，m波

MWCO
molecular weight cutoff 分子量限界

MWD
microwave diathermy マイクロウェーブジアテルミー
molecular weight distribution 分子量分布

10 MWD
ten minutes walking distance 平地を10分間歩行させて最大に歩行できる距離

MWFT
microwave Fourier transform spectroscopy フーリエ変換型マイクロ波分光(計)

MWIA
Medical Women International Association 国際女医協会

MWM
modality worklist management モダリティ・ワークリスト管理

MWN
Medical World News 医学会新聞

MWS
Mallory-Weiss syndrome マロリー・ワイス症候群
Marden-Walker syndrome マーデン・ウォーカー症候群
Mickety-Wilson sndrome ミケティ・ウィルソン症候群
Moersch-Woltman syndrome メルシュ・ヴォルトマン症候群

MWT
myocardial wall thickness 心筋壁肥厚

MWt
molecular weight 分子量

6MWT
six minutes walking test 6分間歩行テスト

M

MX
matrix 基質，母質，マトリックス
mexiletine メキシレチン
Mx
maxwell マクスウェル
minoxidil ミノキシジル
mxd
mixed 混合した，雑多な，異種族間の
MXP
methotrexate prednisone メトトレキサート・プレドニゾン
MXR
mass X-ray 集検用X線
MY
myelocyte 骨髄球
myopia 近視
My
myxedematous 粘液水腫の
MY，My
mayer マイヤー<単位>
My-A
myeloid antigen 骨髄球抗原
My-Ag
myeloid antigen 骨髄球抗原
MyaR
myasthenic reaction 筋無力性反応
Mybl
myeloblast 骨髄芽球
myc
myelocytomatosis 骨髄細胞腫症
Myco
Mycobacterium マイコバクテリウム(属)
Mycol
mycology (真)菌学
MyD，MYD
myotonic (muscular) dystrophy (筋)緊張性ジストロフィ
Myel
myelocyte 骨髄球
myel
myelin ミエリン，髄鞘
myelinated 有髄の
myelogram 脊髄造影図
myeloid 骨髄の，骨髄球様の
myelology 骨髄学

Myelo
myelography 脊髄腔造影(法)
myelo
myelocyte 骨髄球
myel.sched.
myelogram scheduled 脊髄造影図予約済み
MyG
myasthenia gravis 重症筋無力症
MYH11
myosin heavy chain ミオシン重鎖
Myl
myeloblast 骨髄芽球
mylo
mylohyoid 顎舌骨の
MyMD
myotonic muscular dystrophy 筋緊張性ジストロフィ
myo
myocardial 心筋(層)の
myocardium 心筋(層)
myocard
myocardial 心筋(層)の
myocardium 心筋(層)
myo inf
myocardial infarction 心筋梗塞
myol
myology 筋学
myoma
myoma uteri 子宮筋腫
myop
myopia 近視
MyoR
myotonic reaction 筋強直反応
Myringo
myringoplasty 鼓膜形成手術
MYS
myasthenic syndrome 筋無力(症)症候群
MYX
myxoma 粘液腫
MZ
mantle zone 外套層
megaheltz メガヘルツ
mezlocillin メズロシリン
monozygotic 一卵性の
monozygotic twins 一卵性双生児
MZL
mantle zone lymphoma 外套帯リンパ腫

marginal zone lymphocyte 辺縁領域リンパ球

MZPC

mezlocillin メズロシリン

MZR

mizoribine ミゾリビン

N n

N

asparagine	アスパラギン
haploid chromosome number	半数染色体数
loudness	音の大きさ
lymph node metastasis	リンパ節転移
Nähte〈独〉	縫合
Necator	ネカトール(属)
negative	陰性の
Negro	黒人
Neisseria	ナイセリア(属)
Nem	ネム
neomycin	ネオマイシン
neural	中性の
neuraminidase	ノイラミニダーゼ
neurogenic factor	神経因子
neurologist	神経内科医，神経学専門医
neurology	神経学
neuropathy	神経障害，ニューロパシー
Neurose〈独〉＝neurosis	神経症
neutrophil	好中球
newton	ニュートン〈単位〉
niche	ニッシェ，壁の凹み
nicotinamide	ニコチンアミド
nicotine	ニコチン
Nitrobacter	ニトロバクター(属)
nitrogen	窒素
Nocardia	ノカルジア(属)
node	結節
nodule	小結節
none	なし，無
non(-)malignant	非悪性の(腫瘍)，良性の(腫瘍)
Nonne (globulin test)	ノンネ(グロブリン試験)
Nonne test	ノンネテスト
noon	昼，正午
nucleoside	ヌクレオシド
nucleus	核
regional lymph nodes metastasis	所属リンパ節転移

n

index of refraction	屈折率
mean value of n	平均数
nano	ナノ($=10^{-9}$)〈接〉〈単位〉
neutron	中性子

new　新しい
night　夜
normal　正常，規定
nuclear　核の
unit of neutron dosage　中性子線量の単位

^{13}N
nitrogen-13　窒素13

^{15}N
nitrogen-15　重窒素

N，*N*
Avogadro constant〔number〕　アボガドロ(定)数

N，n
nasal　鼻の
nerve　神経
normal　正常，規定
number　番号，数

N，n.
natus〈ラ〉　生来の，先天的な
naris〈ラ〉　外鼻孔
nervus〈ラ〉＝nerve　神経
numerus〈ラ〉＝number　番号，数

N(＋)0-4，N(−)0-4
degree of lymph node metastasis　肉眼的癌リンパ節転移有無程度
lymph node metastasis　肉眼的癌リンパ節転移の程度

n(＋)0-4，n(−)0-4
degree of lymph node metastasis　病理組織学的リンパ節有無程度
lymph node metastasis　病理組織学的リンパ節転移の程度

NA
nalidixic acid　ナリジクス酸
narcotics anonymous〈ラ〉　無名麻薬中毒者
nasal allergy　鼻アレルギー
necrotizing angitis　壊死性血管炎
negative attitude　否定的態度
Negro adult　黒人の成人
neuraminidase　ノイラミニダーゼ
neurologic age　神経学的年齢
neurotic anonymous〈ラ〉　無名神経病者
neutralizing antibody　中和抗体
neutrophil antibody　好中球抗体
no abnormalities　異常なし
nomina anatomica〈ラ〉　解剖学用語
nonalcoholic　非アルコール性の
nonamnionic〔nonamniotic〕　非羊膜の，非羊水の

Nonne-Apelt reaction　ノンネ・アペルト反応
noradrenalin　ノルアドレナリン
not antagonized　拮抗されない
not applicable　適応できない，適切でない
not appropriated　適切でない
not attempted　試みられない
not authorized　認定されていない
not available　利用できない
nuclear antigen　核抗原
nucleic acid　核酸
nucleus accumbens〈ラ〉　側坐核
nucleus ambiguus　(神経)疑核
numerical aperture　開口数
nurse aide　看護助手

Na
Avogadro number〔constant〕　アボガドロ数(定数)
natrium　ナトリウム〈元素〉
sodium　ソジウム(＝ナトリウム)

na, n.a.
non altera〈ラ〉＝no alternative　他法をとるべからず《処》

NAA
α-naphthaleneacetic acid　αナフタレン酢酸
N-acetylarginine　*N*-アセチルアルギニン
N-acetylaspartate　*N*-アセチルアスパラギン酸塩
natural anti-tumor antibody　抗腫瘍自然抗体
neutral amino acid　中性アミノ酸
neutron activation analysis　ニュートロン放射化分析
nicotin(ic) acid amide　ニコチン酸アミド
no apparent abnormalities　はっきりした異常なし

NAAP
N-acetyl-4-aminoantipyrine　*N*-アセチル-4-アミノアンチピリン

NAB
novarsenobenzol　ノバルセノベンゾール

NABA
non-atopic bronchial asthma　非アトピー性喘息

NaBr
sodium bromide　臭化ナトリウム

NAC
accessory nucleus　副神経核
N-acetyl-L-cysteine　*N*-アセチル-L-システイン
nalidixic acid cetrimide agar　ナリジクス酸セトリミド寒天
neoadjuvant chemotherapy　ネオアジュバント化学療法

nitrogen mustard, adriamycin, cyclohexylchloroethylnitrosourea　ニトロゲンマスタード，アドリアマイシン，シクロヘキシルクロロエチルニトロソ尿素
normal axis deviation　正常(電気)軸偏位
nursing audit committee　看護監査委員会

nachm
nachmittags〈独〉　午後に

Nachr
Nachrichten〈独〉　報告

nAChR
nicotinic acetylcholine receptor　ニコチン性アセチルコリン受容体

NACHRI
National Association of Children's Hospitals and Related Institutions　小児病院・関連研究所全国協会

Nachtr
Nachtrag〈独〉　追加，付録

NaCl
sodium chloride　塩化ナトリウム

NACMCF
National Advisory Committee on Microbiological Criteria and Foods　微生物と食品基準諮問委員会

NAcneu
N-acetylneuraminic acid　*N*-アセチルノイラミン酸

Na_2CO_3
sodium carbonate　炭酸ナトリウム

NACOR
National Advisory Committee on Radiation　放射線全国諮問委員会

NACS
neurological and adaptive capacity score　神経的適応能力スコア

NAD
National Association of Deaf　難聴者全国連合
new antigenic determinant　新抗原決定基
nicotinamide adenine dinucleotide　ニコチンアミドアデニンジヌクレオチド
nicotinic acid dehydrogenase　ニコチン酸脱水素酵素，ニコチン酸デヒドロゲナーゼ
no acute distress　急性の病気なし
no additional diagnosis　追加診断なし
no appreciable difference　差を認めない
no appreciable disease　特記すべき疾患なし
non-atopic dermatitis　非アトピー性皮膚炎
nothing abnormal detected　検査結果に異常を認めない

Nad
noradrenaline ノルアドレナリン
NADase
nicotinamide adenine dinucleotidase ニコチンアミドアデニンジヌクレオチダーゼ, NAD アーゼ
19-NADC
19-norandrosterone decanoate 19-ノルアンドロステロンデカノエート
NADDIF
narcotics and dangerous drugs intelligence file 麻薬および危険薬品情報ファイル
NADH
nicotinamide adenine dinucleotide ニコチンアミドアデニンジヌクレオチド
$NADH_2$
reduced nicotinamide adenine dinucleotide 還元型ニコチンアミドアデニンジヌクレオチド
NADH-TR
NADH-tetrazoline reductase NADH テトラゾリン還元酵素
NADL
National Association of Dental Laboratory 歯科技工全国協会
NaDOC
sodium deoxycholate デオキシコール酸ソーダ, デオキシコール酸ナトリウム
NADP
nicotinamide adenine dinucleotide phosphate ニコチンアミドアデニンジヌクレオチドリン酸
NADPH, $NADPH_2$
reduced nicotinamide adenine dinucleotide phosphate 還元型ニコチンアミドアデニンジヌクレオチドリン酸塩
NAdr
noradrenaline ノルアドレナリン
NAE
net acid excretion 総酸排泄(量)
NaE
exchangeable body sodium〔natrium〕 交換可能体内ソジウム(=ナトリウム)
NAEL
National Association of Earmold Laboratories 全国イヤモールド研究所協会
NAEMT
National Association of Emergency Medical Technicians 救急医療に携わる技術者の全国協会
NAF
nafcillin ナフシリン

N

nafoxidine ナフォキシジン
Negro adult female 黒人の成人女性
neutrophil-activating factor 好中球活性化因子

NaF
sodium fluoride フッ化ナトリウム

NAFLD
nonalcoholic fatty liver disease 非アルコール性脂肪肝障害

NAG
N-acetyl-*β*-D-glucosaminidase *N*-アセチル-*β*-D-グルコサミニダーゼ
narrow angle glaucoma 狭(隅)角緑内障
nonagglutinating 非凝集(性)の

NAGA
α-*N*-acetylgalactosaminidase *α*-*N*-アセチルガラクトサミニダーゼ

NAG vibrios
non-agglutinable vibrios ナグビブリオ

NaH
natriuretic hormone ナトリウム利尿ホルモン

$NaHCO_3$
sodium bicarbonate 炭酸水素ナトリウム

NAHSA
National Association of Hearing and Speech Agencies 聴覚言語局全国連合

NAI
neuraminidase inhibition ノイラミニダーゼ阻害
no acute inflammation 急性炎症なし
nutritional assessment index 栄養評価指数

NaI
sodium iodide ヨウ化ナトリウム

NAIL
Neurotics Anonymous International Liaison 無名神経病学者国際連絡

NAIN
non-adrenergic inhibitory nerve 非アドレナリン作動抑制性神経

NAIP
neuronal apoptosis inhibitory protein 神経元アポトーシス抑制蛋白

NAIR
non-adrenergec inhibitory response 非アドレナリン作動(性)抑制反応

NAIT
neonatal alloimmune thrombocytopenia 新生児同種免疫性血小板減少症

NAJ
Nomina Anatomica Japonica〈ラ〉 日本解剖学用語

NaK ATPase
sodium-and potassium-activated adenosine triphosphate — ナトリウムカリウム活性化アデノシン三リン酸

NAL
non-adherent leukocyte — 非付着性白血病

NALD
neonatal adrenoleukodystrophy — 新生児副腎白質ジストロフィ

NALP
neuro adenolysis of the pituitary gland — 脳下垂体アルコールブロック

NALT
nasal-associated lymphoid tissue — 鼻腔関連リンパ組織
nasopharyngeal-associated lymphoid tissue — 上咽頭関連リンパ組織

NAM
Negro adult male — 黒人の成人男性
normal adult male — 健康成人男子

NAMC Survey
National Ambulatory Medical Care Survey — 国民外来医療調査

NAME
nitroarginine methyl ester — ニトロアルギニンメチルエステル

NAME syndrome
nevi, atrial myxoma, myxoid neurofibroma, ephelides syndrome — 母斑・心房粘液腫・粘液性神経線維腫・そばかす症候群，姓名症候群，LAMB症候群

N

NAMH
National Association for Mental Health — 精神衛生全国連合

NAMN
nicotinic acid mononucleotide — ニコチン酸モノヌクレオチド

NAN
N-acetylneuraminic acid — *N*-アセチルノイラミン酸

n.a.n.
nisi alter notetur〈ラ〉 — 気づかれなければ

NANA
N-acetylneuraminic acid — *N*-アセチルノイラミン酸

NANB
non A, non B (hepatitis) — 非A非B型肝炎

NANBNCH
non-A, non-B, non-C hepatitis — 非A非B非C型肝炎

NANBV
non-A, non-B hepatitis virus — 非A非B型肝炎ウイルス

NANC
non-adrenergic, non-cholinergic (nerves) 非アドレナリン作動性,非コリン作動性(神経)

NANDA
North American Nursing Diagnosis Association 北米看護診断協会

N and E
nausea without emesis 嘔吐なしの嘔気

NANM
N-allylnormorphine *N*-アリルノルモルヒネ

NaOH
sodium hydroxide 水酸化ナトリウム

NAON
National Association of Orthopaedic Nurses 整形外科看護師全国協会

NAOT
National Association of Orthopaedic Technologists 整形外科技術者全国協会

NAP
negative after-potential 陰性後電位
nerve action potential 神経活動電位
neuropathy associated protein ニューロパシー関連蛋白
neutrophil alkaline phosphatase 好中球アルカリホスファターゼ
neutrophil attractant protein 好中球走化性蛋白
Nomina Anatomica Paris〈ラ〉 パリ解剖学用語
nucleic acid phosphatase 核酸ホスファターゼ

NAPA
N-acetyl-*p*-aminophenol *N*-アセチル-*p*-アミノフェノール
N-acetyl(-)procainamide *N*-アセチルプロカインアミド
nuclear acidic protein antigen 核酸性蛋白抗原

NAPAN
National Association for Preventions of Addiction to Narcosis 麻薬中毒予防全国連合

NAPAP
N-acetyl-*p*-aminophenol *N*-アセチル-*p*-アミノフェノール

NAPD
no active pulmonary disease 非活動性肺疾患

NaPG
sodium pregnanediol glucuronide プレグナンジオールグルクロン酸ナトリウム

NAPH
naphthyl ナフチル

naph
naphthol ナフトール

NAPM
National Association of Pharmaceutical Manufacturers 医薬品製造者全国協会
NAPNES
National Association for Practical Nurse Education and Service 実践看護教育とサービスの全国連合
NAPT
National Association for Prevention of Tuberculosis 結核予防全国連合
National Association of Physical Therapeutics 物理療法士全国協会
NAPVD
National Association for Prevention of Veneral Disease 性病予防全国連合
NAR
nasal airway resistance 鼻腔抵抗
non albumin rat 無アルブミンラット
NARAL
National Association for Repeal of Abortion Law 堕胎法律廃止全国連合
NARC
narcotic (s) 麻薬
narcotic officer 麻薬管理者
narcotics agent 麻薬取締官
narco
narcotic (s) 麻薬
Nar Inv
narcotic investigation 麻薬監視
narist.
naristillae〈ラ〉 点鼻薬《処》
NAS
nasal 鼻の
neonatal abstinence syndrome 新生児禁断症候群
neonatal air leak syndrome 新生児空気漏出症候群
neuroallergic syndrome 神経アレルギー症候群
no added salt 食塩無添加，無塩
Noise Abatement Society 騒音防止協会
normative aging study 標準年齢研究
NASH
nonalcoholic steatohepatitis 非アルコール性脂肪性肝炎
NAS/NRC
National Academy of Science/National Research Council 米国国立科学アカデミー/国立研究協議会
NAT
N-acetyltransferase *N*-アセチルトランスフェラーゼ

N

natal	出生の
neonatal alloimmune thrombocytopenia	新生児自己免疫性血小板減少症

Nat

nation	国，国民
national	国の，国民の，全国的な
native	生まれつきの，土着の
natural	自然の
nature	自然

Nat.bic.

natrium bicarbonicum〈ラ〉	重曹

NA-test

noradrenaline test	ノルアドレナリン負荷試験

nato

no action	無作用

NATP

neonatal autoimmune thrombocytopenic purpura	新生児自己免疫性血小板減少性紫斑病

Natr

natrium	ナトリウム

NB

nail bed	爪床
Nasenbepinseln〈独〉	点鼻
Negri body	ネグリ(小)体
nephroblastoma	腎芽細胞腫
nervus buccalis	頬神経
neuroblastoma	神経芽細胞腫
newborn	新生児
non-B (hepatitis)	非B型(肝炎)
normoblast	正赤芽球
novobiocin	ノボビオシン
nuclear bag	核袋
nutrient broth	栄養ブロス

Nb

niobium	ニオブ〈元素〉
Nippostrongylus braziliensis	ニッポストロンジルスブラジリエンシス(＝ブラジル鉤虫)

^{95}Nb

radioactive niobium	放射性ニオブ

N/B

neopterin to biopterin (ratio)	ネオプテリン/ビオプテリン(比)

NB, N.B.

nota bene〈ラ〉	よく注意せよ《処》

N

n.B, NB
nichts Besonders<独> 異常なし，特変なし
NBA
N-bromoacetamide *N*-ブロモアセトアミド
NBAS
neonatal behavioral assessment score 新生児行動評価法
Neonatal Behavioral Assessment Standard 新生児行動評価規準
NBB
normal buffer base 正常緩衝塩基
NBC
nocturnal bladder capacity 夜間膀胱容量
nonbacterial conjunctivitis 非細菌性結膜炎
NBCC
nevoid basal cell carcinoma (syndrome) 母斑(様)基底細胞癌(症候群)
NBCCS
nevoid basal cell carcinoma syndrome 母斑(様)基底細胞癌症候群
NBCE
nevus basal cell epithelioma 多発性母斑性基底細胞腫
NBCIE
nonbullous congenital ichthyosiform erythroderma 非水疱型先天性魚鱗様紅皮症
NBCS
newborn calf serum 仔ウシ血清
NBD
nasobiliary drainage 鼻胆管ドレナージ
neurogenic bladder dysfunction 神経因性膀胱機能障害
no brain damage 脳障害なし
NBEI
non-butanol-extractable iodine (syndorome) 非ブタノール抽出ヨウ素(症候群)
NBF
not breast fed 母乳栄養でない
NBI
neutrophil bactericidal index 好中球殺菌指数
no bone injury 骨障害なし
NBICU
Newborn Intensive Care Unit 新生児集中治療部〔病棟〕
NBIE
National Burn Information Exchange 国立熱傷情報交換センター
NB Int
Newborn Intensive (Care) 新生児集中(治療)
NBKS
Nierenbeckenkelchsystem<独> 腎盂腎杯系

N

NBL
not bloody likely　血液らしくない
nbl
normoblast　正赤芽球
NBM
normal bone marrow　正常骨髄
nothing by mouth　絶食
NBME
National Board of Medical Examiners　米国国立医師国家試験実施委員会
normal bone marrow extract　正常骨髄抽出物
NBN
newborn nursery　新生児室
NBOT
National Board of Orthopaedic Technologists　整形外科技術者全国委員会
NBP
needle biopsy prostate　前立腺針生検
neoplastic brachial plexopathy　腫瘍性上腕神経叢疾患
nonbacterial pharyngitis　非細菌性咽頭炎
nonbacterial prostatitis　非細菌性前立腺炎
normal boiling point　正常沸点
NBS
National Bureau of Standards　米国規格標準局
N-bromosuccinimide　*N*-ブロモコハク酸イミド
nevoid basal (cell carcinoma)　母斑(様)基底
no bacteria seen　細菌はみられない
normal blood serum　正常血清
normal bowel sound(s)　正常腸音
normal brain stem　正常脳幹
number of binding site　結合部分
nystagmus blockage syndrome　眼振遮断症候群
NBT
nitroblue tetrazolium (test)　ニトロブルーテトラゾリウム(試験)
normal breast tissue　正常乳腺組織
NBTE
nonbacterial thrombotic endocarditis　非細菌性血栓性心内膜炎
NBTNF
newborn, term, normal, female　新生児・満期・正常・女
NBTNM
newborn, term, normal, male　新生児・満期・正常・男
NBTS
National Blood Transfusion Service　米国輸血サービス

N

NBT T
nitroblue tetrazolium test　ニトロブルーテトラゾリウム試験

NBT test
nitroblue tetrazolium test　ニトロブルーテトラゾリウム試験

NBU
N-nitroso-butylurea　*N*-ニトロソブチルウレア

NBW
noise bandwidth　雑音周波帯
normal birth weight　正常出産時体重

NC
nasal cannula　鼻カニューレ
nasal clearance　鼻クリアランス
natural cytotoxicity　自然細胞傷害
Negro child　黒人小児
neonatal cholestasis　新生児(期)胆汁うっ滞
neural crest　神経堤
neurologic check　神経学的チェック
nevus comedonicus　コメド母斑
nitrocellulose　ニトロセルロース
no casualty　死傷者なし
no change　変化なし
no charge　無料
no complaints　訴えなし
no connection　非結合
noise criteria　音響標準
noncirrhotic　非(肝)硬変の
non-contributory　特記すべきことなし
non corrigent　視力矯正不能
normal control　正常対照
normally closed　正常に閉鎖した
normocephalic　正常頭蓋の
not classified　分類されていない
not cultured　培養されていない
nucleocapsid　ヌクレオカプシド
numerical control　計算管理

nC
nanocurie　ナノキュリー

n.c.
non corrigunt〈ラ〉＝non corrigent　矯正不能

N/C
nuclear cytoplasmic rate　核/細胞質比

N & C
nerves and circulation　神経と循環

NCA
National Council on Alcoholism　アルコール中毒全国委員会
N-carboxyamino acid anhydride　*N*-カルボキシアミノ酸無水物
neurocirculatory asthenia　神経循環性無力症
neutrophil chemotactic activity　好中球遊走活性
nonspecific cross-reacting antigen　非特異的交叉〔差〕反応抗原
nuclear cerebral angiogram　核脳血管造影フィルム

NCAB
National Cancer Advisory Board　国立癌諮問委員会

NCADI
National Clearinghouse for Alcohol and Drug Information　国立アルコール・薬物濫用情報センター

NCAE
National Center for Audio Experimentation　国立音響実験センター

N-CAM
neural cell adhesion molecule　神経細胞接着分子

NcAMP
nephrogenous cyclic adenosine monophosphate　腎原性環状アデノシン一リン酸

NCC
Network Control Center　ネットワーク管理センター
non coronary cusp　大動脈弁無冠尖
nucleated cell count　有核細胞数

NCCH
National Cancer Center Hospital　国立癌センター病院

NCCHD
non-cyanotic congenital heart disease　非チアノーゼ性心疾患

NCCLS
National Committee for Clinical Laboratory Standards　米国臨床検査標準委員会

NCCP
non-cardiac chest pain　非心臓性胸痛

NCC-ST439
NCC-ST439　糖鎖抗原腫瘍マーカー

NCD
N-cadherin　神経細胞カドヘリン
neurocirculatory dystonia　神経循環失調症
no congenital deformities　先天性変形なし
normal childhood diseases　正常小児期疾患

NCd
nucleus caudatus〈ラ〉　尾状核

NCDAI
National Clearinghouse for Drug Abuse Information　国立薬物濫用情報センター

N

NCDC
National Center for Disease Control 国立疾病管理センター
National Communicable Disease Center 国立伝染病センター
NCDO
National Collection of Daily Organism 国立日常微生物収集
NCDV
Nebraska calf diarrhea virus ネブラスカウシ下痢ウイルス
newborn calf diarrhea virus 仔ウシ下痢ウイルス
NCE
negative contrast echocardiography 陰性造影剤心エコー検査(法)
non-cardiac edema 非心(臓)原性浮腫
nonconvulsive epilepsy 痙攣のないてんかん
normochromatic erythrocyte 正色素性赤血球
NCEN
non-cholinergic excitatory nerve 非コリン作動興奮性神経
NCEP
national cholesterol education program コレステロール教育プロジェクト
NCF
nerve cell food 神経細胞栄養物
neutrophil chemotactic factor 好中球走化因子
normal colposcopic finding 正常腟鏡検査所見
NCFPC
National Center for Fish Protein Concentrate 国立魚蛋白凝縮センター
NCFR
National Council on Family Relation 家族関係全国委員会
NCFT
National College of Food Technology 国立食品技術大学
NCGL
nucleus corporis geniculatilateralis 外側膝状体核
NCGS
National Cooperative Gallstone Study 全国協同胆石研究国内協力
NCHCT
National Center for Health Service Research 国立保健医療研究センター
NCHS
National Center for Health Statistics 米国国立保健統計センター
NCHSR & D
National Center for Health Services Research and Development 国立保健サービス研究開発センター

NCI
National Cancer Institute　国立癌研究所
nucleus colliculi inferioris　下丘核
nCi
nanocurie　ナノキュリー〈単位〉
NCIP
nonclassifiable interstitial pneumonia　分類不能の間質性肺炎
NCIPC
National Center for Injury Prevention and Control　国立外傷予防管理センター
NCI powder
naphthalene, creosote, iodoform powder　ナフタリン・クレオソート・ヨードホルム末
NCL
neuronal ceroid lipofuscinosis　神経性セロイドリポフスチノーシス
NCM
nitrocellulose membrane　ニトロセルロース膜
NCMH
National Committee for Mental Hygiene　精神衛生全国委員会
National Committee on Maternal Health　母性健康全国委員会
NCMHE
National Clearinghouse for Mental Health Education　精神衛生教育全国情報センター
NCN
National Council of Nurses　米国看護師協議会
NCNA
National Council on Noise Abatement　騒音防止全国協議会
NCNCA
normochromic normocytic anemia　正色(素)性正赤血球性貧血
NCP
noncollagen protein　非膠原蛋白，非コラーゲン蛋白
NCPE
noncardiogenic pulmonary edema　非心原性肺水腫
NCPF
noncirrhotic portal fibrosis　非硬変性門脈線維症
NCPIE
National Council on Patient Information and Education　患者情報教育全国委員会
NCQA
National Congress of Quality Assurance　質的保障全国会議

N

NCR
nuclear-cytoplasmic ratio 核・細胞質比
NCRP
National Committee on Radiation Protection 放射線防護全国委員会
National Committee on Radiation Protection and Measurements 放射線防護・線量測定全国委員会
National Council on Radiation Protection (and Measurements) 放射線防護(測定)全国協議会
NCS
neocarzinostatin ネオカルチノスタチン
noncoronary sinus 非冠(状)静脈洞
noncured sarcoidosis 非治癒サルコイドーシス
NCSH
National Clearinghouse for Smoking and Health 喫煙と健康のための国内情報センター
NCT
neural crest tumor 神経堤腫瘍
neutron capture therapy 中性子保護療法
noncontact tonometer 非接触型眼圧計
NCTB
neurobehavioral core test battery 神経行動コアテストバッテリー
NCTC
National Collection of Type Culture 国立標準培養収集
NCTR
National Center for Toxicological Research 国立毒物研究センター
NCU
neurological care unit 神経疾患治療部門
nitrogen control unit 窒素コントロール単位
NCV
nerve conduction velocity 神経伝導速度
no commercial value 商品価値なし
noncholera vibrio 非コレラビブリオ(菌)
NCVS
nerve conduction velocity study 神経伝導速度検査
N-CWS
Nocardia rubra cell wall skelton ノカルジアルブラ細胞壁骨格
ND
nalidixic acid ナリジクス酸
nasal deformation 鼻変形
nasal deformity 鼻変形
nasolacrimal duct 鼻涙管
natural death 自然死
neonatal death 新生児死亡

N

neoplastic disease 腫瘍性疾患，新生物性疾患
nerve deafness 神経性難聴
neurotic depression 神経症性うつ病(状態)
neutral density 中性濃度
Newcastle disease ニューカッスル病
New Drug 新薬
next day 翌日
no data データなし
no delay 遅延なし
no disease 病気なし
nondiabetic 非糖尿病(性)の
normal delivery 正常分娩
normal dose 標準量，正常量
not date(d) 日付なし
not detectable 検出不能な
not detected 検出されない
not determined 決定できない
not diagnosed 診断されない
not done 行われない
nothing doing 無行為
nothing done 何もされない
nucleus of Darkschewitsch ダルクシェーヴィチ核
nursing diagnosis 看護診断

Nd
neodymium ネオジミウム〈元素〉

N/D
no defects 欠陥なし

N_d，n_D
refractive index 屈折率

nd，n.d.
numerus digitorum〈ラ〉 指数弁

NDA
National Dental Association 歯科全国連合
new drug application 新薬適用
no data available 利用可能なデータなし
no detectable activity 検出可能な活性なし

NDC
National Drug Code 米国薬剤コード
nondifferentiated cell 非分化細胞

19-NDC
19-nortestosterone decanoate 19-ノルテストステロンデカノエイト

NDCD
National Drug Code Directory 米国薬剤コード集

NDCS
National Deaf Children's Society 難聴児全国協会

N

NDDG
National Diabetes Data Group 全国糖尿病記録グループ
NDE
near death experience 臨死体験
n.d.E, n.d.E.
nach dem Essen〈独〉 食後《処》
NDEA
nitrosodiethylamine ニトロソジエチルアミン
N-nitrosodiethylamine *N*-ニトロソジエチルアミン
NDELA
N-nitrosodiethanolamine *N*-ニトロソジエタノールアミン
n.d.E.z.n.
nach dem Essen zu nehmen〈独〉 食後服用《処》
NDF
neutral detergent fiber 中性デタージェント線維
new dosage form 新投薬様式
Nicolas-Durand-Favre (disease) ニコラ・デュラン・ファーブル(病)
no disease found 何の疾患も見つからず
NDGA
nordihydroguaiaretic acid ノルジヒドログアヤレト酸
NDI
naphthalene diisocyanate ナフタレンジイソシアネイト
nephrogenic diabetes insipidus 腎性尿崩症
NDIR
non-dispersive infrared analyzer 非分散型赤外線分析計
NDMA
nitrosodimethylaniline ニトロソジメチルアニリン
nDNA
native DNA 天然〔未変性〕DNA
N/D NHL
nodular/diffuse non-Hodgkin lymphoma 結節型/び漫〔広汎〕性非ホジキンリンパ腫
NDP
net dietary protein 総〔全〕食事性蛋白
nucleoside 5′-phosphate ヌクレオシド5′-ホスフェート(リン酸)
NDR
neonatal death rate 新生児死亡率
neurotic depressive reaction 神経症性うつ病反応
normal detrusor reflex 正常排尿筋反射
NDS
narrow distal segment 狭末端部
new drug submission 新薬許可出願
normal dog serum 正常イヌ血清

N

NDSB
Narcotic Drugs Supervisory Board　麻薬管理局
NDSC
Network for Detection of Stratospheric Change　成層圏変化検出のためのネットワーク
N-DSK
N-terminal disulfide knot　*N*-ターミナルジスルフィドノット
NDT
neurodevelopmental treatment　神経発達的治療
noise detection threshold　雑音検出閾値
nondestructive testing　非破壊性検査
NDTI
National Disease and Therapeutic Index　全国疾病治療指標
NDV
Newcastle disease virus　ニューカッスル病ウイルス
Nd-YAG
neodymium-yttrium-aluminum-garnet　ネオジミウム・イットリウム・アルミニウム・ガーネット
NE
nausea and emesis　嘔気〔悪心〕と嘔吐
necrotic enteritis　壊死性腸炎
neomycin　ネオマイシン
nephropathia epidemica〈ラ〉　流行性腎症
nerve ending　神経終末
nerve excitability (test)　神経興奮性(検査)
neural excitation　神経興奮
neuroendocrine　神経内分泌の
neuroepithelium　感覚上皮，神経上皮
neurologic examination　神経的検査
neutrophil elastase　好中球エラスターゼ
new edition　新版
new employer　新しい雇用者
no effect　影響なし
no evaluate　評価不能
nonendogenous　非内因性の
norepinephrine　ノルエピネフリン
normal epithelial cell　正常上皮細胞
not enlarged　拡大していない
not evaluated　未評価
not examined　未検査
Ne
neon　ネオン〈元素〉

NEA
neoplasm (carcino) embryonic antigen　胎児性癌抗原
no evidence of abnormality　異常所見なし
non essential amino acid(s)　非必須アミノ酸

NEAA
non essential amino acid(s)　非必須アミノ酸

'neath
beneath　下の
underneath　〜の下に

NEB
neuroendocrine body　神経内分泌体

Neb
nebulization　噴霧

nebul.
nebula〈ラ〉　角膜白濁

NEC
necrotizing enterocolitis　壊死性腸炎
neonatal necrotizing enterocolitis　新生児壊死性腸炎
neuroendocrine cell　神経内分泌細胞
no essential change　本質的な変化なし
nonesterified cholesterol　非エステル化コレステロール
not elsewhere classifiable　他に分類できない
not elsewhere classified　他に分類できない

nec
necessary　必要な

necr
necrosis　壊死

necrol
necrology　死亡統計学

NECT
non-enhanced computed tomography　非強調コンピュータ断層撮影法

NED
no evidence of disease　疾患の徴候なし
no expiration date　失効日付なし
normal equivalent deviation　標準当量偏差

NEEP
negative end-expiratory pressure　終末呼気陰圧

NEF
nephritic factor　腎炎因子
noise exposure forecast　音響曝露予測

NEFA
non-esterified fatty acid　非エステル結合型脂肪酸

NEFG
normal external female genitalia　正常女性外性器〔外陰部〕

NEG
neglect 無視する
Neg
negative 陰性
Negro 黒人
nehi
knee-high 高位膝
NEI
National Eye Institute 国立眼研究所
not elsewhere indicated 他部位に適応されない
nei
non est invents 発見されない
NEJ
neuroeffector junction 神経効果器接合部
NEJM
New England Journal of Medicine ニューイングランド医学雑誌
NEM
N-ethylmaleimide *N*-エチルマレイミド
no evidence of malignancy 悪性(腫瘍)所見なし
not elsewhere mentioned 他部位では認められない
NEMA
National Electrical Manufacturer's Association 国際電気メーカー連合
nema
Nematoda 線虫類
nematode 線虫
nematoid 糸状の，線虫の
nemat
nematology 線虫学
Nemb
Nembutal ネンブタール
NEMD
nonspecific esophageal motor dysfunction 非特異的食道運動機能不全
nemmies
nembutal capsules ネンブタールカプセル
NEMSPA
National Emergency Medical Service Pilot's Association 全国救急ヘリコプターパイロット協会
ne/nd
new edition in preparation-no date can be given 出版日未定の準備中の新刊
neo
neoarsphenamine ネオアルスフェナミン
neonatal 新生児の

neoars
neoarsphenamine　ネオアルスフェナミン
neonat
neonatal　新生児の
neopl
neoplasm　新生物
NEP
negative expiratory pressure　陰性呼気圧
nephrology　腎臓病学
no evidence of pathology　病理学的証拠なし
norepinephrine　ノルエピネフリン
nep
nephrectomy　腎切除(術)，腎摘出術
NEPA
National Environment Policy Act　全国環境政策法
NEPD
no evidence of pulmonary disease　肺疾患の所見なし
NEPH
nephrology　腎臓病学
neph
nephew　甥
nephritis　腎炎
NEPHRO
nephrogram　腎造影〔撮影〕図
NEQ
neuquinon　ノイキノン

NER
no evidence of recurrence　再発の徴候なし
ner, ner.
nerve　神経
nervous　神経(質)の
nervousness　神経質
NERD
no evidence of recurrent disease　再発性疾患の所見なし
ne rep.
ne repeatum〈ラ〉　繰り返さない
NERO
Nutrition Education Research Organization　栄養教育研究組織
nerv
nervous　神経(質)の
nervousness　神経質
NES
Neurobehavioral Evaluation System　神経行動評価システム
nuclear export signal　核外輸送シグナル

NESP
novel erythropoiesis stimulating protein　新赤血球産生刺激蛋白
NESS
non-endocrine short stature　非内分泌性低身長
NET
naso-endotracheal tube　経鼻気管内チューブ
nerve excitability test　神経興奮性検査
neuroectodermal tumor　神経外胚葉腫瘍
neuroexcitability test　神経興奮性検査
norethisterone　ノルエチステロン
net
neutral　中性の
neutralization　中性化
n.et m.
nocte et mane〈ラ〉　夜と朝
NETP
negative extrathoracic pressure　胸郭外陰圧
NETPV
negative extrathoracic pressure ventilation　胸郭外陰圧式の人工呼吸
ne.tr.s.num.
ne tradas sine mummo〈ラ〉　お金を払わなければ渡すな
NETT
nasal endotracheal tube　経鼻気管内チューブ
Neu
neuraminic acid　ノイラミン酸
neu
neurilemma　神経線維鞘
NeuAc
N-acetylneuraminic acid　*N*-アセチルノイラミン酸
NeuGc
N-glycolylneuraminic acid　*N*-グリコリルノイラミン酸
NeuNAc
N-acetylneuraminic acid　*N*-アセチルノイラミン酸
NeuNGc
N-glycolylneuraminic acid　*N*-グリコリルノイラミン酸
neur
neuralgia　神経質
neurasthenia　神経衰弱
neuritis　神経炎
neurology　神経学
Neuro
neurology　神経学，神経内科
neuro
neurologic　神経学の

neurotic	神経(症)の
neurol	
neurologic(al)	神経学の
neurologist	神経科医
neurology	神経学
Neuropath	
neuropathologist	神経病理学者
neuropathology	神経病理学
neurophys	
neurophysiological	神経生理学の
neuropsychiat	
neuropsychiatry	神経精神医学
Neuro-Surg	
neurosurgeon	(脳)神経外科医
neurosurgery	(脳)神経外科(学)
neurs	
neurosis	神経症
neut	
neutral	中性の
neutralize	無力化する，中和する
neutrophil	好中球
Neutro	
neutrophil leukocyte	中性好細胞，好中球
NEXAFS	
near edge X-ray absorption fine structure	X線吸収端微細構造
NEY	
neomycin egg yolk	ネオマイシン卵黄
NEYA	
neomycin egg yolk agar	ネオマイシン卵黄寒天(培地)
NF	
nafcillin	ナフシリン
National Formulary	米国国民医薬品集
Negro female	黒人女性
nephritic factor	腎炎因子
neurofibromatosis	神経線維腫症
neurofilament	神経細線維
neutral fat	中性脂肪
neutral fraction	中性分画
nitrocellulose filter	ニトロセルロースフィルター
nitrofurantoin	ニトロフラントイン
nitrofurazone	ニトロフラゾン
noise factor	雑音因子
nonfiltered	濾過されない
nonfluent	非流暢な
nonfunction	機能しない

Nonne-Froin (syndrome) ノンネ・フロアン(症候群)
nonwhite female 非白人女性
normal flow 正常流(量)
not found 見つからない
nuclear factor 転写因子
nylidrin hydrochloride 塩酸ナイリドリン
nylon fiber ナイロン繊維

nF
nanofarad ナノファラド〈単位〉

NFA
nerve fiber analyzer 視神経線維分析器
non-fecal antigen 非糞抗原
normal fatty acid 直鎖脂肪酸
normal fecal antigen 正常糞便抗原

NFAR
no further action required これ以上治療の必要なし

NFB
National Federation of Blind 盲人全国連合
negative feedback 負のフィードバック
nonfermenting bacteria 非発酵性細菌

NFD
neurofibrillary degeneration 神経原線維変性
no family doctor 家庭医のいない
non-fat dry 無脂肪乾燥ミルク

NFDR
neurofacial-digitorenal (syndrome) 神経顔面指腎(症候群)

NFL
nerve fiber layer 神経線維層

NFLD
nerve-fiber-layer defect 神経線維層欠損

NFLPN
National Federation of License Practitioner Nurses 有資格看護師全国連合

NFLX
norfloxacin ノルフロキサシン

NFOSM
near field optical scanning microscope 走査近視野光学顕微鏡

NFP
national family planning 全国家族計画
natural family planning 自然家族計画
no family physician 家庭医のいない

NFPA
National Fire Protection Association 米国防火協議会

NFPC
nafcillin ナフシリン

N

NFR
no further requirement　これ以上の要求なし
nuclear fast red　核耐性赤色素
NFS
Natural Fertility Study　全国出生調査
NFT
neurofibrillary tangle　神経原線維塊
NFTD
normal full-term delivery　正常満期分娩
NF test
neck flexion test　首曲げテスト
NFTSD
normal, full-term, spontaneous delivery　正常・満期・自然分娩
NFTT
nonorganic failure to thrive　非器質性発育不良
NG
nasogastric　鼻胃の，鼻腔栄養の
nephrography　腎造影撮影法
newgrowth　新生物
nitroglycerin　ニトログリセリン
nitrosoguanidine　ニトロソグアニジン
no good　良くない
no growth　発育のない，培養されない
Ng
Nebengeräusch〈独〉　副雑音
ng
nanogram　ナノグラム（$=10^{-9}$g）〈単位〉
NGA
nutrient gelatin agar　栄養ゼラチン寒天（培地）
NGB
neurogenic bladder　神経因性膀胱
N-Ger
neurological geriatrics　神経（学的）老人学，老人神経学
NGF
nerve growth factor　神経成長因子
NG fdgs
nasogastric feedings　鼻胃経管栄養，鼻腔栄養
NGFR
nerve growth factor receptor　神経細胞増殖因子受容体
NGGR
nonglucogenic/glucogenic ratio　糖非生成/糖生成比
NGI
nuclear globulin inclusion　核グロブリン封入（体）

ng/ml
nanograms per milliliter ナノグラム/ミリリットル
NGNA
N-glycolylneuraminic acid *N*-グリコリルノイラミン酸
NGO
nitroglycerin ointment ニトログリセリン軟膏
Non-Governmental Organizations 民間公益団体
NGR
narrow gauze roll 巻いてある細いガーゼ
NGRS
non-glucose reducing substance 非糖還元性物質
NGS
normal goat serum 正常ヤギ血清
NGSA
nerve growth stimulating activity 神経成長刺激活性
NGSF
nongenital skin fibroblast 非生殖器皮膚線維芽細胞
NGT
nasogastric tube 経鼻胃管，経鼻栄養チューブ
normal glucose tolerance 正常耐糖能
NG tube
nasogastric tube 鼻腔栄養チューブ，経鼻胃管
NGU
non-gonococcal urethritis 非淋菌性尿道炎
NGV
non-gonococcal vulvovaginitis 非淋菌性外陰腟炎
NGZ
no growth zone 菌非発育帯
Nh
nihonium ニホニウム《元素》
NH
natriuretic hormone ナトリウム排泄増加ホルモン
natural hormone 正常抽出ホルモン
neonatal hepatitis 新生児肝炎
nodular histiocyte 小結節性組織球
nonhuman 非人間の
nursing home ナーシングホーム
NH_2
nitrogen mustard ニトロゲンマスタード
NH_3
ammonia アンモニア
NH_4
ammonium アンモニウム
dilute ammonia water 希釈アンモニア水

NHA
nonspecific hepatocellular abnormality　非特異的肝細胞異常
nucleus hypothalamicus anterior〈ラ〉　前視床下核
NHANES
National Health and Nutrition Examination Survey　国民健康栄養検査調査
NHAS
National Hearing Aid Society　国内補聴器協会
NHC
National Health Council　国家健康協議会
Neighborhood Health Center　近隣保健センター
neonatal hypocalcemia　新生児低カルシウム血症
nonhistone chromatin　非ヒストン染色質
nonhistone chromosomal　非ヒストン染色体
nursing home care　ナーシングホームケア
NH_4Cl
ammonium chloride　塩化アンモニウム
NHCP
nonhistone chromosomal protein　非ヒストン染色体蛋白(質)
NHDL
non-high-density lipoprotein　非高比重リポ蛋白
NHDS
National Hospital Discharge Survey　全国病院退院調査
NHE
normal hydrogen electrode　標準水素電極
NHEF
National Health Education Foundation　国立健康教育財団
NHF
National Heart Fund　国立心臓基金
National Hemophilia Foundation　国立血友病財団
NHG
normal human globulin　正常ヒトグロブリン
NHH
neurohypophyseal hormone　神経下垂体ホルモン
NHI
National Health Insurance　国民健康保険制度
National Heart Institute　国立心臓研究所
NHIS
National Health Interview Survey　国民健康問診調査
NHK
normal human kidney　正常ヒト腎臓
NHL
nodular histiocytic lymphoma　結節性組織球性リンパ腫
non-Hodgkin lymphoma　非ホジキン(性)リンパ腫

NHLBI
National Heart Lung Blood Institute　国立心肺血液研究所
NHLI
National Heart and Lung Institute　国立心肺研究所
NHML
non-Hodgkin malignant lymphoma　非ホジキン悪性リンパ腫
NH_3N
ammonia nitrogen　アンモニア窒素
NH_2N-Ox
nitrogen mustard-*N*-oxide　ニトロゲンマスタード-*N*-オキサイド
NHO
National Hospice Organization　全国ホスピス協会
NHP
no histone protein　非細胞核蛋白
non-hemoglobin protein　非ヘモグロビン蛋白
nonhistone protein　非ヒストン蛋白
normal human (pooled) plasma　正常ヒト(保存)血漿
NHPP
nonhistone phosphoprotein　非ヒストン蛋白
normal human pooled plasma　正常ヒト保存血漿
NHR
net histocompatibility ratio　総組織適合性割合
NHS
National Health Service　国民保健制度
normal horse serum　正常ウマ血清
normal human serum　正常ヒト血清
NHT
nonobesity (essential) hypertension　非肥満(本態性)高血圧
NHTS
National Heart Transplantation Study　米国心臓移植調査
NHWM
normal human white matter　正常ヒト蛋白
NI
neuraminidase inhibition　ノイラミニダーゼ阻害
neurological improvement　神経学的改善
no information　情報なし
Noise Index　雑音指数
not identified　無識別
not isolated　分離せず
nursing interview　看護面接
Ni
nickel　ニッケル〈元素〉
NIA
neutrophil-inducing activity　好中球誘導活性

N

no information available 利用できる情報なし

NiA
nicotinic acid ニコチン酸

NIAA
National Institute of Alcohol Abuse 国立アルコール中毒研究所

NIAAA
National Institute on Alcohol Abuse and Alcoholism 国立アルコール濫用・アルコール中毒研究所

NIADDK
National Institute of Arthritis, Diabetes, Digestive and Kidney Diseases 国立関節炎・糖尿病・消化器・腎疾患研究所

NIAID
National Institute of Allergy Infection Disease 国立アレルギー感染症研究所

NIAMD
National Institute of Arthritis and Metabolic Diseases 国立関節炎・代謝疾患研究所

NIC
neonatal intensive care 新生児集中治療

Nic
nicotinyl ニコチニル

NICA
nicotinic acid ニコチン酸

NICC
neonatal intensive care center 新生児集中治療センター

NICE
noninvasive carotid examination 非侵襲性頸動脈検査

NICED
National Institute of Cholera and Enteric Disease 国立コレラ・腸疾患研究所

NICHHD
National Institute of Child Health and Human Development 国立小児健康発育研究所

NICU
neonatal intensive care unit 新生児集中治療管理室〔施設〕
neuro (logical) intensive care unit 神経疾患集中治療室
neurosurgical intensive care unit 神経外科集中治療室
newborn intensive care unit 新生児集中治療部
nonimmunologic contact urticaria 非免疫学的接触蕁麻疹

NID
no identifiable disease 確認できる病気なし
not in distress 痛みなし

NIDA
National Insitute of Drug Abuse 米国国立薬物濫用研究所

NIDD

non insulin dependent diabetes mellitus	非インスリン依存型糖尿病

NIDDM

non insulin dependent diabetes mellitus	インスリン非依存型糖尿病

NIDH

National Institute of Dental Health	国立歯科衛生研究所

NIDR

National Institute of Dental Research	国立歯科研究所

NIE

not included elsewhere	他部位に含まれない

niedr

niedrig〈独〉	低い

NIF

negative inspiratory force	陰性吸気力
neutrophil immobilizing factor	好中球不動化因子
nifedipine	ニフェジピン
nonintestinal fibroblast	非腸管線維芽細胞

nif genes

nitrogen fixation genes	窒素固定遺伝子

NIFS

noninvasive flow study	非侵襲性血流検査

NIg

non-immunoglobulin	非免疫グロブリン

nig.

niger〈ラ〉	黒人，黒い

NIH

National Institutes of Health	国立衛生研究所

NIHF

non-immunologic hydrops fetalis	非免疫性胎児水腫

NIHL

noise-induced hearing loss	騒音起因の聴力不良

Ni.Hos

night hospital	ナイトホスピタル

NIHSS

NIH Stroke Scale	NIH脳卒中スケール

NIL

noise interference level	雑音干渉レベル

nil.

nihil〈ラ〉	無，ゼロ，皆無

nim.

nimus〈ラ〉	多い

NIMH

National Institute of Mental-Health	国立精神衛生研究所

NIMR
National Institute for Medical Research　国立医学研究所
National Institute for Mental Research　国立精神衛生研究所

NINCDS
National Institute of Neurological and Communicative Disorders and Stroke　国立神経病・感染症・脳卒中研究所

NINDS
National Institute of Neuralogical Disorders and Stroke　国立神経疾患・脳卒中研究所［米国］

NIOSH
National Institute of Occupational Safety and Health　国立労働安全衛生研究所

NIP
nipple　乳頭
no infection present　感染歴のない現症
no inflammation present　炎症歴のない現症

NIPPV
nasal intermittent positive pressure ventilation　鼻マスクによる間欠陽圧補助呼吸

NIPTS
noise induced permanent threshold shift　騒音による永久的閾値変動

N

NIR
near infrared　近赤外線の

NIRA
nitrite reductase　亜硝酸塩レダクターゼ〔還元酵素〕

NIRD
non-immune renal disease　非免疫性腎疾患

NIRMP
National Intern and Resident Matching Program　インターン・レジデント調整国家計画

NIRS
near infrared reflectance spectroscopy　近赤外分析法

NIS
no inflammatory signs　炎症徴候なし
non-immune sheep (serum)　非免疫ヒツジ(血清)
nonionic surfactant　非イオン性界面活性剤

NISP
National Information System for Psychology　国立精神病情報システム

NIT
national intelligence test　国民知能検査
NITA
nuclear inclusion type A　核封入体A型
NITD
non-insulin-treated disease　非インスリン治療疾患
nit.ox.
nitrous oxide　亜硝酸化物
nitr.
nitricus〈ラ〉　硝酸の《処》
nitro
nitrocellulose　ニトロセルロース
nitroglycerin　ニトログリセリン
NITTS
noise-induced temporary threshold shift　音刺激による最小可聴閾値の一過性変化
NIV
nodule-inducing virus　小結節誘発性ウイルス
NJ
nasojejunal　鼻空腸の
NK
natural killer (cell)　ナチュラルキラー(細胞)
not known　不明の
nk
neck　頸
NK631
pepleomycin　ペプレオマイシン
N/K
(name) not known　(姓名)不明
NKA
neurokinin A　ニューロキニンA
no known allergies　未既知アレルギー
NKC
non-keratinizing carcinoma　非角化性癌
nonketotic coma　非ケトン性昏睡
NK cell
natural killer cell　ナチュラルキラー細胞
NKDA
no know drug allergy　既知薬物アレルギー
NKF
National Kidney Foundation　国立腎財団
NKH
nonketotic hyperglycemia　ケトン陰性の過血糖
NKHA
nonketotic hyperosmolar acidosis　ケトン陰性の高浸透圧アシドーシス

NKHDC
non-ketotic hyperosmolar diabetic coma — 非ケトン性高浸透圧性糖尿病性昏睡
NKHG
nonketotic hyperglycemia — 非ケトン性高血糖症
NKHHC
nonketotic hyperglycemic-hyperosmolar coma — 非ケトン性高血糖(性)高浸透圧(性)昏睡
NKHOC
nonketotic hyperosmolar coma — 非ケトン性高浸透圧性昏睡
NKHS
nonketotic hyperosmolar syndrome — 非ケトン性高浸透圧症候群
NKR
normal rat kidney — 正常ラット腎
NKT
natural killer T (cell) — ナチュラルキラーT細胞
NKTS
natural killer target structure — ナチュラルキラー標的構造
NL
neural lobe — 神経葉
neutral lipid — 中性脂質
nicht löslich〈独〉 — 不溶性の
nodular lymphoma — 結節性リンパ腫
normal — 正常の
normal libido (coitus and climax) — 正常性欲(・性交・絶頂期)
normal limits — 正常限界
not listed — 登録されていない
Nyhan-Lesch (syndrome) — ナイハン・レッシュ(症候群)
nl
nanoliter — ナノリットル〈単位〉
n.l.
non liquet〈ラ〉 — 明瞭でない
nl., n.l.
non licet〈ラ〉 — 不許可の，不法の，許されていない
NLA
neuroleptanalgesia — 神経弛緩鎮痛
neuroleptanesthesia — 神経遮断麻酔(法)
normal lactase activity — 正常ラクターゼ活性
NLAL
nodule-like alveolar lesion — 小結節様肺胞病変
NLB
needle liver biopsy — 針による肝生検
NLD
nasolacrimal duct — 鼻涙管
necrobiosis lipoidica diabeticorum — 糖尿病性リポイド類壊死(症)

N

necrosis lipoidica diabeticorum〈ラ〉 糖尿病性類脂肪性壊死

NLDA
nodular low density area 小結節低密度領域

NLDL
normal low-density lipoprotein 正常低比重リポ蛋白

NLE
neonatal lupus erythematosus 新生児エリテマトーデス

Nle
norleucine ノルロイシン

NLM
neural larva migrans 神経幼虫移行症
noise level monitor 雑音レベル監視モニタ〔装置〕

NLMC
nocturnal leg muscle cramp 夜間脚筋(肉)痙攣

NLN
no longer needed もはや必要なし

NLNE
National League of Nursing Education 全国看護師教育連合会

NLP
nodular liquefying panniculitis 小結節性溶解脂肪組織炎
no light perception 光覚なし

NLR
nasolacrimal reflex 鼻涙腺反射

NLS
neonatal lupus syndrome 新生児狼瘡症候群

NLT
normal lymphocyte transfer test 正常リンパ球移入試験
not less than ～よりも少なくない

NLX
naloxone ナロキソン

NM
nafamostat mesilate メシル酸ナファモスタット
Negro male 黒人男性
neomycin ネオマイシン
neuromedin ニューロメジン
neuromuscular 神経筋の
nictitating membrane 瞬膜
nitrogen mustard ニトロゲンマスタード
nodular melanoma 結節型黒色腫
nonmalignant 非悪性
nonmotile 運動能力のない
nonwhite male 非白人男性
normetadrenaline ノルメトアドレナリン
normetanephrine ノルメタネフリン
not measurable 測定不可の

not measured　無測定の
not mentioned　無口述の
nuclear medicine　核医学
nuclear membrane　核膜

Nm
Neisseria meningitidis　髄膜炎菌
newton-meter　ニュートンメートル

nM
nachtes Monat〈独〉　翌月《処》
nanomolar　ナノモル(の)

nm
nachmittags〈独〉　午後に《処》
nanometer　ナノメートル〈単位〉
nomenclature　命名法，学名，術語

n/m
no mark　印なし

N & M
nerve and muscle　神経と筋肉

NM, nm
non-motile　非運動性の(細菌)

NM, nm, n & m
nocte et mane〈ラ〉＝night and morning　夜と朝《処》

NMA
neurogenic muscular atrophy　神経性筋萎縮
normeta-adrenaline　ノルメタ・アドレナリン

NMBA
neuromuscular blocking agent　神経筋遮断薬

NMC
neuromuscular control　神経筋制御

NMCD
nephrophtisis-medullary cystic disease　腎結核症・腎髄質嚢胞病

NMCHC
National Material and Child Health Center　国立母子保健センター

NMD
neuromyodysplasia　神経筋異形成症
neuronal migration disorder　神経細胞遊走障害

NMDA
N-methyl-D-aspartate　*N*-メチル-D-アスパラギン酸塩
N-methyl-D-aspartic acid　*N*-メチル-D-アスパラギン酸

NMDP
National Marrow Donor Program　全国骨髄ドナー登録制度

NME
necrotytic migratory erythema　壊死性遊走性紅斑
NMF
natural moist(uriz)ing factor　自然保湿因子
NMGTD
nonmetastatic gestational trophoblastic disease　非転移性妊娠性栄養膜〔絨毛性〕疾患
NMH
neuromuscular hyperexcitability　神経筋興奮亢進
NMI
no mental illness　精神疾患なし
no middle initial　ミドルネームのイニシャルなし
normal male infant　正常男児
NMJ
neuromuscular junction　神経筋接合部
NML
National Medical Library　国立医学図書館
nodular mixed lymphoma　結節性混合性リンパ腫
no man's land　ノーマンズランド
NMM
nodular malignant melanoma　結節性悪性黒色腫(メラノーマ)
NMN
nicotinamide mononucleotide　ニコチンアミドモノヌクレオチド
no middle name　ミドルネームなしの
normetanephrine　ノルメタネフリン
NMNC
nonmercuric noncorrosive　非水銀性非腐蝕性
NMO
nitrogen mustard-*N*-oxide　ナイトロジェンマスタード-*N*-オキシド
nmol
nanomole　ナノモル
NMOR
N-nitrosomorpholine　*N*-ニトロソモルホリン
NMP
normal menstrual period　正常月経周期
nuclear matrix protein　核マトリックス蛋白
nucleoside 5′-monophosphate　ヌクレオシド5′-モノホスフェート〔一リン酸〕
n mque, n.mque.
nocte maneque〈ラ〉=night and morning　夜と朝《処》

N

NMR
Neill-Mooser reaction　ニール・ムーサー反応
neonatal mortality rate　新生児死亡率
nictitating membrane response　瞬目反応
nuclear magnetic resonance　核磁気共鳴
nucleomagnetic resonance　核磁気共鳴
NMR analysis
nuclear magnetic resonance analysis　核磁気共鳴分析
NMR-CT
nuclear magnetic resonance computed tomography　核磁気共鳴断層撮影法
NMRI
nuclear magnetic resonance imaging　核磁気共鳴映像〔画像〕
NMR microscope
nuclear magnetic resonance microscope　核磁気共鳴顕微鏡
NMRS
nuclear magnetic resonance spectroscopy　核磁気共鳴スペクトロスコピー
NMS
neurally mediated syncope　神経反射性失神
neuroleptic malignant syndrome　神経弛緩薬(性)悪性症候群
neuromuscular spindle　神経筋紡錘
normal molecular weight renin substance　正常分子量レニン
normal mouse serum　正常マウス血清
NMSIDS
near-miss sudden infant death syndrome　ニアミス突然乳児死亡症候群
NMT
neuromuscular tension　神経筋緊張
neuromuscular transmission　神経筋伝達
nuclear medicine technology　核医学技術
NMTB
neuromuscular transmission blockade　神経筋伝達遮断
NMTD
nonmetastatic trophoblastic disease　非転移性栄養膜〔絨毛性〕疾患
NMTS
neuromuscular tension state　神経筋緊張状態
NMTT
N-methyltetrazolethiol　*N*-メチルテトラゾールチオール
NMU
neuromuscular unit　神経筋単位
NMV
nasal mask ventilation　鼻マスク人工換気〔呼吸〕法

NN
neonatal — 新生児(期)の
neurinoma — 神経鞘腫
normally nourished — 正常栄養の
nurses' notes — 看護(師)記録

nn.
nervi〈ラ〉 — 神経
nomen novum〈ラ〉 — 新しい名前

n/n
not to be noted — 気づかれない

NNA
normochromic normocytic anemia — 正色(素)性正(赤血)球性貧血

NNAS
neonatal narcotic abstinence syndrome — 新生児麻酔薬禁断症候群

NND
neonatal death — 新生児死亡
New and Nonofficial Drugs — 新非薬局方薬物
nicotinamide nucleotide dehydrogenase — ニコチンアミドヌクレオチド脱水素酵素〔デヒドロゲナーゼ〕

NNDG
dimethyl biguanide — ジメチルビグアニド

NNE
neonatal necrotizing enterocolitis — 新生児壊死性全腸炎
non-neuronal enolase — 非神経細胞(性)エノラーゼ

NNG
nonspecific nonerosive gastritis — 非特異的非びらん性胃炎

NNIS
National Nosocomial Infections Surveillance — 院内感染に関する全国調査

NNM
neonatal mortality — 新生児死亡率
Nicolle-Novy-MacNeal (medium) — ニコル・ノーヴィ・マックニール(培地)
N-nitrosomorpholine — *N*-ニトロソモルホリン

n.nov.
nomen novum〈ラ〉 — 新しい名前

NNR
Nebennierenrinde〈独〉 — 副腎皮質
new and nonofficial remedies — 新非薬局方薬物
not necessary to return — 再来の必要なし

NNS
nonneoplastic syndrome — 非新生物症候群

NNT
nuclei nervi trigemini — 三叉〔差〕神経核

NNW
net national welfare 純国民福祉
NO
narcotics officer 麻薬捜査官
nasal obstruction 鼻閉
neuromyelitis optica〈ラ〉 視神経髄質炎
nitric oxide 一酸化窒素
nitrous oxide 亜酸化窒素
nonobese 非肥満の
normally open 正常に開いた
nursing office 看護師詰所
No
nobelium ノベリウム〈元素〉
N_2O
nitrous oxide (dinitrogen monoxide) 亜酸化窒素，笑気(ガス)
No, No., no.
number 番号，数
numero〈ラ〉 数える，正確に
numerus〈ラ〉＝number 番号，数
No., no.
Nummer〈独〉＝number 番号，数
NOA
no appreciable distance 不感知距離
NOAC
novel oral antico anticoagulants 新規経口凝固薬
NOAEL
no-observed adversed effect level 最大不可逆的作用，無影響量，無毒性量，最大無作用量
NOALA
noise-operated automatic level adjustment 音響レベル自動調節
nob.
nobis〈ラ〉 我々に《処》
NOBT
nonoperative biopsy technique 非手術的生検法
NOC
not otherwise classified ほかに分類されない
noc.
noctis〈ラ〉 夜の
nocturia 夜間多尿(症)
no compl
no complaints 病訴のない，訴えのない
no complications 合併症のない
noct.
noctis〈ラ〉 夜の

N

nocturia　夜間多尿(症)

noct., Noct.
nocte〈ラ〉　夜
nox〈ラ〉　夜

noct.maneq.
nocte maneque〈ラ〉　夜と朝

NOD
nodal rhythm　結節性調律
nodular (melanoma)　結節性(黒色腫)
nonobese diabetes　非肥満性糖尿病
nonobese diabetic　非肥満性糖尿病

NOE
not otherwise enumerated　ほかに摘出されない

NOEL
non-observable effect level　観察できない効果レベル

no ess.abn
no essential abnormalities　本質的な異常なし

NOF
National Osteopathic Foundation　国立骨疾患財団
non-ossifing fibroma　非骨化性線維腫

NOHP
not otherwise herein provided　ここに用意されていない

NOIBN
not otherwise identified by name　名前で個別されない
not otherwise indexed by name　名前で索引されない

NOII
nonocclusive intestinal ischemia　非閉塞性腸(管)虚血

NOK
next of kin　最近親者

NOM
nonsuppurative otitis media　非化膿性中耳炎
normal extraocular movements　正常な外眼運動

nom
nominal　名義上の
nominate　指名する
nominated　指名された
nomination　指名

nom.dub.
nomen dubium〈ラ〉　疑わしい名前《処》

nomen
nomenclature　命名法，学名，学術用語

NOMI
non-occlusive mesenteric ischemia　血管非閉塞性腸間膜虚血症

nom.nov.
nomen novum〈ラ〉　新しい名前《処》

non flam
non flammable — 不燃性の

non-functional ECF
non-functional extracellular fluid — 非機能的細胞外液

NONMEM
nonlinear mixed effect model — 非線型混合効果モデル

non obs.
non obstante〈ラ〉 — 抵抗のない

NON-REM
non-rapid eye movement — ノンレム，非急速眼球運動の

non rep.
non repetatur〈ラ〉 — 繰り返すな，再調剤禁(止)《処》

non repet.
non repetatur〈ラ〉 — 繰り返すな，再調剤禁(止)《処》

nonsegs
nonsegmented (neutrophils) — 非分葉核(好中球)

non seq
non sequitur〈ラ〉 — 従わない

nonspec
nonspecific — 非特異(的)な

non std
non standard — 非標準

nontend
nontender — 圧痛のない

no op
no operation — 非手術

NOPHN
National Organization for Public Health Nursing — 全国公衆衛生看護協会

no p.l.
no perception of light — 光覚なし

NOPTN
National Organ Procurement and Transplantation Network — 移植臓器確保と移植の全国連絡網

NO-PYR
N-nitrosopyrrolidine — *N*-ニトロソピロリジン

NOQNO
2-nonyl-4-hydroxyquinoline-*N*-oxide — 2-ノニル-4-ヒドロキシキノリン-*N*-オキシド

NOR
noradrenaline — ノルアドレナリン
nucleolus organizer region — 仁形成域

nor
normal — 正常な

NORD
National Organization for Rare Disorders　稀少疾患の全国機構
norleu
norleucine　ノルロイシン
norm
normal　正常な
normet
normetanephrine　ノルメタネフリン
normoceph
normocephalic　正常頭蓋の
N or V
nausea and vomiting　嘔気または嘔吐
NOS
nitric oxide synthetase　窒素酸化物合成酵素
not otherwise specified　他に特記事項がなければ
nos
numbers　番号，数
NOSAC
nonsteroidal anti-inflammatory compound　非ステロイド抗炎症化合物
NOSIE
nurses' observation scale for inpatient evaluation　看護師用入院患者評価尺度
no sig
no signature　署名なし
NOT
nocturnal oxygen therapy　夜間酸素療法
nucleus opticus tractus〈ラ〉　視神経束核
NOTT
nocturnal oxygen therapy trial　夜間酸素療法試行
nov.
novum〈ラ〉　新しい
nov.n.
novum nomen〈ラ〉　新しい名前
NOVS
National Office of Vital Statistics　米国人口動態統計局
nov SP, nov.sp.
nova species〈ラ〉, *novum species*〈ラ〉　新種《処》
NO_x
nitrogen oxide　窒素酸化物
noxema
knocks eczema　殴打湿疹
NP
nasal polyp　鼻ポリープ
nasal polypotomy　鼻ポリープ切除術

nasopharyngeal 鼻咽頭の
nasopharynx 鼻咽頭
natriuretic peptide ナトリウム利尿ペプチド
near point 近点《眼》
neopsychiatric 神経精神医学の
nerve palsy 神経麻痺
neuropathology 神経病理学
neuropeptide 神経ペプチド
neurophysin ニューロフィジン
neuropsychiatric 神経精神医学の
neuropsychiatry 神経精神医学
new patient 新患(者)
Niemann-Pick (disease) ニーマン・ピック(病)
nitrogen-phosphorus 窒素リン
nitroprusside ニトロプルシド
nodal point 節点
nodular paragranuloma 小(結)節性側肉芽腫
nonpathologic 非病理的
nonpaying 支払わない
nonphagocytic 非食細胞の
nonpracticing 非開業の
non producing cell 非産生細胞
no phone 電話のない
no progression 進行なし
normal pattern 正常
normal pressure 正常圧
nosocomial pneumonia 院内感染肺炎
not palpable 触れることができない
not performed 無実施
not published 出版されない
nucleoprotein 核蛋白
nucleoside phosphorylase ヌクレオシドホスホリラーゼ
nurse practitioner ナースプラクティショナー
nursing care plan 看護計画
nursing procedure 看護技術

Np
neper ネーパー
neptunium ネプツニウム〈元素〉

n.p.
nomen proprium〈ラ〉 薬名《処》，商品名，固有名
nomine proprio〈ラ〉 特有の名で《処》

NP, np, n.p.
no(thing) particular 異常〔著変〕なし，特記すべきことなし

N

NPA
2-azido-4-nitrophenol　2-アジド-4-ニトロフェノール
nasopharyngeal airwey　鼻咽頭エアウェイ
nasopharyngeal aspirate　鼻咽頭吸引
near point of accommodation　調節近点
nucleus of pretectal area　視蓋前核
p-nitrophenylacetate　*p*-ニトロフェニル酢酸

NPa
nail-patella (syndrome)　爪・膝蓋(症候群)

NPB
nodal premature beat　結節性期外〔早期収縮〕
nonprotein bound　非蛋白結合の
nucleolar precursor body　核小体前駆体

NPC
nasopharyngeal carcinoma　鼻咽頭癌
near point of convergence　輻輳近点
nodal premature contraction　結節性期外収縮
nonparenchymal cell　非実質(性)細胞
nonproductive cough　非湿性咳
nuclear pore complex　核膜孔複合体
nucleus of posterior commissure　後交連核

NPCa
nasopharyngeal carcinoma　鼻咽頭癌

NPCP
National Prostatic Cancer Project　米国前立腺癌研究計画

NPCR
no periodic calibration required　定期的測定不要

NPcult
nasopharyngeal culture　鼻咽頭培養

NPD
native-pooled data method　土着集積データ法
nephrophthisis dextra〈ラ〉　右腎結核
Niemann-Pick disease　ニーマン・ピック病
nitrogen-phosphorus detector　窒素リン検出装置〔剤〕
nocturnal intermittent peritoneal dialysis　夜間間欠的腹膜透析
no pathologic diagnosis　病理的診断なし
5′-nucleotide phosphodiesterase　5′-ヌクレオチドホスホジエステラーゼ

NP detector
nitrogen-phosphorus detector　窒素リン検出装置〔剤〕

NPDL
nodular, poorly differentiated lymphocytic (lymphoma)　結節低分化リンパ球性(リンパ腫)

N

NPDR
nonproliferative diabetic retinopathy　非増殖(性)糖尿病(性)網膜症

NPE
neurogenic pulmonary edema　神経原性肺水腫
neuropsychologic examination　神経心理学(的)検査

NPF
nasopharyngeal fiberscope　鼻咽頭ファイバースコープ
nasopharyngo-fiberscope　上咽頭ファイバースコープ
not provided for　準備されていない

NPG
nonpregnant　妊娠していない

NPGB
p-nitrophenyl guanidinobenzoate　*p*-ニトロフェニルグアニジノベンゾエート

NPH
neutral protamine Hagedorn (insulin)　中性〔中間型〕プロタミンハーゲドルン(インスリン)
normal-pressure hydrocephalus　正常圧水頭症
nucleus pulposus herniation　髄核ヘルニア

NPH insulin
neutral protamine Hagedorn insulin　NPHインスリン

NPI
neuropsychiatric institute　神経精神医学研究所
no present illness　現疾患なし

NPip
N-nitrosopiperidine　*N*-ニトロソピペリジン

NPJT
nonparoxysmal (atrioventricular) junctional tachycardia　非発作性(房室)接合部頻拍(症)

NPM
nothing per mouth　禁食，絶食

NPMA
neural progressive muscular atrophy　神経性進行性筋萎縮症

NPN
nonprotein nitrogen　非蛋白質性窒素

NPO
non per oral　絶食
nothing per os=nil per os　絶食

NPO/HS
nulla per os hora somni〈ラ〉　就寝時経口摂取禁(止)

NPP
normal postpartum　正常分娩後の

4-NPP
4-nitrophenylphosphate　4-ニトロフェニルリン酸

NPPA
nuclear acidic protein antigen　酸性核蛋白抗原

NPPNG
nonpenicillinase-producing *Neisseria gonorrhoeae* 非ペニシリナーゼ産生淋菌
NP polio
nonparalytic poliomyelitis 非麻痺性ポリオ
NPR
net protein ratio 必須蛋白比
non-proliferative retinopathy 非増殖性網膜症
NPr
N-nitrosopyrrolidine *N*-ニトロソピロリジン
n/p r
noise/power ratio 音・圧比
N/P ratio
nucleoplasmic index 核細胞質(＝N/P比)
NPRQ
non-protein respiratory quotient, N-free respiratory quotient 非蛋白(性)呼吸比
NPS
nail-patella syndrome 爪・膝蓋骨症候群
nephrophthisis sinistra〈ラ〉 左腎結核
non-pregnancy serum 非妊娠血清
Nps
nitrophenylsulfenyl ニトロフェニルスルフェニル
NPS1
nail-patella syndrome, type 1 爪・膝蓋骨症候群1型
NPSH
non-protein sulfhydryl (group) 非蛋白スルフヒドリル(基)
NPT
nocturnal penile tumescence 夜間(レム睡眠期に一致してみられる)陰茎勃起
normal pressure and temperature 正常血圧・体温，正常気圧・温度
NPU
net protein utilization 必須蛋白利用
NPV
negative pressure ventilation 陰圧換気
nucleus paraventricularis 室傍核
NPY
neuropeptide Y ニューロペプチドY
NPYR
N-nitrosopyrrolidine *N*-ニトロソピロリジン
4-NQO
4-nitroquinoline 1-oxide 4-ニトロキノリン 1-オキシド
NR
nerve root 神経根
neural retina 神経網膜

neutral red　中性赤(指示薬)
noise reduction　雑音減少
non reactive　無反応(の)
non rebreathing, no respirations　無呼吸，非再呼吸
non responder　非応答者
no radiation　無照射
no reaction　無反応(の)
no recurrence　再発なし
no refill　再調剤禁(止)《処》
no rehearsal　リハーサルなし
no report　報告なし
no respirations　無呼吸，呼吸なし
no response　無反応
normal　正常の
normal range　正常範囲
normal reaction　正常反応
normotensive rat　正常血圧ラット
not recorded　無記録の
nurse　看護師
nutritive ratio　栄養比率
Reynolds number　レイノルズ数

nr
near　近い

n/r
no record　記録なし
not required　要求されない

N

NR, n.r.
non repetatur〈ラ〉=do not repeat　繰り返すな，再調剤禁(止)《処》

Nr, Nr.
Nummer〈独〉=number　番号，数

NRA
no repair action　非修復作用
nuclear reaction analysis　核反応分析

NRAD
no risk after discharge　退院後心配なし

NRBC
normal red blood cell　正常赤血球
nuclear red blood cell　有核赤血球

NRC
National Research Council　国立研究協議会
noise reduction coefficient　雑音減少係数
normal retinal correspondence　網膜正常対応

NRDC
National Research and Development Corporation　国立研究開発財団

NRDS
newborn respiratory distress syndrome　新生児呼吸困難症候群

NREH
normal renin essential hypertension　正常レニン本態性高血圧(症)

n.reit.
ne reiteretur〈ラ〉　再調剤不可《処》

NREM
non-rapid eye movement (sleep)　ノンレム睡眠，非急速眼球運動(睡眠)

NREMS
non-rapid eye movement sleep　ノンレム睡眠，非急速眼球運動睡眠

NRF
normal renal function　正常腎機能

NRGC
nucleus reticularis gigantocelluraris〈ラ〉　巨大細胞網様核

NRH
nodular regenerative hyperplasia　結節性再生性過形成

NRI
nerve root irritation　神経根刺激
nutritional risk index　栄養学的危険指数
nutritional surgical risk index　手術栄養リスク係数

NRIg
normal rabbit immunoglobulin　正常ウサギ免疫グロブリン

NRK
normal rat kidney　正常ラット腎(臓)

NR(O)M
normal range of motion　正常可動域

NRM
nucleus raphe magnus〈ラ〉　大縫線核

NRMP
National Residency Matching Program　全国専門医学研修計画

NRMPI
nonresonant multiphoton ionization　非共鳴多光子イオン化

NRN
no return necessary　再来不要

nRNA
nuclear RNA(=ribonucleic acid)　核(性)RNA(=リボ核酸)

nRNP
nuclear ribonucleoprotein　核リボ核蛋白

NRO
Narcotic Rehabilitation Office　麻薬中毒者回復局

NROM
normal range of motion 正常可動域
NRPG
nucleus reticularis paragigantocellularis〈ラ〉 延髄傍巨大細胞網様核
NRR
net reproduction rate 純再生産率
NRS
nonimmunized rabbit serum 無免疫ウサギ血清
normal rabbit serum 正常ウサギ血清
NRT
Nasenrachentumor〈独〉 上咽頭腫瘍
nicotin replacement therapy ニコチン置換療法
nucleus reticularis tegmenti〈ラ〉 被蓋網様体核
NRV
nucleus reticularis ventralis 腹側網状核
NS
nasal smear 鼻汁塗抹
natural suppressor (cell) 自然抑制T細胞
near side 近傍
nephrosclerosis 腎硬化(症)
nephrotic syndrome ネフローゼ症候群
nervous system 神経系
neurosecretory 神経分泌の
neurosurgeon (脳)神経外科医
neurosurgical (脳)神経外科の
neurosyphilis 神経梅毒
Nissl substance ニッスル小体
nodular sclerosis 結節性硬化(症)
nonsmoker 非喫煙者
nonspecific 非特異的の
nonstimulation 非刺激
nonstructural (protein) 非構造(蛋白)
nonsymptomatic 無症候性の
Noonan syndrome ノーナン症候群
normal saline 生理食塩水
normal serum 正常血清
normal sodium (diet) 正常ナトリウム(食)
no sequelae 続発症なし，後遺症なし
not seen 見られない
not significant 有意差なし
not specified 専門化されていない
not sufficient 十分でない
nuclear sclerosis 核硬化症
nurse station 看護師室，ナースステーション

Ns
nerves 神経
nurse 看護師
ns
nanosecond ナノ秒〈単位〉
no standard 標準なし
NSA
Neurological Society of America 米国神経科学会
Neurosurgical Society of America 米国神経外科学会
normal serum albumin 正常血清アルブミン
no salt added 無塩の
no serious abnormality 重篤な異常なし
NSAA
nonsteroidal antiandrogen 非ステロイド性抗男性ホルモン
NSAD
no signs of acute disease 急性疾患の徴候なし
NSAID(s)
non-steroidal anti-inflammatory drug(s) 非ステロイド性抗炎症薬
NSC
non-service connected 役に立たない結合の
no significant change 大きな変化なし
NSCC
National Society for Crippled Children 全国身障児学会
NSCCA
National Society for Crippled Children and Adults 身体障害児・成人全国協会
NSCDRF
National Sickle Cell Disease Research Foundation 国立鎌状赤血球疾患研究財団
nsCHE
non specific cholinesterase 非特異性コリンエステラーゼ
NSCLC
non-small cell lung carcinoma 非小細胞(性)肺癌
NSCR
National Society for Cancer Relief 癌救助全国協会
NSCU
neonatal special care unit 新生児特殊治療部
NSD
Nairobi sheep disease ナイロビヒツジ病
neonatal staphylococcal disease 新生児ブドウ球菌性疾患
night sleep deprivation 夜間睡眠遮断
noise-suppression device 音響抑制機器
nominal standard dose 公称標準線量

normal spontaneous delivery 正常自然分娩
no significant difference 有意差なし

NSDF
National Sex and Drug Forum 性・薬物全国フォーラム

NSE
neuron-specific enolase 神経特異エノラーゼ
neurosecretory cell 神経分泌細胞
non-specific esterase 非特異的エステラーゼ
normal saline enema 生理食塩水浣腸

nsec
nanosecond ナノ秒

NSF
nephrogenic systemic fibrosis 腎性全身性線維症
nodular subepidermal fibrosis 結節性表皮下線維組織増殖症
non-specific suppressor factor 非特異抑制因子

NSFTD
normal spontaneous full-term delivery 正常自然満期産

NSG
neurosecretory granule 神経分泌顆粒

nsg
nursing 看護，保育

NSGCT
non-seminomatous germ cell tumor 非精上皮腫瘍性睾丸〔精巣〕腫瘍，非セミノーマ〔非精上皮腫〕胚細胞腫瘍

N

NSGCTT
nonseminomatous germ cell testicular tumor 非セミノーマ〔非精上皮腫〕性精巣胚細胞腫瘍

NSGI
non-specific genital infection 非特異的性器感染

NSH
not so hot そんなに熱くない

NSHA
non-spherocytic hemolytic anemia 非球形溶血性貧血

NSHD
nodular sclerosing Hodgkin disease 小結節硬化型ホジキン病

NSHPT
neonatal severe hyperparathyloidism 新生児重症副甲状腺機能亢進症

NSI
noise and sound index 音響指数
non-standard item 非標準項目
no signs of infection 感染の徴候なし
no signs of inflammation 炎症の徴候なし

NSILA
non-suppressive insulin-like activity 非抑制性インスリン様活性
NSK
not specified by kind 種類によって特異化されない
NSLC
non small cell lung cancer 非小細胞性肺癌
NSM
neurosecretory material 神経分泌物質
noise source meter 音源メーター
nonsmoker 非喫煙者
NSMHC
National Society for Mentally Handicapped Children 精神発達遅滞児全国協会
NSMR
National Society for Medical Research 国立医学研究協会
NSN
nephrotoxic serum nephritis 腎毒性血清(性)腎炎
nicotine-stimulated neurophysin ニコチン刺激性ニューロフィジン
NSNA
National Student Nurse Association 全国看護学生連合
NSO
Neosporin ointment ネオスポリン軟膏
not sufficient quantity 非十分量
NSP
neuron specific protein 神経細胞特異的蛋白
non-starch polysaccharide 非デンプン性多糖
n.sp
new species 新種
NSPB
National Society for Prevention of Blindness 国立失明予防協会
NSPF
not specifically provided for 特異的に用意されていない
NSPN
neurosurgery progress note 脳(神経)外科経過記録
NSQ
neuroticism scale questionnaire 神経質尺度質問
NSR
nasal septal reconstruction 鼻中隔再建(術)
neurosensory retina 網膜神経感覚上皮
non-specific release 非特異的遊離
nonsystemic reaction 非全身反応
normal sinus rhythm 正常洞調律

NSRBC
neuraminidase-treated sheep red blood cell ノイラミニダーゼ処理ヒツジ赤血球
NSRH
non-specific reactive hepatitis 非特異性反応性肝炎
NSRP
nerve-sparing radical prostatectomy 神経温存根治前立腺切除術
NSS
normal saline solution 生理食塩水
normal size and shape 正常の大きさと形
not statistically significant 統計学的有意差なし
nutrition(al) support service 栄養維持サービス，栄養補助サービス
NSSL
normal size, shape, and location 正常の大きさ,形,位置
NS sol
normal saline solution 生理食塩水，正常食塩液
NSST
Northwestern sentence structure test ノースウェスタン文章構文テスト
NSSTT
nonspecific ST-T (wave) 非特異的ST-T(波)
NST
non-stress test ノンストレス試験
nucleus of solitary tract 孤束核
nutritional status type 栄養状態型
NST : O, NST(O)
non-shivering thermogenesis : obligatory 非ふるえ熱産生：不可避的
NSTP
nucleus reticularis tegmentalis pontinus〈ラ〉 橋網様被蓋核
NSTT
nonseminomatous testicular tumor 非精上皮腫性精巣〔睾丸〕腫瘍
NST : T, NST(T)
non-shivering thermogenesis : thermoregulatory 非ふるえ熱産生：体温調節性
NSU
neurosurgical unit (脳)神経外科病棟
nonspecific urethritis 非特異性尿道炎
non-specific vaginitis 非特異性腟炎
N surg
neurosurgeon 神経外科医，脳外科医
neurosurgical 神経外科の，脳外科の
NSurg, N.Surg
neurosurgery 神経外科(学)，脳外科(学)

N

NSV
nonspecific vaginitis 非特異性腟炎
NSVD
normal, spontaneous vaginal delivery 正常,自然腟分娩
NSVT
nonsustained ventricular tachycardia 非持続性心室性頻脈
NSX
neurosurgical examination 神経外科検査, 脳外科検査
Nsy
nursery 育児室, 託児所
NT
nasotracheal (tube) 経鼻気管支(チューブ)
neotetrazolium ネオテトラゾリウム(染色)
neural tract tumor 神経系腫瘍
neurotensin ニューロテンシン
neutralization technique 中和手技
neutralization test 中和反応
neutralizing 中和する
nicotine tartrate 酒石酸ニコチン
nontumorous 腫瘍状でない
normal temperature 正常体温
normal tension 正常血圧者
normal tissue 正常組織
normotensive 正常血圧(性)の
nortriptyline ノルトリプチリン
not tested テストなし
Nt
nitron ニトロン
nt
net weight 全(総)重量
nit ニット, ニト〈単位〉
5′NT
5′-nucleotidase 5′-ヌクレオチダーゼ
NT, N & T
nose and throat 鼻と咽喉
NTA
National Tuberculosis Association 全国結核協会
natural thymocytotoxic autoantibody 胸腺細胞傷害性自然自己抗体
nephrotoxic antibody 腎毒性抗体
nitrilotriacetate ニトリロ三酢酸
NTB
nitrotetrazolium blue ニトロテトラゾリウムブルー(染色)
NTBR
not to be resuscitated 蘇生されない

NTC
neotetrazolium chloride 塩化ネオテトラゾリウム(染色)

NTD
neural tube defect 神経管欠損〔欠陥〕
nitroblue tetrazolium dye ニトロブルーテトラゾリウム色素
5′-nucleotidase 5′-ヌクレオチダーゼ

NTDs
neglect tropical disease 顧みられない熱帯病
neural tube defect 神経管欠損〔欠陥〕

NTE
neurotoxic esterase 神経毒性エステラーゼ

ntES
nuclear transfer Embryonic stem cells 体細胞由来胚性幹細胞

NTF
neurotrophic factor 神経成長因子

ntfy
notify 通知する

NTG
nitroglycerin ニトログリセリン
nontoxic goiter 非中毒性甲状腺腫
normal tension glaucoma 正常眼圧緑内障
normal triglyceridemia 正常中性脂肪血

N

NTGO
nitroglycerin ointment ニトログリセリン軟膏

N & thr
nose and throat 鼻と咽喉

NTI
nonthyroid illness 非甲状腺疾患

NTL
netilmicin ネチルミシン

NTM
neothramycin ネオトラマイシン
nontuberculous mycobacteria 非結核性マイコバクテリア

nTM
native tropomyosin 活性〔未変性〕トロポミオシン

NTMI
nontransmural myocardial infarction 非貫壁性心筋梗塞(症)

NTMNG
nontoxic multinodular goiter 非中毒性多結節(性)甲状腺腫

NTN
nephrotoxic nephritis 腎毒性腎炎

NTO
not thrown out 投げ出されない

not tried on 試みられていない

NTP

nitroprusside ニトロプルシド
normal temperature and pressure 常温正常気圧
nucleoside triphosphate ヌクレオシド三リン酸

NT & P

normal temperature and pressure 正常の温度と気圧

19-NTPP

19-nortestosterone phenylpropionate 19-ノルテストステロンフェニルプロピオネイト

NTR

noise-temperature ratio 音・温度比
normotensive rat 正常血圧ラット
nutrition 栄養

NTRDA

National Tuberculosis and Respiratory Disease Association 結核呼吸器疾患全国協会

NTS

nephrotoxic serum 腎毒性血清
not to scale 測定不能
nucleus tractus solitarius 孤束核

NTT

near total thyroidectomy 甲状腺亜全摘(術)

NTV

nerve tissue vaccine 神経組織ワクチン
nervous tissue vaccine 神経組織ワクチン

NTX

naltrexone ナルトレキソン

NTx

neonatal thymectomy 新生児胸腺切除

NU

name unknown 姓名不明

Nu

nucleolus 核小体
nucleus 核

nU

nanounit ナノ単位

nube

nubile 適齢期の

Nuc

nucleoside ヌクレオシド

nuc

nuclear 核の
nucleated 核のある，有核の
nucleus 核

nucl
nucleus　核
NUD
non-ulcer dyspepsia　非潰瘍性消化不良，上腹部不定愁訴機能性胃腸症
NUDS
Northwestern University Disability Scale　ノースウェスタン大学制定障害度
NUG
necrotizing ulcerative gingivitis　壊死性潰瘍性歯肉炎
NUL
no upper limit　上限なし
nullip
nulliparous　未(経)産の
num
number　番号，数
numbered　番号を付された
numerical　数の
Nut
nutrition　栄養
nutr
nutrition　栄養
NUU
mouse uterine unit　マウス子宮単位
NUV
near ultraviolet　近紫外(線)の
NUW
mouse uterine weight　マウス子宮重量
NV
Nasenverstopfung〈独〉　鼻閉
neovascularization　新生血管
neurovascular　神経血管の
neutral value　中和価
new version　新しい見解
new vessel　新生血管
next visit　次回診察
nivalin　ニバリン
non-vaccinated　非接種の，予防接種をしていない
non vegetarian　非菜食主義者
non venereal　非性病の
non-veteran　退役軍人でない，老練でない
non volatile　非揮発性の
normal volunteer　一般ボランティア
nv.
novicincent〈ラ〉　最近の

Nv, NV
naked vision | 肉眼視，裸眼視

N/V, N & V
nausea and vomiting | 悪心〔嘔気〕と嘔吐

Nva
norvaline | ノルバリン

NVAF
nonvalvular atrial fibrillation | 非弁膜症性心房細動

NVB
neurovascular bundle | 神経血管束

NVC
neurovascular compression | 神経脈管圧迫
neurovascular compression syndrome | 神経血管圧迫症候群

NVD
nausea, vomiting, diarrhea | 悪心〔嘔気〕・嘔吐・下痢
neck vein distention | 頸静脈怒張
neovascularization on the disc | 乳頭上新生血管，視神経乳頭部の新生血管
neuro-vascular decompression | 神経血管減圧手術
neurovesicle dysfunction | 神経小胞機能不全
Newcastle virus disease | ニューカッスルウイルス病
nonvalvular (heart) disease | 非弁〔心臓〕疾患
no venereal disease | 性病なし
no venous distention | 静脈拡張なし

NVDC
nausea, vomiting, diarrhea, and constipation | 吐心〔悪心〕・嘔吐・下痢・便秘

NVE
native valve endocarditis | 自己弁心内膜炎
neovascularization elsewhere | 視神経乳頭部位以外の新生血管

NVG
neovascular glaucoma | 血管新生(性)緑内障《眼》

NVI
neovascularization of the iris | 虹彩血管新生《眼》

NVM
nonvolatile matter | 非揮発性物質

NVMA
National Veterinary Medical Association | 米国国立獣医協会

NVP
natural vegetable powder | 自然野菜粉末

NVS
neurological vital sign | 神経性生活徴候

NVSS
normal variant short stature | 変化のない短身

N

NW
naked weight 裸での体重
nasal wash 鼻洗
Nebenwirkung〈独〉 副作用
Norman-Wood (syndrome) ノーマン・ウッド(症候群)

NWB
non weight bearing 免荷

NWR
normotensive Wistar rat 正常血圧ウィスターラット

NWSN
Nocardia water-soluble nitrogen ノカルジア水溶性窒素

NWTS
National Wilms Tumor Study (Group) 全国ウィルムス腫瘍研究(グループ)

Nx
naloxone ナロキソン(麻薬拮抗薬)

Ny
nystagmus 眼振

NYAM
New York Academy of Medicine ニューヨーク医学会

NYBC
New York Blood Center ニューヨーク血液センター

NYD
not yet diagnosed 未診断の
not yet diagnosis 未診断

NYHA
New York Heart Association ニューヨーク心臓協会

NYH-CMC
New York Hospital-Cornell Medical Center ニューヨーク病院・コーネル医学センター

ny.hor
nystagmus horizontalis 水平(性)眼振

NYP
not yet published 未出版の，未刊行の

ny.rot
nystagmus rotatorius 回転(性)眼振

NYS
nystatin ナイスタチン

nyst
nystagmus 眼振

Nysta
electronystagmograph 電気眼振計

NYUMC
New York University Medical Center ニューヨーク大学医学センター

N

ny.und
nystagmus undulans　振子(様)眼振

ny.vert
nystagmus verticalis　垂直(性)眼振

NZ
Nahrungszucker<独>　栄養糖
Nährzucker<独>　滋養糖
normal zone　正常帯，正常範囲

NZB
New Zealand black (mice)　ニュージーランド黒色(マウス)

NZP
nitrazepam　ニトラゼパム

NZW
New Zealand white (mice)　ニュージーランド白色(マウス)

N・Ebl-o
orthochromatic normoblast　正染性正赤芽球

N・Ebl-p
polychromatic normoblast　多染性正赤芽球

O o

O

esophageal orifice	食道入口部
obese	肥満の
obesity	肥満症
objective	客観的な
objective data	客観的情報
objective findings	客観的所見
observation	観察
obstetrics	産科学
occipital	後頭部の
occiput	後頭
occlusal	咬合の
octarius〈ラ〉	パイント
oculus〈ラ〉	眼
odor	匂い
old	古い，年をとった
Onchocerca	オンコセルカ(属)
Oncomelania	片山貝(属)
opening	孔，開口
opening of circuit	回路開始
operator	オペレータ，術者
operon	オペロン
opistan	オピスタン
Opisthorchis	オピストルキス(属)
opium	阿片
oral	経口的，口の
orally	経口的に
orange	オレンジ
orderly	オーダリー
Oriental	東洋人
orthop(a)edic	整形外科の
osteocyte	骨細胞
output	拍出力
oxidative	酸化性の
respiration	呼吸

o

oil	油
optimus〈ラ〉	最適の
orders	指示
os〈ラ〉	骨，口

^{15}O

oxygen-15	酸素15

^{16}O
oxygen-16 酸素16
^{17}O
oxygen-17 酸素17
^{18}O
oxygen-18 酸素18
O_2
oxygen 酸素
O_3
ozone オゾン
$\overline{O}$
without 伴わない
Ö
Ödem〈独〉 浮腫
ö
ödem〈独〉 浮腫
***o*-**
ortho- 真っすぐな《接》
O, o
other(s) その他，他の
OA
Oberarm〈独〉 上腕
obstructive apnea 閉塞性無呼吸
occipital artery 後頭動脈
occipito-anterior 前方後頭位〈胎位〉
occiput anterior 後頭前部
occupationally induced asthma 職業誘発性ぜん息
ocular albinism 眼白子
office automation オフィスオートメーション
old age 老齢
oleic acid オレイン酸
ophthalmic artery 眼動脈
opiate analgesia アヘン剤無痛法
opsonic activity オプソニン活性
optic atrophy 視神経萎縮
optimal allowance 至適許容量
oral alimentation 経口栄養
orotic acid オロチン酸
orthostatic albuminuria 起立性アルブミン尿
osteoarthritis 変形性関節症
oval albumin 卵白アルブミン
overall assessment 総合的な評価
oxalic acid シュウ酸
oa
overall 被膜，診察衣

O & A
observation and assessment　観察と評価

OAA
oxaloacetic acid　オキサロ酢酸

OAAD
ovarian ascorbic acid depletion (method)　卵巣アスコルビン酸減少(法)《検査》

OABP
organic anion-binding protein　有機陰イオン結合蛋白

OAD
obstructive airway disease　閉塞性気道疾患
occlusive arterial disease　閉塞性動脈疾患
overall depth　被膜厚

OADC
oleic acid, albumin, dextrose, catalase medium　オレイン酸・アルブミン・ブドウ糖・カタラーゼ培地

OAE
otoacoustic emission　耳音響放射

OAF
osteoclast activating factor　破骨細胞活性化因子

OAG
Oberarm Gips〈独〉　上腕ギプス
ocular angiography　眼動脈撮影
open angle glaucoma　開放角緑内障

OAGB
Osteopathic Association of Great Britain　イギリス骨疾患協会

OAH
ovarian androgenic hyperfunction　卵巣アンドロゲン性機能亢進
overall height　被膜高

OAJ
open apophyseal joint　開放椎間関節

OAL
overall length　被膜長

OALL
ossification of anterior longitudinal ligament　前縦靱帯骨化症

OALMA
Orthopedic Appliance and Limb Manufactures Association　整形外科矯正器と義肢製造協会

o.alt.hor.
omnibus alternis horis〈ラ〉　1時間おきに《処》

OAM
Office of Aviation Medicine　航空医学診察室
the office of alternative medicine　(米国)代替医療局

OA-MC bypass
occipital artery-middle cerebral artery bypass　大後頭動脈・中大脳動脈バイパス
OAO
off and on　オフとオン，解除と加入
OAP
occlusion d'artère pulmonaire〈仏〉　肺動脈閉鎖
oedeme algu pulmonaire〈ラ〉　急性肺浮腫
ophthalmic artery pressure　眼動脈圧
oscillatory afterpotential　振動性後電位
osteoarthropathy　骨関節症
oxygen at atmospheric pressure　大気圧下の酸素
vincristine(=Oncovin), arabinosylcytosine, prednisone　ビンクリスチン(=オンコビン),アラビノシルシトシン,プレドニゾン
OA-PICA anastomosis
occipital artery-posterior inferior cellebellar artery anastomosis　後頭動脈・後下小脳脳動脈吻合部
OAQPS
Office of Air Quality Planning and Standards　大気質計画標準課
OAR
Office of Air and Radiation　大気放射線局
OARSA
oxacillin aminoglycoside-resistant *Staphylococcus aureus*　オキサシリンアミン配糖体耐性黄色ブドウ球菌
OAS
old age security　老齢保障
oral allergy syndrome　経口〔口腔粘膜〕アレルギー症候群
organic anxiety syndrome　器質性不安症候群
osmotically active substance　浸透性活性物質
OASDHI
Old Age, Survivors, Disability and Health Insurance Social Security　老人・生存者・身障者の健康保険社会保障
OASI
Old-age and Survivor's Insurance　老人と生存者保険
OASM units
ohm, ampere, second and meter units　オーム・アンペア・秒・メートル単位
OASO
overactive superior oblique　過活動上斜筋
OASP
organic acid soluble phosphorus　有機酸可溶性リン
OASR
overactive superior rectus　過活動上直筋

O

OAT
ornithine-8-aminotransferase　オルニチン-8-アミノトランスフェラーゼ
ortho-aminoazotoluene　オルト・アミノアゾトルエン
outside air temperature　外気温度

OAV
oculoauriculovertebral　眼耳脊椎の

OAW
oral airway　(喉頭)エアウェイ
overall width　被膜幅

OB
obese　肥満の
obliterative bronchitis　閉塞性細気管支炎
obstetrics　産科(学)，動物産科学
occult blood　潜血
old bony　古い骨の
olfactory bulb　嗅球
osteoblast　骨芽細胞
output buffer　出力緩衝物

ob
obit　死亡告知

O & B
opium and belladonna　アヘンとベラドンナ

OB, ob.
obit〈ラ〉=he died, she died　死亡した

OB, O.B.
ohne Befund=ohne Besonders=ohne Beschwerde〈独〉　異常所見なし

O

ob, Ob
oblique (position)　斜位

ob, OB, Ob
obstetric　産科の
obstetrical　産科学の
obstetrician　産科医
obstetrics　産科

OBC
ordinary bladder capacity　日常的膀胱容量

OBD
organic brain disease　器質性脳疾患

OBE
castor oil, warm bath, enema　ヒマシ油・温浴・浣腸

OBF
organ blood flow　臓器血流

OBG
obstetrician-gynecologyst　産婦人科医
obstetrics and gynecology　産婦人科学

OBGS
obstetric and gynecologic surgery 産科・婦人科手術
ob-gy
obstetrical-gynecological 産科・婦人科学(の)
OB/GYN, ob-gyn
obsterics and gynecology 産科・婦人科
obstetrician gynecologist 産婦人科医
Obj, obj
object 対象
objective 目的，客観的な
objn
objection 障害
OBL, obl
oblique 斜めの，斜位の
obln
obligation 強制
OBN
occult blood-negative 潜血・陰性
OBP
objective blood pressure 診察時血圧
occult blood-positive 潜血・陽性
ova,blood and parasites 虫卵・潜血・寄生虫
OBRB
outer blood-retinal barrier 外血液・網膜関門
OBRR
obstetric recovery room 産科回復室
obs
obstacle 障害
obs, obs., OBS, Obs
observation 観察
observed 観察された
observer 観察者
obsolete 旧式の，すたれた
obstetrical service 産科(サービス)
obstetrician 産科医
obstetrics 産科学
organic brain syndrome 器質性脳症候群
obsc
obscured 不明瞭な
Obst, obst
obstetrician 産科医
obstetrics 産科学
obstipation 腸閉塞，便秘
obstruct 閉塞する
obstruction 閉塞
obstructive 閉塞の

obstet
obstetric　産科の
Obstruct
obstruction　閉塞
obstructive　閉塞の
obsvd
observed　観察された
obtd
obtained　獲得された
OB-US
obstetrical ultrasound　産科超音波
OBW
observation window　観察窓
OC
obsterical conjugate　産科的結合線
occipital cortex　後頭葉
occlusocervical　咬合面歯頸部の
odor control　臭気管理
Office of Compliance　コンプライアンス事務局
on call　待機して
optic chiasm(a)　視神経交叉〔差〕
oral contraceptive　経口避妊薬
organ culture　器官培養
osteocalcin　オステオカルシン
outer canthus　外斜角
ovarian cancer　卵巣癌
oxitocin　オキシトシン
oxygen closed　酸素閉鎖《麻酔》
oxygen consumed　酸素消費量
O & C, O+C
onset and course (of a disease)　(疾患の)発症および経過
OCA
oculocutaneous albinism　眼皮膚白皮症
olivopontocerebellar atrophy　オリーブ橋小脳萎縮(症)
oral contraceptive agent　経口避妊薬
OCAD
occlusive carotid artery disease　閉塞性頸動脈疾患
O_2 cap
oxygen capacity　酸素容量
OCB
olivo-cochlear bundle　オリーブ蝸牛神経束
Occ
occulusion　閉塞
occ
occipital　後頭の
occiput　後頭

occupation　職業，作業
occurrence　発生，起こること

occ△
occipital triangle　後頭三角

Occ, occ
occasional　ときどきの
occasionally　ときどき

occas
occasional　ときどきの
occasionally　ときどき

OCCC
open-chest cardiac compression　開胸式心臓圧迫

OCC in UTJ
occlusion in utero-tubal junction　子宮卵管結合部閉塞

occip
occipital　後頭の
occiput　後頭

occip.F, occip-F
occipitofrontal　後頭前頭の

occip-F HA
occipitofrontal headache　後頭前頭頭痛

OCCM
open chest cardiac massage　開胸式心マッサージ(法)

OCCPR
open-chest cardiopulmonary resuscitation　開胸式心肺蘇生術

OCC Th, Occ Th, occ.th.
occupational therapy　作業療法

Occup, occup
occupation　職業
occupational　職業の
occupy　占拠する
occupying　占拠している

OCD
obsessive compulsive disorder　強迫性障害
osteochondritis dissecans　離断性骨軟骨炎
ovarian cholesterol depletion　卵巣コレステロール消耗

OCG
omnicardiogram　全心電図
oral cholecystogram　経口胆嚢造影図
oral cholecystography　経口胆嚢造影

OCH
oral contraceptive hormone　経口避妊ホルモン

OCI
ovum capture inhibitor　卵捕獲抑制因子

OCICHS
Organizing Committee of International Congress on Hormonal Steroids — 国際ステロイドホルモン組織委員会

OCL
Occupational Check List — 職業チェックリスト
osteoclast — 破骨細胞

ocl
occlusion — 閉塞，咬合

OCLG
osteoclast-like giant cell — 破骨細胞様巨細胞

OCM
oral contraceptive medication — 経口避妊薬

OCN
oculomotor nucleus — 動眼神経核

OCO
open-close-open — 開放・閉鎖・開放

O.Co.Ag
lack of objectivity, lack of cooperativeness, lack of agreeable — 客観性の欠如・協調性の欠如・無愛想(＝ギルフォード・マーチン人格目録の因子)

OCP
octacalcium phosphate — リン酸オクタカルシウム
ocular cicatricial pemphigoid — 眼類天疱瘡
oral contraceptive pill — 経口避妊薬
ova, cysts and parasites — 虫卵・囊胞・寄生虫

***o*-CPC method**
orthocresolphthalein complexone method — オルトクレゾールフタレインコンプレクソン法

OCR
ocualr countertorsion reflex — 眼球逆回旋反射
ocular counterrolling — 眼球逆回転，眼球反転
oculocardiac reflex — 眼球心臓反射
oculocephalic reflex — 頭位変換眼球反射
oculocephalic response — 眼球脳反応
Office of Civil Right — 市民権利局
optical character reader — 光電式文字読取装置
optical character recognition — 視的性格認知

OCRS
oculocerebrorenal syndrome — 眼脳腎症候群

OCS
ocular conversion symptom — 眼転換症状
open canalicular system — 開放管系
oral contraceptive steroid — 経口避妊ステロイド

11-OCS
11-oxycorticosteroid　11-オキシコルチコステロイド

OCSG
Ovarian Cancer Study Group　卵巣癌研究班

OCSP
orthopaedic examination, special　整形外科検査・特殊

OCT
Object Classification Test　対象分類検査
optical coherence tomography　網膜断層解析装置
oral contraceptive therapy　経口避妊療法
ornithine carbamoyltransferase　オルニチンカルバモイルトランスフェラーゼ
oxytocin challenge test　オキシトシンチャレンジテスト

OCTD
ornithine carbamoyltransferase deficiency　オルニチンカルバモイルトランスフェラーゼ欠損症

OCTT
orocecal transit time　盲腸通過時間

oct.th
occupational therapy　作業療法

octup.
octuplus〈ラ〉　8倍

OCU
observation care unit　観察看護部門

ocul.
oculis〈ラ〉　眼に《処》

ocul.dext.
oculo dextro〈ラ〉　右眼に《処》

oculent.
oculentum〈ラ〉　眼軟膏《処》

ocul.sinist.
oculo sinistro〈ラ〉　左眼に《処》

ocul.utro.
oculo utro〈ラ〉　両眼に《処》

OCV
opacitas corporis vitrei　硝子体混濁
ordinary conversational voice　通常会話声

OCVM
occult vascular malformation　不顕性血管(先天)奇形
ocular cerebral vascular monitor　眼脳血管測定装置

OD
Doctor of Optometry　検眼医
occipital dysplasia　後頭形成異常
occupational dermatitis　職業性皮膚炎
occupational disease　職業病

odds ratio	オッズ比
officer of day	日直医
open drop	開放点滴
optical density	吸光度，光学密度
optical disk	光ディスク
optimal dose	適量
ornithine decarboxylase	オルニチン脱炭酸酵素
orolingual dyskinesia	口舌運動不全
orthostatische dysregulation〈独〉＝ orthostatic disturbance 〔dysfunction〕	起立性調節障害
Osteopathic Doctor	整骨医
outer diameter	外径
out-of-date	旧式の
outside diameter	過量
overdose	過量
oxygen demand	酸素要求量

Od

oculus dexter	右眼

od

oder〈独〉	あるいは，または

o.d.

omni die〈ラ〉	毎日
once a day	1日1回

o/d

on demand	需要に応じて

ODA

occipito-dextra-anterior	右後頭腹側位
osmotic driving agent	浸透圧推進物質

ODAP

vincristine(＝Oncovin), dianhydrogaractitol, adriamycin, cisplatin(＝Platinol)	ビンクリスチン(＝オンコビン), ジアンヒドロガラクチトール, アドリアマイシン, シスプラチン(＝プラチノール)

ODC

ornithine decarboxylase	オルニチン脱炭酸酵素
oxygen dissociation curve	酸素解離曲線
oxyhemoglobin dissociation curve	酸素ヘモグロビン解離曲線

ODCB

orthodichlorobenzene	オルト二塩酸ベンゼン

ODCH

ordinary disease of childhood	小児期一般疾患

ODD

oculo-dento-digital (syndrome)	眼・歯・指(症候群)
oculodentodigital dysplasia	眼歯指形成異常

O

OD'd
overdosed 過量の
ODDS
oculodentodigital syndrome 眼歯指症候群
ODE
Office of Drug Evaluation (米国)薬評価事務局
old dog encephalitis 老犬脳炎
ODG
ophthalmodynamography 眼底血圧検査法
ODGF
osteosarcoma-derived growth factor 骨肉腫由来増殖因子
oding
overdosing 過量の
ODM
ophthalmodynamometer 眼底血圧計
ophthalmodynamometry 眼底血圧測定
ODOD
oculodentoosseous dysplasia 眼歯骨形成異常
odom
odometer 嗅覚計
Odont, odont.
odontogenic 歯の
odontology 歯学
odoram.
odoramentum〈ラ〉 芳香
odorat.
odoratus〈ラ〉 芳香の
odorl
odorless 無臭の
ODP
occipito-dextra-posterior 右後頭背側位
offspring of diabetic parents 糖尿病の親をもつ子供
one dose package 1回量包装
ODQ
on direct questioning 直接質問で
opponens digiti quinti (muscle) 小指対立(筋)
ODSG
ophthalmic Doppler sonogram 眼ド(ッ)プラー超音波図
ODST
overdrive suppression test オーバードライブ抑制試験
ODT
occipitodextra transversa 右後頭横側位，第二頭位
occlusive dressing technique 密封療法
oculodynamic test 眼球動態検査
ODTS
organic dust toxic syndrome 有機粉塵毒性症候群

ODU
optical density unit (s) 光学密度単位

OE
olfactory epithelium 嗅上皮
on examination 診察で
oroesophageal tube feeding 口腔食道経管栄養
orthop (a) edic examination 整形外科検査
otitis externa 外耳炎

Oe
oersted エルステッド〈単位〉

O & E
observation and examination 観察と診察

OEB
Office of Epidemiology and Biostatistics 疫学生物統計学局

OEb
orthochromatic erythroblast 正染性赤芽球

OEC
outer ear canal 外耳道

OEE
osmotic erythrocyte enrichment 浸透圧赤血球強化
outer enamel epithelium 外エナメル上皮

OEF
Osteopathic Educational Foundation 骨疾患教育財団
oxygen extraction fraction 酸素抽出分画

OEIS complex
omphalocele, exstrophy of the bladder, imperforate anus, spine defect complex 臍ヘルニア・膀胱外反(症)・鎖肛・脊髄異常症候群

ÖeK
Ösophaguskrebs〈独〉 食道癌

OEM
opposite ear masked 反対側の耳を遮蔽して

OEP
original endotoxin protein 菌体内毒素蛋白

OER
oxygen enhancement ratio 酸素効果比

o'er
over 過度の

OES
Olympus endoscopy system オリンパス内視鏡システム
optical emission spectroscopy 放出光分光検査法
oral esophageal stethoscope 経口食道聴診器
order entry system 発生源入力システム

oesoph
oesophagus 食道

OET
oral endotracheal tube　経口気管チューブ
oral esophageal tube　経口食道チューブ
OETT
oral endotracheal tube　経口気管チューブ
O.ext.
otitis externa〈ラ〉　外耳炎
OF
occipital-frontal　後頭・前頭
occipitofrontal　後頭前頭の
occipitofrontal diameter　前後径
old face　老人の顔
Ophthalmological Foundation　眼科学財団
optic fundi　眼底
optional form　任意の型
orbitofrontal　眼窩前頭の
orbitofrontal cortex　眼窩前頭皮質
osmotic fragility　浸透圧脆弱性
osteitis fibrosa　線維性骨炎
Osteopathic Foundation　骨疾患財団
Otofurunkel〈独〉　耳癤
o/f, OF, O-F, O/F
oxidation/fermentation (ratio)　酸化・発酵(比)
OFA
oncofetal antigen　腫瘍胎児抗原
OFBM
oxidation-fermentation basal medium　酸化・発酵基礎培地
OFC
occipitofrontal circumference　後頭前頭周囲
orbitofacial cleft　眼窩顔面裂
osteitis fibrosa cystica　嚢胞性線維性骨炎
ofc
office　医院
OFCTAD
occipito-faciocervico-thoraco-abdomino-digital (dysplasia)　後頭・顔・頸・胸郭・腹・指異形成症
OFD
object-film distance　物体・フィルム間距離
occipitofrontal diameter　(頭部)前後径
oral-facial-digital　口・顔面・指
orofaciodigital (dysostosis)　口顔面指(形成不全症)
orofaciodigital (syndorome)　口顔面指(症候群)
OFDS
orofaciodigital syndrome　口顔面指症候群
off
office　医院

Off, off
official 公認の
OF-HA
occipitofrontal headache 後頭前頭頭痛
OFLX
ofloxacin オフロキサシン
OFM
orofacial malformation (先天異常の)口顔奇形
OF rad
occipitofrontal radiation 後頭前頭照射
OG
Obstetrics-Gynecology 産婦人科
ohrengedokuto 黄連解毒湯
optic ganglion 眼神経節
osmolality gap オスモラリティーギャップ
OG-6
(Papanicolaou) orange G-6 counter stain オレンジG- 6 対比染色
OGCT
ovarian germ cell tumor 卵巣生殖細胞腫瘍
OGD
Office of Generic Drug 一般薬品事務室
old granulomatous disease 老年肉芽腫症
OGF
ovarian growth factor 卵巣成長因子
OGH
ovine growth hormone ヒツジ成長ホルモン
OGI
oculogyral illusion 眼ジャイロ錯覚
osteogenesis imperfecta 骨形成不全症
OG stain
orange green stain オレンジグリーン染色
OGT
orogastric tube 経口胃チューブ
OGTT
oral glucose tolerance test 経口ブドウ糖負荷試験
OH
hydroxide 水酸化物
hydroxy ヒドロキシ《接》
hydroxycorticosteroid ヒドロキシコルチコステロイド
hydroxyl group 水酸基
hydroxyl radical ヒドロキシルラジカル
obstructive hypopnea 閉塞性呼吸低下
occipital horn 後頭角
occupational history 職歴

ocular hypertension 高眼圧症
on hand 手近に
open heart 開心術
oral hygiene 口腔衛生
orthostatic hypotension 起立性低血圧
out of hosipital 退院の
Outpatient Hospital 外来病院
oval head 卵型頭

OH^-
hydroxide ion 水酸化イオン

17-OH
17-hydroxycorticosteroid 17-ヒドロキシコルチコステロイド

OH, o.h.
omni hora〈ラ〉=every hour 1時間ごとに《処》

OHA
oral hypoglycemic agent 経口糖尿病薬

3-OHA
3-hydroxyamobarbital 3-ヒドロキシアモバルビタール

OHAHA
ophthalmoplegia-hypotonia-ataxia-hypoacusis-athetosis (syndrome) 眼筋麻痺・緊張低下・運動失調・聴力障害・アテトーゼ（症候群）

OHB_{12}
hydroxycobalamin ヒドロキシコバラミン

O_2Hb
oxyhemoglobin オキシヘモグロビン

OHBA
3-hydroxybutyric acid 3-ヒドロキシ酪酸

OHC
hydroxycholecalciferol ヒドロキシコレカルシフェロール
outer hair cell 外有毛細胞

OH-Cbl
hydroxocobalamin ヒドロキソコバラミン

17-OHCS
17-hydroxycorticosteroid 17-ヒドロキシコルチコステロイド

OHCS, OHCs
hydroxycorticosteroid ヒドロキシコルチコステロイド

OHD
organic hearing disease 器質的聴覚疾患
organic heart disease 器質性心疾患

O

25-OHD$_3$，25(OH)D$_3$
25-hydroxycholecalciferol — 25-ヒドロキシビタミンD$_3$，カルシジオール

6-OHDA
6-hydroxydopamine hydrochloride — 6-ヒドロキシド(ー)パミンヒドロクロライド

18-OH-DOC
18-hydroxy-11-deoxycorticosterone — 18-ヒドロキシ-11-デオキシコルチコステロン

OH-DOC
hydroxydeoxycorticosterone — ヒドロキシデオキシコルチコステロン

OHE
Office of Health Economics — 健康経済研究所

OHF
old healed fracture — 陳旧性治癒骨折
Omsk hemorrhagic fever — オムスク出血熱

OHFA
hydroxy fatty acid — ヒドロキシ脂肪酸

OHG
oral hypoglycemic — 経口血糖降下性の

OHI
ocular hypertension indicator — 眼球高血圧指標
Oral Hygiene Index — 口腔衛生指数

OH IAA
hydroxyindoleacetic acid — ヒドロキシインドール酢酸

OHI-S
Simplified Oral Hygiene Index — 単純化口腔衛生指数

O

OHL
oral hairy leukoplakia — 口腔毛髪状白斑

OHlase
hydroxylase — 水酸化酵素，ヒドロキシラーゼ

ohm-cm
ohm-centimeter — オーム・センチメートル

OHP
hydroxy-progesterone — 水酸化プロゲステロン
hydroxyproline — ヒドロキシプロリン
overhead projector — オーバーヘッドプロジェクタ
oxygen hyperbaric pressure — 高圧酸素療法

17-OHP
17α-hydroxyprogesterone — 17-ヒドロキシプロゲステロン

OHPAA，*o*-HPAA
orthohydroxyphenylacetic acid — オルトヒドロキシフェニル酢酸

OHPP
occluded hepatic portal pressure 遮断時肝側門脈圧
OHRR
open heart recovery room 開心術回復室
OHS
obesity hypoventilation syndrome 肥満換気低下症候群
ocular hypoperfusion syndrome 眼低灌流症候群
open heart surgery 開心術
OHSS
ovarian hyperstimulating syndrome 卵巣過剰刺激症候群
OHT
obesity hypertension 肥満高血圧
ocular hypertension 高眼圧(症)
ocular hypertensive (glaucoma suspect) 眼圧亢進症
orthotopic heart transplant 同所性心臓移植
overhead traction オーバーヘッド牽引
18-OH-THA
18-hydroxy-11-dehydrotetra-hydrocorticosterone 18-ヒドロキシ-11-デヒドロテトラヒドロコルチコステロン

OI
obesity index 肥満指数
objective improvement 客観的改善
obturator internus 内閉鎖筋
opportunistic infection 日和見感染
opsonic index オプソニン指数
orgasmic impairment オルガスム障害
Orientation Inventory 見当識調査票
osteogenesis imperfecta 骨形成不全
otitis interna 内耳炎
oxygeneration index 酸素化係数
oxygen inspired 吸入酸素
oxygen intake 酸素摂取
oxytocin induction オキシトシン分娩誘発
OI congenita
osteogenesis imperfecta congenita 先天性骨形成不全
OICU
obsterics intensive care unit 産科集中監視室
OID
optimal immunomodulating dose 免疫調節適量
organism identification (number) 生物分類(番号)
OIDI
Okinawa Infectious Disease Initiative 沖縄感染症対策イニシアティブ

Oid-Oid disease
distinctive exudative discoid and lichenoid chronic dermatitis — 特異性滲出性円板状苔癬状慢性皮膚炎

OIF
oil immersion field — 油浸域
osteoinducing hormone — 骨誘導因子

OIH
orthoiodohippurate — *o*-ヨード馬尿酸塩
ovulation inducing hormone — 排卵誘発ホルモン

oint
ointment — 軟膏

OIP
organizing interstitial pneumonia — 器質化間質性肺炎

OIPH
Office of International Public Health — 国際公衆衛生局

OIRDA
occipital intermittent rhythmic delta activity — 後頭部間欠性律動性δ波

OISA
Osaka intelligence scale for the aged — 阪大式知能検査

OIT
ovarian immature teratoma — 卵巣未熟奇形腫

OI tarda
osteogenesis imperfecta tarda — 遅発性骨形成不全

OIU
optical internal urethrotomy — 光学内尿道切開(術)

OJ, o.j.
orange juice — オレンジジュース

O

OJB
on the job — 仕事中に

OK
all correct — よろしい
all right — よし
approved — 承諾された
correct — 正しい
old tuberculin Koch — コッホの旧ツベルクリン

ÖK
Ösophaguskrebs〈独〉 — 食道癌

OKA
otherwise known as — さもなければ知られているように

OKAN
optokinetic after-nystagmus — 視運動性後眼振

OKB
Ortho, Kung, B lymphocyte — オルト・クン・Bリンパ球

OKF
Oberkieferfraktur〈独〉 上顎骨骨折

OKK
Oberkiefer Krebs〈独〉 上顎癌

OKmedium
Oka-Katakura medium 岡・片倉培地

OKN
optokinetic nystagmus 視運動性眼振

OKP
optokinetic pattern 視運動性眼振パターン

OKP test
optokinetic pattern test 視運動性眼振パターン検査

OKT
Ollier-Klippel-Trenaunay (syndrome) オリエ・クリッペル・トレノーネイ(症候群)
ornithine-ketoacid transaminase オルニチンケト酸トランスアミナーゼ
Ortho, Kung, T lymphocyte オルト・クン・Tリンパ球

OL
oleandomycin オレアンドマイシン
other location 他の部位

OL, O.L., o.l.
oculus laevus〈ラ〉 左眼

Ol, ol, ol.
oleum〈ラ〉 油《処》

OLA
occipito-laeva-anterior 後頭左前位

OLB
olfactory bulb 嗅球
open-liver-biopsy 開腹下肝生検

OLC
ordinary living conditions 普通生活条件

OLD
obstructive lung disease 閉塞性肺疾患
orthochromatic leukodystrophy 正染性白質萎縮(症)

oleat.
oleatum〈ラ〉 油酸剤《処》

oleores.
oleoresia〈ラ〉 樹脂油《処》

OLF
ossification of ligamentum flavum 黄色靱帯骨化症

olf
olfactory 嗅覚の

OLG
oligodendroglioma 乏突起膠腫

OLGC
osteoclast-like giant cell 破骨細胞様巨細胞
OLH
ovine lactogenic hormone ヒツジ乳腺刺激ホルモン
oll
olla〈ラ〉 壺《処》
OLM
ocular larva migrans 眼幼虫移行症
oleandomycin オレアンドマイシン
ophthalmic laser microendoscope 眼レーザー電子顕微鏡
OLNM
occult lymph node metastasis 不顕性リンパ節転移
ol.oliv.
oleum olivae〈ラ〉 オリーブ油《処》
OLP
occipito-laeva-posterior 後頭左後位
OLR
Otology, Laryngology and Rhinology 耳鼻咽喉科
ol.res.
oleo resin〈ラ〉 油脂《処》
OLRT
on-line real time オンラインリアルタイム
OLT
occipito-laeva-transverse 左後頭横側位《胎位》
occipi tomental transversa 第一頭位
orthotopic liver transplantation 正常位肝移植
OLT, Olt
orthotopic liver transplant 同所性肝移植
OLV
one-lung ventilation 片肺換気
OM
obtuse marginal branch 鈍縁枝
occipitomental 後頭オトガイの
occipitomental diameter 大斜径
occupational medicine 職業医学
oculomotor 動眼神経の
old man〔men〕 老人
oleandomycin オレアンドマイシン
orbitomeatal (line) 眼窩外耳口(線)
osteomalacia 骨軟化症
osteomyelitis 骨髄炎
otitis media 中耳炎
outer membrane 外膜
ovomucoid オボムコイド
ovulation method 排卵法

om.
omni〈ラ〉 ～ごとに《処》
o.m.
omni mane〈ラ〉 毎朝
OMA
Ophthalmic Medical Assistant 眼科医療従事者
otitis media, acuta 急性中耳炎
OMAC
otitis media, acute, catarrhal 中耳炎, 急性カタル性
OMAD
vincristine (=Oncovin), methotrexate, adriamycin, dactinomycin ビンクリスチン(=オンコビン), メトトレキサート, アドリアマイシン, ダクチノマイシン
OMAS
occupational maladjustment syndrome 職業適応障害症候群
otitis media, acute, suppurating 中耳炎, 急性化膿性
OMBL
orbitomeatal basal line 眼窩外耳孔基底線
OMC
open mitral commissurotomy 直視下僧帽弁交連切開術
otitis media chronica 慢性中耳炎
OMCA
otitis media, catarrhal, acute 中耳炎・急性カタル性
OMCC
otitis media, catarrhal, chronic 中耳炎・慢性カタル性
OMCD
outer medullary collecting duct 髄質外層集合管
OMChS
otitis media, chronic, suppurating 中耳炎・慢性化膿性
OMD
ocular muscle dystrophy 眼筋ジストロフィー
oculomandibulodyscephaly 眼下顎頭蓋異常症
3-*o*〔ortho〕-methyldopa 3-*o*-メチルド(ー)パ
organic mental disorder 器質性精神疾患
OM-dopa
3-*o*〔ortho〕-methyldopa 3-*o*-メチルド(ー)パ
OME
otitis media with effusion 滲出性中耳炎
output to maintain erection 勃起維持(静脈)流出量
OMED
Organization Mondial d'Endoscopie Digéstive〈仏〉 世界消化器内視鏡学会

OMED AP
Asian-Pacific Zone of OMED — 世界消化器内視鏡学会アジア太平洋分科会

OMF
oculomandibulofacial syndrome — 後頭下顎顔面症候群

OMFS
oral and maxillofacial surgery — 口腔および顎顔面手術

OMG
ocular myasthenia gravis — 重症眼筋無力症

OMGE
Organization Mondiale de Gastroenterology〈仏〉 — 世界消化器病学会

om.1/4h.
omni quadranta hora〈ラ〉 — 15分ごとに《処》

OMI
old myocardial infarction — 陳旧性心筋梗塞(症)
oocyte maturation inhibitor — 卵細胞成熟抑制因子

OMIPE
Office Mondial d'Information sur les Problémes d'Environnement〈仏〉 — 世界環境問題情報局

OML
orbitomeatal line — 眼窩外耳孔線

OM-line
orbitomeatal line — 眼窩外耳孔線

OMM
ophthalomomandibulomelic (dysplasia, syndrome) — 眼下顎四肢(形成不全)，眼下顎四肢(症候群)
outer mitochondrial membrane — ミトコンドリア外膜

O

om.mane vel noc.
omni mane vel nocte〈ラ〉 — 毎朝または毎夜《処》

OMN
oculomotor nerve (nucleus) — 動眼神経(核)

omn.bid.
omni biduo〈ラ〉 — 2日ごとに

omn.bih.
omni bihora〈ラ〉 — 2時間ごとに

omn.hor.
omni hora〈ラ〉 — 1時間ごとに《処》

omn.2hor.
omni secunda hora〈ラ〉 — 2時間ごとに

omni
omnidirectional — 各方向の
omnirange — 各変域
omnivisual — 各視野

omn.man.
omni mane〈ラ〉 — 毎朝《処》

omn.noct.
omni nocte〈ラ〉=every night　毎夜《処》

omn.quad.hor.
omni quadrante hora〈ラ〉　15分ごとに《処》

omn.quar.hor.
omni quarta hora〈ラ〉　4時間ごとに《処》

omn.sec.hor.
omni secunda hora〈ラ〉　2時間ごとに《処》

omn.tert.hor.
omni tertia hora〈ラ〉　3時間ごとに《処》

OMP
outer membrane protein　外膜蛋白
oxymethylpyrimidine　オキシメチルピリミジン

OMPA
octamethyl pyrophosphoramide　オクタメチルピロホスホラミド(=ペトレックスIII)
otitis media purulenta acuta　急性化膿性中耳炎

OMPC
otitis media purulenta chronica　慢性化膿性中耳炎

om.quad.hor.
omni quadrante hora〈ラ〉　15分ごとに《処》

OMR
operative mortality rate　手術死亡率

OMS
organic mental syndrome　器質精神症候群
organisation mondiale de la santé〈仏〉　世界保健機関
otomandibular syndrome　耳下顎症候群

OMSA
otitis media, suppurative, acute　化膿性急性中耳炎

OMSC
otitis media suppurativa chronica　慢性化膿性中耳炎

OMT
ortho-methyltransferase　*o*-メチルトランスフェラーゼ，オルトメチル転移酵素

OMT, OM/T
oral mucosal transudate　口腔粘膜漏出液

OMU
ocular micrometer unit　接眼ミクロメータ単位

OMV
oronasal mask ventilation　口鼻マスク換気法

OMVC
open mitral valve commissurotomy　直視下僧帽弁交連切開術

ON
optic nerve　視神経
osteonecrosis　骨壊死
overnight　一晩じゅう，徹夜

ON, On, o.n.
omni nocte〈ラ〉 毎夜《処》
ONA
osteonecrosis aseptique〈ラ〉 無菌性骨壊死症
on approv
on approval 到達して
ONB
ortho-nitrobiphenyl *o*-ニトロビフェニル
oncol
oncological 腫瘍学の
oncology 腫瘍学
OND
other neurological disease 他の神経疾患
ONDS
Oriental nocturnal death syndrome 東洋人夜間死亡症候群
ONFH
osteo necrosis of femoral head 大腿骨頭壊死
ONH
optic nerve head 視神経乳頭
optic nerve hypoplasia 視神経乳頭形成不全
ONNI
Office of National Narcotics Intelligence 国家麻薬情報局
ONO
or near offer または近似値で
ONP
ortho-nitrophenyl *o*-ニトロフェニル
operating nursing procedure 手術看護方式
ONPG-GAL
ortho-nitrophenyl-β-galactosidase *o*-ニトロフェニル-β-ガラクトシダーゼ
ONS
Oncology Nursing Society 癌看護協会
ONT
obesity normal tension 肥満正常血圧(者)
ONTG
oral nitroglycerin 経口ニトログリセリン
ONTR
orders not to resuscitate 蘇生させない指示
ony
onymous 名前の明らかな
OO
oophorectomized 卵巣摘出された
oophorectomy 卵巣摘出術
o/o
on account of ～のために

OOB
out of bed — ベッド外で

OOBBRP
out of bed, bathroom privileges — 起床可，入浴可

OOBE
out of body experience — 体験外の

OOC
out of control — 制御できない

OOE
output to obtain erection — 勃起獲得(静脈)流出量

OOL
onset of labor — 分娩開始

OOLR
Ophthalmology, Otology, Laryngology, Rhinology — 眼科学・耳科学・咽喉科学・鼻科学

OOO
out of order — 乱れている，適切でない

OOR
out of room — 部屋から出て

OOTCDE
Office of Over The Counter Drug Evaluations — 非処方箋薬を扱う薬局の監視者

OP
occipital protuberance — 後頭部結節
occipitoparietal — 後頭頭頂の
occiput posterior — 後頭骨後部
old patient (previously seen) — 再来患者
olfactory peduncle — 嗅索
opponens pollicis — 母指対立筋
oropharynx — 中咽頭
orthostatic proteinuria — 起立性蛋白尿
osmotic pressure — 浸透圧
osteoporosis — 骨粗鬆症
ovine prolactin — ヒツジプロラクチン

op.
opus〈ラ〉 — 仕事

o.p.
optimus maximus〈ラ〉 — 最高によい

O & P
ova and parasites — 虫卵と寄生虫

OP, Op, op
operating — 手術している
operation — 手術
operational — 手術の
operation plan — 手術計画
operative — 手術の

O

operative procedure　手術手技
operator　術者
ophthalmic　眼の
ophthalmology　眼科学
opposite　反対の

OP, O/P
outpatient　外来患者

OPA
o-phthalaldehyde　*o*-フタルアルデヒド
oral pharyngeal airway　口腔咽頭エアウェイ
ovarian papillary adenocarcinoma　卵巣乳頭腺癌

OPAL
vincristine (=Oncovin), prednisone, L-asparaginase　ビンクリスチン(=オンコビン), プレドニゾン, L-アスパラギナーゼ

OP amp
operation amplifier　演算増幅器

OPB
outpatient basis　外来患者として

OPC
oculopalatocerebral (syndrome)　眼球口蓋大脳(症候群)
oropharyngeal candidiasis　口腔咽頭カンジダ症
outpatient clinic　外来診療所

OPCA
olivopontocerebellar atrophy　オリーブ橋小脳萎縮症

op.cit.
opus citato〈ラ〉　引用された報告中に

OPCOS
oligomenorrheic polycystic ovary syndrome　希発月経性多嚢胞性卵巣症候群

OPCS
Office of Population, Consensus Survey　人口および世論調査局

OPD
obstetric prediabetes　産科的糖尿病前症
ocular psychosomatic disease　眼・精神身体症
optical path difference　光路差
optical psychosomatic disease　眼精神身体症
oto-palato-digital　耳口蓋指
outpatient department　外来
outpatient dispensary　外来用薬局

o,p′-DDD
2,4′-dichlorodiphenyldichloroethane　2,4′-ジクロロジフェニルジクロロエタン

OpDent
operative dentistry　保存修復学，手術歯科学

OPD syndrome
otopalatodigital syndrome 耳・口蓋・指趾症候群
Ope
operation 手術
open cDNA
open circular DNA 開環状DNA
oper
operate 手術する
operating 手術の
operation 手術
operator 術者
opg
opening 孔
OPH, Oph
obliterative pulmonary hypotension 閉塞性肺低血圧症
OPH, Oph, oph
oculoplethysmograph 眼体積記録器
oculoplethysmography 眼体積記録法
ophtalmoscope 検眼鏡
ophthalmia 眼炎
ophthalmic 眼の
ophthalmology 眼科学
ophthalmoplethysmograph 眼体積変動記録器
ophthalmoscopic 検眼鏡の
oxypolygelatin オキシポリゼラチン
OphD
Doctor of Ophthalmology 眼科医
OphSeg
ophthalmic segment 眼体節
Ophth
ophthalmia 眼炎
ophthalmic 眼の
ophthalmologic 眼科学の
ophthalmologist 眼科医
ophthalmology 眼科学
ophthalmoscope 検眼鏡
Opi-ato
opium alkaloids and atropine オピウムアルカロイドとアトロピン，オピアト
Opi ato inj
opium alkaloids and atropine injection オピアト注
Opi-sco
opium alkaloids and scopolamine オピウムアルカロイドとスコポラミン，オピスコ

OPK
optokinetic 視動性の
OPL
operant preferential looking 有効選択的注視
osmotic pressure lymph リンパ浸透圧
ovine placental lactogen ヒツジ胎盤ラクトゲン
OPLL
ossification of posterior longitudinal ligament 後縦靱帯骨化症
OPM
occult primary malignancy 潜在性原発性悪性腫瘍
ophthalmoplegic migraine 眼筋麻痺性片頭痛
OPMC
Office of Professional Misconduct 職業上不行跡監視局
OPN
optokinetic nystagmus 視運動性眼振
opn
operation 手術
opng
opening 開始
OPP
ortho-phenylphenol *o*-フェニルフェノール
osmotic pressure of plasma 血漿浸透圧
ovine pancreatic polypeptide ヒツジ膵臓ポリペプチド
oxygen partial pressure 酸素分圧
vincristine(=Oncovin), procarbazine, prednisone ビンクリスチン(=オンコビン), プロカルバジン, プレドニゾン

O

opp
opposed 対立した
opposing 対立する
opposite 反対の
opposition 反対
out of print at present 現在印刷されていない
OPPES
oil-associated pneumoparalytic eosinophilic syndrome 油による肺麻痺好酸球増加症症候群
OP-PICA anastomosis
occipital artery-posterior inferior cerebellar artery anastomosis 後頭・後下小脳動脈吻合術
OPPs
Organ Procurement Programs 臓器獲得計画
OPR
Office of Population Research 人口調査局
op.reg.
operative region 手術野

oprg
operating 手術している
OPRT
orotate (orotic acid) phosphoribosyltransferase オロチン酸ホスホリボシル変換酵素〔トランスフェラーゼ〕
orotidylate phosphoribosyltranseferase オロチジレートホスホリボシル変換酵素〔トランスフェラーゼ〕
oprtg
operating 手術している
OPS
osteoporosisi-pseudolipoma syndrome 骨粗鬆症・偽(性)脂肪腫症候群
outpatient service 外来サービス
outpatient surgery 外来手術
OPSA
ovarian papillary serous adenocarcinoma 卵巣乳頭状漿液性腺癌
OPSI (syndrome)
overwhelming postsplenectomy infection (syndrome) 脾摘重篤後感染(症候群)
OPT
orthopantomography オルソパントモグラフィ
ortho-phthalaldehyde *o*-フタルアルデヒド
outpatient 外来患者
outpatient treatment 外来患者治療
Opt, opt, opt.
optical 眼の
optician 眼鏡士
optics 眼，光学
optimus〈ラ〉=optimum, optimal 最適の
optional 随意の
optometrisyt 検眼士
opt.D.
Doctor of Optometry 視力測定士
opthal
ophthalmic 眼科の
ophthalmologist 眼科医
ophthalmology 眼科学
OPV
oral polio virus 経口感染ポリオウイルス
OPWL
opiate withdrawal 阿片剤禁断
Op-Z
opsonized zymosan オプソニン化ザイモザン

OR
odds ratio　オッズ比
operating room　手術室
operations research　オペレーションズリサーチ
optic radiation　視放線
optimum requirement　至適必要量
orientation reflex　オリエンテーション反射
orienting response　指向応答
orthop(a)edic　整形外科の
orthop(a)edist＝orthop(a)edic surgeon　整形外科医
out of range　変域外の
oxygen radical　酸素ラジカル
oxygen requirement　酸素必要量
rate of outflow　流出率

OR, O-R
oxidation-reduction　酸化還元

ORA
older age onset rheumatoid arthritis　高齢発症関節リウマチ

ORANS
Oak Ridge Analytical Systems　オークリッジ分析システム

ORBC
ox red blood cell　ウシ赤血球

orbic
orbicular　輪状の，球型の
orbicularis　輪筋

ORC
ox red cell　ウシ赤血球
oxygen ratio control　酸素比自動コントロール

ORCH
orchiectomy　精巣〔睾丸〕摘除(術)

orch
orchitis　精巣〔睾丸〕炎

ORD
optical rotatory dispersion　旋光分散

Ord, ord, ord.
order　指示
ordered　指示された
orderly　看護師
ordinarius〈ラ〉　通常の
ordinate　縦線
orotidine　オロチジン

OREF
Orthop(a)edic Research and Education Foundation　整形外科における研究と教育のための基金

OR en
oil retension enema 油性停留浣腸
ORF
open reading frame 読み取り枠
Org
orgasmus オルガスムス
org
organ 器官
organic 器官の
organism 生物
organiz
organization 構築
organizational 構築の
ORI
Office of Research Integrity 研究倫理調査室
ori
origin of replication 複製開始遺伝子
ORIF
open reduction and internal fixation 観血的整復兼内固定術
orig
origin 起始
original 起始の
OrJ
orange juice オレンジジュース
ORL
otorhinolaryngologist 耳鼻咽喉医
otorhinolaryngology 耳鼻咽喉科学
ORN
Operating Room Nurse 手術室看護師
Orn
ornithine オルニチン
orn
orange オレンジ
Oro
orotate オロチン酸
orotic acid オロチン酸
Oros
oral osmotic 経口浸透的
ORP
oxidation-reduction potential 酸化還元電位(差)
ORR
Office of Research Resources 研究資源室
ORS
olfactory reference syndrome 嗅覚関連症候群
oral rehydration solution 経口再水加溶液
oral surgeon 口腔外科医

Orthop(a)edic Research Society 整形外科基礎研究会
orthop(a)edic surgery 整形外科

ors.
orationes〈ラ〉 ことば

ORT
ocular radiation therapy 眼放射線療法
operating room technician 手術室技術者
ophthalmic response test 結膜誘発試験
oral rehydration therapy 経口補水療法
Organization for Rehabilitation through Training 訓練によるリハビリテーション機関
orthoptist 視能訓練士

orth
orthopaedics 整形外科

Ortho, ortho
orthochromatic 正染性の
orthop(a)edic 整形外科の
orthop(a)edics 整形外科
orthop(a)ethy 整形外科疾患

orthop
orthopedist 整形外科医

or.X1
oriented to time 時間について見当識のある

or.X2
oriented to time and place 時間と場所について見当識のある

or.X3
oriented to time, place and person 時間・場所・人について見当識のある

OS
Oberschenkel〈独〉 大腿
occupational safety 職業安全
Ohrensausen〈独〉 耳鳴
opening snap 僧帽弁開放音
operating system 基本ソフト
oral surgery 口腔外科学
orthopedic surgeon 整形外科医
orthopedic surgery 整形外科(学)
orthosleep オーソ睡眠, 正睡眠
Osgood-Schlatter (disease) オズグッド・シュラッター(病)
osteogenic sarcoma 骨原性肉腫
osteoid surface 類骨表面
osteopoikilosis 骨斑紋症
osteosarcoma 骨肉腫
osteosclerosis 骨硬化(症)

ouabain sensitive ウアバイン感受性の
overall survival 総生存
oxalosuccinic acid オキザロコハク酸
oxygen saturation 酸素飽和

Os
osmium オスミウム〈元素〉

os
outside 外側

17-OS
17-oxosteroid 17-オキソステロイド

OS, Os, os, O.S.
oculo sinistro〈ラ〉 左眼の
oculus sinister〈ラ〉 左眼

OS, os
osteoscleeosis 骨硬化症

OSA
obstructive sleep apnea 閉塞性睡眠無呼吸

OSAS
obstructive sleep apnea syndrome 閉塞型睡眠無呼吸症候群

O_2sat
oxygen saturation 酸素飽和

OSBT
ovarian serous borderline tumor 卵巣漿液性境界型腫瘍

osc
oscillate 振動する
oscillator 発振器

OSCC
Organ System Coordinating Center 臓器組織共同センター

OSCE
objective structured clinical examination 客観的臨床能力試験

OSCP
oligomycin-sensitivity-conferring protein オリゴマイシン感受性付与蛋白

oscp
oscilloscope オシロスコープ

OSD
outside doctor 外部医師

OSF
obturatoria stapedis fold アブミ骨ひだ閉鎖
osteoclast stimulating factor 破骨細胞刺激因子
outer spiral fiber 外側らせん線維
overgrowth-stimulating factor 過成長刺激因子

OSFM
optical scanning fluorescence microscopy 走査蛍光顕微鏡

O

OSFT
outstretched fingertips 伸展指先
OSG
Oberschenkelgips〈独〉 大腿ギプス
o.s.h.
omni sigula hora〈ラ〉 毎時間《処》
OSHA
Occupational Safety and Health Act 職業安全健康活動
Occupational Safety and Health Administration 米国労働省労働安全保健局
OSI
Office of Scientific Integrity 科学倫理調査室
OSL
optically stimulated luminescence 光励起発光
Osgood-Schlatter lesion オズグッド・シュラッター病変
OSM
oncostatin M オンコスタチンM
oxygen saturation meter 酸素飽和計
Osm, osm, osm.
osmol オスモル，浸透圧当量
osmosis 浸透
osmotic 浸透の
OSMF
oral submucous fibrosis 口腔粘膜下線維症
osmo
osmolality 重量オスモル濃度
osmol
osmole 浸透圧モル
OSR
overall safety rating 全般安全度
OSS
occupational stress syndrome 職業ストレス症候群
osseous 骨性の
OST
oxytocin sensitivity test オキシトシン感受性テスト
oxytocin stress test オキシトシン負荷試験
Osteo
osteopathologist 整骨医
Osteo, osteo
osteoarthritis 変形性関節症
osteomyelitis 骨髄炎
osteopathology 骨病理学
osteopathy 整骨医学
osteoarth
osteoarthritis 変形性関節症

osteocart
osteocartilaginous　骨軟骨の
osteol
osteology　骨学
OSU
Oberschenkelumfang〈独〉　大腿周長
OSUK
Ophthalmological Society of United Kingdom　英国眼科学会
OT
objective test　客観的検査
observe target　観察目標
occupational therapist　作業療法士
occupational therapy　作業療法
ocular tension　眼圧
Oestreicher-Turner (syndrome)　エストリカー・ターナー(症候群)
old term　旧用語
old terminology　旧学術用語
old tuberculin　旧ツベルクリン
old tuberculosis　陳旧性結核
olfactory threshold　嗅閾値
on time　定刻に
operative temperature　作用温度
optic tract　視索
oral tolerance　経口寛容誘導
orientation test　見当識検査
ornithine transcarbamylase　オルニチントランスカルバミラーゼ
orotracheal　気管経由の
orotracheal tube　口腔気管チューブ
overtime　超過時間
oxytocin　オキシトシン
total oxygen content　総酸素含量
5-OT
5-oxytryptamine　5-オキシトリプタミン
OT, Ot, ot, ot.
otitis　耳炎
otolaryngologist　耳鼻咽喉科医
otolaryngology　耳鼻咽喉科学
otologist　耳科医
otology　耳科学
OTA
occupational therapist aid　作業療法士助手
occupational therapy assistant　作業療法助手
Office of Technology Assessment　技術評価事務所

OTAP
occlusive thromboaortopathy 閉塞性凝血性大動脈症
OTAT
ortho-toluidine arsenite test *o*-トルイジン亜砒酸塩試験
OTB
ortho-toluidine boric acid test *o*-トルイジンホウ酸試験
OTB method
ortho-toluidine boric acid method *o*-トルイジンホウ酸法
OTC
ornithine transcarbamylase オルニチントランスカルバミラーゼ
oval target cell 楕円形標的細胞
over the counter 一般薬，市販薬
oxytetracycline オキシテトラサイクリン
OTCA
operative transluminal coronary angiography 術中経管冠(状)動脈造影
OTCD
ornithine transcarbamylase deficiency オルニチントランスカルバミラーゼ欠損症
over the counter drug 大衆薬
OTD
oral temperature device 口腔温度計
organ tolerance dose 臓器許容量
OTE
optically transparent electrode 光透過性電極
OTH
other(s) 他の
O ther
oxygen therapy 酸素療法
OTI
official test insecticide 公認試験殺虫剤
OTNA
osmium tetraoxide-α-naphthylamine 四酸化オスミウム-α-ナフチルアミン
OTO
one time only 1回だけ
OTO, Oto, oto
otolaryngology 耳鼻咽喉科
otology 耳科学
Otol, otol
otologist 耳科医
otology 耳科学
otolar
otolaryngology 耳鼻咽喉科学

_o_-tolidine
orthotolidine　オルトトリジン
otorhinol
otorhinolaryngology　耳鼻咽喉科学
OTR
occupational therapist registered　登録作業療法士
OTS
occipital temporal sulcus　後頭側頭溝
orotracheal suction　口腔気管(チューブ)吸引
OTSG
Office of Surgeon General　一般外科医診察所
OTT
orotracheal tube　口腔気管チューブ
OTTLE
optically transparent thin-layer electrode　光透過性薄層電極
OTU
olfactory tubercle　嗅結節
operational taxonomic unit　分類操作上の単位
OU
Oppenheim-Urbach (syndrome)　オッペンハイム・ウアバッハ(症候群)
O & U
over and under　以上と以下
OU, O.U., o.u.
observation unit　観察室
oculi unitas〈ラ〉　両眼一緒に
oculo utro〈ラ〉　各眼に
oculus uterque〈ラ〉　各眼で
oupt
output　出力
OUR
oxygen uptake rate　酸素吸収速度
OURQ
outer upper right quadrant　外上右1/4(区)
OUS
oculo-urethro-synovite〈仏〉　眼・尿道・滑膜炎
out
outlet　出口
OV
oculovestibular　眼前庭の
office visit　通院
outflow volume　流出量
overventilation　過換気
ovulating　排卵している

Ov, ov.
ovary 卵巣
ovum〈ラ〉 卵
OVA
ovalbumin 卵アルブミン
Ova Ca
ovarian carcinoma 卵巣癌
OVC
ovarian carcinoma 卵巣癌
OvDF
ovarian dysfunction 卵巣機能不全〔機能障害〕
OVG
oil ventriculography 油脳室撮影
oleoventriculography 油脳室撮影
OVH
overhead 頭上
overheat 過熱
OVHD
oval head 卵形の頭
OVIS
Ohio Vocational Interest Survey オハイオ職業興味調査
ovld
overload 過度に負荷する
OVLP
overlap myositis 併発筋炎
OVLT
organum vasculosumlamine terminalis〈ラ〉 第三脳室前腹壁にある終末器官
OVN
ocular vegetative neurosis 眼自律神経症
OVR
oculovestibular reflex 眼前庭反射
OVS
obstructive voiding symptom 尿閉症候群
OVX
ovariectomized 卵巣摘出術を受けた
ovariectomy 卵巣摘出術
O/W
oil in water 水中油型
OW, ow
old woman 老婦人
once weekly 週に1度《処》
open wedge (osteotomy) 楔状骨切り術
orient and west 東洋と西洋
outer wall 外壁
oval window 卵円窓

OWR
Osler-Weber-Rendu (syndrome) オースラー・ウェーバー・ランデュ(症候群)
ovarian wedge resection 卵巣楔切除術
OWVI
Ohio Work Values Inventory オハイオ労働価値調査票
ox
oxide 酸化された
OX3
oriented times three 3種の見当識がある
OX, Ox, O_x
optic chiasm 視交叉〔差〕
orthopaedic examination 整形外科検査
oxacillin オキサシリン
oxalic オキザロ酸の
oxasolone オキサゾロン
oxidant オキシダント
oxygen 酸素
oxymel 薬用シロップ
oxytocin オキシトシン
OXA
oxalic acid オキザロ酸
OXEA
ox erythrocyte antibody ウシ赤血球抗体
OXP
oxaprozin オキサプロジン
oxypressin オキシプレッシン
OXT
oxytocin オキシトシン
OXY, oxy
oxygen 酸素
oxytocin オキシトシン
oxycephs
oxycephalics 尖頭症
oxym
oxymel オキシメル
OY
orange yellow オレンジイエロー
OYL
ossification of yellow ligament 黄色靱帯骨化症
oys
oyster 牡蠣
OZ
opsonized zymosan オプソニン化ザイモザン
oz, oz.
ounce オンス〈単位〉

P p

P

gas partial pressure	気体分圧
mean gas pressure	平均ガス圧
pain	痛み
Pandy reaction	パンディー反応
para	経産
Paragonimus	肺吸虫(属)
parent	親
parental	親の
parental generation	親世代
parietal	頭頂部の
parity	出産歴
parous	経産の
parte〈ラ〉=part	部分
partial pressure	分圧
partus〈ラ〉	分娩
passive	受動の
Pasteurella	パスツレラ(属)
pater〈ラ〉=father	父(親)
patient	患者
pemphigus〈ラ〉	天疱瘡
penicillin	ペニシリン
Penicillium	ペニシリウム(属)
Peptococcus	ペプトコッカス(属)
per-〈ラ〉	～を通して〈接〉
percentile	百分位数
perch	パーチ〈単位〉
percussion	打診
peritoneal dissemination	腹膜播種
peritoneal metastasis	腹膜転移
peritoneum	腹膜
permeability	透過性
peta-	ペタ(=10^{15})〈接〉
peyote	ペヨーテ
pharmacopoeia	薬局方
phenolphthalein	フェノールフタレイン
phenylalanine	フェニルアラニン
Phlebotomus	サシチョウバエ(属)
phon	フォン〈単位〉
phosphate	リン酸塩
phosphoric ester	リン酸エステル
phosphorus	リン〈元素〉
Phthirus	ケジラミ(属)

physiology	生理学
pico-	ピコ(＝10^{-15})〈接〉
pin	ピン，留め針
pink	ピンク，桃色《処》
pint	パイント〈単位〉
placebo	偽薬，プラシボ，プラセボ
plan	計画
plasma	血漿
plasmid	プラスミド
Plasmodium	プラスモジウム(属)
plica	皺襞，ひだ
point	点
poise	ポアズ〈単位〉
poison	毒(物)
polarization	分極
polymyxin	ポリミキシン
pons	橋
poor	弱，貧しい
population	母集団，人口
porcelain	ポーセレン，陶材
porphyrin	ポルフィリン
position	位置，体位，胎向
positive	陽(性)の，正の
post-	後の〈接〉
posterior	後方の，後(ろ)の
posterior (nucleus)	後側核
postpartum	分娩後(の)
power	力
prednisone	プレドニゾン
premolar	小臼歯
presbyopia	老眼
pressure	圧
primary	第一の，原発(性)の
primipara	初産婦
primitive	初期の
probability	確率
probable	有望な
proctos	肛門管
product	産物，生成物，積
progesterone	プロゲステロン，黄体ホルモン
prolactin	プロラクチン，黄体刺激ホルモン
proline	プロリン
promethazine hydrochloride	塩酸プロメタジン
properdin	プロパジン

propionate	プロピオン酸塩
protein	蛋白(質)
Protestant	プロテスタント(の)，新教徒(の)
Proteus	プロテウス(属)
proton	陽子
Providencia	プロビデンシア(属)
provisional	未確定の
proximal	近位の，隣接の
proximum〈ラ〉＝proximal	近い
Pseudomonas	シュードモナス(属)
psychiatrist	精神(科)医
psychiatry	精神医学
psychomotor domain	精神運動領域《医教》
psychosis	精神病
Pulex	ヒトノミ(属)
pulse	脈(拍)
pulumonary	肺(性)の
punctation	赤色斑
punctum proximum〈ラ〉＝near point	(視覚の)近点
pupil	瞳孔
P wave	P波《心電》
pyloroplasty	幽門形成(術)
short arm of a chromosome	染色体短腕

p

papilla	乳頭
past	過去
performance	動作，性能
pigment	色素
polymerase	ポリメラーゼ
predict	予知する
promotor	プロモーター

p.

pars〈ラ〉	部分《処》
partes〈ラ〉	部分《処》
pilula〈ラ〉	丸剤《処》
pondere〈ラ〉＝by weight	重量で《処》
pondus〈ラ〉＝weight	重量
pugillus〈ラ〉	ひと握り《処》
pulverisat〈ラ〉	粉末にした《処》
pulvis〈ラ〉	散剤《処》

^{32}P

radioactive phosphorus	放射性リン

P_{0-3}

peritonial dissemination	腹膜播種の程度

P

P_1
first parental generation 第１親世代
P_2
bisphosphate ビスリン酸
pregnanediol プレグナンジオール
P_3
pregnanetriol プレグナントリオール
P_4
progesterone プロゲステロン
P/3
proximal third (骨の)近位部1/3(区)
***p*-**
para- パラ〈接〉
P-450
cytochrome P-450 チトクロ(ー)ムP450
P, p
page ページ(＝頁)
perforate 穿孔する
perforation 穿孔
polar 極
pole 極
P2, P_2
pulmonary second sound 肺動脈第二音
P-50, P_{50}
oxygen half-saturation pressure of hemoglobin ヘモグロビン50%酸素(化)圧
PA
alveolar pressure 肺胞圧
atrial pressure 心房圧
pancreatic amylase 膵アミラーゼ
panic attack 恐慌発作
paralysis agitans 振戦麻痺
paratyphoid A パラチフスA
particle aggulutination (method) ゼラチン粒子凝集(法), PA(法)
particular average 個々の平均
paternal aunt 父方のおば(＝伯母, 叔母)
pattern analysis パターン解析
performance analysis 動作解析
periarteritis 動脈周囲炎
periodontal abscess 歯周膿瘍
pernicious anemia 悪性貧血
phenylalanine フェニルアラニン
phosphatidic acid ホスファチジン酸
phosphoarginine リン酸アルギニン
photoallergenic 光アレルゲン

physicians assistant	内科医助手
pineapple	パイナップル
pipecolic acid	ピペコリン酸
piromidic acid	ピロミド酸
pituitary adenoma	下垂体腺腫
pituitary-adrenal	下垂体副腎の
plasma adsorption	血漿吸着
plasma aldosterone	血漿アルドステロン
plasmin α_2-antiplasmin complex	プラスミンα_2抗プラスミン複合体
plasminogen activator	プラスミノゲンアクチベータ
platelet aggregation	血小板凝集
polyarteritis	多発(性)動脈炎
position approximate	近似位置
posteroanterior	後前方向
post-operative angina	術後性アンギナ
power amplifier	出力増幅器
prealbumin	プレアルブミン
primary aldosteronism	原発性アルドステロン症
primary amenorrhea	原発性無月経
primary anemia	原発性貧血
proactivator	前賦活体
procainamide	プロカインアミド
prolonged action	遅延作用
prophylactic antibiotic	予防的抗生物質
propionic acid	プロピオン酸
prostate (specific) antigen	前立腺(特異)抗原
protection grade of UV-A	紫外線A波防御度
prothrombin activity	プロトロンビン活性
protrusio acetabuli	股臼底脱出(症)
Pseudomonas aeruginosa	緑膿菌
psoriatic arthritis	乾癬性関節炎
psychoanalysis	精神分析
psychoanalyst	精神分析者
psychogenic aspermia	精神的無精子症
psychological age	精神年齢
pulmonary artery	肺動脈
pulmonary atresia	肺動脈弁閉塞症
pulpo-axial	髄軸の
pyrophosphate arthropathy	ピロリン酸関節症

Pa

arterial pressure	動脈内分圧
pascal	パスカル〈単位〉
protactinium	プロトアクチニウム
pulmonary artery pressure	肺動脈圧

pa
paper　紙，論文

pA_2
affinity constant　親和性定数

p.a.
per abdomen〈ラ〉=for abdomen　腹部に，経腹的に
post applicationem〈ラ〉=after the application　申請後，使用後
pro anno〈ラ〉=for the year　年に

PA，Pa
paranoia　パラノイア

PA，pa
pathology　病理学

PA，p.a.
per annum〈ラ〉=by the year，yearly　年ごとに

P/A，P & A
percussion and auscultation　打診と聴診

PAA
partial agonist activity　部分的作用用薬活性
phenylacetic acid　フェニル酢酸
phosphonoacetic acid　リン酢酸
plasma angiotensinase activity　血漿アンジオテンシナーゼ活性
polyacrylamide　ポリアクリルアミド
polyacrylic acid　ポリアクリル酸
pyridine acetic acid　ピリジン酢酸

p.a.a.
parti affectae applicandus〈ラ〉　病変部に適用《処》

PAAO
Pan-American Association of Ophthalmology　全米眼科学協会

PAB
premature atrial beat　心房性期外収縮
pulmonary artery banding　肺動脈絞扼術

PABA
para-aminobenzoic acid　パラアミノ安息香酸

Pabd
abdominal pressure　腹腔圧

PAC
papular acrodermatitis of childhood　小児丘疹性末端皮膚炎
phenacetin, aspirin, caffeine　フェナセチン・アスピリン・カフェイン
pituitary-adrenal medullary　交感神経・副腎髄質系
plasma aldosterone concentration　血漿アルドステロン濃度

PAC, PAC-1
cisplatin (=Platinol), adriamycin, cyclophosphamide　シスプラチン(=プラチノール),アドリアマイシン,シクロホスファミド

PACAP
pituitary adenylate cyclase activating polypeptide　下垂体アデニン酸シクラーゼ活性ポリペプチド

PACE
cisplatin (=Platinol), adriamycin, cyclophosphamide, etoposide　シスプラチン(=プラチノール),アドリアマイシン,シクロホスファミド,エトポシド
pulmonary angiotensin I converting enzyme　肺アンジオテンシンI変換酵素

PACG
primary angle closure glaucoma　原発性閉塞隅角緑内障

$PaCO_2$
partial pressure of carbon dioxide in artery　動脈血二酸化炭素分圧

$PACO_2$, P_ACO_2
partial pressure of carbon dioxide in alveolar gas　肺胞気二酸化炭素圧

PAcP
prostatic acid phosphatase　前立腺性酸性ホスファターゼ

PACS
picture archiving and communication system　医療画像処理の画像保管通信システム《コン》

PACT
papillary carcinoma of thyroid　甲状腺の乳頭状癌
precardial acceleration tracing　前胸部加速度追跡

P

PAC-V
cisplatin (=Platinol), adriamycin, cyclophosphamide　シスプラチン(=プラチノール),アドリアマイシン,シクロホスファミド

PAD
pelvic adhesive disease　骨盤癒着性疾患
percutaneous abscess drainage　経皮的膿瘍排膿
peripheral arterial disease　末梢(性)動脈疾患
phenacetin, aspirin, desoxyephedrine　フェナセチン・アスピリン・デスオキシエフェドリン
primary affective disorder　原発性情動疾患
primary afferent depolarization　1次求心性線維脱分極
psychoaffective disorder　精神情動疾患
pulsatile assist device　拍動性補助装置

PAd
pulmonary artery diastolic　肺動脈拡張期の

PADP
pulmonary arterial diastolic pressure 肺動脈拡張期圧
PAE
paradoxical air embolism 奇異性空気塞栓症
postantibiotic effect 抗生物質治療効果
p.ae.
partes aequales〈ラ〉 同(等の)部分，等量《処》
paed
paediatrics 小児科学
PAEDP
pulmonary artery end-diastolic pressure 肺動脈拡張終期圧
PAEF
platelet aggregation enhancing factor 血小板凝集増強因子
p.aeq.
partes aequales〈ラ〉 同部分，等量《処》
PAES
positron-induced Auger electron spectroscopy 陽電子励起オージェ電子分光法
PAF
paroxysmal atrial flutter 発作性心房粗動
platelet-activating factor 血小板活性化因子
platelet-aggregating factor 血小板凝集因子
progressive automatic failure 進行性自律神経不全
prostatic antibacterial factor 前立腺抗細菌性因子
pulmonary arteriolovenous fistula 肺動静脈瘻
pulmonary artery flow 肺動脈血流量
PAf
paroxysmal atrial fibrillation 発作性心房細動
PA & F
percussion, auscultation and fremitus 打診・聴診・振とう音
PAF-A
platelet-activating factor of anaphylaxis アナフィラキシー性血小板活性因子
PAFD
pulmonary artery filling defect 肺動脈陰影欠損
PAFI
platelet-aggregating factor inhibitor 血小板凝集因子阻害薬
PAFIB
paroxysmal atrial fibrillation 発作性心房細動
PAG
panarteriography 逆行性上腕動脈造影
pelvic angiogram 骨盤内血管造影
pelvic angiography 骨盤動脈撮影
periaqueductal gray (matter) 中脳中心灰白質
pneumoarthrogram 関節空気造影

post-auricular graft　耳介後部皮弁
pregnancy-associated alpha-glycoprotein　妊娠関連α糖蛋白
pregnancy-associated globulin　妊娠関連グロブリン
Protein Calorie Advisory Group　蛋白カロリー諮問グループ
pulmonary arteriogram　肺動脈造影

PAGE
polyacrylamide gel electrophoresis　ポリアクリルアミドゲル電気泳動

PAgF
platelet-aggregating factor　血小板凝集因子

PAH
p-aminohippurate　パラアミノ馬尿酸塩
p-aminohippuric acid　パラアミノ馬尿酸
partial artificial heart　部分人工心臓
phenylalanine hydroxylase　フェニルアラニン水酸化酵素
polycyclic aromatic hydrocarbon　多環芳香族炭化水素
polynuclear aromatic hydrocarbon　多核芳香性水酸化炭素
postatrophic hyperplasia　萎縮後過形成
pregnancy associated hypertension　妊娠高血圧症
primary afferent hyperpolarization　一次求心性線維過分極
primary alveolar hypoventilation (syndrome)　原発性肺胞低換気(症候群)
pulmonary artery hypertension　肺動脈高血圧
pulmonary artery hypotension　肺動脈低血圧

PAHA
p-aminohippuric acid　パラアミノ馬尿酸

PAHVC
pulmonary alveolar hypoxic vasoconstriction　肺胞低酸素血管攣縮

P

PAI
inferior pulmonary artery　下肺動脈
parathyroid activity index　上皮小体活動係数
plasminogen activator inhibitor　プラスミノゲン活性化抑制因子

PAIC
procedures, alternatives, indications and complications　処置・代替処置・適応と合併症
productive aspergilloma on the inner wall of a cavity　壁在性増殖型アスペルギローマ

PAIDS
pediatric acquired immunodeficiency syndrome　小児後天性免疫不全症候群

PAIF
platelet-aggregation inhibition factor　血小板凝集阻止因子

PAIgG
platelet-associated immunoglobulin G　血小板結合免疫グロブリンG
PAISSR
psychosocial adjustment to illness scale-self-report　疾患への社会心理的適応の自己採点報告
PAIVS
pulmonary atresia with intact ventricular septum　正常心室中隔肺動脈閉鎖
PAJ
paralysis agitans juvenilis　若年性振戦麻痺
PAK
pancreas transplantation after kidney transplantation　腎移植後膵移植
Pseudomonas aeruginosa K　緑膿菌K
PAL
pathology laboratory　病理学検査室
posterior axillary line　後腋窩線
pyogenic abscess of the liver　肝化膿性膿瘍
pyothorax associated lymphoma　膿胸後リンパ腫
pal
palpitation　動悸
PA & Lat
posteroanterior and lateral　後前方と側面
PALM
premature accelerated lung maturation　早発急速進行性肺成熟
PALP
pyridoxal phosphate　ピリドキサ(ー)ルリン酸
palp
palpable　触知可能な
palpate　触診する
palpation　触診
palpitation　動悸
palpi
palpitation　動悸
palpit
palpitation　動悸
PALS
pediatric advanced life support　二次小児救命処置
periarteriolar lymphocyte sheath　細動脈周囲リンパ球鞘
prison-acquired lymphoproliferative syndrome　刑務所罹患リンパ球増殖症候群
PA-LS-ID
pernicious anemia-like syndrome and immunoglobulin deficiency　悪性貧血様症候群と免疫グロブリン欠損

P

Palv
alveolar pressure 肺胞内圧
PAM
penicillin with aluminum monostearate in oil ステアリン酸アルミニウムの油性結晶ペニシリン
periodic acid methenamine silver stain 過ヨウ素酸メセナミン銀染色
pharmaceutical adviser of medicine 医療の薬学的助言者
p-methoxyamphetamine パラメトキシアンフェタミン
pralidoxime プラリドキシム
pregnancy-associated alpha-macroglobulin 妊娠関連αマクログロブリン
primary amebic meningoencephalitis 原発性アメーバ性髄膜脳炎
pulmonary alveolar macrophage 肺胞大食細胞
pulmonary alveolar microlithiasis 肺胞微石症
pulse amplified modulation 脈増幅調節
pulse amplitude modulation パルス振幅変調
2-pyridine aldoxime methiodide ピリジンアルドキシムメチオジド

pam.
pamphlet パンフレット
2-PAM
pralidoxime chloride 塩化プラリドキシム
PAMBA
p-aminomethylbenzoic acid パラアミノメチル安息香酸
PAMC
pterygoarthromyodysplasia congenital 先天性翼状片関節異形成症
PAMD
primary adrenocortical micronodular dysplasia 原発性副腎皮質小結節性形成異常(症)
PAME
primary amebic meningoencephalitis 原発性アメーバ性髄膜脳炎
PAMI
primary angioplasty in myocardial infarction 心筋梗塞治療法比較大規模試験，パミ
PAMP
pathogen-associated molecular pattern 病原体関連分子認識パターン
proadrenomedullin *N*-terminal 20 peptide 降圧作用を有する生理活性物質
pulmonary arterial mean pressure 肺動脈平均圧
PAMS
periodic acid-methenamine silver ペリオジック酸・メテナミン銀

PAN
parents against narcotics 麻薬反対の両親
periarteritis nodosa〈ラ〉 結節性動脈周囲炎
periodic alternating nystagmus 周期交代性眼振
peroxyacetyl nitrate 硝酸ペルオキシアセチル
polyarteritis nodosa 結節性多発動脈炎
positional alcohol nystagmus 体位性アルコール性眼振
puromycin aminonucleoside nephropathy プロマイシンアミノヌクレオシド腎症
puromycin aminonucleoside nephrosis プロマイシンアミノヌクレオシドネフローシス

PANC
pancreas 膵臓

pancreat
pancreatic 膵臓の

PAND
primary adrenocortical nodular dysplasia 原発性副腎皮質結節性形成異常(症)

PANDAS
pediatric autoimmune neuropsychiatric disorders associated with streptococcal infection 連鎖球菌感染症に関連する小児自己免疫神経障害

PANDO
primary acquired nasolacrimal duct obstruction 原発後天性鼻涙管閉塞(症)

Panperi
panperitonitis び漫〔広汎〕性腹膜炎

Pan T
pan T cell antigen 汎T細胞抗原

PAO
peak acid output 最大刺激時酸分泌量
peripheral airway obstruction 末梢性気道閉塞症

PAo
pulmonary artery occlusion (pressure) 肺動脈閉塞(圧)

Pao
ascending aortic pressure 上行大動脈圧

PaO_2
partial pressure arterial oxygen 動脈血酸素分圧

PaO_2, PAO_2
partial pressure alveolar oxygen 肺胞気酸素分圧

PAOA
Pan-American Odontological Association 全米歯科学協会

P

PAOD
peripheral arterial occlusive disease 末梢動脈閉塞疾患
peripheral arteriosclerotic occlusive disease 末梢動脈硬化性閉塞性疾患
popliteal artery occlusive disease 膝窩動脈閉塞性疾患

PAOP
pulmonary artery occlusion pressure 肺動脈閉鎖圧

PAP
pancreatitis associated protein 膵炎関連蛋白質
Papanicolaou (test, class, smear) パパニコロー(検査・分類・染色)
para-amino-propiophenone パラアミノプロピオフェノン
peak airway pressure ピーク気道圧
percutaneous antegrade pyelography 経皮的逆行性腎盂造影
peroxidase-antiperoxidase ペルオキシダーゼ抗ペルオキシダーゼ
placental alkaline phoshatase 胎盤アルカリ性ホスファターゼ
pokeweed antiviral proteins アメリカヤマゴボウ抗ウイルス蛋白
positive after-potential 陽性後電位
positive airway pressure 気道陽圧
pregnancy associated protein 妊娠関連蛋白
primary atypical pneumonia 原発性異型肺炎
prostatic acid phosphatase 前立腺性酸性ホスファターゼ
pulmonary alveolar proteinosis 肺胞蛋白症
pulmonary annuloplasty 肺動脈弁輪形成術
pulmonary arterial pressure 肺動脈圧

Pap
papillary 乳頭の
papilloma パピローマ

pap
papilla 乳頭
papillary adenocarcinoma 乳頭腺癌

PAPA
Parenteral Alimentation Providers Association 経静脈的栄養供給協会

papova
papilloma-polyoma-vacuolating virus パポバウイルス

PAPP
p-aminopropiophenone パラアミノプロピオフェノン
pregnancy-associated plasma protein 妊娠関連血漿蛋白

PAPS
3′-phosphoadenosine-5′-phosphosulfate 3′-ホスホアデノシン-5′-ホスホサルフェート

P

PA/PS
pulmonary atresia/pulmonary stenosis　肺動脈閉鎖(症)/肺動脈弁狭窄(症)

Pap sm
Papanicolaou smear　パパニコロー染色

PAPV
positive airway pressure ventilation　気道内陽圧式人工呼吸

Pa-Pv
pulmonary arterial pressure-pulmonary venous pressure　肺動脈圧・肺静脈圧

PAPVC
partial anomalous pulmonary venus connection　部分的肺静脈還流異常

PAPVD
partial anomalous pulmonary venous drainage　部分的肺静脈還流異常

PAPVR
partial anomalous pulmonary venous return　部分的肺静脈還流異常

PAR
perennial allergic rhinitis　通年性アレルギー性鼻炎
physiological aging rate　生理学的老化率
population attributable risk percent　人口寄与危険度割合
postanesthesia recovery　麻酔後回復
pulmonary arterial resistance　肺動脈抵抗
pulmonary arteriolar resistance　肺細動脈抵抗
pulmonary arteriole resistance　肺小動脈抵抗

PAr
polyarteritis　多発(性)動脈炎

par
paraffin　パラフィン
parallel　平行の

PARA
primary acquired refractory anemia　原発性後天性不応性貧血

Para
number of pregnancies, number of abortions or miscarriages, number of living children　妊娠回数・流産回数・出生児数

para
parathyroidectomy　副甲状腺摘出(術)

Para I
a woman having born one child　出生児 1 人をもつ母親

Para II
a woman having born two children　出生児 2 人をもつ母親

Para III
a woman having born three children　出生児 3 人をもつ母親

para, Para, para.	
paraparesis	不全対麻痺
paraplegia	対麻痺
paraplegic	対麻痺の
parous	経産の
para C	
paracervical	頸傍の
paracent	
paracentesis	穿刺(術), 穿開術
parad	
paradichlorobenzene	パラジクロロベンゼン
paradox	
paradoxical	逆説の
Par.aff.	
pars affecta〈ラ〉	病変部に
para L	
paralumbar	腰傍の
Parapsych	
parapsychology	超心理学
Parasit	
parasitology	寄生虫学
parasym div	
parasympathetic division	副交感神経分割
para T	
parathoracic	胸傍の
paravert	
paravertebral	脊椎傍の
PARC	
perennial allergic rhinoconjunctivitis	通年性アレルギー性鼻結膜炎
parent	
parental	親の
parenteral	非経口の
parenterally	非経口的に
pari	
parietal	頭頂の
Parkin	
Parkinsonism	パーキンソニズム
parot	
parotid	耳下腺の
parox	
paroxysmal	発作性の
PARP	
population attributable risk percent	人口寄与危険率
PARR	
postanesthesia recovery room	麻酔後回復室

P

PaRS
pararectal space 直腸側腔
Part
proteolytically activated receptor for thrombin トロンビンレセプター
part, part.
partial 部分的
partim〈ラ〉 部分的に
partis〈ラ〉 部分の
parturition 分娩
part.aeq.
partes aequales〈ラ〉 同等部
part.bic.
partibus bicitus〈ラ〉 分割量
part.dolent.
partes dolentes〈ラ〉 疼痛部
parti dolenti〈ラ〉 疼痛部位に《処》
partic
particular 特別な
part.vic.
partitis vicibus〈ラ〉 分服で《処》
PARU
postanesthetic recovery unit 麻酔後回復部
parv.
parvus〈ラ〉 短い
PAS
p-aminosalicylate パラアミノサリチル酸
p-aminosalicylate calcium パラアミノサリチル酸カルシウム
p-aminosalicylic acid パラアミノサリチル酸，パス
pan-allergenic state 汎アレルギー状態
Parent Attitude Scale 親態度スケール
periodic acid-Schiff (stain) 過ヨウ素酸シッフ(染色)
peripheral anterior synechia (of iris) 周辺部虹彩前癒着
persistent atrial standstill 持続性心房静止
photoacoustic spectroscopy 光音響分光法
Physician's Activity Study 医師活動調査
pituitary adrenal system 下垂体副腎皮質系
postoperative analgesia service 術後疼痛管理
premature auricular systole 心房(性)期外収縮
professional activity study 職業活動研究
progressive accumulated stress 進行性蓄積ストレス
pulmonary artery stenosis 肺動脈狭窄
superior pulmonary artery 上肺動脈
pas
passage 通過

passenger　通過者

PASA

p-aminosalicylic acid　パラアミノサリチル酸

primary acquired sideroblastic anemia　原発性後天性鉄芽球性貧血

psychological abstracts search and retrieval　精神医学抄録探索・修正

PAS-AB

periodic acid Schiff-Alcian blue combination stain　過ヨウ素酸シッフ・アルシアンブルー複合染色(法)

PASCAL

Pascal　パスカル(＝プログラミング言語)《コン》

PASCC

pseudovascular adenoid squamous cell carcinoma　偽血管性腺様扁平上皮癌

PASCCL

pseudovascular adenoid squamous cell carcinoma of the lung　偽血管性腺様扁平上皮癌

P'ase

alkaline phosphatase　アルカリホスファターゼ

PASH

periodic acid-Sciff hematoxylin　過ヨウ素酸シッフヘマトキシリン

pseudoangiomatous stromal hyperplasia　偽血管腫(性)間質性増殖(症)

PASI

psoriasis area and severity index　乾癬部感受性指数《皮膚》

PASM

periodic acid-silver methenamine　過ヨウ素酸銀メテナミン

pass.

passim〈ラ〉　あちこちに

passive　受け身の

PAST

periodic acid-Schiff technique　過ヨウ素酸シッフ法

past.

pasta〈ラ〉＝paste　泥膏《処》

Past, Past.

Pasteurella　パスツレラ(属)

PAT

paroxysmal atrial tachycardia　発作性心房性頻拍

1-phenyl-5-aminotetrazole　1-フェニル-5-アミノテトラゾール

physician assistant training　医師の助手教育

platelet aggregation test　血小板凝集試験

polyamine acetyltransferase ポリアミンアセチルトランスフェラーゼ
preadmission assessment team 入院前評価チーム
preadmission testing 入院前検査
prophylactic antibiotic treatment 予防的抗生物質治療
pulmonary artery trunk 肺動脈幹

pat
patella 膝蓋骨

PAT, pat
patient 患者

pat, pat.
patent 開存の，特許

PATCO
prednisone, arabinosylcytosine, thioguanine, cyclophosphamide, vincristine (=Oncovin) プレドニゾン，アラビノシルシトシン，チオグアニン，シクロホスファミド，ビンクリスチン(=オンコビン)

PATE
pulmonary artery thromboembolism 肺動脈血栓塞栓症
pulmonary artery thromboendarterectomy 肺動脈血栓動脈内膜剝離

pat.gf
paternal grandfather 父方の祖父

pat.gm
paternal grandmother 父方の祖母

PATH
pituitary adrenotropic hormone 下垂体副腎刺激ホルモン

Path, path.
pathogen 病原体
pathogenesis 病因論
pathogenic 病原性の
pathological 病理学の
pathologist 病理学者
pathology 病理学

Path Dx
pathological diagnosis 病理診断

Path Fx
pathological fracture 病的骨折

pathogen
pathogenesis 病因

pat.med
patent medicine 特許医薬品

pat.T
patellar tenderness 膝蓋骨圧痛

p.aur.
pone aurem〈ラ〉 耳の後

P

PAV
- patch-associated villi　斑点関連絨毛
- Pavulon　パブロン
- percutaneous aortic valvuloplasty　経皮的大動脈弁形成(術)
- poikiloderma atrophicans vasculare　血管性多形皮膚萎縮症
- prolonged atypical vertigo　遅延性非定型的眩暈症
- proportional assist ventilation　気道内流量均衡補償換気法

p/av
- particular average　個々の平均

PAVe
- L-phenylalanine mustard, vinblastine　L-フェニルアラニンマスタード・ビンブラスチン
- procarbazine, Alkeran, vinblastine sulfate　プロカルバジン・アルケラン・硫酸ビンブラスチン

PA-VF
- pulmonary arteriovenous fistula　肺動静脈瘻

PAVM
- pulmonary arteriovenous malformation　肺動静脈奇形，肺動脈，先天異常

PAVN
- paraventricular nucleus　室傍核

PAVNRT
- paroxysmal atrioventricular nodal reviprocal tachycardia　発作性房室結節回帰(性)頻拍

PAW
- peripheral airway　末梢気道
- pulmonary arterial wedge　肺動脈楔入(＝せつにゅう)部

Paw
- airway pressure　気道内圧

P

PAWP
- pulmonary arterial wedge pressure　肺動脈楔入(＝せつにゅう)圧

PB
- palmaris brevis muscle　短掌筋
- pancreaticobiliary　膵胆管の
- paraffin bath　パラフィン浴
- paratyphoid B　パラチフスB
- partial bath　部分清拭
- paucibacillary　少菌型
- Paul-Bunnell test　ポール・バンネル試験
- peripheral blood　末梢血
- peroneus brevis　短腓骨
- *Pharmacopoeia Britannica*〈ラ〉　英国薬局方
- phenobarbital　フェノバルビタール
- phenobarbitone　フェノバルビトン
- phonetically balanced　音声学的にバランスのとれた
- pinealoblastoma　松果体芽腫

pitch balance ピッチバランス
polymyxin B ポリミキシンB
premature beat 期外収縮
pressure breathing 加圧呼吸
protein binding 蛋白結合
protein bound 蛋白結合の
pudendal block 外陰部遮断
punch biopsy パンチ生検

P & B
pain and burning 疼痛と灼熱痛
phenobarbital and belladonna フェノバルビタールとベラドンナ

Pb, Pb.
plumbum〈ラ〉=lead 鉛〈元素〉
presbyopia 老眼
probenecid プロベネシド

P_{BA}
brachial arterial pressure 上腕動脈圧

PBA
percutaneous bladder aspiration 経皮的膀胱吸引
polyclonal B cell activation 多クローン性B細胞活性
polyclonal B cell activator 多クローン性B細胞活性化物質
polyclonal B cell activity 多クローン性B細胞活性
pressure breathing assister 加圧呼吸補助器
prolactin-binding assay プロラクチン結合測定(法)
prune belly anomaly プルーンベリー奇形

PBB
polybrominated biphenyl ポリ臭化ビフェニル

Pb-B
lead level in blood 血中鉛レベル

PBC
peripheral blood cell 末梢血赤血球
point of basal convergence 基礎輻輳点
pregnancy and birth complications 妊娠と出産の合併症
primary biliary cirrhosis 原発性胆汁性肝硬変

PBCL
parafollicular B cell lymphoma 傍濾胞B細胞リンパ腫
physician behavior check list 医師の行動チェックリスト

PBD
percutaneous biliary drainage 経皮的胆道ドレナージ
proliferative breast disease 増殖性乳房疾患

PBE
partial breech extraction 骨盤位介助術
perlsucht bacillus emulsion ウシ結核菌懸濁液

PBF
periflux blood flow 皮膚毛細血管血流量
peripheral blood flow 末梢血流量
placental blood flow 胎盤血流量
pulmonary blood flow 肺血流量
PB-Fe
protein-bound iron 蛋白結合鉄
PBG
porphobilinogen ポルホビリノゲン
PBI
lead intoxication 鉛中毒
penile brachial index ペニスの血圧と上腕動脈収縮期圧との比
prognostic burn index 熱傷予後指数
protein-bound iodine 蛋白結合ヨウ素
PB IgG, PBIgG
platelet-binding IgG 血小板結合免疫グロブリンG
PBK
phosphorylase b kinase ホスホリラーゼbキナーゼ
pseudophakic bullous keratopathy 眼内レンズ性水疱性角膜症
PBL
peripheral blood leukocyte 末梢血白血球
peripheral blood lymphocyte 末梢血リンパ球
peripheral blood mononuclear leukocyte 末梢血単核白血球
PB list
phonetically balanced word list 出現頻度語表
PBM
peripheral blood monocyte 末梢血単核球
peripheral blood mononuclear (cell) 末梢血単核(細胞)
pharmacy benefit management 薬局の利益管理
polyclonal B cell mitogen 多クローン性Bリンパ球マイトゲン
PBMC
peripheral blood mononuclear cell 末梢血単核細胞
PBN
α-phenyl-1-*N*-butylnitrone αフェニル-1-*N*-ブチルニトロン
paralytic brachial neuritis 麻痺性腕神経叢炎
peripheral benign neoplasm 末梢性良性腫瘍
peripheral blood neutrophil 末梢血好中球
polymyxin B sulfate, bacitracin, neomycin 硫酸ポリミキシンB,バシトラシン,ネオマイシン
PBO
placebo 偽薬，プラシボ，プラセボ

PbO
lead monoxide 一酸化鉛
PBP
penicillin-binding protein ペニシリン結合蛋白
peptide-binding protein ペプチド結合蛋白
percutaneous balloon pericardiotomy 経皮的バルーン心嚢(心膜)切開(術)
porphyrin biosynthetic pathway ポルフィリン生合成経路
progressive bulbar palsy 進行性球麻痺
pseudobulbar palsy 仮性球麻痺
PBPI
penile blood pressure index 陰茎血圧指数
PBPK
physiologically based pharmacokinetic model 生理学的薬力学的モデル
PBQ
Preschool Behavior Questionnaire 入学前行動質問票
PBR
premature birth rate 未熟児出生率
PBS
Pharmaceutical Benefits Scheme 薬剤利得計画
phenobarbital sodium フェノバルビタールナトリウム
phosphate-buffered saline リン酸緩衝食塩水
prune belly syndrome プルーンベリー症候群
pulmonary bed sequestration ベッド肺分画
pulmonary branch stenosis 肺枝狭窄(症)
PbS
lead sulfide 硫化鉛
PBSC
penicillin, bacitracin, streptomycin, caprylate ペニシリン,バシトラシン,ストレプトマイシン,カプリル酸塩
peripheral blood stem cell 末梢血幹細胞
PBSCT
peripheral blood stem cell transplantation 末梢血幹細胞移植療法
PBSP
prognostically bad signs during pregnancy 妊娠中予後不良徴候
PBT
Paul-Bunnell test ポール・バンネル試験
picture block (intelligence) test 絵画積木(知能)検査
pulmonary barotrauma 肺の気圧性外傷
PBT_4
protein-bound thyroxine 蛋白結合チロキシン

PBU

α-phenylbutyl urea　*α*フェニルブチル尿素

PBV

cisplatin(=Platinol),bleomycin, vinblastine　シスプラチン(=プラチノール),ブレオマイシン,ビンブラスチン

percutaneous balloon valvuloplasty　経皮的バルーン弁形成(術)

pulmonary blood volume　肺血液量

PBZ

phenylbutazone　フェニルブタゾン

pyribenzamine　ピリベンザミン

PC

Δ′-pyrroline-5-carboxylic acid　Δ′-ピロリン-5-カルボキシル酸

packed cells　濃縮赤血球液

pancreatic cancer　膵癌

paper chromatography　ペーパークロマトグラフィ

paratyphoid C　パラチフスC

parent cell　親細胞

partition chromatography　分配クロマトグラフィ

partition coefficient　分配係数

pelvic cramp　骨盤痙攣

penicillamine　ペニシラミン

penicillin　ペニシリン

pentose cycle　五炭糖サイクル

performance capacity　行動能力

pericarditis constrictiva〈ラ〉　収縮性心膜炎

pericentral region　中心周囲域

petite courbature〈仏〉　小さな痛み

phagocytosis　食菌作用

pharyngitis chronica〈ラ〉　慢性咽頭炎

pheochromocytoma　褐色細胞腫

phone call　電話連絡

phosphate cycle　リン酸サイクル

phosphatidylcholine　ホスファチジルコリン

phosphocreatine　ホスホクレアチン

phosphorylcholine　ホスホリルコリン

photocoagulation　光凝固

phycocyanin　フィコシニアン

plasma concentration　血漿濃度

plasma cortisol　血漿コルチゾール

plasmacytoma　形質細胞腫

platelet concentrate　血小板濃縮液

platelet count　血小板数

Pneumocystis carinii　カリニ肺胞囊虫

pneumotaxic center　呼吸調節中枢

polycentric	多中心の
polyposis coli	大腸ポリポーシス
pondus civile〈ラ〉	常用式重量
popliteal cyst	膝窩嚢胞
portacaval (shunt)	門脈大静脈(シャント)
portal cirrhosis	門脈性肝硬変
postcoital	性交後の
postcricoid	輪状軟骨後面
posterior chamber	後眼房
posterior commissure	後交連
precordium	前胸部
premature contraction	期外収縮
present complaint	主訴
primary care	プライマリケア
primary closure	一次閉鎖
primed lymphocyte	初期リンパ球
procollagen	プロコラーゲン
producing cell	産生細胞
productive cough	湿性痰
proliferative capacity	増殖能
prostatic carcinoma	前立腺癌
protein C	プロテインC
pseudocyst	偽嚢胞
pseudotumor cerebri	偽性脳腫瘍
pulmonary capillary	肺毛細管
pulmonary circulation	肺循環
pulmonic closure (sound)	肺動脈弁閉鎖(音)
Purkinje cell	プルキンエ細胞
pyruvate carboxylase	ピルビン酸カルボキシラーゼ

pc

paracortical area	傍皮質域
percent	パーセント
piece	一部
piriform cortex	梨状葉
plasma cell	形質細胞
point of curve	曲点
pulsating current	拍動流
pyrroline-carboxylic acid	ピロリンカルボキシ酸

6P1C

pain, paresthesia, paleness, pulselessness, palsy, prostration, coldness	疼痛・感覚異常・蒼白・無脈・麻痺・疲労・冷感

PC 1

plasma cell membrane glycoprotein-1	形質細胞膜糖蛋白 1

p.c.

post cibos〈ラ〉=after meal	食後に《処》

P

post cibum〈ラ〉＝after a meal　食後に《処》

P-C

phlogistic corticoid　炎症性コルチコイド

PC, Pc

phenol coefficient　フェノール係数，石炭酸係数

pC, pc

picocurie　ピコキュリー〈単位〉

PCA

pancreatic carcinoma　膵癌
parietal cell antibody　壁細胞抗体
passive cutaneous anaphylaxis　受身皮膚アナフィラキシー
patient care assistant　看護助手
patient-controlled analgesia　患者コントロール下鎮痛法
perchloric acid　過塩素酸
percutaneous carotid arteriogram　経皮的頸動脈造影図
percutaneous coronary angioplasty　経皮的冠(状)動脈形成術
person-centered attitude　人間尊重の態度
plasma cell antigen　形質細胞特異抗原
ponto-cerebellar atrophy　橋小脳萎縮
porous coated anatomic (prosthesis)　多孔性人工関節
portacaval anastomosis　門大静脈吻合
posterior cerebral artery　後大脳動脈
posterior choanal atresia　後鼻孔閉鎖
posterior communicating aneurysm　後交通動脈瘤
posterior communicating artery　後交通動脈
primary cardiac arrest　原発性心停止
pyridonecarboxylic acid　ピリドンカルボン酸

PCA, pCa

prostate cancer　前立腺癌
prostatic carcinoma　前立腺癌

PCAA

pancreas cancer associated antigen　膵癌関連抗原

PCAG

primary closed angle glaucoma　原発性閉塞隅角緑内障

PCB

paracervical block　頸椎傍ブロック
polychlorinated biphenyls　ポリ塩化ビフェニル
procarbazine　プロカルバジン

PCBF

pulmonary capillary blood　肺毛細管血流量

PC-BMP

phosphorylcholine-binding myeloma protein　ホスホリルコリン結合骨髄腫蛋白

P-CBPC
carfecillin sodium, carbenicillin phenyl sodium, carfecillin — カルフェシリンナトリウム，カルベニシリンフェニルナトリウム，カルフェシリン

PCC
percutaneous cecostomy — 経皮的盲腸フィステル形成(術)
peripheral cholangiocarcinoma — 末梢性胆管癌
periscopic concave — 周辺陥凹性
pheochromocytoma — 褐色細胞腫
phosphate carrier compound — リン酸輸送体化合物
plasma catecholamine concentration — 血漿カテコールアミン濃度
plasma cortisol concentration — 血漿コルチゾール濃度
postcricoid cancer — 輪状軟骨後面癌
precoronary care — 早期冠(状)動脈(疾患)治療
premature chromatin condensation — 未熟クロマチン凝縮
premature chromosome condensation — 未熟染色体濃縮
propionyl coenzyme A carboxylase — プロピオニルCoAカルボキシラーゼ
prothrombin-complex concentrate — プロトロンビン複合体濃縮物
prothrombin-complex concentration — プロトロンビン複合体濃度

PCCG
pneumocontrast cytography — 気体膀胱二重造影

PCCP
percutaneous cord cyst puncture — 経皮的臍帯嚢胞穿刺

PCCS
parent-child communication schedule — 親子コミュニケーションスケジュール

PCCU
progressive coronary care unit — 段階冠(状)動脈治療室

PCD
pacer-cardioverter defibrillator — ペースメーカー除細動器
pacing, cardioverting, defibrillating — ペーシング・カルジオバージョン・脱細動
paraneoplastic cerebellar degeneration — 悪性腫瘍に伴う小脳変性
paroxysmal cerebral dysrhythmia — 発作性脳律動異常
percutaneous catheter drainage — 経皮的カテーテルドレナージ
plasma cell dyscrasia — プラズマ細胞疾患
polycystic disease — 多嚢胞性疾患
programmed cell death — アポトーシス

PCDD
polychlorinated dibenzo-*p*-dioxins — ポリ塩化ジベンゾパラジオキシン

PCDF
polychlorinated dibenzofuran — ポリ塩化ジベンゾフラン

PCDUS
plasma cell dyscrasia of unknown significance — 意義不明のプラズマ細胞疾患

PCE
cis-platinum, cyclophosphamide, Eldesine — シスプラチナム,シクロホスファミド,エルデシン
paper chromatoelectrophoresis — 濾紙電気泳動法
polyarthrite chronique évolutive〈仏〉 — 慢性進行性多発関節炎

PCEA
patient-controlled epidural analgesia — 自己調節硬膜外鎮痛(法)

PCEEA
premium curved end to end anastomosis — 分解型彎曲消化管吻合器

PCF
peripheral circulatory failure — 末梢循環不全
pharyngoconjunctival fever — 咽頭結膜熱
posterior cranial fossa — 後頭蓋窩
prothrombin conversion factor — プロトロンビン交換因子

PCFT
platelet complement fixation test — 血小板補体結合試験

PCG
benzyl penicillin — ベンジルペニシリン
paper chromatography — ペーパークロマトグラフィ
paracervical ganglion — 頸傍神経節
penicillin G — ペニシリンG
phonocardiogram — 心音図
plain craniography — 単純頭蓋撮影
pubococcygeus (muscle) — 恥骨尾骨(筋)

PCH
paroxysmal cold hemoglobinuria — 発作性寒冷血色素尿症
primary chronic hepatitis — 原発性慢性肝炎

PChA
posterior choroidal artery — 後脈絡膜動脈

PCHD
polycystic hepatic disease — 多発嚢胞性肝疾患

PchE
pseudocholinesterase — 偽コリンエステラーゼ

PCI
percutaneous cororary intervention — 冠(状)動脈インターベンション
peripheral circulatory impairment — 末梢循環障害
pneumatosis cystoides intestinalis — 腹壁嚢胞状気腫
prophylactic cranial irradiation — 予防的頭蓋照射
protein C inhibitor — プロテインCインヒビター

pCi
picocurie — ピコキュリー〈単位〉

PCIA
particle counting immunoassay 粒子計測免疫測定
PCICHG
Permanent Committee for the International Congress of Human Genetics 国際人類遺伝学会議常置委員会
PCINA
patient-controlled intranasal analgesia 自己調節鼻内鎮痛法
PC-IOL
posterior chamber intraocular lens 眼内後房レンズ
PCIRF
radiologic contrast-induced renal failure 放射線コントラスト(造影剤)誘発性腎不全
PCIS
post-cardiac injury syndrome 心(臓)損傷後症候群
PCK
polycystic kidney 嚢胞腎
PCKD
polycystic kidney disease 多発性嚢胞腎
PCL
plasma cell leukemia 形質細胞白血病
posterior cruciate ligament 後十字靱帯
PCl
picryl chloride 塩化ピクリル
PCLD
polycystic liver disease 多嚢胞性肝疾患
PCLI
posterior chamber lens implant 後眼房レンズ移植
PCM
phase change material 位相変化物質
primary cutaneous melanoma 原発性皮膚黒色腫
protein caloric malnutrition 栄養失調症
protein-carboxyl methylase 蛋白カルボキシルメチラーゼ
pulse-cord modulation 脈拍コード変調
punch-card machine パンチカード機械
PCMB, *p*CMB
parachloromercuribenzoate パラクロロ第二水銀〔メルクリ〕安息香酸塩
PCMBS
p-chloromercuribenzenesulfonic acid パラクロロ第二水銀〔メルクリ〕ベンゼンスルホン酸
PCMF
perceptual cognitive motor function 知覚認識運動機能

P

PCML
primary cutaneous malignant lymphoma — 原発性皮膚悪性リンパ腫

PCMPS
p-chloromercuriphenylsulfonic acid — パラクロロ第二水銀〔メルクリ〕フェニルスルホン酸

PCMR
proportionate cancer mortality ratio — 癌比例死亡率

PCMT
pacemaker circus movement tachycardia — ペースメーカー(興奮)旋回〔輪回〕運動頻拍(脈)

PCN
penicillin — ペニシリン
percutaneous nephrolithotomy — 経皮的腎切石術
percutaneous nephrostomy — 経皮的腎瘻造設術
primary care network — プライマリケア網

PCNA
proliferating cell nuclear antigen — 増殖性細胞核抗原

PCNB
pentachloronitrobenzene — ペンタクロロニトロベンゼン
Permanent Control Narcotics Board — 麻薬永久管理局

***p*-CNB**
p-chloronitrobenzene — パラクロロニトロベンゼン

PCNL
percutaneous nephrostolithotomy — 経皮的腎外瘻切石術

PCNV
Provisional Committee for Nomenclature of Virus — ウイルス命名のための暫定委員会

P_{CO}
carbon monoxide tension — 一酸化炭素分圧
platelet cyclooxygenase — 血小板シクロオキシゲナーゼ
polycystic ovary — 多嚢胞性卵巣
prostaglandin cyclooxygenase — プロスタグランジンシクロオキシゲナーゼ

P_{CO_2}, PCO_2
partial pressure of carbon dioxide — 二酸化炭素〔炭酸ガス〕分圧

PCoA
posterior communicating artery — 後交通動脈

PCO_2A
partial pressure of carbon deoxide in alveolar gas — 肺胞二酸化炭素〔炭酸ガス〕分圧

PCO_2 art
partial pressure of carbon deoxide in artery — 動脈血二酸化炭素〔炭酸ガス〕分圧

PCOD
polycystic ovarian disease — 多嚢胞性卵巣疾患

P

Pcom, P-com
posterior communicating artery　後交通動脈
PCOS
polycystic ovary syndrome　多嚢胞性卵巣症候群
PCP
pentachlorophenol　ペンタクロロフェノール
phenylcyclohexylpiperidine　フェンサイクリジン
1-(1-phenylcyclohexyl) piperidine　1-(1-フェニルシクロヘキシル)ピペリジン
pneumocystitis carinii pneumonia　ニューモシスチス・カリニ肺炎，カリニ肺炎
postoperative constrictive pericarditis　術後収縮性心膜炎
primary care physician　プライマリケア医師
progressive chronic polyarthritis　慢性進行性多発性関節炎
pulmonary capillary pressure　肺毛細血管圧
***p*-CPA, PCPA, *p*CPA**
p-chlorophenylalanine　パラクロロフェニルアラニン
PCPB
percutaneous cardiopulmonary bypass　経皮的心肺バイパス
PC-PFC
polyclonal plaque-forming cell　多クローン性プラーク形成細胞
PCPL
pulmonary capillary protein leakage　肺毛細管蛋白漏出
pcpn.
precipitation　沈殿反応
PCPP
post-centrifugal plasma pheresis　遠心後プラズマフェレーシス
PCPS
percutaneous cardiopulmonary support　経皮的心肺補助
peroral cholangiopancreatoscopy　経口胆道膵管造影(法)
pcpt
perception　知覚
precipitate　沈殿する
precipitation　沈殿反応
PCR
computer-based record　コンピュータに基づく記録
phosphocreatine　ホスホクレアチン
photoconvulsive response　光痙攣反応
plasma clearance rate　血漿クリアランス率
polymerase chain reaction　ポリメラーゼ連鎖反応
principal component regression analysis　主成分回帰分析《統》
protein catabolic rate　蛋白分解酵素

PCRA
percutaneous coronary rotational atherectomy — 経皮的冠(状)動脈回転式粥腫切除術

PCRC
primary colorectal cancer — 原発性結腸直腸癌

PCRI
Papanicolaou Cancer Research Institute — パパニコロー癌研究所

PCS
patient care system — 患者管理機構《医情》
pelvic congestion syndrome — 骨盤うっ血症候群
peroral cholangioscopy — 経口的胆道内視鏡
pharmacogenic confusional syndrome — 薬剤性錯乱症候群
photocalorimetric spectroscopy — 光カロリメトリー分光法
portacaval shunt — 門脈大静脈シャント，門脈大静脈吻合術
postcardiac surgery — 心臓手術後
postcardiotomy syndrome — 心術後症候群
postcholecystectomy syndrome — 胆嚢摘出後症候群
postconcussion syndrome — 脳振とう後症候群
posterior coronary sinus — 後冠(状)動脈洞
precordial stethoscope — 前胸部聴診器
primary cancer site — 原発癌部位
proximal coronary sinus — 近位冠(状)静脈洞
pseudotumor cerebri syndrome — 偽脳腫瘍症候群
punch card system — パンチカード方式

PCs
penicillins — ペニシリン群抗生物質

Pcs
preconscious — 前意識の

PCS，P c/s
primary cesarean section — 一次性帝王切開(術)

PCSM
percutaneous stone manipulation — 経皮的結石操作

PCT
peak concentration time — 最高濃度時間
pharmacologic convulsion therapy — 薬物痙攣療法
photochemotherapy — 光化学治療
picture completion test — 絵画完成テスト
plasmacrit test — プラズマクリットテスト
plasmacytoma — プラズマ細胞腫
platelet hematocrit — 血小板ヘマトクリット
porcine calcitonin — ブタカルシトニン
porphyria cutanea tarda — 晩発性皮膚ポルフィリン症
positron computed tomography — 陽電子断層法
postcoital test — 性交後試験

progestogen challenge test　プロゲストゲンチャレンジ試験
prothrombin consumption time　プロトロンビン消費時間
proximal convoluted tubule　近位曲(尿)細管
pulmonary care team　肺ケアチーム

pct
percent　百分率，パーセント

PCTA
percutaneous coronary transluminal angioplasty　経皮(的)経管的冠(状)動脈形成(術)

PCTFE
polychloro-trifluoroethylene　ポリ塩化三フッ化エチレン

PCU
palliative care unit　緩和ケア病棟
patient care unit　患者管理部門
progressive care unit　段階的患者管理部門
protein-calorie undernutrition　蛋白カロリー低栄養
pulmonary care unit　肺疾患管理部門

p.cut
percutaneous　経皮の

PCV
packed cell volume　血球容積
parietal cell vagotomy　壁細胞迷走神経切断
phenoxymethyl penicillin　フェノキシメチルペニシリン，ペニシリンV
polycythemia vera　真性赤血球増加症
postcapillary venule　毛細血管後小静脈
precentral cerebellar vein　中央前小脳静脈
premature ventricular contraction　心室(性)期外収縮
pressure control ventilation　圧制御調節換気

PCVC
percutaneous central venous catheter　経皮的中心静脈カテーテル

PCWP
pulmonary capillary wedge pressure　肺毛細血管楔入圧

PCZ
pancreozymin　パンクレオザイミン
procarbazine　プロカルバジン

PD
Paget disease　パジェット病，ページェット病
pancreas duct　膵管
pancreaticoduodenectomy　膵頭十二指腸切除
panel discussion　パネルディスカッション
panic disorder　恐慌性障害
paralytic dose　麻痺量
Parkinson disease　パーキンソン病

parkinsonism-dementia complex パーキンソン痴呆症候群
paroxysmal discharge 発作性発射
pediatrics 小児科学
percutaneous deskectomy 経皮的椎間板切除術
per deliquium〈ラ〉 潮解して《処》
peritoneal dialysis 腹膜透析
personality disorder 人格障害
pharmacodynamics 薬力学
photic driving 光駆動
photosensitivity dermatitis 光線過敏症皮膚炎
Pick disease ピック病
pigeon dung 鳩糞便(抗原)
pituitary dwarfism 下垂体性小人症
plasma defect 血漿欠損
pocket dosimeter ポケット線量計
Porak-Durante (syndrome) ポラク・デュラント(症候群)
porphobilinogen deaminase ポルホビリノゲンデアミナーゼ
posterior descending branch 後下行枝
postural drainage 体位ドレナージ
potential difference 電位差
pregnanediol プレグナンジオール
preliminary dressing 仮包帯
present disease 現病
pressor dose 昇圧量
prism diopter プリズムジオプトリー
progression of disease 病気の進行，病気の悪化
protein diet 蛋白食
provisional diagnosis 仮診断
psychodrama 心理劇
psychotic dementia 精神病性痴呆
psychotic depression 精神病的うつ病
pulmonary disease 肺疾患
pulse delay パルス遅延時間
pupillar distance 瞳孔間距離

Pd

palladium パラジウム〈元素〉

pd

papillary distance 乳頭径
period 期間
pound ポンド〈単位〉

pd.

ponderis〈ラ〉 重量の

2-PD

two-point discrimination 2点間識別テスト《神経》

p/d
packs per day　パック/日

pd，p.d.
per diem〈ラ〉　1日あたり，毎日《処》
pro die〈ラ〉　日ごとの
pro dosi〈ラ〉=for a dose　1回量として《処》

PDA
Parenteral Drug Association　非経口薬協会
patent ductus arteriosus　動脈管開存症
patient distress alarm　患者苦痛警告
pediatric allergy　小児アレルギー
personal digital assistants　個人的なジギタル補助具
polymorphous delta activity　多形性δ波
poorly differentiated adenocarcinoma　未分化腺癌
posterior descending (coronary) artery　(冠状動脈)後下行枝
predialyzed human serum　透析前ヒト血清
pulmonary disease anemia　肺疾患(性)貧血
pyrene decanoic acid　ピレンデカン酸

PDAB
paradimethylaminobenzaldehyde　パラジメチルアミノベンズアルデヒド

PDA-division
patent ducts arteriosus division　動脈管切断術

PDase
phosphodiesterase　ホスホジエステラーゼ

PDB
Paget disease of bone　骨パジェット病
p-dichlorobenzene　パラジクロロベンゼン

PDC
padiatric cardiology　小児心臓病
parkinsonism-dementia complex　パーキンソン痴呆症候群
penta-decylcatechol　ペンタデシルカテコール
plasma digoxin concentration　血漿ジゴキシン濃度
poorly differentiated carcinoma　未分化癌
preliminary diagnostic clinic　仮診断クリニック
private diagnostic clinic　民間診断クリニック
probability of detection and conversion　検出と変換の可能性

3-PDC
3-pentadecylcatechol　3-ペンタデシルカテコール

PDCD
primary degenerative cerebral disease　原発性変性脳疾患

PDD
percent depth dose　深部量百分率

P

pervasive developmental disorder 広汎(性)発達障害
photodynamic diagnosis 光力学的診断
photoreceptor drop-down 光感受脱落
primary degenerative dementia 一次性変性痴呆
pyridoxine-deficient diet ピリドキシン欠乏食

Pd.D.
Pedagogiae Doctor 教育学士

PDDB
phenododecinium bromide 臭化フェノドデシニウム

PDE
paroxysmal dyspnea on exertion 発作性労作性呼吸困難
phosphodiesterase ホスホジエステラーゼ
progressive dialysis encephalopathy 進行性透析脳症
pulsed Doppler echocardiography パルス・ド(ッ)プラー心エコー図

PD-ECGF
platelet-derived endothelial cell growth factor 血小板由来内皮細胞増殖因子

Pdet
detrusor P 膀胱利尿筋(内)圧

PDF
peritoneal dialysis fluid 腹膜透析液

PDG
Pharmacopeial Discussion Group 薬局方検討会議
phosphogluconate dehydrogenase ホスホグルコン酸脱水素酵素

PDGA
pteroyl-diglutamic acid プテロイルジグルタミン酸

PDGF
platelet-derived growth factor 血小板由来成長〔増殖〕因子

PDH
past dental history 歯科既往歴
phosphate dehydrogenase リン酸脱水素酵素
pyruvate dehydrogenase ピルビン酸脱水素酵素

PDHC
pyruvate dehydrogenase complex ピルビン酸脱水素酵素複合体

PDI
patient dispensing instruction 患者用服薬指導
periodontal disease index 歯周疾患指数
pharmacological drug interferences 薬理学的薬剤干渉
portable data for imaging 可搬型媒体データ交換規約
proton density image プロトン画像
psychomotor development index 精神運動発達指数

Pdi
transdiaphragmatic pressure 経横隔膜圧

P-diol
pregnanediol プレグナンジオール

PDL
polycystic disease of liver　多嚢胞性肝疾患
prednisolone　プレドニゾロン
primary dysfunctional labor　原発性機能不全(性)肝(臓)
progressively diffused leukoencephalopathy　進行性広汎性白質脳症

Pdl
pudendal　外陰部の

pdl
poundal　ポンダル

PDLC
poorly differentiated lymphocytic lymphoma　低分化リンパ球性リンパ腫

PDLL
poorly differentiated lymphocytic lymphoma　未分化リンパ球性リンパ腫

PDM
polymyositis and dermatomyositis　多発(性)筋炎と皮膚筋炎
pulse duration modulation　パルス幅変調

P-DMEA
phosphoryldimethylethanolamine　ホスホリルジメチルエタノールアミン

PDMS
plasma desorption mass spectrometry　プラズマ脱離マス分光

PDN
prednisone　プレドニゾン

PDPD
protein-deficient pancreatic diabetes　蛋白欠乏性膵性糖尿病

PDPH
post-dural puncture headache　硬膜穿刺後頭痛

PDR
pandevelopmental retardation　全発達遅滞
pediatric radiology　小児放射線学
percentage disappearance rate　消失率
peripheral diabetic retinopathy　末梢性糖尿病網膜症
Physician's Desk Reference　米国医薬品集
plasma disappearance rate　血漿消退率
pleiotropic drug resistance　多相遺伝性薬剤耐性
post-delivery room　分娩後室
post-drug repetition　投薬停止後再発
proliferative diabetic retinopathy　増殖性糖尿病性網膜症

pdr
powder　粉末

PDRc̄VH
proliferative diabetic retinopathy with vitreous hemorrhage　硝子体出血を伴う増殖性糖尿病網膜症

PDS
pain dysfunction syndrome　疼痛機能不全症候群
paroxysmal depolarizing shift　発作性脱分極性シフト
patient data system　患者データシステム
pediatric surgery　小児外科
peritoneal dialysis system　腹膜透析システム
placental dysfunction syndrome　胎盤機能不全症候群
predialyzed human serum　透析前ヒト血清

PDT
percutaneous dilational tracheostomy　経皮的拡張気管切開
pertussis-diphtheria-tetanus　百日咳・ジフテリア・破傷風
photodynamic therapy　光線力学的療法

PDTC
pyrrolidine dithiocarbamate　ピロリジンジチオカルボン酸

PDU
pulsed Doppler ultrasonography　パルスド(ッ)プラー超音波法

PDV
peak diastolic velocity　最大拡張期速度
Valsalva test　バルサルバ試験

PDW
platelet distribution wide　血小板分布幅

PE
cisplatin(=Platinol),etoposide　シスプラチン(=プラチノール),エトポシド
pancreatic extract　膵抽出物
panlobular emphysema　汎小葉型肺気腫
paper electrophoresis　濾紙電気泳動
parallel elastic component　並行弾圧成分
partial epilepsy　部分てんかん
patellofemoral (joint)　膝蓋大腿(関節)
pemphigus erythematosus〈ラ〉　紅斑性エリテマトーデス
penile erection　陰茎勃起
pericardial effusion　心嚢液貯留
peritoneal exudate　腹膜滲出液
phakoemulsification　水晶体乳化
pharmacoepidemiology　薬剤疫学
pharyngoesophageal　咽頭食道の
phenylephrine　フェニレフリン
phosphatidylethanolamine　ホスファチジルエタノールアミン
photographic effect　写真効果
phycoerythrin　フィコエリトリン
physical evaluation　理学的評価
physical examination　理学的検査
plasma epinephrine　血漿エピネフリン
plasma exchange　血漿交換

pleural effusion 胸膜滲出
polyethylene ポリエチレン
polynuclear eosinophil 多核好酸球
portal of entry 侵入門
potential energy 位置エネルギー
powdered extract 粉末エキス
preeclampsia 子癇前症
pressure on expiration 呼気圧
prior to exposure 曝露前に
probable error 確率誤差《統》
pulmonary edema 肺水腫
pulmonary embolism 肺塞栓症
pulmonary embolus 肺塞栓
pulmonary emphysema 肺気腫症
pulmonary eosinophilia 肺好酸球症
pyramidal eminence 錐体隆起
pyrogenic exotoxin 発熱性外毒素

Pe
perylene ペリレン

p.e.
per exemplum〈ラ〉 たとえば

PEA
patient-controlled epidural analgesia 自己調節硬膜外鎮痛
phacoemulsification and aspiration 水晶体超音波乳化吸引術
phenylethylalanine フェニルエチルアラニン
phenylethylalcohol フェニルエチルアルコール
phenylethylamine フェニルエチルアミン
phosphoethanolamine ホスホエタノールアミン

PEB
cisplatin(=Platinol),etoposide, bleomycin シスプラチン(=プラチノール),エトポシド,ブレオマイシン
Physical Evaluation Board 生理的評価委員会

PEb
proerythroblast 前赤芽球

PEBG
phenethyl-biguanide フェネチルビグアナイド

PEC
partial elastic component 部分弾性成分
peduncle of cerebrum 大脳脚
peritoneal exudate cell 腹腔滲出細胞
pleural effusion cell 胸腔滲出細胞
predicted environmental concentration 予測環境濃度

P

PECAM
platelet endothelial cell adhesion molecule 血小板相互間凝集抗原
PECCE
planned extracapsular cataract extraction 計画的白内障嚢外摘出
PECHR
peripheral exudative choroidal hemorrhagic retinopathy 周辺部滲出性脈絡膜出血性網膜症
PE$_{CO_2}$
expired carbon oxide tension 呼気二酸化炭素分圧
PECT
positron emission computed tomography ポジトロンエミッションCT，陽電子放射型コンピュータ断層撮影法
PED
cerebral peduncle 大脳脚
paroxysmal exertion-induced dyskinesia 発作性運動誘発〔誘因〕性ジスキネジー
pediatrician 小児科医
pediatrics 小児科(学)
peduncle 脚
pharyngoesophageal diverticulum 咽頭食道憩室
physical education 体育
postexertional dyspnea 労作後呼吸困難
ped
pedestrian 歩行者
ped.
pedetentim〈ラ〉 徐々に《処》
ped.ed
pedal edema 足浮腫
PEDG
phenylethyldiguanide フェニルエチルジグアニド
Peds, peds
pediatrics 小児科(学)
PEE
end-expiratory pressure 呼気終末圧
predicted energy expenditure 予測基礎代謝量
PEEM
photoemission electron microscope 光電子顕微鏡
PEEP
positive end-expiratory pressure 呼気終末陽圧
PEEPB
positive end-expiratory pressure breathing 呼気終末陽圧呼吸

PEF
peak expiratory flow 最大呼気流量
peritoneal exudate fluid 腹膜滲出液
pharyngoepiglottic fold 咽頭喉頭蓋ひだ
psychiatric evaluation form 精神科評価用紙
pulmonary edema fluid 肺水腫液

PEFR
peak expiratory flow rate 最大呼気速度

PEG
percutaneous endoscopic gastrostomy 経皮内視鏡的胃瘻造設術
pneumoencephalography 気(体)脳造影〔撮影〕法
polyethylene glycol ポリエチレングリコール

PEG-ELS
polyethylene glycol electrolyte lavage solution ポリエチレングリコール電解質液

PEG-J
percutaneous endoscopic gastrojejunostomy 経皮的内視鏡下胃空腸吻合(術)

PEI
cisplatin(=Platinol), etoposide, ifosfamide シスプラチン(=プラチノール), エトポシド, イホスファミド
percutaneous ethanol injection 経皮的エタノール注入
phosphate excretion index リン酸排泄係数
polyethylene-imine ポリエチレンイミン

PEIT
percutaneous ethanol injection therapy 経皮的エタノール注入療法

PEJ
percutaneous endoscopic jejunostomy 経皮的内視鏡下空腸造瘻術

PEK
punctate epithelial keratopathy 点状上皮角膜症

PE-K
phenethicillinum kalium フェネチシリンカリウム

PEL
peritoneal exudate lymphocytes 腹腔滲出液リンパ球

Pel
pelvic 骨盤の

PELS
propionyl erythromycin lauryl sulfate プロピオニルエリスロマイシンラウリル硫酸塩

PEM
peritoneal exudate macrophage 腹腔滲出液大食細胞
polyethylene matrix ポリエチレン基質
positron emission mammography ポジトロンエミッションマンモグラフィ

prescription event monitoring 処方・事象監視
protein energy malnutrition 蛋白エネルギー低栄養
pulmonary endothelial membrane 肺内皮細胞膜

PEMA
phenylethylmalonamide フェニルエチルマロンアミド

PE material
pseudoexfoliation material 偽落屑物質

PEMEC
phenylethylmethylethyl carbonol フェニルエチルメチルエチルカルボノール

PEMF
pulsating electromagnetic field 拍動性電磁場

PEN
peritoneal exudate neutrophil 腹腔滲出好中球

pen
penis 陰茎

Pen, pen
penicillin ペニシリン

PENA
pre-early nuclear antigen 前初期抗原

pend
pendulous 下垂した

PENG
photoelectro-nystagmograph 光電眼振計
photoelectronystagmography 光電眼振法

penic
penicillin ペニシリン

pens
pension 年金

P

pent
penetrate 穿孔する
penetration 穿孔

pento
pentothal ペントタール

PEO
progressive external opthalmoplegia 進行性外眼筋麻痺

PEOS
peroxisomal ethanol oxidizing system ペルオキシソーマルエタノール酸化システム

PEP
peplomycin ペプロマイシン
phosphoenolpyruvate ホスホエノールピルビン酸
phosphoenolpyruvic acid ホスホエノールピルビン酸
polyestradiol phosphate リン酸ポリエストラジオール
polyneuropathy, edema, pigmentation 末梢神経症状・浮腫・色素沈着

positive expiratory pressure 呼気陽圧法
postencephalitic parkinsonism 脳炎後パーキンソン症候群
pre-ejection period 前駆出期

Pep, PEP
peptidase ペプチダーゼ

PEPC
phenethicillin フェネチシリン
phenoxyethyl-penicillin(=phenethicillin) フェノキシエチルペニシリン(=フェネチシリン)

PEPCK
phosphoenolpyruvate carboxykinase ホスホエノールピルベートカルボキシキナーゼ

PEPI
pre-ejection period index 駆出前期指数

PEPP
positive expiratory pressure plateau 呼気陽圧プラトー

peps
pepsin ペプシン

PER
peak ejection rate 左(心)室最大駆出速度
pediatrics emergency room 小児救急室
protein efficiency ratio 蛋白効率比
pudendal evoked response 外陰誘発反応

Per
periodontitis 歯根膜炎
permission 許可

per
perineal 会陰の
period 期間
periodic 周期の
person ヒト

per.an.
per anum〈ラ〉 肛門を通じて《処》

per.bid.
per bidiuum〈ラ〉 2日間《処》

PerCP
peridinin chlorophyll (protein) ペリディニムクロロフィル(蛋白)

percus
percussion 打診

Percuss & ausc
percussion and auscultation 打診法

perf
perfect 完全な
perfected 完成した
perforated 穿孔した

P

perforating 穿孔性の
perforation 穿孔
performed 施行された

PERI
psychiatric epidemiology research interview 精神医学的疫学研究のための面接基準

Peri
pericardium 心膜

peri
perineal 会陰の
perineum 会陰

periap
periapical 歯根端周囲の

Perico
pericoronitis 歯冠周囲炎

Periko
perikoronitis 歯冠周囲炎

perim
perimeter 歯周界，周辺視野計

periodont
periodontology 歯周学

periorb
periorbital 眼窩骨膜の

periph
peripheral 末梢性の
periphery 末梢

periton
peritonsillar abscess 扁桃周囲膿瘍
peritonsillitis 扁桃周囲炎

periumb
periumbilical 臍周囲の

PERK
prospective evaluation of radial keratotomy 角膜切除の予期的評価

PERLA
pupils equal, react to light and accommodation 瞳孔は等しく光線と調節に反応する

perm
permanent 永久の

per.op.emet.
peracta operatione emetici〈ラ〉 嘔吐が終ったときに《処》

perp
perpendicular 垂直，垂直の，直角の

perpad, per.pad
perineal pad 会陰パッド

per.rect.
per rectum〈ラ〉 経直腸的に《処》
PERRLA
pupils are equal and round and reactive to light and accommodation 瞳孔は円形で左右同じ大きさ・対光反射・輻輳反射も正常
PERS
patient evaluation rating scale 患者評価評点スケール
pers
person 個人
personal 個人の
personality 人格
persp
perspiration 発汗
PERT
product-enhanced reverse transcriptase 産物増強性逆転写酵素
psychiatric epidemiology reserch interview 精神医学的疫学研究のための面接基準
pert
pertaining to に属する，～に関する
pertinent 適切な
pertussis 百日咳
per.unc.
period of unconsciousness 意識消失期間
PES
polyethylene sulfonate スルホン酸ポリエチレン
postextrasystolic 期外収縮後の
preepiglottic space 喉頭蓋前域
preexcitation syndrome 早期興奮症候群
programmed electrophysiological stimulation プログラム化された電気生理学的刺激
pseudoexfoliation syndrome 偽(性)剝脱〔落屑〕症候群
Psychiatric Emergency Service 精神科救急サービス
PESP
postextrasystolic potentiation 期外収縮後増強作用
PESS
primary empty sella syndrome 一次的トルコ鞍空虚症候群
PET
peak ejection time 最大駆出時間
polyethylene terephthalate テレフタル酸ポリエチレン
polyethylene tube ポリエチレン管
positron emission tomography 陽電子放射型断層撮影法，ペット
pre-eclamptic toxemia 子癇前妊娠中毒
pre-ejection time 前駆出期時間

P

pet
petrolatum ワセリン
PET-CT
positron emission tomography computed tomography ポジトロンCT
petech
petechiae 点状出血
PET-FDG
positron emission tomography wiht [^{18}F]-labeled fluorodeoxyglucose フッ素18標識陽電子放射型断層撮影(法)
PETN
pentaerythrityl tetranitrate 四亜硝酸ペンタエリスリチル
$PETO_2$
partial pressure of end-tidal oxygen 呼気終末酸素分圧
petr
petroleum 石油
PETT
positron emission transaxial tomography 陽電子放射型横断断層撮影法，ペット
PE tube
polyethylene tube ポリエチレン管
PEUA
pelvic examination under anesthesia 麻酔下骨盤検査
PEV
peak expiratory velocity 最大呼気速度
pulmonary extravascular fluid volume 肺血管外液量
PeV
peripheral vein 末梢静脈
pev
peak electron volts 最大電子ボルト
PEX
plasma exchange 血漿交換
PEx
physical examination 理学的検査
pex, p.ex.
par exemple〈ラ〉 たとえば
per exemplum〈ラ〉 たとえば
PF
pair fed つがい飼育した
parallel fiber 平行線維
pars flaccida〈ラ〉 弛緩部
patellofemoral (joint) 膝蓋・大腿(関節)部
peak flow 最大流量
pemphigus foliaceus〈ラ〉 落葉状天疱瘡
performance factor 行動因子

P

perfusion fluid	灌流液
pericardial fluid	心膜液
peritoneal fluid	腹腔液
permeability factor	透過性因子
personality factor	人格因子
Persönlichkeits-Faktoren-Test〈独〉	人格要素テスト
Physician's Forum	医師討論会
plantar flexion	底屈
plasma filtration	血漿濾過
Plasmodium falciparum	熱帯熱マラリア原虫
platelet factor	血小板因子
pleural fluid	胸水
pre-follicular	濾胞前期
primary failure	一次的無効
protection factor	防御因子
protein fraction	蛋白分画
pseudofolliculus	偽濾胞
pulmonary factor	肺因子
pulmonary flow	肺流量
pulmonary function	肺機能
pulse frequency	脈頻度
Purkinje fiber	プルキンエ線維
purpura fulminans	電撃性紫斑病

Pf

effective filtration pressure	有効濾過圧
Pfeiffer bacillus	パイフェル菌
Pfeifferella	ファイフェレラ属

pF

picofarad	ピコファラド〈単位〉

16PF

sixteen personality factor question	16人格因子〔要素〕検査

PF3

platelet factor 3	血小板第Ⅲ因子

PF4

platelet factor 4	血小板第Ⅳ因子

P/F

oxygenation index	酸素化係数
pass-fail system	合格・不合格システム
pentalogy of Fallot	ファロー五徴症

PFA

paraformaldehyde	パラホルムアルデヒド
perifimbrial adhesion	卵管采周囲癒着
1-phosphofructaldolase	1-ホスホフルクトアルドラーゼ
principal factor analysis	主因子分析
psychological flight avoidance	精神医学的飛行逃避

P

PFB
phosphate-free buffer　リン酸不使用緩衝液
positive feedback　正のフィードバック
pseudofolliculitis barbae　偽(性)白癬性毛瘡
PFC
pelvic flexion contracture　骨盤屈曲拘縮
perfluoro chemicals　ペルフルオロ化合物
pericardial fluid culture　心膜液培養
persistent fetal circulation　胎児循環遺残症
plaque-forming cell　プラーク形成細胞
proximal finger crease　近位指皺襞
pfce
performance　行動
P/F chart
pressure/flow chart　排尿時膀胱内圧/尿流量図
PFCPH
persistent fetal circulation with pulmonary hypertension　肺高血圧(症)を伴う胎児循環遺残(症)
PFD
pancreatic function diagnosis (test)　膵機能診断〔テスト〕
polyostotic fibrous dysplasia　多骨性線維性骨形成異常
p.f.dig.
pulvis foliae digitalis〈ラ〉　ジギタリス葉末《処》
PFE
cisplatin(=Platinol),5-fluorouracil, etoposide　シスプラチン(=プラチノール),フルオロウラシル,エトポシド
PFEAAC
posterior fossa extra-axial arachnoid cyst　後頭蓋窩軸外クモ膜嚢胞
PFFD
proximal femoral focal deficiency　近位大腿骨巣状欠損(症)
PFG
photofluorography　X線螢光撮影法
PFGE
pulsed field gel electrophoresis　パルスフィールド電気泳動法
PFHS
precipitation from homogeneous solution　均一溶液からの沈殿生成
PFI
physical fitness index　体力指数
PFIB
perfluoroisobutylene　ペルフルオロイソブチレン
PFJ
patellofemoral joint　膝蓋・大腿部関節

PFJS
patellofemoral joint syndrome　膝蓋大腿関節症候群
PFK
phosphofructokinase　ホスホフルクトキナーゼ
PFL
cisplatin (=Platinol), 5-fluorouracil, leucovorin　シスプラチン(=プラチノール),フルオロウラシル,ロイコボリン
profibrinolysin　プロフィブリノリジン
PFM
peak flow meter　最大呼気流量計
primary fibromyalgia　原発性線維筋痛
pulse frequency modulation　パルス周波数変調
PFN
partially functional neutrophil　部分機能好中球
plasma fibronectin　血漿フィブロネクチン
PFO
patent foramen ovale　卵円孔開存
PFP
platelet-free plasma　無血小板血漿
PFQ
Personality Factor Questionnaire　人格因子質問票
PFR
peak expiratory flow rate　ピークフロー
peak filling rate　左(心)室最大充満速度
peak flow rate　最大呼気速度
PFS
pressure flow study　圧力尿流試験
primary fibromyalgia syndrome　原発性線維痛症候群
pulmonary function score　肺機能スコア
P-F study, PF Study
Picture-Association Study Assessing Reaction to Frustration　絵画欲求不満テスト
PFT
finger painting test　指書テスト
pancreatic function test　膵機能検査
picture-frustration test　絵画欲求不満試験
posterior fossa tumor　後頭蓋窩腫瘍
prednisone, fluorouracil, tamoxifen　プレドニゾン,フルオロウラシル,タモキシフェン
pulmonary function test　肺機能検査
PFTBE
progressive form of tick-borne encephalitis　進行型ダニ媒介脳炎
PFU
plaque-forming unit　プラーク形成単位

P

pock-forming unit　痘瘡形成単位

Pfu
Pyrococcus furiosus　ピロコッカスフリオサス

PFUO
prolonged fever of unknown origin　原因不明持続熱

PFV
physiological full valve　生理学的完全弁

PG
pancreaticogastrostomy　膵胃吻合
paralysie générale〈仏〉　全身麻痺
parapsoriasis guttata　滴状類乾癬
paregoric　カンフル加アヘンチンキ
parotid gland　耳下腺
partgram　分娩経過図
pentagastrin　ペンタガストリン
pepsinogen　ペプシノゲン
permanent grade　永久段階
phosphatidylglycerol　ホスファチジルグリセロール
phosphogluconate　ホスホグルコネート
phosphoglycerate　ホスホグリセリン酸
pigment granule　色素顆粒
pituitary gonadotropin　下垂体性性腺刺激ホルモン
plasma gastrin　血漿ガストリン
plasma glucose　血漿グルコース
plasma triglyceride　血漿トリグリセリド
postgraduate　卒後の
pregnanediol glucuronide　プレグナンジオールグルクロン酸化合物
pressure of gas　ガス圧
progesterone　プロゲステロン
program guidance　プログラム案内
propyl gallate　没食子酸プロピル
prostaglandin　プロスタグランジン
proteoglycan　プロテオグリカン
pyoderma gangrenosum　壊疽性膿皮症

Pg
plasminogen　プラスミノゲン

pg
page　頁(＝ページ)
picogram　ピコグラム〈単位〉
pregnancy　妊娠

P.G.
Pharmacopeia Germanica〈ラ〉　ドイツ薬局方

PG, Pg, pg, pg.
plurigravida〈ラ〉　経妊婦
pregnant　妊娠した，妊娠の

PGA
phosphoglyceric acid　ホスホグリセリン酸
polyglandular autoimmune (syndrome)　多腺性自己免疫症候群
polyglycolic acid　多グリコール酸
prompt gamma-ray analysis　即発γ線分析
prostaglandin A　プロスタグランジンA
pteroylglutamic acid　プテロイルグルタミン酸

PGAS
persisting galactorrhea-amenorrhea syndrome　持続性乳(汁)漏(出)・無月経症候群
polyglandular autoimmune syndrome　多腺性自己免疫性症候群

PGB
prostaglandin B　プロスタグランジンB

PGC
primordal germ cell　原始生殖細胞
prostaglandin C　プロスタグランジンC

PGD
phosphogluconate dehydrogenase　ホスホグルコン酸脱水素酵素
phosphoglyceraldehyde dehydrogenase　ホスホグリセルアルデヒド脱水素酵素
potential gradient detector　電気勾配検出器
preimplantation genetic diagnosis　着床前遺伝子診断
prostaglandin D　プロスタグランジンD

PGDH
phosphogluconic dehydrogenase　ホスホグルコン酸脱水素酵素

PGE
platelet granule extract　血小板顆粒抽出物
posterior gastroenterostomy　後胃腸吻合(術)
primary generalized epilepsy　原発性全般てんかん
prostaglandin E　プロスタグランジンE

PGEM
prostaglandin E metabolite　プロスタグランジンE代謝産物

PGF
paternal grandfather　父方の祖父
prostaglandin F　プロスタグランジンF

PGG
polyclonal gamma globulin　ポリクローナルγグロブリン
prostaglandin G　プロスタグランジンG

PGH
pituitary gonadotropic hormone　下垂体性性腺刺激ホルモン
pituitary growth hormone　下垂体成長ホルモン
plasma growth hormone　血漿成長ホルモン
porcine growth hormone　ブタ成長ホルモン
prostaglandin H　プロスタグランジンH

P

PGI
phosphoglucoisomerase　グルコースリン酸イソメラーゼ
potassium, glucose, insulin　カリウム・グルコース・インスリン
prostaglandin I　プロスタグランジンI
PGI_2
prostaglandin I_2 (=prostacycline)　プロスタグランジンI_2(=プロスタサイクリン)
PGJ
prostaglandin J　プロスタグランジンJ
PGK
phosphoglycerate kinase　ホスホグリセリン酸キナーゼ
PGL
paragigantocellularis lateralis〈ラ〉　側傍巨大細胞
persistent generalized lymphadenopathy　持続性全身性リンパ節腫脹
PGM
paternal grandmother　父方の祖母
phosphoglucomutase　ホスホグルコムターゼ
phosphoglyceromutase　ホスホグリセロムターゼ
PGN
proliferative glomerulonephritis　増殖性糸球体腎炎
pgn
pigeon　ハト(=鳩)
PGO
phenylglyoxal　フェニルグリオキサール
ponto-geniculo-occipital　橋・膝・後頭(棘波)
PGP
paralysis generalisata progressiva〈ラ〉　進行性全身麻痺
psycho-galvanic phenomenon　精神電流現象
P-gp
P-glycoprotein　P糖蛋白
PGR
population growth rate　人口増加速度
psychogalvanic reflex　精神電流反射
PgR, PGR
progesterone receptor　プロゲステロン受容体
pGRP
procine gastrin releasing peptide　ブタガストリン放出ペプチド
PGS
persistent gross splenomegaly　持続性肉眼的脾腫
pineal gonadal syndrome　松果体性腺症候群
plant growth substance　植物成長物質
postsurgical gastroparesis syndrome　手術後の胃不全麻痺症候群
prostaglandin synthetase　プロスタグランジン合成酵素

PGs
prostaglandins プロスタグランジン類
PGSI
prostaglandin synthetase inhibitor プロスタグランジン合成酵素阻害薬
PGSR
psychogalvanic skin reflex 精神皮膚電流反射
psychogalvanic skin resistance 精神皮膚電流抵抗
psychogalvanic skin response 精神皮膚電流反応
PGT
play group therapy 演劇グループ療法
PGTT
prednisolone-glucose tolerance test プレドニゾロンブドウ糖負荷試験
PGU
peripheral glucose uptake 末梢ブドウ糖取り込み
postgonococcal urethritis 淋疾後尿道炎
PGUT
phosphogalactose-uridyl transferase ホスホガラクトースウリジルトランスフェラーゼ
PGV
proximal gastric vagotomy 近位胃迷走神経切断(術)
PGX
prostaglandin X プロスタグランジンX
PGY
postgraduate year 卒後年
PGYE
peptone, glucose, yeast extract ペプトン・ブドウ糖・酵母抽出物
PH
parathyroid hormone 副甲状腺ホルモン
partially hepatectomized 部分的肝切除された
past history 既往歴
patient history 患者歴
peliosis hepatis 肝臓紫斑病
perianal harpes 肛門周囲ヘルペス
persistent hepatitis 持続性肝炎
personal history 個人歴
phenyl フェニル
plasmapheresis 血漿交換
polycythemia hypertonica 高血圧赤血球増加症
porphyria hepatica 肝性ポルフィリン症
porta hepatis 肝門
portal hepatitis 門脈肝炎
posterior hypothalamus 視床下部後部
previous history 既往歴

primary hyperparathyroidism 原発性上皮小体(機能)亢進(症)
prolyl hydroxylase プロリルヒドロキシラーゼ
prostatic hypertrophy 前立腺肥大
pseudohermaphrodism 偽半陰陽者
pubic hair 恥毛
public health 公衆衛生
pulmonary hypertension 肺高血圧
punctate hemorrhage 点状出血
putaminal hemorrhage 被殻出血

Ph
phalangeal 指(趾)節骨の
pharmacy 薬局，薬学
phenanthrene フェナントレン
Philadelphia chromosome フィラデルフィア染色体

pH
acid-base scale 酸塩基スケール

ph
phase 期，段階，相
phial 小ビン，薬ビン《処》
phon フォン〈単位〉
phosphor リン
phot フォト〈単位〉

PH_3
phosphine ホスフィン

pH_1
isoelectric point 等電点

P/H_3
procaine hydrochloride 塩酸プロカイン

p/h
per hour 1時間あたり

PH，Ph，ph.
pharmacopoeia〈ラ〉 薬局方

Ph，ph
hypopharynx 下咽頭
phosphate リン酸塩，リン酸エステル

pH，P_H
pondus hydrogenii〈ラ〉＝hydrogen ion exponent 水素イオン指数，ピーエイチ〈単位〉

PHA
passive hemagglutination 受身赤血球凝集反応
peripheral hyperalimentation (solution) 末梢高栄養(液)
phenylalanine フェニルアラニン
phytohemagglutinin 植物性血球凝集素
plasma histaminase activity 血漿ヒスタミナーゼ活性

proper hepatic artery 固有肝動脈
pseudohypoaldosteronism 偽性低アルドステロン症
pulse height analyzer 波高分析器

pHa
arterial pH 動脈ピーエイチ

pha
pharmacology 薬理学

phal
phalanges 指(趾)節骨
phalanx 指(趾)節骨

PHA-M, PHA-m
phytohemagglutinin-mucopolysaccharide 植物性血球凝集素ムコ多糖類

PHA-P
phytohemagglutinin-protein 植物性血球凝集素蛋白

Phar
Pharmacopoeia〈ラ〉 薬局方

phar
pharmaceutical 薬学の
pharmacopoeia 薬局方
pharyngeal 咽頭の
pharyngitis 咽頭炎
pharynx 咽頭

PHAR, Phar, phar
pharmacy 調剤部，薬局，薬学

Phar, phar
pharmacist 薬剤師

phar c
pharmaceutical chemistry 薬化学

PHARM, pharm
pharmacist 薬剤師

pharmacol, pharmacol
pharmacological 薬理学の
pharmacology 薬理学

PH art
arterial pH 動脈ピーエイチ

pharyn
pharyngeal 咽頭の

PHAT
passive hemagglutination test 受身赤血球凝集試験

PHB
2,5-dihydroxybiphenyl ジヒドロキシビフェニール
poly-β-hydroxybutyric acid ポリ-β-ヒドロキシ酪酸

Ph.B.
Bachelor of Philosophy 哲学士

Ph B, Ph.B.
British Pharmacopoeia　英国薬局方

Ph BC
phenylbutylcarbinol　フェニルブチルカルビノール

PHC
photocoagulation　光凝固
post-hospital care　退院後のケア
premolar aplasia, hyperhidrosis, and (premature) canities　前臼歯形成不全・多汗症・(壮年性)白毛症
premolar hypodontia, hyperhidrosis and cantities prematura (=Böök syndrome)　前臼歯無歯(症)・多汗症・壮年性白毛症(=ボエーク症候群)
primary health care　プライマリヘルスケア
primary hepatic carcinoma　原発肝癌
primary hepatocellular carcinoma　原発性肝細胞癌
proliferative helper cell　増殖性ヘルパー細胞

Ph.C.
pharmaceutical chemist　薬物化学者

PHCC
pre-hospital coronary care　発症後病院到着前心疾患対策
primary hepatocellular carcinoma　原発性肝細胞癌

PHD
paroxysmal hypnogenic dyskinesia　発作性催眠ジスキネジー
pathological habit disorder　病的習慣疾患
personal health data　個人健康情報
pneumatic hammer disease　振動工具病
pulmonary heart disease　肺心臓疾患, 肺性心

P.H.D.
Public Health Doctor　公衆衛生博士

PhD, ph.D.
Doctor of Philosophy　博士号
philosophiae doctor　医学博士

PhDN
Doctor of Philosophy in Nursing　看護学博士

PHDRS
personal health data recording system　個人医療情報システム

PHE
periodic hearth examination　定期健康診断
preserved human erythrocyte　保存ヒト赤血球
proliferative hemorrhagic enteropathy　増殖性出血(性)腸疾患

Phe
phenylalanine　フェニルアラニン

PHEIC
Public Health Emergency of International — 国際的に懸念される公衆衛生上の緊急事態(WHO)

Phen
phenformin — フェンホルミン

phen
phenobarbital — フェノバルビタール

pheno
phenotype — 表現型

phenolp
phenolphthalein — フェノールフタレイン

phenom
phenomena — 現象〈複数〉
phenomenal — 現象の
phenomenon — 現象〈単数〉

pheo, Pheo
pheochromocytoma — 褐色細胞腫

PHF
paired helical filament — 対らせんフィラメント

PHFG
primary human fetal glia — 一次性ヒト胎児グリア

PHG
portal hypertensive gastropathy — 門脈圧亢進性胃疾患

Ph.G.
Graduate in Pharmacy — 薬学士
Pharmacopoeia Germanica — ドイツ薬局方

PHGA
pteroylheptaglutamic acid — プテロイルヘプタグルタミン酸

PhGABA
β-phenyl-γ-aminobutyric acid — β-フェニル-γ-アミノ酪酸

p-hGH
pituitary human growth hormone — 下垂体性ヒト成長ホルモン

Phgly
phenylglycine — フェニルグリシン

PHH
posthemorrhagic hydrocephalus — 出血後水頭症

PhH
phenylhydrazine — フェニルヒドラジン

PHHI
familial persistent hyperinsulinemic hypoglycemia of infancy — 小児の家族性持続性高インスリン低血糖

PHHL
post-heparin plasma hepatic lipase — ヘパリン加血漿肝性リパーゼ

PHI
pancreatic human insulin — 膵由来ヒトインスリン

passive hemagglutination inhibitor 受身血球凝集抑制物質
past history of illness 既往歴
peptide histidine isoleucine ペプチド・ヒスチジン・イソロイシン
phosphohexose isomerase ホスホヘキソースイソメラーゼ

PHi
intracellular pH 細胞内ピーエイチ

Phi
Philadelphia chromosome フィラデルフィア染色体

phial
phiala〈ギ〉 ビン

phiLC
pseudo light chain 偽L鎖

PHIM
posthypoxic intention myoclonus 低酸素後企図性ミオクローヌス

PHIN
progressive hypertrophic interstitial neuritis 進行性肥厚性間質性神経炎

PHIS
post-head injury syndrome 頭部外傷後症候群

PHIV
portal hypertensive intestinal vasculopathy 門脈圧亢進(症)腸血管症

PHK
platelet phosphohexokinase 血小板ホスホヘキソキナーゼ
postmortem human kidney 死後ヒト腎臓

PHK cells
postmortem human kidney cells 死後ヒト腎細胞

P

PHL
phospholipid リン脂質

PHLA
post-heparin lipolytic activity ヘパリン後脂肪分解活性

PHLPL
post-heparin plasma lipoprotein lipase ヘパリン加血漿リポ蛋白リパーゼ

PHLS
public health laboratory service 公衆衛生研究室サービス

PHM
peptide HM ペプチドHM
phaeohyphomycosis 黒色菌糸症
pulmonary hyaline membrane 肺ヒアリン膜
pulmonary hyaline membrane disease 肺硝子膜症

PhM
pharyngeal musculature 咽頭筋

PHMA
poly-2-hydroxy methacrylate　ポリ-2-水酸化メタクリル酸
PHMB
p-hydroxymercuribenzoic acid　パラヒドロキシメルクリ安息香酸
Phm.B.
Bachelor of Pharmacy　薬学士
Phm.G.
Graduate in Pharmacy　薬学部卒業者
PHN
paroxysmal noctural hemoglobinuria　発作性夜間血色素尿症
passive Heymann nephritis　受身ヘイマン腎炎
post-herpetic neuralgia　帯状疱疹後神経痛
public health nurse　保健師
PHO
pulmonary hypertrophic osteoarthropathy　肺性肥大性骨関節症
phon
phonetics　音声学
phonology　音声学
phono
phonograph　録音図
phos
phosphatase　ホスファターゼ
phosphate　リン酸塩，リン酸エステル
phosphorescence　リン光
phosphorus　リン
phot
photograph　写真
photographic　写真の
photography　写真撮影
photophobia　まぶしがり
photocoag
photocoagulation　光凝固
PHP
persistent hyperphenylalaninemia　持続性高フェニルアラニン血症
pooled human plasma　プールヒト血漿
post-heparin plasma　ヘパリン添加血漿
prepaid health plan　前払い健康保険
primary hyperparathyroidism　一次性副甲状腺機能亢進症，原発性上皮小体機能亢進症
pseudohypoparathyroidism　偽性副甲状腺機能低下症
Public Health Plan　公衆衛生計画
***p*-HPLA, P-HPLA**
p-hydroxyphenylacetic acid　パラヒドロキシフェニル酢酸

P

_p_-HPPA
p-hydroxyphenylpyruvic acid　パラヒドロキシフェニルピルビン酸

PHPS
p-hydroxy-phenyl-salicylamide　パラヒドロキシフェニルサリチルアミド

PHPT
pseudohypoparathyroidism　偽性上皮小体機能低下症

pHPT
primary hyperparathyroidism　原発性上皮小体(機能)亢進(症)

PHPV
persistent hyperplastic primary vitreous　第一次硝子体過形成遺残

PHR
peak heart rate　最大心拍数
photoreactivity　光反応性

phren
phrenic　横隔膜の

PHRI
Public Health Research Institute　公衆衛生研究所

PhRMA
Pharmaceutical Research and Manufacturers Association of America　米国製薬工業協会

PHS
pooled human serum　貯蔵ヒト血清
posthypnotic suggestion　催眠後暗示
primary fibromyalgia syndrome　原発性線維筋肉痛症候群
Public Health Service　公衆衛生局

P

pHSA
polymerized humam serum albumin　重合ヒト血清アルブミン

PHSL
primary hepatosplenic lymphoma　原発性肝脾リンパ腫

PHSN
peritoneum hepato serosa lymph node　腹膜播種・肝転移・漿膜浸潤・リンパ節転移

PHT
phenytoin　フェニトイン
portal hypertension　門脈高血圧症
primary hyperthyroidism　原発性甲状腺機能亢進症
pulmonary hypertension　肺高血圧症

PHTN
portal hypertension　門脈高血圧(症)

PHTS
psychiatric home treatment service　精神科的家庭治療サービス

PHV
persistent hyperplastic vitreous 硝子体過形成遺残
pHv
mixed venous pH 混合静脈ピーエイチ
PHVA
post-hyperventilation apnea 過換気後無呼吸
PHX
pulmonary histiocytosis X 肺原因不明組織球増殖症
PHx
past history 既往歴
PHY
pharyngitis 咽頭炎
physical 身体的な，理学的な
PHY，phy
phytohemagglutinin 植物性血球凝集素
PHYS
physiological 生理学の
PhyS
physiological saline 生理食塩水，生理的食塩
Phys，phys
physician 医師
phys.dis
physical disability 身体障害者
Phys ed
physical education 身体に関する教育
phys exam
physical examination 医学的検査
physio，physio.
physiological 生理学の
physiotherapist 理学療法士
Physiol，physiol
physiological 生理学の
PhysMed，Phys Med
physical medicine 物療医学
PhysTher，phys.ther
physical therapy 物理療法，理学療法
PI
isoelectric point 等電点
pacing impulse ペーシング刺激
pancreatic insufficiency 膵臓機能不全
parasympathetic index 副交感指数
peculiarity index 特性指数
percutaneous injury 経皮損傷
perinatal injury 周生期損傷
per inhalation 吸入により
peripheral iridectomy 周辺虹彩切除(術)

P

permeability index	透過性指数
phagocytic index	食細胞指数
Pharmacopeia Internationalis〈ラ〉	国際薬局方
phosphatidylinositol	ホスファチジルイノシトール
phospholine iodide	ホスホリンアイオダイド
pineal body	松果体
plasma iron	血漿鉄
pneumatosis intestinalis	腸壁気腫
post infectionem〈ラ〉=after infection	感染後の
post-inoculation	接種後の
preload index	前負荷係数
premature infant	早産児，未熟児
prematurity index	早熟指数
present illness	現病歴
primary infarction	原発性梗塞
principal investigator	治験責任医師
proinsulin	プロインスリン
prolactin inhibitor	プロラクチン阻害薬
protamine insulin	プロタミンインスリン
pulmonary incompetence	肺不全，肺動脈弁不全(症)
pulmonary infarction	肺梗塞
pulmonary insufficiency	肺動脈弁閉鎖不全
pulsatility index	拍動指数
pyknosis index	核濃縮指数
Pi	
inorganic phosphate	無機リン
inspiratory pressure	吸気圧
pressure of inspiration	吸気圧
P & I	
protection and indemnity	防御と保護
PI, P/I	
post injury	損傷後の
Pi, PI	
protease inhibitor	蛋白質分解酵素阻害薬
PIA	
plasma insulin activity	血漿インスリン活性
porcine intestinal adenomatosis	ブタ腸腺腫症
postinfarction angina	梗塞後狭心症
preinfarct angina	梗塞前狭心症
PIAPCS	
psycho, inform, acquisition, processing, control system	心理学的情報収集処理管理法
PIAVA	
polydactyly-imperforate anus-vertebral anomalies (syndrome)	多指(趾)(症)・無孔肛門・脊椎骨奇形(症候群)

PIB
partial ileal bypass　部分回腸バイパス術
PIBIDS
photosensitivity, ichthyosis, brittle hair, intellectual impairment, decreased fertility, short stature　光過敏症・魚鱗癬・もろい毛髪・知能障害・生殖能低下・短身長
PIBM
polyisobutylmethacrylate　ポリイソブチルメタクリレート
PIC
Personality Inventory for Children　小児用人格調査票
picibanil　ピシバニール
plasma iron clearance　血漿鉄クリアランス
plasmin α_2-plasmin inhibitor complex　プラスミンα_2プラスミンインヒビター複合体
plasmin-inhibitor (antiplasmin) complex　プラスミン・抗プラスミン複合体
Poison Information Center　毒物情報センター
posterior intermediate curve　後中間彎曲
postinflammatory corticoid　炎症後コルチコイド
postintercourse　性交後の
PICA
posterior inferior cerebellar artery　後下小脳動脈
PICD
primary irritant contact dermatitis　原発性刺激性接触皮膚炎
PICEP
Pharmacy Intervention & Clinical Evaluation Program　薬局参加の医療評価プログラム
PICL
photoinitiated chemoiluminescence　光開始化学発光
pics
pictures　絵，写真
PICSO
pressure-controlled intermittent coronary sinus occlusion　圧調節式間欠冠静脈洞閉塞法
PICT
pancreatic islet cell transplantation　膵島細胞移植術
PICU
pediatric intensive care unit　小児集中治療室
perinatal intensive care unit　周産期集中治療室
psychiatric intensive care unit　精神科集中治療室
pulmonary intensive care unit　肺集中治療室
PID
pain intensity difference　疼痛強度差
pelvic inflammatory disease　骨盤内炎症性疾患
photoionization detector　光イオン化検出器

plasma-iron disappearance rate 血漿鉄消失(率)
prolapsed intervertebral disc 椎間板ヘルニア
proportional, integral, derivative 比例動作・積分動作・微分動作

PIDR
plasma-iron disappearance (rate) 血漿鉄消失率

PIDS
primary immunodeficiency syndrome 原発性免疫不全症候群

PIDT$_{1/2}$
plasma iron disappearance time 1/2 血漿鉄半減時間

PIE
postinfectious encephalomyelitis 感染後脳脊髄(膜)炎
prolactin release inhibiting factor プロラクチン分泌抑制因子
pulmonary infiltration with eosinophilia 肺好酸球増多症
pulmonary interstitial edema 肺間質水腫
pulmonary interstitial emphysema 肺間質性気腫

PIF
peak inspiratory flow 最大吸気量
pectoral island flap 血管茎前胸壁皮弁
permeability increasing factor 透過性増強因子
pigment-inducing factor 色素誘導因子
posterior interbody fusion 後方椎体固定
prolactin release-inhibiting factor プロラクチン放出抑制因子
proliferation inhibiting factor 増殖抑制因子
prostatic interstitial fluid 前立腺間質液

PIFG
poor intrauterine fetal growth 子宮内発育不良

PIFR
peak inspiratory flow rate 最大吸気流量率

PIFT
platelet immunofluorescence test 血小板免疫蛍光検査

PIG
phosphatidylinositol glycan ホスファチジルイノシトールグリカン

pig
pigmented 色素沈着の

pig.
pigmentum〈ラ〉=pigment 色素

Pig, pig
pigmentation 色素沈着

Pig.deg.
pigmentary degeneration 網膜色素変性症

PIGI
pregnancy-induced glucose intolerance 妊娠誘発性ブドウ糖不耐(症)

pigm.
pigmentum〈ラ〉=pigment 色素
pigmt.
pigmentation 色素沈着
pigmentum〈ラ〉=pigment 色素
PIGN
postinfectious glomerulonephritis 感染後性糸球体腎炎
PIH
Diagnostic Personality Inventory for the Handicapped 心身障害児童生徒性格診断検査
phenyl-isopropylhydrazine フェニルイソプロピルヒドラジン
pregnancy induced hypertension 妊娠誘発高血圧
primary intracerebral hemorrhage 原発性脳内出血
prolactin release-inhibiting hormone プロラクチン放出抑制ホルモン
PII
peripheral blood lymphocytes interferon induction test 末梢血リンパ球インターフェロン誘発試験
plasma inorganic iodine 血漿無機ヨウ素
pulmonary incompetence index 肺不全指数
PIIP
portable insulin infusion pump 可搬性インスリン注入ポンプ
PIIS
posterior inferior iliac spine 後下腸骨棘
PIL
patient information leaflet 患者向け服薬指導書
percentage increase in loss 損失の百分率増加
primary intestinal lymphangiesctasia 原発性腸リンパ管拡張(症)
purpose in life test 生きがいテスト
Pil, pil, pil.
pilula〈ラ〉=pill 丸剤《処》
PILN
percutaneous intradiscal laser nucleotomy 経皮的椎間板レーザー髄核切除(術)
pil.pd.
pilulae ponderis〈ラ〉 丸剤重量《処》
PIM
penicillamine-induced myasthenia ペニシラミン誘発筋無力症
PIMS
programmable inplantable medication system プログラム可能な埋込み式薬物システム
PIN
prostatic intraepithelial neoplasia 前立腺上皮内腫瘍
pyridoxine ピリドキシン

pin.
pingnis〈ラ〉 脂肪
ping.
pinguis〈ラ〉 脂肪
PIO$_2$
inspiratory O_2 pressure 吸入気酸素分圧
partial pressure of inspiratory oxygen 吸気酸素分圧
PIOK
poikilocytosis 奇形赤血球(増加)症
PION
posterior ischemic optic neuropathy 後部虚血性視神経炎
PIP
paralytic infantile paralysis 麻痺性小児麻痺
peak inspiratory airway pressure 最大吸気圧
phosphatidylinosytol-diphosphate ホスファチジルイノシトール二リン酸
phosphatidylinosytol-monophosphate ホスファチジルイノシトール一リン酸
piperacillin ピペラシリン
plasma iron pool 血漿鉄プール
present illness program 現病プログラム
proximal interphalangeal 近位指骨間(の)
proximal interphalangeal joint 近位指骨間関節
psychosis, intermittent hyponatremia, polydipsia (syndrome) 精神病・間欠性低ナトリウム血・多渇(症候群)
PIPC
piperacillin ピペラシリン
PIPE
persistent interstitial pulmonary emphysema 持続(性)間質性肺気腫
PIPES
piperazine-*N*, *N'*-bis(2-ethanesulfonic acid) ピペラジン-*N*, *N'*-ビス(2-エタンスルホン酸)
PIPJ
proximal interphalangeal joint 近位指節間関節
PIQ
postero-inferior quadrant 後下象限
PIR
pathologic index rating 重症度分類
piriform (muscle) 梨状(筋)
pir
pillar 柱
P-IRI
plasma immunoreactive insulin 血漿免疫反応性インスリン

PIS
pituitary inhibitory system 下垂体抑制系
primary immunodeficiency syndrome 原発性免疫不全症候群

PISCES
percutaneously inserted spinal cord epidural stimulation 経皮的挿入による脊髄硬膜外刺激

PISP
penicillin G-insensitive *Streptococcus pneumoniae* ペニシリン低感受連鎖球菌性肺炎

PIT
passive immune thrombocytopenia 受動免疫血小板減少症
plasma iron turnover 血漿鉄交代率

pit
Pitocin ピトシン
pituitary 下垂体の

PITC
phenylisothiocyanate フェニルイソチオシアネート

PI test, PI-Test
Persönlichkeit-Interssen Test〈独〉 人格要素テスト，人格関係テスト

PITP
pseudoidiopathic thrombocytopenic purpura 偽(性)特発性血小板減少性紫斑病

PITR
plasma iron turnover rate 血漿鉄交代率

PIV
parainfluenza virus パラインフルエンザウイルス
polydactyly-imperforate anus-vertebral anomalies (syndrome) 多指(趾)・無孔肛門・脊椎骨奇形(症候群)

PIVD
protruded intervertebral disc 椎間板ヘルニア

PIVH
peripheral intravenous hyperalimentation 末梢静脈内過栄養

PIVKA
protein induced by vitamin K absence ビタミンK欠乏誘導蛋白

PIXE
particle induced X-ray emission 荷電粒子励起X線分光法，粒子励起X線分析法

PJ
pancreatic juice 膵液
pancreaticojejunostomy 膵空腸吻合
Peutz-Jeghers (syndrome) ポイツ・ジェガース(症候群)

PJM
postjunctional membrane 後接合部膜

PJP
pancreatic juice protein　膵液蛋白

PJS
Peutz-Jeghers syndrome　ポイツ・ジェガース症候群

pj's
physical jerks　物理的痙攣

PK
Pankreaskrebs〈独〉　膵癌
penetrating keratoplasty　全層角膜移植(術)
pharmacokinetic　薬物動態の
protein kinase　プロテインキナーゼ
psychokinesis　精神運動
psychokinetic　精神運動の
pyruvate kinase　ピルビン酸キナーゼ

pK
dissociation constant　解離定数
equilibrium constant　平衡定数

pk
peck　乾燥容量

PK, P-K
Prausnitz-Küstner　プラウニッツ・キュストナー

PKA
cAMP-dependent protein kinase　cAMP依存性プロテインキナーゼ
prekallikrein activator　プレカリクレイン活性化因子
protein kinase A　プロテインキナーゼA

PKAR
protein kinase activation ratio　プロテインキナーゼ活性化比

PKase
protein kinase　プロテインキナーゼ

PKC
paroxysmal kinesigenic choreoathetosis　発作性運動誘発性舞踏アテトーゼ
protein kinase C　プロテインキナーゼC

PKD
polycystic kidney (disease)　嚢胞腎
proliferative kidney disease　増殖性腎疾患

PKG
Phonokardiogram〈独〉　心音図

PKK
cytokeratin　サイトケラチン
Pankreaskopfkrebs〈独〉　膵頭部癌
prekallikrein　プレカリクレイン

PKM
diphenylhydantoin　ジフェニルヒダントイン

PKN
parkinsonism パーキンソニズム
PKP
penetrating keratoplasty 全層角膜移植(術)
PKR
Prausnitz-Küstner reaction プラウニッツ・キュストナー反応
RNA-dependent protein kinase RNA依存性プロテインキナーゼ
PK reaction
Prausnitz-Küstner reaction プラウニッツ・キュストナー反応
PKS
pericardial knock sound 心膜叩打音
PKT
Prausnitz-Küstner test プラウニッツ・キュストナー試験
PKU
phenylketonuria フェニルケトン尿症
Pkv
peak kilovolt 最大キロボルト
PL
palmaris longus (muscle) 長掌(筋)
pancreatic lipase 膵リパーゼ
peroneus longus 長腓骨筋
phase line 相線
phospholipid リン脂質
photoluminescence フォトルミネセンス法
pilocarpine ピロカルピン
placebo プラセボ，プラシボ，偽薬
placental lactogen 胎盤性ラクトゲン
plasmalemma 細胞膜
plasmin プラスミン
plastic surgeon 形成外科医
plastic surgery 形成外科
polymorphocytic leukemia 多形球性白血病
polymyxin B ポリミキシンB
Posticuslahmung〈独〉 後筋麻痺
preferential looking 選択視
preleukemia 前白血病
primary lysosome 一次リソソーム
primed lymphocytes 初回抗原刺激を受けたリンパ球
product liability 製造物責任，製品保証
prolymphocytic leukemia 前リンパ球性白血病
pulmonary venous pressure 肺静脈圧

punction lumbaire 腰椎穿刺
Purkinje layer プルキンエ層
pyridoxal ピリドキサ(ー)ル
transpulmonary pressure 経肺圧

Pl
pleural dissemination 胸膜播種

pl
picoliter ピコリットル〈単位〉
place 場所
plasma 血漿
plasma cell 形質細胞
plastic 形成性，可塑性
plate，blood platelet 平板・血小板
plexus 叢
plum 倍数
plural 複数の

pl，PL
pleura(l) 胸膜(の)

pl，PL，P.L.
perception of light 光覚
plantar 足底の

pl_{0-1}，Pl_{0-1}
pleural dissemination 胸膜播種性転移の程度

PLA
passive latex agglutination 受身ラテックス凝集反応
peripheral laser angioplasty 末梢レーザー血管形成(術)
phospholipase A ホスホリパーゼA
plasminogen activator プラスミノゲン活性化因子
platelet antigen 血小板抗原
polylactic acid ポリ乳酸
polymer of lactic acid 乳酸ポリマー
potentially lethal arrhythmia 潜在的に致命的な不整脈
product license application 製造許可申請

Pla
left atrial pressure 左房圧

PLA2，PL-A_2
phospholipase-A_2 ホスホリパーゼA_2

PL-AC
N-palmitoyl-araC *N*-パルミトイルアラC

plac.prev.
placenta previa 前置胎盤

plant-flex
plantar flexion 底屈

PLAP
placental alkaline phosphatase 胎盤アルカリホスファターゼ

P

placental leucine aminopeptidase　胎盤性ロイシンアミノペプチダーゼ

pLAR
post late asthmatic response　後遅発型喘息反応

PLase A_2
phospholipase-A_2　ホスホリパーゼA_2

PLAT
cisplatinum（=Platinol）　シスプラチン（=プラチノール）

plat
platinum　白金，プラチナ

plat，Plat
platelet　血小板

platy
platysma　広頸筋

PLB
phospholipase B　ホスホリパーゼB

pLb
prolymphoblast　前リンパ芽球

PL-B
polymyxin B　ポリミキシンB

PLBO
placebo　プラセボ，偽薬，プラシボ

PLC
parenchymal liver cell　肝実質細胞
perivascular lymphocytic cuffing　血管周囲リンパ球浸潤
pharyngolaryngitis chronica〈ラ〉　慢性咽頭喉頭炎
phospholipase C　ホスホリパーゼC
primary liver cancer　原発性肝癌
primary liver carcinoma　原発性肝癌
proinsulin-like component　プロインスリン様成分
protein-lipid complex　蛋白脂質複合体
pseudolymphocytic choriomeningitis　偽（性）リンパ球脈絡髄膜炎

pLc
prolymphocyte　前リンパ球

PLCB
percutaneous large core biopsy　経皮的大核生検

PLCC
primary liver cell cancer　原発性肝細胞癌

PLD
partial lipodystrophy　限局性脂肪ジストロフィ，部分脂質ジストロフィ
phospholipase D　ホスホリパーゼD
platelet defect　血小板欠損（症）
polycystic liver disease　多嚢胞性肝疾患
potential lethal damage　潜在的致死障害

PLDD
percutaneous laser disc decompression — レーザーによる経皮的椎間板減圧術

PLDF
periflux laser Doppler flowmeter — ペリフラックスレーザードード(ッ)プラ流量計

PLDH
plasma lactic dehydrogenase — 血漿乳酸脱水素酵素

PLDR
potential lethal damage repair — 潜在的致死障害回復

PLE
panlobular emphysema — 汎小葉性肺気腫
paraneoplastic limbic encephalopathy — 腫瘍随伴性(大脳)辺縁系脳障害
pleura — 胸膜
polymorphous light eruption — 多形日光疹
protein-losing enteropathy — 蛋白喪失性腸症
pseudolupus erythematosus (syndrome) — 偽エリテマトーデス(症候群)

PLED
periodic lateralized epileptiform discharge — 周期性片側性てんかん様発射

Pleur Fl
pleural fluid — 胸水

PLF
posterolateral fusion — 後側方固定術
psoriatic leukotactic factor — 乾癬性白血球走化因子

PLFS
perilymphatic fistula syndrome — 外リンパフィステル症候群

P

PLG
phonolaryngogram — 音喉頭図

plg, PLg, PLG
plasminogen — プラスミノゲン

PLGA
poly-L-glutamic acid — ポリ-L-グルタミン酸
polymorphous low-grade adenocarcinoma — 多形(性)低分化腺癌

PLGE
protein-losing gastroenteropathy — 蛋白喪失性胃腸症

P-LGV
psittacosis lymphogranuloma venereum — オウム病・性病性リンパ肉芽腫

PLH
placental lactogenic hormone — 胎盤乳腺刺激ホルモン

PLI
planimetric luteal index — 高温相面積指数

PLIF
posterior lumbar interbody fusion　後方椎体間固定術

PLL
poly-L-lysine　ポリ-L-リジン
prolymphocytic leukemia　前リンパ球性白血病

Pll
plexus　叢〈複数〉

PLM
plasma level monitoring　血漿レベルモニター

PLM-Tc
pyrrolidinemetyl-tetracycline　ピロリジンメチルテトラサイクリン

PLN
peripheral lymph node　末梢リンパ節
popliteal lymph node　膝窩リンパ節
posterior lymph node　後リンパ節

Pln
plasmin　プラスミン

PLNC
popliteal lymph node cells　膝蓋リンパ節細胞

PLO
platelet lipoxygenase　血小板リポオキシゲナーゼ
polycystic lipomembranous osteodysplasia　多発嚢胞脂肪膜性骨形成異常

PLP
periodate lysine paraformaldehyde　過ヨウ素酸リジンパラホルムアルデヒド
periodic acid sodium lysin in 2% paraformaldehyde　過ヨウ素酸ナトリウムリジン加2%パラホルムアルデヒド溶液
phospholipase　ホスホリパーゼ
polystyrene latex particle　ポリスチレンラテックス粒子
product liability prevention　製造物責任予防
proteolipid apoprotein　プロテオリピドアポ蛋白
proteolipid protein　プロテオリピド蛋白
pyridoxal phosphate　ピリドキサ(ー)ルリン酸

PL & PD
personal loss and personal damage　個人的損失と個人的障害

PLR
persistent light reaction　残存光反射
pupillary light reflex　瞳孔対光反射

PLS
Papillon-Lefèvre syndrome　パピヨン・ルフェーブル症候群
preleukemic syndrome　前白血球性症候群
Preschool Language Scale　学校前言語スケール

prostaglandin-like substance　プロスタグランジン様物質

pls

please　どうぞ

PlSF

plica stapedis fold　アブミ骨靱帯ひだ

pl.surg

plastic surgery　形成外科医

PLSVC

persistent left superior vena cava　左上大静脈遺残

PLT

platelet　血小板

primed lymphocyte test　感作リンパ球テスト

primed lymphocyte typing　感作リンパ球タイピング

psittacosis-lymphogranuloma-trachoma group microorganism　オウム病・鼠径リンパ肉芽腫・トラコーマ群微生物

plteh

plethoric　多血の

PLTS

platelets　血小板〈複数〉

PLV

live polymyelitis vaccine　ポリオ生ワクチン

phenylalanine, lysine, vasopressin　フェニルアラニン・リジン・バソプレシン

posterior left ventricle　左(心)室後壁

plv.

pulverisat〈ラ〉　粉末にした《処》

pulvis〈ラ〉　散薬，粉末《処》

PLVS

percutaneous left ventricular assist system　体外循環左(心)室補助装置

PLWS

Prader-Labhart-Willi syndrome　プラダー・ラブハート・ウィリ症候群

plx

plexus　叢〈複数〉

PM

pacemaker　ペースメーカー

pagetoid melanocytosis　パジェット(病)様メラニン細胞増加(症)

papillary muscle　乳頭筋

papular mucinosis　丘疹状ムチン沈着症

paramethasone　パラメタゾン

partial meniscectomy　部分的半月板切除

petit mal　小発作

phase modulation　位相変調

phenylalanine and methotrexate フェニルアラニンとメトトレキサート
phlebitis migrans〈ラ〉 移行性静脈炎
physical medicine 物理療法科
plasma membrane 原形質膜
platelet membrane 血小板膜
platelet microsome 血小板ミクロソーム
pneumomediastinum 気縦隔(症)
poliomyelitis ポリオ
polymorphonuclear 多形核の
polymorphs 多形核球
polymyositis 多発性筋炎
pondus medicinale〈ラ〉 薬用ポンド
poor metabolizer 低代謝患者
porokeratosis of Mibelli ミベリ汗孔角化(症)
post menstruum 溶媒添加後
presystolic murmur 収縮前雑音
pretibial myxedema 脛骨前粘液腫
prolactinoma プロラクチン産生腫瘍
promastigote (寄生虫の)前鞭毛期
prostatic massage 前立腺マッサージ
protein methylesterase 蛋白メチルエステラーゼ
pulmonary macrophage 肺大食細胞
pulse modulation 脈変調
puromycin ピューロマイシン
pyridoxamine ピリドキサミン

Pm
mean blood pressure 平均血圧
promethium プロメチウム

pM
picomolar ピコモル〈単位〉

pm
panctum maximum 最大点
picometer ピコメートル〈単位〉
Plasmodium malariae 四日熱(マラリア)原虫
premolar 小臼歯
proper muscle layer 固有筋層
proprial muscle 固有筋

p.m.
primo mane〈ラ〉 早朝に《処》

PM, P.M., p.m.
post meridiem〈ラ〉 午後に《処》
post mortem〈ラ〉 死後に

PMA
4β-phorbol-12β-myristate acetate 4β-ホルボール-12β-ミリスチン酸酢酸塩

P

peroneal muscle atrophy 腓骨筋萎縮症
Pharmaceutical Manufactures Association 米国製薬会社協会
phenylmercuric acetate 酢酸フェニル水銀
phorbol myristate acetate ミリスチン酸酢酸ホルボール
p-methoxyamphetamine パラメトキシアンフェタミン
positive mental attitude 積極的心理的態度
Prinzmetal angina プリンツメタル型狭心症
progressive muscular atrophy 進行性筋萎縮症
pyridylmercuric acetate ピリジル酢酸第二水銀

PMAA
polymetaacrylic acid ポリメタアクリル酸

PMAC
phenylmercuric acetate 酢酸フェニル水銀

PMAF
Pharmaceutical Manufactures Foundation 製薬協会財団

PMase
phosphomonoesterase ホスホモノエステラーゼ

PMA test
primary mental abilities test 基礎知能測定検査

PMB
p-mercuribenzoic acid パラメルクリ安息香酸
polymorphonuclear basophilic leukocyte 多形核好塩基性白血球
postmenopausal bleeding 閉経後出血

PM-B
polymyxin B ポリミキシンB

PMB, P.M.B.
polymorphonuclear basophil 多形核好塩基球

PMBC
peripheral blood mononuclear cell 末梢血単核球

PMBN
polymyxin nonapeptid ポリミキシンノナペプチド

PMBS
p-mercuribenzenesulfonic acid パラメルクリベンゼンスルホン酸

PMC
For Profit Physician Management Company 開業医管理会社
phenylmercuric chloride 塩化フェニル水銀
pleural mesothelial cell 胸膜中皮細胞
pontine micturition center 橋排尿中枢
postmyocarditic cardiomegaly 心筋炎後心肥大
private medical communication 私的医学連絡
pseudomembranous colitis 偽膜性大腸炎

PM clinic
physical medicine clinic　物理療法学外来
PMCO
polarographic myocardial oxygen　ポーラログラフ心筋酸素量
PMD
primary myocardial disease　原発性心筋症
private medical doctor　かかりつけの医師
progressive muscular dystrophy　進行性筋ジストロフィ症
PMDA
Pharmaceuticals and Medical Devices Agency　(独立行政法人)医薬品医療機器総合機構
PMDI
pressurized metered dose inhaler　加圧式定量噴霧吸入器
PM/DM
polmyositis/dermatomyositis　多発性筋炎/皮膚筋炎
PMDS
persistent müllerian duct syndrome　ミュラー管開存症候群
primary myelodysplastic syndrome　原発性脊髄異形成症候群
PME
progressive myoclonus epilepsy　進行性ミオクローヌスてんかん
pulmonary microembolization　肺微小塞栓術
PME, P.M.E.
polymorphonuclear eosinophilic (leukocyte)　多形核好酸性(白血病)
PMEC
pseudomembranous enterocolitis　偽膜性小腸結腸炎
PMF
primary myelofibrosis　原発性骨髄線維症
progressive massive fibrosis　進行性塊状線維症
PMG
phenolphthalein-mono-β-glucuronate　フェノールフタレインモノ-β-グルクロン酸塩
pregnant mare serum gonadotropin　妊馬血清性ゴナドトロピン
PMGCT
primary mediastinal germ-cell tumor　原発性縦隔胚細胞腫瘍
PMH
past medical history　既往歴
phenylmercuric hexachlorophene　ヘキサクロロフェンフェニル水銀
posteromedial hypothalamus　後内側視床下部
previous medical history　既往歴
pure motor hemiplegia　純粋運動性片麻痺
PMHY
past medical history　既往歴

PMI
past medical illness　既往疾病
patient medication instruction　患者向け服薬指導
perioperative myocardial infarction　周術期心筋梗塞
phosphomannose isomerase　ホスホマンノースイソメラーゼ
point of maximum impulse　最大衝動点
point of maximum intensity　最強点
posterior myocardial infarction　後壁心筋梗塞
proportional mortality indicator　全死亡率中の割合
pulmonary gas mixing index　肺内ガス混合指数

PMI, P.M.I.
point of maximal impulse　最大衝動点

PMIM
phase-measurement interferometric microscopy　位相測定干渉顕微鏡

PMIS
postmyocardial infarction syndrome　心筋梗塞後症候群

PML
polymorphonuclear leukocytes　多形核白血球
posterior mitral leaflet　僧帽弁後尖
progressive multifocal leukodystrophy　進行性多巣性白質ジストロフィ
progressive multifocal leukoencephalopathy　進行性多巣性白質脳症
promyelocytic leukemia　前骨髄細胞白血病
pulmonary microlithiasis　肺微石症

PMM
pentamethylmelamine　ペンタメチルメラミン

PMMA
polymethylmethacrylate　ポリメチルメタクリレート

PM-MC flap
pectoralis major myocutaneous flap　大胸筋皮弁

PMMF
pectoralis major myocutaneous flap　大胸筋皮弁

PMN
polymorphonuclear　多形核の
polymorphonuclear neutrophil　多形核好中球
protein manipulation　蛋白操作

PMNCH
partnership for maternal, newborn and child health　妊産婦・新生児・子どもの健康パートナーシップ

PMND
Parkinson syndrome with motor neuron degeneration　運動神経変性を伴うパーキンソン症候群

P

PMNG
polymorphonuclear granulocyte　多形核顆粒球
PMNL
polymorphonuclear leukocyte　多形核白血球
PMNN
polymorphonuclear neutrophil　多形核好中球
PMNR
periadenitis mucosa necrotica reccurens　再発性壊死性粘膜腺周囲炎
PMNs
polymorphonucleocytes　多形核球
PMO
myeloperoxidase　ミエロペルオキシダーゼ
postmenopausal osteoporosis　閉経後の骨粗しょう(鬆)症
PMP
past menstrual period　前月経期
patient management problem　患者マネージ問題
postmortem pancreatogram　剖検膵管像
previous menstrual period　最終月経期
pyridoxamine phosphate　ピリドキサミンリン酸
PMPC
pivmecillinam　ピブメシリナム
PMPO
postmenopausal palpable ovary　閉経後触知可能卵巣
PMPS
postmastectomy pain syndrome　乳房切除後疼痛症候群
PMR
peak metabolic rate　最高代謝率(寒冷時)
perinatal morbidity　周生期罹病率
perinatal mortality rate　周生期死亡率
photomyoclonic reaction　光ミオクローヌス反応
pimaricin　ピマリシン
poliomyeloradiculitis　ポリオ脊髄神経根炎
polymyalgia rheumatica　リウマチ性多発筋痛症
postural miosis reaction　体位性縮瞳反応
proportionate mortality ratio　較正死亡率
proton magnetic resonance　陽子磁気共鳴
PMR, PM & R, PM+R
physical medicine and rehabilitation　物理療法とリハビリテーション
PMRS
Physical Medicine and Rehabilitation Service　物理療法とリハビリテーション科
PMS
perimenstrual syndrome　月経周辺性症候群
periodic movements in sleep　睡眠時周期性運動
phenazine methosulfate　フェナジンメト硫酸

post marketing surveillance 医薬品市販後調査
postmenopausal syndrome 閉経後症候群
pregnant mare serum hormone 妊馬血清ホルモン
premenstrual syndrome 月経前症候群

PMSF
phenylmethylsulfonyl fluoride フェニルメチルスルホニルフッ化物

PMSG
pregnant mare serum gonadotropin 妊馬血清ゴナドトロピン

PMT
pacemaker mediated tachycardia ペースメーカー媒介頻脈
photomultiplier tube 光電子増倍管
premenstrual tension 月経前緊張
pseudosarcomatous myofibroblastic tumor 偽肉腫性筋線維芽細胞腫瘍

PMTC
professional mechanical tooth cleaning プロフェッショナル・メカニカル・トゥース・クリーニング

PMTS
premenstrual tension syndrome 月経前緊張症候群

PMTT
pulmonary mean transit time 肺平均通過時間

PMV
posterior mesencephalic vein 後中脳静脈

PMW
pacemaker wires ペースメーカー線

PMX-B
polymyxin B ポリミキシンB

PN
panangitis nodosa〈ラ〉 結節性汎動脈炎
parenteral nutrition 静脈栄養法
percussion note 打診音
percutaneous nucleotomy 経皮的髄核摘出術
periarteritis nodosa〈ラ〉 結節性動脈周囲炎
peripheral nerve 末梢神経
peripheral neuropathy 末梢神経障害
phosphopyridine nucleotide ホスホピリジンヌクレオチド
phrenic nerve 横隔神経
Polenské number ポレンスケ価
polyarteritis nodosa 結節性多発性動脈炎
polynephritis 多発(性)腎炎
polyneuritis 多発神経炎
polynuclear neutrophyl 多核好中球
pontine nucleus 橋核
positional nystagmus (異常)体位眼振，頭位変換眼振

postnatal 出生後の
practical nurse 准看護師
progress notes 経過記録
psychoneurologist 精神神経科医
psychoneurology 精神神経学
psychoneurotic 精神神経症の
purine nucleoside phosphorylase プリンヌクレオシドホスホリラーゼ
pyelonephritis 腎盂腎炎
pyridoxine ピリドキシン
pyrrolnitrin ピロルニトリン

Pn
pneumatic 空気の
pneumococcus 肺炎球菌
post-hatching days "n" 孵化後日数

pn
pain 痛み
pneumothorax 気胸

P_{N2}
partial pressure of nitrogen 窒素分圧

P5N
pyrimidine-5′-nucleotidase ピリミジン-5′-ヌクレオチダーゼ

P/N
positive to negative 陽性/陰性(比)

p-n
positive-negative 陽性・陰性

PN, Pn, pn
pneumonia 肺炎

PN, P & N
psychiatry and neurology 精神医学と神経(病)学

PNA
Paris Nomina Anatomica パリ解剖学用語《解剖》
peanut agglutinin ピーナッツ凝集
pentose nucleic acid ペントース核酸
percutaneous needle aspiration 経皮的穿刺吸引《生検》

Pna
plasma sodium 血漿ナトリウム

pNA
p-nitroaniline パラニトロアニリン

PNAvQ
positive-negative ambivalent quotient 陰陽二面価比

PNB
perineal needle biopsy 会陰針生検
p-nitrobiphenyl パラニトロビフェニル

P

polymyxin, neomycin, bacitracin ポリミキシン, ネオマイシン, バシトラシン

PNBT
paranitroblue tetrazolium パラニトロブルーテトラゾリウム

PNC
paranasal cancer 鼻傍癌
penicillin ペニシリン
periarteritis nodosa cutaneous 皮膚型結節性動脈周囲炎
peripheral nucleated cell 末梢有核細胞
p-nitrocatechol パラニトロカテコール
polymyxin, neomycin, bacitracin ポリミキシンネオマイシンバシトラシン
postnecrotic cirrhosis 壊死後肝硬変
purine nucleotide cycle プリンヌクレオチドサイクル

PND
paroxysmal nocturnal dyspnea 発作性夜間呼吸困難
postnasal drip 後鼻漏
principal neutralization determinant 主要中和決定因子

pnd
pond ポンド〈単位〉

PNE
plasma norepinephrine 血漿ノルエピネフリン
pneumoencephalogram 気脳図
practical nurse's education 准看護師教育
primary nocturnal enuresis 原発性夜間遺尿症
pseudomembranous necrotizing enterocolitis 偽膜性壊死性全腸炎

PNEC
predicted no-effect concentration 予測無作用濃度

PNET
peripheral neuroectodermal tumor 末梢神経外胚葉腫瘍
permeative neuroectodermal tumor 浸透性神経外胚葉腫瘍
primitive neuroectodermal tumor 未分化神経外胚葉性腫瘍

PNET-MB
permeative neuroectodermal tumor-medulloblastoma 浸透性神経外胚葉腫瘍・髄芽(細胞)腫

pneu
pneumatic 空気の
pneumonia 肺炎

Pneumo, pneumo
pneumoarthrography 関節空気造影法
pneumoencephalography 気脳写
pneumonia 肺炎

Pneumoret
pneumoretroperitoneum 腹膜後気体造影法

pneumoultra
pneumonoultramicroscopic silicovolcanoconiosis　肺微細珪肺，塵肺症
PNF
proprioceptive neuromuscular facilitation　固有受容体神経筋感覚促進法
pnfl
painful　有痛性の
PNG
penicillin G　ペニシリンG
photoelectric-nystagmography　光電眼振計
pneumogram　呼吸曲線
PNH
paroxysmal nocturnal hemoglobinuria　発作性夜間血色素尿症
PNHA
Physicians National Housestaff Association　国内勤務医協会
PNI
peripheral nerve injury　末梢神経障害
postnatal infection　生後感染
prognostic nutritional index　予後からみた栄養指数
psychoneuroimmunology　精神神経免疫学
PNK
polynucleotide kinase　ポリヌクレオチドキナーゼ
PNL
perceived noise level　知覚騒音レベル
percutaneous nephrolithotripsy　経皮的腎結石破砕術
peripheral nerve lesion　末梢神経病変
polymorphonuclear neutrophilic leukocyte　多形核好中球
PNM
perinatal mortality　周生期死亡率
pneumonia　肺炎
postneonatal mortality (syndrome)　出生(直)後新生児死亡(症候群)
pulse number modulation　パルス数変調
PnM
postnatal month　胎児後月齢
PNMA
progressive neural muscular atrophy　進行性神経性筋萎縮症
PNMED
pneumomediastinum　気縦隔
PNMG
persistent neonatal myasthenia gravia　持続性新生児重症筋無力症

PNMT
phenylethanolamine-*N*-methyltransferase フェニルエタノールアミン-*N*-メチルトランスフェラーゼ

PNO
progressive nuclear ophthalmoplegia 進行性核性眼筋麻痺

PNP
peripheral neuropathy 末梢神経障害
pneumoperitoneum 気腹症
polyneuropathy 多発神経症
positive neck pressure 頸部陽圧負荷
psychogenic nocturnal polydipsia 心因性夜間多飲
purine-5′-nucleotidase プリン-5′-ヌクレオチダーゼ
purine nucleotide phosphorylase プリンヌクレオチドリン酸分解酵素
pyridoxine phosphate リン酸ピリドキシン
pyridoxine-5′-phosphate ピリドキシン-5′-リン酸

PNP, P-NP, p-NP
p-nitrophenol パラニトロフェノール

PNPB
positive negative pressure breathing 陽陰圧呼吸

PNPG
p-nitrophenyl-*β*-galactoside パラニトロフェニルガラクトシド
p-nitrophenylglycerin パラニトロフェニルグリセリン

PNPP
p-nitrophenyl phosphate パラニトロフェニルリン酸塩

PNPR
positive negative pressure respiration 陽陰圧呼吸

p-NPS
p-nitrophenyl sulphate パラニトロフェニル硫酸

PNPV
positive negative pressure ventilation 陽陰圧呼吸

PNS
paranasal sinus 副鼻腔
paraneoplastic syndrome 新生物随伴症候群
parasympathetic nervous system 副交感神経
percutaneous nephrostomy 経皮的腎瘻(造設術)
peripheral nerve stimulator 末梢神経刺激装置
peripheral nervous system 末梢神経系

PNT
partial nodular transformation 部分的結節変形
patient 患者
pentamycin ペンタマイシン，ペンタミシン

postnasal tumor　上咽頭腫瘍

pnt
point　点

pnth
pneumothorax　気胸

pnthx
pneumothorax　気胸

PNX
pneumonectomy　肺切除

PNX, Pnx, pnx
pneumothorax　気胸

PO
parieto-occipital　頭頂・後頭の
perioperative　術中の
physician only　医師のみ
posterior　後ろの
preoptic area　視束前野
propylene oxide　酸化プロピレン
pulmonary opening sound　肺開放音
pump-oxygenator　人工心肺装置
pyruvate oxygenase　ピルビン酸酸化酵素

Po
intraocular pressure　眼内圧
opening pressure　初圧
Plasmodium ovale　卵形マラリア原虫
polonium　ポロニウム
poly　多くの
polyp　ポリープ
pulmonary capillary occluded pressure　肺毛細管楔入圧

po'
poor　乏しい

P/O
oxidative phosphorylation ratio　酸化的リン酸化比

p/o
part of　〜の部分

PO, P.O., p.o.
per os〈ラ〉　経口(で)《処》

PO, P/O
phone order　電話指示

PO, P-O, P/O
post(-)operative (state)　術後(の)

PO_2, Po_2
oxygen partial pressure　酸素分圧
oxygen vapor pressure　酸素分圧

P

POA
pancreatic oncofetal antigen — 膵癌胎児抗原
phalangeal osteoarthritis — 指節骨骨関節炎
primary optic atrophy — 原発性視神経萎縮

POACH
prednisone, vincristine (=Oncovin), arabinosylcytosine, cyclophosphamide — プレドニゾン, ビンクリスチン(=オンコビン), アラビノシルシトシン, シクロホスファミド

POAG
primary open angle glaucoma — 原発開放隅角緑内障

PO/AH
preoptic area and anterior hypothalamus — 視索前野と前視床下部

Po ase
peroxidase — ペルオキシダーゼ

POB
phenoxybenzamine — フェノキシベンザミン
phenoxybenzamine hydrochloride — 塩酸フェノキシベンザミン
place of birth — 出生地

POBA
percutaneous old balloon angioplasty — 経皮的旧バルーン動脈形成術

POC
particulate organic carbon — 粒子状有機炭素
postoperative care — 術後ケア
procarbazine, vincristine (=Oncovin), cyclohexylchloroethylnitrosourea — プロカルバジン, ビンクリスチン(=オンコビン), シクロヘキシルクロロエチルニトロソ尿素

P

POCC
procarbazine, vincristine (=Oncovin), cyclohexylchloroethylnitrosourea, cyclophosphamide — プロカルバジン, ビンクリスチン(=オンコビン), シクロヘキシルクロロエチルニトロソ尿素, シクロホスファミド

pocill.
pocillum〈ラ〉 — 小(型)カップ《処》

POCS
postoperative cholangioscopy — 術後胆道鏡

pocul.
poculum〈ラ〉 — カップ《処》

POD
place of death — 死亡場所
polycystic ovarian disease — 多嚢胞卵巣病

POD, P-O-D
postoperative day — 術後日

PODx
preoperative diagnosis 術前診断
POE
pediatric orthopaedic examination 小児整形外科検査
polyoxyethylene ポリオキシエチレン
postoperative endophtalmitis 術後内眼球炎
POEMS
polyneuropathy, organomegaly, endocrinopathy, M protein and skin changes (syndrome) 多発性神経炎・臓器肥大症・内分泌異常症・M蛋白・皮膚病変(症候群)
polyneuropathy, organomegaly, endocrinopathy, M-protein and skin changes syndrome POEMS症候群(=クロウ・深瀬症候群)
POⅠ, Ⅱ, Ⅲ…etc.
postoperative day 1, 2, 3, etc. 第1, 2, 3…術後日
POF
premature ovarian failure 早発卵巣不全(症)
primary ovarian failure 原発性卵巣不全(症)
pyruvate oxidation factor ピルビン酸酸化因子
PofE
portal of entry 侵入門
POG
polymyositis ossificans generalisata 全身性骨化多発性筋炎
POH
poor obstetrical history 不運な産科歴
symbol used in expressing hydroxyl concentration 溶液のアルカリ度を示す記号
POHS
per os hora somni〈ラ〉=through the mouth at the hour of sleep 就寝前経口投与《処》
POIK, poik
poikilocyte 変形〔奇形〕赤血球
poikilocytosis 変形〔奇形〕赤血球症
pois
poison 毒
poisonous 有毒の
POL
polymerized flagellin 重合化フラジェリン, フラジェリン重合体
pol Ⅰ
DNA polymerase Ⅰ DNAポリメラーゼⅠ
pol Ⅱ
DNA polymerase Ⅱ DNAポリメラーゼⅡ
pol Ⅲ
DNA polymerase Ⅲ DNAポリメラーゼⅢ

P

pol ind	
pollen index	花粉指数
Polio	
poliomyelitis	急性灰白髄炎，ポリオ
POLIP	
polyneuropathy, ophthalmoplegia, leukoencephalopathy, and intestinal pseudoobstruction	多発性神経障害・眼筋麻痺・白質脳症・仮性腸閉塞症
POLL, pull.	
pollex〈ラ〉＝thumb	母指
poly	
polyglutamic acid	ポリグルタミン酸
POLY, poly	
polymorphonuclear (leukocyte)	多形核(白血球)
Poly A	
polyadenylic acid	ポリアデニル酸
polyA, poly-A	
polyadenylate	ポリアデニレート
Poly C	
polycytidylic acid	ポリシチジル酸
Poly G	
polyguanilic acid	ポリグアニル酸
poly Glu	
polyglutamic acid	ポリグルタミン酸
polymorph	
polymorphous	多形性の
polys	
polymorphonuclear (leukocytes)	多形核(白血球)〈複数〉
polyso	
polysography	X線重複撮影
Poly T	
polythymidylic acid	ポリチミジル酸
Poly U	
polyuridylic acid	ポリウリジル酸
POM	
pain on motion	運動時痛
prescription only medicine	処方箋必要薬
prisoner of war syndrome	戦争捕虜症候群
POMC	
postoperative maxillary cyst	術後性上顎嚢胞
pro-opiomelanocortin	プロオピオメラノコルチン
POMP	
polyclonal marrow plasmacytosis	多クローン骨髄形質細胞増加
prednisone, vincristine (＝Oncovin), methotrexate, Purinethol	プレドニゾン，ビンクリスチン(＝オンコビン)，メトトレキサート，プリネトール

P

POMR
problem oriented medical record　問題志向型診断記録

POMS
problem-oriented medical system　問題志向型診療システム
profile of mood state　気分状態特性尺度，ポムス

pond.
pondere〈ラ〉　重量で，目方で《処》
ponderosus〈ラ〉　重い

PONR
problem-oriented nursing record　問題志向型看護記録

POP
paroxypropion　パロキシプロピオン
pituitary opioid peptide　下垂体オピオイドペプチド
plasma oncotic pressure　血漿コロイド浸透圧
plasma osmotic pressure　血漿浸透圧
plaster of Paris　ギプス
polycystic ovariann syndrome　多嚢胞卵巣症候群
polymyositis ossificans progressiva　進行性骨化性多発筋炎

POp
postoperative　術後の

pop
popular　人気のある

Pop，pop
popliteal　膝窩の
population　母集団

poplit
popliteal　膝窩の

POPOP
1,4-bis-2-(5-phenyloxazolyl)benzene　1,4-ビス-2-(5-フェニルオキサゾリル)ベンゼン

POPs
persistent organic pollutants　残留性有機汚染物質

POR
problem oriented record　問題志向病歴

por
poorly differentiated adenocarcinoma　低分化型腺癌

P/O ratio
phosphorus/oxygen ratio　P/O比，リン/酸素比

PORH
postocculusive reactive hyperemia　閉塞後反応性充血

port
portable　可搬性の

POS
paraosteal osteosarcoma　傍骨骨肉腫
patient oriented system　患者中心システム
polycystic ovary syndrome　多嚢胞性卵巣症候群

powdered oyster shell	牡蠣末
problem oriented system	問題志向型診療
psychoorganic syndrome	精神・臓器症候群
POS, Pos, pos	
positive	陽性の
Pos, pos	
position	位置，体位
POSC	
preoptic suprachiasmatic area	視束前視交叉〔差〕野
posit.ny	
positional nystagmus	頭位眼振
positron	
positive electron	陽電子
POSM	
patient-operated selected mechanism	患者・手術選択機構
Posm	
plasma osmotic pressure	血漿浸透圧
pos.pr	
positive pressure	陽圧
pos.press	
positive pressure	陽圧
poss	
possibility	可能性
possible	可能な
post	
posterior	後ろの
post mortem	死後の
postmortem examination	病理解剖
post aur.	
post aurem〈ラ〉	耳後の
post cib.	
post cibus〈ラ〉	食後に《処》
postgangl., post gangl.	
postganglionic	神経節後の
postgrad	
postgraduate	卒業後の
Postinoc	
postinoculation	接種後の
post jentac	
post jentaculum〈ラ〉	朝食後《処》
post-op, post op.	
post-operative	術後(の)《処》
post part.	
post partum〈ラ〉＝occurring after childbirth	産後の

P

post prand
post prandium〈ラ〉 夕食後《処》

post sing.sed.liq.
post singulas sedes liquidas〈ラ〉=after every loose stool 毎軟便後に《処》

post.tib.
posterior tibial 後脛骨の

post-transfusion GVHD
post-transfusion graft-versus-host disease 輸血後移植片対宿主病

post traum
post trauma 外傷後の

POT
periostitis ossificans toxica 毒性骨化骨膜炎
purulent otitis media 化膿性中耳炎

pot
potassium カリウム〈元素〉
potential 潜在性の，電位

pot.
potassa〈ラ〉 粗性炭酸カリ《処》
potion〈ラ〉 1服《処》

potass
potassium カリウム〈元素〉

poten
potential 潜在性の

pots
potentiometer 電位差計

POU
placenta, ovaries, uterus 胎盤・卵巣・子宮

POV
peroxidase value 過酸化物価

PoV
portal vein 門脈

POVT
puerperal ovarian vein thrombophlebitis 産床卵巣静脈血栓静脈炎

POW
Powassan (encephalitis) ポワッサン(脳炎)
prisoner of war 戦争捕虜

pow
power 出力

powd
powder 粉末
powdered 粉末にした

POX
peroxidase ペルオキシダーゼ

P

PP

pancreatic peptide	膵ペプチド
pancreatic polypeptide	膵ポリペプチド
paradoxical pulse	奇脈
partial pressure	分圧
past pointing	誤示試験
Payer patch	パイエル板
pentose pathway	五炭糖経路
perfusion pressure	灌流圧
periodic paralysis	周期性四肢麻痺
periportal region	門脈周囲域
peritoneal pseudomyxoma	腹膜偽(性)粘膜腫
pharyngeal posterior	咽頭後(壁)
phthisis pulmonum	肺結核
physical properties	身体的特性
pin prick	ピン痛覚
pipemidic acid	ピペミド酸
Pittsburgh pneumonia agent	ピッツバーグ肺炎因子
placental protein	胎盤蛋白
placenta previa	前置胎盤
plasma pepsinogen	血漿ペプシノゲン
plasma perfusion	血漿灌流
plasmapheresis	血漿交換
polypropylene	ポリプロピレン
posterior pituitary (disease)	下垂体後葉(疾患)
postpill amenorrhea	避妊薬後無月経
presenting part	胎児先進部
private patient	個人的患者
probe puncture	試験穿刺
progressive paralysis	進行麻痺
pro parte	製剤した《処》
propranolol	プロプラノロール
protoporphyria	プロトポルフィリン症
protoporphyrin	プロトポルフィリン
proximal phalanx	基節骨
pseudomyxoma peritonei〈ラ〉	腹膜偽粘液腫
pulse pressure	脈圧
pulsus paradoxus	奇脈
purulent pericarditis	化膿性心膜炎
pyrophosphatase	ピロホスファターゼ
pyrophosphate	ピロリン酸塩

Pp

plasma protein	血漿蛋白
post partum	分娩後(の)
postprandial	食後の
primipara	初産婦

P

pp
polyphosphate　ポリホスフェイト
1-PP
1-phenylpropanol　1-フェニルプロパノール
PP5
placental protein 5　胎盤蛋白 5
P-P
procollagen peptide　プロコラーゲンペプチド
P-5′-P
pyridoxal-5′-phosphate　ピリドキサ(ー)ル-5′-リン酸
PP, P.P.
per primam〈ラ〉=by first　一次の，第Ⅰ期癒合
PP, P.P., Pp, p.p.
per pro〈ラ〉=instead of　〜の代わりに《処》
pluripara〈ラ〉　経産婦
pro paupere〈ラ〉　貧者用として《処》
punctum proximum〈ラ〉=nearest point　近点
PP, P-P
pellagra-preventive　ペラグラ予防の
pp, PP, pp.
pages=page to page　頁〈複数〉，〜頁から〜頁まで
praecipitatus〈ラ〉　沈殿した《処》
pre cipitatus〈ラ〉　沈殿した《処》
PPA
pan paniscus〈ラ〉　ピグミ・チンパンジー
papia papio〈ラ〉　ギニアヒヒ
phenylpyruvic acid　フェニルピルビン酸
pipemidic acid　ピペミド酸
Pittsburgh pneumonia agent　ピッツバーグ肺炎因子
pure pulmonary atresia　真性肺動脈弁閉鎖症
p.p.a.
phiala prius agitata〈ラ〉=the bottle being first shaken　ビンを振盪した後に《処》
PPA, PP & A, pp & a, pp+a
palpation, percussion and auscultation　触診・打診・聴診
PPAA
phenyl-peracetic acid　フェニル過酢酸
PPAF
progressive perivenular alcoholic fibrosis　進行性小〔細〕静脈周囲アルコール性線維症
PPA pos
phenylpyruvic acid positive　フェニルピルビン酸陽性の
PPAR
peroxisome-proliferator-activated receptor　過オキシゾーム増殖活性化受容体

P

PPAS
peripheral pulmonary artery stenosis　末梢性肺動脈狭窄(症)
postpolio atrophy syndrome　ポリオ後萎縮症候群
PPB
positive pressure breathing　陽圧呼吸(法)
ppb
parts per billion　10億分率，10億分の1
PPBS
postprandial blood sugar　食後血糖
PPC
pneumopercardium　気心膜症，心膜気腫
progressive patient care　段階的患者管理
progressive people care　段階的集団ケア
prostatic pressure coefficient　前立腺圧係数
proxymal palmar crease　近位手掌皮膚溝
PPCA
plasma prothrombin conversion accelerator　プラズマプロトロンビン転化促進因子
PPCD
polymorphous posterior corneal dystrophy　多形(性)後角膜ジストロフィ
PPCF
plasma prothrombins conversion factor　プラズマプロトロンビン転化因子
PPCM
postpartum cardiomyopathy　産後心筋症
PPCU
progressive patient care unit　段階的患者管理棟
PPD
paraphenylenediamine　パラフェニレンジアミン
posterior polymorphous dystrophy　多形後部ジストロフィ
postpartum day　産後日
purified protein derivative of tuberculin　精製ツベルクリン蛋白
PPD，Ppd，p.p.d.
packs per day　〜箱/日《処》
PPD，P.P.D.
progressive perceptive deafness　進行性感音性難聴
PPDR
preproliferative diabetic retinopathy　増殖前糖尿病(性)網膜症
PPDS
phonologic programming deficit syndrome　音声プログラミング欠損症候群
PPDS，PPPD-S
purified protein derivative standard (of tuberculin)　精製ツベルクリン蛋白一般用

PPES
palmar-plantar erythrodysesthesia syndrome　手掌・足底紅斑異感覚症候群

PPF
pellagra preventing factor　ペラグラ予防因子
pentagon pyramid flap　五角形ピラミッド皮弁
pirprofen　ピルプロフェン
plasma protein fraction　血漿蛋白
posterior pyramidal fold　後錐体靱帯

PP factor, P.P.factor, P-P factor
pellagra preventive factor　ペラグラ予防因子

PPG
polypropylene glycol　ポリプロピレングリコール
pylorus preserving gastrectomy　幽門保存胃切除術

ppg, ppg.
picopicogram　ピコピコグラム〈単位〉

PPGA
post-pill galactorrhea amenorrhea　ピル後乳汁分泌無月経

ppGpp
guanosine 5′-tetraphosphate　グアノシン5′-四リン酸

PPH
persistent pulmonary hypertension　持続性肺高血圧(症)
posterior pituitary hormone　下垂体後葉ホルモン
postpartum hemorrhage　分娩後出血
primary pulmonary hypertension　原発性肺高血圧症

PPHDF
protein permeable hemodiafiltration　蛋白透過性血液濾過

pphm
parts per hundred million　１億分の１

PPHN
persistent pulmonary hypertension of newborn　新生児肺高血圧残存

PPHP
pseudopseudohypoparathyroidism　偽性偽性上皮小体機能低下症

***P*-PHP, P-PHP**
p-phenylphenol　パラフェニルフェノール

PPI
patient package insert　患者用添付文書
penile pressure index　陰茎動脈(末梢)血圧比
plane position indicator　平面位表示器
post-prostatectomy infection　前立腺摘出後感染
proton pump inhibitor　プロトンポンプ阻害薬
purified porcine insulin　精製ブタインスリン

PPi
inorganic pyrophosphate　無機ピロリン酸塩

PPIE
prolonged postictal encephalopathy — 持続(遷延)性発作後脳障害
PPIM
postperinatal infant mortality — 周生期後乳児死亡率
PPK
palmoplantar keratoderma — 手掌足底(掌蹠)角皮症
palmoplantar keratosis — 手掌足底(掌蹠)角化症
partial panetrating keratoplasty — 部分的全層角膜移植(術)
plasma prekallikrein — 血漿プレカリクレイン
PPL
pars plana lensectomy — 経毛様体扁平部水晶体切除(術)
pasteurisierte Plasmaproteinlösung〈独〉 — 低温滅菌血漿蛋白溶液
penicilloyl polylysine — ペニシロイルポリリジン
phospholipid — リン脂質
prostatic profile length — 前立腺部尿道長
Ppl
pleural pressure — 胸(膜)腔内圧
PPLO
pleuro-pneumonia-like organism — 胸膜肺炎様微生物
PPM
peplomycin, cisplatin (=Platinol), mitomycin C — ペプレオマイシン, シスプラチン(=プラチノール), マイトマイシンC
permanent pacemaker — 永久ペースメーカー
persistent pupillary membrane — 瞳孔膜遺残症
phosphopentomutase — ホスホペントムターゼ
posterior papillary muscle — 後乳頭筋
Propulsiv-Petit-Mal〈独〉 — 前屈小発作
pulse phase modulation — パルス位相変調
PPm
phenolphthalein diphosphate agar medium — フェノールフタレイン二リン酸塩寒天培地
ppm
pulses per minute — 拍動/分
PPM, ppm, ppm.
parts per million — 100万分の1
PPN
partial parenteral nutrition — 部分非経口栄養
peripheral parenteral nutrition — 末梢非経口的栄養
ppn
proportion — 比例
proportional — 比率のとれた
PPNA
peak phrenic nerve activity — 最大横隔神経活動

P

PPNAD
primary pigmented nodular adrenocortical disease　原発(性)色素(性)結節(性)副腎皮質疾患
PPNG
penicillinase-producing *Neisseria gonorrhoeae*　ペニシリナーゼ産生淋菌
PPO
peak pepsin output　最大ペプシン排出量
platelet peroxidase　血小板ペルオキシダーゼ
pleuropneumonia organism　胸膜肺炎微生物
preferred provider organization　医療提供契約
PPOM
Predominantly Profession Ordinary Member　薬剤職能系正会員
PPP
palatopharyngoplasty　口蓋咽頭形成術
palmoplantar pustulosis　掌蹠膿疱症
paraoxypropiophenone　パラオキシプロピオフェノン
pentose phosphate pathway　五炭糖リン酸経路
phenolphthalein in paraffin emulsion　パラフィン乳剤のフェノールフタレイン
pigmented pretibial patches　前脛骨部色素斑
platelet-poor plasma　乏血小板血漿
polluter pays principle　汚染者負担の原則
porcine pancreatic polypeptide　ブタ膵ポリペプチド
portal perfusion pressure　門脈灌流圧
pseudoprecocious puberty　仮性早熟
purified placental protein　精製胎盤蛋白
pustulosis palmaris (et) plantaris　掌蹠膿疱症
PPPA
Poison Prevention Packaging Act　毒性容器防止法
PPPC
phenoxypropyl penicillin　フェノキシプロピルペニシリン
propicillin　プロピシリン
PPPD
porokeratosis palmaris et plantaris disseminata　播種状掌蹠汗孔角化症
pylorus-preserving pancreatoduodenectomy　幽門輪温存膵頭十二指腸切除術
PPPL
pasteurisierte Plasmaproteinlosung 〈独〉　低温滅菌血漿蛋白溶液
Pp/Ps
pulmonary pressure/systemic blood pressure　肺動脈圧/体血圧(比)

P

resistance of PA/resistance of systemic　体肺抵抗比

PPQ

pitch period quotient　ピッチ期間比

PPR

patient-physician relationship　患者医師関係
photopalpebral reflex　光眼瞼反射
Price precipitation reaction　プライス沈降反応

PPRC

Physician Payment Review Committee　医師支払査定委員会

PPRE

peroxisome proliferator activated responsive element　過オキシウム増殖活性化受容体要素

PPRF

paramediane pontine reticular formation　傍正中橋網様体
postpartum renal failure　産後腎不全

PPRibP

phosphoribosylpyrophosphate　ホスホリボシルピロリン酸

PPRP

5-phospho-α-D-ribosylpyrophosphate　5-ホスホ-α-D-リボシルピロリン酸

PPS

pain-producing substance　発痛物質
parapharyngeal space　側咽頭間隙
pepsin　ペプシン
peripheral pulmonic stenosis　末梢性肺動脈狭窄
pneumococcal polysaccharide vaccine　肺炎球菌多糖類ワクチン
polyvalent pneumococcal polysaccharide　多価肺炎球菌多糖類
postperfusion syndrome　体外循環後症候群
postpericardiotomy syndrome　心膜切除後症候群
postpolio syndrome　ポリオ(灰白髄炎)後症候群
postpump syndrome　人工心肺後症候群
primary acquired preleukemic syndrome　原発性後天性前白血病症候群
prospective payment system　予見定額払い方式
pure pulmonary stenosis　純型肺動脈狭窄症

PPS, p.p.s.

pulses per second　パルス/秒

PPSM

plantar-palmar-subungual melanoma　掌蹠爪下黒色腫

PPT

parietal pleural tissue　壁側胸膜組織
partial prothrombin time　部分プロトロンビン時間

plasma prothrombin time　血漿プロトロンビン時間
prone position test　うつむき試験
proximal priority treatment　中枢優先治療

Ppt
pneumoperitoneum　気腹症

ppt
parts per trillion　１兆分の１

PPT 50
population perception threshold 50%　50%感受閾値

PPT, Ppt, ppt
precipitate　沈殿する
precipitation　沈殿反応

Ppt, ppt.
praeparatus〈ラ〉=prepared　準備，調製した《処》

ppta
precipitation　沈殿反応

pptd
precipitated　沈降した，沈殿した

P & P test, P+P-test
prothrombin-proconvertin(-Stuart factor activity) test　プロトロンビン・プロコンバーチン(・スチュワート因子活性)検査

PPTL
postpartum tubal ligation　産後卵管結紮

pptn
precipitation　沈殿反応

PPTS
protein phosphatase　蛋白質脱リン酸酵素

PPTT
prepubertal testicular tumor　思春期前精巣〔睾丸〕腫瘍

PPT vip.pos
pinpric, touch, vibration and position　痛覚・触覚・振動覚・位置覚

PPU
perforated peptic ulcer　穿孔性消化性潰瘍

PPV
paraquat　パラクアット
polyvalent pneumococcal polysaccharide vaccine　多価肺炎球菌多糖ワクチン
positive pressure ventilation　陽圧換気

PPY
pongo pygmaeus〈ラ〉　オランウータン

PQ
atrioventricular conduction (time)　房室伝導時間
permeability quotient　透過性係数
phonation quotient　発声指数
plastoquinone　プラストキノン

pronator quadratus (muscle) 方形回内(筋)
pyrimethamine-quinine ピリメタミンキニーネ

PQ-9
plastoquinone-9 プラストキノン9

PQCT
peripheral quantitative computed tomography 末梢骨定量的CT

PQQ
pyrrolo-quinoline quinone ピロロキノリンキノン

$PQQH_2$
reduced pyrrolo-quinoline quinone 還元ピロロキノリンキノン(2,7,9-トリカルボキシ-1H-ピロロ(2,3-f)キノリン4,5-ジオール)

PQRST
provocative and palliative factor, quality, region, severity, temporal characteristics 誘発および寛解因子・性質・部位・重症度・一時的な特徴
purobucol quantitative regression trial プロブコールの量の違いによる再発試験

PR
Panama red パナマレッド
pars recta 直部
partial remission 部分寛解
partial response 有効
patient relationship 患者関係
pelvic rock 骨盤動揺
percentile rank 百分率階数《統》
perfusion rate 灌流率
peripheral resistance 末梢抵抗
phenol red フェノールレッド
phosphorylase 加リン酸分解酵素
photoreacting 光反応の
photoreaction 光反応
pityriasis rosea バラ色粃糠疹
polymyalgia rheumatica リウマチ性多発筋痛症
polyribosome ポリリボソーム
postural reflex 姿勢反射
pregnancy rate 妊娠率
pressoreceptor 圧受容器
pressure 圧
prevention 予防
PR interval PR間隔《心電》
production rate 産生率
progesterone receptor プロゲステロン受容体
progressive resistance 漸増抵抗

prosthion　プロスチオン
public relation　公的関係
Puerto Rican　プエルトリコ人
pulmonary regurgitation　肺動脈弁閉鎖不全
pulse rate　脈拍数
purplish red　赤紫

Pr

praseodymium　プラセオジミウム〈元素〉
premature　未熟の
prescribe　処方する，命令する
prescription　処方箋
presentation　先進部
prism　プリズム
propafenone　プロパフェノン

pr

pair　対

P & R

pelvic and rectal　骨盤と直腸の
pulse and respiration　脈拍と呼吸

PR，Pr

presbyopia　老眼，老視
proctologist　直腸病専門医
proctology　直腸病学，肛門病学
prolactin　プロラクチン
propyl　プロピル
protein　蛋白

PR，pr，p.r.

per rectum〈ラ〉　直腸から
punctum remotum〈ラ〉　遠点

PR，P/R

pulse/respiration　心拍/呼吸

PRA

5-phosphoribosyl-1-amine　5-ホスホリボシル-1-アミン
plasma renin activity　血漿レニン活性
progesteron receptor assay　プロゲステロン受容体試験
Psoriasis Research Association　乾癬研究協会
Psychological Research Association　心理学研究協会

prac

practice　診療，開業

PRACT

practitioner　開業医

pract

practical　実際的な

praec.

praecipitatus〈ラ〉　沈殿した《処》

praep.
praeparatus〈ラ〉 調製した《処》

pram
perambulator 乳母車

prand.
prandium〈ラ〉 食事《処》

PRAS
pseudo-renal-artery syndrome 偽(性)腎動脈症候群

p.rat.aetat.
pro ratione aetatis〈ラ〉=in proportion to age 年齢相応の，年齢に応じて《処》

PRC
packed red cell 赤血球パック
plasma renin concentration 血漿レニン濃度

prc
procedure 手技

PRCA
pure red cell aplasia 赤芽球癆

prcs
process 過程

PRD
partial reaction of degeneration 部分変性反応
polycystic renal disease 嚢胞腎
postradiation dysplasia 放射線(照射)後形成異常(症)

PRDX
postradiation dysplasia 放射線(照射)後形成異常(症)

PRE
photoreacting enzyme 光反応酵素
pigmented retinal epithelial (cell) 色素網膜上皮(細胞)
progressive resistance exercise 漸増抵抗運動

P

Pre, pre
preliminary 予備の

PREB
pupil record of educational behavior 学習レディネス診断検査

pre-β-Lp
pre-β-lipoprotein プレ-β-リポ蛋白

prec
preceding 前駆の

p rec, p.rec.
per rectum〈ラ〉=through the rectum 直腸から，経直腸

precip
precipitate 沈殿する
precipitation 沈殿反応

precord
precordial 前胸部の

Prec steth
precordial stethoscope 前胸部聴診器
pred
prednisolone プレドニゾロン
PRED, pred
prednisone プレドニゾン
prednis
prednisolone プレドニゾロン
prednisone プレドニゾン
preemies
premature babies 未熟児〈複数〉
preemy
premature baby 未熟児〈単数〉
pref
prefer 好む
preference 好み
prefd
preferred 望まれた
preg
pregnancy 妊娠
pregnant 妊娠した
pregang
preganglionic 節前の
Preinoc
preinoculation 接種前の
prelim
preliminary 予備の
prelim.diag
preliminary diagnosis 暫定診断
prem
premature 早熟の
premature infant 早産児
pre-med
premedication 準備投薬
prenat
prenatal 出生前の
PR enzyme
prosthetic-group removing enzyme 補欠分子族転移酵素
pre-op
preoperative 手術前の
prep
preparation 準備
prepare 準備する
prepare for surgery 手術準備
prepd
prepared 準備された

prepn
preparation 準備
pres
present 現在の
pressure 圧
presby
presbyopia 老視
presbyopic 老視の
presc
prescription 処方，処方箋
preserv
preservation 保存
preserve 保存する
PRESS
prediction residual sum of squares 予備，保存，保護
press
pressure 圧
prev
prevent 予防する
preventative 予防の
previous 以前の
prevent
preventive 予防
prev.hx
previous history 既往歴
PrevMed
preventative medicine 予防医学
pre-voc
pre-vocational 予備教育の
PRF
patient report form 患者報告用紙
personality research form 人格研究用紙
pontine reticular formation 橋網様体
prolactin releasing factor プロラクチン放出因子
pulse recurrence frequency 脈再発頻度
pyrogen-releasing factor 発熱様物質放出因子
pRF
polyclonal rheumatoid factor ポリクローナルリウマチ因子
prF
prefollicular 濾胞前期
prf
proof 証拠
PRFA
plasma recognition factor activity 血漿認識因子活性
p.r.g.
pulvis radix gentianae〈ラ〉 ゲンチアナ根末《処》

PRGC
percutaneous radiofrequency gasserian ganglion coagulation　経皮的ガッセル神経節高周波凝固法
PRGS
phosphoribosylglycineamide synthetase　ホスホリボシルグリシンアミド合成酵素
PRH
preretinal hemorrhage　網膜前出血
prolactin releasing hormone　プロラクチン放出ホルモン
PRI
phosphoribose isomerase　ホスホリボースイソメラーゼ
plexus rectales inferiores　直腸動脈神経叢
PRIF
prolactin release-inhibiting factor　プロラクチン放出抑制因子
PRIH
prolactin release-inhibiting hormone　プロラクチン放出抑制ホルモン

prim
primary　一次性の
prim.diag
primary diagnosis　第一診断
PRIME
procarbazine, iglosamide, methotrexate　プロカルバジン, イグロサミド, メトトレキサート
primip
primipara　初産婦
prim.luc.
prima luce〈ラ〉＝at first light　早朝に
prim.m.
primo mane〈ラ〉＝first in the morning　朝一番に
prin
principal　主要な
princ
principal　主要な
principle　原理
PRIND
prolonged reversible ischemic neurological deficit　遷延性可逆性虚血性神経症候
print
printed　印刷された
printing　印刷中の
prior
priority　優先権
prism
prismatic　プリズムの

P

PRIST	
paper disc radioimmunosorbent test	濾紙放射免疫吸収試験
paper radioimmunosorbent test	ペーパーラジオイムノソルベント試験
priv	
private	私的な
privilege	特典
PRK	
photo-refractive keratectomy	角膜屈折矯正手術
PRL	
photoreceptor membrane	光受容器膜
practical residue limit	実際残留量
prolactin	プロラクチン
PRLN	
pyrrolnitrin	ピロルニトリン
PRM	
paromomycin	パロモマイシン
pertactin	パータクチン
positron remmission microscope	陽電子再放出顕微鏡
preventive medicine	予防医学
primidone	プリミドン
PRMTC	
rolitetracycline	ロリテトラサイクリン
PRN	
polyradiculoneuritis	多発性神経根炎
polyradiculoneuropathy	多発根神経障害
prn, p.r.n.	
pro re nata〈ラ〉=as required	必要に応じて《処》
PRO	
Peer Review Organization	同僚審査機構
projection	突出
pronation	回内
protein	蛋白
prothrombin	プロトロンビン
Pro	
proline	プロリン
pro	
procedure	手技，方法
proceed	続ける
profession	職業
professional	職業の
prophylactic	予防の
prophylaxis	予防
prob	
probability	ありそうな
probably	たぶん

P

problem 問題

Probe

Probeantrotomie〈独〉= Probelaparatomie 試験開腹

Probeauskratzung〈独〉 診査掻爬

Probeexzision〈独〉= Probeinzision 診査切除，試験切開

Probepunktion〈独〉 診査穿刺

Probestück〈独〉 試験切片

Proc

processus〈ラ〉 突起〈単数〉

proc

procedure 方法，手技，処置

proceeding 行為，行動，議事録，会報

process 過程，経験，突起

Procc

processus〈ラ〉 突起〈複数〉

Procs

proceedings 議事録

proct

proctocolonoscopy 直腸肛門大腸鏡検査

proctolitis 直腸肛門炎

proctoplegia 直腸肛門麻痺

proctosigmoidectomy 直腸肛門S状結腸摘出手術

proctosigmoidoscopy 直腸肛門S状結腸鏡検査

PROCT, Proct, proct.

proctologist 直腸病専門医，直腸肛門医

proctology 直腸病学

procto

proctoclysis 直腸灌注

PROCTO, procto

proctology 直腸病学

proctoscopic 直腸鏡検査の

proctoscopy 直腸鏡検査

proc.xiph.

processus xiphoideus〈ラ〉 剣状突起

prod

produced 産生された，産生する

product 産物，生成物

pro dos.

pro dosi〈ラ〉= for a dose １回量として《処》

ProEbl

proerythroblast 前赤芽球

Prof, prof

profession 職業

professional 職業的な

professor 教授

P

PROG
prognathism 顎前突(症)
prog
progenitor 先祖
prognosis 予後
program 計画，プログラム
progress 経過
progressive 進行性の
progn
prognosis 予後
progr
progress 経過，進行する
PROGRES
perindopril protection against recurrent stroke ACE阻害薬の脳卒中再発予防効果における大規模試験
proj
project 突出する
projection 突出
prol
proline プロリン
prolong 延長する
prolonged 延長された
PROLOG
Programming in Logic プロログ
prolong.
prolongatus〈ラ〉 延長された
PROM
passive range of motion 受動可動域
premature rupture of membrane 前期破水
prom
prominent 突出した
promontory 突起
promotion 助長
promotor 促進剤
PROMIS
problem oriented medical information system 問題志向医学情報システム
pron
pronate 回内する
pronation 回内
pron/sup
pronation/supination 回内/回外
prop
proportion 比率
proportional 比率を保った
propranolol プロプラノロール

proph
prophylactic 予防の
PROPLA
prophospholipase A プロホスホリパーゼA
pro rat.aet.
pro ratione aetatis〈ラ〉=according to age 年齢に応じて《処》
pro rect.
pro recto〈ラ〉=by rectum 直腸で，直腸に，肛門に《処》
pros
prostate 前立腺
prosthesis プロテーゼ，人工器官
prosthetic プロテーゼの，人工器官の
prost
prostate 前立腺
prostat
prostatic 前立腺の
prosth
prosthesis プロテーゼ，人工器官
PROT, Prot
Protestant プロテスタント(の)
PROT, prot
protein 蛋白
pro tem.
pro tempore〈ラ〉 当分《処》
prothr.cont
prothrombin content プロトロンビン含量
prothrom
prothrombin プロトロンビン
proth.time
prothrombin time プロトロンビン時間
Pro-thy
prothymocyte 前胸腺細胞
pro-time, pro.time
prothrombin time プロトロンビン時間
PROTO
protoporphyrin プロトポルフィリン
pro ureth.
pro urethra〈ラ〉 尿道に《処》
pro us.ext.
pro usu externo〈ラ〉=for external use 外用《処》
pro vagin.
pro vagina〈ラ〉 腟に《処》
PROVIMI
proteins, vitamins and minerals 蛋白・ビタミン・無機質

Pro-X
prothrombin time　プロトロンビン時間

Prox, prox
proximal　近位の

prox.luc.
proxima luce〈ラ〉=the next morning　翌朝《処》

PRP
panretinal photocoagulation　汎網膜光凝固
pityriasis rubra pilaris　毛孔性紅色粃糠疹
platelet rich plasma　多血小板血漿
pneumo-retroperitoneum　後腹膜気体造影法
polymer of ribosyl and ribitol phosphate　リン酸リボシルとリン酸リビト(ー)ルの重合体
pressure rate product　ダブルプロダクト，圧・率産生物
progressive rubella panencephalitis　進行性風疹全脳炎
proliferative retinopathy photocoagulation　増殖網膜症光凝固(術)

PrP
prion protein　プリオン蛋白

PrP^c^
normal cellular form of prion protein　正常型プリオン蛋白

Pr-Pl-Hb
pyridoxalated plyperized hemoglobin solution　ピリドキサレイテッド・プリペライズド・ヘモグロビン液

PRPP
phosphoribosylpyrophosphate　ホスホリボシルピロリン酸

PRPS
phosphoribosylpyrophosphate synthetase　ホスホリボシルピロリン酸合成酵素

PrP^Sc^
scrapie form of prion protein　異常型プリオン蛋白

PRR
pattern-recognition receptor　パターン認識受容体
population relative risk　人口相対危険度

PRS
Personality Rating Scale　人格評点スケール〔尺度〕
Pierre Robin syndrome　ピエール・ロバン症候群

prs
pairs　対〈複数〉

PRSP
penicillin G-resistant *Streptococcus pneumoniae*　ペニシリンG耐性肺炎球菌
penicillin-resistant *Streptococcus pneumoniae*　ペニシリン耐性肺炎球菌

P

PRT
pendular rotation test　振子様回転検査
phosphoribosyltransferase　ホスホリボシルトランスフェラーゼ
photoradiation therapy　光照射治療
postoperative respiratory treatment　術後呼吸治療
the Picture Rotation Test　絵画空想法

pRTA
proximal renal tubular acidosis　近位尿細管性アシドーシス

PRTase
phosphoribosyltransferase　ホスホリボシルトランスフェラーゼ

PRTH-C
prothrombin time control　プロトロンビン時間コントロール〔対照〕

PRU
unit of peripheral resistance　末梢抵抗単位

PRV
polycythemia rubra vera　真性赤血球増加
pseudorabies virus　仮性狂犬病ウイルス

PRVA
peripheral vein renin activity　末梢静脈レニン活性

PRVC
pressure regulated volume control　圧補正従量式

PRVEP
pattern reversed visual evoked potential　パターン変換視覚誘発電位

PS
chloropicrin　クロロピクリン
pacemaker syndrome　ペースメーカー症候群
paired stimulation　ペア刺激
paradoxical sleep　逆説睡眠
paranoid schizophrenia　妄想型統合失調症
parapharyngeal space　咽頭側間隙
paraspinal　脊髄傍の
parasternal　胸骨傍の
parasympathetic　副交感神経の
pathological stage　病理学的病期
pathologic state　病的状態
patient's serum　患者血清
pediatric surgery　小児外科
Pellegrini-Stieda (syndrome)　ペレグリーニ・シュティーダ(症候群)
perceptual speed　知覚速度
performance status　活動状況
periodic syndrome　周期性症候群

P

peripheral smear　末梢スメア
Pferdestärke〈独〉　馬力
Pharmaceutical Society　薬学会
phenyl sepharose　フェニルセファロース
phosphatidylserine　ホスファチジルセリン
photic stimulation　光刺激
physical status　全身状態
pigeon serum　ハト血清
plasma separation　血漿分離
plastic surgeon　形成外科医
plastic surgery　形成外科
point of symmetry　対称点
polysaccharides　多糖類
polystyrene　ポリスチレン
posterior sagittal diameter of pelvic outlet　骨盤出口後縦径
postmaturity syndrome　過熟妊娠症候群
pregnancy serum　妊娠血清
prescription　処方，投薬
prestimulus　刺激前の
prostatic secretion　前立腺分泌
protein synthesis　蛋白合成
psychiatric　精神医学の
psychomotor seizure　精神運動発作
pulmonary stenosis　肺動脈狭窄(症)
pulmonary surfactant　肺表面活性物質
pulmonic stenosis　肺動脈狭窄症
pyloric stenosis　幽門狭窄(症)
pyriform sinus　梨状陥凹
serum from a pregnant woman　妊婦血清

Ps

pressure systolic　収縮期圧
pseudocyst　偽性嚢胞
psoriasis　乾癬

ps

per secundum〈ラ〉　第II期癒合
picosecond　ピコ秒〈単位〉
pseudo-　偽性の〈接〉

p.s.

post scriptum〈ラ〉　追記

P/S

polyunsaturated fat/saturated fat　多価不飽和脂肪酸/飽和脂肪酸比

P & S

paracentesis and suction　鼓膜切開と吸引
physicians and surgeons　内科医と外科医

P-1-S
0.1% procaine hydrochloride in normal saline — 0.1%塩酸プロカイン食塩液

PS, Ps
prescription — 処方箋
Pseudomonas — シュードモナス属

PS, ps, p.s.
per second — ～/秒，毎秒

PS, P-S
Porter-Silber (chromogens) — ポーター・シルバー(色素原)

PSA
posterior sagittal anorectoplasty — 後縦肛門形成
progressive spinal ataxia — 進行性脊髄失調
prolonged sleep apnea — 遷延性睡眠時無呼吸
prostate-specific antigen — 前立腺特異抗原

PsA
psoriatic arthritis — 乾癬性関節炎

psa, p.s.a.
pone situm affectum〈ラ〉=apply to the affected parts — 病変部に適用《処》

PSAGN
poststreptococcal acute glomerulonephritis — 連鎖球菌後急性糸球体腎炎

ps.an., PSAn, PsAn
psychoanalysis — 精神分析
psychoanalyst — 精神分析者，精神分析専門医
psychoanalytic(al) — 精神分析の
psychoanalyze — 精神分析する

PSAP
prostate specific acid phosphatase — 前立腺特異酸性ホスファターゼ
prostatic serum acid phosphatase — 前立腺性血清酸性ホスファターゼ

PSB
Psychological Strategy Board — 精神医学的戦略委員会

PSBO
partial small bowel obstruction — 部分的小腸閉塞(症)

PSC
pluripotent stem cell — 多能性幹細胞
Porter-Silber chromogen — ポーター・シルバー色素原
posterior subcapsular cataract — 後嚢下白内障
primary sclerosing cholangitis — 原発性硬化性胆管炎
pyriformis sinus cancer — 梨状陥凹癌

psc
pseudocyst — 偽嚢胞

PSCC
posterior subcapsular cataract 後嚢下白内障

PSD
peptone-starch-dextrose ペプトン・デンプン・ブドウ糖
periodic synchronous discharge 周期性同期性放電
placental steroid sulfatase deficiency 胎盤性スルファターゼ欠損症
poststenotic dilatation 狭窄後拡張
psychosomatic disease 心身症

PsD
personality disorder 人格障害

PS detn
particle size determination 粒子サイズ決定

PSE
partial spleen embolization 部分的脾動脈塞栓術
penicillin-sensitive enzyme ペニシリン感受性酵素
portal systemic encephalopathy 門脈体循環性脳障害
postshunt encephalopathy シャント後脳障害
present state examination 現症検査
psychological stress evaluator 心理学的ストレス評価器械（＝ウソ発見器）

PSEC
picosecond ピコ秒
poststress ethanol consumption ストレス後エタノール消費

PSF
phagocytosis-stimulating factor 食細胞刺激因子
point spread function 点広がり関数
posterior stapedial fold 後アブミ骨ひだ
prostacyclin production stimulating factor プロスタサイクリン産生刺激因子
pseudosarcomatous fasci(i)tis 偽肉腫性筋膜炎

p.s.f.
ponds per square foot ポンド/平方フィート

PSG
peak systolic gradient 最大収縮期勾配
polysomnogram 睡眠ポリグラム
polysomnography 睡眠ポリグラフ検査，終夜睡眠ポリグラフ
presystolic gallop 収縮前期奔馬調律
proctosigmoidgraphy 直腸S状結腸X線像

PSGL
P-selectin glycoprotein ligand Pセレクチン糖蛋白リガンド

PSGN
post-streptococcal glomerulonephritis 溶連菌感染後糸球体腎炎

PSH
periarthritis scapulohumeral〈ラ〉 肩甲上腕関節周囲炎

plastic surgical history 形成外科歴
postspinal headache 脊髄後頭痛
pseudo-hypertension 偽高血圧
purpura Schönlein-Henoch シェーンライン・ヘノッホ紫斑病

P & SHy
personal and social history 個人歴と社会歴

PSI
per secundam intentionem〈ラ〉=by second intention 二次の，二期の
problem solving information 問題解決情報
proton spectroscopic imaging プロトンスペクトロスコープ画像
Psychological Screening Inventory 心理学的スクリーニング調査票
psychosomatic inventory 精神身体調査
pulmonary stenoinsufficiency 肺動脈狭窄兼閉鎖不全
pulmonary stenosis and insufficiency 肺動脈狭窄兼閉鎖不全症

psi, p.s.i.
pound(s) per square inch ポンド/平方インチ(=ψ，プサイ)

pSIDS
partially unexplained sudden infant death syndrome 不完全解明乳児突然死症候群

PSIS
posterior sacroiliac spine 後上腸骨棘

PSK
polysaccharide K(=Kureha) ポリサッカライドクレハ，ポリサッカライドK

PSL
parasternal line 胸骨傍線
photo-stimulated luminescence 光刺激発光
potassium, sodium chloride, sodium lactate カリウム・塩化ナトリウム・乳酸ナトリウム
prednisolone プレドニゾロン

PSLS
Prehospital Stroke Life Support 脳卒中病院前救護

PSL sol
potassium, sodium chloride, sodium lactate solution カリウム・塩化ナトリウム・乳酸ナトリウム溶液

PSM
presystolic murmur 収縮前雑音
psychosomatic medicine 心身医学

PSMA
progressive spinal muscular atrophy 進行性脊髄性筋萎縮症
proximal spinal muscular atrophy 近位型脊髄性筋萎縮症

Psmax
maximal safety pressure 最高安全圧
Psmin
minimum safety pressure 最低安全圧
PSM melanoma
palmo-plantar-subungual-mucosal melanoma 掌蹠爪下粘膜黒色腫
PSNS
parasympathetic nervous system 副交感神経系
PSO
physostigmine salicylate ophthalmic サリチル酸フィゾスチグミン点眼(液)
Provider Sponsored Organization 供給者支援組織
proximal subungual onychomycosis 近位爪下爪(甲)真菌症
P sol
partially soluble, partly soluble 部分的に可溶な
PSOM
Predominantly Scientific Ordinary Member 優秀科学者の正規会員
PSOR
psoralen ソラレン
P/sore
pressure sore 床ずれ，褥瘡
PSP
pancreatic spasmolytic polypeptide 膵攣縮寛解ポリペプチド
pancreatic stone protein 膵石蛋白
paralytic shellfish poison 麻痺性貝毒
phenolsulfonphthalein フェノールスルホンフタレイン
positive spike pattern 陽性棘波パターン
progressive supranuclear palsy 進行性核上性麻痺
pseudopregnancy 偽妊娠
psp
posterior subcapsular plague 後被膜下伝染病
PSP, ps.p, p.s.p.
postsynaptic potential シナプス後電位
PSPF
prostacyclin synthesis stimulating plasma factor プロスタサイクリン合成刺激血漿因子
PSP test
phenolsulfonphthalein test フェノールスルホンフタレイン排泄試験
PSQ
Patient Satisfaction Questionnaire 患者満足質問表
postero-superior quadrant 後上象限

PSR
Patellarsehnenreflex〈独〉 膝蓋腱反射
pelvi-spondylite rheumatismal〈仏〉 慢性リウマチ様骨盤脊椎関節強直症
portal systemic resistence 門脈体循環抵抗
proliferative sickle retinopathy 増殖鎌状網膜症
pulmonary stretch receptor 肺伸展受容器

PSRO
Professional Standard Review Organization 職業標準審査機関

PSS
painful shoulder syndrome 有痛性肩症候群
pelvic steal 骨盤静脈流出
physiological saline solution 生理的食塩水
porcine stress syndrome ブタストレス症候群
primary Sjögren syndrome 原発性シェーグレン症候群
progressive systemic sclerosis 進行性全身性硬化症
pure sensory stroke 純粋感覚性脳卒中

PSSO
Professional Standards Service Organization 専門標準検閲機構

PSSP
penicillin susceptible *Streptococcus pneumoniae* ペニシリン感受性肺炎球菌

PST
pancreatic suppression test 膵臓抑制試験
paroxysmal supraventricular tachycardia 発作性上室性頻拍
penicillin, streptomycin, tetracycline ペニシリン,ストレプトマイシン,テトラサイクリン
perfrontal sonic treatment 前頭葉超音波療法
picture story test 絵画物語テスト
poststenotic 狭窄後の
poststimulus time 刺激後時間
prefrontal sonic treatment 前頭葉超音波療法
protamine sulfate test プロタミン硫酸試験

P.St.
punctum sternale〈ラ〉 胸骨穿刺

PST, p.s.t.
platelet survival time 血小板生存時間

PS test
pancreozymin-secretin test パンクレオザイミン・セクレチン試験

PSTH
poststimulus time histogram 刺激後時間ヒストグラム

P

PSTI
pancreatic secretory trypsin inhibitor 膵分泌性トリプシン抑制因子
PSU
photosynthetic unit 光合成ユニット
P subst
protein substance 蛋白物質
PSUR
periodic safety update report 定期安全性最新報告
PSurg, P.surg
plastic surgeon 形成外科医
plastic surgery 形成外科
PSV
pressure support ventilation 圧補助換気
PSVE
progressive subcortical vascular encephalopathy 進行性皮質下血管性脳症
PSVER
pattern-shift visual-evoked response パターンシフト視覚誘発反応
PSVT
paroxysmal supraventricular tachycardia 発作性上室性頻拍(症)
PSW
positive sharp wave 陽性棘波
psychiatric social work 精神科医療ソーシャルワーク
psychiatric social worker 精神科医療ソーシャルワーカー
PSX
pseudoexfoliation 偽(性)剝脱，偽(性)落屑
Psy, psy
psychiatry 精神科，精神医学
psychology 心理学
PSYCH, Psych, psych
psychiatry 精神医学
Psych, psych
psychology 心理学
PSYCHEM
psychiatric chemistry 精神化学
psychiat
psychiatric 精神医学の
psychiatry 精神医学
psycho
psychiatric hospital 精神病院，精神病棟
psychoneurotic personality 精神神経的個性
psychoan
psychoanalysis 精神分析

P

PSYCHOL, psychol.
psychology 心理学
psychomet
psychometrics 精神測定学
psychopath
psychopathic 精神障害の
psychopathological 精神病理の
psychopathol
psychopathological 精神病理の
psychopathology 精神病理学
psychophys
psychophysics 精神物理学
Psychophysiol, psychophysiol.
psychophysiological 精神生理学の
psychophysiology 精神生理学
PsychosMed
Psychosomatic Medicine 精神身体医学
psychosom
psychosomatic 心身の，精神身体の
psychother
psychotherapy 精神療法，心理療法
PSYOP
psychological operations 心理作戦
4P symptom
pain, paralysis, paresthesia, pulselessness 疼痛・麻痺・感覚異常・脈拍喪失の 4 症状
Psy-path, psy-path
psychopathic 精神障害の，精神病質
psy-som
psychosomatic 心身の，精神身体の
Ps-ZES
pseudo-Zollinger-Ellison syndrome 偽(性)ゾリンジャー・エリソン症候群

PT
parathormone パラトルモン，上皮小体ホルモン
parathyroid 上皮小体の
paroxysmal tachycardia 発作性頻拍
pars tensa〈ラ〉 緊張部
passage time 通過時間
percussion tone 打診音
pericardial tamponade 心(膜)タンポナーデ
pertussis toxin 百日咳毒素
pharyngeal tonsil 咽頭扁桃
phenytoin フェニトイン
phonation time 発音持続時間

photophobia まぶしがり，光恐怖
phototoxicity 光毒性
physical therapist 理学療法士
physical therapy 理学療法，物理療法
placebo tablet 偽薬錠
planum temporale 側頭平面
plasma thromboplastin 血漿トロンボプラスチン
pneumothorax 気胸
portio temperature 子宮腟部温度
posterior tibial 後脛骨の
post transfusion〈ラ〉＝after transfusion 輸血後に
precipitation test 沈降反応
pronator teres 円回内筋
propylthiouracil プロピルチオウラシル
protease toxoid プロテアーゼトキソイド
prothrombin time プロトロンビン時間
ptaquiloside プタキロシド
pulmonary thrombosis 肺血栓症
pulmonary toilet 肺洗浄
pulmonary trunk 肺動脈幹
pulmonary tuberculosis 肺結核
pure tone 純音
pyramidal tract 錐体路

Pt
platinum 白金，プラチナ〈元素〉
psychoasthenia 精神衰弱

PT, pt
pint パイント〈単位〉

P

Pt, Pt., pt.
patient 患者

pt, pt.
part 部，部分
perstetur〈ラ〉＝continued 継続せよ《処》
point 点

PTA
pancreas transplantation alone 膵単独移植
parathyroid adenoma 上皮小体腺
percutaneous transluminal angioplasty 経皮経管血管形成術
peritonsillar abscess 扁桃周囲膿瘍
peri-tubal adhesion 卵管周囲癒着
peroxidase labeled antibody ペルオキシダーゼ標識抗体
persistent truncs arteriosus 総動脈管開存
phosphotransacetylase ホスホトランスアセチラーゼ
phosphotungstic acid リンタングステン酸

plasma thromboplastin antecedent　プラズマトロンボプラスチン前駆物質
posttraumatic amnesia　外傷後健忘
prior to admission　入院前(に)
prior to arrival　到着前に
prothrombin activity　プロトロンビン活性
pure tone average　純音平均聴力

PTAC
percutaneous transluminal aortic commissurotomy　経皮(経管)的大動脈弁切開(術)

pt.aequ.
partes aequales〈ラ〉　等分に《処》

PTAH
phosphotangstic acid hematoxylin　リンタングステン酸ヘマトキシリン

PTAP
purified toxoid aluminium phosphate　精製ジフテリアトキソイド

p tase, PTASE
phosphatase　ホスファターゼ

PTB
patellar tendon bearing (cast, orthosis, prosthesis)　膝蓋腱支持装置
patellar tendon bearing cuff suspension below-knee prosthesis　膝蓋腱荷重下腿義足
Posttraumatische Beschwerde〈独〉　頭部外傷後遺症
prior to birth　出生前に
prothrombin　プロトロンビン
pulmonary tuberculosis　肺結核

PTBA
percutaneous transluminal balloon angioplasty　経皮的バルーン血管形成(術)

PTBD
percutaneous transhepatic bile drainage　経皮経肝胆汁ドレナージ
percutaneous transhepatic biliary drainage　経皮経胆道ドレナージ
percutaneous transhepatic bladder drainage　経皮的経肝的胆嚢ドレナージ
percutaneous transluminal ballon dilatation　経皮的バルーン血管拡張(術)

PTBD-EF
percutaneous transhepatic biliary drainageenteric feeding　経皮経肝(的)胆道ドレナージ経腸栄養(法)

PTBE
pyretic tick-borne encephalitis　発熱性ダニ媒介脳炎

PTBS
posttraumatic brain syndrome 外傷後脳症候群

PTB type cast
patella tendon bearing type cast 膝蓋腱部荷重ギプス

PTC
peptichenio ペプチケニオ
percutaneous transhepatic cholangiography 経皮経肝的胆管造影(法)
phenylthiocarbamide フェニルチオカルバミド
phenylthiocarbamoyl フェニルチオカルバモイル
pheochromocytoma, thyroid carcinoma (syndrome) 褐色細胞腫・甲状腺癌(症候群)
plasma thromboplastin component プラズマトロンボプラスチン成分
prior to conception 受胎前に
propionylthiocholine プロピオニルチオコリン
prothrombin complex プロトロンビン複合体
pseudotumor cerebri 偽脳腫瘍

P & TC
Pharmacy and Therapeutics Committee 薬事委員会

PTCA
percutaneous transluminal coronary angioplasty 経皮経管冠(状)動脈形成(術)

PTCCD
percutaneous transhepatic cholecystodrainage 経皮経肝胆嚢ドレナージ

PTCCS
percutaneous transhepatic cholecystoscopy 経皮経肝胆嚢内視鏡

P

PTCD
percutaneous transhepatic cholangial〔cholangio〕drainage 経皮経肝胆道ドレナージ
plasma thromboplastin component deficiency プラズマトロンボプラスチン成分欠損

PTCL
peripheral T cell lymphoma 末梢T細胞型リンパ腫

PTCP
pseudothrombocytopenia 偽血小板減少症

PTCR
percutaneous transluminal coronary recanalization 経皮経管冠(状)動脈内血栓溶解療法
percutaneous transluminal coronary reperfusion 経皮経管冠(状)動脈再灌流

PTCRA
percutaneous transluminal coronary rotational atherectomy 経皮経管的冠(状)動脈回転式粥腫切除術
PTCS
percutaneous transhepatic cholangioscopy 経皮経肝(的)胆道内視鏡
percutaneous transhepatic choledochoscopy 経皮経肝胆道鏡
PTCSL
percutaneous transhepatic choledochoscopic lithotripsy 経皮経肝胆道鏡下胆石破砕術
PTD
permanent total disability 永続的全体障害
personality trait disorder 人格特性障害
prior to delivery 分娩前に
Ptd
phosphatidyl ホスファチジル
PtdCho
phosphatidylcholine ホスファチジルコリン
PtdEth
phosphatidylethanolamine ホスファチジルエタノールアミン
PtdIns
phosphatidylinosytol ホスファチジルイノシトール
PtdSer
phosphatidylserine ホスファチジルセリン
PTE
parathyroid extract 上皮小体抽出物
peritumoral edema 傍腫瘍浮腫
posttraumatic endophthalmitis 外傷後眼内炎
posttraumatic epilepsy 外傷後てんかん
pretibial edema 脛骨前浮腫
pulmonary thromboembolism 肺血栓塞栓症
PTED
pulmonary thromboembolic disease 肺血栓塞栓疾患
PTEG
percutaneous trans-esophageal gastro-tubing 経皮経食道胃管挿入術
PteGlu
pteroylglutamic acid プテロイルグルタミン酸
PteGlu7
pteroylheptaglutamic acid プテロイルヘプタグルタミン酸
PTEN
phosphatase and tensin homolog (deleted from chromosome 10) イノシトールリン脂質脱リン酸化触媒酵素，ピーテン

P

PTES
prothese tibiale a emboitage supracondylien 顆上ソケット下腿義足

PTF
plasma thromboplastin factor プラズマトロンボプラスチン因子
polyvinyl formal sponge ポリビニルホルマールスポンジ
post-tetanic facilitation テタヌス後促進
primary tissue failure 一次性組織損傷

PTF-D
plasma thromboplastin factor D 血漿トロンボプラスチン因子D

PTFE
polytetrafluoroethylene ポリテトラフルオロエチレン

PTFS
posttraumatic fibromyalgia syndrome 外傷後線維筋痛症

PTG
parathyroid gland 上皮小体
plethysmogram 指尖容積脈波
pneumatic tonography 気体眼圧計

PTGA
pteroyltriglutamic acid プテロイルトリグルタミン酸

PTGBD
percutaneous transhepatic gallbladder drainage 経皮経肝胆囊ドレナージ

ptgt
primary target 初目的

PT-GVHD
post-transfusion GVHD 輸血後移植片対宿主病

P

PTH
parathyroid hormone 副甲状腺ホルモン，上皮小体ホルモン
phenylthiohydantoin フェニルチオヒダントイン
post-transfusion hepatitis 輸血後肝炎
prior to hospitalization 入院前に
protionamide プロチオナミド

PTh
primary thrombocythemia 原発性血小板血症

Pth
pathology 病理学
pneumothorax 気胸

PTHBD
percutaneous transhepatic biliary drainage 経皮経肝(的)胆道ドレナージ

PTHC
percutaneous transhepatic cholangiography　経皮経肝(的)胆道造影(法)

PTH-C
C-terminal parathyroid hormone　C末端副甲状腺ホルモン

PTHL
permanent threshold hearing level　永久聴覚閾値

PTH-N
N-terminal parathyroid hormone　N末端副甲状腺ホルモン

PTHrP
parathyroid hormone related protein　副甲状腺ホルモン関連蛋白，上皮小体ホルモン関連蛋白

PTHS
parathyroid hormone secretion　副甲状腺ホルモン分泌，上皮小体ホルモン分泌

PTI
pancreatic trypsin inhibitor　膵トリプシン抑制因子
posterior tympanic isthmus　後鼓膜峡部

PTIC
paratolyl isopropyl carbonyl　パラトリルイソプロピルカルボニル

PT-INR
prothrombin time-international normalize ratio　プロトロンビン時間国際標準比〔値〕

PTK
phototherapeutic keratectomy　治療的角膜表層除去術
protein tyrosine kinase　蛋白(質)チロシンキナーゼ

PTL
perinatal telencephalic leukoencephalopathy　周産期終脳白質脳炎
pharyngotracheal lumen　咽頭気管腔
plasma thyroxin level　血漿チ〔サイ〕ロキシンレベル
posterior tricuspid leaflet　三尖弁後尖

PTLC
precipitation thin-layer chromatography　沈降薄層クロマトグラフィ

PTLD
post-transplant lymphoproliferative disease　移植後リンパ増殖性疾患

PTLS
parathormone-like substance　上皮小体ホルモン様物質

PTM
pentamycin　ペンタマイシン
phenyltrimethylammonium　フェニルトリメチルアンモニウム
physician's therapy mannual　医師の治療マニュアル

post-transfusion mononucleosis 輸血後単核症
post-traumatic meningitis 外傷後髄膜炎
pressure time per minute 圧時間/分

PTMA
phenyltrimethylammonium フェニルトリメチルアンモニウム
phospho-tungsto-molybdic acid リン・タングステン・モリブデン酸

PTMC
paratolyl methyl carbinol パラトリルメチルカルビノール
percutaneous transvenous mitral commissurotomy 経皮経静脈的僧帽弁交連切開術

PTMG
polytetramethyleneglycol ポリテトラメチレングリコール

PTN
pain transmission neuron 痛み伝達ニューロン
phenytoin フェニトイン
pyramidal tract neuron 錐体路ニューロン

PT-N-I
patient-nurse interaction 患者看護師関係

pTNM
post-surgical histopathological classification of TNM 術後病理組織学的分類

PTO
percutaneous obliteration 経皮経肝的食道静脈塞栓術
percutaneous transhepatic obliteration 経皮経肝的閉塞
percutaneous transhepatic obliteration of varices 経皮経肝的食道静脈瘤塞栓術
percutaneous transhepatic obstruction 経皮的経肝的塞栓術
please turn over 裏面〔次頁〕へ続く

PtOH
phosphatidic acid ホスファチジン酸

PTP
percutaneous transhepatic portography 経皮経肝的門脈造影(法)
phospholipid transfer protein リン脂質輸送蛋白
posterior tibial pulse 後脛骨動脈の拍動
post-tetanic potentiation 反復刺激後増強
post-transfusion purpura 輸血後紫斑病
press-through-pack 圧迫包装(=経口薬のパッケージの1つ)
protein tyrosine phosphatase チロシン脱リン酸化酵素

P

Ptp
transpulmonary pressure 経肺圧
PTPA
posterior thalamoperforating artery 後視床穿通動脈
PTPC
percutaneous transhepatic portal catheterization 経皮経肝門脈カテーテル挿入
PTPE
percutaneous transhepatic portal embolization 経皮経肝的門脈造影塞栓術
PTPI
percutaneous transhepatic intraportal infusion therapy 経皮経肝門脈内注入療法
posttraumatic pulmonary insufficiency 外傷後肺不全
PTPM
posttraumatic progressive myelopathy 外傷後進行性脊髄障害
PTPS
postthrombophlebitis syndrome 血栓後症候群
PTPVS
percutaneous transhepatic portal venous sampling 経皮経肝門脈血採取法
PTQ
Parent-Teacher Questionnaire 親・教師質問表
PTR
pan troglodyles〈ラ〉 チンパンジー
paratesticular rhabdomyosarcoma 傍精巣(睾丸)横紋筋肉腫
patellar tendon reflex 膝蓋腱反射
peripheral total resistance 末梢全抵抗
plasma-transfusion reaction 血漿輸血反応
platelet transfusion refractoriness 血小板輸血不応状態
PTr
porcine trypsin ブタトリプシン
PTRA
percutaneous transluminal renal angiography 経皮経管腎動脈造影
percutaneous transluminal renal angioplasty 経皮経管腎動脈形成術
P trx
pelvic traction 骨盤牽引
PTS
painful tonic seizure 有痛性強直性痙攣発作
patellar tendon supracondylar prosthesis 顆上ソケット下腿義足
permanent threshold shift 永久閾値移動

P

phosphotransferase system ホスホトランスフェラーゼ系
postthrombotic syndrome 血栓後症候群
posttraumatic syndrome 外傷後症候群
prosthese tibiale a emboiture supracondylienne〈仏〉 顆上はめ込み脛骨義足

PTS, pts
patients 患者

PTSA
postthymic T-lymphocyte antigen 成熟Tリンパ球特異抗原

PTSD
posttraumatic stress disorder (心的)外傷後ストレス障害

PTT
parenchymal transit time 実質内通過時間
partial thromboplastin time 部分トロンボプラスチン時間
particle transport time 粒子輸送時間
patellar tendon transfer 膝蓋腱移行術
photo-toxic therapy 光毒性治療法
platelet transfusion therapy 血小板輸血療法
posterior tibial transfer 後脛骨移行(術)
pulmonary transit time 肺通過時間

PTTH
prothoracicotropic hormone 前胸腺刺激ホルモン

PTU
phenylthiourea フェニルチオ尿素
propylthiouracil プロピルチオウラシル

PTUCA
percutaneous transluminal ultrasonic coronary angioplasty 経皮経管的超音波冠(状)動脈形成(術)

PTWI
provisional tolerable weekly intake 暫定的1週間許容摂取量

P

PTX
parathyroidectomy 副甲状腺摘出術
pentoxifylline メチルキサンチン(免疫抑制)
phototoxic 光毒の
pneumothorax 気胸

PTX, PTx
parathyroidectomy 上皮小体摘出

PTx, ptx, p.tx
pelvic traction 骨盤牽引

PTZ
pentetrazole ペンテトラゾール
pentylenetetrazol ペンチレンテトラゾール
phenothiazine フェノチアジン

PU
chorionic gonadotropin in pregnancy urine 妊娠尿中絨毛性ゴナドトロピン

pass urine 排尿する
paternal uncle 父方の叔父
pelviureteric 腎盂尿管(移行部)の
pepsin unit ペプシンユニット
peptic ulcer 消化性潰瘍
polyurethan ポリウレタン
power unit パワーユニット
pregnancy urine 妊娠尿
prostatic urethra 尿道前立腺部

Pu
plutonium プルトニウム〈元素〉
purple 紫
putrescine プトレシン

pu
putamen 被殻

pub
pubic 恥骨の
public 公衆の
published 発行された
publisher 発行者，出版社

PUBS
percutaneous umbilical blood sampling 経皮臍帯血採取
purple urine bag syndrome 紫色蓄尿バッグ症候群

PUD
peptic ulcer disease 消化性潰瘍疾患
pudendal 外陰部の

PUD，PuD，Pu D
pulmonary disease 肺疾患

PUE
polyurethan elastomers ポリウレタンエラストマー
pyrexia of unknown etiology 原因不明熱

puerp
puerperium 産褥

PUFA
polyunsaturated fatty acid 多不飽和脂肪酸

pug.
pugillus〈ラ〉 ひとつまみの《処》

PUH
pregnancy urine hormone 妊娠尿ホルモン

PUJ
pelviureteric junction 腎盂尿管移行部

Pul
pulmonary disease 肺疾患

pul
pulpitis 歯髄炎

P

pulvinar 視床枕

PUL, Pul, pul
pulmonary 肺の

PUL, pul
percutaneous ultrasonic lithotripsy 経皮的超音波砕石術

pul.gros.
pulvis grossus〈ラ〉 粗い粉末《処》

PULHEEMS
physical capacity, upper and lower limbs, hearing, eye sight, emotional capacity, mental stability 生理的許容量・上下肢・聴力・視力・感情的許容量・心的安定性

pul ins
pulmonary insufficiency 肺不全

PULM, pulm
pulmonary 肺の

PULM, pulm.
pulmentum〈ラ〉 薄い粥《処》

pul sten
pulmonary stenosis 肺動脈弁狭窄

pul.tenu.
pulvis tenuis〈ラ〉 細かい粉末《処》

pulv
pulverise 粉末化する

PULV, pulv.
pulveres〈ラ〉＝pulvis 粉末《処》

pulv.gros.
pulvis grossus〈ラ〉 粗い粉末《処》

pulv.subtil.
pulvis subtilis〈ラ〉 滑らかな粉末《処》

pulv.tenu.
pulvis tenuis〈ラ〉 細かい粉末《処》

PUN
plasma urea nitrogen 血漿尿素窒素

punct
puncture 穿刺する，穿刺

PUNL
percutaneous ultrasonic nephrolithotripsy 経皮的超音波腎砕石術

PUO
pyrexia of unknown origin 原因不明熱

Puo
purine nucleoside プリンヌクレオシド

PUPPP
pruritic urticarial papules and plaques of pregnancy 妊娠性瘙痒性蕁麻疹様丘疹兼局面症

PUR
polyurethane ポリウレタン
Pur
purine プリン
pur
purulent 化膿の
Pur., pur.
purus〈ラ〉 純粋な
P ura
urethral P 尿道圧
Pura max
maximal Pura 最大尿道圧
purg
purgativus 下剤
PUSC
pontine urine strage center 橋蓄尿中枢
PUT
putamen 被殻
Put
putrescine プトレッシン
PUVA
psoralen-ultraviolet A ソラレン長波長紫外線
PUV angle
posterior urethrovesical angle 後部尿道膀胱角
PV
pancreatic vein 膵静脈
papilloma virus 乳頭腫ウイルス
paraventricular (nucleus) 室傍(核)
paravertebral 脊髄傍の
pemphigus vulgaris 尋常性天疱瘡
peripheral vascular 末梢血管の
peripheral vascular plasma volume 末梢血管血漿量
peripheral vein 末梢静脈
peripheral venous 末梢静脈の
peripheral vessel 末梢血管
pinocytotic vesicle 飲小胞
plasma vaccine 血漿由来ワクチン
plasma viscosity 血漿粘稠度
plasma volume 血漿量
Plasmodium falciparum〈ラ〉 熱帯熱原虫
Plummer-Vinson syndrome プランマー・ビンソン症候群
pneumococcus vaccine 肺炎球菌ワクチン
Polenské value ポレンスケ価
poliovirus ポリオウイルス
polycythemia vera 真性赤血球増加(症)
polyoma virus ポリオーマウイルス

P

polyvinyl ポリビニル
portal vein 門脈
post vaccination〈ラ〉 予防接種後に
pulmonary valve 肺動脈弁（＝右房）
pulmonary vein 肺静脈

Pv
(episcleral) venous pressure （上強膜）静脈圧

pv.
parvus〈ラ〉 小さい

P & V
pyloroplasty & vagotomy 幽門形成術と迷走神経切断術

PV, p.v.
per vaginum〈ラ〉 経腟的に

PVA
polyvinyl acetate ポリ酢酸ビニル
polyvinyl alcohol ポリビニルアルコール

PVB
cisplatin (＝Platinol), vinblastine, bleomycin シスプラチン（＝プラチノール），ビンブラスチン，ブレオマイシン
paravertebral block 脊椎傍ブロック
premature ventricular beat 心室性期外収縮

PVC
polyvinyl chloride ポリ塩化ビニル
postvoiding cystogram 排尿後膀胱造影図
premature ventricular contraction 心室性期外収縮
primary visual cortex 一次視覚皮質
pulmonary venous congestion 肺静脈うっ血

PV_{CO_2}
venous carbon dioxide pressure 静脈二酸化炭素圧

P

PVD
peripheral vascular disease 末梢血管疾患
portal vein dilation 門脈拡張
posterior vitreous detachment 後部硝子体剥離
postvagotomy diarrhea 迷走神経切断後下痢
pulmonary vascular disease 肺血管疾患

PVDc
polyvinyl dichloride ポリ二塩化ビニル

PVDF
polyvinylidene difluoride ポリ二フッ化ビニリデン

PVDT
pertussis vaccine and diphtheria toxoid 百日咳ワクチン・ジフテリアトキソイド

PVE
perivenous encephalomyelitis 静脈周囲脳脊髄炎

periventricular cerebrospinal fluid edema 脳室周囲髄液浮腫
periventricular echodensity 脳室周囲の超音波輝度が高い所見
prosthetic valve endocarditis 人工弁心内膜炎

PVeg.
pemphigus vegetans〈ラ〉 増殖性天疱瘡

Pves
intravesical pressure 膀胱内圧

Pves max
maximal Pves 最大膀胱(内)圧

PVF
portal venous flow 門脈血流量
primary ventricular fibrillation 一次性心室細動
prostatovesicular fluid 前立腺精嚢腺液

PVG
pelvic venography 骨盤静脈造影(法)
pneumoventriculography 気(体)脳室造影(法)

PVH
periventricular hemorrhage 脳室周囲出血
periventricular high intensity 脳室周囲高信号域
pulmonary vascular hypertension 肺血管(性)高血圧(症)

PVI
peripheral vascular insufficiency 末梢血管不全
pressure-volume index 圧・容積係数

PVK
pyruvate kinase ピルビン酸キナーゼ

PVL
periventricular leucomalacia 脳室周囲性白質軟化症
periventricular lucency 脳室周囲低吸収域
purified vaccine lymph 精製痘苗

PVLA
poly-*N*-*p*-vinylbenzyl-lactone-amide ポリ-N-*p*-ビニルラクトンアミド

PVM
pneumonia virus of mice マウス肺炎ウイルス
polyvinylmethyl ether ポリビニルメチルエーテル
proteins, vitamins, minerals 蛋白・ビタミン・ミネラル

PVMed
Preventative Medicine 予防医学

PVN
paraventricular nucleus 室傍核
predictive value of negative test 陰性反応適中度

p.v.n.
per vias naturales〈ラ〉 自然の方法で

PVNS
pigmented villonodular synovitis　色素性絨毛結節性滑膜炎
pvnt
preventive　予防の
PVO
pulmonary venous obstruction (occlusion)　肺静脈閉塞(閉鎖)(症)
PVO_2
mixed venous O_2 pressure　混合静脈血酸素分圧
PvO_2
partial pressure of venous oxygen　静脈酸素分圧
PVOD
peripheral vascular occlusive disease　末梢血管閉塞性疾患
pulmonary vascular obstructive disease　肺血管閉塞(性)疾患
pulmonary veno-occlusive disease　肺静脈閉塞病
PVOV
pulmonic valve opening velocity　肺動脈弁開放速度
PVP
penicillin V potassium　ペニシリンVカリウム
peripheral vein plasma　末梢静脈血漿
peripheral venous pressure　末梢静脈圧
polyvinylpyrrolidone　ポリビニルピロリドン
predictive value of positive test　陽性反応適中度
pulmonary venous pressure　肺静脈圧
PVPC
pivampicillin　ピバンピシリン
PVP-I
povidone-iodine　ポビドンヨード
PVPNO
polyvinyl-pyridine-*N*-oxide　ポリビニルピリジン-*N*-オキシド
PVR
peripheral vascular resistance　末梢血管抵抗
polyomavirus receptor　ポリオーマウイルス受容体
pressure-volume relationship　圧・容積関係
proliferative vitreoretinopathy　増殖性硝子体網膜症
pulmonary valve replacement　肺動脈弁置換術
pulmonary vascular resistance　肺血管抵抗
PVRI
pulmonary vascular resistance index　肺血管抵抗指数
PVS
persistent vegitative state　持続性植物状態
persistent viral syndrome　遷延性(持続性)ウイルス症候群
pigmented villonodular synovitis　色素性絨毛結節性滑膜炎

P

Plummer-Vinson syndrome プランマー・ビンソン症候群
polio virus sensitivity ポリオウイルス感受性
polyvinyl sponge ポリビニルスポンジ
premature ventricular systole 心室性期外収縮
pulmonary vein stenosis 肺静脈狭窄
pulmonic valve stenosis 肺動脈弁狭窄(症)

PVSG
National Polycythemia Vera Study Group 国立真性多血症研究班

PV shunt, P-V shunt
peritoneo(-)venous shunt 腹腔静脈シャント術

PVT
paroxysmal ventricular tachycardia 発作性心室性頻拍(症)
picture vocabulary test 絵画語い発達検査(法)
portal vein thrombosis 門脈血栓症
pressure, volume, temperature 圧力・容積・温度

pvt
private 私的な

PVW
posterior vaginal wall 腟後壁

PW
peristaltic wave 蠕動波
plantar wart 足底疣
posterior wall 後壁
pregnant women 妊婦

pw
pinworms 蟯虫

p/w
parallel with ～と平行に

PW, P-W
Prader-Willi syndrome プラダー・ウィリ症候群

PWA
people with AIDS エイズ患者集団

PWB
partial weight bearing 部分荷重

PWBC
peripheral white blood cell 末梢白血球

PWBRT
prophylactic whole brain radiation therapy 予防的全脳照射療法

PWC
physical working capacity 身体的作業能力
posterior pharyngeal wall cancer 下咽頭後壁癌

PWD
precipitated withdrawal diarrhea 突発性(薬剤)中止下痢(症)

pwd
powder　粉末，散剤
PWE
posterior wall excursion　左心室後壁振幅
PWF
pregnancy without fear　不安のない妊娠
PWI
physiological workload index　生理的作業負荷指数
posterior wall infarct　後壁梗塞
PWLV
posterior wall of left ventricle　左(心)室後壁
PWM
pokeweed mitogen　アメリカヤマゴボウマイトジェン
pulse width modulation　パルス幅変調
Pwmax
maximal working pressure　最大作動圧
PWMI
posterior wall myocardial infarction　後壁心筋梗塞(症)
Pwmin
minimal working pressure　最低作動圧
PWP
pulmonary artery wedge pressure　肺動脈楔入圧
pwr
power　出力
PWS
port wine stain　火炎状母斑，ブドウ酒様血管腫
Prader-Willi syndrome　プラダー・ウィリ症候群
PWT
posterior wall thickness　後壁厚
PWV
posterior wall velocity　後壁速度
pulse wave velocity　脈波伝播速度
PX
pancreatectomized　膵切除された
peroxidase　ペルオキシダーゼ
px
prescription　処方箋
survival rate　生存率
PX，Px
past history　既往歴
physical examination　理学的検査
PX，Px，px
pneumothorax　気胸
prognosis　予後

P

PXA
pleomorphic xanthoastrocytoma 多形性黄色星状膠細胞腫
PXE
pseudoxanthoma elasticum 弾性線維偽黄色腫
PXin
time of arrival 到着時間
PXS
pseudoexfoliation syndrome 偽(性)剝脱(落屑)症候群
PY
person year 人・年
phosphorylated tyrosine リン酸化チロシン
Py
polyoma ポリオーマ
pyridoxal ピリドキサ(ー)ル
pyrimidine ピリミジン
PyC
pyogenic culture 化膿菌培養
Pyd
pyrimidine nucleoside ピリミジンヌクレオシド
PYG
proteose-yeast-glucose プロテオース・イースト・ブドウ糖(ブイヨン)
PYLL
potential years of life lost 潜在的余命損失年数，疾病障害により健康寿命を全うできなかった損失年数
PYP
^{99m}Tc-pyrophosphate テクネチウム99mピロリン酸塩
pyrophosphate ピロリン酸塩
pyph
polyphase 多相
PYR
pyramid 錐体
Pyr, pyr
pyridine ピリジン
pyrimidine ピリミジン
pyruvate ピルビン酸塩
Pyro
pyroglobulin パイログロブリン
pyrophosphate ピロリン酸塩
pyroglu
pyroglutamic acid ピログルタミン酸
PyrP
pyridoxal-5′-phosphate ピリドキサ(ー)ル-5′-リン酸

P

pysed
physical education 医学教育
PYY
peptide YY ペプチドYY
PZ
pancreozymin パンクレオザイミン
prazosin プラゾシン
proliferative zone 増殖帯
PZA
pyrazinamide ピラジナミド
PZC
perphenazine ペルフェナジン
PZ-CCK
pancreozymin-cholecystokinin パンクレオザイミン・コレシストキニン
PZD
partial zona dissection 透明帯開窓〔切開〕法
PZE
piezoelectric ピエゾ電気の
PZI
protamine zinc insulin プロタミン亜鉛インスリン
PZN
periportal zonal necrosis 門脈周囲帯壊死

Q q

Q

cardiac output	心拍出量
coulomb	クーロン
electric quantity	電気量
(urinary) flow rate	尿流量(率)
glutamine	グルタミン
quantitiy	量
quartile	4分割の
quaternary	4原始の，4級の，第4の
question	質問
quinacrine	キナクリン
quinidine	キニジン
quinoline	キノリン
quinone	キノン
quolity	品質
quotient	商，指数，係数
Q-wave	Q波《心電》

q

coefficient of association	協調指数《統》
long arm of a chromosome	染色体長腕
quick	早い

Q

quality factor	(放射線の)線質係数

Q_9

ubichromanol-9	ユビクロマノール9
ubichromenol-9	ユビクロメノール9

$\dot{Q}$

volume flow of blood/unit time	単位時間血(液)流量
volume of blood flow	血(液)流量

Q, q

quart	クォート〈単位〉
quarter	1/4

Q, q, q.

quadque〈ラ〉	～ごとに，おのおの《処》

Q6, Q_6

ubiquinone-6	ユビキノン-6

Q10, Q_{10}

ubiquinone-10	ユビキノン-10

QA

quality assurance	品質保証
quick acting	即効の
quisqualate	キスカル酸

Q & A
question and answer — 質疑応答

QAC
quantitative antiglobulin consumption — 抗グロブリン消費量
quaternary ammonium compound — 第4級アンモニウム化合物

q.a.d.
quaque altera die〈ラ〉＝every other day — 隔日《処》

QALY
quality adjusted life year(s) — QOL補正生存年

q.a.m.
quaque ante meridiem〈ラ〉＝every morning — 毎朝

Q angle
Quatrefage angle — カトルファージュ角

QAP
quality assurance program — 品質保証プログラム

QAP (treatment)
quinidine, atebrin and plasmochin — キニジン・アテブリン・プラスモチン治療，QAP治療

QAS
quality adjusted survival time — QOL補正生存期間
quality assurance standards — 品質保証基準

Q_B
total body clearance — 全身クリアランス

QB
whole blood — 全血

QBCA
quantitative buffy coat analysis — 定量的バフィコート分析

QBV
whole blood volume — 全血(液)量

QC
quality control — 品質管理

Qc
pulmonary capillary blood flow — 肺毛細管血流

QCA
quantitative coronary angiography — 定量的冠動脈造影(法)

QCD
quality control data — 品質管理データ

QCI
quality control information — 品質管理情報

QCL
quality control level — 品質管理水準

QCM
quartz crystal microbalance — 水晶微量天秤法

qcm
quadrat centimeter　平方センチメートル
QCPE
Quantum Chemistry Program Exchange　計算化学プログラム公表機関
QCT
quantitative computed tomography　定量的コンピュータ断層撮影(法)
q.d.
quater in die〈ラ〉=four times a day　1日4回《処》
Qd, q.d.
quaque die〈ラ〉=every day　毎日《処》
QDC
quality delivery cost　品質向上・納期厳守・原価削減
qdm
quadrat decimeter　平方デシメートル
QDR
quantitative digital radiography　定量的デジタルX線撮影(法)
q.d.s.
quater die sumendum〈ラ〉=to be taken four times a day　1日4回服用《処》
QDTA
quantitative differential thermal analysis　温度差解析
q.dx.
quantitas duplex〈ラ〉=a double quantity　2倍量《処》
q.e.d.
quod erat demonstrandum〈ラ〉　明らかになったもの
QEE
quadriceps extension exercise　大腿四頭筋伸展運動
q.e.f.
quod erat faciendum〈ラ〉　行われたもの
q.e.i.
quod erat inveniendum〈ラ〉　発見されたもの
Q-enzyme
1,4-α-glucan branching enzyme　1,4-α-グルカン分枝酵素
QF
query fever　謎の熱
quick freeze　急速冷凍
QFB
Querfingerbreit〈独〉　横指
Querfingerbreite〈独〉　横指幅
Q fever
(Australian) Q fever　(オーストラリア)Q熱

Q-fract
quick fraction 急速分画
q2h
quaque secunda hora〈ラ〉 2時間ごとに《処》
q3h
quaque tertia hora〈ラ〉 3時間ごとに《処》
QH, qh, q.h.
quaque hora〈ラ〉=every hour 1時間ごとに，毎時《処》
QH_2, Q-H_2
ubihydroquinone ユビヒドロキノン=ユビキノール
QHS, q.h.s.
quaque hora somni〈ラ〉=every hour of sleep, each bedtime 毎就寝時に
QI
QI interval 心電図Q波開始からI音節開始までの時間，QI時間
qid, q.i.d.
quater in die〈ラ〉=four times a day 1日4回《処》
qk
quick 速い
QL
quadrilateral 四辺形の
q.l.
quantum libet〈ラ〉=as much as you please 任意量，希望量，好きなだけ《処》
QLH
quality of life and health 生活と健康の質
QLT
quantitative leak test 定量的漏れ試験
qlty
quality 質
qm
quadrat meter 平方メートル
q.m.
quo mondo〈ラ〉 どのような様式で
Qm, q.m.
quaque mane〈ラ〉=every morning 毎朝《処》
Qmax
maximum urinary flow rate 最大尿流量(率)
qmm
quadrat millimeter 平方ミリメートル
Q-M sign
Quénu-Muret sign ケニュ・ミュレー徴候
qn
quotation 引用語句

Qn, q.n.
quaque nocte〈ラ〉=every night　毎夜《処》
QNB
3-quinuclidinyl benzilate　3-キヌクリジニルベンジレート
QNS
quantit(ativel)y not sufficient　量的に不十分，量不足
Qo, QO_2
oxygen consumption　酸素消費量
oxygen quotient　酸素消費率
QOCP
quality of clinical practice　臨床実地の質
QOD, q.o.d.
quaque (altera) die〈ラ〉=every other day　隔日，1日おきに《処》
QOL
quality of life　生活の質
QOPR
quality of pain relief　除痛の質
QOUH
quality of ulcer healing　潰瘍治癒の質
qour.
qourum〈ラ〉=of which　それの
QP
quasti-Pirquet reaction　定量的ピルケー皮内反応
Qp
pulmonary blood flow　肺血流量
q.p.
quantum placet〈ラ〉=as much as desired　任意量，適当量《処》
Q_{PA}
pulmonary arterial flow　肺動脈血流量
QPA
quantitative precipitin analysis　定量沈降分析
QPC
quality of patient care　患者ケアの質
Qpc
pulmonary capillary blood flow　肺毛細血管血流量
q.pl.
quantum placeat〈ラ〉=as much as you please　任意量，希望量，好きなだけ《処》
Qpm, q.p.m.
quaque post meridiem〈ラ〉=each evening　毎夕，毎午後

$\dot{Q}$p/$\dot{Q}$s，$\dot{Q}_P/\dot{Q}_S$
left-to-right shunt ratio　左右シャント比

qq
questionable　疑問のある
questionnaires　アンケート

q.q.
quaque〈ラ〉=each or every　おのおのの，すべての

q.q.d.
quaque quarta die〈ラ〉　4日目ごとに《処》

Qqh，q.q.h.
quaque quarta hora〈ラ〉=every fourth hour　4時間ごとに《処》

QQPR
quantitative and qualitative personal requirement　質的かつ量的個人要求

qq.4 ta hor
quaque quarta hora〈ラ〉=every fourth hour　4時間ごとに《処》

QR
qualification record　資格記録
quantum radiography　量子計数型X線撮影
quick reaction　速反応
quinaldine red　キナルジンレッド

qr
quarter　1/4
quarterly　年4回の，季刊誌

Q.R., q.r.
quantum rectum〈ラ〉　正しい定量《処》

QRDR
quinolone resistance determining regiones　キノロン耐性決定領域

Q

QRGA
quadruple residual gas analyzer　4倍残存気体分析器

QRI
qualitative requirements information　質的要求情報

QRS
initial ventricular complex　初期心室群

QRZ
Quaddelreaktionzeit〈独〉　膨疹反応時間
Quaddelresorptionszeit〈独〉　膨疹吸収時間

QS
QS interval〔pattern〕　QS幅，QS間隔《心電》
quiet sleep　静穏睡眠

$\dot{Q}$s
shunt flow　シャント血流量

q.s.
quantum sufficio, *quantum satis* 〈ラ〉＝a sufficient quantity — 十分量，適量《処》
q.s.ad
quantum satis ad (*de*)〈ラ〉＝to a sufficient quantity — 適量に，十分に《処》
QSAR
quantitative structure-antitumor activity relationship — 定量構造・抗腫瘍活性関係
QSPR
quantitative structure-property relationship — 定量的構造物性相関
$\dot{Q}s/\dot{Q}t$, $\dot{Q}_S/\dot{Q}_T$
right-to-left shunt ratio — 左右シャント比
QSS
quantitative sacroiliac scintigraphy — 定量的仙腸骨シンチグラフィ
Q's sign
Quant's sign — クワント徴候
Q-S test
Queckenstedt-Stookey test — クエッケンステット・ストーキー試験〔検査〕
q.suff.
quantum sufficio〈ラ〉＝as much as suffices — 適量，十分量《処》
QT
QT interval — QT時間《心電》
Queckenstedt test — クエッケンステット試験〔検査〕
Quick test — クイック試験〔検査〕
qt
quantitative — 定量的な
quantity — 量
quart — クォート〈単位〉
$\dot{Q}t$
cardiac output (per minute) — (分時)心拍出量
QTc
corrected QT interval — 補正QT時間
qtd
quartered — 4分(割)された
Q test
Queckenstedt test — クエッケンステット試験〔検査〕
qtnr
questionnaire — 質問事項，アンケート

qtr
quarter 1/4
qua
quadrate 正方形の
quadratus 腰方形筋
quad
quadrangle 四角形
quadriceps 大腿四頭筋
quadrilateral 四辺の
quadriplegic 四肢麻痺患者，四肢麻痺の
quadrip
quadriplegia 四肢麻痺
quadrupl.
quadruplicato〈ラ〉 4倍量に《処》
qual
qualification 資格
qualify 資質化
qualitative 定量的な，質的な
quality 質
qual.anal
qualtitative analysis 定性〔質的〕分析
quals
qualifying examinations 資格試験
qualifying tests 資格試験
quar
quarantine 検疫期間，検疫(所)
quar.pars
quarta pars〈ラ〉 1/4量《処》
quart
quarterly 年4回の，季刊誌
quat.
quater〈ラ〉 4回，4倍
quat.i.d.
quater in die〈ラ〉＝four times a day 1日4回《処》
quest
question 質問
QUF
Querfinger〈独〉 横指
QuF
Queensland fever クイーンズランド熱
qu in
square inch 平方インチ
quinq.
quinque〈ラ〉＝five 5(の)
quint.
quintus〈ラ〉＝fifth 第5の

quot.
quotidie〈ラ〉 毎日(の)
quotid.
quotidie〈ラ〉=daily 毎日の
quot.op.sit
quoties opus sit〈ラ〉=as often as necessary 必要に応じて
QUS
quantitative ultrasound 定量的超音波法
q.v.
quantum vis〈ラ〉=as much as you wish 任意量
quantum volueris〈ラ〉 適量《処》
QVT
quality verification test 品質確認試験
Qw, q.w.
every(=*quaque*〈ラ〉) week 毎週《処》
QWB
quality of well-being scale 健康な生活の質の標準尺度
QWL
quick weight loss 急速減量
q$_x$
mortality rate 死亡率

R r

R

arginine	アルギニン
Behnken unit	ベーンケン単位
drug-resistant plasmid	薬剤耐性プラスミド
gas constant	気体定数
organic radical	有機化合物の基
purine nucleoside	プリンヌクレオシド
race	人種
radioactive	放射線性の，放射能の
radioactive mineral	放射性無機物
radioactive range	放射活性域
radiologist	放射線専門医
radiology	放射線医学
rapid inactivator	迅速不活性型
rate	速度，量
reading	読むこと
real	実際の
Réaumur thermometer	レオミュール温度計
received	受理された
receptor	受容体
recessive	退縮の，劣性の
rechts〈独〉	右の
recruitment phenomenon	補充現象，リクルートメント
rectal	直腸の
rectum	直腸
red	赤(の)，レッド
reductase	リダクターゼ
regimen	規制，治療方式
Reiz〈独〉＝simulus	刺激
relapse	再発
relation	関係
remission	寛解，軽快
represser	抑制因子
resazurin	レサズリン
resectability	切除度
reserpine	レセルピン
resistance	抵抗，耐性
respiration	呼吸
respiratory	呼吸性の
respond	反応する
responder	反応物
response	応答，反応
rest	安静，静止する

resting	安静時の
restricted	制限された
reticulocyte	網赤血球
review	再調査，評論，レビュー
Rhipicephalus	コイタマダニ(属)
Rhizopus	クモノスカビ(属)
Rhus	ウルシ属
rhythm	周期，律動，リズム
rib	肋骨
Richtung	方向
right	右(の)
right eye	右眼
ring finger	環指
roentgen	レントゲン〈単位〉
roentgenologist	放射線学者
rough	粗造な，粗造性
rough colony	粗造型コロニー
routine	ルーチン
rub	摩擦
R wave	R波《心電》
side chain	側鎖

r

coefficient of statistical correlation	統計的相関係数
correlation coefficient	相関関係
radius	半径，橈骨
retard	遅滞する
retarded	遅滞した
ribosomal	リボゾームの
ring	輪
round	丸い
rule	法則

°R

Rankine (scale)	ランキン目盛〈単位〉
Rêaumur (temperature scale)	レ氏(温度目盛)，レオミュール(温度目盛)〈単位〉

R 0-3

resectability	癌切除判定

(R)

rectal	直腸の
right	右

®

resistered trademark	登録商標

R, r

racemic	ラセミ体の
rare	稀な
ratio	比，割合

recht〈独〉= right　右(の)
ribose　リボース

R, R.
Rickettsia　リケッチア(属)
Rinne test　リンネ試験
Rippe〈独〉　肋骨

R, r.
radix〈ラ〉= radical　根《化学》
ramus〈ラ〉　枝
recipe〈ラ〉= take　取れ，飲む，処方する《処》
remotum〈ラ〉　遠い，離れた，遠隔
residuum〈ラ〉= residue　残渣，残留物

RA
airway resistance　気道抵抗
radioactive　放射性の，放射能の
radioactivity　放射能
radionuclide angiography　放射性核種血管造影〔撮影〕法
ragweed antigen　ブタクサ抗原
rate of absorption　吸収速度
Raynaud's (phenomenon)　レイノー(現象)
refractory anemia　不応性貧血
refractory ascites　抗療性腹水
renal artery　腎動脈
renin activity　レニン活性
renin(-)angiotensin　レニン・アンジオテンシン
repeat action　反復作用
reperfusion arrhythmia　再灌流性不整脈
reserve alkaline　アルカリ予備
residual air　残気
retinoic acid　レチノイン酸
rheumatoid arthritis　関節リウマチ
right angle　直角
right atrium　右心房
right auricle　右心耳
Rokitansky-Aschoff (sinus)　ロキタンスキー・アショフ(洞)
room air　室内空気

Ra
radial　橈側の，半径の
radium　ラジウム〈元素〉
rectum above the peritoneal reflection　直腸上部癌

r & a
right and above　右上の

RAA
right acromion anterior (position) 第二横位第一分類(＝RScA)〈胎位〉
right aortic arch 右大動脈弓
RAA, R-A-A
renin(-)angiotensin(-)aldosterone レニン・アンジオテンシン・アルドステロン
RAAS
renin-angiotensin-aldosterone system レニン・アンジオテンシン・アルドステロン系
reticular ascending activating system 網様上行賦活系
RAAW
anterior wall of the right atrium 右房前壁
Rab.U
rabbit unit 家兎単位
RAC
radial artery catheter 橈骨動脈カテーテル
Recombinant DNA Advisory Committee 再結合DNA諮問委員会
Research Advisory Committee 基礎研究諮問委員会
right atrial contraction 右房収縮
rac
racemic ラセミ体の
RACAT
rapid acquisition computed axial tomography 急速撮影コンピュータ体軸断層撮影法
RAD
right atrial dimension 右心房径
right axis deviation 右軸偏位《心電》
roentgen administered dosage X線処理量
roentgen administered dose X線照射量
Rad
radiologist 放射線科医
radiology 放射線医学
radiotherapy 放射線治療
rad, rad.
radial 橈側の，橈骨の
radian ラジアン〈単位〉
radiate 放射する，照射する
radiation 照射
radiation absorbed dose ラド〈単位〉
radical 根《化学》
radicular 神経根の
radiculitis 神経根炎
radius 橈骨，半径
radix〈ラ〉＝root 根

RADA
radioactive 放射性の，放射能の
RADAR
risk assessment of drug-analysis and response レーダー運動
RAD-AR
Risk Benefit Assessment of Drugs Analysis and Response 薬の分析と反応の安全利益評価
RADAS
radiodetection and ranging 放射線の検知と照準
RADCA
right anterior descending coronary artery 右前下行冠(状)動脈
raddef
radiological defence 放射線学的防御
Rad Dx
radiological diagnosis 放射線学的診断
radhaz
radiological hazard 放射線学的障害
radi
radiological inspection 放射線学的視診
radiac
radioactivity-detection-indication-and-computation 放射活性・検出・適応・コンピュータ化
rad.imp
radium implant ラジウム埋没
RADIO
radiotherapy 放射線療法
radiog
radiography 放射線撮影
Radiol
radiologist 放射線専門医
radiology 放射線医学
RADISH
rheumatoid arthritis, diffuse idiopathic skeletal hyperostosis 慢性関節リウマチ・汎発性特発性骨増殖症
radl
radiological 放射線学の
RadLV
radiation leukemia virus 放射線白血病ウイルス
radmon
radiological monitor 放射線監視装置
radn
radiation 照射
rad op
radical operation 根治手術

RADS
reactive airway disease〔dysfunction〕 syndrome　反応性気道疾患〔障害〕症候群
rad/s
radians per second　ラジアン/秒
radsafe
radiological safety　放射線学的安全
RadSO
Radiological Survey officer　放射線調査管理者
rad ther
radiotherapy　放射線治療
RADWASTE
radioactive waste　放射性廃棄物
RAE
right atrial enlargement　右心房拡大
RaE
rabbit erythrocyte　ウサギ赤血球
RAEB
refractory anemia, erythroblastic　赤芽球性不応性貧血
refractory anemia with excess of blasts　芽球増多を伴った不応性貧血
RAEB-t
refractory anemia with excess of blasts in transformation　芽球増多を伴った不応性貧血の白血病化
RAEM
refractory anemia with an excess of myeloblasts　赤芽球増加型不応性貧血
RAF
rapid atrial fibrillation　急速心房細動
repetitive atrial firing　反復性心房興奮
rheumatoid arthritis factor　慢性関節リウマチ因子
ristocetin dependent platelet aggregating factor　リストセチン依存性血小板凝集因子
RAG
radioautogram　ラジオオートグラム
radioisotope angiography　ラジオアイソトープ血管造影法
ragweed　ブタクサ
renal arteriography　腎動脈造影
RAG-1
recombination activating gene-1　組換えアクチベーティング遺伝子1
ⅧR : AG, ⅧRAg, ⅧRAG
factor Ⅷ related antigen　第Ⅷ因子関連抗原

R

RAGE
receptor for advanced-glycation endproduct(s) 高脂血糖症二次産物受容体, AGEレセプター

RAH
regressing atypical histiocytosis 消退型異型組織球増殖(症)
retinal astrocytic hamartoma 網膜神経膠腫性過誤腫
right atrial hypertrophy 右心房肥大

RAHA
rheumatoid arthritis hemagglutination (test) 関節リウマチ凝集(試験)

RAHSA
radioactive human serum albumin 放射性ヒト血清アルブミン

RAI
radioactive interference 放射線活性干渉
radioactive iodine 放射性ヨード
radio-associated impotence 放射線によるインポテンツ

RAID
radioimmunodetection 免疫シンチグラム

RAIU
radioactive iodine uptake 放射性ヨード摂取率

RAL
right ventriculus-aorta-left atrium 心エコー検査のビームの方向

RALG
rabbit antilymphocyte globulin ウサギ抗リンパ球グロブリン

RALPH
renal-anal-lung-polydactyly-hamartoblastoma (syndrome) 腎・肛門・肺・外指・過誤芽腫(症候群)

RALS
remote after-loading system 遠隔操作式後充填方式
remote control after-loading radiotherapy system 遠隔制御式密封小線量治療システム

RALT
routine admisson laboratory test ルーチン入院時検査

R

RALV
rat leukemia virus ラット白血病ウイルス

RAM
random access memory 随時読出し可能メモリ《コン》
rapid alternating movements 急速変換運動
restricted access media 浸透制限充填剤

RAm
mean right atrial pressure 平均右房圧

RAMC
Royal Army Medical Corps 英国軍医団

RAMIg
rabbit anti-mouse immunoglobulin ウサギ抗マウス免疫グロブリン

ramont
radiological monitoring 放射線監視
RAMP
right atrial mean pressure 右心房平均圧
RaMS
radical multiple synovectomy 根治的多関節滑膜切除術
RAN
Resident's Admission Notes レジデント入会記録
ran
random 無作為の
RANA
rheumatoid arthritis-(associated) nuclear antigen 関節リウマチ(関連)核抗原
R-ANP
rat-atrial natriuretic peptide ラット心房性ナトリウム利尿ペプチド
RAO
right anterior oblique (position) 第1斜位，右前斜位
rotational acetabular osteotomy 臼蓋回転骨切り術
RAP
recurrent abdominal pain 再発性腹痛
rehabilitation activities profile リハビリテーション活動側面
renal artery pressure 腎動脈圧
retinal arterial pressure 網膜動脈圧
rheumatoid arthritis precipitate 関節リウマチ沈降素
right acromion posterior (position) 第二横位第二分類(＝RScA)〈胎位〉
right atrial pressure 右心房圧
rap
rapid 速い
rapport 親密
RAPA
radial artery pseudoaneurysm 橈骨動脈偽動脈瘤
rapamycin ラパマイシン
RAPD
random amplified polymorphic DNA 無作為増幅多形デオキシリボ核酸
RAPE
right atrial pressure elevation 右心房圧上昇
RAPM
refractory anemia with partial myeloblastosis 部分的骨髄芽球症を伴う不応性貧血
RAPP
radiologists, anesthesiologists, pathologists and psychiatrists 放射線学者・麻酔学者・病理学者・精神医学者

RAPs
Resident Assessment Protocols　レジデント評価調書
RAR
retinoic acid receptor　レチノイン酸受容体
rar
right arm reclining or recumbent　右側臥位
RARS
refractory anemia with ringed sideroblasts　環状鉄芽球性不応性貧血
RAS
recurrent aphthous stomatitis　再発性アフタ性口内炎
reflection absorption spectroscopy　反射吸収性分光
renal artery stenosis　腎動脈狭窄
renin-angiotensin system　レニン・アンジオテンシン系
reticular activating system　網様体賦活系
rheumatoid arthritis serum　関節リウマチ血清
Rokitansky-Ashoff sinus　ロキタンスキー・アショフ洞
ras.
rasurae〈ラ〉　削片《処》
RAST
radioallergosorbent test　放射アレルゲン吸着試験
RASV
recovered avian sarcoma virus　再生トリ肉腫ウイルス
RAT
repeat action tablet　反復作用錠
right anterior temporal　右側頭葉前部
right anterior thigh　右前下腿
rat
ratio　比
RATG
rabbit anti-human thymocyte globulin　家兎抗ヒトチモサイトグロブリン
RATx
radiation therapy　放射線療法
RAU
radioactive uptake　放射性ヨウ素摂取
recurrent aphthous ulcer　再発性アフタ性潰瘍
RAV
right atrial volume　右心房容積
Rous associated virus　ラウス関連ウイルス
RAW, Raw
airway resistance　気道抵抗
RB
rebreathing　再呼吸
residual body　残存体

R

respiratory bronchiole | 呼吸細気管支
restiform body | 索状体
reticulate body | 網様体
retinoblastoma | 網膜芽細胞腫
retrobulbar | 眼球後の，延髄後の
Riemenbügel〈独〉 | リーメンビューゲル，アブミバンド
right buttock | 右殿部

Rb
rectum below the peritoneal reflection | 下部直腸
rubidium | ルビジウム〈元素〉

RBA
relative binding activity | 相対的結合活性
relative binding affinity | 相対的結合能
rescue breathing apparatus | 救命呼吸維持装置
right basilar artery | 右脳底動脈
right brachial artery | 右上腕動脈
right brow anterior (position) | 右額前位，第二額位〈胎位〉
rose bengal antigen | ローズベンガル抗原

R-band
reverse-band | リバースバンド

RBAP
retinoblastoma associated protein | 網膜芽腫関連蛋白

RBAS
rostral basilar artery syndrome | 前脳底動脈症候群

rBB
right bundle branch | (心臓の)右脚

RBBB
right bundle branch block | 右脚ブロック

RBBsB
right bundle branch system block | 右脚ブロック

RBBX
right breast biopsy examination | 右乳房生検検査

RBC, rbc
red blood cell | 赤血球
red blood cell count | 赤血球数算定
red blood corpuscle | 赤血球

RBC-ADA
red blood cell adenosine deaminase | 赤血球アデノシンデアミナーゼ

RBCD
right border of cardiac dullness | 心濁音域右縁

RBC/P
red blood cell to plasma (ratio) | 赤血球/血漿比

R

RBCV
red blood cell volume 赤血球容積

RBD
rapid-eye-movement sleep behavior disorder レム睡眠時行動障害
right border of dullness 右濁音界

RBE
relative biological effect(iveness) 生物学的効果比

RBELET
relative biological effectiveness linear energy transfer 相対的生物学的効果直線エネルギー移送

RBF
renal blood flow 腎血流量

Rb Imp
rubber base impression ラバーベース印象

RBL
rat basophilic leukemia ラット好塩基球性白血病

RBMT
the Rivermead behavioral memory test リーバーミード行動記憶検査

RBN
retrobulbar neuritis 球後視神経炎

RBOW
rupture fo bag of waters 羊膜破裂，羊膜破水

RBP
retinolbinding protein レチノール結合蛋白
right brow posterior (position) 第二額位〈胎位〉

rBr
reddish brown 赤褐色

RBRF
Reproductive Biological Research Foundation 再生生物学的研究財団

RBRVS
Resource Based Relative Value Scale 財源に基づく相対価表

RBS
rice bran saccharide 米糠糖類
Rutherford backscattering spectroscopy ラザフォード後方散乱分光法

RbSA
rabbit serum albmin ウサギ血清アルブミン

RBT
right brow transverse (position) 第二額位〈胎位〉

RBW
relative biologische Wirksamkeit〈独〉 相対的生物学的効果

RC
radiocarpal 橈骨手根骨の

R

Raymond-Cestan (syndrome)	レイモン・セスタン(症候群)
rectal cancer	直腸癌
red (cell) casts	赤血球円柱
red cell	赤血球
red corpuscle	赤血球
Red Cross	赤十字
referred care	追跡治療
reflection coefficient	反射係数
resistance capacitance	抵抗静電容量
respiration ceases	呼吸停止
respiratory center	呼吸中枢
responder cells	反応細胞
response conditioned	反応状態
retention catheter	留置カテーテル
retrograde cystogram	逆行性膀胱造影
rib cage	胸郭
ristocetin	リストセチン
root canal	(歯)根管
Roussy-Cornil (syndrome)	ルーシー・コーニル(症候群)
routine cholecystectomy	ルーチン胆嚢摘出術

Rc

receptor	受容体

rc.

recenter〈ラ〉	新鮮な《処》
recipe〈ラ〉=take	取れ，(薬を)飲め，処方する《処》

RCA

radionuclide cerebral angiogram	放射性核種脳血管造影図
red cell adherence	赤血球付着
red cell agglutination	赤血球凝集
regulators of complement activation	補体制御系
right carotid artery	右頸動脈
right colic artery	右結腸動脈
right common carotid artery	右総頸動脈
right coronary artery	右冠(状)動脈

Rca, RCa

rectal cancer	直腸癌
rectal carcinoma	直腸癌

rCBF

regional cerebral blood flow	局所脳血流

rCBF study

regional cerebral blood flow study	局所脳血流量測定

rCBV

regional cerebral blood volume	局所脳血流量

RCC

Radiological Control Center	放射線管理センター

R

Rathke cleft cyst ラトケ嚢
renal cell carcinoma 腎細胞癌
right common carotid 右総頸(動脈)
right coronary cusp 右冠尖

RCCA
right common carotid artery 右総頸動脈

RCD
relative (area of) cardiac dullness 相対的心濁音界

RCDA
recurrent chronic dissecting aneurysm 再発性慢性解離性動脈瘤

RCDP
rhizomelic chondrodysplasia punctate 股関節点状骨端形成異常〔異形成〕

RCF
radial centrifugal force 放射状遠心力
relative centrifugal force 比較遠心力

RCG
radioelectrocardiogram 無線心電図
rheocardiogram レオカルジオグラム，心電気図

RCGP
Royal College of General Practitioners 王立一般医協会[英国]

RCI
radionuclide cerebral imaging 放射線同位元素大脳画像法

RCIA
red cell immune adherence 赤血球免疫付着

RCIR
red cell iron renewal 赤血球鉄交代

RCIRR
red cell iron renewal rate 赤血球鉄交代率

RCIT
red cell iron turnover 赤血球鉄交代

RCI-Ut
red cell iron utilization (rate) 赤血球鉄利用(率)

RCL
renal clearance 腎クリアランス

RCLAAT
red *cell-linked* antigen antiglobulin test 赤血球結合抗原抗グロブリン試験

RCM
reinforced clostridial medium 補強クロストリジウム培地
restrictive cardiomyopathy 拘束型心筋症
retinal capillary microaneurysum 網膜微細動脈瘤
right costal margin 右肋骨縁

Royal College of Midwives 英国王立助産師院
RCMRGl
regional cerebral metabolic rate of glucose 局所大脳ブドウ糖代謝率
RCMRO$_2$
regional cerebral metabolic rate of oxygen 局所大脳酸素代謝率
RCN
right caudate nucleus 右尾状核
Royal College of Nursing 英国王立看護院
RCNT
Registered Clinical Nurse Teacher 登録臨床看護教師
RCO
aliphatic acyl radical 脂肪族アシル基
RCOF
ristocetin cofactor リストセチン補助因子
RCP
riboflavin carrier protein リボフラビン担体蛋白
Royal College of Physicians 英国王立内科学院
RCR
relative consumption rate 相対消費率
respiratory control ratio 呼吸調節率
retrocardiac-room 心臓後間腔
RCRA
Resource Conservation and Recovery Act 廃棄物処理に関する法律
RCRC
recurrent colorectal cancer 再発性結腸直腸癌
rcrd
record 記録
RCS
rabbit aorta contracting substance ウサギ大動脈収縮物質
red cell suspension 赤血球浮遊
reticulum cell sarcoma 細網肉腫
right coronary sinus 右冠状静脈洞
Royal College of Surgeons 英国王立外科学会
RCS, R/CS
repeat cesarean section 再帝王切開
RC sign
red color sign 発赤徴候
RCT
radionuclide computed tomography ラジオヌクライドコンピュータトモグラフィ
randomized controlled trial 無作為(比較対照)試験
recirculation time 再循環時間
recycling time 再循環時間

R

red colloidal test　赤色コロイド試験
ristocetin　リストセチン
Rorschach content test　ロールシャッハ内容試験

rct.
rectificatus〈ラ〉　精留した《処》

rctss.
rectificatissim〈ラ〉　最もよく純化した《処》

RCU
recurrent calcium urolithiasis　再発性カルシウム尿石症
red cell iron utilization (rate)　赤血球鉄利用率
remote control unit　遠隔管理室
respiratory care unit　呼吸疾患集中治療部
retrocaval ureter　後大静脈尿管

RCV
radiological chest volume　X線的胸腔容量
red cell volume　赤血球容積

RD
nucleus reticularis dorsalis〈ラ〉　背側網様核
Raynaud disease　レイノー病
recessively inherited form of dystonia　劣性遺伝性ジストニー
recorder　記録者
Registered Dietician　正栄養士
reiter disease　ライター病
renal disease　腎疾患
Rénon-Delille (syndrome)　レノン・デリリュ(症候群)
respiratory disease　呼吸器疾患
response decline　RD現象，反応漸減
reticular dysgenesis　重症免疫不全
retina(l) detachment　網膜剝離
retinal dysplasia　網膜異常形成
Reye disease　ライ病
rheumatic disease　リウマチ性疾患
right deltoid　右三角筋
Riley-Day (syndrome)　ライリー・デイ(症候群)
rubber dam　ラバーダム《歯》

Rd
reading　読むこと

rd
round　丸い
rutherford　ラザフォード〈単位〉

R & D
research and development　研究と開発

RDA
recommended daily allowance　1日許容量
recommended dietary allowance　1日栄養所要量
Respiratory Disease Association　呼吸器疾患協会

right dorso-anterior position 右背前位
RdA
reading age 読書年齢
RDC
research diagnostic criteria 研究用診断基準
RDDP
RNA-dependent DNA polymerase RNA依存DNAポリメラーゼ
RDE
receptor destroying enzyme 受容体破壊酵素
RDEB
recessive dystrophic epidermolysis bullosa 劣性栄養障害性表皮水疱症
RDF
receptor destroying factor 受容体破壊因子
RDGF
retina-derived growth factor 網膜由来成長因子
RDH
ribitdehydrogenase リビット脱水素酵素
rd hd
round head 丸い頭
RDI
recommended daily intake 推奨1日摂取量
redistribution index 再分布指数
relative dose intensity 比較的薬剤強度
RDM
readmission 再入院
rDNA
ribosomal deoxyribonucleic acid リボゾームデオキシリボ核酸
RDO
Radiological Defense Office 放射線学的防御管理室〔管理者〕
RDOD
retinal detachment, oculus dexter 右眼網膜剝離
RDOS
retinal detachment, oculus sinister 左眼網膜剝離
RDP
right dorso-posterior position 右背後位
RDQ
respiratory disease questionnaire 呼吸器疾患質問表
RdQ
reading quotient 読字指数
RDR
reliability diagnostic report 診断報告信頼性
RDRV
rhesus diploid rabies vaccine アカゲザル2倍体細胞株使用狂犬病ワクチン

RDS
respiratory distress syndrome 呼吸困難症候群
reticuloendothelial depressing substance 細網内皮系抑制物質
RDT
regular dialysis treatment 規則的透析治療
RDTE
research, development test and evaluation 検査・発達試験と評価
RDVT
recurrent deep vein thrombosis 再発性深静脈血栓症
RDW
red (blood) cell distribution width 赤血球分布幅
rdy
ready 完了した
RDZ
radiation danger zone 照射危険域
RE
efferent arteriolar resistance 輸出血管抵抗
nucleus reuniens〈ラ〉 再結合核
racemic epinephrine ラセミ体エピネフリン
readmission 再入院
re-education 再教育
reflux esophagitis 逆流性食道炎
regional enteritis 限局性腸炎
renal excretion 腎臓排泄
reticuloendothelial 細網内皮の
reticuloendothelium 細網内皮
right ear 右耳
right eye 右眼
Re
reactance リアクタンス，感応抵抗
rhenium レニウム〈元素〉
re
regarding ～に関して
r/e
rate of (ex)change 交換率
R & E
reseach and education 研究と教育
R+E
round and equal 丸く等しい
RE, R.E.
radium emanation ラジウムエマナチオン
RE, R/E
rectal examination 直腸検査

react
reactance　リアクタンス，感応抵抗
reaction　反応

readm
readmission　再入院

REAL
Revised European-American Classification of Lymphoid Neoplasms　新しいリンパ系腫瘍の欧米分類

REAR
real ear aided response　実耳補聴器装用特性

REB
relative biological effectiveness　相対的生物学的効果比

REC
receptor　受容体

rec
receipt　処方，受領書
recessive　退縮の，劣性の
recipe　処方せよ《処》
recombinant　組換え型
recommend　推薦する
recommendation　推薦
recovery　回復
recur　再発する
recurrence　反復，再発
recurrent　反回の，再発性の

rec.
recens〈ラ〉=fresh, recent　新しい，最近の

rec, REC
record　記録

rec, Rec
recreation　リクリエイション

RECA
right external carotid artery　右外頸動脈

recA
recombinant protein A　遺伝子組換えプロテインA

recd
received　受け取った

recfss
rectificatissimus　最もよく精製した《処》

recg
radioelectrocardiograph　放射線心電図

re.ch
recheck　再びチェックする

Recip, recip.
recipient　受血者，被移植者

reciprocal　相反の，逆の，回帰の

RECIST

response evaluation criteria in solid tumors　固形癌の効果判定基準

recog

recognition　認識

recomm, Recomm

recommend　推薦する
recommendation　推薦

recond

recondition　修理
reconditioning　修理すること

reconstr

reconstruction　再建

recov

recover　回復する
recovery　回復

recr

receiver　受領者

rect, rect.

rectal　直腸の
rectificatus〈ラ〉=rectified　改訂した，矯正した
rectified　矯正
rectum　直腸
rectus muscle　直筋

recumb

recumbent　横臥の，臥床の

recur

recurrence　再発，反復
recurrent　再発(性)の，反回の

red

reduce　整復する，還元する
reduction　整復，還元

redig.in pulv.

redigatur in pulverem〈ラ〉　粉末にする《処》

red.in pulv., Red.in pulv.

reductus in pulverem〈ラ〉=reduced to powder　粉末にした，粉末にせよ《処》

REDOR

rotational echo double resonance　回転エコー二重共鳴

redox

reduction-oxidation　還元・酸化

redsh

reddish　赤い

REDY

recirculating dialysate system　循環吸着式透析液再生装置

REE
rare earth element 希土類元素
resting energy expenditure 安静時消費熱量，安静時エネルギー代謝量

re-ed
re-educate 再教育する
re-education 再教育

reeg
radioelectroencephalography 放射線脳波

re-eval
re-evaluate 再評価する
re-evaluation 再評価

re-ex
re-examination 再試験，再検査

REF
renal erythropoietic factor 腎性造血因子

ref
refer 依頼する，紹介する
reference 参照，文献
referred 依頼された，紹介された
reflex 反射
relief 救助，安心

ref.
referate〈ラ〉 抄録

ref.dent
referring dentist 委託歯科医

ref.doc
referring doctor 依頼医，紹介医

Ref.Dr
referring doctor 依頼医，紹介医

ref.ind
refractive index 屈折率

refl, refl.
reflect 後屈する，反射する
reflection 後屈，反射
reflex 反射

reFP
recombinant fusion protein 遺伝子組換え結合合成蛋白

ref.phys
referring physician 依頼医，紹介医

refr
refrigerator 冷蔵庫

refrig
refrigeration 冷蔵

REG
radioencephalogram 放射性気脳写図

R

radioencephalography 放射性脳写法
rheoencephalography 電流脳写法

Reg, reg, reg.
regarding ～に関して
region 部，部位
register 登録簿，名簿
registerd 登録した，登録された
registration 記載，登録
registry 登録
regular 規則的，規則的な

REGAP
ramus esophago-gastricus ascendens posterior 食道胃上向後枝

reg.cor.
regioni cordis〈ラ〉 心臓の《処》

regen
regenerate 再生する
regeneration 再生

reg.epigast.
regioni epigastricae〈ラ〉 胃窩

reg hepat
regioni hepatis〈ラ〉 肝臓の

reg.rhy
regular rhythm 規則的律動

regs
regions 範囲，領域
regulations 調節，規則

reg.umb.
regio umbilici〈ラ〉＝umbilical region 臍部

reg umbilic
regioni umbillici〈ラ〉 臍の

REH
renin essential hypertension レニン本態性高血圧(症)

R

Reha
rehabilitation リハビリテーション，社会復帰

Rehab, rehab, rehab.
rehabilitate 回復させる
rehabilitation リハビリテーション，社会復帰

rehabil
rehabilitation リハビリテーション，社会復帰

Rehabili
rehabilitation リハビリテーション，社会復帰

REI
renal excretory index　腎排泄係数
rifampicin, ethambutol, isoniazid　リファンピシン,エタンブトール,イソニアジド

REIC
Radiation Effect Information Center　照射効果情報局

REICK
rifampicin, ethambutol, isoniazid, cycloserine, kanamycin　リファンピシン,エタンブトール,イソニアジド,シクロセリン,カナマイシン

REIG
real ear insertion gain　実耳挿入利得

REIR
real ear insertion response　実耳挿入特性

reit.
reiteratur〈ラ〉　反復せよ，再調剤せよ《処》

REL
rate of energy loss　エネルギー消費率〔損失率〕

rel
related　関係した
relation　関係
relative　比較的な，近親の，相対的な
relatively　比較的に
relief　救助，安心

rel hum
relative humidity　相対湿度

reliq, reliq.
reliquus〈ラ〉＝remainder　残り，余り，残余《処》

REM
rapid eye movement　レム，急速眼球運動
reticular erythematous mucinosis　紅色網状ムチン沈着症

rem
remarks　注意，意見
removal　摘出，切除
remove　摘出する，切除する

rem.
remanentia〈ラ〉　残余《処》

REM, rem
roentgen equivalent man〔mammal〕　人体レントゲン線量当量，レム〈単位〉

remab
radiation equivalent manikin absorption　照射当量人体模型吸収

REMD
rapid eye movement (sleep) deprivation　レム睡眠欠損

remg
remaining 残っている
remit
remittent 弛張(性)の
remocon
remote controller 遠隔制御装置
REMP
rapid eye movement period 急速眼球運動期，レム期
REMS
rapid eye movement sleep レム睡眠，急速眼球運動睡眠
REM syndrome
reticular erythematous mucinosis syndrome 網状紅斑性ムチン沈着症候群
REN
renal 腎(臓)の
REOR
real ear occluded response 実耳閉鎖特性
reorg
reorganization 再器質化
reorganize 再器質化する
REO virus
respiratory enteric orphan virus レオウイルス，呼吸器・腸内オーファンウイルス
REP
rational-emotive psychotherapy 合理的・情動的精神療法
reactive eosinophilic pleuritis 反応性好酸球性胸膜炎
retrograde pyelogram 逆行性腎盂造影図
rifampicin リファンピシン
rep
repair 修理する
rep.
repetendum〈ラ〉=to be repeated 繰り返せ
REP, rep
roentgen equivalent physical レプ〈単位〉
REP, rep.
repetatur〈ラ〉=let it be repeated 反復せよ，再調剤せよ《処》
report 報告する
rep.dos.
repetatur dosis〈ラ〉 この量を反復せよ《処》
REPE
re-expansion pulmonary edema 再膨張性肺水腫
repetat.
repetatus〈ラ〉=repeated 繰り返した
repr
representative 代表的な，典型的な
reprint 再印刷，別刷

R

repro
reproduce 複製する
reproduction 複製

reps
repetitions 繰り返し

rep.sem.
repetatur semel〈ラ〉 もう一度繰り返せ《処》

rept
report 報告(する)

rept, rept.
repeat 繰り返す
repetatur〈ラ〉=let it be repeated 反復せよ，繰り返せ《処》

reptd
reported 報告した

Req
requisition 依頼箋《処》

req
request 要求(する)
require 要求する，必要な

RER
renal excretion rate 腎排泄率
replication error DNA複製エラー
respiratory exchange ratio 呼吸交換比
response error relationships 反応量と誤差の関係

rER, RER
rough(-surfaced) endoplasmic reticulum 粗面小胞体《電顕》

RERF
Radiation Effects Research Foundation 放射線影響研究所

RES
recovery evaluation system 機能回復評価システム《リハ》
recurrent erosion syndrome 再発性びらん症候群
respiratory emergency syndrome 呼吸救急症候群
reticuloendothelial system 網(状)内(皮)系，細網内皮系

ReS
reserpine レセルピン
re-suture 再縫合

Res, res
research 研究，調査
researcher 研究者
resect 切除する
resection 切除(術)
reserpine レセルピン
reserve 予備，保存(する)
residence 住居，居住

R

resident レジデント，研修医
residue 残留物，残渣
resistance 抵抗(性)，耐性
resistant 抵抗する
respiratory 呼吸の

resc
rescue 救出する

RESC, resc
resuscitation (救急)蘇生法，意識回復

RESCUE
remote emergency salvage and clean-up equipment 遠隔救急救助浄化設備

Resid vol, resid vol
residual volume 残気量

RESIM
patient simulator for resuscitation training 救急蘇生術訓練用患者シミュレータ
resuscitation simulator for treatment 救急蘇生用訓練シミュレーター

resis
resistance 抵抗(性)，耐性

resist
resistance 抵抗(性)，耐性

Res-N
residual nitrogen 残余窒素

RESP, Resp, resp, resp.
respectively それぞれ
respiration 呼吸，換気
respirator 人工呼吸器
respiratory 呼吸(性)の
respond 反応する
response 応答，反応
responsible 責任のある，反応のある

R

respir
respiration 呼吸，換気
respiratory 呼吸の，換気(の)

REST
Raynaud (phenomenon), esophageal (motor dysfunction), sclerodactly, and telangiectasia (syndrome) レイノー(現象)・食道(運動機能障害)・手指〔足指〕硬化・毛細血管拡張(症候群)
regressive electric shock therapy 逆行性電気ショック治療(法)
regressive electroshock treatment 逆行性電気ショック療法
reticulospinal tract 網様体脊髄路

rest
restrict 制限する
restricted 制限された

restriction　制限

Rest-N

rest nitrogen　残余窒素

resus

resuscitation　(救急)蘇生(法)

RET

rational emotive therapy　理性感情療法

Ret

reticulocyte　網(状)赤血球

ret

rad equivalent therapy　レット〈単位〉

retention　遺残，貯留

retina　網膜

retire　引退する

retired　引退した

return　戻る

RET，ret

retarded　遅滞した，遅延した

reticular　網様の，細網(状)の

retard

retardation　遅滞

retarded　遅滞した，遅延した

ret.cath

retention catheter　留置カテーテル

Ret.diab.

retinopathia diabetica〈ラ〉　糖尿病性網膜症

retic

reticulocyte　網(状)赤血球

retic count

reticulocyte count　網(状)赤血球算定

retic.ct

reticulocyte count　網(状)赤血球数

retics

reticulocytes　網(状)赤血球〈複数〉

retr，retr.

retract　収縮させる，後退させる

retractable　収縮させうる，後退させうる

retracted　収縮した，後退した

retraction　退縮，後退，収縮

Retro.

retroflexio uteri〈ラ〉　子宮後屈

retro

retrograde　逆行の，逆方向の

RETRO.

reverse transcripitase containing oncogenic (virus)　レトロウイルス，逆転写酵素をもつ癌ウイルス

retros
retrogrades 逆行性

REUR
real ear unaided response 実耳裸耳特性

REUS
rectal endoscopic ultrasonography 直腸内視鏡的超音波検査

REV, rev.
reticuloendotheliosis virus 細網内皮症ウイルス
reversal 逆転，反転
reverse 逆の
review 再調査，総説
review 逆転再生
revise 改訂する
revision 改訂
revolution 回転

rev ed
revised edition 改訂版

rev/min
revolutions per minute 回転/分

revocon
remote volume control 遠隔出力制御

Rev of Sym
review of symptoms 症状再調査，病状要約

Rev of Sys
review of systems 系統別再調査

REW
rewind 巻戻し

re-x
re-examination 再検査

Rezi
Rezidiv〈独〉 再発

rezid
rezidivierend〈独〉 再発の

RF
hormone-releasing factor ホルモン放出因子
rapid filling 急速充満期
recognition factor 認識因子
regurgitant fraction 逆流分画
regurgitant fragment 逆流分層
Reitman-Frankel method ライトマン・フランケル法
relative flow rate 比較的流量率
relative function (of the kidney) 相対的腎機能
releasing factor 放出因子
renal failure 腎不全
renal fraction 腎分画
replacement factor 置換因子

replicative form　(ウイルスの)複製型分子
resistance factor　耐性因子
respiratory failure　呼吸不全
respiratory frequency　呼吸頻度，呼吸数
reticular formation　網様体
retroflexed　後転の，反屈の
retroperitoneal fibromatosis　腹膜後線維腫症
reversing factor　逆因子
rheumatic fever　リウマチ熱
rheumatoid factor　リウマチ因子
riboflavin　リボフラビン
risk factor　危険因子
rosette forming　ロゼット形成の

Rf
rate of flow　移動率
rutherfordium　ラザホージウム〈元素〉

RF, rf
radiofrequency　高周波，放射線周波数

RF, R-F
right frontal　右前頭部

RFA
radiofrequency ablation therapy　ラジオ波焼灼療法
right femoral artery　右大腿動脈
right fronto-anterior position　右前頭前位

R factor
releasing factor　解離因子
resistance factor　耐性因子

RFC
radiofrequency current　高周波電流
retrograde femoral catheter　逆行性大腿カテーテル
right frontal craniotomy　右前頭開頭(術)
rosette-forming cell　ロゼット形成細胞

RfD
reference dose　参照量

RFFIT
rapid fluorescent focus inhibition test　急速螢光フォーカス抑制検査

RFFSH
releasing factor of follicle-stimulating hormone　卵胞刺激ホルモン放出因子

RFL
releasing factor of luteinizing (hormone)　黄体化ホルモン放出因子
right fronto-lateral　右前側面

RFLA
rheumatoid factor-like activity　リウマチ様因子活性

RFLC
resistant Friend leukemia cell 耐性フレンド白血病細胞
RFLP
restriction fragment length polymorphism 制限酵素切断片長多型性
RFLPs
restriction fragment length polymorphisms 限定破片長多形性
RFLS
rheumatoid factor-like substance リウマチ因子様物質
Rfm, RFM
rifampicin リファンピシン
rifampin リファンピン
R form
rough form ラフ型
RFP
rifampicin リファンピシン
rifampin リファンピン
right fronto-posterior 右前後方
RFp
right frontal pole 右前頭柱
RFR
refraction 屈折
reject failure rate 拒否失敗率
rfrd
referred 関連した
RFS
rapid frozen section 急速凍結切片
renal function study 腎機能検査
RFT
rat Friend tumor ラットフレンド腫瘍
right fronto-transverse 右前横方向
rosette formation test ロゼット形成試験
RFV
right femoral vein 右大腿静脈
RFW
rapid filling wave 急速充満波
RG
nucleus reticularis gigantocelluraris 〈ラ〉 巨細胞網様核
reading grade 読書学年
right gastric 右胃動脈
right gluteal 右殿筋の，右殿部の
right gluteus 右殿筋
R/G
red/green 赤/緑

RGA
right gastric artery　右胃動脈
RGAS
retained gastric antrum syndrome　幽門洞停留症候群
RGBMT
renal glomerular basement membrane thickness　腎糸球体基底膜疾患
RGC
radio-gas chromatography　放射線ガスクロマトグラフィ
retinal ganglial cells　網膜神経節細胞
retrograde giant contraction　逆行性強収縮
RGE
relative gas expansion　比較的気体膨脹
right gastroepiploic (artery)　右胃大網動脈
RGEA
right gastroepiploic artery　右胃大網動脈
RGG
rabbit gamma globulin　ウサギγグロブリン
RGH
rat growth hormone　ラット成長ホルモン
RGN
registered general nurse　一般正看護師
RGP
retrograde pyelogram　逆行性腎盂造影
rg tp
rough template　粗模型
RH
hormone-releasing hormone　ホルモン放出ホルモン
reactive hyperemia　反応性充血
recurrent herpes　再発性疱疹
redox potential　酸化還元単位
regional heparinization　局所ヘパリン化
regular heparin　通常ヘパリン
regulatory hormone　調節ホルモン
relative humidity　相対湿度
releasing hormone　放出ホルモン
retinal hemorrhage　網膜出血
rib hump　肋骨隆起
Richner-Hanhart (syndrome)　リッチナー・ハンハート(症候群)
right hand　右手
right handed　右利き
right hemisphere　右半球
right hepatic　右肝動脈
right hyperphoria　右上斜位

Rh
rhodium — ロジウム〈元素〉

rh
rheumatic — リウマチ性の

r/h
roentgens per hour — レントゲン/時間

Rh, Rh.
macacus rhesus〈ラ〉 — アカゲザル
Rhipicephalus — コイタマダニ(属)

rh, rh.
rale — ラ音

RHA
rheumatoid arthritis — 関節リウマチ
right hepatic artery — 右肝動脈

Rha
rhamnose — ラムノース

RhA.
rhinitis acuta〈ラ〉 — 急性鼻炎

Rh.aller.
rhinitis allergica〈ラ〉 — アレルギー性鼻炎

Rh.atr.
rhinitis atrophicans〈ラ〉 — 萎縮性鼻炎

RHB
Radiological Health Bulletin — 放射線健康公報
Regional Hospital Board — 地域病院委員会
right heart bypass — 右心バイパス

RHBV
right heart blood volume — 右心血液量

RHC
respiration has ceased — 呼吸停止
right heart catheterization — 右心カテーテル法
right hypochondrium — 右肋下部

Rh classes
Rhesus classes — Rh血液型の分類法

rhCNTF
recombinant human ciliary neurotrophic factor — 遺伝子組換型ヒト毛様体神経成長因子

RHCSA
Regional Hospitals Consultants and Specialist Association — 地域病院顧問・専門医協会

RHD
radioactive health data — 放射性健康データ
relative hepatic dullness — 相対的肝濁音界
rheumatic heart disease — リウマチ性心疾患
round heart disease — 球状心疾患

RhD
Rhesus (hemoloytic) disease — Rh(溶血性)疾患
Rh.DH
rheumatic disease of heart — リウマチ性心疾患
RHE
retinohepatoendocrinologic (syndrome) — 網膜肝内分泌(症候群)
rheo
rheostat — 加減抵抗器
rheol
rheological — 流動学の
rheology — 流動学
rheu fev
rheumatic fever — リウマチ熱
rheum
rheumatic — リウマチ性の
rheumatism — リウマチ
rheumatoid — リウマチ様の
RHF
right (sided) heart failure — 右心不全
Rh.F
rheumatic fever — リウマチ熱
Rh factor, Rh-factor
Rhesus (monkey) factor — Rh因子
Rh.gang.
rhinitis gangrenosa〈ラ〉 — 壊疽性鼻炎
rhG-CSF
recombinant human granulocyte colony-stimulating factor — 遺伝子組換え顆粒球コロニー刺激因子
r-hGH
recombinant human growth hormone — 遺伝子組換えヒト成長ホルモン
Rh.hyper.
rhinitis hypertrophica〈ラ〉 — 肥厚性鼻炎
Rhi
rhinology — 鼻科学
RhIG
Rhesus immune globulin — Rh免疫グロブリン
RhIGIV
Rh immune globulin intravenous — 静脈内Rh免疫グロブリン
rhIL
recombinant human interleukin — 遺伝子組換え型ヒトインターロイキン
Rhin
rhinologist — 鼻科専門医，鼻科医

rhin
rhinitis 鼻炎
rhino
rhinoplasty 鼻形成術，造鼻術
rhinol
rhinological 鼻科学の
rhinologist 鼻科学者
rhinology 鼻科学
rhiz
rhizoma〈ラ〉 根茎《処》
RHL
radiological health laboratory 放射線健康研究室
right hepatic lobe 肝右葉
rhm, Rhm
roentgen per hour per meter ラム〈単位〉
rhMCAF
recombinant human macrophage-monocyte chemotactic and activating factor ヒトマクロファージ走化性および活性化因子
RHO
Regional Hospital Office 地域病院事務局
rhom
rhombic 菱形の
rhomboid 偏菱形
RHPA
reverse hemolytic plaque assay 逆溶血斑測定
RHR
renal hypertensive rat 腎性高血圧ラット
r/hr
roentgens per hour レントゲン/時間
RHS
radial head subluxation 橈骨頭亜脱臼
reticulohistiocytary system 細網組織球系
right-hand side 右手側
Rh.s.
rhinitis simplex〈ラ〉 単純性鼻炎
Rh.s.a.
rhinitis sicca anterior〈ラ〉 乾性前鼻炎
RH syndrome
Ramsay Hunt syndrome ラムゼイ・ハント症候群
RH-TNF
recombinant human tumor necrosis factor ヒト遺伝子組換え型腫瘍壊死因子
Rhu
rheumatology リウマチ学

rHuEPO
recombinant human erythropoietin 遺伝子組換えヒトエリスロポエチン

RHV
right hepatic vein 右肝静脈

Rh.vas.
rhinitis vasomotorica〈ラ〉 血管運動神経性鼻炎

Rhz
Rhizobium 根瘤菌

RI
radio (active) isotope 放射性同位元素，ラジオアイソトープ
regular insulin レギュラーインスリン
respiratory illness 呼吸器疾患
respiratory index 呼吸係数
response increase RI現象，反応増加
ribosome リボゾーム
Röhrer's index ローレル指数

RIA
radioimmunoassay 放射線免疫測定法
reversible ischemic attack 可逆性虚血発作

RIB
riboflavin リボフラビン
right intermediate bronchus 右中間気管支幹(中幹)

rib
D-ribose D-リボース
ribose リボース

RIC
retroactive inhibition 遡及抑制
right internal carotid 右内頸(動脈)

RICA
reight internal carotid artery 右内頸動脈

RI-cisternography
radioisotope cisternography ラジオアイソトープ脳槽〔クモ膜下槽〕造影(法)

RICM
right intercostal margin 右肋骨間縁

RICS
right intercostal space 右肋間腔

RICU
respiratory intensive care unit 呼吸器疾患集中治療室

RID
radial immunodeficiency 放射性免疫不全
radial immunodiffusion 放射状免疫拡散(法)
radio-immunodiffusion 放射免疫拡散

RIE	
radioimmunoelectrophoresis	放射免疫電気泳動法
RIEP	
radio-immunoelectrophoresis	放射免疫電気泳動
rocket immunoelectrophoresis	ロケット免疫電気泳動法
RIF	
resistance inducing factor	抵抗誘発因子
rifampicin	リファンピシン
right iliac fossa	右腸骨窩
right index finger	右示指
rosette inhibition factor	ロゼット形成阻止遺伝子
RIFA	
radioiodinated fatty acid	放射性ヨウ素標識脂肪酸
RIFC	
rat intrinsic factor concentrate	ネズミ内因子濃縮物
RIFMA	
roentgen-isotope-fluorescent method of analysis	レントゲン同位元素螢光解析法
RIg	
rabies immune globulin	狂犬病免疫グロブリン
RI generator	
radioisotope generator	ラジオアイソトープジェネレータ
RIgH	
rabies immune globulin, human	ヒト狂犬病免疫グロブリン
RIH	
right inguinal hernia	右鼠径ヘルニア
RIHSA	
radioiodinated human serum albumin	放射性ヨウ素標識ヒト血清アルブミン(＝RISA)
RI lymphography	
radioisotope lymphography	ラジオアイソトープリンパ造影シンチグラフィ
RIM	
receiving inspection and maintenance	受容・観察・維持
RIMA	
reversible inhibitor of monoamine oxidase	モノアミン酸化酵素阻害薬
right internal mammary artery	右内胸動脈
RI myelography	
radioisotope myelography	ラジオアイソトープミエログラフィ
RIND	
reversible ischemic neurological deficit	可逆性〔回復性〕虚血性神経脱落〔傷害〕，リンド

reversible ischemic neurologic disability　可逆性虚血性神経障害

r in pulv, r.in pulv.

reductus in pulverem〈ラ〉=reduced to powder　粉末にした《処》

RIO

right inferior oblique　右下斜(筋)

RIOJ

recurrent intrahepatic obstructive jaundice　再発性肝内閉塞性黄疸

RIP

radio-immunoprecipitation　同位元素標識免疫沈降反応
radioimmunoprecipitin (test)　放射標識免疫沈降(試験)
reflex inhibiting posture　反射抑制肢位
renin-inhibitory peptide　レニン阻害ペプチド

RIPA

radioimmunoprecipitation　ラジオ免疫沈降法
ristocetin-induced platelet agglutination　血小板リストセチン凝集テスト

RIPS

Research Information Processing System　研究・情報処理組織

RIR

radioisotope renogram　レノグラム
right inferior rectus　右下直(筋)

RI renogram

radioisotope renogram　ラジオアイソトープレノグラム

RIS

radiographic imaging system　放射線画像システム
radioimmunoglobulin scintigraphy　放射性免疫グロブリンシンチグラフィ
radioimmunoscintigraphy　放射免疫シンチグラム
rapid immunofluorescence staining　急速免疫螢光染色法
resonance ionization spectroscopy　共鳴イオン化分光法

RISA

radio-immunosorbent assay　放射性免疫吸着分析
radioiodinated human serum albumin　放射性ヨウ素標識ヒト血清アルブミン

RIST

radioimmunosorbent test　放射免疫吸着試験

RIT

radioimmunoglobulin tehrapy　放射性免疫グロブリン療法
radioimmunotherapy　放射免疫治療
radioiodinated triolein　放射性ヨウ素標識トリオレイン

red cell iron turnover (rate) 赤血球鉄交換率
Rorschach Inkblot Test ロールシャッハ試験

RITA
randomized intervention treatment of angina リタ(＝急性心筋梗塞に関する大規模試験報告書)
right internal thoracic artery 右内胸動脈

RITC
rhodamine isothiocyanate ローダミンイソチオシアネート

RI therapy
radioisotope therapy 放射性同位元素療法

RITR
red cell iron turnover rate 赤血球鉄交替率

RIU
radioactive iodine uptake 放射性ヨウ素(甲状腺)摂取率
red cell utilization 赤血球利用率

RIVC
right inferior vena cava 右下大動脈

RIVD
ruptured intervertebral disc 椎間板ヘルニア

RI venography
radioisotope venography ラジオアイソトープ静脈造影法

RI ventriculography
radioisotope ventriculography ラジオアイソトープ脳室造影法

RI virus
respiratory-illness virus 呼吸器疾患起因ウイルス

RIVS
ruptured interventricular septum 心室中隔破裂

RK
anterior radial keratotomy 角膜放射状切開術
rabbit kidney ウサギ腎臓
radial keratotomy 放射状角膜切開
Rektum Krebs〈独〉 直腸癌
right kidney 右腎

RKH
Rokitansky-Küster-Hauser (syndrome) ロキタンスキー・キュスター・ハウザー(症候群)

RKM
rokitamycin ロキタマイシン

RKY
roentgen kymography エックス線動態撮影法

RL
coarse rales 粗大水泡性ラ音
lateral reticular nucleus 外側網様核

reduction level 還元値，減衰水準
Rekurrenslähmung〈独〉 反回神経麻痺
right lateral 右外側の
right leg 右脚
right lower 右下の
right lung 右肺
Ringer's lactate 乳酸リンゲル液
Roussy-Lévy (syndrome) ルシー・レヴィ(症候群)
total lung resistance 全肺抵抗

Rl
medium rales 中水泡性ラ音

rl
fine rales 細水泡性ラ音

RL_1
few fine rales 少数の小水泡性ラ音

RL_2
moderate number of medium rales 中等量の中水泡性ラ音

RL_3
many coarse rales 多数の粗(大)水泡性ラ音

R/L
right/left 右/左

R & L
right and left 右と左の

R-L
Rechts-Links (Störung)〈独〉 左右(障害)

R-L, R→L
right-left 右から左へ
right to left 右から左へ

RLBCD
right lower border of cardiac dullness 心濁音界右下縁

RLD
related living donor 血縁臓器提供者
retrolabyrinthine deafness 後迷路性難聴
ruptured lumbar disk 腰椎間板ヘルニア

RLE
right lower extremity 右下肢

RLF
replication licensing factor DNA複製ライセンス因子
retained lung fluid 停留肺液
retrolental fibroplasia 水晶体後部線維増殖症
retrolenticular fibroplasia 後水晶体線維形成症
right lateral femoral 右外側大腿の

RLGS
restriction landmark genomic scanning 制限目標遺伝子解析法

RLH
reactive lymphoreticular hyperplasia 反応性リンパ細網細胞増生
RLL
right liver lobe 右肝葉
right lower limb 右下肢
right lower lobe 右下葉
RLLB
right long-leg brace 右長脚副木
RLMD
rat liver mitochondria ラット肝ミトコンドリア
RLN
recurrent laryngeal nerve 反回神経
RLND
regional lymph node dissection 局所リンパ節摘除(術)
retroperitoneal lymph node dissection 後腹膜リンパ節摘除(術)
RLP
remnant-like particles レムナント様リポ蛋白
ribosome-like particle リボゾーム様粒子
RLP-C
remnant lipoprotein cholesterol レムナント様リポ蛋白コレステロール
RLQ
right lower quadrant 右下部1/4区，右下腹部
RLR
right lateral rectus (muscle) 右外直(筋)
RLS
a person who finds difficulty in pronouncing sounds of "R,L,S" 「アール」「エル」「エス」の発語障害者
Reizleitungssystem〈独〉 刺激伝導系
reproductive laparoscopic surgery 生殖(器)の腹腔鏡手術
restless leg syndrome 不穏下肢症候群
Roussy-Levy syndrome ルシー・レヴィ症候群
RLSB
right lower scapular border 右下肩甲骨縁
rl-sh
right-left shunt 右左シャント
R-L Störung
Rechts-Links Störung〈独〉 左右傷害
RLT
reduced liver transplant 縮小肝移植
right lateral thigh 右外側大腿
rltv
relative 相対的
rlv
relieve 安心させる

RLX
right lower extremity 右下肢

RM
radical mastectomy 根治的乳房切断術
ramus marginalis 縁枝
range of motion 可動域
range of movement 可動域
red marrow 赤色骨髄
repetition maximum 反復最大負荷
resistive movement 抵抗運動
respiratory metabolism 呼吸代謝
respiratory movement 呼吸運動
resting metabolism 安静時代謝量
right median 右正中(神経)
Rosenthal-Melkersson (syndrome) ローゼンタール・メルカーソン(症候群)
Rothmann-Makai (syndrome) ロスマン・マケイ(症候群)
rough surfaced microsome 粗面小胞体《電顕》
Rückenmark〈独〉 脊髄

Rm
remission 寛解，軽快

rm
room 部屋，室

r & m
report and memoranda 報告とメモ

RMA
right mentum anterior (position) 第一顔位〈胎位〉

RMAG
rhino-maxillo-aerodynamic-gram 鼻腔・上顎洞気流動態図

Rmax
maximum removal rate 最大除去率

RMB
right main-stem bronchus 右主気管支

RMBF
regional myocardial blood flow 局所心筋血流量

RMC
reflex micturition contraction 反射性排尿収縮
right middle cerebral (artery) 右中大脳(動脈)

RMCA
right middle cerebral artery 右中大脳動脈

RMCAT
right middle cerebral artery thrombosis 右中大脳動脈血栓症

RMD
retromanubrial dullness 後胸骨柄部濁音

R-meter
roentgen-meter レントゲンメーター
r meter, r-meter
radiation meter 放射線量測定器
rate meter 線量率計
RMF
right middle finger 右中指
Rmin
minimum P(＝Pves/Qmax2) 最小抵抗(＝膀胱内圧/最大尿流量２)
RMK
rhesus monkey kidney アカゲザル腎臓
RML
radiation myeloid leukemia 放射性骨髄性白血病
right mediolateral 右中側方
right middle lobe 右中葉
RMLB
right middle lobe bronchus 右中葉気管支
RMLS
right middle lobe syndrome (肺の)右中葉症候群
RMN
Registered Mental Nurse 精神病正看護師
rolling mouse Nagoya 名古屋運動失調性マウス
RMO
regional (of) medical officer 地域医療官，地区検疫官
RMP
resting membrane potential 安静時膜電位
rifampin リファンピン
right mentum posterior (position) 第一顔位(＝頤部後方)〈胎位〉
RMR
relative metabolic rate エネルギー代謝率
right medial rectus (muscle) 右内直(筋)
RMR muscle
right medial rectus muscle 右内直筋
RMS
repetitive motion syndrome 反復運動症候群
rhabdomyosarcoma 横紋筋肉腫
rheumatic mitral stenosis リウマチ性僧帽弁狭窄症
root mean square 実効値
RMSF
Rocky Mountain spotted fever ロッキー山紅斑熱
RMT
right mentum transverse (position) 第一顔位〈胎位〉
right middle temporal 右側頭中部
RMTC
rhesus monkey tissue culture アカゲザル組織培養

R

rmte
remote 遠隔の
RMU
remote maneuvering unit 遠隔操作室
RMV
Reichert-Meissl's value ライヘルト・マイスル価
respiratory minute volume 分時呼吸量
RN
radioactive nuclide 放射性核種
radionuclide 放射性核種
red nucleus 赤核
reflux nephropathy 逆流性腎症
registered nurse (米国の)正看護師
residual nitrogen 残余窒素
Rn
radon ラドン〈元素〉
RNA
radionuclide angiography 放射性核種血管造影
ribonucleic acid リボ核酸
RNAA
radiochemical neutron activation analysis 中性子放射化学分析法
RNAP
RNA polymerase RNA合成酵素
RNase
ribonuclease RNA分解酵素
RND
radical neck dissection 頸部郭清術
reactive neurotic depression 反応性神経性うつ病
retroperitoneal node dissection 後腹膜リンパ節郭清
RNL
regional lymph node 局所リンパ節
RNLC
regional lymph node cell 局所リンパ節細胞
RNMS
Registered Nurse for Mentally Subnormal 精神障害者のため正看護師
RNP
reccurent nerve paralysis 反回神経麻痺
ribonucleic protein リボ核蛋白
ribonucleoprotein リボ核蛋白質
RNP antibody
ribonucleoprotein antibody 抗RNP抗体
RNS
radionuclide scintigraphy 放射核シンチグラフィ
reflex neurovascular syndrome 反射性神経血管症候群

Rnt
roentgenologist 放射線学者，X線専門医
roentgenology 放射線医学，X線医学
RNV
radionuclide venography RI静脈造影
RO
reddish orange 赤橙色
reverse osmosis 逆浸透
right occipital 右後頭部
right occiput 右後頭部
right orifice 右口
routine order 常規の指示
R-O
right occipital 右後頭部
RO, R/O
rule out 除外
ROA
right occiput anterior (position) 第二頭位第一分類〈胎位〉
vibrational Raman optical activity ラマン散乱光の円偏光二色性
ROAD
reversible obstructive airway disease 可逆性閉塞正気道疾患
rob
robertosonian translocation ロバートソン転座
ROC
receptor operated channel 受容体作用チャンネル
resident on call 当直〔待機〕レジデント
ROD
renal osteodystrophy 腎性骨異栄養症
ROE
roentgen レントゲン
ROEF
regional oxygen extraction fraction 局所酸素摂取率
Roent
roentgenologist 放射線学者
Roent, roent
roentgen レントゲン
roentogenology X線医学
r of s
review of systems 系統別再調査
ROI
region of interest 関心部分〔領域〕
ROIH
right oblique inguinal hernia 右斜蝋径ヘルニア
ROL
right occipito-lateral 右後頭側面

ROLC
radiographically occult lung cancer　X線写真オカルト肺癌
ROM
range of motion　関節可動域
read only memory　読出し専用メモリ《コン》
right otitis media　右中耳炎
rupture of membranes　破膜，破水
Rom
Romberg (sign)　ロンベルグ(徴候)
Romb
Romberg (sign)　ロンベルグ(徴候)
ROME
range of motion exercise　(関節)可動域訓練
ROMI
rule out myocardial infarction　心筋梗塞を除外する
ROMSA
right otitis media, suppurative, acute　急性化膿性右中耳炎
ROMSC
right otitis media, suppurative, chronic　慢性化膿性右中耳炎
ROMT，ROM-T
range of motion test　(関節)可動域テスト
ROM WNL
range of motion within nomal limits　可動域正常範囲内
ROP
retinopathy of prematurity　未熟児網膜症
right oblique projection　第一斜位
right occiput posterior (position)　第二頭位第二分類〈胎位〉
Ror
Rorschach (test)　ロールシャッハ(検査)
ROS
review of symptoms　症状再調査
review of systems　系統別再調査
Rosenzweig-PF-Test
Rosenzweig-Picture-Frustration-Test〈独〉　ローゼンツバイク絵画フラストレーションテスト
ROSG
reduced sized orthotopic segmental graft　縮小有茎分節移植片
ROSS
review of subjective symptoms　主観的症状再調査
ROT
remedial occupational therapy　矯正的職業療法
right occiput transverse (position)　第二頭位第二分類〈胎位〉
rule of thumb　経験法則，実験的なやり方

rot, rot.
rotary 回転の
rotate 回転する
rotation 回転，回旋
rotator 回転筋，回旋筋
rot.ny
rotatory nystagmus 回転眼振
rot.nystag
rotatory nystagmus 回転眼振
rotoscol
rotoscoliosos 回転側彎症
rou
rat ovarian unit ラット卵巣単位
rout
routine ルーチン
ROW
rat ovarian weight method ラット卵巣重量法
Rendu-Osler-Weber (syndrome) ランデュ・オースラー・ウェーバー(症候群)
RP
Raynaud phenomenon レイノー現象
reactive protein 反応性蛋白
readiness potential 準備電位
rectal prolapse 直腸脱
red pulp 赤脾髄
refractory period 不応期
relapsing polychondritis 再発性多発性軟骨炎
reporter 報告者
reserpine レセルピン
respirations 呼吸
respiratory rate : pulse rate (index) 呼吸回数：脈拍数(係数)
resting potential 静止電位
restorative proctocolectomy 機能温存直腸結腸切除
rest pain 休息痛
retinitis pigmentosa 色素性網膜炎
retinitis proliferans 増殖性網膜炎
retrograde pyelography 逆行性腎盂造影法
retroperitoneal 後腹膜の
reverse phase 逆相
reverting postmitotics 復帰的分裂終了期
rheumatoid polyarthritis リウマチ様多発(性)関節炎
right parietal 右頭頂部
Rp
pulmonary resistance 肺抵抗
Rezept〈独〉=prescription 処方(箋)，投薬

Rp.
recipe〈ラ〉 処方，処方せよ《処》

R5P
ribose-5-phosphate リボース-5-リン酸
ribulose-5-phosphate リブロース-5-リン酸〔五炭糖〕

R-P
right parietal 右頭頂部

RPA
reverse passive Arthus 逆受動アルツス反応
right pulmonary artery 右肺動脈

RPC
radial peripapillary capillaries 放射状乳頭周囲毛細血管
Radiological Pathological Conference 放射線学的病理学的討論会
recurrent pyogenic cholangiohepatitis 再発性化膿性胆管肝炎
relapsing polychondritis 再発性多発性軟骨炎
remote position control 遠隔位置制御
resident peritoneal cells 腹腔常在細胞
riverse-phase chromatography 逆相クロマトグラフィ

RPCA
reverse passive cutaneous anaphylaxis 逆受身皮膚アナフィラキシー

RPCF test
Reiter (protein complement fixation) test ライター(株蛋白補体結合)試験

RPCGN
rapidly progreesive crescenting glomerulonephritis 急性進行性半月体形成性糸球体腎炎

RPD
retinal pigmentary degeneration 網膜色素変性症

RPE
rating of perceived exertion 知覚度
recurrent pulmonary emboli 再発性肺塞栓
retinal pigment epithelium 網膜色素上皮

RPF
relaxed pelvic floor 弛緩骨盤底部
renal plasma flow 腎血漿流量
retroperitoneal fibrosis 腹膜後線維症

RPG
radiation protection guide 放射線防護基準
retrograde pyelogram 逆行性腎盂造影図

RPGN
rapid(ly) progressive glomerulonephritis 急速進行性糸球体腎炎

Rph
alkali reserve 予備アルカリ

RPHA
reversed passive hemagglutination 逆受身血球凝集反応
RPI
reticulocyte production index 網状赤血球産生指数
RP index
respiratory pulse index 呼吸脈拍比
respiratory (rate)/pulse (rate) index 呼吸(数)/脈拍(数)指数
RPL
radiation physics laboratory 放射線物理学研究室
retropharyngeal lymph node 咽頭後壁リンパ節
RPL-12
infectious lymphoid neoplasma 感染性リンパ様新生物
RPLA
reversed passive latex hemagglutination 逆受身ラテックス血球凝集
RPLND
retroperitoneal lymph node dissection 後腹膜リンパ節郭清
RPM
rapamycin ラパマイシン
retropulsive-petit-mal 背屈小発作
rpm, RPM
revolutions per minute 分時回転数
rotations per minute 1分間回転数
RPN1
ribophorin 1 リボホリン1
RPO
right posterior oblique 右後斜位，前後方向第二斜位
RPP
radical perineal prostatectomy 根治的会陰式前立腺切除(術)
rate-pressure product 圧掛け算値を指標とする数値
reflection photoelectric plethysmograph 反射光電式プレチスモグラフ
retrograde pneumopyelography 逆行性気体腎盂造影法
retropubic prostatectomy 恥骨後前立腺摘出術
Rorschach psychodiagnostic plates ロールシャッハテスト
RPPE
research, program, planning, evaluation 研究・企画・計画・評価
RPR
radius periost reflex 橈骨骨膜反射
rapid plasma reagin (test) 迅速血漿レアギン(テスト)
RPr
retinitis proliferans 増殖性網膜炎
RPRCT
rapid plasma reagin card test 迅速血漿レアギンカードテスト，RPRカードテスト

RPRS
Rorschach prognostic rating scale ロールシャッハ予後評価尺度
Rp/Rs
resistance of PA/resistance of system 体肺抵抗比
RPS
renal pressor substance 腎昇圧物質
RPS, rps, r.p.s.
revolutions per second 毎秒回転数
rounds per second 毎秒回転数
RPSGR
Royal Pharmaceutical Society of Great Britain ロイヤル薬剤師会
RPT
refractory period of transmission 伝達不応期
registered physical technician 公認〔登録〕理学療法士
right posterior temporal 右側頭後部
rotatory pattern test 回転パターンテスト
Rpt
report 報告書, レポート
Rpt, rpt
repeat 繰り返す
RPTA
renal percutaneous transluminal angioplasty 腎経皮経管動脈形成(術)
RPTC
regional poisoning treatment center 地域中毒治療センター
RPTD
ruptured 破裂した
ptd
repeated 繰り返した
reported 報告した
RPU
retropubic urethropexy 恥骨後尿道固定術
RPV
right portal vein 右門脈
right pulmonary vein 右肺静脈
RPVP
right posterior ventricular pre-excitation 右後心室早期興奮症
RQ
respiratory quotient 呼吸商
Rq
residual quotient 残遺指数
RQ, R.Q.
recovery quotient 回復指数

R

RQL
rejectable quality level　限界品質
rqmt
requirement　要求
rqr
require　要求する
requirement　要求
RR
radiation response　放射線効果
recovery room　回復室
relative response　相対的反応
relative risk　相対的リスク
renin release　レニン放出
resistance ratio　耐性率
respiratory reserve　呼吸予備
response rate　反応率
rest room　便所，休憩室
retinal reflex　網膜反射
right rotation　右回転，右回旋
risk ratio　危険比
Riva-Rocci (sphygmomanometer)　リバ・ロッチ血圧計
ruthenium red　ルテニウムレッド
rR
runde Riesenzellen〈独〉　円形巨細胞
Rr.
rami〈ラ〉　枝〈複数〉《解剖》
r & r
rate and rhythm　(脈の)比率とリズム
RR, R/R
respiratory rate　呼吸数
RRA
Radiation Research Associates　放射線研究協力者
radioreceptor activity　放射レセプター活性
radioreceptor assay　放射レセプター測定(法)
RRBC
rabbit red blood cell　ウサギ赤血球
RR & C
record, report and control　記録・報告・調整
RR cells
radiation reaction cells　放射反応細胞
RRD
rhegmatogenous retinal detachment　裂孔原性網膜剝離
RRE
radiation-related eosinophilia　照射関連好酸球増多症
R.R. & E
round regular and equal　瞳孔の正円形と等大

RRF
ragged-red fibers　ラッグドレッド繊維
residual renal function　残存腎機能

RRf
right ring finger　右薬指

RRI
R-R interval　R-R間隔《心電》

RR method
Rantz-Randall method　ランツ・ランダール法

rRNA
ribosomal ribonucleic acid　リボソームリボ核酸，リボソームRNA

RRP
radical retropubic prostatectomy　根治的恥骨後前立腺切除術
relative refractory period　相対不応期

RRpm
respiratory rate per minute　分時呼吸数

RRR
regular rhythm and rate　正常リズムと心拍数
relative risk reduction　相対リスク減少率
renin-release rate　レニン放出率

RRS
retrorectal space　直腸後隙
Richards-Rundle syndrome　リチャーズ・ランデル症候群
Riva-Rocci sphygmomanometer　リバ・ロッチ血圧計

Rrs
(total) respiratory resistance　(全)呼吸抵抗

RRT
relative retention time　比較的停留時間
restamin response test　レスタミン反応テスト

RrTM
respiratory resistance through mouth　口呼吸時の呼吸抵抗

RRU
respiratory resistance unit　呼吸抵抗単位

RRV
rate of rise of voltage　電圧上昇比率
Rhesus rotavirus　アカゲザル・ロタウイルス

RS
random sample　無作為標本
Rauwolfia serpentina　ローウォルフィア・セルペンチーナ
Raynaud syndrome　レイノー症候群
reading of standard　基準の判定
recipient's serum　受血者血清
rectal suppository　直腸坐剤
red softening　赤色軟化

reducing sugar	還元糖
Reed-Sternberg (cell)	リード・スターンバーグ(細胞)
reinforcing stimulus	補強刺激
Reiter syndrome	ライター症候群
renal specialist	腎臓専門医
research summary	研究要約
resistant starch	消化しにくいデンプン
respiratory sound	呼吸音
respiratory system	呼吸器系
response stimulus	反応刺激
Rett syngrome	レット症候群
review of symptoms	症状再調査
review of systems	系統別再調査
Reye syndrome	ライ症候群
rhinal sulcus	嗅脳溝
right septal	右中隔の，右隔壁の
right septum	右中隔，右隔壁
right side	右側
right subclavian	右鎖骨下の
Ringer solution	リンゲル液
Rotor syndrome	ローター症候群

Rs

rating scale	比率目盛

rs

rough-surfaced	粗面の

Rs, RS

rectosigmoid	直腸S状(結腸)部(の)

RSA

rabbit serum albumin	家兎血清アルブミン
rat serum albumin	ラット血清アルブミン
recurrent spontaneous abortion	再発性自然流産
refractory sideroblastic anemia	難治性鉄芽球性貧血
relative specific radioactivity	相対比放射能
respiratory sinus arrhythmia	呼吸性洞性不整脈
reticulum (cell) sarcoma	細網肉腫
right sacrum anterior (position)	第二骨盤位第一分類〈胎位〉
right sarcoanterior	右仙骨前位〈胎位〉
right subclavian artery	右鎖骨下動脈

RSB

intercostal space right sternal border	肋間胸骨右縁
right sternal border	右胸骨縁

RSBT

rhythmic sensory bombardment therapy	律動的感覚衝撃療法

RSC
rat spleen cell ラット脾臓細胞
relative salt concentration 相対塩濃度
right side colon (cancer) 右側結腸(癌)
Royal Society of Chemistry 王立化学協会
RScA
right scapula-anterior (position) 第二横位第一分類(=RAA)〈胎位〉
rsCD23
recombinant soluble CD23 可溶性CD23の遺伝子組換え合成物
R-S cell
Reed-Sternberg cell リード・スタンバーグ細胞
RSCH
rat spinal cord homogenate ラット脊髄ホモジネート
rsch
research 研究，調査
RSCL
Rotterdam symptom check list ロッテルダム症状チェックリスト
RSCN
Registered Sick Children's Nurse 患児の正看護師
RScP
right scapula-posterior (position) 第二横位第二分類(=RAP)〈胎位〉
RSD
reflex sympathetic dystrophy 反射性交感神経性異栄養症
relative standard deviation 相対標準偏差《統》
RSE
rat synaptic ending ラットシナプス終末
RSEP
right somatosensory evoked potential 右体性感覚誘発電位
RSIC
Radiation Standards Information Center 放射線標準情報センター
R-SICU
respiratory-surgical intensive care unit 呼吸器外科集中治療室〔病棟〕
RSIP
rapid-sequence intravenous pyelography 急速(連続)静注腎盂造影法
RSIVP
rapid-sequence intravenous pyelography 急速(連続)静注腎盂造影法
RSL
right sacro-lateral position 右仙骨側位

RSM
regurgitant systolic murmur 逆流性収縮期雑音
ribostamycin リボスタマイシン
RSMIVP
rapid sequence mannitol IVP 急速静注(式)マンニトール負荷腎盂造影法
RSMP
rapid sequence mannitol pyelography 急速静注(式)マンニトール腎盂造影法
RSN
right substantia nigra 右黒質
RSNA
Radiological Society of North America 北米放射線医学会
RSNP
Registered Student Nurse Program 登録看護学生計画
RSO
right salpingo-oophorectomy 右卵管卵巣摘出術
right superior oblique (muscle) 右上斜筋
RSP
rapid sequence pyelography 急速連続腎盂造影法
respirable suspended particulates 呼吸可能な浮遊粒子状物質
right sacrum posterior (position) 第二骨盤位第二分類〈胎位〉
RSPP
relative spinal perfusion pressure 相対的脊髄灌流圧
rsq
rescue 救出する
RSR
regular sinus rhythm 規則的洞律動
response-stimulus ratio 反応・刺激比
right superior rectus (muscle) 右上直(筋)
RS ratio
response-stimulus ratio 応答刺激率
RSRID
reversed single radial immunodiffusion 逆単純放射免疫拡散(法)
RSS
rat stomach strip ラットの胃の線条
rectosigmoidoscope 直腸S状結腸鏡
repetitive stress syndrome 反復ストレス症候群
Russell-Silver syndrome ラッセル・シルヴァー症候群
RSSE
Russian spring-summer encephalitis ロシア春夏脳炎
RSSR
relatively slow sinus rate 相対的緩徐洞調律

RST

radiosensitivity test　放射線感受性試験
right sacrum transverse (position)　第二骨盤位第二分類〈胎位〉
right sarcotransverse　右仙骨横位〈胎位〉
rubrospinal tract　赤核脊髄路

rstr

restricted　制限された

RSU

resin sponge uptake　レジンスポンジ摂取率

RSV

respiratory syncytial virus　呼吸器合胞体ウイルス，RSウイルス
right subclavian vein　右鎖骨下静脈
Rous sarcoma virus　ラウス肉腫ウイルス

RT

rabbit trachea　ウサギ気管
radiation therapy　放射線療法
radiotelemetry　無線遠隔測定装置
radiotherapy　放射線療法
radium therapy　ラジウム療法
rational therapy　合理的療法
reaction time　反応時間
reading test　読書力試験
recovery time　回復時間
recreational therapist　リクリエイション療法士
recreational therapy　リクリエイション療法
rectal temperature　直腸温
rectal tube　直腸カテーテル
reentrant tachycardia　再入頻脈
registered technician　公認〔登録〕技術員〔技師〕
renal transplant(ation)　腎(臓)移植
respiratory tachycardia　呼吸性頻脈
respiratory technology　呼吸技術
respiratory therapist　呼吸療法士
respiratory therapy　呼吸療法
rest tremor　安静時振戦
retension time　停滞時間
reverse transcription　逆転写
right thigh　右大腿
rising test　起立テスト
room temperature　室温
Rubinstein-Taybi (syndrome)　ルビンスタイン・テイビ(症候群)

Rt

total resistance　全抵抗

R

rt
right lateral position 右側臥位
routine ルーチン
R.T
rhathymia, thinking extraversion のんきさと思考的外向
R-T
right temporal 右側頭部
RT, Rt, rt.
right 右(の)
rT3, r-T3
reverse T3(=triiodothyronine) リバーストリヨードチ〔サイ〕ロニン

RTA
renal tubular acidosis 腎尿細管性アシドーシス
renal tubular antigen 腎尿細管抗原
road traffic accident 道路交通災害
RTase
reverse transcriptase 逆転写酸素
RTBD
retrograde transhepatic biliary drainage 逆行性経肝胆道ドレナージ
RTC
rape treatment center 強姦治療センター
renal tubular cell 腎尿細管細胞
return to clinic 再来院
rolitetracycline ロリテトラサイクリン
round-the-clock (therapy) ラウンド・ザ・クロック(療法), 終日療法

RTD
routine test dilution 正規テスト希釈度
RTE
rabbit thymus extract ウサギ胸腺抽出物
renal tubular epithelium 腎尿細管上皮細胞
R test
reductase test 還元酵素試験
RTF
resistance transfer factor 耐性伝達因子
RTG
reference test gain 規準利得
rtg
roentgen レントゲン
RTI
respiratory tract infection 呼吸器感染症
Rti
tissue resistance 組織抵抗

RTK
receptor tyrosine kinase 受容体型チロシンキナーゼ
RTL
red thermoluminescence 赤色熱発光
rtl
rectal 直腸の
rt.lat
right lateral 右外側の
RTM
registered trademark 登録商標
RTN
renal tubular necrosis 腎尿細管壊死
rtn
return 戻ってくる
RTP
radiation therapy planning 放射線治療計画
rapid turnover proteins 迅速交代蛋白
reference test position 規準の位置
renal transplant patient 腎臓移植患者
room-temperature phosphorescence 室温リン光法
RTRR
return to recovery room 回復室に戻る
RTS
real time scan 同時スキャン
Rubinstein-Taybi syndrome ルビンスタイン・テイビ症候群
RTSA
post thymic T-lymphocyte antigen 成熟T細胞特異抗原
rt.scap.bord
right scapular border 右肩甲骨縁
RTTC
Regional Teacher Training Center 地域教育者訓練センター
RTU
real-time ultrasonography 同時〔即時〕超音波検査(法)
RT_3U
iodine-$^{131}T_3$ resin sponge uptake test ヨウ素$^{131}T_3$レジンスポンジ摂取率試験
^{131}I resin uptake ヨウ素$^{131}T_3$レジン摂取率
RTUS
real-time ultrasonography 同時〔即時〕超音波検査(法)
RTV
roentgen television X線テレビジョン
RTVS
room temperature vulcanized silicon 室温加硫シリコン
RTW
return to work 仕事に戻る

RU	
recurrent ulcer	再発性潰瘍
Reflex Umdrehen〈独〉	反射性寝返り運動
residual urine	残尿
resin uptake	レジン摂取量
retrograde urogram	逆行性尿路造影
right upper	右上の
roentgen unit	レントゲン単位
routine urinalysis	ルーチン尿検査
Ru	
ruthenium	ルテニウム〈元素〉
RU, R.U.	
rat unit	ラット単位
RUB	
right upper lobe bronchus	右上葉気管支
rub.	
ruber〈ラ〉=red	赤い
RUE	
right upper extremity	右上肢
RUG	
retrograde urethrogram	逆行性尿道造影図
retrograde urethrography	逆行性尿道造影法
RUL	
right upper lateral	右上外側の
right upper (eye) lid	右上眼瞼
right upper limb	右上肢
right upper lung	右上肺野
RUL, R.U.L.	
right upper lobe	右(肺)上葉
RUM	
residual urine measurement	残尿測定
right upper medial	右上内側の
RUMBA	
real, understandable, measurable, behavioral, achievable	医学教育目標5項目：現実的・理解可能・測定可能・行動で示される・到達可能，ランバ《医教》
R unit	
roentgen unit	レントゲン単位
RUO	
right ureteral orifice	右尿管口
RUP	
right upper pole	右上極
Ru-5-P	
ribulose-5-phosphate	リブロース-5-リン酸塩

rupt
rupture(d) 破裂(した)

rupt'd
ruptured 破裂した

rupt.memb
ruptured membrane 破膜，破水

RUQ
right upper quadrant 右上部1/4区，右上腹部

RUR
resin uptake ratio レジン摂取率

RURTI
recurrent upper respiratory tract infection 再発性上気道感染

RUS
radius, ulna and short finger bones 橈骨・尺骨・短指骨
recurrent ulcerative stomatitis 再発性潰瘍性口内炎

RUSB
right upper scapular border 右上肩甲骨縁
right upper sternal border 右上胸骨縁

RUSS
recurrent ulcerative scarifying stomatitis 再発性潰瘍性乱切口内炎

RUV
residual urine volume 残尿量

RUX
right upper extremity 右上肢

RV
nucleus reticularis ventralis〈ラ〉 腹側網様核
Rauscher virus ローシャーウイルス
recombinant virus 組換えウイルス
rectovaginal 直腸腟の
regurgitant volume 逆流量
renal vein 腎静脈
renal venous 腎静脈の
reovirus レオウイルス
residual volume 残気量
respiratory viral disease 呼吸器ウイルス疾患
retinal vasculitis 網膜血管炎
retroversion 後傾症
retroverted 後傾した
retrovirus レトロウイルス
rheumatoid vasculitis リウマチ性血管炎
rhinitis vasomotor 血管運動性鼻炎
rhinovirus ライノウイルス
right ventricle 右心室
right vision 右眼視力

rimmed vacuole ふちのある空胞
Rotavirus ロタウイルス
rubella vaccine 風疹ワクチン
rubella virus 風疹ウイルス

RVA
rabies vaccine adsorbed 吸着狂犬病ワクチン
reactive volt-ampere 反応性電圧・電流
reentrant ventricular arrhythmia リエントリー心室性不整脈
rib-vertebral angle 肋骨椎体角
right ventricular activation 右(心)室興奮
right ventricular apex (apical) 右(心)室尖(の)
right vertebral artery 右椎骨動脈

RVAD
rib-vertebral angle difference 左右の肋骨椎体角の差
right ventricular assist device 右(心)補助循環装置

RV-angle
rib-vertebral angle 肋骨椎体角

RVAW
right ventricular anterior wall 右(心)室前壁

RVB
red venous blood 赤色静脈血

RVD
respiratory viral disease 呼吸器ウイルス疾患
right ventricular dimension 右(心)室径

RVDO
right ventricular diastolic overload 右(心)室拡張期過負荷

RVDP
right ventricular diastolic pressure 右(心)室拡張期圧

RVDV
right ventricular diastolic volume 右(心)室拡張期容積

RVE
right ventricular enlargement 右(心)室拡大

RVECP
right ventricular endocardial potential 右(心)室心内膜電位

RVEDD
right ventricular end-diastolic diameter 右(心)室拡張終(末)期径

RVEDP
right ventricular end diastolic pressure 右(心)室拡張終(末)期圧

RVEDV
right ventricular end-diastolic volume 右(心)室拡張終期容量

RVEDVI
right ventricular end-diastolic volume index　右(心)室終末拡張期容量係数

RVEF
right ventricular ejection fraction　右(心)室駆出率
right ventricular end-flow　右(心)室終(末)期血流

RVESV
right ventricular end-systolic volume　右(心)室収縮終(末)期容積

RVESVI
right ventricular end-systolic volume index　右(心)室収縮終(末)期容積係数

RVET
right ventricular ejection time　右(心)室駆出時間

Rve-vol
reserve-volume　予備量

RVF
renal vascular failure　腎血管障害
retroversio-flexio (*uteri*)〈ラ〉　(子宮)後傾後屈症
Rift Valley fever　リフト渓谷熱
right ventricular failure　右(心)室不全
right visual field　右視野

RV fist
rectovaginal fistula　直腸腟瘻

RVFP
right ventricular filling pressure　右(心)室充満圧

RVFV
Rift Valley fever virus　リフト渓谷熱ウイルス

RVG
radionuclide ventriculogram　放射性核種心室造影図
radionuclide ventriculography　放射性核種心室造影法
right ventriculography　右(心)室造影

RVH
renal vascular hypertension　腎血管性高血圧
renovascular hypertension　腎血管性高血圧症
right ventricular hypertrophy　右(心)室肥大

RVHD
rheumatic valvular heart disease　リウマチ性弁膜性心疾患

RVI
residual volume index　残気率
right ventricle infarction　右(心)室梗塞

RVID
right ventricular internal dimension　右(心)室内径

RVIT
right ventricular inflow tract　右(心)室流入路

RVLA
reovirus-like antigen　レオウイルス様病原体

RVLM
rostral ventrolateral medulla 吻側延髄腹外側部
RVM
rimmed vacuole myopathy 輪空胞ミオパシー
RVO
relaxed vaginal outlet 弛緩した腟口
right ventricular outflow 右(心)室流出(量)
RVOT
right ventricular outflow tract 右(心)室流出路
RVOTD
right ventricular outflow tract dimension 右(心)室流出路
RVP
renal venous pressure 腎静脈圧
renovascular pressure 腎血管圧
resting venous pressure 安静時静脈血圧
right ventricular pressure 右(心)室圧
RVPRA
renal vein plasma renin activity 腎静脈血漿レニン活性
RVR
rapid ventricular response 急速心室反応
reduced vascular response 減弱血管反応
reduced vestibular response 減弱前庭反応
renal vascular resistance 腎血管抵抗
renal vein renin 腎静脈レニン
repetitive ventricular responses 競合的心室応答
RVRA
renal venous renin assay 腎静脈レニン定量法
RVRC
renal vein renin concentration 腎静脈レニン濃度
RVRI
renal vascular resistance index 腎血管抵抗指数
RVRR
renal vein renin ratio 腎静脈血レニン比
RVS
rabies vaccine, adsorbed 吸着狂犬病ワクチン
retrovaginal space 腟後隙
RVSP
right ventricle systolic pressure 右(心)室収縮期圧
RVSW
right ventricular stroke work 右(心)室拍出仕事量
RVSWI
right ventricular stroke work index 右(心)室1回仕事係数
right ventricular systolic work index 右(心)室1回拍出仕事指数
RVT
renal vein thrombosis 腎静脈血栓症

R

RVTE
recurring venous thromboembolism 再発性静脈血栓塞栓症
RVV
right ventricular volume 右(心)室容積
rubella vaccine-like virus 風疹ワクチン様ウイルス
Russell viper venom ラッセルヘビ毒液
rVV
recombinant vaccinia virus 遺伝子組換えワクシニアウイルス
RVVT
Russell viper venom time ラッセルヘビ毒時間
RW
reaction of Wassermann ワッセルマン反応
respiratory work 呼吸仕事量
Romano-Ward (syndrome) ロマノ・ウォード(症候群)
round window 正円窓
RW, Rw
ragweed ブタクサ
RW, R/W
return to work 仕事に戻る
RW, R-W
Rideal-Walker phenol coefficient test リデール・ウォーカー石炭酸係数試験
ⅧR : WF
factor Ⅷ related von Willebrand factor 第Ⅷ因子フォンウィルブランド因子
Ⅷ related von Willebrand factor 第Ⅷ因子関連フォンウィルブランド因子
RWIS
restraint and immersion stress 拘束水浸ストレス
RWM
round window membrane 正円窓膜
RWP
ragweed pollen ブタクサ花粉
RWS
ragweed sensitivity ブタクサ過敏(性)
RX, RP
recipe 処方
RX, Rx.
drugs 薬
medication 投薬
prescription 処方箋
recipe〈ラ〉=take 服用せよ《処》, 処方, 投薬
therapy 療法
treatment 治療

Rxd
treated — 治療された

RXM
roxithromycin — ロキシスロマイシン

Rxn, RXN, rxn
reaction — 反応

rxns
reactions — 反応〈複数〉

Rx Phys
treating physician — 治療医師

RXT
right exotropia — 右外斜視

R-Y
Roux-en-Y anastomosis — ルーワイ吻合術

RZL
return to zero level — 0〔ゼロ〕域に戻る

RZM
return to zero mark — 0〔ゼロ〕点に戻る

S s

S

area	野，区
entropy	エントロピー，熱力関数
exposure time	曝露時間
Saccharomyces	サッカロミセス(属)
sacral	仙骨の，仙椎の
sacral nerve	仙骨神経
sacral vertebra	仙椎(S 1のように使う)
sacrum	仙骨
sagittal plane	矢状面
saline	塩類の，食塩の
Salmonella	サルモネラ(属)
same	同じ
Sarcocystis	肉胞子虫(属)
saturated	飽和した
saturation	飽和
saturation of hemoglobin	ヘモグロビン飽和度
Schistosoma	住血吸虫(属)
Schizophrenie〈独〉=schizophrenia	統合失調症
Schräge〈独〉	斜位
Schwabach test	シュワバッハ検査
secretion	分泌
secretion granule	分泌顆粒
sedimentation coefficient	沈降係数
senile	老人性の，老年の
sensitive	知覚しうる，感知しうる
septum	中隔，隔壁
serine	セリン
serosa	(胚膜の)漿膜
serous	深達度が漿膜(=s)の癌
Serratia	セラチア(属)
serum	漿液，血清
sevoflurane	セボフルラン
Shigella	赤痢菌(属)
sick	病気の，吐き気がする
siderocyte	シデロサイト，担鉄赤血球
siemens	ジーメンス
sigmoid colon	S状結腸
silicate	ケイ酸塩
silver	銀
single	独身の
sinusitis〈ラ〉	副鼻腔炎
slow inactivator	遅延不活性因子

smooth (bacterial colony)	平滑型(細菌集落)
soft	軟らかい，柔軟な
soil	土壌
solid	固形の，固化した
soluble	可溶な，可溶性
solute	溶質
space	腔，隙，空間
spasm	攣縮，痙攣
specific	特異的
specific activity	比放射能
speed	速度
spherical	球の，球状の
spherical lens	球面レンズ
Spirillum	スピリルム(属)
Spirometra	スピロメトラ(属)
spleen	脾臓，脾
sporadic	散発性の
Sporothrix	スポロトリックス(属)
Sporotrichum	スポロトリクム(属)
S-Romanum	直腸S状部
Staphylococcus	スタヒロコッカス(属)，ブドウ球菌(属)
stimulus	刺激，興奮薬
storage	貯蔵
strained	努力性
Streptobacillus	ストレプトバシラス(属)，連鎖桿菌(属)
Streptococcus	ストレプトコッカス(属)，連鎖球菌(属)
streptomycin	ストレプトマイシン
Strongyloides	ストロンギロイデス(属)，糞線虫(属)
subject	被検者，被験者
subjective	主観の，主観的な
subjective data	主観的情報
subjective finding	自覚所見
substrate	基質
succeeded	成功した
sulcus	溝
sulfur＝sulphur	硫黄
summary	まとめ
supervision	管理，監督
surface	表面
surgeon	外科医
surgery	外科学
surgical	外科的の

suture 縫合
Svedberg unit of sedimentation coefficient 沈降定数のスベドベルグ単位
S-wave S波《心電》
sympathetic 交感の，共感の
synthesis 合成
systole (心)収縮期
thiouridine チオウリジン(＝sU, Srd)
upper margin of sternum 胸骨上縁

s
distance 距離
mercapto メルカプト
satellite 付随体，衛星
sedimentation constant 沈降定数
selection coefficient 淘汰係数
serosal invasion 漿膜層表面浸潤
shunt (blood) シャント血
steady state 安定状態
symmetric 対称的な
thio チオ

S.
signa〈ラ〉 書け，用法《処》

s.
sumat, *sumendus*〈ラ〉＝let him take, to be taken 服用させよ，服用《処》

4S
The Scandinavian Simvastatin Survival Study スカンジナビアシンバスタチン臨床試験

S1
first heart sound 第1心音

S_1
erster Spitzenton〈独〉 心尖第1音

S2
second heart sound 第2心音

S3
third heart sound 第3心音

S4
forth heart sound 第4心音

S II
secondary somesthetic area 二次体性感覚野

S-5900
acetohexamide アセトヘキサミド

S, s
scruple スクループル
second 秒
section 切開，切片，切断

see 見よ
sensation 感覚
series 直列
sign(s) 徴候，符号
singular 単数の
sinister〈ラ〉=left 左の
sinus 洞
sister 看護師，姉妹
son 息子
symmetrical 対称性の

S, S.
Schatten〈独〉=shadow 陰影
Sehschärfe〈独〉=sight 視力

S, s, s.
semis〈ラ〉=half 半分，半《処》

S, s, /S/, /s/
signature 用法指示，署名
signed 署名した

$\bar{S}$, s, $\bar{s}$
sine〈ラ〉=without ～なしの，～を伴わない

SA
salicylic acid サリチル酸
saline 塩類の，食塩水
salivary amylase 唾液(腺型)アミラーゼ
salt added 食塩添加した
sarcoma 肉腫
saturation analysis 飽和分析(法)
scalenus anticus 前斜角(筋)
secondary amenorrhea 続発性無月経
secondary anemia 続発性貧血
second attack 二次発作
semen analysis 精液分析
senile atrophy 老年性萎縮
sensitizing antibody 感作抗体
sensory aphasia 感覚性失語
serum albumin 血清アルブミン
serum aldolase 血清アルドラーゼ
sialic acid シアル酸
sideroblastic anemia 鉄芽球性貧血
single atrium 単心房
single auricle 単心房
sinus arrest 洞停止
sinus arrhythmia 洞性不整脈
skeletal age 骨格年齢
sleep apnea 睡眠時無呼吸
social age 社会年齢

sodium-L-ascorbate ナトリウム-L-アスコルビン酸
soluble in alkaline solution アルカリ性溶液に溶解する
Spanish American スペイン系アメリカ人
specific activity 特異的活性
specific radioactivity 比放射能
sperm abnormality 精子異常
splenic artery 脾動脈
spontaneous abortion 自然流産
Staphylococcus aureus 黄色ブドウ球菌
Stokes-Adams (syndrome) ストークス・アダムス(症候群)
streptavidin ストレプトアビジン
suicide attempt 自殺未遂，自殺企図
sulfonamide スルホンアミド〈=スルファニルアミド〉
supra-abdominal 上腹部の
surface antigen 表面抗原
surface area 体表面積
sustained action 持続作用
sympathetic activity 交感神経活動度
systemic aspergillosis 全身性アスペルギルス症

Sa
samarium サマリウム
saturation 飽和

s.a.
secundum artem〈ラ〉 技術によって，巧妙に《処》

S/A
same as above 上記と同じ

SA，S/A
short arm 短腕

SA，S-A
sinoatrial 洞房の
sinoauricular 洞房の

S & A，S/A
sugar and acetone 糖とアセトン

SAA
serum amyloid A protein 血清アミロイドA蛋白
Stokes-Adams attack ストークス・アダムス発作
surface active agent 界面活性剤

SAARD
slow-acting antirheumatic drug 緩徐作用性抗リウマチ薬

SAB
selective alveolo-bronchography 選択的肺胞気管支造影法
serum albumin 血清アルブミン
sinoatrial〔sinoauricular〕block 洞房ブロック
spontaneous abortion 自然流産

subarachnoid block クモ膜下ブロック

Sab, SAB
Sabouraud (dextrose agar) medium サブロー(ブドウ糖寒天)培地

SABP
spontaneous acute bacterial peritonitis 特発性急性細菌性腹膜炎

SAC
saccharin サッカリン
serum antireticulare cytotoxicum 抗網内細胞毒血清
Specialist Advisory Committee 専門医助言委員会

sac
sacral 仙骨の
sacrum 仙骨

sacch
saccharin サッカリン

SACD
sub-acute combined degeneration 亜急性連合性(脊髄)変性(症)

SACE
serum angiotensin converting enzyme 血清アンジオテンシン変換酵素

SACH
solid ankle cushion heel foot サッチ足

sac-il
sacro-iliac 仙(骨)腸(骨)の

SACSF
subarachnoid cerebrospinal fluid クモ膜下髄液

SACT
sinoatrial conduction time 洞房伝導時間

SAD
schedule for affective disorders (and schizophrenia) 感情障害ならびに統合失調症面接基準
seasonal affective disorder 季節性感情障害
Self-Assessment Depression (scale) 自己評価うつ病(尺度)
single atom detection 原子1個の検出
sino-aortic denervation 洞大動脈除神経

SADQ
Self-Administered Dependency Questionnaire 自己評価依存質問票

SADS
schedule for affective disorder and schizophrenia 感情障害ならびに統合失調症面接基準

SAD test
sugar, acetone, diacetic acid test 糖・アセトン・重酢酸試験

SAE
serious adverse event 重篤な有害事象
signal-averaged electrocardiogram 加算平均心電図法

splenic artery embolization 脾動脈塞栓術

SAEC

serum angiotensin converting enzyme concentration 血清アンジオテンシン変換酵素活性値

SAF

simultaneous auditory feedback 同時聴覚フィードバック

SAFA

soluble antigen fluorescent antibody (test) 可溶性抗原螢光抗体(試験)

SAFM

scanning atomic force microscope 原子間力顕微鏡

SAG

superantigen 超抗原

Swiss(-type) agammaglobulinemia スイス(型)無γグロブリン血症

Sag.d.

sagittal diameter 矢状径

SAGE

Stratospheric Aerosol and Gas Experiment オゾン濃度鉛直分布測定

SAGES

Society of American Gastrointestinal Endoscoping Surgeons 米国胃腸内視鏡外科学会

SAGM

salts-adenine-glucose-mannitol 塩・アデニン・グルコース・マニトール

SAH

S-adenosyl-L-homocysteine S-アデノシル-L-ホモシステイン

subarachnoid hemorrhage クモ膜下出血

systemic arterial hypertension 全身性動脈性高血圧

SAHIOES

Staphylococcus aureus hyperimmunoglobulinemia 黄色ブドウ球菌過免疫グロブリン血症(=E症候群)

SAHS

sleep apnea hypersomnia syndrome 睡眠時無呼吸過眠症候群

SAI

social adequacy index 社会適応指数

social adequacy index of hearing 聴力の社会適応指数

systemic active immunotherapy 全身性能動性免疫療法

SAICAR

5-aminoimidazole-4-*N*-succinocarboxamide ribonucleotide (=succino AICAR) 5-アミノイミダゾール-4-*N*-スクシノカルボキサミドリボヌクレオチド

SAID
sexually acquired immunodeficiency (syndrome) 性行為獲得性〔後天性〕免疫不全(症候群)
speech auto-instructional device 会話自動訓練器

SAIDS
simian acquired immunodeficiency (syndrome) サル後天性免疫不全(症候群)

SAIS
sleep apnea insomnia syndrome 睡眠時無呼吸不眠症候群

SAIT
scholastic aptitude intelligence test 進学適性知能検査

SAK
streptokinase activation ストレプトキナーゼ活性化

SAL
smoldering acute leukemia くすぶり型急性白血病

sal
salicylate サリチル酸塩，サリチル酸エステル
saliva 唾液

sal.
secundum artis leges〈ラ〉 術式に従って《処》

SAL, Sal.
Salmonella サルモネラ(属)

SAL, sal.
saline 塩類の，食塩水

salicyl
salicylate サリチル酸塩，サリチル酸エステル

Salm
Salmonella サルモネラ(属)

Salmiak
sal ammoniac 塩化アンモニウム

SALPI
stage, age, lymphocyte prognostic index 期・年齢・リンパ球予後指数

S

SALT
skin associated lymphoid tissue 皮膚関連リンパ組織

salv
salvage 救出

SAM
S-adenosylmethionine *S*-アデノシルメチオニン
scanning Auger microscope 走査型オージェ電子顕微鏡
senile〔senescence〕 activating mouse 老化促進モデルマウス
surface active material 表面活性物質
sympathetic-adrenal-medullary 交感神経・副腎髄質系
systolic anterior movement (僧帽弁の)収縮期前方運動

SAMA
Student Americans Medical Association　米国医学生協会
SAMBA
Society for Ambulatory Anesthesia　デイケア麻酔に関する学会
SAMe
S-adenosylmethionine　*S*-アデノシルメチオニン
SAMs
self-assembled monolayer　自己集合単分子膜
SAMU
service d'aide médicale urgente〈仏〉　地域緊急医療システム
SAN
sinoatrial node　洞房結節
sinoauricular node　洞房結節
SANA
sinoatrial node artery　洞房結節動脈
speckled anti-nuclear antibody　斑点状抗核抗体
SANC
short-arm navicular cast　手の舟状骨骨折用の肘下ギプス
SANE
severe acoustic noise environment　重度騒音環境
sanit
sanitary　衛生の，保健の
sanitation　衛生
sanit, sanit.
sanitarium＝sanatorium　サナトリウム，健康保養地
S antigen
soluble antigen　可溶性抗原
SAO
aplanchnic artery occlusion　内臓動脈閉塞
small airway obstruction　小気道閉塞
SaO_2
arterial O_2 saturation　動脈血酸素飽和度
arterial oxygen saturation　動脈血酸素飽和度
saturation of arterial blood oxygen　動脈血酸素飽和度
SAP
seminal acid phosphatase　精液酸ホスファターゼ
sensory action potential　知覚活動電位
sensory nerve conduction velocity　知覚神経伝導速度
serum acid phosphatase　血清酸ホスファターゼ
serum alkaline phosphatase　血清アルカリホスファターゼ
serum amyloid P (component)　血清アミロイドP(成分)
Staphylococcus aureus protease　黄色ブドウ球菌蛋白分解酵素
subarachnoid pressure　クモ膜下腔圧
systemic arterial pressure　全身血圧

systolic arterial pressure 収縮期動脈圧

sap

saponification 鹸化

saponify 鹸化する

SAPA

stroma adsorbed protective antigen ストローマ吸着防御抗原

SA-PE

streptavidin-phycoerythrin PE標識ストレプトアビジン

saph

saphenous (vein) 伏在(静脈)

SAPHO

synovitis-acne-pustulosis-hyperostosis osteomyelitis 滑膜炎・痤瘡・膿疱症・骨化過剰骨髄炎

sapon

saponification 鹸化

saponify 鹸化する

SAPS

simplified acute physiology score 救急重症者評価スコア

SAR

seasonal allergic rhinitis 季節性アレルギー性鼻炎

specific absorption rate 信号吸収値

subacute asthmatic response 亜急性喘息反応

Swiss Air Rescue スイス救急飛行隊

synthetic aperture radar マイクロ波合成開口映像システム

Sar

sarcoidosis サルコイドーシス

sarcosine サルコシン

sulpharsphenamine スルファルスフェナミン

SARA

sexually acquired reactive arthritis 性行為感染反応性関節炎

SARC

seasonal allergic rhinoconjunctivitis 季節性鼻アレルギー性結膜炎

sarc

sarcoma 肉腫

S

SARS

severe acute respiratory syndrome 重症急性呼吸器症候群

SARS-CoV

SARS coronavirus サーズコロナウイルス

SART

sinoatrial recovery time 洞房回復時間

SAS

aortic stenosis subaortic stenosis 左(心)室流出路狭窄

saturated ammonium sulphate 飽和硫酸アンモニウム

scalenus anticus syndrome 前斜角筋症候群

self-assessment system 自己研修システム

self-rating anxiety scale	自己評点不安尺度
short-arm splint	肘下の副木
shoulder arm syndrome	肩腕症候群
sleep apnea syndrome	睡眠時無呼吸症候群
small aorta syndrome	小大動脈症候群
social assets scale	社会機能尺度
sodium amylosulfate	アミロ硫酸ナトリウム
space-adaptation syndrome	(宇宙)空間適応症候群
statistical analysis system	統計学的分析システム《コン》
sterile aqueous suspension	無菌水性懸濁液
subaortic stenosis	大動脈弁下部狭窄
subarachnoid space	クモ膜下腔
subaxial subluxation	関節リウマチにおける下位頸椎亜脱臼
supravalvular aortic stenosis	大動脈弁上部狭窄症
surface-active substance	表面活性物質
sympathicoadrenal system	交感神経アドレナリン系

SASA

stereotactic aqua-stream & aspirator	立体的水流吸引器

SASP

salicylazosulfapyridine(=sulfasalazine, salazosulfapyridine)	サリチルアゾスルファピリジン(=スルファサラジン, サラゾサルファピリジン)

SASS

supravalvular aortic stenosis syndrome	大動脈弁上部狭窄症候群

SAST

serum aspartate aminotransferase	血清アスパルテートアミノトランスフェラーゼ

SAT

satellite	付随体, 衛星
scholastic aptitude test	進学適性検査
school ability test	学校能力試験
senior apperception technique	高年用絵画統覚検査
sialic acid transferase	シアル酸転移酵素
speech awareness threshold	語音聴力レベル
spermatogenic activity test	精子形成活動試験
spontaneous autoimmune thyroiditis	突発性自己免疫性甲状腺炎
structural atypism	悪性腫瘍の構造異体
subacute thyroiditis	亜急性甲状腺炎

sat

satisfactory	満足な

SAT, sat.

saturate	深く浸込ませる, 飽和させる
saturation	飽和(度)
saturatus〈ラ〉=saturated	飽和した

S

SAT chromosome
chromosome with satellite 随伴染色体
sat.cond
satisfactory condition 満足状態
sat'd
saturated 飽和した
sat.DNA
satellite deoxyribonucleic acid サテライトデオキシリボ核酸
satis
satisfactory 満足な
SATL
surgical Achilles tendon lengthening 外科的アキレス腱延長
satn
saturation 飽和(度)
sat.sol.
saturated solution 飽和溶液
S. auf 3x tagl n.d.E.z.n.
Signa auf 3 mal täglich nach dem Essen zu nehmen〈独〉 1日3回食後服用
SAV
select-a-vent 通気口選択
supra-annular valve 輪状弁《心外》
SAVE
survival and ventricular enlargement セーブトライアル
SAW
surface acoustic wave 表面弾性波
SAX
X-linked species X染色体種(または表面)抗原
SAXS
small-angle X-ray scattering X線小角散乱
SB
sagittal band (指の)矢状索
sandbag サンドバッグ，砂袋
Schwartz-Bartter (syndrome) シュワルツ・バーター(症候群)
scleral bucking 強膜陥凹
serum bilirubin 血清ビリルビン
shortness of breath 息切れ
shower bath シャワー浴
sideroblast シデロブラスト，担鉄赤芽球
sinobronchitis〈ラ〉 副鼻腔気管支炎
sinus bradycardia 洞性徐脈
small bowel 小腸
soap bath 石鹸清拭
sodium balance ナトリウム平衡
solid body 固体

soybean　大豆
spina bifida　二分脊椎，脊椎破裂
spontaneous breathing　自発呼吸
standard bicarbonate　標準重炭酸塩
stellate ganglion block　星状神経節ブロック
stereotyped behavior　常同性行動，紋切り型行動
sternal border　胸骨縁
Stimmband〈独〉　声帯
sunburn　日光皮膚炎，日焼け
surface-binding (protein)　表面結合(蛋白)

Sb
stibium　アンチモン

sb
stilb　スチルブ

SB, S/B
stillbirth　死産
stillborn　死産

SB, S-B
Stanford-Binet (intelligence test)　スタンフォード・ビネー(知能試験)

Sb, Sb.
strabismus　斜視

SBA
serum bile acid　血清胆汁酸
soybean agglutinin　大豆凝集素
spina bifida aperta　開放二分脊椎
Summary Basis of Approval　新医薬品承認審査概要

SBAG
selective bronchial arteriography　選択的気管支動脈造影法

SBB
Sudan black B stain　ズダンブラックB染色

SBC
serum bactericidal concentration　血清殺菌濃度
sexual behavior center(s)　性行動中枢
solitary bone cyst　孤立性骨嚢腫

SB concentration
standard bicarbonate concentration　標準重炭酸塩濃度

SBD
senile brain disease　老人性〔老年性〕脳疾患

SBE
shortness of breath on exertion　労作時息切れ
subacute bacterial endocarditis　亜急性細菌性心内膜炎

SBF
serum-blocking factor　血清遮断因子
specific blocking factor　特異的遮断因子
splanchnic blood flow　内臓血流量

systemic blood flow　全身血流量，心拍出量

SBH
Sabra hypertensive rat　サブラ高血圧ラット

SBI
soybean (trypsin) inhibitor　大豆(トリプシン)抑制因子
systemic bacterial infection　全身性細菌感染

SBIS
Stanford-Binet Intelligence Scale　スタンフォード・ビネー知能尺度

SBL
soybean lectin　大豆レクチン

SBN
Sabra normotensive strain (rat)　サブラ正常血圧種(ラット)
single-breath nitrogen (test)　窒素1回呼吸法

SBNT
single-breath nitrogen test　一息窒素検査

SBO
small bowel obstruction　小腸閉塞
spina bifida occulta　潜在(性)二分脊椎

Sb_2O_3
antimony trioxide　三酸化アンチモン

Sb_2O_5
antimony pentoxide　五酸化アンチモン

SBOM
soybean oil meal　大豆油食

SBOs
specific behavioral objectives　特定行動目標

SBP
serotonin-binding protein　セロトニン結合蛋白
sex steroid-binding plasma protein　性ホルモン結合血漿蛋白
spontaneous bacterial peritonitis　特発性細菌性腹膜炎
steroid-binding plasma (protein)　ステロイド結合血漿(蛋白)
Sugi basic protein　スギ花粉抗原
systolic blood pressure　収縮期血圧

SBPC
sulfobenzyl penicillin (=sulbenicillin)　スルホベンジルペニシリン(=スルベニシリン)

SBR
small bowel massive resection　小腸大量切除
spleen-to-body-weight ratio　脾臓体重比
strict bed rest　絶対安静
summary basis of reexamination　再審査概要

SBS
shaken baby syndrome　ゆさぶられっ子症候群
short bowel syndrome　短腸症候群
sinobronchial syndrome　副鼻腔気管支症候群

straight back syndrome　ストレートバック症候群

SBT

serum bactericidal test　血清殺菌試験
serum bactericidal titer　血清殺菌力価
single breath test　1回呼吸試験
sulbactam　スルバクタム

SBT，S-B T

Sengstaken-Blakemore tube　センダステークン・ブレークモア管，食道静脈瘤止血用チューブ

SBT/CPZ

sulbactam/cefoperazone　スルバクタム・セフォペラゾン

SBTI

soybean trypsin inhibitor　大豆トリプシン抑制因子

SBTPC

sultamicillin　スルタミシリン

S-B tube，SB Tube

Sengstaken-Blakemore tube　センダスターテン・ブレークモア管，食道静脈瘤止血用チューブ

SBUV

Solar Backscatter Ultraviolet　鉛直分布観測用のオゾン衛生センサー

S by S

symptoms by systems　系統別症状

SC

closure of semilunar valves　半月弁閉鎖
sacrococcygeal　仙尾骨の
same case　同一例
schedule change　スケジュール変更
Schlemm canal　シュレム管
Schüller-Christian (disease)　シュラー・クリスチャン(病)
Schwann cell　シュワン細胞
sciatic　坐骨の
secondary care　二次療法
secretory component　分泌成分
semicircular　半円の
serum complement　血清補体
serum creatinine　血清クレアチニン
sex chromatin　性クロマチン
sickle cell　鎌状赤血球
similarity coefficient　相似係数
skin conductance　皮膚コンダクタンス
Snellen chart　スネレン表
spinal cord　脊髄

S

spleen cell 脾臓細胞
squamous carcinoma 扁平上皮癌
stepped care 段階的治療
stereoscopic campimetry 他眼固視平面視野
sternoclavicular 胸鎖の
sternoclavicular (ligament) 胸鎖靱帯
stimulator cell 刺激細胞
stimulus conditioned 条件刺激
stratum corneum 角質層
Streptococcus ストレプトコッカス(属)
subclavian 鎖骨下の
subcortical 皮質下の
subcutaneous injection 皮下注射
succinylcholine サクシニルコリン
superior colliculus 上丘
suppressor cell 抑制細胞
suppressor cell サプレッサー細胞
synovial cell 関節滑膜固有細胞
systemic candidiasis 全身カンジダ症
systolic click 収縮期クリック

Sc
scandium スカンジウム
schizophrenia 統合失調症

sc
scant 貧しい，不足の
sclera 強膜
subcutaneously 皮下に
sugar coated 糖衣の

sc.
scilicet〈ラ〉 すなわち

SC8109
spironolactone スピロノラクトン

S & C
sclerae and conjunctivae 強膜と結膜

SC，sc
science 科学
scientific 科学的な
subcutaneous 皮下の

SC，s.c.
sine correctione〈ラ〉＝without correction 矯正なしで，訂正なしで

SC，S-C
sickle cell-(hemoglobin) C (disease) 鎌状赤血球(血色素)C(病)

Sc，sc
scapula 肩甲骨
scapular 肩甲骨の

SCA
selective celiac arteriography　選択的腹腔動脈造影
severe congenital anomaly　重症先天奇形
sickle cell anemia　鎌状赤血球貧血
sperm-coating antigen　精子被覆抗原
spino-clavicular angle　棘鎖角
subclavian artery　鎖骨下動脈
superior cerebellar artery　上小脳動脈
suppressor cell activity　抑制細胞活性
surface chemical analysis　表面化学分析

SCAG
selective celiac angiography　選択的腹腔動脈造影

scalp EEG
scalp electroencephalogram　頭皮脳波

SCaM
scanning capacitance microscope　走査型キャパシタンス顕微鏡

SCAN
Schedule for Clinical Assessment of Neuropsychiatry　神経精神科の臨床評価計画

Scand
Scandinavian　スカンジナビアの

SCANIIR
surface composition analysis by neutral and ion impact radiation　中性およびイオン衝撃発光分光

scap
scapula　肩甲骨
scapular　肩甲骨の

scaphocephs
scaphocephalics　狭頭(人種)

SCARMD
severe childhood autosomal recessive muscular dystrophy　劇症小児常染色体劣性筋ジストロフィ

SCAT
sheep cell agglutination test　ヒツジ細胞凝集試験
sheep red cell agglutination test　ヒツジ赤血球凝集反応
sickle cell anemia test　鎌状赤血球貧血検査

scat.
scatula〈ラ〉=box　小箱，箱

SCA test
school and college ability tests　学校・大学能力試験

scat.orig.
scatula originalis〈ラ〉=original package　原箱

SCB
strictly confined to bed　絶対安静

S

SCBF
spinal cord blood flow　脊髄血流量
ScBU
screening bacteriuria　スクリーニング細菌尿
SCC
short-circuit current　短絡電流
short-course chemotherapy　短期化学療法
small cell carcinoma　小細胞癌
small cleaved cell　小付着細胞
squamous cell carcinoma　扁平上皮癌
succinylcholine chloride　スクシニルコリン
SCCA
squamous cell carcinoma　扁平上皮癌
squamous cell carcinoma antigen　扁平上皮癌抗原
SCCB
small cell carcinoma of the bronchus　気管支小細胞癌
SCCH
sternocostoclavicular hyperostosis　胸肋鎖骨過形成症
SCCHN
squamous cell carcinoma of head and neck　頭頸部扁平上皮癌
SCCL
small cell〔oat cell〕 carcinoma of the lung　肺小細胞〔燕麦細胞〕癌
SCD
sickle cell disease　鎌状赤血球病
sister chromatid differentiation　姉妹染色体鑑別
spinocerebellar degeneration　脊髄小脳変性症
sterile connection device　無菌接続装置
subacute coronary disease　亜急性冠(状)動脈疾患
sudden cardiac death　突然心臓死
sudden coronay death　突然冠(状)動脈死
systemic carnitine deficiency　全身性カルニチン欠乏症
Sc.D.
Scientiae Doctor〈ラ〉=Docter of Science　理学博士
SCDA
scapula-dextra anterior position　肩甲右前位
ScDA
scapulo dextra anterior　右肩甲前位〈胎位〉
SCDC
subacute combined degeneration of spinal cord　亜急性連合性脊髄変性症
SCDP
scapulo-dextra posterior position　肩甲右後位

S

SCDS
sudden cardiac death syndrome　心臓性急死症候群

SCE
sister chromatid exchange　姉妹染色分体交換
somatic cell　体細胞
subcutaneous emphysema　皮下気腫

SCEF
stem cell enriched fraction　幹細胞濃縮分画

S cell
syncytium cell　合胞細胞

SCEP
spinal cord evoked potential　誘発脊髄電位

SCF
stem cell factor　幹細胞(刺激)因子
subclavian flap　鎖骨下弁

SCFA
short-chain fatty acid　短鎖脂肪酸

SCFE
slipped capital femoral epiphysis　大腿骨骨頭端線離開
super critical fluid extraction　超臨界流体抽出

SCF-FIA/CL
supercritical fluid flow injection analysis with chemiluminescence　化学発光検出超臨界流体フローインジェクション分析法

SCF/min
standard cubic feet per minute　標準毎分立方フィート

SCG
screening colonography　簡便式大腸X線検査法
serum-chemogram　血清ケモグラム
sodium cromoglycate　クロモグリク酸ナトリウム
superior cervical ganglion　上頸神経節

SCH
Schirmer (test)　シルマー検査
suprachiasmatic　視交叉〔差〕の

Sch
Schizophrenie〈独〉　統合失調症

SCH, sch
succinylcholine　スクシニルコリン

SCHDF
slow continuous hemodiafiltration　緩徐持続的血液濾過透析法

SChE
serum cholinesterase　血清コリンエステラーゼ

sched
schedule　スケジュール，調査表

SCHF
slow continuous hemofiltration　緩徐血液濾過法

schiz
schizophrenia 統合失調症

SCHL
subcapsular hematoma of the liver 肝(臓)被膜下血腫

Schr.
Schriften〈独〉 印刷物，テキスト

SCHUD
slow continuous hemo-ultrafiltration 緩徐持続血液限外濾過法

Schwach
Schwachsinn〈独〉 精神発達遅延

SCI
science citation index 科学引用索引
spinal cord injury 脊髄損傷
stem cell inhibitor 造血幹細胞の可逆的抑制因子
structured clinical interview 構造的臨床面接基準
subconjunctival injection 結膜下注射

sci
subcutaneous injection 皮下注射

Sci, sci
science 科学
scientific 科学的な

SCIA
superficial circumflex iliac artery 浅腸骨回旋動脈

SCID
severe combined immunod efficiency (disease) 重症複合(型)免疫不全症
structured clinical interview for diagnostic and statistic manual of mental disorders(＝DSM) Ⅲ-R DSM(＝精神障害分類診断基準)診断を下すための面接法

SciD
Doctor of Science 理学博士

scint
scintigram シンチグラム

Scinti
scintigram シンチグラム
scintillation シンチレーション

SCIPP
sacrococcygeal-to-inferior pubic point 仙尾下恥骨点

SCIS
severe combined immunodeficiency syndrome 重症複合型免疫不全症候群
Spinal Cord Injury Service 脊髄損傷サービス(科)

SCIU
Spinal Cord Injury Unit 脊髄損傷ユニット(病棟)

SCJ
squamocolumnar junction 扁平円柱上皮接合部
sternoclavicular joint 胸鎖関節
SCK
serum creatine kinase 血清クレアチンキナーゼ
SCL
scleroderma 強皮症，硬皮症
self check list of symptom inventory 自己徴候特性尺度
serum copper level 血清銅レベル
soft contact lens ソフトコンタクトレンズ
symptom checklist 症状チェックリスト
Scl
stem cell leukemia protein 幹細胞白血病蛋白
Scl, scl
sclerosis 硬化(症)
sclerotic 硬化(症)の
SCLA
scapula-laeva anterior position 肩甲左前位
ScLA
left scapulo-latero-anterior position 左肩前位
SCLC
small cell lung cancer 小細胞肺癌
small cell lung carcinoma 小細胞肺癌，肺小細胞癌
SCLD
sickle cell lung disease 鎌状赤血球肺症
SCLE
subacute cutaneous lupus erythematosus 亜急性皮膚型紅斑性狼瘡
Scler
sclerosis 硬化(症)
Sclero
endoscopic sclerotherapy 内視鏡的(食道静脈瘤)硬化療法
sclero
scleroderma 強皮症，硬皮症
SCLP
scapula-laeva posterior position 肩甲左後位
ScLP
left scapulo-posterior position 左肩後位
SCLS
systemic capillary leak syndrome 全身性毛細管漏出症候群
upleural curvilinear lines shadow 胸膜直下の曲線状陰影
SCM
Schwann cell membrane シュワン細胞膜
spondylotic caudal myelopathy 脊椎性尾髄症
State certified midwife (英国の)助産師

S

steatocystoma multiplex　多発性皮脂嚢腫(症)
sternocleidomastoid　胸鎖乳突の
streptococcal cell membrane　連鎖球菌細胞膜

SCMC
sperm-cervical mucus contact test　精子・頸管粘液接触試験
spontaneous cell-mediated cytotoxicity　自発的細胞媒介性細胞傷害性

S-CMC
S-carboxymethylcysteine　*S*-カルボキシメチルシステイン

SCN
suprachiasmatic nucleus　視交叉〔差〕核

SCND
spino-cerebellar negra degeneration　脊髄・小脳路黒核変性

SC node
supraclavicular node　鎖骨上(リンパ)節

SCNS
subcutaneous nerve stimulation　皮下神経刺激

SCO
subcommissural organ　交連下器官

SCOP, scop
scopolamine　スコポラミン

SCOPE
Scientific Committee on Problems of the Environment　環境問題科学委員会

scope
microscope　顕微鏡
oscilloscope　オシロスコープ

Scot virus
Scottish type of influenza virus　インフルエンザウイルスのスコッティー型

SCP
single cell protein　単細胞蛋白質
soluble cytoplasmic protein　可溶性細胞質蛋白
squamous cell papilloma　扁平上皮乳頭腫
submucous cleft palate　粘膜下口蓋裂

scp
scruple　スクループル
spherical candle power　球面燭光

SCPK, S-CPK
serum creatine phosphokinase　血清クレアチンホスホキナーゼ

SCR
silicon controlled rectifier　シリコン制御整流素子
skin conductance response　皮膚コンダクタンス反応
spondylotic caudal radiculopathy　脊椎性尾神経根症

sucralfate　スクラルフェート(＝ショ糖硫酸エステルアルミニウム塩)

SCr
serum creatine　血清クレアチン
serum creatinine　血清クレアチニン

SCR, scr
scruple　スクループル〈単位〉

ScRA
right scapulo-anterior position　右肩甲前位

SCRAM
self-contained radiation monitor　自己内蔵放射線モニター
Support Center for Regulatory Air Models　大気管理支援センター

SCRAP
simple complex reaction-time apparatus　単相性反応・時間装置

script
manuscript　原稿

Scripts, scripts
prescriptions　処方箋

ScRP
right scapulo-posterior position　右肩後位

SCRS
short clinical rating scale　簡易臨床評価尺度

scrup
scruple　スクループル〈単位〉

SCS
spinal cord stimulation　脊髄刺激
surface connecting system　血小板小管系
systolic click syndrome　収縮期クリック症候群

SCSIT
Southern California Sensory Integration Tests　南カリフォルニア感覚統合検査

sc.sp
scapular spine　肩甲(骨)棘

SCT
salmon calcitonin　サケカルシトニン
Sentence Completion Test　文章完成検査
sentence completion test　文章完成テスト
sex chromatin test　性クロマチン検査
sickle cell trait　鎌状赤血球形成傾向
spinal computed tomography　脊髄コンピュータ断層撮影(法)
sugar-coated tablet　糖衣錠

S

scty
security 安全，保障
SCU
self care unit 軽症病棟
shock care unit ショック症集中治療室
Special Care Unit 特別ケア病棟
special care unit 専門別集中治療病棟
SCUBA
self-contained underwater breathing apparatus 自給式潜水器具
SCUCP
small cell undifferentiated carcinoma of the prostate 前立腺未分化小細胞癌
SCUD
septicemic cutaneous ulcerative disease 敗血性皮膚潰瘍性疾患
SCUF
slow continuous ultrafiltration 緩徐持続限外濾過法
SCV
sensory (nerve) conduction velocity 知覚(神経)伝導速度
single concave 単凹面の
smooth, capsulated, virulent 無色の，被嚢のある，毒性のある
squamous cell carcinoma of the vulva 外陰扁平上皮癌
subclavian vein 鎖骨下静脈
SCW
streptococcal cell wall 連鎖球菌細胞壁
SCX
single convex 単凸面の
SD
Sandhoff disease サンドホフ病
Schattendefekt〈独〉 陰影欠損
scleroderma 強皮症
secretion droplet 分泌小滴
self-destroying 自己破壊の
senile dementia 老人〔老年〕性痴呆
septal defect 中隔欠損(症)
septal deviation 中隔彎曲
serological defined 液性抗体により区別される
serologically defined antigen 血清学的識別抗原
serologically detected 血清学的に検出された
serologically determined 血清学的に定量(決定)された
severe dysplasia 重度異形成
shoulder disarticulation 肩(関節)離開
shoulder dislocation 肩(関節)脱臼

Shy-Drager (syndrome) シャイ・ドレーガー(症候群)
soma and dendrite 細胞体樹状突起
sorbitol dehydrogenase ソルビトール脱水素酵素〔デヒドロゲナーゼ〕
sphincter dilatation 括約筋拡張
spondylosis deformans 変形性脊髄症
spontaneous delivery 自然分娩
Sprague-Dawley (rat) スプレーグ・ドーリー(ラット)
spreading depression 拡延性抑制
standard deviation 標準偏差(＝σ)《統》
Stensen duct ステンセン管
streptodornase ストレプトドルナーゼ
stuff development スタッフ能力開発
succinic dehydrogenase コハク酸脱水素酵素
sudden deafness 突発性難聴
sudden death 突然死，急死
superoxide dismutase スーパーオキシドジスムターゼ
surface dose 表面線量
syringe driver 持続皮下注入法
systematic desensitization 系統的脱感作
systolic discharge 収縮期流出

Sd
stimulus discriminative 識別性刺激
stimulus drive 本能的衝動を惹起させる刺激

S/D
sharp/dull 鋭い/鈍い
systolic to diastolic (ratio) (心臓の)収縮期・拡張期(比)

S-D
sickle cell-(hemoglobin) D (disease) 鎌状(赤)血球(血色素)D(病)
strength-duration 強さ・時間

SD, S.D.
skin dose 皮膚線量

SDA
Sabouraud dextrose agar サブローブドウ糖寒天(培地)
sacro-dextra anterior position 右仙骨前位
salt-dependent agglutinin 食塩水依存凝集素
serotonin-dopamine antagonist セロトニンド(ー)パミン拮抗薬
Seventh Day Adventist セブンスデイ教派
sialodacryoadenitis (virus) 唾液涙腺炎(ウイルス)
specific-dynamic action 特殊動的作用
statistical data analysis 統計データ分析プログラム《コン》
steroid-dependent asthma ステロイド依存性喘息

S

succinic dehydrogenase activity　コハク酸脱水素酵素作用
supraduodenal angle　上十二指腸角
survey data analysis　調査データ分析プログラム《コン》

SD antigen
serologically defined antigen　血清学的識別抗原，SD抗原

SDAT
senile dementia of Alzheimer type　アルツハイマー型老年〔老人〕(性)痴呆

SDB
scattered dense body　散在性濃縮体
sleeping disordered breathing　睡眠障害性呼吸
superficial dermal burn　浅達性II度熱傷

SDBP
sitting diastolic blood pressure　坐位拡張期血圧
standing diastolic blood pressure　立位拡張期血圧
supine diastolic blood pressure　背臥位(仰臥位)拡張期圧

SDC
salivary duct carcinoma　唾液腺管癌腫
serum digitalis concentration　血清ジギタリス濃度
serum digoxin concentration　血清ギゴキシン濃度
sodium deoxycholate　デオキシコール酸ナトリウム
splenic dendritic cell　脾樹状細胞
succinyldicholine　スクシニルジコリン

SDD
selective decontamination of the digestive tract　選択的消化管内殺菌(法)
selective digestive (tract) decontamination　選択的消化管内殺菌(法)
slow diastolic depolarization　緩徐拡張期脱分極
sporadic depressive disease　散発性うつ病

SDEEG
stereotactic depth electroencephalogram　定位深部脳波

SDF
soluble dietary fiber　水溶性食物繊維
stroma cell-derived factor　幹細胞分泌因子

SDGF
smooth muscle cell derived growth factor　平滑筋細胞由来増殖因子

SDH
serine dehydrase　セリンデヒドラーゼ
sorbitol dehydrogenase　ソルビトール脱水素酵素
spinal dorsal horn　脊髄後角
subdural hematoma　硬膜下血腫
succinate dehydrogenase　コハク酸脱水素酵素

succinic dehydrogenase　コハク酸脱水素酵素

SDH1

succinate dehydrogenase-1　コハク酸脱水素酵素 1

SDHD

sudden death heart disease　突然死心疾患

SDI

selective dissemination of information　選択的情報サービス

succinic dehydrogenase inhibition　コハク酸脱水素酵素抑制

SDIHD

sudden-death ischemic heart disease　突然死虚血性心疾患

SDL

serum digoxin level　血清ジゴキシンレベル

SDLE

subacute disseminated lupus erythematosus　亜急性播種状エリテマトーデス

SDLT

senile dementia of Lewy body type　レビー小体型老人性痴呆

SDM

sulfadimethoxine　スルファジメトキシン

SDM, sdm

standard deviation of the mean　平均値の標準偏差値

SDMA

Surgical Dressing Manufacturies Association　外科被覆材料製造協会

SDM antigen

serological detectable male antigen　血清学的に検出可能な男性抗原

SDMS

spatial data management system　空間データ管理システム《コン》

SDN

sexually dimorphic nucleus　性的二系核

subdural hematoma　硬膜下血腫

SDP

sacro-dextra posterior position　右仙骨後位

stomach, duodenum, pancreas　胃・十二指腸・膵臓

subdual pressure　硬膜下腔圧

subdural intracranial pressure　硬膜下頭蓋内圧

SD-PC

single donor-platelet concentrate　ヒト血小板濃縮物

SDPS

serial dilution protamine sulfate test　硫酸プロタミン連続希釈試験

SDR

scientific data recorder　科学データ記録器

simple diabetic retinopathy　単純型糖尿病性網膜症

S

SD ratio
systolic/diastolic ratio (心臓の)収縮期・拡張期比

SDS
self directed search 自己診断テスト
self-rating depression scale (抑)うつ性自己評価尺度
sensory deprivation syndrome 感覚妨害症候群
sexual differentiation scale 性分化スケール
Shy-Drager syndrome シャイ・ドレーガー症候群
sodium dodecyl sulfate ドデシル硫酸ナトリウム
somatoform disorder schedule 身体表現性障害スケジュール
speech discrimination score 言語識別スコア
sudden-death syndrome 突然死症候群

Sds, sds
sound 音

SD-SK
streptodornase-streptokinase ストレプトドルナーゼストレプトキナーゼ

SDS-PAGE
sodium dodecyl sulfate-polyacrylamide gel electrophoresis ドデシル硫酸ナトリウムポリアクリルアミドゲル電気泳動

SD spike
SD(=soma-dendritic) spike 細胞体・樹状突起スパイク, SDスパイク

SDT
sacro-dextra transverse position 右仙骨横位
speech detection threshold 語音聴力レベル

SE
exciting sympathin 興奮性シンパチン
saline enema 生理食塩液浣腸
Salmonella enteritis サルモネラ腸炎
sanitary engineering 衛生工学
series elastic component 連続弾性成分
series elastic element 直列弾性要素
sheep erythrocyte ヒツジ赤血球
side effect 副作用
size exclusion 分子量判別上限
soap (suds) enema 石鹸浣腸
special equipment 特殊装置
sphenoethmoidal (suture) 蝶篩骨縫合
spin echo スピンエコー法
spongiform encephalopathy 海綿状脳症
squamous epithelium 扁平上皮
standard error 標準誤差
staphylococcal enterotoxin ブドウ球菌腸内毒素
staphylococcal extract ブドウ球菌エキス

status epilepticus　てんかん重積状態
strong echo　高(輝度)エコー
subendothelial　内皮下の
syncytial endometritis　合胞体細胞性子宮内膜炎

Se
secretion　分泌(型)
secretor　分泌者
secretor gene　分泌遺伝子
selenium　セレン〈元素〉

se
expose to serosa　組織学的漿膜面癌露出度

^{75}Se
selenium-75　セレニウム75

S.E.
Simens-Einheit〈独〉　シーメンス単位

S/E
standardization/evaluation　標準化・評価

S & E
skeletal and extremities　骨格と四肢

SEA
sensitized erythrocyte agglutination (test)　感作赤血球凝集反応
spontaneous electrical activity　自発電気活動
staphylococcal enterotoxine A　ブドウ球菌腸毒素A

SEAMIC
South-East Asian Medical Information Center　東南アジア医学情報センター

SEAPAL
South-East Asia and Pacific Area League against Rheumatism　東南アジアリウマチ連合

SEAT
sheep erythrocyte agglutination test　ヒツジ赤血球凝集テスト

SEB
staphylococcal enterotoxin B　ブドウ球菌腸毒素B

SEBA
staphylococcal enterotoxin B antiserum　ブドウ球菌腸毒素B抗血清

Seb Derm
seborrheic dermatitis　脂漏性皮膚炎

SEC
secretin　セクレチン
secundum〈ラ〉＝according to　〜によれば
Singapore epidemic conjunctivitis　シンガポール流行性結膜炎
sinusoidal endothelial cell　類洞内皮細胞(肝)
size exclusion chromatography　サイズ排除クロマトグラフィ
soft elastic capsule　軟性弾性被膜

Sec
Seconal セコナール
sec
section 切断，切開，切片
sectioned 切開した，切断した
sections (分)節，区画，区分
sec，sec.
second 秒
secondary 第二の，二次的の，二次性の
secretary 秘書
SECG
stress electrocardiography ストレス心電図検査法
SECM
scanning electrochemical microscopy 走査型電気化学顕微鏡
sec.reg.
secundum regulam〈ラ〉 規則に従って《処》
sect，sect.
section 切開，切断
sectioned 切開した，切断した
sections (分)節，区画，区分
SED
Side Effects of Drugs 薬品の副作用
skin erythema dose X線皮膚紅斑量
spondyloepiphyseal dysplasia 脊椎骨端異形成症
staphylococcal enterotoxin D ブドウ球菌腸毒素D
sed.
sedes〈ラ〉＝stool 便
SED，Sed，sed，sed.
sediment 沈渣
sedimentation 沈殿，沈降
sed，sed.
secretary 秘書
sedate 鎮静させる
sedative 鎮静の，鎮静薬
SED congen
spondyloepiphyseal dysplasia congenita 先天性脊椎骨端骨異形成症
sed.rt
sedimentation rate 沈殿率，沈殿速度，沈降速度
SED tarda
spondyloepiphyseal dysplasia tarda 遅発性脊椎骨端骨異形成症
sed.time
sedimentation time 沈殿時間，沈降時間
SEE
staphylococcal enterotoxin E ブドウ球菌腸内毒素E

SEEG
scalp electroencephalogram 頭皮脳波
SEEG, s-EEG
Stereoelektroenzephalographie〈独〉= stereoencephalography 立体(的)脳波(法)
SEER
surveillance, epidemiology and end results 生存率・疫学・最終結果
SEF
sodium excreting factor ナトリウム排泄因子
staphylococcal enterotoxin F ブドウ球菌腸毒素F
SEG
sono-encephalogram 音脳図
Seg
segmentkernige Leukozyten〈独〉 分葉核好中球
seg
segmentation 分割
segmented 分割された
segmented (neutrophil) 分葉核(好中球)
segregate 分離する
segregated 分離された
segregation 分離
Seg, seg
segment 区(域), 分節, 分画, 分割する
SEGS, Segs, segs
segmented neutrophils 分葉核好中球
SEH
European Society of Haematology 欧州血液学会
subependymal hemorrhage 脳室上衣下出血
SEHA
specific emotional hazards of adulthood 成人の特異感情障害
SEHC
specific emotional hazards of childhood 小児期の特異感情障害
sei
expose and invade to serosa 組織学的漿膜面癌露出および浸潤度
SEL
saline exudate *Listeria* 生理食塩水抽出リステリア属
SEM
scanning electron microscope 走査型電子顕微鏡
slow eye movement 遅い眼球運動
standard error of mean 標準偏差, 平均値標準誤差《統》

S

systolic ejection murmur　収縮期駆出性雑音
verbal sample evaluation method　言語標準評価法

sem
semicolon　セミコロン
seminal　精液の

sem.
semen〈ラ〉=seed　精液，種子
semper〈ラ〉　常に

sem, sem.
semi, *semis*〈ラ〉　半分

semel in d.
semel in die〈ラ〉=once a day　1日1回《処》

Semf
seminal fluid　精液

SEMI
subendocardial myocardial infarction　心内膜下心筋梗塞
subendocardial myocardial injury　心内膜下心筋損傷

semih.
semihora〈ラ〉=half an hour　30分

sem.ves.
seminal vesicle　精嚢

SEN
state enrolled nurse　(英国の)準看護師

sen
sensation　感覚
sensitive　感(受)性の

↓sen
decreased sensation　知覚低下，感覚低下
diminished sensation　知覚低下，感覚低下

sens
sensation　感覚
senses　感覚
sensitive　感(受)性の
sensory　感覚の，知覚の

SENS, sens
sensorium　感覚器，感覚中枢

sens, SENS, sens.
sensitivities (test)　感受性(試験)
sensitivity　感受性(試験)，鋭敏度

sense.decr.
sensation decreased　知覚低下した，感覚低下した

sens.lat.
sensu lato〈ラ〉=in the broad sense　広義の

sens.str.
sensu stricto〈ラ〉=in the strict sense　狭義の

SEO
shoulder-elbow orthosis 肩・肘装具
SEP
sensory evoked potential 感覚性誘発電位
septum pellucidum〈ラ〉 透明中隔
sepultus〈ラ〉＝buried 埋葬した
Society of Experimental Psychologist 実験精神科医会
somatosensory evoked potential 体性感覚誘発電位
sperm entry point 精子進入部位
spinal (cord) evoked potential 脊髄誘発電位
surface epithelium 表面上皮
swine enzootic pneumonia ブタ流行性肺炎
systolic ejection period 収縮駆出期
sep
separate 分離する
separated 分離した
separately 別々に
separation 分離
separ.
separatum〈ラ〉＝separately 別々に《処》
SEPS
selenium-containing protein saccharide セレン含有蛋白糖(類)
SEPT
septal nucleus 中隔核
sept, sept.
septem〈ラ〉＝seven 7
septum 中隔
septo
septoplasty (鼻)中隔形成(術)
SEQ
Side-Effects Questionnaire 副作用質問用紙
seq.
sequela〈ラ〉＝that which follows 続発症，後遺症
sequens, *sequentes*〈ラ〉＝the following 次のもの《処》
sequestrum 分裂片，壊死片
Seq, seq
sequence 連鎖，配列順(序)，連続
seq.luce.
sequenti luce〈ラ〉＝the following morning 翌朝，翌日《処》
SER
sensory evoked response 知覚誘発反応
service サービス
smooth-surfaced endoplasmic reticulum 滑面小胞体

S

somatosensory evoked response(s) 体性感覚誘発反応
systolic ejection rate 収縮期駆出率(速度)

Ser
seryl セリル

ser
serial 連続した
serially 連続的に
series 直列，系
serological 血清学的な
serous 漿液(性)の，血清の
serum 漿液，血清

Ser, ser
serine セリン
serology 血清学

SERA
service, education, rehabilitation for addiction 麻薬常習者のためのサービス・教育・リハビリテーション

ser.Cl
serum chloride 血清塩素(イオン)

SERFC
sheep erythrocyte rosette forming capacity ヒツジ赤血球ロゼット形成能

ser.ind
serum index 血清指数

SerK
serine protein kinase 蛋白質中のセリンリン酸化酵素

SERM
selective estrogen receptor modulator 選択的エストロゲン受容体調整

serol
serology 血清学

serosang
serosanguineous 漿液血液状の

Serpins
serine protease inhibitor セリン蛋白質分解酵素阻害因子

serquih.
serquihora〈ラ〉 1時間半

SERRS
surface-enhanced resonance Raman scattering spectroscopy 表面増感共鳴ラマン散乱分光法

SERS
somatosensory evoked response 体性感覚誘発反応
surface enhanced Raman scattering 表面増強ラマン散乱

ser.sect
serial section 連続切片
SERT
serotonin transporter protein セロトニン運搬蛋白
serv.
service(s) サービス
serv, serv.
serva〈ラ〉=keep, preserve 保存せよ《処》
SES
serum enzyme standard 血清酵素標準
socioeconomic status 社会経済状態
subendothelial space 内皮下腔
SEs
staphylococcal enterotoxin 黄色ブドウ球菌エンテロトキシン
sesquih.
sesquihora〈ラ〉=an hour and a half 1時間半
sesquiunc.
sesquiuncia〈ラ〉=an ounce and a half 1オンス半
SESS
secondary empty sella syndrome 続発性トルコ鞍空虚症候群
Sess
sessile 無茎の，無柄の
session 会期，学期，授業時間
SET
systolic ejection time 収縮期駆出時間
single embryo transfer 単一胚移植法
sev
sever 切断する，分離する
several いくつかの
severe 重症の
severed 障害された
SE valve
Starr-Edwards valve スター・エドワーズ弁
SEWHO
shoulder-elbow-wrist-hand-orthosis 肩・肘・手関節・手指装具
SEWO
shoulder-elbow-wrist-orthosis 肩・肘・手関節装具
sex
sexual 性の，性的な，性対象者
SeXO
serum xanthine oxidase 血清キサンチン酸化酵素〔オキシダーゼ〕
s.expr.
sine expression 圧搾しないで《処》

SF

Sabin-Feldman (dye test)	セービン・フェルドマン(色素試験)
safety factor	安全因子
salt free	無塩(の)
scarlet fever	猩紅熱
secondary failure	二次的無効
seizure frequency	発作頻度
seminal fluid	精液
sensitizing factor	感作因子
serum factor	血清因子
serum fibrinogen	血清フィブリノゲン
shunt flow	シャント流量
silicone fluid	液状シリコン
skin fibroblast	皮膚線維芽細胞
skin fluorescence	皮膚螢光
skinned fiber	被覆線維
slow filling	緩徐充満期
soft feces	軟便
sound and flash	音と閃光
sound field	音場
special facility	特別施設
spectrofluorometry	螢光分析測定法
spinal fluid	髄液
spontaneous fracture	自然骨折，特発骨折
stable factor	安定因子
standard form	標準型
Streptococcus faecalis	糞便連鎖球菌，大便連鎖球菌
Streptococcus faecalis broth	SFブイヨン
stress formula	ストレス方式
sulfa preparation	スルファ剤
sulfur hexafluoride	六フッ化硫黄(ガス)
sulphation factor	硫酸化因子
superfamily	スーパーファミリー
suppressor factor	抑制因子
surfactant	表面活性物質
surviving factor	生存因子
synovial fluid	滑液

s.f.

sub finem〈ラ〉	終わりに

SFA

saturated fatty acid	飽和脂肪酸
seminal fluid assay	精液検査
serum folic acid	血清葉酸
superficial femoral artery	表在大腿動脈
suppressive factor of allergy	アレルギーの抑制因子

SFB
surgical foreign body　外科的異物
SFC
spinal fluid count　髄液細胞数算定
spot forming cell　スポット形成細胞
supercritical fluid chromatography　超臨界流体クロマトグラフィ
s.f.c.a.
sub finem conquendi adde〈ラ〉　煮沸の終わりに加えよ《処》
SFD
skin-film distance　皮膚・フィルム(間)距離
small for dates (infant)　在胎週に比して小さい(新生児)＝過少体重(児)
source film distance　線源フィルム間距離
staphylococcal food-borne disease　ブドウ球菌食中毒
SFDE
simultaneous supercritical fluid derivatization and extraction　誘導体化反応超臨界流体抽出
SF def.
silver fork deformity　銀フォーク変形
SFD infant
small-for-dates infant　過小体重児，SFD児
SFE
supercritical fluid extraction　超臨界流体抽出
SFEMG
single-fiber electromyography　単線維筋電図検査(法)
SFFF
salt-free fat-free (diet)　無塩無脂肪(食)
SFFV
spleen focus forming virus　赤芽球性白血病ウイルス
SFG
spotted fever group　紅斑熱群
SFGR
spotted fever group rickettsia　紅斑熱群リケッチア
SFH
schizophrenia family history　統合失調症家族歴
stroma-free hemoglobin　基質遊離血色素
SFHS
stroma-free hemoglobin solution　基質遊離血色素液
SFI
Sexual Functioning Index　性機能指数
Social Function Index　社会機能指数
SFIT
standard family interaction test　標準家族相互作用試験
SFL
synovial fluid lymphocyte　関節液中リンパ球

SFM
scanning force microscopy 原子間力顕微鏡
soluble fibrin monomer 可溶性フィブリンモノマー

SFMC
soluble fibrin monomer complex 可溶性フィブリンモノマー複合体
synovial fluid mononuclear cell 関節滑液内単核細胞

SFNB
stereotactic fine-needle biopsy 定位穿刺生検

S form
smooth form スムーズ型

SFP
screen filtration pressure スクリーン濾過圧
simultaneous foveal perception 中心窩同時視
spinal fluid pressure 脊髄圧
spleen fibrinolytic protease 脾フィブリン溶解蛋白酵素

SFR
skin reacting factor 皮膚反応因子
split function ratio 分腎機能比

s.fr.
spirituus frumenti〈ラ〉=spirit of grain ウイスキー

SFS
small fenestra stapedectomy アブミ骨小開窓
Spiegler-Fendt sarcoid シュピーグラー・フェント類肉腫

SFT
Sabin-Feldman (dye) test セービン・フェルドマン(色素)試験
sensory feedback therapy 感覚フィードバック療法
skinfold thickness 皮脂厚
solitary fibrous tumor 単発性線維性腫瘍

SFTS
severe fever with thrombocytopenia syndrome 重症熱性血小板減少症候群

SF units
Svedberg units of flotation スベドベリ浮上定数

SFV
Semliki Forest virus セムリキ森林ウイルス
shipping fever virus 船積み熱ウイルス
Shope fibroma virus ショープ線維腫ウイルス
squirrel fibroma virus リス線維腫ウイルス
superficial femoral vein 浅大腿静脈

SFW
slow filling wave 緩徐充盈波

SFXR
superficial X-ray 表面X線

SG
secondary glaucoma 続発性緑内障
secretory granule 分泌顆粒
serum globulin 血清グロブリン
serum glucose 血清グルコース
sign 徴候，符号
skin graft 皮膚移植(片)
soluble gelatin 可溶性ゼラチン
substantia gelatinosa 膠様質
Surgeon General 軍医総監
Swan-Ganz catheter スワン・ガンツカテーテル

Sg
segmentkernige Leukozyten<独> 分葉核好中球

S-G
Sachs-Georgi test ザックス・ゲオルギー反応

s-g
subgenus 亜属

SG, Sg, s.g, sg
specific gravity 比重

SGA
short gastric artery 短胃動脈
small-for-gestational-age (infant) 在胎週数に比較して体重の少ない(新生児)＝過少体重(児)
sulfoglycopeptide antigen 硫酸グリコペプチド抗原

SGB
stellate ganglion block 星状神経節ブロック

SGC
Swan-Ganz catheter スワン・ガンツカテーテル

Sg.C.
surgeon captain 外科医長

SG-C
serum gentamicin concentration 血清ゲンタミ〔マイ〕シン濃度

SG cath
Swan-Ganz catheter スワン・ガンツカテーテル

Sg.cr.
Surgeon Commander 軍医中佐

SGD
small group discussion 小人数討議
specific granule deficiency 特殊顆粒欠損症

SGE
secondary generalized epilepsy 二次性全般てんかん
second gas effect 二次ガス効果

SGF
sarcoma growth factor 肉腫成長因子
skeletal growth factor 骨格成長因子

SGFR
single-nephron glomerular filtration rate　単一ネフロン糸球体濾過率
S-GG
subgenera　亜属
SGH
subgaleal hematoma　帽状腱膜下血腫
SGL
serum gastrin level　血中ガストリン値
sgl
single　単一の
SGN
superior gluteal nerve　上殿神経
SGO
Surgeon General Office　外科医全般事務局
Surgery, Gynecology, and Obstetrics　外科・婦人科・産科
S.G.O.
Surgeon-General's Office　米国軍医総監室
SGOMSEC
Scientific Group on Methodologies for Safety Evaluation of Chemicals　化学物質安全性評価法検討会
sGOT, s-GOT
serum glutamic oxaloacetic transaminase　血清グルタミン酸オキサロ酢酸アミノトランスフェラーゼ
SGP
serine glycerophosphatide　セリングリセロホスファチド
soluble glycoprotein　可溶性糖蛋白
sGPT, s-GPT
serum glutamic-pyruvic transaminase　血清グルタミン酸ピルビン酸トランスアミナーゼ
SGR
Sachs-Georgische Reaktion〈独〉　ザックス・ゲオルギー反応
submandibular gland renin　顎下腺レニン
substantia gelatinosa Rolandi　ロランド膠様質

sgs
signs　徴候，符号
SGT
serum gastrin test　血中ガストリン値
Sgt
Schwangerschaft〈独〉　妊娠
SGTH
sex gland trophic hormone　性腺刺激ホルモン(＝ゴナドトロピン)
SGTT
standard glucouce tolerance test　標準耐糖テスト

SGV
salivary gland virus 唾液腺ウイルス
selective gastric vagotomy 選択的胃迷走神経切断

SH
Schönlein-Henoch (disease) シェーンライン・ヘノッホ(病)
semihorizontal position 半水平位《心電》
serum hepatitis 血清肝炎
sex hormone 性ホルモン
sexual harassment 性的嫌がらせ
sham 見かけの
sharp 鋭い
sick in hospital 院内疾患
sinus-histiocytosis 洞組織反応
somatotropic hormone＝somatotropin 成長ホルモン，ソマトトロピン
sperm head 精子頭部
state hospital 州立病院
steroid hormone ステロイドホルモン
streptomycin and isonicotinoylhydrazine ストレプトマイシンとイソニコチン酸ヒドラジド
sulfhydryl スルフヒドリル
sulfhydryl radical スルフヒドリル基，SH基
surgical hernia 外科的ヘルニア
surgical history 外科手術歴
symptomatic hypoglycemia 症候性低血糖(症)
systemic hyperthermia 全身性高熱，全身性高体温

Sh
sheep ヒツジ
Shigella 赤痢菌(属)

SH, Sh, sh
shoulder 肩，ショルダー

SH, S.H.
social history 社会歴

Sh, sh
short 短い

SHA
selective hypoaldosteronism 選択的低アルドステロン症
sensitized hemagglutination 感作血球凝集反応
soluble HL(＝human lymphocyte) antigen 可溶性ヒトリンパ球抗原
staphylococcal hemagglutinating antibody ブドウ球菌(赤)血球凝集抗体
symptomatic hemolytic anemia 症候性溶血性貧血

SHAA
serum hepatitis-associated antigen 血清肝炎関連抗原

S

SHAA-Ab
serum hepatitis-associated antigen-antibody　血清肝炎関連抗原抗体
SHA-Ab
serum hepatitis-associated antibody　血清肝炎関連抗体
SH antigen
serum-hepatitis antigen　血清肝炎，SH抗原
SHARE
Service for Health in Asian and African Region　アジアアフリカ地域健康奉仕
SHAS
Shared Hospital Accounting System　共同利用型病院情報システム
SHAWCO
Students Health and Welfare Centers Organization　学生健康・福祉事務局連合
SHB, S Hb
sulfhemoglobin　スルフヘモグロビン
SHBD
serum X-hydroxy-butyrate dehydrogenase　血清Xヒドロキシブチル酸脱水素酵素
SHBG
sex hormone-binding globulin　性ホルモン結合グロブリン
SHBP
sex hormone binding protein　性ホルモン結合蛋白
SHC
sclerosing hepatic carcinoma　硬化性肝癌
subclavian vein hemodialysis catheter　鎖骨下静脈血透析用カテーテル
SHCO
sulfonated hydrogenerated castor oil　硫酸化水素添加ヒマシ油〔トウゴマ油〕
SHC rat
spontaneous hypercholesterolemia rat　自然発症高脂血症ラット
SHD
simultaneous hydrothermal decomposition　水熱分解同時誘導体化法
syphilitic heart disease　梅毒性心疾患
SHDI
supraoptical hypophysial diabetes insipidus　視交差〔叉〕上核下垂体性尿崩症
SHEENT
skin, head, eyes, ears, nose, throat　皮膚・頭・目・耳・鼻・咽喉
SHEP
Systolic Hypertension in the Eldery Program　米国老年者収縮期型高血圧研究，シェプ

SHF
simian hemorrhagic fever　サル出血(性)熱
SHF, shf
super high frequency　超高周波(数)
SHG
second harmonic generation　光第二高調波発生
synthetic human gastrin　合成ヒトガストリン
SHH
syndrome of hyporeninemic hypoaldosteronism　低レニン血症性低アルドステロン症
SHI
semisynthetic human insulin　半合成ヒトインスリン
Shig
Shigella　赤痢菌(属)
SHIS
shared hospital information system　共同利用型病院情報システム
SHL
sensorineural hearing loss　感覚神経性難聴
sudden hearing loss　特発性聴力損失
shl
shoulder　肩
SHLD, shld
shoulder　肩
shldr
shoulder　肩
SHLM
Society of Hospital Laundry Managers　病院洗濯業者協会
SHM
somatic hypermutation　体細胞超変異
spontaneous hemorrhagic necrosis　特発性出血性壊死
SHML
sinus histiocytosis with massive lymphoadenopathy　リンパ節肥大を伴う洞組織球症
SHMO
Senior Hospital Medical Officer　上級病院医療官
SHMT
serine hydroxymethyltransferase　セリンヒドロキシメチルトランスフェラーゼ
SHN
spontaneous hemorrhagic necrosis　特発性出血性壊死
subacute hepatic necrosis　亜急性肝(臓)壊死
SHO
secondary hypertrophic osteoarthropathy　二次性肥大性骨関節症

sho
shoulder 肩
should
shoulder 肩
SHP
Schönlein-Henoch purpura シェーンライン・ヘノッホ紫斑病
secondary hyperparathyroidism 二次性上皮小体機能亢進(症)
shielded hydrophobic phase シールド疎水性相
surgical hypoparathyroidism 外科(手術)性上皮小体機能低下(症)
SHR
spontaneously hypertensive rat(s) 高血圧自然発症ラット
SHRSP
stroke-prone spontaneous hypertensive rat 脳卒中易発症高血圧自然発症ラット
SHRSP, SHR-SP
spontaneously hypertensive rat, stoke-prone 脳卒中易発症高血圧自然発症ラット
SHS
Schönlein-Henoch syndrome シェーンライン・ヘノッホ症候群
shoulder-hand syndrome 肩手症候群
steely hair syndrome スチール様毛髪症候群
super high speed 超高速
supine hypotensive syndrome 仰臥位低血圧症候群
SHSS
Stanford hypnotic susceptibility scale スタンフォード催眠感受性尺度
SHT
simple hypocalcemic tetany 単純低カルシウム血性テタニー
subcutaneous histamine test 皮下ヒスタミン試験
SHUT
subject's height 被験者の身長
SHV
simian herpes virus サルヘルペスウイルス
SH virus
serum hepatitis virus 血清肝炎ウイルス
SHW
safety, health and welfare 安全・健康・福祉
sitting hepatic window 坐位肝窓(技術)
Shy
thiohypoxanthine チオヒポキサンチン
SI
International System of Unit 国際単位

sacroiliac 仙腸骨の
saline infusion 食塩水注入
saline injection 食塩水注射
saturation index 飽和指数
selectivity index 選択性指数
sensitive index 感受性指標
serious illness 重病
serum insulin 血清インスリン
serum iron 血清鉄
severity index 重症度指数
sex inventory 性項目表
sexual intercourse 性交
similarity index 相似度指数
single injection 単独注射
situs inversus〈ラ〉 内臓転位
small intestine 小腸
smear index 腟スメア指数
special intervension 特別治療
spin-immunoassay スピン免疫(測定)法
spleen index 脾指数
stimulation index 刺激指数
stress incontinence ストレス性失禁
stroke index (1回)心拍出係数
subicteric 亜黄疸
subindex 副索引
sublinguinal 鼠径下
sulfisoxasole(=sulphafurazole) スルフイソキサゾール(=スルファフラゾール)
suppressor index 抑制指数
survey instruction 調査指導
Système International d'Unités〈仏〉= International System of Units 国際単位系，SI単位
systolic index 収縮係数

Si
silicon ケイ素〈元素〉

si
invade to serosa 組織学的漿膜癌滲出度

SI, S.I.
soluble insulin 可溶性インスリン

SIA
Sanitary Institute of America 米国健康研究所
serum inhibitory activity 血清抑制活性
spin immunoassay スピン免疫(測定)法
stimulation-induced analgesia 刺激誘導鎮痛(法)
stress induced analgesia ストレスによる無痛覚症
stress-induced anesthesia ストレス誘発感覚脱出

S

subacute infectious arthritis　亜急性感染性関節炎

Sia
sialic acid　シアル酸

SIADH
syndrome of inappropriate secretion of antidiuretic hormone　抗利尿ホルモン不適合分泌症候群

SIAM
swift increase in alcohol metabolism　アルコール代謝における迅速な増加

sib
sibling　同胞，子孫〈単数〉

SIBC
Association Mondiale des Sociétés d'Anatomie Pathologique de Biologic Clinique〈仏〉　国際臨床病理学会
Société International de Biologie Clinique〈仏〉　国際臨床生物学会

sibs
siblings　同胞，子孫〈複数〉

SIC
serum inhibitory concentration　血清抑制濃度
serum insulin concentration　血清インスリン濃度
serum iron colloid　血清鉄コロイド
siccanin　シッカニン
Société Internationale de Cardiologie〈仏〉　国際心臓学会
Société Internationale de Chirurgie〈仏〉＝International Society of Surgery　国際外科学会

sic.
siccus〈ラ〉＝dry, dried　乾性の《処》

sicc.
siccus〈ラ〉＝dried　乾燥した《処》

SICD
serum isocitric dehydrogenase　血清イソクエン酸脱水素酵素

SICM
scanning ion conductance microscope　走査イオンコンダクタンス顕微鏡

SICOT
Société Internationale de Chirurgie Orthopedique et de Traumatologie〈仏〉＝International Society of Orthopaedic Surgery and Traumatology　国際整形災害外科学会

SICU
Spinal Intensive Care Unit　脊髄集中治療部(病棟)

surgical intensive care unit　外科集中治療部門

SID

Society for Investigative Dermatology　研究的皮膚科学会

source image receptor distance　撮影距離

source isocenter distance　線源アイソセンター間距離

subject identification module　主題同定基準

sudden infant death　乳幼児突然死

suggested indication of diagnosis　診断予想適応症

sulfisomidine　スルフイソミジン

systemic inflammatory disease　全身性炎症性疾患

s.i.d.

spiritus in dedo〈ラ〉　死んだ

sid, s.i.d.

semel in die〈ラ〉＝once a day　１日１回《処》

SIDS

sudden infant death syndrome　乳幼児突然死症候群

SIE

stroke in evolution　進行性脳卒中

SIECUS

Sex Information and Educational Council of United States　米国性情報教育協議会

SIF

serum inhibitory factor　血清抑制因子

somatotropin-inhibiting factor　ソマトトロピン〔成長ホルモン〕阻止因子

SIF cells

small intensely fluorescent cells　小さくて強い螢光を発する細胞

SIg

serum immune globulin　血清免疫グロブリン

sig

signet-ring cell carcinoma　印環細胞癌

SIG, Sig, sig

sigmoidoscope　S状結腸鏡

sigmoidoscopic　S状結腸鏡の

sigmoidoscopy　S状結腸鏡検査(法)

SIg, sIg

surface immunoglobulin　(膜)表面免疫グロブリン，細胞膜免疫グロブリン

Sig, sig

signal　信号，合図，シグナル

signature　用法指示，サイン，署名

signed　サインした，署名した

significant　有意な

S

Sig, sig.
signa〈ラ〉=write, label　表示せよ《処》
signetur〈ラ〉=let it be written　表示させよ《処》

sIgA, S-IgA
secretory immunoglobulin A　分泌型免疫グロブリンA

sig.F.
significant findings　はっきりした所見

sigmo
sigmoidoscopy　S状結腸鏡検査(法)

Sigmoid
sigmoidoscopy　S状結腸鏡検査(法)

sig.n.pro.
signa nomine proprio〈ラ〉=label with the proper name　固有(商品)名で表示せよ

Sig. 1 powder t.i.d.s.
Sig one powder 3 times a day　用法：1日3回1包ずつ服用《処》

Sig.1/3 t.i.d.p.c.Sum.
Signa pars tertia ter in die post cibos Sumenda〈ラ〉=1/3 part 3 times a day after meals, take one third part 3 times daily after meals　用法：1日3回食後1/3ずつ服用《処》

SIH
Société Internationale d'Hematologie〈仏〉=International Society of Haematology　国際血液学会

SIHM
Société Internationale d'Historie de la Médecine〈仏〉　国際医史学会

SIJ
sacroiliac joint　仙腸関節

SI jt
sacroiliac joint　仙腸関節

SIL
sister-in-law　義姉，義妹
Société Internationale de la Lèpre〈仏〉　国際ハンセン病学会
speech interference level　会話妨害レベル
squamous intraepithelial lesion　上皮内扁平病変

SILA
suppressible insulin-like activity　抑制可能インスリン様活性

SI list
seriously ill list　重症患者リスト

sIL-6R
soluble IL-6 receptor　可溶性IL-6受容体

SIM
selected ion monitoring　選択性イオンモニタリング

Society for Industrial Microbiology　産業微生物学会

Sim
simultaneous　同時の

sim
simulant　擬態の
simulation　詐病，仮病

sim.
simul〈ラ〉　ともに《処》

SIMG
Société Internationale de Médecine Générale〈仏〉＝International Society of General Practice　国際一般診療医学会

SIM medium
(hydrogen) sulfide, indole, motility medium　硫化水素・インドール・運動性試験培地，SIM培地

simp.
simplex〈ラ〉＝simple，single　単純な

SIMPL
scientific, industrial and medical photographic laboratories　科学的・産業的・医学的写真研究室

SIMS
second(ary) ion mass spectrometry　二次イオン質量分析法

simu
simulation　詐病，仮病

simula
simulation language　擬態言語

SIMV
synchronized〔synchronous〕intermittent mandatory ventilation　同期式間欠的強制換気

Simva
simvastatin　シンバスタチン

sin, sin.
sine〈ラ〉＝without　～なしの，～を伴わない《処》
sine　サイン
sinister，*sinistra*〈ラ〉＝left　左の
sinus　洞

sine aq.
sine aqua〈ラ〉　水のない《処》

sine conf.
sine confectione〈ラ〉＝without sweetness　甘みなしで《処》

sine express.
sine expressione〈ラ〉　圧搾しないで《処》

SINET
Science Information Network　科学情報ネットワーク

S

sing.
single 独身の，単一の
singular 単一の，単数の
singuli〈ラ〉=each おのおのの
singulorum〈ラ〉=of each それぞれ

sing. auror.
singulis auroris〈ラ〉 毎朝《処》

sinist.
sinister〈ラ〉 左(の)

si non val.
si non valeat〈ラ〉=if it is not strong enough 十分強力でなければ

si n.val.
si non valeat〈ラ〉=if it is not strong enough 十分強力でなければ

SIO
sacroiliac orthosis 仙腸装具

SIOH
supervision, inspection and overhear 超視，視察，偶聴

SIOP
Société Internationale d'Oncologie Pédiatrique〈仏〉=International Society of Paediatric Oncology 国際小児腫瘍学会

si op.sit
si opus sit〈ラ〉=if it is necessary, if necessary, if there is need 必要ならば，必要なとき

SIP
single inline package シングルインラインパッケージ《コン》
slow inhibitory potential 緩徐抑制(性)電位
Society Interamerican Psychology 米国精神医学会
sympathetically independent pain 交感神経非依存性疼痛
synechia iridis posterior 虹彩後癒着

SIPA
shear (stress)-induced platelet aggregation ずり(応力)惹起血小板凝集

SIPE
Société Internationale de Psychopathlogie de l'Expression〈仏〉 国際表現精神病理学会

SIPG
Société Internationale de Pathologie Géographique〈仏〉 国際地理病理学会

SIPI
serum immunoglobulin prognostic index 血清免疫グロブリン予後指数

S

SIPP
severity index of paraquat poisoning パラコート中毒の重症度指数
sIPTH
serum immunoreactive parathyroid hormone 血清免疫反応性上皮小体ホルモン
sir.
sirupi, *sirupus*〈ラ〉 シロップ剤《処》
SIREF
specific immune response-enhancing factor 特異的免疫反応増強因子
SIRF
severely impaired renal function 高度障害腎機能
SIRS
soluble immune response suppressor 可溶性免疫反応抑制因子
systemic inflammatory response syndrome 全身性炎症反応症候群＝サーズ
SIS
sterile injectable suspension 無菌で注射のできる懸濁液
Strategic-Information-System 戦略情報システム
sis
sister 姉，妹，看護師
SISI test
short increment sensitivity index test 短時間増強感覚指数，SISI検査
SISO
sisomicin シソミシン，シソマイシン
SISS
serum inhibitor of streptolysin S ストレプトリシンS血清抑制因子
SiSV
simian sarcoma virus サル肉腫ウイルス
SIT
serum inhibition test 血清抑制試験
Stanford-Intelligenz-Test〈独〉＝Stanford Intelligence Test スタンフォード知能テスト
SITE
suction infusion tissue extractor 吸引灌流組織摘出装置
SITEMSH
Société Internationale de Traumatologie du Ski et de Médecine des Sport d'Hiver〈仏〉＝International Society for Ski Traumatology and Medicine of Winter Sport 国際スキー外傷医学会
sitg
sitting 座っている，坐位の

Sitol
sitological 栄養学の
sitologist 栄養士
sitology 栄養学

sitr
silent treatment 沈黙療法

SITS
Société Internationale de Transfusion Sanguine〈仏〉 国際輸血学会

SIU
Société Internationale d'Urologie〈仏〉=International Society of Urology 国際泌尿器科学会

SI units
Système International d'Unités 国際単位系

SIV
simian immunodeficiency virus サル免疫不全ウイルス

si vir.perm.
si vires permittant〈ラ〉 もし強度が許せば

SIW
self-innicted wound 自損傷

SIX
sulfisoxazole スルフイソキサゾール

SJ, S-J
Stevens-Johnson (syndrome) スティーブンス・ジョンソン（症候群）

SJA
Sophora japonica agglutinin エンジュマメレクチン

SJM
St.Jude Medical valve 二葉円板弁，セイント・ジュード医学弁

SjO_2
saturation of jugular venous blood oxygen 頸静脈血酸素飽和度

SJP
small fiber junctional potential 細線維接合部電位

SJS
Stevens-Johnson syndorome スティーブンス・ジョンソン症候群
Swyer-James symdrome スワイヤー・ジェームス症候群

SjS
Sjögren syndrome シェーグレン症候群

SK
seborrheic keratosis 脂漏性角化症
senile keratosis 老人性角化症
skin 皮膚

solar keratosis 日光性角化症
streptokinase ストレプトキナーゼ
striae keratopathy 線条角膜症

sk
sick 病気
skeletal 骨格の

SKA
streptokinase activation ストレプトキナーゼ活性化

SKAO
supracondylar-knee-ankle orthosis 膝折れ防止用プラスチック短下肢装具

SKA orthosis
supra-knee-ankle orthosis 長下肢装具

SKAT
sex knowledge and attitude test 性知識および態度テスト

sked
schedule 予定，スケジュール

Skel, skel
skeletal 骨格の

SKI
skin 皮膚
Sloan-Kettering Institute スローン・ケタリング研究所

SKL
spleen, kidney, liver 脾・腎・肝

SKM
sarkomycin サルコマイシン

SKSD, SK/SD
streptokinase-streptodornase ストレプトキナーゼ・ストレプトドルナーゼ

sk.tr.
skeletal traction 骨格牽引

sk.trx.
skeletal traction 骨格牽引

sk.tx.
skeletal traction 骨格牽引

SL
salt loser 塩分喪失者
sarcolemma 筋細胞膜
Schwalbe line シュワルベ線
secondary lysosome 二次リソソーム
sensation level 感覚レベル
sensory latency 感覚〔知覚〕潜時
signal level 信号レベル
Sinding Larsen (disease) シンディング・ラーセン(病)
Sjögren-Larsson (syndrome) シェーグレン・ラルソン(症候群)

S

slit-lamp 細隙灯
small leukocyte 小白血球
small lymphocyte 小リンパ球
sodium lactate 乳酸ナトリウム
sound level 音レベル
spleen lymphocyte 脾リンパ球
Stein-Leventhal (syndrome) スタイン・レベンタール(症候群)
streptolysin ストレプトリジン
Strümpell-Lorrain (disease) シュトリュンペル・ローレイン(病)

Sl
sleep 睡眠

sl
slice スライス，切片
slight 軽度の
slow 遅い，緩徐の
slyke スライク

s.l.
saccharum lactis〈ラ〉 乳糖《処》
sensu lato〈ラ〉=in the broad sense 広義の
sensus luminis〈ラ〉 光覚弁

SL, sl
slightly 軽度に，わずかに
sublingual 舌下の

sl., s.l.
secundum legem〈ラ〉=according to the rules 基準〔規則〕に従って《処》

SLA
sacro-laeva anterior position 仙骨左前位
surfactant-like activity 表面活性物質様活性

SLAM
scanning laser acoustic microscope 走査型レーザー音響顕微鏡

SLAP
serum leucine aminopeptidase 血清ロイシンアミノペプチダーゼ

S

SLAR
side looking airborne radar 側視空輸レーダー

SLAT
slide latex agglutination test スライドラテックス凝集試験

SLB
short-leg-brace 神経疾患のリハビリテーション用短下肢装具

sl.blad.inf
slight bladder infection 軽度膀胱感染

SLC
short-leg cast 短下肢装具
sodium-lithium countertransport ナトリウム・リチウム対移送
surrogate light chain 代用L鎖
SLD
serum lactate〔lactic〕 dehydrogenase 血清乳酸脱水素酵素
specific learning disability 特殊学習不適合
spontaneous labyrinthine deviation 自発迷路性偏倚
sld
solid 硬い，固形の
sldf
solidification 固形化
SLDH
serum lactate〔lactic〕 dehydrogenase 血清乳酸脱水素酵素
SLDR
sublethal damage repair 亜致死障害回復
SLE
slit-lamp examination 細隙灯検査
St.Louis encephalitis セントルイス脳炎
systemic lupus erythematosus 全身性エリテマトーデス
SLEA
sheep erythrocyte antibody ヒツジ赤血球抗体
sheep erythrocyte antigen ヒツジ赤血球抗原
SLEV
St.Louis encephalitis virus セントルイス脳炎ウイルス
SLFIA
substrate-labeled fluorescent immunoassay 基質標識蛍光免疫測定法
Slfsyn
self-synchronous 自己同期の
SLHC
St.Luke Hospital Center 聖路加病院
SLI
secretin-like immunoreactivity セクレチン様免疫反応性
somatostatin-like immunoreactivity ソマトスタチン様免疫反応性
stimulation luminous intermittent 間欠発光刺激
SLK
superior limbic keratoconjunctivitis 上(方)輪部角結膜炎
SLKC
superior limbic keratoconjunctivitis 上(方)輪部角結膜炎
SLM
sound level meter 騒音計
supported liquid membrane 含浸型液体膜
SLMV
synaptic like microvesicle シナプス様小胞

S

SLN
supralaryngeal nerve 上喉頭神経
SLO
scanning laser ophthalmoscope レーザー走査型検眼鏡
second look operation 二次手術
streptolysin O ストレプトリジンO
SLOS
Smith-Lemli-Opitz syndrome スミス・レムリ・オピッツ症候群
SLP
sacro-laeva posterior position 仙骨左後位
subluxation of the patella 膝蓋骨亜脱臼
Slp
sex limited protein 性制限蛋白
SLR
straight-leg raising (test) 下肢伸展挙上(試験)
SLR exercise
straight-leg raising exercise 下肢伸展位挙上訓練
SLR test
straight leg raising test 下肢挙上試験
SLS
short-leg splint 短下肢装具，短下肢副子
Sjögren-Larsson syndrome シェーグレン・ラルソン症候群
sodium lauryl sulfate ラウリル硫酸ナトリウム
Stein-Leventhal syndrome スタイン・レベンタール症候群
streptolysin S ストレプトリジンS
SLSEP
short-latency components of the somatosensory evoked potential 短潜時体性知覚誘発電位
SLT
sacro-laeva transverse position 仙骨横位
scanning laser tomography 走査型レーザー断層撮影法
Shiga-like toxin 赤痢菌様毒素
single lung transplant 片肺移植
slt
slight 軽度の
slightly わずかに
SLTA
standard language test of aphasia 失語症の標準テスト
standard list for test of aphasia 失語症検査標準リスト
sly
slowly ゆっくりと
SM
saccadic eye movement 断続性眼球運動

sadomasochism	サドマゾヒズム
Schlafmittel〈独〉	催眠薬, 睡眠薬
semimembranous	半膜様の
Serratia marcescens	霊菌
simple mastectomy	単純乳房切除(術)
sinusitis maxillaris〈ラ〉	上顎洞炎
skim milk	脱脂乳
smoker	喫煙者
smooth muscle	平滑筋
smooth surfaced microsome	滑面小胞体
social maturity scale	社会生活能力検査
sodium morrhuate	肝油脂肪酸ナトリウム
somatomedin	ソマトメジン
Space Medicine	宇宙医学
sphingomyelin	スフィンゴミエリン
spontaneous migration	自然遊走能
sports medicine	スポーツ医学
stapedius muscle	アブミ骨筋
streptomycin	ストレプトマイシン, ストマイ
streptonigrin	ストレプトニグリン
stria medullaris〈ラ〉	髄条
Strümpell-Marie (disease)	シュトリュンペル・マリー(病)
submandibular	下顎骨下の, 顎下の
submucosal	粘膜下の
subnormal	正常以下の
sucrose (mannite) medium	ショ糖(マンニット)培地
suction method	吸引法
superior mesenteric	上腸間膜の
supernatant	上澄みの
surgical margin	切除断端
sustained medication	持続投薬
symptom	症状
synaptic membrane	シナプス膜
synovial membrane	滑膜
systolic murmur	収縮期雑音

Sm

samarium	サマリウム〈元素〉

sm

small	小さい

S/M

sadism/masochism	サディズム/マゾヒズム
sensory to motor	感覚/運動(比)

sm, SM

submucosa	粘膜下

Submucosal=limited to submucosa 深達度が粘膜下層の癌

SMA

sequential multichannel autoanalyzer 連続多重チャンネル自動分析器
sequential multiple analyzer 連続多数〔多種目〕分析器
simultaneous multichannel autoanalyzer 同時多重チャンネル自動分析器
site management associates 治験事務局担当者
smooth muscle antibody 抗平滑筋抗体
smooth muscle autoantibody 平滑筋自己抗体
sometomedin A ソマトメジンA
spinal muscle atrophy 脊髄性筋萎縮症
superior mesenteric artery 上腸間膜動脈
supplementary motor area 補足運動野
synthetic milk adapted 母乳化ミルク

SMA-12/60

Sequential Multiple Analysis-12 different serum tests in 60 minutes 連続多数分析60分12種血清検査

SMA-6

Sequential Multiple Analysis-6 different serum tests 連続多数分析 6 種血清検査

SM-A

somatomedin A ソマトメジンA

Sm Ab

Smith antibody Sm抗体(=可溶性核抗体の一種)

SMABV

superior mesenteric artery blood velocity 上腸間膜動脈血液速度

SMAC

Sequential Multiple Analyzer Computer 連続多項目分析装置，スマック
simultaneous multianalyzer computed 同時分析装置

SMAE

superior mesenteric artery embolus 上腸間膜動脈塞栓

S

SMAF

smooth muscle activating factor 平滑筋活性化因子
specific macrophage activating factor 特異的マクロファージ活性化因子
specific macrophage arming factor 特異的マクロファージ武装化因子
superior mesenteric artery (blood) flow 上腸間膜動脈(血)流量

SMAG

superior mesenteric arteriography 上腸間膜動脈造影

SMAL
serum methyl alcohol level　血清メチルアルコールレベル
small FCC
small follicular center cell　小型濾胞中心細胞
sm.amts
small amounts　少量
sm.an
small animal　小動物
SMANCS
styrene maleic acid neocarzinostatin　スチレンリンゴ酸ネオカルチノスタチン
SMAO
superior mesenteric artery occlusion　上腸間膜動脈閉塞(症)
SMART
stereotactic multiple ark radiotherapy　ライナックでの三次元集光照射システム
SMAS
superficial musculo-aponeurotic system　表在性筋腱膜系
SMA syndrome
superior mesenteric artery syndrome　上腸間膜動脈症候群
SMBG
self monitoring of blood glucose　血糖自己測定
SMBP
serum myelin basic protein　血清ミエリン塩基性蛋白
SMC
sacral micturition center　仙髄排尿反射中枢
smooth muscle cell　平滑筋細胞
System Monitor Center　システムモニターセンター
SM-C
somantomedin C　ソマトメジンC
SMCD
senile macular chorioretinal degeneration　老年性〔老人性〕脈絡網膜黄斑変性症
SMD
senile macular degeneration　老年性〔老人性〕黄斑変性(症)
Spina-malleolen Distanz〈独〉＝spina malleolar distance　腸骨前上棘・顆部間距離，棘踝長
sternocleidomastoid diameter　胸鎖乳突筋直径
submanubrial dullness　胸骨柄下濁音
SMDS
secondary myelodysplastic syndrome　二次性(続発性)骨髄異形成症候群
sudden manhood death syndrome　成人突然死症候群
SME
shape memory effect　形状記憶効果

S

skeletal muscle extract 骨格筋抽出液
stalk-median eminence 下垂体茎中央隆起

SMF
streptozotocin, mitomycin, 5-fluorouracil ストレプトゾトシン, マイトマイシン, フルオロウラシル

SMFM
scanning magnetic force microscope 走査磁力顕微鏡

SMG
submandibular gland 顎下腺

SMH
state mental hospital 州立精神病院

SMI
silent myocardial ischemia 無症候性心筋虚血
simplified menopausal index 簡略更年期指数
supplementary medical insurance 診療保険特別会計

SMIER
Société Médicale Internationale d'Endoscopie et de Radiocinématographie〈仏〉= International Medical Society for Endoscopy and Radiocinematography 国際内視鏡・放射線撮影医学会

SMIg
surface membrane immunoglobulin 表面膜免疫グロブリン

SMIT
Society of Minimally Invasive Therapy 非侵襲治療学会

smk
smoke 喫煙

smkls
smokeless 無煙の

sml
simulate 模倣する
simulation 模倣
simulator 模倣者
small 小さい

SMMC
sternomastoid myocutaneous flap 胸鎖乳突筋皮弁

SMMHC
smooth muscle myosin heavy chain 平滑筋ミオシンH鎖

SMN
second malignant neoplasma 二次悪性新生物
survival motor neuron 生存している運動神経

SMO
senior medical officer 上級医療事務官

Site Management Organization 治験施設支援機関

SMOH
Society of Medical Officer of Health 健康医療事務官協会

SMON
subacute myelo-optico-neuropathy 亜急性脊髄視神経障害，スモン(病)

SMP
sequential management problem 段階的患者管理問題
serum mucoprotein 血清ムコ蛋白
simultaneous macular perception 同時黄斑知覚
slow moving acid protease 遅作用酸性蛋白酵素
submitochondrial particle 亜ミトコンドリア粒子
sulfamethoxypyrazine スルファメトキシピラジン
sympathetically maintained pain 交感神経依存性疼痛

smpx
smallpox 天然痘

SMR
skeletal muscle relaxant 骨格筋弛緩薬
somnolent metabolic rate 睡眠時代謝率
spontaneous rupture of membranes 自然破水
standardized mortality ratio 標準化死亡比
standard metabolic rate 標準代謝率
submucous resection 粘膜下切除術

SMS
scalded mouth syndrome 熱傷様口腔(粘膜)症候群
stiff-man syndrome スティッフマン症候群

Smst
somatostatin ソマトスタチン

SMT
spontaneous mammary tumor 特発性乳腺腫瘍
submucosal tumor 粘膜下腫瘍

SMV
second morning voiding (urine) 起床後2回目の尿
Selbstmord Versuch〈独〉 自殺企図
superior mesenteric vein 上腸間膜静脈

SMVR
supraannular mitral valve replacement 弁輪上僧帽弁置換術

SMWDSep
single, married, widowed, divorced, separated 独身の・結婚した・妻(夫)を失った・離婚した・別居した

SMX
sulfamethoxazole スルファメトキサゾール

S

SMX/TMP
sulfamethoxazole trimethoprim　スルファメトキサゾールトリメトプリム

SMZ
sulfamethoxazole　スルファメトキサゾール

SN
school of nursing　看護学校
scrub nurse　手洗看護師，清潔看護師
sensorineural　感覚神経(性)の
sensory neuron　知覚ニューロン
seronegative　血清陰性の
serotoninergic neuron　セロトニン作働性神経
silicotic nodule　珪肺結節
sinus node　洞結節
spinal needle　脊椎穿刺針
spontaneous nystagumus　自発眼振
student nurse　看護学生
submassive necrosis　亜広汎性壊死
substantia nigra〈ラ〉　黒質
supernatant　上清

Sn
stannum〈ラ〉＝tin　スズ〈元素〉

s.n.
secundum naturam〈ラ〉＝according to nature　自然に従って
suo nomine〈ラ〉　薬名を記して《処》

S/N
signal/noise　信号・雑音(比)

SNA
superior nasal artery　上鼻動脈
sympathetic nervous system activity　交感神経系活性

SNAFu
situational normal, all fouled up　状況は正常で間違いはすべて直っている

SNAP
sensory nerve action potential　感覚神経活動電位

S

SNB
Silverman needle biopsy　シルバーマン針生検

SNC
sistema nervosum centrale〈ラ〉＝central nervous system　中枢神経系
small non-cleaved cell　小型非切れ込み細胞

SNCV
sensory nerve conduction velocity　知覚神経伝導速度

SND
sinus node dysfunction　洞結節機能不全

striatonigral degeneration 線条体黒質変性症

snd
sound 音

SNDF
sperm nucleus-decondensing factor 精子核膨化因子

SNDO
Standard Nomenclature of Diseases and Operations 疾病および手術の標準用語

SNE
severe noise environment 重度騒音環境
subacute necrotizing encephalomyelopathy 亜急性壊死性脳脊髄障害
sympathetic nerve ending 交感神経末端

SNEM
subacute necrotizing encephalo-myelopathy 亜急性壊死性脳脊髄障害

SNERP
sinus node effective refractory period 洞結節有効不応期

SNG
synthetic natural gas 合成自然ガス

SNGBF
single nephron glomerular blood flow 単一ネフロン糸球体血流量

SNGFR
single nephron glomerular filtration rate 単一ネフロン糸球体濾過率

SNGPF
single nephron glomerular plasma flow 単一ネフロン糸球体血漿流量

SNHL
sensorineural hearing loss 感覚神経性難聴

SNI
sequence-number indicator 順序・番号指標

SNM
sulfanilamide スルファニルアミド(=スルホンアミド)

SNMC
Stronger Neo-Minophagen C 強力ネオミノファーゲンC

SNMS
secondary neutral mass spectrometry 二次中性粒子質量分析法

Sno
thioinosine チオイノシン

sno
serial number 続き番号，シリアルナンバー

SNOM
scanning near-field optical microscope 走査型近接場光顕微鏡

s.nom., S.nom.
suo nomine〈ラ〉 薬名を記して《処》
SNP
seronegative polyneuritis 血清反応陰性多発性神経炎
sodium nitroprusside ニトロプルシッド
soluble nucleoprotein 可溶性核蛋白
SNQ
superior nasal quadrant 上鼻側1/4区
SNR
signal-to-noise ratio 信号・雑音比
SNRI
serotonin noradrenaline reuptake inhibitor セロトニン・ノルアドレナリン再取込み阻害薬
snRNA
small nuclear RNA 小核リボ核酸
snRNP
small nuclear RNP 小核リボ蛋白
SNRT
sinus node recovery time 洞結節回復時間
SNS
somatic nervous system 体性神経系
sympathetic nervous system 交感神経系
SNSA
seronegative spondyloarthritides RA因子陰性脊椎関節炎
SNST
sciatic nerve stretch test 坐骨神経伸展検査
SNV
Sin Nombre virus シンノンブレウイルス
spleen necrosis virus 脾臓壊死ウイルス
superior nasal vein 上鼻静脈
SO
Schlatter-Osgood (disease) シュラッター・オスグッド(病)
second opinion 第二の意見，セカンドオピニオン
sham operated 見かけの手術をした
sphincter of Oddi オッディ括約筋
suboccipital 後頭下の
superior oblique (muscle) 上斜筋
supraoptic nucleus 視索上核
supraorbital 眼窩上の
So
socialization 社会化
so
sex offender 性犯罪者
slow twitch oxidative 遅攣縮酸化物

south — 南(の)
special order — 特別注文

so, s.o.
siehe oben〈独〉 — 上記参照，上を見よ

SO_2
sulfur dioxide — 二酸化硫黄

SO_4
sulfate — 硫酸鉛，硫酸エステル

S/O
suspicious of — (〜の)疑い

S & O
salpingo-oophorectomy — 卵管卵巣摘出(術)

SO, S-O
salpingo-oophorectomy — 卵管卵巣摘出(術)

SO_2, So_2
O_2 saturation — 血清酸素飽和度

SOA
speed of advance — 進行速度
speed of approach — 接近速度
symptoms of asthma — 喘息症状

SOAD
sleep, orientation, activity, demand — 睡眠覚醒リズム・見当識・体動〔言動〕・要求〔訴え〕

SOAE
spontaneous oto-acoustic emission — 自動発生耳音響放射

SOAMA
signed out against medical advice — 医学的助言に逆らって自主退院した

SOA-MCA
superficial occipital artery to middle cerebral artery — 浅後頭動脈・中大脳動脈

SOAP
subjective (data), objective (data), assessment and plan — 自覚症状・客観的所見・評価と計画(＝問題志向型システム診療記録様式)

SOB
see order blank — 指図用紙を見よ
shortness of breath — 息切れ
suboccipito-bregmatic — 後頭前頂下の

SOC
short course chemotherapy — 短期化学療法
state of conciousness — 意識状態
syphilitic osteochondritis — 梅毒性骨軟骨炎
System Organ Class — 器官別分類

soc
social — 社会の

society 社会

SOC, SoC
state of consciousness 意識状態

Soc Hist
Social History 社会歴

SOCS
suppressor of cytokine signaling サイトカインシグナル抑制因子

SocSec, Soc.Sec.
Social Security 社会保障

Soc Serv
Social Service 社会サービス

SOD
sulfite oxidase deficiency 亜硫酸化酵素欠損症
superoxide dismutase スーパーオキシドジスムターゼ，超酸化物不均化酵素

Sod
sodomy 獣姦，ソドミー

sod
soda ソーダ
sodium ナトリウム

SODA
substitution, omission, distortion, addition 置換・省略・歪み・付加

sod.bicar
sodium bicarbonate 炭酸水素ナトリウム

sod.chlor.
sodium chloride〈ラ〉 塩化ナトリウム

SODH
sorbitol dehydrogenase ソルビトール脱水素酵素

Sod Pent
sodium pentothal ペントタールナトリウム

SOF
superior orbital fissure 上眼窩裂

S of B
short of breath 息切れ

SOH
tractus supraoptico-hypophysialis〈ラ〉 視神経上核下垂体神経路

SOI
Southern Oscillation Index 南方振動指数

SOL
sacredness of life 生活の神聖さ
sanctity of life 生命の尊厳
soleus ヒラメ筋
space occupying lesion 空間占拠性病変

sol.
solidus〈ラ〉 硬い
solubilis〈ラ〉=soluble 可溶(性)の
solut〈ラ〉 溶かした《処》

SOL, Sol, sd, sol.
solutio〈ラ〉=(a) solution 溶液

solidif
solidification 凝固, 固化

soln
solution 溶液

sol.sat.
solutio saturata〈ラ〉 飽和溶液《処》

solu
solute 溶質

Solut, solut, solut.
solution 溶液

SOLV, solv.
solvatur, *solve*〈ラ〉=dissolve 溶かせ《処》

solv, solv.
solvent 溶媒, 溶材

SOLVD
studies of left ventricular dysfunction 左(心)室機能障害検査, ソルブド

soly
solubility 可溶性

SOM
secretory otitis media 分泌性中耳炎
serous otitis media 滲出性中耳炎
Society of Occupational Medicine 職業医学学会
somatostatin ソマトスタチン
somnolent 傾眠の
superior oblique muscle 上斜筋

som
somatic 身体の, 体幹の
somatology 発育学

somat
somatic 身体の, 体幹の

SOMI
sternal-occipital-mandibular immobilizer 胸骨・後頭骨・下顎骨固定用装具

SO_2MR
systemic oxygen metabolic reserve 系統的酸素代謝予備

SON
superior olivary nucleus 上オリーブ核
supraoptic nuclei 視索上核
supraoptic nucleus 視索上核

S

son an
sonic noise analyzer　騒音分析器
sonar
sound navigation and ranging　ソナー
SOP
small outline package　スモールアウトラインパッケージ《コン》
standard operating procedure　標準操作手技
sop
soprano　ソプラノ
SOPHE
Society of Public Health Educators　公衆衛生教育者協会
S op S, S.op.s, s.op.s.
si opus sit〈ラ〉=if it is necessary　必要ならば《処》
S OP SIT, s.op.sit
si opus sit〈ラ〉=if it is necessary　必要ならば《処》
SOR, S-O-R
stimulus organism reaction　刺激生体反応
Sorb
sorbitol　ソルビトール
Sorb D
sorbitol dehydrogenase　ソルビトール脱水素酵素〔デヒドロゲナーゼ〕
SORD
sorbitol dehydrogenase　ソルビトール脱水素酵素〔デヒドロゲナーゼ〕
SOREMP
sleep(-)onset rapid eye movement (period)　睡眠開始REM(=レム)期, 睡眠発現レム期, 入眠時レム段階
S or S
signs or symptoms　徴候または症状
SOS
speed of sound　音速
stimulation of senses　感覚刺激
succinoxydase system　コハク酸酸化酵素系
SOS, s.o.s.
si opus sit〈ラ〉=if it is necessary　必要ならば《処》
SOT
standard operative temperature　標準作用温度
systemic oxygen transport　全身酸素輸送
SOTD
stabilized optical tracking device　安定化視標追跡器具
SOTT
synthetic medium old tuberculin trichloroacetic acid precipitated　合成培地旧ツベルクリン沈降トリクロロ酢酸

SoU
solar urticaria 日光蕁麻疹
SOx
sulfur oxides 硫黄酸化物，ソックス
SP
sacral promontory 仙骨岬角
sacrum to pubis 仙骨恥骨間の
school phobia 登校拒否症
secretory piece 分泌片
selective photothermolysis 選択的光温度解除
senile plaque 老人斑
septum pellucidum 透明中隔
seropositive 血清陽性の
serum protein 血清蛋白
shunt pressure シャント圧
shunt procedure シャント手技
simple pneumoconiosis 単純じん肺
simulation patient 擬態患者
simultaneous perception 同時視
single phase 単一相
skin potential 皮膚電位
soft palate 軟口蓋
space 腔，隙，空間
speaker スピーカー
spectrophotometer 分光光度計
speech pathology 言語病理学
spike potential 棘波電位
spirometry 肺活量測定(法)
splenomegaly 脾腫
spuri〈ラ〉 偽の《処》
sputum 喀痰
standardized patient or simulated patient 標準模擬患者
standard practice 標準手技
standard procedure 標準手技
staphylococcal protease ブドウ球菌プロテアーゼ
staphylococcal protein A ブドウ球菌蛋白A
static pressure 静止圧
status praesens〈ラ〉 現症
strip package 剝離式包装(薬包)，裸の包装
suboccipital puncture 後頭下穿刺
substance P サブスタンスP，物質P
substance peptide サブスタンスペプチド
sulfopropyl スルホプロピル
summating potential 累加電位
superficial parotidectomy 浅葉耳下腺摘出術

S

suprapubic 恥骨上の
suprapubic pubis 恥骨上結合
suprapubic puncture 恥骨上穿刺
suspected 疑似性
systolic pressure 収縮期血圧

Sp
shampoo 洗髪
sparteine エニシダのアルカロイド
spermine スペルミン
spike 棘波
spinal anesthesia 脊髄麻酔
Spirillum スピリルム(属)
spirometer 肺活量計

sP
senile parkinsonism 老人性パーキンソニズム

sp
space 空，隙，空間
spasm 痙縮，痙攣
special 特別の
speciality 特別
splint 副子

sp.
spiritus〈ラ〉＝spirit(s) 蒸留酒，アルコール

S/P
status post operation 手術後状態

SP，Sp.
Species〈ラ〉 茶剤《処》

SP，Sp，sp
spinal 棘の，棘状突起の
spine 棘，脊椎，脊柱

SP，sp
specialist 専門医，専門家
species 種

SP，S/P
status post〈ラ〉＝no change after その後変化なし，～後の状態 無変化

S

SP，S-P
Smith-Petersen (nail) スミス・ピーターセン(釘)

Sp，sp
sacropubic 仙骨恥骨の

sp，SP
spleen 脾臓

sp，sp.
specific 特異的な，特殊の

SP-1，SP1，SP_1
pregnancy-specific β_1-glycoprotein 妊娠特異(的)β_1糖蛋白質

SPA
single photon absorptiometry 単光子吸収法
skin potential activity 皮膚電位活動
spinal progressive muscular atrophy 脊髄性進行性筋萎縮症
spondylitis ankylopoietica 強直性脊椎炎
spontaneous platelet aggregation 自然血小板凝集
stimulation-produced analgesia 刺激鎮痛法
subject to particular average 特殊平均に属する《統》
suprapatellar amputation 膝蓋骨上切断(術)
suprapubic aspiration 恥骨上膀胱穿刺

SpA, SPA
staphylococcal protein A ブドウ球菌蛋白A

SPAES
superimposed presentation of averaged electrocardiographic signals 心電図信号の平均二重表出

SPAF
stroke prevention in atrial fibrillation 心房細動における脳卒中予防

SPAFS
stroke prevention in atrial fibrillation study 心房細動予防研究

SPAM
scanning photoacoustic microscopy 走査型光音波顕微鏡

SPAMM
spatial modulation of magnetization 磁化の空間調整《画診》

Span
Spanish スペイン人(の), スペイン語(の)

sp.an.
spinal anesthesia 脊椎麻酔, 脊麻

SPARS
spatially resolved spectroscopy 局所的高分解能NMRスペクトル測定法

SPB
supraventricular premature beat 上室性期外収縮

SPBI
serun protein-bound iodine 血清蛋白結合ヨウ素

SPC
salicylamide,phenacetin and caffeine サリチルアミド・フェナセチン・カフェイン
serum phenylalanine concentration 血清フェニルアラニン濃度
single photon counting 単一光子計測
spleen cell 脾臓細胞
Summary of Product Character 製品概要
Supplementary Patent Certificates 特許権補助証明書

S

SPCA
serum prothrombin conversion accelerator — 血清プロトロンビン転化促進因子
short posterior ciliary artery — 短後毛様動脈
SPCAD
serum prothrombin conversion accelerator deficiency — 血清プロトロンビン転化促進因子欠乏症
sp.cd
spinal cord — 脊髄
SPCG
spectral phonocardiogram — スペクトル心電図
SPCM
spectinomycin — スペクチノマイシン
SPD
splenopancreatic disconnection — 脾膵分離
storage pool deficiency — 貯蔵プール欠乏症
storage pool disease — ストレージプール病
SPD, Spd
spermidine — スペルミジン
SPE
septic pulmonary edema — 敗血症性肺水腫
serum protein electrophoresis — 血清蛋白電気泳動(法)
streptococcal pyrogenic endotoxin — 連鎖球菌発熱性内毒素
streptococcal pyrogenic exotoxin — 化膿性連鎖球菌外毒素
sustained physical exercise — 持続性運動負荷
spec
special — 特別な
specialist — 専門医
specific — 特異的な
specification — 専門化
SPEC, spec
specimen — 標本
spec.gr.
specific gravity — 比重
specif
specification — 専門化
specifi
specific — 特異的な
SPECT
single photon emission computed tomography — 単一光子放射型コンピュータ断層撮影法，スペクト
therapy for spontaneous pneumothorax for electrocoagulation under thoracoscopic control — 胸腔鏡下電気凝固法自然気胸治療

SPEP
serum protein electrophoresis　血清蛋白電気泳動
SpEP
spinal evoked potential　脊髄誘発電位
S period
synthesis period　合成期，S期
SPEs
somatosensory evoked potential　体知覚誘発電位
SPF
serum protein fraction　血清蛋白分画
skin protection factor　皮膚防御因子
specific pathogen free　特定病原体非依存状態
spectrophotofluorometer　螢光分光光度計
streptococcal proliferative factor　連鎖球菌増殖因子
Stuart-Prower factor　スチュアート・プラウアー因子
sun protection factor　日光保護因子，日焼け防止指数〈単位〉
sp fl
spinal fluid　脊髄液
SPFX
sparfloxacin　スパルフロキサシン
SPG
sizofiran　シゾフィラン
splenoportography　脾門脈造影
streptococcal protein G　連鎖球菌蛋白G
sucrose phosphate glutamate　グルタミン酸リン酸ショ糖
sp.G
specific gravity　比重
Sp.Gew.
spezifisches Gewicht〈独〉　比重
SP GR, Sp Gr, sp.gr
specific gravity　比重
SPH
secondary pulmonary hemosiderosis　続発性肺血鉄症
sphingomyelin　スフィンゴミエリン
Sph
spherocytosis　球状赤血球症
Sph-1
spherocytosis, Denver type　球状赤血球症，デンバー型
sph, sph.
sphenoidal　蝶形骨洞の
spherical　球状の，球の
sphincter　括約筋
vitrum sphericum〈ラ〉　円柱レンズ

SPHG
stomal polypoid hypertrophic gastritis　吻合部ポリープ状肥厚性胃炎
sphr
spherical　球状の
spheroid　楕円体
SPH-system
septo-preoptico-hypothalamic system　中隔・視束前野・視床下部系
sp.ht
specific heat　比熱
SPI
serum precipitable iodine　血清沈降性ヨウ素
serum protein index　血清蛋白指数
sexual personality index　性的個性指数
Shimoda-shiki Personality Inventory　下田式性格検査
superoxide production index　過酸化物産生指数
SPIDDM
slowly progressive IDDM (=insulin-dependent diabetes mellitus)　緩徐進行型インスリン依存性糖尿病
spif
simplification　単純化
SPIH
superimposed pregnancy-induced hypertension　重加妊娠誘発高血圧
SP indet
species indeterminate　不確定種
SP inquir
species inquired　不確定種
spir
spiral　らせん上の，らせん型の
spiritual　精神の
Spir.
Spirochaeta　スピロヘータ(属)
Spir., spir.
Spiritus〈ラ〉=spirit(s)　アルコール(溶液)，蒸留酒
spir.v.
spiritus vini〈ラ〉=spirit(s) of wine　アルコール，酒精《処》
spiss.
spissus〈ラ〉=dried　乾燥させた《処》
SPIT
systolic pressure-time index　収縮期圧・時間指数
spital
hospital　病院
SPK
simultaneous pancreas and kidney transplantation　膵腎同時移植

superficial punctate keratitis 表在(性)点状角膜炎

spkr
speaker スピーカー

SPL
skin potential level 皮膚電位レベル
sound pressure level 音圧レベル
splanchnic 内蔵の
staphylococcal bacteriophage lysate ブドウ球菌バクテリオファージ製剤
status praesens localis 局所所見

spl
special 特別の
splint 副子

spl, spl.
simplex〈ラ〉=simple 単一の，単純な《処》

SPM
scanning probe microscope 走査プローブ顕微鏡
shocks per minute ショック/分
spiramycin スピラマイシン
suspended particulate material 大気浮遊物質
syllables per minute 音節/分

Spm
spermine スペルミン

SPMA
spinal progressive muscular atrophy 脊髄性進行性筋萎縮症

SPME
solid phase micro extraction 固相微量抽出(法)

SPMP
simultaneous paramacular perception 傍黄斑同時視

SPN
student practical nurse 実務看護学生
supplementary parenteral nutrition 補助的腸管外栄養
sympathetic preganglionic neuron 交感神経節前ニューロン

sp.n.
species novum〈ラ〉=new species 新種

S.Pn.
sinusitis paranasalis〈ラ〉 副鼻腔炎

sp.nov.
species novum〈ラ〉=new species 新種

spnt
spontaneous 自発(的)の，特発(性)の

Sp Ny, Sp.Ny.
spontaneous nystagmus 自発眼振

SPO
stimulated pepsin output 刺激後ペプシン分泌量

S

SpO_2
arterial oxyhemoglobin saturation　動脈性オキシヘモグロビン
pulse oximeter saturation　パルスオキシメーター表示酸素飽和度

sp.o.k.
speech o.k.　発語オーケー

SPoM
scanning potential microscope　走査型電位顕微鏡

spon, spon.
spontan　自然に，特発的に起こった
spontaneous　自発(的)の，自発性の，特発性の

spont
spontaneous　自発(的)の，自発性の，特発性の

spork
spoon and fork　スプーンとフォーク

SPORO
sporatrichosis　スポロトリクム症

spot
spot roentgenography　狙撃X線撮影

SPP
simultaneous peripheral perception　周辺部同時視
suprapubic prostatectomy　恥骨上前立腺切除術

SPP, spp
species　種〈複数〉

Sp Path
speech pathology　言語病理学

SPPS
stable plasma protein solution　安定血漿蛋白溶液

SPR
safe practical requirement　安全実用必要量
skin potential reflex　皮膚電位反射
skin potential response　皮膚電位反応
skin resistance reflex　皮膚抵抗反射
Society for Pediatric Research　小児科研究学会
Society for Physical Research　内科研究学会
surface plasmon resonance　表面プラズモン共鳴

spr
sprain　捻挫

SPRC
Society for Prevention and Relief of Cancer　癌予防救済協会

SPRI
Sjukvardens och Socialv a rdens Planeringsoch Ratinaliserings Institut(s) — 保健福祉サービス計画合理化研究所

SPRITE
signal processing in element — サーモグラフィ検出器の一種

SPROM
spontaneous premature rupture of membrane — 膜自発早期破裂

SPS
Sanitary and Phytosanitary Measures — 衛生植物検疫措置の適用に関する協定
semipermeable surface — 半浸透表面
simple partial seizure — 単純部分発作
sinus premature systole — 洞性早期収縮
sleep promoting substance — 睡眠促進物質
social performance schedule — 社会的遂行能面接基準
Society of Pelvic Surgeons — 骨盤外科医協会
Society of Plastic Surgeons — 形成外科医協会
sodium polyethanol sulfate — ポリエタノール硫酸ナトリウム
specific projection system — 特殊投射系

SpS
sphenoid sinus — 蝶形骨洞

S-P shunt
subduro-peritoneal shunt — 硬膜下腹腔シャント術

SPSS
statistical package for social sciences — 社会科学向け統計解析パッケージ

SPT
Sand play therapy〔technique〕 — 箱庭療法
scamatic projective techniques — 図式的投影法《検査》
secretin-pancreozymin test — セクレチンパンクレオザイミン検査
skin prick tests — 皮膚針刺試験
sleeping period time — 睡眠時間
soft part tumor — 軟部腫瘍
spinal tap — 脊椎穿刺

spt
sputum — 痰

spt.
spiritus〈ラ〉=spirit(s) — 蒸留酒，アルコール(溶液)

SPTI
systolic pressure-time index — 収縮期圧・時間係数

SPTS
subjective posttraumatic syndrome — 自覚的外傷後症候群

S

spts.
spiritus〈ラ〉=spirit(s) 蒸留酒，アルコール(溶液)
SPTT
silicon partial thromboplastin time シリコン部分トロンボプラスチン時間
SPV
selective proximal vagotomy 選択的近位迷走神経切離術
Shope papilloma virus ショープ乳頭腫ウイルス
SP vaccine
small particle vaccine 小粒子ワクチン
SPVD
Society of Prevention of Veneral Disease 性病予防協会
sp.vin.
spiritus vini〈ラ〉=spirit(s) of wine アルコール，酒精《処》
SPW
spinal pressure wave 脊髄圧波
Sp & W
spike and wave complex 棘徐波複合体
SpX
splenectomy 脾摘出術
sp.xr
special x ray (study) 特殊X線(検査)
SPZ
sulfinpyrazone スルフィンピラゾン
SQ
social maturity quotient 社会成熟指数
social quotient 社会性指数
squalene スクアレン
status quo〈ラ〉 現状
stereoquadrophonic 立体4音声の
survey question 調査質問
symptom questionnaire 症状質問票
sq
squamous 扁平な
squamous cell carcioma 扁平上皮癌
square 四角(の)，平方(の)
sq.
sequentia〈ラ〉=the following 次の，下記の
SQ, sq
subcutaneous 皮下の
SQC
statistical quality control 統計的品質管理
SQ cell ca, sq.cell ca.
squamous cell carcinoma 扁平上皮癌

S

sq.cm
square centimeter　平方センチメートル
SQCP
statistical quality control procedure　統計的品質管理手技
sq.epithl
squamous epithelium　扁平上皮
sq.ft
square foot　平方フィート
SQID
superconducting quantum interference device　超伝導量子干渉(計)
sq.in
square inch　平方インチ
sq.m
square meter　平方メートル
sq.mm
square millimeter　平方ミリメートル
sqq, sqq.
sequentia〈ラ〉　続発性の
SQ3R
survey, question, read, review, recite　調査→疑問→読書→評論→叙述
SQUID
superconducting quantum interference device　超伝導量子干渉計
SR
sacroplasmic reticulum　筋小胞体《電顕》
saturation recovery　飽和回復法
scavenger receptor　スカベンジャー受容体
scientific research　科学的研究
secretion rate　分泌率
self-rating　自覚率
sensitization response　感作反応
sex ratio　性比
shunt ratio　シャント率
sigma reaction　シグマ反応
silicone rubber　シリコンゴム
simple reaction　単純反応
sinus rhythm　洞調律
skin resistance　皮膚抵抗
Society of Radiation　放射線学会
soluble, repository　可溶性, 貯蔵型
specific response　特異的反応
speech range　話声域
spontaneous respiration(s)　自発呼吸
stapedial reflex　アブミ骨筋反射

Sternalrand〈独〉	胸骨縁
Sternberg-Reed (cells)	ステルンベルグ・リード(細胞)(＝多核巨細胞)
steroid receptor	ステロイド受容体
stimulation ratio	刺激比
stimulus-response	刺激・反応
stomach rumble	胃鳴音
stretch reflex	伸展反応
sulfonamide-resistant	スルホンアミド抵抗(性)の
superior rectus (muscle)	上直(筋)
sustained release	徐放の
sutures removed	抜糸
systemic reaction	全身反応
systems review	系統別再調査
Sr	
strontium	ストロンチウム〈元素〉
sr	
steradian	ステラジアン〈単位〉
S-R	
stimulus-response theory	刺激反応説，刺激反応理論
SR, Sr	
senior	上級の，年上の
SR, S.R.	
sedimentation rate	(赤血球)沈降速度，赤沈，血沈
SR, S/R	
schizophrenic reaction	分裂症反応
SRA	
right sacro-anterior position	右仙骨部前位，第二骨盤位第一分類〈胎位〉
serum renin activity	血清レニン活性
skin reactive antigen	皮膚反応惹起抗原
startle response audiometry	驚愕反応聴力検査
steroid resistant asthma	ステロイド抵抗性喘息
sulforicinoleic acid	スルホリシノレイン酸
superior rectal artery	上直腸動脈
SRBC	
sheep red blood cell(s)	ヒツジ赤血球
SRBD	
sleep-related breathing disorder	睡眠関連呼吸障害
SRC	
scleroderma renal crisis	強皮症腎クリーゼ
sedimented red cell	沈降赤血球
sensitization response cell	感作反応細胞
sheep red cell	ヒツジ赤血球
skin resistance change	皮膚抵抗変化

spontaneous regression of cancer 癌自然寛解
subrenal capsule assay 腎下被膜効力検定

src
Rous sarcoma oncogene ラウス肉腫オンコジーン

SRCA
specific red cell adherence 特異的赤血球吸着

SR cell
sensitization response cell 感作反応細胞

SRCF
single radio complement fixation 一元放射補体結合(反応)

SRD
sodium-restricted diet ナトリウム制限食
soluble, repository, plus dihydrostreptomycin 可溶性・貯蔵型・添加ジヒドロストレプトマイシン

Srd
thiouridine チオウリジン

SRE
système réticulo-endothélial〈仏〉 (細)網内(皮)系

SRED
single enzyme diffusion 単純酵素拡散
single radial enzyme diffusion 単純放射状酵素拡散法

SREM
sleep with rapid eye movements 急速眼球運動随伴睡眠, レム睡眠

SRF
serum response factor 血清刺激応答因子
severe renal failure 高度腎不全
skin reactive factor 皮膚反応〔惹起〕因子
skin respiratory factor 皮膚呼吸因子
somatotropin releasing factor ソマトトロピン〔成長ホルモン〕放出因子
split renal function 分腎機能
subretinal fluid 網膜下液

SRF-A
slow-reacting factor of anaphylaxis アナフィラキシー緩徐反応因子

SRFC
sheep (red cell) rosette-forming cell ヒツジ(赤血球)ロゼット形成細胞
spontaneous rosette forming cell 自然ロゼット形成細胞

SRFH
somatotropin releasing factor hormone ソマトトロピン〔成長ホルモン〕放出因子ホルモン

SRFOA
slow-reacting factor of anaphylaxis アナフィラキシー緩徐反応因子

SRFS
split renal function study 分腎機能検査
Srg, srg
surgery 外科学
SRH
somatotropin-releasing hormone ソマトトロピン〔成長ホルモン〕放出ホルモン
SRI
severe renal insufficiency 高度腎不全
SRID
single radial immunodiffusion 単純放射状免疫拡散法
SRIF
somatotropin-release-inhibiting factor ソマトトロピン〔成長ホルモン〕放出抑制因子(＝ソマトスタチン)
SRIH
somatotropin release inhibiting hormone ソマトトロピン〔成長ホルモン〕放出抑制ホルモン
SRJ
self-restraint joint 自己制御関節
SRL
skin resistance level 皮膚電気抵抗水準
SRM
search-rescue-medical 捜索・救助・医療
smooth-rough mutation スムースラフミューテイション，SR変異
speed of relative movement 相対運動速度
spontaneous(ly) ruptured membrane 自然破水，自然破膜
superior rectus muscle 上直筋
systolic regurgitant murmur 収縮期逆流性雑音
SRN
state registered nurse (英国の)看護師
subretinal neovascularization 網膜下新生血管
SRNA, sRNA
soluble ribonucleic acid 可溶性リボ核酸
SRNS
steroid-responsive nephrotic syndrome ステロイド反応性ネフローゼ症候群
SRO
sagittal ramus osteotomy 下顎枝矢状骨切り術
SROM
spontaneous(ly) rupture of membrane 自然破膜，自然破水
SRP
right sacro-posterior position 右仙骨部後位
signal recognition particle シグナル〔信号〕認識粒子

signal recognition protein 標識認識蛋白

SRQ-D

self rating questionnaire for depression 抑うつ度自己採点の質問

SRR

skin resistance reflex 皮膚(電気)抵抗反射
skin resistance response 皮膚(電気)抵抗反応
standarized relative risk 標準化相対危険《統》
stillbirth risk rate 死産児率
surgical recovery room 手術回復室

SRRS

social readjustment rating scale 社会再適応評価尺度

SRRSV

Schmidt-Ruppin-Rous sarcoma virus シュミット・ラッピン・ラウス肉腫ウイルス

SRS

schizophrenic residual state 統合失調症残存状態
Silver-Russell syndrome シルバー・ラッセル症候群(＝先天性発育不全)
slow-reacting substance 緩徐反応物質
Social and Rehabilitation Service (米国)社会・リハビリテーション庁
Symptom Rating Scale 症状評点尺度

SRS-A

slow reacting substance of anaphylaxis アナフィラキシー遅延反応物質

SRSV

small round structured virus (軽い食中毒，お腹のかぜウイルスなどの)小型球形ウイルス

SRT

sedimentation rate test (赤血球)沈降速度検査
simple reaction time 単純反応時間
sinus (node) recovery time 洞結節回復時間
social relations test 社会関係検査
speech reception test 言語聴取検査
speech reception threshold 語音聴取閾値
sustained-release theophylline 徐放性テオフィリン
Symptom Rating Test 症状評点試験

SR test

stapedial reflex test アブミ骨筋反射検査

SRV

Schmidt-Ruppin virus シュミット・ラッピンウイルス
small round virus 小円形ウイルス

SRY

sex determining region of Y	Y染色体の性決定領域
Y chromosome-linked sex determining locus	Y染色体連鎖男性決定遺伝子座

SS

saline soak	塩づけ
saline solution	生理食塩水
saliva sample	唾液試料
saturated solution	飽和液
schizophrenia spectrum	統合失調症スペクトル
Schwangerschaft〈独〉	妊娠
scientific staff	学術情報者
scleral spur	強膜岬
semi-soft diet	半軟食
serum sickness	血清病
Sézary syndrome	セザリー症候群
Shigella and *Salmonella* (agar)	赤痢菌サルモネラ(寒天培地)，サルモネラ・シゲラ(培地)
Shigella sonnei	ソンネ赤痢菌，シゲラソンネイ
short stay	短期滞在，短期入院
sho-seiryuto	小青竜湯《漢方》
siblings	同胞，兄弟
sickle cell	鎌(状)血球，鎌状細胞
side to side	側側(＝吻合法の1つ)
sigma score	知能偏差値
Sjögren syndrome	シェーグレン症候群
slow (wave) sleep	徐波睡眠
soap solution	石鹼溶液
soapsuds	石鹼水
Social Security	社会保障，厚生年金
sodium salicylate	サリチル酸ナトリウム
somatostatin	ソマトスタチン(＝GIF)
sonic stimulation	音刺激賦活法
sparingly soluble	わずかに溶ける
special senses	特殊感覚
special services	特別サービス
stable sarcoidosis	安定サルコイドーシス
standard score	標準得点
statistically significant	統計学的に有意な
steady state	定常状態
sterile solution	滅菌溶液
Stickler syndrome	スティックラー症候群
Strachan-Scott (syndrome)	ストラチャン・スコット(症候群)

subaortic stenosis 大動脈弁下部狭窄(症)
subscapularis 肩甲下(筋)
substernal 胸骨下の
suction socket 吸引ソケット
suprasternal notch 胸骨上端
suspended solid 浮遊物質
sweet syndrome 急性熱性好中球性皮膚病

ss
limited to subserosa 組織学的漿膜下癌浸潤度
salt sensitivity 食塩感受性
Sho-Saikoto 小柴胡湯《漢方》
side stream (タバコの)副流煙
single strand 一本鎖
sodium saccharin サッカリンナトリウム
solid state 固形状態
subendothelial space 内皮下間隙
subjects 被検者，被験者〈複数〉
symptoms 症状〈複数〉

ss.
semis〈ラ〉=harf 半量《処》

S.S.
sensu stricto〈ラ〉 厳密な意味で

s.s.
sacrosciatic 仙(骨)坐骨の
sensu stricto〈ラ〉=in the strict sense 狭義の

S-S
semissem〈ラ〉=one-half 1/2，半分
sign-significate theory 場理論

SS，S & S
signs and symptoms 徴候と症状，症候

ss，SS
subserosa 漿膜下
subserosal invasion 漿膜下層組織深達度
subserous 深達度が漿膜下層の癌

ss，$\overline{\text{SS}}$，ss.
semi-〈ラ〉=a half 半分，部分〈接〉
semisse〈ラ〉=a half 半分

ss.，SS
syrupus simplex〈ラ〉=simple syrup 単シロップ《処》

SSA
Sjögren syndrome (antigen) A シェーグレン症候群(抗原)A
skin-sensitizing antibody 皮膚感作抗体
Smith surface antigen スミス表面抗原
smoke-suppressant additive 付加的喫煙抑制
Social Security Administration 社会保障行政

Society for Study of Addiction　アルコールその他危険薬に対する習癖研究学会
special somatic afferent　特殊体性求心性の
sperm-specific antigen　精子特異性抗原
streptococcal superantigen　連鎖球菌スーパー抗原
sulfasarazine　スルファサラジン
sulfosalicylic acid　スルホサリチル酸

SS-A antibody
anti Sjögren syndrome A antibody　シェーグレン症候群A抗体

SS agar
Shigella and *Salmonella* agar　赤痢菌サルモネラ菌寒天(培地)

SSAV
simian sarcoma-associated virus　サル肉腫関連ウイルス

SSB
short spike bursts　短棘分節運動
single side band　単側波帯
single stranded DNA-binding protein　一本鎖DNA結合蛋白質
Sjögren syndrome B　シェーグレン症候群B
Society for Study of Blood　血液研究学会

SS-B antibody
anti Sjögren syndrome B antibody　シェーグレン症候群B抗体

SSBG
sex steroid-binding globulin　性ステロイド結合グロブリン

SSC
standard saline citrate　標準クエン酸食塩水
superior semicircular canal　上半規管

SSc
systemic sclerosis　全身性硬化症

SSCA
sensitized sheep cell agglutination (test)　感作ヒツジ(赤)血球凝集(反応)

SSCCS
slow spinal cord compression syndrome　遅発脊髄圧迫症候群

SSCF
sleep stage change frequency　睡眠段階変化頻度

SSCP
single stranded conformation polymorphism　単鎖〔一本鎖〕DNA高次構造多型解析(法)

SSCr
stainless steel crown　ステンレス鋼歯冠

SSD
screening for somatoform disorder　身体表現障害スクリーニング
social service department　医療社会事業部
solid state detector　半導体検出器

source-skin distance 線源・皮膚間距離
source surface distance 線源・表面間距離
sudden sniffing death コカイン中毒突然死

SSd
saikosaponin-d サイコポニンD

ssDNA, SSDNA
single stranded deoxyribonucleic acid 一本鎖〔単鎖〕デオキシリボ核酸

SSE
saline solution enema 食塩水浣腸
skin self-examination 皮膚自己検査
soap solution enema 石鹸水浣腸
soapsuds enema 石鹸浣腸
subacute spongiform encephalopathy 亜急性海綿状脳症
system system engineering 体系体系工学

SSEA
sensitized sheep erythrocyte agglutination 感作ヒツジ赤血球凝集(反応)
stage-specific embryonic antigen ステージ特異的胎児抗原

SSEH
spontaneous spinal epidural hematoma 特発性脊椎硬膜外血腫

SS enema
saline solution enema 食塩水浣腸

SSEP
short latency somatosensory evoked potential 短潜時体性知覚誘発電位
somatic sensory electric potential 体性知覚誘発電位

S̄ seq.
sine sequela〈ラ〉=without sequel 続発症なしに《処》

SSF
soluble suppressor factor 可溶性抑制因子

SS factor
smooth selecting factor 均一性選択因子

SSHL
severe sensorineural hearing loss 高度感覚神経性難聴

SSI
segmental spinal instrumentation 分節性脊椎固定術
small scale integration 小規模集積回路
streptomyces subtilisin inhibitor ストレプトミセススブチリシンインヒビター
symptom-sign inventory 症状・徴候調査票

SSII
Safran Student's Interest Inventory サフラン学生興味調査票

SSKI
saturated solution potassium iodide ヨウ化カリウム飽和液

S

SSL
skin surface lipid 皮膚表面脂質
supraglottic subtotal laryngectomy 声門上喉頭部分摘出
SSLI
serum sickness-like illness 血清病様疾患
SSM
social stratification and mobility scale 社会成層と流動尺度
specific substance MARUYAMA 結核菌体抽出物質＝丸山ワクチン
superficial spreading melanoma 表在拡大型黒色腫
SSMS
saturated solution of magnesium sulfate 硫酸マグネシウム(＝$MgSO_4$)飽和溶液
spark source mass spectrometry 火花放電イオン化固体質量分析法
SSN
somatostatin neuron ソマトスタチンニューロン
s.sn., s.s.n
signetur suo nomine〈ラ〉＝let it be labeled with its own name その名前を表示せよ，氏名を記入せよ《処》
sub suo nomine〈ラ〉 薬名を記して《処》
ss notch
sacrosciatic notch 仙坐骨切痕
SSNS
steroid-sensitive nephrotic syndrome ステロイド過敏ネフローゼ症候群
SSO
special sense organ 特殊感覚器
Sso_2
computed arterial oxygen saturation コンピュータ表示動脈血酸素飽和度
SSP
Sanarelli-Shwartzman phenomenon サナレリ・シュワルツマン現象
scintiphoto-splenoportography 閃光写真脾門脈造影法
silver spike point ツボ圧迫低周波療法
silver spike point electrode 銀棘点電極
small spherical particle 小球状粒子
spasmodic spinal paralysis 痙性脊髄麻痺
spastic spinal paralysis 痙性脊髄麻痺
subacute sclerosing panencephalitis 亜急性硬化性全脳炎
subspecies 亜種
SSPE
subacute sclerosing panencephalitis (virus) 亜急性硬化性全脳炎(ウイルス)

S

SSPG
steady state plasma glucose 定常状態血漿ブドウ糖
SSPI
steady state plasma insulin 定常状態血漿インスリン
SSPL
saturation sound pressure level 最大出力音圧レベル
SSPPD
subtotal stomach-preserving pancreaticoduodenectomy 全胃温存膵頭十二指腸切除術
SSPS
Shalling-Sifneos Personality Scale 失感情症のふるい分けテスト
side-to-side portacaval shunt 側側門脈大静脈シャント
SSR
steroid-resistant rejection ステロイド抵抗性拒絶(反応)
sympathetic skin response 交感神経皮膚反応
SSRE
shear stress responsive element ずり応力応答成分
SSRI
selective serotonin re(-)uptake inhibitor 選択的セロトニン再取込み阻害薬
SSRIs
selective serotonin re(-)uptake inhibitors 選択的セロトニン再取込み阻害薬
ssRNA
single-stranded RNA 一本鎖RNA
SS-RTP
solid-surface room-temperature phosphorescence 固相表面室温リン光
SSS
scalded skin syndrome 熱傷様皮膚症候群
secondary Sjögren syndrome 二次性〔続発性〕シェーグレン症候群
septic severity score 敗血症重症度スコア
sick sinus syndrome 洞(機能)不全症候群
small sharp spike 小鋭棘波
specific soluble substance 特異性可溶性物質
sterile saline soak 無菌性の塩づけ
superior sagittal sinus 上矢状静脈洞
systemic sicca syndrome 全身性乾燥症候群
sss
stratum superstratum〈ラ〉 層を重ねて《処》
SSSS
staphylococcal scalded skin syndrome ブドウ球菌性熱傷様皮膚症候群
SSST
superior sagittal sinus thrombosis 上矢状静脈洞血栓(症)

S

SSSV
superior sagittal sinus (blood) velocity　上矢状(静脈)洞(血流)速度
SST
sagittal sinus thrombosis　矢状(静脈)洞血栓症
social skills training　社会生活技能訓練
somatosensory thalamus　体性感覚視床
SSTR
somatostatin receptor　ソマトスタチン受容体
s.str.
sensu stricto〈ラ〉=in the strict sense　狭義の
SSV
sheep seminal vesicle　ヒツジ精嚢
simian sarcoma virus　サル肉腫ウイルス
s.s.v.
sub signo veneni〈ラ〉　毒薬標を貼って《処》
SSX
sulfisoxazole　スルフイソキサゾール
ST
esotropia〈ラ〉　内斜視
heat stable enterotoxin　耐熱性内毒素
Salmonella typhi　チフス菌
Salmonella typhimurium　ネズミチフス菌
scapulothoracic　肩甲胸郭の
Schiøtz tonometry　シェッツ眼圧測定計
sclerotherapy　硬化療法
scutum tympanicum〈ラ〉　鼓室蓋
sedimentation time　沈降時間
semitendinosus　半腱様(筋)
sensitivity training　感受性訓練
serum transferrin　血清トランスフェリン
shock therapy　ショック療法
silent thyroiditis　無症候性甲状腺炎
silent treatment　沈黙療法
simulation test　シミュレーションテスト
sinus tachycardia　洞頻脈
sinus tympani　鼓室洞
skin temperature　皮膚温度
skin test　皮膚試験〔反応〕
slight trace　極微量
speech therapist　言語療法士
sphincter tone　括約筋張筋
standardized test　標準化試験
standard treatment　標準的治療
striatum　線条(体)
ST-segment　(心電図の)ST部分《心電》

sulfamethoxazole-trimethoprim スルファメトキサゾールトリメトプリム
sulfathiazol スルファチアゾール
sun-reactive skin type 太陽に反応する皮膚の型
supportive psychotherapy 支持的精神療法
surface tension 表面張力
surgical therapy 外科的療法
survival time 生存時間
syncytiotrophoblast 合胞体層
Szondu test ソンディテスト

St
stabkernige Leukozyten〈独〉 桿状核白血球
Stanton number スタントン数
sternum 胸骨
stoke ストーク
subtype 亜型

st
stage (of disease) 病期
standing 立位の
status 状態，持続
sterile 生殖不能の，滅菌の
stimulation 刺激
stimuli 刺激〈複数〉
stone 結石，石
straight まっすぐな
strength 強さ，強度
stretch 伸ばす

S-T
sickle cell thalassemia 鎌状赤血球サラセミア

ST, st
stimulus 興奮薬，刺激薬
stomach 胃

ST, S.T.
speech therapy (department) 言語療法(分野)

St, st.
stent〈ラ〉=let them stand 立てよ《処》
stet〈ラ〉=let it stand 立てよ《処》

STA
Science and Technology Agency 科学技術庁
serum thrombotic accelerator 血清血栓形成促進因子
serum tobramycin assay トブラマイシン定量(法)
stand(ing) at attention 直立姿勢(をとる)
superficial temporal artery 浅側頭動脈

sta
stationary 一定の，変化のない

Stab
stab leukocyte 桿状核(白血)球
stab
stabilizer 安定剤
stabs
stabkernige〈独〉=staff or band neutrophils 桿(状)核(白血)球
staflo
stable-flow 安定流
Stage A
active stage 活動期
Stage H
healing stage 治癒過程期
Stage S
scarred stage 瘢痕期
STAI
state-trait anxiety inventory 状態・特性不安質問検査
STA-MCA
(anastomosis between) superficial temporal artery and middle cerebral artery 浅側頭動脈・中大脳動脈(吻合術)(=ST-MC)
superficial temporal artery-middle cerebral artery (anastomosis) 浅側頭動脈・中大脳動脈(吻合術)
superior temporal artery-middle cerebral artery 上側頭動脈・中大脳動脈
stand
standard 標準の
standardized 標準化された
standard
standardization 標準化，力価決定
standardized 標準化された
Stan Psych
Standard Psychiatric Nomenclature 標準精神医学用語集
STAP
Stimulus-Triggered Acquisition of Pluripotency 刺激惹起性多能性獲得
STA-PCA
superficial temporal artery to posterior cerebral artery 浅側頭動脈・後大脳動脈
STAP cells
Stimulus-Triggered Acquisition of Pluripotency cells 刺激惹起性多能性獲得細胞
Stapes mob
stapes mobilization アブミ骨可動術
staph
staphylococcal ブドウ球菌(性)の

STAPH, staph, Staph.
Staphylococcus スタヒロコッカス(属), ブドウ球菌(属)

Staph.aur
Staphylococcus aureus 黄色ブドウ球菌

Stap.mob
stapes mobilization アブミ骨可動術

STA-SCA
superficial temporal artery-superior cerebellar artery 浅側頭動脈・上小脳動脈

STAT
signal transduction and activator of transcription (細胞内)信号伝達と転写活性因子

stat
electrostatic 電気的に安定な
statistics 統計(学)

stat., Stat
statim〈ラ〉=immediately すぐさま, ただちに, 直接に, 至急で

statist
statistical 統計(学)の
statistics 統計(学)

stat.p.c.
statium post cibos〈ラ〉=immediately after meals 食直後

stats
statistics 統計(学)

status
status epilepticus 痙攣重積発作

Stb, stb.
stillborn 死産の

STBS
suspension TRIS-buffered saline トリス緩衝食塩水浮遊液

STC
sensitivity time control 感受性時間調節管理《超音波》
serum theophylline concentration 血清テオフィリン濃度
sexually transmitted condition 性行為感染状態
soft tissue calcification 軟部組織石灰化
Stroke Treatment Center 脳卒中治療センター
strychnine ストリキニン

ST cell
suppressor T cell サプレッサーT細胞

STD
sexual(ly) transmitted disease 性(行為)感染症
skin test dose 皮膚試験(用)量
sodium tetradecyl sulfate テトラデシル硫酸ナトリウム

S

source-tumor distance　線源・腫瘍間距離
standard test dose　標準試験(用)量，標準検査(用)量

std
saturated　飽和した
standard　標準の
standardization　標準化
standardized　標準化された

Std.
Stunde〈独〉　時間

stdg
standing　立位の，立っている

Std TF
standard tube feeding　標準経管栄養

STEF
simple test of evaluating hand function　上肢機能評価の簡易テスト

STEL
short-term exposure level　短期曝露限界

STEM
scanning transmission electron microscope　走査透過型電子顕微鏡

STEN, S-TEN
staphylococcal toxic epidermal necrolysis　ブドウ球菌(性)中毒性表皮壊死融解症

ster
sterile　生殖不能の，不妊の，滅菌の
sterilization　滅菌
sterilize　滅菌する
sterilizer　滅菌器

sterad
steradian　ステラジアン〈単位〉

STEREO
stereopsis　立体視

Stereo, stereo
stereogram　立体写真
stereoscopy　立体撮影
stereotaxic instrument　定位脳手術装置

stern.punct
sternal puncture　胸骨穿刺

S test
secretin test　セクレチンテスト

Stetho
stethoscope　聴診器

STF
serum thymic factor　血清胸腺因子

serum thymus factor 血清胸腺因子
special tube feeding 特殊経管栄養

stf
staff 幹部

STG
short-term goals 短期目標
split thickness graft 中間層皮弁

stg
stage 段階，病期
staging 病期分類する

STGC
syncytiotrophoblastic giant cell(s) 合胞体性巨細胞

STH
somatotropic hormone(=somatotropin) 成長ホルモン(=ソマトトロピン)
steroid hormone ステロイドホルモン
subtotal hysterectomy 子宮亜全摘

S-Thal
sickle (cell) thalassemia 鎌状赤血球サラセミア

SThM
scanning thermal microscope 走査型熱顕微鏡

STI
serum trypsin inhibitor 血清トリプシン抑制因子
soybean trypsin inhibitor 大豆トリプシン抑制因子
systolic time interval 収縮期間隔，収縮時間隔

STIC
serum trypsin inhibitor(y) capacity 血清トリプシン抑制能

stillat
stillatim〈ラ〉=by drops 滴下で

Still B, stillb.
stillborn 死産の

stim
stimulate 刺激する
stimulation 刺激
stimulus 刺激薬，興奮薬

stimn
stimulation 刺激

STIR
short TI inversion recovery 短反転時間回復

STJ
subtalar joint 距骨下関節

STK
streptokinase ストレプトキナーゼ

STL
septal tricuspid leaflet 三尖弁中隔炎
serum theophylline level 血清テオフィリン濃度レベル

S

STLV
simian T cell leukemic virus　サルT細胞白血病ウイルス

STM
scanning tunneling microscope　走査型トンネル顕微鏡
short-term memory　短期記憶
spectro-temporal mapping　一時的分光作画
streptomycin　ストレプトマイシン

STMC
synovial tissue mononuclear cell　関節滑液膜単核細胞

ST-MC
(anastomosis between) superficial temporal artery and middle cerebral artery　浅側頭動脈・中大脳動脈(吻合術)(＝STA-MCA)

STN
subthalamic nucleus　視床下核

STNR
symmetrical tonic neck reflex　対称性緊張性首反射

STNS
sham transcutaneous nerve stimulation　見かけの経皮的神経刺激

STO
sodium triphosphate　三リン酸ナトリウム
sterno-turnover　胸骨翻転術

STOF
systemic toxic organ failure　全身菌毒性臓器不全

stom
stomach　胃

sto.map
stomach map　胃地図

stomat
stomatology　口腔学

stom.lav
stomach lavage　胃洗浄

STOP
surgical termination of pregnancy　妊娠中絶手術
Swedish Trial in Old Patients with Hypertension　スウェーデン老年者高血圧降圧薬有用性調査，ストップ

STP
scanning tunneling potentiometry　走査トンネル電位計
serenity-tranquillity-peace　晴朗・静穏・平和
sodium thiopental　チオペンタールナトリウム
standard temperature and pulse　正常体温・正常脈拍
supracondylar tibial prosthesis　顆上頸骨装具
symptomatic thrombocytopenic purpura　症候性血小板減少性紫斑病

S

STP, s.t.p.
standard temperature and pressure　標準温度・標準気圧

STPD
standard temperature and pressure, dry　標準温度・標準気圧・標準乾燥状態

STPF
stabilized temperatur platform furnace　温度の安定した平板炉

St pr., St.pr.
status praesens〈ラ〉=present status　現症

STPS
specific thalamic projection system　特異的視床投射系
standard temperature and pressure, saturated　標準温度・気圧・飽和

STQ
superior temporal quadrant　上耳側1/4

STR
soft tissue relaxation　軟部組織弛緩

Str
striatum　線条(体)

str
straight　まっすぐな
strain　株，ひずみ
strength　強さ，強度
stretch　伸ばす
strong　強い
structural　構造の
structure　構造

STR, str.
Streptococcus　ストレプトコッカス(属)，連鎖球菌(属)

Strab, strab.
strabismus　斜視

strep
streptomycin　ストレプトマイシン

STREP, Strep, strep.
Streptococcus　ストレプトコッカス(属)，連鎖球菌(属)

strept.
Streptococcus　ストレプトコッカス(属)，連鎖球菌(属)

streptoc.
Streptococcus　ストレプトコッカス(属)，連鎖球菌(属)

strobed
stroboscopically illuminated　ストロボスコープで照明された
stroboscopically measured　ストロボスコープで計測された

strobo
stroboscope　ストロボスコープ

STRT
skin temperature recovery time　皮膚温度回復時間

struc
structural　構造の
structure　構造，構成

struct
structural　構造の
structure　構造，構成

STS
scanning tunneling spectroscopy　走査トンネル分光法
serological test for syphilis　梅毒血清反応
short-term storage　短期貯蔵
simplified trypticase serum medium　簡易トリプチケース血清培地
standard test for syphilis　梅毒標準検査
standard two-stage method　標準二段階法
steroid sulfatase　ステロイドスルファターゼ

STSG
split-thickness skin graft　中間層植皮

STSS
staphylococcal toxic shock syndrome　ブドウ球菌性中毒性ショック症候群
streptococcal toxic shock syndrome　連鎖球菌毒ショック症候群
subjective tinnitus severity scale　耳鳴重症度評価法

STT
sensitization test　感作試験
serial thrombin time　連続トロンビン時間
skin temperature test　皮膚温度検査
spinothalamic tract　脊髄視床路

S

sttg
sitting　坐位の，座っている

STU
skin test unit　皮膚試験単位

stu
student　学生

STUMP
stromal tumors of unknown malignant potential　潜在悪性度不明基質腫瘍

STV
short-term variability　胎児心迫数基線細変動

superior temporal vein　上側頭静脈
STX
saxitoxin　サキシトキシン
sulfamethoxazole　スルファメトキサゾール
S.typhi
Salmonella typhi　(腸)チフス菌
S.typhi.
Salmonella typhosa〈ラ〉　チフス菌
STZ
streptozocin　ストレプトゾシン
streptozotocin　ストレプトゾトシン
SU
salicyluric acid　サリチル尿酸
sensation unit　感作単位
serologic tests for syphilis　梅毒の血清学的検査
skin unit　皮膚単位
solar urticaria　日光蕁麻疹
strontium unit　ストロンチウム単位
sulfonylurea　スルホニル尿素
sulfur unit　硫黄単位
supine　背臥の，仰臥の
sU
thiouridine　チオウリジン
SU 4885
metopyrone　メトピロン
s.u.
siehe unten〈独〉　下を見よ，下記参照
su, su.
subject　被験者，被検者
sumat〈ラ〉　とらせよ《処》
sumendum〈ラ〉　摂取せよ《処》
surgeon　外科医
surgery　外科(学)
surgical　外科的な，外科の
SUA
serum uric acid　血清尿酸
single umbilical artery　単一臍動脈
SUB, sub
substitute　代理(人)
subac
subacute　亜急性の
Subara, Subara.
Subarachnoidealblutung〈独〉＝subarachnoid hemorrhage〔bleeding〕　クモ膜下出血

S

Sub.AS
subaortic stenosis 大動脈弁下狭窄症
subclav
subclavian 鎖骨下の
subclavicular 鎖骨下の
subclin
subclinical 無症状の，不顕性の
subcr
subcreptiant 亜捻髪音の
subcrep，subcrep.
subcrepitant 亜捻髪音の
subcu，subcu.
subcutaneous 皮下の
subcutaneously 皮下に
subcut，subcut.
subcutaneous 皮下(の)
subcutaneously 皮下に
Subdura，Subdura.
subdurales Hämatom〈独〉＝subdural hematoma 硬膜下出血，硬膜下血腫
sub fin.coct.
sub finem coctionis〈ラ〉 沸騰の終りに《処》
subgen
subgenus 亜属
SUBI
the Subjective Well-being Inventory 心の健康自己評価質問用紙
subind.
subinde〈ラ〉＝immediately after 直後に
subj
subject 被験者，被検者
subjective 自覚的な
subjective angle 主観的視角
subl
sublimation 昇華
sublime 昇華する
sublingual 舌下の
subl.
sublimis〈ラ〉 表在性の，高所の
subl，subl.
sublimatus〈ラ〉＝sublimate 昇華する，昇華した
subling
sublingual 舌下の
sublux
subluxation 亜脱臼
submand
submandibular 下顎骨下の，顎下の

SubN
subthalamic nucleus 視床下核
suboccip
suboccipital 後頭下の
suborb.stim
suborbital stimulation 眼窩下刺激
subq
subsequent 次の
Sub-Q, subq, sub-q
subcutaneous 皮下の
subsc
subscapular 肩甲下の
subscap
subscapular 肩甲下の
subsp, subsp.
subspecies 亜種
subst
substance 物質
substitute 代理(人)
substd
substandard 標準以下の
subt.
subtilis〈ラ〉 細末の《処》
suc
succeed 成功する
success 成功
successor 成功者
succinyl スクシニル(基)
suc.
succus〈ラ〉=juice 液，汁
Succ
succinate コハク酸塩
succinic コハク酸の
succ
succinylcholine スクシニルコリン
succinyl CoA
succinyl coenzyme A スクシニル補酵素A
SUCM
simultaneous urethral cystometry 同時性尿道膀胱内圧測定
SUD
skin unit dose 皮膚単位量
subjective unit of disturbance 不安階層表
sudden unexpected death 予測不能突然死，内因性急死
sudden unexplained death 原因不明突然死
SUDEP
sudden unexpected death in epilepsy てんかん患者の突然死

SUDH
succinodehydrogenase　スクシノデヒドロゲナーゼ
SUDI
sudden unexpected death of infant　小児の突然不慮死
SUDS
sudden unexplained death syndrome　原因不明突然死症候群
suf
sufficient　十分な
suff
sufficient　十分な
sug
sugar　砂糖，糖
suggest　示唆する
sug.
sugatur〈ラ〉　吸わせよ《処》
sugend.
sugendus〈ラ〉　吸わせるべき《処》
SUI
stress urinary incontinence　ストレス性尿失禁
SUID
sudden unexpected infant death　不慮乳幼児突然死
sudden unexplained infant death　原因不明乳幼児突然死
sulf
sulfaricus　硫酸(塩)の
sulfate　硫酸(塩)の
sulfatis　硫酸(塩)の
sulfur　硫酸(塩)の
sulf, sulf.
sulfate　硫酸塩，硫酸エステル
sulfa
sulfanilamide(＝sulfonamide)　スルファニルアミド(＝スルホンアミド)
sulph
sulphate　硫酸塩
sum
summary　要約
summation　加重，総和
sum.
sumat〈ラ〉＝let (the patient) take　服用させよ《処》
sume〈ラ〉＝take　服用する，取る《処》
sumendum〈ラ〉＝let (the patient) take　服用させよ《処》
1 sum.
unum sumatur〈ラ〉＝to be taken at once　頓用，頓服《処》

SUMP
Suzuki universal micro-printing (method) 鈴木万能微細印象法＝スンプ法
sum tal
sumattalem〈ラ〉 同量を服用《処》
SUN
serum urea nitrogen 血清尿素窒素
SUO
syncope of unknown origin 原因不明失神
SUP, sup, sup.
superficial 浅い，表在(性)の
superior 上(方)の
supination 回外
supinator (muscle) 回外(筋)
supine 背臥の，仰臥の
supra〈ラ〉＝above, over 上の
super
supervisor 監督，指導者
superf
superficial 浅い，表在(性)の
superfic
superficial 浅い，表在(性)の
supp
suppurative 化膿性の
supp, supp., Supp.
suppositorium〈ラ〉＝suppository 坐薬
suppl
supplement 付録，追加
supplemental 予備の
supplementary 補充の，補足の
SUPPORT
study to understand prognoses and preferences for outcomes and risks of treatments サポート(＝予後と治療結果のための患者選択および治療の危険性を理解するための研究)
suppos.
suppositorium〈ラ〉＝suppository 坐薬
Suppos.rect.
Suppositoriae rectales〈ラ〉 肛門坐薬《処》
Suppos.ureth.
Suppositoriae urethrales 尿道坐薬
supp.rect.
suppositoria rectalia〈ラ〉 肛門坐薬《処》
supps
supplements 補足，増刊

supp.ureth.
suppositoria urethralis〈ラ〉 尿道坐薬
Su-Pr
streptococcal protein 連鎖球菌性蛋白
supra cit.
supra citato〈ラ〉＝citer above 上記の，上に引用した
supra pat
suprapatellar 膝蓋骨上の
Su-Ps，SU-PS
streptococcal polysaccharide 連鎖球菌ポリサッカリド
supt
superintendent 局長，管理者
supv
supervision 管理，監督
supervisor 管理人，監督者
sur
surface 表面
sur cdr
surgeon commander 外科医長
SURG，Surg，surg.
surgeon 外科医
surgery 外科(学)，手術(法)
surgical 外科(的)の，外科手術(上)の
SURS
solitary ulcer of rectum syndrome 孤立性直腸潰瘍症候群
surv
survey 調査する
surveyor 調査者
survill
surveillance 調査
SUS
stained urinary sediment 染色(済み)尿沈渣
sus，SUS
suppressor-sensitive (mutant) サプレッサー感受性変異体，抑圧遺伝子感受性変異体
susc
susceptibility 感(受)性
susceptible 感(受)性のある
susp
suspension 一時的停止，懸吊
sut
suture 縫合(術)，縫合線
SUTI
symptomatic urinary tract infection 症候性尿路感染(症)
SUUD
sudden unexpected unexplained death 原因不明予測不能突然死

SUV
small unilamellar vesicle　小単薄層小胞，小型単層小胞
SUX
succinylcholine　スクシニルコリン
SUZI
subzonal injection　透明帯下注入法
subzonal (sperm) insertion　透明帯下(精子)注入法
SV
common ventricle　単心室
saphenous vein　伏在静脈
sarcoma virus　肉腫ウイルス
scalp vein　頭皮静脈
secretory vesicle　分泌小胞
selective gastric vagotomy　選択的胃迷走神経切離術
selective vagotomy　選択的迷走神経切離術
semilunar valve　半月弁
seminal vesicle　精嚢
semivertical position　半垂直位心電図
Sendai virus　仙台ウイルス
severe　重症の
Shope virus　ショープウイルス
simian virus　サルウイルス
single ventricle　単心室
single vibration　単振動
sinus venosus　静脈洞
snake venom　ヘビ毒
Spielmeyer-Vogt (disease)　シュピールマイアー・フォークト(病)
splenic vein　脾静脈
spontaneous ventilation　自発呼吸，自発換気
stria vascularis〈ラ〉　血管条
stroke volume　1回拍出量
subclavian vein　鎖骨下静脈
sulcus vocali〈ラ〉　声帯溝症
supraventricular　上室(性)の
systolic volume　収縮期容量
Sv
sievert　シーベルト〈単位〉
synaptic vesicle　シナプス小胞
sv
survey　調査する
SV40
simian virus 40　サルウイルス40
s.v.
spiritus vini〈ラ〉=spirit(s) of wine　アルコール，酒精《処》

S/V
slender value 痩身値
survivability/vulnerablity 生存性・脆弱性比

SVA
selective visceral angiography 選択的臓器動脈造影
special visceral afferent (nerve) 特殊内臓求心性(神経)

SVAS
subvalvular aortic stenosis 大動脈弁膜下狭窄
supravalvular aortic stenosis 大動脈弁上部狭窄

SV(E)C
stereovector electro cardiogram 立体ベクトル心電図

SVC
sorting vertical conveyer コンベア系院内搬送システム
stereovector cardiogram 立体ベクトル心電図
subclavian vein catheterization 鎖骨下静脈カテーテル挿入
subclavian vein compression 鎖骨下静脈圧迫
superior vena cava 上大静脈
suprahepatic vena cava 肝上位上大静脈
supraventricular contraction 上室性期外収縮

SVCCS
superior vena cava compression syndrome 上大静脈圧迫症候群

SVCG
spatial vectorcardiogram 空間ベクトル心電図
superior venacavography 上大静脈造影

SVCO
superior vena cava obstruction 上大静脈閉塞

SVCP
Special Virus Cancer Program 特殊ウイルス癌計画

SVC-RPA shunt
superior vena cava-right pulmonary artery shunt 上大静脈・右肺動脈シャント(術)

SVCS
superior vena cava syndrome 上大静脈症候群

SVD
simple vertex delivery 自然経腟分娩
sinus venous defect 静脈洞欠損症
spontaneous vaginal delivery 自然腟分娩
swine vesicular disease ブタ水疱病

SVE
special visceral efferent (nerve) 特殊内臓遠心性(神経)
Streptococcus viridans endocarditis ビリダンス連鎖球菌(性)心内膜炎

SVECG
stereovector-electrocardiogram 立体ベクトル心電図

SVG
saphenous vein graft　伏在静脈移植片
s.v.g.
spiritus vini gallici〈ラ〉=brandy　ブランデー
S.V.gal.
spiritus vini gallici〈ラ〉=brandy　ブランデー
SVI
slow virus infection　遅発性ウイルス感染症
sludge volume index　汚泥容量指標
stroke volume index　1回拍出係数
SVLP
Special Virus-Leukemia Program　特殊ウイルス・白血病計画
SVM
seminal vesicle microsome　精嚢ミクロソーム
SVN
Student Vocational Nurse　看護師訓練中学生
Svo_2
(mixed) venous oxgen saturation　(混合)静脈血酸素飽和度
SVP
small volume parenteral　少量注射
SVPB
supraventicular premature beat　上室性期外心拍
SVPC
supraventricular premature contraction　上(心)室性期外収縮
SVR
slow vertex response　頭頂部緩反応
stimulated volume rate　刺激液量
systemic vascular resistance　全身血管抵抗，体血管抵抗
systolic vascular resistance　収縮期血管抵抗
s.v.r.
spiritus vini rectincatus〈ラ〉　希釈アルコール《処》
SVRI
systemic vascular resistance index　全身(体循環)血管抵抗指数
SVS
slit ventricle syndrome　スリット脳室症候群
SVT
sinoventricular tachyarrhythmia　洞室頻拍症
subclavian vein thrombosis　鎖骨下静脈血栓
supraventricular tachyarrhythmia　上(心)室性不整頻拍
supraventricular tachycardia　上(心)室性頻拍
s.v.t.
spiritus vini tenuis〈ラ〉　ブランデー《処》
SVTP
sound, velocity, temperature, pressure　音・速度・温度・圧

S

SW
salt water 塩水
Schwartz-Watson (test) シュワルツ・ワトソン(試験)
sea water 海水
short wave 短波
slow wave 徐波
social worker ソーシャルワーカー
stab wound 刺創
sterile water 滅菌水
stroke work 1回拍出仕事(量)
Sturge-Weber (syndrome) スタージ・ウェーバー(症候群)

sw
sweet 甘い
swelling 腫脹

S & W
spike and wave complex 棘徐波複合体

SWC
spike and wave complex 棘徐波複合(体)

SWD
short wave diathermy 短波ジアテルミー，短波透熱量法
sine wave diathermy サイン〔正弦〕波ジアテルミー

SW dia.
short wave diathermy 短波ジアテルミー
sine wave diathermy 正弦〔サイン〕波ジアテルミー

S & W enema
soap and water enema 石鹸水浣腸

SWFI
sterile water for injection 注射用滅菌水〔無菌水〕

SWG
silk worm gut 絹糸
standard wire gauge 標準針金測径器

SWI
sterile water for injection 注射用滅菌水
stroke work index 1回拍出仕事係数
surgical wound infection 手術創感染

SWM
segmental wall motion 局所壁運動

SWMA
segmental wall motion amplitude 局所壁運動振幅

SWOG
South Western Oncology Group サウスウェスタン癌研究班

SWR
serum Wassermann reaction 血清ワッセルマン反応

SWS
slow wave sleep　徐波睡眠
Sturge-Weber syndrome　スタージ・ウェーバー症候群
SWS cone pigment
short wave sensitive cone pigment　青錐(状)体色素
SWT
septal wall thickness　中隔壁厚
Sx
medical sign(s) and symptom(s)　医学徴候と症候
Sx, sx
sign(s)　徴候
symptom(s)　症状
SXA
single-energy X-ray absorptiometry　単エネルギーX線吸収測定装置
Sx Hx
social history　社会歴
SXL
short-arc xenon lamp　短弧キセノン燈
SXM
scanning probe microscope　走査型探査顕微鏡
SXR
soft X-ray region　軟X線域
SXS
stellar X-ray spectra　星状X線スペクトル
sx & sx
sign(s) and symptom(s)　徴候と症状，症候
SXT
stable X-ray transmitter　安定X線伝導体
SY
syphilis　梅毒
SYA
subacute yellow atrophy　亜急性黄色萎縮
sycate
symptom cause test　症候作因試験
SYD
see your doctor　かかりつけ医を訪ねよ
Sym, sym
symmetric　対称性の
symmetrical　対称性の
symmetry　対称，対称性
symptoms　症状
symb
symbol　記号
symbolic　記号の，象徴的な

symp
sympathetic 共感の，交感の
symptom(s) 症状
sympat
sympathetic 共感の，交感の
sympath
sympathetic 共感の，交感の
symp.sys
sympathetic system 交感(神経)系
sympt
symptom(s) 症状
SYN
synchronous 同調
synthetic 合成の
Syn
synchondrosis 軟骨結合
syn
synergist 共力(協力)薬
synergy 共力(協力)作用
synonym 同意語，類語
synovial 髄液の
synovitis 髄膜炎
sync
synchronous 同調の，同期性の
synch
synchronous 同調の，同期性の
synchro
synchronization 時間的一致，心拍同期特定時の撮影《画診》
synchronized IMV
synchronized〔synchronous〕 intermittent mandatory ventilation 同期的間欠的強制換気(＝SIMV)
synd
syndrome 症候群
Syn FI
synovial fluid 髄液
synopt
synoptiscope 両眼視機能検査鏡，シノプチスコープ
synov
synovectomy 滑膜切除(術)
synovial 髄液の
synovitis 髄膜炎
synth
synthetic 合成の

syph
syphilis 梅毒
syphilitic 梅毒性の
syphilologist 梅毒学者
syphilology 梅毒学

syr
syrup 糖蜜，シロップ

SYS
stretching-yawning syndome ストレッチングあくび症候群

sys
system 系(統)，器官系
systemic 全身性の

syst
systemic 全身性の
systole 収縮期

Syst, syst, syst.
systolic (心)収縮期(性)の

syst.m.
systolic murmur (心)収縮期雑音

SZ
streptozo(to)cin ストレプトゾ(ト)シン

Sz
skin impedance 皮膚インピーダンス

sz
size 大きさ

SZ, Sz
schizophrenia 統合失調症

Sz, sz
seizure 発作

SZD
streptozo(to)cin diabetes ストレプトゾ(ト)シン糖尿病

T t

T

intermittent hypertropia	間欠性上斜視
intraocular tension	眼圧
primary tumor	原発腫瘍
ribosylthymidine	リボシルチミジン
ribosylthymine	リボシルチミン
tablespoon	大さじ《処》
tablespoonful	大さじ１杯の《処》
Taenia	条虫(属)，テニア(属)
tamoxifen	タモキシフェン
tau〈ギ〉	タウ
T-bandage	T包帯
temporal	側頭部の
temporary	一過性の
tender	圧痛のある
tenderness	圧痛
tension	圧，緊張
tera-	テラ(=10^{12})《接》
term	用語
tesla	テスラ〈単位〉
testosterone	テストステロン
tetracycline	テトラサイクリン
Tetrahymena	テトラヒメナ(属)
T-fiber	T線維
theophylline	テオフィリン
therapeutic plan	治療計画
therapist	療法士
thoracic	胸(椎)の
thoracic vertebra(e)	胸椎
thorax〈ラ〉	胸郭
threonine	スレオニン
thrombus	血栓
thymidine	チミジン
thymine	チミン
thymus	胸腺
thymus-derived (lymphocyte)	胸腺由来(リンパ球)
thyroid	甲状(腺)の
thyroxine	チ〔サイ〕ロキシン
tidal gas	１回換気
tidal volume	１回換気量
time period	時間間隔
timing	タイミング
tincture	チンキ(剤)

tissue	組織
tocopherol	トコフェロール
tone	緊張
topical	局所的な
total	全，総，完全な
toxicity	毒性
Toxoplasma	トキソプラズマ(属)
trace	痕跡の，微量の
Transformation zone	移行帯
transition point	移行点
transmittance	透過率
transverse	横の，横断の
transverse colon	横行結腸
tray	皿
Treponema	トレポネーマ(属)
Triatoma	トリアトーマ(属)
Trichinella	トリキネラ(属)
Trichomonas	トリコモナス
Trichophyton	白癬菌(属)
tricuspid	三尖弁
Trypanosoma	トリパノソーマ(属)
tuberculin	ツベルクリン
tuberculosis	結核(症)
tumor	腫瘍
T wave	T波《心電》
type	型

t

tabulated	錠剤になった
tales〈ラ〉	同量の《処》
target	目標
teaspoon	茶さじ，小さじ《処》
teaspoonful	茶さじ１杯の《処》
teeth	歯〈複数〉
ter〈ラ〉	３回《処》
terminal	終末の，末端の
title	標題
transferred	伝達された
translocation	転座
tropical	熱帯の

2,4,5-T

2,4,5-trichlorophenoxyacetic acid	2,4,5-トリクロロフェノキシ酢酸

3T

triage-treatment-transportation	選別・応急処置・後方搬送

T_1

monoiodothyronine	モノヨードチ〔サイ〕ロニン

tricuspid first heart sound 三尖弁第Ⅰ心音

T_1〔T_2…〕，T1〔T2…〕
first thoracic vertebra, second thoracic vertebra, etc. 第一胸椎・第二胸椎…など

T_2
diiodothyronine ジヨードチ〔サイ〕ロニン
transverse relaxation time 横緩和時間
tricuspid second heart sound 三尖弁第Ⅱ心音

T_3
triiodothyronine トリヨードチ〔サイ〕ロニン

T_4
thyroxine (=tetraiodothyronine) チ〔サイ〕ロキシン(=テトラヨードチ〔サイ〕ロニン)

T1/2
reaction half-time 反応半減期
symbol for half-life of radioactive isotope 放射性アイソトープの半減期記号

T+
increased tension 緊張増加，(眼)圧上昇

T_{+1}, T_{+2}…
intraocular tension (眼)圧の増大度

T−
decreased tension 緊張減少，(眼)圧低下

T↑
tension increased (眼)圧上昇

T↓
tension decreased (眼)圧低下

T↓↓
testicles both descended 両側睾丸下降した

T/
than ～より
then それから

T, *T*
absolute temperature 絶対温度

T, *t*
tritium トリチウム，三重水素(=^3H)

T, t
temperature 温度，体温
tertiar- 第三の〈接〉
tertiary 第三の，３番目の
time 時間

T, t, t.
temporal 一過性の
temporary 一過性の

T

$t_{1/2}$, t1/2
half-life 半減期
half time 半減期

TA
alkaline tuberculin アルカリ性ツベルクリン
arterial tension 動脈圧
axillary temperature 腋窩(体)温
target area 標的域
technical assistance 技術協力
technology assessment 技術事前評価
temporal arteritis 側頭動脈炎
tendon of Achilles アキレス腱
therapeutic abortion 治療的流産
thyroglobulin agglutination チ〔サイ〕ログロブリン凝集
thyroglobulin antibody チ〔サイ〕ログロブリン抗体
thyroid antibody 甲状腺抗体
thyroid autoantibody 甲状腺自己抗体
tibialis anterior 脛骨前面
titratable acid 滴定酸
traffic accident 交通事故
transactional analysis 交流分析
transaldolase トランスアルドラーゼ
transfer agent 伝達因子
transplantation antigen 移植抗原
tricuspid atresia 三尖弁閉鎖症
triggered activity 誘発活動
truncus arteriosus 総動脈幹
tryptophan acid (method) トリプトファン過塩素酸(試験)
tryptophan acid (reaction) トリプトファン過塩素酸(反応)
typhus abdominalis 腸チフス

Ta
appearance time 出現時間
tantalum タンタル〈元素〉

T.a.
tinctura amara〈ラ〉 苦味チンキ《処》

T & A
tonsillectomy and adenoidectomy 扁桃摘出(術)とアデノイド摘出(術)
tonsills and adenoid(s) 扁桃とアデノイド

TA, T.A.
tension artérielle〈仏〉 動脈圧
toxin-antitoxin 毒素・抗毒素

TAA
thioacetamide チオアセタミド

thoracic aorta aneurysm 胸部大動脈瘤
tumor-associated antibody 腫瘍関連抗体
tumor associated antigen 腫瘍関連抗原

TAAA
thoracoabdominal aortic aneurysm 胸膜部大動脈瘤

TAAIDS
transfusion-associated aquired immunodeficiency syndrome 輸血・関連後天性免疫欠損症候群

TAB
therapeutic abortion 治療的流産
typhoid, paratyphoid A, and paratyphoid B (vaccine) 腸チフス・パラチフスA・パラチフスB(混合ワクチン)

Tab
table 表

TAB, tab, tab., Tab.
tabella〈ラ〉=tablet 錠剤《処》

TABC
typhoid-paratyphoid A, B and C (vaccine) 腸チフス・パラチフスABC(ワクチン)

Tab/D
tablets daily 1日の錠剤用量

TABDT
antityphoid, anti A and B paratyphoid, antidiphtheria, antitetanus 抗腸チフス・抗パラチフスAとB・抗ジフテリア・抗テタヌス混合ワクチン

TABP
type a behavior pattern タイプa 行動型

tabs
tablets 錠(剤)《処》

TAC
tetracaine, epinephrine, cocaine テトラカイン・エピネフリン・コカイン
thyroid-adrenocortical (syndrome) 甲状腺・副腎皮質(症候群)
triallylcyanurat トリアリルシアヌール酸
truncus arteriosus communis 総動脈幹

TACE
transarterial chemoembolization 経動脈性化学塞栓術
transcatheter arterial chemoenbolization 肝動脈化学塞栓療法
trianinsyl chlorethylene トリアニンジル塩化エチレン

tach
tachycardia 頻脈, (心)頻拍

tachy, tachy.
tachycardia 頻脈, (心)頻拍

T

TACK
Na-tosyl-L-arginyl-chloromethyle ketone | Na-トシル-L-アルギニルクロロメチルケトン

TAD
thiamine allyl disulfide | チアミンアリルジスルフィド
6-thioguanine, arabinosylcytosine, daunorubicin | 6-チオグアニン,アラビノシルシトシン,ダウノルビシン
transient acantholytic dermatosis | 一過性棘融解性皮膚症

TAE
total adominal evisceration | 胸部臓器全摘術
transcatheter arterial embolization | 経カテーテル肝動脈塞栓術
tris, acetic acid, EDTA | トリス・酢酸・エチレンジアミンテトラ酢酸(緩衝液)

TAF
target aiming function | 集中維持機能
T cell activating factor | T細胞活性化因子
tissue angiogenesis factor | 組織脈管形成因子
T lymphocyte activating factor | Tリンパ球活性化因子
toxoid-antitoxin floccules | トキソイド・抗毒素沈降物
trypsin, aldehyde, fuchsin | トリプシン・アルデヒド・フクシン
tumor angiogenesis factor | 腫瘍血管形成因子

TAf
Tuberkulin Albumose frei〈独〉 | ツベルクリン・アルブミン陰性

TAG
thymine, adenine, guanine | チミン・アデニン・グアニン
tumor associated glycoprotein | 腫瘍関連糖蛋白

TaG
tantalum gauze | タンタルムガーゼ

tägl
täglich〈独〉 | 毎日《処》

TAH
temperature, altitude, humidity | 温度・標高・湿度
total abdominal hysterectomy | 腹式子宮全摘術
total artificial heart | 完全人工心臓
transabdominal hysterectomy | 経腹式子宮摘出(術)

TAHBSO
total abdominal hysterectomy, bilateral salpingo-oophorectomy | 腹式子宮全摘術・両卵管卵巣摘出術

TAHRI
Tobacco and Health Research Institute | タバコと健康研究所

T

TAI
tissue antagonist of interferon　インターフェロン組織拮抗物質
transcatheter arterial infusion　経カテーテル動注療法

TAL
tachypleus tridentatus amoebocyte lysate　カブトガニ由来の分解質
tendo-Achillis lengthening　アキレス腱延長術
thymic alymphoplasia　胸腺リンパ形成不全(症)

Tal
talose　タロース

talc.
talcum〈ラ〉=powder　粉末，散(剤)《処》

tal.dos.
tales doses〈ラ〉=such doses　同量《処》

TALL, T-ALL
T cell adult lymphocyte leukemia　T細胞成人急性白血病
T cell-type acute lymphocytic leukemia　T細胞急性リンパ性白血病

TAM
tamoxifen　タモキシフェン
teenage mother　10代の母親
toxoid-antitoxin mixture　トキソイド・抗毒素合剤
transient abnormal myelopoiesis　一過性異常骨髄造血症
tunneling acoustic microscope　トンネル音響顕微鏡

t-AMCHA, TAMCHA
trans-4-aminomethyl cyclohexane carboxylic acid　トラネキサム酸

TAME
tosyl-arginine methyl ester　トシルアルギニンメチルエステル

TAMI
thrombolysis angioplasty myocardial infarction　血栓融解心筋梗塞血管形成術

TAN
total adenine nucleotides　全アデニンヌクレオチド
total ammonia nitrogen　全アンモニア窒素

T

tan
tangent　タンジェント

TANe
toluenesulfonylarginine methyl ester　トルエンスルホニルアルギニンメチルエステル

TANI
total axial lymph-node irradiation　総リンパ節軸照射

T antigens
tumor antigens　腫瘍抗原

TAO
thromboangiitis obliterans 閉塞性血栓性血管炎
triacetyloleandomycin トリアセチルオレアンドマイシン

TAP
total acid phosphatase 総酸性リン酸分解酵素
transporter associated with antigen processing 抗原作用に関係する担体
tricuspid annuloplasty 三尖弁縫縮術
trypsin activation protein トリプシン活性化蛋白

Tap
transport protein (細胞内)輸送蛋白

TAPC
talampicillin タランピシリン

TAPL
tractus arteriosus posterolateralis (脊髄)後側動脈路

TAPP
transabdominal preperitoneal herniorrhaphy 経腹腔前腹膜ヘルニア縫合術

TAPVC
total anomalous pulmonary venous connection 総肺静脈灌流異常症

TAPVD
total anomalous pulmonary venous drainage 総肺静脈灌流異常症

TAPVR
total anomalous pulmonary venous return 総肺静脈灌流異常症

4ta qq.hor.
quarta quaque hora〈ラ〉＝every fourth hour 4時間ごとに《処》

TAQW
transient abnormal Q waves 一過性異常Q波《心電》

TAR
airway resistance through nose 経鼻気道抵抗
Takada-Ara reaction 高田・荒反応
thrombocytopenia-absent radius 血小板減少・橈骨欠損症候群
tissue (tumor) air ratio 組織(腫瘍)空中線量比
total abortion rate 総流産率
total ankle replacement 人工足関節全置換術

TARA
total articular replacement arthroplasty 全関節置換関節形成(術)
tumor-associated rejection antigen 腫瘍関連拒絶抗体

tart
tartaric 酒石(酸)の

T

tart.a.
tartaric acid 酒石酸
TAS
tetanus antitoxic serum 破傷風抗毒素血清
tumor-associated substance 腫瘍関連物質
TASA
tumor-associated cell surface antigen 腫瘍関連細胞表面抗原
T'ase
tryptophan synthetase トリプトファン合成酵素
TAST
trans-acoustic sending technique 経聴道超音波発信法
TAT
tetanus antitoxin 破傷風抗毒素
thematic apperception test 絵画(主題)統覚検査
thrombin-antithrombin (Ⅲ complex) トロンビンアンチトロンビン(Ⅲ複合体)
thromboplastin activation (test) トロンボプラスチン活性化(試験)
thyrosine aminotransferase チ〔サイ〕ロシンアミノトランスフェラーゼ
tumor activity test 腫瘍活性試験
TAT, T.A.T.
toxin-antitoxin 毒素・抗毒素
TATA
tumor associated transplantation antigen 腫瘍関連移植抗原
TATD
thiamin-8-(methy-6-acetyl-dihydrotyoctate)-disulfide チアミン-8-(メチル-6-アセチル・ジヒドロチオクテート)-ジスルフィド
TA test
thyroglobulin aggregation test チ〔サイ〕ログロブリン凝集試験
TAT reaction
toxin-antitoxin reaction 毒素・抗毒素反応
TATST
tetanus antitoxin skin test 破傷風抗毒素皮膚試験
tave
octave 音階
TAVI
transcatheter aortic valveimplantation 経カテーテル大動脈弁留置術
TAVR
transcatheter aortic valve replacement 経カテーテル大動脈弁置換術

T

Ta-wave
auricular T wave　心房性T波

taxon
taxonomy　分類学

TB
Taschenband〈独〉　仮声帯
Taussig-Bing (syndrome)　タウシヒ・ビング(症候群)
terminal bar　閉鎖堤
terminal bronchiole　終末細気管支
thromboxane B　トロンボキサンB
thymol blue　チモールブルー
toluidine blue　トルイジンブルー
total base　総塩基
total bilirubin　総ビリルビン(量)
tracheobronchitis　気管気管支炎
tub bath　入浴
tuberculosis　結核(症)

T_b
body temperature　体温

Tb
biological half-life　生物学的半減期
terbium　テルビウム〈元素〉

TB, Tb
tubercle bacillus　結核菌

TBA
T-bandage　T字包帯
testosterone-binding affinity　テストステロン結合親和性
thioacetazone　チオアセタゾン
thiobarbituric acid　チオバルビツール酸
thyroxine-binding albumin　チ〔サイ〕ロキシン結合アルブミン
to be added　加えるべき《処》
total bile acid　総胆汁酸
traditional birth attendant　伝統的産婆
trypsin-binding activity　トリプシン結合活性
tubercle bacillus　結核菌
tumor-bearing animal　担癌動物

TBAB
transbronchial needle aspiration biopsy　経気管支針生検

TBAC
transbronchial aspiration cytology　経気管支吸引細胞診

TBA reaction
thiobarbituric acid reaction　チオバルビツール酸反応

TBARS
thiobarbituric acid reactive substance　チオバルビツール酸反応物質

TBB
tenor, baritone, bass　テノール・バリトン・バス
transbronchial biopsy　経気管支生検
TBBC
total B_{12} binding capacity　総〔全〕B_{12}結合能
TBBM
total body bone mineral　全身骨ミネラル
TBBMC
total body bone mineral content　全身骨塩量
TBBMD
total body bone mineral density　全身骨塩密度
TBC
target-binding capacity　標的結合能
thrombocyte　栓球，血小板
thyroxine binding capacity　チ〔サイ〕ロキシン結合能
thyroxine-binding coagulin　チ〔サイ〕ロキシン結合凝固素
total body calcium　全〔総〕カルシウム量
total body clearance　全〔総〕クリアランス
tubercidin　ツベルシジン
Tbc
tubercle bacillus　結核菌
Tbc, TbC
tuberculosis　結核(症)
TBCI
T_3 binding capacity index　トリヨード・チ〔サイ〕ロニン結合能指数
tbcn.
tuberculin　ツベルクリン
TBE
tick-borne encephalitis　ダニ媒介脳炎
tris, borate, EDTA　トリス・ホウ酸・エチレンジアミンテトラ酢酸(緩衝液)
tuberculin bacillus emulsion　菌乳剤ツベルクリン
TB-E
toluidine blue-eosin　トルイジンブルーエオジン
TBF
total body fat　全体脂肪(量)
total body fluid　全体液(量)
tumor blood flow　腫瘍血流(量)
TBFB
tracheobronchial foreign body　気管気管支異物
TBG
testosterone-binding globulin　テストステロン結合グロブリン
thyroxine-binding globulin　チ〔サイ〕ロキシン結合グロブリン

TBG cap
thyroxine-binding capacity　チ〔サイ〕ロキシン結合能
TBGI
thyroxine-binding globulin index　チ〔サイ〕ロキシン結合グロブリン指数
TBGP
total blood granulocyte pool　全血顆粒球数
TBH
total body hematocrit　全身ヘマトクリット
total-body hyperthermia　全身高熱療法
TBI
^{131}I-thyro-binding index　ヨード131甲状腺結合指数
tooth brushing instruction　歯磨き指導
(serum) total bilirubin　(血清)総ビリルビン
total body irradiation　全身照射
TBIA
thyroid stimulating hormone brinding inhibiting activity　甲状腺刺激ホルモン結合阻害活性
TBII
thyrotropin binding inhibitory immunoglobulin　TSH結合抑制性免疫グロブリン
TBIL
total bilirubin　総ビリルビン(量)
T bili
total bilirubin (assay)　総ビリルビン(定量法)
TBI-test
thyroxine-binding-index test　チ〔サイ〕ロキシン結合指数試験
TBK
total body kalium〔potassium〕　全カリウム量
TBL
tracheobronchial lymph node　気管気管支リンパ節
tbl, Tbl
table　表
tablet　錠(剤)《処》
TBLB
transbronchial lung biopsy　経気管支肺生検
TBLC
term birth, living child　満期産生存小児
TBLI
term birth, living infant　満期産生存乳幼児
TBM
toluidine blue metachromasia　トルイジンブルー異染色
tuberculous meningitis　結核性髄膜炎
tubule basement membrane　尿細管基底膜

TBN
bacillus emulsion 菌乳剤
total body nitrogen 全身窒素
TBNA
total body neutron activation 全身ニュートロン活性化
transbronchial needle aspiration 経気管支吸引細胞診
TBNAA
total body neutron activation analysis 全身ニュートロン活性化分析
TBNAB
transbronchial needle aspiration biopsy 経気管支針吸引生検
TBP
testosterone-binding protein テストステロン結合蛋白
throxine binding protein チ〔サイ〕ロキシン結合蛋白
true boiling point 真沸騰点
tuberculous peritonitis 結核性腹膜炎
TBPA
thyroxine binding prealbumin チ〔サイ〕ロキシン結合プレアルブミン
TBPE
tetra-bromphenolphthalein ethyl ester テトラブロムフェノールフタレインエチルエステル
TB-RD
tuberculosis-respiratory disease 結核・呼吸器疾患
TBS
total body surface 全身表面(積)
tracheobronchoscopy 気管気管支鏡検査(法)
tribromosalicylanilide トリブロモサリチルアニリド
tuberculosis sanatorium 結核療養所
tbs
tablespoon 大さじ《処》
TBSA
total body surface area 全身表面積
TBSI
Tanaka Binet scale of intelligence 田中・ビネー式知能検査
tbsp
tablespoonful 大さじ１杯の《処》
TBT
tolbutamide test トルブタミド試験
tracheobronchial toilet 気管気管支洗浄
tracheobronchial tree 気管気管支枝
TBTC
tributyltin chloride 塩化トリブチルスズ
TBTO
tributyltin oxide 酸化トリブチルスズ

TBV
total blood volume 全血液量
tubercle bacillus vaccine 結核菌ワクチン
TBW
total body water 全身水分量
total body weight 総体重
TBWA
total body water 全身水分量
TBX
total-(whole) body irradiation 全身照射
TBZ
tetrabenazine テトラベナジン
thiabendazole チアベンダゾール
TC
target cell 標的細胞
T cell cloning method T細胞クローン法
temperature compensation 温度代償
teratocarcinoma 奇形癌
terminal care ターミナルケア，(終)末期医療
tetracycline テトラサイクリン
thermal conductivity 熱伝導性
thiocarbanilidin チオカルバニリジン
thoracic cage 胸郭
throat culture 咽頭培養
thyrocalcitonin チ〔サイ〕ロカルシトニン
ticlopidine チクロピジン
time constant 時定数
tissue culture 組織培養
to contain 含む(こと)
toluene-2,4-diisocyanate トルエン-2,4-ジイソシアネイト
tonic contraction 強直収縮
total calcium 総カルシウム量
total cholesterol 総コレステロール量
total colectomy 全結腸切除(術)
total colonoscopy 全結腸鏡検査(法)
transcobalamin トランスコバラミン
transcortin トランスコルチン
transcutaneous 経皮的な
transverse colon 横行結腸
trauma center 外傷センター
true cord 声帯
Tubencatarrh〈独〉 耳管カタル
tuberculin ツベルクリン
tubocurarine ツボクラリン

tubocurarine chloride 塩化ツボクラリン
tumor cell 腫瘍細胞
type crossmatch 血液型交叉〔差〕試験

Tc
cytotoxic T cell 細胞傷害性T細胞
technetium テクネチウム〈元素〉
tocainide トカイニド

TC_{50}
median toxic concentration 50%中毒濃度
toxic concentration fifty 50%中毒濃度

T/C
to consider 考慮する

T & C
type and crossmatch 血液型と交叉〔差〕試験

^{99m}Tc
technetium-99m テクネチウム99m

TC, T/C, Tc, t.c.
telephone call 電話連絡

TCA
taurocholic acid タウロコール酸
terminal cancer 末期癌
thyrocalcitonin チ〔サイ〕ロカルシトニン
total circulating albumin 総循環アルブミン
tricarboxylic acid (cycle) トリカルボン酸(回路)
trichloroacetate トリクロル酢酸塩
trichloroacetic acid トリクロル酢酸
trichloroethanol トリクロロエタノール
tricyclic antidepressant 三環系抗うつ薬
tricyclic antipsychotics 三環系抗精神病薬

TCAD
tricyclic antidepressant 三環系抗うつ薬

TCA method
trichloracetic acid method トリクロル酢酸法, TCA法

TCB
transcatheter biopsy 経カテーテル生検

TcB
transcutaneous bilirubinometry 経皮的ビリルビン濃度測定法

TCBP
tetrahymena calcium-binding protein テトラヒメナカルシウム結合蛋白

TCBS
thiosulfate-citrate-bile salts-sucrose (agar) チオ硫酸・クエン酸・胆汁酸・ショ糖培地

TCC
terminal complement complex 補体最終活性化分子
thromboblast(ic) cell component 血小板母細胞成分

transitional cell carcinoma　移行上皮癌
trichlorocarbanilide　トリクロロカルバニリド

TCCA
transitional cell cancer associated (virus)　移行上皮癌関連(ウイルス)

TCCAV
transitional cell cancer associated virus　移行上皮癌関連ウイルス

TCCFI
transcranial color flow image　経頭蓋超音波カラーフロー断層像

TCCL
T cell chronic lymphocytic (leukemia)　T細胞性慢性リンパ球性(白血病)

TCD
thermal conductivity detector　熱伝導性検出器
tissue culture dose　組織培養量
total cardiac dimension　全心臓容積
transcranial doppler sonography　経頭蓋ド(ッ)プラー超音波走査法
transcranial doppler ultrasonography　経頭蓋骨ド(ッ)プラー超音波検査法
transverse cardiac diameter　心臓横径
tumor control dose　腫瘍治癒線量
tumor cure dose　腫瘍治癒線量

TCD_{50}
50% tissue culture (dose)　50%組織培養(量)

TCDD
2,3,7,8-tetrachlorodibenzo-*p*-dioxin　2,3,7,8-テトラクロロジベンゾパラジオキシン
time-controlled drug delivery　時間制御方式薬剤投与(装置)

TCDT
transcranial color doppler tomography　経頭蓋骨超音波カラード(ッ)プラー断層法

TCE
T cell clonal excess　T細胞クローン過剰
tetrachlorodiphenylethane　テトラクロロジフェニルエタン
tetrachloroethylene　テトラクロロエチレン
transcatheter chemo-embolization　制癌剤動注兼塞栓療法
trichloroethylene　トリクロロエチレン

T cell
thymus(-derived) cell　胸腺(由来)細胞

TCES
transcutaneous cerebral electric stimulation　頭蓋経皮電気刺激法

T

TCF
screening total colonoscopy 全大腸内視鏡検診
total coronary flow 全冠(状動脈)血流量
tumor cytolytic factor 腫瘍細胞溶解因子
TCFU
trichlorofluoromethane トリクロロフルオロメタン
TCGF
T cell growth factor T細胞増殖因子
TCGF-R
T cell growth factor receptor T細胞増殖因子受容体
TCGP
taeniae coli muscle of guinea-pig モルモット結腸紐筋
TCH
tanned cell hemagglutination タンニン酸処理赤血球凝集(反応)
total circulating hemoglobin 全循環ヘモグロビン
Tch
teaching 教育する
T.CH
total cholesterol 総コレステロール
TChE
total cholinesterase 総コリンエステラーゼ
T-CHO
total cholesterol 総コレステロール
Tchr
teacher 教育者，教師
TCI
target controlled infusion 目標調節式注入法
transient cerebral ischemia 一過性脳虚血
TCID
tissue culture infective dose 組織培養感染量
$TCID_{50}$
median tissue culture infective dose 50%組織培養感染量
50% tissue culture infection dose 50%組織培養感染量
TCIE
transient cerebral ischemic episode 一過性脳虚血発作
TCIPA
tumor cell induced platelet aggregation 腫瘍細胞誘発血小板凝集
TCL
tibial collateral ligament 内側側副靱帯
TCLL
T cell chronic lymphatic leukemia 慢性T細胞リンパ性白血病
T cell chronic lymphocytic leukemia 慢性T細胞リンパ球性白血病
TCM
tissue culture medium 組織培養培地

Tc^{99m}
technetium-99m　テクネチウム99m
TCN
tetracycline　テトラサイクリン
TCNE
tetracyanoethylene　テトラシアノエチレン
TcNM
tumor with node metastasis　リンパ節転移を伴う腫瘍
TC+NP
throat culture+nasopharyngeal culture　咽頭培養と鼻咽頭培養
TCNS
transcutaneous nerve stimulator　経皮的神経刺激装置
Tco_2
total carbon dioxide　総〔全〕二酸化炭素
TCP
teacher-child-parent　教師・子・親
total circulating potein　全循環蛋白
trichlorophenol　トリクロロフェノール
tricresyl phosphate　リン酸トリクレシル
$TcPaO_2$
transcutaneous arterial oxygen pressure　経皮内動脈血酸素分圧
TCPC
total cavopulmonary connection　完全大静脈肺動脈結合
$tcPco_2$
transcutaneous carbon dioxide pressure　経皮的二酸化炭素分圧
TCP/IP
Transmission Control Protocol/Internet Protocol　ティーシーピーアイピー〈コン〉
$tcPO_2$
transcutaneous blood oxygen monitoring　経皮酸素分圧監視
$tcPo_2$
transcutaneous oxygen pressure　経皮的酸素分圧
TCPR
T cell proliferative reaction　T細胞増殖反応
TCPS
total cavopulmonary shunt　完全大静脈肺動脈吻合
TCR
T cell antigen receptor (gene)　T細胞抗原受容体(遺伝子)
T cell reactivity　T細胞反応性
T cell receptor　T細胞受容体
transcallosal response　経胼胝体応答

T & CrM
type and cross-matching 血液型と交叉〔差〕試験
TCS
traumatic cervical syndrome 外傷性頸部症候群
TCSA
tetrachlorosalicylanilide テトラクロロサリチルアニリド
TCT
thrombin clotting time トロンビン凝固時間
thyrocalcitonin チ〔サイ〕ロカルシトニン
tracheal cytotoxin 気管上皮細胞毒素
transcranial brain tomography 経頭蓋脳断層法
Tct.
tinctura〈ラ〉 チンキ《処》
TCUK
tissue culture urokinase 組織培養ウロキナーゼ
TCV
thoracic cage volume 胸郭容量
TCVA
thromboembolic cerebral vascular accident 血栓塞栓性脳血管障害
TD
table of distribution 分布表
tardive dyskinesia 遅発性ジスキネジア，晩期運動障害
T cell dependent T細胞依存の
Terminaldruck〈独〉 終圧
test dose 試験的用量
therapy discontinued 治療中止(された)
thiodrol チオドロール
thoracic duct 胸管
threshold dose 閾値量
threshold of detectability 検出(可能)閾値
threshold of discomfort 不快感閾値
threshold tone decay 一時的閾値変動
thymus dependent (cell) 胸腺依存(細胞)
tic douloureux 三叉〔差〕神経痛
timed disintegration 定時崩壊
tocopherol deficient トコフェロール欠乏の
tolerance dose 耐容量
torsion dystonia 捻転ジストニー
total disability 完全廃疾
total discrimination 完全識別，総合識別
total dose 全量，総投与量
toxic dose 中毒量
tracheal diameter 気管(直)径

transdermal 経皮の
transient depolarization 一過性脱分極
transverse diameter 横径
traveller's diarrhea 旅行者下痢症
tumor dose 腫瘍量
typhoid dysentery チフス様赤痢，腸チフス

Td
doubling time 倍加時間

TD_{50}
median toxic dose 50%毒性量
toxic dose 50 50%中毒量

t.d.
tales doses〈ラ〉=such doses 同量《処》
temporal dextra〈ラ〉 右側頭に

TD, Td
tetanus-diphtheria (toxoid) 破傷風・ジフテリア(トキソイド)

TD, T/D
treatment discontinued 治療中止

TDA
thymus-dependent antigen 胸腺依存抗原
thymus-dependent area 胸腺依存領域
thyroid stimulating hormone displacing activity 甲状腺刺激ホルモン代替活性
thyrotropin displacement activity 甲状腺刺激物質

TDA antigen
thymus-dependent antigen 胸腺依存性抗原

T dap
tetanus-diphtheria-pertussis vaccine 破傷風・ジフテリア・百日咳三種混合ワクチン

TDB
total disability benefit 全障害者医療補助金
Toxicology Data Bank 毒物データバンク(の一種)

TDC
thymic dendritic cell 胸腺樹状細胞
total dietary calories 全食事カロリー

TDD
thoracic duct drainage 胸管ドレナージ
total digitalizing dose 総ジギタリス飽和量

t.d.d.
ter de die〈ラ〉=three times a day 1日3回《処》

TDDA
thoracic duct drainage 胸管ドレナージ

TDE
tetrachlorodiphenylethane テトラクロロジフェニルエタン

total digestible energy　全消化(可能)カロリー

TDF
testis-determining factor　精巣決定因子
thinking disturbance factor　思考障害因子
thoracic duct fistula　胸管瘻
thoracic duct flow　胸管流量
time dose (and) fractionation (factor)　時間線量分割(因子)
tissue-damaging factor　組織障害因子
total dietary fiber　総食物繊維量
tumor degenerating factor　腫瘍変性因子

TDH
thermostable direct hemolysin　耐熱性直接溶血毒
traumatic dislocation of hip　外傷性股関節脱臼

TDI
thought disorder index　思考障害指数
tolerable daily intake　1日耐容摂取量
toluene diisocyanate　トルエンジイソシアネート
tolylene diisocyanate　トリレンジイソシアネート
total-dose infusion　全量注入
total-dose insulin　インスリン総投与量
triacetyldiphenolisatin　トリアセチルジフェノールイサチン

TDL
thoracic duct lymphocytes　胸管リンパ球
thymus-dependent lymphocytes　胸腺依存リンパ球

TDM
therapeutic drug monitoring　薬剤血中濃度モニタリング
trehalose dimycolate　トレハロースジミコレート

TDN
total digestible nutrients　全消化(可能)栄養分

t-DNA
transfer deoxyribonucleic acid　転移デオキシリボ核酸

TDO
thermo-disc-oxygenator　熱交換器内蔵人工肺

TDP
ribothymidine 5′-diphosphate　リボチミジン 5′-二リン酸
thermal death point　熱死点
thiamine diphosphate　チアミン二リン酸
thoracic duct pressure　胸管圧
thymidine diphosphate　チミジン二リン酸

TdP
Tanzen der Patella〈独〉　膝蓋(骨)跳動
torsade de pointes〈仏〉　特有の心電図波形をみる心室性頻拍の特殊型

TDPR
T lymphocyte dependent proliferative response　Tリンパ球依存幼若化反応

TDR
Special Programme for Research and Training in Tropical Diseases　熱帯病研究と訓練特別計画
time dose relationship　時間線量関係
total daily requirement　１日のエネルギー必要量

TdR
thymidine　チミジン

Tdr
thymine deoxyriboside　チミンデオキシリボシド

TDS
temperature, depth, salinity　温度・深さ・塩分
thiamine disulfide　チアミンジスルフィド
total dissolved solid　全溶解固形物

t.d.s.
ter die sumendum〈ラ〉　１日３回服用《処》

TDT
tentative discharge tomorrow　明日仮退院
thermal death time　加熱致死時間
transverse diameter of thorax　胸郭横径
tumor-doubling time　腫瘍２倍時間

TdT
terminal deoxynucleotidyl transferase　終末デオキシリボヌクレオチド転換酵素

TDT, TdT
tone decay test　聴力疲労試験

TDTH
delayed-type hypersensitivity effector T cell　遅延型過敏反応のエフェクターT細胞

TDZ
thymus dependent zone　胸腺依存帯
tinidazole　チニダゾール

T_E
expiratory phase time　呼息総時間

TE
echo time　エコー時間《画診》
expiratory time　換気時間
tennis elbow　テニス肘
test ear　試験耳，検査耳
tetracycline　テトラサイクリン
threshold energy　閾値エネルギー
thromboembolism　血栓塞栓症
thymic epithelium　胸腺上皮
thymus epithelial (cell)　胸腺上皮(細胞)

thyrotoxic exophthalmos	甲状腺中毒性眼球突出症
time estimation	時間推定
tissue equivalent	組織当量
tonic extension	強直性伸展
tonsillectomy	扁桃摘出(術)
tonsils excised	扁桃切除(された)
tooth extracted	抜歯(された)
total estrogen (excretion)	総エストロゲン(排出)
trace element	微量元素
tracheoesophageal	気管食道の
treadmill exercise	トレッドミル運動
triethyleneglycol	トリエチレングリコール
Tuberkulineinheit〈独〉	ツベルクリン単位
tumor echo	腫瘍エコー

T_e

effective half-life	有効半減期

Te

tellurium	テルル〈元素〉
tetanic (contraction)	テタニー性(攣縮)

T & E

testing and evaluation	試験と評価
training and experience	研修と経験

T-e

erythrocyte triiodothyronine	赤血球トリヨードチ〔サイ〕ロニン

TE, Te

tetanus	破傷風

TE, T & E

trial and error	試行錯誤

TEA

tanned erythrocyte aggulutination test	タンニン酸処理赤血球凝集反応
tetraethylammonium	テトラエチルアンモニウム
thermal energy analyzer	熱エネルギー分析器
thromboendarterectomy	血栓内膜摘除術
total exchange albumin	総交替アルブミン
tracheal-esophageal airway	気管・食道エアウェイ
triethanolamine	トリエタノールアミン

TEAB

tetraethylammonium bromide	臭化テトラエチルアンモニウム

TEAC

tetraethyl ammonium chloride	塩化テトラエチルアンモニウム

TEAE

triethylaminoethyl	トリエチルアミノエチル

TEAS
transcutaneous electric(al) acupoint stimulation　経皮的ツボ電気刺激療法，経皮通電経穴刺激法
teasp
teaspoonful　茶さじ1杯の《処》
TeBG
testosterone binding globulin　テストステロン結合グロブリン
TEBG, TeBG
testosterone-estradiol-binding globulin　テストステロン・エストラジオール結合グロブリン
TEC
thymic epithelial cell(s)　胸腺上皮細胞
thyroid epithelial cell(s)　甲状腺濾胞上皮細胞
total electron count　総電子数
total (blood) eosinophil count　総(血中)好酸球数
total exchange capacity　総交換能力
tec
technic　技術
technical　技術的
technician　技術者
technological　技術の
technology　技術
T & EC
Trauma and Emergency Center　外傷救急センター
tech
technical　技術の
technician　技師
technique　技術
techn
technician　技師
TECV
traumatic epiphyseal coxa vara　外傷性骨端性内反股
TED
threshold erythema dose　閾値紅斑量
thromboembolic disease　血栓塞栓(性)疾患
thyroid eye disease　甲状腺性眼病
tracheoesophageal dysraphism　気管食道癒合不全
TEE
thermic effect of exercise　運動の熱効果
trans-esophageal echocardiography　経食道的心臓超音波検査，経食道心エコー(検査)法《画診》
tyrosine ethyl ester　チロシンエチルエステル
TEEP
tetraethylpyrophosphate　テトラエチルピロリン酸

TEER
transepithelial electrical resistance　細胞膜抵抗
TEF
tracheoesophageal fistula　気管食道瘻
Teff
time of effective half-life　有効半減期
teflon
tetrafluoro-ethylene　テトラフルオロエチレン
TEG
thromboelastogram　トロンボエラストグラム
thromboelastograph　トロンボエラストグラフ
thromboelastography　トロンボエラストグラフィ
TEIC
teicoplanin　テイコプラニン
TEL
tetraethyl lead　テトラエチル鉛
TELE, Tele, tele
telemetry　テレメトリ，遠隔測定(法)
tele ci
telecurietherapy　遠隔照射療法
tele Co
telecobalt therapy　コバルト遠隔照射療法
TEM
transanal endoscopic microsurgery　経肛門内視鏡下顕微手術
transmission electron microscope　透過(型)電(子)顕(微鏡)
transmission electron microscopy　透過(型)電(子)顕(微鏡)法
triethanolamine　トリエタノールアミン
triethylenemelamine　トリエチレンメラミン
temp
temporal　側頭の
temporary　一過性の，一時的な
Temp, temp, temp.
temperature　温度，体温
temp dext.
tempori dextro〈ラ〉　右側頭へ
TEMPO
tetramethylpiperidine-*N*-oxide　テトラメチルピペリジン-*N*-オキシド
tempry
temporary　一時的な，一過性の
TEN
total excretory nitrogen　総排泄窒素
toxic epidermal necrolysis　中毒性表皮融解症
toxic epidermolytic necrolysis　中毒性表皮融解壊死型薬疹
ten
tense　緊張した

tension 緊張，張力，圧

tend

tender 圧痛のある

tenderness 圧痛

tendon 腱

tenot

tenotomy 切腱術

TENS

transcutaneous electrical (nerve) stimulation 経皮的電気(神経)刺激

tens

tension 緊張，張力，圧

tent

tentative 暫定的な

tent-diag

tentative diagnosis 暫定的診断

TEOAE

transiently evoked otoacoustic emission 瞬間的誘発耳音響放射

TEP

expiratory pause time 呼気休止時間

tetraethylpyrophosphate テトラエチルピロリン酸

totally extraperitoneal herniorrhaphy 腹腔鏡下ヘルニア修復術のうち腹膜外到達法

TEPA

tespamin テスパミン

triethylenephosphoramide トリエチレンホスホラミド

TEPP

tetraethylpyrophosphate テトラエチルピロリン酸

TER

thymal epithelial reticulocyte 胸腺上皮性細網細胞

ter

tertiary 第三の

ter.

tere〈ラ〉 研和せよ《処》

term

terminal 終末の，末端の，電極の

ter.sim.

tere simu〈ラ〉 ともに研和せよ《処》

tert

tertiary 第三の

TES

N-tris(hydroxymethyl)methyl-2-aminoethanesulfonic acid *N*-トリス(ヒドロキシメチル)メチル-2-アミノエタンスルホン酸

time controlled explosion system	放出開始時間制御型経口投与システム
time to end-systole	収縮末期までの時間
transcutaneous electrical stimulation	経皮的電気刺激
treatment of emergent symptom	緊急症状処置

TESE

testicular sperm extraction	精巣内精子回収

TESPA

triethylenethiophosphoramide	トリエチレン・チオホスホラミド

TEST

tubal embryo stage transfer	卵管胎芽期移植

TET

teacher of electrotherapy	電気療法師
tetanus toxin	破傷風毒素
total ejection time	総駆出時間
total exchangeable thyroxin(e)	総交換可能チ〔サイ〕ロキシン
treadmill exercise test	トレッドミル運動試験
tubal embryo transfer	卵管胎芽移植

Tet

tetralogy of Fallot	ファロー四徴(症)

Tet, tet

tetanus	破傷風

TETA

triethylenetetramine	トリエチレンテトラミン
triethylenetetramine dihydrochloride	二塩酸トリエチレンテトラミン

TETD

tetraethylthiuram disulfide	二硫化テトラエチルジザルフィド

tetra

tetraplegia	四肢麻痺

tetrac

tetraiodothyroacetic acid	テトラヨウ素サイロ酢酸

tet.tox.

tetanus toxoid	破傷風トキソイド

TEV

talipes equinovarus	内反足

TEWL

transepidermal water loss	経表皮水分喪失

TF

tactile fremitus	触覚振盪音
temperature factor	温度因子
tetralogy of Fallot	ファロー四徴(症)
thymidine factor	チミジン因子
thymus factor	胸腺因子

tissue factor 組織因子
tonic flexor 強直性屈筋
total flow 全流量
transcription factor 転写因子
transfer factor 転移因子，伝達因子
transfer function 伝達関数
tube feeding 経管栄養
tube feeding via a nasoduodenal tube 非経口的栄養補給
tuberculin filtrate ツベルクリン濾液

T/F
Fallot tetrad ファロー四徴(症)
Fallot tetralogy ファロー四徴(症)
true or false 正または誤《医教》

TF, Tf
transferrin トランスフェリン

TF, t.f.
tuning fork 音叉

TFA
topical fluoride application 局所フッ化物塗布
total fatty acids 総脂肪酸
trifluoroacetic acid トリフルオロ酢酸

TFC
triangular fibrocartilage 三角線維軟骨

TFD
target-to-film distance 目標とフィルム間の距離

TFE
tetrafluoroethylene テトラフルオロエチレン
trifluoroethanol トリフルオロエタノール

Tf-Fe
transferrin-bound ferritin トランスフェリン結合フェリチン

TFLX
tosufloxacin トスフロキサシン

TFM, Tfm
testicular feminization (syndrome) 睾丸性〔精巣性〕女性化(症候群)

TFN
total fecal nitrogen 総便中窒素
transferrin トランスフェリン

TFNH
transient familial neonatal hyperbilirubinemia 一過性家族性新生児高ビリルビン血症

TFP
treponemal false-positive トレポネーマ偽陽性
tubular fluid divided by plasma concentration 血漿濃度により分離される尿細管液

TFPI
tissue factor pathway inhibitor　凝固組織因子発現阻害因子
TFPZ
trifluoperazine　トリフルオペラジン
TFR
total fertility rate　総特殊出生率
transferrin receptor　トランスフェリン受容体
TFS
testicular feminization syndrome　睾丸性女性化症候群，精巣性女性化症候群
thyroid function studies　甲状腺機能検査
TFT
tetracycline fluorescence test　テトラサイクリン螢光試験
thrombus formation time　血栓形成時間
thymol flocculation test　チモール綿状反応
thyroid function test　甲状腺機能検査
trifluorothymidine　トリフルオロチミジン
TFX
thymic factor X　胸腺因子X
TG
tendon graft　腱移植(片)
testosterone glucuronide　テストステロングルクロニド
tetraglycine　テトラグリシン
thermogravimetry　熱重量測定
thioglycollate　チオグリコール酸
thioguanine　チオグアニン
tomography　断層撮影法
toxic goiter　中毒性甲状腺腫
treated group　治療群
triacylglycerol　トリアシルグリセロール
trigeminal (neuralgia)　三叉〔差〕(神経痛)
triglyceride　トリグリセリド
tumor growth　腫瘍成長
tympanogram　チンパノグラム
6-TG
6-thioguanine　6-チオグアニン
T & G
tongue and groove　舌と歯溝
TG, Tg
thyroglobulin　チ〔サイ〕ログロブリン
TGA
thermogravimetric analysis　温度比重測定解析
thyroglobulin antibody　チ〔サイ〕ログロブリン抗体
total gonadotropin activity　総ゴナドトロピン活性
transient global amnesia　一過性全健忘(症)
transposition of great arteries　大血管転位症

tumor glycoprotein assay 腫瘍糖蛋白定量(症)

TgAb
(anti-)thyroglobulin antibody (抗)チ〔サイ〕ログロブリン抗体

TGB
thyroid-binding globulin 甲状腺結合グロブリン
tongued, grooved and beaded 舌の・歯溝の・数珠状の

TGC
thioglycollate チオグリコール酸
time gain compensation 時間利得補償回路
truncus gastrocolica〈ラ〉 胃腸幹

TGC medium
thioglycollate medium チオグリコール酸塩培地

TGE
theoretical growth evaluation 理論的成長評価
transmissible gastroenteritis 伝染性胃腸炎

TGE-AGAR
tryptone glucose extract milk agar トリプトングルコースエキスミルク寒天

TGF
therapeutic gain factor (照射)治療可能比
transforming growth factor トランスフォーミング増殖因子
tubuloglomerular feedback 尿細管糸球体フィードバック
tumor growth factor 腫瘍成長因子

TGFA
triglyceride fatty acid トリグリセリド脂肪酸

TGF-β
transforming growth factor-beta β型トランスフォーミング増殖因子

TGG
turkey gamma globulin 七面鳥γグロブリン

TGGE
temperature gradient gel electrophoresis 温度勾配ゲル電気泳動

TGHA
thyroglobulin hemagglutination チ〔サイ〕ログロブリン血液凝集反応

TGL
triglyceride lipase トリグリセリドリパーゼ
triglycerides トリグリセリド
tuberculin, globulinous 結核菌10%食塩浮遊液中の含有グロブリン量

tgl
täglich〈独〉 1日に，毎日《処》

T

TGP
tabacco glycoprotein タバコ糖蛋白
TGR
thioguanosine チオグアノシン
TGT
thromboplastin generation test トロンボプラスチン生成試験
tolbutamide-glucagon test トルブタミド・グルカゴン試験

tgt
target 標的
TGV
thoracic gas volume 胸腔内ガス容量
transposition of the great vessels 大血管転位症
TGY
trypsine, glucose, yeast (agar) トリプトン・ブドウ糖・酵母(寒天培地)

TH
ethionamide エチオナミド
tetrahydrocortisol テトラヒドロコルチゾール
thalamic hemorrhage 視床出血
theophylline テオフィリン
thrill 振戦
thyroid hormone 甲状腺ホルモン
thyrosine hydroxylase チ〔サイ〕ロシン水酸化酵素
thyrotropic hormone 甲状腺刺激ホルモン
total hysterectomy 子宮全摘出(術)
triple-helical region 三重らせん構造部
tyrosine hydroxylase チ〔サイ〕ロシン水酸化酵素
Th
thalamus 視床
thenar 母指球の
therapy 療法，治療
thigh 大腿
thoracic 胸椎の
thorium トリウム〈元素〉
throat 喉頭，喉
thrombin トロンビン
thyroid 甲状(腺)の
TH_4
tetrahydrofolate テトラヒドロ葉酸
TH，Th
helper T cell ヘルパーT細胞
TH，Th，th
thoracic 胸郭の，胸部の
thorax 胸郭

T

THA
terminal hepatic artery — 固有肝動脈
total hip arthroplasty — (人工)股関節全置換術
total hydroxyapatite — 総ヒドロキシアパタイト

ThA
thoracic aorta — 胸部大動脈

THA, T.H.A.
1,2,3,4-tetrahydro-5-aminoacridine — 1,2,3,4-テトラヒドロ-5-アミノアクリジン

thal, Thal
thalassemia — サラセミア，地中海性貧血

THAM
trihydroxymethyl-aminomethane — トリヒドロキシメチルアミノメタン
tromethamine — トロメタミン

THAN
transient hyperammonemia of newborn — 新生児一過性高アンモニア血症

thanat
thanatology — 死学

THARIES
total hip articular replacement by internal eccential shells — 股関節表面全置換術

THb
tidal hemoglobin — 循環ヘモグロビン量
total hemoglobin — 総ヘモグロビン量

THBF
total hepatic blood flow — 総肝血流量

Thbs
thrombospondin-1 — トロンボスポンジン 1

THC
δ-9-tetrahydrocannabinol — δ-9-テトラヒドロ〔四水酸化〕カンナビノール
tetrahydrocortisol — テトラヒドロコルチゾール
tetrahydrocortisone — テトラヒドロコルチゾン
thiocarbanidin — チオカルバニジン
thrombin hirudin complex — トロンビンヒルジン複合体
transhepatic cholangiogram — 経肝胆管造影図
transhepatic cholangiography — 経肝胆管造影法
transplantable hepatocellular carcinoma — 移植可能肝細胞癌

Thc
helper T cell — ヘルパーT細胞

THD
total harmonic distortion — 全高調波ひずみ(率)
transverse heart diameter — 心横径

T

Thd
ribothymidine リボチミジン
THDOC
tetrahydrodeoxycorticosterone テトラヒドロデオキシコルチコステロン
THE
tetrahydrocortisone テトラヒドロコルチゾン
tropical hypereosinophilia 熱帯性好酸球増加症
theor
theoretical 理論の，理論的な
ther
therapeutic 治療の
thermometer 体温計，温度計
THER, ther
therapy 療法，治療
THERAP
therapeutic 治療の
ther.ex
therapeutic exercise 治療的運動
therm
thermal 熱の
th.ex
therapeutic exercise 治療的運動
THF
tetrahydrocortisol テトラヒドロコルチゾール
tetrahydrofluorenone テトラヒドロフルオレノン
tetrahydrofolic (acid) テトラヒドロ葉酸
tetrahydrofuran テトラヒドロフラン
thymic humoral factor 胸腺体液性因子
ThF
helper T cell factor ヘルパーT細胞因子
THFA
tetrahydrofolic acid テトラヒドロ葉酸
tetrahydrofurfuryl alcohol テトラヒドロフルフリルアルコール
Thg
thyroglobulin チ〔サイ〕ログロブリン
THGL
thyroglobulin チ〔サイ〕ログロブリン
THH
telangiectasia hereditaria haemorrhagica 出血性遺伝性毛細血管拡張症
THI
temperature humidity index 温・湿指数
trihydroxy-indole トリヒドロキシインドール

THI, Thi
thiamin チアミン
Thio
thiosulfate チオ硫酸塩
Thio-TEPA, thio-TEPA, Thiotepa, thiotepa
thiotriethylene phosphoramide チオトリエチレンホスホルアミド
THL
true histiocytic lymphoma 真性細網肉腫
THM
trihalomethane トリハロメタン
THO
ribosylthymin リボシルチミン
tyrosine hydroxylase チロシン水酸化酵素
THOMIS
Total Hospital Operating and Medical Information System 総合病院運営と医学情報システム
Thor
thoracic surgery 胸部外科
Thor, thor.
thoracic 胸郭の
thorax 胸郭
THP
Tamm-Horsfall protein タム・ホースフォルムコ蛋白(質), 糖蛋白
tetrahydropapaveroline テトラヒドロパパベロリン
tissue hydrostatic pressure 組織静水圧
Total Health Promotion Plan 総合健康推進計画
total hydroxyproline 総ヒドロキシプロリン
trihexyphenidyl トリヘキシフェニジル
THP-ADM
tetrahydropyranyl adriamycin テトラヒドロピラニルアドリアマイシン
THPP
2,4,6-trihydroxypropiophenone 2,4,6-トリヒドロキシプロピオフェノン
THPP, ThPP
thiamine pyrophosphate チアミンピロリン酸
THQ
tetrahydroxy-quinone テトラヒドロキシキノン
THR
target heart rate 目標心拍数
total heart replacement 人工心臓全置換術
total hip joint replacement 人工股関節全置換術
transhepatic resistance 経肝抵抗

T

Thr
threonine トレオニン
thr
thrill 振戦
thyroid 甲状腺の
thyroidectomy 甲状腺摘出〔切除〕(術)
THRF
thyrotrop(h)ic hormone-releasing factor 甲状腺刺激ホルモン放出因子
throm
thrombosis 血栓症
thrombus 血栓
Thromb, thromb
thrombosis 血栓症
thrombus 血栓
thrombo
thrombosis 血栓症
THS
tetrahydrodeoxycortisol テトラヒドロデオキシコルチゾール
tetrahydro-11-desoxycortisol テトラヒドロ-11-デスオキシコルチゾル
tetrahydrosteroid テトラヒドロステロイド
Tolosa-Hunt syndrome トロサ・ハント症候群
Th.Surg.
thoracic surgery 胸部外科
THT
teacher of hydrotherapy 水治療指導員
THTH
thyrotrop(h)ic hormone 甲状腺刺激ホルモン
TH/TS
heper T cell/suppressor T cell ヘルパーT細胞/サプレッサーT細胞比
THU
tetrahydrouridine テトラヒドロウリジン
THUG
thyroid uptake gradient 甲状腺摂取勾配
THVO
terminal hepatic vein obliteration 終末肝静脈閉塞
Thx
thomboxane トロンボキサン
Thy
thymine チミン
thymocyte 胸腺細胞
thy
thymectomy 胸腺摘出〔切除〕(術)

thymus 胸腺

Thy-1
a kind of T cell antigen T細胞抗原の一種

thym.turb.
thymol turbidity チモール混濁

THYSA
thymus specific antigen 胸腺T細胞特異抗原

THZ
thiazolidomycin チアゾリドマイシン

THz
terahertz テラヘルツ

TI
inspiratory time 吸気時間
inversion time 反転時間
therapeutic index 治療指数
thoracic index 胸郭指数
thymus independent 胸腺非依存性
time interval 時間間隔
tissue invasiveness 組織浸潤性
transverse diameter between ischia 坐骨横径
tricuspid incompetence 三尖弁機能不全
tricuspid insufficiency 三尖弁閉鎖不全症

Ti
titanium チタン〈元素〉

TI, Ti
tumor-inducing (plasmid) 腫瘍誘発プラスミド

TIA
thymus-independent area 胸腺非依存(領)域
transient (cerebral) ischemic attack 一過性(脳)虚血(性)発作
turbidimetric immunoassay 免疫比濁法

TIAFT
The International Association of Forensic Toxicologist 国際法中毒学協会

TIAg
thymus-independent antigen 胸腺非依存性抗原

TIAH
total implantation of artificial heart 人工心臓完全移植
totally implanted artificial heart 全埋没人工心臓

TIA-IR
transent ischemic attack-incomplete recovery 一過性虚血発作・不完全回復

Ti antigen
thymus-independent antigen 胸腺非依存性抗原

tib
tibia 脛骨
tibial 脛骨の

TIBC
total iron binding capacity　総鉄結合能

tib.-fib.
tibia-fibula　脛骨・腓骨

TIC
ticarcillin　チカルシリン
trypsin inhibitory capability (assay)　トリプシン抑制能(検定法)

TICAD
Tokyo International Conference on African Development　アフリカ開発会議

TICU
trauma intensive care unit　外傷集中治療室

TID
thermionic ionization detector　熱イオン化検出器
tubulo-interstitial disease　尿細管・間質性疾患

tid, t.i.d.
ter in die〈ラ〉　1日3回《処》

t.i.d.s.
ter in die sumenda〈ラ〉　1日3回服用《処》

TIE
transient ischemic episode　一過性虚血発作

TIF
tumor-inducing factor　腫瘍誘発因子
tumor-inhibiting factor　腫瘍抑制因子

TIFA
Todd insecticidal generator　トッド殺虫ガス発生器

TIFPB
thrombin increasing fibrinopeptide B　トロンビン増加性フィブリノペプチドB

TIG, TIg
tetanus immune globulin　破傷風免疫グロブリン

TIL
tumor infiltrating lymphocytes　腫瘍集合リンパ球

TIM
triosephosphate isomerase　三炭糖リン酸イソメラーゼ

TIMI
thrombolysis in myocardial infarction　心筋梗塞の血栓溶解

TIMP
tissue inhibitor of metalloproteinases　メタロプロテナーゼインヒビター

TIN
tubulo-interstitial nephritis　尿細管間質性腎炎
tubulointerstitial nephropathy　尿細管間質性腎障害

t.i.n.
ter in nocte〈ラ〉　夜間3回《処》

tinc
tincture チンキ(剤)《処》
tinct.
tinctura〈ラ〉=tincture チンキ(剤)《処》
T_3 Index
triiodothyronine index トリヨードチ〔サイ〕ロニン指数
ting
tingling 刺痛
TINU
tubulointerstitial nephritis uveitis syndrome 間質性腎炎・ブドウ膜炎症候群
TIO
trans-ileocolic obliteration of gastroesophageal varices 経回腸静脈的食道胃静脈瘤塞栓術
TIP
inspiratory pause time 吸気休止時間
TIP
terminal interface processor 端末中間処理
thermal inactivation point 熱不活性化点
translation inhibitory protein 翻訳阻止蛋白
tumor inducing principle 腫瘍誘発物質
TIPBn
transurethral incision of prostate and bladder neck 経尿道的前立腺・膀胱頸部切開術
TIPC
ticarcillin チカルシリン
Ti plasmid
tumor-inducing plasmid 腫瘍誘発性プラスミド
TIPP
the injury prevention program 事故防止プログラム
TIPPS
tetraiodophenolphthalein sodium テトラヨードフェノールフタレインナトリウム
TIPS
transjugular intrahepatic portosystemic shunt 経皮的肝内門脈シャント術
TIR
terminal innervation ratio 終末神経支配比
Toll-interleukin-1 receptor Toll/インターロイキン1受容体
total immunoreactive (insulin) 総免疫反応性(インスリン)
TIS
transdermal infusion system 経皮注入システム
trypsin insoluble segment トリプシン不溶セグメント
tumor *in situ* 上皮内腫瘍

T

TISP
total immunoreactive serum pepsinogen 全免疫反応性血清ペプシノゲン

TISS
therapeutic intervention scoring system 医療処置点数制

TIT
Treponema (*pallidum*) immobilization test 梅毒トレポネーマ不動化試験
triiodothyronine トリヨードチ〔サイ〕ロニン

TI/TE
inspiratory-expiratory phase time ratio 吸気相・呼気相時間比

TITH, TITh
triiodothyronine トリヨードチ〔サイ〕ロニン

titr
titrate 滴定する

TIU
thyroid iodine uptake 甲状腺ヨウ素摂取率

TIUV
total intrauterine volume 総子宮内容積

TIVA
total intravenous anesthesia 完全静脈麻酔

TIVC
thoracic inferior vena cava 胸部下大静脈

TJ
terajoule テラジュール
triceps jerk 三頭筋反射
Troell-Junet (syndrome) トロエル・ジェネー(症候群)

Tj
tight junction 密着帯，閉鎖帯

TJO
transjugular retrograde obliteration for gastric varices 経頸静脈的逆行性胃静脈瘤塞栓術

TJR
total joint replacement 全関節置換術

TK
killer T cell キラーT細胞，細胞傷害性T細胞
tachykinin タキキニン
thymidine kinase チミジンキナーゼ
transketolase トランスケトラーゼ

TK1
soluble thymidine kinase 可溶性チミジンキナーゼ

TK2
mitochondrial thymidine kinase　ミトコンドリア性チミジンキナーゼ

TKA
total knee arthroplasty　全膝関節置換術
transketolase activity　トランスケトラーゼ活性

TKD
thymidine kinase deficient　チミジンキナーゼ欠乏の
tokodynamometer　子宮娩出力測定器

TKG
tokodynamograph　子宮娩出力記録表
tokodynamography　子宮娩出力測定法

TKm, TKM
thymidine kinase, mitochondrial　ミトコンドリア性チミジンキナーゼ

TKO
to keep open　開けたまま(にすること)

TKP
total knee prosthesis　全人工膝関節

TKR
total knee (joint) replacement　人工膝関節全置換術

TKS
thymidine kinase, soluble　可溶性チミジンキナーゼ

TL
team leader　チームリーダー
temporal lobe　側頭葉
thermal lens spectroscopy　熱レンズ分光法
thermolabile　熱不安定の
thermoluminescence　熱ルミネッセンス
threat to life　生命を脅かす
thrombolysis　血栓溶解
thymic(-derived) lymphocyte　胸腺(由来)リンパ球
thymic lymphoma　胸腺リンパ腫
thymus leukemia　胸腺白血病
time lapse　時間の経過
time limited　時間制限のある
tolerance level　許容レベル
total lipids　全脂質
total lung (capacity)　全肺(活量)
transmission loss　透過損失

Tl
thallium　タリウム〈元素〉

^{201}Tl
thallium-201　タリウム201〈元素〉

T-L
thymus(-dependent) lymphocyte　胸腺(依存)リンパ球

TL, T.L.
tubal ligation 卵管結紮
TLA
tissue lactase activity 組織ラクターゼ活性
translaryngeal aspiration 経喉頭吸引
translumbar aortography 経腰的大動脈造影撮影法
TLAA
T lymphocyte-associated antigen Tリンパ球関連抗原
T lam
thoracic laminectomy 胸椎椎弓切除
TL antigen
thymus leukemia antigen 胸腺白血病抗原
TLC
tender loving care 優しく親切な看護
thin-layer chromatography 薄層クロマトグラフィ
tibial collateral ligament 内側側副靱帯
T lymphocyte clone Tリンパ球クローン
total L-chain concentration 総L鎖濃度
total lung capacity 全肺気量
total lung compliance 総肺コンプライアンス
total lymphocyte count 総リンパ球数
triple lumen catheter 三孔式カテーテル
TLCA
taurolithocholic acid タウロリトコール酸
TL-CFC
T lymphocyte colony-forming cell Tリンパ球コロニー形成細胞
TLCK
Nα-tosyl-L-lysyl chloromethyl ketone *Nα*-トシル-L-リジルクロロメチルケトン
TLD
thermoluminescence dosimeter 熱螢光線量計
thermoluminescent dosimetry 温度発光線量計
thoracic lymph duct 胸管
threshold load of dyspnea 呼吸困難の自覚閾値
tumor lethal dose 腫瘍致死量
TLD_{95}
tumor lethal dose ninety-five 95%腫瘍致死線量
TLE
temporal lobe epilepsy 側頭葉てんかん
thin-layer electrophoresis 薄層電気泳動
total lipid extract 全脂質抽出物
TLG
thyroid lymphography 甲状腺リンパ造影
TLI
total lymph-node irradiation 全身リンパ節放射線照射
trypsin-like immunoactivity トリプシン様免疫活性

TLK
thermal laser keratoplasty　熱レーザー角膜形成
TLN
transperitoneal haparoscopic nephrectomy　経腹膜腹腔鏡下腎摘出
TLP
total larngopharyngectomy　咽頭喉頭部全摘出
TLR
tonic labyrinthine reflex　緊張性迷路反射
Toll-like receptor　Toll様受容体
TLS
tight lens syndrome　タイトレンズ症候群
tumor lysis syndrome　腫瘍溶解症候群
TLSO
thoraco-lumbo-sacral orthosis　胸腰仙骨部専用コルセット
TLT
tryptophan load test　トリプトファン負荷試験
TLV
total lung volume　全肺容積
TLVSW
total left ventricular stroke work　全左(心)室拍出仕事量
TM
standard mean temperature　標準平均温度
tarsometatarsal (joint)　足根中足骨の
tarsometatarsal (joint)　足根中足関節
temperature by mouth　口腔温
temperature meter　温度計
temporalis muscle　側頭筋
temporal mandibular　側頭下顎骨の
temporal muscle　側頭筋
temporomandibular　顎の，側頭下顎骨の
teres major (muscle)　大円(筋)
terramycin　テラマイシン
thrombomodulin　トロンボモジュリン
time-motion (technique)　時間・運動(手技)
tobramycin　トブラマイシン
total mastectomy　全乳房切断術
trademark　商標，トレードマーク
transcendental meditation technique　瞑想方法
transmediastinal　経縦隔の
transmembrane　細胞膜貫通
transport mechanism　輸送機序
tropical medicine　熱帯医学
tropomyosin　トロポミオシン
tubular myelin　管状ミエリン
tumor　腫瘍

tympanic membrane 鼓膜

Tm
maximum tubular clearance 最大尿細管クリアランス
maximum tubular glucose (reabsorptive capacity) 尿細管ブドウ糖(再吸収能)最大量
melting temperature (生体高分子の)融解温度
memory T cell 記憶T細胞
muscle temperature 筋肉温度
thulium ツリウム〈元素〉
tubular excretory mass 尿細管最大排泄量
tubular transport maximum 尿細管最大輸送量

t.m.
total massa〈ラ〉 全量《処》

T & M
time and material 時間と材料
type and crossmatch 血液型と交叉〔差〕試験

TM, Tm
maximal tubular excretory capacity 最大尿細管排泄能

TMA
tetramethylammonium テトラメチルアンモニウム
thrombotic microangiopathy 血栓性微小血管障害
thyroid microsomal antibody 甲状腺ミクロソーム抗体
trimethoxyamphetamine トリメトキシアンフェタミン
trimethoxyphenyl-aminopropane トリメトキシフェニルアミノプロパン
trimethylamine トリメチルアミン
trimethyl-aminooxide トリメチルアミノオキシド
trimethyl arsenate トリメチルヒ素化合物

TMAb
thyroid microsomal antibody 甲状腺ミクロソーム抗体

TMAI
tetramethylammonium iodide ヨウ化テトラメチルアンモニウム

T-max, T_{max}
maximum daily temperature 日内最高体温
time of maximum concentration 最高濃度時間
time to the peak concentration 最高血中濃度到達時間

T

TMB
tetramethylbenzidine テトラメチルベンジジン

TMB-4
trimedoxime トリメドキシム

TMBA
trimethylbenzanthracene トリメチルベンズアントラセン

TMC
tonsillar mononuclear cells 扁桃単核細胞

tracheal mucous clearance 気管粘液クリアランス

TMCA
trimethylcolchicinic acid トリメチルコルヒチン酸

TMCD
tetramethyl-cyclobutanediol テトラメチルシクロブタンジオール

TMD
trochanter malleolar distance 下肢長

TmD
diodrast tubular excretory mass ダイオドラスト尿細管排泄最大量

TME
teacher of medical electricity 医学電気学指導員
total metabolizable energy 総代謝可能エネルギー
transmissible mink encephalopathy 伝達可能ミンク脳症

TMF
thymocyte mitogenic factor 胸腺細胞有糸分裂因子

TmG
transport maximum glucose ブドウ糖最大移送値

Tm_G, TmG, Tmg
maximum tubular glucose (reabsorptive capacity) 尿細管ブドウ糖(再吸収能)最大量

TMI
transmural myocardial infarction 壁内心筋梗塞

TMIF
tumor-cell migratory inhibition factor 腫瘍細胞遊走抑制因子

TMJ
temporomandibular joint 顎関節

TMJ-PDS
temporomandibular joint-pain dysfunction syndrome 顎関節疼痛性機能不全症候群

TMJS
temporomandibular joint syndrome 顎関節症候群

TM jt.
temporomandibular joint 顎関節

TML
terminal motor latency 終末運動潜時
tetramethyl lead テトラメチル鉛

T-ML
T cell malignant lymphoma T細胞悪性リンパ腫

TM line
tuberculum maxillare line 上顎結節線

TMMG
teacher of massage and medical gymnastics マッサージと医学体操の指導員

TMNG
toxic multinodular goiter | 中毒性多結節性甲状腺腫

TMO
trimethadione | トリメタジオン

T-MOP
6-thioguanine, methotrexate, vincristine (=Oncovin), prednisone | 6-チオグアニン，メトトレキサート，ビンクリスチン(=オンコビン)，プレドニゾン

TMP
ribothymidine5′-phosphate | リボチミジン5′リン酸
thiamine monophosphate | チアミン一リン酸
thymidine monophosphate | チミジン一リン酸
transmembrane potential | 膜内外電位差
transmembrane (hydrostatic) pressure | 膜内外静水圧(差)
trimethaphan | トリメタファン
trimethoprim | トリメトプリム
trimethyl-phosphate | トリメチルリン酸
4,5′,8-trimethylpsoralen | 4,5′,8-トリメチルプソラレン

TmPAH
tubular excretory mass of PAH (=para-aminohippurate) | 尿細管パラアミノ馬尿酸塩再吸収極量

TMPD
tetramethyl-*p*-phenylenediamine | テトラメチル-*p*-フェニレンジアミン

TMPP
trithioparamethoxyphenylpropene | トリチオパラメトキシフェニルプロペン

TMP-SMX
trimethoprim-sulfamethoxazole | トリメトプリム・サルファメトキサゾール

TMR
tissue-maximum dose ratio | 組織最大線量比
topical magnetic resonance | 局所磁気共鳴
transmyocardiac revascularization | 心筋内血管新生術
transmyocardial revascularization laser | レーザー心臓血管新生術

TMRITC
tetramethylrhodamine isothiocyanate | テトラメチルロダミンイソチオシアネート

TMS
tetramethylsilane | テトラメチルシラン
thallium myocardial scintigraphy | タリウム心筋シンチグラフィ
transcranial magnetic stimulation | 経頭蓋脳磁気刺激
trimethylsilyl | トリメチルシリル(基)

TMST
treadmill stress test　トレッドミルストレス試験
TMT
mamillothalamic tract　乳頭体視床路
tarsometatarsal (joint)　足根中足(関節)
treadmill test　トレッドミル試験
tympanic membrane thermometer　鼓膜体温計
Tmt, tmt.
treatment　治療
TMTC
too many to count　多すぎて数えきれない
TMTD
tetramethyl-thiuram disulfide　二硫化テトラメチルチウラム
TM test
treadmill test　トレッドミル試験
TmTs
trans-mucosal therapeutic system　経粘膜治療システム
TMU
tetramethylurea　四メチル尿素，テトラメチルウレア
TMV
tobacco mosaic virus　タバコモザイクウイルス
tracheal mucous velocity　気管粘液速度
TMZ
transformation zone　化成帯，転換帯
TN
talonavicular　距舟状骨の
team nursing　チーム看護の
temperature normal　体温正常
tenascin　テネイシン
total nitrogen　総窒素
trigeminal neuralgia　三叉〔差〕神経痛
trigeminal nucleus　三叉〔差〕神経核
trochlear nucleus　滑車神経核
Tn
thoron　トロン
transposon　トランスポゾン
T_4N
normal serum thyroxin(e)　正常血清チ〔サイ〕ロキシン
T/N
tar and nicotine　タールとニコチン
TN, Tn
normal intraocular tension　正常眼圧
TNBS
trinitrobenzenesulfonic acid　トリニトロベンゼンスルホン酸

T

TNC
thymic nurse cell 胸腺栄養細胞
too numerous to count 多すぎて数えきれない
troponin C トロポニンC

TNCB
2,4,6-trinitrol-1-chlorobenzene トリニトロール塩化ベンゼン

TND
term normal delivery 満期正常分娩

TNDM
transient neonatal diabetes mellitus 一過性新生児糖尿病

TNF
tumor necrosis factor 腫瘍壊死因子

TNFR
tumor necrosis factor receptor TNF受容体

TNF-sR1
TNF soluble receptor 1 可溶性TNF受容体

TNG
tongue 舌
toxic nodular goiter 中毒性結節性甲状腺腫
trinitroglycerol トリニトログリセロール

Tng
tonography トノグラフィ
training 研修

TNH
transient neonatal hyperammonemia 一過性新生児高アンモニア血症

TNI
total nodal irradiation 全リンパ節照射
troponin I トロポニンI

TNM
tetranitromethane テトラニトロメタン
tumor nodes metastasis (classification) 腫瘍リンパ節転移(分類)

TNMR
tritium nuclear magnetic resonance トリチウム核磁気共鳴

tNMU
tonic neuromuscular unit 持続性神経筋単位

TNP
trinitrophenyl トリニトロフェニル基

TNPG
trinitrophloroglucinol トリニトロフロログルシノール

TNR
tonic neck reflex 緊張性頸反射

TNS
2-*p*-toluidinylnaphthalene-6-sulfonic acid　2-*p*-トルイジニルナフタレン-6-スルホン酸
transcutaneous nerve stimulation　経皮的神経刺激
transcutaneous neural stimulation　経皮的神経刺激
Tullie-Niebörg syndrome　タリー・ニーベルク症候群
tumor necrosis serum　腫瘍壊死血清

tns
tension　緊張，張力，圧

tnsn
tension　緊張，張力，圧

TNSV
tobacco necrosis satellite virus　タバコ壊死サテライトウイルス

TNT
tetranitroblue tetrazolium　テトラニトロブルーテトラゾリウム
2,4,6-trinitrotoluene　2,4,6-トリニトロトルエン
trinnitrotoluene　トリニトロトルエン
troponin T　トロポニンT

TNTC, t.n.t.c.
too numerous to count　多すぎて数えきれない

TNV
tabacco necrosis virus　タバコ壊死ウイルス

TNZ
thermoneutral zone　温熱中間帯

TO
oral temperature　口腔体温
target organ　標的器官
temperature, oral　口腔温
thromboangiitis obliterans　閉塞性血栓血管炎
thrown out　抜け出された
tinctura opii〈ラ〉　アヘンチンキ《処》
total obstruction　完全閉塞
total oestrogens　総発情ホルモン
tubo-ovarian　卵管卵巣の

TO_2
oxygen transport rate　酸素輸送率

t.o.
turn over　裏をみよ

TO, T.O., T/O, t.o.
telephone order　電話指示

TOA
tubo-ovarian abscess　卵管卵巣膿瘍

T

TOAP
thioguanine, vincristine (=Oncovin), arabinosylcytosine, prednisone — チオグアニン,ビンクリスチン(=オンコビン),アラビノシルシトシン,プレドニゾン

TOB
tobramycin — トブラマイシン

tob
tobacco — タバコ

TOBEC
total body electorical conductivity — 全身電気伝導度測定法

TOC
table of contents — 目次
total organic carbon — 総有機炭素

TOCP
triorthocresyl phosphate — リン酸トリオルトクレジル

TOCST
total correlation spectroscopy — 全相関分光法

TOD
tension of oculus dexter — 右眼圧
time of delivery — 出産時
total oxygen demand — 総酸素要求量

TOEFL
Test of English as a Foreign Language — 米国留学のための英語力試験

TOET
tympanic orifice of eustachian tube — 耳管鼓室開口部

TOF
tetralogy of Fallot — ファロー四徴(症)
time of flight — 飛行時間
train-of-four (ratio) — 四連反応(比)

T of A
transposition of aorta — 大動脈転位(症)

T of F
tetralogy of Fallot — ファロー四徴(症)

TOFMS
time of flight mass spectrometry — 飛行時間型質量分析法

T

tog
together — ともに

TOH
tyrosine hydroxylase — チロシンヒドロキシラーゼ

tol
tolerance — 耐性, 許容度
tolerate — 耐える

tolb
tolbutamide — トルブタミド

TOLD
Test of Language Development　言語発達試験
TOM
triacethyl-oleandomycin　トリアセチルオレアンドマイシン
TOMHS
treatment of mild hypertension study　中等度高血圧治療研究
tomo., Tomo
tomogram　断層撮影図
tomography　断層撮影
TOMS
total ozone mapping spectrometer　全オゾン分布分光器
tonoc
tonight　今夜
tonoct
tonight　今夜
TO number
turnover number　代謝回転数
TOP
association areas of temporal, occipital and parietal lobes of cerebral hemisphere　大脳半球の側頭・後頭・頭頂葉の連合野
temporal, occipital, parietal　側頭・後頭・頭頂の
termination of pregnancy　妊娠中絶
tissue oncotic pressure　組織コロイド浸透圧
top
topically　局所的に
TOPS
take off pound sensibly　上手にやせる会
TOPV
trivalent oral poliovirus vaccine　三価経口ポリオウイルスワクチン
TORCH
toxoplasma, rubella, cytomegalo-and herpes-virus (syndrome)　トキソプラズマ・風疹・サイトメガロ・ヘルペス・ウイルス（症候群）
T or R
tenderness or rebound　圧痛または反跳圧痛
Torr, torr
Torricelli　トール〈単位〉
TOS
tension of oculus sinster　左眼圧
thoracic outlet syndrome　胸郭出口症候群
tricuspidal opening snap　三尖弁開放音
Tos, tos
tosyl　トシル（基）

TOSCA
Toxic Substance Control Act　毒性物質管理法
TOSS
total suppression of spinning side bands　核磁気共鳴の低速回転で生じる側波帯の除去法《画診》
tot
total　全，総，完全の
Total, total
total gastrectomy　胃全摘術
tot.prot.
total protein　全〔総〕蛋白(量)
t.o.w.
to other ward　他病棟へ
TOWER
testing, orientation, work, evaluation, rehabilitation　検査・治療方針決定・作業・評価・社会復帰
tox, Tox, tox.
toxemia　毒血症
toxic　中毒(性)の，毒(性)の
toxicity　毒性
toxicologist　毒物学者
toxicology　中毒学，毒物学
toxin　毒素，トキシン
TOXIN
toxicology information network　毒物情報システム
TOXLINE
toxicology information on-line　オンライン毒物情報システム
TOXO, Toxo
toxoplasmosis　トキソプラズマ症
TP
posterior tibial　後脛骨(筋)の
p-terphenyl　*p*-テルフェニル
temperature and pressure　温度と気圧
terminal phalanx　末節骨
testosterone propionate　プロピオン酸テストステロン
tetanus-pertussis　破傷風・百日咳
thiamphenicol　チアンフェニコール
threshold potential　閾値電位
thrombocytopenic purpura　血小板減少性紫斑病
thrombophlebitis　血栓性静脈炎
thymic polypeptide　胸腺ポリペプチド
thymidine phosphorylase　チミジンホスホリラーゼ
thymus protein　胸腺蛋白
tibialis posterior　脛骨後面
ticlopidine　チクロピジン
tiopronin　チオプロニン

tissue pressure 組織圧
toilet paper トイレットペーパー
total pancreatectomy 膵全摘(出)術
total paralysis 全身麻痺
total parotidectomy 耳下腺全摘出術
total phosphorus 総リン
total protein 全〔総〕蛋白(量)
transforming principle 形質転換因子
transverse process 横突起
Treponema pallidum 梅毒トレポネーマ
triosephosphate トリオースリン酸
tryptophan トリプトファン
tuberculin precipitation ツベルクリン沈殿
tuberculosis pulmonum 肺結核
tympanoplasty 鼓室形成術

Tp
physical half-time 物理学的半減期
tampon タンポン
thrombopoietin トロンボポエチン
toxoplasma トキソプラズマ
toxoplasmosis トキソプラズマ病
trichophytia pompholyciformis〈ラ〉 汗疱状白癬

6-TP
6-thiopurine 6-チオプリン

TP, T−P
temporoparietal 側頭頭頂の

T & P, T+P
temperature and pulse 体温と脈拍

TPA
12-*o*-tetradecanoylphorbol-13-acetate 12-*o*-テトラデカノイル-13-アセトイルホルボル酢酸
Third-Party Administrators 医療保険事務代行
tissue polypeptide antigen 組織ポリペプチド抗原
total parenteral alimentation 全非経口的栄養法
Treponema pallidum agglutination (test) 梅毒トレポネーマ凝集(試験)
tumor(-derived) polypeptide antigen 腫瘍(由来)ポリペプチド抗原

tPA, t-PA
tissue plasminogen activator 組織性プラスミノゲンアクチベータ

TPAL
tractus arteriosus posterolateralis〈ラ〉 後脊髄動脈

TPB
tetraphenyl borate テトラフェニルホウ酸
tryptone phosphate broth リン酸トリプトンブロス

TPBF
total pulmonary blood flow　全肺血流量
TPC
thromboplastic plasma component　血栓形成促進性血漿成分
total plasma catecholamines　全血漿カテコールアミン
total plasma cholesterol　全血漿コレステロール
treatment planning conference　治療計画カンファレンス
Treponema pallidum complement (fixation test)　梅毒トレポネーマ補体(結合試験)
TPCF test
Treponema pallidum complement fixation test　梅毒トレポネーマ補体結合試験
TPCK
N-tosyl-L-phenylalanyl chloromethyl ketone　*N*-トシル-L-フェニルアラニルクロロメチルケトン
TPCV
total packed cell volume　濃縮血球量
TPD
temporary partial disability　一過性部分的廃疾
thiamine propyl disulfide　二硫化チアミンプロピル
tip palmar distance　指尖手掌間距離
two point discrimination　2点(間)識別テスト
two point distinction　2点(間)識別
TPDCV
6-thioguanine, procarbazine, dibromodulcitol, cyclohexylchloroethylnitrosourea, vincristine　6-チオグアニン,プロカルバジン,ジブロモダルシトール,シクロヘキシルクロロエチルニトロソ尿素,ビンクリスチン
TPE
therapeutic plasma exchange　治療的血漿交換
time to peak ejection　ピーク駆出までの時間
tropical pulmonary eosinophilia　熱帯肺好酸球症
typhoid-paratyphoid enteritis　腸チフス・パラチフス腸炎
t.pedis
tinea pedis〈ラ〉　足部白癬(＝水虫)
TPEPS
tooth-pulp-evoked potentials　歯髄誘発電位
TPF
thymus permeability factor　胸腺透過性因子
TPFR
time to peak filling rate　心拡張期最大充満までの時間
TPG
therapeutic play group　治療的演劇グループ
transmembrane potential gradient　膜内外電位差勾配

tryptophan-peptone-glucose (broth) トリプトファン・ペプトン・ブドウ糖(ブロス)

TPH
thromboembolic pulmonary hypertension 血栓塞栓性肺高血圧
transplacental hemorrhage 経胎盤出血

TPHA
Treponema pallidum hemaggulutination assay 梅毒トレポネーマ血球凝集反応

TPHA test
Treponema pallidum hemagglutination test 梅毒トレポネーマ感作赤血球凝集試験

TPI
tissue perfusion index 組織灌流係数
title-page index 標題ページ索引
toe pressure index 足指血圧と上腕動脈収縮期圧との比
Tokyo University personality inventory 東大式人格表
Treponema pallidum immobilization (test) 梅毒トレポネーマ不動化(試験)
triose phosphate isomerase トリオーズホスフェイトイソメラーゼ
triphosphoinositide トリホスホイノシチド

TPIA
Treponema pallidum immobilization adherence 梅毒トレポネーマ不動化付着
Treponema pallidum immune adherence (test) 梅毒トレポネーマ免疫付着(試験)

TPI test
Treponema pallidum immobilization test 梅毒トレポネーマ不動化試験

TPK
tau protein kinase タウ蛋白キナーゼ

TPL
thromboplastin トロンボプラスチン
total phospholipid 総リン脂質
total profile length 全尿道長

Tpl
transplantation 移植

TPM
temporary pacemaker 一時的ペースメーカー
thrombophlebitis migrans 遊走性血栓性静脈炎
triphenylmethane トリフェニルメタン

T

TPMB
Treponema pallidum methylene blue test　梅毒トレポネーマ・メチレンブルー試験

TPMP
triphenylmethyl phosphonium　トリフェニルメチルホスホニウム

TPN
thalamic projection neuron　視床投射神経細胞
total parental nutrition　総静脈栄養，非経腸栄養法
total parenteral nutrition　中心静脈栄養(法)(＝高カロリー輸液)
triphosphopyridine nucleotide　トリホスホピリジンヌクレオチド

TPNH
reduced triphosphopyridine nucleotide　還元型トリホスホピリジンヌクレオチド

TPO
thrombopoietin　トロンボポエチン
thyroid peroxidase　甲状腺ペルオキシダーゼ
tryptophan peroxidase　トリプトファンペルオキシダーゼ

TPOAb
anti-thyroid peroxidase antibody　抗甲状腺ペルオキシダーゼ抗体
thyroid peroxidase antibody　甲状腺ペルオキシダーゼ抗体

TPP
testosterone phenylpropionate　テストステロン・フェニルプロピオネート
thiamine pyrophosphatase　チアミンピロホスファターゼ
thiamine pyrophosphate　チアミンピロリン酸
triphenyl phosphate　リン酸トリフェニル
true precocious puberty　真性早熟

TPp
tidal plasma protein　循環血漿蛋白量

TP & P
time, place and person　時間・場所・人

TPPN
total peripheral parenteral nutrition　完全静脈非経口栄養法

TPQs
threshold planning quantities　限界計画値

TPR
testosterone production rate　テストステロン産生率
tissue peak ratio　組織ピーク線量比
total peripheral resistance　全末梢血管抵抗
total pulmonary resistance　全肺血管抵抗
tumor-peak dose ratio　組織ピーク線量比

TPR, T.P.R.
temperature, pulse and respiration 体温・脈拍・呼吸
T : P ratio
thyroid/plasma ratio 甲状腺：血漿比
TPS
trypsin トリプシン
tumor polysaccharide substance 腫瘍多糖類物質
TPT
tetraisopropylthitan テトライソプロピルチタン
tetraphenyl tetrazolium テトラフェニルテトラゾリウム
total protein tuberculin 全蛋白ツベルクリン
triphenyltin トリフェニルスズ
typhoid-paratyphoid (vaccine) 腸チフス・パラチフス(ワクチン)
TPTHS
total parathyroid hormone secretion (rate) 全〔総〕上皮小体ホルモン分泌(率)
TPTX
thyroid parathyroid extraction 甲状腺・副甲状腺摘出
TPTZ
tripyridyltriazine トリピリジルトリアジン
TPV
terminal portal vein 終末門脈枝
tetanus-pertussis vaccine 破傷風・百日咳ワクチン
total plasma volume 全血漿量
TPVR
total peripheral vascular resistance 全末梢血管抵抗
total pulmonary vascular resistance 全肺血管抵抗
TPZ
thioproperazine チオプロペラジン
TQ
tocopherolquinone トコフェロールキノン
tourniquet 駆血帯
TQC
total quality control 総合的品質管理
TR
repetition time 繰り返し時間《画診》
Takada-Ara reaction 高田・荒反応
Takata reaction 高田反応
teaching and research 教育と研究
tegmental reticular system 天蓋網状系
terminal stimulus 終末刺激
tetrazolium reduction テトラゾリウム還元
Texas red テキサスレッド
therapeutic radiology 治療的放射線医学

therapeutic ratio 治療可能比
thyroid hormone receptor 甲状腺ホルモン受容体
total resistance 全抵抗
total response 全反応
trabecular meshwork 強角膜線維柱帯
trachea 気管
transfusion reaction 輸血反応
translational research 橋渡し研究
transparent region 透明領域《超音波》
tricuspid regurgitation 三尖弁閉鎖不全症
troy 金衡
tuberculin reaction ツベルクリン反応
Tuberkulin Rückstand〈独〉 新ツベルクリン
tubular reabsorption 尿細管再吸収
tubular rising 耳管隆起
turbidity reducing 混濁度低下
turnover rate 交代速度

Tr
transferrin トランスフェリン
transillumination rate 透光率
triamcinolone トリアムシノロン
trophoblast 栄養膜
trypsin トリプシン

t_r
radiologic half-life 放射線学的半減期

tr
trachea 気管
traction 牽引
trauma 外傷
treatment 治療
tremor 振戦
trityl トリチル(基)

tr.
tritura〈ラ〉 研磨せよ《処》

T & R
tenderness and rebound 圧痛および反跳圧痛

TR, T(R)
temperature, rectal 直腸温

TR, Tr
trachoma トラコーマ

Tr, tr
trace 痕跡
transfer 移入，伝達

TRA
terminal repeat array 反復配列

T

Texas red conjugated streptavidin テキサスレッド標識ストレプトアビシン
transaldolase トランスアルドラーゼ
trans-retinoic acid トランスレチノイン酸
tumor rejection antigen 腫瘍拒絶抗原
tumor-resistant antigen 腫瘍抵抗性抗原

TRAb
thyroid stimulating hormone receptor antibody 甲状腺刺激ホルモン受容体抗体
thyrotropin チ〔サイ〕ロトロピン受容体抗体
TSH receptor antibody 抗TSHレセプター自己抗体

trach
trachea 気管
trachoma トラコーマ

Trach, trach
tracheotomy 気管切開(術), 気切

trach.asp.
tracheal aspiration 気管吸引

TRACP
tartarate resistant acid phosphatase 酒石酸抵抗性酸ホスファターゼ

tract
traction 牽引

TRAIDS
transfusion-related AIDS 輸血関連(性)エイズ

train
training 研修

TRALI
transfusuin-related acute lung injury 輸血関連急性肺障害, トラリ

TRAM
Treatment Response Assessment Method 治療反応評価法

Tr.am.
tinctura amara〈ラ〉 苦味チンキ《処》

TRAMPCOL
6-thioguanine, rubidomycin, arabinosylcytosine, methotrexate, prednisolone, cyclophosphamide, vincristine (=Oncovin) 6-チオグアニン, ルビドマイシン, アラビノシルシトシン, メトトレキサート, プレドニゾロン, シクロホスファミド, ビンクリスチン (=オンコビン)

trans
transaction 処理, 会報
transfer 運搬する, 移入する
transformer トランス, 変圧器

transilluminate ～に光を通過させる
transverse 横の，横断の

trans D, trans.d.
transverse diameter 横径

transm
transmission 伝達，媒介

transpl
transplant 移植組織(片)
transplantation 移植(術)

trans.sec.
transverse section 横断面

trans.sect.
transverse section 横断面

transv.proc.
transverse process 横突起

trany
transparency 透明度

TRAP
tartrate-resistant acid phophatase 酒石酸抵抗性酸ホスファターゼ
6-thioguanine, rubidomycin, arabinosylcytosine, prednisone 6-チオグアニン，ルビドマイシン，アラビノシルシトシン，プレドニゾン

trap
trapezius (muscle) 僧帽(筋)

TRAS
transplant renal artery stenosis 移植腎動脈狭窄(症)

trau
trauma 外傷
traumatic 外傷性の

TRAV
transient recurrent atypical vertigo 一過性再発性非定型的眩暈症

TRB
terbutaline テルブタリン

TRBF
total renal blood flow 全腎血流量

TRC
tanned red cell タンニン酸処理赤血球
tanned red cell aggultination test タンニン酸処理感作赤血球凝集反応
tissue repair cells 組織修復細胞
total respiratory conductance 総呼吸コンダクタンス

TRCA
tanned red cell agglutination タンニン酸処理赤血球凝集(反応)

T

TRCH
tanned red cell hemagglutination　タンニン酸処理赤血球凝集反応

trch
trachea　気管
tracheotomy　気管切開術
trachoma　トラコーマ

TRCHII
tanned red cell hemagglutination inhibition immunoassay　タンニン酸処理赤血球凝集抑制免疫学的検定(法)

TRCI
total red cell iron　循環全赤血球鉄

TRCV
total red-cell volume　全赤血球容積

TRD
tongue retaining device　舌保持器
tractional retinal detachment　牽引性網膜剝離

TRDN
transient respiratory distress of the newborn　一過性新生児呼吸促迫

TRDS
transient respiratory distress syndrome　一過性呼吸促迫症候群

TRE
thymic reticuloepithelial　胸腺網状上皮の
thyroid hormone response element　甲状腺ホルモン反応要素
tissue polypeptide antigen responsive promoter elements　組織ポリペプチド抗原反応推進要素

treat
treatment　治療，処理

trem
trembling　ふるえ

tremb
trembling　ふるえ

TREND
tropical environment data　熱帯環境データ

Trend
Trendelenburg (position)　トレンデレンブルク(体位)

Trep
Treponema　トレポネーマ(属)

TRF
T cell replacing factor　T細胞代替因子
telomeric repeat binding factor　テロメア結合蛋白
thyrotrop(h)in-releasing factor　甲状腺刺激ホルモン放出因子

Trf
Trommelfell〈独〉　鼓膜

TRFC
total rosette-forming cell　総〔全〕ロゼット形成細胞
Trfell
Trommelfell〈独〉　鼓膜
TRFR
tubular rejection fraction rate　尿細管排泄率
TRG
transient reflecting grating technique　過渡反射格子法
trg
training　研修
trgt
target　標的
TRH
thyrotropin-releasing hormone　甲状腺刺激ホルモン放出ホルモン
TRHR
thyrotropin-releasing hormone receptor　甲状腺刺激ホルモン放出ホルモン受容体
TRI
total red cell iron　全赤血球鉄
total response index　全反応指数
toxic release inventory　有害物質放出目録
trichloroethylene　トリクロロエチレン
tri
triceps　三頭(筋)
T_3RIA
triiodothyronine radioimmunoassay　トリヨードチ〔サイ〕ロニン放射(標識)免疫検定(法)
TRIAC
triiodothyroacetic acid　トリヨウ化チロ酢酸
Triam
triamcinolone　トリアムシノロン
TRIC
trachoma inclusion conjunctivitis (agent)　トラコーマ封入体(性)結膜炎(因子)
tricaphos
tricalcium phosphate　リン酸トリカルシウム
Trich, trich.
Trichomonas　トリコモナス(属)
Tricho
trichomoniasis　トリコモナス症
trid.
triduum〈ラ〉　3 日間《処》
trig
trigeminy　三段脈
trigger　引き金，トリガー

trigonal　三角の

TRIG, Trig, trig.
triglyceride　トリグリセリド

trig.pnt.
trigger point　ひきがね点，発痛点

trig.pt.
trigger point　ひきがね点，発痛点

trip
triple　三倍の
triplet　三倍にする
triplication　三倍化

trir.
tritura〈ラ〉　粉にする，砕く《処》

TRIS, Tris, tris
tris (hydroxymethyl)-aminomethane　トリス・ヒドロキシメチル・アミノメタン
tris (hidroxymethyl)methylamine　トリス・ヒドロキシメチル・メチルアミン

tri sten
tricuspid stenosis　三尖弁狭窄

TRIT
triiodothyronine　トリヨードチ〔サイ〕ロニン
trithyronine　トリサイロニン

trit.
triturare〈ラ〉　咀嚼する，粉にする
tritus, *tritura*〈ラ〉=triturate　研磨した，研磨せよ，粉砕する《処》

TRITC
tetramethyl-rhodamine isothiocyanate　テトラメチルローダミンイソチオシアネイト

TRI test
tetrazolium reduction inhibition (test)　テトラゾリウム還元阻止(試験)

trityl-
triphenylmethyl-　トリフェニルメチル〈接〉

TRK
transketolase　トランスケトラーゼ

TRL
triglyceride-rich lipoproteins　トリグリセリド豊富リポ蛋白

TRM
trichomycin　トリコマイシン

TRMC
trapezius myocutaneous flap　僧帽筋皮弁

TRML
terminal　末端，端末

trmt
treatment　処置，治療
tRNA, t-RNA
transfer RNA(=ribonucleic acid)　転移リボ核酸，転移RNA
tRNA-aa
aminoacyl transfer RNA　アミノアシルt-RNA
TRNG
tetracycline-resistant *Neisseria gonorrhoeae*　テトラサイクリン耐性淋菌
truncus arteriosus〈ラ〉　総動脈幹
TRO
to return to office　外来に再来する
troch.
trochanter　転子
trochischi〈ラ〉　トローチ《処》
trochiscus〈ラ〉=troche　トローチ，口内錠《処》
trop
tropic　熱帯の
tropical　熱帯の
Trop Med
tropical medicine　熱帯医学
TRP
total refractory period　完全不応期
tricho-rhino-phalangeal (syndrome)　毛髪・鼻・指(症候群)
tubular reabsorption of phosphate　尿細管無機リン再吸収量
Trp
tryptophan　トリプトファン
%TRP
% tubular reabsorption of phosphate　尿細管リン再吸収率
TRPA
tryptophan-rich prealbumin　トリプトファン豊富プレアルブミン
TRPF
total renal plasma flow　全腎血漿流量
tr pl, TrPl
treatment plan　治療計画
trp operon
tryptophan operon　トリプトファンオペロン
TRPRS
tryptophanyl-trans ribonucleic acid synthetase　トリプトファニル転移リボ核酸合成酵素
TRPT
theoretical renal phosphorus threshold　理論的腎臓リン閾値
TRQ
tinnitus reaction questionnaire　耳鳴に関する質問

TRR
total renal resistance 全腎血管抵抗
TRS
total reducing sugars 総〔全〕還元糖
total renin substrate 総レニン基質
treatment response scale 治療反応性尺度
tubuloreticular structure 管網状構造
TrS
traumatic surgery 外傷外科(学)
trs
transfer 移送する，転移する
T_3-RSU
triiodothyronine resin sponge uptake T_3レジンスポンジ摂取率
TRSV
tobacco-ringspot virus タバコ環状斑ウイルス
TRT, trt
treatment 治療，療法
TRU
turbidity reducing unit 混濁度低下単位
T_3RU
triiodothyronine resin uptake (test) トリヨードチ〔サイ〕ロニン摂取(検査)
TRUS
transrectal ultrasonography 経直腸超音波検査法《画診》
TRV
tobacco rattle virus タバコごろごろウイルス
TRW
tubular reabsorption of water 尿細管水分再吸収
TRX, trx
traction 牽引
TRXF
total reflection X-ray fluorescence 全反射螢光X線分析法
TRY, Try
tryptophan トリプトファン
Try H
tryptophan hydroxylase トリプトファン水酸化酵素
Tryp
tryptophan トリプトファン
TS
nucleus tractus solitarius〈ラ〉 孤束核
Tay-Sachs (disease) テイ・サックス(病)
teaching strategies 教授方略《医教》
temperature sensitive 温度感受性の
terminal sensation 末端感覚
terminal stimulus 終末刺激
thermosonimetry 熱音響測定

thermostable	温度安定の
thoracic surgery	胸部外科(学)
thrombospondin	トロンボスポンジン
thymidine synthetase	チミジン合成酵素
tocopherol supplemented	トコフェロールを補充(添加)した
toe signs	母趾徴候
total solids	全固形物
Tourette syndrome	トゥーレット症候群
toxic substance	中毒性物質
tracheal sound	気管音
Transplantation Society	移植学会
transsexual	性転換(者)
transverse section	横断面
transverse sinus	横洞
trauma score	外傷表
treadmill score	トレッドミルスコア
tricuspid stenosis	三尖弁狭窄症
triple strength	3倍の強さ
tropical sprue	熱帯スプルー
tubal stenosis	耳管狭窄症
tuberous sclerosis	結節性硬化(症)
tumor specific	腫瘍特異的な
Turner syndrome	ターナー症候群
type-specific (antibodies)	型特異性(抗体)

Ts

skin temperature	皮膚温度
suppressor T cell	抑制性T細胞，サプレッサーT細胞
tosyl	トシル(基)

t.s.

temporal sinistra〈ラ〉	左側頭

T/S

thyroid serum (radioiodine) ratio	甲状腺血清放射ヨード比

t/s

third stage	第3期

T & S

type and screen	血型判定スクリーン

TS, T.S.

test solution	試験検査溶液

TSA

p-toluenesulfonic acid (test)	*p*-トルエンスルホン酸(試験)
therapeutic substances act	治療薬物効果
trichostatin A	トリコスタチンA
tumor-specific antibody	腫瘍特異抗体

T

tumor-specific antigen 腫瘍特異抗原
tumor-surface antigen 腫瘍表面抗原
tumor-susceptible antigen 腫瘍感受性抗原
type-specific antibody 型特異性抗体

T_4SA
thyroxin(e)-specific activity チ〔サイ〕ロキシン特異的活性

TSAb
thyroid stimulating antibody 甲状腺刺激抗体

TSAC
title, subtitle and caption 標題・副題と見出し

TSANZ
Thoracic Society of Australia and New Zealand オーストラリア・ニュージーランド胸部医学会

TSAP
total serum acid phosphatase 血清総酸性リン酸分解酵素

Tsaph
temperature in the saphenous vein 小伏在静脈温度

TSB
total serum bilirubin 総血清ビリルビン
total spinal block 全脊椎麻酔
trypticase soy broth トリプチケースソイブロス

TSBA
total serum bile acids 総血清胆汁酸

TSBAb
thyroid stimulating blocking antibody 甲状腺刺激遮断抗体

TSBB
transtracheal selective bronchial brushing 経気管的選択的気管支擦過

TSC
technetium sulfur colloid テクネチウムイオウコロイド
Therapeutic Social Club 治療社会クラブ
thiosemicarbazide チオセミカルバジド
thiosemicarbazone チオセミカルバゾン
thymic stromal cells 胸腺上皮細胞
total static compliance 総〔全〕静的コンプライアンス
tuberous sclerosis complex 結節硬化症

TSCA
Toxic Substances Control Act (米国)有害物質規制法

TSD
target skin distance 焦点皮膚間距離
Tay-Sachs disease タイ・サックス病

TSE
testicular self-examination 精巣自己検査

TSEB
total skin electron beam 全身電子線照射療法

Tsect, T sect., T-sect.
transverse (cross) section 横断面
TSES
target symptom evaluation scale 目標症候評価基準
T-set
tracheotomy set 気管切開セット
TSF
thrombopoiesis-stimulating factor 血小板造血刺激因子
thymocyte stimulating factor 胸腺細胞刺激因子
triceps skinfold 三頭筋皮下脂肪
triceps skinfold thickness 上腕三頭筋部の脂肪の厚さ
TsF
suppressive T cell factor 抑制性T細胞因子
TSG
tumor-specific glycoprotein 腫瘍特異性糖蛋白
TSGP
tumor-specific glycoprotein 腫瘍特異性糖蛋白
TSH
thyroid stimulating hormone 甲状腺刺激ホルモン
TSHR
thyroid stimulating homone receptor 甲状腺刺激ホルモン受容体
TSH-RF
thyroid-stimulating hormone-releasing factor 甲状腺刺激ホルモン放出ホルモン
TSH-RH
thyroid-stimulating hormone-releasing hormone 甲状腺刺激ホルモン放出ホルモン
TSH test
thyroid stimulating hormone test 甲状腺刺激ホルモン試験
TSI
thyroid stimulating immunoglobulin 甲状腺刺激性免疫グロブリン
tricuspid stenoinsufficiency 三尖弁狭窄兼閉鎖不全症
triple sugar(=lactose, glucose, sucrose)iron (agar medium) 三糖(=乳糖・ブドウ糖・ショ糖)鉄(寒天培地)
trophic state index 栄養状態指数
TSIA
triple sugar iron agar 三糖鉄寒天(培地)
TSI agar medium
triple sugar iron agar medium 三糖鉄寒天培地
T-sign
Thomson sign トムソン徴候
Tsk
T cell specific tyrosine kinase T細胞特異的チロシンキナーゼ
TSL
terminal sensory latency 終末知覚潜時

TSLS
toxic shock like syndrome　劇症A型溶連菌感染症
TSM
type-specific M (protein)　型特異的M(蛋白)
ts mutant
temperature-sensitive mutant　温度感受性突然変異体
ts mutation
temperature-sensitive mutation　温度感受性突然変異
TSO
thromboangiitis obliterans　閉塞性血栓性血管炎
TSP
thermo-spray ionization　サーモスプレー吸入法
thrombin-sensitive protein　トロンビン感受性蛋白
thyroid-stimulating　前下垂体甲状腺刺激
thyroid-stimulating pituitary　甲状腺刺激下垂体
total serum protein　総血清蛋白
transduodenal sphincteroplasty　経十二指腸括約筋形成術
trisodium phosphate　リン酸三ナトリウム
tropical spastic paraparesis　熱帯性痙性脊髄麻痺
tsp
teaspoon　茶さじ，小さじ《処》
teaspoonful　茶さじ１杯の《処》
TSPA
thiophosphoramide　チオホスホルアミド(＝チオテパ)
triethylene thiophosphoamide　トリエチレンチオリン酸アミド
TSPAP
total serum prostatic acid phosphatase　総血清前立腺性酸ホスファターゼ
T-spine
thoracic spine　胸椎
TSPR
total systemic peripheral resistance　全身血管抵抗
TSR
testosterone-sterilized (female) rat　テストステロン不妊(雌)ラット
total systemic resistance　総体循環抵抗，全体循環抵抗
transient situational reaction　一過性状況反応
T : S ratio
thyroid/serum ratio　甲状腺：血清比
TSS
sodium tetradecyl sulfate　テトラデシル硫酸ナトリウム
time sharing system　時間分割システム
toxic shock syndrome　中毒性ショック症候群
tropical splenomegaly syndrome　熱帯性脾腫症候群

T

tumor-specific substance　腫瘍特異物質

TSSA

tumor-specific (cell) surface antigen　腫瘍特異性(細胞)表面抗原

TSSE

toxic shock syndrome exotoxin　中毒性ショック症候群外毒素

TSST

toxic shock syndrome toxin　中毒性ショック症候群毒素

TSST-1

toxic shock syndrome toxin type-1　中毒性ショック症候群1型

TST

thromboplastin screening test　トロンボプラスチンスクリーニング試験

total sleep time　総睡眠時間

toxic shock toxin　毒素性ショック毒素

treadmill stress test(ing)　トレッドミルストレス検査

tumor skin test　腫瘍皮膚試験

TSTA

toxoplasmin skin test antigen　トキソプラズマ皮膚試験抗原

tumor-specific tissue antigen　腫瘍特異性組織抗原

tumor-specific transplantation antigen　腫瘍特異性移植抗原

T-state

tension state　緊張状態

TSTI

tumor-specific transplantation immunity　腫瘍特異性移植免疫

TSU

triple sugar urea (agar)　3種の糖尿素(寒天)

TSV

total stomach volume　総〔全〕胃容量

TSVR

total systemic vascular resistance　全体血管抵抗

TT

tablet triturate〈ラ〉　湿製錠剤《処》

tactile tension　(眼)触診緊張度

tendon transfer　腱移行(術)

tensor tympani muscle　鼓膜張筋

terminal tendon　終腱

test tube　試験管

tetanus toxoid　破傷風トキソイド

tetrazol　テトラゾール

thrombin time　トロンビン時間

thrombotest　トロンボテスト

thymol turbidity　チモール混濁

tibial tuberosity　脛骨粗面

tilt table　斜面台，傾斜台

toilet training 排便訓練
tolerance test 負荷試験
total thyroxine 総チ〔サイ〕ロキシン
total time 全時間，総時間
transit time 血液通過時間
transthoracic 経胸(郭)の
transtracheal 経気管の
trophoblastic tumor 栄養膜腫瘍
tuberculin tested ツベルクリン検査された
tumor thrombus 腫瘍血栓

TT_3
total triiodothyronine 総トリヨードチ〔サイ〕ロニン

TT_4
total thyroxine 総チ〔サイ〕ロキシン

T & T
time and temperature 時間と温度
touch and tone 脈と心音

TTA
tetanus toxoid antibody 破傷風トキソイド抗体
thenoyltrifluoroacetone テノイルトリフルオロアセトン
transtracheal aspirates 経気管吸引物
transtracheal aspiration 経気管吸引
trifluorothenoylacetone トリフルオロテノイルアセトン
tumor transplantation antigen 腫瘍移植抗原

TTAG
tubotympano aerodynamicgraphy 耳管鼓室気流動態法

TTBV
total trabecular bone volume 総海綿骨量

TTC
Teacher Training Center 教師訓練センター《医教》
tetrazolium chloride 塩化テトラゾリウム
triphenyltetrazolium chloride 塩化トリフェニルテトラゾリウム

TTC reduced method
triphenyltetrazolium chloride reduced method TTC還元法

TTC test
triphenyltetrazolium-chloride test 塩化トリフェニールテトラゾリウム試験

TTD
temporary threshold drift 一過性閾値変動
tetraethyl-thiuram disulfide 二硫化テトラエチルチウラム
threshold tone decay 閾値音減衰
tissue tolerance dose 組織耐量

transfusion transmitted diseases 輸血による伝染病
transient tic disorder 一過性チック疾患
transverse thoracic diameter 横胸径，胸部横径

TTD test
threshold tone decay test 閾値音減衰検査

TTE
transthoracic echocardiography 経胸壁心臓超音波検査

T_4-test
1251-tetraiodothyronine resin sponge uptake test テトラヨウ素〔サイ〕ロニンレジンスポンジ取り込み試験

TTF
tensor tympani fold 鼓膜張筋ひだ

TTFB
4,5,6,7-tetrachloro-2-trifluoromethylbenzimidazole 4,5,6,7-テトラクロロ-2-トリフルオロメチルベンゾイミダゾール

TTH
thyrotrop(h)ic hormone 甲状腺刺激ホルモン

TTh
tritiated thymidine トリチウムチミジン

TTHM
total trihalomethane 総トリハロメタン

TTI
tension-time index 張力時間係数
transtracheal insufflation 経気管通気(法)

TTJV
transtracheal jet ventilation 経気管ジェット換気

TTL
total thymic lymphocyte 総胸腺リンパ球

TTLC
true total lung capacity 真総肺活量

TTM
tensor tympani muscle 鼓膜張筋

TTN
Technology Transfer Network 技術移転ネットワーク
transient tachypnea of newborn 新生児一過性多〔頻〕呼吸(症)

TTNA
transthoracic needle aspiration 経胸針吸引

TTNB
transient tachypnea of newborn 新生児一過性多〔頻〕呼吸(症)
transthoracic needle (aspiration) biopsy 経胸針(吸引)生検

TTO
to take out 持ち出す(ために)

TTOT
transtracheal oxygen therapy 経気管的酸素療法

T

TTP
ribothymidine 5′-triphosphate リボチミジン5′-三リン酸
thrombotic thrombocytopenic purpura 血栓性血小板減少性紫斑病
thymidine (5′-)triphosphate チミジン(5′-)三リン酸
TTP-HUS
thrombotic thrombocytopenic purpura and hemolytic uremic syndrome 血栓性血小板減少性紫斑病と溶血性尿毒症症候群
TTR
transthoracic resistance 経胸郭抵抗
transthyretin トランスサイレチン
triceps tendon reflex 三頭筋腱反射
TTS
tarsal tunnel syndrome 足根管症候群
temporal threshold shift 一過性閾値変動
transdermal therapeutic system 経皮吸収治療システム
transverse tubular system 横行小管系
TTT
the tree test バウムテスト，樹木画による人格診断法
thymol turbidity test チモール混濁試験
tolbutamide toleranee test トルブタミド負荷試験
TTT line
Twining-tuberculum sella torcular line トワイニングの鞍結節と内後頭隆起を結ぶ線
TTTS
twin to twin transfusion syndrome 双胎間輸血症候群
TTTT
test tube turbidity test 試験管混濁試験
TTV
tracheal transport velocity 気管輸送速度
transfusion transmitted virus 輸血感染ウイルス
TTVP
temporary transvenous pacemaker 一時的経静脈ペースメーカー
TTX
tetrodotoxin テトロドトキシン
TTY
teletypewriter テレタイプライター《コン》
T-type
tetany type テタニー型
TU
thermal unit 熱単位
thiouracil チオウラシル
thyroidal uptake 甲状腺摂取
Todd units トッド単位

transurethral　経尿道の
turbidity unit　混濁単位

T_3U
triiodothyronine upake (test)　トリヨードチ〔サイ〕ロニン摂取(検査)
triiodothyronine uptake ratio　トリヨードチ〔サイ〕ロニン摂取率

TU, T.U.
toxic unit　中毒単位，毒物単位
tuberculin unit　ツベルクリン単位

TUB
tubouterine (junction)　卵管子宮(接合部)

tub
tubing　挿管
tubular adenocarcinoma　管状腺癌

tub 1
tubular adenocarcinoma, well differentiated type　管状腺癌の高分化型

tub 2
moderately differentiated type　管状腺癌の中分化型

tuberc, tuberc.
tuberculosis　結核(症)

TUC
transurethral coagulation　経尿道的凝固術

TUE
transurethral extraction　経尿道的摘出

TUEP
transurethral evaporation of prostate　経尿道的前立腺蒸散術

TUF
transurethral fulguration　経尿道的焼灼術

TUG
total urinary gonadotropin　全〔総〕尿(中)性腺刺激ホルモン

TUI
transurethral incision　経尿道切開(術)

TUIBN
transurethral incision of bladder neck　経尿道的膀胱頸(部)切開

TUIP
transurethral incision of prostate　経尿道的前立腺切開

TUL
transurethral lithotripsy　経尿道的結石破砕術
transurethral ureterolithotripsy　経尿道的尿管結石砕石術

TULIP
transurethral ultrasound-guided laser induced prostatectomy　経尿道的超音波誘導下レーザー前立腺切除術

TULS
transurethral laser surgery — 経尿道的レーザー外科
tum
tummy — 胃，おなか，(幼児語で)ぽんぽん
tumor — 腫瘍
TUMT
transurethral microwave thermotherapy — 経尿道的温熱療法
TUR
transurethral (electro-)resection — 経尿道的(電気)切除術
tur
turgor — ツルゴール
Tu.R.
Tuberkulin Reaktion〈独〉 — ツベルクリン反応
TURB
transurethral resection of bladder (tumor) — 経尿道的膀胱(腫瘍)切除
turb
turbid — 濁った，混濁した
turbidity — 混濁
turbinate — 鼻甲介
turbid
turbidity — 混濁
TURBN
transurethral resection of bladder neck — 経尿道的膀胱頸切除術
TUR-Bt, TURBT
transurethral resection of bladder tumor — 経尿道的膀胱腫瘍切除術
TURCaP
transurethral resection of carcinoma of prostata — 経尿道的前立腺癌切除術
TURF
trans urethral radiofrequency heating — 経尿道的光線照射高熱療法
turg
turgor — トルゴール，ツルゴール
TURP
transurethral resection of prostate — 経尿道的前立腺切除術
turp
turpentine — テルペンチン(＝マツヤニ由来精油)
TURS
transurethral resection syndrome — 経尿道的切除症候群
tus.
tussis〈ラ〉 — せき《処》

tuss.urg.
tussi urgente〈ラ〉 せきの発作時《処》
TUU
transureteroureterostomy 経尿管尿管吻合(術)
TUUN
transureteroureteronephrostomy 経尿管尿管腎吻合(術)
TUV
total urine volume 全尿量
TUVP
transurethral electro-vaporization of prostate 経尿道的前立腺電気蒸散術
TV
talipes varus 内転足
television テレビ
tetrazolium violet テトラゾリウム紫
thoracic vertebrae 胸椎
tickborne virus ダニ媒介ウイルス
tidal volume 1回換気量
total volume 総〔全〕容量，総体積
toxic vertigo 中毒性めまい
transvenous 経静脈の
trial visit 試験診察
Trichomonas vaginalis 腟トリコモナス
trichomoniasis vaginitis 腟トリコモナス症，トリコモナス性腟炎
tricuspid valve 三尖弁
trivalent 三価の
truncal vagotomy 幹迷走神経切断術
tuberculin volutin ツベルクリンボルチン
tubulovesicles 管状小胞
typhus vaccine 発疹チフスワクチン
TVC
third ventricle cyst 第三脳室囊胞
timed vital capacity 時間肺活量
triple voiding cystography 三段排尿膀胱造影法
TVD
toxic vapor damper 毒蒸気減衰器
toxic vapor detector 毒蒸気検出器
transmissible virus dementia 伝達可能ウイルス性痴呆
TV epilepsy
television epilepsy テレビてんかん
TVH
total vaginal hysterectomy 腟式全子宮摘出(術)
TVL
tenth value layer 1/10の価層

TVP
tensor veli palatini 口蓋帆張(筋)
textured vegetable protein 植物組織蛋白
transvenous pacemaker 経静脈ペースメーカー
transvesical prostatectomy 経膀胱的前立腺切除
tricuspid (valve) prolapse 三尖弁逸脱(症)
TV pacemaker
transvenous pacemaker 経静脈ペースメーカー
TVR
tonic vibration reflex 緊張性振動性反射
total vascular resistance 全血管抵抗
tricuspid valve replacement 三尖弁置換術
TVS
trans-vaginal sonography 経腟超音波検査法
TVSS
tactile vision substitution system 視覚補綴システム
TVT
tunica vaginalis testis 精巣鞘膜
TVU
total volume urine 全〔総〕尿量
TW
terminal web 終末ウェブ《電顕》
total (body) water 全身水分
TWA
time weighted average concentration 時間荷重平均濃度
TWAR
Taiwan acute respiratory 台湾急性呼吸
Twb
wet bulb temperature 湿球温度
TWBC
total white blood cells 全白血球，総白血球
TWE
tepid water enema ぬるま湯浣腸，微温湯浣腸
T1WI
T1 weighted image T１強調画像
T2WI
T2 weighted image T２強調画像
TWIMC
to whom it may concern これにかかわる人に
TWL
transepidermal water loss 経表皮水分喪失
TWO
this week only 今週かぎり
TX
thyroidectomy 甲状腺摘出(術)，甲状腺切除(術)

transplantation 移植

Tx

therapy 療法
thymectomized 胸腺除去
transfusion 輸液，輸血
triton X トリ〔ライ〕トンX

T & X

type and crossmatch (血液)型と交叉〔差〕(適合)試験

TX，Tx，tx

treatment 治療

Tx，TX

thromboxane トロンボキサン

Tx，tx，tx.

traction 牽引

TxA_2

thromboxane A_2 トロンボキサンA_2

TxA，TXA

thromboxane A トロンボキサンA

TXB

thromboxane B トロンボキサンB

TxB_2

thromboxane B_2 トロンボキサンB_2

TXP

toxopyrimidine トキソピリミジン

TXRF

total reflection X-ray fluorescence spectrometry 全反射螢光X線分析法

TY

Toyomycin トヨマイシン

Ty

thyroxine チ〔サイ〕ロキシン
type 型
tyramine チラミン

Tymp

tympanicity 鼓音性
tympanitic 鼓音(性)の
tympany 鼓腸，(打診の)鼓音

tymp

tympanic 鼓膜の，鼓室の

tymp. memb.

tympanic membrane 鼓膜

TYMV

turnip yellow mosaic virus カブラ黄斑モザイクウイルス

typ，typ.

typical 代表的な，典型的な

TypeⅣ-C
type four collagen　Ⅳ型コラーゲン

Tyr
tyrosine　チロシン

Tys
sclerotylosis　硬化性角皮症

U u

U

- *acidum uricum*〈ラ〉＝uric acid　尿酸
- enzyme unit　酵素単位
- International Unit　国際単位
- *ulcus*〈ラ〉＝ulcer　潰瘍の
- ulnar　尺骨の，尺側の
- ultralente (insulin)　ウルトラレンテ(インスリン)
- umbilicus　臍
- unable　不可能な
- uncertain　不確実な
- understandable　理解できる
- unit (s)　単位
- university　大学
- unknown　不明の，未知の
- upper　上の，上位の
- uracil　ウラシル
- uranium　ウラン，ウラニウム〈元素〉
- uridine　ウリジン
- uridylic acid　ウリジル酸
- urinary　尿の
- urine　尿(の)
- urologist　泌尿器科医
- urology　泌尿器科(学)
- *utendus*〈ラ〉　用いられる
- uterus　子宮
- uvula　口蓋垂

u

- unclassified　分類不能の
- unified atomic mass unit　統一原子質量単位
- unter〈独〉　下の

u.

- *usus*〈ラ〉　用法《処》

1/U

- one fingerbreadth above umbilicus　臍上１指幅

U/1

- one fingerbreadth below umbilicus　臍下１指幅

U/2

- upper one-half　(長骨の)上部1/2(区)

U/3

- upper third　(長骨の)上部1/3(区)

U, u

- ulna　尺骨
- urea　尿素

urethra　尿道

UA

ultra-audible (sound)　可聴域外の(音響)
ultrasonic arteriogram　超音波動脈撮影図
umbilical artery　臍動脈(の)
unaggregated　非凝集の，非塊状の
unstable angina　不安定狭心症
Unterarm〈独〉　前腕
upper airway　上気道
upper arm　上腕
urethra　尿道
uridylic acid　ウリジル酸
urinary aldosterone　尿(中)アルドステロン
urine aliquot　尿部分標本
urocanic acid　ウロカニン酸
uterine aspiration　子宮吸引

u.a.

usque ad〈ラ〉　～まで《処》

U/A

uterine activity　子宮活動

UA，U/A

uric acid　尿酸

UA，U/A，Ua

urinalysis　尿検査，検尿

UAA

uracil,adenine,adenine(=termination codon)　ウラシル・アデニン・アデニン(=終止コドン)

UAB

under arm brace　アンダーアームブレス

UAC

umbilical artery catheter　臍動脈カテーテル
upper airway congestion　上気道うっ血

UA/C

uric acid-creatinine (ratio)　尿酸/クレアチニン(比)

UAD

upper airway disease　上気道疾患

UAE

unilateral absence of excretion　片側排泄欠如
urine albumin excrete　尿中アルブミン排泄量

UAEM

University Association for Emergency Medicine　救急医療大学協会

UAF

ut aliquid Hat〈ラ〉　ともに生じたある物

UAG
uracil, adenine, guanine (=termination codon) ウラシル・アデニン・グアニン(=終止コドン)
UAGA
Uniform Anatomical Gift Act 統一臓器提供運動
UAI
uterine activity integral 子宮活動間隔
uterine activity interval 子宮活動間隔
UA & M
urinalysis and microscopy 尿検査と顕微鏡検査(法)
UAN
uric acid nitrogen 尿酸窒素
UAO
upper airway obstruction 上気道閉塞
UAP
unstable angina pectoris 不安定狭心症
urinary alkaline phosphatase 尿アルカリホスファターゼ
UAR
upper airway resistance 上気道抵抗
UAS
upper abdominal surgery 上腹部手術
UASA
upper airway sleep apnea 上気道(性)睡眠(時)無呼吸(症)
UAU
uterine activity unit 子宮活動単位
UAVC
univentricular atrioventricular connection 単心室房室結合
UB
umbound bilirubin 非抱合型ビリルビン
uric blood 尿潜血
urinary bladder 膀胱
UB, Ub
upper back 上背部
UBA
Umweltbundesamt〈独〉 ドイツの環境保護庁
undenatured bacterial antigen 非変質性細菌性抗原
unit of biological activity 生物学的活性単位
UBBC
unsaturated (vitamin) B_{12} binding capacity 不飽和(ビタミン)B_{12}結合能
UBC
unsaturated binding capacity 不飽和結合能
UBE
upper body ergometer 上半身エルゴメーター

UBF
uterine blood flow　子宮血流量
UBFV
uterine artery blood flow velocity　子宮動脈血流速度
UBG, Ubg
urobilinogen　ウロビリノゲン
UBI
ultraviolet blood irradiation　紫外線血液照射(法)
UBL
undifferentiated B cell lymphoma　未分化B細胞リンパ腫
UBM
ultrasound biomicroscope　生体超音波顕微鏡
urothelial basement membrane　尿路上皮基底膜
Ubn
urobilin　ウロビリン
UBP
ureteral back pressure　尿管後方圧
UBT
urea broth test　尿素呼気テスト
UC
ulcerative colitis　潰瘍性大腸炎
ultracentrifugal　超遠心(分離)の
umbilical cholesterol　臍(血)コレステロール
umbilical cord　臍帯
unchanged　不変の
unclassifiable　分類不能の
unconscious　無意識の，意識のない，意識不明の
under coating　下塗層
undifferentiated carcinoma　未分化癌
unesterified cholesterol　非エステル化コレステロール
unsatisfactory condition　不満足状態
urea clearance　尿素クリアランス
urethral catheterization　尿道カテーテル法
urinary catheter　尿道カテーテル
urine concentration　尿濃度
uterine contraction　子宮収縮
uc
usual care　通常治療
U & C
urethral and cervical (cultures)　尿道および子宮頸の(培養)
usual and customary　普通かつ慣例的な
UC, U/C
urine culture　尿培養
UCA
ultracentrifugal analysis　超遠心分析

ultraclean air　超清浄空気

UCB
unconjugated bilirubin　未〔非〕抱合ビリルビン

UCBC
umbilical cord blood culture　臍帯血(液)培養

UCBR
unconjugated bilirubin　未〔非〕抱合ビリルビン

UCC
United Cancer Council　米国癌審議会
urgent care center　緊急治療センター

UCD
usual childhood disease　小児期通常疾患

UCE
urea cycle enzymopathy　尿素サイクル酵素疾患

UCF
ultracentrifuge　超遠心分離

UCG
retrograde urethrocystography　逆行性尿道膀胱造影
ultrasonic cardiogram　心エコー図
ultrasound cardiogram　超音波カルジオグラム
ultrasound cardiography　超音波心臓検査法
urethrocystography　尿道膀胱造影法
urinary chorionic gonadotropin　尿(中)絨毛性ゴナドトロピン

UCHD
usual childhood disease　小児期通常疾患

UCHI
usual childhood illness　小児期通常疾患

UCHS
uncontrolled hemorrhagic shock　未処置の出血性ショック

UCI
umbilical cord implantation　臍帯埋没療法
urethral catheter in　尿道カテーテル挿入
urinary catheter in　尿路カテーテル挿入
usual childhood illness　小児期通常疾患

UCL
ulnar collateral ligament　(肘関節の)内側側副靱帯
uncomfortable loudness level　不快音量域値
upper control limit　上方管理限界

UCL, U Cl
urea clearance (test)　尿素クリアランス(検査)

UCLL
uncomfortable loudness level　不快音レベル

UCLP
unilateral cleft of lip and palate　片側口唇口蓋裂

UCM
unclassified cardiomyopathy　型不明心筋症

UCO
urethral catheter out　尿道カテーテル抜去
urinary catheter out　尿路カテーテル抜去
UCP
urethral closure pressure　尿道閉鎖圧
urinary coproporphyrin　尿(中)コプロポルフィリン
urinary C peptide　尿(中)Cペプチド
UCPA
United Cerebral Palsy Association　米国脳性麻痺協会
UCP max
maximum urethral closure pressure　最高尿道閉鎖圧
UCPP
urethral closure pressure profile　尿道閉鎖圧曲線
UCPT
urinary coproporphyrin test　尿(中)コプロポルフィリン検査
UCR
unconditioned reflex　無条件反射
unconditioned response　無条件反応
UCRE
urine creatinine　尿クレアチニン
UCS
unconditioned stimulation　無条件反射
unconditioned stimulus　無条件刺激
uterine compression syndrome　子宮圧迫症候群
UC & S
urine culture and sensitivity　尿培養と感受性
UCS, Ucs
unconscious　無意識の，意識のない，意識不明の
UCT
ultrasonic cardiotomogram　超音波心断層図
ultrasound cardiotomogram　超音波心断層図
unchanged conventional treatment　不変在来治療
UCTD
unclassifiable connective tissue disease　分類不能の結合組織疾患
undifferentiated connective tissue disease　未分化結合組織疾患
UCTS
undifferentiated connective tissues syndrome　未分化結合組織症候群
UCU
urinary care unit(s)　泌尿器治療ユニット
UCV
uncontrolled variable　自由度

UD
ulcerative dermatosis 潰瘍性皮膚病
ulcus duodeni 十二指腸潰瘍
ulnar deviation 尺側偏位〔偏差〕
underdeveloped 体格不良の
undifferentiated 未分化の
unipolar depression 単極性うつ病
unit dose 単位量
urethral discharge 尿道排泄物
urethral drainage 尿道ドレナージ
uridine diphosphate ウリジン二リン酸
uroporphyrinogen decarboxylase ウロポルフィリノゲンデカルボキシラーゼ
uterine delivery 子宮分娩
uterine distention 子宮拡張

ud
undifferentiated (carcinoma) 未分化型(癌)

u.d.
ut dictum〈ラ〉 指示どおり

UDC
undeveloped countries 低開発国
uninhibited detrusor (muscle) capacity 非抑制排尿(筋)容量
Universal Decimal Classification 国際十進分類法
usual disease of childhood 小児期通常疾患

UDCA
ursodeoxycholic acid ウルソデオキシコール酸

UDD
unit dose dispensing 1回量分配

udf
und die folgende〈独〉 次のように

UDI
urinary diagnostic index 泌尿器疾患診断指数

UDN
ulcerated dermal necrosis 潰瘍性皮膚壊死

UDO
undetermined origin 未確定原因
unwilling drop-out 不本意な脱落《統》

UDP
unassisted diastolic pressure 無補助拡張期圧
unit dose package 1回量包装
uridine diphosphate ウリジン二リン酸
uridine 5′-diphosphate ウリジン5′-二リン酸

5′-UDP
uridine 5′-diphosphate ウリジン5′-二リン酸

UDPG
uridine diphosphate glucose　ウリジン二リン酸グルコース
uridine diphosphate glucuronic acid　ウリジン二リン酸グルクロン酸

UDPGA
uridine diphosphate glucuronate　ウリジン二リン酸グルクロン酸
uridine diphosphoglucuronic acid　ウリジン二リン酸グルクロン酸

UDPGal, UDP-Gal, UDPgal
uridine diphosphate galactose acid　ウリジン二リン酸ガラクトース

UDP-Glc, UDP-glc
uridine diphosphate glucose　ウリジン二リン酸グルコース

UDPGT
uridine diphosphate glucuronyl transferase　ウリジン二リン酸グルクロン酸転移酵素

UDS
ultra-Doppler sonography　超音波ド(ッ)プラー法
unconditioned stimulus　無条件刺激
unscheduled DNA synthesis　不定期DNA合成
urodynamic study　尿水力学検査

UDT
undescended testicle　停留精巣〔睾丸〕

UE
ultrasonic endoscope　超音波内視鏡
uncertain etiology　不確定な病因
under elbow　肘下の
undetermined etiology　原因不明の病因
uninvolved epidermis　非罹患表皮
upper esophagus　上部食道
upper extremities　上肢

UEA
upper extremity arterial　上肢動脈性の

UEA-1
Ulex Europian agglutinin I　ヨーロッパ産ハリエニシダ凝集素 I

UEG
ultrasonic encephalogram　超音波脳造影
unifocal eosinophilic granuloma　単病巣好酸球(性)肉芽腫

UEP
unit evolutionary period　単位進化時間

UES
undifferentiated embryonal sarcoma　未分化の胎芽肉腫
upper esophageal sphincter　上部食道括約筋

UESP
upper esophageal sphincter pressure　上部食道括約筋圧
UESR
upper esophageal sphincter relaxation　上部食道括約筋弛緩
Uext, U/ext, u/ext
upper extremity　上肢
UF
ultrafiltrate　限外濾過物
ultrafiltration　限外濾過
ultrasonic frequency　超音波周波数
uncertainty factor　不確定因子
universal feeder　共通供給者
unknown factor　未知因子
until finished　終わるまで
urea formaldehyde　ホルムアルデヒド尿素
urinary formaldehyde　尿(中)ホルムアルデヒド
UFA
unesterified (free) fatty acid　非エステル化(遊離)脂肪酸
UFCa
ultrafiltrable calcium　限外濾過性カルシウム
UFCT
ultrafast computed tomography　超高速コンピュータ断層撮影(法)
UFM
uroflowmetry　尿流量測定
UFMG
uroflowmetrogram　尿流曲線
UFMg
ultrafiltrable magnesium　限外濾過性マグネシウム
UFP
ultrafiltration pressure　限外濾過圧
UFR
ultrafiltration rate　限外濾過率
urine filtration rate　尿濾過率
UFV
ultrafiltration volume　限外濾過量
UG
upward gaze　上方注視
urethrogram　尿道造影
urethrography　尿道造影撮影法
urinary glucose　尿中グルコース
urogastrone　ウロガストロン
urogenital　(泌)尿生殖器の, 尿性器の
uteroglobulin　子宮グロブリン

Ug.
unguentum〈ラ〉, Unguentum〈独〉= ointment　軟膏《処》

U/G
general urinalysis　一般検尿

UGA
under general anesthesia　全身麻酔(法)下で
uracil, guanine, adenine (= termination codon)　ウラシル・グアニン・アデニン(=終止コドン)
urogenital atrophy　尿生殖器萎縮(症)

UGAA
urethritis gonorrhoica anterior acuta　急性淋菌性前部尿道炎

UGD
urogenital diaphragm　尿生殖隔膜

U-gen
urobilinogen　ウロビリノゲン

UGF
unidentified growth factor　未確認成長因子
urinary gonadotropin fragment　尿中ゴナドトロピン分画

UGH
uveitis-glaucoma-hyphema (syndrome)　ブドウ膜炎・緑内障・前房出血(症候群)

UGH+
uveitis-glaucoma-hyphema plus vitreous hemorrhage (syndrome)　ブドウ膜炎・緑内障・前房出血および硝子体出血(症候群)

UGI
upper gastrointestinal　上部胃腸の
upper gastrointestinal (tract)　上部消化(管)の

UGIB
upper gastrointestinal bleeding　上部消化管出血

UGIH
upper gastrointestinal (tract) hemorrhage　上部消化(管)出血

UGIS
upper gastrointestinal series　上部消化管(X線)造影

UGIT
upper gastrointestinal tract　上部消化管

UGP
urinary gonadotropin peptide　尿中ゴナドトロピンペプチド

UGPA
urethritis gonorrhoica posterior acuta　急性淋菌性後部尿道炎

UGPP
uridyldiphosphate glucose pyrophosphorylase　ウリジル二リン酸グルコースピロリン酸分解酵素

UGS
urogenital sinus 尿生殖洞
UGT
uridine diphosphate glucuronosyltransferase ウリジン二リン酸グルクロン酸転移酵素
urogenital tuberculosis 泌尿生殖器結核
UH
umbilical hernia 臍ヘルニア
upper half 上半分
UHD
unstable hemoglobin disease 不安定ヘモグロビン病
UHF
ultra-high frequency (wave) 超高周波，極超短波
Ultrahochvakuum〈独〉 超高(度)真空
UHFV
ultrahigh-frequency ventilation 超高頻度人工換気法
UHL
unilateral hilar lymph node enlargement 一側性肺門リンパ節腫大
universal hypertrichosis lanuginosa 全身性胎生毛性多毛(症)
UHMW
ultrahigh molecular weight 超高分子量
UHMWPE
ultrahigh molecular weight polyethylene 超高分子ポリエチレン
UHR
underlying heart rhythm 基礎心拍リズム
universal hip replacement 人工骨頭置換術
UHT
ultrahigh temperature 超高温
UHV
ultrahigh vacuum 超高(度)真空
UHV, uhv
ultrahigh voltage 超高電圧
UI
Ulcer Index 潰瘍指数
ultrasound imaging 超音波画像
urinary incontinence 尿失禁
uroporphyrin isomerase ウロポルフィリンイソメラーゼ
uroporphyrinogen isomerase ウロポルフィリノゲンイソメラーゼ
u.i.
ut infra〈ラ〉 下のように《処》
UIBC
unbound iron-binding capacity 遊離鉄結合能

unsaturated iron binding capacity　不飽和鉄結合能

UIC
uninhibited contraction　(膀胱の)無抑制性収縮

UICC
Unio - International Contra Cancer〈ラ〉=L'Union Internationale Contre le Cancer〈仏〉　国際対癌協会

UICC classification
union international counter cancer classification　国際対癌連合分類

UICPA
Union Internationale de Chimie Pure et Appliquée〈仏〉　純粋応用化学国際連合

UICT
Union Internationale Contre la Tuberculose〈仏〉　国際結核予防連合

u.i.d.
uno in die〈ラ〉　毎日1回《処》

UID/S
unilateral interfacetal dislocation or subluxation　片側小関節面脱臼または亜脱臼

UIEP
urine immunoelectrophoresis　尿免疫電気泳動(法)

UIES
International Union for Health Education　国際保健教育連合

UIHSU
Union Internationale d'Hygiène et de Médecine Scolaires et Universitaires〈仏〉　国際学校保健連合

UIMC
Union Internationale des Services Médicaux des Chemins de Fer　国際鉄道医療連合

UIP
Union Internationale de Phlébologie〈仏〉　国際静脈外科連合
unusual interstitial pneumonitis　非通常型間質性肺炎
usual interstitial pneumonia　通常型間質性肺炎
usual interstitial pneumonia (of Liebow)　(リーボウの)通常型間質性肺炎
usual interstitial pneumonitis　通常(型)間質性肺炎

UIPPA
International Union of Pure and Applied Physics　国際純粋応用物理学連合

UIPVT
Union Internationale contre le Péril Vénérien et les Tréponématoses〈仏〉　国際性病予防連合

UIQ
upper inner quadrant　上内1/4区(＝四半部)

UISAE
Union Internationale des Sciences Anthropologiques et Ethnologiques〈仏〉　人類科学・人種科学国際連合

UISB
International Union of Biological Science　国際生物科学連合
Union Internationale des Sciences Biologiques〈仏〉　国際生物科学連合

UISE
Union Internationale de Secours aux Enfants〈仏〉　国際児童福祉連合

UISN
International Union of Nutritional Science　国際栄養科学連合
Union Internationale des Science de la Nutrition〈仏〉　国際栄養科学連合

UJ
universal joint (syndrome)　自在関節(症候群)

UK
unknown　不明の，未知の
urinary kallikrein　尿(中)カリクレイン
urine potassium　尿(中)カリウム
urokinase　ウロキナーゼ

UKA
unicompartmental knee arthroplasty　片側人工膝関節置換術

UKa
urinary kallikrein　尿(中)カリクレイン

UKF
Unterkieferfraktur〈独〉　下顎骨骨折

UK IC
urokinase intracoronary　ウロキナーゼ冠注

UKK
Unterkieferkrebs〈独〉　下顎癌

U

UKT
United Kingdom Transplant　英国移植協会

UKW
Ultrakurzwellen〈独〉　超短波

UL
unauthorized leave　無許可休暇
undifferentiated lymphoma　未分化リンパ腫

upper lid 上眼瞼
upper limb 上肢
upper limit 上限
upper lobe 上葉

Ul
Ulcer Index 潰瘍指数

Ul-Ⅰ-Ⅳ
ulcer Index Ⅰ-Ⅳ 潰瘍指数Ⅰ～Ⅳ(度)

U & L, U/L
upper and lower 上および下

U & LC
upper and lower case 上と下の場合

ULDH
urinary lactic acid dehydrogenase 尿(中)乳酸脱水素酵素

UlF
ultra-low frequency 超低周波

ULL
uncomfortable loudness level 不快音量レベル

ULLE
upper lid, left eye 上眼瞼・左眼

ULN
upper limits of normal 正常値の上限

uln
ulna(r) 尺骨(の)

ULO
upper limb orthosis 上肢矯正器具

ULP
upper limb prosthesis 上肢(人工)装具，上義肢

ULPE
upper lobe pulmonary edema 上葉肺水腫

ULQ
upper left quadrant 上左部1/4区(＝四半部)，左上象限

ULR
guaifenesin, phenylpropanolamine, and phenylephrine グアイフェネシン・フェニルプロパノールアミン・フェニレフリン

ULRE
upper lid, right eye 上眼瞼・右眼

ULS
ultrasonic laparoscope 超音波腹腔鏡

ULT
ultrahigh temperature 超高温

ult
ultimate 最終の，最後の

U

ult.praes.
ultimum praescriptus〈ラ〉 最後の処方《処》

ULV
ultra-low volume (spray) 超微量(散布)

UM
Mache unit マッヘ単位
unmarried 未婚の
untere Muschel〈独〉 下鼻甲介
upper motor (neuron) 上位運動(ニューロン)
uracil mustard ウラシルマスタード
uromorulin ウロモルリン

UMA
urinary muramidase activity 尿(中)ムラミダーゼ活性

Umax
maximum urinary osmolality 最大尿浸透圧

umb
umbilical 臍の
umbilicus 臍

umb.reg.
umbilical region 臍部

UMCD
uremic medullary cystic disease 尿毒症性髄質嚢胞病

UMG
uretero-manometrography 尿管内圧検査法

UMHP
World Organization of Science for the History of Pharmacy 世界薬学史学会機構

UMIN
university medical information network 大学医療情報ネットワーク, ユーミン

UMLS
Unified Medical Language System 統合型の医学用語システム

UMN
upper motor neuron 上位運動ニューロン

UMNB
upper motor neurogenic bladder 上位運動神経因性膀胱(障害)

UMNL
upper motor neuron lesion 上位運動ニューロン障害

UMP
uridine monophosphate ウリジン一リン酸

UMPK
uridine monophosphate kinase ウリジン一リン酸キナーゼ

UMS
urethral manipulation syndrome 尿道操作症候群

UN
ulnar nerve 尺骨神経

undernoutrished 低栄養の
United Nations 国際連合
urea nitrogen 尿素窒素
urinary nitrogen 尿窒素

un
unable 不可能な

u.n.
usu noto〈ラ〉 周知の方法で《処》

U_{Na}
urinary concentration of sodium 尿中ナトリウム濃度

UNa
urinary natrium (sodium) 尿中ナトリウム

unab
unabridged 要約しない

unacc
unaccompanied ～を伴わない

UNAIDS
A joint response to HIV/AIDS 国連エイズ計画

unan
unanimous 一致した

UNARCO
United Nations Narcotics Commission 麻薬協議会国際連合

unc
unconscious 意識のない，無意識の

UNCED
United Nation Conference on Environment and Development 国連環境開発会議

uncert
uncertainties 不確実(性)

unchg
unchanged 不変の

unclas
unclassified 分類不能の

uncod
uncovered 矯正されない

uncomp
uncompensated 非代償(性)の
uncomplicated 合併症のない

uncompl
uncomplicated 合併症のない

uncon
unconscious 無意識の，意識のない

uncond
unconditioned 無条件の

uncond.ref
unconditioned reflex 無条件反射
uncond.resp
unconditioned response 無条件反応
uncoop
uncooperative 非協力的な
UNCOR, uncor
uncorrected 補正〔矯正〕していない
uncorr
uncorrected 補正〔矯正〕していない
UnCS, unCS
unconditioned stimulus 無条件刺激
unct.
unctus〈ラ〉 塗抹した《処》
UNCV
ulnar nerve conduction velocity 尺骨神経伝導速度
UNDCP
United Nations International Drug Control Programme 国連薬物統制計画
undet
undetermined 決定されていない，不明の
undet.etiol.
undetermined etiology 原因不明の
undet.orig.
undetermined origin 原因不明の，起源不明の
UNDP
United Nations Development Programme 国連開発計画
UNEP
United Nations Environment Program 国連環境計画
UNESCO
United Nations Educational, Scientific and Cultural Organization 国連教育科学文化機関，ユネスコ
UNFDAC
United Nations Fund for Drug Abuse Control 薬物乱用規制国際連合基金
unfin
unfinished 未完の
UNFPA
United Nations Funds for Population Activities 人口活動国際連合基金
UNG, ung.
unguentum〈ラ〉 軟膏《処》

ungt.
unguentum〈ラ〉　軟膏《処》
UNICEF
United Nations International Children's Emergency Fund　国連児童基金
unicorp
unicorporated　単一提携の
unif
uniform　単一型
uniformity　単一型の
unilat
unilateral　片側(性)の
unis
unisexual　単一性の
univ
universal　世界的な，普遍的な
universally　世界的に，普遍的に
Univ, univ
university　大学
UNK, unk
unknown　不明の
unkn
unknown　不明の
unof
unofficial　非公式の，非局方の
unoff
unofficial　非公式の，非局方の
UNOS
United Network for Organ Sharing　米国臓器移植ネットワーク
UNP
ulnar nerve palsy　尺骨神経麻痺
unqual
unqualified　品質化されていない
unrem
unremitting　非再燃性の
unremit
unremitting　非再燃性の
unrep
unreported　未報告の
unrepresented　未提示の
UNRRA
United Nations Relief and Rehabilitation Administration　救済と社会復帰国際連合機関
uns
unsatisfactory　不満足な

UnS, un.s.
unconditioned stimulus 無条件刺激
***uns*-, uns**
unsymmetrical 非対称的な
unsat
unsatisfactory 不満足な
unsaturated 不飽和の
UNSCEAR
United Nations Scientific Committee on Effects of Atomic Radiation 原子爆弾の放射線の影響に関する国際連合科学委員会
unst
unstable 不安定な
unsteady ふらふらする
unsw
unsweetened 甘味を加えていない
unsym
unsymmetrical 非対称の
Unters
Untersuchung〈独〉 検査
UNTS
unilateral nevoid telangiectasia syndrome 片側性母斑性毛細血管拡張症候群
UNX
uninephrectomy 片腎切除(術)
UO
undetermined origin 原因不明の
ureteral orifice 尿管口
urinary output 尿路排出
urine output 尿排出
UO, U/O
under observation 観察下(の)
U/O adeq
urine output adequate 尿量適量
UOD
ultimate oxygen demand 最終酸素需要
UOP
urinary output 尿路排出
UOQ
upper outer quadrant 上外1/4区(＝四半部)
UOsm
urinary osmolality 尿重量オスモル濃度，尿浸透圧
Uosm
urinary osmolality 尿(容量)浸透圧
UP
ulcerative proctitis 潰瘍性直腸炎

ultrahigh purity	超高純度
umbilical portion	臍部
under proof	保証付きの
unipolar	単極の
Unna-Pappenheim (stain)	ウンナ・パッペンハイム(染色)
upper quahile	上位1/4区
upright posture	立位
ureteropelvic	尿管腎盂の，尿管骨盤の
uridine phosphorylase	ウリジンホスホリラーゼ
urinary protein	尿蛋白
urine gonadotropin	尿中ゴナドトロピン
urine protein	尿蛋白
uroporphyrin	ウロポルフィリン
uvulopalatopharyngoplasty	口蓋垂口蓋咽頭形成術

Up

hyperosmolar urea and prostaglandin	高濃度尿素とプロスタグランジン

up

unproof	未証明
unproofed	未証明の

U/P

concentration in urine and plasma	尿中・血漿中濃度
urine-plasma ratio	尿・血漿比

UPA, u-PA

urokinase (type) plasminogen activator	ウロキナーゼ型プラスミノゲンアクチベータ

UPA-R

urokinase plasminogen activator receptor	ウロキナーゼ型プラスミノゲンアクチベータ受容体

UPC

universal product code	全般的生産コード
unknown primary carcinoma	原発癌不明

UPD

urinary production (rate)	尿産生(率)

UPG

uroporphyrinogen	ウロポルフィリノゲン

UPI

University Personality Inventory	学生精神健康調査
uteroplacental insufficiency	子宮胎盤(機能)不全(症)
uteroplacental ischemia	子宮胎盤虚血

UPIGO

Union Professionnelle Internationale des Gynécologistes et Obstétriciens 〈仏〉	産科婦人科国際専門家連合

UPJ
ureteropelvic junction　腎盂尿管接合部

UPL
upper left　上左(象限)
upper leg　大腿

UPLIF
unilateral posterior lumbar interbody fusion　片側後方腰椎椎体固定(術)

UPmax
maximum urethral pressure　最高尿道内圧

up OOB ad lib
up out of bed ad libitum　自由にベッドから出て立ってよい

UPOR
usual place of residence　通常居住地

UPP
urethral pressure profile　尿道内圧曲線
urethral pressure profilometry　尿道内圧測定
uvulopalatoplasty　口蓋垂口蓋形成術

upper GI
upper gastrointestinal series　上部消化管撮影

upper GI series
upper gastrointestinal series　上部消化管X線検査

UPPP
uvulopalatopharyngoplasty　軟口蓋咽頭形成術

UPPRA
upright peripheral plasma renin activity　立位末梢血漿レニン活性

UPS
ultraviolet photoelectron spectroscopy　紫外線光電子分光鏡検査(法)
uroporphyrinogen synthetase　ウロポルフィリノゲン合成酵素
uterine progesterone system　子宮プロゲステロン系

UPSC
uterine papillary serous carcinoma　子宮乳頭状漿液細胞癌

UPSIT
University of Pennsylvania smell identification test　ペンシルベニア大学嗅覚鑑定試験

UPT
urine pregnancy test　尿妊娠検査

upt
uptake　摂取率《核医学》

UPTD
unit pulmonary toxic dose　肺毒性単位

UQ
ubiquinone　ユビキノン
upper quadrant　上位部1/4区(＝四半部)，上象限
urine quantity　尿量

UR
unconditional response　無条件反応
unconditioned reflex　無条件反射
unit risk　ユニットリスク
unrelated　無関係の
upper respiratory　上部呼吸器の
uridine　ウリジン
urinal　蓄尿器，蓄尿ビン
urinary retention　尿うっ滞
utilization review　医療費内容審査

u/r
upper right　上右(象限)

UR，Ur，Ur.
urologist　泌尿器科医
urology　泌尿器科(学)

UR，Ur，ur
urinary　尿の，泌尿器の
urine　尿

ura
urethral　尿道の

Ura，URA
uracil　ウラシル

ur anal，ur.anal.
urinalysis　尿検査，検尿
urine analysis　尿分析

uranog
uranographer　口蓋図
uranographic　口蓋図の
uranography　口蓋図

URC
upper rib cage　上胸部

URD
undifferentiated respiratory disease　鑑別診断不可呼吸器疾患
unrelated donor　非血縁ドナー
unspecific respiratory disease　非特異的呼吸器疾患
upper respiratory disease　上部気道疾患，上部呼吸器疾患

Urd，URD
uridine　ウリジン

Urd-5′-P
uridine 5′-monophosphate　ウリジン5′-一リン酸

Urd-5′-P2
uridine 5′-diphosphate　ウリジン5′-二リン酸
Urd-5′-P3
uridine 5′-triphosphate　ウリジン5′-三リン酸
ure
ureteral　尿管の
Urea N
urea nitrogen　尿素窒素
URED
unable to read　読字不能
ureth
urethra　尿道
urethral　尿道の
URF
uterine relaxing factor　子宮弛緩因子
urg
urgent　緊急の
URI
upper respiratory illiness　上部気道疾患
upper respiratory tract infection　上部気道感染(症)
urinary 17-KS
urinary 17-ketosteroid　尿中17-ケトステロイド
urinary 17-OHCS
urinary 17-hydroxycorticosteroid　尿中17-ヒドロキシコルチコステロイド
urinary 17-OS
urinary 17-oxosteroid　尿中17-オキソステロイド
URL
uniform resource locator　ユーアールエル(=インターネット上の情報の住所)
UR & M
urinalysis, routine and microscopic　尿検査・通常および顕微鏡法
URO
uroporphyrin　ウロポルフィリン
uro, Uro, URO
urological　泌尿器(科)の
urology　泌尿器科(学)
UROgen
uroporphyrinogen　ウロポルフィリノゲン
uro-gen
urogenital　(泌)尿生殖器の，尿性器の
Urol, urol, urol.
urologist　泌尿器科医
urology　泌尿器科(学)
URQ
upper right quadrant　上右部1/4区(=四半部)

URT
upper respiratory tract 上部呼吸器，上部気道
uterine resting tone 安静時子宮緊張度
URTI
upper respiratory tract illness 上部呼吸器疾患
upper respiratory tract infection 上部気道感染症
URVD
unilateral renovascular disease 片側性腎血管疾患
US
ultrasonic 超音波の
ultrasonic examination 超音波検査
ultrasonography 超音波検査(法)
ultrasound 超音波
ultrasound imaging 超音波診断法《画診》
unconditioned stimulation 無条件刺激
unconditioned structure 無条件構造，絶対構造
unknown significance 意義不明
Unterschenkel〈独〉 下腿
upper segment 上部
urine sugar 尿糖
Usher syndrome アッシャー症候群
us
usu 用いよ《処》
u.s.
ut supra〈ラ〉 前と同じ
USAFH
United States Air Force Hospital 米国空軍病院
USAH
United States Army Hospital 米国陸軍病院
USAHC
United States Army Health Clinic 米国陸軍診療所
USAIDR
United States Army Institute of Dental Research 米国陸軍歯科研究所
USAIDS
United States Agency for International Development 米国国際開発庁
USAMEDS
United States Army Medical Service 米国陸軍医療サービス
USAN
United States Adopted Names (Council) 米国公用名，米国承認名
USAP
unstable angina pectoris 不安定狭心症

USB
universal serial bus　ユーエスビー(＝PCインターフェイス)
upper sternal border　上部胸骨縁
USBS
United States Bureau of Standards　米国規格局
USBuStand
United States Bureau of Standards　米国規格局
USCVD
unsterile controlled vaginal delivery　非滅菌管理経腟分娩
USD
United States Dispensatory　米国薬局方注解
USDEA
United States Drug Enforcement Agency　米国薬効局
USDHEW
United States Department of Health, Education and Welfare　米国健康教育福祉局
USE
ultrasonic echography(＝ultrasonography)　超音波検査(法)
USERID
user identification　使用者確認
us.ext.
usus externus〈ラ〉　外用《処》
usf
und so fort〈独〉　などなど
USFMS
United States foreign medical (school) student　米国外国医科(大学)学生
USG
ultrasonogram　超音波検査図《画診》
ultrasonography　超音波診断(法)《画診》
USH
usual state of health　通常の健康状態
USI
urinary stress incontinence　緊張性尿失禁, ストレス(性)尿失禁
us.int.
usus internus〈ラ〉　内用《処》
USMC
United States Medicinal Chemistry　米国医薬化学連合
USMH
United States Marine Hospital　米国海兵隊病院

USMLE
United States Medical Licensing Examination　米国医学資格審査方式の1つ
USN
ultrasonic nebulizer　超音波ネブライザー
USO
unilateral salpingo-oophorectomy　片側卵管卵巣摘出
USOGH
usual state of good health　通常の健康良好状態
USOH
usual state of health　通常の健康状態
USP
United States Pharmacop(o)eia　米国薬局方
upper sternal border　胸骨上縁
US pat
United States patent　米国特許
USPDI
United States Pharmacop(o)eia Drug Information　米国薬局方薬品情報
USPhar, US phar
United States Pharmacop(o)eia　米国薬局方
USPHS
United States Public Health Service　米国公衆衛生局
USPU
United States Pharmacop(o)eia Unit　米国薬局方単位
USR
unheated serum reagin (test)　非加熱血清レアギン(試験)
USS
ultrasound scanning　超音波スキャニング
ust.
ustus〈ラ〉　焦性の，焼かれた
US tip
ultrasound tip　超音波チップ
USU
Unterschenkelumfang〈独〉　下腿周長
USUCVD
unsterile uncontrolled vaginal delivery　非滅菌自然経腟分娩
USVH
United States Veterans Hospital　米国在郷軍人病院
USW
ultrashort wave　超短波
ultrasonic wave　超音波
usw.
und so weiter〈独〉　その他

UT
Ullrich-Turner (syndrome) ウルリッヒ・ターナー(症候群)
universal time 万国時間
Unna-Thost (syndrome) ウンナ・トースト(症候群)
untested 未検査の
untreated 未治療の
urinary tract 尿路
urticaria 蕁麻疹

UTBG
unbound TBG(=thyroxin-binding globulin) 非結合チ〔サイ〕ロキシン結合グロブリン，非結合TBG

UTC
coordinated universal time 協定世界時

UTD
up to date 最近の

ut dic.
ut dictum〈ラ〉=as directed 指示どおり(に)《処》

ut dict.
ut dictum〈ラ〉=as directed 指示どおり(に)《処》

utend.
utendus〈ラ〉 使用される，用いられる
utendus〈ラ〉 使用せよ《処》

utend.mor.sol.
utendus more solito〈ラ〉 通常方法で使用せよ《処》

ut ft
ut flat〈ラ〉 作られるように《処》

UTI
urinary tract infection 尿路感染(症)
urinary trypsin inhibitor 尿(中)トリプシン抑制〔阻害〕物質

ut.inf.
ut infra〈ラ〉 下記のように《処》

UTIs
urinary tract infections 尿路感染症

UTJ
utero-tubal junction 子宮卵管境界

UTLD
Utah Test of Language Development 言語発達ユタ検査

U

UTM
urinary tract malformation 尿路奇形

UTO
upper tibial osteotomy 上部脛骨切り術

UTOC
upper thoracic outlet compression (syndrome) 上(部)胸郭出口圧迫(症候群)

UTP
unilateral tension pneumothorax 片側(性)緊張(性)気胸
uridine triphosphate ウリジン三リン酸

5′-UTP
uridine 5′-triphosphate ウリジン5′-三リン酸

UTS
Ullrich-Turner syndrome ウルリッヒ・ターナー症候群
ulnar tunnel syndrome 尺骨トンネル症候群
ultimate tensile strength 超張力
ultrasound 超音波

ut supr.
ut supra〈ラ〉 上記のように《処》

UTZ
ultrasound 超音波

UU
urinary urea 尿中尿素
urine urobilinogen 尿(中)ウロビリノゲン

UUD
uncontrolled unsterile delivery 自然非滅菌分娩

UUE
use until exhausted 消耗するまで使う，排泄されるまで使う

UUN
urinary urea nitrogen excretion 尿中尿素窒素排泄
urine urea nitrogen 尿中尿素窒素

UUO
unilateral ureteral occulusion 片側尿管閉塞(症)

UUP
urine uroporphyrin 尿(中)ウロポルフィリン

UV
ulcus ventriculi 胃潰瘍
ultraviolet 紫外(線)の
ultraviolet light 紫外線(光)
umbilical cord 臍帯
umbilical vein 臍静脈
ureterovesical 尿管膀胱の
urinary volume 尿路排泄量
urine volume 尿量

U_v
Uppsala virus ウプサラウイルス

UVA
ultraviolet A (ray) 長波長紫外線，紫外線A
ureterovesical angle 尿管膀胱角

UVAC
uterine vacuum aspirating curette 子宮真空吸引掻爬器

UVASER
ultraviolet amplification by stimulated emission of radiation　照射放出刺激による紫外線増幅
UVB
ultraviolet B (ray)　中波長紫外線，紫外線B
UVC
ultraviolet C (ray)　短波長紫外線，紫外線C
umbilical venous catheter　臍静脈カテーテル
UVCY
ultraviolet-cut & non-cyanopsia　紫外線削除・非青視
UVEB
unifocal ventricular ectopic beat　一焦点心室異所性拍動
UVER
ultraviolet-enhanced reactivation　紫外線増強再活性化
UV fistula
ureterovaginal fistula　尿管腟瘻
UVG
urethrovesicography　尿道膀胱撮影
UVH
univentricular heart　単心室
UVI
ultraviolet irradiation　紫外線放散，紫外線照射
UVJ
ureterovesical junction　尿管膀胱移行(結合)部
UVJ-stenosis
ureterovesical junction stenosis　尿管膀胱移行(結合)部狭窄
UVL
ultraviolet light　紫外線(光)
UV lamp
ultraviolet lamp　紫外線殺菌灯
UV light
ultraviolet light　紫外線
UV method
ultraviolet method　紫外部測定法
UV/MV
umbilical vein to maternal vein　臍静脈・母体静脈
UVP
ultraviolet photometry　紫外線光度計測(法)，紫外線測光
U
UV/P
concentration of solute urine　尿中溶質濃度
UVR
ultraviolet radiation　紫外線照射
UV ray
ultraviolet ray　紫外線

UV-reactivation
ultraviolet light reactivation 紫外線回復

UVSC
ultraviolet solar constant 紫外線太陽恒数

UV therapy
ultraviolet therapy 紫外線療法

UW
unilateral weakness 片側(性)脱力

U/WB
unit of whole blood 全血単位

UWD
Urbach-Wiethe disease ウルバッハ・ヴィーテ病

UWL
unstirred water layer 攪拌されにくい水の層

UWM
unwed mother 未婚の母

UWT
urea washout test 尿素洗い出し試験

UX
uranium X(=proactinium) ウランX(=プロアクチニウム)

Ux
urinalysis 尿検査, 検尿

ux.
uxor〈ラ〉 妻

UX_1
uranium X_1 ウラニウム〔ウラン〕X_1

V v

V

coefficient of variation	変動〔変異〕係数《統計》
corneal vascularization	角膜内血管進入
unipolar chest lead	単極胸部導出〔誘導〕《心電》
vaccinated	予防接種を受けた
vaccine	ワクチン
vagina	腟，鞘
valine	バリン
vanadium	バナジウム〈元素〉
variable	可変の，不定の，可変部
varicella	水痘
vegetarian	菜食主義者
vegetation	増殖(症)，生長，成長
vehicle	基剤，賦形剤
ventilation	換気(量)
ventilator	人工呼吸器，換気装置，ベンチレータ(ー)
ventricular (wave)	心室(波)
vermiform process	虫垂
vertebral	椎骨の
vertex sharp transient	頭蓋頂鋭波《脳波》
vertical	垂直，垂直の
vestibular	前庭の，前房の
vial	バイアル，小ビン
vires	力〈複数〉
virgin	処女の，初めての
virulence	菌力，毒力，発病力
virulent	有毒の，毒性の
vis	力〈単数〉
visit	訪問，来院
visitor	訪問者
visual	視覚の
vitamin	ビタミン
vitreous	硝子(体)の，ガラス(状)の
vitrum〈ラ〉	ビン《処》
volt	ボルト〈単位〉
voltage	電圧
volume of a gas	気体の容積・体積
vomiting	嘔吐，吐き出したもの

v

vaccerine	ワセリン
vaccum	吸引する，真空(化)，減圧
vaccum tube	吸引管

value	値
vapor	蒸気
vascular invasion	リンパ管侵襲
vein invasion	静脈侵襲
venule	小静脈，細静脈
verification of cure	治癒の証明
vessel	血管
vicinal	隣接の
viscosity	粘稠度
visibility	可視性
von〈独〉	フォン(＝姓につける前置詞)

v.

vespere〈ラ〉＝in the evening	晩に《処》
vide〈ラ〉＝see	見よ，参照せよ《処》

V_0

initial velocity	初速度

V_{0-3}

vascular invasion	(癌細胞の)脈管浸潤の有無と程度

V_1

ophthalmic division of fifth cranial nerve	第5脳神経眼枝

V_2

maxillary division of fifth cranial nerve	第5脳神経上顎枝

V_3

mandibular division of fifth cranial nerve	第5脳神経下顎枝

$\dot{V}$

gas volume/unit time (flow velocity)	単位時間あたりのガス量〔気流〕(速度)

$\bar{v}$

mixed venous blood	混合静脈血
venous admixture	混合静脈血

v^-

viral	ウイルス(由来)の〈接〉

V, v

(roman numeral) five	(ローマ数字の) 5
valve	弁
variation	変異，変動，変種
velocity	速度(＝m/s)
venous	静脈の
venous blood	静脈血
ventral	腹側の
ventricle	室，心室，脳室
ventricular	心室の，脳室の

verbal	言語の，口頭の，口述の
vertex	頭(蓋)頂，頂
very	非常に
violet	紫，バイオレット
virus	ウイルス
voice	声の
volume	容積，体積，容量

V, V.

Vibrio	ビブリオ(属)
vision	視覚，視力
visual acuity	視力

V, *V*

vector	ベクトル，媒介者

V, v, v.

vena〈ラ〉=vein	静脈
versus〈ラ〉=towards, in that direction	～対～，～に対して

+V, +v

positive vertical divergence	実性垂直性開散

VA

alveolar volume	肺胞容量〔容積〕
anatomical volume	解剖学的容積
vacuum aspiration	真空吸引(法)
valve area	弁口面積
vancomycin	バンコマイシン
variant angina	異型狭心症
vascular access	バスキュラーアクセス
vasodilator agent	血管拡張薬
(nucleus) ventralis anterior	前腹側(核)
ventricular aneurysm	心室動脈瘤
ventricular arrhythmia	心室性不整脈
ventroanterior	腹側前部の
vertebral artery	椎骨動脈
vestibular asymmetry	前庭左右不均衡
Veterans Administration	退役軍人管理〔運営〕
vinca alkaloid	アルカロイド
viral antigen	ウイルス性抗原
visual agnosia	視覚失認
visual aid	視覚補助
visual axis	視軸
vitamin A	ビタミンA
voltaic alternative	電気交流

Va

arterial gas volume	動脈血ガス量

V.a.

Verdacht auf〈独〉	～の疑い

VA, Va
visual acuity 視力
VA, va
volt ampere ボルトアンペア
VA, V-A
ventriculo-atrial (心)室(心)房の
$\dot{V}_A$, V_A
alveolar ventilation per minute 分時肺胞換気量
volume of alveolar gas 肺胞気容積〔容量〕
VAA
Vaccination Assistance Act ワクチン接種協力機構
vasoactive amine 血管作用性アミン
virus associated antigen ウイルス関連抗原
VAB
veno-arterial bypass (大腿)静動脈バイパス(術)
vinblastine sulfate, actinomycin D, bleomycin 硫酸ビンブラスチン,アクチノマイシンD,ブレオマイシン
vincristine, actinomycin D, bleomycin ビンクリスチン,アクチノマイシンD,ブレオマイシン
VAB-6
vinblastine, actinomycin D, bleomycin, cisplatin, cyclophosphamide ビンブラスチン,アクチノマイシンD,ブレオマイシン,シスプラチン,シクロホスファミド
VAB-II
vinblastine sulfate, actinomycin D, bleomycin, platinum 硫酸ビンブラスチン,アクチノマイシンD,ブレオマイシン,プラチナム
VAB-VI
cyclophosphamide, vinblastine sulfate, actinomycin D, bleomycin, platinum シクロホスファミド,硫酸ビンブラスチン,アクチノマイシンD,ブレオマイシン,プラチナム
VABCD
vinblastine, adriamycin, bleomycin, cyclohexylchloroethylnitrosourea, dacarbazine ビンブラスチン,アドリアマイシン,ブレオマイシン,シクロヘキシルクロロエチルニトロソ尿素〔ウレア〕,ダカルバジン
VABES
vasoablative endothelial sarcoma (血管)内皮肉腫
VABP
ventroarterial bypass pumping 腹側動脈バイパスポンピング
VAC
ventriculoarterial connection 心室動脈結合

ventriculoatrial condition 室房状態
ventriculoatrial conduction 室房伝導
vincristine, actinomycin D, cyclophosphamide ビンクリスチン,アクチノマイシンD,シクロホスファミド
vincristine, adriamycin, cisplatin ビンクリスチン,アドリアマイシン,シスプラチン
vincristine, adriamycin, cyclophosphamide ビンクリスチン,アドリアマイシン,シクロホスファミド

vac
vaccine ワクチン
vacuum 真空(化), 吸引する, 減圧

VACA
vincristine, actinomycin D, cyclophosphamide, adriamycin ビンクリスチン,アクチノマイシンD,シクロホスファミド,アドリアマイシン

vacc
vaccination 予防接種, 種痘(法)
vaccine ワクチン

VAcc, VA_{cc}
visual acuity with correction 矯正視力

VAC system
Virus Adansonian Cryptogram System ウイルス命名システム

VAD
vascular access device 血管接近装置
ventricular assist device 補助人工心臓
vincristine, adriamycin, dexamethasone ビンクリスチン,アドリアマイシン,デキサメタゾン
vitamin A deficiency ビタミンA欠乏(症)

VaD
vascular dementia 血管性痴呆

V Ad
vocational adjustment 職業適応

VADA
vincristine, adriamycin, dexamethasone, actinomycin D ビンクリスチン,アドリアマイシン,デキサメタゾン,アクチノマイシンD

VADCS
ventricular atrial distal coronary sinus 心室心房遠位冠(状)静脈洞

Vadj
vocational adjustment 職業適応

V Adm
Veterans Administration 退役軍人局

VAE
venous air embolism　静脈空気塞栓症

VAFAC
vincristine, adriamycin, 5-fluorouracil, methotrexate (= Amethopterine), cyclophosphamide　ビンクリスチン,アドリアマイシン,フルオロウラシル,メトトレキサート(=アメトプテリン),シクロホスファミド

VAG
vertebral angiography　橈骨血管造影
vertebral arteriography　橈骨動脈造影

vag.
vaginitis　膣炎，腱鞘炎

VAG, Vag, vag.
vagina　膣，鞘
vaginal　膣の

Vagg
vaginae　(滑液)梢

VAG HYST, Vag hyst, vag.hyst.
vaginal hysterectomy　膣式子宮摘出(術)，膣式子宮切除(術)

VAGM
vein of Galen aneurysmal malformation　ガレン静脈動脈瘤性奇形

VAH
vertebral ankylosing hyperostosis　椎骨強直性骨増殖症
Veterans Administration Hospital　在郷軍人病院
virilizing adrenal hyperplasia　男性化副腎過形成
volatile aromatic hydrocarbons　揮発性芳香族炭化水素

VAHBE
ventricular atrial His bundle electrocardiogram　心室心房ヒス束心電図

VAHS
virus-associated hemophagocytic syndrome　ウイルス関連血球貪食症候群

VAIN
vaginal intraepithelial neoplasia　膣上皮内新生物

VAIVT
vascular access intervention therapy　経皮的バスキュラーアクセス拡張術

VAKT
visual, association, kinesthetic, tactile　視覚・連想・運動感覚・触覚

val
value　値
valued　価値のある
valve　弁

VAL, Val, val.
valine　バリン
VALE
visual acity, left eye　視力・左眼
VAM
ventricular arrhythmia monitor　心室不整脈モニター(監視装置)
vinblastine, adriamycin, mitomycin-C　ビンブラスチン,アドリアマイシン,マイトマイシンC
VP-16, adriamycin, methotrexate　エトポシド,アドリアマイシン,メトトレキサート
VAMC
Veterans Administration Medical Center　在郷軍人病院
VAMP
vesicle associated membrane protein　小嚢関連膜蛋白
vincristine, actinomycin, methotrexate, prednisone　ビンクリスチン,アクチノマイシン,メトトレキサート,プレドニゾン
vincristine, adriamycin, 6-mercaptopurine, prednisolone　ビンクリスチン,アドリアマイシン,6-メルカプトプリン,プレドニゾロン
vincristine, adriamycin, methylprednisolone　ビンクリスチン,アドリアマイシン,メチルプレドニゾロン
vincristine, amethopterin, 6-mercaptopurine, prednisolone　ビンクリスチン,アメトプテリン,6-メルカプトプリン,プレドニゾロン
vincristine, amethopterin, 6-mercaptopurine, prednisone　ビンクリスチン,アメトプテリン,6-メルカプトプリン,プレドニゾン
VAN
value added network　付加価値通信網《コン》
ventricular aneurysmectomy　心室動脈瘤切除(術)
vincristine, adriamycin, nimustine hydrochloride　ビンクリスチン,アドリアマイシン,塩酸ニムスチン
V antigen
viral antigen　ウイルス抗原
VAOD
visual acuity, oculus dexter　視力・右眼
VA↓OD
visual acuity decreased, oculus dexter　視力低下・右眼
VAOS
visual acuity, oculus sinister　視力・左眼

VA↓OS
visual acuity decreased, oculus sinister　視力低下・左眼

VAOU
visual acuity, oculi unitas　視力・両眼

VA↓OU
visual acuity decreased, oculi unitas　視力低下・両眼

VAP
vaginal acid phosphatase　膣酸ホスファターゼ
variant angina pectoris　異型狭心症
vincristine, adriamycin, prednisone　ビンクリスチン,アクチノマイシン,プレドニゾン
vincristine, adriamycin, procarbazine　ビンクリスチン,アドリアマイシン,プロカルバジン

VAPA
vincristine, adriamycin, prednisone, arabinosylcytosine　ビンクリスチン,アドリアマイシン,プレドニゾン,アラビノシルシトシン

VAPCS
ventricular atrial proximal coronary sinus　心室心房近位冠(状)静脈洞

VA_{ph}
visual acuity with pinhole　針穴視力

VA-PICA
vertebral artery-posterior inferior cerebellar artery aneurysm　椎骨後下小脳動脈分岐部動脈瘤

vapor
vaporization　蒸気化

VAPS
visual analogue pain scale　可視的アナログ式疼痛評価,バップス
volume assisted pressure support　呼吸量確保圧サポート，バップス

$\dot{V}_A/\dot{Q}c$
alveolar ventilation perfusion ratio　換気血流比

VAR
visual aural range　視聴域
volt-ampere reactive　電圧・電流反応性

var
variable　可変の，不定の
variant　変異株，変異体，変種
variation　変異，変動
varicose　静脈瘤の，結節状構造の
varicosities　静脈瘤様腫脹，結節状構造
variety　変種
various　種々の

varying 変化する

VARE
visual acuity, right eye 視力・右眼

VAS
vesicle attachment site 小嚢付着部位
visual analogue scale 視覚アナログ尺度《心理》

Vas
vascular 血管の

vas bund
vascular bundle 血管束

VASC
Visual-Auditory Screening (test for) Children 小児用視覚聴覚スクリーニング(検査)

VASC, vasc
vascular 血管の

VAsc, VA$_{sc}$
visual acuity without correction 裸眼視力

vas.dis
vascular disease 血管疾患

vasec
vasectomy 血管切除術

V-A shunt
ventriculoatrial shunt 脳室心房シャント

vasodil
vasodilatation 血管拡張

VAS RAD
vascular radiology 血管放射線(医)学

VAST
vibroacoustic stimulation test 振動・音刺激試験

vas vit.
vas vitreum〈ラ〉 ガラス管

VAT
ventricle, atrium, trigger 心房同期型心室ペーシング
ventricular activation time 心室興奮時間
visual action time 視覚活動時間
visual actoin therapy 視覚活動療法

VATER
vertebral defects, anal atresia, tracheoesophageal fistula, and radial defects 脊椎奇形・鎖肛・気道食道瘻・橈骨欠損

VATH
vinblastine, adriamycin, thiotepa ビンブラスチン,アドリアマイシン,チオテパ
vinblastine, adriamycin, thiotepa, Halotestin ビンブラスチン,アドリアマイシン,チオテパ,ハロテスチン

VATS
video-assisted thoracic surgery　胸腔鏡下手術

VAV
VP-16(=etoposide), adriamycin, vincristine　エトポシド, アドリアマイシン, ビンクリスチン

VAZ
vena azygos〈ラ〉　奇静脈, 右縦胸静脈

VB
vagina bulbi　眼球鞘
venous blood　静脈血
Veronal buffer　ベロナール緩衝液
vertebrobasilar (arteries)　椎骨脳底(動脈)
viable birth　生存可能出生
vinblastine　ビンブラスチン
vinblastine, bleomycin　ビンブラスチン, ブレオマイシン
virus buffer　ウイルス緩衝
vitamin B　ビタミンB
voided bladder　排尿(後)膀胱

VBA
vincristine, bischloroethylnitrosourea, adriamycin　ビンクリスチン, ビスクロロエチルニトロソ尿素, アドリアマイシン

VBAC
vaginal birth after cesarean section　帝王切開後の経腟出産

VBAI
vertebrobasilar artery insufficiency　椎骨脳底動脈(循環)不全(症)

VBAIN
vertebrobasilar artery insufficiency nystagmus　椎骨脳底動脈(循環)不全(性)眼振

VBAP
vincristine, bischloroethylnitrosourea, adriamycin, prednisone　ビンクリスチン, ビスクロロエチルニトロソ尿素, アドリアマイシン, プレドニゾン

VBC
vincristine, bleomycin, cisplatin　ビンクリスチン, ブレオマイシン, シスプラチン

VBD
Veronal-buffered diluent　ベロナール緩衝液賦形

VBDS
vanishing bile duct syndrome　胆管消失症候群

VBE
Veronal buffered saline containing EDTA　EDTA含有ベロナール緩衝液

VBG
vagotomy and Billroth gastroenterostomy 迷走神経切断とビルロート胃腸吻合(術)
vein bypass graft 静脈バイパス移植
venous blood gas 静脈血液ガス
Veronal buffered glycerol グリセリン含有ベロナール緩衝液
vertebrobasilar artery 椎骨脳底動脈
vertical-banded gastroplasty 垂直帯胃形成術

VBI
vertebrobasilar insufficiency 椎骨脳底動脈循環不全
vertebrobasilar ishemia 椎骨脳底動脈虚血

VBL
vinblastine ビンブラスチン

VBM
vinblastine, bleomycin, methotrexate ビンブラスチン,ブレオマイシン,メトトレキサート
vincristine, bleomycin, methotrexate ビンクリスチン,ブレオマイシン,メトトレキサート

VBMCP
vincristine, bischloroethylnitrosourea, melphalan, cyclophosphamide, prednisone ビンクリスチン,ビスクロロエチルニトロソ尿素,メルファラン,シクロホスファミド,プレドニゾン

VBOS
Veronal buffered oxalated saline ベロナール緩衝シュウ酸塩加生(理)食(塩)水

VBP
vagal body paraganglioma 迷走神経傍神経節腫
venous blood pressure 静脈圧
ventricular premature beat 心室期外収縮
vinblastine, bleomycin, cisplatin (=Platinol) ビンブラスチン,ブレオマイシン,シスプラチン(=プラチノール)

VBR
ventricular-brain ratio 脳室・脳比

VBS
Veronal buffered saline ベロナール緩衝生食水
vertebral basilar (artery) system 椎骨脳底(動脈)系

Vbt
vinblastine ビンブラスチン

V

VC
acuity of color vison 色覚能
vascular change 血管(性)変化
vasoconstriction 血管収縮
vasoconstrictor 血管収縮薬

vena cava 大静脈
venereal case 性病症例
venous capillary 静脈性毛細血管
ventricular contractions 心室収縮
vertebral canal 脊柱管
villous capillary 絨毛毛細管《電顕》
vincristine ビンクリスチン
vinyl chloride 塩化ビニル
visual cortex 視覚皮質
vital capacity 肺活量
vitamin C ビタミンC
vomitting center 嘔吐中枢
vowel-consonant 母音・子音
VP-16(=etoposide), carboplatin エトポシド, カルボプラチン

%VC
percent vital capacity パーセント肺活量

VC, V_c, Vc
pulmonary capillary blood volume 肺毛細(血)管血液量

VC, v.c.
vocal cord 声帯

V/C, V-C
ventilation-circulation (ratio) 換気・循環(比)

VCA
vancomycin, colistin, anisomycin バンコマイシン, コリスチン, アニソマイシン
viral capsid antigen ウイルス粒子抗原

VCAM
vascullar cell adhesion molecule 血管内皮細胞接着分子

VCAP
vincristine, cyclophosphamide, adriamycin, prednisone ビンクリスチン, シクロホスファミド, アドリアマイシン, プレドニゾン

VCC
vasoconstrictor center 血管収縮中枢

VCD
vacuum constriction device 陰圧式勃起補助用具
vena colica dextra〈ラ〉 右結腸静脈
vocal cord dysfunction 声帯機能異常

VCE
vagina, ectocervix and endocervix 腟・子宮腟部・子宮頸内膜

Vcepv
vitrum cum epistomio vitreo〈ラ〉 ガラス栓のついたビン《処》

VCF
vaginal contraceptive film 腟内避妊用フィルム
velocity of circumferential fiber shortening (左(心)室)内周短縮速度

vincristine, cyclophosphamide, 5-fluorouracil　ビンクリスチン, シクロホスファミド, フルオロウラシル

Vcf
circumferential fiber shortening velocity　円周方向短縮速度

VCG
vectorcardiogram　ベクトル心電図
vectorcardiography　ベクトル心電図法
voiding cystogram　排尿時膀胱造影〔撮影〕図
voiding cystography　排尿時膀胱造影〔撮影〕(法)
voiding cystourethrogram　排尿時膀胱尿道造影〔撮影〕図

VCI
volatile corrosion inhibitor　揮発性腐食防止剤

V-cillin
penicillin V　ペニシリンV

vCJD, v-CJD
variant form of Creutzfeldt-Jakob disease　変異型クロイツフェルト・ヤコブ病, バリアント型CJD

VCL
visual comfort light　視快適光

VCM
vancomycin　バンコマイシン
vena colica media〈ラ〉　中結腸静脈
vinyl chloride monomer　塩化ビニル単量体〔モノマー〕
volume compensation method　容積補償法

VCMP
vincristine, cyclophosphamide, melphalan, prednisone　ビンクリスチン, シクロホスファミド, メルファラン, プレドニゾン
vincristine, cyclophosphamide, 6-mercaptopurine, prednisolone　ビンクリスチン, シクロホスファミド, 6-メルカプトプリン, プレドニゾロン

V_{CNS}
volume of central nervous system　中枢神経系容積〔体積〕

$\dot{V}co$
carbon monoxide　一酸化炭素排出量

Vco_2
carbon dioxide elimination　二酸化炭素排出量

VCP
vincristine, cyclophosphamide, prednisone　ビンクリスチン, シクロホスファミド, プレドニゾン

VCQ
vincristine, carboquone, adriamycin　ビンクリスチン, カルボコン, アドリアマイシン

VCR
vasoconstriction rate 血管収縮率
vincristine ビンクリスチン
vincristine sulfate 硫酸ビンクリスチン

VCS
vasoconstrictor substance 血管収縮物質
vena cava superior〈ラ〉 上大静脈
vena cava superior syndrome 上大静脈閉塞症候群
vesicocervical space 膀胱子宮頸腔

VCSA
viral cell surface antigen ウイルス細胞表面抗原

VCSF
ventricular cerebrospinal fluid 脳室髄液

VCT
venous clotting time 静脈血凝固時間

VCU
voiding cystourethrogram 排尿時膀胱尿道造影〔撮影〕図

VCUG
vesicoureterogram 膀胱尿管造影〔撮影〕図
voiding cystourethrogram 排尿時膀胱尿道造影〔撮影〕図
voiding cystourethrography 排尿時膀胱尿道造影〔撮影〕法

VCV
ventricular conduction velocity 心室伝導速度
volume controlled ventilation 従量式調節換気
vowel-consonant-vowel 母音・子音・母音

VD
dead space volume 死腔量
vapor density 蒸気密度
vascular dementia 脳血管性痴呆
vasodilation 血管拡張
vasodilator 血管拡張薬
venereal disease 性病
venous dilatation 静脈拡張
ventrodorsal 腹背側の
vessel disease 血管疾患
virus diarrhea ウイルス性下痢
visus dexter 右眼視力
vitamin D ビタミンD
volume of distribution 分配量

Vd
apparent volume of distribution みかけの分布容積

vd
double vibrations 重複振動
void 無効な，排尿する
voided 排尿した

vd.
vide〈ラ〉＝see　見よ，参照せよ《処》

V.d.
visus dextra〈ラ〉　右眼視力

V & D
vomiting and diarrhea　嘔吐と下痢

＋VD
positive vertical divergence　陽性垂直性開散

－VD
negative vertical divergence　陰性垂直性開散

VD, V_D
volume of dead space　死腔量，死腔容積

V_DA
alveolar dead space volume　肺胞死腔量
ventilation of alveolar dead space　肺胞死腔換気量
volume of alveolar dead space　肺胞死腔量

VDA
venereal disease awareness　性病注意
vigorous diagnostic approach　積極的診断法
visual discriminatory acuity　識別視力

VDAC
voltage-dependent anion-(selective) channel　電圧依存性陰イオン(選択性)チャンネル

Vd alv
alveolar dead space　肺胞死腔

V_Dan
ventilation of anatomic dead space　解剖学的死腔換気
volume of anatomic dead space　解剖学的死腔容積

Vd anat
anatomic dead space　解剖学的死腔

VDAVP
4-valine-8-D-arginine vasopressin　バリン・アルギニン・バソプレシン

VDB
Venereal Disease Branch　性病分局
voltage-dependent block　膜電位依存性抑制

VdB
van den Bergh (test)　ファンデンベルグ(試験)

VDBCC
vincristine, dactinomycin, bleomycin, cisplatin, cyclophosphamide　ビンクリスチン,ダクチノマイシン,ブレオマイシン,シスプラチン,シクロホスファミド

VDBT
vasucular dementia of Binswanger type　ビンスワグナー型血管性痴呆

VDC
vasodilator center　血管拡張中枢
Venereal Disease Clinic　性病クリニック(外来)
VDCCs
voltage-dependent calcium channels　膜電位依存性カルシウムチャンネル
VDD
vincristine, doxorubicin, dexamethasone　ビンクリスチン,ドキソルビシン,デキサメタゾン
vitamin D dependent (rickets)　ビタミンD依存性(くる病)
VDDR
vitamin D-dependent rickets　ビタミンD依存性くる病
v.d.E
vor dem Essen〈独〉　食前
VDEL
Venereal Disease Experimental Laboratory　性病実験研究所〔検査室〕
VDEM
vasodepressor material　血管拡張物質
VDG
venereal disease, gonorrhea　淋病
vdg.
voiding　排尿時の
VDH
valvular disease of the heart　心(臓)弁膜症，弁膜性心疾患
vascular disease of heart　心血管疾患
VDL
visual detection level　視覚検出レベル
VDM
vasodepressor material　血管抑制物質
vasodilator material　血管拡張物質
VDN
vindesine　ビンデシン
VDP
ventricular premature depolarization　心室早期脱分極
vinblastine, dacarbazine, cisplatin (= Platinol)　ビンブラスチン,ダカルバジン,シスプラチン(=プラチノール)
vincristine, daunorubicin, prednisone　ビンクリスチン,ダウノルビシン,プレドニゾン
Vd p
physiologic dead space　生理学的死腔
VDR
venous diameter ratio　静脈(直)径比

V

VDRL
venereal disease research laboratory (test) 性病研究所梅毒検査法
Venereal Disease Research Laboratories 米国性病研究所

VDRR
vitamin D-resistant rickets ビタミンD抵抗性くる病

VDS
vasodilator substance 血管拡張物質
venereal disease-syphilis 性病・梅毒
ventrale derotation spondylodese 腹側頸椎癒着術
vindesine ビンデシン

v.d.S
vor dem Schlafen〈独〉 就寝前《処》

v.d.schlaf.
vor dem Schlafen (gehen)〈独〉= *hora decubitus*〈ラ〉 就床時《処》

Vdss
volume of distribution steady state (薬物の血中)分布容量

VDT
visual display terminal 視覚表示端末装置
visual distortion test 視覚ひずみ検査

VDT/I
ventricle, double, trigger/inhibit 心房同期型心室ペーシング

VDT syndrome
visual display terminal syndrome VDT症候群

VDU
video display unit ビデオ表示装置
visual display unit 視覚表示装置

VDV
ventricular diastolic volume 心室拡張期容積

V_D/V_T, VD/VT
ratio of dead space (gas) to tidal (gas) volume 死腔気体容量の1回換気量率

V_E
expired gas volume per minute 分時換気量
minute ventilation 分時換気量
respiratory minute volume 毎分呼吸量
volume airflow per unit of time 単位時間あたりの気流容積〔容量〕
volume of expired gas 呼気ガス量

VE
esophageal lead 食道導出〔誘導〕
vacuum extraction 吸引分娩
vacuum extractor 吸引分娩器
vaginal examination 膣検

vascular ectasia　血管拡張症
Venezuelan encephalitis　ベネズエラ脳炎
venous extension　静脈伸展
ventricular elasticity　心室弾性
ventricular escape　心室(性)逸脱〔補足〕
ventricular extrasystole　心室性期外収縮
vesicular exanthema　小水疱疹
viral encephalitis　ウイルス(性)脳炎
visual efficiency　視力効率
vitamin E　ビタミンE
Voegtlinsche Einheit〈独〉　フェークトリン単位
volume ejection　体積駆出
voluntary effort　随意的努力

VE, Ve
ventilation　換気(量)，呼吸数

VEA
ventricular ectopic activity　心室異所性活動
ventricular ectopic arrhythmia　心室異所性不整脈
virus envelope antigen　ウイルス外膜抗原

VEB
ventricular ectopic beat　心室性期外収縮

VEC
video-enhanced contrast　ビデオコントラスト増強

VECG
vector electrocardiogram　ベクトル心電図

VECGF
vascular endothelial cell growth factor　血管内皮増殖因子

VECP
visually evoked cortical potential　視覚誘発脳皮質電位，視覚誘発脳波

vect
vector　ベクター，媒介動物

VED
vacuum extraction delivery　吸引分娩
ventricular ectopic depolarization　心室異所性脱分極

VEDP
ventricular end-diastolic pressure　心室拡張終期圧

VEDV
ventricular end-diastolic volume　心室拡張終期容積

VEE
Venezuelan equine encephalomyelitis (virus)　ベネズエラウマ脳脊髄炎(ウイルス)

vee dee
venereal disease　性病

V-EEG
vigilance-controlled electroencephalogram 覚醒調節脳波
VEF
ventricular ejection fraction 心室駆出分画
visually evoked field 視覚誘発野
VEG
ventriculoencephalography 脳室造影〔撮影〕法
veg
vegetable 野菜
vegetarian 菜食主義者
vegetarianism 菜食主義
Veg, veg
vegetation 組織増殖
vegetations 増殖(症), 疣(＝ゆう)腫, 生長, 成長
VEGF
vascular endothelial growth factor 血管内皮増殖因子
vehic.
vehiculum〈ラ〉 賦形薬(剤), 媒介者, 便薬《処》
vel, vel.
velocity 速さ, 速度
Velcro
Velcro rale ベルクロラ音
veloc, veloc.
velocity 速度, 速さ
VEM
vasoexcitor material 腎昇圧物質
vergence eye movements 両眼離反眼運動
vincristine, cyclophosphamide, mitomycin-C ビンクリスチン, シクロホスファミド(＝エンドキサン), マイトマイシンC
VEMP
vincristine, cyclophosphamide (＝Endoxane), 6-mercaptopurine, prednisolone ビンクリスチン, シクロホスファミド(＝エンドキサン), 6-メルカプトプリン, プレドニゾロン
vincristine, cyclophosphamide (＝Endoxane), 6-mercaptopurine, prednisone ビンクリスチン, シクロホスファミド(＝エンドキサン), 6-メルカプトプリン, プレドニゾン
vincristine, cyclophosphamide, methotrexate, prednisone ビンクリスチン, シクロホスファミド(＝エンドキサン), メトトレキサート, プレドニゾン

ven
venereal 性病の
venomous 毒の
ventral 腹側の，腹の，腹部の
ventricle 室，心室，喉頭室

Ven, ven.
venous 静脈の

Vend
van den Bergh test ファンデンベルグ試験

Vene.Sek.
Venen-Sektion〈独〉 静脈切開

VENP
vincristine, cyclophosphamide (= Endoxane), Natulan, prednisolone ビンクリスチン，シクロホスファミド(＝エンドキサン)，ナツラン，プレドニゾロン
vincristine, cyclophosphamide (= Endoxane), Natulan, prednisone ビンクリスチン，シクロホスファミド(＝エンドキサン)，ナツラン，プレドニゾン

vent
ventilate 換気する
ventilation 換気
ventilator 換気装置，人工呼吸器，ベンチレータ(ー)
ventral 腹側の，腹部の，腹の

VENT, vent
ventricle 室，心室，脳室
ventricular 心室の，脳室の

vent.fib
ventricular fibrillation 心室細動

ventr
ventral 腹側の，腹の，腹部の

ventric
ventricle 室，心室，脳室
ventricular 心室の，脳室の

ventric.fib
ventricular fibrillation 心室細動

VEOG
vector-electro-oculography ベクトル眼電位図計

VEP
vincristine, cyclophosphamide (= Endoxane), prednisolone ビンクリスチン，シクロホスファミド(＝エンドキサン)，プレドニゾロン
visual evoked potential 視覚誘発電位

VEPA

vinblastine, etoposide, prednisone, adriamycin　ビンブラスチン，エトポシド，プレドニゾン，アドリアマイシン

vincristine, cyclophosphamide (＝Endoxane), prednisolone, adriamycin　ビンクリスチン，シクロホスファミド（＝エンドキサン），プレドニゾロン，アドリアマイシン

VEPA-B

vinblastine, etoposide, prednisone, adriamycin, bleomycin　ビンブラスチン，エトポシド，プレドニゾン，アドリアマイシン，ブレオマイシン

VEPF

vascular endothelial cell proliferation factor　血管内皮細胞増殖因子

VER

visual(ly) evoked response　視覚(性)誘発反応

voiding flow rete　排尿流量，排尿流速

Vergl

Vergleiche〈独〉　比較

vert

vertebra　椎骨，椎

vertebral　(脊)椎骨の

vertical　垂直の

vertigo　めまい

vert.comp.

vertebral compression　脊椎圧迫

vertical compression　垂直(性)圧迫

vert.compr.

vertebral compression　脊椎圧迫

vertical compression　垂直(性)圧迫

VES

velocity sedimentation erythrocyte　赤血球沈降速度，赤沈，血沈

ventricular extrasystole　心室性期外収縮

ves

vessel　管，血管

VES, ves.

vesica〈ラ〉＝vesica　膀胱，胆嚢

vesicle　小(水)疱，小嚢

vesicular　小胞(性)の，小水疱(性)の

vesic

vesicle　小嚢，小(水)疱

vesicular　小胞(性)の，小嚢(状/性)の

vesp.

vesper〈ラ〉　夕方，夕刻に《処》

vest
vestibular 前庭の
vestibule 前庭

ves.ur.
vesica urinaria〈ラ〉 膀胱

VESV
ventricular end-systolic volume 心室収縮終期容積
vesicular exanthema of swine virus ブタ水疱性発疹ウイルス

Vet
veteran 退役軍人
veterinary 獣医(学)の

V et, v.et.
vide etiam〈ラ〉 ～もまた参照せよ《処》

Vet Adm
Veterans Administration 退役軍人局

Vet Admin
Veterans Administration 退役軍人局

Vet.M.B.
Bachelor of Veterinary Medicine 獣医学士

vet med
veterinary medicine 獣医学

Vet Sci
veterinary science 獣医科学

VF
left leg 左脚
ventilatory failure 換気不全
ventricular fluid 脳室(随)液
ventricular flutter 心室粗動
vestibular function 前庭機能
vitamin F ビタミンF
vitreous fluorophotometry 硝子体螢光光度測定(法)
voice frequency 声の周波数

Vf
video frequency 映像周波数

VF, Vf
visual field 視野

VF, Vf, v.f.
ventricular fibrillation 心室細動

VF, V.F.
vocal fremitus 声音振盪

VFA
volatile fatty acid 揮発性脂肪酸

V factor
verbal comprehension factor 言語〔語句〕理解力因子

V

VFAM
vincristine, 5-fluorouracil, adriamycin, mitomycin-C — ビンクリスチン,フルオロウラシル,アドリアマイシン,マイトマイシンC

Vfb
ventricular fibrillation — 心室細動

VFC
ventricular function curve — 心室機能曲線

VFD
ventricular filling period — 心室充満期
visual feedback display — 視覚フィードバック画面表示

VFDF
very fast death factor — 超急速死要因

VFI
visual fields intact — 視野無(損)傷

Vfib, V fib.
ventricular fibrillation — 心室細動

VFL
ventricular flutter — 心室粗動

VFP
ventricular filling pressure — 心室充満(期)圧
ventricular fluid pressure — 脳室(髄)液圧

VFS
vascular fragility syndrome — 血管脆弱症候群

VFT
venous filling time — 静脈充満時間
ventricular fibrillation threshold — 心室細動閾値

VG
valeur globulaire〈仏〉 — 赤血球係数, 容量指数
van Gieson (stain) — ファンギーソン染色
ventricular gallop — 心室(性)奔馬調律
ventricular gradient — 心室勾配《心電》
ventriculography — 脳室造影〔撮影〕
vitamin G — ビタミンG
Vogelgesicht〈独〉 — 鳥様顔貌
volume of gas — 気体容積, 気体体積

v.g.
verbi gratia〈ラ〉 — たとえば

V & G
vagotomy and gastroenterotomy — 迷走神経切断および胃腸切開(術)

VG, V/G
very good — とても良い

VGAD
vein of Galen aneurysmal dilatation — ガレン静脈動脈瘤性拡張

VGCC
voltage-gated calcium channel　電位開放カルシウムチャンネル

VGH
very good health　非常に良い健康状態

vgl.
vergleiche〈独〉　比較の

VGM
vein graft myringoplasty　静脈移植鼓膜形成(術)
ventriculogram　脳室造影〔撮影〕図

VGP
viral glycoprotein　ウイルス(性)糖蛋白

V_H
H chain(=heavy-chain) variable region　H鎖可変領域
variable heavy-chain domain　可変部H鎖ドメイン

VH
vaginal hysterectomy　経腟子宮摘出術
venous hematocrit　静脈(血)ヘマトクリット
ventricular hypertrophy　心(室)肥大
Veterans Hospital　在郷軍人病院
viral hepatitis　ウイルス性肝炎
vitamin H　ビタミンH

vh
very high　とても高い

v/h
vulnerability/hardness　脆弱性・硬度比

VHD
valvular heart disease　弁膜性心臓疾患
viral hematodepressive disease　ウイルス性血液低下疾患

VHDA
very high density area　超高濃度陰影部分《画診》

VHDL
very-high-density lipoprotein　超高比重リポ蛋白

VHF
very high frequency　超高頻度
viral hemorrhagic fever　ウイルス性出血熱

VHF/UHF
very high and ultrahigh frequency　高周波と超高周波

VHL
von Hippel-Lindau disease　フォンヒッペル・リンダウ病

V_I
inspired gas volume per minute　吸気分時換気量

VI
vaginal irrigation　腟内洗浄
venous incompetence　静脈(弁)不全

ventilation index 換気指数
virginium ビルギニウム
virtual instruments 仮想装置
virulence 菌力，毒力
viscosity index 粘(稠)度指数
visual impairment 視覚障害
visual inspection 視診
visually impaired 視力障害の
vitality index 活力指数
vitamin I ビタミンI
volume index 容積指数
volume of inspired gas 吸気ガス量

Vi
inspired volume 吸気量
virulent 有毒の，毒性の

v.i.
via intermedia(*tis*)〈ラ〉=intermediate way 中間の方法で
vide infra〈ラ〉 下を見よ

VIA
virus-inactivating agent ウイルス不活性化剤
virus infection-associated antigen ウイルス感染に伴う抗原

Vi antigen
virulence antigen 毒力抗原，ビルレンス抗原

VIB
Vocational Interest Blank 職業興味記入用紙《心理》

vib
vibrate 振動する
vibratory 振動の

VIB, vib, vib.
vibration 振動

VIC
Values Inventory for Children 小児用価値調査票
vaporizer in(side) circuit 回路内気化器
vasoinhibitory center 血管抑制中枢
visual communication (therapy) 視覚コミュニケーション(療法)
voice intensity controller 声強度調節装置

vic
vicinal 隣接の

vic.
vices〈ラ〉=times ～回，～倍

VICA
velocity internal carotid artery 内頸動脈速度

VID
vaginal intraepithelial dysplasia 腟上皮内異形成(症)

visible iris diameter　可視虹彩(直)径

vid.

vide〈ラ〉=see　見よ，参照せよ《処》

VIF

virus-induced interferon　ウイルス誘導インターフェロン

VIG

vaccinia immune globulin　ワクシニア免疫グロブリン

vinblastine, ifosfamide, gallium (nitrate)　ビンブラスチン，イホスファミド，(硝酸)ガリウム

VIM

video intensification microscopy　ビデオ増幅顕微鏡

Vim

nucleus ventralis intermedius　視床腹中間核

vim

vinum〈ラ〉=wine　ブドウ酒，ワイン《処》

VIN

vaginal intraepithelial neoplasia　腟上皮内癌

vulvar intraepithelial neoplasia　外陰(部)上皮内新生物

vulvar intraepithelial neoplasm　外陰(部)上皮内新生物

Vin

vinyl ether　ビニルエーテル

VIN Ⅲ

vulvar carcinoma in situ　上皮内外陰部腫瘍

vin, vin.

vinum〈ラ〉=wine　ワイン，ぶどう酒《処》

VINR

virus induced necrotic region　ウイルスによる壊死巣

VIO

Veterinary Investigation Office　獣医学研究所

VIP

vasoactive intestinal peptide　血管活性腸ペプチド

vasoactive intestinal polypeptide　血管作動性腸管ポリペプチド

vasoinhibitory peptide　血管抑制(性)ペプチド

venous impedance plethysmography　静脈インピーダンス体積(変動)記録法

ventilation-infusion-pump　換気・輸液・ポンプ

very important person　最重要人物

vinblastine, ifosfamide, cisplatin (=Platinol)　ビンブラスチン，イホスファミド，シスプラチン(=プラチノール)

visual identification point　視同定点

voluntary interruption of pregnancy　自発的妊娠中絶

VP-16, ifosfamide, cisplatin (=Platinol)　エトポシド，イホスファミド，シスプラチン(=プラチノール)

V

VIP-oma
vasoactive intestinal polypeptide (secreting) tumor　血管活性腸ポリペプチド(分泌性)腫瘍
vipre
visual precision　視明瞭度
VIPS
very important person syndrome　最重要人物症候群
VIQ
verbal intelligence quotient　語句〔言語〕的知能指数
Vocational Interest Questionnaire　職業興味質問表
VIR
virology　ウイルス学
vir.
viridis〈ラ〉=green　緑色の
virulent　有毒の，毒性の
virol
virology　ウイルス学
VIS
vaginal irrigation smear　膣洗浄塗抹(標本)，膣洗浄スメア
venous insufficiency syndrome　静脈不全症候群
vertebral irritation syndrome　椎骨刺激症候群
vocational interest schedule　職業興味スケジュール
vis
vision　視覚
visiting　訪問の
visitor　訪問者
visual　視覚の
VISC
vitreous infusion suction cutter　硝子体注入吸引カッター
visc
visceral　内臓の
viscosity　粘(稠)度，粘性，粘着性
viscous　粘着性の
VIT
venom immunotherapy　毒素免疫療法
vit
vital　生体の，生命の，生活の
vitrectomy　硝子体切除(術)
vit.
vitellus〈ラ〉=york of an egg　卵黄
Vit, vit
vitamin　ビタミン
vitreous　ガラス質〔状〕の，(眼の)硝子体(液)の

vit Bcx
vitamin B complex　ビタミンB群
VIT CAP, vit.cap.
vital capacity　肺活量
vitel.
vitellus〈ラ〉＝york of an egg　卵黄
VITIES
voltammetry at interface between two immiscible electrolyte solution　2つの混合できない電解質溶液の界面電解電量計
vit.ov.
vitellus ovi〈ラ〉　卵黄《処》
vit.ov.sol.
vitello ovi solutus〈ラ〉　卵黄に溶解した《処》
vit P
vitamin P　ビタミンP
vit PP
pellagra-preventive vitamin　ビタミンPP，ペラグラ予防ビタミン
vitr
vitreous　ガラス質〔状〕の，(眼の)硝子体(液)の
vitr, vitr.
vitreous　ガラス質〔状〕の，(眼の)硝子体(液)の
vitreus〈ラ〉　ガラス製の，透明な
vitrum〈ラ〉　ガラス
vit rec
vital record　生命記録
Vit U
Cabagin＝Vitamin U　キャベジン(＝ビタミンU)
vivi
vivisection　生体解剖，生体実験
viz, viz.
videlicet〈ラ〉＝namely　すなわち，換言すれば
VJ
ventriculojugular (shunt)　脳室頸静脈(シャント)
vitamin J　ビタミンJ
Vogel-Johnson agar　フォーゲル・ジョンソン寒天(培地)
VJC
ventriculojugulocardiac (shunt)　脳室頸静脈心臓(シャント)
VK
Vitalkapazität〈独〉　肺活量
vitamin K　ビタミンK
Vogt-Koyanagi (syndrome)　フォーグト・小柳(症候群)

VKC
vernal keratoconjunctivitis　春季角結膜炎
VKG
Vektorkardiogramm〈独〉　ベクトル心電図
VKH
Vogt-Koyanagi-Harada (syndrome)　フォークト・小柳・原田(症候群)

V_L
L chain variable region　L鎖の可変領域〔部〕
variable light-chain domain　可変部L鎖ドメイン
VL
left arm　左腕
vena lienalis〈ラ〉　脾静脈
venerische(s) Leiden〈独〉　性病
ventralis lateralis (nucleus)　腹外側(核)
ventrolateral (nucleus)　腹外側(核)の
Verdauungs-leukozytose〈独〉　食事性白血球増加(症)
visceral leishmaniasis　内臓リーシュマニア症
vision, left　左視覚，左眼視力
vitamin L　ビタミンL
Vl
Versuchsleiter〈独〉　実験者
VLA
vanillacetic acid　バニル酢酸
vanillactic acid　バニル乳酸
very late activation　最晩期活性化
very low altitude　超低高度
virus-like agent　ウイルス様因子
VLAP
visual laser-assisted prostatectomy　直視下レーザー(補助)前立腺切除術

VLB
vinblastine　ビンブラスチン
vincaleukoblastine　ビンカロイコブラスチン
VLBR
very low birth rate　非常に低い出生率
VLBW
very low birth weight　超低出生(時)体重
VLCD
very low calorie diet　超低カロリー食
VLCFA
very long chain fatty acid　極長鎖脂肪酸
VLD
very low density　超低比重
VLDL
very low density lipoprotein　超低比重リポ蛋白

VLDLC
very low density lipoprotein cholesterol — 超低比重リポ蛋白コレステロール
VLDLP
very low density lipoprotein — 超低比重リポ蛋白
VLDS
verbal language developmental scale — 言語発達基準
VLDTG, VLD-TG
very low density lipoprotein triglyceride — 超低比重リポ蛋白トリグリセリド
VLE
vision left eye — 左視覚，左眼視力
VLED
very low energy diet — 超低カロリー食
VLF
very low frequency — 超低周波(数)
VLFA
very long chain saturated fatty acid — 極長鎖飽和脂肪酸
VLG
ventral nucleus of the lateral geniculate body — 外側膝状体の腹側核
VLH
ventrolateral nucleus of the hypothalamus — 視床下部の腹外側核
VLIA
virus-like infections agent — ウイルス様感染因子
VLM
visceral larva migrans — 内臓幼虫移行症
VLN
very low nitrogen — 超低窒素
VL nucleus
ventrolateral nucleus — 腹外側核
VLP
vincristine, L-asparaginase, prednisone — ビンクリスチン,L-アスパラギナーゼ,プレドニゾン
virus-like particle — ウイルス様粒子
VLR
very low range — 超低域
VLSI
very-large-scale integrated circuit — 超大規模集積回路
vltge
voltage — 電位
VL thalamotomy
ventrolateral thalamotomy — 視床腹外側核破壊術
vlv
valve — 弁

valvular 弁の

VM
vasomotor 血管運動(性)の
vasomotor nerve 血管運動神経
ventilation maxima〈仏〉 最大換気
ventralis medialis 内側腹側
ventricular mass 心室筋(重)量
ventricular muscle 心室筋
ventromedial 腹内側の
ventromedian nucleus 腹内側核
Verner-Morrison (syndrome) バーナー・モリソン(症候群)
vestibular membrane 前庭膜
viral myocarditis ウイルス性心筋炎
vitamin M ビタミンM

Vm
maximal uptake velocity 最大取り込み速度
voltmeter 電圧計

vm.
ventralis medialis〈ラ〉 腹側正中
vormittags〈独〉 午前に

V/m
volts per minute ボルト/分

Vm, VM
viomycin バイオマイシン

VMA
vanillylmandelic acid バニリルマンデル酸

VMAD
vincristine, methotrexate, adriamycin, actinomycin D ビンクリスチン, メトトレキサート, アドリアマイシン, アクチノマイシンD

Vmax
maximum velocity (of shortening) 最大収縮速度, Vマックス

VMC
vasomotor center 血管運動神経中枢

VMCG
vector magnetocardiogram ベクトル心磁図

VMCP
vincristine, melphalan, cyclophosphamide, prednisone ビンクリスチン, メルファラン, シクロホスファミド, プレドニゾン

VMD
veterinary medicine doctor 獣医

vMDV
virulent Marek disease virus マレク病ウイルス

VMetP
vincristine, methotrexate, prednisolone　ビンクリスチン, メトトレキサート, プレドニゾロン
VMGT
Visual Motor Gestalt Test　視覚運動ゲシュタルト検査
VMH
ventromedial hypothalamic (neurons, nuclei)　腹内側視床下部(ニューロン/核)
VMI
Visual-Motor Integration (test)　視覚・運動統合(検査)
VMIT
Visual-Motor Integration Test　視覚・運動統合検査
VMN
ventromedial nuclei　腹内側核
ventromedial nucleus　腹内側核
VMP
vincristine, 6-mercaptopurine, prednisolone　ビンクリスチン, 6-メルカプトプリン, プレドニゾロン
vincristine, 6-mercaptopurine, prednisone　ビンクリスチン, 6-メルカプトプリン, プレドニゾン
VMR
vasomotor rhinitis　血管運動性鼻炎
VMS
vena mesenterica superior　上腸間膜静脈
Visual Memory Score　視覚記憶スコア《心理》
visual memory span　視覚記憶スパン
VMST
Visual-Motor Sequencing Test　視覚・運動順序検査《心理》
VMT
vasomotor tone　血管運動緊張
ventilatory muscle training　換気〔呼吸〕筋訓練
VN
vesical neck　膀胱頸(部)
vestibular nucleus　前庭核
virus neutralization　ウイルス中和
virus neutralizing　ウイルス中和(性)の
visceral nucleus　内臓核
vitronectin　ビトロネクチン
V.n.
vitrum nigrum〈ラ〉　黒色ビン
VNA
Visiting Nurses Association　訪問看護師協会
VNC
vesical neck constriction　膀胱頸部狭窄
VNR
ventral nerve root　前(神経)根

vitronectin receptor | ビトロネクチン受容体

VNRC
Vegetation Nutritional Research Center | 植物性栄養研究センター

VNS
vegetative nervous system | 植物神経系
villonodular synovitis | 絨毛結節性滑膜炎

VNTR
variable number of tandem repeat | 縦列反復の可変数

VO
verbal order | 口頭指示
(ventricular) volume overload | (心室)容積過負荷

V_0
standard volume | 標準容積(体積)

Vo
void volume | 排出量

vo
verso | 裏，背面

Vo_2
oxgen uptake | 酸素摂取量
oxygen consumption | 酸素消費量

V/O, v.o.
verbal order | 口頭指示

V.o.a.
nucleus ventralis oralis anterior | 前吻側腹側核

VOC
vaporizer outside circuit | 回路外気化器

voc
vocational | 職業の

vocab, vocab.
vocabulary | 語彙

VOD
veno-occlusive disease | 肝中心静脈閉塞症
venous occlusive disease | 静脈閉塞(性)疾患
visio, oculus dexter (*dextra*)〈ラ〉 | 右眼視覚

vol
volar | 手のひらの，足の裏の
volumetric | 容量の
voluntary | 随意的な
volunteer | ボランティア

vol%
volume per cent | 容積百分率，体積百分率

VOL, vol, vol.
volume | 容積，容量，体積，巻

vol, vol.
volatilis〈ラ〉 | 揮発性の《処》

Vol Adm
voluntary admission　自発的入院

volt
volatile　揮発性の

voly
voluntary　随意の

VOM
vinyl chloride monomer　塩化ビニルモノマー
volt-ohm-milliammeter　ボルト・オーム・ミリアンペア計

vom.
vomitus〈ラ〉　嘔吐

v-onc
viral oncogene　ウイルス癌遺伝子

VOP
venous occlusion plethysmography　静脈閉塞体積(変動)記録法

V.o.p.
nucleus ventralis oralis posterior　後吻側腹側核

VOR
vestibulo-ocular reflex　前庭眼反射
vestibulo-ocular response　前庭動眼反応
visual omnirange　視全方位式無線標識

vorm, vorm.
vormals〈独〉　以前に
vormittags〈独〉　午前に

VOS
visio oculus sinister〈ラ〉　左眼視覚
visus oculi sinistri〈ラ〉　左眼視力

vos.
vitello ovi solutus〈ラ〉　卵黄に溶解した《処》

VOT
voice onset time　声発現時間

VOU
visio , oculi utriusque〈ラ〉　両眼の視覚

VP
physiological volume　生理学的容積
porphyria variegata〈ラ〉＝variegate porphyria　異型ポルフィリン症
vascular permeability　血管透過性
vasopressin　バソプレシン
velopharyngeal　口蓋帆咽頭の
venipuncture　静脈穿刺
venous (volume) plethysmograph　静脈体積(変動)記録器
venous pressure　静脈圧
ventricular pacing　心室ページング
vibrio parahaemolyticus　腸炎ビブリオ

vincristine, prednisone	ビンクリスチン,プレドニゾン
viral protein	ウイルス(性)蛋白
vitamin P	ビタミンP
Voges-Proskauer (test, reaction)	フォーゲス・プロスカウアー(試験/反応)
Voges-Proskauer semisolid agar medium	フォーゲス・プロスカウエル半固形寒天培地
volume pressure	容積圧
vulnerable period	易損期, 受攻期

Vp

plasma volume	血漿量
ventricular premature (beats)	心室性期外収縮

↑VP

increased venous pressure	静脈圧上昇

↓VP

decreased venous pressure	静脈圧低下

Vp.

Versuchsperson〈独〉	被検者

VP-16

etoposide	エトポシド

V/P

vapor to liquid	蒸気液体比
ventilation and perfusion	換気と灌流

V & P

vagotomy and pyloroplasty	迷走神経切断兼幽門形成術

V-P

ventriculo-peritonial (shunt)	脳室腹腔シャント術

VP, vp

vapor pressure	蒸気圧

VP, V/P

ventriculoperitoneal	脳室腹腔の

VP, V-P

vincristine, prednisolone	ビンクリスチン,プレドニゾロン

VPA

valproic acid	バルプロ酸
vascular plasminogen activator	血管性プラスミノゲン活性化物質

V-PAGE

vertical PAGE(=polyacrylamid gel electrophoresis)	垂直型アクリルアミドゲル電気泳動

VPB

ventricular premature beat	心室性期外収縮

VPBCPr
vincristine, prednisone, vinblastine, chlorambucil, procarbazine　ビンクリスチン,プレドニゾン,ビンブラスチン,クロラムブシル,プロカルバジン

VPC
vapor-phase chromatography　蒸気相クロマトグラフィ
ventricular premature contraction　心室性期外収縮
volume percent　容積百分率

VPCA
vincristine, prednisone, cyclophosphamide, arabinosylcytosine　ビンクリスチン,プレドニゾン,シクロホスファミド,アラビノシルシトシン

VPCMF
vincristine, prednisone, cyclophosphamide, methotrexate, 5-fluorouracil　ビンクリスチン,プレドニゾン,シクロホスファミド,メトトレキサート,フルオロウラシル

VPCT
ventricular premature contraction threshold　心室(性)期外収縮閾値

VPD
vapor phase decomposition　気相分解
ventricular premature depolarization　心室(性)期外脱分極

VPDIA
vena pancreaticoduodenalis inferior anterior〈ラ〉　下前膵十二指腸静脈

VPF
vascular permeability factor　血管透過性因子

VPG
velopharyngeal gap　口蓋帆咽頭裂
venting percutaneous gastrostomy　排出用経皮胃造瘻(術)

VPI
vapor phase inhibitor　気相抑制因子
vegetable peroxidase inhibitants　植物性ペルオキシダーゼ抑制物質
velopharyngeal insuffcient　口蓋咽頭機能不全，口蓋咽頭形成不全
velopharyngeal insufficiency　口蓋帆咽頭不全(症)
ventral posterior inferior　腹側後下(核)
virus structural protein　ウイルス構造蛋白
Vocational Preference Inventory　職業選択調査表

VPJ
verrucae planae juvenites〈ラ〉　若年性扁平疣贅

VPL
(nucleus) ventralis posterolateralis　腹側後外側(核)
ventral posterolateral (nucleus)　腹側後外側(核)

VPLS
ventilation perfusion lung scan　肺換気血流スキャン
VPM
(nucleus) ventralis posteromedialis　腹側後内側(核)
ventral posteromedial (nucleus)　腹側後内側(核)
ventroposteromedial thalamic nucleus　腹側後内側視床核
vpm
vibrations per minute　1分あたりの振動
VPN
ventral pontine nucleus　橋腹側核
VPP
viral porcine pneumonia　ウイルス性ブタ肺炎
vitamin PP　ビタミンPP
VPR
Voges-Proskauer reaction　フォーゲス・プロスカウアー反応
volume-pressure response　容積圧反応
V-P ratio
ventilation-perfusion ratio　換気・灌流比
VPRC
volume of packed red cell　血液に対する赤血球の容積%
VPS
valvular pulmonic stenosis　肺動脈弁狭窄(症)
ventricular premature systole　心室性期外収縮
ventro-peritoneal shunt　脳室腹腔シャント
VPS, vps, v.p.s.
vibrations per second　振動数/秒
VP shunt, v-p shunt, V-P shunt
ventriculo(-)peritoneal shunt　脳室腹腔シャント
VP test, V-P test
Voges-Proskauer test　フォーゲス・プロスカウアー検査〔試験〕
VPW
ventricular pressure wave　心室圧波
VQ
ventilation/perfusion per minute　分時肺換気血流比
ventilation quotient　換気率
voice quality　声質
V/Q
ventilation/perfusion (lung scan)　肺換気/血流(肺スキャン)
ventilation-perfusion quotient〔ratio〕　換気灌流商〔比〕
VQFP
vincristine, carboquone, 5-fluorouracil, prednisolone　ビンクリスチン,カルボコン,フルオロウラシル,プレドニゾロン

VR
double valve replacement 弁置換術
right arm electrode for electrocardiogram 心電図用右腕電極
valve replacement 弁置換
variable response 可変反応
variotin バイオチン
vascular resistance 血管抵抗
venous return 静脈還流
ventilation rate 換気率
ventilation ratio 換気比
ventilation reserve rate 換気予備率
ventricular rate 心室レート，心室拍動数
ventricular response 心室反応
ventricular rhythm 心室リズム，心室律動
vestibular recruitment 前庭漸増現象
virtual reality 仮想現実
vision, right 右眼視覚
vocational rehabilitation 職業リハビリテーション
volume residue 残気量

VR，vr，v.r.
ventral root (脊髄神経)前根

VR，V.R.
vocal resonance 声帯共鳴

VRBC
red blood cell volume 赤血球容積

VRC
venous renin concentration 静脈(血)レニン濃度
ventral (nerve) root, cervical 前(神経)根・頸髄

VRCP
vitreoretinochoroidopathy 硝子体網膜脈絡膜症

VRC_1〔VRC_2, VRC_3, etc.〕
ventral root, cervical, by number 第1〔2,3…〕頸髄前根

VRD
ventricular radial dysplasia 心室橈骨異形成(症)，心室橈骨形成異常(症)
vinrosidine ビンロシジン
viral respiratory disease ウイルス性呼吸器疾患
von Recklinghausen disease フォンレックリングハウゼン病

VRE
vancomycin-resistant enterococcus バンコマイシン耐性腸球菌

VR & E
vocational rehabilitation and education 職業リハビリテーション教育

V region, V-region
variable region 可変部領域
VRG
vertical ring gastroplasty 垂直輪異形成(術)
VRI
viral respiratory infection ウイルス呼吸器感染(症)
VRL
ventral (nerve) root, lumbar 腰髄の前(神経)根
VRL_1〔VRL_2, VRL_3, etc.〕
ventral (nerve) root, lumbar, by number 第1〔2,3…〕腰髄前(神経)根
VRMS
van Riper auditory memory span ヴァンライパー聴覚記録期間
VRNA
viral ribonucleic acid ウイルスリボ核酸
VRO
varus rotational osteotomy 内反捻転骨切り術
VROM
voluntary range of motion 随意的可動範囲
VRR
ventral root reflex 前根反射
ventral root response 前根応答
VRS
verbal rating scale (痛みの)口頭評価尺度
Vocational Rehabilitation Services 職業リハビリテーションサービス
volume reduction surgery 肺容量減少手術
VRSA
vancomycin-resistant *Staphylococcus aureus* バンコマイシン耐性黄色ブドウ球菌
VRT
ventral (nerve) root, thoracic 前(神経)根・胸髄
vertical radiation topography 垂直照射断層撮影(法)
visual recognition threshold 視認識閾値
(Benton) Visual Retention Test (ベントン)視覚記銘力検査
VRT_1〔VRT_2, VRT_3…etc.〕
ventral root, thoracic, by number 第1〔2,3…〕胸髄前根
VRV
ventricular residual volume 心室残気量
VS
vaccinatoin scar 予防接種痕
vaccine serotype ワクチンの血清型
vagal stimulation 迷走神経刺激
vaginal smear 腟スミア
vasospasm 血管攣縮
ventricles 胃

ventricular septum　心室中隔
vertically selective　垂直選択的な
vertical subluxation　垂直性亜脱臼
very sensitive　非常に感受性の高い
vesicular sound　肺胞音，小水泡音
vesicular stomatitis (virus)　水疱性口内炎(ウイルス)
vital sign　生命徴候
Vogt-Spielmeyer (syndrome)　フォーグト・シュピールマイヤー(症候群)
volumetric solution　定量液

v.s.
vibration seconds　振動秒
vide supra〈ラ〉=see above　上を見よ《処》

VS, V.S.
veterinary surgeon　獣(医)外科医

Vs, VS
venae sectio〈ラ〉=venesection, venisection　静脈切開
visus sinister〈ラ〉　左眼視力

vs, vs.
single vibration　単一振動《循環》
venesection　瀉血
versus〈ラ〉=against　対
very soluble　超易溶性

vs, v/s
visited　訪問した
visitors　訪問者

V.S., V/S, v.s.
vital sign(s)　バイタルサイン

VSA
variant-specific surface antigen　変株特異的表面抗原

VSAG
viral superantigen　ウイルススーパー抗原

VSB
vestigial side-band　残留側波帯

V.s.B.
venae sectio brachii〈ラ〉　上腕静脈切開
venaesectio brachii〈ラ〉　肘静脈からの瀉血

vsby
visibility　視認性

VSC
voluntary surgical contraception　自発的手術(的)避妊

VSD
ventricular septal defect　心室中隔欠損症
virtually safe dose　実質的安全用量

VSF
vascular stromal fraction 間質血管細胞群
VSG
variable surface glycoprotein 可変性表面糖蛋白
variant surface glycoprotein 変株表面糖蛋白
vitesse de sédimentation globulaire 〈仏〉 血沈，赤血球沈降速度
VSHD
ventricular septal heart defect 心室中隔欠損(症)
VSI
very seriously ill 重篤疾患
VSM
vascular smooth muscle 血管平滑筋
vistamycin ビスタマイシン
VSMC
vascular smooth muscle cells 血管平滑筋細胞
VSN
vital signs normal 生命徴候正常
vsn
vision 視覚
VSO
very special old とても古い
VSOK
vital sign OK バイタルサインOK
VSP
ventricular septal perforation 心室中隔穿孔
VSR
ventricular septal rupture 心室中隔破裂
vestibulospinal reflex 前庭脊髄反射
VSS
visual sexual stimulation 視覚性的刺激
vital signs stable 生命徴候安定
V/S/S
vital signs stable バイタルサイン安定
VSSA
virus-specific surface antigen ウイルス特異的表面抗原
VST
ventral spinothalamic tract 腹側脊髄視床路
VSTA
virus-specific transplantation antigen ウイルス特異的移植抗原
VSULA
vaccination scar, upper left arm 予防接種痕・左上腕
VSV
vesicular stomatitis virus 水疱性口内炎ウイルス
volume support ventilation 量支持換気

VSW
ventricular stroke work 心室１回仕事量

V_T
physiological dead space in percent of tidal volume 1回換気量に対する生理学的死腔のパーセンテージ
tidal volume 1回換気量

VT
gas volume unit time ガス容積単位時間
tetrazolium violet テトラゾリウム紫
vacuolating toxin 空胞化毒素
vacuum tube 真空管
variable time 可変時間
variotin バリオチン
vasotocin バソトシン
ventricular tachyarrhythmia 心室性不整頻拍
ventricular tachycardia 心室頻拍
Verhaltenstherapie〈独〉 行動療法
verotoxin ベロ毒素

Vt
pulmonary parenchymal tissue volume 肺実質組織量

V.T
vitamin T ビタミンT

V & T
volume and tension (of pulse) 脈容積と脈圧

VT, V_T
total ventilation 全〔総〕換気

VT, Vt
tidal volume 1回換気量

VT, V.T.
vacuum tuberculin 真空ツベルクリン

vT, v.T.
vom Tausend〈独〉 千分の，千分率，パーミル

V_TA
alveolar tidal volume 肺胞1回換気量

VTA
ventral tegmental area (神経の)腹側被蓋部(野)

VTE
venous thromboembolism 静脈性血栓塞栓症
vicarious trial and error 代理的試行錯誤

VTEC
verotoxin (producing) *Escherichia coli* ベロ毒素産生大腸菌

V-test
Voluter test ヴォルーター試験

VTG
volume thoracic gas　容積胸腔ガス
VTH
vaginal total hysterectomy　腟式子宮全摘出術
VTI
volume thickness index　容積厚さ指数
VTM
mechanical tidal volume　機械的１回換気量
VT-NS
ventricular tachycardia nonsustained　非持続性心室頻拍
VTP
voluntary termination of pregnancy　自発的妊娠中絶
VTR
videotape recorder　ビデオレコーダー
Vtr
volume trriger　吸気トリガー流量
vtr.
vitrum〈ラ〉　ガラス
VTS
vesicular transport system　小胞輸送システム
VT-S
ventricular tachycardia sustained　持続性心室頻拍
VT/VF
ventricular tachycardia/ventricular fibrillation　心室頻拍/心室細動
VTVM
vacuum tube voltmeter　真空管電圧計
VTX, vtx
vertex　頭蓋頂，頭頂，頂
VU
varicose ulcer　静脈瘤性潰瘍
very urgent　非常に緊急の
vitamin U　ビタミンU
v.u.
von untem〈独〉　下方から
VU, vu
volume unit　音量単位
VUE
villitis of unknown etiology　原因不明の絨毛炎
VUG
voiding up to urethrography　排尿時膀胱尿道造影
VUJ
vesicoureteral junction　膀胱尿管接合〔分岐〕部
VUR
vesicoureteral reflux　膀胱尿管逆流(現象)

VUV
vaccum ultraviolet　真空紫外線
VV
vaccinia virus　ワクチニアウイルス
vagina and vulva　膣と外陰部
varicose vein(s)　拡張蛇行静脈
venovenous bypass　静脈静脈短絡路
ventricular volume　心室容積
verruca vulgaris　尋常性疣贅(＝ゆうぜい)，いぼ
viper venom　クサリヘビ毒素
voided volume　排尿量
Vv.
vitrum viride〈ラ〉　緑色のビン《処》
V/V
volume per volume　容量/容量
V & V
vulva and vagina　外陰部と膣
VV，Vv，vv.
veins　静脈
venae〈ラ〉　静脈〈複数〉
vv，v.v.
vice versa〈ラ〉＝order changed　順序入れ替え，逆に
VVA
venous-to-venous anastomosis　静脈・静脈吻合〔術〕
Vicia villosa agglutinin　ビロードクサフジ凝集素
VVB
venovenous bypass　静脈静脈バイパス
VVC
vulvovaginal candidiasis　陰門膣カンジダ症
VVD
vaginal vertex delivery　経膣頭頂位分娩
vascular volume of distribution　血管容積分布
VV fistula
vesicovaginal fistula　膀胱膣瘻
VVFR
vesicovaginal fistula repair　膀胱膣瘻再建
VVH
veno-venous hemofiltration　静脈・静脈血液濾過
VVI
ventricle-ventricle-inhibited　心室抑制型ペーシング
vocal velocity index　声帯速度指数
V/VI
grade five on a six-grade basis　(心雑音) 6 段階の 5 度
VVL
Vicia villosa lectin　ビロードクサフジレクチン

VV lig
varicose vein ligation 拡張蛇行静脈結紮
VVOR
visual vestibuloocular reflex 視覚的前庭眼反射
VVQ
verbalizer-visualization questionnaire 言語化・視覚化質問表
VVR
vasovagal reflex 血管迷走神経反射
VVS
vesicovaginal space 膀胱腟腔
vulvar vestibulitis syndrome 外陰部腟前庭炎
VW, V.W., v.w.
vessel wall (脈)管壁，血管壁
V/W, v/w
volume per weight 容積/重量
V wave
vertex sharp transient wave 頭(蓋)頂一過性鋭波
VWD
ventral wall defect 腹壁欠損(症)
vWD, VWD
von Willebrand'(s) disease フォンヴィレブランド病
VWF
velocity wave form 速度波形
vibration white finger 振動白(色)指，白ろう病
vWF, VWF
von Willebrand factor フォンヴィレブランド病因子
vWS, vWs
von Willebrand syndrome フォンヴィレブランド症候群
VX
varix 静脈瘤
Vx, vx
vertex 頭蓋頂，頭頂，頂
VZ
varicella zoster 水痘帯状疱疹
VZIG
varicella zoster immunoglobulin 水痘帯状疱疹免疫グロブリン
VZIg
varicella zoster immune globulin 水痘帯状疱疹免疫グロブリン
VZV
varicella zoster virus 水痘帯状疱疹ウイルス
V・s
volt-second ボルト・秒

W w

W

tryptophan	トリプトファン
tungsten（＝wolfram）	タングステン〈元素〉
ward	病棟
watt	ワット〈単位〉
weakness	筋力低下，脱力
Weber	ウェーバー
Weber test	ウェーバー検査
wehnelt	ウェーネルト
weight	重量
west	西（の）
western	西部の
white (blood) cell	白血球
white epithelium	白色上皮
whole (response)	全（反応）
width	広さ
Wistar (rat)	ウィスター（ラット）
wolfram	ウォルフラン〈元素〉
word fluency	（発）語流暢，能弁《心理》
work	仕事
Wuchereria	糸状虫

w

wall	壁
warm	温かい
weather	気象
wet	湿った
wine	ワイン，ぶどう酒
woman	女性
wrong	誤った

5W

when, where, why, what, work	いつ・どこで・なぜ・なにが・おこるのか

W＋

weakly positive	弱陽性の

W，w

water	水
weak	弱い
white	白（い）
wide	幅
widow(ed)	未亡人（になった）
widower	男やもめ，寡夫
wound	創傷

W, w, w.
wife　妻
Woche〈独〉=week　週

W, w/, $\overline{w}$, w.
with　〜を伴った

WA
Wiskott-Aldrich (syndrome)　ヴィスコット・オールドリッチ(症候群)

W/A
weakness or atrophy　脱力又は萎縮
white adult　白人成人

WA, W/A
when awake　覚醒時に

WAAVP
World Association for the Advancement of Veterinary Parasitology　世界獣医寄生虫学協会

WAB
Western Aphasia Battery (Test)　ウェスタン失語(症)統合検査
World Association for Buiatrics　国際牛疾病協会

WABT
Western Aphasia Battery Test　ウェスタン失語(症)統合検査

WACH
wedge adjustable cushioned heel (shoe)　ウェッジ調整クッションヒール(靴)

WAF
weakness, atrophy, fasciculation　脱力・萎縮・線維束攣縮
white adult female　白人成人女性

WAG
wearable artificial glomerulus　着用式人工糸球体

WAGR
Wilms (tumor), aniridia, genitourinary (abnormalities) and (mental) retardation　ウィルムス(腫)・無虹彩・尿路(奇形)・(精神)発達遅滞

WAHVM
World Association for the History of Veterinary Medicine　世界獣医学史協会

WAIHA
warm-type autoimmune hemolytic anemia　温式自己免疫性溶血性貧血

WAIS
Wechsler adult intelligence scale　ウェクスラー成人知能検査

WAIS-R
Wechsler Adult Intelligence Scale Revised　ウェクスラー成人知能スケール〔検査〕改訂版

WAK
wearable artificial kidney　携行式人工腎臓

WALK
weight activated locking knee　体重負荷によるロッキング膝

WAM
white adult male　白人成人男性

WAP
wandering atrial pacemaker　遊走性心房ペースメーカー
whole abdominopelvic irradiation　総腹骨盤照射

WAPT
Weidel Auditory Processing Test　ワイデル聴覚処理検査

WaR
Wassermann reaction　ワッセルマン反応

WAR, w.a.r.
without additional reagents　追加試薬なしに

WARDS
Welfare of Animals Used for Research in Drugs and Therapy　薬物および治療法の研究に使用される動物の福祉

WARF, Warf
warfarin　ワルファリン

WARI
wheezing associated respiratory infection　呼吸器感染に伴うぜん鳴

WAS
Ward Atmosphere Scale　病棟雰囲気尺度
weekly activity summary　週活動サマリー
whiplash associated disorder　鞭打ちに伴う疾患
Wiskott-Aldrich syndrome　ウィスコット・オールドリッチ症候群
World Association for Sexology　世界性科学会

WASO
wakefulness after sleep onset　睡眠開始後覚醒

WASP
Weber Advanced Spatial Perception (test)　ウェーバー高等空間知覚(テスト)
World Association of Societies of Pathology, Anatomic and Clinical　世界解剖・臨床病理学会

Wass
Wassermann test　ワッセルマン検査

WAT
weight, altitude, temperature　体重・身長・体温
white adipose tissue　白色脂肪組織
word association test　語連想検査

WAVA
World Association of Veterinary Anatomists　世界獣医解剖学協会

WAVFH
World Association of Veterinary Food Hygienists　世界獣医食品衛生学協会

WAVMI
World Association of Veterinary Microbiologists, Immunologists and Specialists in Infectious Diseases　世界獣医微生物学・免疫学・伝染病学協会

WAVP
World Association of Veterinary Pathologists　世界獣医病理学協会

WAVPPB
World Association of Veterinary Physiologists, Pharmacologists and Biochemists　世界獣医生理学・薬理学・生化学協会

WB
stored whole blood-CPD　CPD加保存血液
waist belt　(拘束)胴ベルト
washable base　洗浄可能基剤
washed bladder　洗浄された膀胱
water bottle　水筒
Wechsler-Bellevue (Scale)　ウェクスラー・ベルビュー(尺度)《心理》
weight bearing　重量を支える
well baby　健康乳(幼)児
Western blot　ウェスタンブロット
wet bulb　湿球
whole blood　全血
whole body　全身
Willowbrook (virus)　ウィロウブルック(ウイルス)

WB, Wb
weber　ウェーバー〈単位〉
weightbearing　荷重

WBA
wax bean agglutinin　ワックスビーン凝集原
wole body activity　全身活動

WBACT
whole blood activated clotting time　全血活性化凝固時間

WBAPTT
whole-blood activated partial thromboplastin time　全血活性化部分トロンボプラスチン時間

WBAT
weightbearing as tolerated　耐荷重

WBC
weightbearing with crutches　クラッチ〔松葉杖〕使用時の荷重

well baby care　健康乳幼児〔赤ん坊〕ケア，育児相談〔保育〕
well baby clinic　健康乳幼児〔赤ん坊〕クリニック，育児相談外来
white blood cell (count)　白血球(数)
white blood corpuscle　白血球

WBC diff
white blood count and differential　白血球数と分画

WBC/hpf
white blood cells per high-power field　高拡大野あたりの白血球(数)

WBCT
whole blood clotting time　全血凝固時間

WBDS
whole body digital scanner　全身デジタルスキャナー

WBE
Weißbroteinheit〈独〉　白パン単位
whole-body extract　全身抽出物

WBF
whole blood folate　全血葉酸

WB-F
fresh whole blood CPD　CPD加新鮮血液

WBGT
wet-bulb globe temperature (index)　湿球黒球温度(指標)
wet-bulb globe thermometer　湿球黒球湿度

WBH
whole blood hematocrit　全血ヘマトクリット
whole-body hyperthermia　全身高熱

WBI
whole body irradiation　全身放射線照射

WBM
whole boiled milk　完全煮沸ミルク

WBN
well born nursery　健康乳児保育室
white blood nitrogen　白血球窒素
whole blood nitrogen　全血窒素
wide band noise　広帯域雑音

WBPTT
whole blood partial thromboplastin time　全血部分トロンボプラスチン時間

WBQC
wide-base quad cane　広基部四脚杖

WBR
whole body radiation　全身照射
whole body retention　全身貯留

W

WBRS
Ward Behavior Rating Scale 病棟行動評点尺度
WBRT
whole-blood recalcification time 全血カルシウム再沈着時間
whole-brain radiation therapy 全脳放射線治療
WBS
Wechsler-Bellevue Scale ウェクスラー・ベルビュースケール
whole body scan 全身スキャン
whole body shower 全身シャワー
Wiedemann-Beckwith syndrome ヴィーデマン・ベックウィズ症候群
withdrawal body shakes 禁断症状による体の震え
wound-breaking strength 創開離強度
WBT
waking body temperature 覚醒時体温
wet-bulb temperature 湿球温度
WBTF
Waring Blender tube feeding ウェアリングブレンダー〔フードプロセッサ〕使用経管栄養
WBTT
weightbearing to tolerance 耐荷重
WBUS
weeks by ultrasound 超音波検査での(妊娠)週
WBV
whole blood volume 全血量
WC
ward confinement 病棟分娩
water closet 便所
Weber-Christian (syndrome) ウェーバー・クリスチャン(症候群)
wet compress 湿布
white (cell) cast 白血球円柱
white cell 白血球
white count 白血球数
whooping cough 百日咳
work capacity 仕事能力
writer's cramp 書痙，書字痙攣
WC, WC'
whole complement 全補体
WC, w.c.
wound check 創傷チェック
WC, W/C
wheelchair 車椅子
white child 白人小児

W

WCC
Walker carcinosarcoma cell　ウォーカー癌肉腫細胞
well-child care　健康児保育
white cell count　白血球数
WCD
Weber-Christian disease　ウェーバー・クリスチャン病
WCE
white coat effect　白衣効果
WCED
World Commission on Environment and Development　世界環境開発委員会
WCGS
Western Collaborative Group Study　ウェスタン・コラボライティブ・グループ・スタディ
WCH
white coat hypertension　白衣高血圧(症)
WCICCM
World Congress on Intensive and Critical Care Medicine　世界集中治療医学会
WCL
Wenckebach cycle length　ウェンケバッハ周期長
whole-cell lysate　全細胞溶解産物
word connection list　(単)語連結リスト
W/cm²
watts per centimeter squared　ワット/cm²
WCOT
wall coated open tubular　壁被覆開口管の
WCPT
World Confederation for Physical Therapy　世界物理療法学会
WCR
Walthard cell rest　ワルタルド細胞遺残
WCRP
World Climate Research Program　世界気候観測計画
WCS
Wisconsin Compression System　ウィスコンシン圧縮システム
WCST
Wisconsin Card-Sorting Test　ウィスコンシンカード分類検査
WD
wallerian degeneration　ウォーラー変性
well developed　体格の良い
well differentiated　よく分化した
wet dressing　湿布，罨法
Whipple disease　ウィップル病

Whitney Damon (dextrose) ホィットニー・デーモン(デキストロース)
Wilson disease ウィルソン病
with disease 疾患のある
withdrawal dyskinesia 禁断症状による運動障害
without dyskinesia ジスキネジーを伴わない
Wolman disease ウォルマン病
wrist disarticulation 手根関節離断〔離開〕(術)

Wd
ward 病棟，共同病室
wolffian duct ウォルフ管

W→D
wet-to-dry (傷の経過が)湿から乾へ

W/D
warm and dry 暖かで乾燥した
withdrawal 離脱症状・退薬症状・禁断症状

WD, wd
wound 創傷，外傷
wounded 傷ついた，負傷した，傷心の

WDCA
well-differentiated carcinoma 高分化型癌(腫)

WDCC
well-developed collateral circulation よく発達した側副循環

WDHA
watery diarrhea-hypokalemia-achlorhydria (syndrome) 水様下痢・低カリウム血症・無胃酸(症候群)

WDHH
watery diarrhea-hypokalemia-hypochlorhydria (syndrome) 水様下痢・低カリウム血症・無塩酸(症候群)

WDHHA
watery diarrhea, hypochlorhydria, hypokalemia, and alkalosis 水様下痢・低塩酸・低カリウム血・アルカローシス

WDI
warfarin dose index ワルファリン用量指数

WDL
well-differentiated lymphocyte よく分化したリンパ球

w-DLE
widespread discoid lupus erythematosus 広範囲円板状エリテマトーデス

WDLL
well-differentiated lymphatic lymphoma よく分化したリンパ性リンパ腫
well-differentiated lymphocytic lymphoma よく分化したリンパ球性リンパ腫

WDPM
well-differentiated papillary mesothelioma　高分化型乳頭状中皮腫

WDS
watery diarrhea syndrome　水様下痢症候群
withdrawal symptoms (syndrome)　禁断症状(症候群)

wds
wounds　創傷，外傷

WDWN
well developed, well nourished　体格がよく栄養良好な

WDWNBM
well-developed, well-nourished black male　体格がよく栄養良好な黒人男性

WDWNWF
well-developed, well-nourished white female　体格がよく栄養良好な白人女性

WDWNWM
well-developed, well-nourished white male　体格がよく栄養良好な白人男性

WE
wax ester　ろうエステル
western encephalitis　西部脳炎
western encephalomyelitis　西部脳脊髄炎
whiskey equivalent　ウイスキー換算で
Williams-Eagle (agar)　ウィリアムス・イーグル(寒天)
wound of entry　入口創

WEE
western equine encephalitis　西部ウマ脳炎

WEEV
western equine encephalitis virus　西部ウマ脳炎ウイルス

WEF
war emergency formula　戦時緊急処方

wef
with effect from　～からの効果を伴った

WEG
water-ethyleneglycol　水・エチレングリコール

Weil-Felix
Weil-Felix reaction　ヴァイル・フェリックス反応

WER
wheal erythema reaction　膨疹紅斑反応

WES
wall-echo shadow　壁反響性陰影
Work Environment Scale　仕事環境尺度《心理》

WESR

Westergren erythrocyte sedimentation rate	ウェスターグレン赤血球沈降率
Wintrobe erythrocyte sedimentation rate	ウィントローブ赤血球沈降率

WF

warm front	温暖前線
Waterhouse-Friderichsen (syndrome)	ウォーターハウス・フリーデリクセン(症候群)
Wistar-Furth	ウィスター・ファース
word fluency (test)	(発)語流暢(検査)

Ⅷ WF

factor Ⅷ related von Willebrand factor	第Ⅷ因子関連フォンヴィレブランド因子

WF, W/F, wf

white female	白人女性

WF, W-F

Weil-Felix (reaction, test)	ヴァイル・フェリックス(反応/検査)

WFAPS

World Federation of Association of Pediatric Surgeons	世界小児外科学会連盟

WFE

Williams flexion exercises	ウィリアムズ屈曲運動

WFH

World Federation of Healing	世界治療連盟
World Federation of Hemophilia	世界血友病学会

WFI

water for injection	注射用蒸留水

WFL

within functional limits	機能範囲内

WFMH

World Federation for Mental Health	世界精神衛生連盟

WFN

World Federation of Neurology	世界神経学連盟

WFNMB

World Federation of Nuclear Medicine and Biology	世界核医学連盟

WFNRS

World Federation of Neuroradiological Societies	世界神経放射線学会連合

WFNS

World Federation of Neurological Surgeons	脳神経外科世界連合
World Federation of Neurosurgical Societies	国際脳神経外科学会

WF-O
will follow in office | 医院で経過を追う

WFOT
World Federation of Occupational Therapists | 世界作業療法学連盟

WFP
World Food Program | 世界食糧計画

WFPHA
World Federation of Public Health Association | 世界公衆衛生協会連盟

WFPMM
World Federation of Proprietary Medicine Manufacturers | 世界大衆薬製造協会

WFR
Weil-Felix reaction | ワイル・フェリックス反応
wheal-and-flare reaction | 膨疹・潮紅反応

WFSA
World Federation of Societies of Anaesthesiologists | 世界麻酔学会連合

WFSICCM
World Federation of Societies of Intensive and Critical Care Medicine | 世界集中治療医学会連合

WFUMB
World Federation for Ultrasound in Medicine and Biology | 世界超音波医学学術連合

WG
water gauge | 水ゲージ
Wegener granulomatosis | ウェゲナー肉芽腫症(＝多発血管炎肉芽腫症)
wire guide | ワイヤーガイド
Wright-Giemsa (stain) | ライト・ギムザ(染色)

WGA
wheat germ agglutinin | 小麦胚凝集素

WGO
Weltgesundheitsorganisation〈独〉 | 世界保健機関

WH
walking heel (cast) | 歩行用踵(ギプス)
well healed | 治癒良好な
well-hydrated | 十分水分補給された
Werdnig-Hoffmann (syndrome) | ウェルドニッヒ・ホフマン(症候群)
whole homogenate | 全ホモジネート
wound healing | 創傷治癒
wound hormone | 創傷ホルモン

wh
whisper ささやく
whispered ささやいた
white 白い

WHA
warmed, humidified air 暖房加湿空気
World Health Assembly 世界保健総会

WHAMES
weight, hight, appearance, mentality, emotion and sexual devolopment 体重・身長・外貌・知性・性発育

wh ch
wheelchair 車椅子
white child 白人小児

WHD
Werdnig-Hoffmann disease ウェルドニッヒ・ホフマン病

WHHL
Watanabe heritable hyperlipidemic rabbit 遺伝性家族性高コレステロール血症モデルウサギ

WHNR
well-healed, no residuals 治癒良好・残遺なし

WHNS
well healed, nonsymptomatic 治癒良好で無症状の
well-healed, no sequelae 治癒良好・後遺症なし

WHO
World Health Organization 世界保健機関
wrist-hand orthosis 手関節背屈装具

whp
whirlpool 渦流

WHPB
whirlpool bath 渦流浴

whpl
whirlpool 渦流

WHR
waist-hip circumference ratio ウェスト・ヒップ周囲比

Whr
watt hour ワット時

WHS
Werdnig-Hoffmann syndrome ウェルドニッヒ・ホフマン症候群

WHV
woodchuck hepatitis virus ウッドチャック肝炎ウイルス

WHVP
wedged hepatic vein pressure 楔入(部)肝静脈圧
wedged hepatic venous pressure 楔入(部)肝静脈圧

WHYMPI
Westhaven Yale Multidimensional Pain Inventory — ウエストヘイヴン・イェール多次元痛み項目表

WI
walk-in (patient) — 予約なしの来院(患者)
water ingestion — 水摂取
watershed infarction — 境界域梗塞
waviness index — うねり指数
Wistar (rat) — ウィスター(ラット)

WI-38
Wistar Institute 38 — ウィスターインスティテュート38

W/I
within — 内部の，以内の

WIA
walking imagined analgesia — 歩行想定除痛〔麻酔〕
wounded in action — 動作中の受傷

WIC
women, infants, and children — 婦人・乳児・小児

wid., Wid.
widow — 未亡人
widowed — 未亡人〔男やもめ〕になった
widower — 男やもめ

Widal
Widal reaction — ウィダール反応

WII
Work Information Inventory — 仕事情報調査票《心理》

WILD
What I Like to Do — (学生興味調査票の)私がしたい事

WIPI
Word Intelligibility by Picture Identification — 絵画同定による単語了解度

WIPO
World Intellectual Property Organization — 世界知的所有権機関

WIQ
Waring Intimacy Questionnaire — ウェアリング親密性質問票

WIS
wafer inspection system — (光学式の)異物検査装置
Wechsler Intelligence Scale — ウェクスラー知能評価尺度

WISC
Wechsler intelligence scale for children — ウェクスラー児童用知能検査

WISC-R
Wechsler Intelligence Scale for Children-Revised — ウェクスラー小児用知能スケール改訂版
WIT
warm ischemic time — 温阻血時間
water-induced thermotherapy — 水誘発温熱療法
WITT
Wittenborn (psychiatric rating scale) — ウィッテンボーン(精神症状評価尺度)
W-J
Woodcock-Johnson (Psychoeducational Battery) — ウッドコック・ジョンソン(心理学的学習統合検査)
WJPB
Woodcock-Johnson Psychoeducational Battery — ウッドコック・ジョンソン心理的学習統合検査
WK
Wernicke-Korsakoff (syndrome) — ウェルニッケ・コルサコフ(症候群)
wet Kata — 湿カタ寒暖計
Wilson-Kimmelstiel (syndrome) — ウィルソン・キンメルシュティール(症候群)
wk
week — 週
well known — よく知られた，既知の
work — 仕事
/wk
per week — /週
WK, wk
weak — 弱い
WKD
Wilson-Kimmelstiel disease — ウィルソン・キンメルシュティール病
WK dis.
Wilson-Kimmelstiel disease — ウィルソン・キンメルシュティール病
WKF
well-known fact — よく知られた事実
wkly
weekly — 毎週
WKS
Wernicke-Korsakoff syndrome — ウェルニッケ・コルサコフ症候群
wks
weeks — 週
WKY
Wistar-Kyoto rats — ウィスター・京都ラット

WL
waiting list 待ちリスト
waterload (test) 水負荷(試験)
wavelength 波長
weight loss 体重減少
work load 仕事負荷

WLE
wide local excision 広範囲局所切除(術)

WLF
whole lymphocyte fraction 全リンパ球分画

WLI
weight-length index 体重・身長指数

WLM
work-level month 月の仕事水準

WLN
within limit of normal 正常範囲内

WLR
within-list recognition リスト内再認

WLS
wet lung syndrome 湿性肺，水腫肺症候群

WLT
water load test 水負荷試験
whole lung tomography 全肺断層撮影(法)

WM
Waldenström macroglobulinemia ワルデンシュトレームマクログロブリン血(症)
wall motion 壁運動
ward manager 病棟主任
warm, moist 温暖・湿潤な
Wernicke-Mann (hemiplegia) ヴェルニッケ・マン(片麻痺)
wet mount ウェットマウント
whole milk 全乳
Wilson-Mikity (syndrome) ウィルソン・ミキティ(症候群)
woman milk 母乳

wm
whole mount 全組織標本

WM, W/M
white male 白人男性

WMA
wall motion abnormalities 壁運動異常
wall-motion abnormality 壁運動異常
World Medical Association 世界医師会

WMC
weight-matched control 体重をマッチさせたコントロール

WMD
warm moist dressing (sterile) 暖かい(滅菌した)湿布
WME
Williams medium E ウィリアムズ培地E
WMF
white married female 白人既婚女性
Wm flex.ex.
Williams flexion exercises ウィリアムズ屈曲運動
WML
white matter lesion (cerebral) (大脳)白質損傷
WMLA
World Medical Law Association 世界医事法学会
WMM
white married male 白人既婚男性
WMO
World Meteorological Organization 世界気象機関
WMP
warm moist pack (unsterile) 温湿パック(非滅菌の)
weight management program 体重管理プログラム
WMR
work metabolic rate 仕事代謝率
World Medical Relief 世界医療援助
WMS
wall-motion study 壁運動研究
Wechsler Memory Scale ウェクスラー記憶尺度
Wms flex.ex.
Williams flexion exercises ウィリアムズ屈曲運動
WMSI
wall motion score index 壁運動評点指数
WMX
whirlpool, massage, exercise 渦流・マッサージ・運動
WN
wave number 波数
WN, W/N
well nourished 栄養良好な
WNAP
whole nerve action potential 全神経活動電位
WND, wnd
wound 創傷, 外傷
WNE
West Nile encephalitis 西ナイル脳炎
WNF
well-nourished female 栄養良好な女性

WNL
within normal limits 正常範囲内

WNLS
weighted nonlinear least squares　加重非線形最小二乗(法)
WNM
well-nourished male　栄養良好な男性
WNPW
wide, notched P wave　幅広い切痕のあるP波
WNV
West Nile virus　西ナイルウイルス
WNWD
well nourished, well developed　栄養良好で体格の良い
WO
wash(-)out　洗い出し，ウォッシュアウト
water-in-oil emulsion adjuvant　油中水型乳剤アジュバント
W/O
water in oil　油中水(型)，油中水滴(型)(乳剤)
WO, wo
weeks old　週齢
WO, W/O
written order　書かれた指示，文章での指示，命令書
W/O, w/o
without　～を伴わない，～なしの，～せずに
WOB
work of breathing　呼吸の仕事(量)
WOC
without compensation　代償なしで
WOE
wound of entry　入口創，射入創
WOFL
wound fluid　創液，滲出液
WOIEP
World Office of Information on Environmental Problems　世界環境問題情報局
WOIH
Council of World Organizations Interested in the Handicapped　世界身体障害者機構
WONCA
World Organization of National Colleges, Academies and Academic Association of General Practitioners/Family Physicians　世界家庭医学会議
WOP
without pain　痛みを伴わない

WOR
Weber-Osler-Rondu (syndrome) ウェーバー・オスラー・ロンデュ(症候群)

WOS
West of Scotland Coronary Prevention Study ウォス・スタディ

WOSCOPS
West of Scotland Coronary Prevention Study 一次予防のための大規模試験

W/O type
water in oil type 油中水型

WOU
women's outpatient unit 女性外来部，婦人科外来

WOW
water-in-oil-in-water emulsion adjuvant 水中油中水型乳剤アジュバント，多重乳剤アジュバント

WOWS
Weak Opiate Withdrawal Scale 弱アヘン剤離脱尺度

WOX
wound of exit 出口創，射出熱

WP
water packed 水を入れた
weakly positive 弱陽性の
wedge pressure 楔入(部)圧
wettable powder 可溶性パウダー
whirpool 渦流
white pulp 白(色)脾髄

W/P
water/powder (ratio) 水/粉(比)

WP, Wp
working point 顕微鏡の焦点，作働点

WP, W/P
whirlpool 渦(巻き)

WP, WPk
wet pack 湿布

WPA
World Psychiatric Association 世界精神医学連合

WPAI
Wilson-Patterson Attitude Inventory ウィルソン・パターソン態度調査票《心理》

WPB
whirlpool bath 渦流浴

WPC
water pollution control 水質汚染管理

WPCA
water pollution control act 水質汚染管理活動

WPCC
Western Pharmaceutical and Chemical Corporation — 西部薬局・化学協会

WPCU
weighted patient care unit — 肥満患者治療部

WPFM
Wright Peak Flow Meter — ライト最大流量計

WPk
wet pack — 湿布

WPM, w.p.m.
word(s) per minute — 毎分～語，語/分《電信》

WPN
white (mucosa with) punctation — 斑点のある白い(粘膜)

WPPSI
Wechsler Preschool and Primary Scale of Intelligence — ウェクスラー就学前・小学生用知能尺度

WPRS
Wittenborn Psychiatric Rating Scale — ウィッテンボーン精神症状評点尺度

WPSI
Wittenborn Psychiatric Symptoms Inventory — ウィッテンボーン精神症状評価項目表

WPT
warbled pure tone — 震純音
water provocative test — 水負荷試験

WPW
Wolff-Parkinson-White (syndrome) — ウォルフ・パーキンソン・ホワイト(症候群)

WR
water retention — 水(分)貯留
weak response — 弱反応
whole response — 全反応
wide range — 広域，広範囲
wiping reflex — 払いのけ反射
work rate — 仕事率，仕事速度

WR-2721
ethiofos — エチオフォス

W-R
Waaler-Rose test — ワーラー・ローズ試験〔反応〕

WR, Wr
Wassermann reaction — ワッセルマン反応

WR, Wr, wr
weakly reactive — 弱反応性の

WR, Wr, wr, wr.
wrist — 手首，手関節，手根

W/R, W/r
with respect to　～に関して

Wr_a
Wright antigen　ライト抗原

WRAML
Wide Range Assessment of Memory and Learning　記憶と学習の広範囲評価

WRAT
Wide Range Achievement Test　広範囲達成検査《心理》

WRBC
washed red blood cell(s)　洗浄赤血球

WRC
washed red cell(s)　洗浄赤血球
water-retention coefficient　水分貯留係数

WRE
whole ragweed extract　全ブタクサ抽出物

w ref
with reference　～を参照して

W-response
whole response　全反応

WREST
wide range employment sample test　広範囲雇用サンプル検査《心理》

WRF
World Rehabilitation Fund　世界リハビリテーション基金

WRIOT
wide range interest-opinion test　広範囲興味意見検査

WRIPT
wide range intelligence and personality test　広範囲知能人格検査

WRK
Woodward reagent K　ウッドワード試薬K

WRMT
Woodcock Reading Mastery Test　ウッドコック読み熟達総合テスト

WRS
Wiedemann-Rauten-Strauch syndrome　ウィーデマン・ラウテン・ストラウク症候群

WRVP
wedged renal vein pressure　楔入(部)腎静脈圧

WS
Waardenburg syndrome　ワーデンブルグ症候群
Wallenberg syndrome　ワーレンベルグ症候群
Warthin-Starry (stain)　ウォーシン・スターリー(染色法)
watermelon stomach　スイカ状の胃

water soluble	水溶性の
water swallow	水嚥下
Werner syndrome	ヴェルナー症候群
Westphal-Strümpell (syndrome)	ヴェストファル・シュトリュンペル(症候群)
West syndrome	ウェスト〔ウエスト〕症候群
wet swallow	水と一緒の嚥下
Wilder silver (stain)	ワイルダー銀(染色)
Williams syndrome	ウィリアムズ症候群
Wirbelsäule〈独〉	脊柱
workshop	ワークショップ
work simplification	仕事単純化

W & S

wound and skin	創傷と皮膚

W-s

watt seconds	ワット秒

WSA

water soluble adjuvant	水溶性アジュバント
water-soluble antibiotic(s)	水溶性抗生物質
World Health Statistics Annual	世界健康統計年報

WSAVA

World Small Animal Veterinary Association	世界小動物獣医学協会

WSB

wheat soy blend	麦ダイズ混合

WSD

water seal drainage	静水柱圧利用排液

WSDI

Wahler self-description inventory	ワーラー自己記述調査票

W-sec

watt seconds	ワット秒

WSL

Wesselsbron (virus)	ヴェッセルスブロン(ウイルス)

WSR

Westergren sedimentation rate	ウェスターグレン沈降率

WSRF

end-stage renal failure	末期腎不全

WSSDT

Washington Speech Sound Discrimination Test	ワシントン会話音鑑別検査《心理》

WSSFN

World Society for Stereotaxic and Functional Neurosurgery	国際定位脳手術学会

WT

walking tank	歩行用ボンベ

wall thickness 壁の厚さ
water temperature 水温
wild type 野生型
Wilms tumor ウィルムス腫瘍
wisdom teeth 智歯，親知らず
work therapy 作業療法

wt.
white 白い，白人

%wt
weight percent 質量百分率

WT，Wt，wt.
weight 重量，重さ，体重

wt.b.
weight bearing 重量を支える

WTd
diastolic left ventricular posterior wall thickness 左(心)室後壁拡張期厚

W-T-D
wet-to-dry 湿から乾へ

WTE
whole time equivalent 総時間等量

WTF
weight transferral frequency 体重移動頻度

WTO
World Trade Organization 世界貿易機関

WTPCF
whole treponema pallidum complement fixation test 全トレポネマ・パリズム補体結合試験

WTs
systolic left ventricular posterior wall thickness 左(心)室後壁収縮期厚

WU
Word Understanding 単語理解《心理》

W/U，w/u
work-up 検査

WUSCT
Washington University Sentence Completion Test ワシントン大学文章完成試験〔検査〕《心理》

WV
walking ventilation 歩行時肺換気量
whispered voice ささやき声

W_v
variable dominant spotting (mouse) 変異多数斑紋(マウス)

W/V
weight per volume 容積あたり重量

w/v
percent "weight in volume" 容積(中)重量パーセンテージ
WVA
World Veterinary Association 世界獣医師会
WVI
Work Values Inventory 作業価値調査表《心理》
WV-MBC
walking ventilation to maximal breathing capacity (ratio) 歩行時肺換気量・分時最大換気〔呼吸〕量(比)
WVPA
World Veterinary Poultry Association 世界獣医家禽学協会
WW
Weight Watchers 体重を気にする人，(食事療法で)減量に努めている人
wet weight 湿潤重量，透析前体重量
W→W
wet-to-wet 湿から湿へ
w/w
percent "weight in weight" 重量(中)重量パーセンテージ
W/W, w/w
weight (of solute) per weight (of solvent) (溶液)重量あたりの(溶質)重量
WWAC
walk with aid of cane 杖の助けを借りて歩く
WWI
World of Work Inventory 作業世界調査表《心理》
W/wo
with or without ～を伴うまたは伴わない
WWTP
wastewater treatment plant 廃水処理プラント
WWW
world wide web 全世界情報網(＝インターネット通信網の１つ)
WX, W/X
wound of exit 出口創，射出創
WxB
wax bite ワックスバイト《歯》
WxP
wax pattern ワックス型《歯》
WY
women years 婦人年，女性年
WY/NRT
Weidel Yes/No Reliability Test ワイデル・イエス/ノー信頼度検査

WZa
wide zone alpha (hemolysis) 広範囲アルファ(溶血)

X x

X

androgenic (zone)	アンドロゲン産生(帯)
break	切断(する)
cross-bite	交差〔交叉〕咬合
crossed with	交差〔交叉〕した
crossmatch	交差〔交叉〕(適合)試験
decimal scale of potency or dilution	効能や希釈の十進法スケール
exophoria	外斜位《眼》
exophoric	外斜位の《眼》
extra	余分の，特別の
female sex chromosome	女性(性)染色体
intermittent exotropia	間欠性外斜視《眼》
Kienböck unit (of X-ray exposure)	(X線曝露の)キーンベック単位
magnification	拡大
multiplication	乗法，乗じる
nervus vagus	迷走神経
reactance	誘導抵抗
removal of	～の除去
respirations	呼吸《麻酔》
start of anesthesia	麻酔開始
(roman numeral) ten	(ローマ数字の)10
times	～回，～倍
transverse	横径の，横断の，横軸の
xanthosine	キサントシン
X descent	X谷
Xenopsylla	ネズミノミ(属)
xerophthalmia	眼球乾燥(症)
xerose bacillus	乾燥菌
X-unit	エックス単位，X(線)単位

x

axis	軸
lateral axis	横軸
mole fraction	モル分率
specific acoustic reactance	特異聴力感応抵抗

Χ, χ

chi〈ギ〉	(ギリシャ文字の)カイ

X, x

exposure	曝露，露呈，露髄
extremity	先端，極端，肢
unknown	不明，未知
xanthine	キサンチン

$\overline{X}$, x
except ～を除いて
sample mean サンプル平均

$\overline{X}$, $\overline{x}$
except ～を除いて
sample mean サンプル平均値の記号《統》

XA
xanthurenic acid キサンツレン酸

Xa
activated factor X 活性因子X
chiasma 交叉〔差〕

Xaa
unknown amino acid 未知のアミノ酸

xact
exactly 正確に，厳密に

XAFS
X-ray absorption fine structure X線吸収微細構造法

X : Ag
factor X antigen 第X因子抗原

XAL
xenon arc lamp キセノンアークランプ

Xam
examination 試験，検査

X-A mixture
xylene-alcohol mixture キシレン・アルコール混合物

Xan
xanthine キサンチン

XANES
X-ray absorption near edge structure X線吸収端近傍構造法

Xanth, xanth.
xanthomatosis 黄色腫症

Xao
xanthosine キサントシン

XAT
X-ray analysis trial X線解析試験

x-axis
horizontal axis 水平軸

***x* axis of Fick**
transverse axis of Fick フィックの横軸《眼》

X-Bein
genu valgum 外反膝

X-Bell
extractum belladonnae〈ラ〉 ベラドンナエキス《処》

XBM
out-patient basal metabolism rate 外来患者基礎代謝率

XBT
xylose breath test キシロース呼吸試験
XC
excretory cystogram 排出性膀胱造影〔撮影〕図
xylene diisocyanate キシレンジイソシアネイト
Xc
reactance リアクタンス
X-C
X-chromosome X染色体
XCCE
extracapsular cataract extraction (水晶)嚢外白内障摘出(術)
xch
exchange 交換する
X-chrome
a sex-determinant chromosome 性決定染色体
X-copool
extractum scopoliae〈ラ〉 ロートエキス《処》
XCT
X-ray computed tomography X線CT
XD
xanthoma disseminatum 播種性黄色腫
X-line dominant 伴性優性《遺伝》
4Xd
four times a day 1日4回《処》
X & D
examination and diagnosis 検査と診断
x'd
X-rayed X線を照射した，X線撮影をした
XDFHom
Diploma of the Faculty of Homeopathy ホメオパシー学修了証書
XDH
xanthine dehydrogenase キサンチン脱水素酵素，キサンチンデヒドロゲナーゼ
X disease
morbid symptoms of unknown origin 原因不明の病的症状
XDP
xanthine diphosphate キサンチン二リン酸
xeroderma pigmentosum 色素性乾皮症
X-ray diffraction powder X線回折粉末
XDR
transducer 変換器，トランスデューサー
XDT
defibrillation threshold 除細動閾値
diversional therapy 気晴らし療法

X

Xe
xenon　キセノン〈元素〉
XECT, XeCT, Xe-CT
xenon-enhanced computed tomography　キセノン増強コンピュータ連動断層撮影(法)
X-ed
crossed　交差〔叉〕した，交差〔叉〕性の
XEF
excess ejection fraction　過大駆出率
XEG
X-ray emission gage　X線放射計器
XEMS
X-ray fluorescence element mapping spectrometer　螢光X線マッピング装置
xeno
xenodiagnosis　キセノン診断
xenodiagnostic　キセノン診断の
xenograph　キセノン写真
xenographic　キセノン写真の
xenography　キセノン写真
XEQ
execute　実行する《コン》
Xero
xeromammography　乾式乳房撮影(法)
XES
X-ray emission spectra　X線放出スペクトル
X-ray energy spectromerty　X線エネルギー分光計
X-ray energy spectrometer　X線エネルギー分光計
X-ray energy spectroscopy　X線エネルギー分光学
XF
extra fine　超微細の
xerophthalmic fundus　眼球乾燥症の眼底
X-factor
heme　ヘム
hemin　ヘミン
Xfmr
transformer　トランス，変圧器
xg
crossing　交叉〔差〕
Xg antigen
Xg blood group (antigen)　Xg血液型(抗原)
XGP
xanthogranulomatous pyelonephritis　黄色肉芽腫性腎盂腎炎
XH
extra hard　超硬度の
extra heavy　超重量の

extra high — 超高度の

XHIM
X-linked high IgM syndrome — X(染色体)連鎖高IgM血症

XIC, Xic
X inactivation center — X(染色体)不活化中心

Xid
X-linked immunodeficiency — 伴性免疫不全症

XIH
idiopathic hypercalcuria — 特発性高カルシウム尿症

XIM
X-ray intensity meter — X線照度計

XIP
X-ray in plaster (examination) — ギプス固定のままでのX線写真

xiph
xiphoid — 剣状の

XIST
X inactive center specific transcript — X(染色体)不活性中心特異転写(物)

X-ized
crystallized — 結晶化した

XKO
not knocked out — ノックアウトされていない

XL
excess lactate — 過剰乳酸
xylose lysine — キシロースリジン(培地)

XLA
X-linked agammaglobulinemia — 伴性無γグロブリン血症

XLD
xylose, lysine, deoxycholate — キシロース・リジン・デオキシコール酸塩(培地)

X-leg
crossleg — 外反膝

XLFDP
crosslinked fibrin degradation product — 架橋フィブリン分解生成物

XLH
X-linked hypophosphatemia — 伴性低リン酸(塩)血(症)

XLHM
X-linked hyper IgM syndrome — 伴性高IgM症候群

XLI
X-linked ichthyosis — 伴性劣性魚鱗癬, X(染色体)連鎖魚鱗癬

XLJR
X-linked juvenile retinoschisis — 伴性若年性網膜分離(症)

XLMR
X-linked mental retardation 伴性精神遅滞
XLP
X-linked lymphoproliferative syndrome 伴性劣性リンパ増殖症候群
X-Lp
X-lipoprotein X-リポ蛋白
XLR
X-linked recessive 伴性劣性の
XLS
X-linked recessive lymphoproliferative syndrome X(染色体)連鎖リンパ球増殖性症候群
XLSA
X-linked sideroblastic anemia 伴性劣性鉄芽球性貧血
XM
cross-match(ing) 交叉〔差〕(適合)試験
X_m
magnetic susceptibility 磁化率
X-mas
Christmas (factor) クリスマス(因子)
X-match
cross-match 交叉〔差〕(適合)試験
X-matching
cross-matching 交叉〔差〕(適合)試験
X-MFT
X-ray maxillo-mucosal function test X線上顎粘膜機能試験
XMM
xeromammography 乾式乳房撮影(法)
XMP
xanthine monophosphate キサンチン一リン酸
xanthosine monophosphate キサントシン一リン酸
XN
night blindness 夜盲(症)
Xn
Christian キリスト教徒
XNA
xenogeneic natural antibody 異種自然抗体
XO
gonadal dysgenesis of Turner type ターナー型性器発育異常，ターナー型生殖器発育不全
presence of only one sex chromosome 性染色体が1つだけ存在
xanthine oxidase キサンチン酸化酵素，キサンチンオキシダーゼ
XOAN
X-linked ocular albinism, Nettleship ネトルシップ伴性眼白子(症)

X-off
transmitter off　トランスミッターオフ《コン》
XOM
entraocular movements　眼球運動，外眼(筋)運動
X-on
transmitter on　トランスミッターオン《コン》
XOP
X-ray out of plaster　ギプスを外した状態でのX線写真
XOR
exclusive operating room　専用手術室
45XO syndrome
Turner syndrome　ターナー症候群
XP
exophoria　外斜視
xeroderma pigmentosum　色素性乾皮症
Xp
short arm of chromosome X　X染色体短腕
Xp, X-p, XP
X-ray photograph　X線写真
X-ray photography　X線検査(法)
XPN
xanthogranulomatous pyelonephritis　黄色肉芽腫性腎盂腎炎
X prep.
X-ray preparation　X線準備
X-protein
antigammaprotein　抗ガンマ蛋白
XPS
X-ray photoelectron spectroscopy　X線光電子分光法
X-ray photoemission spectroscopy　X線発光分光学
XP-T
exophoria-tropia　外斜位斜視
Xq
long arm of chromosome X　X染色体長腕
XR
xeroradiographic equipment　ゼロラジオグラフィ装置
xeroradiography　ゼロラジオグラフィ
xerox radiography　ゼロックス放射線図
X-linked recessive　伴性劣性の《遺伝》
XR, xr
X-ray　X線
X-ray
radiograph　放射線写真(の)
XRD
X-ray diffraction　X線回折

X

XRF
X-ray fluorescence　X線螢光
XRM
X-ray microanalyzer　X線微小解析器
XRMR
X-linked recessive mental retardation　伴性劣性精神(発達)遅滞
XRN
X-linked recessive nephrolithiasis　X(染色体)連鎖劣性腎石症
XRO
xenoradiography　キセノン放射線写真
XRPM
X-ray projection microscope　X線放射顕微鏡
XRPT
X-ray and photofluorography technician　X線・螢光写真技術者
XRT
X-ray radiation treatment　X線照射治療
X-ray technician　X線技術者
X-ray therapy　X線〔放射線〕療法
XS
corneal scar　角膜の瘢痕
cross-section　断面
xiphisternum　剣状突起
Xs
excess　過剰
xs
chiasma　交叉〔差〕
XSA
cross-sectional area　断面積
xenograph surface area　異種移植片表面積
XSCID
X-linked severe combined immunodeficiency　伴性劣性重症複合免疫不全症
X scopol
extractum scopoliae〈ラ〉　ロートエキス《処》
X-sect, x sect.
cross-section　断面
XS-LIM
exceeds limits (of procedure)　(手技の)限界を超える
XSLR
crossed straight leg raising (sign)　交差〔叉〕下肢伸展挙上(徴候)
XSP
xanthoma striatum palmare　手掌線条黄色腫
XSPG
X-linked spastic palaplegia　X(染色体)連鎖性痙性対麻痺

45X syndrome
Turner syndrome　ターナー症候群
XT
exotropia〈ラ〉　外斜視
exotropia　外斜視
exotropic　外斜視(性)の
Xta
chiasmata　交叉〔差〕
chiasmate　染色体交叉〔差〕〈複数〉
Xtal
crystal　結晶，水晶，結晶(性)の
XTE
xeroderma, talipes and enamel (defect)　乾皮症・彎足・エナメル質(欠損)
XTM
xanthoma tuberosum multiplex　多発性結節性黄色腫
XTP
xanthosine triphosphate　キサントシン三リン酸
XTV
X-ray television　X線テレビ
XU
excretory urogram　排出性尿路造影〔撮影〕図
Xu, XU
X-unit　X(線)単位
xul
xylulose　キシルロース
XUV
extreme ultraviolet　極紫外線
xvse
transverse　横径の，横断の，横軸の
X walk
cross-walk　交叉〔差〕歩行
XX
normal female chromosome type　正常女性染色体型《遺伝》
46 XX
46 chromosomes, 2X chromosomes (= normal female)　46染色体・2本のX染色体，正常女性の染色体
xxh
double extra hard　2倍硬度
double extra heavy　2倍質量
XXX
triple X syndrome, triple X female, super-female syndrome　トリプルX症候群
XX〔XXX, XXXX…〕
double〔triple/quadruple…〕 strength　2倍〔3倍/4倍…〕強度(＝強度の倍数)

X

49 XXXXY
49 chromosomes, 4X and 1Y chromosomes (=XXXXY syndrome) — 49染色体・４本のX染色体と１本のY染色体(=XXXXY症候群)

47 XXY
47 chromosomes, 2X and 1Y chromosomes (=Klinefelter syndrome) — 47染色体・２本のX染色体と１本のY染色体(=クラインフェルター症候群)

XXYsyndrome
Klinefelter syndrome — XXY症候群, クラインフェルター症候群

XY
normal male chromosome type — 正常男性染色体型《遺伝》
normal male sex chromosome type — 正常男性(性)染色体型

46 XY
46 chromosomes, 1X and 1Y chromosome (normal male) — 46染色体=XY染色体(=正常男性の染色体)

47 XY+21
47 chromosomes, male, additional chromosome 21 (=Down syndrome, chromosome 21 trisomy) — 47染色体・男性・21染色体が１本多い(=ダウン症候群, 21染色体トリソミー)

Xyl
xylose — キシロース

XYL, Xyl
Xylocaine — キシロカイン

Xyl & cort.
Xylocaine and cortisone — キシロカインとコルチゾン

47 XYY
47 chromosomes, 1X and 2Y chromosomes (=XYY xyndrome) — 47染色体・１本のX染色体と２本のY染色体(=XYY症候群)

X-zone
adrenal cortex inner — 副腎皮質内層

Y y

Y
male sex chromosome 男性(性)染色体，Y染色体
pyrimidine nucleoside ピリミジンヌクレオシド
tyrosine チロシン
Y descent Y谷
years 年
yellow 黄色の
Yersinia エルシニア(属)
yield 収量，収率
young 若い，若年の
yttrium イットリウム〈元素〉

y
longitudinal axis 縦軸

^{90}Y
yttrium-90 イットリウム90

YA
Yersinia arthritis エルシニア(属)関節炎

Y/A
years ago ～年前
years of age ～歳，年齢～歳

YAC
yeast artificial chromosome 酵母人工染色体

YACP
young adult chronic patient 若年成人慢性患者

YADH
yeast alcohol dehydrogenase 酵母アルコール脱水素酵素

YAG
yttrium-aluminium-garnet (laser) イットリウム・アルミニウム・ガーネット(レーザー)，ヤグ(レーザー)

***y* axis of Fick**
longitudinal axis of Fick フィックの縦軸《眼》

Yb
ytterbium イッテルビウム〈元素〉

Y/B
yellow/blue 黄色・青色の

Y band
iliofemoral band 腸骨大腿骨帯

YBC
yeast biochemical card 酵母同定用カード

Y-BOCS
the Yale-Brown obsessive compulsive scale エール・ブラウン強迫行為〔強迫性障害〕薬効評価尺度

Y body
fluorescent spot seen on long arm of chromosome 染色体長腕の螢光斑
YBr
yellowish brown 黄褐色の
YBT
Yerkes-Bridges Test ヤークス・ブリッジズ検査《心理》
YC
Y-chromosome Y染色体
YCB
yeast carbon base 酵母炭素塩基
Y chrom
male sex chromosome 男性染色体
YCT
Yvon coefficient test イヴォン係数試験
yd
yard ヤード(=約0.9m)〈単位〉
yd^2
square yard 平方ヤード
y day
yesterday 昨日
YDES
yin deficiency-yang excess syndrome 陰欠乏・陽過剰症候群
YE
yeast extract 酵母抽出物
yellow enzyme 黄色酵素
yearb
yearbook 年鑑
YEG
yeast extract glucose 酵母抽出ブドウ糖
YEH_2
reduced yellow enzyme 還元型黄色酵素
YEI
Yersinia enterocolitica infection エルシニア・エンテロコリチカ感染
Yel, yel
yellow 黄色(の)
yelsh
yellowish 黄色い
YEPD
yeast extract-peptone dextrose 酵母抽出ペプトン・ブドウ糖
ye.s.
yellow spot 黄斑(網膜)
YF
yellow fever 黄熱病

YFA
young female arteritis 若年女性動脈炎
YFI
yellow fever immunization 黄熱病予防接種
YFV
yellow fever virus 黄熱ウイルス
YG test, Y-G test
Yatabe-Guilford personality test 矢田部・ギルフォード性格検査《心理》
YHMD
yellow hyaline membrane disease 黄色ヒアリン膜症
YHT
Young-Helmholtz theory ヤング・ヘルムホルツ説
YJV
yellow jacket venom スズメバチ毒
Yk
York (antibody) ヨーク(抗体)
YLC
youngest living child 最年少生存児
YLF
yttrium lithium fluoride イットリウムリチウムフッ化物
YM
yeast,mannitol (medium) 酵母・マンニトール(培地)
YMA
yeast morphology agar 酵母形態学培地
YMB
yeast malt broth 酵母麦芽ブイヨン
YMT
Yaba monkey tumor ヤバサル腫瘍
YMWA
Young Moslem Women Association 若い回教婦人協会
YNB
yeast nitrogen base 酵母窒素塩基
YNS
yellow nail syndrome 黄色爪症候群
YO, Y/O, y/o
years old 年齢，～歳の
YOB
year of birth 生年，誕生年
YOD
year of death 死亡年
YORA
younger-onset rheumatoid arthritis 若年発症性慢性関節リウマチ
YP
yeast phase 酵母相

yield pressure 産出圧

YPA
yeast, peptone, adenine sulfate 酵母・ペプトン・硫酸アデニン

YPK
yellowish pink 黄色味がかったピンク色

YPLL
years of potential life lost 生存可能損失年

YPM
Yersinia pseudotuberculosis-derived mitogen エルシニアスーパー抗原性外毒素

Yr
younger より若い

yr
year 年

yrb
yearbook 年鑑

YRD
Yangtze River disease 揚子江病

yrs
years 年

YS
Yoshida sarcoma 吉田肉腫

YS, ys, y.s.
yellow spot (網膜の)黄斑

YS, y.s.
yolk sac 卵黄包，卵黄嚢

YSC
yolk sac carcinoma 卵黄包〔嚢〕癌

ysh
yellowish 黄色い

YSS
Yale scale score エール目盛り得点，エール・スケールスコア

YST
yolk sac tumor 卵黄包〔卵黄嚢〕腫瘍

YT, yt
yttrium イットリウム〈元素〉

Yuppie flu
young urban professional people flu ヤッピー感冒

YVS
yellow vernix syndrome 黄色ニス症候群

Y-Wye
wybutine ワイブチン

YY syndrome
Klinefelter syndrome — YY症候群，クラインフェルター症候群

Z z

Z

atomic number	原子数
benzyloxycarbonyl	ベンジルオキシカルボニル(基)
equivalent weight	当価重量
glutamic (acid)	グルタミン(酸)
impedance	インピーダンス
intermediate disk (=Z line, Z disk)	中間版(=Z線/Z板)
ionic charge number	イオン電荷数
no effect	効果なし
proton number	陽子数
standardized deviate	調整標準化偏差値
standard score	標準得点
Zahl〈独〉	数
Zeit〈独〉	時，時間
zero	ゼロ
zone	帯，区域，ゾーン
Zuckung〈独〉	単収縮，攣縮
Zwischenwirbelscheibe〈独〉	椎間板
zymosan	ザイモサン，酵母細胞壁成分

z

catalytic amount	触媒量
standard normal deviate	標準偏差

Z, Z-

zusammen〈独〉	複合，いっしょに，総計で

Z, Z', Z''

increasing degree of contraction	収縮漸増を表す記号

ZA

zygomatic arch	頬骨弓

za

zikka〈独〉=about	約《処》

zam

examination	(食道胃)試験

ZAP

zymosan-activated plasma	ザイモサン活性化血漿

ZA Ra

Zondek-Aschheimsche Reaktion〈独〉	ツォンデック・アッシュハイム反応

ZAS

zymosan-activated serum	ザイモサン活性化血清

***z* axis of Fick**

vertical axis of Fick	フィックの垂直軸

ZB
zebra body ゼブラ小体
z.B.
zum Beispiel〈独〉 たとえば
ZC
zona compacta 緻密層
ZCP
zinc chloride poisoning 塩化亜鉛中毒
ZD
zero discharge ゼロ発射
zinc deficient 亜鉛欠乏の
ZD, Z/D
zero defects 無欠点，無欠陥
ZDDP
zinc dialkyldithiophosphate ジアルカリジチオリン酸亜鉛
z.d.E, z.d.E.
zwischen dem Essen〈独〉，*inter cibos*〈ラ〉=between meals 食間(に)《処》
Z-disk
Zwischenscheibe〈独〉=intermediate disk 中間板
Z-DNA
zigzag left-handed double-helical deoxyribonucleic acid 左巻き二重鎖らせんDNA
ZDS
zinc depletion syndrome 亜鉛枯渇症候群
ZDV
zidovudine ジドブジン
zE
zum Exempel〈独〉 たとえば，例題
ZE, Z-E
Zollinger-Ellison (syndrome) ゾリンジャー・エリソン(症候群)
Zea
trans-zeatin ゼアチン
ZEEP
zero end-expiratory pressure 呼気終末0〔ゼロ〕圧，呼気終末平圧
ZES
Zollinger-Ellison syndrome ゾリンジャー・エリソン症候群
Z-ESR
zeta erythrocyte sedimentation rate ゼータ赤血球沈降速度
ZF
zero frequency ゼロ頻度
zona fasciculata (副腎皮質の)束状帯，索状帯

ZFY
Y-linked zinc finger protein　Y染色体性ジンクフィンガー蛋白

ZG
zona glomerulosa　(副腎皮質の)球状帯
zymogen granule　酵素原顆粒《電顕》

Z/G
zoster immunoglobulin　帯状疱疹免疫グロブリン

ZGM
zinc glycinate marker　グリシン酸亜鉛マーカー

ZI, z.i.
zona incerta　(神経)不確帯

ZIFT
zygote intrafallopian transfer　受精卵輸卵管内注入法，体外受精卵卵管内移植法

ZIG, ZIg
zoster immunoglobulin　帯状疱疹免疫グロブリン

ZIG-V
venous zoster immunoglobulin　静脈帯状疱疹免疫グロブリン

ZIM
zimelidine　ジメリジン

ZINEB
zinc ethylenebis　エチレンビス亜鉛

ZIP
zoster immune plasma　帯状疱疹免疫血漿，帯状疱疹免疫プラズマ

ZIRAM
zinc dimethyldithiocarbamate　ジメチルジチオカルバメイト亜鉛

ZK
Zungen Krebs〈独〉　舌癌

ZKi
Zentrum der Kinderheilkunde〈独〉　小児療育センター

ZKS
zentrale Koordination Störung〈独〉　中枢性協調障害

ZLA
isotope with atomic number Z and atomic weight A　原子記号Zおよび原子量Aの同位元素

Z-line
zigzag line　食道胃粘膜接合部，ジグザグ線

ZLS
Zimmerman-Laband syndrome　ツィマーマン・レーバンド症候群

ZM
Zimmerman reaction　ツィマーマン(発色)反応

Zm
zygomaxillare　頬骨上顎骨

zm
zoom　ズーム

ZMA
zinc meta-arsenite　メタヒ酸亜鉛

ZMC
zygomatic　頬骨の
zygomatic maxillary complex　頬骨上顎骨複合体
zygomaxillary complex　頬骨上顎骨複合体

ZMH
Zungenmandelhypertrophie〈独〉　舌扁桃肥大

ZN
Ziehl-Neelsen (method, stain)　チール・ネールゼン(法/染色)

Zn
zinc　亜鉛〈元素〉

z.n.
zu nehmen〈独〉　服用《処》

ZnO
zinc oxide　酸化亜鉛

ZnOE
zinc oxide-eugenol (white zinc)　酸化亜鉛・ユージノール

ZnP
zinc protoporphyrin　亜鉛プロトポルフィリン

ZNS
Zentralnervensystem〈独〉　中枢神経系
Ziehl-Neelsen stain　チール・ネールゼン染色(法)
zonisamide　ゾニサミド

ZnTT
zinc sulfate turbidity test　硫酸亜鉛混濁試験，クンケル試験

ZO
Zichen-Oppenheim (syndrome)　ジッヘン・オッペンハイム(症候群)
Zuelzer-Ogden (syndrome)　ズルジャー・オグデン(症候群)

ZOE
zinc oxide-eugenol (white zinc)　酸化亜鉛・ユージノール

Zoo C
Zoological Code　動物命名規約

Zool
zoological　動物学の
zoology　動物学

zos
zoster　帯状疱疹，ヘルペス

Z

zosteriform 帯状疱疹状の

ZP
zona pellucida 透明帯

ZPA
zone of polarizing activity 分極活性ゾーン

ZPC
zero point of charge 電荷の零〔ゼロ〕点
zopiclone ゾピクロン

ZPG
zero population growth 人口のゼロ成長

ZPI
zinc-protamine-insulin 亜鉛プロタミンインスリン

ZPLS
Zimmerman Preschool Language Scale ツィマーマン就学前言語スケール

ZPN
impedance pneumogram インピーダンス呼吸運動描画器

ZPO
zinc peroxide 過酸化亜鉛

ZPP
zinc protoporphyrin 亜鉛プロトポルフィリン

ZPT
zinc pyrithione ピリチオン亜鉛

ZR
zona reticularis (副腎皮質)網状体

Zr
zircon ジルコン
zirconium ジルコニウム〈元素〉

ZS
Zellweger syndrome ツェルヴェガー症候群

ZSB
zero stool (since) birth 出生後便通なし

ZSM
zonisamide ゾニサミド

ZSO
zinc suboptimal 次善(量)亜鉛

ZSPT
zona-free hamster egg sperm penetration test 透明帯除去ハムスター卵子を用いる精子侵入〔貫通〕試験

ZSR
zeta sedimentation rate〔ratio〕 ゼータ沈降速度率〔比〕

ZST
zinc sulfate turbidity test 硫酸亜鉛混濁試験
zinc sulphate test 硫酸亜鉛混濁試験

ZT
Ziehen test　チーエン試験
zinc turbidity　亜鉛混濁反応

Zt
Zeit〈独〉　時，時間

ZTP
zero temperature plasma　0度血漿

ZTS
zymosan-treated serum　ザイモサン処理血清

ZTT
zinc sulfate turbidity test　硫酸亜鉛混濁試験

Zuck
Zuckung〈独〉　痙攣，攣縮

Zugg
Zuggurtungs-osteosynthesis　ワイヤーによる圧迫固定

Zus
Zusammenfassung〈独〉　まとめ

zus
zusammen〈独〉　集める

ZVD
zentraler Venendruck〈独〉　中心静脈圧

ZW
zeruminales Wasser〈独〉　耳垢水

zw
zuwischen〈独〉　～の間

Zwang
Zwangsneurose〈独〉　強迫神経症

zw.d.E
zwischen dem Essen〈独〉，*inter cibos*〈ラ〉=between meals　食間(に)《処》

zy，Zy
zygion　ジギオン
zymosan　ザイモサン

ZyC
zymosan complement　ザイモサン補体(試薬)

zygo
zygomatic　頬骨の
zygomaticus　頬骨

Zylo
Zyloprim　ザイロプリム

zymol
zymology　発酵学，酵素学

ZZ
Zellenzahl〈独〉　細胞数
zweieiige Zwillinge〈独〉　二卵(性)双生児

zz
zigzag　ジグザグ

zZ, z.Z.
zur Zeit〈独〉　今のところ，現在

zz, Zz., zz.
zinzer〈独〉, *zingiber*〈ラ〉＝ginger　ショウガ

数字・記号

0-L
0-low titer　ゼロ低価

0-mu
anucleolate mutation　無核突然変異

1,25(OH)$_2$D$_3$
1,25-dihydroxycholecalciferol　1,25-ジヒドロキシコレカルシフェロール

1,3-DPG
1,3-diphosphoglycerate　1,3-ジホスホグリセレート

1,5-AG
1,5-anhydroglucitol　1,5-アンヒドログルシトール

1-BN(2)
1-bromo-naphthol(2)　ブロモナフトール

1-PP
1-phenylpropanol　1-フェニルプロパノール

1/d
once a day　1日1回《処》

1/U
one fingerbreadth above umbilicus　臍上1指幅

^{1}H
hydrogen(=protium)　水素1(=プロチウム)

1 sum.
unum sumatur〈ラ〉=to be taken at once　頓用，頓服《処》

1α-OHCC
1α-hydroxycholecalciferol　1αヒドロキシコレカルシフェロール

2,3-DPG
2,3-diphosphoglycerate　2,3-ジホスホグリセレート

2,4,5-T
2,4,5-trichlorophenoxyacetic acid　2,4,5-トリクロロフェノキシ酢酸

2,4-D
2,4-dichlorophenoxyacetic acid　2,4-ジクロロフェノキシ酢酸

2,4-DAA
2,4-diaminoanisole　2,4-ジアミノアニソール

2,7-FAA
N,*N'*-2,7-fluorenyl-enebis acetamide　*N*,*N'*-2,7-フルオレニルエネビアセトアミド

2-AAF
2-acetylaminofluorene　2-アセチルアミノフルオレン

記号・数字

2-FAA
N-2-fluorenylacetamide　*N*-2-フルオレニルアセトアミド

2-PAM
pralidoxime chloride　塩化プラリドキシム

2-PD
two-point discrimination　2点間識別テスト

2/d
twice a day　1日2回《処》

2DE, 2-DE
two-dimensional echocardiogram　断層心エコー図，二次元エコー図
two-dimensional echocardiography　断層心エコー図法，二次元エコー図法

2DF
2-deoxy-L-fucose　2-デオキシ-L-フコース

2DG, 2-DG
2-deoxy-D-glucose　2-デオキシ-D-グルコース

^{2}H
hydrogen-2(=deuterium)　水素2，重水素(=ジューテリウム)

2HPP
two hours postprandial (blood sugar)　食後2時間の(血糖値)

2ME
2-mercaptoethanol　2-メルカプトエタノール

2′-CMP
cytidine-2′-monophosphate　シチジン-2′-一リン酸

3-HMC
3-hydroxymethyl-β-carboline　3-ヒドロキシメチル-β-カルボリン

3-HT
3-hydroxytyramine　3-ヒドロキシチラミン(ドパミン)

3-MC
3-methylcholanthrene　3-メチルコラントレン

3-MECA
3-methylcholanthrene　3-メチルコラントレン

3-MT
3-methoxytyramine　3-メトキシチラミン

3-OHA
3-hydroxyamobarbital　3-ヒドロキシアモバルビタール

3-PDC
3-pentadecylcatechol　3-ペンタデシルカテコール

3AP, 3-AP
3-acetylpyridine　3-アセチルピリジン

3C
continuity, conprehensiveness, coordination — 継続性・包容力・協調性
convenience, composition, competence — 便利性・親切・信頼

3DE, 3-DE
three-dimensional echocardiogram — 三次元エコー図
three-dimensional echocardiography — 三次元エコー図法

3DPA
3-deoxypentonic acid — 3-デオキシペントン酸

3E
education, enforcement, engineering — プライバシー保守の3大条件：教育・法的規制・技術
effort, eating, emotion — 狭心症誘発の3大因子：労作・食事・情動

^{3}H
hydrogen-3 (=tritium) — 水素3，三重水素(=トリチウム)

^{3}H-TdR
tritiated thymidine — トリチウム化チミジン

3M
meningitis, measles, mumps — 脳膜炎・風疹・流行性耳下腺炎

3T
triage-treatment-transportation — 選別・応急処置・後方搬送

3′-CMP
cytidine-3′-monophosphate — シチジン-3′-一リン酸

3β-DH
3β-oxyhydro dehydrogenase — 3β水酸化脱水素酵素

4-CLTA
4-chlorotestosterone acetate — 4-クロロテストステロン酢酸

4-CLTC
4-chlorotestosterone capronate — 4-クロロテストステロンカプロン酸

4-CLTP
4-chlorotestosterone propionate — 4-クロロテストステロンプロピオン酸

4-HAQO
4-hydroxyaminoquinoline-L-oxide — 4-ヒドロキシアミノキノリンL-オキサイド

4-MU
4-methylumbelliferone — 4-メチルウンベリフェロン

4-NPP
4-nitrophenylphosphate — 4-ニトロフェニルリン酸

記号・数字

4-NQO
4-nitroquinoline 1-oxide — 4-ニトロキノリン 1-オキシド

4CV
four chamber view — 四腔断面

4F
fat, forty〔fifty〕, female and fertile — 太った・40代〔50代〕・女性，生殖力のある

4G×6H×10D
four grains times six hours times ten days — 4グレン×6時間×10日

4MMPD
4-methoxy-meta-phenylenediamine — 4-メトキシ-メタ-フェニレンジアミン

4P symptom
pain, paralysis, paresthesia, pulselessness — 疼痛・麻痺・感覚異常・脈拍喪失の4症状

4S
The Scandinavian Simvastatin Survival Study — スカンジナビアシンバスタチン臨床試験

4ta qq.hor.
quarta quaque hora〈ラ〉＝every fourth hour — 4時間ごとに《処》

4Xd
four times a day — 1日4回《処》

4×d
four times a day — 1日4回《処》

5-AS
5-aminosalicylic acid — 5-アミノサリチル酸

5-Aza
5-azacytidine — 5-アザシチジン

5-azaC
5-azacytidine — 5-アザシチジン

5-AzCdR
5-aza-2′-deoxycytidine — 5-アザ-2′-デオキシシチジン

5-AzCR
5-azacytidine — 5-アザシチジン

5-AzU
5-azauracil — 5-アザウラシル

5-AzUR, 5-AZUR
5-azauridine — 5-アザウリジン

5-FC
5-fluorocytosine — 5-フルオロシトシン

5-FU
5-fluorouracil — フルオロウラシル

5-FUDR
5-fluoro-2′-deoxyuridine — 5-フルオロ-2′-デオキシウリジン

5-HETE
5-hydroxy-eicosatetraenoic acid — 5-ヒドロキシ-エイコサテトラエン酸

5-HIAA
5-hydroxyindoleacetic acid — 5-ヒドロキシインドール酢酸

5-HT
5-hydoroxytriptamine(=serotonin) — 5-ヒドロキシトリプタミン(=セロトニン)

5-HTP
5-hydroxytryptophan — 5-ヒドロキシトリプトファン(=セロトニン前駆体)

5-MOP
5-methoxypsoralen — 5-メトキシソラレン

5-OT
5-oxytryptamine — 5-オキシトリプタミン

5hmCyt
5-hydroxymethyl cytosine — 5-ヒドロキシメチルシトシン

5hmdCyd
5-hydroxymethyl deoxycytidine — 5-ヒドロキシメチルデオキシシチジン

5hmdUrd
5-deoxymethyl deoxyuridine — 5-ヒドロキシメチルデオキシウリジン

5hmUra
5-hydroxymethyl uracil — 5-ヒドロキシメチルウラシル

5W
when, where, why, what, work — いつ・どこで・なぜ・なにが・おこるのか

5′-DFUR
5′-deoxy-5-fluorouridine — デオキシフルオロウリジン

5′-UDP
uridine 5′-diphosphate — ウリジン5′-二リン酸

5′-UTP
uridine 5′-triphosphate — ウリジン5′-三リン酸

5′NT
5′-nucleotidase — 5′-ヌクレオチダーゼ

6-APA
6-aminopenicillanic acid — 6-アミノペニシラン酸

6-AzU
6-azauracil — 6-アザウラシル

6-AzUR, 6-AZUR
6-azauridine — 6-アザウリジン

6-CP
6-chloropurine — 6-クロロプリン

6-HD
6-hydroxydopamine — 6-ヒドロキシド(ー)パミン

6-MP
6-mercaptopurine — 6-メルカプトプリン

6-MPR
6-mercaptopurine ribonucleoside — 6-メルカプトプリンリボヌクレオシド

6-MTI
6-methylthioinosine — 6-メチルチオイノシン

6-OHDA
6-hydroxydopamine hydrochloride — 6-ヒドロキシド(ー)パミンヒドロクロライド

6-TG
6-thioguanine — 6-チオグアニン

6-TP
6-thiopurine — 6-チオプリン

6MWT
six minutes walking test — 6分間歩行テスト

6P1C
pain, paresthesia, paleness, pulselessness, palsy, prostration, coldness — 疼痛・感覚異常・蒼白・無脈・麻痺・疲労・冷感

7-ACA
7-amino-cephalosporinic acid — 7-アミノセファロスポリン酸

7D
seven D=①birth defect, ②abnormal development, ③behavioral deviations, ④neurological disorder, ⑤immunodeficiencies, ⑥generalized debilitation, ⑦premature death — 7つのD=①出生欠陥 ②異常発達 ③行動偏倚 ④神経異常 ⑤免疫不全 ⑥全身無気力 ⑦早産死

8-ME
8-mercaptoguanosine — 8-メルカプトグアノシン

10 MWD
ten minutes walking distance — 平地を10分間歩行させて最大に歩行できる距離

11-OCS
11-oxycorticosteroid — 11-オキシコルチコステロイド

^{11}C
carbon-11 — 炭素11

11β-OHSD
11β-hydroxysteroid dehydrogenase — 11βヒドロオキシステロイド脱水素酵素

11β-hydroxysteroid dehydrogenase　11βヒドロオキシステロイド脱水素酵素

^{12}C
carbon-12　炭素12

^{13}C
carbon-13　炭素13

^{13}N
nitrogen-13　窒素13

^{14}C
carbon-14　炭素14

^{15}N
nitrogen-15　重窒素

^{15}O
oxygen-15　酸素15

^{16}O
oxygen-16　酸素16

16PF
sixteen personality factor question　16人格因子〔要素〕検査

17-K
17-ketosteroid(s)　17-ケトステロイド

17-KGS
17-ketogenic steroid(s)　17-ケトン生成ステロイド

17-KS
17-ketosteroid(s)　17-ケトステロイド

17-OH
17-hydroxycorticosteroid　17-ヒドロキシコルチコステロイド

17-OHCS
17-hydroxycorticosteroid　17-ヒドロキシコルチコステロイド

17-OHP
17α-hydroxyprogesterone　17-ヒドロキシプロゲステロン

17-OS
17-oxosteroid　17-オキソステロイド

^{17}O
oxygen-17　酸素17

17α-OHP, 17-α-OH-P
17α-hydroxyprogesterone　17αヒドロキシプロゲステロン

18-OH-DOC
18-hydroxy-11-deoxycorticosterone　18-ヒドロキシ-11-デオキシコルチコステロン

数字・記号

18-OH-THA
18-hydroxy-11-dehydrotetra-hydrocorticosterone — 18-ヒドロキシ-11-デヒドロテトラヒドロコルチコステロン

^{18}O
oxygen-18 — 酸素18

19-NADC
19-norandrosterone decanoate — 19-ノルアンドロステロンデカノエート

19-NDC
19-nortestosterone decanoate — 19-ノルテストステロンデカノエイト

19-NTPP
19-nortestosterone phenylpropionate — 19-ノルテストステロンフェニルプロピオネイト

24,25$(OH)_2D_3$
24,25-dihydroxycholecalciferol — 24,25-ジヒドロキシコレカルシフェロール

25-HCC
25-hydroxycholecalciferol — 25-ヒドロキシコレカルシフェロール

25-OHD_3, 25$(OH)D_3$
25-hydroxycholecalciferol — 25-ヒドロキシビタミンD_3, カルシジオール

^{32}P
radioactive phosphorus — 放射性リン

45X syndrome
Turner syndrome — ターナー症候群

45XO syndrome
Turner syndrome — ターナー症候群

46 XX
46 chromosomes, 2X chromosomes (= normal female) — 46染色体・2本のX染色体, 正常女性の染色体

46 XY
46 chromosomes, 1X and 1Y chromosome (normal male) — 46染色体=XY染色体(=正常男性の染色体)

47 XXY
47 chromosomes, 2X and 1Y chromosomes (=Klinefelter syndrome) — 47染色体・2本のX染色体と1本のY染色体(=クラインフェルター症候群)

47 XY+21
47 chromosomes, male, additional chromosome 21 (=Down syndrome, chromosome 21 trisomy) — 47染色体・男性・21染色体が1本多い(=ダウン症候群, 21染色体トリソミー)

47 XYY
47 chromosomes, 1X and 2Y chromosomes(＝XYY xyndrome) — 47染色体・１本のX染色体と２本のY染色体(＝XYY症候群)

49 XXXXY
49 chromosomes, 4X and 1Y chromosomes(＝XXXXY syndrome) — 49染色体・４本のX染色体と１本のY染色体(＝XXXXY症候群)

^{56}Co
cobalt-56 — コバルト56

^{57}Co
cobalt-57 — コバルト57

^{58}Co
cobalt-58 — コバルト58

^{59}FE
radioactive iron — 放射性鉄

^{60}Co
cobalt therapy — コバルト(60)治療
cobalt-60 — コバルト60

^{67}Ga
gallium-67 — ガリウム67

^{67}Ga-gallium citrate
gallium-67-gallium citrate — ガリウム67・クエン酸ガリウム

^{75}Se
selenium-75 — セレニウム75

^{81m}Kr
krypton-81m — クリプトン81m

^{90}Y
yttrium-90 — イットリウム90

^{95}Nb
radioactive niobium — 放射性ニオブ

^{99}Mo
molybdenum-99 — モリブデン99

^{99m}Tc
technetium-99m — テクネチウム99m

^{111}In-DTPA
indium-111 diethylene triamine pentaacetic acid — インジウム111ジエチレントリアミン五酢酸

^{123}I
iodine-123 — ヨウ素123

^{123}I-HSA
iodine-123 human serum albumin — 放射性ヨウ素123標識ヒト血清アルブミン

^{125}I
iodine-125 — ヨウ素125

radioactive infarct particle	放射性塞栓粒子
^{125}IT$_3$RSU	
iodine-125 triiodothyronine resin sponge uptake	ヨウ素125トリヨードチ〔サイ〕ロニンレジン摂取率
^{129}Cs	
cesium-129	セシウム129
^{131}Cs	
cesium-131	セシウム131
^{131}I	
iodine-131	ヨウ素131
radioactive iodine	放射性ヨウ素
^{131}I-AA	
iodine-131 aggregated albumin	ヨウ素131標識凝集アルブミン
^{131}I-adosterol	
iodine-131 adosterol	ヨウ素131アドステロール
^{131}I-HSA	
iodine-131 human serum albumin	放射性ヨウ素131標識ヒト血清アルブミン
^{131}I-MAA	
iodine-131 macroaggregate albumin	ヨウ素131標識大凝集アルブミン
^{131}I-MIBG	
iodine-131 metaiodobenzylguanidine	ヨウ素131メタヨウ化ベンジルグアニジン
^{131}I-PVP	
iodine-131 polyvinylpyrrolidone	ヨウ素131ポリビニルピロリドン
^{131}I-PVP test	
iodine-131 polyvinylpyrrolidone test	ヨウ素131ポリビニルピロリドン試験，ゴルドン試験
^{131}I-RB	
iodine-131 rose bengal	ヨウ素131ローズベンガル
^{131}IT$_3$RSU	
iodine-131 triiodothyronine resin sponge uptake	ヨウ素131トリヨードチ〔サイ〕ロニンレジン摂取率
^{192}Ir	
iridium-192	イリジウム192
^{201}Tl	
thallium-201	タリウム201〈元素〉
^{252}Cf	
californium-252	カリフォルニウム252
Ⅷ:C	
factor Ⅷ coagulant activity	第Ⅷ因子凝固活性
ⅧCAG	
factor Ⅷ coagulant antigen	第Ⅷ因子凝固抗原

ⅧR : AG, ⅧRAg, ⅧRAG
factor Ⅷ related antigen 第Ⅷ因子関連抗原
ⅧR : WF
Ⅷ related von Willebrand factor 第Ⅷ因子関連フォンヴィレブランド因子
factor Ⅷ related von Willebrand factor 第Ⅷ因子フォンヴィレブランド因子
Ⅷ WF
factor Ⅷ related von Willebrand factor 第Ⅷ因子関連フォンヴィレブランド因子
/d
daily 毎日の
per day /日
/HPF, /hpf
per high-power field 強拡大の一視野(あたり)
/min
per minute 毎分，1分間に
/wk
per week /週
//bars
parallel bars 平行棒
%^{59}Fe util
^{59}Fe utilization 鉄(＝^{59}Fe)の赤血球利用率
%LC
percent labeled cell 標識細胞百分率
%LM
percent labeled mitosis 標識分裂細胞百分率
%TRP
% tubular reabsorption of phosphate 尿細管リン再吸収率
%VC
percent vital capacity パーセント肺活量
%wt
weight percent 質量百分率
＋V, ＋v
positive vertical divergence 実性垂直性開散
＋VD
positive vertical divergence 陽性垂直性開散
－VD
negative vertical divergence 陰性垂直性開散
'cap
handicapped 身体障害のある
'cept
accept 受容
except 例外
'gram
radiogram X線写真

数字・記号

'neath
beneath　下の
underneath　～の下に

Å
Angström unit　オングストローム(単位)

°A
degree absolute　絶対温度

©
Copyright, All Rights Reserved　著作権，コピーライト

°C
degree Celsius　摂氏(温度)
degree centigrade　摂氏度

°F
degree Fahrenheit　華氏(温度)

°R
Rankine (scale)　ランキン目盛〈単位〉
Réaumur (temperature scale)　レ氏(温度目盛)，レオミュール(温度目盛)〈単位〉

@bs.
at bedside　ベッドサイドにて，臨床にて

$\dot{M}_0$
mean life　平均寿命

$\bar{O}$
without　伴わない

Ö
Ödem〈独〉　浮腫

ö
ödem〈独〉　浮腫

ÖeK
Ösophaguskrebs〈独〉　食道癌

ÖK
Ösophaguskrebs〈独〉　食道癌

$\dot{Q}$
volume flow of blood/unit time　単位時間血(液)流量
volume of blood flow　血(液)流量

$\dot{Q}p/\dot{Q}s$, $\dot{Q}_P/\dot{Q}_S$
left-to-right shunt ratio　左右シャント比

$\dot{Q}s$
shunt flow　シャント血流量

$\dot{Q}s/\dot{Q}t$, $\dot{Q}_S/\dot{Q}_T$
right-to-left shunt ratio　左右シャント比

$\dot{Q}t$
cardiac output (per minute)　(分時)心拍出量

(R)
rectal　直腸の
right　右

®
resistered trademark　登録商標

$\dot{S}$ seq.
sine sequela〈ラ〉=without sequel　続発症なしに《処》

$\overline{\dot{S}S}$, $\overline{SS}$, $\dot{S}\dot{S}$
semis〈ラ〉=one-half　1/2, 半分

$\overline{S}$, s, $\overline{s}$
sine〈ラ〉=without　～なしの, ～を伴わない

$\dot{V}$
gas volume/unit time (flow velocity)　単位時間あたりのガス量〔気流〕(速度)

$\dot{V}_A/\dot{Q}c$
alveolar ventilation perfusion ratio　換気血流比

$\dot{V}_A$, V_A
alveolar ventilation per minute　分時肺胞換気量
volume of alveolar gas　肺胞気容積〔容量〕

$\overline{v}$
mixed venous blood　混合静脈血
venous admixture　混合静脈血

v^-
viral　ウイルス(由来)の〈接〉

$\overline{X}$, $\overline{x}$
except　～を除いて
sample mean　サンプル平均値の記号《統》

$\overline{X}$, x
except　～を除いて
sample mean　サンプル平均

×2〔3…〕d
times two〔three…〕days　×2〔3…〕日

×3〔4…〕
times three, times four, …　3回〔倍〕, 4回〔倍〕…

↓sen
decreased sensation　知覚低下, 感覚低下
diminished sensation　知覚低下, 感覚低下

↑VP
increased venous pressure　静脈圧上昇

↓VP
decreased venous pressure　静脈圧低下

ギリシャ文字

α-Bgt, ABgT
alpha-bungarotoxin αブンガロトキシン
α-bungarotoxin αブンガロトキシン
α-chy
α-chymotrypsin αキモトリプシン
α-$ETCO_2$
difference between arterial to end-tidal CO_2 tension 動脈・終末呼気炭酸ガス分圧較差
α-GD
α-glycerophosphate dehydrogenase αグリセロホスフェイトデヒドロゲナーゼ
α-HBD
α-hydroxybutyrate dehydrogenase αヒドロキシ酪酸脱水素酵素
α-HCH
α-hexachlorocyclohexane αヘキサクロロシクロヘキサン
α-HH
alpha-hydrazinohistidine αヒドラジノヒスチジン
α-KG
alpha-ketoglutarate αケトグルタレート
α-LP
alpha-lipoprotein αリポ蛋白
α-MMT
alpha-methyl-m-tyrosine αメチル-m-チロシン
α-MPT
α-methyl-p-thyrosine αメチル-p-チロシン
α-T
α-tocopherol αトコフェロール
$α_1$-AG
$α_1$-acidglycoprotein $α_1$酸性糖蛋白
$α_1$-M
$α_1$-microglobulin $α_1$ミクログロブリン
$α_1$-MG
$α_1$-microglobulin $α_1$マイクログロブリン
$α_1$-microglobulin $α_1$ミクログロブリン
$α_1$AC
$α_1$-antichymotrypsin $α_1$アンチキモトリプシン
$α_1$AT, $α_1$-AT
alpha1-antitrypsin $α_1$抗トリプシン，$α_1$アンチトリプシン
$α_1$-antitrypsin $α_1$抗トリプシン，$α_1$アンチトリプシン

ギリシャ文字

α_2-M
α_2-macroglobulin　α_2マクログロブリン

α_2-PI
α_2-plasmin inhibitor　α_2プラスミン阻害物質〔インヒビター〕

α_2AT，α_2-AT
α_2-antitrypsin　α_2抗トリプシン，α_2アンチトリプシン

αAT，AAT
alpha antitrypsin　α抗トリプシン

αFUC，α-FUC
alpha-fucosidase　αフコシダーゼ

αf，α-f
alpha-fetoprotein　αフェトプロテイン

αHCD，α-HCD
alpha-heavy chain disease　α重鎖病
α heavy chain disease　α重鎖病

αIB，α-IB，AIB
alpha-isobutyric acid　αイソ酪酸
α-isobutyric acid　αイソ酪酸

αMM，α-MM
alpha-methyl mannoside　αメチルマンノシド

β
β ray　ベータ線

β-a
β-alanine　βアラニン

β-AIB
β-aminoisobutyric acid　βアミノイソ酪酸

β-Ala
β-alanine　βアラニン

β-BuTX
β-bungarotoxin　βブンガロトキシン

β-EP
β-endorphin　βエンドルフィン

β-Est
β-esterase　βエステル分解酵素

β-gal
β-galactosidase　βガラクトシダーゼ

β-GL
β-glucuronidase　βグルクロニダーゼ

β-HCG
Beta-human chorionic gonadotropin　βヒト絨毛性ゴナドトロピン

β-HG，BHG
beta-hydroxyglutamic acid　β水酸化グルタミン酸

β-LP
β-lipoprotein　βリポ蛋白

β-LPH
β-lipotropic hormone　β脂肪刺激放出ホルモン
β-M
β-methasone　βメタゾン
β-MD
β-metyldigoxin　メチルジゴキシン
β-T
β-tocopherol　βトコフェロール
β-T-3
β-tocotrienol　βトコトリエノール
β-TG
β-thromboglobulin　βトロンボグロブリン
β-TGdR
β-2′-deoxythioguanosine　β 2′-デオキシチオグアノシン
β-VLDL
β-migrated very-low-density lipoprotein　β超低比重リポ蛋白
β/A4
β-A-four　βA 4 蛋白
$β_2$-MG
$β_2$-microglobulin　$β_2$ミクログロブリン
$β_2$-m, $β_2$M, $β_2$-M
$β_2$-microglobulin　$β_2$ミクログロブリン
βHS, β-HS
β hemolytic streptococcus　β溶血性連鎖状球菌
βray
beta ray　ベータ線, β線
Γ-T
Γ-tocopherol　Γトコフェロール
γ
immunoglobulin　免疫グロブリン
microgram　マイクログラム
photon　光子
γ ray　ガンマ線
γ-BHC
gamma benzene hexachloride　γ六塩酸ベンゼン
γ-EP
γ-endorphin　γエンドルフィン
γ-GT
γ-glutamyltransferase　γグルタミルトランスフェラーゼ
γ-GTP
γ-glutamyl transpeptidase　γグルタミルトランスペプチダーゼ

ギリシャ文字

γ-HCD
γ-heavy chain disease | γH鎖病
γ-LPH
γ-lipotropic hormone | γ脂肪刺激放出ホルモン
γ-Sm, γ-SM
γ-seminoprotein | γセミノプロテイン
γA
immunoglobulin A | 免疫グロブリンA
γAbu
γ-aminobutyric acid | γアミノ酪酸
γD
immunoglobulin D | 免疫グロブリンD
γE
immunoglobulin E | 免疫グロブリンE
γG
immunoglobulin G | 免疫グロブリンG
γM
immunoglobulin M | 免疫グロブリンM
γOz
gamma-oryzanol | γオリザノール
γ-oryzanol | γオリザノール
ΔEh
redox potential difference | 酸化還元電位差
ΔIRI/ΔBS
immunoreactive insulin/blood sugar insulinogenic index | インスリン原性指数
δ
double bond | 二重結合
δ-ALA
δ-aminolevulinic acid | δアミノレブリン酸
δ-ALA-S
δ-aminolevulinic acid synthetase | δアミノレブリン酸合成酵素
δ-T
delta-tocopherol | δトコフェロール
ε-ACA
epsilon-aminocaproic acid | イプシロン〔ε〕アミノカプロン酸
κ
magnetic susceptibility | 磁化率
κ chain
kappa chain | κ鎖
λ
decay constant | 崩壊定数
microliter | マイクロリットル
wavelength | 波長

ギリシャ文字

μ	
micro-	マイクロ(=10^{-6})〈接〉
micrometer	マイクロメートル〈単位〉
micron	ミクロン
μA	
microampere	マイクロアンペア〈単位〉
μb	
microbar	マイクロバール〈単位〉
μbar, μ-bar	
microbar	マイクロバール〈単位〉
μC	
microcoulomb	マイクロクーロン〈単位〉
μC hr.	
microcurie-hour	マイクロキュリー時間〈単位〉
μc.h.	
microcurie hour	マイクロキュリー時間〈単位〉
μCi	
microcurie	マイクロキュリー〈単位〉
μCi-hr	
microcurie hour	マイクロキュリー時間〈単位〉
μcoul	
microcoulomb	マイクロクーロン〈単位〉
μF, μf	
microfarad	マイクロファラッド〈単位〉
μg	
microgram	マイクログラム〈単位〉
μH	
microhenry	マイクロヘンリー〈単位〉
μHCD	
μ heavy chain disease	μ重鎖病
μIU	
micro-international unit	マイクロ〔μ〕国際単位
μl	
μliter	マイクロリットル〈単位〉
μm	
micrometer	マイクロメートル〈単位〉
μmg	
micromilligram	マイクロミリグラム〈単位〉
μmm	
micromillimeter	マイクロミリメートル〈単位〉
μmol	
micromol	マイクロモル〈単位〉
μN	
nuclear magneton	核磁子
μR	
microroentgen	マイクロレントゲン

μs
microsecond マイクロ秒〈単位〉
μsec
microsecond マイクロ秒〈単位〉
μU
microunit マイクロ単位
μV
microvolt マイクロボルト〈単位〉
μW
microwatt マイクロワット〈単位〉
μ_x
force of mortality 死力
$\mu\gamma$
microgamma(=picogram) マイクロガンマ(=ピコグラム)(=10^{-12}g)
$\mu\mu$
micromicro マイクロマイクロ(=10^{-6})
micromicron マイクロミクロン〈単位〉
$\mu\mu$c
micromicrocurie マイクロマイクロキュリー〈単位〉
$\mu\mu$F
micromicrofarad マイクロマイクロファラッド〈単位〉
$\mu\mu$g
micromicrogram マイクロマイクログラム〈単位〉
$\mu\Omega$
microhm マイクロオーム〈単位〉
ν
kinematic viscosity 運動粘性率
neutrino ニュートリノ
o
omicron オミクロン
ρ-factor
rho factor ρ因子
Σ
sum 総計，合計
syphilis 梅毒
σ
standard deviation 標準偏差
surface tension 表面張力
ΦLC
pseudo light chain 偽L鎖遺伝子
χ^2
chi square カイ2乗

ψ

pseudouridine シュードウリジン

wavelength 波長

ω

angular velocity 角速度

略語逆引き

用語一覧

あ

アイナー　**INAH**
アイルランド・スウェーデン・ニューヨーク型ソケット　**ISNY socket**
アインシュタイン　**E**
アインスタイニウム　**E, Es**
アウラノフィン　**AF**
アエロバクター　**AERO**
アエロバクター(属)　**A**
アーガイル・ロバートソン　**Arg-Rob**
アーガイル・ロバートソン(瞳孔)　**AR**
アカゲザル　**MMU, Rh, Rh.**
アカゲザル・ロタウイルス　**RRV**
アカゲザル2倍体細胞株使用狂犬病ワクチン　**RDRV**
アカゲザル腎臓　**RMK**
アカゲザル組織培養　**RMTC**
アカデミック臨床研究機関　**ARO**
アガリクスビスポラスアグルチニン　**ABA**
アガロース　**AG**
アガロースゲル(内)電気泳動(法)　**AGE**
アカントケイロネマ(属)　**A**
アキレス腱　**AT, TA**
アキレス腱延長術　**ATL, ETA, TAL**
アキレス腱反射　**AJ, A-J, ASR, ATR**
アキレス腱反射検査　**ART**
アキレス腱反射弛緩相時間　**ART**
アキレス(腱)反射時間　**ARZ**
アクセレリン・コンバルチン　**ACC**
アクチニウム　**Ac**
アクチニウムエマナチオン　**AC Em**
アクチノバシラス(属)　**A**
アクチノマイシン　**ACT, act**
アクチノマイシンD　**ACD, ACM-D, AMD**
アクチノマイシンD, ビンクリスチン, シスプラチン(=プラチノール)　**AVP**
アクチノマイシンD, フルオロウラシル, シクロホスファミド　**ACFUCY**
アクチノマイシンD, ブレオマイシン, ビンクリスチン　**ABV**
アクチノミセス(属)　**A, A.**
アクチノン　**An**
アクチバトール　**FKOA**
アクチン　**A, ACT**
アクチン結合蛋白　**ABP**
アクトミオシン　**AM**
アクラシノマイシン　**ACM**
アクラルビシン　**ACR**
アクラルビシン, プレドニゾロン　**AP**
アクリジンオレンジ(試験)　**AO**
アクリジンオレンジ診断　**AO diag**
アクリフラビン　**ACR**
アクリルアミドゲル　**AGE**
アクリルの　**Acr**
アクロマイシン　**ACM**
アコニターゼ　**AC, ACO**
アコニチン　**AC**
アコニット・ベラドンナ・クロロホルム塗膏　**ABC**
アコニット・ベラドンナ・クロロホルム軟膏　**ABC**
アザグアニン　**AZG, azg.**
アザチオプリン　**AZ, AZP**
アザロマイシンF　**AZL**
アジアアフリカ地域健康奉仕　**SHARE**
アジア医化学連合　**AFMC**
アジア医学生協会　**ARMSA**
アジア医師連絡協議会　**AMDA**
アジアインフルエンザウイルス　**A_2**
アジアオーストラリア脳神経外科学会　**AASNS**
アジアオセアニア医師会連合　**CMAAO**
アジアオセアニア核医学生物学連盟　**AOFNMB**
アジアオセアニア神経学会　**AOAN**
アジアオセアニア内分泌学会連合　**FESAO**
(日本)アジア救ライ協会　**JALMA, JLMA**
アジア獣医師会連合　**FAVA**
アジア消化器病学会　**AAG**
アジア小児外科学会　**AAPS**
アジア製薬業連盟　**FAPA**
アジア太平洋眼科学アカデミー　**APAO**

アジア太平洋血液学会 **APSH**
アジア太平洋歯学連盟 **APDF**
アジア太平洋心臓学会 **APSC**
アジア太平洋物理医学リハビリテーション連盟 **APLPMR**
アジア太平洋免疫学会連合 **FIMSA**
アジア労働衛生会議 **AAOH**
アシクロビル **ACV**
アシドαナフチルアセテートエステラーゼ **ANAE**
アシドーシス **acid**
アジドチミジン **AZT**
アジドデオキシチミジン **AZT**
アシネトバクター(属) **A**
アジュバント **adj**
アジュバント関節炎 **AA**
アジュバント病 **AD**
アジリジニルベンゾキノン **AZQ**
アシル基脱水素酵素 **GAD**
アシルキャリア蛋白 **ACP**
アシルコエンザイムAコレステロールアシルトランスフェラーゼ **ACAT**
アシル担体蛋白 **ACP**
アース **E**
アスカリス(属) **A**
アスコルビン酸(=ビタミンC) **AsA, ASC**
アスコルビン酸因子 **AAF**
アスター黄色ウイルス **AYV**
アスタチン **At**
アズテック法 **AZTEC**
アステロコッカス(属) **A**
アストラップ法 **AS**
アストラブルーエオジン **AB-E**
アズトレオナム **AZT**
アストロミシン **ASTM**
アスパラギナーゼ **Asp, asp.**
アスパラギナーゼ,ビンクリスチン,ダウノルビシン,プレドニゾン **AVDP, avdp**
アスパラギン **Asn, asn, Asx, B, N**
アスパラギン酸 **Asp, asp., Asx, B, D**
アスパラギン酸アミノ基転移酵素 **aspAT**
アスパラギン酸アミノトランスフェラーゼ **ASAT, AST**
アスパラギン酸塩 **asp**
アスパルテートカルバミール転移酵素 **ATCase**
アスピリン **ASP**
アスピリン・カフェイン・フェナセチン **ACP**
アスピリン(=アセチルサリチル酸)・フェナセチン・カフェイン **APC**
アスピリン・フェナセチン・カフェイン錠(剤) **APC tabs**
アスピリン・フェナセチン・カフェインとコデイン **APCC**
アスピリン過敏喘息 **ASA**
アスピリン心筋梗塞研究 **AMIS**
アスピリン腸溶錠 **EA**
アスピリン誘発(性)喘息 **AIA**
アスベスト小体 **AB**
アスペルギルス(属) **A**
アスポキシシリン **ASPC**
アズールA **aA**
アズールB **aB**
アズールC **aC**
アズレン **AZL**
アセスメント **A, asmt**
アセタゾールアミド **AC**
アセチル **Ac**
アセチル-L-リシンメチルエステル **ALME, ALMe**
アセチルアセトネート **acac**
アセチルアミノフルオレン **FAA**
アセチルアルギニンメチルエステル **AAME**
アセチルキタサマイシン **A-LM, ALM**
アセチルグリシル-L-リジンメチルエステル **AGLMe**
アセチルコエンザイムA **AcCoA, Ac CoA, CoAAc**
アセチルコリン **AC, ac, AcCh, Ac Ch, ACH, ACh, Ach**
アセチルコリンエステラーゼ **AcCHS, AChE**
アセチルコリン受容体 **AcChR, AChR**
アセチルコリン受容体抗体 **AChRAb**
アセチルコリン受容体蛋白 **AChRP**
アセチルサリチル酸(=アスピリン) **ASA**
アセチルシステイン **AC**
アセチルスピラマイシン **Ac-SPM, ACSPM, A-SPM**
アセチルスルファニールク

ロライド **ASC**
アセチルノイラミン酸 **ANA**
アセチルピペラジン **AP-2**
アセチル補酵素A **CoAAc, AcCoA, Ac CoA**
アセチル補酵素〔コエンザイム〕A カルボキシラーゼ **ACC**
アセチルメチルカルビノール **AMC**
アセチルロイコマイシン **A-LM**
アセチレン **acetl**
アセットロケーション **AL**
アセテート **Ac**
アセテートキナーゼ **AK**
アセトアセテート **AcAc**
アセトアミノフェン **AAP**
アセトキシプレグネノロン **AOP**
アセト酢酸 **AA, AcAc**
アセトバクタースボキシダンス因子 **ASF**
アセトヘキサミド **AH, S-5900**
アセトン **A, ace, ace., Acet, acet., Me**
アセトン/水 **AC/W**
アセトン抽出血清 **Aero, aero**
アセメタシン **ACM**
アゾトバクター(属) **A**
アゾバクター(属) **Az**
アゾベンアルソン酸 **ABA**
アダム(=解剖学用コンピュータソフト) **ADAM**
アダムス・ストークス(症候群) **AS, A-S**
アダムス・ストークス症候群 **Ad-St**
アダムス・ストークス発作 **ASA**
アチーブメントテスト **AT**
アッシャー症候群 **US**
アッシュハイム・ツォンデック(妊娠)(検査) **AZ, A.-Z., Az**
アッシュハイム・ツォンデック(妊娠)検査 **AZT**
アッシュハイム・ツォンデック(妊娠)反応 **AZR**
アディー・ホームズ(症候群) **AH**
アデニル酸 **A, AA**
アデニルシクラーゼ **AC**
アデニレイトキナーゼ **Adkin**
アデニレートエネルギーチャージ **AEC**
アデニレートキナーゼ **AK**
アデニレートサイクラーゼ刺激活性 **ACSA**
アデニレートシクラーゼ **AC**
アデニレートシクラーゼ阻害物質〔阻害薬〕 **ACI**
アデニレートシクラーゼ毒素 **ACT**
アデニロコハク酸 **AMP-S**
アデニン **A, Ade**
アデニン・ウラシル・グアニン(=開始コドン) **AUG**
アデニン・チミン・グアニン **ATG**
アデニンアラビノシド **ara-A, Ara-A**
アデニンアラビノシド-5′-一リン酸 **Ara-AMP**
アデニンおよびチミン型 **AT type**
アデニン二リン酸 **APP**
アデニンホスホリボシルトランスフェラーゼ **APRT**
アデニンホスホリボシルトランスフェラーゼ欠損症 **APRT deficiency**
アデノイド **ade, AV**
アデノイド咽頭結膜炎 **APC**
アデノイド摘出兼扁桃摘出術 **A & T**
アデノウイルス **Adeno-virus, ADV, AD virus, APC-virus**
アデノウイルス2型 **Ad2**
アデノウイルス関連ウイルス **AAV**
アデノ衛星ウイルス **ASV**
アデノ関連ウイルス **AAV**
アデノシルB12 **Ado B12**
アデノシルコバラミン **Ado Ccl**
アデノシン **A, Ado**
アデノシン-5′-一リン酸 **Ado-5′-P**
アデノシン-5′-二リン酸 **Ado-5′-P2, ADP**
アデノシン-5′-三リン酸 **Ado-5′-P3**
アデノシン-5-二リン酸グルコース **ADPG**
アデノシン-5′-ホスホサルフェート **APS**
アデノシン5′-一リン酸 **AMP, A5MP**

アデノシン一リン酸 **AMP**
アデノシンキナーゼ **ADK**
アデノシン三リン酸 **ADT, AMP-P-P, ATP**
アデノシンデアミナーゼ **ADA, ADD**
アデノシントリホスファターゼ **ATPase**
アデノシン二リン酸 **ADP**
アデノシンバソプレシン **AVP**
アデノシン四リン酸 **A tetra P**
アデノシンリン硫酸 **APS**
アデノーマ **A**
アデノ様ウイルス **ALV**
アテノロール **ATEN**
アテローム血栓性脳梗塞 **ABI, ATBI**
アテローム(性動脈)硬化(症) **AS, ATHSC, Athsc, athsc., ATS**
アテローム硬化性心血管疾患 **ACVD, ASCVD**
アト(=10^{-18}) **a.**
アドソン手技 **Adson's M**
アトピー咳嗽 **AC**
アトピー型喘息 **ABA**
アトピー性角膜結膜炎 **AKC**
アトピー性呼吸器疾患 **ARD**
アトピー性皮膚炎 **AD**
アドミッタンス **A**
アトムプローブ **AP**
アトムプローブ電界イオン顕微鏡 **AP-FIM**
アドリアマイシン **Adria**
アドリアマイシン(=ドキソルビシン：DOX, DXR) **ADM, ADR, Adr, AM**
アドリアマイシン,シクロホスファミド,エトポシド **ACE**
アドリアマイシン,シクロホスファミド,ビンクリスチン(=オンコビン),アラビノシルシトシン,プレドニゾン **ACOAP**
アドリアマイシン,シクロホスファミド,ビンクリスチン(=オンコビン),フルオロウラシル **ADCONFU**
アドリアマイシン,シクロホスファミド,ビンクリスチン(=オンコビン),プレドニゾン **ACOP**
アドリアマイシン,シクロホスファミド,ビンクリスチン(=オンコビン),プレドニゾン,プロカルバジン **ACOPP**
アドリアマイシン,シクロホスファミド,メトトレキサート **ACM**
アドリアマイシン,シタラビン,6-メルカプトプリン,プレドニゾロン **ACMP**
アドリアマイシン,シタラビン,シクロホスファミド(=エンドキサン),プレドニゾロン **ACEP**
アドリアマイシン,ジメチルトリアゼノイミダゾールカルボキサミド **ADIC**
アドリアマイシン,ビンクリスチン **AV**
アドリアマイシン,ビンクリスチン(=オンコビン),アラビノシルシトシン,プレドニゾン **ADOAP**
アドリアマイシン,ビンクリスチン,イホスファミド,プレドニゾロン **AVIP**
アドリアマイシン,ビンクリスチン,プレドニゾロン **AdVP**
アドリアマイシン,ビンクリスチン,プロカルバジン **AVP**
アドリアマイシン,ビンブラスチン,メトトレキサート **AVM**
アドリアマイシン,フルオロウラシル **AF**
アドリアマイシン,ブレオマイシン,シクロホスファミド,マイトマイシンC **ABCM**
アドリアマイシン,ブレオマイシン,シスプラチン,放射線療法 **ABCX**
アドリアマイシン,ブレオマイシン,ダカルバジン,ビンブラスチン **ABDV**
アドリアマイシン,ブレオマイシン,ビンブラスチン,ダカルバジン **ABVD**
アドリアマイシン,ブレオマイシン,プレドニゾン **ABP**
アドリアマイシン,プレドニゾン,ビンクリスチン(=オンコビン) **APO**
アドリアマイシン,ロイケラン,ビンクリスチン(=オンコビン),メトトレキサート,アクチノマイシンD,ダカルバジン

ALOMAD
アドレナリン **A, Ad, AD, Adr, adr, adren, adren.**
アドレナリン作動性ニューロン **AN**
アドレナリン受容体結合体 **ARB**
アドレナリンプロタルゴール **ad-pro**
アトロピン **A, AT, atrop, atrop.**
アトロピン昏睡療法 **ACT**
アナフィラキシー **A**
アナフィラキシー緩徐反応因子 **SRF-A, SRFOA**
アナフィラキシー好酸球遊走因子 **ECF-A**
アナフィラキシー性血小板活性因子 **PAF-A**
アナフィラキシー遅延反応物質 **SRS-A**
アナフィラキシーの炎症(性)因子 **IFA, IF-A**
アナフィラトキシン **AT**
アナポリスリンパ芽球グロブリン **ALG**
アナログ・デジタル(変換) **A/D, A-D**
アナログ・デジタル・アナログ記録 **adar**
アナログ・デジタルデータ記録システム **ADRS**
アナログ・デジタル **AD, A/D**
アナログ・デジタル変換器 **ADC**
アナログ・デジタル変換コンピュータ **adcom**
アニオンギャップ **AG**
アニソ化プラスミノーゲンストレプトキナーゼ **ASPAC**
アニリン **anil**
アニリン・イオウ・ホルムアルデヒド **ASF**
アニリンゲンチアナバイオレット **AGV**
(蚊)アノフェレス(属) **A, A.**
アーノルド・キアリ(症候群) **AC**
アパシェ **APACHE**
アパルシリン **APPC**
アビシン・ビオチン結合法 **ABC method**
アビジン・ビオチン(ペルオキシダーゼ)複合体 **ABC**
アヒル肝炎ウイルス **DHBV**
アヒル胚狂犬病ワクチン **DEV**
アービン症候群 **IS**
アフィニティ精製抗体 **AIA**
アプガースコア **Apgar score, APS**
アブシジン酸 **ABA**
アブシディア(属) **A**
アプドーマ **APUDoma**
アブミ骨可動術 **Stapes mob, Stap.mob**
アブミ骨筋 **SM**
アブミ骨筋反射 **SR**
アブミ骨筋反射検査 **SR test**
アブミ骨小開窓 **SFS**
アブミ骨靱帯ひだ **PlSF**
アブミ骨ひだ閉鎖 **OSF**
アブミバンド **RB**
アフラトキシン **AF, AFT**
アフラトキシンB **AFB**
アフラトキシンG **AFG**
アフリカ・ミドリザル腎細胞 **GMK**
アフリカ医学研究財団 **AMRF**
アフリカウマ病 **AHS**
アフリカ開発会議 **TICAD**
アフリカバーキットリンパ腫 **ABL**
アフリカブタコレラウイルス **ASFV**
アフリカミドリザル **AGM**
アプリジン **AP**
アプリン酸 **AP**
アベコース **Abe**
アーベルソン白血病ウイルス **AMuLV**
アヘン剤無痛法 **OA**
アヘンチンキ **TO**
アヘンとベラドンナ **O & B**
アボガドロ(定)数 **N,** ***N***
アボガドロ数(定数) **Na**
アポ酵素 **AE**
アポスチルブ **asb**
アポ蛋白 **Apo**
アポトーシス **PCD**
アポトーシス阻害 **Bcl-2**
アポモルヒネ **APO**
アポリポ蛋白 **Apo**
アマクリン細胞 **AM**
アマルガム **AAA**
アミオダロン **AMD**
アミオダロン誘発性甲状腺中毒症 **AIT**
アミカシン **AMK**
アミタール **AMY**
アミトプテリン **AMT**
アミトリプチリン **AMI, AMP, AMT, AT**
アミノアシラーゼ1 **ACY1**
アミノアシル **aa, AA**
アミノアシルt-RNA **tRNA-aa**

アミノアシル転移リボ核酸 **aa-tRNA**
アミノアセトニトリル **AAN**
アミノアセトン **AA**
アミノイソ酪酸 **AIB**
アミノイミダゾールカルボキサミド **AIC**
アミノイミダゾールカルボキサミドリボ核酸 **AICAR**
アミノエチル・イソチウロニウム **AET**
アミノ吉草酸 **AVA**
アミノ基転移酵素 **ATs**
アミノグリコシド **AGs**
アミノグルテチミド **AGL**
アミノサイクロヘキシルペニシリン **AC-PC**
アミノサイジン **AMD**
アミノ酢酸ジヒドロキシアルミニウム **DAA**
アミノサリチル酸 **ASA**
アミノ酸 **AA**
アミノ酸活性化酵素 **AAAE**
アミノ酸酸化酵素 **AAO**
アミノデオキシカナマイシン **ADKM**
アミノデオキシカナマイシン(＝ベカナマイシン) **AKM**
アミノデオキシカナマイシンB **DKB**
アミノトランスフェラーゼ **AT**
アミノトリアゾール **AT, ATA**
アミノヌクレオチド **AN**
アミノ配糖体 **AG, AGs**
アミノ馬尿酸塩 **AH**
アミノヒドロキシプロパン二リン酸塩 **APD**
アミノヒドロキシベンジルペニシリン **AMPC**
アミノピリン **AP**
アミノフィリン・フェノバルビタール・エフェドリン **APE**
アミノプテリン **AMP**
アミノペプチダーゼ **AP**
アミノペプチダーゼN **AMPN, APN**
アミノベンジルペニシリン **ABPC**
アミノ酪酸アルミニウム **ALGLYN**
アミノレブリン酸 **ALA, ALA, Ala**
アミノレブリン酸合成酵素 **ALAS**
アミノレブリン酸合成酵素2 **Alas-2**
アミノレブリン酸脱水素酵素 **ALAD**
(α)アミラーゼ **AMS**
アミラーゼ **Am, AMY, Amy, amyl**
アミラーゼクリアランス **Cam**
アミラーゼクレアチニンクリアランス比 **ACCR, Cam/Ccr**
アミル基 **AM, am, Am**
アミロイドA(蛋白) **AA**
アミロイドA蛋白 **AA protein**
アミロイドE(蛋白) **AE**
アミロイドL蛋白 **AL protein**
アミロイドアンギオパシー **AA**
アミロイド小体 **CA**
アミロイド症に伴う脳出血 **HCHWA**
アミロイド前駆体蛋白 **APP**
アミロイド物質 **AS**
アミログルコシダーゼ **AMG**
アミロ硫酸ナトリウム **SAS**
アミン前駆物質摂取と脱炭酸 **APUD**
アムホテリシン **AMPH**
アムホテリシンB **AMPH, AMPH-B**
アメトプテリン **AM**
(体内寄生性)アメーバ(属) **E**
アメーバ原虫 **EH**
アメーバ性髄膜脳炎 **AME**
アメーバ性肉芽腫性脳炎 **GAE**
アメリカ→米国も参照
アメリカ人 **AM, Am, Amer**
アメリカの **AM, Am, Amer**
アメリカヤマゴボウ抗ウイルス蛋白 **PAP**
アメリカヤマゴボウマイトジェン **PWM**
アメリシウム **Am**
アモキサピン **AX**
アモキシシリン **AMPC, AM-PC, AMX**
アラインメント **AL, al**
アラキドン酸 **AA, $C_{20=4}$**
アラタ体 **CA**
アラニン **A, Ala**
アラニンアミノトランスフェラーゼ **AAT, ALAT, ALT**
アラニントランスアミナーゼ **ALAT**
アラバミン **Ab**
アラビノシル-5-フルオロシチジン **ara-FC**
アラビノシルウラシル(＝

ウラシルアラビノシド） **ara-U, Ara-U**
アラビノシルシトシン **aC**
アラビノシルシトシン（＝シトシンアラビノシド） **Ara C, Ara-C, ara-C**
アラビノース **Ara**
アリザリン赤 **AZR**
アリザリンイエロー **AZY**
アリザリンレッドS **ARS**
アリューシャン病 **AD**
アリューシャン病ウイルス **ADV**
アリル **Ar**
アリルアミダーゼ **AA**
アリルスルファターゼA **ARSA, ASA**
アリルスルファターゼB **ARSB**
「アール」「エル」「エス」の発語障害者 **RLS**
アルカリゲネス（属） **A**
アルカリ性ツベルクリン **TA**
アルカリ性プロテアーゼ阻害剤 **API**
アルカリ性溶液に溶解する **SA**
アルカリ性リン酸分解酵素 **AL-Pase**
アルカリ（性）の **Alk, alk**
アルカリホスファターゼ **AKP, Alk phos., alk.phos., Alk PO_4, alk.p'tase, ALP, AL-Pase, AP, KA, P'ase**
アルカリホスファターゼ抗アルカリホスファターゼ（複合体） **APAAP**
アルカリ予備 **AR, RA**
アルカロイド **VA**
アルギナーゼ欠損症 **AD**
アルギ（ニ）ノコハク酸 **ASA**
アルギニン **Arg, R**
アルギニンインスリン負荷試験 **AITT**
アルギニンバソトシン **AVT**
アルギニンバソプレシン **AVP**
アルギニン負荷試験 **ATT**
アルギ（ニ）ノコハク酸合成酵素 **ASS**
アルギ（ニ）ノコハク酸合成酵素欠損症 **ASD**
アルギ（ニ）ノコハク酸リアーゼ欠損症 **ALD**
アルキル化剤 **AA**
アルキルベンゼンスルホン酸塩 **ABS**
アルコール **Alc, alc, alcoh, sp., spir.v., sp.vin., s.v.**
アルコール（溶液） **Spir., spir., spt., spts.**
アルゴル **ALGOL**
アルコール・エーテル・アセトン溶液 **AEA solution**
アルコール・クロロホルム・エーテル（混合液） **ACE**
アルコール・ホルマリン・酢酸 **AFA**
アルコール・薬物・交通安全国際委員会 **ICADTS**
アルコール・薬物中毒研究財団 **ADARF**
アルコール依存症者更生会 **AA**
アルコール（性）ケトアシドーシス **AKA**
アルコール使用調査票 **AUI**
アルコール性肝炎 **AH**
アルコール性肝硬変 **AC**
アルコール性肝疾患 **ALD**
アルコール性心疾患 **AHD**
アルコール性膵炎 **AIP**
アルコールその他危険薬に対する習癖研究学会 **SSA**
アルコール代謝における迅速な増加 **SIAM**
アルコール脱水素酵素 **ADH**
アルコール中毒児スクリーニング検査 **CAST**
アルコール中毒者更生国際医師団 **IDAA**
アルコール性中毒性小脳変性 **ACD**
アルコール中毒全国委員会 **NCA**
アルコールデヒドロゲナーゼ **AD, ADH**
アルコールと麻薬に関する指導進歩のための協会 **AAIAN**
アルコール（性）の **alcoh**
アルコール誘発クッシング類似症候群 **APCS**
アルコール離脱 **AW**
アルゴン **A**
アルゴンプラズマ凝固法 **APC**
アルゴンレーザー虹彩切開（術） **ALI**
アルゴンレーザー光凝固（術） **ALP**
アルシアンブルー **AB**
アルシアンブルー染色

AB
アルジオキサ　**ALDA**
アルスフェナミン　**AR, Ars, ars**
アルゼンチン出血(性)熱　**AHF**
アルツハイマー型痴呆　**ATD, DAT**
アルツハイマー型痴呆の機能的評価　**FAST**
アルツハイマー型老年〔老人〕(性)痴呆　**SDAT**
アルツハイマー神経原線維変性　**ANC**
アルツハイマー神経線維変化　**ANT**
アルツハイマー病　**AD**
アルツハイマー様老年性痴呆　**ALSD**
アルツハイマー(型)老人性痴呆　**ASD**
アルデヒド脱水素酵素　**AlDH, ALDH**
アルデヒドフクシン　**AF**
アルドース還元酵素　**AR**
アルドース還元酵素阻害剤　**ARI**
アルドステロン　**ALD, aldo**
アルドステロン産生腺腫　**APA**
アルドステロン刺激因子　**ASF**
アルドステロン刺激ホルモン　**ASH**
アルドステロン分泌欠損　**ASD**
アルドステロン分泌率　**ASR**
アルドステロン誘発性蛋白　**AIP**
アルドラーゼ　**ALD, Ald**
アルトロース　**Alt**
アルバート・アインシュタイン医科大学　**AECM**
アルファカルシドール　**ALF**
アルファフェトプロテインの標準化日本委員会　**JSCA**
アルブミン　**A, AL, ALB, Alb, alb**
アルブミン,カゼイン,レシチン　**ACL**
アルブミン・カルシウム・マグネシウム　**acm**
アルブミン・グロブリン比　**ALB/GLOB**
アルブミン・ブドウ糖・カタラーゼ　**ADC**
アルブミン/クレアチニン比　**ACR, A/R ratio**
アルブミン/グロブリン(比)　**A-G, A/G**
アルブミン/コアグリン比　**A/C ratio**
アルブミンクリアランス　**alb.C, CAlb, C alb, Calb, C.alb**
アルブミン排泄率　**AER**
アルボウイルス　**ABV, Arbo, ARBO**
アルミゲル　**AL Gel**
アルミニウム　**AI, Al**
アルミニウムアジュバント　**ALUM**
アルミニウム沈降破傷風トキソイド　**APT**
アレルギー　**A, AI, ALG, alg., algy, ALL, all**
アレルギー情報協会　**AIA**
アレルギー性　**ALG**
アレルギー性気管支肺アスペルギルス症　**ABPA**
アレルギー性気管支肺真菌症　**ABPM**
アレルギー性呼吸器疾患　**ARD**
アレルギー性湿疹性接触皮膚炎　**AECD**
アレルギー性接触皮膚炎　**ACD**
アレルギー性喘息　**AA**
アレルギー性肉芽腫性血管炎　**AGA**
アレルギー性鼻炎　**AR, Rh.aller.**
アレルギー専門医　**A**
アレルギー増強因子　**EFA**
アレルギー治療医学　**ARM**
アレルギーと免疫学　**A & I**
アレルギーの　**ALG**
アレルギーの特異的抗原検査　**FAST**
アレルギーの抑制因子　**SFA**
アレン視覚検査　**AVT**
アロイン・ベラドンナ・ストリキニーネ　**ABS**
アロキサン　**ALX**
アロース　**All**
アロテトラハイドロアルドステロン　**allo-THA**
アロテトラハイドロコルチコステロン　**allo-THC**
アンケート　**qq, qtnr**
アンジオテンシノゲン　**ATNG**
アンジオテンシノゲン　**AGT, Aogen**
アンジオテンシン　**A, ANG**
アンジオテンシンⅠ　**A-Ⅰ, AI, ANG Ⅰ**
アンジオテンシンⅡ　**A-Ⅱ, ANG Ⅱ**
アンジオテンシンⅡ受容体拮抗薬　**ARB**

アンジオテンシンIII **A-III**
アンジオテンシンI変換酵素 **AICE**
アンジオテンシン感受性検査 **AST**
アンジオテンシン関連ペプチド **ARP**
アンジオテンシン変換酵素 **ACE**
アンジオテンシン変換酵素阻害物質〔阻害薬〕 **ACEI**
アンジオテンシン様物質 **ALS**
アンソニーノーバン研究センター **ANRC**
アンダーアームブレス **UAB**
アンチトキシン **antitox**
アンチトロンビン **AT**
アンチトロンビンIII **AT-III**
アンチピリン **AP**
アンチマイシン **ant**
アンチマイシンA **Ant A**
アンチモン **Sb**
アンテナ **ant**
アンドロゲン(分泌)過剰症 **HA**
アンドロゲン過剰症・インスリン抵抗性・黒色表皮腫(症候群) **HAIR-AN**
アンドロゲン産生(帯) **X**
アンドロゲン指数 **AI**
アンドロゲン受容体 **AR**
アンドロスタノロン **AS**
アンドロステロン **A, ANDRO**
アンドロロジー国際学会 **CIDA**
アンピシリン **A, ABPC, AM, AMP**
アンヒドロ・グルシトール **AG**
アンフェタミン **A, AMP, AMPH, amphet, amphetamine, AMT**
アンフェタミン面接評点尺度 **AIRS**
アンプル **amp, AMP, amp, ampul.**
アンペア **A, A, a, a., amp**
アンペア・時 **amp-hr**
アンペア・ボルト・オーム **AVO**
アンペア計 **AM**
アンペア時 **Ah**
アンペア数 **amp**
アンペア秒 **AS, AS, a-s, a.s.**
アンモニア **AMM, amm, ammon,** NH_3
アンモニア・銅・砒素 **ACA**
アンモニア窒素 NH_3N
アンモニウム NH_4
あいまいな **amb**
あざ **BMK, bmk**
あちこちに **pass.**
あなたの情報と案内の参考に **FYIG**
あなたの情報の参考に **FYI**
あらゆる危険に対して **AAR**
ありそうな **prob**
あるいは **od**
ある物 **Etw**
上げる **elev**
亜鉛 **Zn**
亜鉛化インスリン懸濁液 **IZS**
亜鉛華ユージノールセメント F_2
亜鉛欠乏の **ZD**
亜鉛枯渇症候群 **ZDS**
亜鉛混濁反応 **ZT**
亜鉛プロタミンインスリン **ZPI**
亜鉛プロトポルフィリン **ZnP, ZPP**
亜黄疸 **SI**
亜急性壊死性脳脊髄障害 **SNE, SNEM**
亜急性黄色萎縮 **SYA**
亜急性海綿状脳症 **SSE**
亜急性肝(臓)壊死 **SHN**
亜急性感染性関節炎 **SIA**
亜急性冠(状)動脈疾患 **SCD**
亜急性硬化性全脳炎 **SSP**
亜急性硬化性全脳炎(ウイルス) **SSPE**
亜急性甲状腺炎 **SAT**
亜急性骨髄単球性白血病 **MLS**
亜急性細菌性心内膜炎 **SBE**
亜急性脊髄視神経障害 **SMON**
亜急性喘息反応 **SAR**
亜急性の **subac**
亜急性播種状エリテマトーデス **SDLE**
亜急性皮膚型紅斑性狼瘡 **SCLE**
亜急性連合性脊髄変性症 **SCDC**
亜急性連合性(脊髄)変性(症) **SACD**
亜型 **St**
亜広汎性壊死 **SN**
亜酸化窒素 **NO,** N_2O
亜酸化窒素・酸素・イソフルレン麻酔 **GOI**
亜酸化窒素・酸素・エンフルラン麻酔 **GOE**

亜酸化窒素・酸素・神経遮断麻酔併用法 **GONLA**
亜酸化窒素・酸素・セボフルレン麻酔法 **GOS**
亜酸化窒素・酸素・ハロタン麻酔 **GOF**
亜酸化窒素・酸素・ペントレン麻酔法 **GOP**
亜硝酸塩レダクターゼ〔還元酵素〕 **NIRA**
亜硝酸アミル **AN**
亜硝酸化物 **nit.ox.**
亜硝酸ジサイクロヘキシルアミン **DCHN**
亜種 **SSP, subsp, subsp.**
亜属 **s-g, S-GG, subgen**
亜脱臼 **sublux**
亜致死障害回復 **SLDR**
亜捻髪音の **subcr, subcrep, subcrep.**
亜ミトコンドリア粒子 **SMP**
亜硫酸ビスマス培地 **BS**
亜硫酸化酵素欠損症 **SOD**
阿片 **O**
阿片剤禁断 **OPWL**
明日 **cr., crst.**
明日仮退院 **TDT**
明日退院 **DT**
明日の **crast.**
明日の夕方 **cr.vesp., CV, c.v.**
開けたまま(にすること) **TKO**
開けたままにせよ **KO, K/O**
合図 **Sig, sig**
愛の対象 **LO**
曖昧な **equiv**
青 **Bl, bl**
赤(の) **R**
赤い **redsh, rub.**
赤池情報量基準 **AIC**
赤紫 **PR**
赤/緑 **R/G**
明るい **brt**
明らかな **app, appar, cl, mfst**
明らかに **app**
明らかになったもの **q.e.d.**
悪性(腫瘍) **malig**
悪性萎縮性丘疹症 **MAP**
悪性栄養膜奇形腫 **MTT**
悪性外耳炎 **MEO**
悪性カルチノイド症候群 **MCS**
悪性関節リウマチ **MRA**
悪性間葉性腫瘍 **MMT**
悪性(腫瘍)関連変化 **MAC**
悪性奇形腫 **MT**
悪性胸水 **MPE**
悪性胸膜中皮腫 **MPM**
悪性(体液性)高カルシウム血症 **HHM**
悪性高血圧 **MHT**
悪性高体温(症) **MH**
悪性高熱(症) **MH**
悪性高熱症の疑い(がある) **MHS**
悪性黒子黒色腫 **LMM**
悪性黒色腫 **MM**
悪性持続性頭位眩暈症 **MPPV**
悪性腫瘍関連体液性高カルシウム血症 **MAHH**
悪性腫瘍に伴う高カルシウム血症 **MAH**
悪性腫瘍に伴う小脳変性 **PCD**
悪性腫瘍の異型度 **G**
悪性腫瘍の構造異体 **SAT**
悪性(腫瘍)所見なし **NEM**
悪性腎硬化症 **MN**
悪性腎新生物 **MRN**
悪性線維性組織球腫 **MFH**
悪性組織球増殖(症) **MH**
悪性中胚葉混合腫瘍 **MMMT**
悪性乳頭状中皮腫 **MPM**
悪性の **M, mal., malig**
悪性貧血 **PA**
悪性貧血様症候群と免疫グロブリン欠損 **PA-LS-ID**
悪性末梢神経鞘腫瘍 **MPNST**
悪性ミュラー管混合腫瘍 **MMMT**
悪性リンパ腫 **ML**
握手 **HG**
握力 **GP, HG**
握力計 **dyn**
浅い **sup, SUP, sup., superf, superfic**
朝 **M, m., mng, mo′**
朝(に) **man.**
朝いちばんで **man.pr., man.prim.**
朝一番に **prim.m.**
朝と夕方 **m.et v., M.u.A., m.u.a**
朝と夜 **m.et n., M & N**
朝に **m., matut.**
朝のこわばり **MS**
朝早く **lucp., luc.prim., m.p.**
足 **F, f, Ft, ft**
足首/上腕血圧指数 **AAI**
足治療士連合 **FBP**
足の裏の **vol**
足の外科学博士 **DSC**

足の拇指　**GT**
足浮腫　**ped.ed**
与えて書け　**D.S., d.s.**
与えよ　**D, d., dand., d.d., dent., det., dtr., exhib.**
与える　**D, d.**
値　**v, val**
温かい　**w**
温めた　**calef.**
温めよ　**calef.**
暖かい(滅菌した)湿布　**WMD**
暖かで乾燥した　**W/D**
頭　**cap, hd**
頭のいい　**brt**
頭・目・耳・鼻・咽喉　**HEENT**
新しい　**n, nov., rec.**
新しい胸部X線撮影装置　**AMBER**
新しい見解　**NV**
新しい雇用者　**NE**
新しい属と種　**gen.et sp.nov.**
新しい名前　**nn., n.nov., nom.nov., nov.n.**
新しいリンパ系腫瘍の欧米分類　**REAL**
圧　**P, PR, pres, press, T, ten, tens, tns, tnsn**
圧掛け算値を指標とする数値　**RPP**
圧痕　**Imp, imp, impr**
圧挫症候群　**CS**
圧搾　**expn**
圧搾しないで　**s. expr., sine express.**
(眼)圧上昇　**T+, T ↑**
圧上昇時間　**DAZ**
圧受容器　**PR**
圧時間/分　**PTM**
圧縮　**compr, comprn, expn**
圧縮ガス協会　**CGA**
圧縮空気　**CA**
圧縮された　**compd, compr**
圧縮錠(剤)　**CT**
圧縮錠剤粉末　**CTT**
圧縮性の　**comp**
圧縮せよ　**compr.**
圧縮増幅　**CA**
圧縮できる　**comp**
圧縮分光列　**CSA**
圧縮率　**CR**
圧制御調節換気　**PCV**
圧調節式間欠冠静脈洞閉塞法　**PICSO**
圧痛　**DE, T, tend**
圧痛および反跳圧痛　**T & R**
圧痛のある　**T, tend**
圧痛のない　**nontend**
圧痛または反跳圧痛　**T or R**
(眼)圧低下　**T ↓, T−**
(眼)圧の増大度　**$T_{+1}, T_{+2}\cdots$**
圧迫(症)　**compr, comprn**
圧迫された　**compd, compr**
圧迫症候群　**CS**
圧迫する　**comp**
圧迫で指が痛みを感ずる　**DTP**
圧迫包装(＝経口薬のパッケージの１つ)　**PTP**
圧平眼圧計　**App.T**
圧補助換気　**PSV**
圧補正従量式　**PRVC**
圧力・容積・温度　**PVT**
圧力尿流試験　**PFS**
圧力の時間微分　**dP/dT**
圧・容積関係　**PVR**
圧・容積係数　**PVI**
圧・率産生物　**PRP**
悪化　**aggrav**
悪化させる　**aggrav**
悪化指数　**DI**
集められた　**agg**
集める　**zus**
熱い　**H**
熱(い〔温かい〕水)と冷(たい水)　**h & c, H & C**
姉　**sis**
油　**o, Ol, ol, ol.**
油による肺麻痺好酸球増加症症候群　**OPPES**
甘い　**dulc., sw**
甘みなしで　**sine conf.**
余り　**reliq, reliq.**
雨水　**aq.pluv.**
誤りの　**err**
誤った　**w**
洗い出し　**WO**
粗い　**gros.**
粗い粉末　**pul.gros., pulv.gros.**
粗模型　**rg tp**
現す　**exh**
安産　**GD**
安心　**ref, rel**
安心させる　**rlv**
安全　**scty**
安全・健康・福祉　**SHW**
安全域　**MS**
安全因子　**FS, SF**
安全実用必要量　**SPR**
安全認定食品添加物　**GRAS**
安静　**R**
安静時エネルギー代謝量　**REE**
安静時子宮緊張度　**URT**
安静時消費熱量　**REE**
安静時静脈血圧　**RVP**
安静時振戦　**RT**
安静時代謝量　**RM**
安静時の　**R**
安静時の消費エネルギー　**Mets**

安静時膜電位　**RMP**
安息香酸ナトリウムカフェイン　**Cnb**
安息香酸　**BzOH**
安息香酸エステル　**B, benz, benz.**
安息香酸エストラジオール　**EB**
安息香酸塩　**B, benz, benz.**
安定X線伝導体　**SXT**
安定因子　**SF**
安定化視標追跡器具　**SOTD**
安定血漿蛋白溶液　**SPPS**
安定剤　**stab**
安定サルコイドーシス　**SS**
安定状態　**s**
安定流　**staflo**
按摩　**mass, mass.**
暗室試験　**DRT**
暗視野　**DG**
暗順応　**DA**
罨法　**cat, cat., WD**

い

イヴォン係数試験　**YCT**
イエカ(属)　**C**
イエーガー視力表　**J1-J3**
イオタ　**i**
イオン化されない血色素　**HHB**
イオン感受領域効果トランジスタ　**ISFET**
イオン干渉クロマトグラフィ　**IIC**
イオン干渉試薬　**IIR**
イオン強度　**I**
イオン交換　**IC, IEX**
イオン交換クロマトグラフィ　**IEC**
イオンサイクロトロン共鳴　**ICR**
イオン散乱分光法　**ISS**
イオン選択電極　**ISE**
イオン相互作用試薬　**IIR**
イオン中和分光　**INS**
イオン定数　**K**
イオン電荷数　**Z**
イオン表面散乱　**ISS**
イギリス→英国も参照
イギリス骨疾患協会　**OAGB**
イギリス熱単位　**BTHU**
イーグル・ハンクスアミノ酸培地(培養液)　**EHAA**
イーグル基礎培地　**BME**
イーグル基本培地　**EBM**
イサチンβチオセミカルバゾン　**IBT**
(車)イス　**CH**
イズロン酸　**Ido U, Ido UA**
イセパミシン　**ISP**
イソ　**i**
イソアミラーゼ　**isoamy**
イソクエン酸脱水素酵素　**ICD, ICDH, IDH**
イソソルビド 5-モノニトレート　**ISMN**
イソニアジド・メタスルホン酸　**INMS**
イソニコチン酸ヒドラジド　**IHMS**
イソニコチン酸ヒドラジド(=イソニアジド)　**INH**
イソニコチン酸ビドラジド　**INAH**
イソブチル基　**isobu**
イソブチルシアノアクリレート　**IBC, IBCA**
イソプリノシン　**IPS**
イソフルレン　**I**
イソプレナリン　**ISP**
イソプロテレノール　**IP, IPR, ISO**
イソプロピリデンアミノベンジルペニシリン(=ヘタシリンカリウム)　**IPABPC**
イソプロピルノルアドレナリン(=イソプロテレノール)　**IPNA**
イソプロピルアルテレノール　**IPA**
イソプロピルアンフェタミン　**IMP**
イソ酪酸　**IBA**
イソロイシル　**ILE, Ile**
イソロイシン　**I, ILE, Ile, ILEU, Ileu, ileu**
イタコン酸　**ITA**
イタリック体　**ital**
イタリック体で印刷する　**ital**
イダルビシン　**IDA, IDR**
イッテルビウム　**Yb**
イットリウム　**Y, YT, yt**
イットリウム・アルミニウム・ガーネット(レーザー)　**YAG**
イットリウム 90　**^{90}Y**
イットリウムリチウムフッ化物　**YLF**
イディオタイプ　**Id**
イドクスウリジン　**IDU, IDUR**
イドース　**Ido**
イートン・ランバート症候群　**EL, ELS**
イートン・ランバートの筋無力症症候群　**MSEL**
イヌ　**D**
イヌ(の)ジステンパー　**CD**
イヌ(の)ジステンパーウイルス　**CDV**
イヌ(の)ジステンパー脳炎　**CDE**
イヌ腎(臓)組織培養　**DKCT**
イヌ赤血球　**DRBC**
イヌ赤血球抗血清　**ADRIS**
イヌ単位　**DU**
イヌ伝染性肝炎(ウイルス)　**HCC**
イヌの　**C**
イヌの重症筋無力症　**CMG**
イヌリン　**In**
イヌリンクリアランス　**CIN, Cin, c.in.**
イヌリン除去率　**E_{IN}**
イノシトール　**Ino**
イノシトールリン酸　**InsP, IP, IPs**
イノシトールリン酸化触媒酵素　**PTEN**
イノシル　**Ino**
イノシン　**I, Ino**
イノシン 5′-(モノ〔一〕)リ

ン酸 **Ino-5′-P**
イノシン5′-三リン酸 **ITP**
イノシン5′-二リン酸 **IDP**
イノシン一リン酸 **IMP**
イノシン5′-ジ〔二〕リン酸 **Ino-5′-P2**
イノシン5′-トリ〔三〕リン酸 **Ino-5′-P3**
イノシン酸 **IMP**
イノシン酸ピロホスホリラーゼ **IAP**
イノシン二リン酸 **IDP**
イノシンホスホリラーゼ **IP**
イノシンモノリン酸 **IMP**
イプシロン〔ε〕アミノカプロン酸 **ε-ACA**
イブニングケア **E-care**
イブプロフェン **IBU**
イブラヒム・ベック(病) **IB**
イホスファミド **Ifex, IFOS, IFX**
イホスファミド,カルボプラチン,エトポシド **ICE**
イホスファミド,シスプラチン(=プラチノール),アドリアマイシン **IPA**
イホスファミド,メスナによる尿道保護,アドリアマイシン,シスプラチン **IMAC**
イホスファミド・メスナによる尿道保護・メトトレキサート・エトポシド **IMVP-16**
イホスファミド・メスナによる尿道保護・メトトレキサート・フルオロウラシル **IMF**
イホスファミド,メトトレキサート,ビンクリスチン **IMV**
イボテン酸 **ibo**
イミダゾール酢酸リボヌクレオチド **IAAR**
イミダゾール焦性ブドウ酸 **IPA**
イミノ二酢酸 **IDA**
イミプラミン **IMI, IMIP, IMP**
イミペネム/シラスタチンナトリウム **IPM/CS**
イムノブロッティング **IB**
イメージ増倍管 **II**
イメージ板 **IP**
イヤホン **EAR**
イラストレーター **il**
イリジウム **Ir**
イリジウム192 **^{192}Ir**
イリニウム **Il**
イリノイ言語学習能力診断検査 **ITPA**
インクブロット試験(=ロールシャッハテスト) **IBT**
インジウム **In**
インジウム111ジエチレントリアミン五酢酸 **^{111}In-DTPA**
インジゴ **ind, ind.**
インジゴカルミン **IC**
インジゴカルミンテスト **iCT, ICT**
インスリン **I, in, In, INS, ins**
インスリン・グルカゴン **I-G**
インスリン・トランスフェリン・エタノラミン・セレニウム **ITES**
インスリン・プロタミン亜鉛 **IPZ**
インスリン依存性糖尿病 **IDD, IDDM**
インスリン応答 **IR**
インスリン感受性指数 **ISI**
インスリン痙攣療法 **iCT, ICT**
インスリン原性指数 **ΔIRI/ΔBS**
インスリン昏睡治療 **iCT, ICT**
インスリン受容体基質 **IRS**
インスリンショック療法 **IST**
インスリン総投与量 **TDI**
インスリン耐性試験 **ITT**
インスリン単位 **IE**
インスリン治療 **IT**
インスリン低血糖試験 **IHT**
インスリン抵抗性 **IR**
インスリン抵抗性糖尿病 **IRDM**
インスリン転写因子 **bHLM, IPF**
インスリン反応性要素 **IRE**
インスリン非依存型糖尿病 **NIDDM**
インスリン非依存性糖尿病 **IID, IIDM**
インスリン必要量 **IR**
インスリン頻回注射療法 **iCT, ICT, MIIT, MIT**
インスリン分解活性 **IDA**
インスリン分泌 **IS**
インスリン分泌試験 **IST**
インスリン分泌指数 **II**
インスリン誘発最大酸分泌 **IPAO**
インスリン様活性 **ILA**

インスリン様活性物質 **ILAS**
インスリン様成長因子 **IGF，ILGF**
インスリン様成長因子結合蛋白 **IGFBP**
インスリン様物質 **ILM**
インスリンレセプター **IR**
インセンティブスパイロメータ **IS**
インセンティブスパイロメトリー **IS**
インターα トリプシンインヒビター **ITI**
インダクタンス係数 **induc**
インダニルカルベニシリン(=カリンダシリン) **ICBPC**
インターフェイス・メッセージ・プロセッサ **IMP**
インターフェロン **IF，IFN，INF，ITF**
インターフェロン刺激反応因子 **ISRE**
インターフェロン制御因子 **IRF**
インターフェロン組織拮抗物質 **TAI**
インターフェロン単位 **IFU**
インターフェロン様物質 **ILS**
インタープレスサービス，国際報道機関 **IPS**
インターベンショナルラジオロジー **IVR**
インターロイキン **IL**
インターロイキン1β変換酵素 **ICE**
インターロイキン2誘導T細胞チロシンキナーゼ **Itk**
インターン **INT，Int**
インターン・レジデント調整国家計画 **NIRMP**
インターンと医学生の協会 **AIMES**
インチ **in，in，ins**
インチ・オンス **in.oz.**
インチ・ポンド **in.lb.，in-lb**
インディアン小児肝硬変 **ICC**
インデックスメディクス **IM，I.M.**
インドシアニングリーン **ICG**
インドメタシン **IMT，IND，indo，INDO，indocin**
インドール-3-アセトニトリル **IAN**
インドール-3-カルビノール **I-3-C**
インドールアミン **IA**
インドールグリセロリン酸塩 **InGP**
インドール酢酸 **IAA**
インドール酸 **IA**
インパルス **IMPL**
インパルス/秒 **IPS**
インピーダンス **Z**
インピーダンス胃電図 **IE**
インピーダンス角 **IA**
インピーダンス呼吸運動描画器 **ZPN**
インピーダンス静脈波計 **IPG**
インピーダンス心拍出量 **ICO**
インピーダンスプレチスモグラフィ **IPG**
インフォームドアセント **IA**
インフォームドコンセント **IC**
インフュージョンポンプ **IP**
インフルエンザ **flu**
インフルエンザウイルスのスコッティー型 **Scot virus**
インフルエンザウイルスワクチン **IVV**
インフルエンザ菌B型 **HIB，HITB**
インフルエンザ菌由来の制限エンドヌクレアーゼ **Hind** II〔III〕
インレー **inl**
インポテンス **IMP，Impo**
いくつかの **sev**
いくらか **etw**
いつ・どこで・なぜ・なにが・おこるのか **5W**
いっしょに **Z，Z-**
いのちの電話連盟 **FIND**
いぼ状表皮異形成 **EV**
いぼ **VV**
入口創 **WE，WOE**
以上と以下 **O & U**
以前結婚したことのある人 **FMP**
以前に **fmrly，vorm，vorm.**
以前の **fmr，frmr，prev**
以前は **form**
以内の **W/I**
生かす **anim**
生きがいテスト **PIL**
生きている **l，L，LIV**
生きており活動している **L & A**
行かせる **mitt，mitt.**
出雲急性期脳卒中病院前診断チェックリスト **IPAS**
位相測定干渉顕微鏡 **PMIM**

位相変化物質　**PCM**
位相変調　**PM**
位置　**l, locn, P, Pos, pos**
位置エネルギー　**PE**
囲繞性心内膜側心室切開術　**EEV**
医院　**ofc, off**
医院で経過を追う　**WF-O**
医用放射線化学資格認定書　**DMR, D.M.R.**
医用放射線診断資格認定書　**DMRD, D.M.R.D.**
医学　**M, MED, Med, med., meds, MEDS**
医学・獣医学研究所　**IMVS**
医学・生物学的電子工学　**MBE**
医学イラストレーター協会　**AMI**
医学会員　**F.phy.S.**
医学会新聞　**MWN**
（米国）医学関連文献分析検索システム　**MEDLARS**
医学基礎用語集　**MALIMET**
医学教育　**ME, pysed**
医学教育学士　**MSPE, M.S.P.E.**
医学教育勧告審議会　**ACME**
医学教育研究協会　**ASME**
医学教育責任者　**DME**
医学教育認定書　**Dip.Phys.Edu.**
医学教育プログラム　**MEDPRO**
医学教育目標５項目：現実的・理解可能・測定可能・行動で示される・到達可能　**RUMBA**
医学教育連絡委員会　**LCME**
医学記録管理者　**MRA**
医学訓練センター　**MTC**
医学研究委員会単位　**MRCU**
医学研究協議会　**MEDRESCO**
医学研究室　**med lab**
医学研究所　**IOM**
医学研究情報システム　**MRIS**
医学研究所有資格者　**LInstPhys**
医学研究審議会　**MRC**
医学研究センター　**MRC**
医学研究団体　**MRC**
医学研究博士　**D.Med.Sc.**
医学研究用動物補充基金　**FRAME**
医学検査技士　**FIMLT**
医学研修生　**INT, Int**
医学校　**Acad Med**
医学校環境ストレス　**MSES**
医学航空便　**MAP**
医学国際協会　**MEDICO**
医学国際職業協会　**APIM**
医学雑誌編集者国際委員会　**ICMJE**
医学（博）士　**MD, M.D.**
医学士　**B.M., B.Med., BMS, B.M.S., B.S.Med., D en M, D.Med., D.Ph.Sc., M.B., M.Med, MSD, M.S.Med**
医学歯学部門　**MED-DENT**
医学試験　**ME**
医学事項索引用見出し　**MeSH**
医学情報サービス　**MIS**
医学情報システム　**MIS**
医学神経精神病研究部門　**MNRU**
医学生　**medic, medix, MS**
医学生教育システム　**MEDICATES**
医学総管理者　**MDG**
医学徴候と症候　**Sx**
医学治療ユニット　**MTU**
医学的空気排除　**MAE**
医学的経過観察　**MFU**
医学的検査　**phys exam**
医学的助言に逆らって　**AMA, a.m.a.**
医学的助言に逆らって自主退院した　**SOAMA**
医学的助言に逆らって退院した　**DAMA, disch.AMA**
医学的中毒性環境　**MTE**
医学的調査　**MS**
医学的排泄　**medevac**
医学的排泄物　**MD**
医学的リハビリテーション　**MR**
医学電気学指導員　**TME**
医学図書館協会　**MLA**
医学の　**M, MED, Med, med.**
医学博士　**PhD, ph.D., Dr Med, Dr.Med.**
医学判断学　**MDM**
医学微生物学学際委員会　**MEMIC**
医学部　**Med Sch**
医学文献索引　**MI**
医学文献司書　**M.R.I.**
医学文献集　**IM, I.M., Ind.Med.**
医学放射線治療医免許　**D.M.R.T.**

医学報道進歩のための研究所　IAMC
医科学国際組織委員会　COIMS
医科学士　Med.Sc.D.
医科大学　Med Sch
医科大学入学試験　MCAT
医科大学の外来診療　MUPK
医科展示者協会　MEA
医原病　DOMP
医事記録ファイル　MRF
医事記録用紙　MRF
医事法制士資格認定書　DMJ
医師　d, doc, D.Ph.Sc., Dr., medic, Phys, phys
医師活動調査　PAS
医師国家試験合格者　DNB
医師支払査定委員会　PPRC
医師生涯教育　CME
医師討論会　PF
医師の行動チェックリスト　PBCL
医師の指示簿　DOB
医師の実践要綱　CP
医師の助手教育　PAT
医師の治療マニュアル　PTM
医師のみ　PO
医師免許証所有者　ML, M.L.
医薬の　med, med.
医薬品　med, med.
医薬品安全試験基準　GLP
(英国)医薬品安全性研究所　DSRU
医薬品・医薬部外品・化粧品・医療機器の製造販売後安全管理の基準　GVP
(独立行政法人)医薬品医療機器総合機構　PMDA
日米EU医薬品規制調和国際会議　ICH
医薬品規制用語集　MEDDRA
医薬品市販後調査　PMS
医薬品情報　DI
医薬品情報基準　GPP
医薬品製造者全国協会　NAPM
医薬品庁　MCA
医薬品の供給および品質管理に関する日本の基準　JGSP
医薬品の使用経験　DE
医薬品の製造と品質管理に関する規準　GMP
医薬品の製造販売後の調査および試験の実施に関する基準　GPSP
医薬品の便益性とリスクを科学的に評価解析することを目的とした国際財団　IMBRF
医薬用の　ad us.med.
医用ガス分析器　MGA
医用工学　BME
医用生体工学　MBE
医用電子機器　ME
医用電子工学　ME
医用電子工学と生物電子工学　ME & BE
医用の　M
医用放射線・電子学資格認定書　DMRE
医用マイクロコンピュータクラブ　MMC
医用硫酸デキストラン　MDS
医療　MT
医療衛生サービス責任者　DMSS
医療援助　medicaid
医療介護　medicare
医療監査計画　MAP
医療管理計画グループ　MMPG
医療器械進歩のための協会　AAMI
医療機関における医薬品管理規範　GDP
医療機器事故報告制度　MDR
医療技術　Med Tech, med.tech.
医療技術学士　BMT
医療技術士　B.S.Med.Tech.
医療記録技術　MRT
医療記録部門　MRD
医療訓練器具勧告委員会委員　FACMTA
医療研究用加速器　MRR
医療サービス責任者　DGMS, DMS
医療サービスの副支配人　ADMS
医療実施者単位　MPU
医療質的査定機構　MQRO
医療(費)支払い　MP
医療市民行動計画　MedCAP
医療事務員　MO
医療事務主任　CMO
医療社会事業部　SSD
医療従事者勧告サービス　EMAS
医療情報　MEDINFO
医療情報管理システム協会　HIMSS
医療情報システム　MEDIS
医療情報システム開発センター　MEDIS-DC
医療情報代理業　MIIA
医療情報担当者　MR
医療情報ネットワーク

MINET
医療処置点数制 **TISS**
医療人権センター
COML
医療設備研究と開発研究所
MERDI
医療宣伝機関協会
AMAA
医療専門家 **medex**
医療相談連絡事務所
MCLO
医療装備管理事務所
MEMO
医療ソーシャルワーカー
MSW
医療提供契約 **PPO**
医療データシステム
MDS
医療と義務 **MD**
医療と法の消費者組織
COML
医療内部被曝線量
MIRD
医療における技術評価
MTA
医療の **M**
医療の薬学的助言者
PAM
医療費内容審査 **UR**
医療奉仕活動
MEDSAC
医療奉仕団 **MSC**
医療法人 **MedC**
医療法律学 **med juris**
医療保健サービス責任者
DMHS
医療保険事務代行 **TPA**
医療補助者 **medicaid**
医療用具放射線局[米国]
CDRH
医療用廃棄物 **MW**
医療予備隊 **MEDRC**
依存病者 **IP**
依頼医 **ref.doc, Ref.Dr, ref.phys**
依頼された **ref**
依頼する **ref**
依頼箋 **Req**
委員 **commn**
委員会 **BD, Bd, bd, comm, commn**
委員会制定栄養規則
CAC
委託看護師 **CN**
委託歯科医 **ref.dent**
委任 **comm, commn**
易結晶化フラグメント
Fc, FC, Fc
易損期 **VP**
易熱・熱安定抗原
LS antigen
易熱性毒素 **HLT**
胃 **ST, st, stom, tum, VS**
胃アルコールデヒドロゲナーゼ **GADH**
胃液 **GF**
胃液検査 **GA**
胃カメラ **GC, GT**
胃下部 1/3 **A**
胃冠(状)静脈 **CV**
胃窩 **reg.epigast.**
胃潰瘍 **Gastric ul, GU, MG, UV**
胃癌 **CV, GC, MK**
胃癌抗原 **GCA**
胃筋電図記録 **EGG**
胃機能抑制ポリペプチド
GIP
胃鏡検査 **GCY**
胃空腸吻合術 **GJ**
胃血流量 **GBF**
胃形成術 **GP**
胃健剤 **MM**
胃酸分泌 **GAS**
胃十二指腸潰瘍 **GDU**
胃十二指腸動脈 **GDA**
胃十二指腸の **GD**
胃上部 **C**
胃上部 1/3 区 **C**
胃周囲の血行遮断 **GD**
胃食道圧勾配 **GEPG**
胃食道逆流 **GER, GOR**
胃食道逆流疾患 **GERD**
胃食道の **GE**
胃情動の **GE**
胃腫瘍関連抗原 **GATT**
胃砂時計状収縮 **HCS**
胃切開術 **gastro**
胃切除術 **GR, MR**
胃全摘術 **Total, total**
胃洗浄 **stom.lav**
胃造瘻術 **GT**
胃大網動脈 **GEA**
胃チューブ **GT, MT**
胃中部 **M**
胃中部 1/3 区 **M**
胃地図 **sto.map**
胃腸炎 **GE**
胃腸幹 **TGC**
胃腸管 **GI, GIT**
胃腸管治療システム
GITS
胃腸系 **GIS**
胃腸出血 **GIH**
胃腸症状 **GIS**
胃腸膵臓内分泌系 **GEP**
胃腸膵の **GEP**
胃腸造影図 **GIS**
胃腸装置 **GIA**
胃腸通過時間 **GITT**
胃腸内細菌叢 **GIBF**
胃腸内視鏡検査 **GE**
胃腸の **GI**
胃腸病学 **GAS, gastroenterol, GE**
胃腸吻合術 **GE, GIA**
胃内ガス **GIS**
胃内視鏡法 **GFS**
胃内に **ig, IG**
胃内の **ig, IG**
胃内容排出 **GE**
胃内容排出時間 **GET**
胃内容物排出速度 **GER**
胃内容排出遅延 **DGE**

胃粘膜　**GM**
胃粘膜血流量　**GMBF**
胃粘膜バリア　**GMB**
胃の　**gast**
胃の運動性　**GM**
胃バイパス手術　**GBS**
胃半切除・迷走神経切断（術）　**H & V**
胃ファイバースコープ　**FGS，GFB，GFS**
胃フィステル　**GF**
胃壁在細胞　**GPC**
胃ポリープ　**GP**
胃鳴音　**SR**
胃抑制ペプチド　**GIP**
胃容量　**GV**
胃X線透視撮影　**MDL，M.D.L**
胃・十二指腸・膵臓　**SDP**
胃・十二指腸潰瘍　**MDG**
胃瘻造設術　**GT**
異化遺伝子活性化蛋白　**CAP**
異化代謝産物モジュール因子　**CMF**
異形吸虫(属)　**H**
異形接合体　**Ht**
異形接合の　**HET**
異型移行　**AT**
異型移行帯　**aT，AT**
異型狭心症　**VA，VAP**
異型結核(症)　**ATB**
異型血管　**aV**
異型上皮　**ATP**
異型腺腫様過形成　**AAH**
異型の　**atyp**
異型ポルフィリン症　**VP**
異型リンパ球　**ATL**
異好性移植抗原　**HTA**
異所　**dysto**
異所性骨化　**HO**
異所性焦点　**EF**
異所性心房性頻拍　**EAT**
異所性脱分極　**ED**
異所性の　**ect**
異所の　**aber**
異常　**abnor，abnorm，AN**
異常型プリオン蛋白　**PrP^Sc**
異常キラー細胞　**AK**
異常左軸偏位　**ALAD，ALA-D**
異常子宮出血　**AUB**
異常静脈還流　**AVR**
異常所見　**ACF**
異常所見なし　**NEA，OB，O.B.**
異常耐糖能　**AGT**
異常蛋白血症を伴う血管リンパ芽球性リンパ節症　**AILD**
異常糖負荷試験　**AGTT**
異常なし　**NA，n.B，NB**
異常〔著変〕なし，特記すべきことなし　**NP，np，n.p.**
異常の　**A，AB，ABN，Abn，abn，abnor，abnorm**
異常不随意運動　**AIM**
異常不随意運動疾患　**AIMD**
異常不随意運動尺度　**AIMS**
異常プロトロンビン　**APT**
異種移植片表面積　**XSA**
異種甲状腺刺激因子　**HTF**
異種自然抗体　**XNA**
異種族間の　**mxd**
異種発生の　**heterog**
異性関係(尺度)　**HR**
異性の　**isom**
異染性脳白質変性症　**MLD**
異染性白質異常症　**ML**
異物　**CA，FB，for bod**
異物感　**FKG**
(光学式の)異物検査装置　**WIS**
移行上皮癌　**TCC**
移行上皮癌関連(ウイルス)　**TCCA**
移行上皮癌関連ウイルス　**TCCAV**
移行性静脈炎　**PM**
移行帯　**T**
移行点　**T**
移住医師　**DP physician**
移植　**Tpl，TX**
移植(術)　**transpl**
移植(片)　**gr**
移植学会　**TS**
移植可能肝細胞癌　**THC**
移植可能なインスリン放出装置で糖尿病を治療する国際研究グループ　**ISG-IID**
移植抗原　**TA**
移植後リンパ増殖性疾患　**PTLD**
移植腎動脈狭窄(症)　**TRAS**
移植臓器確保と移植の全国連絡網　**NOPTN**
移植素材生体提供者　**LRD**
移植組織(片)　**transpl**
移植片浸潤性リンパ球　**GIL**
移植片対宿主　**GVH，GvH**
移植片対宿主疾患　**GVHD**
移植片対宿主反応　**GVH，GVHR**
移植片対白血病細胞反応　**GVL**
移送する　**trs**

移動　**Amb, amb., ambul, displ**
移動式冠（状動脈）疾患管理部門　**MCCU**
移動手術室　**MR**
移動する　**amb, ambul**
移動性の　**Amb, amb., mob**
移動度　**mob, mobil**
移動標的指示薬　**MTI**
移動率　**Rf**
移入　**Tr, tr**
移入する　**trans**
萎縮　**atr, atrop, atrop.**
萎縮（症）　**A**
萎縮後過形成　**PAH**
萎縮した　**contr**
萎縮する　**A**
萎縮性鼻炎　**AR, Rh.atr.**
偉大な　**g**
椅子とベッド　**CB**
硫黄　**S**
硫黄酸化物　**SOx**
硫黄単位　**SU**
意気消沈した　**depr**
意義不明　**US**
意義不明のプラズマ細胞疾患　**PCDUS**
意見　**rem**
意識　**CS, CS, Cs, cs**
意識回復　**RESC, resc**
意識している　**CS, CS, Cs, cs**
意識障害　**DOC**
意識障害分類（＝3-3-9度方式）　**JCS**
意識消失　**LOC**
意識消失期間　**per.unc.**
意識状態　**SOC, SOC, SoC**
意識のある　**CS, CS, Cs, cs**
意識のない　**UC, UCS, Ucs, unc, uncon**
意識不明の　**UC, UCS, Ucs**
意識変容状態　**ASC**
意識レベル　**LOC**
維持　**M, MR**
維持血液透析　**MHD**
維持電解質溶液　**MES**
維持平均時間　**MTBM**
維持量　**M, MD**
遺残　**ret**
遺伝　**hered**
遺伝学　**GEN, gen, genet**
遺伝決定率　**DGD**
遺伝子組換え型ヒトインターロイキン　**rhIL**
遺伝子組換え型ヒト毛様体神経成長因子　**rhCNTF**
遺伝子組換え顆粒球コロニー刺激因子　**rhG-CSF**
遺伝子組換え結合合成蛋白　**reFP**
遺伝子組換え微生物　**GEMs**
遺伝子組換えヒトエリスロポエチン　**rHuEPO**
遺伝子組換えヒト成長ホルモン　**r-hGH**
遺伝子組換えプロテインA　**recA**
遺伝子組換えワクシニアウイルス　**rVV**
遺伝子実験委員会　**COGENE**
遺伝子操作　**GM**
遺伝子ターゲット　**GT**
遺伝子治療　**GT**
遺伝子頻度　**Gf**
遺伝性圧脆弱性神経疾患　**HPSN**
遺伝性アデノーマ〔扁平腺腫〕症候群　**HFAS**
遺伝性運動知覚〔運動感覚性〕ニューロパシー　**HMSN**
遺伝性オパール様〔乳白色〕象牙質　**HOD**
遺伝性過血糖症　**HH**
遺伝性家族性高コレステロール血症モデルウサギ　**WHHL**
遺伝性果糖不耐症　**HFI**
遺伝性感覚運動（性）ニューロパシーIII型　**HSMN III**
遺伝性感覚性ニューロパシー　**HSN**
遺伝性球状赤血球症　**HS**
遺伝性血管運動神経症性浮腫　**HAE**
遺伝性血管（運動）神経性浮腫　**HANE**
遺伝性血管浮腫　**HAE**
遺伝性高血圧　**GH**
遺伝性高血圧ラット　**GHR**
遺伝性口唇状赤血球症　**Hst**
遺伝性高赤血球膜ホスファチジルコリン（＝レシチン）溶血性貧血　**HPCHA**
遺伝性高胎児ヘモグロビン症　**HPFH**
遺伝性骨爪異形成症　**HOOD**
遺伝性コプロポルフィリン症　**HC, HCP**
遺伝性コポルフィリン症　**HCP**
遺伝性失調性多発性神経炎　**HAP**
遺伝性出血〔溶血〕性毛細（血）管拡張症　**HHT**
遺伝性腎炎　**HN**
遺伝性腎炎蛋白　**HNP**
遺伝性進行性ジストニア　**HPD**

い

遺伝性腎性尿崩症　**CNDI**
遺伝性膵(臓)炎　**HP**
遺伝性爪甲・骨異形成(症候群)　**HOODS**
遺伝性代謝障害　**IMD**
遺伝性楕円赤血球症　**HE**
遺伝性多発神経炎性失調(症)　**HAP**
遺伝性多発性軟骨性外骨症　**HMCE**
遺伝性知覚性自律神経性ニューロパシー　**HSAN**
遺伝性低リン血症性くる病　**HHRH**
遺伝性乳癌遺伝子1〔2〕　**BRCA1〔2〕**
遺伝性熱変性奇形赤血球　**HPP**
遺伝性の　**hered**
遺伝性梅毒　**LH**
遺伝性白質変性症　**GLD**
遺伝性非球状赤血球性溶血性貧血　**HNSHA**
遺伝性皮膚悪性黒色腫　**HCMM**
遺伝性非ポリープ性結腸直腸癌　**HNPCC**
遺伝性び漫性白質脳症　**HDLS**
遺伝性表皮形成異常　**IED**
遺伝性部位特異的結腸癌　**HSSCC**
遺伝性慢性腎炎　**HCN**
遺伝性毛細血管脆弱症　**HCF**
遺伝性有汗性外胚葉形成異常症　**HHED**
遺伝性幽門狭窄　**HPS**
遺伝性溶血性症候群　**HHS**
遺伝性溶血性貧血　**HHA**
遺伝性良性上皮内異角化症　**HBID**
遺伝的有意線量　**GSD**
遺伝と環境　**H and E, H & E, H & E**
遺伝の　**genet**
遺伝網膜芽細胞腫の炎症に関する転写因子　**DRTF**
緯度　**lat, lat.**
家・樹木・人物描画試験　**HTP**
息　**br, br., brth**
息切れ　**SB, SOB, S of B**
息こらえ　**BH**
息こらえ発作　**BHS**
息をする　**br**
閾値エネルギー　**TE**
閾値音減衰　**TTD**
閾値音減衰検査　**TTD test**
閾値紅斑量　**TED**
閾値電位　**TP**
閾値の知覚度　**LS**
閾値量　**TD**
育児室　**Nsy**
育児相談〔保育〕　**WBC**
育児相談外来　**WBC**
幾分　**etw**
石　**C, st**
石のような　**lapid.**
急いで　**Ce**
板　**BD, Bd, bd**
痛み　**P, pn**
痛みが持続する間　**dur.dol.**
痛みがやわらぐまで　**donec dol.exulav.**
痛み伝達ニューロン　**PTN**
痛みなし　**NID**
痛みの程度の5段階評価　**FRS**
痛みを伴わない　**WOP**
一塩基の　**monobas**
一元放射補体結合(反応)　**SRCF**
一次求心性線維過分極　**PAH**
一次救命処置　**BLS, LSFA**
一次視覚皮質　**PVC**
一次心臓救命処置　**BCLS**
一次性心室細動　**PVF**
一次性組織損傷　**PTF**
一次性帝王切開(術)　**PCS, P c/s**
一次性の　**prim**
一次性ヒト胎児グリア　**PHFG**
一次性副甲状腺機能亢進症　**PHP**
一次性変性痴呆　**PDD**
一次的トルコ鞍空虚症候群　**PESS**
一次的無効　**PF**
一次の　**PP, P.P.**
一次ビームとして中性原子を用いる表面分析法　**FAB**
一次閉鎖　**PC**
一次予防のための大規模試験　**WOSCOPS**
一次リソソーム　**PL**
一時的閾値変動　**TD**
一時的経静脈ペースメーカー　**TTVP**
一時的停止　**susp**
一時的な　**temp, tempry**
一時的な位置　**loc.tens.**
一時的分光作画　**STM**
一時的ペースメーカー　**TPM**
一焦点心室異所性拍動　**UVEB**
一部　**pc**
一枚　**f**
一卵性双生児　**EZ, MZ**
一卵性の　**MZ**
一価経口ポリオウイルスワ

クチン　MOPV
一過性閾値変動　TTD, TTS
一過性異常Q波　TAQW
一過性異常骨髄造血症　TAM
一過性家族性新生児高ビリルビン血症　TFNH
一過性棘融解性皮膚症　TAD
一過性(脳)虚血(性)発作　TIA
一過性虚血発作　TIE
一過性虚血発作・不完全回復　TIA-IR
一過性呼吸促迫症候群　TRDS
一過性黒内障　AF
一過性再発性非定型的眩暈症　TRAV
一過性状況反応　TSR
一過性新生児高アンモニア血症　TNH
一過性新生児呼吸促迫　TRDN
一過性新生児糖尿病　TNDM
一過性全健忘(症)　TGA
一過性脱分極　TD
一過性チック疾患　TTD
一過性の　T, T, t, t., temp, tempry
一過性脳虚血　TCI
一過性脳虚血発作　TCIE
一過性部分的廃疾　TPD
一過性卵細胞質隆起　FC
一酸化炭素　CO
一酸化炭素拡散能　Duco
一酸化炭素血色素　COHB, COHb, COHgB
一酸化炭素肺拡散能　DCCO, DLCO
一酸化炭素排出量　Vco
一酸化炭素分圧　Pco
一酸化炭素ヘモグロビン　COHB, COHb, COHgB, HBCO, HbCO
一酸化窒素　NO
一酸化鉛　PbO
一緒に沸騰させよ　coq.sim.
一斉同時通信　CSMA/CD
一息窒素検査　SBNT
一側性肺門リンパ節腫大　UHL
一致した　unan
一対の　gem
一定　C
一定圧　CP
一定の　sta
一定率　FR
一滴ずつ　guttat.
一般医学　GM
一般医学会員　FCGP
一般医学クリニック　GMC
一般医学の　GM
一般医卒後修練連合機関　JCPTGP
一般医認定書　DGM
一般医療　gen prac, GMS
一般医療協会　AGP
一般因子　G factor
一般開業医　GP
一般学習能力　G
一般看護ケア　GNC
一般看護審議会　GNC
一般教育目標　GIO
一般外科医　GS
一般外科医診察所　OTSG
一般外科医認定書　DGS
一般外科学　GS
一般研究　GR
一般健康質問票　GHQ
一般検尿　U/G
一般歯科医学校　AGD
一般手技　gen.proc
一般手術室　GOR
一般集中治療室　GICU
一般診療(所)　GP
一般正看護師　RGN
一般性腺刺激活性　GGA
一般体性遠心神経　GSE
一般体性求心神経　GSA
一般体性求心性　GSA
一般的義務のある医療事務官　GDMO
一般内科外科学　GM & S
一般内科外科の　GM & S
一般内臓遠心神経　GVE
一般内臓遠心性　GVE
一般内臓求心神経　GVA
一般内臓求心性　GVA
一般の　allgem, GEN, gen, gen'l, gnrl
一般病院　GH
一般ボランティア　NV
一般薬　OTC
一般薬品事務室　OGD
一般予防医学　GPM
一般臨床研究センター　GCRC
一般臨床サービス　GCS
一服せよ　f.p.
(水剤の)一服量　H, Ht.
(頓服水剤の)一服量　haust.
一本鎖　ss
一本鎖DNA結合蛋白質　SSB
一本鎖RNA　ssRNA
一本鎖〔単鎖〕デオキシリボ核酸　ssDNA, SSDNA
溢血　extrav
偽りの　F
犬　D

い

今のところ **zZ, z.Z.**
妹 **sis**
色 **C, col**
色のついた **C, col**
引退した **ret**
引退する **ret**
引用語句 **qn**
引用された報告中に **op.cit.**
引用した場所に **in loc.cit., loc.cit.**
引用する **cit**
印環細胞癌 **sig**
印刷された **print**
印刷中の **print**
印刷物 **Schr.**
印象 **Imp, imp, impr**
因子 **F, Fac**
咽頭 **phar**
咽頭・喉頭・結膜炎ウイルス **Adeno-virus, APC-virus**
咽頭炎 **phar, PHY**
咽頭気管腔 **PTL**
咽頭筋 **PhM**
咽頭結膜熱 **PCF**
咽頭後(壁) **PP**
咽頭喉頭蓋ひだ **PEF**
咽頭喉頭部 **HP**
咽頭喉頭部全摘出 **TLP**
咽頭後壁リンパ節 **RPL**
咽頭食道憩室 **PED**
咽頭食道の **PE**
咽頭の **phar, pharyn**
咽頭培養 **TC**
咽頭培養と鼻咽頭培養 **TC+NP**
咽頭扁桃 **PT**
咽頭扁桃〔アデノイド〕切除・口蓋扁桃切除 **Ade-Loto**
咽頭扁桃〔アデノイド〕切除・口蓋扁桃摘出術 **Ade-Lec**
咽頭扁桃肥大 **ade**
(病)院内 **IH**
院内感染 **HOI**
院内感染に関する全国調査 **NNIS**
院内感染肺炎 **NP**
院内外科医 **HS**
院内疾患 **SH**
院内侵入接触 **HAPC**
院内(感染性)肺炎 **HAP**
陰圧換気 **NPV**
陰圧式勃起補助用具 **VCD**
陰イオン・フェリチン **AF**
陰萎 **IMP, Impo**
陰影 **S, S.**
陰影欠損 **FD, SD**
陰核 **clit**
陰核切除 **clit**
陰核の **clit**
陰極 **CA, Ca, Cath, Cath., K, K., Ka, KA, Ka, ka**
陰極開放強直 **COTE, COTe**
陰極開放拘縮 **KOC**
陰極開放収縮 **CaOC, COC, KOZ**
陰極開放性クローヌス **COC, COCL, COCl**
陰極開放濃度 **KOC**
陰極継続痙攣 **CADTe**
陰極持続 **KD**
陰極持続強縮 **KDT**
陰極持続強直 **KDTe**
陰極線 **CR**
陰極線オシロ(グラフ) **CRO**
陰極線オシロスコープ **CRO**
陰極線管 **CRT**
陰極の **C, CA, Ca, KA, Ka, ka**
陰極閉鎖 **KC**
陰極閉鎖間代収縮 **CCCl**
陰極閉鎖強直 **CaCTe, KCT, KCTe, KST**
陰極閉鎖(時)収縮 **CACC, CaCC**
陰極閉鎖収縮 **CCC, KCC**
陰極閉鎖攣縮 **KSZ**
陰欠乏・陽過剰症候群 **YDES**
陰茎 **pen**
陰茎海綿体(血)圧 **ICP**
陰茎海綿体筋 **BC muscle**
陰茎血圧指数 **PBPI**
陰茎動脈(末梢)血圧比 **PPI**
陰茎勃起 **PE**
陰性 **Neg**
陰性吸気力 **NIF**
陰性後電位 **NAP**
陰性呼気圧 **NEP**
陰性垂直性開散 **−VD**
陰性造影剤心エコー検査(法) **NCE**
陰性の **N**
陰性反応適中度 **PVN**
陰電子 $\mathbf{e^-}$
陰部肛門直腸症候群 **GAR**
陰部単純ヘルペス **HSG**
陰部ヘルペス〔疱疹〕 **HG**
陰門腟カンジダ症 **VVC**
陰陽二面価比 **PNAvQ**
飲小胞 **PV**
飲酒家 **alcoh**
飲料 **bev**

う

ヴァイル・フェリックス（反応/検査） **WF, W-F**
ヴァイル・フェリックス反応 **Weil-Felix**
ウアバイン感受性の **OS**
ヴァンライパー聴覚記録期間 **VRMS**
ウイスキー **s.fr.**
ウイスキー換算で **WE**
ヴィスコット・オールドリッチ（症候群） **WA**
ウィスコット・オールドリッチ症候群 **WAS**
ウィスコンシン圧縮システム **WCS**
ウィスコンシンカード分類検査 **WCST**
ウィスター・ファース **WF**
ウィスター（ラット） **W, WI**
ウィスター・京都ラット **WKY**
ウィスターインスティテュート 38 **WI-38**
ウィスターラット（の）ライディヒ細胞腫瘍 **LTW**
ウィダール反応 **Widal**
ウィッテンボーン（精神症状評価尺度） **WITT**
ウィッテンボーン精神症状評価項目表 **WPSI**
ウィッテンボーン精神症状評点尺度 **WPRS**
ウィップル病 **WD**
ヴィーデマン・ベックウィズ症候群 **WBS**
ウィーデマン・ラウテン・ストラウク症候群 **WRS**
ウィリアムス・イーグル（寒天） **WE**
ウィリアムズ屈曲運動 **WFE, Wm flex.ex., Wms flex.ex.**
ウィリアムズ症候群 **WS**
ウィリアムズ培地 E **WME**
ウイルス **V, v**
ウイルス外膜抗原 **VEA**
ウイルス学 **VIR, virol**
ウイルス癌遺伝子 **v-onc**
ウイルス緩衝 **VB**
ウイルス感染に伴う抗原 **VIA**
ウイルス関連血球貪食症候群 **VAHS**
ウイルス関連抗原 **VAA**
ウイルス抗原 **V antigen**
ウイルス構造蛋白 **VPI**
ウイルス呼吸器感染（症） **VRI**
ウイルス細胞表面抗原 **VCSA**
ウイルススーパー抗原 **VSAG**
ウイルス性肝炎 **VH**
ウイルス性血液低下疾患 **VHD**
ウイルス性下痢 **VD**
ウイルス性抗原 **VA**
ウイルス性呼吸器疾患 **VRD**
ウイルス性出血熱 **VHF**
ウイルス性心筋炎 **VM**
ウイルス性ブタ肺炎 **VPP**
ウイルス（性）蛋白 **VP**
ウイルス中和 **VN**
ウイルス中和（性）の **VN**
ウイルス（性）糖蛋白 **VGP**
ウイルス特異的移植抗原 **VSTA**
ウイルス特異的表面抗原 **VSSA**
ウイルスによる壊死巣 **VINR**
ウイルス（由来）の **v-**
ウイルス（性）脳炎 **VE**
ウイルス不活性化剤 **VIA**
ウイルス命名システム **VAC system**
ウイルス命名のための暫定委員会 **PCNV**
ウイルス誘導インターフェロン **VIF**
ウイルス様因子 **VLA**
ウイルス様感染因子 **VLIA**
ウイルス様粒子 **VLP**
ウイルスリボ核酸 **VRNA**
ウイルス粒子抗原 **VCA**
ウィルソン・キンメルシュティール（症候群） **WK**
ウィルソン・キンメルシュティール病 **WKD, WK dis.**
ウィルソン・ミキティ（症候群） **WM**
ウィルソン・パターソン態度調査票 **WPAI**
ウィルソン中枢回路 **CTW**
ウィルソン病 **WD**
ウィルムス（腫）・無虹彩・尿路（奇形）・（精神）発達遅滞 **WAGR**
ウィルムス腫瘍 **WT**
ウィロウブルック（ウイルス） **WB**
ウィントローブ赤血球沈降率 **WESR**
ウェアリング親密性質問票 **WIQ**

ウェアリングブレンダー〔フードプロセッサ〕使用経管栄養　**WBTF**
ウェクスラー・ベルビュー（尺度）　**WB**
ウェクスラー・ベルビュースケール　**WBS**
ウェクスラー児童用知能検査　**WISC**
ウェクスラー就学前・小学生用知能尺度　**WPPSI**
ウェクスラー小児用知能スケール改訂版　**WISC-R**
ウェクスラー成人知能検査　**WAIS**
ウェクスラー成人知能スケール〔検査〕改訂版　**WAIS-R**
ウェクスラー知能評価尺度　**WIS**
ウェゲナー肉芽腫症　**WG**
ウェスターグレン赤血球沈降率　**WESR**
ウェスターグレン沈降率　**WSR**
ウェスタン・コラボライティブ・グループ・スタディ　**WCGS**
ウェスタン失語（症）統合検査　**WAB, WABT**
ウェスタンブロット　**WB**
ウェスト・ヒップ周囲比　**WHR**
ウェスト〔ウエスト〕症候群　**WS**
ヴェストファル・シュトリュンペル（症候群）　**WS**
ウエストヘイヴン・イェール多次元痛み項目表　**WHYMPI**
ウェクスラー記憶尺度　**WMS**
ウェッジ調整クッションヒール（靴）　**WACH**
ヴェッセルスブロン（ウイルス）　**WSL**
ウェットマウント　**WM**
ウェーネルト　**W**
ウェーバー・クリスチャン（症候群）　**WC**
ウェーバー・クリスチャン病　**WCD**
ウェーバー　**W, WB, Wb**
ウェーバー・オスラー・ロンデュ（症候群）　**WOR**
ウェーバー検査　**W**
ウェーバー高等空間知覚（テスト）　**WASP**
ウェルドニッヒ・ホフマン（症候群）　**WH**
ウェルドニッヒ・ホフマン症候群　**WHS**
ウェルドニッヒ・ホフマン病　**WHD**
ヴェルナー症候群　**WS**
ウェルニッケ・コルサコフ（症候群）　**WK**
ウェルニッケ・コルサコフ症候群　**WKS**
ウェルニッケ・マン（片麻痺）　**WM**
ウェンケバッハ周期長　**WCL**
ウォーカー癌肉腫細胞　**WCC**
ウォーシン・スターリー（染色法）　**WS**
ウォス・スタデイ　**WOS**
ウォーターハウス・フリーデリクセン（症候群）　**WF**
ウォッシュアウト　**WO**
ウォーラー変性　**WD**
ヴォルーター試験　**V-test**
ウォルフ・パーキンソン・ホワイト（症候群）　**WPW**
ウォルフ管　**Wd**
ウォルフラン　**W**
ウォルマン病　**WD**
ウサギγグロブリン　**RGG**
ウサギ気管　**RT**
ウサギ胸腺抽出物　**RTE**
ウサギ血清アルブミン　**RbSA**
ウサギ抗マウス免疫グロブリン　**RAMIg**
ウサギ抗リンパ球グロブリン　**RALG**
ウサギ腎臓　**RK**
ウサギ赤血球　**RaE, RRBC**
ウサギ大動脈収縮物質　**RCS**
ウシアルブミン　**BA**
ウシインスリン　**BI**
ウシ海綿状脳症　**BSE**
ウシ下垂体抽出液　**BPE**
ウシ型マイコバクテリア　**MB**
ウシガンマグロブリン　**BGG**
ウシキモトリプシン　**BCTR**
ウシ血色素　**BHb**
ウシ血漿アルブミン　**BPA**
ウシ血清アルブミン　**BSA**
ウシ血清腎炎　**BSA nephritis**
ウシ甲状腺刺激ホルモン　**BTSH, B-TSH**
ウシ視床下部由来成長因子　**HDGF**
ウシ心臓滲出肉汁　**BHIB**
ウシ膵臓トリプシン抑制因子　**BPTI**
ウシ膵（臓）ポリペプチド　**BPP**

ウシ成長ホルモン　**BGH**
ウシ赤血球　**BRBC, ORBC, ORC**
ウシ赤血球抗体　**OXEA**
ウシ胎仔血清　**FBS, FCS**
ウシ胎仔腎　**EBK**
ウシ大動脈内皮　**BAE**
ウシ大動脈内皮細胞　**BAE**
ウシ膣炎ウイルス　**BVV**
ウシトリプシノーゲン　**BTg**
ウシトリプシン　**BTr**
ウシ乳頭腫ウイルス　**BPV**
ウシの　**bov**
ウシの感染性角結膜炎　**IBK**
ウシ肺疫　**CBPP**
ウシ白血病ウイルス　**BLV**
ウシパピローマウイルス　**BPV**
ウシ・ブタインスリン　**BPI**
ウシヘルペスウイルス　**BHV**
ウシ流産菌輪テスト　**ABR test**
ウッドコック・ジョンソン(心理学的学習統合検査)　**W-J**
ウッドコック・ジョンソン心理的学習統合検査　**WJPB**
ウッドコック読み熟達総合テスト　**WRMT**
ウッドチャック肝炎ウイルス　**WHV**
ウッドワード試薬K　**WRK**
ウプサラウイルス　**U_v**
ウマ　**H**
ウマ肝アルコール脱水素酵素　**HLALD**
ウマ血清　**HoS, HS**
ウマ血清アルブミン　**HSA**
ウマ抗破傷風トキソイドグロブリン　**HoaTTG**
ウマ抗ヒト芽球グロブリン　**EAHLG**
ウマ抗ヒト胸腺グロブリン　**HAHTG**
ウマ抗ヒト胸腺細胞グロブリン　**HATG**
ウマ抗リンパ球グロブリン　**EALG**
ウマ成長ホルモン　**EGH**
ウマ赤血球　**HRBC, HRC**
ウマ伝染性貧血　**EIA**
ウマ脳炎　**EE**
ウマバエ　**G**
ウマ鼻肺炎　**ERP**
ウマ鼻肺炎ウイルス　**ERV**
ウマヘルペスウイルス　**EHV**
ウマ免疫グロブリン　**Holg**
ウマ流産ウイルス　**EAV**
ウラシル　**U, Ura, URA**
ウラシル・アデニン・アデニン(＝終止コドン)　**UAA**
ウラシル・アデニン・グアニン(＝終止コドン)　**UAG**
ウラシル・グアニン・アデニン(＝終止コドン)　**UGA**
ウラシルマスタード　**UM**
ウラニウム　**U**
ウラニウム〔ウラン〕X_1　**UX_1**
ウラン　**U**
ウランX(＝プロアクチニウム)　**UX**
ウリジル酸　**U, UA**
ウリジル二リン酸グルコースピロリン酸分解酵素　**UGPP**
ウリジン　**U, UR, Urd, URD**
ウリジン5′-一リン酸　**Urd-5′-P**
ウリジン5′-二リン酸　**5′-UDP, UDP, Urd-5′-P2**
ウリジン5′-三リン酸　**Urd-5′-P3**
ウリジン5′-三リン酸　**5′-UTP**
ウリジン一リン酸　**UMP**
ウリジン一リン酸キナーゼ　**UMPK**
ウリジン三リン酸　**UTP**
ウリジン二リン酸　**UD, UDP**
ウリジン二リン酸ガラクトース　**UDPGal, UDP-Gal, UDPgal**
ウリジン二リン酸グルクロン酸　**UDPG, UDPGA**
ウリジン二リン酸グルクロン酸転移酵素　**UDPGT, UGT**
ウリジン二リン酸グルコース　**UDPG, UDP-Glc, UDP-glc**
ウリジンホスホリラーゼ　**UP**
ウルシ属　**R**
ウルソデオキシコール酸　**UDCA**
ウルトラレンテ(インスリン)　**U**
ウルバッハ・ヴィーテ病　**UWD**
ウルリッヒ・ターナー(症

候群） UT
ウルリッヒ・ターナー症候群 UTS
ウロガストロン UG

ウロカニン酸 UA
ウロキナーゼ UK
ウロキナーゼ型プラスミノゲンアクチベータ UPA, u-PA
ウロキナーゼ型プラスミノゲンアクチベータ受容体 UPA-R
ウロキナーゼ冠注 UK IC
ウロビリノゲン UBG, Ubg, U-gen
ウロビリン Ubn
ウロポルフィリノゲン UPG, UROgen
ウロポルフィリノゲンイソメラーゼ UI
ウロポルフィリノゲン合成酵素 UPS
ウロポルフィリノゲンデカルボキシラーゼ UD
ウロポルフィリン UP, URO
ウロポルフィリンイソメラーゼ UI
ウロモルリン UM
ウンナ・トースト（症候群） UT
ウンナ・パッペンハイム（染色） UP
ウシ結核菌懸濁液 PBE
うがい剤 GARG, garg.
うがいさせる ft.garg.
う歯 C
う蝕（になる） DK
う蝕歯・喪失歯・充填歯係数 dmf index, DMF Index
う蝕歯・要抜去歯・充填歯指数 def index
うっ血型心筋症 CCM
うっ血した cong.
うっ血性右（心）不全 CRVF
うっ血性心筋症 COCM
うっ血性心疾患 CHD
うっ血性心不全 CCF, CHF
うつ状態の depr
うつ状態評価尺度 DSI
（抑）うつ性自己評価尺度 SDS
うつ病 D
うつ病項目表 DI
うつむき試験 PPT
うねり指数 WI
うぶ毛性多毛症 HL
うちくるぶし IM
うつ病 depr
右眼 Od, R, RE
右眼圧 TOD
右眼角膜異物 FBCOD
右眼視覚 VOD, VR
右眼視力 RV, VD, V.d.
右眼に ocul.dext.
右眼網膜剝離 RDOD
右額後位 FDP, FDT
右額前位 RBA
右額前位（胎児） FDA
（心臓の）右脚 rBB
右脚 RL
右脚ブロック RBBB, RBBsB
右口 RO
右心カテーテル法 RHC
右心血液量 RHBV
右心耳 RA
右心室 RV
右心室肥大 HVD
右心バイパス RHB
右心発育不全〔低形成〕症候群 HRHS
右心不全 RHF
右心房 RA
右心房圧 RAP
右心房圧上昇 RAPE
右心房拡大 RAE
右心房径 RAD
右心房肥大 RAH
右心房平均圧 RAMP
右心房容積 RAV
右耳鼓膜 MTAD
右（心）室１回仕事係数 RVSWI
右（心）室１回拍出仕事指数 RVSWI
右（心）室圧 RVP
右（心）室拡大 RVE
右（心）室拡張期圧 RVDP
右（心）室拡張期過負荷 RVDO
右（心）室拡張期容積 RVDV
右（心）室拡張終（末）期圧 RVEDP
右（心）室拡張終（末）期径 RVEDD
右（心）室拡張終期容量 RVEDV
右（心）室駆出時間 RVET
右（心）室駆出率 RVEF
右（心）室径 RVD
右（心）室梗塞 RVI
右（心）室興奮 RVA
右（心）室終（末）期血流 RVEF
右（心）室収縮期圧 RVSP
右（心）室収縮終（末）期容積 RVESV
右（心）室収縮終（末）期容積係数 RVESVI
右（心）室終末拡張期容量係数 RVEDVI
右（心）室充満圧 RVFP
右（心）室心内膜電位 RVECP

右(心)室尖(の) **RVA**
右(心)室前壁 **RVAW**
右(心)室造影 **RVG**
右(心)室内径 **RVID**
右室二腔心 **DCRV**
右(心)室拍出仕事量 **RVSW**
右(心)室肥大 **RVH**
右(心)室不全 **RVF**
右(心)室容積 **RVV**
右(心)室流出(量) **RVO**
右(心)室流出路 **RVOT, RVOTD**
右(心)室流入路 **RVIT**
右軸偏位 **RAD**
右腎 **RK**
右腎結核 **NPD**
右旋性 **D**
右旋性(の) **D, d, dex**
右旋性・左旋性 **DL**
右旋(性)の **dext.**
右側 **RS**
右側結腸(癌) **RSC**
右側に向かって **dext.**
右(心)房(に) **AD**
右房収縮 **RAC**
右房前壁 **RAAW**
右(心)補助循環装置 **RVAD**
右腕の血圧 **BPRA**
生まれた **B, geb**
生まれつきの **Nat**
(航空)宇宙医学 **AM**
宇宙医学 **SM**
乳母車 **pram**
烏口肩峰靱帯 **CAL**
烏口鎖骨靱帯 **CCL**
烏口上腕の **CB**
上および下 **U & L, U/L**
上外 1/4 区(＝四半部) **UOQ**
上と下の場合 **U & LC**
上に引用した **supra cit.**
上の **sup, SUP, sup., U**
上半分 **UH**
上左(象限) **UPL**
上右(象限) **u/r**
上を見よ **so, v.s.**
植込み型自動心臓除細動器 **IACD**
植込み型除細動器 **ICD**
植込み型心臓除細動器・除細動器カテーテル **ICDC**
植込み型心臓除細動器・心房頻脈ペーシング **ICD-ATP**
植込み型補聴器 **IHA**
魚蛋白濃度 **FPC**
受け取った **recd**
受け身の **pass.**
受身血球凝集抑制物質 **PHI**
受身赤血球凝集試験 **PHAT**
受身赤血球凝集反応 **PHA**
受身皮膚アナフィラキシー **PCA**
受身ヘイマン腎炎 **PHN**
受身ラテックス凝集反応 **PLA**
動き **mtn**
後(ろ)の **P**
後ろの **PO, post**
臼でついて細かくした **cont, cont., contus.**
渦(巻き) **WP, W/P**
薄い粥 **PULM, pulm.**
(〜の)疑い **S/O**
疑わしい **d**
疑わしい名前 **nom.dub.**
(肘関節の)内側側副靱帯 **UCL**
内くるぶし **MM, mm**
内と外(の) **I & E**
内ひき **add, ADD**
訴えなし **NC**
訴えのない **no compl**
訴えられた **compl**
腕と肩 **A & sh, A & SH**
埋込み型除細動器 **AICD, AID**
裏 **vo**
裏面〔次頁〕へ続く **PTO**
裏をみよ **t.o.**
上澄みの **SM**
運動 **E, Ex, ex, exer, mtn, MVMT, mvt**
運動エネルギー **K, KE**
運動過剰(症)の衝動障害 **HID**
運動過多性心臓症候群 **HHS**
運動感受性 **MS**
運動機能テスト **MFT**
運動共鳴ラーマン分光法 **KRRS**
運動産生刺激 **MPS**
運動死 **DIA**
運動時換気量増加 **EH**
運動識別精度 **MDA**
運動時呼吸困難 **DE, DOE**
運動指数 **EI, MI**
運動時痛 **POM**
運動疾患 **MD**
運動失語 **MA**
運動失調毛細血管拡張病 **AT**
運動指標得点 **MIS**
運動終板 **MEP**
運動神経成長因子 **MNGF**
運動神経伝導速度 **MCV, MNCV**
運動神経変性を伴うパーキンソン症候群 **PMND**
運動制限 **EL, LOM**

運動潜時　**ML**
運動喪失　**LOM**
運動単位　**MU**
運動単位活動電位
　MUAP
運動単位電位　**MUP**
運動電位　**MP**
運動ニューロン疾患
　MND
運動粘性率　ν
運動年齢テスト　**MAT**
(自発)運動能力のある
　M
運動能力のない　**NM**
運動の最大域　**FROM**
運動の熱効果　**TEE**
運動皮質　**MCx**
運動分析システム　**MAS**
運動誘発アナフィラキシー
　EIAn
運動誘発喘息　**EIA**
運動療法　**KT**
運搬する　**trans**
運搬波送出両側波帯
　BSB

え

(喉頭)エアウェイ　**OAW**
エアートラッピング　**AT**
エアートラッピング指数　**ATI**
エアロゾル再呼吸法　**ARM**
エアロゾル粒子の平均粒子径　**MMAD**
エイコサペンタエン酸　**EPA**
エイズ　**AIDS**
エイズ医学基金　**AMF**
エイズ患者集団　**PWA**
エイズ関連疾患　**ARD, ARDS**
エイズ関連症候群　**ARC**
エイズ関連状態　**ARC**
エイズ関連レトロウイルス　**ARV**
エイベルソン(白血病)ウイルス　**AbLV**
エウスタキオ管圧　**ETP**
エウスタキオ管の　**eust.**
エオジン好性指数　**EI**
エオジンメチレンブルー培地　**EMB agar**
エキシマレーザー　**Eximer Laser**
エキス　**Ex., Ext., ext, ext., Extr.**
エキソヌクレアーゼ　**EXO**
エクオリン　**AQ**
エクサ(=10^{18})　**E**
エグザフス　**EXAFS**
エクスターン　**ext, ext.**
エグゼルフス　**EXELFS**
エクセルプタ・メディカ財団　**EMF**
エコーウイルス　**ECHO**
エコーウイルス・ライノウイルス・感冒ウイルス　**ERC**
エコー時間　**TE**
エコナゾール　**ECZ**
エコー脳写　**echo, EEG**
エコープラナー像　**EPI**
エシェリキア(属)　**E, E., *Esch.***
エステトロール　**E_4**
エステラーゼ　**ES**
エステラーゼA4　**ESA-4**
エステラーゼD　**ESD, EsD**
エステラーゼ単位　**EU**
エステラーゼ賦活剤　**ES-Act**
エステル　**E**
エステル型/総コレステロール(比)　**EC/TC**
エステル型コレステロール　**EC, Echo**
エステル分解酵素　**ES**
エステル分解酵素阻止因子　**EI**
エストラジオール　**E_2, E-diol**
エストラジオール(=E_2)　**ED, Ed**
エストラジオール結合指数　**EBI**
エストラジオール結合蛋白　**EBP**
エストラジオール産生率　**EPR**
エストラジオールシクロペンチルプロピオネート　**ECP**
エストラジオール受容体　**ER**
エストラムスチン　**EM**
エストラムスチン結合蛋白　**EMBP**
エストリオール　**E_3, Es**
エストリオール(=E_3)　**ET, Et**
エストリオール/クレアチニン(比)　**E/C**
エストリカー・ターナー(症候群)　**OT**
エストロゲン　**E**
エストロゲン・クレアチニン比　**E/C**
エストロゲン刺激性ニューロフィジン　**ESN**
エストロゲン受容体　**ER, ESTR**
エストロゲン受容体試験　**ERA**
エストロゲン受容体蛋白　**ERP**
エストロゲン受容体免疫細胞化学分析　**ER-ICA**
エストロゲン消退出血　**EWB**
エストロゲンフィードバック検査　**F-test**
エストロゲン・プロゲステロン　**EP**
エストロゲン補充療法　**ERT**
エストロン　**E_1, Eo, EO**
エスベム　**ESVEM**
エスペラマイシン　**EPM**
エタクリン酸　**EA**
エタノール　**E**
エタノールゲル化試験　**EGT**
エタノール代謝率　**EMR**
エタンヒドロキシ二リン酸(=エチドロン酸ナトリウム)　**EHDP**
エタンブトール　**EB, EMB**
エチオナミド　**ETH, TH**
エチオフォス　**WR-2721**
エチニルエストラジオール　**EE**

エチニルエストラジオールメチルエーテル **EEME**
エチニルエストレノール **ETEL**
エチニルノルテストステロン(＝ノルエチンドロン) **ETNT**
エチル **E**
エチルアミノケトン **EAI**
エチルアルコール **ETOH, EtOH**
エチルエタン硫酸 **EES**
エチル基 **Et**
エチルコハク酸エリスロマイシン **EES**
エチルトリメチロールトリメタン三硝酸 **ETTN**
エチルニトロニトロソグアニジン **ENNG**
エチルノルエピネフリン **ENE, E.N.E.**
エチルノルスプラレニン **ENS**
エチルビニルエーテル **EVE**
エチルメタンスルホン酸 **EMP, EMS**
エチレンオキサイドガス **EOG**
エチレンオキシド **ETOX**
エチレングリコールジメタクリル酸 **EDMA**
エチレングリコールビス(2-アミノエチルエーテル)四酢酸 **EGTA**
エチレンクロルヒドリン **ECH**
エチレンジアミン **ED, EDA, EN**
エチレンジアミン四グルタミン酸 **EDTG**
エチレンジアミン四酢酸 **EDTA, ETA**
エチレンジアミン四酢酸依存性偽血小板減少症 **EP**
エチレンジアミン四酢酸カルシウム二ナトリウム **CA EDTA**
エチレンジアミン四酢酸セタブロン **EDTAC**
エチレンジアミン四酢酸ナトリウム **ETAA**
エチレンビス亜鉛 **ZINEB**
エチレンビニルアルコール **EVA**
エックス線動態撮影法 **RKY**
エックス単位 **X**
エッセンス **Ess, ess.**
エーディエーエム **ADAM**
エディ熱板試験 **EHPT**
エディンガー・ヴェストファル(核) **E-W**
エデト酸カルシウム二ナトリウム **CaEDTA, CaEdTA**
エーテル **E, eth**
エーテルクロロホルム(混合液) **E-C**
エーテルクロロホルム混合物 **EC mix**
エーテルとクロロホルム **EC**
エトキシカルボニルエトキシジヒドロキノリン **EEDQ**
エトキシ蟻酸無水物 **EFA**
エトキシスクレロール **AS**
エトスクシミド **ESM**
エトポシド **EPEG, VP-16**
エトポシド,アドリアマイシン,シスプラチン(＝プラチノール) **EAP**
エトポシド,アドリアマイシン,ビンクリスチン **VAV**
エトポシド,アドリアマイシン,メトトレキサート **VAM**
エトポシド,イホスファミド,シスプラチン(＝プラチノール) **VIP**
エトポシド,カルボプラチン **VC**
エトポシド,シクロホスファミド,ヒドロキシダウノマイシン,ビンクリスチン(＝オンコビン) **ECHO**
エトポシド,ビンブラスチン,アドリアマイシン **EVA**
エトポシド,フルオロウラシル,シスプラチン(＝プラチノール) **EFP**
エトポシド,メトトレキサート,アクチノマイシンD,シトロボラム因子 **EMA-CO**
エトポシド,メトトレキサート-ロイコボリン,アクチノマイシンD,シクロホスファミド,ビンクリスチン(＝オンコビン) **EMA-CO**
エドモンストン・ザグレブ(ワクチン) **EZ**
エーナ解剖学名 **JNA**
エナメル質 **E**
エニアック **ENIAC**
エニシダのアルカロイド **Sp**
エネルギー **E**
エネルギー消費 **EE**
エネルギー消費率〔損失率〕 **REL**

エネルギー性力学的心不全 **EDHI**
エネルギー損失広域微細構造 **EXELFS**
エネルギー代謝率 **RMR**
エネルギー動的心不全 **EDCI**
エネルギー分散X線分光法 **EDX**
エネルギー分散型X線分光法 **EDS**
エネルギー率 **EQ**
エノキサシン **ENX**
エノシタビン,アクラルビシン,ビンクリスチン(=オンコビン),6-メルカプトプリン,プレドニゾロン **BAOMP**
エノラーゼ **Eno, ENOL**
エバンスブルー **EB**
エバンスブルー・クリアランス試験 **CT-1824**
エピアロプレグナノロン **EAP**
エピアンドロステロン **EA**
エピスター法 **EPISTAR**
エピソード **epis**
エーピーティー(=胃排出検査の1つ) **APT**
エピネフリン **E, EP, epi, Epi, EPI, Epin, epineph**
エピネフリン負荷試験 **ETT**
エピルビシン,ブレオマイシン,ビンブラスチン **EBV**
エフェクターT細胞/標的細胞比 **E/T**
エフェクター細胞 **EC**
エフェクター細胞対標的細胞 **E/T**
エフェドリン **EPD, ephed**
エプシロン **e**
エプスタイン・マッキントッシュ・オクスフォード(吸入器) **EMO**
エプスタイン・マッキントッシュ・オクスフォード吸入器 **EMO inhaler**
エプスタインバーウイルス **EBV**
エポキシド **EP**
エボラ出血熱 **EHF**
エミアト **EMIAT**
エムデン・マイヤーホフ(経路) **E-M**
エムデン・マイヤーホフ・パルナス経路 **EMP pathway**
エムデン・マイヤーホフ経路 **EMP, EM pathway**
エメリー・ドレフュス(型)筋ジストロフィ **EDMD**
エモリー血管形成術・外科的比較試験 **EAST**
エヤン・ヴィダル(症候群) **HW**
エーラース・ダンロス症候群 **ED, EDS**
エラスターゼ **El**
エラスターゼトキソイド **ET**
エラスターゼ様蛋白 **ELP**
エラスターゼ抑制能 **EIC**
エラスチカ・ワンギーソン(染色) **EVG**
エラスチカヘマトキシリンエオジン **EHE**
エラストマー潤滑剤 **ELA**
エリキシル **Elx**
エリキシル(剤) **EL, El, el, elix**
エリジペロスリックス **ERY, Ery**
エリジペロトリックス(属) **E**
エリス・ファン・クレフェルト症候群 **EC**
エリスロポエチン **EP, EPo, EPO**
エリスロポ(イ)エチン感受性細胞 **ESC**
エリスロポエチン感受性細胞 **ERC**
エリスロポエチン産生酵素 **EPE**
エリスロポエチン受容体 **EPOR**
エリスロマイシン **E, EM**
エリスロマイシンエストレート **EM-E**
エリスロマイシン局所用溶液 **ETS**
エリスロマイシンプロピオネート **EMP**
エリテマトーデス(細胞) **LE**
エリテマトーデス/扁平苔癬 **LE/LP**
エリテマトーデス因子 **LEF, LE factor**
エリテマトーデス細胞 **LE cell**
エリテマトーデス試験 **LE test**
エリテマトーデス標本 **LE prep**
エール・スケールスコア **YSS**
エール・ブラウン強迫行為〔強迫性障害〕薬効評価尺度 **Y-BOCS**
エルカトニン **ECT**
エルキャット **LCAT**

え

エルキャット〔LCAT〕欠損症 **LCAT deficiency**
エルグ **e, erg**
エルゴカルシフェロール＝ビタミンD_2 **D_2**
エルゴステロールの選択的生合成阻害薬 **EBI**
エルシニア(属) **Y**
エルシニア・エンテロコリチカ感染 **YEI**
エルシニア(属)関節炎 **YA**
エルシニアスーパー抗原性外毒素 **YPM**
エルステッド **Oe**
エルビウム **Er**
エルブ・シャルコー(症候群) **EC**
エール目盛り得点 **YSS**
エールリッヒ癌 **EC**
エールリッヒ細胞破壊ウイルス **ED virus**
エールリッヒ単位 **EU**
エールリッヒ腹水癌 **EAC**
エールリッヒ腹水腫瘍 **EAT**
エールリッヒ腹水腫瘍細胞 **EATC**
エレクトロスプレーイオン化 **ESI**
エレベーター **elev**
エンカウンターグループ **EG**
エンケファリン **ENK**
エンザイム **enz**
エンジュマメレクチン **SJA**
エンテロウイルス **EV**
エンテロキナーゼ **EK**
エンテロバクター(属) **E**
エンテロモナス(属) **E**
エンドキサン **ENX, Ex, ex**
エンドセリン **ET**
エンドセリン変換酵素 **ECE**
エンドトキシン **ET, Et, Ex**
エンドトキシン様活性 **ELA**
エンドペルオキシド **EP**
エンドミセス(属) **E**
エンドリマックス(属) **E**
エンドルフィン **Ep**
エントロピー **S**
エンビオマイシン **EVM**
エンフルレン **E**
エンラマイシン **EDC**
えら **Gl, gl**
会陰 **peri**
会陰針生検 **PNB**
会陰切開術 **epis**
会陰の **per, peri**
会陰パッド **perpad, per.pad**
映像周波数 **Vf**
絵 **pics**
壊死 **necr**
壊死後肝硬変 **PNC**
壊死性潰瘍性歯肉炎 **NUG**
壊死性血管炎 **NA**
壊死性腸炎 **NE, NEC**
壊死性遊走性紅斑 **NME**
壊死により電解質とステロイドが産生される心臓病 **ESCN**
壊死片 **seq.**
壊疽 **gangr**
壊疽性肉芽腫 **GG**
壊疽性膿皮症 **PG**
壊疽性鼻炎 **Rh.gang.**
永久閾値移動 **PTS**
永久段階 **PG**
永久聴覚閾値 **PTHL**
永久の **perm**
永久ペースメーカー **PPM**
永続的全体障害 **PTD**
英国 **Brit**
英国・アイルランド外科医協会 **ASGBI**
英国医学協会 **BMA**
英国医学研究委員会 **MRC-UK**
英国医学研究協議会 **BMRC**
英国医学雑誌 **BMB, BMJ**
英国医学生連盟 **BMSA**
英国医師・外科医会員 **FCPS**
英国医師会員有資格者 **LRCP**
英国移植協会 **UKT**
英国一般医学会員 **FRCGP**
英国王立看護院 **RCN**
英国王立外科学会 **RCS**
英国王立助産師院 **RCM**
英国王立内科学院 **RCP**
英国解剖学会 **B.A.S.**
英国眼科学会 **BOA, OSUK**
英国眼科協会員 **FBOA**
英国癌征圧運動 **BCC**
英国協同臨床グループ **BCCG**
英国軍医団 **RAMC**
英国形成外科医協会 **BAPS**
英国外科医協会 **BSTA**
英国外科医師会員有資格者 **LRCS**
英国外科学会会員 **FRCS**
英国外科学雑誌 **Br.J.Surg.**
英国外科獣医師会員 **MRCVS**
英国公衆保健衛生院会員 **FRIPHH**
英国国営医療 **BNHS**

英国国際健康教育学会 **BSIHE**
英国骨疾患学会 **BOA**
英国催眠治療学会 **BSH**
英国産業衛生学会 **BOHS**
英国産婦人科医師会員 **FRCOG**
英国産婦人科学会認定書 **DRCOG**
英国産婦人科学資格〔免状〕 **DORCG**
英国歯科医会会員 **FDSRCS**
英国歯科医師会 **BDA**
英国歯科矯正学会 **BSSO**
英国耳鼻咽喉科学会 **BLROA**
英国獣医学雑誌 **BVJ**
英国獣医学会 **BVA**
英国小児科学会 **BPA**
英国小児外科医協会 **BAPS**
英国人 **Br, Brit**
英国心臓協会 **BCS**
英国身体障害者リハビリテーション審議会 **BCRD**
英国制御監視委員会 **BCIC**
英国整形外科学会 **BOA**
英国精神医学会 **BPsS**
英国精神科学会会員 **FBPsS**
英国卒後医学連盟 **BPMF**
英国体育協会 **BAPT**
英国調剤医薬品集 **BPC, B.P.C.**
英国てんかん協会 **BEpA**
英国内科・外科学会員 **FRFPS**
英国内科医・外科医分科会員有資格者 **LRFPS**
英国内科学会会員 **FRCP**
英国内科学会 **Ba Phys Med**
英国難聴学会 **BAHOH**
英国難聴者協会 **BDA**
英国熱量単位 **BTU**
英国(人)の **Br, Brit**
英国泌尿器外科医協会 **BAUS**
英国皮膚科・梅毒学会 **BADS**
英国皮膚科学会 **BDA**
英国標準の **B.S.**
英国物理療法士会員 **FBCP**
英国法医科学会 **BAFS**
英国法医学会 **BAFM**
英国放射線単位・測定委員会 **BCRUM**
英国麻薬委員会 **CND**
英国薬局 **BDH**
英国薬局方 **BP, B.P., BPh, B.Ph., PB, Ph B, Ph.B.**
英国予防医学会 **BMPS**
英国臨床細胞学会 **BSCC**
英国聾唖者協会 **BDDA**
映画 **MP**
栄養 **NTR, Nut, nutr**
栄養維持サービス **NSS**
栄養学 **Sitol**
栄養学的危険指数 **NRI**
栄養学の **Sitol**
栄養教育研究組織 **NERO**
栄養士 **Sitol**
栄養指数 **EQ**
栄養失調症 **PCM**
栄養士認定書 **DN**
栄養障害性表皮水疱症 **EBD**
栄養状態型 **NST**
栄養状態指数 **TSI**
栄養ゼラチン寒天(培地) **NGA**
栄養糖 **NZ**
栄養と補水 **F & W**
栄養評価指数 **NAI**
栄養比率 **NR**
栄養不良関連糖尿病 **MRDM**
栄養ブロス **NB**
栄養補給 **fdg**
栄養補助サービス **NSS**
栄養膜 **Tr**
栄養膜腫瘍 **TT**
栄養良好 **eutroph.**
栄養良好で体格の良い **WNWD**
栄養良好な **WN, W/N**
栄養良好な女性 **WNF**
栄養良好な男性 **WNM**
栄養良好の **eutroph.**
影響 **influ**
影響(力) **infl**
影響なし **NE**
影響を与える **influ**
影響を及ぼす **influ**
鋭敏度 **sens, SENS, sens.**
衛生 **sanit**
衛生(学) **H, Hyg, hyg**
衛生学技士 **EST**
衛生学士 **B.Hyg., MSH, M.S.Sc**
衛生学修士 **M.Hyg.**
衛生学認定書 **DSSc**
衛生学博士 **DHy, D.Hy., Dr.Hy.**
衛生技師 **Hyg, hyg**
衛生工学 **SE**
衛生士 **Hyg, hyg**
衛生施設局 **DS**
衛生植物検疫措置の適用に関する協定 **SPS**
衛生的な **Hyg, hyg**
衛生の **sanit**
衛生部隊 **MC**

え

衛星 **s, SAT**
衛生学の **Hyg, hyg**
描いた **del.**
易う蝕性 **CS**
疫学 **epdm, EPDML, EST**
疫学者 **epdm, EPDML**
疫学生物統計学局 **OEB**
疫学の **epdm, EPDML**
(溶)液 **Lsg**
液 **J, j, jc, jc., suc.**
液(体) **L**
液化石油ガス **LPG**
液化天然ガス **LNG**
液(体)クロマトグラフィ **LC**
液状(の) **LIQ, Liq, liq.**
液状シリコン **SF**
液状膜 **LM**
液性(の) **F, FL, Fl, fl, fld**
液性因子 **H**
液性抗体により区別される **SD**
液性の **fluid.**
液相・固相クロマトグラフィ **LSC**
液相・液相クロマトグラフィ **LLC**
液相エピタキシ **LPE**
液体 **fl.**
液体(の) **F, LIQ, Liq, liq.**
液体液体分布 **LLD**
液体酸素 **lox**
液体試料中の全炭酸 **DIC**
液体シンチレーションカウンター **LSC**
液体水素 **LH_2**
液体窒素 **LN_2**
液体ヘリウム **LHe**
液体膜 **LM**
液量オンス **FL OZ, fl oz, fl.oz.**
腋下加圧角 **APA**
腋窩 **A, Ax, ax**
腋窩・大腿動脈バイパス **AF bypass, A-F.Bypass**
腋窩・大腿バイパス **AX-F**
腋窩(体)温 **TA**
腋窩温度 **AT**
腋窩中線 **MAL**
腋窩の **A, Ax, ax**
腋窩リンパシンチグラフィ **AXL**
腋毛 **AH**
枝 **br, R, r., Rr.**
円 **cir, cir.**
円回内筋 **PT**
円蓋 **F, FX**
円形巨細胞 **rR**
円形脱毛症 **AA**
円形メジャー **CM**
円周状の **cir, cir., Circ, circ**
円周平均速度 **mVCF**
円周方向短縮速度 **Vcf**
円錐角膜 **KC**
円錐角膜線 **KCL**
円錐切除(術) **coniz**
円柱 **C, cyl**
円柱上皮 **C, CE**
円柱(状)の **C**
円柱レンズ **C, cyl, sph, sph.**
円筒鏡型エネルギー分光器 **CMA**
円二色性 **CD**
円板状エリテマトーデス〔紅斑性狼瘡〕 **DLE**
延髄呼吸化学受容器 **MRC**
延髄後の **RB**
延髄傍巨大細胞網様核 **NRPG**
延髄網様体 **BRF**
延長 **E, elong, ext, ext.**
延長された **prol, prolong.**
延長する **prol**
延命効果 **DOL**
炎症 **inf, inf., infl, inflam, inflamm**
炎症過程 **infl proc**
炎症後コルチコイド **PIC**
炎症性関節疾患 **IJD**
炎症性コルチコイド **P-C**
炎症性線状疣状表皮母斑 **ILVEN**
炎症性総排出腔性ポリープ **ICP**
炎症性腸疾患 **IBD**
炎症性腸症候群 **IBS**
炎症性乳頭状過形成(症) **IPH**
炎症性ネフローゼ腎炎 **INN**
炎症性の **inflam, inflamm**
炎症性類線維ポリープ **IFP**
炎症徴候なし **NIS**
炎症の徴候なし **NSI**
炎症歴のない現症 **NIP**
遠位運動潜時 **DML**
遠位型脊髄性筋萎縮症 **DSMA**
遠位冠(状)静脈洞 **DCS**
遠位頬側正中咬合の **MODB**
遠位口唇切歯の **DLAI**
遠位指節間関節 **DIP(J)**
遠位指節骨 **DP**
遠位手掌皮膚溝 **DPC**
遠位指皺襞 **DFC**
遠位正中咬合の **MOD**
遠位腸管 **DI**
遠位尿細管 **DCT, DT**

遠位尿細管アシドーシス　**dRTA**
遠位の　**D, d., dis, dist**
遠位脾腎静脈吻合術　**DSRS**
遠位部 1/3 区　**D/3**
遠隔　**R, r.**
遠隔位置制御　**RPC**
遠隔管理室　**RCU**
遠隔救急救助浄化設備　**RESCUE**
遠隔出力制御　**revocon**
遠隔照射療法　**tele ci**
遠隔制御式密封小線量治療システム　**RALS**
遠隔制御装置　**remocon**
遠隔操作式後充填方式　**RALS**
遠隔操作室　**RMU**
遠隔測定(法)　**TELE, Tele, tele**
遠隔転移　**DM**
遠隔の　**dis, rmte**
遠見視力　**DVA**
遠心(面)頬側咬合面の　**DBO**
遠心(面)頬(面)歯髄(面)の　**DBP**
遠心(面)頬(面)の　**DB**
遠心後プラズマフェレーシス　**PCPP**
遠心(面)歯頸(面)の　**DC**
遠心(面)歯肉(面)の　**DG**
遠心(面)唇(面)　**DLA, DLa**
遠心性環状紅斑　**EAC**
遠心性の　**eff, effer**
遠心(面)舌(面)歯髄(面)の　**DLP**
遠心舌側咬合(面)の　**DOL**
遠心(面)舌(面)の　**DL**
遠心の　**cent, cent., dist**
遠心分離　**cfg**
遠心分離クロマトグラフィ　**CPC**
遠心面切端面の　**DI**
遠心面舌面咬合面の　**DOL**
遠心力　**cf, G**
遠視　**H, HY, Hy**
遠視性乱視　**ASH, AsH, As.H, HA**
遠視の　**H, HY, Hy**
遠点　**PR, pr, p.r.**
鉛直分布観測用のオゾン衛生センサー　**SBUV**
塩化(物)　**Cl**
塩化亜鉛中毒　**ZCP**
塩化アンモニウム　**ACK, NH_4Cl, Salmiak**
塩化エチルベンジル　**EBC**
塩化カリウム　**KCl**
塩化カルシウム　**$CaCl_2$**
塩化銀　**AgCl**
塩化シアノゲン　**CK**
塩化ジメチルツボクラリン　**DME**
塩化水銀安息香酸塩　**CMB**
塩化水素　**HCL**
塩化水素酸　**HCL**
塩化水素酸の　**Hydrochl**
塩化セチルピリジニウム　**CPC**
塩化第二鉄　**$FeCl_3$**
塩化ツボクラリン　**TC**
塩化テトラエチルアンモニウム　**TEAC**
塩化テトラゾリウム　**TTC**
塩化トリフェニルテトラゾリウム　**TTC**
塩化トリフェニールテトラゾリウム試験　**TTC test**
塩化トリブチルスズ　**TBTC**
塩化ナトリウム　**NaCl, sod.chlor.**
塩化ネオテトラゾリウム(染色)　**NTC**
塩化バリウム　**$BaCl_2$**
塩化ピクリル　**PCl**
塩化ビニル　**VC**
塩化ビニル単量体〔モノマー〕　**VCM**
塩化ビニルモノマー　**VOM**
塩化フェニル水銀　**PMC**
塩化物　**chl, chlorid.**
塩化プラリドキシム　**2-PAM**
塩化マグネシウム　**$MgCl_2$**
塩化メチルベンゾール　**MBC**
塩化メチルロザニリン　**MRC**
塩基　**B, b.**
塩基イオン定数　**K_b, K_b**
塩基球からのヒスタミン放出　**HRB**
塩基欠乏　**BD**
塩基性胎児蛋白　**BFP**
塩基性蛋白　**BP**
塩基性フェトプロテイン　**BEP**
塩基対　**bp, b.p.**
塩酸　**HCL**
塩酸エタフェノン　**ETF**
塩酸ジカルベトキシサイアミン　**DECT**
塩酸デスオキシエフェドリン　**DOE**
塩酸デソキシピリドキシン　**DPD**
塩酸ドキサプラム　**DH**
塩酸ドキシサイクリン　**DOTC**

塩酸ナイリドリン **NF**
塩酸の **mur**
塩酸フェノキシベンザミン **POB**
塩酸プロカイン **H_3, P/H_3**
塩酸プロメタジン **P**
塩酸モルヒネ **morph.hydr**
塩水 **SW**
塩水浴 **bal.mar., BM, B.M., b.m.**
塩素 **Cl**
塩素遊離の **FFC**
塩分喪失者 **SL**
塩類の **S, SA, SAL, sal.**
塩・アデニン・グルコース・マニトール **SAGM**
演劇グループ療法 **PGT**
演算増幅器 **OP amp**
縁枝 **RM**
(辺)縁の **marg**
嚥下させよ **deglut.**
嚥下せよ **deglut.**

お

オウム病・性病性リンパ肉芽腫　**P-LGV**
オウム病・鼠径リンパ肉芽腫・トラコーマ群微生物　**PLT**
オキサシリン　**MPIPC, OX, Ox, O_x**
オキサシリンアミン配糖体耐性黄色ブドウ球菌　**OARSA**
オキサゾロン　**OX, Ox, O_x**
オキサプロジン　**OXP**
オキザロコハク酸　**OS**
オキサロ酢酸　**OAA**
オキザロ酸　**OXA**
オキザロ酸の　**OX, Ox, O_x**
オキシダント　**OX, Ox, O_x**
オキシテトラサイクリン　**OTC**
オキシトシン　**OC, OT, OX, Ox, O_x, OXT, OXY, oxy**
オキシトシン感受性テスト　**OST**
オキシトシンチャレンジテスト　**OCT**
オキシトシン負荷試験　**OST**
オキシトシン分娩誘発　**OI**
オキシプレッシン　**OXP**
オキシヘモグロビン　**O_2Hb**
オキシポリゼラチン　**OPH, Oph, oph**
オキシミオグロビン　**MbO_2**
オキシメチルピリミジン　**OMP**
オキシメル　**oxym**
オクタメチルピロホスホラミド(=ペトレックスIII)　**OMPA**
オークリッジ分析システム　**ORANS**
オージェ電子分光法　**AES**
オージオグラム　**audio**
オージオメーター　**audio**
オシロスコープ　**oscp, scope**
オズグッド・シュラッター(病)　**OS**
オズグッド・シュラッター病変　**OSL**
オースチン・ムーア補綴　**A-M PR**
オステオカルシン　**OC**
オーストラリア・ニュージーランド胸部医学会　**TSANZ**
オーストラリア医学研究所員　**FAIP**
オーストラリア医師会員　**MRACP**
オーストラリア肝炎関連抗原　**AUHAA**
オーストラリア血清肝炎　**AuSH, AuSh**
オーストラリア抗原　**AA, AU, Au, AuAg, Au-Ag**
オーストラリア抗原蛋白　**AuP**
オーストラリア抗原放射免疫定量　**AAR**
オーストラリア国際血圧実態調査　**ANBPS**
オーストラリア歯科医会会員　**FACDS**
オーストラリア病院管理研究所員　**FAIHA**
オーストラリア放射線科学会員　**FCRA**
オスミウム　**Os**
オスモラリティーギャップ　**OG**
オスモル　**Osm, osm, osm.**
オースラー・ウェーバー・ランデュ(症候群)　**OWR**
オーソ睡眠　**OS**
オゾン　**O_3**
オゾン濃度鉛直分布測定　**SAGE**
オーダリー　**O**
オッズ比　**OD, OR**
オッディ括約筋　**SO**
オッペンハイム・ウアバッハ(症候群)　**OU**
オトガイ舌筋　**GG**
オトガイ舌骨　**GH**
オートラジオグラフィ　**AR, ARG**
オートラジオグラム　**ARG**
オハイオ職業興味調査　**OVIS**
オハイオ労働価値調査票　**OWVI**
オーバードライブ抑制試験　**ODST**
オーバーヘッド牽引　**OHT**
オーバーヘッドプロジェクタ　**OHP**
オピアト　**Opi-ato**
オピアト注　**Opi ato inj**
オピウムアルカロイドとアトロピン　**Opi-ato**
オピウムアルカロイドとスコポラミン　**Opi-sco**
オピスコ　**Opi-sco**
オピスタン　**O**
オフィスオートメーション　**OA**
オプソニン化ザイモザン

Op-Z, OZ
オプソニン活性　**OA**
オプソニン指数　**OI**
オフとオン　**OAO**
オブラート嚢
cap.amyl.
オブラートに入れて
ad cap.amyl.

オフロキサシン　**OFLX**
オピストルキス(属)　**O**
オペレーションズリサーチ
OR
オペレータ　**O**
オペロン　**O**
オボムコイド　**OM**
オミクロン　***o***
オーム・アンペア・秒・メートル単位
OASM units
オーム・センチメートル
ohm-cm
オムスク出血熱　**OHF**
オランウータン　**PPY**
オランダ型アミロイド(沈着)症を伴う(遺伝性)脳出血　**HCHWA-D**
オリエ・クリッペル・トレノーネイ(症候群)
OKT
オリエンテーション反射
OR
オリゴマイシン感受性付与蛋白　**OSCP**
オリーブ蝸牛神経束
OCB
オリーブ橋小脳萎縮(症)
OCA
オリーブ橋小脳萎縮症
OPCA
オリーブ油　**ol.oliv.**
オリンパス内視鏡システム
OES
オルガスム障害　**OI**
オルガスムス　**Org**
オルソパントモグラフィ
OPT
オルト・クン・Tリンパ球　**OKT**
オルト・アミノアゾトルエン　**OAT**
オルト・クン・Bリンパ球
OKB
オルト二塩酸ベンゼン
ODCB
オルトクレゾールフタレインコンプレクソン法
***o*-CPC method**
オルトトリジン
***o*-tolidine**
オルトヒドロキシフェニル酢酸　**OHPAA, *o*-HPAA**
オルトメチル転移酵素
OMT
オルニチン　**Orn**
オルニチン-8-アミノトランスフェラーゼ　**OAT**
オルニチンカルバモイルトランスフェラーゼ
OCT
オルニチンカルバモイルトランスフェラーゼ欠損症
OCTD
オルニチンケト酸トランスアミナーゼ　**OKT**
オルニチン脱炭酸酵素
OD, ODC
オルニチントランスカルバミラーゼ　**OT, OTC**
オルニチントランスカルバミラーゼ欠損症
OTCD
オルブライト遺伝性骨ジストロフィ　**AHO**
オレアンドマイシン
OL, OLM, OM
オレイン酸　**$C_{18=1}$, OA**
オレイン酸・アルブミン・ブドウ糖・カタラーゼ培地　**OADC**
オレイン酸エタノールアミン　**EO**
オレイン酸エタノールアミン・加アミドトリゾ酸メグルミン　**EOMA**
オーレオスライシン
ARTN, ATHR
オーレオマイシン　**AM**
オレンジ　**O, orn**
オレンジG-6対比染色
OG-6
オレンジイエロー　**OY**
オレンジグリーン染色
OG stain
オレンジジュース　**OJ, o.j., OrJ**
オロチジレートホスホリボシル変換酵素〔トランスフェラーゼ〕　**OPRT**
オロチジン　**Ord, ord, ord.**
オロチン酸　**OA, Oro**
オロチン酸ホスホリボシル変換酵素〔トランスフェラーゼ〕　**OPRT**
オングストローム(単位)
Å
オンコスタチンM　**OSM**
オンコセルカ(属)　**O**
オンス　**oz, oz.**
オンライン医学関連文献分析システム
MEDLARS on-Line, MEDLINE
オンライン毒物情報システム　**TOXLINE**
オンラインリアルタイム
OLRT
ビンクリスチン(＝オンコビン),メトトレキサート,アドリアマイシン,ダクチノマイシン
OMAD
おいしい　**dulc.**
おおよそ　**aprx, etw**

おおよその **appr, appr., approx, approx.**
お金を払わなければ渡すな **ne.tr.s.num.**
おくび **eruct**
おなか **tum**
おのおの **Q, q, q.**
おのおのの **AA, aa., q.q., sing.**
おのおのを同量 **AA, aa.**
おもな **CH, Ch, ch, m**
おもな核の異常 **MAKA**
および **et**
およびその他 **et al.**
およびそれに続くもの **et seq.**
汚染指数 **CI**
汚染者負担の原則 **PPP**
汚染除去因子 **DF**
汚泥容量指標 **SVI**
尾の **CD, Cd, cd**
欧州医薬品庁 **EMEA**
欧州監視評価計画 **EMEP**
欧州分子生物学協会 **EMBO**
啞(＝おし) **M, m.**
起こりがちな **incd, incdt, incid**
起こること **occ**
悪寒・発熱・寝汗 **CFNS**
悪心〔嘔気〕・嘔吐・下痢 **NVD**
悪心〔嘔気〕と嘔吐 **N/V, N & V**
悪阻指数 **EI**
終わりに **s.f.**
終わるまで **UF**
置き換える **displ**
甥 **neph**
王水 **aq.r.**
王立医学会員[英国] **MRSM**
王立一般医協会[英国] **RCGP**
王立エディンバラ医師会員[英国] **MRCPE**
王立化学協会 **RSC**
王立外科学会会員[英国] **MRCS**
王立健康協会員[英国] **MRSH**
王立産婦人科学会会員 **MRCOG**
王立内科学会会員 **MRCP**
凹形の **CC, Cc**
凹面の **CC, Cc, cv**
応急処置 **FA**
応答 **R, RESP, Resp, resp, resp.**
応答刺激率 **RS ratio**
応答なし **DNR**
応用化学 **AC**
応用化学雑誌 **JAC**
応用寄生虫学・昆虫学認定書 **DAP & E**
応用骨疾患学会 **AAO**
応用された **appl**
応用心理分析協会 **AAP**
応用生物学者協会 **AAB**
応用放射線学連合委員会 **JCAR**
欧州医薬化学連合 **EFMC**
欧州頸動脈外科研究者グループ **ECST**
欧州外科的研究協会 **ESSR**
欧州血液学会 **ESH, SEH**
欧州口腔病学研究会 **GERSO**
欧州行動療法学会 **EABT**
欧州呼吸器学会 **ERS**
欧州歯科産業連盟 **FIDE**
欧州歯列矯正学会 **EOS**
欧州心臓学会 **ESC**
欧州生化学会連合 **FEBS**
欧州製薬団体連合会 **EFPIA**
欧州透析移植学会議 **EDTA**
欧州糖尿病研究協会 **EASD**
欧州脳行動学会 **EBBS**
欧州臨床化学会議 **ECCC**
欧州臨床検査標準委員会 **ECCLS**
欧州臨床調査研究協会 **ESCI**
殴打湿疹 **noxema**
黄褐色の **YBr**
黄色(の) **Yel, yel**
黄色・青色の **Y/B**
黄色酵素 **YE**
黄色腫症 **Xanth, xanth.**
黄色靱帯骨化症 **OLF, OYL**
黄色爪症候群 **YNS**
黄色蛋白 **FP**
黄色肉芽腫性腎盂腎炎 **XGP, XPN**
黄色ニス症候群 **YVS**
黄色の **flav., lut., Y**
黄色ヒアリン膜症 **YHMD**
黄色ブドウ球菌 **SA, Staph.aur**
黄色ブドウ球菌エンテロトキシン **SEs**
黄色ブドウ球菌過免疫グロブリン血症(＝E 症候群) **SAHIOES**
黄色ブドウ球菌蛋白分解酵素 **SAP**
黄体 **CL, CL, cl., c.l.**
黄体化ホルモン **LH**
黄体化〔黄体形成〕ホルモ

ン・卵胞刺激ホルモン放出因子　**LH/FSH-RF**
黄体化ホルモン放出因子　**RFL**
黄体化未破裂卵胞(症候群)　**LUF**
黄体化未破裂卵胞症候群　**LUFS**
黄体期欠損　**LPD**
黄体形成ホルモン　**LH**
黄体形成〔黄体化〕ホルモン放出因子　**LRF**
黄体形成〔黄体化〕ホルモン放出ホルモン　**LHRH, LRH**
黄体形成〔黄体化〕ホルモン放出因子　**LHRF**
黄体刺激ホルモン　**CLSH, LH, LSH, LTH, LTP, P**
黄体刺激ホルモン放出因子　**LHRF**
黄体刺激ホルモン抑制因子　**LTHIF**
黄体乳腺刺激ホルモン　**LMT(H)**
黄体(機能)不全　**CLI**
黄体ホルモン　**CLH, P**
黄疸　**ict., j, jaund, jaund., JD**
黄疸指数　**ict.ind, II**
黄疸出血性レストスピラ　**LI**
黄疸性血清肝炎　**ISH**
黄疸(性)の　**IC, iCT, ICT**
黄疸発生物　**IG**
黄熱ウイルス　**YFV**
黄熱病　**YF**
黄熱病予防接種　**YFI**
(網膜の)黄斑　**YS, ys, y.s.**
黄斑　**Mac**
黄斑(網膜)　**ye.s.**
黄斑上増殖　**EMP**
黄緑野菜　**GYV**
黄連解毒湯　**OG**
嘔気〔悪心〕と嘔吐　**NE**
嘔気または嘔吐　**N or V**
嘔吐　**V, vom.**
嘔吐が終ったときに　**per.op.emet.**
嘔吐症状　**eE**
嘔吐中枢　**EC, VC**
嘔吐と下痢　**V & D**
嘔吐なしの嘔気　**N and E**
横臥の　**recumb**
横隔神経　**PN**
横隔(膜)神経刺激　**DNS**
横隔膜　**D, diaph, DPH**
横隔膜刺激　**DS**
横隔膜(面)心筋梗塞　**DMI**
横隔膜電気刺激性呼吸　**EPR**
横隔膜の　**DI, phren**
横胸径　**TTD**
(骨盤出口の)横径　**BI**
横径　**TD, trans D, trans.d.**
横行結腸　**T, TC**
横行小管系　**TTS**
横指　**FB, fb, QFB, QUF**
横指幅　**QFB**
横足根関節　**MTJ**
横断の　**T, trans, X, xvse**
横断面　**CSA, trans.sec., trans.sect., TS, Tsect, T sect., T-sect.**
横突起　**TP, transv.proc.**
横洞　**TS**
横紋筋肉腫　**RMS**
扇形注入器での灌注法　**FD**
大渦巻き　**LWP**
大型単層状小胞　**LUV**
大型濾胞中心細胞　**large FCC**
大きい　**amp., ampl., Lg, lg., Lge, lge, Mag, mag, magn., maj, mass, mass.**
大きさ　**dim, dim., sz**
大きな変化なし　**NSC**
大さじ　**T, tbs**
大さじ1杯　**cochl.mag.**
大さじ1杯の　**tbsp**
大(型)中性アミノ酸　**LNAA**
大粒錠剤　**bol**
大(型)転換細胞　**LTC**
大幅なサンプル・バイアスシフト法　**ESBS**
大(型)網(状)赤血球　**LR**
多い　**nim.**
多くの　**g, Po**
多すぎて数えきれない　**TMTC, TNC, TNTC, t.n.t.c.**
覆い・覆い取り試験　**CUT**
岡・片倉培地　**OKmedium**
沖縄感染症対策イニシアティブ　**OIDI**
送れ　**M, m., mitt, mitt., mt.**
遅らせる　**dly**
遅れた　**dlyd**
行われたもの　**q.e.f.**
行われない　**ND**
雄　**M, m**
遅い　**sl**
遅い眼球運動　**SEM**
穏やかな　**MOD, mod**
穏やかに　**lenit.**
夫　**H, husb, husb.**
夫と妻　**H/W**

音　Sds, sds, snd
音と閃光　SF
音の大きさ　N
音の強さの弁別検査　IDL test
音レベル　SL
音・圧比　n/p r
音・温度比　NTR
音・速度・温度・圧　SVTP
頤(おとがい)　M, m.
頤後位の　MP
頤前方位　MA
頤(=オトガイ)の　ment
頤右後位　MDP
男で東洋人　m/o
男の子　Fel, fel
男やもめ　W, w, wid., Wid.
同じ　do., ead., S
同じく　id.
同じ(治療を)継続せよ　CS
同じ場所〔個所〕で　ib., ibid.
各々の　a, E, ea
覚え書き　memo
重い　H, hv, hvy, pond.
重さ　WT, Wt, wt.
親　P
親子コミュニケーションスケジュール　PCCS
親細胞　PC
親知らず　WT
親世代　P
親態度スケール　PAS
親の　P, parent
親・教師質問表　PTQ
音圧レベル　SPL
音喉頭図　PLG
音階　tave
音楽効果　M & E
音楽療法　MT
音響　acous
音響・振動研究所　ISVR
音響陰影　AS
音響快適度指数　ACI
音響光学変調フィルター　AOTF
音響指数　NSI
音響性耳内筋反射　AR
音響線追跡　ART
音響の　acst
音響曝露予測　NEF
音響標準　NC
音響抑制機器　NSD
音響量比　AQ
音響レベル自動調節　NOALA
音源　A
音源メーター　NSM
音叉　TF, t.f.
音刺激による最小可聴閾値の一過性変化　NITTS
音刺激賦活法　SS
音場　SF
音声学　phon
音声学的にバランスのとれた　PB
音声振盪　frem
音声プログラミング欠損症候群　PPDS
音節/分　SPM
音速　SOS
音脳図　SEG
音量　VU, vu
音量不快レベル　LDL
音量レベル　LL
温式自己免疫性溶血性貧血　WAIHA
温浸せよ　dig.
温浸法　INF, Inf, inf
温湿パック(非滅菌の)　WMP
温水　aq.cal.
温阻血時間　WIT
温暖・湿潤な　WM
温暖前線　WF
温度　T, t, Temp, temp, temp.
温度・標高・湿度　TAH
温度・深さ・塩分　TDS
温度安定の　TS
温度因子　TF
温度感受性突然変異　ts mutation
温度感受性突然変異体　ts mutant
温度感受性の　TS
温度眼振の視性抑制の欠如　FFS
温度計　ther, TM
温度勾配ゲル電気泳動　TGGE
温度差解析　QDTA
温度代償　TC
温度と気圧　TP
温度の安定した平板炉　STPF
温度パターン　CP
温度発光線量計　TLD
温度比重測定解析　TGA
温湯に可溶な　HWS
温熱中間帯　TNZ
温熱で治療〔処理〕した　HT
温熱療法　HT
温パック　HP, H.P.
温浴　HTB
温和な　mit.
温・湿指数　THI
女の　G

か

(ギリシャ文字の)カイ **X, χ**
カイ2乗 **χ^2**
ガイガー・ミュラー管 **GM tube**
ガイガー・ミュラー計数管 **GM, GM counter**
カイザー・パーマネント(治療食) **K-P**
カイザー・フライシャー輪 **FLR**
カイゼル・フライシャー輪 **KFR**
ガイダンスバリュー **GV**
カイロマイクロン **chylo**
カイロミクロン **CM**
ガウス **B, G, Gs**
ガウス単位 **B**
カウプ・ダベンポート指数 **KI**
カウフマン・ピーターソン(塩基) **KP**
カウフマン心理・教育アセスメントバッテリー **K-ABC**
カウフマン発育尺度〔スケール〕 **KDS**
カウンターフロー遠心分離 **CCE**
カウント/時 **cph**
カウント/秒 **CPS**
カウント/分 **cpm**
ガウンとタオル **G & T**
カオリン・セファリン凝固時間 **KCCT**
カオリン加部分トロンボプラスチン時間 **K-PTT**
カオリン凝固時間 **KCT**
カサガイヘモシアニン **LH**
カシン・ベック病 **KB**
ガス **G**
ガス圧 **PG**
ガス液体クロマトグラフィ **GLC**
カスガマイシン **KSM**
ガスクロマトグラフィ **GC**
ガスクロマトグラフィ・燃焼炉・同位体質量分析システム **GC/C/IRMS**
ガスクロマトグラフィ気道電子捕獲検出法 **GC-ECD**
ガスクロマトグラフィ質量分析コンピュータ **GCMS-CPU**
ガスクロマトグラフィ質量分析システム **GCMS**
ガスクロマトグラフィ質量分離図 **GCMF**
ガス交換 **GEX**
ガス固体クロマトグラフィ **GSC**
カスト **CAST**
カースドマン・スタイナート(症候群) **CS**
ガストリン **G**
ガストリン分泌細胞 **G cell, G-cell**
ガストリン放出ペプチド **GRP**
ガストリン放出ホルモン **GRP**
ガス容積単位時間 **VT**
ガーゼ **carbas.**
カゼイン **CN**
カゼインキナーゼII **CK II**
ガーゼ交換 **GW**
カダシル **CADASIL**
カタツムリレクチン **HPL**
カダベリン **Cad**
カタラーゼ **CAT**
カタール **kat**
ガッタパーチャ **GP**
カッツ適応スケール **KAS**
カッパ **K**
カッパ・ブンガロ毒素 **KBgT**
カッパーバンド **CuB**
カップ **pocul.**
カテコール-*O*-メチル基転移酵素阻害薬 **COMT inhibitor**
カテコール(アミン) *O*-メチルトランスフェラーゼ **CMT**
カテコール *O*-メチルトランスフェラーゼ **COMT**
カテコールアミン **CA, CAT**
カテコールアミンと代謝産物 **CAT-MET**
カテコールメチルトランスフェラーゼ **CCMT**
カテーテル **Cath., cath.**
カテーテル関連細菌尿 **CAB**
カテーテル関連敗血症 **CRS**
カテーテル採取尿 **CSU**
カテーテル挿入状態の膀胱 **CB**
カテーテル尿 **cath**
カテーテル尿残渣 **CUS**
カテーテル法 **Cath, Cath.**
カテーテル誘発痙攣 **CIS**
カテーテルを挿入する **Cath., cath.**
ガードナー症候群 **GS**
ガードナー人格調査分析 **GAP**
ガドペンテト酸 **Gd-DTPA**
カドミウム **Cad, Cd**
カドミウムシェル **CDS**

カドミウム試験 **Cd-probe**
カトリック(の) **C, Cath, Cath.**
ガドリニウム **Gd**
カトルファージュ角 **Q angle**
カナダ医学生インターン連盟 **CAMSI**
カナダ医学微生物学会 **CAMM**
カナダ医師会 **CMA**
カナダ移植可能細動除去器研究 **CIDS**
カナダ看護師協会 **AIC, CNA**
カナダ関節炎リウマチ学会 **CARS**
カナダ胸部疾患学会 **CTS**
カナダ結核病学会 **CTA**
カナダ公衆衛生学会 **CPHA**
カナダ国家 TNM 分類委員会 **CNC**
カナダ国家精神衛生協会 **CNCMH**
カナダ歯科学会 **CDA**
カナダ歯科研究財団 **CDRF**
カナダ歯科研究所協議会 **CDLC**
カナダ女医連合 **FMWC**
カナダ小児疾患研究学会 **CSSDC**
カナダ心理学協会員 **FCPA**
カナダ整形外科医協会 **C.O.A.**
カナダ精神健康協会 **CMHA**
カナダ生物学会連合 **CFBS**
カナダ赤十字社 **CRACS**
カナダ大学看護学生協会 **CUNSA**
カナダ農業農産食品省 **AAFC**
カナダ病理学者協会 **CAP**
カナダ放射線医学会 **CAR**
カナダリウマチ学会 **CRA**
カナマイシン **K, KM**
カナマイシン・バンコマイシン **KV**
カナマイシン・バンコマイシン入り血液寒天培地 **KVLBA**
カナマイシンアセチルトランスフェラーゼ **KAT**
カニクイザル **MFA**
カニクイザルの腎 **CMK**
カネンドマイシン **ADK, KDM**
カハール間質核 **INC**
カハール(間質)細胞 **ICC**
カフ圧迫時末梢静脈圧上昇率 **CORRP**
カフェイン **caf**
ガフキー号数 **G**
カプセル(剤) **cap, cap., caps., capsul.**
カプセル化 **encap**
カプセルに入れられた **encap**
カプセルに入れる **encap**
カブトガニ由来の分解質 **TAL**
カブトガニレクチン **LPA**
カプトプリル **CAP**
カブラ黄斑モザイクウイルス **TYMV**
カプラン・ズルジャー(症候群) **KZ**
カブリ(=冠血管形成術とバイパス術の血管新生比較調査) **CABRI**
カプリルヒドロキサム酸 **CHA**
カプレオマイシン **CAP, CM, CPM, CPRM**
カプロン酸 **CA**
カポジ水痘様疹 **KVE**
カポジ肉種 **KS**
カポジ肉腫関連ヘルペスウイルス **KSHV**
カポジ肉腫と日和見感染 **KS/OI**
カーマ **K**
ガマ単位 **BU**
カーメン単位 **KU**
ガラクターゼ活性物質 **Gal-Act**
ガラクツロン酸 **GalU, GalUA**
ガラクトース一リン酸 **gal-1-P**
ガラクトキナーゼ **GALK, GK**
ガラクトサミン **GalN, $GalNH_2$**
ガラクトシダーゼ **GAL**
ガラクトシル **GAL**
ガラクトース **Gal, gal.**
ガラクトース・オキシダーゼ・シッフ反応 **GOS**
ガラクトース-1-リン酸ウリジルトランスフェラーゼ **GALT**
ガラクトースオキシダーゼ **GO**
ガラクトース負荷試験 **GalTT, GAL TT**
ガラクトセレブレシド **GC**
カラゲニン **CA**
ガラス **vitr, vitr., vtr.**
ガラス管 **vas vit.**
ガラス質〔状〕の **Vit,**

vit, vitr, vitr, vitr.
ガラス製の **vitr, vitr.**
ガラス線維補強プラスチック **FRP**
ガラス栓のついたビン **Vcepv**
ガラス(状)の **V**
カラット **C, ct**
ガラニン **GAL**
カラムクロマトグラフィ **CC**
ガランサミン **GT**
カリウム **ACK, K, Kal, pot, potass**
ガリウム **Ga**
カリウム・塩化ナトリウム・乳酸ナトリウム **PSL**
カリウム・塩化ナトリウム・乳酸ナトリウム溶液 **PSL sol**
カリウム・グルコース・インスリン **PGI**
カリウム・チタン・リン酸 **KTP**
ガリウム 67 **^{67}Ga**
ガリウム 67・クエン酸ガリウム **^{67}Ga-gallium citrate**
カリクレイン **Ka, KK**
カリクレイン・キニン・キニノゲン・キニナーゼ **KKKK**
カリクレイン・キニン系 **KK system**
カリクレイン・トリプシン阻害因子 **KTI**
カリクレイン単位 **KU**
カリクレイン抑制単位 **K, KIU**
カリニ肺炎 **PCP**
カリニ肺胞嚢虫 **PC**
カリフォルニア心理検査 **CPI**
カリフォルニア脳炎 **CE**
カリフォルニア脳炎ウイルス **CEV**
カリフォルニウム **Cf**
カリフォルニウム 252 **^{252}Cf**
カリフラワーモザイクウイルス **CaMV, CLMW**
カリマトバクテリウム(属) **C**
ガリレオ **gal**
カリンダシリン=カルベニシリンインダニルエステル **CIPC**
カール・パーセル・メイブーム・ギル法 **CPMG**
カルシウム **Ca**
カルシウム・マグネシウムを含まない **CMF**
カルシウムイオン **Ca^{2+}**
カルシウム依存性蛋白キナーゼ **CDPK**
カルシウム依存性蛋白分解酵素 **CDP**
カルシウム依存性中性プロテアーゼ **CANP**
カルシウム依存性調節蛋白 **CDR**
カルシウム依存性プロテアーゼ **CAF**
カルシウム拮抗薬 **CA, CCB**
カルシウムクリアランス/クレアチニンクリアランス(比) **Cca/Ccr**
カルシウム結合蛋白 **CABP, CaBP**
カルシウム結合蛋白(質) **CBP**
カルシウム骨指数 **CaBI**
カルシウム試験 **CAL**
カルシウム遮断薬 **CB**
カルシウム沈着 **calcif**
カルシウム排泄 **CaE**
カルシウムピロリン酸二水和物 **CPPD**
カルシウム負荷試験 **CaTT**
カルシウム賦活因子 **CAF**
カルシウム不含タイロード液 **CFT**
カルシウム不含リン酸緩衝食塩水 **CFBS**
カルシウム誘発カルシウム放出 **CICR**
カルシウム流入ブロッカー **CEB**
カルジオタコメータ **CTM**
カルジオリ〔ライ〕ピン **CL**
カルジオリ〔ライ〕ピン蛍光(抗体) **CLF**
カルジオリ〔ライ〕ピン自然レシチン **CNL**
カルジオリ〔ライ〕ピン絮状〔綿状〕テスト **CFT**
カルジオリ〔ライ〕ピン補体結合 **CCF**
カルシジオール **25-OHD_3, 25(OH)D_3**
カルシトニン **CT**
カルシトニン遺伝子関連ペプチド **CGRP**
カルジノフィリン **CZ**
カルシノーマ 125(卵巣癌腫瘍マーカー) **CA125**
カルシノーマ 19-9(膵癌腫瘍マーカー) **CA19-9**
カルシノーマ 50(膵癌・胆嚢癌腫瘍マーカー) **CA50**
ガルスアデノ様ウイルス **GAL**
カルタゲナー症候群 **KS**
カルチノイド腫瘍 **cd**

カルチノイド症候群 **CS**
カルニチンアシル転移酵素 **CAT**
カルニチンパルミトイル転移酵素〔トランスフェラーゼ〕欠損症 **CPT deficiency**
カルニチンパルミトイルトランスフェラーゼ **CPT**
カルバジルキノン **CQ**
ガルバーニ現象 **galv.**
ガルバーニ電流の **Galv, galv**
カルバマゼピン **CBZ**
カルバマゾール **CBZ**
カルバミルリン酸合成酵素欠損症 **CPS**
カルバモイル **Cbm**
カルバモイルリン酸合成酵素欠損症 **CPSD**
カルビマゾール **CGI**
カルフェシリン **CFPC, P-CBPC**
カルフェシリンナトリウム,カルベニシリンフェニルナトリウム **P-CBPC**
カルベニシリン **CB, CBCN**
カルボキシヘモグロビン **COBH**
カルボキシベンジルペニシリン=カルベニシリン **CBPC**
カルボキシメチル **CM**
カルボキシメチルセルロース **CMC, CM-cellulose, COMC**
カルボキシメチルセルロースナトリウム **CMC-Na**
カルボキシル運搬蛋白質 **CCP**
カルボコン **CQ**
カルボニルサリチルアミド **CSA**
カルボニルシアニド-*m*-クロロフェニルヒドラゾン **CCCP**
カルボニルシアニド-*p*-トリフルオロメトキシフェニルヒドラゾン **FCCP**
カルボプラチン,ドキソルビシン,シクロホスファミド **CDC**
(塩化)カルボベンゾキシ **Cbz**
カルボマイシン **CRM**
カルボールフクシン **CF**
カルマン(症候群) **KAL**
カルマン症候群 **KS**
カルムスチン,ビンクリスチン(=オンコビン),プロカルバジン,プレドニゾン **BOPD**
カルメット・ゲラン・ウシ結核菌(ワクチン) **BCG**
カルメット・ゲラン桿菌(ワクチン) **BCG**
カルモジュリン **CaM**
カルモナム **CRMN**
カルノフスキー行動〔活動〕評価スケール **KPS**
カルモフール **HCFU**
カレハ嗅覚小島 **IsC**
ガレン静脈動脈瘤性拡張 **VGAD**
ガレン静脈動脈瘤性奇形 **VAGM**
カロリー **C, c, cal**
カロリー計算 **Cal Ct, cal.ct**
カロリー制限された **CR**
カロリンスカ人格尺度 **KSP**
ガロン **C, cong., gal, gal.**
ガロン/秒 **g/s**
ガロン/分 **gal/min, g/m**
カーン・シンボルテスト(=作業式投影法) **KTSA**
ガングリオン **G, gang, gangl, Ggl**
ガンシクロビル **GANC, GCV**
カンジダ(属) **C, CAN**
カンジダ菌 **CA**
カンジダ爪(甲)真菌症 **CO**
カンジダ代謝性抗原 **CMA**
カンタベリーアルコール中毒スクリーニング検査 **CAST**
カーン知能検査 **KIT**
ガンディー・ナンタ病 **GN**
カンデラ **cd**
カンフル加アヘンチンキ **PG**
カンボジア国立マラリアセンター **CNM**
ガンマ **Gm**
ガンマ線 **γ, GR**
かかと穿刺血液ガス **HSBG**
かかりつけ医を訪ねよ **SYD**
かかりつけの医師 **PMD**
かぜウイルス **CC-Virus**
かたさき **A**
かたまりにする **agl**
かたより試験 **DT**
からっぽ **MT**
下位運動(ニューロン) **LM**
下位運動ニューロン **LMN**
下位運動ニューロン病変 **LMNL**

か

下位垂直帝王切開(術) **LVCS**
下咽頭 **HP, Ph, ph**
下咽頭癌 **HPC**
下咽頭後壁癌 **PWC**
下右(部)1/4区 **LRQ**
下オリーブ核 **IO**
下外部1/4区 **LOQ**
下角 **IA**
下眼瞼 **LL**
下眼瞼・右眼 **LLOD, LLRE**
下眼瞼・左眼 **LLLE, LLOS**
下顎運動路軌跡記録装置 **MKG**
下顎開反射 **JOR**
下顎癌 **UKK**
下顎挙出器具 **MAP**
下顎骨 **mand**
下顎骨下の **SM, submand**
下顎骨骨折 **UKF**
下顎骨枝 **Mr**
下顎骨疼痛症候群 **MPDS**
下顎骨の **mand**
下顎枝矢状骨切り術 **SRO**
下顎(骨)整形外科整復器具 **MORA**
下顎(骨)体 **Mb**
下顎(骨)反射 **MR**
下顎反射 **JJ**
下丘 **IC**
下丘核 **NCI**
下気道 **LRT**
下気道疾患 **LRI, LRTI**
下記の **f, ff, fol, sq.**
下記のように **ut.inf.**
下限 **LL**
下限以下の **BLL**
下行結腸 **D, DC**
下行大動脈 **DAo, DecAo, Desc AO**
下行(性)の **desc**
下行の **desc**
下降 **desc**
下十二指腸角 **IDA**
下肢 **LE, L/E, L ext., l/ext, lx, lx.**
下肢挙上試験 **SLR test**
下肢伸展位挙上訓練 **SLR exercise**
下肢伸展挙上(試験) **SLR**
下肢切断(術) **LEA**
下肢長 **BL, TMD**
下斜筋 **IO**
下垂 **desc**
下垂萎縮肩症候群 **DSS**
下垂した **pend**
下垂体 **HY, hyp**
下垂体アデニン酸シクラーゼ活性ポリペプチド **PACAP**
下垂体オピオイドペプチド **POP**
下垂体茎中央隆起 **SME**
下垂体後葉 **DYN, HHL**
下垂体後葉(疾患) **PP**
下垂体後葉ホルモン **PPH**
下垂体性小人症 **PD**
下垂体性性腺刺激ホルモン **PG, PGH**
下垂体成長ホルモン **PGH**
下垂体性ヒト成長ホルモン **p-hGH**
下垂体切除(術) **hyp**
下垂体切除術 **HE**
下垂体切除性アロキサン糖尿病(患者) **HAD**
下垂体腺腫 **PA**
下垂体前葉 **ALH, ALP, Ant pit., ant.pit., AP, HVL**
下垂体前葉抽出物 **APE**
下垂体前葉反応 **APR, HVR**
下垂体前葉ホルモン **APH**
下垂体前葉類似物質 **APL**
下垂体中葉 **HML**
下垂体摘出術を受けた **HPX, HX**
下垂体の **pit**
下垂体副腎刺激ホルモン **PATH**
下垂体副腎の **PA**
下垂体副腎皮質系 **PAS**
下垂体抑制系 **PIS**
下膵十二指腸動脈 **IPDA**
下前膵十二指腸静脈 **VPDIA**
下前腸骨棘 **AIIS**
下前頭回 **IFG**
下側右心房 **LLRA**
下側頭動脈 **ITA**
下大静脈 **IVC, IVS**
下腿 **BK, BKTT, US**
下腿外方捻転 **Latero**
下腿周長 **USU**
下腿切断 **BKA, BK AMP**
下腿内方捻転 **Medio**
下腿歩行可能ギプス **BKWP**
下中隔右心房 **LSRA**
下直筋 **IR**
下腸間膜静脈 **IMV**
下腸間膜神経節 **IMG**
下腸間膜動脈 **IMA, IRA**
下殿神経 **IGN**
下塗層 **UC**
下内(部)1/4区 **LIQ**
下(方)の **INF, inf, infer**
下半(分) **LH**
下半身陰圧 **LBNP**
下半身陽圧負荷 **LBPP**

下背部(痛)　**LB**
下背部屈曲　**LBB**
下背部痛　**LBP**
下肺　**LL**
下肺動脈　**PAI**
下鼻甲介　**inf.turb, UM**
下鼻側(部)1/4区　**INQ**
下鼻動脈　**INA**
下部歯間の　**IDI, IdI**
下部消化管クローン病　**LICD**
下部食道(圧)　**LEP**
下部食道括約筋　**LES**
下部食道括約筋圧　**LESP**
下部正中　**LML**
下部直腸　**Rb**
下部尿路腫瘍　**LUTT**
下腹部手術　**LAS**
下腹壁動脈　**IEA**
下壁心筋梗塞　**Inf.MI**
下壁心筋梗塞(症)　**IMI**
下方から　**v.u.**
下方管理限界　**LCL**
下方注視　**DG**
下方と上方の　**L & U**
下方プリズム基底　**BD**
下葉　**LL**
下葉気管支　**LLB**
化学　**chem**
化学・温熱・放射線療法　**CHR**
化学・細菌・核の　**CBN**
化学・細菌・放射能・核の　**CBRN**
化学・細菌・放射能機関　**CBRA**
化学・細菌・放射能研究室　**CBRL**
化学・細菌・放射能の　**CBR**
化学・細菌・放射能要素　**CBRE**
化学・生物学活性度　**CBA**
化学・生物学事故防止計画　**CBAICP**
化学・生物学の　**CB**
化学・生物兵器戦　**CBW**
化学イオン化(法)　**CI**
化学エネルギー　**CE**
化学学士　**B.C.S.**
化学活性　**A**
化学気相成長法　**CVD**
化学結合効果　**CBE**
化学合成培地　**CDM**
化学構造自動構造決定システム　**CHEMICS**
化学士　**B.C., B.Ch., B.S.Ch**
化学者　**chem**
化学者と薬学者　**C & D**
化学受容器引金帯　**CTZ**
化学情報およびデータシステム　**CIDS**
化学情報検索システム　**CIS**
化学抄録サービス　**CAS**
化学抄録サービス源索引　**CASSI**
化学製造工業　**CPI**
化学・生物・放射性物質・核　**CBRN**
化学戦　**CW**
化学走性　**CT, CTX**
化学走性活性　**CTA**
化学走性産出因子　**CGF**
化学抽出物　**CA**
化学的交感神経切除(術)　**CS**
化学的酸素必要量　**COD**
化学的純粋　**CP**
化学的生物学的放射線医学的　**CBR**
化学的分析のためのX線電子分光法　**ESCA**
化学伝達物質　**CM**
化学伝達物質遊離抑制薬　**ICMR**
化学と化学技術　**C & CT**
化学の　**chem, cml**
化学媒体　**CM**
化学発光　**CL**
化学発光検出超臨界流体フローインジェクション分析法　**SCF-FIA/CL**
化学発光酵素免疫(測定)法　**CLEIA**
化学発光免疫測定〔分析〕法　**CLIA**
化学物質安全性データシート　**MSDS**
化学物質安全性評価法検討会　**SGOMSEC**
化学物質頻回曝露感度症候群　**MCSS**
化学兵器　**CW**
化学平衡を考慮した因子分析法　**FAEC**
化学遊走　**CM**
化学療法　**Chem, chem, chemo, Chemother, CT**
化学療法係数　**CHI**
化学療法係数〔指数〕　**CC**
化学療法指数　**CI**
化学療法誘発(性)嘔気〔嘔吐〕　**CINE**
化合物　**C, cmpd, CO, COMP, COMP., compd, compd., CP, CPD, cpd, cpds**
化成帯　**TMZ**
化膿菌培養　**PyC**
化膿性汗腺炎　**HS**
化膿性急性中耳炎　**OMSA**
化膿性心膜炎　**PP**
化膿性中耳炎　**POT**
化膿性の　**supp**
化膿性連鎖球菌外毒素　**SPE**
化膿の　**pur**
火炎状母斑　**PWS**

火傷患者収容室　**BU**
加圧　**compr，comprn**
加圧呼吸　**PB**
加圧呼吸補助器　**PBA**
加圧式定量噴霧吸入器　**PMDI**
加減抵抗器　**rheo**
加算平均心電図法　**SAE**
加算平均誘発電位　**AEP**
加重　**sum**
加重非線形最小二乗(法)　**WNLS**
加水分解　**H**
加速(度)　**AC，ac，Acc，acc，accel**
加速器質量分析計　**AMS**
加速時間　**AcT**
加速性心室固有リズム　**AIVR**
加速増殖野　**AGA**
加速〔促進〕度(現象)　**a.**
加速凍結乾燥　**AFD**
加速歩行　**fest**
加速力　**G forces，G-forces**
加熱・換気・空調　**HVAC**
加熱・換気・冷却　**HV & C**
加熱気管切開カラー　**HTC**
加熱致死時間　**TDT**
加熱と換気　**HTVT**
加熱プローブユニット　**HPU**
加リン酸分解酵素　**PR**
加齢(性)黄斑変性(症)　**ARMD**
加齢研究進歩のための協会　**AAAR**
可及的速やかに　**AEC**
可逆性虚血性神経障害　**RIND**
可逆性〔回復性〕虚血性神経脱落〔傷害〕　**RIND**
可逆性虚血発作　**RIA**
可逆性閉塞正気道疾患　**ROAD**
可視虹彩(直)径　**VID**
可視性　**v**
可視的アナログ式疼痛評価　**VAPS**
可塑性　**pl**
可聴域外の(音響)　**UA**
可聴閾値下　**IA**
可聴周波数　**af，audio**
可聴胎児心音　**FHH**
可動域　**RM**
(関節)可動域訓練　**ROME**
可動域正常範囲内　**ROM WNL**
(関節)可動域テスト　**ROMT，ROM-T**
可動遺伝要素　**MGE**
可動化　**mob**
可動性　**mob，mobil**
可動制限母趾　**HL**
可動性の　**mob**
可動性ブロッカー付き一側肺換気用気管内チューブ　**ETMB**
可動性腕支持用具　**MAS**
可撓性モード　**F mode**
可撓(性)の　**flex，flx**
可能性　**poss**
可能な　**poss**
可搬型媒体データ交換規約　**PDI**
可搬性インスリン注入ポンプ　**PIIP**
可搬性超低温液化ガス容器　**LGC**
可搬性の　**port**
可変時間　**VT**
可変性表面糖蛋白　**VSG**
可変の　**V，var**
可変反応　**VR**
可変部　**V**
可変部 H 鎖ドメイン　V_H
可変部 L 鎖ドメイン　V_L
可変部領域　**V region，V-region**
可溶性　**S，soly**
可溶性，貯蔵型　**SR**
可溶性・貯蔵型・添加ジヒドロストレプトマイシン　**SRD**
可溶性 CD23 の遺伝子組換え合成物　**rsCD23**
可溶性 IL-6 受容体　**sIL-6R**
可溶性 TNF 受容体　**TNF-sR1**
可溶性アコニターゼ　**ACO-S**
可溶性インスリン　**SI，S.I.**
可溶性核抗原　**ENA**
可溶性核蛋白　**SNP**
可溶性抗原　**S antigen**
可溶性抗原螢光抗体(試験)　**SAFA**
可溶性細胞質蛋白　**SCP**
可溶性ゼラチン　**SG**
可溶性チミジンキナーゼ　**TK1，TKS**
可溶性糖蛋白　**SGP**
可溶性パウダー　**WP**
可溶性ヒトリンパ球抗原　**SHA**
可溶性フィブリンモノマー　**SFM**
可溶性フィブリンモノマー複合体　**SFMC**
可溶性免疫反応抑制因子　**SIRS**
可溶性抑制因子　**SSF**
可溶性リボ核酸　**SRNA，sRNA**
可溶性リンゴ酸脱水素酵素　**MDH1，MDHS**
可溶な　**S**
可溶(性)の　**sol.**
仮声帯　**FC，TB**

(房水流出率の)仮性C値 **Cps**
仮性球麻痺 **PBP**
仮性狂犬病ウイルス **PRV**
仮性早熟 **PPP**
仮説 **hyp, hypoth**
仮説の **hyp**
仮想現実 **VR**
仮想装置 **VI**
花粉指数 **pol ind**
改良型亜全胃温存膵頭十二指腸切除術 **MSSPPD**
価値に応じて **ad val.**
価値のある **val**
果汁 **FJ**
果糖 **Fru**
果糖-一リン酸 **F-1-P, F1P**
果糖6-リン酸 **F-6-P, F6P**
果糖負荷試験 **FTT**
画像交換フォーマット **GIF**
画像の保存と運送 **ISAC**
画像ファイリングシステム **IS & C**
画像保管管理システム **PACS**
芽球化因子 **BF**
芽球増多を伴った不応性貧血 **RAEB**
芽球増多を伴った不応性貧血の白血病化 **RAEB-t**
科 **DPT**
科学 **SC, sc, Sci, sci**
科学イオン化質量分析 **CI-MS**
科学引用索引 **SCI**
科学技術庁 **STA**
科学技術データ委員会 **CODSAT**
科学士 **BS**
科学情報ネットワーク **SINET**
科学的・産業的・医学的写真研究室 **SIMPL**
科学的研究 **SR**
科学的根拠に基づいた医学 **EBM**
科学的診断学士 **MSD**
科学的な **SC, sc, Sci, sci**
科学データ記録器 **SDR**
科学倫理調査室 **OSI**
架橋壊死 **BN**
架橋肝壊死 **BHN**
架橋剤 **DSS**
架橋フィブリン分解生成物 **XLFDP**
臥位の **LY, ly, ly.**
臥床の **recumb**
変える **mod, mod.**
家禽ペストウイルス **FPV**
家事 **hskpg.**
家族 **F, Fam, fam**
家族関係全国委員会 **NCFR**
家族計画 **FP, FPP**
家族計画センター **FPC**
家族性アミロイド多発性ニューロパシー **FAP**
家族性アルツハイマー病 **FAD**
家族性異常アポB血症 **FDB**
家族生活・性教育計画 **FLSEP**
家族性筋萎縮性側索硬化症 **FALS**
家族性痙性対麻痺 **FSP**
家族性血球貪食リンパ組織球症 **FEL**
家族性血漿蛋白過剰過サイロキシン血症 **FDH**
家族性原発性肺高血圧 **FPPH**
家族性高コレステロール血症 **FH, FHC, FHLDL**
家族性高トリグリセリド血症 **FHTG**
家族性黒内障性白痴 **FAI**
家族性混合性高脂血症 **FCHL**
家族性脂質異常高血圧 **FDH**
家族性若年性腎症 **FJN**
家族性若年性大腸ポリポーシス **FJPC**
家族性周期性四肢麻痺 **Fam per.par.**
家族性自律神経障害 **FD**
家族性滲出性硝子体網膜症 **FEVR**
家族性成長ホルモン欠損症 **IGHD**
家族性大腸腺腫症 **FAC, FAP**
家族性大腸ポリポーシス **FPC**
家族性多発性内分泌新生物 **FMEN**
家族性地中海熱 **FMF**
家族性低βリポ蛋白血症 **FHBLP**
家族性低カルシウム尿性高カルシウム血症 **FHH**
家族性低形成貧血 **FHA**
家族性内臓筋障害 **FVM**
家族性脳血管痴呆症 **CADASIL**
家族性片麻痺性片頭痛 **FHM**
家族評価書式 **FEF**
家族福祉のための協会 **AFW**
家族療法 **FT**
家族歴 **FA, Fa, fam.hist, FH, F Hx, FHx**
家族歴あり **FHP**

家畜の　**dom**
家畜用の　**ad us.vet.**
家庭医　**fam.doc, Fam phys, fam phys, FD, FMD, FP, GP**
家庭医学　**FP**
家庭医学開業医　**FP**
家庭医助手　**AHP**
家庭医のいない　**NFD, NFP**
家庭医療計画　**FMP**
家庭血糖モニター　**HBGM**
(青年期病歴上の)家庭生活・教育水準・活動・薬物使用・性的行動・自殺観念/企図　**HEADSS**
家庭治療　**HC**
家庭内健康管理　**HHC**
家庭の　**dom**
家庭訪問　**HV**
家庭〔在宅〕用経腸高カロリー輸液　**HEH**
家兎血清アルブミン　**RSA**
家兎抗ヒトチモサイトグロブリン　**RATG**
家兎単位　**KE, Rab.U**
荷重　**WB, Wb**
荷電粒子励起X線分光法　**PIXE**
華氏(温度)　**°F, FAHR, Fahr, F.F**
書かれた指示　**WO, W/O**
書かれたように調剤せよ　**DAW**
書け　**S.**
掛け算　**mult**
渦流　**whp, whpl, WP**
渦流・マッサージ・運動　**WMX**
渦流浴　**WHPB, WPB**
過運動性心症候群　**HKH-syndrome**
過塩素酸　**PCA**
過オキシウム増殖活性化受容体要素　**PPRE**
過オキシゾーム増殖活性化受容体　**PPAR**
過ヨウ素酸リジンパラホルムアルデヒド　**PLP**
過活動児童〔小児〕症候群　**HACS**
過活動上斜筋　**OASO**
過活動上直筋　**OASR**
過換気　**HV, hypervent, OV**
過換気後無呼吸　**PHVA**
過換気症候群　**HVS**
過屈曲損傷　**HF inj**
過血糖性糖原分解因子　**HGF**
過形成　**H**
過形成関節症　**HOA**
過形成細胞　**HC**
過形成性過分泌性胃疾患　**HHG**
過形成節　**HN**
過形成点　**HPF**
過形成胞状結節　**HAN**
過去　**p**
過呼吸　**HV, hypervent**
過誤　**E, err**
過酸化亜鉛　**ZPO**
過酸化ジクミル　**DCP**
過酸化脂質　**LPO**
過酸化水素　**diox, H_2O_2**
過酸化物価　**POV**
過酸化物産生指数　**SPI**
過小体重児　**LFG infant, SFD infant**
過伸展損傷　**HE inj.**
過剰　**Ex, ex, Xs**
過剰運動性症候群　**HMS**
過剰栄養　**hyperal**
過剰塩基　**BE**
過剰換気　**EV**
過剰相対リスク　**ERP**
過剰側方(外側)圧迫症候群　**ELPS**
過剰昼間睡眠　**EDS**
過剰乳酸　**XL**
過剰熱産生　**EHP**
過熟妊娠症候群　**PS**
過成長刺激因子　**OSF**
過大駆出率　**XEF**
過大体重児　**HFD infant, LFD infant, LGA infant**
過程　**prcs, proc**
過度に負荷する　**ovld**
過度の　**o'er**
過渡反射格子法　**TRG**
過熱　**OVH**
過反応性マラリア性脾腫　**HMS**
過半数　**maj**
過敏(性)結腸　**IC**
過敏症　**A, HS**
過敏性　**A, HS**
過敏性胃症候群　**ISS**
過敏性頸動脈洞症候群　**HCSS**
過敏性血管炎　**HA, HV**
過敏性大腸症候群　**ICS**
過敏性腸疾患　**IBD**
過敏性(大)腸症候群　**IBS**
過敏性肺(臓)炎パネル　**HSP**
過敏性肺疾患　**HLD**
過敏性肺臓炎　**HP**
過敏性排尿症候群　**IVS**
過敏性肺胞炎　**HA**
過敏毒阻害剤　**AI**
過敏の　**hypersens**
過分極双極細胞　**HPBC**
過分葉好中球　**HYPP**
過マンガン酸カリウム　**$KMnO_4$**
過免疫抗天然痘 γ グロブ

リン **HAGG**
過ヨウ素酸銀メテナミン **PASM**
過ヨウ素酸シッフ(染色) **PAS**
過ヨウ素酸シッフ・アルシアンブルー複合染色(法) **PAS-AB**
過ヨウ素酸シッフヘマトキシリン **PASH**
過ヨウ素酸シッフ法 **PAST**
過ヨウ素酸ナトリウムリジン加2%パラホルムアルデヒド溶液 **PLP**
過ヨウ素酸メセナミン銀染色 **PAM**
過量 **OD**
過量の **OD'd, oding**
寡夫 **W, w**
窩 **cav, F**
課 **C**
蝸牛 **C**
蝸牛核 **CN**
蝸牛核活動電位 **CANAP**
蝸牛電位 **CP**
蝸牛瞳孔反応 **CPR**
蝸牛内直流電位 **EP**
蝸牛内電位 **EP**
蝸牛内の **i coch**
蝸牛マイクロフォニックス・スパイラログラフィ **CMS**
蝸牛マイクロホン作用 **CM**
蝸電計 **EcochG, ECochG**
蝸電図 **EcochG, ECochG**
蝸電図(検査)法 **EcochG, ECochG**
顆間の **intercond**
顆上顎骨装具 **STP**
顆上ソケット下腿義足 **PTES, PTS**
顆上はめ込み脛骨義足 **PTS**
顆粒 **G, GRN**
顆粒円柱 **GC**
顆粒化 **gran**
顆粒球 **GR**
顆粒球・赤血球・巨核球・大食細胞コロニー形成単位 **GEMM-CFU**
顆粒球・大食細胞 **GM**
顆粒球・大食細胞コロニー形成細胞 **GM-CFC**
顆粒球・大食細胞コロニー形成ユニット **GM-CFU**
顆粒球・大食細胞コロニー刺激因子 **GM-CSF**
顆粒球：赤芽球比 **G：E**
顆粒球凝集 **Ga**
顆粒球系/赤芽球系(比) **G/E**
顆粒球減少性アンギナ **AA**
顆粒球抗体検出螢光(法) **GIFT**
顆粒球交替率 **GTR**
顆粒球コロニー刺激因子 **G-CSF**
顆粒球消失率 **GDR**
顆粒球染色体分裂像 **Gm**
顆粒球増多促進因子 **GPF**
顆粒球特異抗核因子 **GSANF**
顆粒球特異抗核抗原 **GS-ANA**
顆粒球の辺縁部プール **MGP**
顆粒球半減時間 **GDRT 1/2**
顆粒球物質 **GS**
顆粒球マクロファージコロニー形成単位 **CFU-GM**
顆粒球免疫螢光検査 **GIFT**
顆粒球様システイン物質 **GS**
顆粒球抑制リンパ球(＝LGL様細胞) **GIL**
顆粒形成時間 **GT**
顆粒細胞 **GC**
顆粒細胞腫 **GCT**
顆粒層 **GL, GRL**
顆粒の **gran**
顆粒膜細胞 **GC**
顆粒リンパ球増多症 **GLPD**
下位と上位の **L & U**
介在する **intermed**
介在ニューロン **IN**
介在配列(＝イントロン) **IVS**
介在腹部圧迫・心肺蘇生 **IAC-CPR**
外因子 **EF**
外因性アレルギー肺胞炎 **EAA**
外因性中耳炎 **EOM**
外因性の **exog**
外因性プラスミノゲン賦活体 **EPA**
外陰(部)上皮内新生物 **VIN**
外陰部遮断 **PB**
外陰部腟前庭炎 **VVS**
外陰部と腟 **V & V**
外陰部の **Pdl, PUD**
外陰扁平上皮癌 **SCV**
外陰誘発反応 **PER**
外エナメル上皮 **OEE**
外果 **LM**
外果ひだ **LMF**
外界の **ext, ext.**
外眼(筋)運動 **XOM**
外眼角耳孔線 **CML**
外眼筋 **EOM**
外眼筋無傷 **EOMI**
外観 **asp**

外気温度　**OAT**
外血液・網膜関門　**OBRB**
外径　**ED, OD**
外限界膜　**ELM**
外頸・内頸動脈　**EC-IC**
外頸動脈　**EC, ECA**
外国医学校卒業者試験教育委員会　**ECFMG**
外国医科大学卒業生　**FMG**
外国の　**for**
外後頭隆起点　**In**
外骨症　**exos**
外耳　**EE**
外耳炎　**EO, OE, O.ext.**
外耳道　**EAC, EAM, OEC**
外耳道保存鼓室形成手術　**CAT**
外耳の　**ext.aud**
外斜位　**EXO, X**
外斜位斜視　**XP-T**
外斜位の　**X**
外斜角　**OC**
外斜視　**XP, XT**
外斜視(性)の　**XT**
外傷　**inj, tr, trau, WD, wd, wds, WND, wnd**
外傷(部位)　**les**
外傷一次救命救急処置　**BTLS**
外傷救急センター　**T & EC**
外傷外科(学)　**TrS**
外傷後眼内炎　**PTE**
外傷後健忘　**PTA**
外傷後症候群　**PTS**
外傷後進行性脊髄障害　**PTPM**
外傷後髄膜炎　**PTM**
(心的)外傷後ストレス障害　**PTSD**
外傷後線維筋痛症　**PTFS**
外傷後てんかん　**PTE**
外傷後の　**post traum**
外傷後脳症候群　**PTBS**
外傷後肺不全　**PTPI**
外傷死　**DOI**
外傷重症度係数　**ISI**
外傷重症度スコア　**ISS**
外傷集中治療室　**TICU**
外傷性頸部症候群　**TCS**
外傷性股関節脱臼　**TDH**
外傷性骨端性内反股　**TECV**
外傷性の　**trau**
外傷性肺浮腫　**IPE**
外傷センター　**TC**
外傷表　**TS**
外生殖器　**EG**
外性器　**EG**
外旋　**ER, ext.rot**
外側　**os**
外側咽頭壁　**LPW**
外側延髄症候群　**LMS**
外側核　**L**
外側陥凹狭窄(症)　**LRS**
外側陥凹症候群　**LRS**
外側広(筋)　**LVL**
外側視床下部　**LH**
外側膝状核　**LGN**
外側膝状体　**LGB**
外側膝状体核　**NCGL**
外側膝状体の腹側核　**VLG**
外側静脈洞　**LVS**
外側静脈洞血栓症静脈炎　**LST**
外側脊髄視床路　**LST, LST tract**
外側仙骨静脈　**LSV**
外側前庭脊髄路　**LVST**
外側側副靭帯　**FCL, LCL**
外側腟壁　**LVW**
外側の　**lat, lat.**
外側半月(板)切除(術)　**lat.men.**
外側毛帯　**LL**
外側網様核　**RL**
外側翼状突起　**LPP**
外側翼突筋　**LPM**
外側らせん線維　**OSF**
外直(筋)　**LR**
外腸骨静脈　**EIV**
外腸骨動脈　**EIA**
外的経路阻害物　**EPI**
外的動脈加圧強化法　**EECP**
外的力学的効率　**EME**
外転(筋)　**ABD, Abd, abd, abd.**
外転運動　**ABD, Abd, abd, abd.**
外転症　**EV, ev**
外転する　**ABD, Abd, abd, abd.**
外套細胞リンパ腫　**MCL**
外套層　**MZ**
外套帯リンパ腫　**MZL**
外内側　**LM**
外尿道括約筋　**EUS**
外尿道括約筋筋電図測定　**EUS emg**
外尿道口　**EUM**
外妊　**EP**
外反膝　**X-Bein, X-leg**
外反〔外転〕母趾　**HAV**
外反母趾　**HA, HV**
外反母趾角　**HVA**
外胚葉性形成異常(異形成)・欠指・黄斑変性(症候群)　**EEM**
外皮　**env, INTEG**
外鼻孔　**N, n.**
外部医師　**OSD**
外部精密査定　**EQA**
外部抵抗　**ER**
外部の　**ext, ext.**
外部放射線照射療法　**EBRT**
外壁　**OW, ow**

外方プリズム基底　**BO**
外膜　**ADV, OM**
外膜蛋白　**EMP, OMP**
外有毛細胞　**OHC**
外用　**ad us.ext., ad us.exter., pro us.ext., us.ext.**
外用のみ　**FEUO**
外用薬と有色化粧品　**ext & cc**
外来　**CL, Cl, CLIN, Clin, clin., OPD**
外来患者　**MOP, OP, O/P, OPT**
外来患者基礎代謝率　**XBM**
外来患者治療　**OPT**
外来患者として　**OPB**
外来抗体に対する異型抗体　**HAMA**
外来サービス　**OPS**
外来手術　**OPS**
外来小児科学会　**APA**
外来診療所　**OPC**
外来に再来する　**TRO**
外来(通院)の　**ambul**
外来〔通院〕の　**Amb, amb.**
外来病院　**OH**
外来用薬局　**OPD**
外リンパフィステル症候群　**PLFS**
会員　**mem**
会期　**Sess**
会議　**conf, cong, cong.**
会計年度　**FY**
会社　**INC, Inc, Inc., inc.**
会報　**bull, bull., proc, trans**
会話音声　**CV**
会話自動訓練器　**SAID**
会話妨害レベル　**SIL**
回外　**ever, sup, SUP, sup.**
回外(筋)　**sup, SUP, sup.**
回帰の　**Recip, recip.**
回使用中間面　**GUI**
回旋　**rot, rot.**
回旋筋　**rot, rot.**
回旋枝　**CB, CIX, CX**
回旋した　**circum**
回旋性線状魚鱗癬　**ILC**
回虫　**Asc**
回虫抗原　**AA**
回腸　**I, IL**
回腸S状結腸吻合　**ISA**
回腸結腸動脈　**ICA**
回腸肛門吻合(術)　**IAA**
回腸(囊)肛門吻合術　**IPAA**
回腸直腸吻合術　**IRA**
回腸バイパス　**IB**
回腸分節　**IS**
回転　**REV, rev., rot, rot.**
回転/分　**rev/min**
回転エコー二重共鳴　**REDOR**
回転(性)眼振　**ny.rot**
回転眼振　**rot.ny, rot.nystag**
回転筋　**rot, rot.**
回転する　**rot, rot.**
回転側彎症　**rotoscol**
回転と多振動の結合した分光測定　**CRAMPS**
回転の　**rot, rot.**
回転パターンテスト　**RPT**
回内　**PRO, pron**
回内/回外　**pron/sup**
回内する　**pron**
回復　**rec, recov**
回復期　**conv**
回復期(の)　**CS**
回復期患者　**CS**
回復期の　**conv**
回復させる　**Rehab, rehab, rehab.**
回復時間　**RT**
回復指数　**RQ, R.Q.**
回復した　**m**
回復室　**RR**
回復室に戻る　**RTRR**
回復状態　**CS**
回復する　**recov**
回復良好　**GR**
回盲接合部　**ICJ**
回路　**cct, cir, cir., Circ, circ**
回路外気化器　**VOC**
回路開始　**O**
回路条件抑制因子　**CCI**
回路内気化器　**VIC**
快適域値　**CL**
快適大きさ曲線　**MCL**
快適な　**comf**
改善　**Imp, imp, impr, IMPRV, impvt**
改善した　**Imp, imp, impr**
改善する　**Imp, imp, impr**
改訂　**REV, rev.**
改訂した　**rect, rect.**
改訂する　**REV, rev.**
改訂長谷川式簡易知能評価スケール　**HDS-R**
改訂版　**rev ed**
改良する　**imv**
改良タイロード液　**MTS**
海外医学校卒業生医師試験　**FMGEMS**
海外協力リハビリテーション救助要請　**CORRA**
海外視力障害者のための米国財団　**AFOB**
海水　**aq.mar., SW**
海水浴　**bal.mar., BM, B.M., b.m.**
(脳の)海馬　**H**

海馬 **HC, HIP, HIPP**
(脳の)海馬釆(=さい) **FH**
海馬シナプス血漿膜 **HSPM**
海馬錐体細胞 **HPC**
海綿状脳症 **SE**
海綿静脈洞 **CS**
海綿静脈洞血栓症 **CST**
海綿静脈洞浸潤 **CSI**
界面活性剤 **SAA**
皆無 **nil.**
咳嗽反射 **CR**
絵画完成テスト **PCT**
絵画空想法 **PRT**
絵画語い発達検査(法) **PVT**
絵画創作(=性格テストの1つ) **MAPS**
絵画積木(知能)検査 **PBT**
絵画(主題)統覚検査 **TAT**
絵画同定による単語了解度 **WIPI**
絵画物語検査 **BGT**
絵画物語テスト **PST**
絵画欲求不満試験 **PFT**
絵画欲求不満テスト **P-F study, PF Study**
開眼 **EO**
開眼効果 **EO**
開眼失行 **ALO**
開環状DNA **open cDNA**
開胸式心臓圧迫 **OCCC**
開胸式心肺蘇生術 **OCCPR**
開胸式心マッサージ(法) **OCCM**
開業 **prac**
開業医 **PRACT**
開業医管理会社 **PMC**
開業医連合[英国] **MPU**
開業外科医助手 **A.H.S.**
開業免許 **L**
開業有資格者 **Lic Med**
開口 **O**
開口数 **NA**
開散 **div, div.**
開心術 **OH, OHS**
開心術回復室 **OHRR**
開始 **opng**
開始因子 **IF**
開存の **pat, pat.**
開頭(術) **crani**
開発業務受託機関 **CRO**
開発する **dev**
開腹(術) **LAP, lap, lap.**
開腹下肝外胆管ドレナージ **LBD**
開腹下肝生検 **OLB**
開放・閉鎖・開放 **OCO**
開放角緑内障 **OAG**
開放管系 **OCS**
開放性伸展 **ER**
開放椎間関節 **OAJ**
開放点滴 **OD**
開放二分脊椎 **SBA**
解雇された **dism**
解雇する **dism**
解除 **canc**
解除と加入 **OAO**
解像力 **def**
解答 **ans**
解剖 **dissec**
解剖(学) **An, Anat, anat**
解剖学的死腔 **ADS, Vd anat**
解剖学的死腔換気 **$V_D$an**
解剖学的死腔容積 **$V_D$an**
解剖学的な **Anat, anat**
解剖学的容積 **VA**
解剖学用語 **NA**
解剖(学)と生理(学) **A & P**
解剖(学)の **Anat, anat**
解離 **dissoc**
解離因子 **R factor**
解離する **dissoc**
解離性胸部大動脈瘤 **DTAA**
解離性上斜視 **DHT**
解離性脳動脈瘤 **CDA**
解離促進因子 **DAF**
解離定数 **K, K_d, pK**
塊 **mas., mass, mass.**
塊状の **mass, mass.**
概括重症度 **GSR**
潰瘍指数 **UI, Ul**
潰瘍指数Ⅰ～Ⅳ(度) **Ul-Ⅰ-Ⅳ**
潰瘍性大腸炎 **CU, UC**
潰瘍性直腸炎 **UP**
潰瘍性皮膚壊死 **UDN**
潰瘍性皮膚病 **UD**
潰瘍治癒の質 **QOUH**
潰瘍の **U**
顧みられない熱帯病 **NTDs**
顔 **F**
顔マスク **FM**
顔を伏せている **fc ly**
踵・膝・脛(試験) **HKS**
鏡 **mir**
牡蠣 **oys**
牡蠣末 **POS**
各眼で **OU, O.U., o.u.**
各眼に **OU, O.U., o.u.**
各自の **E**
各視野 **omni**
各変域 **omni**
各方向の **omni**
角 **c.**
角化棘細胞腫 **KA**
角化係数 **CI**
角化症パッチ **KP**
角化上皮 **K**
(屈曲)角形成 **Ang,**

ang.
角結膜炎　**KC**
角結膜炎を伴うアトピー性皮膚炎　**ADKC**
角視力　**AV**
角質化落屑性扁平化生　**KDSM**
角質細胞増殖因子　**KGF**
角質層　**SC**
角速度　**ω**
角膜・強膜・結膜　**csc**
角膜異栄養(症)　**CD**
角膜移植(片)　**CT**
角膜炎　**Kera**
角膜炎・魚鱗癬・難聴症候群　**KID**
角膜屈折矯正手術　**PRK**
角膜(曲率)計　**K**
角膜後面〔裏面〕沈着物　**KP**
角膜混濁　**CO**
角膜ジストロフィ　**CD**
角膜切除の予期的評価　**PERK**
角膜前涙液層破壊時間　**BUT**
角膜内血管進入　**V**
角膜内皮変性症　**ECD**
角膜内レンズ　**ICL**
角膜の大きさ　**CS**
角膜の瘢痕　**XS**
角膜白濁　**nebul.**
角膜放射状切開術　**RK**
角膜網膜電位　**CRP**
拡延　**Dil, dil.**
拡延性抑制　**SD**
拡散圧　**DP**
拡散強調画像　**DWI**
拡散係数　**D**
拡散定数　**D**
拡散能(力)　**D**
拡散箱　**DC**
拡散量　**D**
拡大　**Dil, dil., enl., exp, Mag, mag, magnif, X**
拡大根治乳房切除　**ERM**
拡大された　**enlgd**
拡大した　**enl.**
拡大していない　**NE**
拡大する　**enl., Mag, mag**
拡大難治性突然変異システム　**ARMS**
拡張　**dil, dilat**
拡張型心筋症　**DCM**
拡張〔弛緩〕期　**diast**
拡張期　**D**
拡張期圧　**DP**
拡張期圧時間係数　**DPTI**
(左(心)室)拡張期径　**DD**
拡張期血圧　**DBP**
(僧帽弁)拡張期後退速度　**DDR**
拡張期雑音　**DM, DS**
拡張期終期　**ED**
拡張期充満　**DFP**
拡張期心室内容積　**DVV**
拡張期大動脈圧　**DAP**
拡張〔弛緩〕期の　**dias, diast**
拡張期奔馬律　**dg**
拡張した　**dil, dist**
拡張終(末)期圧　**EDP**
拡張終(末)期径　**EDD**
拡張終期雑音　**LSM**
拡張終(末)期心室容量　**EDV**
拡張終(末)期(部分)長　**EDL**
拡張終(末)期負荷　**EDL**
拡張終(末)期(心臓)壁厚　**EDWTH**
拡張終(末)期容積　**EDV**
拡張終(末)期容積指数　**EDVI**
拡張初期雑音　**EDM**
拡張心　**EH**
拡張する　**dil, dilat**
拡張性の　**dist**
(頸管)拡張(子宮)掻爬(術)　**D & C**
拡張蛇行静脈　**VV**
拡張蛇行静脈結紮　**VV lig**
拡張中期雑音　**MDM**
拡張と吸引　**D & E**
(頸管)拡張(子宮)内容除去(術)　**D & E**
拡張末期径　**Dd**
学位　**D, d**
学位記　**dpl.**
学業成績年齢　**AA**
学習計画　**LS**
学習(能力)障害　**LD**
学習能力評価〔推定値〕　**ELP**
学習レディネス診断検査　**PREB**
学術情報者　**SS**
学術用語　**nomen**
学生　**stu**
学生健康・福祉事務局連合　**SHAWCO**
学生精神健康調査　**UPI**
学部　**Dept, dept**
学名　**nm, nomen**
学力考査　**AT**
学力指数　**AQ, A.Q.**
学力年齢　**AA**
核　**N, Nu, nuc, nucl**
核医学　**NM**
核医学技術　**NMT**
核異常指数　**DI**
核異性体転位　**IT**
核黄疸　**KI**
核外輸送シグナル　**NES**
核間眼筋麻痺　**INO**
核共鳴時の　**D**
核グロブリン封入(体)　**NGI**
核抗原　**NA**
核硬化症　**NS**
核細胞質(＝N/P 比)　**N/P ratio**

核酸　**NA**
核酸性蛋白抗原　**NAPA**
核酸ホスファターゼ　**NAP**
核小体　**Nu**
核小体前駆体　**NPB**
核磁気共鳴　**NMR**
核磁気共鳴映像〔画像〕　**NMRI**
核磁気共鳴顕微鏡　**NMR microscope**
核磁気共鳴スペクトロスコピー　**NMRS**
核磁気共鳴断層撮影法　**NMR-CT**
核磁気共鳴の低速回転で生じる側波帯の除去法　**TOSS**
核磁気共鳴分析　**NMR analysis**
核磁子　**μN**
核耐性赤色素　**NFR**
核袋　**NB**
核蛋白　**NP**
核内封入体　**INI**
核の　**n, nuc**
核のある　**nuc**
核脳血管造影フィルム　**NCA**
核濃縮指数　**KI, KPI, PI**
核反応分析　**NRA**
核封入体A型　**NITA**
核マトリックス蛋白　**NMP**
核膜　**NM**
核膜孔複合体　**NPC**
核リボ核蛋白　**nRNP**
核(性)RNA(＝リボ核酸)　**nRNA**
核・細胞質比　**NCR**
核/細胞質比　**N/C**
覚醒時体温　**WBT**
覚醒時に　**WA, W/A**
覚醒時膀胱容量　**ABC**
覚醒調節脳波　**V-EEG**
覚醒反応　**AR**
喀出する　**expt, expt.**
喀痰　**SP**
隔日　**q.a.d., QOD, q.o.d.**
隔日治療　**ADT**
隔日に　**alt.die., alt.dieb., dieb.alt.**
隔日療法　**ADT**
隔時に　**alt.h., alt.hor.**
隔週の　**biw**
隔壁　**S**
隔夜に　**alt.noc., alt.noct.**
隔離症・小耳症・裂(症候群)　**HMC**
隔離ベッド　**IB**
撹拌されにくい水の層　**UWL**
確実因子　**CF**
確定物質　**DS**
確認された　**C**
確認できる病気なし　**NID**
確率　**P**
確率誤差　**PE**
獲得された　**obtd**
獲得性免疫寛容　**AIT**
顎下腺　**SMG**
顎下腺レニン　**SGR**
顎下の　**SM, submand**
顎間固定　**IMF**
顎関節　**TMJ, TM jt.**
顎関節症候群　**TMJS**
顎関節疼痛性機能不全症候群　**TMJ-PDS**
顎顔面・口腔外科資格認定書　**DMFOS**
顎顔面口腔外科認定書　**Dip.MFOS**
(下)顎顔面骨形成不全(症)　**MFD**
顎口虫　**G**
顎舌骨の　**mylo**
顎前突(症)　**PROG**
顎二腹筋　**DM**
顎の　**TM**
数　**N, n, N, n., No, No., no., No., no., nos, Nr, Nr., num, Z**
数の　**num**
数える　**No, No., no.**
片側口唇口蓋裂　**UCLP**
片側小関節面脱臼または亜脱臼　**UID/S**
片側排泄欠如　**UAE**
片側〔半側〕不全麻痺　**HP**
片肺移植　**SLT**
片肺換気　**OLV**
片麻痺性片(側)頭痛　**HPM**
片耳　**AU, A.U., a.u., aur.**
片山貝(属)　**O**
肩　**SH, Sh, sh, shl, SHLD, shld, shldr, sho, should**
肩(関節)脱臼　**SD**
肩(関節)離開　**SD**
肩・肘・手関節・手指装具　**SEWHO**
肩・肘・手関節装具　**SEWO**
肩・肘装具　**SEO**
固い　**h, hrd**
固く充填されたカプセル　**HFC**
固める　**agl**
型　**T, Ty**
(血液)型と交叉〔差〕(適合)試験　**T & X**
型特異性(抗体)　**TS**
型特異性抗体　**TSA**
型特異的M(蛋白)　**TSM**
型不明心筋症　**UCM**
硬い　**dur., lapid., sld, sol.**
形　**F, f**

塊をつくれ **ft.mas.**
傾き **grad**
傍らの **JUXT, juxt**
合衆国の **AM, Am, Amer**
合併した **inc, inc.**
合併症 **CM, Cm, cm, COMP, comp, compic, compl, compl., Complic, complic**
合併症のない **no compl, uncomp, uncompl**
学会 **ACAD, acad**
学期 **Sess**
学校・大学能力試験 **SCA test**
学校前言語スケール **PLS**
学校能力試験 **SAT**
括約筋 **sph, sph.**
括約筋拡張 **SD**
括約筋張筋 **ST**
活性 **A, a, act, activ**
活性因子X **Xa**
活性化 **A, a**
活性化D因子＝補体第3成分プロアクチベータ転換酵素 **D**
活性化T細胞 **ATC**
活性化(賦活)凝固凝血時間 **ACT**
活性化凝固時間 **ACT**
活性化胸腺細胞 **ATC**
活性化する **actv**
活性化第II因子(＝トロンビン) **F II a**
活性型プロテインC **APC**
活性化による細胞死 **AICD**
活性化部分トロンボプラスチン時間 **APTT**
活性酸素種 **AOS**
活性代謝率 **AMR**
活性炭 **AC**
活性炭吸着塩素化合物 **AOCL**
活性炭血液灌流〔吸着〕 **CHP**
活性〔未変性〕トロポミオシン **nTM**
活性プロトロンビン複合物質 **APCC**
活性ペプシン **AP**
活性ワクチン **L vaccine**
活動 **A, a, act**
活動期 **Stage A**
活動亢進の **hyper A, hyperact.**
活動させる **anim**
活動(型)サルコイドーシス **AS**
活動指数 **AI**
活動状況 **PS**
活動睡眠 **AS**
活動性の **A, a, act**
活動性慢性肝炎 **ACH**
活動低下の **hypo A, hypoact**
活動電位 **AP**
活動電位持続(時間) **APD**
活動電位波高 **APA**
活動度 **A, a, act, activ**
活発な抵抗 **AR**
活用する **imv**
活力指数 **VI**
喀血 **hemop**
滑液 **SF**
滑液包内の **isy**
滑車神経核 **TN**
滑膜 **SM**
滑膜炎・痤瘡・膿疱症・骨化過剰骨髄炎 **SAPHO**
滑膜切除(術) **synov**
滑面小胞体 **SER, SM**
褐色(の) **Br, Br., brn**
褐色細胞腫 **BAT, PC, PCC, pheo, Pheo**
褐色細胞腫・甲状腺癌(症候群) **PTC**
株 **str**
壁 **w**
壁運動 **WM**
壁運動異常 **WMA**
壁運動研究 **WMS**
壁運動評点指数 **WMSI**
壁の厚さ **WT**
壁の凹み **N**
鎌(状)血球 **SS**
鎌状(赤)血球(血色素)D(病) **S-D**
鎌状細胞 **SS**
鎌状赤血球 **SC**
鎌状赤血球(血色素)C(病) **SC, S-C**
鎌状赤血球形成傾向 **SCT**
鎌状赤血球サラセミア **S-T, S-Thal**
鎌状赤血球肺症 **SCLD**
鎌状赤血球病 **SCD**
鎌状赤血球貧血 **SCA**
鎌状赤血球貧血検査 **SCAT**
鎌状赤血球ヘモグロビン **Hb S**
鎌状赤血球ヘモグロビンC **HbSC**
上小脳脚交叉 **DSC**
紙 **pa**
紙袋に入れて **ad chart.**
紙巻タバコ **cig**
紙巻タバコ喫煙者 **CS**
紙巻タバコ喫煙本数/日 **c/d**
粥に混ぜて **in pulm.**
硝子質の **HYLO**
体 **B**
仮診断 **PD**

か

仮診断クリニック　**PDC**
仮包帯　**PD**
軽い　**lev, lev.**
軽く　**levit.**
川崎病　**KD, KS**
丸剤　**p., Pil, pil, pil.**
丸剤塊　**mas.pil., m.p.**
丸剤重量　**pil.pd.**
丸剤に金箔せよ　**deaur.pil.**

丸剤をつくれ　**f.pil., f.pil., ft.pil.**
丸薬　**glob**
甘味を加えていない　**unsw**
汗腺膿瘍　**HS**
汗疱状白癬　**Tp**
完成した　**perf**
完成していない　**inc, inc.**
完全右脚ブロック　**CRBBB**
完全栄養　**CDD**
完全円　**CR**
完全かつ検証可能で不可逆的な解体　**CVID**
完全寛解　**CR**
完全左脚ブロック　**CLBBB**
完全識別　**TD**
完全煮沸ミルク　**WBM**
完全静脈非経口栄養法　**TPPN**
完全静脈麻酔　**TIVA**
完全人工心臓　**TAH**
完全心ブロック　**CHB**
完全制御　**CR**
完全大血管転位〔転換〕症　**complete TGA**
完全大静脈肺動脈結合　**TCPC**
完全大静脈肺動脈吻合　**TCPS**
完全電気変性反応　**CRD**
完全な　**C, comp, compl, cpl, int, int., perf, T**
完全に良くかつ十分な　**FGF**
完全の　**tot**
完全廃疾　**TD**
完全不応期　**TRP**
完全フロイントアジュバント　**CFA**
完全閉塞　**TO**
完全房室ブロック　**CAVB, complete A-V block**
完了・計算問題・語彙・追跡　**CAVF**
完了した　**rdy**
完了した拍動　**CS**
肝(臓)　**L, LIV**
肝アルコール脱水素酵素　**LADH**
肝アルコールデヒドロゲナーゼ　**LADH**
肝移植片　**LG**
肝右葉　**RHL**
肝炎　**hep, HEP**
肝炎・伝染性単核症　**HIM**
肝炎関連(ウイルス)　**HA**
肝炎関連抗原　**HAA**
肝カタラーゼ　**HC**
肝化膿性膿瘍　**PAL**
肝外血流量　**EHBF**
肝外性門脈高血圧症　**EHPH**
肝外胆管　**EHBD**
肝外胆道閉鎖症　**EHBA**
肝外閉塞　**EHO**
肝外閉塞性黄疸　**EOJ**
肝芽細胞腫　**HBL**
肝癌細胞　**HCC, HTC**
肝癌組織培養　**HTC**
肝灌流液　**LP**
肝灌流指数　**HPI**
肝機能検査　**LFT**
肝機能検査図表　**HG**
肝頸静脈逆流　**HJR**
肝血管遮断　**HVE**
肝血漿流量　**HPF**
肝血流量　**HBF, LBF**
肝結合蛋白　**HBP**
肝/血漿(濃度比)　**L/P**
肝コンピュータ断層撮影吸収度　**HCTD**
肝硬変(症)　**LC**
肝(臓)左葉　**LLL**
肝左葉　**LHL**
肝再生血清因子　**LRSF**
肝細胞癌　**HC, HCC**
肝細胞機能　**HF**
肝細胞形成異常　**LCD**
肝細胞刺激因子　**HSF**
肝細胞腫瘍　**LCT**
肝細胞接着分子　**L-CAM**
肝細胞腺腫　**HCA**
肝細胞増殖因子　**HGF**
肝細胞膜抗原　**LMA, LMP**
肝細胞膜抗体　**LMA**
肝細胞膜自己抗体　**LMA**
肝細胞容積分画　**HVF**
肝細網内皮細胞　**HREC**
肝鎖骨の　**Hep/Clav**
肝上位上大静脈　**SVC**
肝実質細胞　**PLC**
肝脂質超酸化反応　**HLP**
肝(臓)疾患　**LD**
肝腫大　**HP**
肝腎症候群　**HRS**
肝・腎・脾　**LKS**
肝・腎・脾・膀胱　**LKSB**
肝・腎・脾触知不能　**LKS non.pal.**
肝腎ミクロソーム　**LKM**
肝腎ミクロソームの　**LKM**
肝静脈　**HV**
肝静脈圧勾配　**HVPG**
肝静脈自由圧　**HVFP**

肝静脈の　**HV**
肝静脈流出　**HVE**
肝静脈流出遮断　**HVOO**
肝親和性門脈血因子　**HPBF**
肝生検　**LB**
肝赤血球産生性ポルフィリン症　**HEP**
肝性コプロポルフィリン症　**HCP**
肝性脳症　**HE**
肝性ポルフィリン症　**PH**
肝性リパーゼ　**HL**
肝腺腫　**HA**
肝臓　**H**
肝臓クリニック　**LC**
肝臓(原)形質膜　**LPM**
肝臓残留因子　**LRF**
肝臓紫斑病　**PH**
肝臓の　**reg hepat**
肝代謝　**HM**
肝中心静脈閉塞症　**VOD**
肝(性)トリグリセリドリパーゼ　**HTGL**
肝(臓)と鉄　**L & I**
肝(臓)と脾(臓)　**L & S, L+S**
肝・鉄・赤色骨髄　**LIRBM**
肝特異抗原　**LSA**
肝特異的膜リポ蛋白　**LSP**
肝動脈　**HA**
肝動脈化学塞栓療法　**TACE**
肝動脈血流　**HABF**
肝動脈持続動注法　**CHAI**
肝動脈塞栓形成(法)　**HAE**
肝動脈塞栓形成法　**HAE**
肝動脈の化学的塞栓形成(法)　**HACE**
肝動脈(血)流量　**HAF**
肝内下大静脈遮断(操作)　**IIVC**
肝内結石　**IHGS**
肝内胆管　**IHBD**
肝内胆汁　**C bile**
肝内胆汁うっ滞　**IC, IHC, IHPC**
肝内胆道閉鎖　**IHA**
肝内抵抗　**IHR**
肝内門脈高血圧　**IHPH**
肝内門脈閉塞症　**IPO**
肝内リンパ球　**IHL**
肝(性)の　**HEP**
肝脳疾患　**HCD**
肝脳脊髄炎ウイルス　**HEV**
肝拍動図　**HPT**
肝ヒドロキシメチルグルタリルコエンザイムA　**HMG-CoA**
肝(臓)被膜下血腫　**SCHL**
肝脾腫大　**HSM**
肝・脾・腎　**LSK**
肝・脾・腎巨大症　**LSKM**
肝ブドウ糖産生　**HGP**
肝ブドウ糖排出量　**HGO**
肝(機能)不全　**HI**
肝(臓)分画上昇　**LVER**
肝閉塞門脈圧　**HOPP**
肝ホスホリラーゼホスファターゼ　**LPP**
肝門　**PH**
肝門脈　**HPV**
肝門脈ガス　**HPVG**
肝門脈サブトラクション血管造影法　**HPSA**
肝由来グリセリドリパーゼ　**HGL**
肝油脂肪酸ナトリウム　**SM**
肝流出　**HOF**
肝レンズ核変性(症)　**HLD**
含浸型液体膜　**SLM**
含水化合物　**hyd**
含有する　**cont, cont., contag, contg**
含量　**cont, cont., contag, contg**
(歯)冠　**Cr**
冠　**cap**
冠貫通酵素　**CPE**
冠血管抵抗　**CVR**
冠血流　**CF**
冠血流(量)　**CBF**
冠状静脈洞血流量　**CSBF**
冠状縫合　**CS**
冠(状)動脈インターベンション　**PCI**
冠(状動脈)疾患〔不全〕看護　**CCN**
冠(状動脈)疾患管理における回復訓練プログラム　**CCTP**
冠(状動脈)疾患集中治療室　**CCU, CICU**
冠(状)動脈疾患集中治療　**ICC**
冠(状)静脈洞　**CS**
冠(状)静脈洞流量　**CSF**
冠(状)静脈洞刺激　**CSS**
冠(状)動脈　**CA**
冠(状)動脈回旋枝　**CCA**
冠(状)動脈回転式粥腫切除術　**CRA**
冠(状)動脈危険因子　**CRF**
冠(状)動脈狭窄指数　**CSI**
冠(状)動脈形成試験　**ACME**
冠(状)動脈外科研究　**CASS**
冠(状)動脈血栓　**CT**
冠(状)動脈血流予備量　**CFR**
冠(状)動脈硬化　**CS**
冠(状)動脈硬化指数　**CAI**
冠(状)動脈硬化性心疾患

CASHD
冠(状)動脈疾患　**CAD**
冠(状)動脈疾患集中治療部門　**ICCU**
冠(状)動脈性心(臓)疾患　**CAHD**
冠(状)動脈性心疾患　**CHD**
冠(状)動脈造影法　**CAG**
冠(状)動脈塞栓　**CAE**
冠(状)動脈内血栓溶解療法　**iCT, ICT**
冠(状)動脈内超音波(検査)　**ICUS**
冠(状)動脈の解離性動脈瘤　**DACA**
冠(状)動脈バイパス　**CAB**
冠(状)動脈バイパス移植(術)　**CBG**
冠(状)動脈バイパス手術　**CABS**
冠(状)動脈バイパス術　**CABG, CABGS**
冠(状)動脈左主幹部疾患　**LMCAD**
冠(状)動脈閉塞(症)　**CAO**
冠(状)動脈閉塞性疾患　**CAOD**
冠(状)動脈瘤　**CAA**
冠(状)動脈攣縮　**CAS**
冠(状)の　**COR, Cor**
冠不全　**CI**
冠不全〔疾患〕看護　**CCN**
冠(状)静脈洞リズム〔調律〕　**CS rhythm**
冠(疾患)リハビリテーションプログラム　**CRP**
(雑誌の)巻　**Jahrg**
巻　**VOL, vol, vol.**
看護　**BSC, nsg**
看護・理解・研究　**CURE**
看護学会員　**FCNA**
看護学士　**BN, B.NSc., B.Sc.Nurs., BSN, B.S.Nurs., DNSc, M.N., M.S.N**
看護学修士　**MSN**
看護学生　**SN**
看護学博士　**PhDN**
看護学校　**SN**
看護学校卒業生　**Gns**
看護監査委員会　**NAC**
看護管理学士　**BSNA**
看護管理認定書　**DNSA**
看護技術　**NP**
看護教育医師　**DNE**
看護教育学士　**B.S.Nurs.Ed., M.S.N.Ed**
看護教育責任者　**DNE**
看護(師)記録　**NN**
看護計画　**NP**
(英国の)看護師　**SRN**
看護師　**NR, Ns, Ord, ord, ord., S, s, sis**
看護師訓練中学生　**SVN**
看護師室　**NS**
看護師長　**HN**
看護師詰所　**NO**
看護師認定書　**DN**
看護師用入院患者評価尺度　**NOSIE**
看護上の同僚　**AN**
看護助手　**NA, PCA**
看護診断　**ND**
看護面接　**NI**
陥凹　**depr, Imp, imp, impr**
陥凹性病変に伴う皺襞集中　**FC**
浣腸　**EN, en, en., ENEM, enem**
浣腸(剤)　**E**
浣腸剤をつくれ　**ft.enem.**
浣腸(剤を注入)せよ　**inj.enem.**
乾カタ寒暖計　**DK**
乾球　**DB**
乾球温　**DB**
乾球温度　**DBT**
乾式乳房撮影(法)　**Xero, XMM**
乾(燥)性角結膜炎　**KCS**
乾性ガス分別濃度　**F**
乾性前鼻炎　**Rh.s.a.**
乾性調合カプセル剤　**DFC**
乾性の　**sic.**
乾癬　**Ps**
乾癬研究協会　**PRA**
乾癬性関節炎　**PA, PsA**
乾癬性白血球走化因子　**PLF**
乾癬部感受性指数　**PASI**
乾燥アガロースフィルム被覆　**DAFO**
乾燥菌　**X**
乾燥外科包帯　**DSD**
乾燥血液斑点　**DBS**
乾燥減量　**LOD**
乾燥させた　**spiss.**
乾燥した　**sicc.**
乾燥重量　**DW**
乾燥性脂肪遊離組織　**DFFT**
乾燥脱脂乳　**DSM**
乾燥凍結　**FD**
乾燥凍結ブタ真皮　**LPS**
乾燥被覆包帯　**DD**
乾燥無菌包帯　**DSD**
乾燥滅菌　**DHS**
乾燥容量　**pk**
乾皮症・彎足・エナメル質(欠損)　**XTE**
乾量クォート　**dq**
乾量パイント　**dp**
患児の正看護師　**RSCN**
(男性/女性)患者　**AEG, aeg.**

患者　**KKe, P, PAT, pat, PNT, Pt, Pt., pt., PTS, pts**
患者・手術選択機構　**POSM**
患者医師関係　**PPR**
患者関係　**PR**
患者看護師関係　**PT-N-I**
患者管理機構　**PCS**
患者管理部門　**PCU**
患者苦痛警告　**PDA**
患者ケアの質　**QPC**
患者血清　**PS**
患者コントロール下鎮痛法　**PCA**
患者情報教育全国委員会　**NCPIE**
患者中心システム　**POS**
患者データシステム　**PDS**
患者と病院教育の供給源の予測　**CPHER**
患者に服用させよ　**CAP, cap, cap.**
患者に持たせよ　**habt.**
患者入院(滞在)期間　**LOPS**
患者評価評点スケール　**PERS**
患者報告用紙　**PRF**
患者マネージ問題　**PMP**
患者満足質問表　**PSQ**
患者向け服薬指導　**PMI**
患者向け服薬指導書　**PIL**
患者用添付文書　**PPI**
患者用服薬指導　**PDI**
患者歴　**PH**
患部に　**dolent part.**
眼　**E, O, Opt, opt, opt.**
眼(内)圧　**IOP, IOT**
眼圧　**OT, T**
眼圧亢進症　**OHT**
眼炎　**OPH, Oph, oph, Ophth**
眼下顎四肢(形成不全)　**OMM**
眼下顎四肢(症候群)　**OMM**
眼下顎頭蓋異常症　**OMD**
眼角間距離　**ICD**
眼科(医)　**Auge**
眼科医　**DOS, OphD, Ophth, opthal**
眼科医コンタクトレンズ学会　**CLAO**
眼科医療従事者　**OMA**
眼科学　**OP, Op, op, OPH, Oph, oph, Ophth, opthal**
眼科学・耳科学・咽喉科学・鼻科学　**OOLR**
眼科学研究協会　**ARO**
眼科学財団　**OF**
眼科学の　**Ophth**
眼科資格〔免状〕　**D.O.**
眼科認定医　**DOMS**
眼科の　**opthal**
眼科分析公定法[米国]　**AOAC**
眼窩外耳口(線)　**OM**
眼窩外耳孔基底線　**OMBL**
眼窩外耳孔線　**OML, OM-line**
眼窩下縁外耳孔線　**IOML**
眼窩下刺激　**suborb.stim**
眼窩間距離　**IOD**
眼窩顔面裂　**OFC**
眼窩骨膜の　**periorb**
眼窩上の　**SO**
眼窩前頭の　**OF**
眼窩前頭皮質　**OF**
眼球運動　**EOM, XOM**
眼球運動記録　**EMR**
眼球運動記録装置　**EMRS**
眼球運動計　**EMG**
眼球運動測定器　**EMMA**
眼球外運動　**EOM**
眼球間距離　**IGD**
眼球乾燥(症)　**X**
眼球乾燥症の眼底　**XF**
眼球逆回旋反射　**OCR**
眼球逆回転　**OCR**
眼球口蓋大脳(症候群)　**OPC**
眼球高血圧指標　**OHI**
眼球後の　**RB**
眼球鞘　**VB**
眼球人工電位　**EAP**
眼球心臓反射　**OCR**
眼球電図　**EOG**
眼球動態検査　**ODT**
眼球突出　**Ex, ex, exoph**
眼球突出・脛骨前粘液水腫・骨関節症(ばち状指)症候群　**EMOS**
眼球突出・限局性粘液水腫・変形関節(症候群)　**EMO**
眼球突出・甲状腺機能亢進症因子　**EHC**
眼球突出惹起作用　**EPA**
眼球突出反応　**EPR**
眼球突出誘発因子　**EPF, EPS**
眼球内異物　**IOFB**
眼球内の　**IO**
眼球脳反応　**OCR**
眼球反転　**OCR**
眼筋ジストロフィー　**OMD**
眼筋麻痺・緊張低下・運動失調・聴力障害・アテトーゼ(症候群)　**OHAHA**
眼筋麻痺性片頭痛　**OPM**
眼鏡士　**Opt, opt, opt.**
眼鏡で矯正　**c gl, c.gl.**
眼外科学士　**M.S.Opthal**

眼外科学認定書 **DChO**
眼研究財団 **ERF**
眼瞼形成(術) **bleph**
眼瞼痙攣 **BS**
眼硬化係数 **K**
眼ジャイロ錯覚 **OGI**
眼白子 **OA**
眼耳脊椎の **OAV**
眼自律神経症 **OVN**
眼神経節 **OG**
眼脂 **AB**
眼振 **Ny, nyst**
眼振遮断症候群 **NBS**
眼振方向優位性 **DP**
眼歯骨形成異常 **ODOD**
眼歯指症候群 **ODDS**
眼歯指形成異常 **ODD**
眼前庭の **OV**
眼前庭反射 **OVR**
眼精神身体症 **OPD**
眼精疲労 **Asth, asth.**
眼体積記録器 **OPH, Oph, oph**
眼体積記録法 **OPH, Oph, oph**
眼体積変動記録器 **OPH, Oph, oph**
眼体節 **OphSeg**
眼低灌流症候群 **OHS**
眼底 **FO, OF**
眼底血圧計 **ODM**
眼底血圧検査法 **ODG**
眼底血圧測定 **ODM**
眼転換症状 **OCS**
眼ド(ッ)プラー超音波図 **ODSG**
眼動脈 **OA**
眼動脈圧 **OAP**
眼動脈撮影 **OAG**
眼内圧 **Po**
眼内移動 **IOT**
眼内筋 **IOM**
眼内後房レンズ **PC-IOL**
眼内レンズ **IOL**
眼内レンズ移植 **IOLI**
眼内レンズ性水疱性角膜症 **PBK**
眼軟膏 **oculent.**
眼の **OP, Op, op, OPH, Oph, oph, Ophth, Opt, opt, opt.**
眼脳血管測定装置 **OCVM**
眼脳腎症候群 **OCRS**
眼皮膚白皮症 **OCA**
眼部帯状ヘルペス **HZO**
眼放射線療法 **ORT**
眼由来増殖因子 **EDGF**
眼幼虫移行症 **OLM**
眼類天疱瘡 **OCP**
眼レーザー電子顕微鏡 **OLM**
眼・耳・鼻・咽喉 **EENT, E.E.N.T.**
眼・精神身体症 **OPD**
眼・尿道・滑膜炎 **OUS**
桿(状)核(白血)球 **stabs**
桿菌 **B, B., Bac, Bac.**
桿剤 **BACILL**
桿状核(白血)球 **Stab**
桿状核白血球 **St**
寒天ゲル拡散試験〔検査〕 **ADT**
寒天ゲル拡散法 **AGD**
寒天ゲル沈殿試験 **AGPT**
寒天ゲル二重拡散法 **AGDD**
寒天コロニー形成単位 **ACFU**
寒冷凝集素 **CA**
寒冷凝集素症候群 **CAS**
寒冷凝集素病 **CAD**
寒冷凝集反応 **CA**
寒冷式円錐切除(術) **CKC**
寒冷昇圧(の) **CP**
寒冷昇圧検査 **CPT**
寒冷昇圧試験 **CPT**
寒冷赤血球凝集素(価) **CHA**
寒冷赤血球凝集素テスト **CHA**
寒冷沈降物 **cryo**
寒冷の **frig.**
寒冷不溶性グロブリン **CIG**
寒冷療法 **cryo**
換気 **RESP, Resp, resp, resp., respir, vent**
換気(の) **respir**
換気(量) **V, VE, Ve**
換気・灌流比 **V-P ratio**
換気・循環(比) **V/C, V-C**
換気・輸液・ポンプ **VIP**
換気灌流商〔比〕 **V/Q**
換気〔呼吸〕筋訓練 **VMT**
換気血流比 $\dot{V}_A/\dot{Q}c$
換気亢進 **HV**
換気時間 **TE**
換気指数 **VI**
換気する **vent**
換気装置 **V, vent**
換気速度係数 **AVI**
換気調節 **AC**
換気と灌流 **V/P**
換気比 **VR**
換気不全 **VF**
換気予備比 **BRR**
換気予備率 **VR**
換気予備量 **BR**
換気率 **VQ, VR**
換言すれば **viz, viz.**
間隔 **int, int.**
間欠カテーテル法 **IC**
間欠性外斜視 **X**
間欠性急性ポルフィリン症 **IAP**
間欠清潔カテーテル挿入

ICC
間欠性色素黒化 **IPD**
間欠性上斜視 **H, T**
間欠性大動脈閉塞症 **IAO**
間欠性の **INT, Int, int**
間欠性跛行 **IC**
間欠性閉塞隅角緑内障 **IACG**
間欠性ヘパリン化 **IH**
間欠性律動性δ波 **IRDA**
間欠的陰圧換気 **INPV**
間欠的陰圧呼吸法 **INPB**
間欠的陰圧補助的換気 **INPB**
間欠的強制換気 **IDV**
間欠的強制換気(法) **IMV**
間欠的頸椎牽引 **ICTX**
間欠的頸部牽引 **iCT, ICT**
間欠的腹膜透析(法) **IPD**
間欠的膀胱洗浄 **IBI**
間欠的補助換気 **IAV**
間欠的陽圧 **IPP**
間欠的陽圧呼吸 **IPPB, IPPR**
間欠的陽圧(吹入)酸素療法 **IPPO**
間欠的陽圧人工換気(法) **IPPV**
間欠的陽陰圧換気法 **IPNPV**
間欠的陽陰圧呼吸 **IPNPB**
間欠発光刺激 **SLI**
間欠流遠心白血球アフェレーシス **IFCL**
間欠流遠心法 **IFC**
間(質)細胞 **IC**
間擦性黄色腫 **ITX**
間質液 **IF, ISF, ISW**
間質血管細胞群 **VSF**
間質細胞 **ISC**
間質細胞液 **ISCF**
間質細胞刺激ホルモン **ICSH**
間質細胞腫瘍 **iCT, ICT**
間質(性)疾患 **ID**
間質性角膜炎 **IK**
間質性腎炎 **IN**
間質性腎炎・ブドウ膜炎症候群 **TINU**
間質性肺炎 **IP, ISP**
間質性肺気腫 **IPE**
間質性肺疾患 **ILD**
間質性肺線維症 **IPF**
間質性肺臓炎 **IPn**
間質性放射線肺炎 **IRP**
間質性リンパ性肺炎 **ILP**
間質組織 **IT**
間質レーザー光凝固 **ILP**
間接クームス試験 **iCT, ICT**
間接螢光狂犬病抗体(検査) **IFRA**
間接螢光抗体 **IFA**
間接螢光抗体検査 **IFAT**
間接抗グロブリン試験 **IAGT, IAT, IDAT**
間接抗グロブリンロゼット形成反応 **IARR**
間接最大呼吸量 **IMBC**
間接自傷〔自損〕行為 **ISDB**
間接視神経損傷症候群 **IONIS**
間接赤血球凝集(反応) **IH**
間接赤血球凝集抗体 **IHA**
間接的血圧測定システム **IBPMS**
間接的な **ind, ind.**
間接熱量測定 **IC**
間接の **ind, ind.**
間接ビリルビン **IB, I-Bil, IDBR**
間接プラーク形成細胞 **IPFC**
間接法 **IDM**
間接放射性核種膀胱造影(法) **IRC**
間接放射免疫標識定量法 **IRIA**
間接膜免疫螢光(検査) **IMI**
間接ミクロ血球凝集 **IMH**
間接免疫螢光法 **IIF**
間接免疫ペルオキシダーゼ **IIP**
間入性早期期外収縮 **IPVC**
間葉系間質細胞 **MSC**
間葉系腫瘍 **GIMT**
嵌入 **Impx**
嵌入した **Imp, imp**
寛解 **R, Rm**
寛骨臼 **acetab**
幹細胞(刺激)因子 **SCF**
幹細胞濃縮分画 **SCEF**
幹細胞白血病蛋白 **Scl**
幹細胞分泌因子 **SDF**
幹部 **stf**
幹迷走神経切断術 **TV**
感応電流の **far**
感覚 **S, s, sen, sens**
感覚/運動(比) **S/M**
感覚器 **SENS, sens**
感覚減退 **hypes**
感覚刺激 **SOS**
感覚上皮 **NE**
感覚神経活動電位 **SNAP**
感覚神経性難聴 **SHL, SNHL**
感覚神経(性)の **SN**
感覚性失語 **SA**
感覚性誘発電位 **SEP**
感覚〔知覚〕潜時 **SL**
感覚〔知覚〕脱失〔消失〕の

か

A
感覚中枢　SENS, sens
感覚低下　↓ sen
感覚低下した　sense.decr.
感覚鈍麻　hypes
感覚の　sens
感覚フィードバック療法　SFT
感覚妨害症候群　SDS
感覚誘発電位　EP_s
感覚レベル　SL
感光乳剤層　Em
感作因子　SF
感作血球凝集反応　SHA
感作抗体　SA
感作試験　STT
感作赤血球凝集反応　SEA
感作単位　SU
感作反応　SR
感作反応細胞　SRC, SR cell
感作ヒツジ(赤)血球凝集(反応)　SSCA
感作ヒツジ赤血球凝集(反応)　SSEA
感作リンパ球テスト　PLT
感作リンパ球タイピング　PLT
感受性(試験)　sens, SENS, sens.
感受性訓練　ST
感受性時間調節管理　STC
感受性指標　SI
感情　emot
感情障害ならびに統合失調症面接基準　SAD, SADS
感(受)性　susc
感(受)性の　sen, sens
感(受)性のある　susc
(接触)感染　contag
感染　INF, inf, inf., infect
感染管理看護師　ICN
感染後性糸球体腎炎　PIGN
感染後の　PI
感染後脳脊髄(膜)炎　PIE
感染細胞蛋白　ICP
感染した　INF, inf, inf.
感染していない　FFI
感染症　ID, infec.dis
感染症に伴う血球貪食症候群　IAHS
感染症部門　IDS
(米国)感染症防止担当協会　APIC
感染する　INF, inf, inf.
感染性　INF, inf, inf.
感染性ウシ鼻・気管炎　IBR
感染性ウシ鼻・気管炎ウイルス　IBRV
感染性核酸　INA
感染〔伝染〕性肝炎　IH
感染性気管支炎　IB
感染性心内膜炎　IE
感染性単核球症　INFM, inf mono
感染性単核細胞症　MI
感染性腸疾患　IBD
感染性の　contag
感染性膿疱性(外陰)腟炎　IPV
感染性ヒト肝炎　IHH
感染性リンパ様新生物　RPL-12
感染赤血球　IRBC
感染増強因子　IPF
感染対策委員会　ICC
感染対策チーム　iCT, ICT
感染多重度　moi, MOI
感染単位　iu
感染の　INF, inf, inf., infect
感染の徴候なし　NSI
感染部位　IA
感染予防　IP
感染量　ID
感染歴のない現症　NIP
感知しうる　S
感応　I
感応抵抗　Re, react
感冒　CC
感冒ウイルス　CC-Virus
感冒研究組織　CCRU
頑癬　EM
鉗子分娩　FD, F.D.
慣習に従って　a.u.
管　D, ves
管外遊出　extrav
管共鳴反応　CRR
管腔　l, L, lum
管腔拡張用金属ステント　EMS
管腔内ソマトスタチン　ILSS
管腔内超音波　ILUS
管腔内ホチキス　ILS
管状小胞　TV
管状腺癌　tub
管状腺癌の高分化型　tub 1
管状腺癌の中分化型　tub 2
管状ミエリン　TM
管成長因子　DGF
管電圧波高値　kVp
(腺)管内癌　IDC
管内増殖　IDP
(腺)管内乳頭状癌　IPC
(腺)管内乳頭状膵癌　IPNP
管内癒着　ITA
(脈)管壁　VW, V.W., v.w.
管壁細胞　LC
管網状構造　TRS

管理 **adm, Adm, ctl, mgmt, mgt, mng, S, supv**
管理された環境での経過時間 **CET**
管理者 **adm., ADM, supt**
管理人 **mgr, supv**
関係 **R, rel**
関係した **rel**
関心部分〔領域〕 **ROI**
関心領域 **ADI, AOI**
関節 **art, artic, artt, J, jnt, JT, jt**
関節位置覚 **JPS**
関節運動の最大域 **FRJM**
関節液中リンパ球 **SFL**
関節炎 **arth**
関節炎衝撃測定尺度 **AIMS**
関節炎とリウマチ性疾患 **ARD**
関節炎の **arth**
関節炎リウマチ研究審議会 **ARCR**
関節炎リウマチ財団 **ARF**
関節滑液内単核細胞 **SFMC**
関節滑液膜単核細胞 **STMC**
関節滑膜固有細胞 **SC**
関節可動域 **ROM**
関節可動性制限 **LJM**
関節吸引 **jt.asp**
関節近傍の **JA**
関節空気造影 **PAG**
関節空気造影法 **Pneumo, pneumo**
関節拘縮 **JC**
関節受動(術) **mob**
関節上腕靭帯の上腕骨剝離 **HAGL**
関節切開(術) **arthr, arthrot**
関節(腔)内の **IA, i.a.**
関節軟骨石灰症 **ACC, CCA**
関節(性)の **artic**
関節包 **B, Bb**
関節包内骨折 **IC fx**
関節面大転子間距離 **ATD**
関節リウマチ **RA, RAHA, RHA**
関節リウマチ因子 **RAF**
関節リウマチ(関連)核抗原 **RANA**
関節リウマチ凝集(試験) **RAHA**
関節リウマチ血清 **RAS**
関節リウマチ沈降素 **RAP**
関節リウマチにおける下位頸椎亜脱臼 **SAS**
関節リウマチ・汎発性特発性骨増殖症 **RADISH**
関節離断(術) **disart, disartic**
関連医師 **AfP, AfPh**
(〜に)関連した **assocd, assoc'd**
関連した **affil, rfrd**
監査 **insp, insp., INSPEC**
監査する **insp**
監査役 **INSPEC**
監察医 **ME**
監視 **montrg**
監督 **S, super, supv**
監督者 **supv**
緩下薬 **Lax, lax**
緩下薬乱用症候群 **LAS**
緩徐拡張期脱分極 **SDD**
緩徐血液濾過法 **SCHF**
緩徐作用性抗リウマチ薬 **SAARD**
緩徐持続血液限外濾過法 **SCHUD**
緩徐持続限外濾過法 **SCUF**
緩徐持続的血液濾過透析法 **SCHDF**
緩徐充盈波 **SFW**
緩徐充満期 **SF**
緩徐進行型インスリン依存性糖尿病 **SPIDDM**
緩徐の **sl**
緩徐反応物質 **SRS**
緩徐抑制(性)電位 **SIP**
緩衝 **bfr**
緩衝塩基 **BB**
緩衝剤溶解性物質 **BSBC**
緩衝された **bf**
緩衝指数 **BI**
緩衝蒸留水 **BDW**
緩衝食塩水 **BS, BSS**
緩衝リンゲル液 **bfR sol**
緩速語音聴取検査 **DSTT**
緩和ケア病棟 **PCU**
緩和バルビツレート療法 **MBT**
還元 **red**
還元・酸化 **redox**
還元型黄色酵素 **YEH_2**
還元型グルタチオン **GSH**
還元型トリホスホピリジンヌクレオチド **TPNH**
還元型ニコチンアミドアデニンジヌクレオチド **$NADH_2$**
還元型ニコチンアミドアデニンジヌクレオチドリン酸塩 **NADPH, $NADPH_2$**
還元型フラビン・リン酸塩 **FPH_2**
還元酵素試験 **R test**
還元ジホスホピリジンヌクレオチド(＝NADH) **DPNH**

還元する **red**
還元値 **RL**
還元鉄 **Fer.red.**
還元糖 **RS**
還元ピロロキノリンキノン(2,7,9-トリカルボキシ-1H-ピロロ(2,3-f)キノリン4,5-ジオール) **$PQQH_2$**
還元フラビンアデニンジヌクレオチド **$FADH_2$**
還元ヘモグロビン **HHb**
環境 **environ.**
環境影響評価 **EIA**
環境衛生規準 **EHC**
環境管理単位 **ECU**
環境技術情報センター **AMTIC**
環境研究室 **ERL**
環境上の抵抗 **ER**
環境制御装置 **ECS**
環境タバコ煙 **ETS**
環境と遺伝 **E & H**
環境の **environ.**
環境保健サービス **EHS**
環境保護庁 **EPA**
環境問題科学委員会 **SCOPE**
環境療法 **MT**
環状DNA **cDNA**
環状GMP **cGMP**
環状切除(術) **CIR，cir，CIRC，Circ，circ**
環状切除された **CIR，cir，Circ，circ**
環状層化整列システム **APAS**
環状鉄芽球性不応性貧血 **RARS**
環状肉芽腫 **GA**
環状ヌクレオチドホスホジエステラーゼ **CNPase**
環指 **R**
環軸間隙 **AAD，AAI**
環軸関節不全脱臼 **AAS**
環軸関節融合 **AAF**
環軸歯突起間距離 **ADD**
環軸椎回旋位固定 **AARF**
環軸椎前方亜脱臼 **AAS**
環軸椎脱臼 **AAD**
環軸椎の **AD**
(正中)環軸の **AD**
環(椎)軸(椎)の **AA**
環切(術) **CIR，cir，CIRC，Circ，circ**
環椎後頭骨の **AO**
環椎後頭骨変位 **AOD**
環椎歯突起間距離 **ADI**
癌 **CA，Ca，ca，Can**
癌外膜浸潤 **A**
癌外膜浸潤の程度(病理組織所見) **A，a**
癌肝転移 **H**
癌看護協会 **ONS**
癌家系症候群 **CES**
癌関連血清抗原 **CASA**
癌関連ポリペプチド抗原 **CAPA**
癌監視システム **CSS**
癌危険ランキングと情報システム **CHRIS**
癌救助全国協会 **NSCR**
癌凝固性因子 **CCF**
癌研究所 **ICR**
癌研究対策アジア連合 **AFOCC**
癌自然寛解 **SRC**
癌切除判定 **R 0-3**
癌胎児抗原倍増時間 **CEA-DT**
癌胎児性抗原 **CEA**
癌胎盤性アルカリホスファターゼ **CPALP**
癌治療におけるQOL診断法 **CARES-SF**
癌治療部門 **DCT**
癌とポリオ研究基金 **CPRF**
癌の局所療法 **LCT**
癌の研究と治療のための欧州共同体 **EORTC**
癌の病期分類と結果報告のための国際委員会 **ICPR**
癌の病期分類と結果報告のための日本委員会 **JJC**
癌の病期分類と予後の報告のための米国連合委員会 **AJC**
癌破壊因子 **CBF**
癌比例死亡率 **PCMR**
癌予防救済協会 **SPRC**
簡易心機図法 **MCG-S**
簡易新薬申請 **ANDA**
簡易精神症状スケール **BPRS**
簡易知能テスト **MMST**
簡易トリプチケース血清培地 **STS**
簡易臨床評価尺度 **SCRS**
簡潔な国際化学物質評価証書 **CICAD**
簡便式大腸X線検査法 **SCG**
簡便精神医学的評価尺度 **BPRS**
簡略 **BV**
簡略外傷重症度尺度 **AIS**
簡略更年期指数 **SMI**
観血的整復兼内固定術 **ORIF**
観察 **O，obs，obs.，OBS，Obs**
観察下(の) **UO，U/O**
観察看護部門 **OCU**
観察記録 **IR**
観察された **obs，obs.，OBS，Obs，obsvd**
観察室 **OU，O.U.，o.u.**

観察者　**obs, obs., OBS, Obs**
観察できない効果レベル　**NOEL**
観察と診察　**O & E**
観察と評価　**O & A**
観察窓　**OBW**
観察目標　**OT**
韓国抗原　**KA**
顔貌・心拍数・足底刺激に対する反射・筋の緊張・呼吸のスコア　**Apgar score**
顔面　**F**
顔面・肩甲・上腕型筋ジストロフィ　**FSH**
顔面痙攣　**FS**
顔面肩甲上腕型筋ジストロフィ　**FSHD, FSMD**
顔面肩甲上腕の　**FSH**
顔面ジスキネジア　**FD**
顔面神経　**FN**
顔面神経洞　**FS**
顔面神経麻痺　**FP**
顔面測定　**FM**
顔面の　**fac.**
顔面播種状粟粒性狼瘡　**LMDF**
顔面板　**fc pl**
灌注　**IRRG, irrg, irrig**
灌流圧　**PP**
灌流液　**PF**
灌流率　**PR**
(陰茎海綿体の)灌流量と内圧記録　**DICC**
鑑別凝集試験　**DAT**
鑑別血球計算　**diff**
鑑別刺激　**DS**
鑑別診断　**DD, DDX, diff.diag**
鑑別診断不可呼吸器疾患　**URD**
鑑別適性試験　**DAT**
鑑別滴定量　**DT**
鑑別の　**diff**
S-カルボキシメチルシステイン　**S-CMC**

き

キアスマ　**CH**
ギガ(＝10^9)　**G**
ギガオーム(＝$10^9\Omega$)　**GΩ**
ギガサイクル　**Gc**
ギガ電子ボルト　**GeV, Giv**
ギガベケレル　**GBq**
ギガヘルツ　**GHz**
ギガワット　**GW**
キサンチン　**X, x, Xan**
キサンチン一リン酸　**XMP**
キサンチンオキシダーゼ　**XO**
キサンチン酸化酵素　**XO**
キサンチン脱水素酵素　**XDH**
キサンチンデヒドロゲナーゼ　**XDH**
キサンチン二リン酸　**XDP**
キサンツレン酸　**XA**
キサントシン　**X, Xao**
キサントシン一リン酸　**XMP**
キサントシン三リン酸　**XTP**
キシルロース　**xul**
キシレン・アルコール混合物　**X-A mixture**
キシレンジイソシアネイト　**XC**
キシロカイン　**XYL, Xyl**
キシロカインとコルチゾン　**Xyl & cort.**
キシロース　**Xyl**
キシロース・リジン・デオキシコール酸塩(培地)　**XLD**
キシロース呼吸試験　**XBT**
キシロースリジン(培地)　**XL**
キース・ウェジナー　**KW**
キース・ウェジナー・バーカー(本態性高血圧症)　**KWB**
キース・ウェジナー分類　**KW classification**
キスカル酸　**QA**
キーストン双眼鏡視覚調査　**KTVS**
キセノン　**Xe**
キセノンアークランプ　**XAL**
キセノン写真　**xeno**
キセノン写真の　**xeno**
キセノン診断　**xeno**
キセノン診断の　**xeno**
キセノン増強コンピュータ連動断層撮影(法)　**XECT, XeCT, Xe-CT**
キセノン放射線写真　**XRO**
キーセルバッハ部位　**LK**
キタサマイシン　**KM**
キッズ　**KIDS**
キナクリン　**Q**
キナーゼ活性化因子　**KAF**
キナルジンレッド　**QR**
ギニアヒヒ　**PPA**
キニジン　**Q**
キニジン・アテブリン・プラスモチン治療　**QAP (treatment)**
キニノゲン　**Kgn**
キヌタ・アブミ骨関節　**IS**
キヌタ骨　**I**
キヌタ骨長突起　**LPI**
キヌレン酸　**KA**
キネトカルジオグラム　**KCG**
キノリン　**Q**
キノロン耐性決定領域　**QRDR**
キノン　**Q**
ギプス　**Gi, POP**
ギブズ・ヘルムホルツ方程式　**G+H**
ギプス固定のままでのＸ線写真　**XIP**
ギブズ自由エネルギー　**G, G**
ギプス包帯　**C**
ギプスを外した状態でのＸ線写真　**XOP**
ジベレル酸　**GA**
キーホールリンペット〔鍵穴付着〕ヘモシアニン　**KLH**
キメラ　**chi**
キモトリプシノゲン　**ChTg**
キモトリプシン　**CT**
キモトリプシン単位　**CU**
キモトリプシン様蛋白　**CLP**
キモトリプシン抑制活性　**CIA**
キャサヌール森林熱　**KFD**
キャサヌール森林病　**KFD**
キャットフォード視力測定器　**CVAA**
キャップ結合蛋白質　**CBP**
ギャップジャンクション　**GJ**
キャベジン(＝ビタミンU)　**Vit U**
キャンドル時間　**C hr, c hr, chr**
キャンバーウェル家族評価尺度　**CFI**
キューサー　**CUSA**
キュリー　**C, c, Ci**

キュリウム **Cm**
キュリー時間 **C hr, c hr, chr, Ci-hr**
キュリー単位 **CI**
キュンチャー(針) **K**
キュンチャー釘 **K nail**
キラー(細胞) **K**
キラー・ヘルパー因子 **KHF**
キラーT細胞 **TK**
キラー細胞 **K cell**
キラル誘導化試薬 **CDA**
ギラン・バレー症候群 **GBS, G-BS**
ギラン・バレー(症候群) **GB**
ギリシャ語 **Gk**
ギリシャ語の **G**
ギリシャ人 **Gk**
キリスト教医学協会 **CMS**
キリスト教徒 **Xn**
キルシュナー針金〔鋼線〕 **K wire**
ギルバート **Gb, F**
ギルフォード・マーチン人格目録 **GAMIN**
キロ(=10^3) **k**
キロアンペア **kA**
キロ塩基 **kb**
キロ塩基対 **kbp, kbs**
キロガウス **kG**
キロカロリー **kcal**
キロカロリー(=kcal) **Cal**
キロキュリー **kCi**
キログラム **kg, kilo**
キログラム・カロリー **kg cal**
キログラム・メートル **kg・m**
キログラム/秒 **kgps, kg/s**
キロサイクル **kc**
キロサイクル/秒 **kcps, kc.p.s., kc/s**
キロジュール **KJ**
キロダルトン **kd**
キロ電子ボルト **keV, kev**
キロ透過性係数 **K**
キロニュートン **kN**
キロバイト **KB**
キロパスカル **kPa**
キロ秒 **ks**
キロベクレル **kBq**
キロベース **kb**
キロベース対 **kbs**
キロヘルツ **kHz**
キロボルト・アンペア **kVA**
キロポンド **kp**
キロメガサイクル **kMc**
キロメガサイクル/秒 **kMcps**
キロメートル **kilo, km**
キロメートル/秒 **kmps, km/s**
キロリットル **kl**
キロレントゲン **kR**
キロワット **kW**
キロワット時 **kWh, kW-hr**
キング・アームストロング単位 **KAU**
キング・アームストロング単位 **KA unit**
キング・アームストロング単位 **KA**
キングスベリー・クラーク法 **KC method**
キーンズ・セイアー・シャイ(症候群) **KSS**
キーンズ・セイアー症候群 **KSS**
(X線曝露の)キーンベック単位 **X**
キンメルスティール・ウィルソン(症候群) **KW**
きれいな **cl, clr**
切った **inc, inc.**
切る **incid.**
企業内中核安全性情報 **CCSI**
企図振戦 **IT**
危急状態 **CC**
危急状態管理 **CC**
危険 **haz**
危険因子 **RF**
危険期間の **ARP**
危険な **haz**
危険な実験作業室 **hot labo**
危険比 **RR**
危険リスト **DL**
危篤(的)の **crit**
気圧 **ATM, atm**
気圧計 **bar**
気圧計の **bar**
気圧の **B, bar**
気温 **AT**
気管 **TR, tr, trach, trch**
気管・食道エアウェイ **TEA**
気管音 **TS**
気管気管支異物 **TBFB**
気管気管支炎 **TB**
気管気管支鏡検査(法) **TBS**
気管気管支枝 **TBT**
気管気管支洗浄 **TBT**
気管気管支リンパ節 **TBL**
気管吸引 **trach.asp.**
気管(直)径 **TD**
気管経由の **OT**
気管支 **Br, Br., bronch**
気管支炎 **BR, Br, bronch**
気管支可逆性指数 **BRI**
気管支拡張(症) **bronchiect**
気管支拡張症 **BE**

き

気管支拡張薬　**BD**
気管支活性亢進　**BH**
気管支癌　**BC**
気管支関連リンパ組織　**BALT**
気管支鏡　**BF, BFS, BFs, Bronch, bronch., BS**
気管支鏡検査　**BRO**
気管支鏡検査医　**Bronch**
気管支鏡検査法　**BF**
気管支鏡的な　**Bronch**
気管支鏡の　**Bronch**
気管支鏡(検査)法　**Bronch, bronch.**
気管支胸膜の　**BP**
気管支胸膜瘻　**BPF**
気管支痙攣　**BSp**
気管支血管模様　**BVM**
気管支血流量　**BBF**
気管支原発癌　**BGCA**
気管支枝　**B**
気管支小細胞癌　**SCCB**
気管支食道科(学)　**BE**
気管支声　**BRPH, Brph, brph**
気管支(肺胞)洗浄(法)　**BAL**
気管支洗浄　**BL**
気管支(肺胞)洗浄液　**BALF**
気管支喘息　**BA**
気管支造影　**BG**
気管支造影図　**bronch**
気管支造影法　**broncho**
気管支動脈　**BrA**
気管支動脈圧　**BAP**
気管支動脈造影　**BAG**
気管支動脈塞栓術　**BAE**
気管支動脈(内)注入(療法)　**BAI**
気管支動脈内注入(療法)　**BAI**
気管支の　**B, Bron**
気管支肺アスペルギルス症　**BPA**
気管支肺異形成(症)　**BPD**
気管支肺洗浄　**BPL**
気管支肺胞大食細胞　**BAM**
気管支肺胞の　**BA, BV**
気管支反応亢進　**BHR**
気管支反応性亢進　**BH**
気管支ファイバースコープ　**FOB**
気管支ファイバースコープ検査　**FB**
気管支噴霧吸入　**BAI**
気管支(肺胞)洗浄　**BAW**
気管上皮細胞毒素　**TCT**
気管食道の　**TE**
気管食道癒合不全　**TED**
気管食道瘻　**TEF**
気管支リンパ節　**BLN**
気管切開(術)　**Trach, trach**
気管切開術　**trch**
気管切開セット　**T-set**
気管内　**IT**
気管内吸引　**ETS**
気管内心拍動波　**ITCG**
気管内チューブ　**ETT, IT**
気管内の　**E, endo, endo-trach**
気管内麻痺　**ITN**
気管粘液クリアランス　**TMC**
気管粘液速度　**TMV**
気管(支)肺胞細胞　**BAC**
気管分岐部下縁　**B**
気管支誘発試験　**BPT**
気管輸送速度　**TTV**
気胸　**pn, pnth, pnthx, PNX, Pnx, pnx, PT, Pth, PTX, PX, Px, px**
気候変動に関する政府間パネル　**IPCC**
気骨導聴力差　**AB gap, A-B gap**
気心膜症　**PPC**
気象　**w**
気腫　**EM, emph, emphys**
気質　**M**
気縦隔　**PNMED**
気縦隔(症)　**PM**
気切　**Trach, trach**
気相分解　**VPD**
気相抑制因子　**VPI**
気息性　**B**
気速指数　**AVI**
気体眼圧計　**PTG**
気体酸素　**GO, GO_2, GOX**
気体体積　**VG**
気体窒素　**GN**
気体定数　**R**
気体の容積・体積　**V**
気体分圧　**P**
気体膀胱二重造影　**PCCG**
気体容積　**VG**
気づかれない　**n/n**
気づかれなければ　**n.a.n.**
気道　**aw, aw.**
気道圧　**AWP**
気道コンダクタンス　**Caw, Gaw**
気道抵抗　**AR, AWR, RA, RAW, Raw**
気道内圧　**Paw**
気道内圧緩和換気　**APRV**
気道内陽圧式人工呼吸　**PAPV**
気道内流量均衡補償換気法　**PAV**
気道反応係数　**ARI**
気道反応性　**AR**
気道平滑筋　**ASM**
気道閉塞　**AWO**
気道閉塞・出血・危急状

況,膿瘍排膿・内視鏡・異物,迅速な処理・誠実な(医師の態度) **ABCDEFGH**
気道陽圧 **PAP**
気導 **AC, A.C., LL**
気導(時間)/骨導(時間) **AC/BC**
気導骨導差 **AB gap, A-B gap**
気導と骨導 **A & BC**
気導または交流 **AC**
気(体)脳室造影(法) **PVG**
気脳写 **Pneumo, pneumo**
気脳写(像) **AEG**
気脳図 **PNE**
気脳造影〔撮影〕図 **AEG**
気(体)脳造影〔撮影〕法 **PEG**
気晴らし療法 **XDT**
気分・見当識・判断・情動・内容 **MOJAC**
気分および/または感情 **M/A**
気分状態特性尺度 **POMS**
気腹症 **PNP, Ppt**
気休め薬 **ADT**
気流限界区域 **FLS**
希釈 **dil, dilut.**
希釈アルコール **s.v.r.**
希釈アンモニア水 **NH_4**
希釈血液塊溶解時間 **DBCLT**
希釈した **dil, dilut., dl**
希釈する **dilut.**
希釈せよ **Dil, dil.**
希釈力価 **DS**
希釈量 **DV**
希土類元素 **REE**
希発月経性多囊胞性卵巣症候群 **OPCOS**
希薄 **Dil, dil.**
希望量 **q.l., q.pl.**
技師 **tech, techn**
技術 **tec, tech**
技術移転ネットワーク **TTN**
技術協力 **TA**
技術事前評価 **TA**
技術者 **tec**
技術的 **tec**
技術によって **s.a.**
技術の **tec, tech**
技術の法則に従いつくれ **FSAR**
技術評価事務所 **OTA**
奇異性空気塞栓症 **PAE**
奇形 **abnor, abnorm, deform**
奇形癌 **TC**
奇形赤血球(増加)症 **PIOK**
奇静脈 **AV, A-V, VAZ**
奇胎 **M**
奇脈 **PP**
季刊誌 **qr, quart**
季節性アレルギー性鼻炎 **SAR**
季節性感情障害 **DAS, SAD**
季節性鼻アレルギー性結膜炎 **SARC**
紀元後 **AD**
客観的な **Obj, obj**
昨日 **y day**
拮抗(作用)的な **antag, antag.**
既往疾病 **PMI**
既往歴 **Anamn, PH, PHI, PHx, PMH, PMHY, prev.hx, PX, Px**
既婚・未婚・寡婦・離婚 **MSWD**
既婚の **M, m**
既知の **wk**
既知薬剤アレルギー **KDA**
既知薬物アレルギー **NKDA**
記憶 **M, m**
記憶T細胞 **Tm**
記憶指数 **MQ**
記憶喪失性貝中毒 **ASP**
記憶と学習の広範囲評価 **WRAML**
記号 **symb**
記号の **symb**
記載 **Reg, reg, reg.**
記載して投与せよ **d et s**
記述する **descr**
記録 **Arch, doc, rcrd, rec, REC**
記録・報告・調整 **RR & C**
記録者 **RD**
記録なし **n/r**
起源不明の **undet.orig.**
起床可,入浴可 **OOBBRP**
起床後2回目の尿 **SMV**
起始 **orig**
起始の **orig**
起電力 **E**
起立性アルブミン尿 **OA**
起立性蛋白尿 **OP**
起立性調節障害 **OD**
起立性低血圧 **OH**
起立テスト **RT**
黄色い **yelsh, ysh**
黄色味がかったピンク色 **YPK**
基 **GP, gp**
基幹病院 **BH**
基剤 **V**
基準局 **B.S.**
基準〔規則〕に従って **sl., s.l.**
基準の判定 **RS**
基質 **MX, S**

基質蛋白　**MP**
基質定数　**Ks**
基質標識螢光免疫測定法　**SLFIA**
基質分解メタロプロテイナーゼ　**MMPs**
基質遊離血色素　**SFH**
基質遊離血色素液　**SFHS**
基質由来腐敗加速因子　**DAF-S**
基節骨　**PP**
基線　**B，BL**
基礎　**Found，found.**
基礎医学認定書　**Dip.BMS**
基礎エネルギー消費量　**BEE**
基礎研究諮問委員会　**RAC**
基礎酸素燃焼　**BOF**
基礎酸分泌量　**BAO**
基礎人格評価表　**BPI**
基礎心拍リズム　**UHR**
基礎体温　**BBT**
基礎体温表　**BTC**
基礎胎児心拍数　**BFHR**
基礎代謝　**BM**
基礎代謝率　**BMR**
基礎知能測定検査　**PMA test**
基礎的休息活動周期　**BRAC**
基礎の　**fund**
基礎培地　**BM**
基礎皮膚抵抗　**BSR**
基礎輻輳点　**PBC**
基礎分泌最高酸濃度　**BAC**
基礎分泌量　**BSV，BSVR**
基礎ペプシン分泌量　**BPO**
基礎ロールシャッハスコア　**BRS**
基底核　**BN**
基底細胞　**BC**
基底細胞過形成　**BCH**
基底細胞癌　**BCC**
基底細胞形成不全　**BCH**
基底細胞上皮腫　**BCE**
基底細胞母斑　**BCN**
基底細胞母斑症候群　**BCNS**
基底層　**BL**
基底点　**BA**
基底の　**bas，bas.**
基底板　**BL**
基底部高　**H of F**
基底膜　**BM**
基底膜帯　**BMZ**
基底膜肥厚　**BMT**
基底膜様物質　**BMLM**
基底(細胞)融解変性　**BLD**
基部の　**bas，bas.**
基本曲線　**BC**
基本周期　**BCL**
基本小体　**EB**
基本心拍数　**BHR**
基本ソフト　**OS**
基本多細胞単位　**BMU**
基本的線維芽成長因子　**bFGF**
基本的沈殿物と水　**BS & W**
基本的な膵(臓)トリプシン阻害剤　**BPTI**
基本電位リズム　**BER**
基本洞周期長　**BSCL**
基本の　**c**
寄稿　**Beitr**
寄生虫学　**Parasit**
寄与危険度　**AR**
寄与危険度割合　**ARP**
規準の位置　**RTP**
規準利得　**RTG**
規制　**R**
規則　**regs**
規則的　**Reg，reg，reg.**
規則的透析治療　**RDT**
規則的洞律動　**RSR**
規則的な　**Reg，reg，reg.**
規則的に便通がある　**BOR**
規則的律動　**reg.rhy**
規則に従って　**sec.reg.**
規定　**n，N，n**
亀裂　**Fiss，fiss**
偽悪性高熱症(患者)　**MHS**
偽陰性の　**FN，Fneg**
偽エリテマトーデス(症候群)　**PLE**
偽血管腫(性)間質性増殖(症)　**PASH**
偽血管性腺様扁平上皮癌　**PASCC，PASCCL**
偽血小板減少症　**PTCP**
偽コリンエステラーゼ　**PchE**
偽高血圧　**PSH**
偽(性)腎動脈症候群　**PRAS**
偽声帯　**FVC**
偽性偽性上皮小体機能低下症　**PPHP**
偽性上皮小体機能低下症　**PHPT**
偽性低アルドステロン症　**PHA**
偽性伝達物質　**FT**
偽性の　**ps**
偽性脳腫瘍　**PC**
偽性嚢胞　**Ps**
偽性副甲状腺機能低下症　**PHP**
偽(性)ゾリンジャー・エリソン症候群　**Ps-ZES**
偽(性)特発性血小板減少性紫斑病　**PITP**
偽動脈瘤　**FA**
偽肉腫性筋線維芽細胞腫瘍　**PMT**

偽肉腫性筋膜炎　**PSF**
偽妊娠　**PSP**
偽脳腫瘍　**PTC**
偽脳腫瘍症候群　**PCS**
偽嚢胞　**PC, psc**
偽(性)白癬性毛瘡　**PFB**
偽半陰陽者　**PH**
偽(性)剥脱　**PSX**
偽(性)剥脱(落屑)症候群　**PXS**
偽(性)剥脱〔落屑〕症候群　**PES**
偽閉経療法　**GnRH agonist therapy**
偽膜性壊死性全腸炎　**PNE**
偽膜性小腸結腸炎　**PMEC**
偽膜性大腸炎　**PMC**
偽薬　**ADT, P, PBO, PL, PLBO**
偽薬錠　**PT**
偽陽性の　**FP**
偽(性)落屑　**PSX**
偽落屑物質　**PE material**
偽(性)リンパ球脈絡髄膜炎　**PLC**
偽濾胞　**PF**
偽L鎖　**phiLC**
偽L鎖遺伝子　**ΦLC**
幾何学の　**geom**
幾何標準誤差　**GSE**
幾何級数　**GP**
幾何平均　**GM**
幾何平均値　**GMT**
揮発性脂肪酸　**VFA**
揮発性の　**vol, vol., volt**
揮発性腐食防止剤　**VCI**
揮発性芳香族炭化水素　**VAH**
期　**ph**
期外収縮　**ES, Extra, PB, PC**
期外収縮後増強作用　**PESP**
期外収縮後の　**PES**
期間　**D, d., pd, per**
期限が切れた　**exp, Exp, EXP**
期待回復時間　**ETR**
期待誤差　**EE**
期待されている　**exp, expt, expt.**
期待値　**E**
期・年齢・リンパ球予後指数　**SALPI**
稀少疾患の全国機構　**NORD**
義(理の)兄弟　**BIL**
義姉　**SIL**
義肢　**AFL**
義父　**FIL**
義妹　**SIL**
義理の母　**M/L**
義理の娘　**DIL**
(神経)疑核　**NA**
疑似性　**SP**
疑問のある　**qq**
器官　**org**
器官系　**sys**
器官の　**org**
器官培養　**OC**
器官別分類　**SOC**
器械　**appl**
器具　**app, appar, appl, batt, Inst, inst**
器質化間質性肺炎　**OIP**
器質化肺炎を伴う閉塞性細気管支炎　**BOOP**
器質性心疾患　**OHD**
器質精神症候群　**OMS**
器質性精神疾患　**OMD**
器質性脳疾患　**OBD**
器質性脳症候群　**obs, obs., OBS, Obs**
器質性不安症候群　**OAS**
器質的聴覚疾患　**OHD**
輝度　**B**
機械　**Inst, inst**
(胆石の)機械式砕石法　**MBL**
機械操作による心(蔵)血管データ分析　**card amp**
機械的1回換気量　**VTM**
機械的炎症　**MI**
機械的換気補助　**MVA**
機械的関節装置　**MJA**
機械的刺激　**MS**
機械的な　**mech**
機械的肺換気法　**MV**
機械的腰痛(症)　**MLBP**
機械的療法　**mecano**
機械(的)療法　**Mechano, mechano**
機器中性子放射化分析法　**INAA**
機構　**mech**
機序　**mech**
機能　**A, a, F, fct, fn, funct**
機能温存直腸結腸切除　**RP**
機能回復評価システム　**RES**
機能検査　**FS**
機能検査依頼　**FTR**
機能検査報告　**FTR**
機能試験　**FT**
機能しない　**NF**
機能する　**fn, funct**
機能的細胞外液　**FECF**
機能性胃腸障害　**FGID**
機能性子宮出血　**FUB**
機能性終末神経支配比　**FTIR**
機能性ディスペプシア　**FD**
機能性難聴　**FHL**
機能性の　**funct**
機能喪失　**lf**

機能喪失平均時間 **MTBFL**
機能的・解剖学的負荷 **FAL**
機能的MRI **FMRI**
機能的顎矯正装置 **FKOA**
機能的活性 **FA**
機能的経皮的神経刺激 **FTNS**
機能的頸部郭清術 **FND**
機能的好気性障害 **FAI**
機能的残気量 **FiO_2, FR, FRC**
機能的循環補助 **MCA**
機能的自立度評価法 **FIM**
機能的神経筋刺激 **FNS**
機能的短縮 **FS**
機能的腸障害〔疾患〕 **FBD**
機能的追求 **fi**
機能的電気刺激 **FES**
機能的尿道長 **FPL**
機能的評価選別質問 **FASQ**
機能的不応期 **FRP**
機能的膀胱容量 **FBC**
機能ナトリウム分泌 **EFNa**
機能範囲内 **WFL**
機能評価項目表 **FAI**
機能不全 **MAL**
機能不全性子宮出血 **DUB**
機能不全性(子宮)出血 **DFB**
機能不全レベル **LOI**
擬態患者 **SP**
擬態言語 **simula**
擬態の **sim**
聴こえない **inaud**
議事録 **proc, Procs**
傷ついた **WD, wd**
吉草酸ベタメタゾンクリーム **BV**
拮抗 **antag, antag.**
拮抗(作用) **antag, antag.**
拮抗された **A**
拮抗されない **NA**
拮抗する **antag, antag.**
喫煙 **smk**
喫煙者 **SM**
喫煙縮合物 **CSC**
喫煙と健康に関する活動 **ASH**
喫煙と健康のための国内情報センター **NCSH**
逆因子 **RF**
逆位 **inv**
逆受身血球凝集反応 **RPHA**
逆受身皮膚アナフィラキシー **RPCA**
逆受身ラテックス血球凝集 **RPLA**
逆受動アルツス反応 **RPA**
逆浸透 **RO**
逆説睡眠 **PS**
逆説の **paradox**
逆相 **RP**
逆相クロマトグラフィ **RPC**
逆単純放射免疫拡散(法) **RSRID**
逆転 **REV, rev.**
逆転再生 **REV, rev.**
逆転した **iv**
逆転写 **RT**
逆転写酸素 **RTase**
逆転写酵素をもつ癌ウイルス **RETRO.**
逆に **vv, v.v.**
逆の **Recip, recip., REV, rev.**
逆比率換気 **IRV**
逆方向の **retro**
逆溶血斑測定 **RHPA**
逆流性収縮期雑音 **RSM**
逆流性食道炎 **RE**
逆流性腎症 **RN**
逆流分画 **RF**
逆流分層 **RF**
逆流量 **RV**
逆ローテーションシステム **CRS**
脚 **L ext., l/ext, Lg, lg., PED**
脚間(核) **IP**
脚長 **BL**
脚長差 **LLD**
脚ブロック **BBB, bun.br.blk.**
客観性の欠如・協調性の欠如・無愛想(=ギルフォード・マーチン人格目録の因子) **O.Co.Ag**
客観的改善 **OI**
客観的検査 **OT**
客観的情報 **O**
客観的所見 **O**
客観的進歩発展 **ado**
客観的な **O**
客観的臨床能力試験 **OSCE**
逆行性 **retros**
逆行性気体腎盂造影法 **RPP**
逆行性強収縮 **RGC**
逆行性経肝胆道ドレナージ **RTBD**
逆行性上腕動脈造影 **PAG**
逆行性腎盂造影 **RGP**
逆行性腎盂造影図 **REP, RPG**
逆行性腎盂造影法 **RP**
逆行性大腿カテーテル **RFC**
逆行性電気ショック治療(法) **REST**
逆行性電気ショック療法

REST
逆行性尿道造影図　RUG
逆行性尿道造影法　RUG
逆行性尿道膀胱造影
UCG
逆行性尿路造影　RU
逆行性膀胱造影　RC
逆行の　retro
(脳の)弓状核　Ar
弓状核　ARC
弓状係蹄渦巻指紋　ALW
弓状彎曲の　circum
牛眼　buphth.
牛(酪)乳　BM
牛乳　CM, KM
牛乳アレルギー　CMA
牛乳蛋白　CMP
丘疹状ムチン沈着症　PM
旧学術用語　OT
旧式の　obs, obs., OBS, Obs, OD
旧ツベルクリン　OT
旧用語　OT
臼蓋回転骨切り術　RAO
臼蓋指数　AI
臼蓋迫害角　AI
臼歯　M
臼歯列指数　DI
休暇　Lv, lv
休憩室　RR
休息痛　RP
吸引　asp
吸引管　v
吸引灌流組織摘出装置
SITE
吸引灌流チップ　AI tip
吸引する　v, vac
吸引ソケット　SS
吸引分娩　VE, VED
吸引分娩器　VE
吸引法　SM
吸角　C, c
吸気　I, Insp, insp, Inspir, inspir
吸気/呼気時間比
I/E ratio
吸気圧　Pi
吸気ガス量　VI
吸気休止時間　TIP
吸気筋　IM
吸気筋訓練　IMT
吸気後休止時間　EIP
吸気酸素分圧　FiO_2, PIO_2
吸気〔吸入〕酸素分画濃度
FIO_2
吸気時間　TI
吸気相・呼気相時間比
TI/TE
吸気相・呼気相比　I/E
吸気相/呼気相時間比
I/E
吸気中枢　IC
吸気抵抗　IR
吸気トリガー流量　Vtr
吸気の　Insp, insp, Inspir, inspir
吸気肺活量　IVC
吸気分時換気量　V_I
吸気末プラトー　EIP
吸気陽性気道圧　IPAP
吸気予備(量)　IR
吸気流量率(速度)　IFR
吸気量　Vi
吸光度　A, E, OD
吸光度単位・フルスケール
AUFS
吸収　ABs, absorp
吸収・分泌・代謝・排出
ADME
吸収係数　AC, CA
吸収する〔した〕　asp
吸収速度　RA
吸収度　A
吸収軟膏　AO
吸収不良(症候群)　MA
吸収不良症候群　MAS
吸収率　CA
吸収率較差　DAR
吸収量　*D*
吸収力　a.
吸湿性コンデンサー湿度調節器　HCH
吸水薬罨法　HP
吸息　I
吸着狂犬病ワクチン
RVA, RVS
吸着交叉〔差〕疫電気泳動法
ACIE
吸入　I, insuf, insuf.
吸入(法)　INH, inh, inhal
吸入気酸素分圧　PIO_2
吸入酸素　OI
吸入〔吸気〕酸素濃度
FIO_2
吸入試験　IT
吸入により　PI
吸入療法　IT
求心神経遮断性疼痛症候群
DPS
求心神経遮断疼痛症候群
DAP
求心性の　aff, aff.
急激なGによる失神
G-LOC
急死　SD
急性アレルギー性脳炎
AAE
急性胃腸炎　AGE
急性胃粘膜病変　AGML
急性胃病変　AGL
急性咽頭結膜熱　APCF
急性ウイルス性肝炎
AVH
急性壊死性潰瘍性歯肉炎
ANUG
急性壊死性出血性脳症
ANHE
急性壊死性膵炎　ANP
急性炎症性脱髄性多発根神経炎　AIDP
急性炎症性多発根ニューロパシー　AIP
急性炎症なし　NAI

急性黄色(肝)萎縮(症)
AYA
急性横断性脊髄炎　**ATM**
急性横断性ミエロパシー
ATM
急性灰白髄炎　**Polio**
急性潰瘍性歯肉炎　**AUG**
急性カタル性結膜炎
CCA
急性かつ広範な阻血性筋壊死　**AMIM**
急性化膿性耳下腺炎
ASP
急性化膿性中耳炎
APOM, OMPA
急性化膿性閉塞性胆管炎
ASOC
急性化膿性右中耳炎
ROMSA
急性過敏性症候群　**AHS**
急性顆粒球(性)白血病
AGL
急性肝炎　**AH**
急性換気不全　**AVF**
急性冠血管梗塞　**ACI**
急性間欠性ポルフィリン症
AIP
急性感作性リンパ球増加(症)　**AIL**
急性間質性腎炎　**AIN**
急性間質性肺炎　**AIP**
急性感染症　**AID**
急性感染性多発神経炎
AIP
急性感染(性)脳炎　**AIE**
急性冠(状)動脈閉塞(症)
ACO
急性冠(状)(動脈)(機能)不全(症)　**ACI**
急性肝不全　**ALF**
急性期　**AP**
急性期蛋白　**APP**
急性気道感染症　**ARI**
急性狭隅角緑内障
ANAG
急性巨核芽球性白血病
AMKL
急性局所性脳浮腫
AFCE
急性頸部外傷症候群
ACTS
急性好酸球性肺炎　**AEP**
急性高山病　**AMS**
急性喉頭気管気管支炎
ALTB
急性後部多発性板状色素上皮症　**APMPPE**
急性硬膜外血腫　**AEDH**
急性硬膜下血腫　**ASDH**
急性呼吸器感染症　**ARI**
急性呼吸器疾患　**ARD, ARI, ARTI**
急性呼吸切迫症候群
ARDS
急性呼吸不全　**ARF, ARI**
急性骨髄芽球性白血病
AML
急性骨髄性白血病　**AML**
急性骨髄性白血病での遺伝子　**HRX**
急性骨髄線維症　**AMF**
急性骨髄単球性白血病
AMML, AMMoL, MLA
急性昏迷状態　**ACS**
急性細菌性心内膜炎
ABE
急性錯乱状態　**ACS**
急性左(心)室不全
ALVF
急性散在性脳炎　**ADE**
急性散在性脳脊髄炎
ADEM
急性糸球体腎炎　**AGN**
急性時集中治療　**AIT**
急性疾患の徴候なし
NSAD
急性十二指腸潰瘍　**ADU**
急性十二指腸粘膜病変
ADML
急性出血性結膜炎　**AHC**
急性出血性膵炎　**AHP**
急性出血性脳脊髄炎
AHE
急性出血性白質脳炎
AHLE
急性出血性膀胱炎　**AHC**
急性術後腎不全
APORF
急性腫瘍融解症候群
ATLS
急性条件下壊死　**ACN**
急性小脳失調(症)　**ACA**
急性自律神経ニューロパシー　**AAN**
急性腎盂腎炎　**APN**
急性腎炎　**AN**
急性心筋梗塞　**AMI**
急性心筋不全　**AMI**
急性神経根刺激　**ANRI**
急性神経刺激　**ANI**
急性心血管(疾患)　**ACV**
急性進行性半月体形成性糸球体腎炎　**RPCGN**
急性心(臓)疾患　**AHD**
急性心不全　**AHF**
急性腎不全　**ARF**
急性前骨髄球性白血病
APL, AProL, A ProL
急性全身性結核　**AGT**
急性全身性紅斑性狼瘡
ASLE
急性前脊髄障害　**AASCI**
急性前ブドウ膜炎　**AAU**
急性相　**AP**
急性巣状脳虚血　**AFCI**
急性増殖　**AP**
急性側索硬化症　**ALS**
急性粟粒結核(症)　**AMT**
急性単芽球性白血病
AMOL, AMoL
急性単球性白血病
AML, AMOL,

AMoL, AMonoL
急性単純性膀胱炎　AUC
急性胆嚢炎　AC
急性中耳炎　AOM, OMA
急性中毒性脳症　ATE
急性転化　BC
急性毒性表皮剝脱　EAT
急性特発性心膜炎　AIP
急性特発性汎自律神経失調症　AIPD
急性尿細管壊死　ATN
急性尿道症候群　AUS
急性熱性好中球性皮膚病　SS
急性熱性呼吸器疾患　AFRD, AFRI
急性粘膜皮膚眼(症候群)　AMO
急性粘膜病変　AML
急性の　a, AC, ac
急性脳炎症候群　AES
急性脳梗塞　ACI
急性脳症候群　ABS
急性脳脊髄膜炎　ACM
急性の病気なし　NAD
急性肺炎　AP
急性肺障害　ALI
急性肺性心　CPA
急性肺浮腫　OAP
急性肺胞障害　AAI
急性播種性表皮壊死症　ADEN
急性白血病　AL
急性パニック特性尺度　API
急性汎自律神経失調症　APD
急性(期)反応因子　APRF
急性(期)反応(性)物質　APR
急性鼻炎　RhA.
急性皮質壊死　ACN
急性皮膚エリテマトーデス　ACLE
急性皮膚筋炎　AD
急性非リンパ芽球性白血病　ANLL
急性非リンパ性白血病　ANLL
急性不安発作　AAA
急性封入体脳炎　AIE
急性不応性心筋虚血　ARMI
急性分娩時胎児仮死　AIFD
急性分類不能白血病　AUL
急性閉塞隅角緑内障　AACG, ACAG
急性閉塞性化膿性胆管炎　AOSC
急性ヘルペス性歯根口内炎　AHGS
急性ポリオ脳炎　APE
急性未分化白血病　AUL
急性網膜壊死　ARN
急性溶血性貧血　AHA
急性腰部外傷症候群　ALTS
急性溶連菌感染後糸球体腎炎　APSGN
急性リウマチ熱　ARF
急性両耳性中耳炎　BOMA
急性淋菌性後部尿道炎　UGPA
急性淋菌性前部尿道炎　UGAA
急性リンパ芽球性白血病　ALbL
急性リンパ芽球(性)白血病　ALL
急性リンパ球性白血病　CALL
急性リンパ性白血病　ALL
急性リンパ球性白血病共通抗原(＝CD 10)　CALLA
急性リンパ肉腫細胞性白血病　ALSL
急性連鎖球菌後糸球体腎炎　APSGN
急性労作性横紋筋融解(症)　AER
急性狼瘡(性)心膜炎　ALP
急性濾胞性結膜炎　CFA
急速眼球運動　REM
急速眼球運動期　REMP
急速眼球運動随伴睡眠　SREM
急速眼球運動睡眠　REMS
急速螢光フォーカス抑制検査　RFFIT
急速減量　QWL
急速撮影コンピュータ体軸断層撮影法　RACAT
急速充満期　RF
急速充満波　RFW
急速(連続)静注腎盂造影法　RSIP, RSIVP
急速静注(式)マンニトール腎盂造影法　RSMP
急速静注(式)マンニトール負荷腎盂造影法　RSMIVP
急速進行性糸球体腎炎　RPGN
急速心室反応　RVR
急速心房細動　RAF
急速単収縮　FT
急速凍結切片　RFS
急速分画　Q-fract
急速変換運動　RAM
急速免疫螢光染色法　RIS
急速冷凍　QF
急速連続腎盂造影法　RSP
急迫する　exprim.
級　Cl

き

救急　emer, emerg
救急医師　EP
救急医療　EMS
救急医療技術員　EMT
救急医療サービス　EHS
救急医療システム　EMS, EMSS
救急医療大学協会　UAEM
救急医療チーム　EMT
救急医療に携わる技術者の全国協会　NAEMT
救急医療部　DEM, Dem
救急外来患者　EOP
救急観察用ベッド　EOB
救急患者収容治療室　ACU
救急管理研究施設　ECRI
救急公共情報　EPI
救急サービス　ES
救急産院と新生児保護　EMIC
救急室開胸　ERT
救急室開腹　ERL
救急車　Amb, amb.
救急重症者評価スコア　SAPS
救急司令本部　EOH
救急蘇生術訓練用患者シミュレータ　RESIM
救急蘇生用訓練シミュレーター　RESIM
救急治療室　ER
救急治療部　ED, ETU
救急病棟　EW
救急部　EU
救急部での死亡　DIE
救急ベッドサービス　EBS
救済と社会復帰国際連合機関　UNRRA
救出　salv
救出する　resc, rsq
救助　ref, rel
救命呼吸維持装置　RBA
球海綿体反射　BCR
球海綿体反応　BCR
球型の　orbic
球後視神経炎　RBN
球状・線維状の　G-F
球状アクチン　G-actin
球状心疾患　RHD
球状赤血球症　Sph
球状赤血球症，デンバー型　Sph-1
(副腎皮質の)球状帯　ZG
球状の　Glob, S, sph, sph., sphr
球の　S, sph, sph.
球面燭光　scp
球面レンズ　S
給食　fdg
鳩糞便(抗原)　PD
嗅閾値　OT
嗅覚関連症候群　ORS
嗅覚計　odom
嗅覚の　olf
嗅球　OB, OLB
嗅結節　OTU
嗅索　OP
嗅上皮　OE
嗅電図　EOG
嗅脳溝　RS
頬骨上顎骨　Zm
去痰の　exp, expec., expect., expt, expt.
去痰薬　expect., expt, expt.
巨核芽球　MKB
(骨髄)巨核球　MEG, meg
巨核球　Mgk
巨核球コロニー形成刺激因子　M-CSF
巨核球コロニー形成単位　CFU-M, CFU-Meg
巨核球コロニー刺激因子　Meg-CSF, MK-CSF
巨核球増幅因子活性　MK-POT
巨核球由来成長因子　MKDGF
巨細胞腫　GCT
巨細胞性間質性肺炎　GIP
巨細胞性封入体病　CMID
巨細胞動脈炎　GCA
巨細胞網様核　RG
巨赤芽球性貧血　MA
巨(大)赤芽球(性)の　meg
巨大陰性T波　GNT
巨大細胞封入体病　CID
巨大細胞封入体病(CID)ウイルス　CID virus
巨大細胞網様核　NRGC
巨大左房　GLA
巨大色素有毛母斑　GPHN
巨大軸索形成　GAF
巨大軸索ニューロパシー　GAN
巨大セロトニン含有ニューロン　GSCN
巨大セロトニンニューロン　GSN
巨大ド(ー)パミン含有細胞　GDC
巨大な　M
巨大乳頭結膜炎　GPC
巨大微少終板電位　GMEPP
巨大濾胞リンパ腫　GFL
居住　Res, res
居住環境　habit
拒否失敗率　RFR
挙睾(筋)反射　CR
挙上　elev
虚血スコア　IS
虚血性冠(状動脈)疾患　ICD
虚血性冠(状動脈)心疾患　ICHD
虚血性脚疾患　ILD

虚血性急性腎不全　**IARF**
虚血性血栓性脳血管疾患　**ITCVD**
虚血性骨壊死　**INB**
虚血性細胞変化　**ICC**
虚血性四肢疾患　**ILD**
虚血性視神経疾患　**ION**
虚血性心左(心)室機能不全　**ILVD**
虚血性心疾患　**IHD**
虚血性腎症　**IRD**
虚血性大腸炎　**IC**
虚血性腸疾患　**IBD**
虚血性脳血管性頭痛　**ICVH**
虚血性脳梗塞　**IBI**
虚弱　**debil.**
虚弱した　**debil.**
虚脱度　**CI**
許可　**Per**
許可条件　**COA**
許容しうる適格レベル　**aql**
許容しうる品質標準　**aql**
許容できる危険率　**AHR**
許容度　**tol**
許容レベル　**TL**
魚鱗癬・頬・眉(症候群)　**ICE**
距骨下関節　**STJ**
距舟状骨の　**TN**
距離　**dis, dist, s**
距離試験　**DT**
極端　**X, x**
鋸歯状の　**Dent, dent.**
兄弟　**B, br, bro, SS**
共因子　**CoF**
共役因子　**CF, F**
共役の　**conjug.**
共感の　**S, symp, sympat, sympath**
共振　**cons**
共調　**coor, CoOrd, coord**
共通供給者　**UF**
共通抗原　**CA**
共通データ処理組織　**CDPS**
共通の　**com**
共通肺静脈腔　**CPVC**
共通房室管孔　**CAVC**
共通房室弁口　**AV canal, A-V canal, AV communis, A-V communis**
共同　**conjug.**
共同音当量レベル　**CNEL**
共同血液センター審議会　**CCBC**
共同健康協会　**CHA**
共同指向初期治療　**COPC**
共同生活で感染する肺炎　**CAP**
共同選択企画　**COP**
共同体健康サービス　**CHS**
共同体精神健康センター　**CMHC**
共同の　**conjug.**
共同病室　**Wd**
共同利用型病院情報システム　**SHAS, SHIS**
共分散分析　**ANCOVA**
共鳴イオン化分光法　**RIS**
共鳴過度　**Hyp**
共役　**conjug.**
共有度係数　**M**
共力(協力)作用　**syn**
共力(協力)薬　**syn**
仰臥位　**BKLY**
仰臥位低血圧症候群　**SHS**
仰臥の　**SU, sup, SUP, sup.**
狂犬病免疫グロブリン　**RIg**
供給者支援組織　**PSO**
供血者血球浮遊液　**DC**
供血者血清　**DS**
供血者の血漿　**DP**
京都大学 iPS 細胞研究所　**CiRA**
協会　**Assn, assn., assoc, assoc.**
協調　**coor, CoOrd, coord**
協調指数　**q**
協定世界時　**UTC**
協力　**coop**
協力する　**coop**
協力的な　**coop**
狭(隅)角緑内障　**NAG**
狭義の　**sens.str., s.s., s.str.**
狭窄後拡張　**PSD**
狭窄後の　**PST**
狭心症　**ang.pect, AP**
狭心症誘発の 3 大因子：労作・食事・情動　**3E**
狭頭(人種)　**scaphocephs**
狭末端部　**NDS**
恐慌性障害　**PD**
恐慌発作　**PA**
恐怖調査スケジュール　**FSS**
胸(部)　**C, CH, Ch, ch**
胸囲　**BG, BU, CC**
胸郭　**RC, T, TC, TH, Th, th, Thor, thor.**
胸郭横径　**TDT**
胸郭外陰圧　**NETP**
胸郭外陰圧式の人工呼吸　**NETPV**
胸郭外陰圧補助呼吸　**CNPV**
胸郭外持続陰圧　**CNETP, EENETP**
胸郭外持続陰圧換気

CNETPV
胸郭指数 TI
胸郭出口症候群 TOS
胸郭の TH, Th, th, Thor, thor.
胸郭の前後径 APDT
胸郭容量 TCV
胸管 TD, TLD
胸管圧 TDP
胸管ドレナージ TDD, TDDA
胸管留置管排液 CTD
胸管流量 TDF
胸管リンパ球 TDL
胸管瘻 TDF
胸腔鏡下交感神経遮断術 ETS
胸腔鏡下手術 VATS
胸腔鏡下電気凝固法自然気胸治療 SPECT
胸腔滲出細胞 PEC
胸腔内 IT
胸(膜)腔内圧 IPP, Ppl
胸腔内ガス容量 TGV
胸腔内気体量 IGV
胸骨 St
胸骨・後頭骨・下顎骨固定用装具 SOMI
胸骨縁 SB, SR
胸骨下の SS
胸骨下部左縁 LLLSB, LLSB
胸骨左縁 LSB
胸骨上縁 S, USP
胸骨上端 SS
胸骨穿刺 P.St., stern.punct
胸骨中線 MSL
胸骨柄下濁音 SMD
胸骨傍線 PSL
胸骨傍の PS
胸骨翻転術 STO
胸三角筋部皮弁 DP flap
胸左腕 CL
胸鎖関節 SCJ
胸鎖靱帯 SC
胸鎖乳突筋直径 SMD
胸鎖乳突筋皮弁 SMMC
胸鎖乳突の SCM
胸鎖の SC
胸式呼吸 cost resp
胸水 PF, Pleur Fl
胸腺 T, thy
胸腺T細胞特異抗原 THYSA
胸腺依存(細胞) TD
胸腺依存抗原 TDA
胸腺依存性抗原 TDA antigen
胸腺依存帯 TDZ
胸腺依存領域 TDA
胸腺依存リンパ球 TDL
胸腺因子 TF
胸腺因子X TFX
胸腺栄養細胞 TNC
胸腺(依存)リンパ球 T-L
胸腺(由来)細胞 T cell
胸腺細胞 Thy
胸腺細胞刺激因子 TSF
胸腺細胞傷害性自然自己抗体 NTA
胸腺細胞有糸分裂因子 TMF
胸腺樹状細胞 TDC
胸腺上皮 TE
胸腺上皮(細胞) TE
胸腺上皮細胞 TEC, TSC
胸腺上皮性細網細胞 TER
胸腺除去 Tx
胸腺体液性因子 THF
胸腺蛋白 TP
胸腺摘出〔切除〕(術) thy
胸腺透過性因子 TPF
胸腺内 i.t.
胸腺白血病 TL
胸腺白血病抗原 TL antigen
胸腺非依存(領)域 TIA
胸腺非依存性 TI
胸腺非依存性抗原 TIAg, Ti antigen
胸腺ポリペプチド TP
胸腺網状上皮の TRE
胸腺由来(リンパ球) T
胸腺(由来)リンパ球 TL
胸腺リンパ形成不全(症) TAL
胸腺リンパ腫 TL
胸(包)帯 CS
胸椎 BW, BWS, D, D-spine, T, T-spine, TV
胸椎椎弓切除 T lam
胸椎の Th
胸痛 CP
胸(椎)の T
胸部 Br
胸部X線 CX
胸部X線(フィルム) CXR
胸部X線像 CR
胸部横径 TTD
胸部下大静脈 TIVC
胸部下部食道 Ei
胸部下部と腹部食道 E
胸部外科 Thor, Th.Surg.
胸部外科(学) TS
胸部疾患医認定書 DCD
胸部疾患結核病医認定書 DCTD
胸部上部食道 Iu
胸部臓器全摘術 TAE
胸部大動脈 ThA
胸部大動脈瘤 TAA
胸部中部食道 Im
胸部と右腕 CR
胸部と左足 CF
胸部の TH, Th, th
胸部誘導 BWA
胸部理学療法 CPT

胸壁　**CW**
胸壁外カウンターパルゼーション法　**ECP**
胸壁外心臓圧迫　**ECP**
胸壁外心臓圧迫法　**ECC**
胸壁外心肺蘇生　**ECPR**
胸壁コンプライアンス　**Ccw**
胸傍の　**para T**
胸膜　**PLE**
胸膜(の)　**pl, PL**
胸膜滲出　**PE**
胸膜中皮細胞　**PMC**
胸膜直下の曲線状陰影　**SCLS**
胸膜内カテーテル　**IC**
胸膜肺炎微生物　**PPO**
胸膜肺炎様微生物　**PPLO**
胸膜播種　**Pl**
胸膜播種性転移の程度　**pl_{0-1}, Pl_{0-1}**
胸膜部大動脈瘤　**TAAA**
胸腰仙骨部専用コルセット　**TLSO**
胸肋鎖骨過形成症　**SCCH**
莢膜抗原　**K**
強化インスリン療法　**ICIT, IIT**
強化経静脈性腎盂造影法　**IIVP**
強化水溶液　**FA**
強角膜線維柱帯　**TR**
強拡大視野　**HPF, hpf**
強拡大の一視野(あたり)　**/HPF, /hpf**
強心剤　**CC**
強制　**obln**
強制吸気　**FI**
強制呼気(呼出)法　**FET**
強制収容所症候群　**KZS**
強制収容所神経症　**KZ-Neurose**
強制選択視　**FPL**
強制利尿　**FD**
強直持続時間　**Dt**
強直収縮　**TC**
強直性屈筋　**TF**
強直性伸展　**TE**
強直性脊椎炎　**AS, SPA**
強直性脊椎関節炎　**AS**
強直性脊椎骨化過剰　**ASH**
強度　**st, str**
強度/持続時間比　**I/T**
強迫神経症　**Zwang**
強迫性障害　**OCD**
強皮症　**SCL, sclero, SD**
強皮症腎クリーゼ　**SRC**
強膜　**sc**
強膜陥凹　**SB**
強膜岬　**SS**
強膜硬性係数　**K**
強膜と結膜　**S & C**
強力鎮静薬　**DS**
強力な　**fort.**
強力ネオミノファーゲンC　**SNMC**
教育　**ed, educ, Instr**
教育学士　**Pd.D.**
教育可能な精神遅滞　**EMR**
教育開発　**ED**
教育計画　**E**
教育された　**ed**
教育試験サービス　**ETS**
教育指数　**EQ**
教育者　**ed, Tchr**
教育省　**MOE**
教育する　**Tch**
教育と研究　**TR**
教育年齢　**EA**
教育の　**ed, educ**
教育の一般認可　**GCE**
教育用テレビ　**ETV**
教官　**Instr**
教室　**DPT**
教師　**Tchr**
教師・子・親　**TCP**
教師訓練センター　**TTC**
教授　**Prof, prof**
教授方略　**TS**
教授面接　**MTP**
教養のある　**intell**
境界　**LIM**
境界域梗塞　**WI**
境界型人格障害　**BPD**
境界群　**B group**
境界(型)ブドウ糖負荷試験　**BGTT**
境界領域高血圧ラット　**BHR**
境界例の診断面接基準　**DIB**
頬咽頭の　**BPh**
頬(面)遠心(面)の　**BD**
頬縁　**MB**
頬(面歯)頸(面)の　**BC**
頬骨　**zygo**
頬骨弓　**ZA**
頬骨骨折　**JBF**
頬骨上顎骨複合体　**ZMC**
頬骨の　**ZMC, zygo**
頬神経　**NB**
頬(面)唇(面)の　**BLa**
頬軸位頸面の　**BAC**
頬軸位の　**BA**
頬(面)軸(面)歯肉(面)の　**BAG**
頬(面)(歯)髄(面)の　**BP**
頬側近心面の　**BM**
頬側咬合面の　**BO**
頬側歯肉面の　**BG**
頬側舌面の　**BL**
頬(側)の　**B, Bucc**
頬鼻(側)の　**BN**
(骨)橋　**Br**
橋　**P**
橋核　**PN**
橋(加工)義歯　**Br**
橋小脳萎縮　**PCA**
橋中心性髄鞘融解症　**CPM**

橋蓄尿中枢　**PUSC**
橋排尿中枢　**PMC**
橋腹側核　**VPN**
橋保存鼓室乳突削開術　**IBM**
橋網様体　**PRF**
橋網様被蓋核　**NSTP**
橋・膝・後頭(棘波)　**PGO**
興味　**int，int.**
興味深い　**int，int.**
凝塊　**coag**
凝血　**go**
凝血酵素　**Hpx**
凝血退縮　**CR**
凝結　**flocc**
凝固　**COAG，coag，solidif**
凝固因子　**CF**
凝固時間　**CLT，cl T，cl.time，coag.time，CT**
凝固組織因子発現阻害因子　**TFPI**
凝固帯　**KB**
凝固第Ⅰ因子(＝フィブリノゲン)　**F Ⅰ**
凝固第Ⅱ因子(＝プロトロンビン)　**F Ⅱ**
凝固第Ⅲ因子(＝組織トロンボプラスチン)　**F Ⅲ**
凝固第Ⅳ因子(＝カルシウムイオン)　**F Ⅳ**
凝固第Ⅴ因子(＝不安定因子)　**F Ⅴ**
凝固第Ⅶ因子(＝安定因子)　**F Ⅶ**
凝固第Ⅷ因子　**F Ⅷ**
凝固第Ⅷ因子フォンウィルブラント因子活性　**F Ⅷ RWA，F Ⅷ R：WA**
凝固第Ⅸ因子　**F Ⅸ**
凝固第Ⅺ因子　**F Ⅺ**
凝固第Ⅻ因子(接触因子)　**F Ⅻ**
凝固第ⅩⅢ因子(フィブリン安定化因子)　**F ⅩⅢ**
凝固第Ⅹ因子(スチュアート因子)　**F Ⅹ**
凝固第Ⅷ因子関連抗原　**F Ⅷ R AG，F Ⅷ R：AG**
凝固第Ⅷ因子凝固活性　**F Ⅷ：C**
凝固第Ⅷ因子凝固抗原　**F Ⅷ CAG**
凝固第Ⅷ因子フォンウィルブラント因子　**F Ⅷ R：WF**
凝固点　**FP**
(熱)凝固ヒト免疫グロブリンG　**AHG**
凝集　**aggreg，flocc**
凝集(作用)　**aggl，Agglut，agglut，agglut.，AGL**
凝集・架状検査　**AFT**
凝集アルブミン　**AA**
凝集した　**agg，aggl，Agglut，agglut，agglut.**
凝集する　**agg，aggl，aggr**
凝集反応　**aggl，Agglut，agglut，agglut.，AGL，COA**
凝集ヒトγグロブリン　**AHGG**
凝集ヒトグロブリン　**AHG**
凝集物　**agg，aggr**
(溶液の)凝集〔濃縮〕力　**CS**
凝集力　**CS**
凝乳酵素　**lab**
矮小体軀(症)　**D**
矯正　**rect，rect.**
矯正(術)　**cor，cor.**
矯正されない　**uncod**
矯正した　**rect，rect.**
矯正視力　**VAcc，VA_{cc}**
矯正心理学者協会　**ACP**
矯正治療士　**CT**
矯正治療部　**CTD**
矯正で　**cc，c.c.**
矯正的職業療法　**ROT**
矯正なしで　**SC，s.c.**
矯正の　**cor，cor.**
矯正不能　**n.c.**
蟯虫　**pw**
蟯虫(属)　**E**
鏡映描写法　**MDT**
競合　**compet**
競合結合定量(法)　**CBA**
競合する医療プラン　**CMP**
競合蛋白結合(性)の　**CPB**
競合蛋白結合分析　**CPBA**
競合蛋白質結合放射測定法　**CPBA**
競合的心室応答　**RVR**
競争排除　**CE**
驚愕反応聴力検査　**SRA**
曲光度　**DS**
曲線下領域　**AUC**
曲直線輪郭　**CLP**
曲点　**pc**
局　**bur**
局在性進行食道癌　**LAEC**
局所気管麻酔(法)　**LTA**
局所酸素摂取率　**ROEF**
局所磁気共鳴　**TMR**
局所腫瘍温熱(療法)　**LTH**
局所照射　**Lx，LX**
局所所見　**SPL**
局所心筋血流量　**RMBF**
局所性骨溶性高カルシウム血症　**LOH**
局所性脳損傷　**FBI**
局所大脳酸素代謝率

RCMRO₂
局所大脳ブドウ糖代謝率 **RCMRGl**
局所的アデノシンキナーゼ **FAK**
局所適応症候群 **LAS**
局所的血管内凝固 **LIC**
局所的高分解能 NMR スペクトル測定法 **SPARS**
局所的興奮状態 **LES**
局所的な **T**
局所的に **top**
局所的熱平衡 **LTE**
局所の **lo, LO, loc**
局所(大)脳血流(量) **LCBF**
局所脳血流 **rCBF**
局所脳血流量 **rCBV**
局所脳血流量測定 **rCBF study**
局所脳ブドウ糖消費量 **LCGU**
局所脳ブドウ糖代謝率 **LCMRG**
局所フッ化物塗布 **TFA**
局所壁運動 **SWM**
局所壁運動振幅 **SWMA**
局所ヘパリン化 **RH**
局所麻酔(法) **LA**
局所麻酔薬共融物 **EMLA**
局所リンパ管炎リーシュマニア(症) **LLL**
局所リンパ節 **RNL**
局所リンパ節細胞 **RNLC**
局所リンパ節摘除(術) **RLND**
局長 **supt**
局部組織前位縫合皮弁 **LTAF**
極 **P, p**
極小開頭血腫洗浄除去法 **HITT**
極紫外線 **XUV**
極端な **ext, ext.**
極長鎖脂肪酸 **VLCFA**
極長鎖飽和脂肪酸 **VLFA**
極低周波 **ELF**
極低周波磁場 **ELFMF**
極微量 **ST**
極量 **MD**
棘 **SP, Sp, sp**
棘下筋 **IS**
棘踝長 **SMD**
棘口吸虫(属) **E**
棘孔 **FS**
棘鎖角 **SCA**
棘状突起の **SP, Sp, sp**
棘徐波複合(体) **SWC**
棘徐波複合体 **Sp & W, S & W**
棘の **SP, Sp, sp**
棘波 **Sp**
棘波電位 **SP**
極めて純粋な **exf**
均一酵素免疫測定法 **HEI**
均一制限因子 **HRF**
均一性選択因子 **SS factor**
均一溶液からの沈殿生成 **PFHS**
均等脳波反応 **AER**
近位胃迷走神経切断(術) **PGV**
近位型脊髄性筋萎縮症 **PSMA**
近位冠(状)静脈洞 **PCS**
近位曲(尿)細管 **PCT**
近位指骨間(の) **PIP**
近位指骨間関節 **PIP**
近位指皺襞 **PFC**
近位指節間関節 **PIPJ**
近位手掌皮膚溝 **PPC**
近位爪下爪(甲)真菌症 **PSO**
近位大腿骨巣状欠損(症) **PFFD**
近位尿細管性アシドーシス **pRTA**
近位の **P, Prox, prox**
(骨の)近位部 1/3(区) **P/3**
近(心)遠心の **MD**
近見時の上斜位 **H'**
近見時の上斜視 **HT'**
近見時の内斜視 **ET'**
近心頰側咬合の **MBO**
近心頰側歯髄の **MBP**
近心頰側の **MB**
近心歯頸の **MC**
近心側頭硬化症 **MTS**
近心の **M**
近心面切端の **MI**
近似 **approx**
近似位置 **PA**
近似致死濃度 **ALC**
近似分裂病 **BS**
近紫外(線)の **NUV**
近視 **M, MY, myop**
近視性乱視 **Am, am, ASM, AsM, As.M.**
近視(性)の **M**
近視複合乱視 **MAs**
近視優勢の乱視 **AMP**
近親の **rel**
近赤外線の **NIR**
近赤外分析法 **NIRS**
近接様効果 **ID**
(視覚の)近点 **P**
近点 **NP, PP, P.P., Pp, p.p.**
近傍 **NS**
近隣保健センター **NHC**
金 **Au, aur.**
金塩療法 **GST**
金衡 **TR**
金属 **M, met**
金属・酸化シリコン半導体 **MOS**
金属感応成分 **MRE**

き

金属キレート親和性クロマトグラフィ **MCAC**
金属性異物 **MFB**
金属(性)の **met, met.**
金チオリンゴ酸ナトリウム **GST**
金のインレー **G**
金標識抗原検出法 **GLAD**
菌が付着・侵入している細胞 **CBO**
(真)菌学 **Mycol**
菌株 **colet**
菌形指数 **MI**
菌自動同定法 **BAIT**
菌状息肉症 **MF**
菌状息肉症/セザリー症候群 **MF/SS**
菌体外毒素 **EXT**
菌体内毒素蛋白 **OEP**
菌乳剤 **TBN**
菌乳剤ツベルクリン **TBE**
菌非発育帯 **NGZ**
菌力 **V, VI**
筋 **MM, mm, Ms, musc, musc.ligt, mus-lig**
筋異栄養(症) **MD**
筋萎縮性側索硬化症 **ALS, LAS**
筋(肉)カルニチン欠乏(症) **MCD**
筋学 **myol**
筋(肉)活動 **MA**
筋(肉)活動電位 **MAP**
筋曲光率 **MD**
筋強直反応 **MyoR**
筋緊張性ジストロフィ **MD, MMD, MyMD**
筋緊張低下・精神障害・性機能不全〔低下〕・肥満(症候群) **HHHO**
筋緊張低下・精神障害・肥満(症候群) **HHO, H_2O**
筋機能検査 **MFT**
筋群 **MG**
筋(肉)血流量 **MBF**
筋原線維の **MF**
筋(肉)検査 **MT**
筋痙攣 **Msp**
筋骨格の **MuS**
筋細胞膜 **SL**
筋ジストロフィ **MD**
筋ジストロフィ協会 **MDA**
筋ショック因子 **MSF**
筋小胞体 **SR**
筋上皮(細胞) **ME**
筋収縮性頭痛 **MCH**
筋弛緩薬 **MR**
筋伸展反射 **MR**
筋(肉)刺激 **M stim**
筋受容体 **MR**
筋神経接合部 **MNJ**
筋神経の **MN**
筋腎代謝症候群 **MNMS**
筋性大動脈弁下部狭窄(症) **MSS**
筋層 **ML**
筋層ジストロフィ **dy**
筋層の **m**
筋注 **IMI**
筋電位 **MP**
筋電図 **EMG**
筋電図検査 **EMG**
筋電図の高低振幅比 **H/L**
筋(肉)と腱 **MT**
筋頭 **cap**
筋肉 **M, M, m., MM, mm, Ms, musc**
筋肉温度 **Tm**
筋肉クレアチンキナーゼ **MCK**
筋肉検査 **ME**
筋肉内(注射) **IM, im, I.m.**
筋肉内ガンマグロブリン **IMGG**
筋肉内注射 **IMI**
筋肉内免疫グロブリン **IGIM, IMIG**
筋肉ヘモグロビン **Mb**
筋(性)の **musc**
筋の交感神経の活動 **MSA**
筋(肉)バランス **MB**
筋反応検査〔試験〕 **MRT**
筋皮弁 **MC**
筋ホスホリラーゼ欠損症 **MPD**
筋膜 **F**
筋無力(症)症候群 **MYS**
筋無力性反応 **MyaR**
筋(肉)毛細(血)管基底膜 **MCBN**
筋(肉)毛細(血)管基底膜肥厚 **MCBNT**
筋力 **MMst, mm st, mmst., mm str, MS, M str**
筋力計 **dyn**
筋力低下 **W**
筋・筋膜疼痛症候群 **MPD, MPS**
筋・筋膜疼痛症候群 **MPDS**
禁忌 **contra**
禁忌の **contra**
禁食 **NPM**
禁断症状(症候群) **WDS**
禁断症状による運動障害 **WD**
禁断症状による体の震え **WBS**
銀 **Ag, arg., S**
銀棘点電極 **SSP**
銀染色仁形成体部 **AgNOR**
銀フォーク変形 **SF def.**
緊急 **emer, emerg**
緊急医療システム **EMS**

緊急外傷収容部門　**ETU**
緊急症状処置　**TES**
緊急〔救急〕心疾患治療　**ECC**
緊急〔救急〕心疾患治療部　**ECCU**
緊急生命維持装置　**ELSS**
緊急対応能力　**EC**
緊急治療センター　**UCC**
緊急の　**urg**
緊急放送システム　**EBS**
緊急用飲用水殺菌剤　**EDWGT**
緊急呼び出し　**EM**
緊張　**T, ten, tens, tns, tnsn**
緊張減少　**T−**
緊張時間　**A, ASZ**
緊張した　**ten**
緊張状態　**T-state**
緊張性頸反射　**TNR**
(筋)緊張性ジストロフィ　**MyD, MYD**
緊張性振動性反射　**TVR**
緊張性尿失禁　**USI**
緊張性迷路反射　**TLR**
緊張増加　**T＋**
緊張部　**PT**

く

グアイフェネシン・フェニルプロパノールアミン・フェニレフリン **ULR**
グアニジノエチル・メルカプト酢酸 **GEMSA**
グアニジノ化合物 **GC**
グアニジノコハク酸 **GSA**
グアニジノ酢酸 **GAA**
グアニジノ酪酸 **GBA**
グアニジン **G, Gdn**
グアニル酸 **G**
グアニル酸キナーゼ **GUK**
グアニル酸シクラーゼ **GC**
グアニン **G, Gua**
グアニン・シトシン型 **GC type**
グアニン・シトシン含有量 **GC content**
グアネチジン **GN**
グアノシン **G, GUO, Guo**
グアノシン(5′-)二リン酸 **GDP**
グアノシン二リン酸-D-マンノース **GDP-D-mannose**
グアノシン二リン酸マンノース **GDPM**
グアノシン(5′-)三リン酸 **GTP**
グアノシン三リン酸 **GRTP**
グアノシン 5′-四リン酸 **ppGpp**
グアノシン 5′-リン酸 **GMP**
グアノシン結合脾臓細胞 **G-SC**
グアヤレチン酸 **GA**
クイック試験〔検査〕 **QT**
クイーンズランド熱 **QuF**
クエッケンステット・ストーキー試験〔検査〕 **Q-S test**
クエッケンステット試験〔検査〕 **QT**
クヴェーム・シルツバッハ(試験) **KS**
クエッケンステット試験〔検査〕 **Q test**
クエン酸 **CA**
クエン酸リン酸ブドウ糖 **CPD**
クエン酸塩 **cit**
クエン酸塩ブドウ糖液 **ACDS**
クエン酸回路 **CC**
クエン酸カルシウム尿素 **CCC**
クエン酸合成酵素 **CS**
クエン酸処理ヒト全血 **CWHB**
クエン酸抽出物 **CAE**
クエン酸ヒドロキシキノリン **HQC**
クエン酸ブドウ糖 **ACD**
クエン酸マグネシウム **Mag.cit**
クエン酸リン酸ブドウ糖液 **CPD solution**
クォート **Q, q, qt**
クーゲル・ストロフ(症候群) **KS**
クーゲルベルク・ヴェランデル(病) **KW**
クサリヘビ毒素 **VV**
グジュロ・ブラン(症候群) **GB**
クーダー職業選好記録 **KPR-V**
クーダー選好記録 **KPR**
クーダーテスト **KT**
クーダー動作性検査 **KPT**
グッドパスチャー症候群 **GP, GPS, GS**
クッパーマン指数 **KI**
クニッツ膵臓トリプシンインヒビター **KPTI**
クプファー細胞 **KC**
クマシーブリリアントブルー **CBB**
クーマーマイシン **CMRM**
クームス試験 **CT**
クモザル **ASP**
クモノスカビ(属) **R**
クモ膜下腔 **SAS**
クモ膜下腔圧 **SAP**
クモ膜下出血 **SAH, Subara, Subara.**
クモ膜下髄液 **SACSF**
クモ膜下ブロック **SAB**
クライストチャーチ染色体 **Ch, CH**
クライハウエル・ベトケ(試験) **K-B**
クライン・レビン症候群 **KL**
クラインフェルター・ラインフェンスタイン・オルブライト(症候群) **KRA**
クラインフェルター症候群 **KS, XXYsyndrome, YY syndrome**
クラーク・ハッドフィールド(症候群) **CH**
クラス A 麻薬 **class A's**
クラス B 麻薬 **class B's**
クラス M 麻薬 **class M's**
クラス X 麻薬 **class X's**
グラスゴーコーマスケール **GCS**
グラスゴー転帰尺度〔スケール〕 **GOS**
クラッチ〔松葉杖〕使用時の

荷重　**WBC**
グラディエントエコー　**GRE**
クラドスポリウム(属)　**C**
クラブラン/チカルシリン　**CVA/TIPC**
クラブラン酸　**CVA, CVD**
クラブラン酸/アモキシシリン　**CVA/AMPC**
クラミジア(属)　**C**
クラミジアの外膜複合体　**COMC**
グラミシジン　**GRD**
グラミシジンA　**GA**
グラミシジンJ　**GR-J, GRMN-J**
(重量の)グラム　**Gm, gm**
グラム　**g, grm**
グラム/100 mL　**Gm%, gm%**
グラム/cc　**gm/cc**
グラム/ミリリットル　**g%**
グラム/リットル　**G/L, g/l, gm/l**
グラムイオン　**g-ion**
グラム陰性桿菌　**GNB, GNR**
グラム陰性桿菌性髄膜炎　**GNBM**
グラム陰性球菌　**GNC**
グラム陰性菌　**GNB, gr−**
グラム陰性双球菌　**GND**
グラム陰性の　**Gm−, GN**
グラム陰性ブロス　**GN broth**
グラムカロリー　**cal, g cal, g-cal, gm cal**
グラム染色(法)　**GS**
グラムセンチメートル　**g-cm**
グラムパーセント　**g%**
グラム分子重量　**GMW**
グラム分子容量　**GMV**
グラムメートル　**g-m, gm-m**
グラムモル　**g-mol**
グラム陽性桿菌　**GPB**
グラム陽性球菌　**GPC**
グラム陽性菌　**gr＋**
グラム陽性線維　**GPF**
グラム陽性の　**G＋, Gm＋, GP, GrP**
クラリスロマイシン　**CAM**
グリア成熟因子　**GMF**
グリア成長因子　**GGF**
グリア線維酸性蛋白　**GFAP**
グリア促進因子　**GPF**
クリアランス　**C, CL, clnc, Cx**
クリアランス率　**C**
グリオキサル酸　**G**
グリオキザルビスグアニルヒドラゾン　**GAG**
クリオ〔寒冷〕グロブリン　**CG**
クリオグロブリン　**Cry**
クリオ〔寒冷〕グロブリン血(症)　**CG**
クリオ免疫グロブリン　**cryo-Ig**
クリグラー鉄寒天(培地)　**KIA**
グリコキサラーゼ　**GLO**
グリコケノデオキシコール酸　**GCDC**
グリコーゲン　**G, glyco**
グリコゲン合成単位　**GU**
グリコーゲン指数　**GI**
(ペプチド中の)グリココル　**Gly**
グリココール酸　**GC**
グリコサミノグリカン　**GAG**
グリコサミノグリカン分解酵素　**GL enzyme**
グリコシル化ヘモグロビン　**G-HB**
グリコシレーション阻害因子　**GIF**
グリコデオキシコール酸　**GDC**
グリコヘモグロビン　**GHB**
グリコリル　**Gl**
グリコールメタアクリレート　**GMA**
グリコレーション増強因子　**GEF**
グリシリジン　**GL**
グリシリジン鉄コロイド　**GIC**
グリシル　**Gly**
グリシルグリシン　**GG**
グリシレチン酸　**GA**
グリシン　**G, Gly**
グリシンアミドリボヌクレオチド　**GAR**
グリシンエチルエステル　**GEE**
グリシン過多糖蛋白(質)　**GRG**
グリシンキシリッド　**GX**
グリシン酸亜鉛マーカー　**ZGM**
グリシンリッチβグリコプロテイン　**GBG**
グリシンリッチγグリコプロテイン(血清蛋白成分)　**GGG**
グリース・ロミジン試薬　**GR**
クリスタルバイオレット　**CV**
クリスチャン・ウェーバー(症候群)　**CW**
クリスパー(クリスパーインターフィアランス)　**CRISPRi**

クリスマス(因子)
X-mas
クリスマス因子 **CF**
グリセオフルビン **GRF**
グリセライト **gly, glyc.**
グリセリド **glyc**
グリセリルグアヤコール塩 **GG**
グリセリン **glyc**
グリセリン(=グリセロール) **glc**
グリセリン-1-リン酸酸化酵素 **GPO**
グリセリン一ステアリン酸エステル **GMS**
グリセリン浣腸 **GE**
グリセリン含有ベロナール緩衝液 **VBG**
グリセリン基 **gl**
グリセリン水 **GW**
グリセリンと水 **G&W**
グリセリンと水浣腸 **GWE**
グリセルアルデヒド **Dg**
グリセルアルデヒド-3-リン酸 **G3P, G-3-P**
グリセルアルデヒド-3-リン酸脱水素酵素 **G-3-PD**
グリセルアルデヒド-3-リン酸デヒドロゲナーゼ **GAPDH**
グリセルアルデヒド還元酵素 **GAR**
グリセロホスフェートデヒドロゲナーゼ **GDH**
グリセロホスホリルコリン **GPC**
グリセロール **gly**
グリセロールエステルヒドロラーゼ **GEH**
グリセロールキナーゼ **GK**
グリセロール三リン酸 **Glycerol-3-P**
グリセロール脱水素酵素 **GDH**
グリセンチン **GLI**
グリチルリジン鉄コロイド **GIF**
グリチルリチン **GR**
クリッペル・テレノー・ウェーバー症候群 **KTWS**
クリッペル・テレノー症候群 **KT syndrome**
クリーナーマイクロアナリシス **CMA**
クリニカルエンジニアリング **CE**
グリニッジ標準時 **GMT, G.M.T.**
クリニテストとアセテスト **C&A**
クリニミール **CML**
クリプトコックス(属) **C**
クリプトン **Kr**
クリプトン 81 m **^{81m}Kr**
クリペル・フェーユ(症候群) **KF**
クリペル・フェーユ症候群 **KFS**
クリミア・コンゴ出血熱 **CCHF**
クリーム **crem., Crm**
クリューバー・バレラ染色 **KB**
クリューバー・ビューシー症候群 **KBS**
グリーン(の) **g, grn**
クリンダマイシン **CC, CLDM, CLM, CM**
グリーンティーポリフェノフラクション **GTP**
グル音 **G**
グルカゴン **GN**
グルカゴン・インスリン(療法) **GI**
グルカゴン活性 **GLA**
グルカゴン分泌 **GS**
グルカゴン免疫反応性 **GI**
グルカゴン様ペプチド **GLP-1**
グルカゴン様免疫反応物質 **GLI**
グルクロニド **glucur**
グルクロン酸 **GA, GlcU, GlcUA, Glc-UA, GluA**
グルコース-1,6-二リン酸 **G-1,6-P**
グルココルチコイド **GC**
グルココルチコイド感応部位 **GRE**
グルココルチコイド結合蛋白 **GBP**
グルココルチコイド奏効性アルドステロン症 **GSH**
グルココルチコステロイド **GCS**
グルコサミン **GlcN**
グルコシル化最終産物 **AGEs**
グルコース **G, g, Glu, GLU, glu., gluc**
グルコース・インスリン・塩化カリウム **GIK**
グルコース・インスリン・カリウム溶液 **GIK**
グルコース・ガラクトース吸収不全 **GGM**
グルコース・グルカゴン・トリプトアミド負荷試験 **GGtt**
グルコース・トリス・EDTA **GTE**
グルコース・フルクトース・キシリトール混合液 **GFX**
グルコース/生理食塩水 **G/NS**

グルコース/窒素比 **G/N r**
グルコース(=ブドウ糖)/窒素比 **GN, G/N**
グルコース-1-リン酸 **Glu-1-p, G1P**
グルコース-6-ホスファターゼ **G6Pase**
グルコース-6-リン酸 **G6P**
グルコース-6-リン酸脱水素酵素 **G6PD, G-6PD, G-6-PD, G6PDH**
グルコース-6-リン酸デヒドロゲナーゼ **GPD**
グルコース閾値の異常 **AGT**
グルコース一リン酸 **GMP**
グルコースオキシダーゼ **glu.ox., GO, g.o.**
グルコースオキシダーゼ/ペルオキシダーゼ法 **GOD/POD**
グルコースコントロールインスリン注入システム **GCIIS**
グルコース産生 **GP**
グルコース消費指数 **GCI**
グルコースゼラチンベロナール緩衝液 **GGVB**
グルコース注入率 **GIR**
グルコース反応 **GR**
グルコースリン酸イソメラーゼ **GPI, PGI**
グルコースリン酸イソメラーゼ欠乏症 **GPID**
グルコース六リン酸脱水素酵素 **G6DP**
グルコース輸送担体 **GLUT**
グルコン酸 **GlcA**
グルコン酸カリウム **KGL**
グルコン酸カルシウム **Ca gluc**
グルシニウム(=ベリリウム) **Gl**
グルタチオン **GSH**
グルタチオン・インスリントランスヒドロゲナーゼ **GIT**
グルタチオン-S-変換酵素 **GST**
グルタチオン-S-変換酵素胎盤型 **GST-P**
グルタチオン還元酵素 **GR, GSR, GSSG-R**
グルタチオン合成酵素欠乏症 **GSD**
グルタチオン重炭酸加リンゲル液 **GBR**
グルタチオンペルオキシダーゼ **GP, GPX, GSH-P**
グルタチオンペルオキシダーゼ1 **GPX1**
グルタチオンペルキオシダーゼ **GSHPx**
グルタミニル **Gln**
グルタミル **Glu**
グルタミルトランスペプチダーゼ **GT, GTP**
グルタミン **GIN, Gln, Glu, Glx, Q**
グルタミン(酸) **Z**
グルタミン・リジン・チロシン **GLT**
グルタミン合成酵素 **GS**
グルタミン酸 **E, GL, Glu, Glx**
グルタミン酸・リジン・アラニン・チロシン **GLAT**
グルタミン酸エステル **glu**
グルタミン酸塩 **glu**
グルタミン酸オキサロ酢酸トランスアミナーゼ **GOT**
グルタミン酸脱水素酵素 **GDH, GLDH**
グルタミン酸デカルボキシラーゼ **GAD**
グルタミン酸デヒドロゲナーゼ **GLD**
グルタミン酸ナトリウム **MSG**
グルタミン酸ピルビン酸トランスアミナーゼ **GPT**
グルタミン酸リン酸ショ糖 **SPG**
グルタミントランスペプチダーゼ活性蛋白 **GAP**
グルタメートγセミアルデヒド合成酵素 **GSAS**
グルタメートデヒドロゲナーゼ **GDH**
グルタールアルデヒド **GA**
クルチッキー細胞癌(腫) **KCC**
クルツケ身体障害スケール **KDSS**
グルテン感受性過敏腸障害 **GSE**
グループ医療保険 **HIPC**
グループ環境スケール **GES**
クループ関連ウイルス **CAV**
グループ仕事 **GW**
グループ適応療法 **GAT**
グループリーダー **GL**
グループ療法 **GP TH, GpTh, Gp Th, GT**
クレアチニン **CR, Cr, cr, cr., CRE, Crea, creat, Crt, CRTNN**
クレアチニンクリアランス **CC, Ccr, CrCl, Crcl**

クレアチニン身長比 **CHI**
クレアチン **cr, creat**
クレアチンキナーゼ **CK**
クレアチンキナーゼアイソエンザイム **CK-ISO**
クレアチンキナーゼ心筋由来アイソザイム **CK-MB**
クレアチンキナーゼ脳由来アイソザイム **CK-BB**
クレアチンホスホキナーゼ **CPK**
クレアチンホスホキナーゼMBアイソザイム **CPK-MB**
クレアチンリン酸 **cp, CP, CrP, Crp**
クレアチン・リン酸キナーゼ心筋束 **CPK-MB**
グレイ **Gy**
グレーヴス病 **GD**
クレシールバイオレット **CV**
クレスト(＝皮下石灰沈着症・レイノー症状・食道障害・手指硬化・多発性毛細血管拡張症)(症候群) **CREST**
クレゾールレッド **CR**
グレード **gr**
クレブシエラ(属) **K, Kleb(s)**
クレブス・ヘンゼライト(サイクル) **KH**
クレブス・リンゲル重炭酸塩緩衝剤 **KRBB**
クレブス・リンゲルヘペス **KRH**
クレブス・リンゲルリン酸(緩衝溶液) **KRPS**
クレブス・リンゲルリン酸緩衝液 **KRP**
クレブス・レフラー桿菌 **KL bac**
クレブス・ヘンゼライト溶液 **KHS**
クレペリン・モレル(病) **KM**
グレーン **gr**
クレンジング浣腸 **CE**
グレンブラッド・ストランベリー症候群 **GS**
クロイツバイン脂肪腫症候群 **KLS**
クロイツフェルト・ヤコブ症候群 **CJS**
クロイツフェルト・ヤコブ病 **CJD**
クロキサシリン **CLX, CX**
クロキツネザル **LMA**
クロージングボリュウム **CV**
グロス **G**
グロスウイルス **GV**
グロスウイルス抗原 **GSA**
グロス細胞表面抗原 **GCSA**
クロストリジウム **CL, CI, Clostr**
クロストリジウム(属) **C**
グロス白血病ウイルス **GLV**
クロテナガザル **HCO**
クロトン油 **Co**
クロナゼパム **CZP**
クロニジン **CL**
クローニング阻止因子 **CLIF**
クローヌス **C, Cl, cl**
クローヌス指数 **CI**
クロノルキス **Clon**
グローバル診断法 **GAS**
グローバルファンド日本委員会 **FGFJ**
グロビンインスリン **GI, G.I.**
クロフィブレート **CLOF**
グローブ寒暖計 **GT**
グロブリン **G, Glob**
グロブリン/アルブミン係数 **G/A quotient**
グロブリン過剰血紫斑病 **HGP**
グロブリン結合インスリン **GBI**
グロボイド白質ジストロフィ **GLD**
グロー放電質量分析法 **GDMS**
グロー放電ランプ **GDL**
クロマチン結合蛋白(質) **CBP**
クロム **Cr**
クロム放出試験〔検査〕 **CRT**
クロムミョウバン・ヘマトキシリン・フロキシン **CHP**
クロモグリク酸ナトリウム **SCG**
クロモグリク酸二ナトリウム **DSC, DSCG**
クロモトロープ酸 **CTA**
クロモバクテリウム(属) **C, CHR, Chr, Chrbac**
クロモマイシン **CHRM**
クロモマイシンA 3 **CHRM**
クロラムフェニコール **C, CAP, CHL, CP**
クロラムフェニコールアセチル転移酵素 **CAT, CATase**
クロラムブシル **CHL, CLB**
クロラムブシル,ビンブラスチン,プロカルバジン,プレドニゾン **ChlVPP, ClVPP**
クロルキノール **CHQ**

クロルジアゼポキシド **CDE，CDZ**
クロルテトラサイクリン **CTC**
クロルニトロフェン **CNP**
クロルプロマジン **Ch，CP，CPZ**
クロロアセトフェノン **CAP，CN**
クロロエチル・シクロヘキシル・ニトロソウレア **CCNU**
クロロキニジンとプリマキン **CP**
クロロキン **CQ**
クロロキン・キニーネ **CQ**
クロロキン耐性熱帯熱マラリア原虫 **CRPF**
クロロキンとプリマキン **CP**
クロロキンマスタード **CQM**
クロロクルオリン **Chl**
クロロ酢酸アルデヒド **CAA**
クロロ酢酸エステル分解酵素 **CAE**
クロロジアリルアセトアミド **CDAA**
クロロチアジド **CHTZ，CT，CTZ**
クロロトリアジン **CTZ**
クロロピクリン **PS**
クロロフェニル・ジメチルウレア **CMu**
クロロフェニルアラニン **CPA**
クロロフェノキシイソ酪酸エチル **CPIB**
クロロブタノール **Chlb**
クロロフルオロカーボン **CFC**
クロロフルオロメタン **CFM**
クロロプレン **chloro**
クロロベンジリデンマロノニトリル **CS**
クロロホルム **Chl，chl，chlor**
クロロホルムエーテル **CE，C-E**
クロロホルムエーテル混合物 **CE mix**
クロロマイセチン **CM**
クロロメチルメチルエーテル **CMME**
クロロメチルメチルエーテルの発癌性 **CMME**
クーロン **C，Q**
クーロン/ボルト **C/V**
クローン化阻止因子 **CIF**
クローン生存率 **CA**
クローン阻止因子 **CIF**
クローン病 **CD**
クローン病の活性指標 **CDAI**
クーロン毎キログラム **C/kg**
クワシオルコル・マラスムス症候群 **KMS**
クワント徴候 **Q's sign**
クンケル試験 **ZnTT**
くし型電極 **IDE**
くすぶり型急性白血病 **SAL**
くるぶし **ank**
くるぶし奇形矯正 **AFO**
くるぶし反射 **AJ，A-J**
区 **A，S**
区(域) **Seg，seg**
区域 **Z**
区画 **sec，sect，sect.**
区分 **sec，sect，sect.**
区別する **dist**
区別の **diff**
苦味チンキ **T.a.，Tr.am.**
郡 **Co**
組換え型 **rec**
駆血帯 **TQ**
駆出音 **ES**
駆出期 **Ep**
駆出期雑音 **EM**
駆出時間 **ET**
駆出性クリック **EC**
駆出性収縮期雑音 **ESM**
駆出前期指数 **PEPI**
駆出短縮 **FS**
駆出分画 **EF**
駆出率 **EF**
繰り返さない **ne rep.**
繰り返し **reps**
繰り返し時間 **TR**
繰り返した **repetat.，rptd**
繰り返してもよい **MR**
繰り返す **do.，rept，rept.，Rpt，rpt**
繰り返すな **non rep.，non repet.，NR，n.r.**
繰り返せ **rep.，rept，rept.**
空 **sp**
空(腸)回腸の **JI**
空(腸)回腸バイパス(術) **JIB**
空回腸吻合(術) **JI**
空間 **S，SP，sp**
空間最大ベクトル **MSV**
空間周波数特性 **MTF**
空間占拠性病変 **SOL**
(宇宙)空間適応症候群 **SAS**
空間データ管理システム **SDMS**
空間の生物学的観察 **BIOS**
空間ベクトル心電図 **SVCG**
空気 **ATM，atm，atmos**
空気清浄法改正条例

CAAA
空気速度　**AV, Av**
空気伝導　**LL**
空気の　**atmos, Pn, pneu**
空虚トルコ鞍　**ES**
空虚トルコ鞍症候群　**ESS**
空中線量　**E**
空中発生の　**abn**
空腸　**JEJ, Jej, jej**
空腸胃重積(症)　**JGI**
空腸空腸吻合(術)　**JJ**
空腸経管栄養　**JTF**
空腸憩室炎　**JD**
空腸内の　**IJ**
空洞　**cav**
空腹期の消化管強収縮運動　**IMC**
空腹時(検査)　**F**
空腹時ガストリンレベル　**FGL**
空腹時血漿グルコース　**FPG**
空腹時血漿脂質　**FPL**
空腹時血清レベル　**FSL**
空腹時血糖　**BFS, FB, FBS, FGB, FSG**
空腹時血糖値　**FBG, FBS**
空腹時総胆汁酸　**FTBA**
空胞化毒素　**VT**
偶然の　**accid**
偶発故障率　**CFR**
偶発疾患死　**DID**
偶発性低体温　**AH**
隅角底　**AR**
腔　**cav**
腔内　**icav**
腔内ラジウム(療法)　**ICR**
草　**herb**
薬　**D, RX, Rx.**
薬製造教育情報協会　**MEDIA**
薬とアルコールの委員会　**CODA**
薬と化粧品の色　**D & C color**
薬に反対する母親　**MADs**
薬の　**MED, Med, med.**
薬の分析と反応の安全利益評価　**RAD-AR**
(米国)薬評価事務局　**ODE**
薬を続けよ　**cont.rem.**
果物　**frt**
果物と野菜　**FV**
果物野菜貯蔵研究協会　**FVPRA**
砕いた　**contrit.**
砕く　**trir.**
口顔面指(形成不全症)　**OFD**
口顔面指(症候群)　**OFD**
口呼吸時の呼吸抵抗　**RrTM**
口の　**O**
口・顔面・指　**OFD**
屈曲　**f, fl, flex, flx**
屈曲・伸展障害　**flex-ext inj.**
屈曲させる　**flex**
屈曲した　**F, flex**
屈曲時における内旋　**IRF**
屈筋　**flex**
屈折　**RFR**
屈折異常　**am, am.**
屈折度　**D, dptr, DS**
屈折(左右)不同(症)　**Anisometr**
屈折率　**n, N_d, n_D, ref.ind**
国　**Nat**
国の　**Nat**
首曲げテスト　**NF test**
頸　**nk**
組　**Cl**
組換えアクチベーティング遺伝子１　**RAG-1**
組換えウイルス　**RV**
組換え型ヒト白血球インターフェロンA　**IFLrA**
曇った　**cl**
暗い　**dk**
久里浜式アルコール症選別検査　**KAST**
車椅子　**WC, W/C, wh ch**
黒い　**bk, Bl, bl, blk, nig.**
加えよ　**ad., add.**
加える　**admov.**
加えるべき　**TBA**
軍医総監　**SG**
軍医中佐　**Sg.cr.**
軍の　**mil**
軍用ショック治療ズボン　**MAST**
軍歴　**MH**
訓練によるリハビリテーション機関　**ORT**
訓練によるリハビリテーションのための米国組織　**AORTF**
訓練療法　**ET**
群　**G, g, GP, gp, grp**
群特異性抗原　**GAG**
群特異的抗原　**GSA**
群特異的な　**GS, gs**
群特別成分　**GC**
薫煙　**FUM**
薫煙する　**FUM**
薫蒸　**FUM**
薫蒸する　**FUM**

け

ゲイ関連免疫不全疾患 **GRID**
ケイ酸塩 **S**
ケイ素 **Si**
ケカビ(属) **M**
ゲージ **ga.**
ケジラミ(属) **P**
ケースカンファレンス **CC**
ケースワーカー **CW**
ケトアシドーシス **KA**
ケトアジピン酸 **Ka**
ケトイソ吉草酸 **KIV**
ケトエノール顆粒 **KEG**
ケトグルタラメート **KGM**
ケトコナゾール **KCZ**
ゲートコントロール説 **GCT**
ケトーシス型高グリシン血症 **KH**
ケトース **keto**
ケトステロイド **KS**
ケトチフェン **K**
ケトフェニルブタゾン **KPB**
ケト酪酸 **KB**
ケトン **keto**
ケトン・アルコール(結合物) **ketol**
ケトン/抗ケトン(比) **K/A, K：A**
ケトン陰性の過血糖 **NKH**
ケトン陰性の高浸透圧アシドーシス **NKHA**
ケトン体血症 **keto**
ケトン生成ステロイド **KGS**
ケトン体 **KB**
ケトン対抗ケトン **k/a**
ケトン尿 **keto**
ケトンの **keto**
ケニュ・ミュレー徴候 **Q-M sign**
ケノデオキシコール酸 **CDC, CDCA**
ケープ試験 **CAPE**
ケフラーゴールド1 **KG-1**
ケフリン,ゲンタマイシン,カルベニシリン **KGC**
ケラタン硫酸 **KS**
ケラチノサイト変性値 **DK**
ケラチン **K**
ケラチン・ミオシン・エピデルミン・フィブリン **KMEF**
ゲラン・スターン(症候群) **GS**
ケル因子 **K**
ケル陰性 **k**
ゲル拡散 **GD**
ゲル拡散法 **GFT**
ゲルクロマトグラフィ **GC**
ケル血液型 **K**
ゲル浸透性クロマトグラフィ **GPC**
ゲルストマン・シュトロイスラー・シャインカー症候群 **GSS**
ゲル電気泳動 **GE**
ゲル内沈降反応 **GDP**
ケルビン **K**
ケルマ **K, kerma**
ゲルマニウム **Ge**
ケルマン超音波白内障破砕吸引術 **KPE**
ケルマン法 **KEP**
ケル陽性 **k**
ゲル濾過 **GF**
ケローセン・アルコール・酢酸ジオキサン **KAAD**
ゲンスレン・エルプ症候群 **GE**
ゲンタマイシン **GE, GM**
ゲンタミシン **GM**
ゲンタミ〔マイ〕シン・バンコマイシン・ナイスタチン **GVN**
ケンダル化合物E(＝コルチゾン) **KE**
ゲンチアナ根末 **p.r.g.**
ゲンチアナ紫 **GV**
ケント乳児発育尺度〔スケール〕 **KIDS**
下剤 **CATH, Cath, Cath., cath., cathar, purg**
下痢 **d, Lax, lax**
下痢性貝毒 **DSP**
下痢と嘔吐 **D & V**
毛のはえぎわ **HL**
外科 **Chir, chir.**
外科(学) **CH, su, su., SURG, Surg, surg.**
外科・婦人科・産科 **SGO**
外科医 **D.Surg., S, su, su., SURG, Surg, surg.**
外科医全般事務局 **SGO**
外科医長 **Sg.C., sur cdr**
外科学 **S, Srg, srg**
外科学士 **B.Chir, B.Sur., CB**
外科学修士 **M.S.**
外科学博士 **D.Ch.**
外科修士 **CM, C.M.**
外科集中治療部門 **SICU**
外科手術(上)の **chirurg., SURG, Surg, surg.**
外科手術歴 **SH**
外科(手術)性上皮小体機能低下(症) **SHP**

外科的アキレス腱延長　**SATL**
外科的異物　**SFB**
外科的な　**su, su.**
外科的の　**S**
外科的ヘルニア　**SH**
外科的療法　**ST**
外科(的)の　**chirurg., SURG, Surg, surg.**
外科の　**su, su.**
外科博士　**M.Ch.**
外科被覆材料製造協会　**SDMA**
外科有資格者　**LCh**
仮病　**sim, simu**
解毒　**detox, DTX**
解毒センター　**detoxcen**
刑務所罹患リンパ球増殖症候群　**PALS**
形(状)　**fm**
形式　**F, f**
形状　**F, f**
形状記憶効果　**SME**
形質細胞　**pc, pl**
形質細胞腫　**PC**
形質細胞特異抗原　**PCA**
形質細胞白血病　**PCL**
形質細胞膜糖蛋白１　**PC 1**
形質転換因子　**TP**
形成　**fmn**
形成(物)　**frmn**
形成外科　**PL, PS, PSurg, P.surg**
形成外科医　**PL, pl.surg, PS, PSurg, P.surg**
形成外科医協会　**SPS**
形成外科のための米国耳鼻科学会　**AOSPS**
形成外科歴　**PSH**
形成性　**pl**
形態　**fig**
形態学　**morph**
形態学的な　**morph**
形態的死因不明死　**MUD**
形容詞　**adj**
系　**ser**
系(統)　**col, sys**
系統的酸素代謝予備　**SO_2MR**
系統的多臓器失調　**MSOF**
系統的脱感作　**SD**
系統別再調査　**Rev of Sys, r of s, ROS, RS, SR**
系統別症状　**S by S**
芸術療法　**AT**
(直)径　**D, d.**
係数　**C, c, coef, coeff, I, Q**
係蹄　**LH**
契約外科医　**CS**
計画　**P, prog**
計画出産外来　**BCC**
計画的白内障嚢外摘出　**PECCE**
計器　**G**
計算　**calc, caln, ct**
計算化学プログラム公表機関　**QCPE**
計算可能　**compu**
計算可能の　**compu**
計算管理　**NC**
計算機制御　**DDC**
計算した　**calcd**
計算者　**compu**
計算収縮値　**CCR**
計算する　**calc**
計算速度　**CR**
計測誤差　**EOM**
計測システム標準インターフェイス　**GPIB**
計量　**mensur**
珪肺結節　**SN**
経営　**mgmt, mgt**
経営サービス組織　**MSO**
経営者　**exec, exec.**
経横隔膜圧　**Pdi**
経カテーテル肝動脈塞栓術　**TAE**
経カテーテル生検　**TCB**
経カテーテル大動脈弁置換術　**TAVR**
経カテーテル大動脈弁留置術　**TAVI**
経カテーテル動注療法　**TAI**
経回腸静脈的食道胃静脈瘤塞栓術　**TIO**
経肝胆管造影図　**THC**
経肝胆管造影法　**THC**
経肝抵抗　**THR**
経過　**c, cse, prog, progr**
経過記録　**PN**
経管栄養　**TF**
経気管吸引　**TTA**
経気管吸引物　**TTA**
経気管ジェット換気　**TTJV**
経気管支吸引細胞診　**TBAC, TBNA**
経気管支生検　**TBB**
経気管支肺生検　**TBLB**
経気管支針吸引生検　**TBNAB**
経気管支針生検　**TBAB**
経気管挿管法　**ET**
経気管通気(法)　**TTI**
経気管的酸素療法　**TTOT**
経気管的選択的気管支擦過　**TSBB**
経気管の　**TT**
経気管肺換気法　**ITPV**
経胸郭抵抗　**TTR**
経胸針吸引　**TTNA**
経胸針(吸引)生検　**TTNB**
経胸(郭)の　**TT**
経胸壁心臓超音波検査　**TTE**
経頸静脈的逆行性胃静脈瘤

塞栓術　**TJO**
経験　**proc**
経験法則　**ROT**
経口(で)　**PO, P.O., p.o.**
経口〔口腔粘膜〕アレルギー症候群　**OAS**
経口胃チューブ　**OGT**
経口栄養　**OA**
経口感染ポリオウイルス　**OPV**
経口寛容誘導　**OT**
経口気管チューブ　**OET, OETT**
経口血糖降下性の　**OHG**
経口再水加溶液　**ORS**
経口食道チューブ　**OET**
経口食道聴診器　**OES**
経口浸透的　**Oros**
経口胆道膵管造影(法)　**PCPS**
経口胆嚢造影　**OCG**
経口胆嚢造影図　**OCG**
経口腸管洗浄液　**CCS**
経口的　**O**
経口的胆道内視鏡　**PCS**
経口的に　**O**
経口糖尿病薬　**OHA**
経口ニトログリセリン　**ONTG**
経口避妊ステロイド　**OCS**
経口避妊ホルモン　**OCH**
経口避妊薬　**BCP, OC, OCA, OCM, OCP**
経口避妊療法　**OCT**
経口ブドウ糖負荷試験　**OGTT**
経口補水療法　**ORT**
経肛門内視鏡下顕微手術　**TEM**
経喉頭吸引　**TLA**
経済学　**econ**
経済の　**econ**
経産　**P**
経産の　**P, para, Para, para.**
経産婦　**M, multip., Multip, PP, P.P., Pp, p.p.**
経産婦の　**MP, multip., Multip**
経十二指腸括約筋形成術　**TSP**
経食道的心臓超音波検査　**TEE**
経静脈 DSA　**IVDSA**
経静脈栄養　**IVN**
経静脈性脂肪負荷テスト　**IFTT**
経静脈性腎盂造影法　**IVP**
経静脈性胆道造影(法)　**IVC**
経静脈性胆嚢撮影法　**IVC**
経静脈性デジタルサブトラクション血管造影　**IVDSA**
経静脈的栄養供給協会　**PAPA**
経静脈内シクロホスファミド(療法)　**IVCY**
経静脈の　**TV**
経静脈ペースメーカー　**TVP, TV pacemaker**
経静脈輸液　**IVF**
経縦隔の　**TM**
経頭蓋ド(ッ)プラー超音波走査法　**TCD**
経胎盤出血　**TPH**
経胆管的胆道超音波検査(法)　**IDUS**
経中心静脈栄養　**IVH**
経直腸　**p rec, p.rec.**
経直腸超音波検査法　**TRUS**
経直腸的に　**per.rect.**
経腸栄養　**EN**
経腸的高カロリー栄養　**EH**
経腟子宮摘出術　**VH**
経腟超音波検査法　**TVS**
経腟的に　**PV, p.v.**
経腟頭頂位分娩　**VVD**
経聴道超音波発信法　**TAST**
経度　**long**
経動脈 DSA　**IADSA**
経動脈性化学塞栓術　**TACE**
経頭蓋骨超音波カラード(ッ)プラー断層法　**TCDT**
経頭蓋骨ド(ッ)プラー超音波検査法　**TCD**
経頭蓋超音波カラーフロー断層像　**TCCFI**
経頭蓋脳磁気刺激　**TMS**
経頭蓋脳断層法　**TCT**
経内腔直腸超音波検査　**ELUS**
経尿管尿管腎吻合(術)　**TUUN**
経尿管尿管吻合(術)　**TUU**
経尿道切開(術)　**TUI**
経尿道的温熱療法　**TUMT**
経尿道的凝固術　**TUC**
経尿道的結石破砕術　**TUL**
経尿道的光線照射高熱療法　**TURF**
経尿道的焼灼術　**TUF**
経尿道的(電気)切除術　**TUR**
経尿道的切除症候群　**TURS**
経尿道的前立腺・膀胱頸部切開術　**TIPBn**
経尿道的前立腺癌切除術　**TURCaP**
経尿道的前立腺蒸散術

TUEP
経尿道的前立腺切開
TUIP
経尿道的前立腺切除術
TURP
経尿道的前立腺電気蒸散術
TUVP
経尿道的超音波誘導下レーザー前立腺切除術
TULIP
経尿道的摘出　TUE
経尿道的尿管結石砕石術
TUL
経尿道的膀胱頸(部)切開
TUIBN
経尿道的膀胱頸切除術
TURBN
経尿道的膀胱腫瘍切除術
TUR-Bt, TURBT
経尿道的膀胱(腫瘍)切除
TURB
経尿道的レーザー外科
TULS
経尿道の　TU
経妊婦　PG, Pg, pg, pg.
経粘膜治療システム
TmTs
経肺圧　PL, Ptp
経皮吸収治療システム
TTS
経皮経管冠(状)動脈形成(術)　PTCA
経皮経管冠(状)動脈再灌流
PTCR
経皮経管冠(状)動脈内血栓溶解療法　PTCR
経皮経管血管形成術
PTA
経皮経管腎動脈形成術
PTRA
経皮経管腎動脈造影
PTRA
経皮(経管)大動脈弁切開術
PTAC
経皮経肝胆汁ドレナージ
PTBD
経皮経肝胆道鏡　PTCS
経皮経肝胆道鏡下胆石破砕術　PTCSL
経皮経肝(的)胆道造影(法)
PTHC
経皮経肝(的)胆道ドレナージ　PTHBD
経皮経肝胆道ドレナージ
PTCD
経皮経肝(的)胆道ドレナージ経腸栄養(法)
PTBD-EF
経皮経肝(的)胆道内視鏡
PTCS
経皮経肝胆嚢ドレナージ
PTCCD, PTGBD
経皮経肝胆嚢内視鏡
PTCCS
経皮経管的冠(状)動脈回転式粥腫切除術
PTCRA
経皮(的)経管的冠(状)動脈形成(術)　PCTA
経皮経肝的食道静脈塞栓術
PTO
経皮経肝的食道静脈瘤塞栓術　PTO
経皮経肝的胆管造影(法)
PTC
経皮経管的超音波冠(状)動脈形成(術)　PTUCA
経皮経肝的閉塞　PTO
経皮経肝的門脈造影(法)
PTP
経皮経肝的門脈造影塞栓術
PTPE
経皮経肝門脈カテーテル挿入　PTPC
経皮経肝門脈血採取法
PTPVS
経皮経肝門脈内注入療法
PTPI
経皮経静脈的僧帽弁交連切開術　PTMC
経皮経食道胃管挿入術
PTEG
経皮経胆道ドレナージ
PTBD
経皮臍帯血採取　PUBS
経皮酸素分圧監視　$tcPO_2$
経皮損傷　PI
経皮注入システム　TIS
経皮通電経穴刺激法
TEAS
経皮的エタノール注入
PEI
経皮的エタノール注入療法
PEIT
経皮的拡張気管切開
PDT
経皮的ガッセル神経節高周波凝固法　PRGC
経皮的カテーテルドレナージ　PCD
経皮的冠(状)動脈回転式粥腫切除術　PCRA
経皮的冠(状)動脈形成術
PCA
経皮的肝内門脈シャント術
TIPS
経皮的逆行性腎盂造影
PAP
経皮的旧バルーン動脈形成術　POBA
経皮的経肝的塞栓術
PTO
経皮的経肝的胆嚢ドレナージ　PTBD
経皮的頸動脈造影図
PCA
経皮的結石操作　PCSM
経皮的臍帯嚢胞穿刺
PCCP
経皮的酸素分圧　$tcPo_2$
経皮的腎外瘻切石術
PCNL
経皮的神経刺激　TNS
経皮的神経刺激装置

TCNS
経皮的腎結石破砕術
PNL
経皮的腎切石術　PCN
経皮的心肺バイパス
PCPB
経皮的心肺補助　PCPS
経皮的腎瘻(造設術)
PNS
経皮的腎瘻造設術　PCN
経皮的髄核摘出術　PN
経皮的穿刺吸引　PNA
経皮的挿入による脊髄硬膜外刺激　PISCES
経皮的大核生検　PLCB
経皮的大動脈弁形成(術)
PAV
経皮的胆道ドレナージ
PBD
経皮的中心静脈カテーテル
PCVC
経皮的超音波砕石術
PUL, pul
経皮的超音波腎砕石術
PUNL
経皮的椎間板切除術　PD
経皮的椎間板レーザー髄核切除(術)　PILN
経皮的ツボ電気刺激療法
TEAS
経皮的電気(神経)刺激
TENS
経皮的電気刺激　TES
経皮的な　TC
経皮的内視鏡下胃空腸吻合(術)　PEG-J
経皮的内視鏡下空腸造瘻術
PEJ
経皮的二酸化炭素分圧
$tcPco_2$
経皮的膿瘍排膿　PAD
経皮的バスキュラーアクセス拡張術　VAIVT
経皮的バルーンカテーテルによる狭窄弁開大術
BV
経皮的バルーン血管拡張(術)　PTBD
経皮的バルーン血管形成(術)　PTBA
経皮的バルーン心嚢(心膜)切開(術)　PBP
経皮的バルーン弁形成(術)
PBV
経皮的ビリルビン濃度測定法　TcB
経皮的膀胱吸引　PBA
経皮的盲腸フィステル形成(術)　PCC
経皮的レーザー冠(状)動脈形成術　ELCA
経皮内視鏡的胃瘻造設術
PEG
経皮内動脈血酸素分圧
$TcPaO_2$
経皮の　p.cut, TD
経表皮水分喪失
TEWL, TWL
経鼻胃管　NGT,
NG tube
経鼻栄養チューブ　NGT
経鼻気管支(チューブ)
NT
経鼻気管内チューブ
NET, NETT
経鼻気道抵抗　TAR
経腹腔前腹膜ヘルニア縫合術　TAPP
経腹式子宮摘出(術)
TAH
経腹的に　p.a.
経腹膜的　IP, ip, i.p.
経腹膜的に　IP, ip, i.p.
経腹膜腹腔鏡下腎摘出
TLN
経胼胝体応答　TCR
経膀胱的前立腺切除
TVP
経毛様体扁平部水晶体切除(術)　PPL
経腰的大動脈造影撮影法
TLA
脛骨　tib
脛骨・腓骨　tib.-fib.
脛骨後面　TP
脛骨前粘液腫　PM
脛骨前浮腫　PTE
脛骨前面　TA
脛骨粗面　TT
脛骨内捻　ITT
脛骨の　tib
軽快　R, Rm
軽鎖　LC
軽鎖(病)　L-chain
軽鎖I　LCI
軽鎖沈着病　LCDD
軽鎖病　LCD
軽症病棟　MCU, SCU
軽睡眠　LS
軽度異形成　MD
軽度拡張型うっ血性心筋症
MDCM
軽度鶏卵継代　LEP
軽度高フェニルアラニン血(症)　MHPA
軽度膵炎　MIP
軽度に　SL, sl
軽度の　sl, slt
軽度扁平上皮内病変
LGSIL
軽度膀胱感染
sl.blad.inf
軽度リンパ腫　LGL
軽メロミオシン　LMM
痙縮　sp
痙性脊髄麻痺　SSP
痙攣　conv, S, sp, Zuck
痙攣重積発作　status
痙攣ショック療法　CST
痙攣性疾患　CD
痙攣のないてんかん
NCE
痙攣を引き起こす薬量
CD

傾斜磁場エコー　**GE**
傾斜台　**TT**
傾眠の　**SOM**
携行式人工腎臓　**WAK**
携行用ホルターモニター　**AHM**
携帯型自己腹腔透析　**CPRD**
携帯式血圧測定監視法　**ABPM**
携帯式血圧測定法　**ABPM**
継続管理　**FL up, fl up, FU, F/U, f/u**
継続教育　**CE**
継続教育単位　**CEU**

継続させよ　**contin.**
継続された　**cont'd**
継続する　**CONT, cont.**
継続する〔した〕　**contin.**
継続性・包容力・協調性　**3C**
継続せよ　**contin., KO, K/O, pt, pt.**
継続的喫煙者　**CS**
憩室　**D**
螢光　**FL, fluores**
螢光X線マッピング装置　**XEMS**
螢光眼底（血管）造影（法）　**FAG**
螢光狂犬病抗体　**FRA**
螢光（眼底）血管造影（法）　**FA**
螢光検定（法）　**FA**
螢光抗核抗体（法）　**FANA**
螢光酵素免疫法　**FIA**
螢光抗体　**FA**
螢光抗体（法）　**FA**
螢光抗体価　**FTA**
螢光抗体検査　**FAT**
螢光抗体法　**FAT, IFL**
螢光酵素免疫法　**FIA**
螢光色素蛋白　**APC, APCY**
螢光指数　**FI**
螢光小体　**F body**
螢光像増倍管　**IA**
螢光測定（法）　**fluor**
螢光単位　**FU**
螢光定量　**FA**
螢光トレポネーマ抗体吸収　**FTA-AB**
螢光トレポネーマ抗体吸収（試験）　**FTA-ABS**
螢光トレポネーマ抗体試験　**FTA**
螢光の　**FL, fluor, fluores**
螢光倍増音信号デジタル化診断用X線装置　**IIDR**
螢光発色セルソーター　**FACS**
螢光標識血清蛋白　**FLSP**
螢光標識抗体　**FLA**
螢光分光光度計　**SPF**
螢光分析測定法　**SF**
螢光偏光免疫（学）検定　**FPIA**
頸（静脈）　**jug**
頸（部）　**cerv, cerv., CX, Cx, cx.**
頸管粘液　**CM**
頸管粘液結晶形成　**CMC**
頸（椎）胸椎　**CTV**
頸神経　**C**
頸軸面の　**CA**
頸静脈　**JV**
頸静脈圧　**JV, JVP**
頸静脈圧迫（試験）　**jug.comp.**
頸静脈カテーテル　**JVC**
頸静脈血酸素飽和度　**SjO_2**
頸静脈孔　**JF**
頸静脈孔症候群　**JFC, JFS**
頸静脈鼓室傍神経節腫　**JTP**
頸静脈怒張　**JVD, NVD**
頸静脈二腹筋（リンパ節）　**JD**
頸静脈の　**JV**
頸静脈波　**JV, JVP**
頸（部）腟液　**CVF**
頸椎　**C, CS, C sp, C-spine, CV, HW, HWS**
頸椎・腰椎牽引　**C & L trx**
頸椎および骨盤牽引　**C & P trx**
頸椎牽引　**C trx**
頸椎症性脊髄症　**CSM**
頸椎椎間板ヘルニア　**CDH, HNP**
頸椎椎弓切除（術）　**C lam**
頸椎の分節　**C1-7**
頸椎傍ブロック　**PCB**
頸動脈　**CA**
頸動脈音血管像　**CPA**
頸動脈海綿静脈洞（瘻）　**CC**
頸動脈海綿静脈洞瘻　**CCF**
頸動脈化学受容体刺激　**CCRS**
頸動脈可聴周波数分析　**CAA**
頸動脈球傍神経節腫　**CBP**
頸動脈ステント留置術　**CAS**
頸動脈撮影法　**CAG**
頸動脈鞘　**CS**
頸動脈小体　**CB**
頸動脈造影法　**CAG**
頸動脈体神経遮断　**CBD**
頸動脈洞　**CS**
頸動脈洞圧　**CSP**
頸動脈洞圧試験　**CSP test**

頸動脈洞過敏症候群 **CSHS**
頸動脈洞刺激 **CSS**
頸動脈洞症候群 **CSS**
頸動脈洞神経 **CSN**
頸動脈洞神経刺激(装置) **CSNS**
頸動脈洞反射 **CSR**
頸動脈洞マッサージ **CSM**
頸動脈内の **IC**
頸動脈内膜切除〔剝離〕術 **CEA**
頸動脈の **car**
頸動脈波 **CAP, Car, Carot**
頸動脈拍動トレーシング〔記録法〕 **CPT**
頸(部)の **C, cer, cerv, cerv., CX, Cx, cx.**
頸の **jug**
頸部郭清術 **RND**
頸部交感神経節 **GCSN**
頸部刺激 **CS**
頸部縦隔探査 **CME**
頸部食道 **Ce**
頸部脊椎症 **CS**
頸部内頸動脈 **CICA**
頸部に巻きついた臍帯 **CAN**
(子宮)頸部粘液 **CM**
頸部陽圧負荷 **PNP**
頸傍神経節 **PCG**
頸傍の **para C**
頸・胸・腰仙椎装具 **CTLSO**
頸・胸・腰椎装具 **CTLO**
頸・胸椎装具 **CTO**
警告反応 **AR**
経食道心エコー(検査)法 **TEE**
隙 **S, SP, sp**
劇症A型溶連菌感染症 **TSLS**
劇症ウイルス性肝炎 **FVH**
劇症肝炎 **FH**
劇症肝不全 **FHF**
劇症小児常染色体劣性筋ジストロフィ **SCARMD**
劇薬 **DD**
劇薬取締法 **DDA**
欠陥 **impair**
欠陥なし **N/D**
欠陥のある **def**
欠落 **def**
欠失 **Def, def., del**
欠損 **def, Def, def., defic**
欠損(症) **defic**
欠損の **abs**
欠損のある **defic**
欠乏 **def, defic**
欠乏(症) **Def, def., defic**
欠陥 **def**
月経 **CTa, Cta, cta, men, meno, menstru**
月経がある **menst, menstru**
月経丸薬 **M-pill**
月経期 **MP**
月経期外出血 **IMB**
月経困難症 **dysme, DYSM**
月経周辺性症候群 **PMS**
月経前緊張 **PMT**
月経前緊張症候群 **PMTS**
月経前症候群 **PMS**
月経前に **a.m.**
月経年齢 **MA**
月経の **menst, menstru**
月経の終了 **FMP**
月経誘発 **MI**
月経量 **MBL**
月経歴 **MH**
月報 **MR**
月曜日 **M, MON, Mon**
月齢 **Lm**
血圧 **BD, BL PR, bl.pr, BP, B.P.**
血圧計 **BPG**
血圧記録器 **BPR**
血圧昇圧癌化学療法 **IHC**
血圧上昇 **BPI**
血圧センサー固定圧 **HDP**
血圧測定システム **BPMS**
血圧低下 **BPD**
血圧と脈拍 **BP & P**
血液力学側面図 **HP**
血液 **B, b, BL, BL, bl, Bld, bid.**
血液・脳脊髄液関門 **BCSFB**
血液・リンパ系 **BLS**
血液一酸化炭素 **BCO**
血液(病)学 **Hem, HEMAT, hemat., Hematol, hematol.**
血液学 **haematol**
血液学者 **haematol, Hematol, hematol.**
血液型 **BLT, BIT, BT**
(ダッフィの)血液型因子 **FY**
血液型抗原 **BGAg**
血液型交叉〔差〕試験 **TC**
血液型と交叉〔差〕試験 **T & M, T & C, T & CrM**
血液型物質 **BGS**
血液型分類 **BGC**
血液顆粒細胞特異的活動 **BGSA**
血液緩衝塩基 **BBB**

け

血液寒天(培地) **BA**
血液寒天平板 **BAP**
血液灌流 **DHP, HP**
血液希釈値 **BDV**
血液吸着 **HA**
血液凝固時間 **BCT**
血液血清学的試験 **BST**
血液研究学会 **SSB**
血液検査 **BLT**
血液検査のため朝食延食 **HB/BW**
血液産生率 **BPR**
血液酸素 **BO_2**
血液酸素レベル依存 **BOLD**
血液神経関門 **BNB**
血液前駆細胞 **HPC**
血液センター **BC**
血液像 **BB, BlB**
血液喪失 **BL**
血液通過時間 **TT**
血液透析 **HD**
血液透析室 **HDU**
血液透析誘発性一過性白血球減少症 **HTL**
血液透析誘発性低酸素血症 **HH**
血液二酸化炭素 **BCO_2**
血液に対する赤血球の容積% **VPRC**
血液尿素窒素 **BUN**
血液粘性亢進網膜症 **HVR**
血液の **b-y**
血液脳関門 **BBB, B.B.B., BHS, HEB**
血液培養 **BC, BLC, BL C, BlC, bl.cult**
血液バンク **BB, Bld Bnk**
血液比重 **Gb**
血液病専門医 **Hematol, hematol.**
血液容量 **BLV, Bl vol**
血液らしくない **NBL**
血液量 **BV**
血液リンパ生成成長因子 **HLGF**
血液濾過 **HF**
血液濾過透析 **HDF**
血液濾過療法 **HFT**
血液ワッセルマン **BW**
血縁者間生体腎移植でのドナー血輸血 **DSBT**
血縁者間軟層輸血 **DSBCT**
血縁臓器提供者 **RLD**
血型判定スクリーン **T & S**
血液寒天基礎培地 **BAB**
血管 **BV, v, ves**
血管運動緊張 **VMT**
血管運動神経 **VM**
血管運動神経性鼻炎 **Rh.vas.**
血管運動神経中枢 **VMC**
血管運動性鼻炎 **RV, VMR**
血管運動(性)の **VM**
血管外腫瘤 **EVM**
血管外の **EV**
血管外肺腫瘤 **ELM**
血管外肺水分量 **EVLW**
血管外皮細胞腫 **HPC**
血管拡張 **vasodil, VD**
血管拡張症 **VE**
血管拡張中枢 **VDC**
血管拡張物質 **VDEM, VDM, VDS**
血管拡張薬 **VA, VD**
血管活性腸ペプチド **VIP**
血管活性腸ポリペプチド(分泌性)腫瘍 **VIP-oma**
血管逆転症 **BVI**
血管筋脂肪腫 **AML**
血管茎前胸壁皮弁 **PIF**
血管作動性腸管ポリペプチド **VIP**
血管作用性アミン **VAA**
血管疾患 **vas.dis, VD**
血管実質組織反応 **AMTR**
血管写 **AG, Angio, angio**
血管写(像) **AG, ANG, Ang, ang., Angio, angio**
血管腫・血小板減少症候群 **HTS**
血管周囲細胞腫 **HPC**
血管周囲リンパ球浸潤 **PLC**
血管収縮 **VC**
血管収縮中枢 **VCC**
血管収縮物質 **VCS**
血管収縮薬 **VC**
血管収縮率 **VCR**
血管条 **SV**
血管神経性浮腫 **ANE**
血管新生(性)緑内障 **NVG**
血管脆弱症候群 **VFS**
血管性多形皮膚萎縮症 **PAV**
血管性痴呆 **VaD**
血管性プラスミノゲン活性化物質 **VPA**
血管接近装置 **VAD**
血管切除術 **vasec**
血管造影〔撮影〕(法) **AG, Angio, angio**
血管造影〔撮影〕図 **AG, ANG, Ang, ang., Angio, angio**
血管束 **vas bund**
血管抵抗 **VR**
血管透過性 **VP**
血管透過性因子 **VPF**
血管内 **IV**
血管内異物 **IVFB**
血管内液 **IVF**
血管内気管支肺胞腫瘍 **IBAT**

け

血管内気管支肺胞上皮腫瘍 **IVBAT**
血管内凝固 **IVC**
血管内凝固・線溶(症候群) **ICF**
血管内消費性凝固障害 **IVCC**
血管内赤血球凝集 **IEA, IRCA**
血管内超音波 **IVUS**
血管内乳頭状内皮過形成 **IPEH**
血管内皮 **BVE**
血管内皮細胞接着分子 **VCAM**
血管内皮細胞増殖因子 **VEPF**
血管内皮細胞由来過分極因子 **EDHF**
血管内皮細胞由来弛緩因子 **EDRF**
血管内皮細胞由来収縮因子 **EDCF**
血管内皮増殖因子 **VECGF, VEGF**
血管内皮白血球粘着物質 **ELAM**
血管の **Vas, VASC, vasc**
血管非閉塞性腸間膜虚血症 **NOMI**
血管平滑筋 **VSM**
血管平滑筋細胞 **VSMC**
血管壁 **VW, V.W., v.w.**
血管(性)変化 **VC**
血管放射線(医)学 **VAS RAD**
血管迷走神経反射 **VVR**
血管免疫芽球性リンパ節症 **AIBL, AIL**
血管容積分布 **VVD**
血管抑制中枢 **VIC**
血管抑制物質 **VDM**
血管抑制(性)ペプチド **VIP**
血管攣縮 **VS**
血胸 **HTX**
血球 **BK**
(赤)血球吸着(現象) **HAD, HAd**
(赤)血球凝集(反応) **H**
(赤)血球凝集抑制抗体 **HIA**
血球凝集抑制反応 **HI**
(赤)血球凝集抑制免疫定量(法) **HII**
(赤)血球凝集抑制モルヒネ試験 **HIMT**
血球計 **hemocyt**
血球計算板 **hemocyt**
血球算定(法) **BC**
血球貪食細胞性リンパ組織球増多(症) **HLH**
血球貪食症候群 **HPS**
血球容積 **PCV**
血行動態拡張反応 **HER**
血算 **BC**
血小板 **plat, Plat, PLT, PLTS, TBC**
血小板因子 **PF**
血小板活性化因子 **PAF**
血小板顆粒抽出物 **PGE**
血小板凝集 **PA**
血小板凝集因子 **PAF, PAgF**
血小板凝集因子阻害薬 **PAFI**
血小板凝集試験 **PAT**
血小板凝集増強因子 **PAEF**
血小板凝集阻止因子 **PAIF**
血小板結合免疫グロブリンG **PB IgG, PBIgG, PAIgG**
血小板欠損(症) **PLD**
血小板減少・橈骨欠損症候群 **TAR**
血小板減少性紫斑病 **TP**
血小板抗原 **PLA**
血小板シクロオキシゲナーゼ **PCO**
血小板小管系 **SCS**
血小板数 **PC**
血小板生存時間 **PST, p.s.t.**
血小板造血刺激因子 **TSF**
血小板相互間凝集抗原 **PECAM**
血小板第Ⅲ因子 **PF3**
血小板第Ⅳ因子 **PF4**
血小板濃縮液 **PC**
血小板分布幅 **PDW**
血小板ヘマトクリット **PCT**
血小板ペルオキシダーゼ **PPO**
血小板母細胞成分 **TCC**
血小板ホスホヘキソキナーゼ **PHK**
血小板補体結合試験 **PCFT**
血小板膜 **PM**
血小板ミクロソーム **PM**
血小板免疫螢光検査 **PIFT**
血小板輸血不応状態 **PTR**
血小板輸血療法 **PTT**
血小板由来成長〔増殖〕因子 **PDGF**
血小板由来内皮細胞増殖因子 **PD-ECGF**
血小板リストセチン凝集テスト **RIPA**
血小板リポオキシゲナーゼ **PLO**
血色素 **Hb, hemo, Hg, HGB, Hgb, hGB, hgb.**
血色素 α 鎖 **HB A**
血色素 β 鎖 **HBB**
血色素 γ 鎖A **HBG1**

血色素 γ 鎖G　**HBG2**
血色素 δ 鎖　**HBD**
血色素 ε 鎖　**HBE**
血色素 ζ 鎖　**HBZ**
血色素異常症　**HP**
血色素結合能　**HbBC**
血色素減少症　**hypo**
血色素電気泳動　**HE**
血色素濃度　**HC**
血漿　**P, pl**
血漿アルドステロン　**PA**
血漿アルドステロン濃度　**PAC**
血漿アンジオテンシナーゼ活性　**PAA**
血漿インスリン活性　**PIA**
血漿エピネフリン　**PE**
血漿ガストリン　**PG**
血漿カテコールアミン濃度　**PCC**
血漿灌流　**PP**
血漿吸着　**PA**
血漿クリアランス率　**PCR**
血漿グルコース　**PG**
血漿欠損　**PD**
血漿交換　**PE, PEX, PH, PP**
血漿コルチゾール　**PC**
血漿コルチゾール濃度　**PCC**
血漿コロイド浸透圧　**POP**
血漿ジゴキシン濃度　**PDC**
血漿消退率　**PDR**
血漿浸透圧　**OPP, POP, Posm**
血漿成長ホルモン　**PGH**
血漿蛋白　**Pp, PPF**
血漿チ〔サイ〕ロキシンレベル　**PTL**
血漿鉄　**PI**
血漿鉄クリアランス　**PIC**
血漿鉄交代率　**PIT, PITR**
血漿鉄消失(率)　**PID**
血漿鉄消失率　**PIDR**
血漿鉄半減時間　**PIDT**$_{1/2}$
血漿鉄プール　**PIP**
血漿トリグリセリド　**PG**
血漿トロンボプラスチン　**PT**
血漿トロンボプラスチン因子D　**PTF-D**
血漿ナトリウム　**Pna**
血漿乳酸脱水素酵素　**PLDH**
血漿尿素窒素　**PUN**
血漿認識因子活性　**PRFA**
血漿粘稠度　**PV**
血漿濃度　**PC**
血漿濃度により分離される尿細管液　**TFP**
血漿ノルエピネフリン　**PNE**
血漿比重　**GP**
血漿ヒスタミナーゼ活性　**PHA**
血漿フィブロネクチン　**PFN**
血漿プレカリクレイン　**PPK**
血漿プロトロンビン時間　**PPT**
血漿分離　**PS**
血漿ペプシノゲン　**PP**
血漿無機ヨウ素　**PII**
血漿免疫反応性インスリン　**P-IRI**
血漿薬物濃度　**Cp**
血漿輸血反応　**PTR**
血漿由来ワクチン　**PV**
血漿量　**PV, Vp**
血漿レニン活性　**PRA**
血漿レニン濃度　**PRC**
血漿レベルモニター　**PLM**
血漿濾過　**PF**
血栓　**T, throm, Thromb, thromb**
血栓形成時間　**TFT**
血栓形成促進性血漿成分　**TPC**
血栓後症候群　**PTPS, PTS**
血栓症　**throm, Thromb, thromb, thrombo**
血栓症に伴うヘパリン誘因性血小板減少症　**HITT**
血栓性血小板減少性紫斑病　**TTP**
血栓性血小板減少性紫斑病と溶血性尿毒症症候群　**TTP-HUS**
血栓性疾患における抗血小板療法の有効性を調査解析している国際的な機関　**APT**
血栓性静脈炎　**TP**
血栓性微小血管障害　**TMA**
血栓塞栓(性)疾患　**TED**
血栓塞栓症　**TE**
血栓塞栓性脳血管障害　**TCVA**
血栓塞栓性肺高血圧　**TPH**
血栓内膜摘除術　**TEA**
血栓融解心筋梗塞血管形成術　**TAMI**
血栓溶解　**TL**
血清　**BS, S, ser**
血清Xヒドロキシブチル酸脱水素酵素　**SHBD**
血清アスパルテートアミノトランスフェラーゼ　**SAST**
血清アミロイドA蛋白　**SAA**
血清アミロイドP(成分)　**SAP**

血清アルカリホスファターゼ **SAP**
血清アルドラーゼ **SA**
血清アルブミン **SA, SAB**
血清アンジオテンシン変換酵素 **SACE**
血清アンジオテンシン変換酵素活性値 **SAEC**
血清イソクエン酸脱水素酵素 **SICD**
血清因子 **SF**
血清インスリン **SI**
血清インスリン濃度 **SIC**
血清陰性の **SN**
血清塩素(イオン) **ser.Cl**
血清学 **Ser, ser, serol**
血清学的識別抗原 **SD, SD antigen**
血清学的な **ser**
血清学的に検出可能な男性抗原 **SDM antigen**
血清学的に検出された **SD**
血清学的に定量(決定)された **SD**
血清肝炎 **SH, SH antigen**
血清肝炎ウイルス **SH virus**
血清肝炎関連抗原 **SHAA**
血清肝炎関連抗原抗体 **SHAA-Ab**
血清肝炎関連抗体 **SHA-Ab**
血清キサンチン酸化酵素〔オキシダーゼ〕 **SeXO**
血清胸腺因子 **FTS, STF**
血清グルコース **SG**
血清グルタミン酸オキサロ酢酸アミノトランスフェラーゼ **SGOT, S-GOT**
血清グルタミン酸ピルビン酸トランスアミナーゼ **SGPT, S-GPT**
血清クレアチニン **SC, SCr**
血清クレアチン **SCr**
血清クレアチンキナーゼ **SCK**
血清クレアチンホスホキナーゼ **SCPK, S-CPK**
血清グロブリン **SG**
血清血栓形成促進因子 **STA**
血清ケモグラム **SCG**
血清ゲンタミ〔マイ〕シン濃度 **SG-C**
血清酵素標準 **SES**
血清コリンエステラーゼ **SChE**
血清殺菌試験 **SBT**
血清殺菌濃度 **SBC**
血清殺菌力価 **SBT**
血清酸素飽和度 **SO_2, So_2**
血清酸ホスファターゼ **SAP**
血清ジギタリス濃度 **SDC**
血清刺激応答因子 **SRF**
血清ギゴキシン濃度 **SDC**
血清ジゴキシンレベル **SDL**
血清指数 **ser.ind**
血清遮断因子 **SBF**
血清総酸性リン酸分解酵素 **TSAP**
血清胆汁酸 **SBA**
血清蛋白 **SP**
血清蛋白結合ヨウ素 **SPBI**
血清蛋白指数 **SPI**
血清蛋白電気泳動 **SPEP**
血清蛋白電気泳動(法) **SPE**
血清蛋白分画 **SPF**
血清沈降性ヨウ素 **SPI**
血清テオフィリン濃度 **STC**
血清テオフィリン濃度レベル **STL**
血清鉄 **SI**
血清鉄コロイド **SIC**
血清銅レベル **SCL**
血清トランスフェリン **ST**
血清トリプシン抑制因子 **STI**
血清トリプシン抑制能 **STIC**
血清乳酸脱水素酵素 **SLD, SLDH**
血清尿酸 **SUA**
血清尿素窒素 **SUN**
血清の **ser**
血清反応陰性多発性神経炎 **SNP**
血清ヒアルロニダーゼ単位 **HUS**
血清病 **SS**
血清病様疾患 **SSLI**
血清ビリルビン **SB**
血清フィブリノーゲン **SF**
血清フェニルアラニン濃度 **SPC**
血清プロトロンビン転化促進因子 **SPCA**
血清プロトロンビン転化促進因子欠乏症 **SPCAD**
血清補体 **SC**
血清ミエリン塩基性蛋白 **SMBP**
血清ムコ蛋白 **SMP**
血清メチルアルコールレベル **SMAL**
血清免疫グロブリン **SIg**
血清免疫グロブリン予後指数 **SIPI**

血清免疫反応性上皮小体ホルモン **sIPTH**
血清葉酸 **SFA**
血清陽性の **SP**
血清抑制因子 **SIF**
血清抑制活性 **SIA**
血清抑制試験 **SIT**
血清抑制濃度 **SIC**
血清レニン活性 **SRA**
血清ロイシンアミノペプチダーゼ **SLAP**
血清ワッセルマン反応 **SWR**
血中アイソトープクリアランス **BIC**
血中アルコール **BA**
血中アルコール含量 **BAC**
血中アルコール濃度 **BAC**
血中アルコールレベル **BAL**
血中ガス含量 **C**
血中ガストリン値 **SGL, SGT**
血中ガスの濃度を示す記号 **C**
血中グルコース **BG, BGlu**
血中単核球 **BMC**
血中単球 **BM**
血中鉛レベル **Pb-B**
血中二酸化炭素分圧 **B-PCO_2**
血中尿酸 **BUA**
血沈 **Bl Skg, SR, S.R., VES**
血沈,赤血球沈降速度 **VSG**
血糖 **BG, BGlu, BlS, BS, B.S., BZ**
血糖自己測定 **SMBG**
血糖上昇係数 **GI**
血糖レベル **BSL**
血尿 **hem**
血尿測定 **HUM**
血嚢胞点 **HCS**
血餅退縮 **CR**
血餅溶解時間 **BLT**
血友病 **hemo**
血流(量) **BF**
血流エネルギー **BFE**
血流速度 **BFR**
血(液)流量 **$\dot{Q}$**
血(液)量 **BLV, Bl vol**
(循環)血(液)量増加 **BE, BVE**
(循環)血(液)量増量薬 **BVE**
決定 **determin, detn**
決定器官 **CO**
決定されていない **undet**
決定的ではない **INC, inc, inc.**
決定できない **ND**
結核(症) **T, TB, Tbc, TbC, tuberc, tuberc.**
結核・呼吸器疾患 **TB-RD**
結核菌 **MTB, TB, Tb, TBA, Tbc**
結核菌10%食塩浮遊液中の含有グロブリン量 **TGL**
結核菌体抽出物質＝丸山ワクチン **SSM**
結核菌ワクチン **TBV**
結核呼吸器疾患全国協会 **NTRDA**
結核症・胸部疾患認定書 **DTCD**
結核性髄膜炎 **TBM**
結核性腹膜炎 **TBP**
結核予防全国連合 **NAPT**
結核療養所 **TBS**
結局は **inf, inf.**
結合 **bind, conn, connex, jnt, junct**
結合(部) **J**
結合エストロゲン **CE**
結合血清鉄 **BSI**
結合織筋痛症 **FM**
結合織肥満細胞 **CTMC**
結合した **geb, inc, inc.**
結合状態密度 **JDOS**
結合組織 **CT, IT**
結合組織炎 **FIB, iCT, ICT**
結合組織病〔疾患〕 **CTD**
結合組織マッサージ **CTM**
結合の **comb, conn**
結合〔抱合〕型ビリルビン **CB**
結合部早期収縮 **JPS**
結合物 **conn**
結合部分 **NBS**
結合ペプチド免疫反応 **CPR**
結合遊離比 **B/F**
結婚 **marr, matr.**
結婚した **M, m**
結婚している・独身の・やもめの・離婚した **MSWD**
結婚(年月)日 **DOM**
結婚歴 **MH**
結紮 **Lig, lig, lig., ligg, ligg.**
結紮糸 **Lig, lig, lig., ligg, ligg.**
結紮する **Lig, lig, lig.**
結紮凍結療法 **LC therapy**
結紮法 **Lig, lig, lig., ligg, ligg.**
結晶 **crys, cryst, Xtal**
結晶(性)亜鉛インスリン **CZI**
結晶インスリン **CI**

結晶化　**cryst, crystn**
結晶化した　**cryst, X-ized**
結晶性アミノ酸　**CAA**
結晶性の　**cryst**
結晶性卵アルブミン　**CEA**
結晶(性)の　**Xtal**
結晶性の　**crys**
結石　**C, st**
結石生成指数　**LI**
結節　**N**
結節型/び漫〔広汎〕性非ホジキンリンパ腫　**N/D NHL**
結節型黒色腫　**NM**
結節間眼筋麻痺　**INOP**
結節間溝　**BG**
結節間の　**IT**
結節硬化症　**TSC**
結節腫　**G, gang, gangl, Ggl**
結節状構造　**var**
結節状構造の　**var**
結節性(黒色腫)　**NOD**
結節性悪性黒色腫(メラノーマ)　**NMM**
結節性期外〔早期収縮〕　**NPB**
結節性期外収縮　**NPC**
結節性硬化(症)　**NS, TS**
結節性紅斑　**EN**
結節性混合性リンパ腫　**NML**
結節性再生性過形成　**NRH**
結節性組織球性リンパ腫　**NHL**
結節性多発性動脈炎　**PN**
結節性多発動脈炎　**PAN**
結節性調律　**NOD**
結節性動脈周囲炎　**PAN, PN**
結節性汎動脈炎　**PN**
結節性表皮下線維組織増殖症　**NSF**
結節性補充収縮　**JE, JEB**
結節性リンパ腫　**NL**
結節低分化リンパ球性(リンパ腫)　**NPDL**
結腸運動係数　**CMI**
結腸肛門吻合(術)　**CAA**
結腸切除(術)　**CR**
結腸造ろう(術)　**colost**
結腸直腸癌　**CC**
結腸直腸外科(学)　**CRS**
結腸直腸手術　**CRS**
結腸直腸線癌　**CRA**
結腸直腸の　**CP**
結腸直腸吻合(術)　**CRA**
結腸と直腸の遺伝性腺腫症　**HACR**
結腸フィステル形成(術)　**colost**
結膜　**conj**
結膜・強膜　**CS**
結膜炎　**CJ**
結膜下注射　**SCI**
結膜と強膜　**C & S**
結膜分泌物　**CS**
結膜誘発試験　**ORT**
結論　**conc**
楔合した　**Imp, imp**
楔状骨切り術　**OW, ow**
楔状束　**FC**
楔入(部)圧　**WP**
楔入(部)肝静脈圧　**WHVP**
楔入(部)腎静脈圧　**WRVP**
(永久歯の)犬歯　**C**
(乳歯の)犬歯　**c**
犬歯の　**C**
元気でいきいきした状態　**A & W**
元気な　**F**
元素の　**elem**
幻覚　**hallu, halluc**
幻覚・錯覚・妄想　**HID**
幻覚剤　**hallu**
幻覚を起こさせる　**hallu**
幻覚を生ずる　**hallu**
幻聴　**GH**
見当識検査　**OT**
見当識調査票　**OI**
言語化・視覚化質問表　**VVQ**
言語識別スコア　**SDS**
言語障害児のための協会　**AFASIC**
言語聴取検査　**SRT**
言語治療学士　**B.Sp.Thy.**
言語年齢　**LA**
言語の　**V, v**
言語発達基準　**VLDS**
言語発達試験　**TOLD**
言語発達ユタ検査　**UTLD**
言語標準評価法　**SEM**
言語病理学　**SP, Sp Path**
言語〔語句〕理解力因子　**V factor**
言語療法(分野)　**ST, S.T.**
言語療法士　**ST**
肩甲下(筋)　**SS**
肩甲下の　**subsc, subscap**
肩甲間部　**ISR**
肩甲胸郭の　**ST**
肩甲(骨)棘　**sc.sp**
肩甲骨　**Sc, sc, scap**
肩甲骨関節窩・上腕の　**GH**
肩甲骨の　**Sc, sc, scap**
肩甲上腕関節周囲炎　**PSH**
肩甲左後位　**SCLP**
肩甲左前位　**SCLA**
肩甲右後位　**SCDP**
肩甲右前位　**SCDA**

肩鎖関節　**ACJ**
肩手症候群　**SHS**
肩峰　**A**
肩峰関節　**AC jt.**
肩峰骨頭間距離　**AHI**
肩峰鎖骨の　**AC, A.C., A-C, A/C**
肩腕症候群　**SAS**
研究・情報処理組織　**RIPS**
研究　**invest, Res, res, rsch**
研究・企画・計画・評価　**RPPE**
研究資源室　**ORR**
研究者　**F, Res, res**
研究者主導研究　**IIR, IIS, IIT**
研究所　**Inst, inst**
研究所の治験審査委員会　**IRB**
研究的皮膚科学会　**SID**
研究と開発　**R & D**
研究と教育　**R & E**
研究皮膚科学会　**IDS**
研究用診断基準　**DCR, RDC**
研究用新薬届　**IND**
研究要約　**RS**
研究倫理調査室　**ORI**
研修　**Tng, train, trg**
研修医　**HO, Res, res**
研修と経験　**T & E**
研磨した　**trit.**
研磨せよ　**tr., trit.**
研和せよ　**ter.**
限　**L**
限外希釈　**LD**
限外希釈法　**LDA**
限外濾過　**UF**
限外濾過圧　**UFP**
限外濾過性カルシウム　**UFCa**
限外濾過性マグネシウム　**UFMg**
限外濾過物　**UF**
限外濾過法　**ECUM**
限外濾過率　**UFR**
限外濾過量　**UFV**
限界　**LIM, lim**
限界計画値　**TPQs**
限界死　**L+**
限界品質　**RQL**
(手技の)限界を超える　**XS-LIM**
限局型若年性歯周炎　**LJP**
限局疾患　**LD**
限局性脛骨前粘液水腫　**LPM**
(肝)限局性結節性過形成　**FNH**
限局性脂肪ジストロフィ　**PLD**
限局性腸炎　**RE**
限局性〔偏心性〕内膜肥厚　**EIT**
限局性の　**loc**
限局性播種性エリテマトーデス　**L-DLE**
限定栄養食　**DFD**
限定された　**def**
限定する　**def**
限定破片長多形性　**RFLPs**
剣状突起　**proc.xiph., XS**
剣状の　**xiph**
原因不明　**CU, CUD**
原因不明アミロイド　**AUO**
原因不明胸痛　**CPUE**
原因不明骨髄様化生　**AMM**
原因不明持続熱　**PFUO**
原因不明失神　**SUO**
原因不明心筋疾患　**MDUO**
原因不明性組織球増殖症　**HX**
原因不明突然死　**SUD**
原因不明突然死症候群　**SUDS**
原因不明乳幼児突然死　**SUID**
原因不明熱　**FUO, PUE, PUO**
原因不明の　**E.U., undet.etiol., undet.orig., UO**
原因不明の絨毛炎　**VUE**
原因不明の単クローン性免疫グロブリン症　**MGUS**
原因不明の病因　**UE**
原因不明の病的症状　**X disease**
原因不明予測不能突然死　**SUUD**
原位置に　***in situ***
原核生物系統学に関する国際委員会　**ICSP**
原形質膜　**PM**
原稿　**Ms, script**
原子　**AT, at, at.**
原子１個の検出　**SAD**
原子間力顕微鏡　**AFM, SAFM, SFM**
原子記号Ｚおよび原子量Ａの同位元素　**ZLA**
原子軌道　**AO**
原子吸光(分析)　**AA**
原子吸光測定　**AAS**
原子吸収スペクトル測光法　**AAS**
原子質量単位　**amu**
原子数　**Z**
原子生物学的化学　**ABC**
原子の　**at, at.**
原子爆弾の放射線の影響に関する国際連合科学委員会　**UNSCEAR**
原子番号　**at.no.**
原子物理学・生物工学・コンピュータ・情報処理・

け

電子工学・精密化学・遺伝子操作 **ABCDEFG**
原子容量 **at vol**
原子量 **A, at.wt., A.W.**
原子量単位 **AWU, awu**
原子レベル分解能顕微鏡 **ARM**
原始生殖細胞 **PGC**
原疾患死 **DOD**
原発開放隅角緑内障 **POAG**
原発型〔分類不能型〕免疫不全症 **CVID**
原発肝癌 **PHC**
原発癌部位 **PCS**
原発癌不明 **UPC**
原発後天性鼻涙管閉塞(症) **PANDO**
原発(性)色素(性)結節(性)副腎皮質疾患 **PPNAD**
原発腫瘍 **T**
原発性アメーバ性髄膜脳炎 **PAM, PAME**
原発性アルドステロン症 **PA**
原発性異型肺炎 **PAP**
原発性肝癌 **PLC**
原発性肝細胞癌 **PHC, PHCC, PLCC**
原発性肝脾リンパ腫 **PHSL**
原発性機能不全(性)肝(臓) **PDL**
原発性血小板血症 **PTh**
原発性結腸直腸癌 **PCRC**
原発性硬化性胆管炎 **PSC**
原発性甲状腺機能亢進症 **PHT**
原発性梗塞 **PI**
原発性後天性前白血病症候群 **PPS**
原発性後天性鉄芽球性貧血 **PASA**
原発性後天性不応性貧血 **PARA**
原発性骨髄線維症 **PMF**
原発性シェーグレン症候群 **PSS**
原発性刺激性接触皮膚炎 **PICD**
原発性視神経萎縮 **POA**
原発性縦隔胚細胞腫瘍 **PMGCT**
原発性情動疾患 **PAD**
原発性上皮小体機能亢進症 **PHP**
原発性上皮小体(機能)亢進(症) **PH, pHPT**
原発性心筋症 **IMD, PMD**
原発性心停止 **PCA**
原発性脊髄異形成症候群 **PMDS**
原発性線維筋痛 **PFM**
原発性線維筋肉痛症候群 **PHS**
原発性線維痛症候群 **PFS**
原発性全般てんかん **PGE**
原発性胆汁性肝硬変 **PBC**
原発性腸リンパ管拡張(症) **PIL**
原発性脳内出血 **PIH**
原発性肺高血圧症 **PPH**
原発性肺胞低換気(症候群) **PAH**
原発性皮膚悪性リンパ腫 **PCML**
原発性皮膚黒色腫 **PCM**
原発性貧血 **PA**
原発性副腎皮質結節性形成異常(症) **PAND**
原発性副腎皮質小結節性形成異常(症) **PAMD**
原発性閉塞隅角緑内障 **PACG, PCAG**
原発性変性脳疾患 **PDCD**
原発性慢性肝炎 **PCH**
原発性慢性巨赤芽球性貧血 **ICMA**
原発性無月経 **PA**
原発性免疫不全症候群 **PIDS, PIS**
原発性夜間遺尿症 **PNE**
原発性卵巣不全(症) **POF**
原発巣不明癌 **CUPS**
原発(性)の **P**
原箱 **scat.orig.**
原爆障害調査委員会 **ABCC**
原理 **princ**
眩惑快不快限界域 **BCD**
健康 **hlth.**
健康,教育,福祉 **HEW**
健康・事故保険 **H & A Ins**
健康維持 **HM**
健康医療事務官協会 **SMOH**
健康管理・倫理・人間の価値に関する国際研究機関 **IIHCEHV**
健康危険度評価 **HRA**
健康教育学士 **BPHE, B.S.H.Ed.**
健康局 **DH**
健康記録 **hel rec**
健康記録協会 **AHR**
健康記録情報医療管理協会 **IHRIM**
健康経済研究所 **OHE**
健康資源管理局 **HRG**
健康志向の体育 **HOPE**
健康疾病評点尺度 **HSRS**
健康児保育 **WCC**

健康状態観察調査　HIS
健康情報システム　HIS
健康成人男子　NAM
健康組織審議会　COHO
健康チェック検査　HCT
健康調査表　MDI
健康適応検査　HIT
健康で生存している　A & H
健康と安全のガイド　HSG
健康と環境　HEV
健康と損害保険　H & Ins
健康な生活の質の標準尺度　QWB
健康に関連した生活の質　HRQOL
健康乳(幼)児　WB
健康乳児保育室　WBN
健康乳幼児〔赤ん坊〕クリニック　WBC
健康乳幼児〔赤ん坊〕ケア　WBC
健康表　BH
健康評価検査　HAE
健康評価のための質問　HAQ
健康奉仕雇用者同盟　COHSE
健康保険計画　HIP
健康保険研究所　HII
健康保険登録委員会　HIRB
健康保養地　sanit, sanit.
健康余命　DFLE
健常者　HS
牽引　tr, tract, TRX, trx, Tx, tx, tx.
牽引性網膜剝離　TRD
現行喫煙者　CS
現在　zZ, z.Z.
現在印刷されていない　opp
現在の　cur, pres
現在の愁訴　CC
現状　SQ
現疾患なし　NPI
現症　HOPI, SP, St pr., St.pr.
現症以前　BP
現症検査　PSE
現象　D, dev, devel, dvlp, phenom, phenom
現象の　phenom
現代医学用語　CMT
現病　PD
現病プログラム　PIP
現病歴　HP, HPC, HPI, HPP, PI
堅固　h
検疫(所)　quar
検疫官　MOH
検疫期間　quar
検眼医　OD
検眼鏡　OPH, Oph, oph, Ophth
検眼鏡の　OPH, Oph, oph
検眼士　Opt, opt, opt.
検査　Ex, ex, exam, Unters, W/U, w/u, Xam
検査(室)(データ)　LB
検査・治療方針決定・作業・評価・社会復帰　TOWER
検査・発達試験と評価　RDTE
検査結果に異常を認めない　NAD
検査した　Ex, ex
検査室　LAB, Lab, lab
検査室手技　lab.proc.
検査室操作　lab.proc.
検査室報告　LR
検査する　exam
検査せず　DNT
検査(室)データ　LD, Ld
検査と診断　X & D
検査日時　Ad
検査日　DOE
検査不能　CNT
検査耳　TE
検出(可能)閾値　TD
検出可能な活性なし　NDA
検出限界以下　BDL
検出されない　ND
検出と変換の可能性　PDC
検出不能な　ND
検者　exam
検討　eval
検討する　eval
検尿　UA, U/A, Ua, ur anal, ur.anal., Ux
減圧　v, vac
減少　dcr, dim, dim., dimin
減少(する)　DC, D/C, d/c
減少させる　decr, dim, dim.
減少した　dec, decr, dim, dim., dimin
減少する　dcr, dec, decr
減弱血管反応　RVR
減弱前庭反応　RVR
減衰振子様回転検査　DPRT
減衰水準　RL
減衰全反射　ATR
減衰の長さ　AL
減数分裂活性化ステロール　MAS
減数分裂抑制物質　MPS
減速(度)　decel
(食事療法で)減量に努めて

いる人　**WW**
嫌気性グラム陰性桿菌　**AGNR**
絹糸　**SWG**
絹糸で清掃する　**floss**
腱　**tend**
腱移行(術)　**TT**
腱移植(片)　**TG**
腱交叉〔差〕　**ChT**
腱鞘炎　**vag.**
厳重な監視　**CS**
厳密な　**d，lit，lit.**
厳密な意味で　**S.S.**
厳密に　**xact**
顕化　**sap，sapon**
顕化する　**sap，sapon**
顕在性不安(検査)　**MAS**
顕性遠視　**H.m.**
顕性の　**manif**
顕微鏡　**micr，scope**
顕微鏡因子　**MF**
顕微鏡下精巣上体精子吸引法　**MESA**
顕微鏡検査法　**MIC，mic，micr，micro**
顕微鏡スライド　**MS**
顕微鏡的な　**MIC，mic，micro**
顕微鏡の　**MIC，mic，micro，mkr**
顕微鏡の焦点　**WP，Wp**
顕微鏡(的)陽性・培養(的)陰性　**MPCN**
懸吊　**susp**

こ

コアグラーゼ　**coag**
コアグラーゼ陰性ブドウ球菌　**CNS**
コアグラーゼ陽性ブドウ球菌　**CPS**
コイタマダニ(属)　**R, Rh, Rh.**
コイルプラネット遠心(法)　**CPC**
コエンザイム　**CO, Co**
コエンザイムA　**CoA**
コエンザイムF　**CoF**
コエンザイム〔補酵素〕Q(=ユビキノン)　**CoQ**
コエンザイムR　**CoR**
コカイン　**C, coc, coke**
コカイン中毒突然死　**SSD**
コカインとヘロイン　**C & H**
コカインとモルヒネ　**C & M**
コクサッキー(ウイルス)　**C**
コクサッキーA　**CA**
コクサッキーBウイルス　**CBV**
コクサッキーウイルス　**Cox-V, CV, C virus, C-virus**
コクシエラ(属)　**C**
コクシジオイデス(属)　**C**
コクラン共同計画　**CC**
コクレフェル症候群　**KS**
コケーン症候群　**CS**
コサイン　**cos**
コシュランド・ネメシー・フィルマーモデル　**KNF model**
コセカント　**cosec**
コタンジェント　**cot, cotan**
コッパー・レパート(培地)　**KR**
コップ　**C, c**
コップ1杯　**cyath.**
コッヘル・デブレ・セメレーニュ(症候群)　**KDS**
コッホ・ウィークス菌　**KW**
コッホ桿菌　**BK**
コッホの旧ツベルクリン　**OK**
コデイン　**COD**
コデイン含有フィオリナール　**Fior Ċ Cod**
コードファクター　**CF**
コナダニ(属)　**A**
ゴナドトロピン　**Gn**
ゴナドトロピン刺激検査　**G-test**
ゴナドトロピン負荷試験　**HCG test, hCG test, HMG test**
ゴナドトロピン放出ホルモン　**GmRH**
ゴナドトロピンレセプター結合抑制因子　**GnRBI**
ゴニオスコピー　**Gonio**
コーネル医学指数　**CMI**
コハク酸塩　**Succ**
コハク酸酸化酵素系　**SOS**
コハク酸脱水素酵素　**SD, SDH**
コハク酸脱水素酵素1　**SDH1**
コハク酸脱水素酵素作用　**SDA**
コハク酸脱水素酵素抑制　**SDI**
コハク酸の　**Succ**
コバラミン　**Cbl**
コバラミン結合蛋白(質)　**CBP**
コバルト　**Co**
コバルト・クロム・タングステン・ニッケル　**Co-Cr-W-Ni**
コバルト・クロム・モリブデン〔水鉛〕　**Co-Cr-Mo**
コバルト56　**^{56}Co**
コバルト57　**^{57}Co**
コバルト58　**^{58}Co**
コバルト60　**^{60}Co**
コバルト遠隔照射療法　**tele Co**
コバルトグラフ　**CO-graphy**
コバルト(60)治療　**^{60}Co**
コバルト反応　**CoR**
コバルトプロトポルフィリン　**COPP**
コピー　**CY, cy**
コピーライト　©
コブラ因子　**CoF**
コブラ毒因子　**CoVF, CVF**
コブラ毒素　**CT**
コプロトポルフィリン　**COPP**
コプロポルフィリノゲン　**COPROgen**
コプロポルフィリン症　**COPRO, CP**
コボル　**COBOL**
コメド母斑　**NC**
ゴモリメテナミン銀染色　**GMS**
コモンマーモセット　**CJA**
コラーゲン　**Col**
コランジル　**DH**
コリシン　**col, Col**
コリーズ骨折　**Colles'fx.**
コリスチメテート,ニスタチン,バンコマイシン　**CNV**
コリスチン　**CL, CS**
コリスチン・デキストロマ

イシン軟膏 **CDS**
コリスチン・ノナペプチド **CLNP**
コリネバクテリム(属) **C**
コリマイシン **COM**
ゴリラ **GGO**
コリン **Ch, Cho**
コリンアセチラーゼ **ChA, Ch-A**
コリンアセチル基転移酵素 **CAT**
コリンアセチル転移酵素 **ChAT, CHAT**
コリンアセチルトランスフェラーゼ **CHAC, ChAc**
コリンアセチル基転移酵素試験 **CAT**
コリンエステラーゼ **CEA, ChE, CHS**
コリンオキシダーゼ **CO**
コリンキナーゼ **CK**
コリングリセロリン脂質 **CGP**
コリン欠乏低メチオニン **CDM**
コリン作動性分化因子 **CDF**
コルサコフ症候群 **KS**
コール酸 **CA**
ゴルジ **Go**
ゴルジ関連小胞体リソソーム **GERL**
ゴルジ腱紡錘 **GTO**
ゴルジ細胞 **GC**
ゴルジ装置 **GA**
ゴルジ体 **GC**
コルステロール **CHO**
コルチコステロイド **CS, CTS**
コルチコステロイド結合グロブリン **CBG**
コルチコステロイド結合蛋白(質) **CBP**
コルチコステロン **Compound B**
コルチコトロピン様中葉ペプチド **CLIP**
コルチゾール **Col, Compound F**
コルチゾール結合グロブリン **CBG**
コルチゾール産生率 **CPR**
コルチゾールブドウ糖負荷試験 **CGTT**
コルチゾール分泌率 **CSR**
コルチゾン **Compound E, COR, cort, cort., E**
コルチゾン経口ブドウ糖負荷試験 **COGTT**
コルチゾン耐性〔抵抗性〕胸腺細胞 **CRT**
コルチゾン抵抗性胸腺細胞 **CRT**
コルチゾンブドウ糖負荷試験 **CGTT**
ゴールデンモンガベイ **CGA**
ゴルドナール症候群 **GS**
ゴールドブラット高血圧(症)腎 **KGHT**
ゴールドマン視野計 **GP**
ゴルドン試験 **^{131}I-PVP test**
コルヒチン **CLC**
コレ・シカール(症候群) **CS**
コレカルシフェロール **CC, D_3**
コレシストキニン **CCK, CK**
コレシストキニン・オクトペプチド **CCK-OP**
コレシストキニン・パンクレオザイミン **CCK-PZ, CK-PZ**
コレシストキニン様免疫反応性 **CCKLI**
コレステリルエステル転送蛋白 **CETP**
コレステリン **chol**
コレステリンエステル **chol-ester**
コレステリン肉芽腫 **CG**
コレステロール **C, Ch, CHOL, Chol, chol, choles, cholest**
コレステロール・レシチン(試験) **CL**
コレステロール/リン脂質(比) **C/P, C/PL**
コレステロールエステル **CE, ChE, CHOL E, CHOL EST, Chol est., chol.est.**
コレステロールエステル化活性 **CEA**
コレステロールエステル水解酵素 **CEH**
コレステロールエステル転送蛋白 **CETP**
コレステロールオキシダーゼ **CoD**
コレステロール教育プロジェクト **NCEP**
コレステロール結石 **CS**
コレステロール蓄積症 **CESD**
コレステロール低下脂質 **CLL**
コレステロール尿酸リン脂質指数 **CUPI**
コレステロール飽和指数 **CSI**
コレラ菌毒素 **CTox**
コレラ腸毒素 **CT**
コレラ毒素 **CT**
コロイド金曲線溶液 **GOLDSOL**
コロイド抗原 **CA**

コロイド状金 **CG**
コロイド静水圧勾配 **CHPG**
コロイド状の **coll**
コロイド浸透圧 **COP, CP**
コロイド鉄 **CI**
コロジオン **collod.**
コロナウイルス **CoV**
コロニー **COL, col**
コロニー形成因子抗原 **CFA**
コロニー形成活性 **CSA**
コロニー形成活性化因子 **CSF**
コロニー形成細胞 **CFC**
コロニー形成試験 **CFE**
コロニー形成阻止活性 **CIA**
コロニー形成単位 **CFU**
コロニー形成(性)の **CF**
コロニー推進活動 **CPA**
コロニー数 **CC**
コロニー阻止 **CI**
コロニー阻止因子 **CIF**
コロボーム・心奇形・魚鱗癬・精神遅滞・聴力異常 **CHIME**
コロラドダニ熱 **CTF**
コロラドダニ熱ウイルス **CTF virus**
コロンビア樹脂 **CR39**
コロンビア大学知能成熟度表 **CMMS**
コロンビウム(=ニオブ) **Cb**
コンカナバリンA **Con A**
コンカナバリンA加培養細胞の上清 **CAS**
コングルチニン **Cg**
コンゴーレッド **CoR, Cor, CR**
コンゴーレッド係数 **CI**
コンジローマ **Con**
コンストラクションマネジメント **CM**
コンダクタンス **G, g**
コンタクトレンズ **CL**
コンタクトレンズ(ハード/ソフト) **CL(H/S)**
コンタクトレンズ製造業者協会 **CLMA**
コンタクトレンズ取扱い者協会 **ACLP**
コンデンサ **cond**
コンドロイチン **Ch**
コンドロイチン四硫酸 **c-4-s**
コンドロイチン硫酸 **ChS, CS**
コンドロイチン硫酸・蛋白 **CS-P**
コンドロイチン硫酸A **CSA**
コンパクトディスク **CD**
コンピュータ **cmptr**
コンピュータ応用簡易知能スケール **CADS**
コンピュータ管理指導 **CMI**
コンピュータ教育応用研究所 **CEARC**
コンピュータ局所像 **CT**
コンピュータグラフィックス **CG**
コンピュータサーモグラフィシステム **CTS**
コンピュータ支援教育 **CBE**
コンピュータ支援診断学 **CADs**
コンピュータ支援設計/アラインメント制御方法 **CAD/CAM**
コンピュータ軸位断層法 **CAT**
コンピュータ自動測定・管理 **CAMAC**
コンピュータ出力マイクロフィルム **COM**
コンピュータ援用設計・コンピュータ援用製造 **CAD/CAM**
コンピュータ処理X線映像法 **CR**
コンピュータ診断システム **CAD**
コンピュータ制御X線回折器 **CCXD**
コンピュータ(補助)断層撮影 **CAT**
コンピュータ断層撮影(法) **CT, CTT**
コンピュータ断層装置 **ACTA scanner**
コンピュータ断層(撮影)メトリザマイド脊髄撮影(法) **CTMM**
コンピュータで計算された **CC**
コンピュータデータ登録キーボード **CDEK**
コンピュータ統合生産 **CIM**
コンピュータ内蔵携行型鎮痛自己調節投与用輸液ポンプ **CADD-PCA**
コンピュータ内蔵携行型薬物投与用輸液ポンプ **CADD**
コンピュータに保存された救急記録 **COSTAR, CO-STAR**
コンピュータに基づく記録 **PCR**
コンピュータによるX線濃度測定 **CXD**
コンピュータによる学習システム **CMTL**
コンピュータの入出力ポート **I/O, I&O**
コンピュータ表示動脈血酸素飽和度 **Sso_2**
コンピュータ腹部断層撮影

CAT
コンピュータ分析脳波 **CEEG**
コンピュータ補助学習 **CAI, CAL**
コンピュータ補助自己評価 **CASA**
コンピュータ補助体軸断層撮影(法) **CAAT**
コンピュータ補助多変量解析システム **CAMPAS**
コンピュータ補助知覚検査 **CASE**
コンピュータ補助糖尿病指導(システム) **CADI**
コンピュータ補助による評価 **CAA**
コンピュータ補助ミエログラフィ **CAM**
コンピュータ補助モニターシステム **CAMS**
コンピュータ補助による新薬申請 **CANDA**
コンピュータ利用学習支援システム **CBT**
コンプライアンス **C, Co**
コンプライアンス事務局 **OC**
コンプレックス **C, Cx**
コンベア系院内搬送システム **SVC**
ゴールドマン・ホジキン・キャッツ方程式 **GHK**
ここに用意されていない **NOHP**
ことば **ors.**
この時点で **h.t.**
この量を与えよ **d.t.d.**
この量を反復せよ **rep.dos.**
これ以上治療の必要なし **NFAR**
これ以上の要求なし **NFR**
これにかかわる人に **TWIMC**
子ウシ血清 **CS**
小(型)カップ **pocill.**
(軽い食中毒,お腹のかぜウイルスなどの)小型球形ウイルス **SRSV**
小型個体撮像素子 **CCD**
小型単層小胞 **SUV**
小型非切れ込み細胞 **SNC**
小型薬包紙 **chartul**
小型濾胞中心細胞 **small FCC**
小さじ **t**
小さじ1杯 **cochl.min., coch.med.**
小島 **is**
小鼻 **AN**
小箱 **cist., scat.**
小ビン **ph, V**
小人 **D**
小麦胚凝集素 **WGA**
五角形ピラミッド皮弁 **PPF**
五酸化アンチモン $\mathbf{Sb_2O_5}$
五炭糖経路 **PP**
五炭糖サイクル **PC**
五炭糖リン酸経路 **PPP**
午後 **a**
午後に **nachm, nm, PM, P.M., p.m.**
午前(中)に **AM, A.M., a.m., vm., vorm, vorm.**
古玄蒼朮 **AL**
古典的 **C**
古典的経路 **CP**
古典的条件づけ **CC**
古典的補体反応経路 **CCP**
仔ウシ胸腺 **CT**
仔ウシ胸腺抽出物 **CTE**
仔ウシ血清 **NBCS**
仔ウシ下痢ウイルス **NCDV**
仔ウシ小腸ホスファターゼ **CIP**
仔ハムスター腎細胞株21 **BHK 21**
呼気 **EXP, exp., expir**
呼気・吸気比 **E/I**
呼気圧 **PE**
呼気ガス **E**
呼気ガス内酸素濃度 $\mathbf{FeO_2}$
呼気ガス量 $\mathbf{V_E}$
呼気気道陽圧 **EPAP**
呼気休止時間 **TEP**
呼気終(末)期圧 **EEP**
呼気終(末)期食道圧 **EEEP**
呼気終(末)期肺容積 **EELV**
呼気終末0〔ゼロ〕圧 **ZEEP**
呼気終末圧 **PEE**
呼気終末酸素分圧 $\mathbf{PETO_2}$
呼気終末二酸化炭素〔炭酸ガス〕濃度 $\mathbf{FETCO_2}$, $\mathbf{ET_{CO_2}}$
呼気終末平圧 **ZEEP**
呼気終末陽圧 **PEEP**
呼気終末陽圧呼吸 **PEEPB**
呼気二酸化炭素分圧 $\mathbf{PE_{CO_2}}$
呼気の **exp, expir**
呼気肺活量 **EVC**
呼気閉塞指数 **CVI**
呼気陽圧呼吸 **EPAP**
呼気陽圧プラトー **PEPP**
呼気陽圧法 **PEP**
呼気予備量 **ERV**
呼吸 **br, br., brth, O, R, RESP,**

こ

Resp, resp, resp., respir, RP, X
呼吸/秒　BPS
呼吸/分　BPM
呼吸(数)/脈拍(数)指数　RP index
呼吸運動　RM
呼吸音　br.snds, Br sounds, br.sounds, BS, B.S., b.s., RS
呼吸回数：脈拍数(係数)　RP
呼吸可能な浮遊粒子状物質　RSP
呼吸器　BA
呼吸器・腸内オーファンウイルス　REO virus
呼吸器ウイルス疾患　RV, RVD
呼吸器感染症　RTI
呼吸器感染に対する多種ワクチン　MVRI
呼吸器感染に伴うぜん鳴　WARI
呼吸器系　RS
呼吸器系の伸展性　CRS
呼吸器外科集中治療室〔病棟〕　R-SICU
呼吸器合胞体ウイルス　RSV
呼吸器疾患　RD, RI
呼吸器疾患起因ウイルス　RI virus
呼吸器疾患協会　RDA
呼吸器疾患質問表　RDQ
呼吸器疾患集中治療室　RICU
呼吸技術　RT
呼吸救急症候群　RES
呼吸曲線　PNG
呼吸係数　RI
呼吸交換比　RER
呼吸困難　Dp, dysp
呼吸困難指数　DI
呼吸困難症候群　RDS
呼吸困難の　dysp
呼吸困難の自覚閾値　TLD
呼吸困難のためベッド頭部を上げる　HOB up SOB, HOB UP SOB
呼吸細気管支　RB
呼吸時間　ET
呼吸仕事量　RW
呼吸疾患集中治療部　RCU
呼吸商　RQ
呼吸数　FR, fR, RF, RR, R/R, VE, Ve
呼吸する　br
呼吸性洞性不整脈　RSA
呼吸性の　R
呼吸性頻脈　RT
呼吸装置　BA
呼吸速度　BR
呼吸代謝　RM
呼吸中枢　EC, RC
呼吸調節中枢　PC
呼吸調節率　RCR
(全)呼吸抵抗　Rrs
呼吸抵抗単位　RRU
呼吸停止　CB, RC, RHC
呼吸なし　NR
呼吸に伴う覚醒　AAR
呼吸(性)の　RESP, Resp, resp, resp.
呼吸の　Res, res, respir
呼吸の仕事(量)　WOB
呼吸頻度　FR, fR, RF
呼吸不全　RF
呼吸脈拍比　RP index
呼吸容量　BC
呼吸予備　RR
呼吸量確保圧サポート　VAPS
呼吸療法　RT
呼吸療法士　RT
呼息　E, EXP, exp., expir
呼息する　exp
呼息総時間　T_E
呼息の　exp, expir
固化　solidif
固化した　S
固形化　sldf
固形癌の効果判定基準　RECIST
固形状態　ss
固形の　S, sld
固視反射テスト　FRT
固相螢光免疫測定法　FIAX
固相表面室温リン光　SS-RTP
固相微量抽出(法)　SPME
固体　SB
固定　fxg
固定液　FF
固定関心領域法　FROI
固定された　fxd
固定した　f
固定術　F, fus
固定する　immobi
固定的分裂終了期　FP
固定内部強化　fi
固有括約筋機能不全(障害)　ISD
固有括約筋欠損(症)　ISD
固有肝動脈　PHA, THA
固有筋　pm
固有筋層　pm
固有筋層(まで)　mp
固有受容体神経筋感覚促進法　PNF
固有心拍数　IHR
固有層　LP
固有層リンパ球　LPL
固有の　inher

固有名　**n.p.**
固有(商品)名で表示せよ　**sig.n.pro.**
股関節・膝装具(副子)　**HKO**
股関節骨関節炎　**HOA**
(人工)股関節全置換術　**THA**
股関節点状骨端形成異常〔異形成〕　**RCDP**
股関節の屈曲・外転・外旋　**FABER**
股関節の屈曲・外転・外旋・伸展試験　**FABERE**
股関節の屈曲・内転・内旋・伸展試験　**FADIRE**
股関節表面全置換術　**THARIES**
股関節部　**H**
股関節離断(術)　**HD**
股臼底脱出(症)　**PA**
股・膝・足関節装具　**HKAO**
孤束核　**NST, NTS, TS**
孤立性骨嚢腫　**SBC**
孤立性収縮期高血圧(症)　**ISH**
孤立性直腸潰瘍症候群　**SURS**
故人　**D, d, dec, decd, dec'd**
故障木解析法　**FTA**
故障モード効果分析　**FMEA**
枯草菌　**BS**
枯草熱　**HF**
(冠状動脈)後下行枝　**PDA**
後発射　**AD**
個々の　**E, indiv, INDIV**
個々の平均　**PA, p/av**
個人　**pers**
個人医療情報システム　**PHDRS**
個人カウンセリング　**IC**
個人健康情報　**PHD**
個人生涯リスク　**ILR**
個人的患者　**PP**
個人的損失と個人的障害　**PL & PD**
個人的なジギタル補助具　**PDA**
個人の　**indiv, INDIV, pers**
個人の病歴　**IMR**
個人療法　**ind.th.**
個人歴　**PH**
個人歴と社会歴　**P & SHy**
個別有効量　**IED**
雇用　**emp, empl**
雇用者　**emp, empl**
誇張　**exag**
誇張する　**Ex, ex, exag**
(打診の)鼓音　**Tymp**
鼓音性　**Tymp**
鼓音(性)の　**Tymp**
鼓索　**CT**
鼓室蓋　**ST**
鼓室形成術　**TP**
鼓室洞　**ST**
鼓室の　**tymp**
鼓腸　**Tymp**
鼓膜　**MT, TM, Trf, Trfell, tymp.memb.**
鼓膜形成手術　**Myringo**
鼓膜切開と吸引　**P & S**
鼓膜体温計　**TMT**
鼓膜張筋　**TT, TTM**
鼓膜張筋ひだ　**TTF**
鼓膜の　**tymp**
語彙　**vocab, vocab.**
語音聴取閾値　**SRT**
語音聴力レベル　**SAT, SDT**
語学研究所　**LL**
語句〔言語〕的知能指数　**VIQ**
(発)語流暢　**W**
(発)語流暢(検査)　**WF**
(単)語連結リスト　**WCL**
語連想検査　**WAT**
語/分　**WPM, w.p.m.**
誤嚥性肺炎　**AP**
誤差　**E, err**
誤差原因除去　**ECR**
誤示試験　**PP**
護身術　**DOH**
顧問医　**CP**
口　**o**
口蓋咽頭機能不全　**VPI**
口蓋咽頭形成術　**PPP**
口蓋咽頭形成不全　**VPI**
口蓋挙(筋)　**LP**
口蓋図　**uranog**
口蓋垂　**U**
口蓋垂口蓋咽頭形成術　**UP**
口蓋垂口蓋形成術　**UPP**
口蓋図の　**uranog**
口蓋帆咽頭の　**VP**
口蓋帆咽頭不全(症)　**VPI**
口蓋帆咽頭裂　**VPG**
口蓋帆挙(筋)　**LVP**
口蓋帆張(筋)　**TVP**
口蓋披裂　**CP**
口蓋扁桃　**FT**
口蓋扁桃肥大　**GMH**
口蓋(破)裂　**CP**
口蓋裂　**Cl Pal, Cl pal., cl.pal., GS**
(先天異常の)口顔奇形　**OFM**
口顔面指症候群　**OFDS**
口腔咽頭エアウェイ　**OPA**
口腔咽頭カンジダ症　**OPC**
口腔インプラント国際会議

ICOI
口腔衛生 OH
口腔衛生指数 OHI
口腔および顎顔面手術
OMFS
口腔温 TM, TO
口腔温度計 OTD
口腔学 stomat
口腔気管(チューブ)吸引
OTS
口腔気管チューブ OT, OTT
口腔外科医 D.Surg., ORS
口腔外科学 OS
口腔外科学修士 MDS
口腔外科学博士 D.D.S.
口腔外科免許医 L.D.S.
口腔食道経管栄養 OE
口腔洗浄剤 Collut.
口腔体温 TO
口腔内う蝕原性検査 ICT
口腔粘膜下線維症
OSMF
口腔粘膜漏出液 OMT, OM/T
口腔毛髪状白斑 OHL
口径 cal
口述した dict
口述する dict
口述の V, v
口臭防止剤 ABB
口唇口蓋裂 CLP
口唇単純ヘルペス HSL
口唇の La
口授どおりに m.dict.
口舌運動不全 OD
口蹄疫病 FMD
口頭指示 VO, V/O, v.o.
口頭の V, v
(痛みの)口頭評価尺度
VRS
口内錠 troch.
口鼻マスク換気法 OMV
工学士 B.M.E.
工業化学 AC
工業用加メチルエタノール
IMS
工業用テレビ ITV
公共死亡率防御国際連合
IUPM
公共団体 Inst, inst, Instn
公称標準線量 NSD
公衆 gen pub
公衆衛生 PH
公衆衛生・熱帯医学士
MPHTM
公衆衛生学士 BPH, BSPH, MSPH
公衆衛生学資格認定書
DPH
公衆衛生学修士 MPH
公衆衛生学博士 DPH
公衆衛生看護学士
BSPHN
公衆衛生監視員協会連合
AAPHI
公衆衛生監視者協会
APHI
公衆衛生技官 MOH
公衆衛生教育学士
M.Ph.Ed., MSPHE
公衆衛生教育者協会
SOPHE
公衆衛生局 DPH, PHS
公衆衛生計画 PHP
公衆衛生研究室サービス
PHLS
公衆衛生研究所 PHRI
公衆衛生工学研究所協会
AIPHE
公衆衛生工学士
MPHE, MSPHE
公衆衛生証明書 CPH
公衆衛生博士 P.H.D.
公衆の pub
公衆保健学博士 Dr.P.H.
公衆保健歯科認定書
DPHD
公的関係 PR
公認医療管理・臨床助手
CMAAC
公認〔登録〕技術員〔技師〕
RT
公認健康安全支部
AHSB
公認試験殺虫剤 OTI
公認助産師 CNM
公認入院計画 CHAP
公認の Off, off
公認〔登録〕理学療法士
RPT
公平な F
公報 bull, bull.
勾配 grad
勾配ゲル電気泳動 GGE
孔 F, For, Forr, O, opg
巧妙に s.a.
広域 WR
広域学位論文索引 CDI
広基部四脚杖 WBQC
広義の sens.lat., s.l.
広頸筋 platy
広帯域雑音 WBN
広帯域超音波減衰率
BUA
広汎型若年性歯周炎
GJP
広汎心内膜切除術
EERP
広汎性間質性線維症
DIF
広汎〔び漫〕性間質性肺疾患
DILD
広汎性間質性肺石灰化
DIPC
広汎性(腺)管内要素 EIC
広汎〔び漫〕性強皮症 DS
広汎性血管内凝固 DIC
広汎性の D
広汎〔び漫〕性閉塞性肺症候群 DOPS

広汎〔び漫〕性皮膚リーシュマニア症　**DCL**
広汎〔び漫〕性片側(性)亜急性視神経網膜炎　**DUSN**
広汎性発赤　**DR**
広汎〔び漫〕性未分化(型)リンパ腫　**DUL**
広汎〔び漫〕性メザンギウム硬化(症)　**DMS**
広汎〔び漫〕性メザンギウム増殖　**DMP**
広汎(性)発達障害　**PDD**
広背筋皮弁　**LDMC**
広範囲　**WR**
広範囲アルファ(溶血)　**WZa**
広範囲円板状エリテマトーデス　**w-DLE**
広範囲興味意見検査　**WRIOT**
広範囲局所切除(術)　**WLE**
広範囲雇用サンプル検査　**WREST**
広範囲照射野　**EF**
広範囲達成検査　**WRAT**
広範囲知能人格検査　**WRIPT**
広範囲の　**ext, ext.**
広範な看護施設　**ECF**
甲状腺・副甲状腺摘出　**TPTX**
甲状腺・副腎皮質(症候群)　**TAC**
甲状腺：血漿比　**T：P ratio**
甲状腺：血清比　**T：S ratio**
甲状腺亜全摘(術)　**NTT**
甲状腺外頸部放射性活動　**ENR**
甲状腺外チロキシン　**ETT**
甲状腺機能検査　**TFS, TFT**
甲状腺機能亢進症　**HT**
甲状腺結合グロブリン　**TGB**
甲状腺血清放射ヨード比　**T/S**
甲状腺抗体　**TA**
甲状腺刺激下垂体　**TSP**
甲状腺刺激抗体　**TSAb**
甲状腺刺激遮断抗体　**TSBAb**
甲状腺刺激性免疫グロブリン　**TSI**
甲状腺刺激物質　**TDA**
甲状腺刺激ホルモン　**TH, THTH, TSH, TTH**
甲状腺刺激ホルモン結合阻害活性　**TBIA**
甲状腺刺激ホルモン試験　**TSH test**
甲状腺刺激ホルモン受容体　**TSHR**
甲状腺刺激ホルモン受容体抗体　**TRAb**
甲状腺刺激ホルモン代替活性　**TDA**
甲状腺刺激ホルモン放出因子　**THRF, TRF**
甲状腺刺激ホルモン放出ホルモン　**TRH, TSH-RF, TSH-RH**
甲状腺刺激ホルモン放出ホルモン受容体　**TRHR**
甲状腺自己抗体　**TA**
甲状腺髄様癌　**MCT, MTC**
甲状腺性眼病　**TED**
甲状腺摂取　**TU**
甲状腺摂取勾配　**THUG**
甲状腺切除(術)　**TX**
甲状腺中毒性眼球突出症　**TE**
甲状腺(機能)低下(症)に伴う無汗性外胚芽形成異常症　**HEDH**
甲状腺摘出〔切除〕(術)　**thr, TX**
甲状腺の　**thr**
甲状腺の乳頭状癌　**PACT**
甲状腺ペルオキシダーゼ　**TPO**
甲状腺ペルオキシダーゼ抗体　**TPOAb**
甲状腺ホルモン　**TH**
甲状腺ホルモン受容体　**TR**
甲状腺ホルモン反応要素　**TRE**
甲状腺ミクロソーム抗体　**McAb, TMA, TMAb**
甲状腺ヨウ素摂取率　**TIU**
甲状腺リンパ造影　**TLG**
甲状腺濾胞上皮細胞　**TEC**
甲状(腺)の　**T, Th**
叩打痛　**KS**
交換(する)　**exch, exch.**
交換可能体内ソジウム(＝ナトリウム)　**NaE**
交換する　**xch**
交換性カリウム　**Ke**
(新生児の)交換輸血　**BET**
交換輸血　**BEx, ET**
交換率　**r/e**
交感(神経)系　**symp.sys**
交感神経・副腎髄質系　**PAC, SAM**
交感神経アドレナリン系　**SAS**
交感神経依存性疼痛　**SMP**
交感神経活動度　**SA**
交感神経系　**SNS**
交感神経系活性　**SNA**

交感神経節前ニューロン **SPN**
交感神経非依存性疼痛 **SIP**
交感神経皮膚反応 **SSR**
交感神経末端 **SNE**
交感の **S，symp，sympat，sympath**
交互(性)の **A**
交互の **ALT，alt**
(冷温)交互〔交代〕浴 **CB**
交叉〔差〕 **CH，int，int.，Xa，xg，xs，Xta**
交叉〔差〕価 **COV**
交叉〔差〕緩和マジック角度回転法 **CPMAS**
交叉〔差〕(適合)試験 **XM，X-match，X-matching**
交叉〔差〕した **X**
交叉〔差〕気免疫拡散 **CEID**
交叉〔差〕反応(性)蛋白 **CRP**
交叉〔差〕反応(性)物質 **CRM**
交叉〔差〕反応(性)物質陰性 **CRM−**
交叉〔差〕反応(性)物質陽性 **CRM+**
交叉〔差〕歩行 **X walk**
交差〔叉〕下肢伸展挙上(徴候) **XSLR**
交差〔叉〕咬合 **X**
交差〔叉〕(適合)試験 **X**
交差〔叉〕した **X-ed**
交差〔叉〕性の **X-ed**
交代運動率 **AMR**
交代おおい試験 **ACT**
交代する **A，ALT，alt**
交代性外斜視 **ADS，AXT**
交代性共同性内斜視 **ACCS**
交代性上斜視 **DVD**
交代性内斜視 **ACS**
交代速度 **TR**
交代(性)の **A，ALT，alt**
交代プリズムおおい試験 **APCT**
交代浴 **CB**
交通事故 **MVA，TA**
交通性水頭症 **CH**
交流 **AC，A.C.，ac，a/c**
交流・直流 **AC-DC，ac/dc**
交流分析 **TA**
交連下器官 **SCO**
光学 **Opt，opt，opt.**
光学者協会 **AOP**
光学電子顕微鏡 **LEM**
光学内尿道切開(術) **OIU**
光学密度 **DO，OD**
光学密度単位 **ODU**
光(感)覚 **LS**
光覚 **L，LP，LPerc，pl，PL，P.L.**
光覚なし **NLP，no p.l.**
光覚のみ **LPO**
光覚弁 **l.s.，s.l.**
光(学)顕(微鏡) **LM**
光合成ユニット **PSU**
光差 **LD**
光子 **γ**
光錐 **LC，LK**
光線過敏症皮膚炎 **PD**
光線性角化症 **AK**
光線力学的療法 **PDT**
光速 **c**
光電眼振計 **PENG，PNG**
光電眼振法 **PENG**
光電式文字読取装置 **OCR**
光電子顕微鏡 **PEEM**
光電子増倍管 **PMT**
光毒性 **PT**
光毒性治療法 **PTT**
光毒の **PTX**
光度 **I**
光路差 **OPD**
向流クロマトグラフィ **CCC**
向流電気泳動法 **ES**
好異種抗体 **HA**
好塩基球 **B，bas，bas.，baso**
好塩基球化学走性因子 **BCF**
好塩基球コロニー形成単位 **CFU-Ba**
好塩基球脱顆粒試験 **BDT**
好塩基性の **B**
好塩基性リンパ球 **baso**
好気性菌数の測定 **APC**
好酸球 **E，Eo，EO，eo.，EOS，Eos，eos.，Eosins，eosins.**
好酸球顆粒内蛋白 **ECP**
好酸球コロニー形成細胞 **EO-CFC**
好酸球コロニー形成単位 **CFU-Eo，CFU-EO**
好酸球コロニー刺激因子 **Eo-CSF**
好酸球刺激プロモーター **ESP**
好酸球浸潤肺臓炎 **EP**
好酸球性白血病 **EoL**
好酸球走化因子 **ECA**
好酸球増加症 **EO**
好酸球増多・筋肉痛症候群 **EMS**
好酸球増多症候群 **HES，HS**
好酸球蛋白Ｘ **EP-X**
好酸球肉芽腫 **EG**
好酸球ペルオキシダーゼ **EPO**

こ

好酸球遊走因子　**ECF**
好酸球由来神経毒　**EDN**
好酸球由来抑制因子　**EDI**
好酸性細胞指数　**AI**
好酸性の　**Eo**
好中球　**N, neut, Neutro**
好中球・赤血球・マクロファージ・巨核球コロニー形成単位　**CFU-GEMM**
好中球アルカリホスファターゼ　**NAP**
好中球エラスターゼ　**NE**
好中球活性化因子　**NAF**
好中球抗体　**NA**
好中球コロニー形成単位　**CFU-G**
好中球殺菌指数　**NBI**
好中球走化因子　**NCF**
好中球走化性蛋白　**NAP**
好中球不動化因子　**NIF**
好中球遊走因子　**LE**
好中球遊走活性　**NCA**
好中球誘導活性　**NIA**
好中球由来結晶誘発走化性因子　**CCF**
考慮する　**T/C**
行為　**A, a, act, proc**
行動　**B, beh, mtn, pfce, proc**
行動異常　**BD**
行動因子　**PF**
行動科学研究室　**BESRL**
行動型　**BP**
行動検査　**BT**
行動疾患　**BD**
行動主義　**beh**
行動生物学における伝達　**CBB**
行動治療進歩のための協会　**AABT**
行動の　**B**
行動能力　**PC**
行動パターン　**BP**
行動反応聴覚検査　**BOA**
行動評価尺度　**BRS**
行動療法　**BT, VT**
合格・不合格システム　**P/F**
合計　**Σ**
合剤　**co., mist**
合成　**CO, S**
合成音比率　**CNR**
合成期　**S period**
合成自然ガス　**SNG**
合成低残渣食　**LRD**
合成の　**compo, SYN, synth**
合成培地旧ツベルクリン沈降トリクロロ酢酸　**SOTT**
合成ヒトガストリン　**SHG**
合成物　**compo**
合同全地球海洋潮流研究　**JGOFS**
合法的に　**leg**
合法の　**leg**
合胞細胞　**S cell**
合胞体細胞性子宮内膜炎　**SE**
合胞体性巨細胞　**STGC**
合胞体層　**ST**
合理的・情動的精神療法　**REP**
合理的療法　**RT**
抗アクチン抗体　**AAA**
抗悪性貧血(因子)　**APA, APAF**
抗インスリン血清　**AIS**
抗インスリン抗体　**AIA**
抗インスリン自己抗体　**IAA**
抗ウイルス因子　**AVF**
抗ウイルス抗体　**AVA**
抗ウイルス蛋白　**avp**
抗ウイルスリンパ球血清　**ALS**
抗炎症(性)の　**AIF**
抗炎症(性)非ステロイド(性)の　**AIN**
抗ガス壊疽血清　**AGGS**
抗カルジオリピン　**aCL**
抗カルジオリピン抗体　**ACA**
抗ガンマ蛋白　**X-protein**
抗肝腎ミクロソーム抗体　**LKMAb**
抗核因子　**ANF**
抗核抗体　**ANA, ANEA**
抗核小体抗体　**ANoA**
抗キモトリプシン　**ACT**
抗狂犬病血清　**ARS**
抗胸管リンパ球グロブリン　**ATDLG**
抗胸腺細胞ガンマグロブリン　**ATGAM**
抗胸腺細胞グロブリン　**ATG**
抗胸腺細胞血清　**ATS**
抗基底膜抗体　**anti-BM antibody**
抗凝血性の　**AC, anti-coag**
抗凝血薬　**AC**
抗凝固薬　**anti-coag**
抗凝固療法　**ACT**
抗グロブリン　**AG**
抗グロブリン検査〔試験〕　**AGT**
抗グロブリン消費検査〔試験〕　**AGCT**
抗グロブリン消費量　**QAC**
抗血管内皮細胞抗体　**AECA**
抗血小板血漿　**APP**
抗血小板抗体　**APA**
抗血清　**AS**
抗血栓性持続濾過システム　**ACUS**

抗血友病A因子 **AHA**
抗血友病因子 **AHF**
抗血友病因子A **AHF(-)A**
抗血友病因子B **AHF(-)B**
抗血友病グロブリン **AHG**
抗血友病グロブリンA **AHG**
抗血友病グロブリンF **AHF**
抗原 **AG, Ag**
抗原感受性細胞 **ASC**
抗原結合細胞 **ABC**
抗原結合の **AB**
抗原結合能 **ABC**
(免疫グロブリンGの)抗原結合フラグメント **FAB, Fab**
抗原結合リンパ球 **ABL**
抗原決定基 **AD**
抗原抗体(複合体) **Ag-Ab**
抗原抗体テスト **AGB**
抗原抗体反応 **AAR**
抗原抗体反応阻止試験 **AARIT**
抗原作用に関係する担体 **TAP**
抗原提示細胞 **APC**
抗原反応(性)細胞 **ARC**
抗原表示細胞 **A cell**
抗原頻度 **Af**
抗痙攣指数 **ACI**
抗痙攣薬 **AED**
抗甲状腺ペルオキシダーゼ抗体 **TPOAb**
抗甲状腺ミクロソーム抗体 **McAb**
抗甲状腺薬 **ATD**
抗好酸球血清 **AES**
抗好中球血清 **ANS**
抗好中球細胞質抗体 **ANCA**
抗高血圧薬 **AHD**
抗酵母因子 **AYF**
抗サイログロブリン **ATG**
抗サイログロブリン抗体 **ATA**
抗細菌活性 **ABA**
抗細網性細胞傷害血清 **ACS**
抗酸(菌) **AF**
抗酸化剤 **Ao**
抗酸(性)(桿)菌 **AFB**
抗シュードモナスヒト血漿 **APHP**
抗心筋抗体 **AMA**
抗心筋自己抗体 **AHMA**
抗出血因子 **ABF**
抗糸球体基底膜 **anti-GBM**
抗糸球体抗体 **AGA**
抗重力 **AG**
抗神経炎因子 **ANF**
抗脂肪肝の **AFL**
抗酒剤アルコール反応 **AAR**
抗真菌薬 **FLCZ**
抗蛇毒液 **ASV**
抗腫瘍自然抗体 **NAA**
抗腫瘍免疫 **ATI**
抗スタフィロリジン **ASTA**
抗スタフィロリジン反応 **ASTR**
抗ストレプトキナーゼ **ASK**
抗ストレプトコッカルポリサッカライド **ASP**
抗ストレプトザイム検査 **ASTZ**
抗ストレプトドルナーゼ **ASD**
抗ストレプトリジン **AS, ASL**
抗ストレプトリジンO **ASLO, ASO**
抗ストレプトリジンO(力価) **ASTO**
抗ストレプトリジンOテスト **ASLOT**
抗ストレプトリジンO力価 **ASOT**
抗ストレプトリジン検査 **AST**
抗ストレプトリジン反応 **ASR**
抗ストレプトリジン力価 **AST**
抗セントロメア抗体 **ACA**
抗生物質関連偽膜性結腸炎 **AAPC, AAPMC**
抗生物質関連大腸炎 **AAC**
抗生物質治療効果 **PAE**
抗生物質と化学療法の学際的学会 **ICAAC**
抗生物質と臨床療法 **AM & CT**
抗赤血球自己抗体 **AEA**
抗精神病薬 **Major**
抗線維素溶解試験 **AFT**
抗線(維素)溶(解)酵素反応 **AFR**
抗体 **AB, Ab, ab, AB, Ab, ab, ABO, aby, AK**
抗体依存(性)細胞性細胞毒性 **ADCC**
抗体依存性細胞傷害 **ADCC**
抗体依存性細胞媒介性細胞傷害作用 **ADCMC**
抗体依存増進 **ADE**
抗体感作赤血球 **EA**
抗体関与免疫 **AMI**
抗体形成(性)の **AF**
抗体欠損(性)症候群 **ADS**
抗体欠乏症候群 **AMS**
抗体産生細胞 **ABPC,**

AFC, APC
抗体産生前駆細胞 **APCP**
抗体産生(性)の **AF**
抗体媒介細胞毒性 **AMC**
抗体被覆細菌 **ACB**
抗体分泌細胞 **ASC**
抗体補体結合感作(ヒツジ)赤血球 **EAC**
抗腸チフス・抗パラチフスAとB・抗ジフテリア・抗テタヌス混合ワクチン **TABDT**
抗デオキシリボヌクレアーゼB **ADN-B**
抗テタニー剤 **AT.10**
抗てんかん作用の **AE**
抗てんかん薬 **AE, AED**
抗トキソプラズマ抗体 **ATA**
抗トリプシン **AT**
抗毒素 **antitox**
抗毒素単位 **AE, AU**
抗破傷風血清 **ATS**
抗ヒアルロニダーゼ **AH, AHD, AHU**
抗ヒアルロニダーゼ(力)価 **AHT**
抗ヒアルロニダーゼ試験 **AHT**
抗ヒアルロニダーゼ反応 **AHP**
抗ヒスタミン剤 **AH**
抗ヒスタミン性の **AH**
抗ヒスタミン薬 **AH**
抗ヒトγグロブリン **AHGG**
抗ヒト胸腺血清 **AHTS**
抗ヒト胸腺細胞グロブリン **AHTG, ATG**
抗ヒト胸腺細胞血漿 **AHTP**
抗ヒトグロブリン **AHG**
抗ヒト成長ホルモン **anti-HGH**
抗ヒトリンパ球(グロブリン) **AL**
抗ヒトリンパ球グロブリン **AHLG**
抗ヒトリンパ球血清 **AHLS**
抗脾(臓)細胞グロブリン **ASPG**
抗フィブリノゲン **A-F**
抗フィブリノリシン **AFL**
抗プラスミン **AP**
抗不安薬 **Minor**
抗ヘビ毒 **ASTO**
抗平滑筋抗体 **ASMA, SMA**
抗便秘剤 **ACR**
抗補体活性 **ACA**
抗補体の **AC**
抗補体免疫螢光 **ACIF**
抗補体免疫酵素検査 **ACIE**
抗マウスリンパ球血清 **AMLS**
抗マクロファージグロブリン **AMG**
抗マクロファージ〔大食細胞〕血清 **AMS**
抗マラリアキャンペーン **AMC**
抗ミオシン抗体 **AMA**
抗ミトコンドリア抗体 **AMA**
抗ミュラー因子 **AMF**
抗ミュラー管ホルモン **AMH**
抗免疫グロブリン **AIG**
抗免疫グロブリン抗体 **AIA**
抗モルヒネ投与量 **AMD**
抗網内細胞毒血清 **SAC**
抗葉酸物質拮抗因子 **CF**
抗溶血性因子 **AHF**
抗溶血性グロブリン **AHG**
抗ラット胸腺細胞血清 **ATS**
抗リウマチ薬 **ARDs**
抗リン脂質抗体 **APL**
抗リン脂質抗体症候群 **APS**
抗リンパ芽球グロブリン **ALG**
抗リンパ球グロブリン **ALG**
抗リンパ球血漿 **ALP**
抗リンパ球血清 **ALS**
抗リンパ球抗体 **ALA**
抗利尿物質 **ADS**
抗利尿ホルモン **ADH, adh**
抗利尿ホルモン不適合分泌 **ISADH**
抗利尿ホルモン不適合分泌症候群 **SIADH**
抗利尿ホルモン分泌異常 **IADH**
抗利尿ホルモン分泌異常症候群 **IADHS**
抗療性腹水 **RA**
抗連鎖球菌抗体価 **ASOT**
抗連鎖球菌ヒアルロニダーゼ **ASH**
抗A型肝炎抗体 **anti HA**
抗B型肝炎e抗体 **anti HBe**
抗B型肝炎コア抗体 **anti HBc**
抗B型肝炎表面抗体 **anti HBs**
抗HIV免疫血清グロブリン **HIVIG**
抗RNP抗体 **RNP antibody**
抗TSHレセプター自己抗体 **TRAb**
攻撃ウイルス基準 **CVS**

攻撃誘導試験　**HCT**
更年期　**meno**
更年期角化腫　**KC**
更年期指数　**MI**
更年期障害　**meno**
更年期症候群　**CS**
更年期の　**meno**
肛門括約筋　**AS**
肛門管　**P**
肛門坐薬　**Suppos.rect., supp.rect.**
肛門周囲皮膚　**E**
肛門周囲ヘルペス　**PH**
肛門性器間距離　**AGD**
肛門に　**pro rect.**
肛門病学　**PR, Pr**
肛門部空腸吻合(術)　**HPE**
肛門を通じて　**per.an.**
効果　**eff**
効果あるまで加えよ　**ad effect.**
効果的な　**eff**
効果なし　**Z**
効果発現時間　**IRT**
効能や希釈の十進法スケール　**X**
効率　**EFF**
効率のよい　**eff**
拘縮　**C, contr**
拘束型心筋症　**RCM**
拘束した　**conf**
拘束水浸ストレス　**RWIS**
咽頭側間隙　**PS**
後アブミ骨ひだ　**PSF**
後胃腸吻合(術)　**PGE**
後遺症　**seq.**
後遺症なし　**NS**
後腋窩線　**PAL**
後下行枝　**PD**
後下象限　**PIQ**
後下小脳動脈　**PICA**
後下腸骨棘　**PIIS**
(視床)後外側(核)　**LP**
後冠(状)動脈洞　**PCS**
後眼房　**PC**
後眼房レンズ移植　**PCLI**
後過分極電位　**AHP**
後胸骨柄部濁音　**RMD**
後期アレルギー反応　**LAR**
後期後発射　**LAD**
後期反応　**LPR**
後期陽性成分　**LPC**
後筋麻痺　**PL**
後屈　**refl, refl.**
後屈する　**refl, refl.**
後脛骨移行(術)　**PTT**
後脛骨動脈の拍動　**PTP**
後脛骨(筋)の　**TP**
後脛骨の　**post.tib., PT**
(子宮)後傾後屈症　**RVF**
後傾した　**RV**
後傾症　**RV**
後交通動脈　**PCA, PCoA, Pcom, P-com**
後交通動脈瘤　**PCA**
後交連　**PC**
後交連核　**NPC**
後(続)効果　**AE**
後骨髄球　**ME**
(脊髄)後根　**DR, dr, dr.**
後根神経節　**DRG**
(脊髄)後根侵入部　**DREZ**
後根電位　**DRP**
後根反射　**DRR**
後鼓膜峡部　**PTI**
後(続)作用　**AE**
後索刺激装置　**DCS**
後索内側毛帯　**DCML**
後十字靱帯　**PCL**
後上象限　**PSQ**
後上腸骨棘　**PSIS**
後視床穿通動脈　**PTPA**
後縦肛門形成　**PSA**
後縦靱帯骨化症　**OPLL**
後水晶体線維形成症　**RLF**
後錐体靱帯　**PPF**
後前方向　**PA**
後前方と側面　**PA & Lat**
後脊髄動脈　**Asp, TPAL**
後接合部膜　**PJM**
後側核　**P**
(脊髄)後側動脈路　**TAPL**
後側方固定術　**PLF**
後大静脈尿管　**RCU**
後大脳動脈　**PCA**
後退　**retr, retr.**
後退させうる　**retr, retr.**
後退させる　**retr, retr.**
後退した　**retr, retr.**
後中間彎曲　**PIC**
後中脳静脈　**PMV**
後遅発型喘息反応　**pLAR**
後天性巨細胞性封入体病　**ACID**
後天性心疾患　**AHD**
後天性腎性尿崩症　**ANDI**
後天性嚢胞性腎疾患　**ACDK**
後天性表皮水疱症　**EBA**
後天性免疫出血性疾患　**AIHD**
後天性免疫不全症候群　**AIDS**
後天性免疫不全病　**AID**
後天性溶血性貧血　**AHA**
後転の　**RF**
後頭　**O, occ, occip**
後頭・顔・頸・胸郭・腹・指異形成症　**OFCTAD**
後頭・後下小脳動脈吻合術　**OP-PICA anastomosis**

後頭・前頭　**OF**
後頭オトガイの　**OM**
後頭蓋窩　**PCF**
後頭蓋窩腫瘍　**PFT**
後頭蓋窩軸外クモ膜嚢胞　**PFEAAC**
後頭下顎顔面症候群　**OMF**
後頭角　**OH**
後頭下穿刺　**SP**
後頭下の　**SO, suboccip**
後頭形成異常　**OD**
後頭骨後部　**OP**
後頭三角　**occ △**
後頭前頂下の　**SOB**
後頭前頭周囲　**OFC**
後頭前頭照射　**OF rad**
後頭前頭頭痛　**occip-F HA, OF-HA**
後頭前頭の　**occip.F, occip-F, OF**
後頭前部　**OA**
後頭側頭溝　**OTS**
後頭頭頂の　**OP**
後頭動脈　**OA**
後頭動脈・後下小脳脳動脈吻合部　**OA-PICA anastomosis**
後頭の　**occ, occip**
後頭左後位　**OLP**
後頭左前位　**OLA**
後頭部間欠性律動性 δ 波　**OIRDA**
後頭部結節　**OP**
後頭部の　**O**
後頭葉　**OC**
後内側視床下部　**PMH**
後乳頭筋　**PPM**
後脳　**ME**
後嚢下白内障　**PSC, PSCC**
後半遠位皮質尿細管　**LDCT**
後発射　**AF**
後被膜下伝染病　**psp**
後鼻孔閉鎖　**PCA**
後鼻漏　**PND**
後吻側腹側核　**V.o.p.**
後部虚血性視神経炎　**PION**
後部硝子体剝離　**PVD**
後部尿道膀胱角　**PUV angle**
後腹膜気体造影法　**PRP**
後腹膜の　**RP**
後腹膜リンパ節郭清　**RND, RPLND**
後腹膜リンパ節摘除(術)　**RLND**
後壁　**PW**
後壁厚　**PWT**
後壁拡張期後退速度　**DPWV**
後壁梗塞　**PWI**
後壁心筋梗塞(症)　**PMI, PWMI**
後壁速度　**PWV**
後方散乱係数　**BSF**
後方椎体間固定術　**PLIF**
後方椎体固定　**PIF**
後方の　**P**
後放電　**AF**
後脈絡膜動脈　**PChA**
後無顆粒島状皮質　**AID**
後迷路性難聴　**RLD**
後リンパ節　**PLN**
(脊柱)後彎(症)　**kyph**
厚生年金　**SS**
厚生労働省　**MHLW**
厚生労働大臣　**MH**
恒久性レンズ形角質増加症　**HLP**
恒常温水　**CHW**
紅色の　**E**
紅色網状ムチン沈着症　**REM**
紅斑　**eryth**
紅斑性エリテマトーデス　**PE**
紅斑熱群　**SFG**
紅斑熱群リケッチア　**SFGR**
紅斑量　**ED**
虹彩角膜内皮(症候群)　**ICE**
虹彩クリップレンズ　**ICL**
虹彩血管新生　**NVI**
虹彩後癒着　**SIP**
虹彩切除　**IR**
虹彩突起　**IP**
虹彩と瞳孔　**I/P**
虹彩部分欠損・鎖肛症候群　**CAS**
咬筋　**MA, MM**
咬筋硬直　**MMR**
咬合　**ocl**
咬合の　**O**
咬合面歯頸部の　**OC**
航空医学　**Aeromed, AM**
航空医学技術者　**AVT**
航空医学協会　**AMA, ASMA**
航空医学研究室　**AML**
航空医学研究所　**IAM**
航空医学診察室　**OAM**
航空医学装備研究室　**AMEL**
航空医学避難管理センター　**AECC**
航空医療指導者協会　**AMDA**
航空機内医療サポートシステム　**IMSS**
航空避難医療　**Amd Evac**
降圧作用を有する生理活性物質　**PAMP**
降圧薬　**AHD**
高アルファリポ蛋白血症　**HALP**
高アンドロゲン症　**HA**
高圧　**HP, HT, h.t.**

こ

高圧液体親和性クロマトグラフィ **HPLAC**
高圧換気 **HPV**
高圧浣腸 **HE**
高圧機械呼吸 **HPMV**
高圧酸素 **HO**
高圧酸素(療法) **HPO**
高圧酸素療法 **HBO, HOD, HOT, OHP**
高圧神経症候群 **HPNS**
高圧帯 **HPZ**
高位鉗子分娩 **HFD**
高位脛骨骨切り術 **HTO**
高位膝 **nehi**
高位前方切除術 **HAR**
高閾値機械受容器 **HTM**
高右心耳 **HRA**
高運動性群 **HMG**
高(輝度)エコー **SE**
高エネルギーイオン化放射能 **HEIR**
高エネルギーイオン散乱 **HEIS**
高エネルギーリン酸塩 **HEP**
高エネルギー可視光線 **HEV light**
高栄養 **hyperal**
高栄養輸液 **HA**
高栄養溶液 **HAS**
高オルニチン血症・高アンモニア血症・ホモシトリン血症(症候群) **HHH**
高温 **HT**
高温水 **HTW**
高温相面積指数 **PLI**
高温短時間(殺菌)法 **HTST**
高温熱 **HT**
高ガストリン血症性過塩酸症 **HH**
高カルシウム血症・骨溶解・T 細胞症候群 **HOTS**
高カロリー **HC**
高カロリー輸液 **TPN**
高可撓性 **hiflex**
高拡大野あたりの白血球(数) **WBC/hpf**
高眼圧(症) **OH, OHT**
高解像度心電図 **HRE**
高解像度心電図検査法 **HRE**
高解像度電子顕微鏡 **HREM**
高解像度〔高分解能〕透過型電子顕微鏡 **HRTEM**
高感度コリメーター **HS**
高圧酸素治療 **HBO**
高輝度網膜電図 **BF ERG**
高緊張 **HT, h.t.**
高グロブリン血(性)紫斑病 **HGP**
高血圧 **HBP, hptn, HT, HTN, hyperten**
高血圧(症) **HPN, hpn., hypn**
高血圧(性)クリーゼ **HTC**
高血圧検出・追跡プログラム **HDFP**
高血圧自然発症ラット **SHR**
高血圧症 **HTA**
高血圧情報インパクト **IHI**
高血圧性血管疾患 **HTVD, HVD**
高血圧性心血管疾患 **HAVD, HCVD, HTCVD**
高血圧性腎硬化(症) **HN**
高血圧性心疾患 **HCD, HHD, HTHD**
高血圧性腎症 **HTN**
高血圧性動脈硬化症 **HAS**
高血圧性動脈硬化性心血管疾患 **HASCVD**
高血圧性動脈硬化性心疾患 **HASCHD, HASHD**
高血圧性の **HTN, hypertens**
高血圧性脳(内)出血 **HICH**
高血圧性肺血管疾患 **HPVD**
高血圧赤血球増加症 **PH**
高血圧と蛋白尿 **HP**
高血圧と動脈硬化性心疾患 **H & ASHD**
高血圧の境界(域) **BH**
高血圧の診断と治療に関する米国合同委員会 **JNC**
高血圧プラス蛋白尿 **HP**
高血管内皮細胞 **HEC**
高血糖指数 **HI**
高血糖性高浸透圧性非ケトン性(昏睡) **HHNK**
高血糖性高浸透圧性非ケトン性症候群 **HHNKS**
高コレステロールおよびトコフェロール欠乏(症) **HCTD**
高コレステロール血症 **HC**
高抗原腫瘍 **HAT**
高校生人格質問表 **HSPQ**
高高度網膜出血 **HARH**
高高度網膜障害 **HAR**
高山〔高所〕病 **HHCS**
高酸素 **HO**
高酸素(症)・高炭酸ガス(症)の **HHPC**
高酸素(症)・炭酸(ガス)正常状態の **HNC**
高酸素圧 **HOP**
高酸素分圧 **HPPO**
高出生時体重 **HBW**
高次精神〔知能〕機能 **HIF**

高周波 **RF，rf**
高周波域 **HFR**
高周波数 **HF**
高周波数型疲労 **HFF**
高周波通過フィルター **HPF**
高周波電流 **HFC，RFC**
高周波と超高周波 **VHF/UHF**
高周波療法 **fulg**
高所恐怖症 **acro**
高所の **subl.**
高所脳浮腫 **HACE**
高所肺水腫 **HAPE, HAPO**
高脂血症 **HL**
高脂血糖症二次産物受容体 **RAGE**
高脂肪(食) **HF**
高純度の **HP**
高振幅徐波 **HVS**
高振幅性収縮 **HAPC**
高浸透圧食塩水 **HS**
高浸透圧性高血糖性非ケトン性(症候群) **HHN**
高浸透圧性非ケトン性昏睡 **HNC，HNKC, HONK**
高浸透圧性非ケトン性糖尿病昏睡 **HNKDC**
高浸透圧性非ケトン性糖尿病状態 **HNKDS**
高浸透性造影剤 **HOCA，HOCM**
高照射応答 **HIR**
高親和性コリン輸送 **HAChT**
高性能 **HP**
高性能イオンクロマトグラフィ **HPIC**
高性能液体クロマトグラフィ **HPLC**
高性能サイズ除外クロマトグラフィ **HPSEC**
高性能情報処理通信 **HPCC**
高性能の再現性 **HiFi**
高性能薄層クロマトグラフィ **HPTLC**
高性能微粒子フィルター **HEPA filter**
高性能膜 **HPM**
高性能毛細管電気流動 **HPCE**
高線維食 **HFD**
高線量群 **HDG**
高速イオン散乱分光法 **HEIS**
高速液体クロマトグラフィ **HSLC**
高速回転式粥腫切除術 **HSRA**
高速向流クロマトグラフィ **HSCCC**
高速撮影グラディエントエコー **MP-RAGE**
高速撮影法 **FLASH**
高速軸索原形質輸送 **FAT**
高速親和性クロマトグラフィ **HPAC**
高速スピンエコー法 **FSE**
高速先端分析法 **HPFA**
高速走査法 **HSS**
高速電子衝撃質量分析法 **FAB-MS**
高速度 **HV**
高速鉛療法 **HVLT**
高速フーリエ変換 **FFT**
高代謝患者 **EM**
高炭酸ガス換気反応 **HCVR**
高炭水化物(食) **HCD, Hi CHO**
高炭水化物低線維(食) **HCLF**
高脂血糖症二次産物 **AGE**
高蛋白 **HP**
高蛋白(食) **HiPro, Hi Prot**
高蛋白食 **HPD**
高蛋白補給 **HPS**
高窒素 **HN**
高張食塩エピネフリン **HSE**
高張乳酸加食塩液 **HLS**
高張乳酸加リンゲル液 **HLS**
高鉄ダイアミン・アルシアンブルー染色 **HID-AB stain**
高電圧 **HV**
高電圧電気泳動 **HVE**
高電圧透過型電子顕微鏡 **HVTEM**
高電圧濾紙電気泳動法 **HVPE**
高電位 **HV**
高電子移動度トランジスター **HEMT**
高電子密度無晶性物質 **EDAM**
高トリグリセリド血症 **HTG**
高度 **ALT，alt**
高度感覚神経性難聴 **SSHL**
高度危険妊娠 **HRP**
高度形成異常(症) **HGD**
高度鶏卵継代(ウイルス) **HEP**
高度研究計画 **ARP**
高度集中治療室 **HCU**
高度障害腎機能 **SIRF**
高度硝子体牽引 **MVR**
高度腎不全 **SRF，SRI**
高度に **mkdly**
高度の **mkd**
高度爆発性の **HE**
高度不安 **HA**
高度免疫抗痘瘡 γ グロブリン **HAGG**
高度網膜周囲増殖 **MPP**

高度網膜周囲退縮　**MPR**
高度落屑性上皮内病変　**HGSIL**
高透過性浮腫　**HPE**
高等研究計画局　**ARPA**
高糖質（食）　**HCD, Hi CHO**
高内皮細静脈　**HEV**
高年用絵画統覚検査　**SAT**
高粘（稠）度症候群　**HSV**
高能力　**HP**
高能力鉄蛋白　**HiPIP**
高濃度尿素とプロスタグランジン　**Up**
高反応レベルレーザー治療　**HLLT**
高配向熱分解黒鉛　**HOPG**
高比重ポリエチレン　**HDP**
高比重リポ蛋白　**HDL, HDLP**
高比重リポ蛋白コレステロール　**HDL cholesterol**
高比重リポ蛋白の測定　**HDL determination**
高頻度　**HF**
高頻度（人工）換気〔呼吸〕法　**HFV**
高頻度胸壁圧迫法　**HFCWC**
高頻度（染色体）組換え（株）　**Hfr**
高頻度繰り返し周波数　**HPRF**
高頻度ジェット換気〔呼吸〕（法）　**HFJV**
高頻度振動　**HFO**
高頻度振動換気法〔呼吸法〕　**HFOV**
高頻度（形質）導入　**Hft**
高頻度陽圧呼吸〔換気〕　**HFPPV**
高分解能 CT　**HRCT**
高分解能光学顕微鏡検査　**HRLM**
高分解能コリメーター　**HR**
高分解能電子顕微鏡法　**HREM**
高分解能の　**HR**
高分化型癌（腫）　**WDCA**
高分化型乳頭状中皮腫　**WDPM**
高分子　**MM**
高分子化学国際誌　**IJPAC**
高分子キニノゲン　**HMK, HMW kininogen**
高分子性外在性変質感受性蛋白　**LETS protein**
高分子量　**HMW**
高分子量成分　**HMWC**
高分子レニン抽出物　**HMS**
高ヘパリン量　**HHD**
高密度　**HD**
高密度細管システム　**DTS**
高密度デポジット糸球体腎炎　**DDD**
高免疫グロブリンE　**HIE**
高免疫血清　**HIS**
高用量群　**HDG**
高容量・低圧　**HVLP**
高容量吸引〔吸収〕器　**HVE**
高溶解性　**HR**
高麗人参　**GP**
高リポ蛋白血症　**HL, HLP**
高流量血液透析　**HF**
高レニン本態性高血圧（症）　**HREH**
高齢者・盲者・身体障害者への援助　**AABD**
高齢者高血圧欧州共同研究　**EWPHE**
高齢者のための医療介助　**MAA**
高齢発症関節リウマチ　**ORA**
高 IgE 血症　**hyper-IgE**
高 IgE 症候群　**HIES**
高 IgM 型免疫不全（症候群）　**HIGMI**
強姦治療センター　**RTC**
梗塞　**inf, inf.**
梗塞（症）　**inf, inf., infarct**
梗塞後狭心症　**PIA**
梗塞サイズ指標　**ISI**
梗塞前狭心症　**PIA**
鉤頭虫症　**Acanth**
鉤頭虫の　**Acanth**
喉頭　**LAR, lar, lx, lx., Th**
喉頭（科）医　**larng, Laryngol**
喉頭炎　**laryn**
喉頭蓋　**Epi, epig**
喉頭蓋前域　**PES**
喉頭蓋の　**epig**
喉頭（科）学　**LAR, lar, larng, Laryng, Laryngol**
喉頭（科）学の　**larng**
喉頭癌　**KKK**
喉頭気管気管支炎　**LTB**
喉頭気管食道の　**LTE**
喉頭気管麻酔　**LTA**
喉頭鏡検査（法）　**laryn**
喉頭筋　**LM**
喉頭室　**ven**
喉頭切開（術）　**LF**
喉頭切除（術）　**LG**
喉頭前庭　**LV**
喉頭の　**laryn**
喉頭ファイバースコープ　**LF**
硬化　**indur**

こ

硬化(症) **Scl, scl, Scler**
硬化性萎縮性苔癬 **LSA**
硬化性角皮症 **Tys**
硬化性肝癌 **SHC**
硬化(症)の **Scl, scl**
硬化療法 **ST**
硬結 **indur**
硬鶏眼 **HD**
硬口蓋 **HP**
硬膏 **emp.**
硬皮症 **SCL, sclero**
硬便 **HF**
硬膜外 **Epi**
硬膜外・輸液併用利尿排石法 **EID**
硬膜外圧 **EDP**
硬膜外液 **EDF**
硬膜外血液斑 **EBP**
硬膜外血腫 **EDH, Epidura**
硬膜外性脊髄圧迫 **ESCC**
硬膜外脊髄電気刺激法 **ESES**
硬膜外の **ED**
硬膜外麻酔 **Ep, Epid**
硬膜下腔圧 **SDP**
硬膜下血腫 **SDH, SDN, Subdura, Subdura.**
硬膜下出血 **Subdura, Subdura.**
硬膜下頭蓋内圧 **SDP**
硬膜下腹腔シャント術 **S-P shunt**
硬膜上頭蓋腔圧 **EDP**
硬膜穿刺後頭痛 **PDPH**
硬膜動静脈瘻 **DAVF**
硬 X 線画像分析〔分光〕計 **HXIS**
腔 **S, SP**
較差 **D**
較差干渉コントラスト(顕微鏡) **DIC**
較正 **CAL**
較正死亡率 **PMR**
鉱質 **min**
鉱質コルチコイド **MC, M-C**
鉱物質除去 **demin**
鉤虫(属) **A**
構音指数 **AI**
構成 **compo, struc, struct**
構成体 **form**
構造 **constit, str, struc, struct**
構造的臨床面接基準 **SCI**
構造の **str, struc, struct**
構築 **organiz**
構築の **organiz**
構内情報通信網 **LAN**
酵素 **E, enz**
酵素・抗体比 **E/A ratio**
(国際生化学連合の)酵素委員会 **EC**
酵素学 **fermentol, zymol**
酵素活性〔反応性〕のある **EA**
酵素基質 **ES**
酵素欠乏症 **ED**
酵素原顆粒 **ZG**
酵素単位 **EU, U**
酵素の **enz, F**
酵素番号 **EC, EC number**
(固相)酵素免疫測定法 **ELISA**
酵素免疫測定法 **EIA**
酵素抑制物質 **EI**
酵母・ペプトン・硫酸アデニン **YPA**
酵母・マンニトール(培地) **YM**
酵母アルコール脱水素酵素 **YADH**
酵母形態学培地 **YMA**
酵母細胞壁成分 **Z**
酵母人工染色体 **YAC**
酵母相 **YP**
酵母炭素塩基 **YCB**
酵母窒素塩基 **YNB**
酵母抽出物 **YE**
酵母抽出ブドウ糖 **YEG**
酵母抽出ペプトン・ブドウ糖 **YEPD**
酵母同定用カード **YBC**
酵母麦芽ブイヨン **YMB**
睾丸性〔精巣性〕女性化(症候群) **TFM, Tfm, TFS**
膠原 **Col**
膠原病 **CD, CTD, CVD**
膠原病性間質性肺炎 **CD-IP**
膠着補体結合反応 **CCAT**
膠嚢 **cap gel.**
膠様質 **SG**
膠様の **coll**
興奮 **agit**
興奮・収縮 **EC**
興奮した **agit**
興奮収縮連関 **ECC**
興奮性アミノ酸輸送体 **EAATs**
興奮性シナプス後電位 **EPSP**
興奮性シンパチン **SE**
興奮性接合部電位 **EJP**
興奮分泌連関 **E-S coupling**
興奮薬 **S, ST, st, stim**
講義 **lect, Lect**
講師 **lect, Lect**
声強度調節装置 **VIC**
声の **V, v**
声の周波数 **VF**
声発現時間 **VOT**
氷 **aq.aster., aq.astr.**

氷の　glac
国産の　dom
国際アルコール・薬物依存協会　ICAA
国際アルコール中毒防止委員会　ICPA
国際アレルギー学会　AIA, IAA
国際アレルギー協会　CIA
国際医学教育局　DIME
国際医学研究　IMR
国際医学情報センター　IMIC
国際医学生協会連盟　FIAEM, IFMSA
国際医学図書司書会議　ICML
国際医学博物館協会　IAMM
国際医史学アカデミー　IAHM
国際医史学会　SIHM
国際一般診療医学会　SIMG
国際一般名　INN
国際遺伝学会議　ICG
国際遺伝学連合　IGF
国際医薬品卸連盟　IFPW
国際医用生体工学連合　IFMBE
国際医用電子工学連合　IFME
国際医療科学組織会議　CIOMS
国際医療救援　MERI
国際医療経済学会　iHEA
国際医療情報学会　IMIA
国際インプラント研究者チーム　ITI
国際ウイルス学会議　ICV
国際ウイルス命名委員会　ICTV
国際ウイルス命名法　ISVN
国際うつ病予防治療委員会　ICPD
国際エイズ会議　ICA
国際エイズ学会　IAS
国際衛生学・予防医学・社会医学連盟　IFHPSM
国際栄養科学連合　IUNS, UISN
国際横紋筋腫研究会　IRS
国際応用心理学会　IAAP
国際オージオロジー学会　AUDI
国際音声学協会　API
国際音声協会　IPA
国際音声言語医学会　IALP
国際温泉気候学会　ISMH
国際外陰部疾患学会　ISSVD
国際解剖学用語委員会　IANC
国際解剖学連合　IFAA
国際科学技術センター　ISTC
国際科学財団　IFS
国際化学物質安全性カード　ICSC
国際化学物質安全性計画　IPCS
国際化学療法学会　ICC, ISC
国際学術連合　ICSU
国際家族計画連盟　IPPF
国際家畜増殖獣医学協会　AIVPA, IVAAP
国際学校保健連合　UIHSU
国際眼科学会連盟　IFOS
国際眼科コンタクトレンズ会議　ICLCO
国際柑橘類ウイルス学者機構　IOCV
国際環境医学・生物学協会　AIMBE
国際環境医学生物学協会　IAMBE
国際環境情報源照合システム　INFOTERRA
国際癌研究機構　IARC
国際癌研究協同体　CANCIRCO
国際癌研究データバンク　ICRDB
国際看護索引　INI
国際看護師協会　ICN
国際眼財団　IEF
国際肝臓研究協会　IASL
国際癌胎児性蛋白質学会　ISOBM
国際癌治療増感研究協会　IASCT
国際感度指数　ISI
国際眼内レンズ学会　IIIC
国際癌予見予防研究会　DEPCA
国際気管食道科学会　IBES
国際脚足学会　CIP
国際牛疾病協会　WAB
(ユネスコ)国際教育局　IBE
国際胸部内科医外科医アカデミー　IACPS
国際緊急援助隊医療チーム　JMTDR
国際禁欲学会　ICS
国際軍事医薬委員会　ICMMP
国際形成外科学連合　IPRS
国際形成外科学連合アジア太平洋部会　APIPRS
国際系統細菌学委員会　ICSB
国際外科医師会員　FICS

国際外科学連盟　**IFSC**
国際外科学会　**ICS, SIC**
国際血液学標準化委員会　**ICSH**
国際血液学会　**ISH, SIH**
国際結核肺疾患予防連合　**IUATLD**
国際結核予防連合　**IUAT, UICT**
国際血栓止血学会　**ISTH**
国際結腸・直腸病学会　**ISSDCR**
国際血友病学会　**IHS**
国際原子力機関　**IAEA**
国際原子力情報システム　**INIS**
国際顕微鏡学会　**IFSH**
国際口腔インプラント学士会　**ICOI**
国際航空宇宙医学アカデミー　**IAASM**
国際口腔顎顔面外科学会　**IAOMS**
国際口腔外科学会　**IAOS**
国際口腔病学会　**ASI**
国際高血圧学会　**ISH**
国際公衆衛生局　**OIPH**
国際抗生物質学情報センター　**ICIA**
国際交通医学会　**ITMA**
国際交通災害医学会　**IAATM**
国際抗てんかん連盟　**ILAE**
国際行動発達学会　**ISSBD**
国際骨髄移植登録　**IBMTR**
国際骨髄腫基金　**IMF**
国際混濁単位　**IOU**
国際細菌命名規約　**IJSB**
国際細胞学会　**IAC**
(ユネスコ)国際細胞研究機構　**ICRO**
国際細胞生物学会議　**ICCB**
国際細胞生物連合　**IFCB**
国際産(科)婦人科(学会)連合　**FIGO**
国際歯科医師会　**ICD**
国際歯科医療管理協会　**ILDPA**
国際歯科学会員　**FICD**
国際歯顎顔面放射線学会　**IADMFR**
国際歯学生協会　**AIED, IADS**
国際歯学連盟　**FDI**
国際歯科研究学会　**IADR**
国際磁気共鳴医学会　**ISMRM**
国際色彩照明方式委員会　**ICI**
国際色素細胞会議　**IPCC**
国際実験動物委員会　**ICLA**
国際実験動物科学会議　**ICLAS**
国際疾病・傷害および死因統計分類　**ICDID**
国際疾病および死因分類　**ICDCD**
国際疾病分類　**ICD, ISCD**
国際失明予防学会　**IAPB**
国際失明予防協会　**AIPC**
国際児童青年精神医学会　**IACAPAP**
国際児童福祉連合　**UISE**
国際耳鼻咽喉科学会議　**ICO**
国際耳鼻咽喉科学会連合　**IFOS**
国際社会福祉協議会　**ICSW**
国際社会保障協会　**ISSA**
国際斜視学会　**ISA**
国際集団精神療法学会　**IAGP**
国際手術研究会連合　**IFORS**
国際十進分類法　**UDC**
国際腫瘍疾患分類　**CIDO**
国際腫瘍疾病分類　**ICDO**
国際循環器(外科)学会　**ISC**
国際純粋・応用生物物理学機構　**IOPAB**
国際純粋・応用物理学連合　**IUPAP**
国際純粋応用物理学連合　**UIPPA**
国際純正・応用化学連合　**IUPAC**
国際女医会　**AIFM**
国際女医協会　**MWIA**
(WHOの)国際障害分類　**ICIDH**
国際消化器外科学会　**CICD**
国際小児科学会　**IPA**
国際小児学会　**AIP**
国際小児眼科学会　**ISPO**
国際小児歯科学会　**IAPD**
国際小児腫瘍学会　**SIOP**
国際小児腎研究　**ISKDC**
国際小児脳神経外科学会　**ISPN**
国際小児ホスピス　**CHI**
国際消費者機構　**CI**
国際静脈学会　**IUP**
国際静脈外科連合　**UIP**
国際職業安全衛生情報センター　**CIS**
国際植物命名規約　**Bot.c**
国際助産師連盟　**ICM**
国際女性心身医学会産科婦人科学会　**ISPOG**
国際自律神経研究会　**ISNR**
国際心理学者協会　**ICP**
国際神経化学会　**ISN**
国際神経芽細胞腫病期分類

INSS
国際神経外科医レーザー連合 LANSI
国際神経精神薬理学会 CINP
国際神経病理学会 ISN
国際人口科学研究連合 IUSSP
国際心身医学会 ICPM
国際心臓学会 SIC
国際腎臓学会 ISN
国際心臓血管学会 ICVS
国際心臓研究学会 ISHR
国際心臓病学会 ISC
国際心臓連盟 ICF
国際身体障害者年 IYDP
国際身体障害者リハビリテーション学会 ISRD
国際心肺移植学会 ISHLT
国際人類遺伝学会議常置委員会 PCICHG
国際膵移植登録 IPTR
国際膵島移植登録 ITR
国際スキー外傷医学会 SITEMSH
国際頭痛学会 IHS
国際ステロイドホルモン組織委員会 OCICHS
国際スポーツ体育学会 CIEPS
国際生化学・分子生物学連合 IUBMB
国際生化学連合 IUB
国際整形災害外科学会 SICOT
国際精神腫瘍学会 IPOS
国際精神神経内分泌学会 ISPNE
国際精神遅滞研究協会 IASSMD
国際精神分析学会 IPA
国際精神療法医学連盟 FIPM, IFMP, IFP
国際性病予防連合 IUVDT, UIPVT
国際生物科学連合 IUBS, UISB
国際生物学事業計画 IBP
国際生物気象学会 ISB
国際生命情報科学会 ISLIS
国際製薬団体連合会 IFPMA
国際生理科学連合 IUPS
国際接触皮膚炎研究グループ ICDRG
国際喘息協会 INTERASMA
国際前立腺症状スコア IPSS
国際大学協会 IAU
国際大学結腸・直腸外科医学会 ISUCRS
国際対癌協会 UICC
国際対癌連合分類 UICC classification
国際大気汚染防止団体連合会 IUAPPA
国際代謝異常眼疾患学会 ISMED
国際体力医学連盟 FIMS
国際体力研究委員会 ICPFR
国際単位 IE, IU, SI, U
国際単位系 SI, SI units
国際知的障害研究協会 IASSID
国際知的障害者育成会連盟 ILSMH
国際聴覚学会 IHS
国際地理学連合 IGU
国際地理眼科学会 ISGEO
国際地理病理学会 SIPG
国際定位脳手術学会 WSSFN
国際的に懸念される公衆衛生上の緊急事態（WHO） PHEIC
国際鉄道医療連合 UIMC
国際てんかん協会 IBE
国際電気生理筋運動学会 ISEK
国際電気標準委員会 IEC
国際電気メーカー連合 NEMA
国際電子顕微鏡学会 IFSEM
国際天文学連合 IAU
国際統計協会 ISI
国際同種療法協会 IHL, LHI
国際疼痛学会 IASP
国際糖尿病連合 IDF
国際糖尿病連盟 FID
国際毒物学連合 IUTOX
国際毒物学会 IST
国際トラコーマ予防機構 IOAT
国際度量衡委員会 CIPM
国際度量衡局 BIPM
国際内科学会 ISIM
国際内視鏡・放射線撮影医学会 SMIER
国際乳癌研究グループ IBCSG
国際乳児生存研究 ISIS
国際人間工学会 IEA
国際熱尺度〔スケール〕 ITS
国際熱傷学会 ISBI
国際熱帯医学マラリア会議 CIMTP, ICTMM
国際の intl
国際脳研究機構 IBRO
国際脳神経外科学会 WFNS
国際肺癌学会 IASLC
国際発展のための機関

こ

AID
国際反核医師の会 IPPNW
国際犯罪学会 ISC
国際ハンセン病学会 ILA，SIL
国際鼻科学会 IRS
国際比較白血病および関連疾患学会 IACRLRD
国際微生物学者連合 IAMB
国際微生物学会協会 IAMLT
国際微生物学会連合 IUMS
国際泌尿器科学会 SIU
国際皮膚科学会議 ICD
国際皮膚科学会連盟 ICD
国際病院安全管理協会 IAHS
国際病院連盟 FIH，IHF
国際病期分類 INSS
国際表現精神病理学会 SIPE
国際標準化機構 ISO
国際標準値 INR
国際標準逐次刊行物番号 ISSN
国際標準図書番号体系 ISBI
国際標準品 IRP
国際病理学会 IAP
国際物理医学・リハビリテーション学会 FIMPR
国際物理医学会 FIMP
国際物理療法学リハビリテーション学会連盟 IFPMR
国際物理療法学連盟 IFPM
国際不妊学会連合 IFFS
国際プラネタリウム協会 IPS
国際プレゼンテーション協会 IPS
国際分析科学会議 ICAS
国際ヘルスケア質向上協会 ISQUA
国際法医学会 IALM
国際法科学協会 IAFS
国際放射線医学会議 ICR
国際放射線学教育・情報委員会 ICRE
国際放射線学会 ISR
国際放射線技士学会 ISRRT
国際放射線単位測定委員会 ICRU
国際放射線防護委員会 ICRP
国際胞虫症学会 IAHD
国際法中毒学協会 TIAFT
国際法毒物学協会 IAFT
国際保健規則(WHO) IHR
国際保健・体育・リクリエイションスポーツ・ダンス協議会 ICHPER-SD
国際保健医療研究協力委員会 CHRD
国際保健教育連合 IUHE，UIES
国際保健局 IHD
国際補綴矯正学会 ISPO
国際母乳連盟 LLLI
国際麻薬統制委員会 INCB
国際麻薬取締官協会 INEOA
国際脈管学連合 IUA
国際脈管学会 ICA
国際ミリ単位 IMU，ImU
国際民族心理学会 ISNAE
国際メートル法 IMS
国際免疫学会連合 IUIS
国際薬学生連盟 IPSF
国際薬学連盟 FIP
国際薬剤疫学学会 ICPE，ISPE
国際薬草学協議会 ICBM
国際薬理学連合 IUPHAR
国際薬局方 IP，PI
国際有害化学物質登録制度 IRPTC
国際輸血学会 SITS
国際夢研究所 IIDR
国際腰椎学会 ISSLS
国際養豚獣医学協会 IPVS
国際ラジウム単位 IRU
国際ラット単位 IRU
国際リウマチ連盟 ILAR
国際リハビリテーション医学会 IRMA，ISPRM
国際流行疫学協会 IEA
国際理論・応用力学連合 IUTAM
国際臨床化学連合 IFCC
国際臨床検査技師協会 IAMLT
国際臨床視覚電気生理学会 ISCEV
国際臨床生物学会 SIBC
国際臨床病理学会 ISCP，SIBC
国際リンパ学会 ISL
国際連合 UN
国際労働衛生学会 ICOH
国際労働機関 ILO
国際老年精神医学会 IPA
国際老年病学会 IAG
国際ロールシャッハ協会 IRS

国内勤務医協会　**PNHA**
国内補聴器協会　**NHAS**
国民　**Nat**
国民外来医療調査　**NAMC Survey**
国民健康栄養検査調査　**NHANES**
国民健康栄養状態調査　**HANES**
国民健康保険制度　**NHI**
国民健康問診調査　**NHIS**
国民総生産　**GNP**
国民知能検査　**NIT**
国民の　**Nat**
国民保健制度　**NHS**
国立アルコール・薬物濫用情報センター　**NCADI**
国立アルコール中毒研究所　**NIAA**
国立アルコール濫用・アルコール中毒研究所　**NIAAA**
国立アレルギー感染症研究所　**NIAID**
国立医学研究協会　**NSMR**
国立医学研究所　**NIMR**
国立医学図書館　**NML**
国立魚蛋白凝縮センター　**NCFPC**
国立音響実験センター　**NCAE**
国立外傷予防管理センター　**NCIPC**
国立鎌状赤血球疾患研究財団　**NSCDRF**
国立癌化学療法サービスセンター　**CCNSC**
国立癌研究所　**NCI**
国立眼研究所　**NEI**
国立癌諮問委員会　**NCAB**
国立関節炎・代謝疾患研究所　**NIAMD**
国立関節炎・糖尿病・消化器・腎疾患研究所　**NIADDK**
国立癌センター病院　**NCCH**
国立血友病財団　**NHF**
国立研究開発財団　**NRDC**
国立研究協議会　**NRC**
国立健康教育財団　**NHEF**
国立骨疾患財団　**NOF**
国立コレラ・腸疾患研究所　**NICED**
国立歯科衛生研究所　**NIDH**
国立歯科研究所　**NIDR**
国立疾病管理センター　**NCDC**
国立失明予防協会　**NSPB**
国立小児健康発育研究所　**NICHHD**
国立食品技術大学　**NCFT**
国立神経疾患・脳卒中研究所［米国］　**NINDS**
国立神経病・感染症・脳卒中研究所　**NINCDS**
国立腎財団　**NKF**
国立真性多血症研究班　**PVSG**
国立心臓基金　**NHF**
国立心臓研究所　**NHI**
国立心肺血液研究所　**NHLBI**
国立心肺研究所　**NHLI**
国立精神衛生研究所　**NIMH, NIMR**
国立精神病情報システム　**NISP**
国立伝染病センター　**NCDC**
国立毒物研究センター　**NCTR**
国立日常微生物収集　**NCDO**
国立熱傷情報交換センター　**NBIE**
国立標準培養収集　**NCTC**
国立保健医療研究センター　**NCHCT**
国立保健サービス研究開発センター　**NCHSR & D**
国立母子保健センター　**NMCHC**
国立薬物濫用情報センター　**NCDAI**
国立労働安全衛生研究所　**NIOSH**
国連エイズ計画　**UNAIDS**
国連開発計画　**UNDP**
国連環境開発会議　**UNCED**
国連環境計画　**UNEP**
国連教育科学文化機関　**UNESCO**
国連児童基金　**UNICEF**
国連の国際農業開発基金　**IFAD**
国連薬物統制計画　**UNDCP**
黒鉛・ベンザルコニウム・ヘパリン　**GBH**
黒鉛療法　**GrTr**
黒鉛炉原子化プラズマ発光分析法　**FAPES**
黒鉛炉原子吸光法　**GFAAS**
黒鉛炉非熱励起分光分析　**FANES**
黒球温　**GT**
黒光　**BL**
黒人　**bk, Bl, bl, blk, N, Neg, nig.**
黒人小児　**NC**
黒人女性　**BF, B/F, b/f, NF**

黒人男性　**BM, B/M, NM**
黒人の　**B**
黒人の成人　**NA**
黒人の成人女性　**NAF**
黒人の成人男性　**NAM**
黒子・心房粘液腫・粘膜皮膚の粘液腫・青色母斑症候群　**LAMB syndrome**
黒子症・心電図異常・眼間隔開離・肺動脈狭窄・性器奇形・発育遅滞・難聴症候群　**LEOPARD syndrome**
黒死(病)　**BD**
黒色アスペルギルス　**AN**
黒色丘疹性皮膚病　**DPN**
黒色菌糸症　**PHM**
黒色腫　**mel**
黒色腫関連抗原　**MAA**
黒色腫転移　**MM**
黒色の　**B, bk, Bl, bl, blk**
黒色表皮(肥厚)症　**AN**
黒色ビン　**V.n.**
黒色分芽菌症　**CBM**
黒色縫合絹糸　**BSS**
黒質　**SN**
黒内障性家族性白痴　**AFI**
黒皮症　**DM**
極超短波　**UHF**
穀草　**G, g**
心の健康自己評価質問用紙　**SUBI**
試みられていない　**NTO**
試みられない　**NA**
答え　**A**
答え(る)　**ans**
国家健康協議会　**NHC**
国家保健福祉局　**DNHW**
国家麻薬情報局　**ONNI**
国境なき医師団　**MSF**
骨　**B, o**
骨移植(片)　**BG**
骨塩定量評価　**BMS**
骨塩量　**MD**
骨塩量〔骨密度〕測定　**BMD**
骨壊死　**ON**
骨芽細胞　**OB**
骨学　**osteol**
骨格筋弛緩薬　**SMR**
骨格筋抽出液　**SME**
骨格筋の　**MS**
骨格牽引　**sk.tr., sk.trx., sk.tx.**
骨格成長因子　**SGF**
骨格と四肢　**S & E**
骨格年齢　**SA**
骨格の　**sk, Skel, skel**
骨幹　**diaph**
骨幹端　**metaph**
骨幹の　**diaph**
骨関節症　**OAP**
骨吸収刺激因子　**BRSF**
骨虚血性壊死　**INB**
骨グラ蛋白質　**BGP**
骨形成促進蛋白　**BMP**
骨形成不全　**OI**
骨形成不全症　**OGI**
骨形成率　**BFR**
骨形態発生蛋白　**BMP**
骨原性肉腫　**OS**
骨硬化(症)　**OS, os**
骨細胞　**O**
骨疾患教育財団　**OEF**
骨疾患研究学士　**M.Sc.Ost**
骨疾患財団　**OF**
骨疾患出版協会　**AOP**
骨障害なし　**NBI**
骨髄　**BM, MAR**
骨髄異形成症候群　**DMPS, MDS**
骨髄移植　**BMT**
骨髄壊死　**BMN**
骨髄炎　**OM, Osteo, osteo**
骨髄外プラズマ細胞腫　**EMP**
骨髄芽球　**Mbl, Mybl, Myl**
骨髄学　**myel**
骨髄(様)化生　**MM**
骨髄肝性プロトポルフィリン症　**EHP, EHPP**
骨髄基質細胞抗原　**BST1**
骨髄球　**MY, Myel, myelo**
骨髄球抗原　**My-A, My-Ag**
骨髄球様の　**myel**
骨髄腔　**MC**
骨髄(顆粒球)系/赤芽球系細胞(比)　**M/E, M : E**
骨髄細胞　**BMC**
骨髄細胞腫症　**myc**
骨髄酸性ホスファターゼ　**BMAP**
骨髄産生率　**MPR**
骨髄腫グロブリンA　**Mg-A**
骨髄腫グロブリンG　**Mg-G**
骨髄腫形態得点　**MMS**
骨髄腫促進得点　**MPS**
骨髄性化生を伴う骨髄硬化症　**MMM**
骨髄性白血病　**ML**
骨髄性ポルフィリン症　**EPP**
骨髄線維症　**MF**
骨髄線維症(性)骨硬化(症)　**MOS**
骨髄増殖性疾患　**MD, MPD**
骨髄単芽球白血病　**MMoL**
骨髄単核球　**BMMC**
骨髄単核細胞　**MMNC**
骨髄(性)単球(性)白血病　**MML**

こ

骨髄単クローン形質細胞増加症　**MOMP**
骨髄内圧　**BMP**
骨髄軟膜細胞　**BM-BC**
骨髄の　**myel**
骨髄の好酸性線維組織球性（部位）　**EFHBM**
骨髄非貪食細胞　**BM-NPC**
骨髄肥満細胞　**BMMC**
骨髄放出率　**MRR**
骨髄由来の　**B**
骨髄由来マクロファージ　**BMDM, BMM**
骨髄抑制　**BMD**
骨折　**F, Fr, frac, Fract, fract, FX, Fx, fx, FXR**
骨折部位　**FS**
骨性の　**OSS**
骨接合　**BC**
骨粗鬆症　**OP**
骨粗鬆症・偽（性）脂肪腫症候群　**OPS**
骨損傷　**BI**
骨体　**COR**
骨端　**epiph**
骨伝導　**BC**
骨と関節　**BJ, B/J, B & J**
骨（伝）導　**KL**
骨導　**BC**
骨内鉱質含有量　**BMC**
骨内注入（輸液）　**IOI**
骨内の　**endos, endost**
骨軟化症　**OM**
骨軟骨の　**osteocart**
骨肉腫　**OS**
骨肉腫由来増殖因子　**ODGF**
骨年齢　**BA**
骨パジェット病　**PDB**
骨斑紋症　**OS**
骨盤位　**BEL**
骨盤位介助術　**PBE**
骨盤入口の対角線結合径　**CD**
骨盤うっ血症候群　**PCS**
骨盤屈曲拘縮　**PFC**
骨盤痙攣　**PC**
骨盤外科医協会　**SPS**
骨盤牽引　**P trx, PTx, ptx, p.tx**
骨盤静脈造影（法）　**PVG**
骨盤静脈流出　**PSS**
骨盤帯付き長下肢装具　**HKAFO**
骨盤出口後縦径　**PS**
骨盤出口縦径　**AP**
骨盤動脈撮影　**PAG**
骨盤動揺　**PR**
骨盤と直腸の　**P & R**
骨盤内炎症性疾患　**PID**
骨盤内径　**CD**
骨盤内血管造影　**PAG**
骨盤内静脈うっ血症候群　**IVCS**
骨盤の　**Pel**
骨盤癒着性疾患　**PAD**
骨皮質指数　**IBA**
骨病理学　**Osteo, osteo**
骨マトリックス・グラ蛋白　**MGP**
骨密度　**BMD**
骨由来成長因子　**BDGFs**
骨誘導因子　**OIF**
骨（塩）量　**BMD**
骨量測定法　**MD**
骨・関節・筋　**BJM**
骨・関節外科医協会　**ABJS**
異なる　**diff, fgn**
粉にする　**trir., trit.**
好み　**pref**
好む　**pref**
細かい粉末　**pul.tenu., pulv.tenu.**
細かく切った　**conc.**
米糠糖類　**RBS**
暦の　**Chron, chron.**
殺された　**kd**
壊れやすい　**frag**
今週かぎり　**TWO**
今晩　**hoc vesp., h.v.**
今夜　**h.n., tonoc, tonoct**
今夕　**h.v.**
困難　**dx, h**
困難な　**diff, hrd**
昆虫学　**Entom.**
根　**R, r., rad, rad., rad, rad.**
（歯）根管　**RC**
根茎　**rhiz**
根治手術　**rad op**
根治的会陰式前立腺切除（術）　**RPP**
根治的多関節滑膜切除術　**RaMS**
根治的恥骨後前立腺切除術　**RRP**
根治的乳房切断術　**RM**
根治的左頸部郭清（術）　**LND, LRND**
根治的左乳房切断（術）　**LRM**
根治度　**C**
根瘤菌　**Rhz**
混合　**mix.**
混合受身凝集法　**MPHA**
混合感染　**m**
混合寒冷グロブリン血（症）　**MC**
混合機能酸化酵素　**MFO**
混合凝集反応　**MAR**
混合結合組織病　**MCTD**
混合抗グロブリン反応　**MAR**
混合効率　**ME**
混合呼吸器ワクチン　**MRV**
混合コロニー形成単位　**CFU-mix**
混合細菌毒素　**MBT**
混合細胞型　**MC**

混合細胞凝集反応
MCAR
混合細胞結節性(リンパ腫)
MC-N
混合した **mxd**
混合して錠剤とせよ
ft.mas.div.in pil.
混合静脈血 $\bar{v}$
混合静脈血酸素分圧
PVO_2
混合静脈酸素飽和
MVOS
混合静脈の **MV**
混合静脈ピーエイチ
pHv
混合しラベルに記入せよ
mis.et sig.
混合神経活動電位
MNAP
混合神経伝達速度
MNCV
混合人工授精 **CAI**
混合性過誤腫 **MH**
混合性器発育異常 **MGD**
混合性皮膚(細胞)白血球反応 **MSLR**
混合性免疫不全〔疾患〕
CID
混合赤血球吸着試験
MHA
混合せよ **F.M.，f.m.**
混合白血球培養 **MLC**
混合白血球反応 **MLR**
混合ビタミン **multivits**
混合物 **M，m，m.，mist，mix.，mixt.**
混合物をつくれ **F.M.，f.m.，ft.mist.，m.ft.，M.ft.**
混合本態性寒冷グロブリン血症 **MECG**
混合免疫螢光検査法
MIF
混合乱視 **Mis Astig**
混合リンパ球腫瘍細胞
MLTC
混合リンパ球腫瘍細胞反応
MLTR
混合リンパ球相互作用
MLI
混合リンパ球濃度 **MLC**
混合リンパ球培養 **MLC**
混合リンパ球反応 **MLR**
混成国際的診断面接
CIDI
混成の **compo**
混濁 **turb，turbid**
混濁角膜症候群 **CCS**
混濁した **ged，turb**
混濁単位 **TU**
混濁度低下 **TR**
混濁度低下単位 **TRU**
混和して作れ **m.f.，M.f.**
混和し丸剤塊とせよ
m.f.mass.pil.
混和し丸剤とせよ
M et f.pil.，m.f.pil.
混和し散剤1包とし同量12包とせよ
M.f.pulv.D.t.d.XII
混和し散剤12包とせよ
M.f.pulv.XII
混和し散剤とせよ
M et f.pulv.，m.f.pulv.，M.f.pulv.，M.ft.pulv.
混和し常法に従ってつくれ
m.ft.l.a.，M.ft.l.a.
混和し使用法を記入して与えよ **M.D.S.，m.d.s.**
混和し水剤とせよ
M.f.mist.，M.f.mixt.，m.f.sol.
混和してつくれ **m.f.，M.f.，m.ft.，M.ft.**
混和し軟膏をつくれ
m.f.ung.，M.f.ung.
混和し用法を記せ
m.et sig.
混和する **M，m，m.**
混和物 **M，m，m.**
痕跡 **Tr，tr**
痕跡の **T**
壺音性の **amph**

さ

サイクリック AMP 結合蛋白 **CAP**
サイクリック AMP 受容蛋白 **CRP**
サイクリック AMP, サイクリック〔環状〕アデノシン 3′,5′-リン酸 **cAMP**
サイクリックグアノシン 3′,5′-一リン酸 **cGMP**
サイクリン依存キナーゼ **CDK**
サイクリン依存キナーゼ 2 **CDKN2**
サイクル **C, C, c, cyc**
サイクル/時 **cph**
サイクル/秒 **CPS, CS, C.S., C/S, c/s**
サイクル/分 **c.min., c/min, c/min., cpm**
サイクロデキストリン **CyD**
サイクロトロン **CYC, cyc**
サイクロヘキサール **CH**
サイコポニンD **SSd**
サイズ排除クロマトグラフィ **SEC**
サイトカイン **CK**
サイトカインシグナル抑制因子 **SOCS**
サイトカイン依存性好中球走化性 **CINC**
サイトカラシン B **CB**
サイトケラチン **PKK**
サイトメガロウイルス **CHV, CMV**
ザイモサン **Z, zy, Zy**
ザイモサン活性化血漿 **ZAP**
ザイモサン活性化血清 **ZAS**
ザイモサン処理血清 **ZTS**
ザイモサン補体(試薬) **ZyC**
ザイロプリム **Zylo**
サイン **Sig, sig, sin, sin.**
サインした **Sig, sig**
サイン〔正弦〕波ジアテルミー **SWD**
サウスウェスタン癌研究班 **SWOG**
サキシトキシン **STX**
サクシニルコリン **SC**
サクランボ赤色斑(点) **CRS**
サケカルシトニン **SCT**
ササゲマメ・モザイクウイルス **CPMV**
ササゲマメ萎黄病斑状ウイルス **CCMV**
サシチョウバエ(属) **P**
サッカリン **SAC, sacch**
サッカリンナトリウム **ss**
サッカロミセス(属) **S**
ザックス・ゲオルギー反応 **S-G, SGR**
サーズコロナウイルス **SARS-CoV**
サッチ足 **SACH**
サディズム/マゾヒズム **S/M**
サテライトデオキシリボ核酸 **sat.DNA**
サドマゾヒズム **SM**
サナトリウム **sanit, sanit.**
サナレリ・シュワルツマン現象 **SSP**
サバンナモンキー **CAE**
サービス **SER, serv.**
サブスタンス P **SP**
サブスタンスペプチド **SP**
サブラ高血圧ラット **SBH**
サブラ正常血圧種(ラット) **SBN**
サフラン学生興味調査票 **SSII**
サプレッサーT 細胞 **ST cell, Ts**
サプレッサー感受性変異体 **sus, SUS**
サプレッサー細胞 **SC**
サブロー(ブドウ糖寒天)培地 **Sab, SAB**
サブローブドウ糖寒天(培地) **SDA**
サポート(=予後と治療結果のための患者選択および治療の危険性を理解するための研究) **SUPPORT**
サマリウム **Sa, Sm**
サーモグラフィ検出器の一種 **SPRITE**
サーモスプレー吸入法 **TSP**
サラセミア **thal, Thal**
サリチルアゾスルファピリジン(=スルファサラジン, サラゾサルファピリジン) **SASP**
サリチルアミド・フェナセチン・カフェイン **SPC**
サリチル酸 **SA**
サリチル酸エステル **sal, salicyl**
サリチル酸塩 **sal, salicyl**
サリチル酸ナトリウム **SS**
サリチル酸フィゾスチグミン点眼(液) **PSO**
サリチル尿酸 **SU**
サル **M**
サル T 細胞白血病ウイル

ス　**STLV**
サルウイルス　**SV**
サルウイルス 40　**SV40**
サル核内封入体因子
MINIA
サルコイドーシス　**Sar**
サル後天性免疫不全(症候群)　**SAIDS**
サルコシン　**Sar**
サルコマイシン　**SKM**
サル細胞　**MC**
サル出血(性)熱　**SHF**
サル腎(臓)　**MK**
サル腎(臓)細胞　**MKC**
サル腎(臓)組織培養
MKTC
サル赤血球(受容体)
MRBC
サル肉腫ウイルス
SiSV, SSV
サル肉腫関連ウイルス
SSAV
サルの細胞適合因子
MAC
サルヘルペスウイルス
SHV
サル免疫不全ウイルス
SIV
サルモネラ(属)　**S, SAL, Sal., Salm**
サルモネラ・シゲラ(培地)
SS
サルモネラ腸炎　**SE**
サンドバッグ　**SB**
サンドホフ病　**SD**
サンプル平均　$\overline{\mathbf{X}}$, **x**
サンプル平均値の記号
$\overline{\mathbf{X}}$, $\overline{\mathbf{x}}$
ジクロロベンジジン
DCB
スクシニルコリン　**succ**
ささやいた　**wh**
ささやき声　**WV**
ささやく　**wh**
さじ1杯　**coch., coch.amp., cochl.**
さじ2杯　**cochl.duo**
さもなければ知られているように　**OKA**
去る　**Lv, lv**
左角　**LA**
左眼　**L, LE, OL, O.L., o.l., OS, Os, os, O.S.**
左眼圧　**TOS**
左眼遠視　**LHT**
左眼角膜異物　**FBCOS**
左眼視覚　**VOS**
左眼斜視　**LHT**
左眼視力　**LV, L.V., VL, VLE, VOS, Vs, VS**
左眼に　**ocul.sinist.**
左眼の　**OS, Os, os, O.S.**
左眼網膜剝離　**RDOS**
左脚　**LB, LBB, LL, VF**
左脚後枝ヘミブロック
LPH
左脚前枝ブロック
LAFB
左脚前枝ヘミブロック
LAH, LAHB
左脚ブロック
LABBB, LBBB
左心室後壁振幅　**PWE**
左耳鼓膜　**MTAS**
左(心)室　**LV**
左(心)室1回仕事係数
LVSWI
左(心)室圧　**LVP**
左(心)室圧力　**LVT**
左(心)室過活動　**LVO, LVOA**
左(心)室拡大　**LVE**
左(心)室拡張(終(末))期(圧)　**$\mathbf{LV_D}$, LVd**
左(心)室拡張期圧
LVDP
左(心)室拡張期内(径)
LVID, LVIDD
左(心)室拡張期容積
LVDV
左(心)室拡張終(末)期圧
LVEDP, LVEP
左(心)室拡張終(末)期径
LVDd, LVEDD
左(心)室拡張終(末)期周径
LVEDC
左(心)室拡張終(末)期の
LVED
左(心)室拡張終(末)期領域
LVEDa
左(心)室カテーテル法
LHC
左(心)室機能　**LVF**
左(心)室機能障害検査
SOLVD
左(心)室機能不全　**LVD**
左(心)室脚ブロック
lt.vent.BBB
左(心)室急速充満時間
$\mathbf{LVT_1}$
左(心)室虚血　**LVI**
左(心)室緊張　**LVS**
左(心)室駆出　**LVE**
左(心)室駆出時間
LVET
左(心)室駆出時間指数
LVETI
左(心)室駆出率　**LVEF**
左(心)室駆出量　**LVSV**
左(心)室径　**LVD, LVDI**
左(心)室血液量　**LHBV**
左(心)室交感神経節切除(術)　**LCSG**
左(心)室梗塞容積　**LVIV**
左(心)室後壁　**PLV, PWLV**
左(心)室後壁(厚)
LVPW
左(心)室後壁厚
LVPWT

左(心)室後壁拡張期厚 **WTd**
左(心)室後壁収縮期厚 **WTs**
左(心)室最大駆出速度 **PER**
左(心)室最大充満速度 **PFR**
左(心)室耳 **LA, LAA**
左(心)室(拍出)仕事量 **LVSW**
左(心)室仕事量係数〔指数〕 **LVWI**
左(心)室収縮期圧 **LVSP**
左(心)室収縮期駆出 **LVSO**
左(心)室収縮期指数 **LVSI**
左(心)室収縮終(末)期径 **LVESD, LVIDs**
左(心)室収縮終(末)期容積 **LVESV**
左(心)室収縮終(末)期容積指数 **LVESVI**
左(心)室収縮終(末)期領域 **LVESa**
左(心)室充満圧 **LVFP**
左(心)室初期拡張期圧 **LVIDP**
左(心)室心筋重量 **LVM, LVMM**
左(心)室心内膜(半分) **LVEndo**
左(心)室心内膜下心筋虚血 **LVSEMI**
左(心)室前駆出期 **LVPEP**
左(心)室前壁 **LVAW**
左(心)室造影 **LVG**
左(心)室束枝ブロック **LVFB**
左(心)室体積 **Lvmas, LV mass**
左(心)室中隔壁 **LVSW**

左室低形成 **HLV**
左(心)室低形成症候群 **HLHS**
左室低形成症候群 **HLVS**
左(心)室動脈瘤 **LVA**
左(心)室動脈瘤切除(術) **LVA**
左(心)室(拡張期)内径 **LVID, LVIDd**
左(心)室内径(拡張終(末)期) **LVID(ed)**
左(心)室内径(収縮終(末)期) **LVID(es)**
左(心)室バイパスポンプ **LVBP**
左(心)室拍出仕事量 **LVW**
左(心)室拍出力指数 **LVSPI**
左(心)室ピーク収縮期圧 **LVPSP**
左(心)室ピーク充満率 **LVPFR**
左(心)室肥大 **HVG, LVH**
左(心)室負荷 **LHS**
左(心)室不全 **LHF, LVF**
左(心)室(機能)不全(症) **LVI**
左(心)室分時流量 **LVMF**
左(心)室壁 **LVW**
左(心)室壁運動(異常) **LVWM, LVWMA**
左(心)室壁運動指数 **LVWMI**
左(心)室壁厚 **LVWT**
左(心)室房 **LA**
左(心)室房容積 **LAV**
左(心)室房容積変化 **LAVC**
左(心)室補助循環装置 **LVAD**

左(心)室容積 **LVV**
左(心)室流出路 **LVOT**
左(心)室流出路狭窄 **SAS**
左(心)室流出路径 **LVOTD**
左(心)室拡張終(末)期容積 **LVEDV**
左(心)室収縮終(末)期径 **LVDs**
左軸偏位 **LAD**
左腎(臓) **LK**
左腎結核 **NPS**
左前斜位(の) **LAO**
左旋性アルファ・アセチル・メタドール **LAAM**
左旋性の **lev, lev.**
左側 **LHs, LS**
左側結腸(癌) **LSC**
左側呼気終末圧 **LEEP**
左方の **Lt, lt., lt**
左(心)房圧 **LAP**
左房圧 **Pla**
左(心)房異常 **LAA**
左(心)房拡大 **LAE**
左(心)房拡張終(末)期容積 **LAEDV**
左(心)房過負荷 **LAO**
左(心)房径 **LAD**
左(心)房形成不全 **HLA**
左(心)房経壁圧 **LATP**
左(心)房血管新生 **LANV**
左(心)房血栓 **LAT**
左(心)房後壁 **LAPW**
左(心)房自然エコーコントラスト **LASEC**
左(心)房収縮 **LAC**
左(心)房収縮終(末)期容積 **LAESV**
左(心)房大動脈(比) **LA : A, La : A**
左(心)房粘液腫 **LAM**
左(心)房の(圧) **LA**

さ

左(心)房排出指数　**LAEI**
左(心)房肥大　**LAH**
左(心)房壁　**LAW**
左(心)房(球状)弁血栓　**LABVT**
左(心)房ボール〔球〕(状)弁　**LABV**
左右(障害)　**R-L**
左右(比)　**L/R**
左右シャント　**LR-SH, L-R shunt**
左右シャント比　$\dot{Q}p/\dot{Q}s$, $\dot{Q}_P/\dot{Q}_S$, $\dot{Q}s/\dot{Q}t$, $\dot{Q}_S/\dot{Q}_T$
左右傷害　**R-L Störung**
左右の肋骨椎体角の差　**RVAD**
左右肺独立換気　**DLV**
左右不同(の)　**A, a**
左腕　**LA, VL**
左腕の血圧　**BPLA**
左(耳)・温(刺激)　**LW**
坐位拡張期血圧　**SDBP**
坐位肝窩(技術)　**SHW**
坐位の　**sitg, sttg**
坐骨横径　**TI**
坐骨海綿体筋　**IC muscle**
坐骨収納型大腿義足　**CAT-CAM**
坐骨神経伸展検査　**SNST**
坐骨脊柱間　**BISP**
坐骨恥骨軟骨結合　**IPS**
坐骨の　**SC**
坐剤をつくらせる　**ft.suppos.**
坐薬　**supp, supp., Supp., suppos.**
作業　**A, occ**
作業価値調査表　**WVI**
作業世界調査表　**WWI**
作業の自動化　**FA**
作業不能　**DB**
作業療法　**MT, OCC Th, Occ Th, occ.th., oct.th, OT, WT**
作業療法士　**OT**
作業療法士助手　**OTA**
作業療法助手　**OTA**
作図家　**il**
作働点　**WP, Wp**
作用　**A, a, act, eff**
作用温度　**OT**
作用機序　**MOA**
砂糖　**sug**
砂浴　**BA, bal.arenae**
(較)差　**diff**
差　**D**
差スペクトル　**DS**
差分吸収ライダー　**DIAL**
差分光法　**DS**
差を認めない　**NAD**
座長　**c, chm**
挫傷した　**colat**
挫滅〔壊死〕組織除去　**deb**
挫・裂・切・刺創　**CLIP**
詐病　**sim, simu**
(連)鎖　**CH**
鎖骨　**Cl, cl, clav, clav.**
鎖骨下静脈　**SCV, SV**
鎖骨下静脈圧迫　**SVC**
鎖骨下静脈カテーテル挿入　**SVC**
鎖骨下静脈血栓　**SVT**
鎖骨下静脈血透析用カテーテル　**SHC**
鎖骨下動脈　**ASC, SCA**
鎖骨下の　**SC, subclav**
鎖骨下弁　**SCF**
鎖骨上(リンパ)節　**SC node**
鎖骨中線　**MCL**
再印刷　**repr**
再灌流性不整脈　**RA**
再灌流を伴う心筋虚血　**MIR**
再教育　**RE, re-ed**
再教育する　**re-ed**
再器質化　**reorg**
再器質化する　**reorg**
再建　**reconstr**
再結合 DNA 諮問委員会　**RAC**
再結合核　**RE**
再検査　**re-ex, re-x**
再呼吸　**RB**
再循環時間　**RCT**
再試験　**re-ex**
再審査概要　**SBR**
再生　**regen**
再生する　**regen**
再生生物学的研究財団　**RBRF**
再生トリ肉腫ウイルス　**RASV**
再生不良性急性白血病　**HAL**
再生不良性貧血　**AA, apla, APLA**
再調査　**R, REV, rev.**
再調剤禁(止)　**non rep., non repet., NR, NR, n.r.**
再調剤せよ　**reit., REP, rep.**
再調剤不可　**n.reit.**
再帝王切開　**RCS, R/CS**
再入院　**RDM, RE, readm**
再入頻脈　**RT**
再燃　**exac**
再発　**R, rec, recur, Rezi**
再発する　**rec**
再発性アフタ性潰瘍　**RAU**
再発性アフタ性口内炎　**RAS**
再発性壊死性粘膜腺周囲炎　**PMNR**

再発性潰瘍　**RU**
再発性潰瘍性口内炎　**RUS**
再発性潰瘍性乱切口内炎　**RUSS**
再発性化膿性胆管肝炎　**RPC**
再発性カルシウム尿石症　**RCU**
再発性肝内閉塞性黄疸　**RIOJ**
再発性結腸直腸癌　**RCRC**
再発性自然流産　**RSA**
再発性疾患の所見なし　**NERD**
再発性上気道感染　**RURTI**
再発性静脈血栓塞栓症　**RVTE**
再発性深静脈血栓症　**RDVT**
再発性多発性軟骨炎　**RP, RPC**
再発性の　**rec**
再発性肺塞栓　**RPE**
再発性びらん症候群　**RES**
再発性腹痛　**RAP**
再発性疱疹　**RH**
再発性慢性解離性動脈瘤　**RCDA**
再発なし　**NR**
再発(性)の　**recur**
再発の　**rezid**
再発の徴候なし　**NER**
再評価　**re-eval**
再評価する　**re-eval**
再分布指数　**RDI**
再縫合　**ReS**
再膨張性肺水腫　**REPE**
再来院　**RTC**
再来患者　**OP**
再来の必要なし　**NNR**
再来不要　**NRN**
在郷軍人病　**LD**
在郷軍人病院　**VAH, VAMC, VH**
在宅介護　**HH**
在宅介助(者)　**HH**
在宅看護　**HN**
在宅経管(栄養)　**HTB**
在宅経管栄養　**HTF**
在宅経管栄養法　**HEN**
在宅経腸栄養法　**HEEA, HEEH**
在宅頸椎牽引ユニット　**HCTU**
在宅抗生物質注射療法　**HPAT**
在宅酸素療法　**HOT**
在宅子宮モニタリング　**HUM**
在宅自動化腹膜透析　**HAPD**
在宅出産経験　**HOME**
在宅静脈抗生物質療法　**HIVAT**
在宅静脈内高カロリー栄養法　**HIVH**
在宅人工換気療法　**HMV**
在宅人工呼吸　**HCV**
在宅成分栄養法　**HEEH**
在宅中心静脈栄養法　**HPN**
在宅治療　**HT**
在宅における高カロリー輸液　**HTPN**
在宅入院制度　**HAD**
在宅腹膜透析　**HPD**
在宅プロトロンビン時間モニタリング　**HPTM**
在宅薬剤注入療法　**HDIT**
在宅輸液療法　**HIT**
在胎月齢　**GA**
在胎週数に比較して体重の少ない(新生児)＝過少体重(児)　**SGA**
在胎週に比して小さい(新生児)＝過少体重(児)　**SFD**
在胎年齢　**CA**
在来型血液透析　**CV**
災害　**Acc, acc**
災害救援医療チーム　**DMAT**
(赤十字の)災害時活動　**DS**
災害弱者　**CWAP**
災害ストレス障害　**DSD**
災害ストレス反応　**DSR**
材料　**mat, mtl**
砕石術　**litho**
財源に基づく相対価表　**RBRVS**
財団　**Found, found.**
採血せよ　**mitt.sang.**
採集する　**coll**
細管式等速電気泳動法　**IP**
細管状構造体　**MTS**
細顆粒　**FG**
細菌　**B, bact**
細菌学　**bact, bacti**
細菌学者　**bact, bacter**
細菌学的指数　**BI**
細菌学認定書　**Dip.Bac.**
細菌学の　**bact, bact.**
細菌クロロフィル　**BChL**
細菌抗原複合体　**BAC**
細菌除去装置　**ARD**
細菌性静脈内蛋白　**BIP**
細菌性心内膜炎　**BE**
細菌性白色下痢　**BWD**
細菌性ホスファチジルエタノールアミン　**BPE**
細菌増殖検出器　**BACTEc**
細菌乳濁液　**BE**
細菌尿スクリーニング　**BST**
細菌(性)の　**bact**
細菌培養炉液　**BCF**
細菌はみられない　**NBS**

さ

細菌鞭毛限局抗原 **H antigens**
細菌命名規約 **Bac.C.**
細菌抑制検査 **BIA**
細血管障害性溶血性貧血 **MHA**
細隙結合 **GJ**
細隙灯 **SL**
細隙灯検査 **SLE**
細孔電流 **AC**
細糸 **F, fil, MF**
細静脈 **v**
細水泡性ラ音 **rl**
細切した **c, c.**
細線維 **MF**
細線維接合部電位 **SJP**
細腸管針 **FIN**
細動 **Fib, fib, fibr, fibrill**
細動脈周囲リンパ球鞘 **PALS**
細動を除去する **defib**
細微粒子 **fines**
細胞異型度 **CAT**
細胞依存性抗体 **CDA**
細胞依存ヘルパー因子 **chf**
細胞栄養層 **CT**
細胞外液 **ECF, ECW**
細胞外液腔 **ECS**
細胞外液量 **ECFV, EFV**
細胞外マトリックス〔基質〕 **ECM**
細胞介在リンパ球融解〔溶解〕(反応) **CML**
細胞外組織 **ECT**
細胞回転周期特異性薬剤 **CCS**
細胞外の **EC**
細胞外容量 **ECV**
細胞化学的生物検定法 **CBA**
細胞学 **cytol**
細胞学的な **cytol**
細胞顆粒アミノペプチダーゼ **APM**
細胞間陰性電位 **INP**
細胞間腔 **ICS, IS**
細胞間螢光 **ICF**
細胞間結合蛋白 **ICBP**
細胞間結合物質 **ICS**
細胞間質液腔 **IFS**
細胞間質液量 **IFV**
細胞間接着分子 **ICAM**
細胞寒天平板 **CAP**
細胞指向性阻害物質 **CDI**
細胞質 **Cyt**
細胞質作用 **CP**
細胞質内膜 **ICM**
細胞質膜 **CM**
細胞質(内)免疫グロブリン **cIg**
細胞質免疫グロブリン **CyIg**
細胞質(内)免疫グロブリンM **cIgM**
(抗癌剤の)細胞周期非特異性薬剤 **CCNS**
細胞傷害試験 **CTA**
細胞傷害試験培地 **CTM**
細胞傷害指数 **CI**
細胞毒性(試験) **CT**
細胞傷害性 T 細胞 **Tc, TK**
細胞傷害性 T 細胞分化因子 **CTDF**
細胞傷害性 T リンパ球 **CTL**
細胞傷害性単位 **CU**
細胞傷害度スコア **CIS**
細胞診活動指数 **CAI**
細胞診断学 **cytol**
細胞数 **cc, ZZ**
細胞性癌遺伝子 **c-onc**
細胞性免疫 **CI**
細胞性免疫不全症候群 **CIDS**
細胞接着分子 **CAM**
細胞洗浄透析 **CWD**
細胞増殖 **CP**
細胞体・樹状突起スパイク **SD spike**
細胞体質 **CSK**
細胞体樹状突起 **SD**
細胞体積 **CV**
細胞調製施設 **FiT**
細胞抽出物 **CE**
細胞治療 **CT**
細胞通過 **CP**
細胞毒性因子 **CTF**
細胞毒性抗体 **CA**
細胞毒性リンパ球 **CL**
細胞内液 **ICF, IF**
細胞内液量 **ICFV, IFV**
細胞内結合蛋白 **ICBP**
細胞内限局性壊死 **FCD**
細胞内混濁 **CIC**
細胞内水分量 **ICW**
細胞内蛋白分解 **IP**
細胞内の(濃度) **IC**
細胞内ピーエイチ **PHi**
細胞内遊離カルシウム濃度 $[Ca^{2+}]_i$
細胞内容量 **ICV**
細胞内レチノイン酸結合蛋白 **CRABP**
細胞粘着因子 **CAF**
細胞媒介性細胞障害 **CMC**
細胞媒介免疫 **CMI**
細胞媒介免疫反応 **CMIR**
細胞培養 **CC**
細胞培養培地 **CCM**
細胞バンク **CB**
細胞病変作用 **CPE**
細胞表面(抗原) **Cs**
細胞表面因子 **CSF**
細胞表面抗原 **CSA**
細胞表面蛋白 **CSP**
細胞表面変調 **CSM**
細胞付加型脂肪移植 **CAL**

細胞分裂因子　**CDF**
細胞分裂周期　**CDC**
細胞壁　**CW**
細胞壁骨格　**CWS**
細胞壁透析　**CWD**
細胞変性現象　**CP**
細胞変性効果　**CPE**
細胞膜　**CM, PL**
細胞膜貫通　**TM**
細胞膜抵抗　**TEER**
細胞膜免疫グロブリン　**SIg, sIg**
細胞(内)免疫グロブリン　**C-Ig**
細胞融解因子　**CF**
細胞溶解単位　**LU**
細胞容積　**CV**
細胞レチノール結合蛋白　**CRBP**
細末の　**subt.**
細網組織球系　**RHS**
細網内皮　**RE**
細網内皮系抑制物質　**RDS**
細網内皮症ウイルス　**REV, rev.**
細網内皮の　**RE**
細網肉腫　**RCS, RSA**
細網肉腫・組織球性リンパ腫　**HL**
細網(状)の　**RET, ret**
菜食主義　**veg**
菜食主義者　**V, veg**
最下部1/4区　**LQ**
最近親者　**NOK**
最近の　**nv., UTD**
最強点　**PMI**
最古の　**eld**
最後野　**AP**
最後に　**in extrem., inf, inf.**
最後の　**ult**
最後の1/4　**LQ**
最後の処方　**ult.praes.**
最高　**M, Max, max, max., Max**
最高安全圧　**Psmax**
最高胃液分泌量　**MSV**
最高確率数値　**MPN**
最高血中濃度　**CMAX**
最高血中濃度到達時間　**T-max,** T_{max}
最高酸素濃度　**MAC**
最高酸分泌量　**MAO**
最高随意圧　**MVP**
最高総胆汁酸　**MTBA**
最高代謝率(寒冷時)　**PMR**
最高によい　**o.p.**
最高尿素クリアランス　**Cm**
最高尿道内圧　**UPmax**
最高尿道閉鎖圧　**UCP max**
最高の　**max, max., Max**
最高濃度　**Cp**
最高濃度時間　**PCT, T-max,** T_{max}
最高排尿速度　**MVR**
最高ペプシン活性　**MPA**
最高ペプシン分泌量　**MPO**
最高膀胱随意圧　**MBVP**
最小　**m., MIN, min.**
最小1日必要量　**MDR**
最小閾値　**MT**
最小壊死量　**MND**
最小角分解能　**MAR**
最小可聴音圧　**MAP**
最小感染量　**MID**
最小丘疹量　**MPD**
最小許容濃度　**MAC**
最小記録一式　**MDS**
最小検出可能濃度　**MDC**
最小検出可能量　**MDQ**
最小甲状腺機能正常型グレーブス病　**MEGD**
最小抗生物質濃度　**MAC**
最小公倍数　**LCM**
最小紅斑量　**MED**
最小殺菌濃度　**MBC, MCC**
最小殺菌レベル　**MBL**
最小殺原虫濃度　**MPC**
最小時間間隔　**MTI**
最小識別臭気　**MIO, M.I.O.**
最小重量　**min wt**
最小侵襲手術　**MIS**
最小侵襲治療法　**MIT**
最小蕁麻疹量　**MUD**
最小赤血球凝集量　**MHD**
最小接触技術　**MCT**
最小阻止濃度　**MHK**
最小致死濃度　**MLC**
最小致死量　**DLM, LFD, MFD, MLD**
最小中毒　**MTD**
最小聴域　**MAF**
最小抵抗(＝膀胱内圧/最大尿流量2)　**Rmin**
最小毒性量　**LOAEL**
最小の　**MIN, min.**
最小肺胞(麻酔)濃度　**MAC**
最小発育阻止濃度　**MGC, MIC**
最小発育阻止量　**MID**
最小繁殖単位　**MRU**
最小反応値　**Drm, d.r.m.**
最小反応量　**MRD**
最小光毒(性)紅斑(線)量　**MPED**
最小光毒量　**MPD**
最小病変糸球体腎炎　**MLGN**
最小偏倚ヘパトーマ　**MDH**
最小マイコプラズマ殺菌濃度　**MPC**
最小麻酔濃度　**MAC**
最小有意差　**LSD**
最小有効中毒量　**LETD**

最小有効尿濃度　**MEUC**
最小有効濃度　**MEC**
最小有効量　**LED, MAD, MED**
最小溶血量　**MHD, M.H.D.**
最小抑制濃度　**CMI**
最小量　**MD**
最小レベルの毒性ライン　**MTL**
最少必須培地　**MEM**
最初に　**a.p.**
最初の　**inl**
最初の発作　**FA**
最重要人物　**VIP**
最重要人物症候群　**VIPS**
最終規則的月経　**LRMP**
最終月経　**IR, LR**
最終月経期　**LMP, PMP**
最終酸素需要　**UOD**
最終診断　**Final Dx**
最終正常月経　**LNMP**
最終電気痙攣閾値　**FET**
最終の　**ult**
最終沸点　**FBP**
最終目標　**f**
最新医薬全集　**MDE**
最大　**M, Max, max, max., Max**
最大１日許容摂取量　**MDPI**
最大１日摂取許容量　**MADI**
最大安静時肛門圧　**MRAP**
最大域　**FR**
最大運動換気　**MEV**
最大運動負荷試験法　**METT**
最大エントロピー法　**MEM**
最大横隔神経活動　**PPNA**
最大不可逆的作用　**NOAEL**
最大解析対象集団　**FAS**
最大拡散能力　**MDC**
最大拡張期速度　**PDV**
最大可動域　**FROM**
最大換気　**VM**
最大換気〔呼吸〕　**MB**
最大換気有効率　**MRE**
最大眼球速度　**MES**
最大換気量　**MBC, MVV1**
最大灌流圧　**MPP**
最大吸気圧　**MIP, PIP**
最大吸気流量率　**MIFR, PIFR**
最大吸気量　**IC, MIC, PIF**
最大凝集比　**MAR**
最大強度　**FS**
最大許容摂取量　**MPI**
最大許容線量　**MAD**
最大許容濃度　**MAC, M.A.C, MPC, MTC**
最大許容(線)量　**MPD, M.P.D.**
最大許容レベル　**MPL**
最大キロボルト　**Pkv**
最大駆出時間　**PET**
最大屈曲角度　**AGF**
最大クリアランス　**Cm, Cm.**
最大結合能　**Bmax**
最大効果　**ME**
最大公約数　**GCF, GCM, GCN**
最大呼気圧　**MEP**
最大呼気速度　**MEFR, PEFR, PEV, PFR**
最大呼気中間流量　**FMF**
最大呼気フローボリウム曲線　**MEFV**
最大呼吸効果投与量　**DER MX**
最大呼気流量　**FEF, MEF, PEF**
最大呼気流量計　**PFM**
最大細胞濃度　**MCC**
最大左(心)室房　**LA-MAX**
最大雑音区　**MNA**
最大作動圧　**Pwmax**
最大酸素消費量　**MOC**
最大酸素摂取量　**MOI**
最大〔最高〕酸濃度　**MAC**
最大弛緩率　**MRR**
最大刺激　**MS**
最大刺激検査　**MST**
最大刺激時酸分泌量　**PAO**
最大持続換気量　**MSVC**
最大シャント血流面積　**MSFA**
最大シャント血流面積係数　**MSFAI**
最大収縮期勾配　**PSG**
最大収縮速度　**Vmax**
最大手術血液準備量　**MSBOS**
最大出力音圧レベル　**SSPL**
最大使用可能周波数　**MUF**
最大衝動点　**MPI, PMI, PMI, P.M.I.**
最大静脈血酸素消費量　**MVO_2, MVO_2**
最大静脈酸素飽和　**MVO**
最大除去率　**Rmax**
最大食道圧　**MaxEP**
最大神経伝達速度　**MNCV**
最大身長　**GL**
最大伸展角度　**AGE**
最大心拍数　**MHR, MPR, PHR**
最大随意(的)収縮　**MVC**
最大耐性　**MTP**
最大耐用量　**MTD**
最大中間呼気流速　**MMFR**

最大中間呼気流量 **MMEF, MMF**
最大中毒濃度 **MTC**
最大点 **pm**
最大電気ショック(性発作) **MES**
最大電子ボルト **pev**
最大投与量 **MD**
最大取り込み速度 **Vm**
最大努力 **ME**
最大トレッドミル検査 **MTT**
最大トレッドミルストレス検査 **MTST**
最大尿意 **MDV**
最大尿細管クリアランス **Tm**
最大尿細管排泄能 **TM, Tm**
最大尿浸透圧 **Umax**
最大尿素クリアランス **Cm**
最大尿素合成率 **MRUS**
最大尿道圧 **MUP, Pura max**
最大尿(中)濃度 **MUC**
最大尿濃度 **CMU**
最大尿流量(率) **Qmax**
最大尿流量率 **MFR**
最大の **M, max, max., Max**
最大濃度 **MC**
最大非中毒量 **HNTD**
最大病院利益 **MHB**
最大閉鎖圧 **MCP**
最大ペプシン排出量 **PPO**
最大膀胱(内)圧 **Pves max**
最大膀胱容量 **MBC**
最大無作用量 **NOAEL**
最大溶血点 **HMP**
最大利得 **FOG**
最大流量 **PF**
最大流量率 **MFR**
最大量 **D MX, MD**
最大露光許容量 **MPE**
最長発声時間 **MPT**
最低 **m.**
最低安全圧 **Psmin**
最低合格指数 **MPI**
最低合格水準 **MPL**
最低作動圧 **Pwmin**
最低の **l, L**
最低濃縮時間 **LCT**
最低濃度 **LC**
最低有用高周波 **LUHF**
最適の **o, Opt, opt, opt.**
最年少生存児 **YLC**
最年長の **eld**
最晩期活性化 **VLA**
催眠(状) **HYP, Hyp**
催眠(状態) **hypno**
催眠後暗示 **PHS**
催眠術 **hypho, hypno., hypnot**
催眠術者 **hypnot**
催眠術の **hypho, hypno.**
催眠状態下の直達暗示 **DSUH**
催眠法 **hypho, hypno., hypnot**
催眠薬 **hypho, hypno., SM**
臍(血)コレステロール **UC**
臍周囲の **periumb**
臍静脈 **UV**
臍静脈・母体静脈 **UV/MV**
臍静脈カテーテル **UVC**
臍帯 **UC, UV**
臍帯血 **CB**
臍帯血単核細胞 **CBMC**
臍帯血(液)培養 **UCBC**
臍帯血リンパ球 **CBL**
臍帯埋没療法 **UCI**
臍(＝さい)腸間膜憩室 **MD**
臍動脈(の) **UA**
臍動脈カテーテル **UAC**
臍の **umb**
臍部 **reg.umb., umb.reg., UP**
臍ヘルニア **UH**
臍ヘルニア・巨舌・巨人(症候群) **EMG**
臍ヘルニア・巨舌・巨人症候群 **EMG syndrome**
臍ヘルニア・膀胱外反(症)・鎖肛・脊髄異常症候群 **OEIS complex**
鰓骨格生殖器(症候群) **BSG**
鰓神経炎 **BN**
最近の **rec.**
細網内皮系 **RES**
杯 **C, c**
杯細胞 **GC**
作戦中死亡 **KIA**
作話症 **confab**
削片 **ras.**
昨年 **LY, ly, ly.**
索 **Cd**
索引・ページ・表題のついた **IPT**
索引とページを示した **I & P**
索状体 **RB**
索状帯 **ZF**
酢剤 **A**
酢酸 **AA, ac a, acet.**
酢酸アルコール・ホルマリン **AAF**
酢酸ゲンチアナバイオレット **AGV**
酢酸コルチゾン **CA**
酢酸シプロテロン **CPA, CTA**
酢酸セルロース **CA, CDA**
酢酸セルロース空洞線維

CAHF
酢酸抽出性フェロ蛋白 **AEP**
酢酸デオキシコルチコステロン **DCA, DOCA**
酢酸デスオキシコルチコステロン **DCA**
酢酸の **ace, ace.**
酢酸ヒドロキシコルチコステロン **HC**
酢酸ヒドロコルチゾン **HC, HCA**
酢酸フェニル水銀 **PMA, PMAC**
酢酸ベタメタゾン **BA**
酢酸メチルプレドニゾロン **MPA**
酢酸メドロキシプロゲステロン塩 **MPA**
酢酸メレンゲストロール **MGA**
酢酸酪酸セルロース **CAB**
酢酸ロイプロリド,ビンブラスチン,アドリアマイシン,マイトマイシンC **L-VAM**
錯体化学国際会議 **ICCC**
錯乱した **conf, confus**
指図 **Inst, inst**
指図用紙を見よ **SOB**
刷子縁 **BB**
刷子縁膜 **BBM**
刷子縁膜小胞 **BBMV**
殺菌 **disin**
殺菌・透過性増強蛋白 **BPI**
殺菌剤 **disin, germi**
殺菌指数 **BI**
殺菌濃度 **BC**
殺真菌剤 **fungi**
雑音 **B, br, M, m, Ms**
雑音因子 **NF**
雑音干渉レベル **NIL**
雑音検出閾値 **NDT**
雑音減少 **NR**
雑音減少係数 **NRC**
雑音指数 **NI**
雑音周波帯 **NBW**
雑音レベル監視モニタ〔装置〕 **NLM**
雑誌 **Ann, ann, Annls, Arch, J, Jour, jour, jrl, jrnl**
雑誌引用報告 **JCR**
雑種 **H of sp, hyb**
雑種第一代 **F_1**
雑種第二代 **F_2**
雑性乱視 **Mis Astig**
雑多な **misc, mxd**
雑録 **Misc**
撮影距離 **SID**
錯覚 **ill**
擦過傷 **Abr, abr, abras**
擦剤 **lin, lin., linim**
里親 **FM**
寒い **c**
皿 **T**
三角(筋) **Delt**
三角形の **Delt**
三角線維軟骨 **TFC**
三角の **trig**
三価経口ポリオウイルスワクチン **TOPV**
三価の **TV**
三環系抗うつ薬 **TCA, TCAD**
三環系抗精神病薬 **TCA**
三孔式カテーテル **TLC**
三叉〔差〕(神経痛) **TG**
三叉〔差〕神経(=第Ⅴ脳神経)運動核 **Mot Ⅴ**
三叉〔差〕神経核 **NNT, TN**
三叉〔差〕神経痛 **TD, TN**
三酸化アンチモン **Sb_2O_3**
三心房心 **CTA**
三次元エコー図 **3DE, 3-DE**
三次元エコー図法 **3DE, 3-DE**
三重水素(=トリチウム) **^3H**
三重水素(=^3H) **T, *t***
三重らせん構造部 **TH**
三硝酸グリセリン **GTN**
三尖弁 **T, TV**
三尖弁逸脱(症) **TVP**
三尖弁開放音 **TOS**
三尖弁機能不全 **TI**
三尖弁狭窄 **tri sten**
三尖弁狭窄兼閉鎖不全症 **TSI**
三尖弁狭窄症 **TS**
三尖弁後尖 **PTL**
三尖弁前尖 **ATL**
三尖弁第Ⅰ心音 **T_1**
三尖弁第Ⅱ心音 **T_2**
三尖弁置換術 **TVR**
三尖弁中隔炎 **STL**
三尖弁閉鎖症 **TA**
三尖弁閉鎖不全症 **TI, TR**
三尖弁縫縮術 **TAP**
三炭糖リン酸イソメラーゼ **TIM**
三段排尿膀胱造影法 **TVC**
三段脈 **trig**
三糖(=乳糖・ブドウ糖・ショ糖)鉄(寒天培地) **TSI**
三糖鉄寒天培地 **TSIA, TSI agar medium**
三頭(筋) **tri**
三頭筋腱反射 **TTR**
三頭筋反射 **TJ**
三頭筋皮下脂肪 **TSF**
三倍化 **trip**
三倍にする **trip**
三倍の **trip**
三リン酸ナトリウム

STO
参考書　biblio
参照　Cf., cf., ref
参照せよ　v., vd., vid.
参照量　RfD
残遺指数　Rq
残気　RA
残気率　RVI
残気量　Resid vol, resid vol, RV, VR
残渣　R, r., Res, res
残存光反射　PLR
残存腎機能　RRF
残存体　RB
残尿　RU
残尿測定　RUM
残尿量　RUV
残余　reliq, reliq., rem.
残余窒素　Res-N, Rest-N, RN
残留性有機汚染物質　POPs
残留側波帯　VSB
残留物　R, r., Res, res
産(科病)院　Mat
産科　ob, OB, Ob, OB/GYN, ob-gyn
産科(サービス)　obs, obs., OBS, Obs
産科(学)　OB
産科・婦人科学(の)　ob-gy
産科・婦人科手術　OBGS
産科医　ob, OB, Ob, obs, obs., OBS, Obs, Obst, obst
産科回復室　OBRR
産科学　O, obs, obs., OBS, Obs, Obst, obst
産科学士　BAO
産科学修士　AOM
産科学的真結合線　CO, CVO
産科学の　ob, OB, Ob
産科集中監視室　OICU
産科超音波　OB-US
産科的結合線　OC
産科的糖尿病前症　OPD
産科の　ob, OB, Ob, obstet
産科婦人科国際専門家連合　UPIGO
産業　indust
産業・科学・医学の波長　ISM
産業医学　Ind-Med, IT
産業衛生財団　IHF
産業看護研究所　INI
産業人口　IP
産業の　IND, indust
産業微生物学会　SIM
産業保健医認定書　DIH
産後心筋症　PPCM
産後腎不全　PPRF
産後の　post part.
産後日　PPD
産後卵管結紮　PPTL
産出圧　YP
産児制限　BC
産床卵巣静脈血栓静脈炎　POVT
産褥　puerp
産生細胞　PC
産生された　prod
産生する　prod
産生率　PR
産物　P, prod
産物増強性逆転写酵素　PERT
産婦人科　OG
産婦人科医　OBG, OB/GYN, ob-gyn
産婦人科学　OBG
産婦人科学士　MOG
産婦人科学卒業証書　D.C.O.G.
産婦人科資格〔免状〕　D.G.O.
産婦人科認定書　Dip.G. & O.
散(剤)　talc.
散在(性)硬化(症)　DS
散在性単神経炎　MNM
散在性濃縮体　SDB
散剤　p., pwd
散剤にせよ　fp, f.p.
散剤をつくれ　ft.pulv.
散発性うつ病　SDD
散発性の　S
散布剤　conspers.
散布せよ　consperg.
散薬　plv.
算術指数　ArQ
算定数値　compu
酸　A, AC, ac
酸塩基検査〔調査/試験〕　ABL
酸塩基スケール　pH
酸塩基平衡　ABB, ABC
酸化・発酵(比)　o/f, OF, O-F, O/F
酸化・発酵基礎培地　OFBM
酸化亜鉛　ZnO
酸化亜鉛・ユージノール　ZnOE, ZOE
酸化アルミニウム　ALOX
酸化エチレン　EO, ETHO
酸化型グルタチオン　GSSG
酸化カルシウム　CaO
酸化還元　OR, O-R
酸化還元単位　RH
酸化還元電位　E, Eo^+
酸化還元電位(差)　ORP
酸化還元電位差　ΔEh
酸化された　ox
酸化性の　O
酸化的リン酸化比　P/O

酸化トリブチルスズ　**TBTO**
酸化プロピレン　**PO**
酸化ヘモグロビン　**HBO, HbO**
酸化防止剤　**Ao**
酸化マグネシウム　**MgO**
酸化マグネシウム(懸濁液)　**MOM**
酸化抑制剤　**BHA**
酸化リチウム　**Li_2O**
酸価　**AN**
酸性雨被害調達データベース　**ADS**
酸性核蛋白抗原　**NPPA**
酸性化滴　**acid**
酸性血清試験陽性の遺伝性赤血球多核　**HEMPAS**
酸性デタージェント繊維　**ADF**
酸性糖蛋白　**AGP**
酸性と中性　**a/n**
酸性ホスファターゼ　**acid phos, acid PO_4, acid p'tase**
酸性ホスファターゼ 1　**ACP1**
酸性ホスファターゼ 2　**ACP2**
酸性マルターゼ欠損　**AMD**
酸性ムコ多糖類　**AMP, AMPS**
酸性リン酸分解酵素　**ACP**
酸素　**O_2, OX, Ox, O_x, OXY, oxy**
酸素 15　**^{15}O**
酸素 16　**^{16}O**
酸素 17　**^{17}O**
酸素 18　**^{18}O**
酸素解離曲線　**ODC**
酸素化係数　**OI, P/F**
酸素含(有)量　**Co_2**
酸素吸収速度　**OUR**
酸素供給量　**DO_2**
酸素効果比　**OER**
酸素消費率　**Qo, QO_2**
酸素消費量　**OC, Qo, QO_2, Vo_2**
酸素摂取　**OI**
酸素摂取量　**Vo_2**
酸素抽出分画　**OEF**
酸素低親和性突然変異ヘモグロビン　**Hb Kansas**
酸素比自動コントロール　**ORC**
酸素必要量　**OR**
酸素分圧　**OPP, PO_2, Po_2**
酸素閉鎖　**OC**
酸素ヘモグロビン解離曲線　**ODC**
酸素飽和　**OS, O_2sat**
酸素飽和計　**OSM**
酸素輸送率　**TO_2**
酸素要求量　**OD**
酸素容量　**O_2 cap**
酸素ラジカル　**OR**
酸素療法　**O ther**
酸と塩　**AS**
酸(性)の　**A, a**
酸のイオン化〔解離〕定数　**K_a, K_a**
酸バランス調節　**ABC**
酸(性)ホスファターゼ　**ACP, Ac-Pase, AC-PH, AP**
酸を示す記号　**HA**
酸・塩基(比)　**A/B**
暫定診断　**prelim.diag**
暫定的 1 週間許容摂取量　**PTWI**
暫定的診断　**tent-diag**
暫定的な　**a.i., tent**

し

コンピュータ補助によるシミュレーション外科 **CASS**
ジアシルグリセロール **DAG, DG**
ジアセチルチアミン **DAT**
ジアセチルモノキシム **DAM**
ジアセチルモルヒネ **DAM**
ジアゼパム **DIAZ, DZ, DZP**
ジアゼパム結合阻害物質 **DBI**
ジアゾアセチル-DL-ノルロイシンメチルエステル **DAN**
ジアゾウラシル **DU**
ジアゾオキソノルロイシン **DON**
ジアゾ反応陽性物質 **DPM**
ジアゾビシクロオクタン **DABCO**
ジアテルミー **D, Dia, dia., diath**
ジアトリゾエート **DTZ**
シアナミド **Cy**
シアノ B_{12} **CN-B_{12}**
シアノアセトヒドラジド **CAH**
シアノコバラミン **CN-Cbl, CNCBL**
シアノフェンホス **CYP**
ジアミノジフェニルスルホン **DADPS**
ジアミノジフェニルスルホン(=ダプソン) **DDS, DDSO**
ジアミノピメリン酸 **DAP**
ジアミノフェニルインドール **DAPI**
ジアミノプロピオン酸 **DPR**
ジアミノベンゼン **DAB, DMB**
ジアミノベンジジン **DAB**
ジアミノ酪酸 **DBU**
ジアミン酸化酵素 **DAO**
ジアミンジクロロプラチナ **DDP**
ジアルカリジチオリン酸亜鉛 **ZDDP**
シアル酸 **SA, Sia**
シアル酸転移酵素 **SAT**
ジアルジア(属) **G**
シアン **CN, CY, Cy, cy**
シアン化水素 **HCN**
シアン化水素酸 **HCN**
シアン化物 **CYN**
シアン感受性因子 **CSF**
シアン基 **CN**
シアン酢酸ヒドラジド **CAH**
ジアンヒドロガラクチタル,アドリアマイシン,シスプラチン(=プラチノール) **DAP**
シアンメトヘモグロビン **CMG, HiCN, MHbCN**
ジイソアミロキシ・チオカルバニリド **DAT**
ジイソブチルフェノキシポリエトキシエタノール **DBPPEE**
ジイソプロピルアミン **DIP**
ジイソプロピルアミン・ジクロロアセテート **DADA**
ジイソプロピルアミンジクロロアセテート **DIPA-DCA**
ジイソプロピルフルオロリン酸 **DEP, DFP, DIFP**
ジイソプロピルホスホフルオリデート **DIPF**
シェーグレン・ラルソン(症候群) **SL**
シェーグレン・ラルソン症候群 **SLS**
シェーグレン症候群 **SjS, SS**
シェーグレン症候群(抗原)A **SSA**
シェーグレン症候群A抗体 **SS-A antibody**
シェーグレン症候群B **SSB**
シェーグレン症候群B抗体 **SS-B antibody**
ジェー血液因子 **J**
ジェー酸 **J-acid**
ジエタノールアミン **DEA**
ジエチル・ニトロフェニルチオリン酸 **DNPT**
ジエチルアミノエタノール **DEAE**
ジエチルアミノエタノールサリチル酸 **DEAE**
ジエチルアミノエチル **DEAE**
ジエチルアミノエチルデキストラン **DEAE-D**
ジエチルカルバマジン **DEC**
ジエチルスチルベストロール **DES**
ジエチルトリプタミン **DET**
ジエチルトリプタミン・ジメチルトリプタミン・ジプロピルトリプタミンなどの幻覚剤 **big D**
ジエチルニトロサミン

DENA
ジエチルパラニトロフェニルチオホスフェイト **DNTP**
ジエチルバルビツール酸 **DEBA**
ジエチルピロカルボネート **DEPC, DPC**
ジエチルブタンジオル **DEB**
ジエチルプロパンジオール **DEP**
ジエチル硫酸 **DES**
ジエチルリンゴ酸 **DEM**
ジエチレングリコール **DEG**
ジエチレントリアミン五酢酸 **DTPA**
ジエチレンホスホラミド **DEPA**
シェッツ眼圧測定計 **ST**
ジェネリック製薬工業協会 **GPIT**
シェプ **SHEP**
ジェファーソン医科大学 **JMC**
ジエポキシブタン **DEB**
ジェームズタウンキャニオンウイルス **JCV**
ジェリー・スロウウイルス **JSV**
ジェンキンス活動調査 **JAS**
シェーンライン・ヘノッホ(病) **SH**
シェーンライン・ヘノッホ紫斑病 **PSH, SHP**
シェーンライン・ヘノッホ症候群 **SHS**
ジオキシストレプトマイシン **DOSM**
ジオプトリー **D, diop, dipt, dptr**
シカ出血(性)熱 **HFD**
ジギオン **zy, Zy**
ジギタリス **DIG, dig**
(内因性)ジギタリス様物質 **DIS**
ジギタリス様物質 **DLS**
ジギタリス葉末 **p.f.dig.**
ジグザグ **zz**
ジグザグ線 **Z-line**
シグナル **Sig, sig**
シグナル〔信号〕認識粒子 **SRP**
シグマ反応 **SR**
シクラシリン **ACPC**
シクラゾシン **cyc**
シクラミン酸カルシウム **CC**
ジグリセリド **DG, DAG**
ジグリセリドリパーゼ **DGL**
ジグルクロニド非結合性ビリルビン **DBu**
シクロオキシゲナーゼ **CO, COX**
シクロカーボ・チアミン **CCT**
ジクロキサシリン **DCL, DX**
シクロスポリン **CS, CSP, cy**
シクロスポリンA **CA, CSA, CsA, CYA**
シクロセリン **CS**
シクロセリン・セホキシチン・果糖寒天培地 **CCFA**
シクロデキストリン誘起室温リン光 **CI-RTP**
シクロプロパン **CYCLO, Cyclo, cyclo**
シクロヘキサミド **CX, CXD**
シクロヘキサンジメタノール **CHDM**
シクロヘキシミド **CHX**
シクロヘキシルアデノシン **CHA**
シクロヘキシルアミノエタンスルホン酸 **CHES**
シクロヘキシルアミノプロパンスルホン酸 **CAPS**
シクロヘキシルアミン **CHA**
シクロヘキシルクロロエチルニトロソウレア,シクロホスファミド,ビンクリスチン,ブレオマイシン **CCVB**
シクロヘキシルクロロエチルニトロソウレア,シクロホスファミド,ビンクリスチン,プロカルバジン,プレドニゾン **CCVPP**
シクロヘキシルクロロエチルニトロソ尿素,アドリアマイシン,ビンブラスチン **CAVe**
シクロヘキシルクロロエチルニトロソ尿素,シクロホスファミド,ビンクリスチン **CCV**
シクロヘキシルクロロエチルニトロソ尿素,ビンクリスチン(=オンコビン),プレドニゾン **CCOP**
シクロヘキシルクロロエチルニトロソ尿素,ビンブラスチン,ブレオマイシン **CVB**
シクロヘキシルクロロエチルニトロソ尿素,プロカルバジン,メトトレキサート **CPM**
シクロペンタジエン **CPD**
シクロペンテノフェナントレン **CPP**

し

シクロホスファミド **CP, CPA, CPM, CTX, Ctx, CY, CYC, CYCLO, Cyclo**
シクロホスファミド,アドリアマイシン,エトポシド **CAE**
シクロホスファミド,アドリアマイシン,シスプラチン(=プラチノール) **CAP**
シクロホスファミド,アドリアマイシン,ジメチルトリアゼノイミダゾールカルボキサミド **CyADIC**
シクロホスファミド,アドリアマイシン,ダカルバジン **CAD, CADIC**
シクロホスファミド,アドリアマイシン,ビンクリスチン **CAV**
シクロホスファミド,アドリアマイシン,ビンクリスチン,シスプラチン(=プラチノール),エトポシド **CAV-P-VP**
シクロホスファミド,アドリアマイシン,ビンクリスチン,プレドニゾン **CAVP**
シクロホスファミド,アドリアマイシン,フルオロウラシル **CAF**
シクロホスファミド,アドリアマイシン,フルオロウラシル,ビンクリスチン,プレドニゾン **CAFVP**
シクロホスファミド,アドリアマイシン,フルオロウラシル,プレドニゾン **CAFP**
シクロホスファミド,アドリアマイシン,ブレオマイシン,ビンクリスチン(=オンコビン),プレドニゾン **CABOP, CA-BOP**
シクロホスファミド,アドリアマイシン,プレドニゾン **CAP**
シクロホスファミド,アドリアマイシン,プロカルバジン,ブレオマイシン,ビンクリスチン(=オンコビン),プレドニゾン **CAP-BOP**
シクロホスファミド,アドリアマイシン,メトトレキサート **CAM**
シクロホスファミド,アドリアマイシン,メトトレキサート,エトポシド,ビンクリスチン(=オンコビン) **CAMEO**
シクロホスファミド,アドリアマイシン,メトトレキサート,フルオロウラシル **CAMF**
シクロホスファミド,アドリアマイシン,メトトレキサート,ブレオマイシン **CAMB**
シクロホスファミド,アドリアマイシン,メトトレキサート,プロカルバジン **CAMP**
シクロホスファミド,エトポシド,シスプラチン(=プラチノール) **CEP**
シクロホスファミド,エトポシド,ビンクリスチン **CEV**
シクロホスファミド,シクロヘキシルクロロエチルニトロソ尿素,メトトレキサート **CCM**
シクロホスファミド,シスプラチン(=プラチノール) **CP**
シクロホスファミド,シスプラチン(=プラチノール),エトポシド **CPV**
シクロホスファミド,シスプラチン(=プラチノール),ビスクロロエチルニトロソ尿素 **CPB**
シクロホスファミド,シスプラチン,フルオロウラシル,エストラムスチン **CCFE**
シクロホスファミド,ノバントロン,フルオロウラシル **CNF**
シクロホスファミド,ハロテスチン,ビンクリスチン(=オンコビン),プレドニゾン **CyHOP**
シクロホスファミド,ビスクロロエチルニトロソ尿素,エトポシド **CBV**
シクロホスファミド,ヒドロキシダウノマイシン,ビンクリスチン(=オンコビン),プレドニゾン **CHOP**
シクロホスファミド,ヒドロキシダウノルビシン,ビンクリスチン(=オンコビン) **CHO**
シクロホスファミド,ヒドロキシダウノルビシン,ビンクリスチン(=オンコビン),プレドニゾン,ブレオマイシン **CHOP-B**
シクロホスファミド,ヒドロキシダウノルビシン,ビンクリスチン(=オンコビン),プレドニゾン,放射線 **CHOR**
シクロホスファミド,ヒドロキシ尿素,アクチノマ

し

イシンD,メトトレキサート,ビンクリスチン(=オンコビン),シトロボラム因子,アドリアマイシン　**CHAM-OCA**
シクロホスファミド,ビンクリスチン(=オンコビン),L-フェニルアラニンマスタード,アドリアマイシン　**CONPADRI I**
シクロホスファミド,ビンクリスチン(=オンコビン),L-フェニルアラニンマスタード,アドリアマイシン,メトトレキサート　**CONPADRI II**
シクロホスファミド,ビンクリスチン(=オンコビン),L-フェニルアラニンマスタード,アドリアマイシン,メトトレキサート,強化ドキソルビシン　**CONPADRI III**
シクロホスファミド,ビンクリスチン,アドリアマイシン　**CVA**
シクロホスファミド,ビンクリスチン,アドリアマイシン,ジメチルトリアゼノイミダゾールカルボキサミド　**CY-VA-DIC**
シクロホスファミド,ビンクリスチン,アドリアマイシン,ビスクロロエチルニトロソ尿素,メトトレキサート,プロカルバジン　**CVA-BMP**
シクロホスファミド,ビンクリスチン(=オンコビン),アラビノシルシトシン,プレドニゾン　**COAP**
シクロホスファミド,ビンクリスチン,プレドニゾン　**CVP**
シクロホスファミド,ビンクリスチン(=オンコビン),プレドニゾン　**COP**
シクロホスファミド,ビンクリスチン,プレドニゾン,アドリアマイシン　**CVPA**
シクロホスファミド,ビンクリスチン(=オンコビン),プレドニゾン,アドリアマイシン　**COPA**
シクロホスファミド,ビンクリスチン,プレドニゾン,ダウノルビシン　**CVPD**
シクロホスファミド,ビンクリスチン(=オンコビン),プレドニゾン,ビスクロロエチルニトロソ尿素,メクロルエタミン　**COPBM**
シクロホスファミド,ビンクリスチン(=オンコビン),プレドニゾン,ブレオマイシン　**COP-BLEO**
シクロホスファミド,ビンクリスチン(=オンコビン),プレドニゾン,ブレオマイシン,アドリアマイシン,マツラン　**COP-BLAM**
シクロホスファミド,ビンクリスチン,プレドニゾン,プロカルバジン　**CVPP**
シクロホスファミド,ビンクリスチン(=オンコビン),プロカルバジン,プレドニゾン　**COPP**
シクロホスファミド,ビンクリスチン(=オンコビン),メチルクロロエチル-シクロヘキシルニトロソ尿素　**COM**
シクロホスファミド,ビンクリスチン(=オンコビン),メチルクロロエチル-シクロヘキシルニトロソ尿素,ブレオマイシン　**COMB**
シクロホスファミド,ビンクリスチン,メトトレキサート　**CVM**
シクロホスファミド,ビンクリスチン(=オンコビン),メトトレキサート　**COM**
シクロホスファミド,ビンクリスチン(=オンコビン),メトトレキサート,アラビノシルシトシン　**COMA**
シクロホスファミド,ビンクリスチン(=オンコビン),メトトレキサート,シトシンアラビノシド　**COMCA**
シクロホスファミド,ビンクリスチン(=オンコビン),メトトレキサート,プレドニゾン　**COMP**
シクロホスファミド,ビンクリスチン(=オンコビン),メトトレキサート,ロイコボリン,アラビノシルシトシン　**COMLA**
シクロホスファミド,フルオロウラシル,シトキサントロン　**CFM**
シクロホスファミド,フルオロウラシル,プレドニゾロン　**CFP**
シクロホスファミド,フルオロウラシル,プレドニ

ゾン,タモキシフェン **CEPT**
シクロホスファミド,ブレオマイシン,プロカルバジン,プレドニゾン,アドリアマイシン **CBPPA**
シクロホスファミド,プレドニゾン **CP**
シクロホスファミド,ヘキサメチルメラミン,アドリアマイシン,*cis*-ジアミンジクロロプラチナ **CHAD**
シクロホスファミド,ヘキサメチルメラミン,アドリアマイシン,シスプラチン(=プラチノール) **CHAP**
シクロホスファミド,ヘキサメチルメラミン,フルオロウラシル **CHF**
シクロホスファミド,メクロルエタミン,ビンクリスチン(=オンコビン),プロカルバジン,プレドニゾロン **C-MOPP**
シクロホスファミド,メトトレキサート,エトポシド,デキサメタゾン **CMED**
シクロホスファミド,メトトレキサート,シクロヘキシルクロロエチルニトロソ尿素 **CMC**
シクロホスファミド,メトトレキサート,フルオロウラシル **CMF**
シクロホスファミド,メトトレキサート,フルオロウラシル,タモキシフェン **CMF-TAM**
シクロホスファミド,メトトレキサート,フルオロウラシル,ヒドロキシ尿素 **CMFH**
シクロホスファミド,メトトレキサート,フルオロウラシル,ビンクリスチン **CMFV**
シクロホスファミド,メトトレキサート,フルオロウラシル,ビンクリスチン,プレドニゾン **CMFVP**
シクロホスファミド,メトトレキサート,フルオロウラシル,プレドニゾン **CMFP**
シクロホスファミド,メトトレキサート,フルオロウラシル,プレドニゾン,タモキシフェン,ハロテスチン **CMFPTH**
シクロホスファミド,硫酸ビンブラスチン,アクチノマイシンD,ブレオマイシン,プラチナム **VAB-Ⅵ**
シクロホスファミド,ルビダゾン,ビンクリスチン(=オンコビン),プレドニゾン **CROP**
シクロホスファミド・プラチノール **Ctx-Plat**
ジクロラール尿素 **DCU**
ジクロルフェナミド **DI**
ジクロルフェノールインドフェノール **DPIP**
ジクロロアセテート **DCA**
ジクロロイソプレナリン **DCI**
ジクロロイソプロテレノール **DCI**
ジクロロ酢酸 **DCA**
ジクロロジフェニルジクロロエタン **DDD**
ジクロロジフェニルトリクロロエタン(=クロロフェノタン) **DDT**
ジクロロジフェニルメチルカルビノール **DMC, DCPC**
ジクロロフェニルジメチル尿素 **DCMC**
ジクロロフェン **G_4**
ジクロロメタン **DCM**
ジクロロメトトレキサート **DCM**
ジケトピペラジン **DKP**
シゲラソンネイ **SS**
ジゴキシン **Dig**
ジゴキシン様免疫反応物 **DLIS**
シコチアミン **CCT**
ジシクロヘキシル **DCH**
ジシクロヘキシルカルボジイミド **DCC, DCCI**
ジジム **D, di**
ジスキネジーを伴わない **WD**
シスジアミン-1,1-シクロブタンジカルボシレイトプラチナム **CBDCA**
シスジアミンジクロロプラチナ,ビンデシン,ブレオマイシン **DVB**
シスタチオニン **Cys**
シスチン **C, Cys**
シスチン・グアニン **CG**
シスチンアミノペプチダーゼ **CAP**
シスチン還元酵素 **H-Cys**
シスチントリプチケース寒天培地 **CTA**
システアミン **Cyst**
システイン **C, Cys**
システムモニターセンター **SMC**
ジステンパーウイルス **DV**
シスプラチナム,シクロホスファミド,エルデシン **PCE**

し

シスプラチン **CDDP, Cis, *cis*-DDP, CP**
シスプラチン(＝プラチノール) **PLAT**
シスプラチン(＝プラチノール),アドリアマイシン,シクロホスファミド **PAC, PAC-1, PAC-V**
シスプラチン(＝プラチノール),アドリアマイシン,シクロホスファミド,エトポシド **PACE**
シスプラチン(＝プラチノール),エトポシド **PE**
シスプラチン(＝プラチノール),エトポシド,イホスファミド **PEI**
シスプラチン(＝プラチノール),エトポシド,ブレオマイシン **PEB**
シスプラチン,シクロホスファミド,アドリアマイシン **CISCA**
シスプラチン,ビンクリスチン(＝オンコビン),ブレオマイシン **COB**
シスプラチン(＝プラチノール),ビンクリスチン(＝オンコビン),ペプレオマイシン **COP**
シスプラチン,ビンブラスチン,エトポシド,ブレオマイシン **CVEB**
シスプラチン(＝プラチノール),ビンブラスチン,ブレオマイシン **PVB**
シスプラチン,フルオロウラシル **CF**
シスプラチン(＝プラチノール),フルオロウラシル,エトポシド **PFE**
シスプラチン(＝プラチノール),フルオロウラシル,ロイコボリン **PFL**
シスプラチン,フルオロウラシル,ロイコボリンカルシウム **CFL**
シスプラチン(＝プラチノール),ブレオマイシン,ビンブラスチン **PBV**
シスプラチン(＝プラチノール),ペプレオマイシン,マイトマイシンC **CPM**
シスプラチン,ベペシド **CV**
シスプラチン,メトトレキサート,ビンブラスチン **CMV**
ジスプロシウム **Dy**
ジスルファニルアミドフェノールフタレイン **DSP**
ジセチアミン **DCET**
ジソピラミド **DP**
シゾフィラン **SPG**
シソマイシン **SISO**
シソミシン **SISO**
シダ状模様 **FLP**
シダ葉現象 **FLP**
シタラビン **Cy**
シタラビン,アドリアマイシン,チオグアニン **CAT**
ジチオエリトリトール **DTE**
ジチオトレイトール **DTT**
ジチオプロピルチアミン **DTPT**
シチジル・シチジル・アデニル **C-C-A**
シチジン **C, CR, Cyd**
シチジン二リン酸コリン **CD-choline**
シチジン 2′-一リン酸 **2′-CMP**
シチジン 3′-一リン酸 **3′-CMP**
シチジン 5′-一リン酸 **Cyd 5′-P**
シチジン 5′-二リン酸 **CDP, Cyd 5′-P2**
シチジン 5′-二リン酸グリセロール **CDP glycerol**
シチジン 5′-二リン酸コリン **CDP choline**
シチジン 5′-三リン酸 **Cyd 5′-P3**
シチジン一リン酸 **CMP**
シチジン三リン酸 **CTP**
シッカニン **SIC**
ジッヘン・オッペンハイム(症候群) **ZO**
ジデオキシアデノシン **ddA**
ジデオキシイノシン **DDI**
ジデオキシシチジン **ddC**
シデロサイト **S**
シデロブラスト **SB**
シトシン **C, Cyt**
シトシン・シトシン・グアニン・グアニン **CCGG**
シトシンアラビノシド **CA**
シトシンアラビノシド,ダウノルビシン **CAD**
シトシン二リン酸 **CDP**
ジドブジン **ZDV**
シトロバクター(属) **C**
シナプス後電位 **PSP, ps.p, p.s.p.**
シナプス小胞 **Sv**
シナプス膜 **SM**
シナプス様小胞 **SLMV**
ジニトロオルトクレゾール **DNOC**

ジニトロクレゾール **DN, DNC**
ジニトロクロロベンゼン **DNCB**
ジニトロナフトール **DNN**
ジニトロフェニル・鍵穴アオガイヘモシアニン **DNP-KLH**
ジニトロフェニル蛋白法 **DNP method**
ジニトロフェニルヒドラジン **DNPH**
ジニトロフェニルモルヒネ **DNPM**
ジニトロフェノール **DNP, DNP, Dnp**
ジニトロブチルフェノール **DNBP**
ジニトロフルオロベンゼン **DFB**
ジニトロベンゼン **DNB, D.N.B.**
シノキサシン **CINX**
シノプチスコープ **synopt**
ジパラヒドラジノフェニルスルホン **DHPS**
ジパルミトイルホスファチジルコリン **DPPC**
ジヒドララジン **DHZ**
ジヒドロアロプレノロール **DHA**
ジヒドロイソコデイン **DHIC**
ジヒドロウリジン **D**
ジヒドロエルゴクリプチン **DHE, DHEC**
ジヒドロエルゴコルニン **DHO**
ジヒドロエルゴタミン **DHE**
ジヒドロエルゴトキシン **DHT**
ジヒドロキシプロポキシメチルグアニン **DHPG**
ジヒドロキシアセトン **DHA**
ジヒドロキシアデニン **DHA, DHOA**
ジヒドロキシグルタミン酸アルミニウム **DAG**
ジヒドロキシコプロスタン酸 **DHCA**
ジヒドロキシジブチルエーテル **DHBE**
ジヒドロキシジプロピルニトロソアミン **DHPN**
ジヒドロキシトリプタミン **DHT**
ジヒドロキシビフェニール **PHB**
ジヒドロキシフェニルアラニン **DOPA, Dopa**
ジヒドロキシフェニル酢酸 **DOPAA**
ジヒドロキシフェニルセリン **DOPS**
ジヒドロキシプロピルテオフィリン **DHT**
ジヒドロキシプロピルメチルグアニン **DHPG**
ジヒドロキシマンデル酸 **DMA, DOMA**
ジヒドロキシメチルフラトリジン **FT**
ジヒドロクロロチアジド **DCT**
ジヒドロストレプトマイシン **DHSM, DS, DST**
ジヒドロタキステロール **DHT**
ジヒドロチミン **DHT**
ジヒドロデスオキシストレプトマイシン **DOSM**
ジヒドロテストステロン **DHT**
ジヒドロピリジン **DHP**
ジヒドロプテリジン還元酵素 **DHPR**
(7,8-)ジヒドロ葉酸 **DHF**
ジヒドロ葉酸 **FH_2**
ジヒドロ葉酸還元酵素 **DHFR**
ジピリダモール **DIP, DPM**
ジピリダモール・タリウム画像 **DTI**
ジピロメテン **DPM**
ジフ **GIF**
ジフェニドール **DFN**
ジフェニル-*p*-フェニレンジアミン **DPPD**
ジフェニルアミン **DPA**
ジフェニルアミン反応 **DPA reaction**
ジフェニルオキサゾール **DPO**
ジフェニルクロルアルシン **AD, DA**
ジフェニルヒダントイン **DPH, PKM**
ジフェニルヘキサトリエン **DPH**
ジフェニルメタンジイソシアネート **MDI**
ジフェノール酸 **DPA**
ジフェンヒドラミン **DPH**
ジブカイン数 **DN**
ジブチリルサイクリックAMP(＝アデノシン一リン酸) **DBcAMP**
ジブチルヒドロキシトルエン **BHT**
ジフテリア **DI, Dip, dip, diph**
ジフテリア・破傷風 **diph-tet, diph/tet**
ジフテリア・破傷風・百日咳(ワクチン) **DTP**
ジフテリア破傷風毒素 **DTT**

ジフテリア・百日咳・破傷風(ワクチン) **DPT**
ジフテリア・百日咳・破傷風・ポリオ **DPTP**
ジフテリア・百日咳・破傷風・ポリオ・麻疹 **DPTPM**
ジフテリア・百日咳免疫 **DPI**
ジフテリア抗毒素 **DAT**
ジフテリアトキソイド **diph-tox**
ジフテリア毒素 **DT, DTX**
ジフテリア毒素 A **DTA**
ジフテリア毒素感受性 **DTS**
ジフテリアと破傷風の混合ワクチン **DT**
ジフテリア破傷風ワクチン **DT-VAC**
ジフテリア標準毒素 **DTN**
ジプラミトイルレシチン **DPL**
ジフルオロジフェニルトリクロロエタン **DFDT**
ジフルオロメチルオルニチン **DFMO**
ジフルドロコルチゾン吉草酸一般クリーム **DFV**
ジプロピオン酸塩 **DP**
ジプロピオン酸ベクロメタゾン **BDP**
ジプロピオン酸ベクロメタゾンエアゾール **BDA**
ジプロピオン酸ベクロメタゾンクリーム **BMD**
ジプロピルアセテート **DPA**
ジプロピルトリプタミン **DPT**
シプロフロキサシン **CPFX**
ジブロモエタン **DBE**
ジブロモサリチルアニリド **DBS**
ジブロモダルシトール,アドリアマイシン,ビンクリスチン,タモキシフェン,ハロテスチン **DAVTH**
ジブロモダルシトール,アドリアマイシン,ビンクリスチン,ハロテスチン **DAVH**
ジブロモマンニトール **DBM**
ジベカシン **DKB**
ジベナミン **DBA**
ジペプチジルアミノペプチダーゼ **DAP**
ジペプチジルペプチダーゼ **DPP**
ジヘマトポルフィリンエーテル **DHE**
シーベルト **Sv**
ジベンコジド **DBC**
ジベンジルエチレンジアミン **DBED**
ジベンズアントラセン **DBA**
ジホスゲン **DP**
ジホスホイノシチド **DPI**
ジホスホグリセレート **DPG**
ジホスホグリセレートホスファターゼ **DPGP**
ジホスホグリセレートムターゼ **DPGM**
ジホスホチアミン **DPT**
ジホスホピリジンヌクレオチダーゼ **DPNase**
ジホスホピリジンヌクレオチド **DPN**
シミュレーションテスト **ST**
ジメタジオン **DMO**
シメチジン **CIM**
ジメチルトリアゼノイミダゾールカルボキサミド **DTIC**
ジメチルアセトアミド **DMAC**
ジメチルアデノシン **DMA**
ジメチルアミノエタノール **DMAE**
ジメチルアミン **DMA**
ジメチルアルギニン **DMA**
ジメチル・イミノジ酢酸 **HIDA**
ジメチルエーテル **DME**
ジメチルオキサゾリジン **DMO**
ジメチルオキシアルファメチルフェネチラミン **DOM**
ジメチルカルビノール **DMC**
ジメチルグアニルグアニジン **DMGG**
ジメチルグリシン **DMG**
ジメチルシステイン **DMC**
ジメチルジチオカルバメイト亜鉛 **ZIRAM**
ジメチルジチオカルバメート **DDC**
ジメチルステロン **DMS**
ジメチルスルホン酸 **DMS**
ジメチルスルホキシド **DMS, DMSO**
ジメチルスルホン **$DMSO_2$**
ジメチルチアゾールジフェニルテトラゾリウム臭酸塩 **MTT**
ジメチルチオウレア **DMTU**
ジメチルテレフタル酸 **DMT**

し

ジメチルトリプタミン　**DMT**
ジメチルニトロサミン　**DMN, DMNA**
ジメチルビグアニド　**DMBG, NNDG**
ジメチル砒素酸　**DMAA**
ジメチルヒドラジン　**DMH**
ジメチルフェニルピペラゾニウム　**DMPP**
ジメチルフタル酸　**DMP**
ジメチルポリシオキサン　**DMPS**
ジメチルホルムアミド　**DMF, DMFA**
ジメチル硫酸　**DMS**
ジメチルリン酸　**DMP**
ジメトキシ-メチルアンフェタミン　**DOM**
ジメトキシフェニルエチルアミン　**DMPE, DMPEA**
ジメトキシフェニルペニシリン　**DMPPC**
ジメリジン　**ZIM**
ジメルカプトコハク酸　**DMSA**
ジメルカプロール　**DMP**
ジーメンス　**S**
シーメンス単位　**S.E.**
シャイ・ドレーガー(症候群)　**SD**
シャイ・ドレーガー症候群　**SDS**
ジャクソン・プラット(ドレーン)　**JP**
ジャクソン職業興味調査　**JVIS**
ジャクソン人格調査表　**JPI**
ジャドキンス左(冠(状)動脈用カテーテル)　**JL**
ジャドキンス右(冠(状)動脈用カテーテル)　**JR**
ジャネー病　**JD**
ジャノッティ・クロスティ症候群　**G-C syndrome**
シャリエール計測板　**Ch**
シャルコー・マリー・トゥース病　**CMT, CMTD**
シャルコー・ライデン結晶　**CLC**
シャワー浴　**SB**
シャント圧　**SP**
シャント血　**s**
シャント血流量　$\dot{Q}s$
シャント後脳障害　**PSE**
シャント手技　**SP**
シャント率　**SR**
シャント流量　**SF**
シュウ酸　**OA**
シュウ酸カルシウム　**ca.ox.**
ジュウテリウム　**D**
シュードモナス(属)　**P**
シュードウリジン　ψ
シュードモナス属　**PS, Ps**
シュトリュンペル・マリー(病)　**SM**
シュトリュンペル・ローレイン(病)　**SL**
ジュニア　**jr**
ジューニアス・クーント病　**JKD**
シュピーグラー・フェント類肉腫　**SFS**
シュピールマイアー・フォークト(病)　**SV**
シュミット・ラッピン・ラウス肉腫ウイルス　**SRRSV**
シュミット・ラッピンウイルス　**SRV**
シュラー・クリスチャン(病)　**SC**
シュラッター・オスグッド(病)　**SO**
シュラップネル膜　**M flac, M.flac., m.flac.**
ジューリング疱疹状皮膚炎　**DHD**
ジュール　**J**
ジュール/クーロン　**J/C**
シュレム管　**SC**
シュワバッハ検査　**S**
シュワルツ・バーター(症候群)　**SB**
シュワルツ・ワトソン(試験)　**SW**
シュワルベ線　**SL**
シュワン細胞　**SC**
シュワン細胞膜　**SCM**
ショウガ　**zz, Zz., zz.**
ジョサマイシン　**JM**
ショック/分　**SPM**
ショック症集中治療室　**SCU**
(抗)ショックパンツ　**MAST**
ショック療法　**ST**
ショ糖(マンニット)培地　**SM**
ジヨードチ〔サイ〕ロニン　$\mathbf{T_2}$
ジヨードチ〔サイ〕ロ酢酸　**DIAC**
ジヨードチロシン　**DIT**
ジヨードヒドロキシフェニルピルビン酸　**DIHPPA**
ショープウイルス　**SV**
ショープ線維腫ウイルス　**SFV**
ショープ乳頭腫ウイルス　**SPV**
ショルダー　**SH, Sh, sh**
ジョン・ホプキンス医学研究所　**JHMI**
ジョン・ホプキンス大学医

学部　**JHUSM**
ジョン・ホプキンス大学衛生学公衆衛生学科　**JHUSHPH**
ジョン・ホプキンス病院　**JHH**
ジョーンズ・モート(型)反応　**JMR**
ジョンソン・ケニースクリーニングテスト　**JKST**
ジョーンミルトンハーゲン(抗体)　**JMH**
ジラ　**JIRA**
ジラウリルホスファチジルコリン　**DLPC**
シラミ媒介回帰熱　**LBRF**
シリアルナンバー　**sno**
シリコンゴム　**SR**
シリコン制御整流素子　**SCR**
シリコン半導体を応用した電気化学センサー　**CHEMFET**
シリコン部分トロンボプラスチン時間　**SPTT**
ジル　**gi, Gl, gl**
ジルコニウム　**Zr**
ジルコン　**Zr**
シールド疎水性相　**SHP**
シルバー・ラッセル症候群(＝先天性発育不全)　**SRS**
シルバーマン針生検　**SNB**
ジルベール症候群　**GS**
シルマー検査　**SCH**
シロエリマンガベイ　**CTL**
シロップ　**syr**
シロップ剤　**sir.**
シロテナガザル　**HLA**
シンガポール流行性結膜炎　**SEC**
シングルインラインパッケージ　**SIP**
シンチグラム　**scint, Scinti**
シンチレーション　**Scinti**
シンディング・ラーセン(病)　**SL**
シンノンブレウイルス　**SNV**
シンバスタチン　**Simva**
ジェムの　**gem**
しばしば起こる　**freq**
しぼった母乳　**EBM**
し(嗜)眠状態　**DRS**
口腔外科学修士　**M.Ch.D.**
子癇(＝しかん)　**eclamp**
子癇前症　**PE**
子癇前妊娠中毒　**PET**
子宮　**U**
子宮亜全摘　**STH**
子宮圧迫症候群　**UCS**
子宮外妊娠　**EUP, GEU**
子宮拡張　**UD**
子宮活動　**U/A**
子宮活動間隔　**UAI**
子宮活動単位　**UAU**
子宮下部帝王切開(術)　**LCCS**
子宮間質過形成　**HIU**
子宮吸引　**UA**
子宮鏡下卵管内精子注入法　**HIT**
子宮筋腫　**myoma**
子宮筋電法　**EHG**
子宮グロブリン　**UG**
子宮頸癌　**CC**
子宮頸管癌　**CACX, CaCx**
子宮頸癌ワクチン　**HPVV**
子宮頸管乾燥塗抹標本　**CDS**
子宮頸管粘液貫通　**CMP**
子宮頸管粘液検査　**CMT**
子宮頸管粘液接触テスト　**CMCT**
子宮頸上皮内癌　**IE Ca cx**
子宮頸部上皮内腫瘍　**CIN**
子宮頸部粘液　**CMS**
子宮頸部粘液抽出物　**CME**
子宮血流量　**UBF**
子宮後屈　**Retro.**
子宮弛緩因子　**URF**
子宮収縮　**UC**
子宮収縮負荷試験　**CST**
子宮真空吸引搔爬器　**UVAC**
子宮全摘出(術)　**TH**
子宮胎盤虚血　**UPI**
子宮胎盤(機能)不全(症)　**UPI**
子宮体部癌　**KK**
子宮腟部温度　**PT**
子宮底・結合間距離　**FSA**
子宮底結合間距離　**FSD**
子宮底の高さ　**H of F**
子宮摘出術　**hys., HYST, hyst.**
子宮摘出術と放射線照射　**H & R**
子宮摘出と不妊術　**H & S**
子宮動脈血流速度　**UBFV**
子宮内　**IU**
子宮内圧　**IUP**
子宮内圧モニター　**IPM**
子宮内異物　**IUFB**
子宮内隔膜　**IUD**
子宮内ガス　**IUG**
子宮内器具　**IUD**
子宮内死亡　**IUD**
子宮内死亡胎児　**DFU**
子宮内スメアテスト

EST
子宮内成長率　**IUGR**
子宮内胎児仮死　**IUFD**
子宮内胎児死(亡)　**FDIU, IUFD**
子宮内胎児発育　**IUG**
子宮内胎児発育遅延　**IUFGR**
子宮内胎児輸血　**IUFT**
子宮内で　**in ut**
子宮内妊娠　**IUG, IUP**
子宮内妊娠分娩　**IUPD**
子宮内発育遅延児　**IUGR**
子宮内発育不良　**PIFG**
子宮内避妊器具　**ICD, IUCD**
子宮内付着　**IUA**
子宮内プロゲステロン避妊システム　**IPCS**
子宮内膜　**IUM**
子宮内膜症　**EM**
子宮内膜掻爬術　**Aus**
子宮内輸血　**IUT**
子宮内容除去術　**Aus**
子宮乳頭状漿液細胞癌　**UPSC**
子宮嚢胞過形成　**HCU**
子宮プロゲステロン系　**UPS**
子宮分娩　**UD**
子宮娩出力記録表　**TKG**
子宮娩出力測定器　**TKD**
子宮娩出力測定法　**TKG**
子宮卵管境界　**UTJ**
子宮卵管結合部閉塞　**OCC in UTJ**
子宮卵管造影法　**HGS, HSG, HSP, hystero**
子孫　**desc, sib, sibs**
支持構造　**Found, found.**
支持的精神療法　**ST**
支払わない　**NP**
支配・交叉〔差〕(遺伝)　**CO**
支配性社会的外向　**As**
支配人　**Dir**
止血穿刺閉鎖器具　**HPCD**
氏名を記入せよ　**s.sn., s.s.n**
仕事　**op., W, wk**
仕事環境尺度　**WES**
仕事情報調査票　**WII**
仕事速度　**WR**
仕事代謝率　**WMR**
仕事単純化　**WS**
仕事中に　**OJB**
仕事中に受傷した　**IOD**
仕事に戻る　**RTW, RW, R/W**
仕事能力　**WC**
仕事負荷　**WL**
仕事率　**WR**
四亜硝酸ペンタエリスリチール　**PETN**
四塩化炭素　**carbon tet**
四角(の)　**sq**
四角形　**quad**
四腔断面　**4CV**
四酢酸鉛シッフ　**LTAS**
四酸化オスミウム-α-ナフチルアミン　**OTNA**
四肢　**ext, ext.**
四肢形成　**AER**
四肢血液量　**LBF**
四肢血管抵抗　**LVR**
四肢麻痺　**quadrip, tetra**
四肢麻痺患者　**quad**
四肢麻痺の　**quad**
四辺形の　**QL**
四辺の　**quad**
四メチル尿素　**TMU**
市販後の調査実施基準　**GPSP**
市販薬　**OTC**
市民権利局　**OCR**
市民航空医学協会　**CAMA**
示唆する　**sug**
示差眼圧測定　**DT**
示差寒暖分析　**DTA**
示差走査熱量測定　**DSC**
示指　**In, ind, ind.**
示指固有伸筋　**EIP**
(固有)示指伸筋　**EIP**
矢状径　**Sag.d.**
(指の)矢状索　**SB**
矢状(静脈)洞血栓症　**SST**
矢状面　**S**
死　**D, d., EOL**
死因　**CM, COD**
死学　**thanat**
死腔　**D, DS**
死腔気　**D**
死腔気体容量の1回換気量率　**V_D/V_T, VD/VT**
死腔容積　**VD, V_D**
死腔量　**VD, VD, V_D**
死後に　**PM, P.M., p.m.**
死後の　**post**
死後ヒト腎細胞　**PHK cells**
死後ヒト腎臓　**PHK**
死産　**DD, SB, S/B**
死産児率　**SRR**
死産の　**Stb, stb., Still B, stillb.**
死傷(者)　**Cas**
死傷者処理所　**CCS**
死傷者なし　**NC**
死体　**cdv, DB**
死体(の)　**CAD, Cad**
死体処理センター　**CDC**
死体提供者　**CD**
死の　**mort**
死亡　**Exit, EXP, exp., M, m.**
死亡告知　**ob**
死亡時間　**DT**
死亡した　**D, d, D,**

d., dec, decd, dec'd, OB, ob.
死亡している **M, m.**
死亡数 **mort, mortal**
死亡統計学 **necrol**
死亡年 **YOD**
死亡場所 **POD**
死亡(年月)日 **DOD**
死亡埋葬 **D & B**
死亡未熟女児 **IDFC**
死亡未熟男児 **IDMC**
死亡率 **D/T, mor, mort, mortal, MR, q_x**
死亡率の相違性の研究 **IDS**
死亡率比 **MR**
死滅細胞内細菌 **KICB**
死滅(微)生物 **KO**
死滅麻疹ワクチン(ウイルス) **KMV**
死滅〔死菌〕ワクチン **KV**
死力 μ_x
死んだ **D, d., s.i.d.**
糸球体(腎の) **G**
糸球体圧 **GP**
糸球体基底膜 **GBM**
糸球体近接細胞(数) **JGC**
糸球体近接の **JG**
糸球体血漿流量 **GPF**
糸球体硬化 **GS**
糸球体高血圧 **GHT**
糸球体細尿管腎炎 **GlTN**
糸球体刺激ホルモン **GSH**
糸球体指数 **GI**
糸球体上皮細胞 **GEC**
糸球体腎炎 **GN**
糸球体尿細管腎炎 **GTN**
糸球体尿細管調節 **GTB**
糸球体毛細血管壁 **GCW**
糸球体濾過 **GF**
糸球体濾過亢進 **GHF**
糸球体濾過量 **GFR**
糸状虫 **W**
糸状虫仔虫 **Mf, mf**
糸状の **fil, nema**
至急 **Cito !**
至急調剤せよ **cito disp. !**
至急で **stat., Stat**
至適許容量 **OA**
至適必要量 **OR**
次亜ヨウ素酸 **HOI**
次亜ヨウ素酸塩 **HIO**
次回診察 **NV**
次元フーリエ変換 **DFT**
次善(量)亜鉛 **ZSO**
耳炎 **OT, Ot, ot, ot.**
耳下顎症候群 **OMS**
耳下腺 **PG**
耳下腺混合腫瘍 **MPT**
耳下腺全摘出術 **TP**
耳下腺の **parot**
耳下点・鼻下点間距離 **DSAN**
耳介 **A, aur., auric**
耳介後部皮弁 **PAG**
耳介皺 **ELC**
耳介内の **IA, i.a.**
耳科医 **OT, Ot, ot, ot., Otol, otol**
耳科学 **OT, Ot, ot, ot., OTO, Oto, oto, Otol, otol**
耳管圧 **ETP**
耳管カタル **TC**
耳管狭窄症 **TS**
耳管鼓室開口部 **TOET**
耳管鼓室気流動態法 **TTAG**
耳管通気 **LD**
耳管の **eust.**
耳管隆起 **TR**
耳口蓋指 **OPD**
耳孔挿入式補聴器 **IE**
耳後の **post aur.**
耳垢水 **CW, ZW**
耳垂プレチスモグラフ **APG**
耳性眼瞼反射 **APR**
耳性瞬目反射 **APR**
耳瘻 **OF**
耳内連絡 **CIA**
耳鼻咽喉医 **ORL**
耳鼻咽喉科 **HNO, OLR, OTO, Oto, oto**
耳鼻咽喉科医 **OT, Ot, ot, ot.**
耳鼻咽喉科学 **HNOH, ORL, OT, Ot, ot, ot., otolar, otorhinol**
耳鼻咽喉科資格認定書 **DLO**
耳鼻科 **ENT**
耳鳴重症度評価法 **STSS**
耳鳴に関する質問 **TRQ**
耳・口蓋・指趾症候群 **OPD syndrome**
自我発達スケール〔尺度〕 **EDS**
自家感作性皮膚炎 **ASD**
自家骨髄移植 **AuBMT**
自家骨髄 **ABM**
自家骨髄移植(療法) **ABMT**
自家輸血返血法 **ATS**
自覚症状・客観的所見・評価と計画(=問題志向型システム診療記録様式) **SOAP**
自覚所見 **S**
自覚的外傷後症候群 **SPTS**
自覚的な **subj**
自覚率 **SR**
自給式潜水器具 **SCUBA**
自己癌細胞刺激誘導キラー細胞 **ATLAK**
自己研修システム **SAS**
自己抗体 **AAbs**

し

自己混合リンパ球反応 **AMLR**
自己集合単分子膜 **SAMs**
自己診断テスト **SDS**
自己制御関節 **SRJ**
自己測定血圧 **ABP**
自己徴候特性尺度 **SCL**
自己調節硬膜外鎮痛 **PEA**
自己調節硬膜外鎮痛(法) **PCEA**
自己調節鼻内鎮痛法 **PCINA**
自己同期の **Slfsyn**
自己内蔵・運搬可能な医療器械 **MUST**
自己内蔵放射線モニター **SCRAM**
自己破壊の **SD**
自己評価依存質問票 **SADQ**
自己評価うつ病(尺度) **SAD**
自己評点不安尺度 **SAS**
自己不溶性免疫複合体 **AISIC**
自己弁心内膜炎 **NVE**
自己免疫(性)血小板減少(症) **AT**
自己免疫疾患 **AID**
自己免疫性肝炎 **AIH**
自己免疫性血小板減少性紫斑病 **AITP, ATP**
自己免疫性高脂血症 **AIH**
自己免疫性甲状腺炎 **AIT, AITD**
自己免疫性好中球減少症 **AIN**
自己免疫性精巣炎 **AIAO**
自己免疫性プロゲステロン皮膚炎 **APD**
自己免疫性無精子症性睾丸炎 **AIAO**
自己免疫性溶血性貧血 **AHA**
自己免疫多内分泌カンジダ症候群 **APECS**
自己免疫多内分泌病・カンジダ症・外胚葉ジストロフィ **APECED**
自己免疫の **AI**
自己免疫プロゲステロン皮膚炎 **AIPD**
自己免疫(性)補体結合 **AICF**
自己免疫(性)溶血(性)疾患 **AHD**
自己免疫(性)溶血性貧血 **AIHA**
自在関節(症候群) **UJ**
自殺完遂 **CS**
自殺企図 **SA, SMV**
自殺未遂 **SA**
自殺予防研究センター **CSSP**
自然 **Nat**
自然家族計画 **NFP**
自然経腟分娩 **SVD**
自然血小板凝集 **SPA**
自然骨折 **SF**
自然細胞傷害 **NC**
自然死 **DND, ND**
自然成長ホルモン **IGH**
自然対数 **ln**
自然腟分娩 **SVD**
自然に **spon, spon.**
自然に従って **s.n.**
自然の **Nat**
自然の方法で **p.v.n.**
自然破水 **SMR, SRM, SROM**
自然発症高脂血症ラット **SHC rat**
自然破膜 **SRM, SROM**
自然非滅菌分娩 **UUD**
自然分娩 **SD**
自然保湿因子 **NMF**
自然野菜粉末 **NVP**
自然遊走能 **SM**
自然抑制T細胞 **NS**
自然流産 **SA, SAB**
自然ロゼット形成細胞 **SRFC**
自損傷 **SIW**
自動DNA分析装置 **HUGA**
自動運動 **AE**
自動音量調節 **AVC**
自動介助運動 **AAE**
自動化学生物学的監視機構 **ACBWS**
自動化検診 **AMHT**
自動化検診システム **AMHTS**
自動感作抗体試験 **ART**
自動感度調節 **AGC**
自動既往症 **AMH**
自動記録水晶電気眼圧計 **ARCET**
自動血圧計の測定センサーが動脈を探す方式 **APS**
自動健診施設 **AMHTS**
自動車事故 **AA, MVA**
自動信号処理器 **ASP**
自動迅速化学測定装置 **ARCA**
自動診断取得情報検索システム **ADMIRES**
自動制御装置 **auto**
自動生体細胞分析分離装置 **ABCAS**
自動ゼロ設定 **AZS**
自動総合健診システム **AMHTS**
自動体外式除細動器 **AED**
自動台車搬送システム **ACT**
自動的輝度調節 **ABC**
自動的生物研究室 **ABL**

し

自動的に作用する甲状腺小結節　**AFTN**
自動デジタルデータ過誤記録機　**adder**
自動デジタルデータ集合システム　**ADDAS**
自動デジタルデータ取得と記録　**addar**
自動データ連接　**ADL**
自動発生耳音響放射　**SOAE**
自動発声処理分析器　**AVTA**
自動腹膜灌流　**APD**
自動放射標識免疫検定　**ARIA**
自動明聴調節　**ARC**
自動臨床検査分析器　**ACA**
自発換気　**SV**
自発眼振　**SN，Sp Ny，Sp.Ny.**
自発呼吸　**SB，SR，SV**
自発性の　**spon，spon.，spont**
自発的細胞媒介性細胞傷害性　**SCMC**
自発的手術(的)避妊　**VSC**
自発的抵抗運動　**ARE**
自発的入院　**Vol Adm**
自発的妊娠中絶　**VIP，VTP**
自発電気活動　**SEA**
自発(的)の　**spnt，spon，spon.，spont**
自発迷路性偏倚　**SLD**
自閉症児行動評価表　**BRIAC**
自由エネルギー　**F**
自由音場　**FF**
自由電子レーザー　**FEL**
自由度　**DF，D/F，df，d.f.，UCV**
自由な　**F**
自由に　**adlib.，ad lib.，Ad lib.**
自由にベッドから出て立ってよい　**up OOB ad lib**
自由門脈圧　**FPP**
自由誘導減衰　**FID**
自由連想　**FA**
自立生活　**IL**
自律訓練法　**AT**
自律神経系　**ANS**
地場焦点核磁気共鳴法　**FONAR**
弛緩　**Lax，lax**
弛緩期　**D**
弛緩骨盤底部　**RPF**
弛緩した腟口　**RVO**
弛緩性の　**flac**
弛緩性皮膚　**CL**
(鼓膜)弛緩部　**M flac，M.flac.，m.flac.**
弛緩部　**PF**
弛緩不能症　**ACH**
弛張(性)の　**remit**
私的医学連絡　**PMC**
私的な　**priv，pvt**
児童　**Ch，ch**
児童絵画統覚検査　**CAT**
児童用不安尺度　**CMAS**
(胎)児頭　**FH**
児頭骨盤不適合　**CPD**
使用後　**p.a.**
使用される　**utend.**
使用者確認　**USERID**
使用せよ　**utend.**
使用前に振盪せよ　**agit.esu.**
使用人　**emp，empl**
刺激　**R，S，st，st，stim，stimn**
刺激・反応　**SR**
刺激液量　**SVR**
刺激(作用)過多症候群　**HSS**
刺激後時間　**PST**
刺激後時間ヒストグラム　**PSTH**
刺激後ペプシン分泌量　**SPO**
刺激細胞　**SC**
刺激指数　**SI**
刺激惹起性多能性獲得　**STAP**
刺激惹起性多能性獲得細胞　**STAP cells**
刺激する　**stim**
刺激性および感作原性低分子物質　**MSIS**
刺激生体反応　**SOR，S-O-R**
刺激前の　**PS**
刺激鎮痛法　**SPA**
(心臓)刺激伝導系　**ICS**
刺激伝導系　**RLS**
刺激反応説　**S-R**
刺激反応理論　**S-R**
刺激比　**SR**
刺激物質　**E substance**
刺激薬　**ST，st，stim**
刺激誘導鎮痛(法)　**SIA**
刺激誘発者　**FS**
刺創　**SW**
刺痛　**ting**
姉妹　**S，s**
姉妹染色体鑑別　**SCD**
姉妹染色分体交換　**SCE**
(一)肢　**ext，ext.，extr，extrem**
肢　**X，x**
肢体不自由者　**crip**
肢帯(型)筋異栄養(症)　**LGMD**
肢帯(型)筋ジストロフィ　**LG，LGMD**
肢端黒子型黒色腫　**ALM**
(四)肢誘導　**EA**
事故　**Acc，acc，accid，acdt**
事故・健康保険　**A & H ins**

事故死　**DAI**
事故死と四肢切断　**ad & d**
事故死の　**ACK**
事故で緊急を要す　**A & E**
事故にあったが健康である　**A & H**
事故(年月)日　**D/A**
事故防止プログラム　**TIPP**
事故誘発の　**AI**
事象関連緩徐脳電位　**ERSP**
事象関連電位　**ERP**
事象関連反応　**ERR**
事前評価　**A, asmt**
事務用共通処理言語　**COBOL**
青春期視床下部症候群　**HPS**
姿勢反射　**PR**
思考(散乱)した　**incoher**
思考障害因子　**TDF**
思考障害指数　**TDI**
思考内容　**COT**
思春期前精巣〔睾丸〕腫瘍　**PPTT**
指欠損・外胚葉性形成異常・口唇口蓋裂症候群　**EEC syndrome**
指向応答　**OR**
指骨間の　**IPH**
指示　**dir, dir., indic, o, Ord, ord, ord.**
指示音以上の音圧　**DBRN**
指示された　**Ord, ord, ord.**
指示した方法で　**m.dict., mor.dict.**
指示的な　**dir**
指示どおり　**u.d.**
指示どおり(に)　**ut dic., ut dict.**
指示どおり調剤せよ　**DAD**
指示どおりに　**mod praesc, mod.praesc**
指示のとおり　**m.d., md, md.**
指示のとおり用いられるべし　**m.d.u.**
指伸筋　**ED**
指書テスト　**PFT**
指静脈開存圧　**FVOP**
指数　**exp, I, In, ind, ind., Q**
指数〔係数〕・メディクス　**Ind.Med.**
指数弁　**CF, c.f., FC, FZ, nd, n.d.**
指尖手掌間距離　**FPD, TPD**
指尖床間距離　**FFD**
指尖脈波曲線　**FSG**
指尖容積脈波　**PTG**
指節間(関節)　**IP**
指節間角化症　**IPK**
指節間関節　**IPJ**
指(趾)節骨　**phal**
指節骨骨関節炎　**POA**
指(趾)節骨の　**Ph**
指定の場所に　**l.c.**
指定部位　**Ep**
指導者　**super**
指導書　**IB**
指導的組織精神医学　**DO**
指標　**bar, indic**
指名　**nom**
指名された　**nom**
指名する　**nom**
指紋　**dactygram**
指紋学　**dacty**
指紋型　**FPP**
指紋検査法　**dacty**
指紋術　**dacty**
施行された　**perf**
施設内生命安全委員会　**IBC**
持続　**D, d., st**
持続,〜の間　**dur, dur.**
持続(性)陰圧　**CNP**
持続(性)陰圧換気　**CNPV**
持続インスリン点滴静注　**CIVII**
持続温熱腹膜灌流　**CHPP**
持続可能な開発のための環境保全イニシアティブ　**ECOISD**
持続(性)間質性肺気腫　**PIPE**
持続血液濾過法　**CHF**
持続作用　**SA**
持続酸素療法　**COT**
持続静脈高栄養法　**C-IVH**
持続睡眠　**DS**
持続睡眠療法　**DS**
持続する　**CONT, cont., contin.**
持続性運動負荷　**SPE**
持続性肝炎　**PH**
持続性貫壁性刺激物質　**LATS**
持続性機械的人工呼吸　**CMV**
持続性吸息中枢　**APC**
持続性血液濾過透析　**CHDF**
持続性甲状腺刺激(ホルモン)　**LATS**
持続性甲状腺刺激物質　**LAST, LATS**
持続性甲状腺刺激物質保護体　**LATS-P**
持続性高フェニルアラニン血症　**PHP**
持続性サルファ剤　**LSF**
持続性植物状態　**PVS**

持続性神経筋単位 **tNMU**
持続性心室頻拍 **VT-S**
持続性新生児重症筋無力症 **PNMG**
持続性心房静止 **PAS**
持続性全身性リンパ節腫脹 **PGL**
持続性肉眼的脾腫 **PGS**
持続性乳(汁)漏(出)・無月経症候群 **PGAS**
持続性肺高血圧(症) **PPH**
持続性部分てんかん **EPC**
持続(遷延)性発作後脳障害 **PPIE**
持続性陽圧呼吸 **CDP**
持続他動運動 **CPM**
持続注入 **CI**
持続注入排泄尿路造影図 **CIXU**
持続的加温エアロゾル **CHA**
持続的気道陽圧法 **CPAP**
持続的携帯型腹膜透析 **CAPD**
持続的血液浄化療法 **CBP**
持続的周期腹膜透析 **CCPD**
持続的静脈・静脈血液濾過 **CVVH**
持続的腎置換療法 **CRRT**
持続的遂行能検査 **CPT**
持続的電気的反応能 **CERA**
持続的陽圧換気 **CMV**
持続的陽圧換気法 **CPPV**
持続的陽圧呼吸(法) **CPPB**
持続点滴静注 **CIV**
持続動静脈血液透析 **CAVHD**
持続動静脈血液透析濾過 **CAVHDF**
持続動静脈血液濾過 **CAVH**
持続投薬 **SM**
持続(性)の **cont, cont.**
持続脳室ドレナージ **CVD**
持続皮下インスリン注入(療法) **CSII**
持続皮下インスリン注入ポンプ **CSIIP**
持続皮下注入法 **CSA, SD**
持続ヘパリン化 **CH**
脂血症浄化因子 **LCA**
脂(肪)向性因子 **LTF**
脂質研究センター **LRC**
脂質研究センター冠(状)動脈一次予防試験 **LRC-CPPT**
脂質合成 **LS**
脂質蓄積型ミオパシー **LSM**
脂質転送蛋白 **LTP**
脂質動員 **LM**
脂質動員因子 **LMF**
脂質動員物質 **FMS**
脂質動員ホルモン **FMH, LMH**
脂質誘発高血糖 **FIH**
脂質輸送蛋白 **LTP**
脂肪 **ax., F, pin., ping.**
脂肪過多・高温・過小月経・耳下腺症候群 **AOP-syndrome**
脂肪肝 **FL**
脂肪肝・腎症候群 **FLKS**
脂肪肝細胞 **FLC**
脂肪幹〔間質〕細胞 **ASCs**
脂肪結合シアル酸(=シアリン酸) **LBSA**
脂肪血症清浄化因子 **LCF**
脂肪細胞 **Ad**
脂肪酸 **FA**
脂肪酸アルコール・プロピレングリコール **FAPG**
脂肪酸結合蛋白 **FABP**
脂肪酸合成酵素 **FAS**
脂肪酸受容体 **FAA**
脂肪酸分解酵素 **CPT**
脂肪腫性血管周囲〔血管外皮〕細胞腫 **LHPC**
脂肪親和性因子 **LTF**
脂肪線条 **FS**
脂肪族アシル基 **RCO**
脂肪塞栓症候群 **FES**
脂肪組織・造血組織比 **F.H.**
脂肪組織抽出物 **ATE**
脂肪組織への脂肪酸転入率 **FIAT**
脂肪体 **LB**
脂肪蓄積係数 **CR**
脂肪貯蔵細胞 **FSC**
脂肪微粒子 **LM**
脂肪負荷試験 **FTT**
脂肪由来幹細胞 **ADSC**
脂肪抑制 **ChemSat**
脂漏性角化症 **SK**
脂漏性皮膚炎 **Seb Derm**
時間 **d.Z, hr, hrs, Std., T, t, Z, Zt**
時間・運動(手技) **TM**
時間・場所・人 **TP & P**
時間・場所・人について見当識のある **or.X3**
時間荷重平均濃度 **TWA**
時間間隔 **T, TI**
時間推定 **TE**
時間制御方式薬剤投与(装置) **TCDD**
時間制限のある **TL**

時間線量関係　**TDR**
時間線量分割(因子)　**TDF**
時間的一致　**synchro**
時間と温度　**T & T**
時間と材料　**T & M**
時間と場所について見当識のある　**or.X2**
時間に対する心室圧の微分値　**dp/dt**
時間について見当識のある　**or.X1**
時間の終りに　**hor.un.spatio**
時間の経過　**TL**
時間肺活量　**TVC**
時間分割システム　**TSS**
時間利得補償回路　**TGC**
時定数　**TC**
時,時間　**H, h**
時・分・秒　**HMS**
笑気ガス・酸素・エーテル　**GOE**
舐剤　**conf.**
舐汁　**linct**
紫外線　**UV light, UV ray**
紫外線(光)　**UV, UVL**
紫外線A　**UVA**
紫外線A波防御度　**PA**
紫外線B　**UVB**
紫外線C　**UVC**
紫外線回復　**UV-reactivation**
紫外線血液照射(法)　**UBI**
紫外線光電子分光鏡検査(法)　**UPS**
紫外線光度計測(法)　**UVP**
紫外線削除・非青視　**UVCY**
紫外線殺菌灯　**UV lamp**
紫外線照射　**UVI, UVR**
紫外線増強再活性化　**UVER**
紫外線測光　**UVP**
紫外線太陽恒数　**UVSC**
紫外線放散　**UVI**
紫外線療法　**UV therapy**
紫外(線)の　**UV**
紫外部測定法　**UV method**
紫色蓄尿バッグ症候群　**PUBS**
視運動性眼振　**OKN, OPN**
視運動性眼振パターン　**OKP**
視運動性眼振パターン検査　**OKP test**
視運動性後眼振　**OKAN**
視快適光　**VCL**
視角中心視野測定　**AC**
視覚　**V, V., vis, vsn**
視覚・運動順序検査　**VMST**
視覚・運動統合(検査)　**VMI**
視覚・運動統合検査　**VMIT**
視覚・連想・運動感覚・触覚　**VAKT**
視覚アナログ尺度　**VAS**
視覚運動ゲシュタルト検査　**VMGT**
視覚活動時間　**VAT**
視覚活動療法　**VAT**
視覚記憶スコア　**VMS**
視覚記憶スパン　**VMS**
(ベントン)視覚記銘力検査　**VRT**
視覚検出レベル　**VDL**
視覚コミュニケーション(療法)　**VIC**
視覚失認　**VA**
視覚障害　**VI**
視覚性的刺激　**VSS**
視覚的前庭眼反射　**VVOR**
視覚の　**V, vis**
視覚皮質　**VC**
視覚ひずみ検査　**VDT**
視覚表示装置　**VDU**
視覚表示端末装置　**VDT**
視覚フィードバック画面表示　**VFD**
視覚補助　**VA**
視覚補綴システム　**TVSS**
視覚誘発電位　**VEP**
視覚誘発脳波　**VECP**
視覚誘発脳皮質電位　**VECP**
視覚(性)誘発反応　**VER**
視覚誘発野　**VEF**
視蓋前核　**NPA**
視交叉〔差〕　**OX, Ox, O_x**
視交叉〔差〕核　**SCN**
視交差〔叉〕上核下垂体性尿崩症　**SHDI**
視交叉〔差〕の　**SCH**
視索　**OT**
視索上核　**SO, SON**
視床　**Th**
視床下核　**STN, SubN**
視床下部　**H, HT, Ht, Hth, Hyp, hyp, HYPOTH**
視床下部・下垂体・甲状腺軸　**HHTA**
視床下部・下垂体・甲状腺の　**HPT**
視床下部・下垂体・性腺の　**HPG**
視床下部・下垂体・副腎(軸)　**HPA**
視床下部・下垂体・副腎軸　**HHAA**
視床下部・下垂体・副腎の　**HHA**
視床下部・下垂体・副腎皮質系　**HPA**

し

視床下部・下垂体・副腎皮質の　**HPA**
視床下部・神経下垂体複合体　**HNC**
視床下部下垂体系　**HPS**
視床下部血流量　**HBF**
視床下部後部　**PH**
視床下部神経下垂体系　**HNS**
視床下部性無月経　**HA**
視床下部前部　**AH**
視床下部抽出物　**HE**
視床下部の腹外側核　**VLH**
視床下部腹内側(核)　**HVM**
視床下部分泌因子　**HSA**
視床下部放出因子　**HypRF**
視床下部放出ホルモン　**HRH**
視床出血　**TH**
視床枕　**pul**
視床投射神経細胞　**TPN**
視床内側部　**MT**
視床腹外側核破壊術　**VL thalamotomy**
視床腹中間核　**Vim**
視神経　**ON**
視神経萎縮　**OA**
視神経交叉〔差〕　**OC**
視神経上核下垂体神経路　**SOH**
視神経髄質炎　**NO**
視神経線維分析器　**NFA**
視神経束核　**NOT**
視神経乳頭　**ONH**
視神経乳頭陥凹比　**C/D**
視神経乳頭形成不全　**ONH**
視神経乳頭部位以外の新生血管　**NVE**
視神経乳頭部の新生血管　**NVD**
視軸　**VA**
(医学的)視診　**MI**
視診　**insp, insp., INSPEC, VI**
視診・触診・打診・聴診　**IPPA**
視診する　**insp**
視全方位式無線標識　**VOR**
視束交叉〔差〕　**CH, CO**
視束前視交叉〔差〕野　**POSC**
視束前野　**PO**
視索前野と前視床下部　**PO/AH**
視聴域　**VAR**
視聴覚　**audio, audiovis, AV**
視聴覚(教育)器具　**audio, audiovis, AVA**
視聴覚(教育)器具事務局　**BAVA**
視聴覚教育部　**AVID, BAVE**
視聴覚研究協会　**AVRA**
視聴覚個別指導　**AVT**
視聴覚性的刺激　**AVSS**
視聴覚(教育)センター　**AVC**
視的性格認知　**OCR**
視同定点　**VIP**
視動性の　**OPK**
視認識閾値　**VRT**
視認性　**vsby**
視能訓練士　**ORT**
視標追跡検査　**ETT**
視放線　**OR**
視明瞭度　**vipre**
視野　**CV, F, F., f, fd, fld, VF, Vf**
視野刺激　**FS**
視野無(損)傷　**VFI**
視野良好　**GVF**
視力　**av., S, S., V, V., VA, Va**
視力・右眼　**VAOD, VARE**
視力・左眼　**VALE, VAOS**
視力・両眼　**VAOU**
視力回復のためのアイバンク　**EBSR**
視力矯正資格認定書　**DOrth**
視力矯正不能　**NC**
視力検定学士　**DO**
視力効率　**VE**
視力障害者への援助　**AB, A/B**
視力障害の　**VI**
視力測定学士　**B.S.Opt., D.Opt., M.Opt**
視力測定士　**B.Opt., DOS, opt.D.**
視力調節　**Acc, ACC, acc**
視力低下・右眼　**VA ↓ OD**
視力低下・左眼　**VA ↓ OS**
視力低下・両眼　**VA ↓ OU**
痔(核)　**hem, Hemo**
歯学　**Odont, odont.**
歯学博士　**DMD, D.M.D.**
歯科医　**DDM, den, Dent, dent.**
(英国)歯科医会会員　**FDS**
歯科医学　**den**
歯科医学士　**DDSc, D.D.Sc.**
歯科医師団　**DC**
歯科医術　**den**
歯科医療サービス　**MDS**
歯科衛生士　**B.S.Dent, Den Hyg, DH**
歯科衛生認定書　**DDH**

歯科学　Dent, dent.
歯科学士　B.D.Sc., B.Sc.Dent, M.D.Sc, M.S.Dent
歯科学博士　DDSc, D.D.Sc.
歯科学免許医　L.D.Sc.
歯科既往歴　PDH
歯科技工士　DT
歯科技工全国協会　NADL
歯科矯正認定書　DDO
歯科外科博士　M.Ch.D.
歯科研究行動科学協会　BSDR
歯科口腔外科学士　B.Ch.D., B.D.S.
歯科公衆衛生認定書　DDPH
歯科材料商連合　DTF
歯科手術　DS
歯科手術室　DOR
歯科情報管理基金　FDD
歯科全国連合　NDA
歯科治療審議会　CDT
歯科の　den, Dent, dent.
歯科病院協会　ADH
歯科文献索引　IDL
歯科文書財団　DDF
歯冠周囲炎　Perico, Periko
歯冠と架工義歯　Cr & Br
歯間溝　IDG
歯矯正資格認定書　DOrth
歯外科認定書　Dip.Ds.
歯頸(面)舌(面)軸(面)の　CLA
歯根端周囲の　periap
歯根膜炎　Per
歯状回　DG
歯状核・赤核・淡蒼球・ルイ体萎縮症　DRPLA
歯状の　Dent, dent.
歯周界　perim
歯周学　periodont
歯周疾患指数　PDI
歯周膿瘍　PA
歯軸の　GA
歯髄炎　pul
歯髄誘発電位　TPEPS
歯槽骨切除(術)　Alvx, ALVX
歯槽突起切除　Alvx, ALVX
歯槽の　ALV, alv, alv.
歯肉　G, ging.
歯肉炎　G
歯肉癌　GK
歯肉形成　Gply
歯肉軸の　GA, G/A
歯肉指数　GI
歯肉切除　Gvty
歯肉舌面軸の　GLA
歯肉の　G, g
歯(性)の　Dent, dent.
滋養糖　NZ
(食道胃)試験　zam
試験　exp, exper, Xam
試験・意見・忠告　EOA
試験開腹　Probe
試験官　E, Ex, ex, exam
試験管　TT
試験管混濁試験　TTTT
試験管内で　in vit., IV, i.v.
試験検査溶液　TS, T.S.
試験室　BZ
試験診察　TV
試験切開　Probe
試験切片　Probe
試験穿刺　PP
試験的用量　TD
試験と評価　T & E
試験耳　TE
試行間間隔　ITI
試行錯誤　TE, T & E
試料直接導入法　DSI
資格　qual
資格記録　QR
資格試験　quals
資質化　qual
資料　info, infor
飼育　fdg
辞書　dict
辞典　dict
嗜好に適した酸味を加えよ　ad grat.acid
嗜癖　addict
嗜癖研究センター特性尺度　ARCI
嗜癖重症度指数　ASI
磁化の空間調整　SPAMM
磁化率　$\varkappa$, k, X_m
磁気　Mag, mag
磁気画像(診断)法　MSI
磁気強度　I
磁気共鳴　MR
磁気共鳴映像法　MRI
磁気共鳴血管造影法　MRA
磁気共鳴コンピュータ画像診断法　MR-CT
磁気共鳴断層撮影法　MR-CT, MRT
磁気共鳴胆道撮影(法)　MRC
磁気共鳴分光画像(法)　MRSI
磁気共鳴マンモグラフィ　MRM
磁気心臓ベクトル　MHV
(核)磁気スペクトロスコピー　MRS
磁気ディスク　MD
磁気テープ　MT
磁気の　Mag, mag
磁気流体力学　MHD
磁気力　I
磁束(密度)　*J*

磁力顕微鏡 **MFM**
篩骨(洞) **eth**
篩骨上顎板 **EMP**
篩骨(洞)の **eth**
塩づけ **SS**
式 **F**
色覚 **C**
色覚異常 **CCD**
色覚能 **VC**
色彩 **col**
色視 **CV**
色素 **p, pig., pigm., pigmt.**
色素顆粒 **CMG, PG**
色素希釈法 **DDG, DDT**
色素結合能 **DBC**
色素試験 **DT**
色素指数 **CI, FI**
色素失調(症) **IP**
色素性乾皮症 **XDP, XP**
色素性絨毛結節性滑膜炎 **PVNS, PVS**
色素性網膜炎 **RP**
色素沈着 **Pig, pig, pigmt.**
色素沈着の **pig**
色素網膜上皮(細胞) **PRE**
色素誘導因子 **PIF**
色調・循環・体温・動き **CCTM**
色度座標による国際表色系 **CIE**
色盲 **CVD**
色盲の **CB**
識別 **ID, iden**
識別閾(値) **JND**
識別〔弁別〕刺激 **DS**
識別視力 **VDA**
識別〔弁別〕スコア **DS**
識別する **dist, iden**
識別性刺激 **Sd**
識別力 **DP**

(円柱レンズの)軸 **A**
軸 **AX, Ax, ax, x**
軸位遠位頸面の **ACD, ADC**
軸位遠位咬合面の **ADO**
軸位遠位歯肉面の **ADG**
軸位遠位切歯面の **ADI**
軸位遠位面の **ad**
軸位近心咬合面の **AMO**
軸位頸面の **AC**
軸位(面)咬合(面)の **AO**
軸位口唇舌面の **ALAL, ALaL, A La L**
軸位正中遠位の **AMD**
軸位切歯面の **AI**
軸位舌面咬合面の **ALO**
軸(面)近心(面)歯頸(面)の **AMC**
軸(面)近心(面)歯肉(面)の **AMG**
軸(面)近心(面)の **AM**
軸(面)頬(面)歯肉(面)の **ABG**
軸(面)頬(面)舌(面)の **ABL**
軸(面)頬(面)の **AB, ab**
軸傾度 **AX grad**
軸索 **ax, cx**
軸索起始部 **IS**
軸索終末 **AT**
軸索分岐 **AA**
軸(面)唇(面)歯肉(面)の **ALAG, ALaG**
軸(面)唇(面)の **ALA, ALa, A La**
軸(面)歯髄(面)の **AP**
軸(面)歯肉(面)の **AG**
軸(面)舌(面)歯頸(面)の **ALC**
軸(面)舌(面)歯肉(面)の **ALG**
軸(面)舌(面)の **AL**
軸性の **a., A, a, ax**

(電気)軸偏位 **AD**
軸面頬面頸面の **ABC**
軸面近位切歯面の **AMI**
軸面の **a., A, a**
静かに注ぐ **dec**
下の **'neath, lr, u**
下のように **u.i.**
下を見よ **s.u., v.i.**
(足骨の)下1/3 **L/3**
従わない **non seq**
七面鳥γグロブリン **TGG**
失感情症のふるい分けテスト **SSPS**
失禁 **incont**
失禁患者援助協会 **HIP**
失禁の **INC, inc, inc., incont**
失血 **BL**
失見当(識)の **DS**
失行(症) **apr, aprax**
失効した **exp, Exp, EXP**
失効日付なし **NED**
失語症 **APH, aph**
失語症検査標準リスト **SLTA**
失語症の標準テスト **SLTA**
失調(症) **incont**
失調性片麻痺 **AH**
失読症 **dyslex**
失認 **AGN, agn**
失敗した **F**
失敗の原因 **COF**
(避妊)失敗率 **FR**
実験 **E, exp, exper, expt, expt.**
実験医学・外科学研究所 **IEMS**
実験支援組織 **ESS**
実験室 **LAB, Lab, lab**
実験室ブランチ補体結合(試験) **LBCF**

実験者　E, Vl
実験心理学研究所　IEP
実験精神科医会　SEP
実験単位　EU
実験的アレルギー性筋炎　EAM
実験的アレルギー性心筋炎　EAM
実験的アレルギー性神経炎　EAN
実験的アレルギー性精巣炎　EAAO, EAO
実験的アレルギー性脳脊髄炎　EAE
実験的アレルギー性ブドウ膜炎　EAU
実験的糸球体腎炎　EGN
実験的自己免疫性胸腺炎　EAT
実験的自己免疫性筋炎　EAM
実験的自己免疫性甲状腺炎　EAT
実験的自己免疫性重症筋無力症　EAMG
実験的自己免疫精巣炎　EAO
実験的腸球菌心内膜炎　EEE
実験的なやり方　ROT
実験的方法　LP
実験動物飼育者協会　LABA
実験の　E, exp, exper, expt, expt., exptl
実行する　exec, exec., XEQ
実行の　exec, exec.
実効温度　ET
実効遮蔽　EM
実効線量　E, ED
実効値　RMS
実効輻射温　ER
実在する　exist
実際残留量　PRL
実際的な　pract
実際にやって示す　dem
実際の　R
実耳挿入特性　REIR
実耳挿入利得　REIG
実耳閉鎖特性　REOR
実耳補聴器装用特性　REAR
実耳裸耳特性　REUR
実質外域　EPZ
実質性角膜炎　KP
実質的安全用量　VSD
実質内域　IPZ
(臓器)実質内出血　IPH
実質内通過時間　PTT
実性垂直性開散　+V, +v
実践看護教育とサービスの全国連合　NAPNES
実存する　exist
実測重炭酸塩　a.Bic
実測水素イオン濃度　apH
実測炭酸ガス分圧　$aPco_2$
実務看護学生　SPN
室　An, V, v, ven, VENT, vent, ventric
室温　ATPD, ATPS, RT
室温加硫シリコン　RTVS
室温と圧　ATP
室温リン光法　RTP
(心)室間の　IV
室上稜　CSV
室内気温　IAT
室内空気　RA
室房状態　VAC
室房伝導　VAC
(心)室(心)房の　VA, V-A
室傍(核)　PV
室傍核　NPV, PAVN, PVN
疾患　D, dis, disord, Dz, Erkrkg, Krkh, M, m.
疾患あるいは損傷　I or I
疾患のある　WD
疾患の徴候なし　NED
疾患への社会心理的適応の自己採点報告　PAISSR
疾患予防・環境管理局　BDPEC
疾病　dis, Dz, M, m.
疾病因子　DF
疾病および手術の標準用語　SNDO
疾病原因　D Ety
疾病行動質問票　IBQ
疾病障害により健康寿命を全うできなかった損失年数　PYLL
疾病対象血清　DCS
疾病と共存して生きる　LWD
疾病予防計画　DPP
疾病率と死亡率の週報　MMWR
悉無律(=しつむりつ)　ANG, ANL, AON
湿カタ寒暖計　WK
(傷の経過が)湿から乾へ　W→D
湿から乾へ　W-T-D
湿から湿へ　W→W
湿球　WB
湿球温度　Twb, WBT
湿球黒球温度(指標)　WBGT
湿球黒球湿度　WBGT
湿疹　Ez
湿疹・喘息・枯草熱(の複合症状)　EAHF
湿疹性アレルギー性接触皮膚炎　EACD
湿潤重量　WW

し

湿性痰　**PC**
湿性肺　**WLS**
湿製錠剤　**TT**
湿度　**h, humi**
湿度指数　**HI**
湿度制御システム　**MCS**
湿熱　**MH**
湿布　**cat, cat., comp, fo, WC, WD, WP, WPk, WPk**
質　**qlty, qual**
質疑応答　**Q & A**
質的かつ量的個人要求　**QQPR**
質的な　**qual**
質的保障全国会議　**NCQA**
質的要求情報　**QRI**
質問　**Q, quest**
質問事項　**qtnr**
質量　**M, m, mas., mass, mass.**
質量百分率　**%wt**
質量分析　**FAB, MS**
質量分析法　**MS**
膝下　**BK**
膝外側角　**FA, FTA**
膝蓋・大腿(関節)部　**PF**
膝蓋・大腿部関節　**PFJ**
膝蓋腱移行術　**PTT**
膝蓋腱荷重下腿義足　**PTB**
膝蓋腱支持装置　**PTB**
膝蓋腱反射　**KJ, kj, KK, Kk, PSR, PTR**
膝蓋腱部荷重ギプス　**PTB type cast**
膝蓋骨　**pat**
膝蓋骨亜脱臼　**SLP**
膝蓋骨圧痛　**pat.T**
膝蓋骨上切断(術)　**SPA**
膝蓋骨上の　**supra pat**
膝蓋骨脱臼　**DLP**
膝蓋靱帯　**LP**
膝蓋靱帯の長さ　**LT**
膝蓋大腿(関節)　**PE**
膝蓋大腿関節症候群　**PFJS**
膝蓋(骨)跳動　**TdP**
膝蓋軟骨軟化症　**CMP**
膝蓋リンパ節細胞　**PLNC**
膝関節装具　**KO**
膝関節離断(術)　**KD**
膝窩下バイパス(術)　**IPB**
膝窩腱　**Hams**
膝窩動脈閉塞性疾患　**PAOD**
膝窩の　**Pop, pop, poplit**
膝窩リンパ節　**PLN**
膝胸位　**KCP**
膝屈曲筋　**Hams, HS**
膝窩嚢胞　**PC**
膝腱　**HS**
膝上切断術　**AKA, AK amp., A/K Amp, Ak amp.**
膝神経節帯状疱疹　**GHZ**
膝前方痛　**AKP**
膝(関節)内障　**IDK**
膝内障　**IDK**
島　**is**
示された　**indic**
示した　**I**
示している　**ind, ind.**
示す　**ind, ind.**
湿った　**w**
下田式性格検査　**SPI**
写真　**phot, pics**
写真効果　**PE**
写真撮影　**phot**
写真専門家連合　**JPEG**
写真の　**phot**
社会　**soc**
(米国)社会・リハビリテーション庁　**SRS**
社会化　**So**
社会科学向け統計解析パッケージ　**SPSS**
社会関係検査　**SRT**
社会機能指数　**SFI**
社会機能尺度　**SAS**
社会経済状態　**SES**
社会再適応評価尺度　**SRRS**
社会サービス　**Soc Serv**
社会進歩指標　**ISP**
社会生活技能訓練　**SST**
社会生活能力検査　**SM**
社会性指数　**SQ**
社会成熟指数　**SQ**
社会精神衛生協会　**ASMH**
社会成層と流動尺度　**SSM**
社会適応指数　**SAI**
社会的遂行能面接基準　**SPS**
社会年齢　**SA**
社会の　**soc**
社会福祉　**C'wealth**
社会福祉学士　**DSW**
社会復帰　**Reha, Rehab, rehab, rehab., rehabil, Rehabili**
社会保障　**SocSec, Soc.Sec., SS**
社会保障行政　**SSA**
社会歴　**SH, S.H., Soc Hist, Sx Hx**
射出創　**WX, W/X**
射出熱　**WOX**
射精　**Ej**
射創　**GSW**
射入創　**WOE**
斜位　**ob, Ob, S**
斜位の　**OBL, obl**
斜視　**Sb, Sb., Strab, strab.**
斜の　**diag, diag.**
斜面台　**TT**

煮沸 **boil, Coct, coct.**
煮沸する **ferv.**
煮沸せよ **bull, bull., c, c., coq.**
煮沸の終わりに加えよ **s.f.c.a.**
遮断因子 **BF**
遮断抗体 **BA**
遮断時肝側門脈圧 **OHPP**
遮断周波数 **COF**
遮蔽曲線 **MC**
遮蔽試験 **CT**
遮蔽レベル較差 **MLD**
瀉下性の **cathar**
瀉下(性)の **CATH, Cath, Cath., cath.**
瀉血 **vs, vs.**
瀉血せよ **f.va.**
尺側手根屈筋 **FCU**
尺側手根伸(筋) **ECU**
尺側の **U**
尺側偏位〔偏差〕 **UD**
尺度 **G**
灼熱脚症候群 **BF**
灼熱足症候群 **BFS**
若年(発症)型〔性〕糖尿病 **JD, JDM**
若年型〔性〕糖尿病 **JOD**
若年性喉頭乳頭腫(症) **JLP**
若年女性動脈炎 **YFA**
若年性(の) **J**
若年性萎縮症 **JA**
若年性黄色肉芽腫 **JXG**
若年性顆粒膜細胞腫瘍 **JGCT**
若年性関節炎 **JA**
若年性関節リウマチ **JRA**
若年性喉頭乳頭腫 **JLP**
若年性黒内障(性)精神遅滞 **JAI**
若年性自己免疫性重症筋無力症 **JAMG**
若年性歯周炎 **JP**
若年性踵骨骨折 **JCF**
若年性進行麻痺 **juve para**
若年性振戦麻痺 **PAJ**
若年成人慢性患者 **YACP**
若年性成人発症型糖尿病 **MODY**
若年性全身(完全)麻痺 **JGP**
若年性足底皮膚症 **JPD**
若年性〔型〕糖尿病 **JODM**
若年性特発(性)(脊椎)側彎(症) **JIS**
若年性熱帯膵(臓)炎症候群 **JTPS**
若年性パーキンソニズム **JP**
若年性鼻咽頭血管線維腫 **JNPAF**
若年性皮膚筋炎 **JDMS**
若年性皮膚筋炎/多発(性)筋炎 **JDMS/PM**
若年性扁平疣贅 **VPJ**
若年性ホルモン **JH**
若年性慢性関節炎 **JCA**
若年性慢性骨髄性白血病 **JCML**
若年性慢性多発(性)関節炎 **JCP**
若年(性)の **juv, juv., juve**
若年の **Y**
若年発症性慢性関節リウマチ **YORA**
若年ミオクロニーてんかん **JME**
弱 **P**
弱アヘン剤離脱尺度 **WOWS**
弱視 **Asth, asth.**
弱毒化された **AT**
弱反応 **WR**
弱反応性の **WR, Wr, wr**
弱陽性の **W+, WP**
尺骨 **U, u**
尺骨(の) **uln**
尺骨神経 **UN**
尺骨神経伝導速度 **UNCV**
尺骨神経麻痺 **UNP**
尺骨トンネル症候群 **UTS**
尺骨の **U**
手関節 **WR, Wr, wr, wr.**
手関節背屈装具 **WHO**
手技 **Man, MANIP, manip, prc, pro, proc**
手芸療法 **MAT**
手根 **WR, Wr, wr, wr.**
手根管 **CT**
手根管減圧(術) **CTD**
手根管症候群 **CTS**
手根関節離断〔離開〕(術) **WD**
手根中手骨 **CM**
手根中手骨関節 **CMJ**
手根中手骨(間)の **CMC**
手根トンネル **CT**
手術 **OP, Op, op, Ope, oper, opn**
手術(法) **SURG, Surg, surg.**
手術栄養リスク係数 **NRI**
手術回復室 **SRR**
手術看護方式 **ONP**
手術計画 **OP, Op, op**
手術後状態 **S/P**
手術後の胃不全麻痺症候群 **PGS**
手術歯科学 **OpDent**
手術室 **OR**
手術室看護師 **ORN**

し

手術室技術協会　**AORT**
手術室技術者　**ORT**
手術している　**OP, Op, op, oprg, oprtg**
手術死亡率　**OMR**
手術手技　**OP, Op, op**
手術準備　**prep**
手術する　**oper**
手術前の　**pre-op**
手術創感染　**SWI**
手術できない　**inop**
手術の　**OP, Op, op, oper**
(外科)手術日　**DOS**
手術法　**MO**
手術野　**AO, op.reg.**
手掌・足底紅斑異感覚症候群　**PPES**
手掌線条黄色腫　**XSP**
手掌足底(掌蹠)角化症　**PPK**
手掌足底(掌蹠)角皮症　**PPK**
手足子宮(症候群)　**HFU**
手・足・性器(症候群)　**HFG**
手段的日常生活動作　**IADL**
手動の　**MO**
手動弁　**HB, HM, mm, m.m.**
手根(骨)の　**Ca**
手浴　**HW**
手腕振動症候群　**HAVS**
主因子分析　**PFA**
主栄養　**MF**
主冠(状)動脈　**MCA**
主観的視角　**subj**
主観的症状再調査　**ROSS**
主観的情報　**S**
主観的な　**S**
主観の　**S**
主(要)血清学的抗原　**MSA**
主細静脈　**MV**
主腎動脈狭窄(症)　**MRAS**
主成分回帰分析　**PCR**
主訴　**CC, COMP, comp, compl, compl., complt, HK, PC**
主訴の病歴　**HCC**
主題同定基準　**SID**
主知覚核　**MSN**
主任　**CS**
主肺動脈　**MPA**
主婦　**HW, h.w.**
主要塩基性蛋白　**MBP**
主要組織遺伝子複合体　**MHC**
主要組織適合抗原　**MHA**
主要組織適合抗原系　**MHS**
主要組織適合部位　**MHR**
主要中和決定因子　**PND**
主要な　**prin, princ**
主要免疫原性部位　**MIR**
主流煙　**MS**
寿命　**LSp, L sp.**
寿命研究　**LSS**
取捨選択の　**Eclec, eclec**
受血者　**Recip, recip.**
受血者血清　**RS**
受攻期　**VP**
受診　**HV**
受傷(年月)日　**DI, D/I**
受精　**fert**
受精因子　**FF, F factor**
受精管理調査諮問委員会　**CIFC**
受精させた　**fer'd, fertd.**
受精させる　**impreg**
受精指数　**FI**
受精した　**fer'd, fertd.**
受精能(因子)　**F**
受精能獲得抑制因子　**DF**
受精日　**GD**
受精卵輸卵管内注入法　**ZIFT**
受胎　**fert**
受胎させる　**impreg**
受胎前に　**PTC**
受動可動域　**PROM**
受動の　**P**
受動免疫化学療法　**AICT**
受動免疫血小板減少症　**PIT**
受容　**'cept**
受容・観察・維持　**RIM**
受容器　**A**
受容された歯科医療　**ADR**
受容体　**A, R, Rc, REC**
受容体作用チャンネル　**ROC**
受容体破壊因子　**RDF**
受容体破壊酵素　**RDE**
受容体型チロシンキナーゼ　**RTK**
受理された　**R**
受領者　**recr**
受領書　**rec**
酒石酸　**tart.a.**
酒石酸エチレンジアミン　**EDT**
酒石酸エルゴタミン　**ET**
酒石酸抵抗性酸ホスファターゼ　**TRACP, TRAP**
酒石酸ニコチン　**NT**
酒石酸リゼルグ酸ジエチラミン　**LSD 25**
酒石(酸)の　**tart**
酒精　**spir.v., sp.vin., s.v.**
授業時間　**Sess**
授乳(期)　**lac, lact**
授乳期無月経法　**LAM**
授乳している　**lact**

授乳ラット血清因子
LRSF
腫脹　**sw**
腫瘍　**T, TM, tum**
腫瘍2倍時間　**TDT**
腫瘍移植抗原　**TTA**
腫瘍エコー　**TE**
腫瘍壊死因子　**TNF**
腫瘍壊死血清　**TNS**
腫瘍学　**oncol**
腫瘍学の　**oncol**
腫瘍活性試験　**TAT**
腫瘍感受性抗原　**TSA**
腫瘍関連移植抗原
TATA
腫瘍関連拒絶抗体
TARA
腫瘍関連抗原　**TAA**
腫瘍関連抗体　**TAA**
腫瘍関連細胞表面抗原
TASA
腫瘍関連糖蛋白　**TAG**
腫瘍関連物質　**TAS**
腫瘍拒絶抗原　**TRA**
腫瘍血管形成因子　**TAF**
腫瘍血栓　**TT**
腫瘍血流(量)　**TBF**
腫瘍抗原　**T antigens**
腫瘍細胞　**TC**
腫瘍細胞破壊因子　**CBF**
腫瘍細胞遊走抑制因子
TMIF
腫瘍細胞誘発血小板凝集
TCIPA
腫瘍細胞溶解因子　**TCF**
腫瘍集合リンパ球　**TIL**
腫瘍状でない　**NT**
腫瘍随伴性(大脳)辺縁系脳障害　**PLE**
腫瘍性疾患　**ND**
腫瘍性上腕神経叢疾患
NBP
腫瘍成長　**TG**
腫瘍成長因子　**TGF**
腫瘍胎児抗原　**OFA**
腫瘍多糖類物質　**TPS**
腫瘍致死量　**TLD**
腫瘍治癒線量　**TCD**
腫瘍抵抗性抗原　**TRA**
腫瘍糖蛋白定量(症)
TGA
腫瘍特異抗原　**TSA**
腫瘍特異抗体　**TSA**
腫瘍特異性移植抗原
TSTA
腫瘍特異性移植免疫
TSTI
腫瘍特異性組織抗原
TSTA
腫瘍特異性糖蛋白
TSG, TSGP
腫瘍特異性(細胞)表面抗原
TSSA
腫瘍特異的な　**TS**
腫瘍特異物質　**TSS**
腫瘍皮膚試験　**TST**
腫瘍表面抗原　**TSA**
腫瘍変性因子　**TDF**
腫瘍(由来)ポリペプチド抗原　**TPA**
腫瘍誘発因子　**TIF**
腫瘍誘発性プラスミド
Ti plasmid
腫瘍誘発物質　**TIP**
腫瘍誘発プラスミド
TI, Ti
腫瘍溶解症候群　**TLS**
腫瘍抑制因子　**TIF**
腫瘍量　**TD**
腫瘍リンパ節転移(分類)
TNM
腫瘤・圧痛・反跳圧痛なし
MTR-0
種　**SP, sp, SPP, spp**
種子　**sem.**
種々の　**var**
種々の生理活性ペプチド
MBP
種痘(法)　**vacc**
種痘群の余分発生率
EIRV
種痘様水疱症　**HV**
種類　**GEN, gen**
種類によって特異化されない　**NSK**
樹状上皮T細胞　**DETC**
樹状上皮ランゲルハンス細胞　**DLC**
樹状突起　**D**
樹状突起棘　**DS**
樹枝状血管　**bV**
樹枝状細胞　**DC**
樹脂油　**oleores.**
樹木画による人格診断法
TTT
十二指腸　**D, duod**
十二指腸液　**Df**
十二指腸潰瘍　**DG, DU, UD**
十二指腸球部　**DB**
十二指腸ゾンデ　**DS**
十二指腸内視鏡　**DFS**
十二指腸内刺激　**IDS**
十二指腸内の　**ID**
十二指腸粘膜　**DM**
十二指腸の　**duod**
十二指腸ファイバースコープ　**FDS**
十分強力でなければ
si non val., si n.val.
十分水分補給された
WH
十分でない　**NS**
十分で軟らかな(食事)
FS
十分な　**suf, suff**
十分な水で煮沸せよ
coq in sa.
十分な量を随意に　**clqs.**
十分に　**q.s.ad**
十分量　**q.s., q.suff.**
収集　**coll**
収集する　**coll**
収縮　**C, contr, contra, retr, retr.**

し

(心)収縮期　**S**
収縮期　**syst**
(心臓の)収縮期・拡張期(比)　**S/D**
(心臓の)収縮期・拡張期比　**SD ratio**
収縮期圧　**Ps**
収縮期圧・時間係数　**SPTI**
収縮期圧・時間指数　**SPIT**
収縮期間隔　**STI**
収縮期逆流性雑音　**SRM**
収縮期駆出時間　**SET**
収縮期駆出性雑音　**SEM**
収縮期駆出率(速度)　**SER**
収縮期クリック　**SC**
収縮期クリック症候群　**SCS**
(左(心)室)収縮期径　**DS**
収縮期血圧　**SBP, SP**
収縮期血管抵抗　**SVR**
(心)収縮期雑音　**syst.m.**
収縮期雑音　**SM**
(僧帽弁の)収縮期前方運動　**SAM**
収縮期動脈圧　**SAP**
(心)収縮期(性)の　**Syst, syst, syst.**
収縮期平均駆出勾配　**MSEG**
収縮期容量　**SV**
収縮期流出　**SD**
収縮駆出期　**SEP**
収縮係数　**SI**
収縮後期雑音　**LSM**
収縮させうる　**retr, retr.**
収縮させる　**retr, retr.**
(心)収縮(持続)時間　**DS**
収縮時間　**CT**
収縮時間隔　**STI**
収縮した　**contr, retr, retr.**
収縮終(末)期径　**ESD**
収縮終(末)期ストレス　**ESS**
収縮終(末)期の圧　**ESP**
収縮終(末)期容量　**ESV**
収縮終(末)期期隆起　**ESS**
収縮する　**contr**
収縮性心膜炎　**CP, PC**
収縮前期奔馬調律　**PSG**
収縮前雑音　**PM, PSM**
収縮漸増を表す記号　**Z, Z', Z''**
収縮中期クリック　**MSC**
収縮電位複合体　**CEC**
収縮末期　**ES**
収縮末期径　**Ds**
収縮末期までの時間　**TES**
収縮要素　**CC, CE**
収縮力　**CF**
収束　**conv, converg**
収束イオンビーム　**FIB**
収束電子線回折法　**CBED**
収容力　**cy**
収率　**Y**
収量　**Y**
州　**Co**
州立精神病院　**SMH**
州立病院　**SH**
充血　**H**
充血した　**cong.**
充血単位　**HU**
住居　**Res, res**
住血吸虫(属)　**S**
周囲　**circum, environ.**
周囲の　**amb, environ.**
周期　**C, cy, R**
周期交代性眼振　**PAN**
周期性呼吸を伴う傾眠症　**HPB**
周期性四肢麻痺　**PP**
周期性症候群　**PS**
周期性同期性放電　**PSD**
周期性白皮症　**ap**
周期性片側性てんかん様発射　**PLED**
周期性無呼吸を伴う傾眠症　**HPA**
周期的経静脈高カロリー輸液　**Cyc-IVH, I-IVH**
周期(性)の　**C, c.**
周期の　**per**
周(囲)径　**cir, cir., Circ, circ**
周(囲)径の　**cir, cir., Circ, circ**
周産期集中治療室　**PICU**
周産期終脳白質脳炎　**PTL**
周術期心筋梗塞　**PMI**
周生期後乳児死亡率　**PPIM**
周生期死亡率　**PMR, PNM**
周生期損傷　**PI**
周生期罹病率　**PMR**
周知の方法で　**u.n.**
周長　**cir, cir., Circ, circ**
周長の　**cir, cir., Circ, circ**
周波　**C, c**
周波数　**cy, F, freq**
周波数/秒　**c/s**
周波数依存減衰　**FDA**
周波数追跡反応　**FFR**
周波数偏移キーイング　**FSK**
周波数変調　**FM**
周波数弁別域　**DLF**
周辺陥凹性　**PCC**
周辺虹彩切除(術)　**PI**
周辺視野計　**perim**
周辺部虹彩前癒着　**PAS**
周辺部滲出性脈絡膜出血性網膜症　**PECHR**
周辺部同時視　**SPP**

し

臭化エチジウム　**EB**
臭化カリウム　**KBr**
臭化水銀水酸化プロパン　**BMHP**
臭化水素酸　**HBr**
臭化デカメトニウム　**C10**
臭化テトラエチルアンモニウム　**TEAB**
臭化ドデシルトリメチルアンモニウム　**DTAB**
臭化ナトリウム　**NaBr**
臭化パラブロモフェナシル　**BPB**
臭化フェノドデシニウム　**PDDB**
臭化物　**brom.**
臭化ヘキサメトニウム　**C_6**
臭化ペンタメトニウム　**C_5**
臭化メチル　**MB**
臭化リチウム　**LiBr**
臭気管理　**OC**
臭素　**Br**
臭素化合物　**brom.**
臭素クレゾールグリーン　**BCG**
柔軟な　**S**
重加妊娠誘発高血圧　**SPIH**
重回帰分析　**MLR**
重クロム酸ナトリウム　**bichrome**
重合化フラジェリン　**POL**
重合ヒト血清アルブミン　**pHSA**
重鎖　**HC, H chain**
重心　**COG**
重心図　**EGG**
重症いびき症候群　**HSD**
重症眼筋無力症　**OMG**
重症〔危急〕患者看護　**CCN**
重症〔危急〕患者管理部門　**CCMU**
重症患者リスト　**SI list**
重症〔危急〕管理医学　**CCM**
重症急性呼吸器症候群　**SARS**
重症虚血肢　**CLI**
重症筋無力症　**MG, MyG**
重症〔危急〕時間　**CH**
重症先天奇形　**SCA**
重症治療室　**CCU**
重症度指数　**SI**
重症度分類　**PIR**
重症熱性血小板減少症候群　**SFTS**
重症の　**sev, SV**
重症複合型免疫不全症候群　**SCIS**
重症複合(型)免疫不全症　**SCID**
重症免疫不全　**RD**
重症ヤマアラシ状魚鱗癬　**IHG**
重水　**D_2O**
重水素(＝ジューテリウム)　**D, ^{2}H, hh**
重曹　**DHO, Nat.bic.**
重炭酸イオン　**HCO_3^-**
重炭酸塩　**BC, bicarb**
重窒素　**^{15}N**
重度異形成　**SD**
重度騒音環境　**SANE, SNE**
重篤疾患　**VSI**
重篤な異常なし　**NSA**
重篤な有害事象　**SAE**
重病　**SI**
重複振動　**vd**
重複切痕　**DN**
重メロミオシン　**HMM**
重役　**Dir**
重有機化合物　**HOC**
重要な　**Imp, imp**
重陽子　**D, d, *d***
重力　**G, g, gr, grav.**
重力加速度　**G**
重力除去した　**g.e., g-e**
重力スケール〔尺度〕　**g scale**
重力で引き起される意識喪失　**GLOC**
重力ドレナージ(法)　**DD**
重粒子線癌治療装置　**HIMAC**
重量　**p., W, WT, Wt, wt.**
(溶液)重量あたりの(溶質)重量　**W/W, w/w**
重量オスモル濃度　**osmo**
重量(中)重量パーセンテージ　**w/w**
重量単位　**G**
重量で　**p., pond.**
重量の　**pd.**
重量モル濃度　**m**
重量を支える　**WB, wt.b.**
修飾頸部郭清術　**MND**
修飾性抗リウマチ薬　**DMARDS**
修飾物質蛋白　**MP**
修飾率　**MR**
修正係数　**MF**
修正左前斜位　**mLAD**
修正した　**mod, mod.**
修正実効温度　**CET**
修正する人　**mods**
修正大血管転位　**CTGA**
修正大血管転位〔転換〕症　**corrected TGA, Cor.TGA**
修正洞結節回復時間　**CSNRT**
修復　**MR**
修理　**recond**
修理する　**rep**
修理すること　**recond**
従業員健康年金連合

し

FEHB
従属物　Dep, dep.
従属変数　DV
従来型インスリン療法　CIT
従来の換気法　CV
従量式調節換気　VCV
終圧　ED, FP, TD
終(末)期腎疾患　ESRD
終(末)期腎不全　ESRF
終(末)期陽圧呼吸　EPPB
終腱　TT
終日療法　RTC
終板電位　EPP
終末一般経路　FCP
終末ウェブ　TW
終末運動潜時　TML
終末肝静脈閉塞　THVO
終末呼気陰圧　NEEP
終末細気管支　TB
終末刺激　TR, TS
終末神経支配比　TIR
終末知覚潜時　TSL
終末デオキシリボヌクレオチド転換酵素　TdT
終末の　t, term
終末門脈枝　TPV
終夜睡眠ポリグラフ　PSG
習慣性顔面痙攣　HFS
習慣〔慣例〕に従って　ad us.
週　W, w, w., wk, wks
週活動サマリー　WAS
週に1度　OW, ow
週齢　WO, wo
就床時　v.d.schlaf.
就寝時(に)　HS, h.s., h.som.
就寝時経口摂取禁(止)　NPO/HS
就寝時刻　BT
就寝〔就眠〕時に　hor.decub.
就寝時に　h.d., hor.decu., hor.som.
就寝前　v.d.S
就寝前経口投与　POHS
集学的治療　MDT
集検用X線　MXR
集光レンズ　cond
集合　agg, aggreg, assby
集合管　CT
集合容積　coll vol
集積　agg
集積回路　IC
集積血液量　CBV
集団　M, m, mas., mass, mass.
集団合致等級分類　GCR
集団治療　GP TH, GpTh, Gp Th, GT
集中維持機能　TAF
集中観察室　IOU
集中観察治療部門　ITOU
集中呼吸管理　IRC
集中呼吸管理治療部　IRCU
集中する　conc, concentr, concn
集中暖房装置　CHU
集中治療　IC, IT
集中治療回復室　CCRU
集中治療看護部　ICN
集中治療施設　ICF
集中治療室　IOU
集中治療棟　ICW
集中治療部〔室〕　ICU
集中治療部門　ITU
集中的通常療法　iCT, ICT
集中的な　intens
集中免疫抑制　IIS
絨毛癌　CC, CCA, Ch-ca
絨毛間隙　IVS
絨毛結節性滑膜炎　VNS
絨毛上皮癌　CE
絨毛上皮腫　Ch-ep, chorio
絨毛性甲状腺刺激ホルモン　hCT
絨毛性ゴナドトロピン　CGH
絨毛性性腺刺激ホルモン　CG, CGT
絨毛性成長ホルモンプロラクチン　CGP
絨毛性ソマトマンモトロピン　CS
絨毛穿刺　CVS
絨毛毛細管　VC
愁訴　COMP, comp, compl, compl., complt
愁訴リスト　BL
銃創　GSW
(小)銃弾　bul
獣医　M.V., VMD
獣医衛生認定書　DVH
獣医科学　Vet Sci
獣医学　vet med
獣医学・牧畜学士　B.V.Sc. & AH
獣医学教官・研究者協会　AVTRW
獣医学研究所　VIO
獣医学公衆保健認定医　DVPH
獣医学士　B.Vet.Med., B.Vet.Sci., BVM, BVS, B.V.Sc., Vet.M.B.
獣医学博士　DVM, DVSc
獣医外科学士　B.Vet.Sur., BVS
獣医内科学・外科学士　BVMS
獣医(学)の　Vet
獣医用の　ad us.vet.
獣姦　Sod

獣(医)外科医　**VS, V.S.**
獣外科医ロイヤル大学協会　**ARCVS**
獣外科学博士　**D.V.S.**
獣内科外科学博士　**DVMS**
獣放射線医学博士　**DVR**
縦隔　**Med**
縦隔移動　**MS**
縦隔疾患　**MD**
縦(直)径　**LD**
縦走筋　**LM**
縦列反復の可変数　**VNTR**
宿主依存性変異　**HCM, HCV, HIM**
宿主回復　**HCR**
宿主対移植片(疾患)　**HVG**
宿主対移植片反応　**HVGR**
宿主防御因子　**HDF**
縮小肝移植　**RLT**
縮小する　**decr**
縮小有茎分節移植片　**ROSG**
十進法の　**dec**
出血　**BL, bl, bleed, haemorrh, hem, hemorr, hemorrh**
出血・微細動脈瘤　**HMA**
出血因子　**HF**
出血後水頭症　**PHH**
出血時間　**bl.time, bl.x, BT**
出血性遺伝性毛細血管拡張症　**THH**
出血性ショック脳症　**HSE**
出血性ショック脳症症候群　**HSES**
出血性大腸炎　**HC**
出血性ネフローゼ腎炎　**HNN**
出血性の　**hemorr**
出血性びらん性胃炎　**HEG**
出血性網膜症　**HR**
出血とショック　**H & S**
出血と滲出液　**H and E, H & E**
出血熱　**HF**
出現時間　**Ta**
出現頻度語表　**PB list**
出現率　**IN, incid**
出産　**Del, del., dlvr, dy, GEN, gen**
出産/分　**BPM**
出産時　**TOD**
出産指示　**d/o**
出産した　**dld**
出産調節薬　**BCM**
出産の　**dd**
出産歴　**P**
出生・死・結婚　**BDM**
出生/分　**BPM**
出生(直)後新生児死亡(症候群)　**PNM**
出生後の　**PN**
出生後便通なし　**ZSB**
出生児１人をもつ母親　**Para Ⅰ**
出生児２人をもつ母親　**Para Ⅱ**
出生児３人をもつ母親　**Para Ⅲ**
出生時体重　**BBW, BW, BWt, GG**
出生時低体重　**LBW**
出生時低体重児　**LBWI, LOWBI**
出生時発育指数　**DBI**
出生前に　**PTB**
出生前の　**AN, prenat**
出生地　**BP, BPL, POB**
出生調節　**BC**
出生の　**NAT**
出生(年月)日と出生地　**DPOB**
出生率　**IN**
出生歴　**BH**
出版されない　**NP**
出版社　**pub**
出版日未定の準備中の新刊　**ne/nd**
出発日　**DOD**
出力　**oupt, pow, pwr**
出力緩衝物　**OB**
出力増幅器　**PA**
術後(の)　**PO, P-O, P/O, post-op, post op.**
術後ケア　**POC**
術後呼吸治療　**PRT**
術後収縮性心膜炎　**PCP**
術後性アンギナ　**PA**
術後性上顎嚢胞　**POMC**
術後胆道鏡　**POCS**
術後疼痛管理　**PAS**
術後内眼球炎　**POE**
術後の　**POp**
術後日　**POD, P-O-D**
術後病理組織学的分類　**pTNM**
術語　**nm**
術式に従って　**sal.**
術者　**O, OP, Op, op, oper**
術前化学療法　**iCT, ICT**
術前血液希釈　**HD**
術前自家血保存　**DP**
術前診断　**PODx**
術中の　**PO**
術中腹腔内化学療法　**HIIC**
術中経管冠(状)動脈造影　**OTCA**
術中血管造影(法)　**IVA**
術中出血回収　**BS**
術中照射療法　**IOR, IORT**
術中胆管造影図　**IOC, IOCG**
術中超音波検査　**IOS**

術中動脈内フィブリン溶解療法 **IIFT**
術中微小針吸引術 **IOFNA**
術中放射線照射 **IOR**
術中放射線療法 **IORT**
術直後人工装具装着 **IPPF**
術野 **fld**
需要に応じて **o/d**
巡回 **cir, cir., Circ, circ**
春季角結膜炎 **VKC**
准看護師 **LPN, PN**
純音 **PT**
純音平均聴力 **PTA**
純化した **dep.**
純型肺動脈狭窄症 **PPS**
純国民福祉 **NNW**
純再生産率 **NRR**
純水 **aq.pur.**
純粋運動性片麻痺 **PMH**
純粋応用化学国際連合 **UICPA**
純粋感覚性脳卒中 **PSS**
純粋な **Pur., pur.**
循環 **C, c, CC, cir, cir., Circ, circ**
循環器集中治療部〔室〕 **CICU**
循環吸着式透析液再生装置 **REDY**
循環虚脱 **CC**
循環系平均充満圧 **MFP**
循環血液量 **CBV**
循環血漿蛋白量 **TPp**
循環血漿量 **CPV**
循環血中免疫複合体 **CIC**
循環血中リンパ球 **CBL**
循環時間 **CT**
循環時間延長 **CTD**
循環している **Circ, circ**
循環する **Circ, circ**
循環全赤血球鉄 **TRCI**
循環の **cir, cir., Circ, circ**
循環ヘモグロビン量 **THb**
順行性腎盂造影 **AP**
順序・番号指標 **SNI**
順序入れ替え **vv, v.v.**
順応 **A, a, a., Acc, ACC, acc, accom**
順応した **adj**
順応した小児 **AC**
順応する **adj**
(英国の)准看護師 **SEN**
准看護師教育 **PNE**
准教授 **AP**
準備 **Ppt, ppt., prep, prepn**
準備された **prepd**
準備されていない **NPF**
準備する **prep**
準備中 **in prep**
準備電位 **RP**
準備投薬 **pre-med**
瞬間的誘発耳音響放射 **TEOAE**
瞬時圧 **IP**
瞬時最大努力 **BME**
瞬時心臓死 **ICD**
瞬時薄層クロマトグラフィ **ITLC**
瞬膜 **NM**
瞬目・点頭・逓拝・痙攣 **BNS, BNS Krampf**
瞬目反応 **NMR**
女性 **F, Fe, fe, w**
女性(の) **fem**
女性外来部 **WOU**
女性(性)染色体 **X**
女性年 **WY**
女性の **F, fem**
処女の **V**
処女膜 **MI**
処置 **Man, MANIP, manip, proc, trmt**
処置・代替処置・適応と合併症 **PAIC**
処方 **F, form, presc, PS, rec, Rp., RX, RP, RX, Rx.**
処方(箋) **Rp**
処方・事象監視 **PEM**
処方した方法で **mod praesc, mod.praesc, MP, m.p.**
処方集 **F**
処方する **Pr, R, r., rc.**
処方せよ **rec, Rp.**
処方箋 **Pr, presc, PS, Ps, px, RX, Rx., Scripts, scripts**
処方箋とともに与えよ **dCf**
処方箋必要薬 **POM**
処方どおりに **e.m.p.**
処方を記して **cf**
処方を記して与えよ **dtr.c.for.**
処理 **trans, treat**
初(期)圧 **IP**
初圧 **AD, ID, Po**
初回抗原刺激を受けたリンパ球 **PL**
初回診断 **ID**
初回量 **ID**
初期 **beg**
初期B細胞抗原 **BP-1**
初期胸部照射 **ICI**
初期抗原 **EA**
初期勾配指数 **ISI**
初期故障率 **DFR**
初期手術可能性 **IOC**
初期心室群 **QRS**
初期睡眠障害 **ISD**
初期精神的発達 **IPE**
初期の **inl, P**
初期の癌での染色体のロス

LOH
初期沸点　IBP
初期羊水穿刺　EA
初期リンパ球　PC
初経　FMP
初産婦　P, Pp, primip
初節　IS
初速　IV
初速度　V_0
初潮　FMP
初妊婦　grav.1, grav.İ
初年度計画　FYP
初発エコー　IE
初発尿意　FDV
初発膀胱充満感　FS
初歩の　elem
初目的　ptgt
助言　Adv
助言する　adv.
助言の　Adv
助産師　MW
(英国の)助産師　SCM
助産師有資格者　LM
助手　assist, Asst, asst
助長　prom
所属リンパ節転移　N
書痙　WC
書字痙攣　WC
書籍目録テスト　BKT
書面で　in litt.
徐々に　grad., ped.
徐波　SW
徐波睡眠　SS, SWS
徐波睡眠時に持続性棘徐波を示すてんかん　CSWS
徐放性テオフィリン　SRT
徐放の　SR
徐脈　brady
徐脈頻脈症候群　BST, BTS
除外　excl, RO, R/O
除外した　exc
除去する　excl
除去率　E, ER
除細動　DF
除細動閾値　DFT, XDT
除脂肪体重　LBM
除痛の質　QOPR
(二)硝酸イソソルビド　ISDN
架〔線〕出限界　Lf
架状沈殿物　floc
架状沈殿物にする　floc
架状反応　floc
架〔線〕状反応単位　Lf
署名　S, s, /S/, /s/, Sig, sig
署名した　S, s, /S/, /s/, Sig, sig
署名なし　no sig
蒸気　v
蒸気圧　VP, vp
蒸気液体比　V/P
蒸気化　vapor
蒸気相クロマトグラフィ　VPC
蒸気密度　VD
蒸気浴　bal.vap., BAL VAP, b.v.
蒸発　evapn
蒸発させよ　evap.
蒸発した　evap
蒸発する　evap
蒸留　dist
蒸留した　dest., dist
蒸留酒　sp., spt., spts.
蒸留水　aq.dest., Aq dest, DDW, DW, D/W
蒸留水処理　DHT
蒸留水にてつくれ　f.op.aq.dest.
蒸留　destil
蒸留する　dest.
蒸留せよ　dist.
小円形ウイルス　SRV
小鋭棘波　SSS
小カロリー　c, cal
小核リボ核酸　snRNA
小核リボ蛋白　snRNP
小管膜小嚢　CMV
小臼歯　B, P, pm
小気道閉塞　SAO
小規模集積回路　SSI
小球状の　Glob
小球状粒子　SSP
小結晶セルロース三酢酸塩　MCT
小結節　N
小結節硬化型ホジキン病　NSHD
小結節性組織球　NH
小結節性溶解脂肪組織炎　NLP
小結節低密度領域　NLDA
小結節誘発性ウイルス　NIV
小結節様肺胞病変　NLAL
小骨盤腔内持続温熱灌流療法　CHMPP
小冊子　man
小柴胡湯　ss
小細胞癌　SCC
小細胞肺癌　SCLC
小手術服　MSS
小指　L
小指外転筋　ADM, ADQ
小指球(の)　Hy
小指伸筋　EDM, EDQ
小指対立(筋)　ODQ
小静脈　v
小水泡音　VS
小水疱疹　VE
小水疱(性)の　VES, ves.
小舌の　ling
小青竜湯　SS
小(結)節性側肉芽腫　NP

小大動脈症候群　**SAS**
小単薄層小胞　**SUV**
小腸　**SB, SI**
小腸大量切除　**SBR**
小腸ファイバースコープ　**FIS**
小腸閉塞　**SBO**
小動物　**sm.an**
小動脈　**a.**
小動脈瘤　**MA**
小頭(蓋)症　**MC**
小頭人種　**microcephs**
小人数討議　**SGD**
小児　**Ch, ch, J**
小児アレルギー　**PDA**
小児うつ病目録　**CDI**
小児栄養　**CN**
小児科　**K. KL**
小児科(学)　**PED, Peds, peds**
小児科医　**DPM, PED**
小児科外来診療協会　**AAPS**
小児科学　**paed, PD**
小児科学士　**B.Ped.**
小児科研究学会　**SPR**
小児癌研究グループ　**CCSG**
小児期一般疾患　**ODCH**
小児期筋ジストロフィ　**CMD**
小児期疾患　**CD**
小児気質性格　**CBC**
小児期自閉症評価点スケール〔尺度〕　**CARS**
小児期多嚢胞病〔疾患〕　**CPD**
小児期通常疾患　**UCD, UCHD, UCHI, UCI, UDC**
小児期の特異感情障害　**SEHC**
小児期慢性非特異性下痢　**CNDC**
小児期慢性良性好中球減少症　**CBN**
小児虐待および放置　**CA/N**
小児救急室　**PER**
小児丘疹性末端皮膚炎　**PAC**
小児教育心理学認定書　**DCEP**
小児期リウマチ疾患　**CRD**
小児外科　**PDS, PS**
小児血液財団　**CBF**
小児血液疾患　**CHD**
小児後天性免疫不全症候群　**PAIDS**
小児疾患　**ChD, CHD**
小児疾患包括的管理　**IMCI**
小児脂肪便症　**CD**
小児集中治療室　**PICU**
小児人格質問表　**CPQ**
小児神経学　**CHN**
小児神経軸索萎縮(症)　**INAD**
小児神経軸索ジストロフィ　**INAD**
小児心臓病　**PDC**
小児心理学　**CP**
小児整形外科検査　**POE**
小児精神(科)医　**CP**
小児精神医学　**CHP, CP**
小児直腸　**CR**
小児の痛みの程度を判定する指標　**CHEOPS**
小児の家族性持続性高インスリン低血糖　**PHHI**
小児の突然不慮死　**SUDI**
小児の両親認識　**CCP**
小児病院・関連研究所全国協会　**NACHRI**
小児病院医療センター　**CHMC**
小児病棟　**CW**
小児福祉研究所　**ICW**
小児放射線学　**PDR**
小児保健資格〔免状〕　**D.C.H.**
小児保護基金　**CDF**
小児慢性水疱症　**CBDC**
小児用価値調査票　**VIC**
小児用座席拘束装置　**CRD**
小児用視覚聴覚スクリーニング(検査)　**VASC**
小児用人格調査票　**PIC**
小児用耐性容器　**CRP**
小児用包括的評価尺度　**CGAS**
小児療育センター　**ZKi**
小児レフサム病　**IR**
小の　**min**
小脳　**ME**
小脳橋角(部)　**CPA**
小脳内核細胞　**ICNC**
小脳プルキンエ細胞　**CPC**
小嚢　**VES, ves., vesic**
小嚢関連膜蛋白　**VAMP**
小嚢(状/性)の　**vesic**
小嚢付着部位　**VAS**
小白血球　**SL**
小病院　**INF, inf**
小付着細胞　**SCC**
小伏在静脈温度　**Tsaph**
小発作　**PM**
小胞子菌(属)　**M**
小胞体　**ER**
小胞(性)の　**VES, ves., vesic**
小胞輸送システム　**VTS**
小(水)疱　**VES, ves., vesic**
小葉外終末乳管　**ETD**
小葉上皮内癌　**LCIS**
小葉組織崩壊　**LD**
小葉中心性肺気腫　**CE**
小葉内終末管　**ITD**
小葉肺胞腫瘍　**LATu**
小リンパ球　**SL**
小粒子ワクチン

SP vaccine
上衣腫　**EP**
上衣の　**EP**
上位 1/4 区　**UP**
上位運動(ニューロン)　**UM**
上位運動神経因性膀胱(障害)　**UMNB**
上位運動ニューロン　**UMN**
上位運動ニューロン障害　**UMNL**
上位の　**U**
上位部 1/4 区(＝四半部)　**UQ**
上咽頭関連リンパ組織　**NALT**
上咽頭腫瘍　**NRT, PNT**
上咽頭ファイバースコープ　**NPF**
上右部 1/4 区(＝四半部)　**URQ**
上オリーブ核　**SON**
上下限　**BUL**
上眼窩裂　**FOS, SOF**
上眼瞼　**UL**
上眼瞼・右眼　**ULRE**
上眼瞼・左眼　**ULLE**
上眼瞼挙(筋)　**LPS**
上顆　**E**
上顎癌　**OKK**
上顎結節線　**TM line**
上顎骨　**max, max., Max**
上顎骨骨折　**OKF**
上顎洞　**MS**
上顎洞炎　**SM**
上顎洞根本手術　**C-L op**
上顎(骨)の　**max, max., Max**
上丘　**SC**
上気道　**UA**
上気道うっ血　**UAC**
上気道疾患　**UAD**
上気道(性)睡眠(時)無呼吸(症)　**UASA**
上気道抵抗　**UAR**
上気道閉塞　**UAO**
上級医療事務官　**SMO**
上級外傷患者蘇生コース　**ATLS**
上級の　**SR, Sr**
上級病院医療官　**SHMO**
上記参照　**s.o.**
上記と同じ　**S/A**
上記の　**supra cit.**
上記のように　**ut supr.**
上(部)胸郭出口圧迫(症候群)　**UTOC**
上胸部　**URC**
上義肢　**ULP**
上限　**UL**
上限なし　**NUL**
上頸神経節　**SCG**
上交叉〔差〕域内基礎部分　**MBSC**
上向結腸　**AC**
上向大動脈　**ACS AO**
上向(性)と下向(性)の　**A & D, A and D**
上行結腸　**A**
上行性の　**asc**
上行性網様体賦活系　**ARAS**
上行大動脈　**AA, AAo, AO, AscAo, ASCAO**
上行大動脈圧　**Pao**
上行大動脈嚢性中心壊死　**CMN-AA**
上喉頭神経　**SLN**
上鼓室　**At**
上左部 1/4 区(＝四半部)　**ULQ**
上十二指腸角　**SDA**
上小脳動脈　**SCA**
上上肢後面形成シーネ(副子)　**LAPMS**
上矢状静脈洞　**SSS**
上矢状静脈洞血栓(症)　**SSST**
上矢状(静脈)洞(血流)速度　**SSSV**
上耳側 1/4　**STQ**
上肢　**UE, Uext, U/ext, u/ext, UL**
上肢機能固定器　**FAB**
上肢機能評価の簡易テスト　**STEF**
上肢矯正器具　**ULO**
上肢筋緊張反応　**ATR**
上肢(人工)装具　**ULP**
上肢動脈性の　**UEA**
上(心)室性期外収縮　**SVPC**
上室性期外収縮　**SPB, SVC**
上室性期外心拍　**SVPB**
上(心)室性頻拍　**SVT**
上(心)室性不整頻拍　**SVT**
上室(性)の　**SV**
上斜位　**H, HP**
上斜筋　**SO, SOM**
上斜視　**HT**
上象限　**UQ**
上手にやせる会　**TOPS**
(腸骨の)上前棘　**Ant.sup.spine**
上前棘　**ant.sup.sp.**
上清　**SN**
上側頭静脈　**STV**
上側頭動脈・中大脳動脈　**STA-MCA**
上大静脈　**SVC, VCS**
上大静脈・右肺動脈シャント(術)　**SVC-RPA shunt**
上大静脈圧迫症候群　**SVCCS**
上大静脈症候群　**SVCS**
上大静脈造影　**SVCG**
上大静脈閉塞　**SVCO**
上大静脈閉塞症候群

VCS
上直(筋) **SR**
上直腸動脈 **SRA**
上直筋 **SRM**
上腸間膜静脈 **SMV, VMS**
上腸間膜動脈 **SMA**
上腸間膜動脈血液速度 **SMABV**
上腸間膜動脈症候群 **SMA syndrome**
上腸間膜動脈造影 **SMAG**
上腸間膜動脈塞栓 **SMAE**
上腸間膜動脈閉塞(症) **SMAO**
上腸間膜動脈(血)流量 **SMAF**
上腸間膜の **SM**
上殿神経 **SGN**
上内 1/4 区(＝四半部) **UIQ**
上(方)の **sup, SUP, sup.**
上半規管 **SSC**
上半身エルゴメーター **UBE**
上背部 **UB, Ub**
上肺動脈 **PAS**
上発光顕微鏡 **ELM**
上皮 **EP, ep, EPI, epith**
上皮異形成症 **ED**
上皮抗原 **EA**
上皮細胞 **EC, EPC, EP cell, epith, ep's**
上皮細胞間の **IE**
上皮細胞膜抗原 **EMA**
上皮小体 **PTG**
上皮小体活動係数 **PAI**
上皮小体(機能)亢進(症) **HPT, HPTH**
上皮小体(機能)亢進性ホルモン **HPTH**
上皮小体腺 **PTA**
上皮小体抽出物 **PTE**
上皮小体摘出 **PTX, PTx**
上皮小体の **PT**
上皮小体ホルモン **PT, PTH**
上皮小体ホルモン関連蛋白 **PTHrP**
上皮小体ホルモン分泌 **PTHS**
上皮小体ホルモン様物質 **PTLS**
上皮性腫瘍 **ET**
上皮成長因子 **EGF**
上皮成長因子受容体〔レセプター〕 **EGFR, EGF-R**
上皮内外陰部腫瘍 **VIN** Ⅲ
上皮内癌 **CIS, IEC**
上皮内腫瘍 **TIS**
上皮内の **IE**
上皮内白血球 **IEL**
上皮内扁平病変 **SIL**
上皮内リンパ球 **IEL**
上皮の **EP, ep, EPI, epith**
上皮病巣形成単位 **EFFU**
上皮由来弛緩因子 **EpDRF**
上皮様の **EP**
上鼻静脈 **SNV**
上鼻側 1/4 区 **SNQ**
上鼻動脈 **SNA**
上部 **US**
(長骨の)上部 1/2(区) **U/2**
(長骨の)上部 1/3(区) **U/3**
上部胃腸の **UGI**
上部気道 **URT**
上部気道感染(症) **URI**
上部気道感染症 **URTI**
上部気道疾患 **URD, URI**
上部胸骨縁 **USB**
上部脛骨切り術 **UTO**
上部呼吸器 **URT**
上部呼吸器疾患 **URD, URTI**
上部呼吸器の **UR**
上部歯間の **IdS**
上部消化管 **UGIT**
上部消化管 X 線検査 **upper GI series**
上部消化管撮影 **upper GI**
上部消化管出血 **UGIB**
上部消化管(X 線)造影 **UGIS**
上部消化管内視鏡 **GIF, GTF**
上部消化(管)出血 **UGIH**
上部消化(管)の **UGI**
上部食道 **UE**
上部食道括約筋 **UES**
上部食道括約筋圧 **UESP**
上部食道括約筋弛緩 **UESR**
上腹部 **epigast, ER**
上腹部手術 **UAS**
上腹部の **epig, SA**
上腹部不定愁訴 **NUD**
上方管理限界 **UCL**
上方注視 **UG**
上方プリズム基底 **BU**
上葉 **UL**
上葉肺水腫 **ULPE**
上(方)輪部角結膜炎 **SLK, SLKC**
上腕 **AE, OA, UA**
上腕囲・胸囲・身長 **ACH**
上腕ギプス **OAG**
上腕筋囲 **AMC**
上腕骨 **hum., humer**

上腕骨橈骨(骨)癒合症 **HRS**
上腕三頭筋部の脂肪の厚さ **TSF**
上腕静脈切開 **V.s.B.**
上腕神経炎 **BN**
上腕動脈(圧) **BA**
上腕動脈(血)圧 **BrAP**
上腕動脈圧 **BAP, P_{BA}**
上腕動脈経由による脳血管撮影 **BGA**
上腕動脈造影法 **BAG**
上腕の **br, branch**
少菌型 **PB**
少女 **gal**
少数 **dec**
少数の **dec**
少数の小水泡性ラ音 **RL_1**
少量 **LD, sm.amts**
少量群 **LDG**
(治療薬を)少量ずつ頻繁に投与せよ **csc**
少量注射 **SVP**
少量に **frust.**
少量の **ex paul**
少量ヘパリン **LDH**
正午 **M, m., N**
(医師)生涯教育認定評価プログラム **CEARP**
成就指数 **AQ**
床上安静 **BR**
抄録 **ref.**
抄録化と目録化 **A & I**
条件 **cond, condn**
条件回避反応 **CAR, CER**
条件刺激 **CS, SC**
条件情動反応 **CER**
条件詮索反射 **COR**
条件詮索反射聴力検査 **CORA**
条件詮索反応聴力検査 **COR(-audiometry)**
条件付け **C**
条件付け場所嗜好(試験) **CPP**
条件反射 **cond.ref, CR**
条件反応 **cond.resp., CR**
条虫(属) **T**
状況は正常で間違いはすべて直っている **SNAFu**
状態 **cond, condn, st**
状態・特性不安質問検査 **STAI**
状態密度 **DOS**
承諾 **Co**
承諾された **OK**
承認された品質標準 **aql**
昇圧量 **PD**
昇華 **subl**
昇華した **subl, subl.**
昇華する **subl, subl, subl.**
松果体 **epiph, PI**
松果体芽腫 **PB**
松果体性腺症候群 **PGS**
省 **Dept, dept**
省略 **ABB, abbr**
乗じる **X**
乗法 **X**
消炎性コルチコイド **AC, APC**
消化 **dig.**
消化エネルギー **DE**
消化可能な蛋白 **DP**
消化管 **GIT, GI tract**
消化管間移動複合 **IMC**
消化管感染 **GII**
消化管間葉系腫瘍 **GIST**
消化管関連リンパ系組織 **GALT**
消化管出血 **GIH**
消化管端・端吻合 **EEA**
消化管内視鏡 **GIF**
消化管ホルモン **GIH**
消化管リンパ装置 **GALS**
消化器癌 **GICA**
消化器癌抗原 **GICA**
消化器系 **GIS**
消化器系学会の合同学術集会 **DDW**
消化器腫瘍 **GIT**
消化器病 **DD**
消化吸収率 **CD**
消化させる **dig.**
消化しにくいデンプン **RS**
消化障害 **indig**
消化性潰瘍 **PU**
消化性潰瘍疾患 **PUD**
消化不良 **dysp, indig**
消失時間 **DT**
消失率 **PDR**
消退型異型組織球増殖(症) **RAH**
消毒 **disin**
消毒薬 **disin**
消費者安全担当官 **CSO**
消費者保護と環境健康サービス **CPEHS**
消費性凝固障害 **CC**
消耗症 **MAR**
消耗するまで使う **UUE**
症候 **SS, S & S, sx & sx**
症候群 **synd**
症候作因試験 **sycate**
症候性血小板減少性紫斑病 **STP**
症候性低血糖(症) **SH**
症候性尿路感染(症) **SUTI**
症候性溶血性貧血 **SHA**
症状 **CS, SM, ss, Sx, sx, Sym, sym, symp, sympt**
症状・徴候調査票 **SSI**
症状再調査 **Rev of Sym, ROS, RS**
症状質問票 **SQ**

症状チェックリスト SCL
症状評点試験 SRT
症状評点尺度 SRS
症例 c, Cs, cs
症例検討会 CC
症例対照研究 CCS
症例治療検討会 CTC
症例の今までの経過 CH
症例ファイル CF
症例報告書 CRF
症例報告書の変更・修正記録 CLF
笑気(ガス) N_2O
笑気エーテル麻酔 GOE
笑気フローセン麻酔 GOF
笑気ペントレン麻酔 GOP
商 Q
商業的性労働者 CSW
商品価値なし NCV
商品名 n.p.
商標 TM
章 CH, Ch, ch, chap
紹介医 ref.doc, Ref.Dr, ref.phys
紹介された ref
紹介する ref
常温正常気圧 NTP
常規の指示 RO
常習者 AD
常染色体性優性魚鱗癬 ADI
常染色体優性遺伝多発性嚢胞性腎疾患 ADPKD
常染色体(性)優性の AD
常染色体劣性遺伝 AR
常染色体劣性遺伝多発性嚢胞腎 ARPKD
常染色体劣性遠位型筋ジストロフィ ARDMD
常染色体劣性の AR
常体温 abs.feb.
常同性行動 SB
常法で m.s.
常法に従って L.A., l.a.
常法に従ってつくれ f.l.a., F.L.A
常法によりつくれ FSA, f.tl.a., ft.s.a.
常用式(重量) avdp, avoir
常用式重量 PC
常用式ポンド lb av.
常用者 AD
常用ソフトコンタクトレンズ DWSCL
情意領域 A
情緒 emot
情緒的に EM
情緒の emot
情緒不安定性格疾患 EUCD
情緒不安定パーソナリティ〔人格〕障害 EPD
情動 emot
情動因子 EF
情動指数 EQ
情動疾患クリニック ADC
情動障害 ED
情動的に EM
情動の emot
情報 inf, inf., info, infor
情報 DNA I-DNA
情報検索 IR
情報交換用米国標準コード ASCII
情報収集自由法 FOIA
情報・生産・システム IPS
情報伝達実験 INTREX
情報伝達リボ核酸 iRNA, mRNA
情報内容 IC
情報なし NI
情報ネットワークシステム INS
掌蹠爪下黒色腫 PPSM
掌蹠爪下粘膜黒色腫 PSM melanoma
掌蹠膿疱症 PPP
焼灼術 caut
焼灼する caut
焼灼法 caut
焦性の ust.
焦性ブドウ酸 BTS
焦点 foc
(レンズの)焦点距離 F
焦点距離 f, FD, F.D., FL
焦点形成単位 FFU
焦点の f, foc
焦点皮膚間距離 TSD
焦点皮膚距離 FHA, FHD
(X 線写真の)焦点フィルム間距離 FSD
焦点フィルム間距離 FFD
硝酸銀 $AgNO_3$
硝酸セルロース cell nitr
硝酸の nitr.
硝酸ペルオキシアセチル PAN
硝子円柱 HC
硝子細胞 HC
硝子体過形成遺残 PHV
硝子体螢光光度測定(法) VF
硝子体混濁 OCV
硝子体出血を伴う増殖性糖尿病網膜症 PDRc̄VH
硝子体切除(術) vit
硝子体注入吸引カッター VISC
(眼の)硝子体(液)の Vit, vit, vitr, vitr, vitr.
硝子体網膜脈絡膜症 VRCP
硝子(体)の V

し

証拠　evid, prf
証拠文書　doc
証書　chiro
証明された　C, CERT, Cert, cert, cert.
証明されたように　i.q.e.d.
証明書　CERT, Cert, cert, cert., CTF
証明する　CERT, Cert, cert, cert.
象徴的な　symb
猩紅熱　SF
傷害　dam, inj
傷害する　inj
傷害なし　FOD
傷害(年月)日　DI, D/I, DOI
傷心の　WD, wd
照射　rad, rad., radn
照射関連好酸球増多症　RRE
照射危険域　RDZ
照射効果情報局　REIC
照射する　rad, rad.
照射当量人体模型吸収　remab
照射放出刺激による紫外線増幅　UVASER
照射野　fd
蒸解　dig.
蒸留酒　Spir., spir.
障害　dis, disord, dist, dx, impair, objn, obs
障害(のある)　hcap, HCAP, hcp, HCP
障害された　impair, sev
障害されていない　int, int.
障害者のための歯科学院　ADH
障害調整生存年数　DALY
障害調整平均余命　DALE
静注ヒスタミン試験　IHT
静(脈)注(射)薬物乱用(者)　IVDU
静注用免疫グロブリン製剤　IVIG
(大腿)静動脈バイパス(術)　VAB
静脈　V, v, v., VV, Vv, vv., VV, Vv, vv.
静脈・静脈血液濾過　VVH
静脈・静脈吻合〔術〕　VVA
(上強膜)静脈圧　Pv
静脈圧　VBP, VP
静脈圧上昇　↑VP
静脈圧低下　↓VP
静脈移植鼓膜形成(術)　VGM
静脈インピーダンス体積(変動)記録法　VIP
静脈栄養法　PN
静脈拡張　VD
静脈拡張なし　NVD
静脈確保(せよ)　KVO
静脈還流　VR
静脈空気塞栓症　VAE
静脈(直)径比　VDR
静脈血　V, v, VB
静脈血液ガス　VBG
静脈血凝固時間　VCT
(混合)静脈血酸素飽和度　Svo_2
静脈酸素分圧　PvO_2
静脈周囲脳脊髄炎　PVE
静脈充満時間　VFT
静脈静脈短絡路　VV
静脈静脈バイパス　VVB
静脈侵襲　v
静脈伸展　VE
静脈性血栓塞栓症　VTE
静脈性腎盂造影　IP
静脈性腎盂造影(法)　IP
静脈性閉塞性性機能障害　CVOD
(経)静脈性尿路造影〔撮影〕法　IVU
静脈性毛細血管　VC
静脈切開　cutdown, Vene.Sek., Vs, VS
静脈切開(術)　CD
静脈穿刺　VP
静脈帯状疱疹免疫グロブリン　ZIG-V
静脈体積(変動)記録器　VP
静脈洞　SV
静脈洞欠損症　SVD
静脈内 Rh 免疫グロブリン　RhIGIV
静脈内局所交感神経遮断　IRS
静脈内局所麻酔　IRA
静脈内心電図　IVECG
静脈内注射　IV
静脈内(急速)点滴腎盂撮影(法)　DIVP
静脈内の　IV
静脈内ブドウ糖負荷試験　IGTT, IVGTT
静脈内平滑筋腫　IVL
静脈内免疫グロブリン　IGIV
静脈内輸液　IVT
静脈二酸化炭素圧　PV_{CO_2}
静脈の　V, v, Ven, ven.
静脈バイパス移植　VBG
静脈(弁)不全　VI
静脈不全症候群　VIS
静脈閉塞(性)疾患　VOD
静脈閉塞体積(変動)記録法　VOP
静脈(血)ヘマトクリット　VH
静脈用ピギーバック

IVPB
静脈瘤　**VX**
静脈瘤性潰瘍　**VU**
静脈瘤内注入　**IVI**
静脈瘤内注入法　**IV**
静脈瘤の　**var**
静脈瘤様腫脹　**var**
静脈(血)レニン濃度　**VRC**
静脈路確保　**IV route**
衝撃　**Impx**
衝撃変動　**IM**
衝突活性化分離法　**CAD**
衝突誘起の解離　**CID**
衝動　**D, IMPL**
漿状　**dpl.**
漿液　**S, ser**
漿液血液状の　**serosang**
漿液(性)の　**ser**
漿剤　**MUC**
(胚膜の)漿膜　**S**
漿膜下　**ss, SS**
漿膜下層組織深達度　**ss, SS**
漿膜層表面浸潤　**s**
(滑液)鞘　**Vagg**
鞘　**V, VAG, Vag, vag.**
錠(剤)　**tabs, tbl, Tbl**
錠剤　**cp, TAB, tab, tab., Tab.**
錠剤になった　**t**
踵脛(検査)　**H → S, HTS**
踵膝(検査)　**HTK**
踵膝(試験)　**HK, H-K**
踵・膝蓋骨　**HP, H → P**
食(事)　**cib.**
食塩感受性　**ss**
食塩水　**SA, SAL, sal.**
食塩水依存凝集素　**SDA**
食塩水浣腸　**SSE, SS enema**
食塩水注射　**SI**
食塩水注入　**SI**
食塩添加した　**SA**
食塩の　**S**
食塩無添加　**NAS**
食間薬　**BM**
食後　**n.d.E, n.d.E.**
食後２時間の(血糖値)　**2HPP**
食後血糖　**PPBS**
食後に　**p.c., post cib.**
食後の　**Pp**
食後服用　**n.d.E.z.n.**
食細胞刺激因子　**PSF**
食細胞指数　**PI**
食事　**C, c., c, c., prand.**
食事間隔　**IMI**
食事サービス　**FS**
食事室　**DR**
食事性蛋白摂取　**DPI**
食事性白血球増加(症)　**VL**
食事と再梗塞の実験　**DART**
食事誘発性熱源　**DIT**
食前　**v.d.E**
食前と就寝時　**AC & HS**
食前に　**AC, a.c.**
食中毒　**FP**
食直後　**stat.p.c.**
食堂　**DR**
食道　**E, ES, Eso, esoph, oesoph**
食道・胃・十二指腸　**ESD**
食道圧　**EP**
食道胃管エアウェイ〔気道〕　**EGTA**
食道胃十二指腸内視鏡検査　**EGD**
食道胃上向後枝　**REGAP**
食道胃接合部　**EGJ, EG junction, J**
食道胃切除　**EG**
食道胃粘膜接合部　**Z-line**
食道運動性　**EM**
食道下部　**LES**
食道癌　**ÖeK, ÖK, Ce, EC, EK**
食道静脈瘤圧　**IOVP**
食道静脈瘤止血用チューブ　**SBT, S-B T, S-B tube, SB Tube**
食道静止圧　**EST**
食道体部　**EB**
食道通過時間　**ETT**
食道電気内圧曲線　**EPT**
食道導出〔誘導〕　**VE**
食道内バルーン拡張　**IEBD**
食道内バルーンカテーテル　**EBC**
食道入口部　**O**
食道の　**esoph**
食道破裂　**ER**
食道ファイバースコープ　**EF**
食道噴門接合部　**ECJ, e-c junction, EC-junction**
食道閉鎖式エアウェイ　**EOA**
食品・栄養委員会　**FNB**
食品・殺虫剤・生産物安全局　**BFPPS**
食品・薬品・化粧品条例　**FD & C**
食品・薬品・法律研究所　**FDLI**
食品・薬品研究室　**F & DL**
食品・薬品公務員協会　**AFADO**
食品安全応用栄養センター　**CFSAN**
食品栄養サービス　**FNS**
食品研究活動センター　**FRAC**
食品照射の検知法に関する

研究計画　**ADMIT**
食品助言サービス　**FAS**
食品添加物に関する合同専門家委員会　**JECFA**
食品の危害分析・重要管理点監視方式　**HACCP**
食品法律と薬品情報　**FL & DI**
食物依存性運動誘発アナフィラキシー　**FDEIA**
食物性中毒性無白症　**ATA**
食物摂取　**ingest**
食物繊維　**DF**
食物認識訓練　**FAT**
食欲　**app**
(国連の)食糧農業機関　**FAO**
植物　**Bot, bot.**
植物学の　**Bot, bot.**
植物神経系　**VNS**
植物性栄養研究センター　**VNRC**
植物性血球凝集素　**PHA, PHY, phy**
植物性血球凝集素蛋白　**PHA-P**
植物性血球凝集素ムコ多糖類　**PHA-M, PHA-m**
植物成長物質　**PGS**
植物性ペルオキシダーゼ抑制物質　**VPI**
植物組織蛋白　**TVP**
植物標本室　**Hb**
触診　**palp**
触診・打診・聴診　**PPA, PP & A, pp & a, pp+a**
(眼)触診緊張度　**TT**
触診する　**palp**
触知可能な　**palp**
触媒　**cat, cat.**
触媒定数　**Kc, Kcat, Ko**
触媒量　**z**
褥瘡　**decub., P/sore**
燭　**C, c, ca**
職業　**occ, Occup, occup, pro, Prof, prof**
職業安全　**OS**
職業安全健康活動　**OSHA**
職業医学　**OM**
職業医学学会　**SOM**
職業活動研究　**PAS**
職業興味記入用紙　**VIB**
職業興味質問表　**VIQ**
職業興味スケジュール　**VIS**
職業上不行跡監視局　**OPMC**
職業ストレス症候群　**OSS**
職業性皮膚炎　**OD**
職業選択調査表　**VPI**
職業態度〔意識〕尺度　**JAS**
職業チェックリスト　**OCL**
職業知識テスト　**KOT**
職業適応　**V Ad, Vadj**
職業適応障害症候群　**OMAS**
職業的な　**Prof, prof**
職業的病院活動委員会　**CPHA**
職業の　**Occup, occup, pro, voc**
職業病　**OD**
職業標準審査機関　**PSRO**
職業誘発性ぜん息　**OA**
職業リハビリテーション　**VR**
職業リハビリテーション教育　**VR & E**
職業リハビリテーション局　**DVR**
職業リハビリテーションサービス　**VRS**
職歴　**OH**
食間(に)　**i.c., z.d.E, z.d.E., zw.d.E**
食間間隔　**IMI**
食間に　**int.cib.**
食菌作用　**PC**
触覚振盪音　**TF**
燭光　**CP**
燭光時　**C hr, c hr, chr**
徐脈　**B**
汁　**J, j, jc, jc., suc.**
印　**mrkr**
印なし　**n/m**
印を付けた　**mkd**
白(い)　**W, w**
白い　**alb., wh, wt.**
白黒　**b & w**
白パン単位　**WBE**
人格　**pers**
人格因子　**PF**
人格因子質問票　**PFQ**
人格関係テスト　**PI test, PI-Test**
人格研究用紙　**PRF**
人格障害　**PD, PsD**
人格特性障害　**PTD**
人格評点スケール〔尺度〕　**PRS**
人格要素テスト　**PF, PI test, PI-Test**
人口　**P**
人口・エイズに関する地球規模問題イニシアティブ　**GII**
人口および世論調査局　**OPCS**
人口活動国際連合基金　**UNFPA**
人口寄与危険度割合　**PAR**
人口寄与危険率　**PARP**
人口増加速度　**PGR**

人口相対危険度　**PRR**
人口調査局　**OPR**
人口統計　**demogr**
人口統計学者　**demogr**
人口統計の　**demogr**
人口と環境の審議会　**COPE**
人口のゼロ成長　**ZPG**
人工　**art，art.**
人工栄養乳製品　**CM**
人工換気　**AV**
人工甘味料　**AS**
人工器官　**pros，prosth**
人工器官の　**pros**
人工気胸(法)　**AP**
人工鉱物繊維　**MMMF**
人工硬膜　**DMP**
人工肛門　**Afta**
人工肛門形成(術)　**colost**
人工股関節全置換術　**THR**
人工呼吸　**AR**
人工呼吸器　**RESP，Resp，resp，resp.，V，vent**
人工骨頭置換術　**UHR**
人工膝関節全置換術　**TKR**
人工受精　**art.insem，KB**
人工授精　**AI**
人工心臓　**AH**
人工腎臓　**AK**
人工心臓完全移植　**TIAH**
人工心臓全置換術　**THR**
人工心肺　**AHL**
人工心肺後症候群　**PPS**
人工心肺装置　**PO**
人工膵島　**AEP**
人工足関節全置換術　**TAR**
人工蘇生器　**CPR**
人工太陽灯　**HS**
人工多能性幹細胞　**iPS**
人工知能　**AI**
人工妊娠中絶　**KA**
人工の　**art，art.，artif**
人工破水　**ARM，AROM**
人工ペースメーカーによる心室リズム　**APVR**
人工ペースメーカー誘導心室調律　**APIVR**
人工弁心内膜炎　**PVE**
人工(的)勃起　**AE**
人工流産　**AA**
人種　**R**
人体計測(法)　**anthropom.**
人体内レントゲン当量　**INREM**
人体曝露評価計画　**HEAL**
人体レントゲン線量当量　**REM，rem**
人道的心理学協会　**AHP**
人乳　**BM，MM**
人乳リゾチーム　**HML**
人物画知能検査　**DAM**
人物画テスト　**DAP**
人物描写テスト　**DAP**
人類　**mort，mortal**
人類科学・人種科学国際連合　**UISAE**
人類学　**anthro，Anthrop**
人類学者　**anthro**
心因性夜間多飲　**PNP**
心(臓)移植　**CTx**
心運動亢進症　**HHS，HKH-syndrome**
心運動図　**KCG**
心エコー検査　**ECHO**
心エコー検査のビームの方向　**RAL**
心エコー図　**ECHO，echo，UCG**
心音　**HS，HT，h.t.**
心音図　**PCG，PKG**
心横径　**THD**
心(臓)カテーテル法　**CC**
心外膜　**Epi，EPI**
心外膜の　**EP**
心拡大　**CE**
心拡張期最大充満までの時間　**TPFR**
心窩部　**ER**
心窩部(胃部)不快感症候群　**EDS**
心気症　**Hs**
心気症の　**hypo**
心気症の患者　**hypo**
心(臓)胸郭(比)　**CT**
心胸郭係数　**CTR**
心胸郭比　**CTR**
心胸郭面積比　**CTAR**
心胸比　**C/T**
心筋　**CM**
心筋(層)　**myo，myocard**
心筋βアドレナリン作用性受容体　**MBAR**
心筋エネルギー欠乏状態　**MEDS**
心筋炎　**MC**
心筋炎後心肥大　**PMC**
心筋灌流画像　**MPI**
心筋灌流シンチグラフィ　**MPS**
心筋血流量　**MBF**
心筋梗塞　**MCI，MI，myo inf**
心筋梗塞研究部門　**MIRU**
心筋梗塞後症候群　**PMIS**
心筋梗塞治療法比較大規模試験　**PAMI**
心筋梗塞の血栓溶解　**TIMI**
心筋梗塞の再閉塞予防に関する研究システム　**J-MIC**

心筋梗塞を除外する **ROMI**
心筋酸素(消費) **MO_2**
心筋酸素消費量 **MOC, MVO_2, MVO_2**
心筋疾患 **MD**
心筋収縮状態 **MCS**
心筋収縮力 **MCF**
心筋症 **CM, CMP**
心筋傷害 **MD**
心筋線維症 **MF**
心筋代謝率 **MMR**
心筋内血管新生術 **TMR**
心筋(層)の **myo, myocard**
心筋壁肥厚 **MWT**
心筋抑制因子 **MDF**
心機図 **MCG**
心機能指数 **CFI**
心腔内シャント **IS**
心(臓)血管回復室 **CVRR**
心(臓)血管機能障害スコア **CVD**
心(臓)血管系 **CVS**
心(臓)血管外科(学) **CVS**
心(臓)血管呼吸器(系) **CVR**
心(臓)血管コンピュータ断層撮影 **CVCT**
心(臓)血管疾患 **CVD**
心血管疾患 **CD, VDH**
心血管疾患管理室 **CCU**
心(臓)血管状態 **CV starus**
心(臓)血管腎疾患 **CVRD**
心(臓)血管腎性の **CVR**
心(臓)血管造影法 **CAG**
心血管造影分析システム **CAAS**
心(臓)血管抵抗 **CVR**
心(臓)血管の **cardiov, CV**
心(臓)血管不全 **CVF**
心(臓)血管モニター **CVM**
心係数 **CI**
心原性ショック **CGS, CS**
心原性脳塞栓症 **CBE**
心原性肺水腫 **CPE**
心(臓)交感神経 **CSN**
心(臓)呼吸 **CR**
心(臓)呼吸(器)の **cardio-resp**
心(臓)呼吸(性)の **CR, C-R**
心サイクル **HC**
心雑音 **HM, m**
心仕事 **CW**
心仕事係数 **CWI**
心身医学 **PSM**
心身症 **PSD**
心身障害児童生徒性格診断検査 **PIH**
心身の **psychosom, psy-som**
心身リハビリテーション協会 **APMR**
心(臓)周期 **CC**
心室 **V, v, ven, VENT, vent, ventric**
心室(波) **V**
心室1回仕事量 **VSW**
心室圧波 **VPW**
心室異所性活動 **VEA**
心室異所性脱分極 **VED**
心室異所性不整脈 **VEA**
心室(性)逸脱〔補足〕 **VE**
心室拡張期容積 **VDV**
心室拡張終期圧 **VEDP**
心室拡張終期容積 **VEDV**
心室間孔 **IVF**
心室(性)期外収縮 **PCV**
心室期外収縮 **VBP**
心室(性)期外収縮閾値 **VPCT**
心室(性)期外脱分極 **VPD**
心室機能曲線 **VFC**
心室筋 **VM**
心室筋(重)量 **VM**
心室駆出分画 **VEF**
心室グラディエント **G**
心室勾配 **VG**
心室興奮時間 **VAT**
心室細動 **vent.fib, ventric.fib, VF, Vf, v.f., Vfb, Vfib, V fib.**
心室細動閾値 **VFT**
心室残気量 **VRV**
心室収縮 **VC**
心室収縮終期容積 **VESV**
心室充満(期)圧 **VFP**
心室充満期 **VFD**
心室心房遠位冠(状)静脈洞 **VADCS**
心室心房近位冠(状)静脈洞 **VAPCS**
心室心房ヒス束心電図 **VAHBE**
心室性期外収縮 **PVB, PVC, PVS, VE, VEB, VES, Vp, VPB, VPC, VPS**
心室性不整頻拍 **VT**
心室性不整脈 **VA**
心室早期脱分極 **VDP**
心室粗動 **VF, VFL**
心室弾性 **VE**
心室遅延電位の陽性基準であるフィルター処理後のQRS **FQRS**
心室中隔 **IVS, VS**
心室中隔欠損 **ISD, IVSD**
心室中隔欠損(症) **VSHD**
心室中隔欠損症 **VSD**

し

心室中隔厚　**IS，IVST**
心室中隔振幅　**IVSE**
心室中隔穿孔　**VSP**
心室中隔前部　**IVSA**
心室中隔破裂　**RIVS，VSR**
心室電図　**EVG**
心室伝導速度　**VCV**
心室橈骨異形成(症)　**VRD**
心室橈骨形成異常(症)　**VRD**
心室動脈結合　**VAC**
心室動脈瘤　**VA**
心室動脈瘤切除(術)　**VAN**
心室内伝導障害　**IVCD**
心室内伝導遅延　**IVCD**
心室の　**V，v，VENT，vent，ventric**
心室拍動数　**VR**
心室反応　**VR**
心室頻拍　**VT**
心室頻拍/心室細動　**VT/VF**
心室不整脈モニター(監視装置)　**VAM**
心室ペーシング　**VP**
心室(性)奔馬調律　**VG**
心室容積　**VV**
心室抑制型ペーシング　**VVI**
心室リズム　**VR**
心室律動　**VR**
心室レート　**VR**
心(臓)疾患　**CD，HD**
心疾患　**H**
心(臓)疾患管理室　**CCU**
心(臓)疾患集中治療部〔室〕　**CICU**
心疾患資料連絡協議会　**ICHD**
心疾患歴　**HDH**
心術後症候群　**PCS**
心(臓)循環訓練　**HCT**
心磁図　**MCG**
心(臓)滲出液　**HI**
心尖第１音　**S_1**
心尖拍動　**AB**
心尖拍動図　**ACG，APCG**
心尖部第一音　**M_1**
心尖部第二音　**M_2**
心尖部肥大　**APH**
心(臓)促進中枢　**CAC**
心(臓)損傷後症候群　**PCIS**
心(臓)蘇生(術)　**CR**
心(臓)蘇生チーム　**CRT**
心臓　**H，HT**
心臓・肝臓・腎臓　**HLK**
心臓・肺・腹　**HLA**
心臓足首血管指数　**CAVI**
心臓移植　**HT，HTX**
心臓横径　**TCD**
心臓外来モニター部門　**CAMU**
心臓(病)学　**CARD，card，cardio，Cardiol，cardiol，CARDOOL**
心臓危険指数　**CRI**
心臓キモグラフ　**CKG**
心臓キモグラフ法　**CKG**
心臓外科　**CAS**
心臓外科集中治療部〔室〕　**CSICU**
心臓後間腔　**RCR**
心臓細胞条件下培地　**HCM**
心臓縦(直)径　**LD**
心臓手術後　**PCS**
心臓神経症　**CN**
心臓性急死症候群　**SCDS**
心臓性の　**C**
心臓性不整脈抑制治験　**CAST**
心臓性不調律　**CD**
心臓絶縁　**CF**
心臓先天(性)奇形　**CMH**
心臓(血管)造影(法)　**ACG**
心臓同種移植片動脈硬化(症)　**CAA**
心臓と肺　**H & L**
心臓と肺正常　**H & L OK**
心臓内注射　**ICI**
心臓内の　**IC，i card**
心臓(病)(性)の　**card**
心臓の　**reg.cor.**
心臓反応因子　**HRF**
心臓病　**HD**
心臓病学認定書　**Dip.Card.**
心臓病専門医　**cardiol**
心臓リハビリテーション　**CR**
心(膜)タンポナーデ　**PT**
心弾動図　**BCG，BKG**
心弾動図(法)　**BCG**
心濁音域右縁　**RBCD**
心濁音界　**CD**
心濁音界左縁　**LBCD**
心濁音界左下縁　**LLBCD**
心濁音界右下縁　**RLBCD**
心注　**ICI**
心停止　**CA**
心電気図　**RCG**
心電計　**ECG，EKG**
心電図　**CEG，ECG，EK，EKG**
心電図Ｑ波開始からＩ音節開始までの時間　**QI**
心電図解析標準　**CSE**
心電図上の反応　**ECR**
心電図信号の平均二重表出　**SPAES**
心電図対数　**ECL**
心電図(検査)法　**ECG**
心電図用右腕電極　**VR**
心動作不整　**DAH**
心動図　**MCG**

心(臓)内カテーテル記録(法)　**ICR**
心内血栓　**ICT**
心内膜　**End, END**
心内膜炎　**EC**
心内膜下心筋梗塞　**SEMI**
心内膜下心筋損傷　**SEMI**
心内膜活性率　**EVR**
心内膜床欠損(症)　**ECCD, ECD**
心内膜心筋線維症　**EMF**
心内膜切除術　**ER**
心内膜線維弾性症　**ECFE, EF, EFE**
心内膜の　**EN, endo**
心嚢液貯留　**PE**
心拍/呼吸　**PR, P/R**
(1回)心拍出係数　**SI**
(分時)心拍出量　**$\dot{Q}$t**
心拍出量　**CO, Q, SBF**
心拍出量/心係数　**CO/CI**
心拍数　**bpm, HF, HR, HRT**
心拍数範囲　**HRR**
心拍同期特定時の撮影　**synchro**
心拍動と同期した身体加速　**BAAH**
心拍変動　**HRV**
心肺運動負荷試験　**CPX**
心肺(同時)移植　**H-L Tx**
心肺係数　**HLR**
心肺血(液)量　**CPBV**
心肺蘇生(法)　**HLR**
心肺蘇生術　**CPR**
心肺蘇生のABC(気道確保・呼吸・循環)手順　**ABC**
心肺停止(状態)　**CPA**
心肺の　**CP, CR, C-R**
心肺脳蘇生術　**CPCR**
心肺脳蘇生法　**CCPR**
心肺バイパス　**CPB**
心肺予備力　**CPR**
心(室)肥大　**VH**
心ブロック　**HB**
心不全　**card.insuff, CF, CI, HF**
心(臓)弁膜症　**VDH**
心房　**A, A**
心房・心室の　**A/V**
心房・ヒス束時間　**AH interval**
心房圧　**PA**
心房拡張期駆馬音　**ADG**
心房(性)期外収縮　**PAS**
心房頸動脈の　**AC**
心房細動　**AF, Af, AFI, AFib, A fib., At Fib, at.fib., ATR FIB, atr.fib., AUR FIB, aur.fib.**
心房細動における脳卒中予防　**SPAF**
心房細動予防研究　**SPFA**
心房(性)収縮期雑音　**ASM**
心房心室同期型(ペースメーカー)　**DDD**
心房心室ユニバーサルペーシング　**DDD**
心房性T波　**Ta-wave**
心房性期外収縮　**AES, APB, APC, APCs, PAB**
心房性収縮波　**A waves**
心房性早期収縮　**APS**
心房性ナトリウム利尿因子　**ANF**
心房性ナトリウム利尿ペプチド　**ANP**
心房性ナトリウム利尿ポリペプチド　**ANP**
心房性頻拍　**AT**
心房性奔馬性(リズム〔律動〕)　**AG, ag**
心房性有効不応期　**AERP**
心房粗動　**AF, AFL**
心房中隔　**AS, IAS**
心房中隔一次孔欠損　**ASD-Ⅰ**
心房中隔欠損　**ASHD, ISD**
心房中隔欠損(症)　**IASD**
心房中隔欠損症　**ASD**
心房中隔切除術　**ASR**
心房中隔二次孔欠損　**ASD-Ⅱ**
心房中隔瘤　**IASA**
心房調律　**AP**
心房電図　**EAG**
心房同期型心室ペーシング　**VAT, VDT/I**
心房同期型ペースメーカー　**ASVIP**
心房内伝導障害　**IACD**
心房内の　**IA, i.a.**
心房の　**aur., auric**
心房の・頸動脈の・心室の　**ACV**
心房不全　**AI**
心房弁狭窄　**AS**
心房抑制型ペーシング　**AAI**
心膜　**Peri**
心膜液　**PF**
心膜液培養　**PFC**
心膜気腫　**PPC**
心膜叩打音　**PKS**
心膜切除後症候群　**PPS**
心(機能)抑制中枢　**CIC**
心(臓)抑制中枢　**CIC**
心容積　**HV**
心(臓)容量　**CV**
心(臓)リハビリテーション部(病棟)　**CRU**
心理学　**Psy, psy, Psych, psych, PSYCHOL, psychol.**
心理学研究協会　**PRA**

心理学士 **B.Ps., B.Psych., M.Ps**
心理学資格認定書 **D.Psy.**
心理学者協会 **AP**
心理学的情報収集処理管理法 **PIAPCS**
心理学的スクリーニング調査票 **PSI**
心理学的ストレス評価器械（＝ウソ発見器） **PSE**
心理学博士 **D.Psy.Sci.**
心理劇 **PD**
心理作戦 **PSYOP**
心理分析進歩のための協会 **AAP**
心理療法 **psychother**
心理療法進歩のための協会 **AAP**
心(臓)/体重(比) **H/BW**
仁形成域 **NOR**
申請後 **p.a.**
迅速血漿レアギン(テスト) **RPR**
迅速血漿レアギンカードテスト **RPRCT**
迅速交代蛋白 **RTP**
迅速不活性型 **R**
迅速分別染色 **DQ**
迅速攣縮性解糖の **FG**
迅速攣縮性酸化解糖の **FOG**
伸筋 **ext, ext., extens**
伸縮性ポリテトラフルオロエチレン **EPTFE, E-PTFE**
伸長因子 **EF**
伸張式食道ステント **EES**
伸展 **Dil, dil., E, ext, ext., extens**
伸展した **extd**
伸展時における内旋 **IRE**
伸展時の外旋 **ERE**
伸展する **ext, ext.**
伸展性・速度・酸素化・圧 **CROP**
伸展反応 **SR**
伸展指先 **OSFT**
身障者用ペンション **DP**
身体 **B**
身体傷害 **BI**
身体障害児・成人全国協会 **NSCCA**
身体障害児援助協会 **AACC**
身体障害者 **HP, phys.dis**
身体障害者組織学会 **COPH**
身体障害者のための器具研究委員会 **CRAD**
身体障害者用電話 **HC telephone**
身体障害のある **'cap**
身体的作業能力 **PWC**
身体的特性 **PP**
身体的な **PHY**
身体に **corp.**
身体に関する教育 **Phys ed**
身体の **som, somat**
身体表現障害スクリーニング **SSD**
身体表現性障害スケジュール **SDS**
身体ヘマトクリット/静脈血ヘマトクリット(比) **bh/vh**
身長 **BL, H, h, Hgt, Ht, KL**
身長/体重(比) **H/BW**
身長年齢 **HA**
信号 **Sig, sig**
信号・雑音(比) **S/N**
信号・雑音比 **SNR**
信号吸収値 **SAR**
(細胞内)信号伝達と転写活性因子 **STAT**
信号レベル **SL**
信頼期間 **CIs**
侵襲性活性検査 **IAT**
侵襲性腺管癌 **IDC**
侵入門 **PE, PofE**
神経 **N, n, N, n., ner, ner., nn., Ns**
神経アレルギー症候群 **NAS**
神経因子 **N**
神経因性膀胱 **NGB**
神経因性膀胱機能障害 **NBD**
神経炎 **neur**
神経温存根治前立腺切除術 **NSRP**
神経科医 **neurol**
神経外胚葉腫瘍 **NET**
神経学 **N, neur, Neuro, neurol**
神経学専門医 **N**
神経学的改善 **NI**
神経学的チェック **NC**
神経学的年齢 **NA**
神経学の **neuro, neurol**
神経芽細胞腫 **NB**
神経下垂体ホルモン **NHH**
神経活動電位 **NAP**
神経管欠損〔欠陥〕 **NTD, NTDs**
神経顔面指臀(症候群) **NFDR**
神経筋異形成症 **NMD**
神経筋緊張 **NMT**
神経筋緊張状態 **NMTS**
神経筋興奮亢進 **NMH**
神経筋遮断薬 **NMBA**
神経筋制御 **NMC**
神経筋接合部 **MNJ, NMJ**
神経筋単位 **NMU**
神経筋電図法 **ENMG**
神経筋伝達 **NMT**

神経筋伝達遮断　**NMTB**
神経筋の　**MN，NM**
神経筋紡錘　**NMS**
神経系　**NS**
神経系腫瘍　**NT**
神経系肉芽腫性血管炎　**GANS**
(脳)神経外科(学)　**Neuro-Surg**
神経外科(学)　**NSurg，N.Surg**
(脳)神経外科医　**Neuro-Surg，NS**
神経外科医　**N surg**
神経外科検査　**NSX**
神経外科集中治療室　**NICU**
(脳)神経外科の　**NS**
神経外科の　**N surg**
(脳)神経外科病棟　**NSU**
神経血管圧迫症候群　**NVC**
神経血管減圧手術　**NVD**
神経血管束　**NVB**
神経血管の　**NV**
神経元アポトーシス抑制蛋白　**NAIP**
神経原性肺水腫　**NPE**
神経原線維塊　**NFT**
神経原線維変性　**NFD**
神経効果器接合部　**NEJ**
神経膠腫条件下培養基　**GCM**
神経膠腫由来成長因子　**GDGF**
神経行動コアテストバッテリー　**NCTB**
神経行動評価システム　**NES**
神経興奮　**NE**
神経興奮性(検査)　**NE**
神経興奮性検査　**NET**
神経根　**NR**
神経根炎　**rad，rad.**
神経根刺激　**NRI**
神経根の　**rad，rad.**
神経細線維　**NF**
神経細胞栄養物　**NCF**
神経細胞カドヘリン　**NCD**
神経細胞接着分子　**N-CAM**
神経細胞増殖因子受容体　**NGFR**
神経細胞特異的蛋白　**NSP**
神経細胞遊走障害　**NMD**
神経弛緩鎮痛　**NLA**
神経弛緩薬(性)悪性症候群　**NMS**
神経質　**ner，ner.，nerv，neur**
神経疾患集中治療室　**NICU**
神経疾患治療部門　**NCU**
神経疾患のリハビリテーション用短下肢装具　**AFO，SLB**
神経質尺度質問　**NSQ**
神経支配　**innerv**
神経支配された　**innerv**
神経遮断麻酔(法)　**NLA**
神経終板電流　**EPC**
神経終末　**NE**
神経循環失調症　**NCD**
神経循環性無力症　**NCA**
神経症　**N，neurs**
神経障害　**N**
神経鞘腫　**NN**
神経症性うつ病(状態)　**ND**
神経症性うつ病反応　**NDR**
神経上皮　**NE**
神経小胞機能不全　**NVD**
神経心理学(的)検査　**NPE**
神経衰弱　**neur**
神経性過食症　**BN**
神経性筋萎縮　**NMA**
神経性食思不振症　**AN**
神経性食欲不振症　**anorex**
神経精神医学　**neuropsychiat，NP**
神経精神医学研究所　**NPI**
神経精神医学の　**NP**
神経精神科の臨床評価計画　**SCAN**
神経性進行性筋萎縮症　**NPMA**
神経精神疾患研究協会　**ARNMDI**
神経性生活徴候　**NVS**
神経性セロイドリポフスチノーシス　**NCL**
神経成長因子　**NGF，NTF**
神経成長刺激活性　**NGSA**
神経性難聴　**ND**
神経生理学の　**neurophys**
神経節　**G，gang，gangl，Ggl，Ggll**
神経接合部外膜アセチルコリン受容体　**EJR**
神経節後の　**postgangl.，post gangl.**
神経節細胞　**GC**
神経節遮断薬　**GBA**
神経節の　**gang，gangl**
神経線維腫症　**NF**
神経線維鞘　**neu**
神経線維層　**NFL**
神経線維層欠損　**NFLD**
神経組織ワクチン　**NTV**
神経堤　**NC**
神経堤腫瘍　**NCT**
神経的検査　**NE**
神経的適応能力スコア　**NACS**
神経電図(検査)法　**ENG**

神経伝導速度　**NCV**
神経伝導速度検査　**NCVS**
神経と筋肉　**N & M**
神経特異エノラーゼ　**NSE**
神経毒性エステラーゼ　**NTE**
神経と循環　**N & C**
神経内科　**Neuro**
神経内科医　**N**
神経内分泌細胞　**NEC**
神経内分泌体　**NEB**
神経内分泌の　**NE**
神経(質)の　**ner, ner., nerv**
神経(症)の　**neuro**
神経梅毒　**NS**
神経発達的治療　**NDT**
神経反射性失神　**NMS**
神経病理学　**Neuropath, NP**
神経病理学者　**Neuropath**
神経分泌顆粒　**NSG**
神経分泌細胞　**NSE**
神経分泌の　**NS**
神経分泌物質　**NSM**
神経ペプチド　**NP**
神経麻痺　**NP**
神経脈管圧迫　**NVC**
神経網膜　**NR**
神経葉　**NL**
神経幼虫移行症　**NLM**
神経(学的)老人学　**N-Ger**
唇口症候群　**COS**
唇切縁の　**LAI, LaI**
唇側歯頸の　**LAC, LaC**
唇側歯肉の　**LAG, LaG**
振戦　**TH, thr, tr**
振戦痴呆　**dt's**
振戦麻痺　**PA**
振戦せん(＝譫)妄　**DT, DTs, Dt's, dt's**
振動　**VIB, vib, vib.**
振動・音刺激試験　**VAST**
振動工具病　**PHD**
振動数/秒　**cps, c/s, VPS, vps, v.p.s.**
振動する　**osc, vib**
振動性後電位　**OAP**
振動の　**vib**
振動白(色)指　**VWF**
振動秒　**v.s.**
振幅　**am, am., amp**
(声の)振幅動揺指数　**APQ**
振幅変調　**AM**
振幅変調と周波数変調の比　**am/fm**
侵入防止システム　**IPS**
浸液に　**ad baln.**
浸剤　**inf., INF, Inf, inf**
浸剤をつくれ　**ft.infus.**
浸漬せよ　**M**
浸潤　**INF**
浸潤癌　**IC**
浸潤性小葉癌　**ILC**
浸潤性腺管癌　**IDC**
浸潤度　**INF**
浸水足　**IF**
浸透　**Osm, osm, osm.**
浸透圧　**OP**
浸透圧クリアランス　**Cosm**
浸透圧推進物質　**ODA**
浸透圧脆弱性　**OF**
浸透圧赤血球強化　**OEE**
浸透圧当量　**Osm, osm, osm.**
浸透圧モル　**osmol**
浸透性活性物質　**OAS**
浸透制限充填剤　**RAM**
浸透性神経外胚葉腫瘍　**PNET**
浸透性神経外胚葉腫瘍・髄芽(細胞)腫　**PNET-MB**
浸透の　**Osm, osm, osm.**
浸軟　**mac.**
真核細胞開始因子　**eIF**
真空(化)　**v, vac**
真空管　**VT**
真空管電圧計　**VTVM**
真空吸引(法)　**VA**
真空紫外線　**VUV**
真空ツベルクリン　**VT, V.T.**
真空で　**i vac**
真空内の　**i vac**
真結合線　**CV**
真珠腫　**chole**
真性グロブリン溶解　**ECL**
真性グロブリン溶解時間　**ECLT, ELT**
真性細網肉腫　**THL**
真性赤血球増加　**PRV**
真性赤血球増加(症)　**PV**
真性赤血球増加症　**PCV**
真性早熟　**TPP**
真性肺動脈弁閉鎖症　**PPA**
真総肺活量　**TTLC**
真皮　**Cor**
真沸騰点　**TBP**
陣痛・分娩・回復・(出)産後　**LDRP**
陣痛室　**LR**
陣痛と出産　**L & D, L+D**
深胃・縦断の　**DG-L**
深吸気時気管支拡張　**BFDI**
深呼吸　**DB**
深在脈　**DP**
深指屈筋　**FDP**
深睡眠　**DS**
深達性II度熱傷　**DDB**
深達度が漿膜下層の癌　**ss, SS**

深達度が漿膜(＝s)の癌　S
深達度が粘膜下層の癌　sm, SM
深腸骨回旋動脈　DCIP
深部X線治療　DXRT
深部X線　DXR
深部腱反射　DTR
深部散乱層　DSL
深部静脈血栓症　DVT
深部(海)水温温度測定器　BT
深部脳刺激　DBS
深部脳波　DEEG, depth EEG
深部脳波検査(法)　DEEG
深部皮膚熱傷　DDB
深部(線)量　E_d
深部量百分率　PDD
深夜　mdnt
進化　evol
進学適性検査　SAT
進学適性知能検査　SAIT
進行型ダニ媒介脳炎　PFTBE
進行した　adv.
進行した乳癌　ABC
進行する　progr
進行性外眼筋麻痺　PEO
進行性塊状線維症　PMF
進行性核上性麻痺　PSP
進行性核性眼筋麻痺　PNO
進行性感音性難聴　PPD, P.P.D.
進行性球麻痺　PBP
進行性筋萎縮症　PMA
進行性筋ジストロフィ　DMP
進行性筋ジストロフィ症　PMD
進行性広汎性白質脳症　PDL
進行性骨化性多発筋炎　POP
進行性指掌角化症　KTPP
進行性小〔細〕静脈周囲アルコール性線維症　PPAF
進行性自律神経不全　PAF
進行性神経性筋萎縮症　PNMA
進行性膵炎　ADP
進行性脊髄失調　PSA
進行性脊髄性筋萎縮症　PSMA
進行性全身性硬化症　PSS
進行性全身麻痺　PGP
進行性多巣性白質ジストロフィ　PML
進行性多巣性白質脳症　PML
進行性蓄積ストレス　PAS
進行性透析脳症　PDE
進行性の　prog
進行性脳卒中　SIE
進行性肥厚性間質性神経炎　PHIN
進行性皮質下血管脳症　PSVE
進行性風疹全脳炎　PRP
進行性ミオクローヌスてんかん　PME
進行速度　SOA
進行なし　NP
進行麻痺　PP
進展　evol
進歩した冠(状)動脈治療　ACT
進歩した生命情報システム　ALIS
診査　Ex, ex, exam, expl
診査医　ME
診査開腹　exp.lap
診査する　expl
診査切除　Probe
診査穿刺　Probe
診査掻爬　Probe
診査の　expl
診察衣　oa
診察〔検査〕されずに帰った　LWBS
診察時血圧　OBP
診察で　OE
診断　D, DG, dg, Diag, diag., DX, Dx, dx
診断学的面接基準　DIS
診断画像　DI
診断関連グループ　DRG
診断群分類包括評価　DPC
診断群別定額支払方式　DRG/PPS
診断計画　D
診断されない　ND
診断情報システム　DIS
診断する　DG, dg, diag
診断センター　DC
診断的印象　Dx Imp
診断的機能検査　DFT
診断的腹腔洗浄法　DPL
診断(上)の　DG, dg, diag
診断不可能　GOK
診断報告信頼性　RDR
診断未確定　DU
診断未決定　DU
診断予想適応症　SID
診療　prac
診療科　MD
診療記録管理者　MRA
診療所　CL, Cl, CLIN, Clin, clin., Disp., disp., INF, inf
診療短時間予約　MSA
診療保険特別会計　SMI

尋常性魚鱗癬　**IV**
尋常性天疱瘡　**PV**
尋常性疣贅(＝ゆうぜい)　**VV**
靱帯　**L, Lgt, lgt., lgts, Lig, lig, lig., ligg, ligg., ligs**
靱帯の　**musc.ligt, mus-lig**
新医薬品再審査申請のための市販後調査実施に関する基準　**GPMSP**
新医薬品承認審査概要　**SBA**
新患(者)　**NP**
新規経口抗凝固薬　**NOAC**
新教徒(の)　**P**
新抗原決定基　**NAD**
新種　**nov SP, nov.sp., n.sp, sp.n., sp.nov.**
新生血管　**NV**
新生児　**NB**
新生児・満期・正常・男　**NBTNM**
新生児・満期・正常・女　**NBTNF**
新生児一過性高アンモニア血症　**THAN**
新生児一過性多〔頻〕呼吸(症)　**TTN, TTNB**
新生児壊死性全腸炎　**NNE**
新生児壊死性腸炎　**NEC**
新生児エリテマトーデス　**NLE**
新生児黄疸　**IN**
新生児肝炎　**NH**
新生児期　**INF, inf, inf.**
新生児期家族性永続性高インスリンによる低血糖症　**FHHI**
新生児胸腺切除　**NTx**
新生児禁断症候群　**NAS**
新生児空気漏出症候群　**NAS**
新生児行動評価規準　**NBAS**
新生児行動評価法　**NBAS**
新生児呼吸窮迫症候群　**IRDS**
新生児呼吸困難症候群　**NRDS**
新生児自己免疫性血小板減少症　**NAT**
新生児自己免疫性血小板減少性紫斑病　**NATP**
新生児室　**NBN**
新生児紫斑病　**MMN**
新生児死亡　**ND, NND**
新生児死亡率　**NDR, NMR, NNM**
新生児重症副甲状腺機能亢進症　**NSHPT**
新生児集中(治療)　**NB Int**
新生児集中治療　**ICN, NIC**
新生児集中治療管理室〔施設〕　**NICU**
新生児集中治療センター　**NICC**
新生児集中治療部　**NICU**
新生児集中治療部〔病棟〕　**NBICU**
新生児出血　**HN**
新生児出血性疾患　**HDN**
新生児術後痛判定用スコア　**CRIES**
新生児(期)胆汁うっ滞　**NC**
新生児単純ヘルペス　**HSN**
新生児チアノーゼ　**CN**
新生児低カルシウム血症　**NHC**
新生児同種免疫性血小板減少症　**NAIT**
新生児特殊治療部　**NSCU**
新生児吐血　**HN**
新生児(期)の　**NN**
新生児の　**neo, neonat**
新生児膿痂疹　**IN**
新生児肺高血圧残存　**PPHN**
新生児剝脱性皮膚炎　**DEN**
新生児副腎白質ジストロフィ　**NALD**
新生児ブドウ球菌性疾患　**NSD**
新生児麻酔薬禁断症候群　**NNAS**
新生児メレナ　**MN**
新生児溶血性疾患　**HDN, MHN**
新生児狼瘡症候群　**NLS**
新生物　**neopl, NG**
新生物随伴症候群　**PNS**
新生物性疾患　**ND**
新生マウス流行性下痢症ウイルス　**EDIM virus**
新赤血球産生刺激蛋白　**NESP**
新鮮液状血漿　**FP**
新鮮ガス流　**FGF**
新鮮血清　**FS**
新鮮水　**fw, f.w.**
新鮮水傷害　**FWD**
新鮮凍結血漿　**FFP**
新鮮凍結の　**FF**
新鮮な　**rc.**
新鮮薬草の　**herb.recent.**
新属　**gen.nov.**
新ツベルクリン　**TR**
新投薬様式　**NDF**
新版　**NE**
新非薬局方薬物　**NND, NNR**
新薬　**ND**

新薬許可出願　**NDS**
新薬調査　**IND**
新薬適用　**NDA**
腎(臓)移植　**RT**
腎(臓)移植(術)　**KT**
腎移植(片)　**KT**
腎移植後膵移植　**PAK**
腎盂腎炎　**PN**
腎盂腎杯系　**NBKS**
腎盂尿管移行部　**PUJ**
腎盂尿管接合部　**UPJ**
腎盂尿管(移行部)の　**PU**
腎炎　**neph**
腎炎因子　**NEF, NF**
腎下被膜効力検定　**SRC**
腎芽細胞腫　**NB**
腎機能検査　**RFS**
腎クリアランス　**RCL**
腎血管圧　**RVP**
腎血管障害　**RVF**
腎血管性高血圧(症)　**RVH**
腎血管抵抗　**RVR**
腎血管抵抗指数　**RVRI**
腎血漿流量　**RPF**
腎血流量　**RBF**
腎原性環状アデノシンーリン酸　**NcAMP**
腎経皮経管動脈形成(術)　**RPTA**
腎結核症・腎髄質嚢胞病　**NMCD**
腎硬化(症)　**NS**
腎細胞癌　**RCC**
腎糸球体基底膜疾患　**RGBMT**
腎昇圧物質　**RPS, VEM**
腎(臓)重量　**KW**
腎疾患　**RD**
腎疾患集中治療室　**KICU**
腎疾患に続発する高血圧(症)　**HSRD**
腎症候性出血熱　**HFRS**
腎静脈　**RV**
腎静脈圧　**RVP**
腎静脈血漿レニン活性　**RVPRA**
腎静脈血栓症　**RVT**
腎静脈血レニン比　**RVRR**
腎静脈の　**RV**
腎静脈レニン　**RVR**
腎静脈レニン定量法　**RVRA**
腎静脈レニン濃度　**RVRC**
腎髄質嚢胞症　**MCD**
腎切除(術)　**nep**
腎性高血圧ラット　**RHR**
腎性骨異栄養症　**ROD**
腎性全身性線維症　**NSF**
腎性造血因子　**REF**
腎性尿崩症　**NDI**
腎造影撮影法　**NG**
腎造影〔撮影〕図　**NEPHRO**
腎臓　**K**
腎臓移植患者　**RTP**
腎臓専門医　**RS**
腎臓提供者　**KD**
腎臓排泄　**RE**
腎臓病学　**NEP, NEPH**
腎(臓)蛋白　**KP**
腎(臓)治療　**KT**
腎澄明細胞肉腫　**CCSK**
腎摘出術　**nep**
腎毒性血清　**NTS**
腎毒性血清(性)腎炎　**NSN**
腎毒性抗体　**NTA**
腎毒性腎炎　**NTN**
腎(臓)特異(的)蛋白　**KSP**
腎動脈　**RA**
腎動脈圧　**RAP**
腎動脈狭窄　**RAS**
腎動脈造影　**RAG**
腎内逆流　**IRR**
腎尿細管壊死　**RTN**
腎尿細管抗原　**RTA**
腎尿細管細胞　**RTC**
腎尿細管上皮細胞　**RTE**
腎尿細管性アシドーシス　**RTA**
腎(臓)の　**REN**
腎(臓)パンチ　**KP**
腎(臓)パンチ検査　**KPT**
腎杯　**K**
腎排泄係数　**REI**
腎排泄率　**RER**
腎不全　**RF**
腎分画　**RF**
腎(臓)・肝(臓)・脾臓　**KLS**
腎・肛門・肺・外指・過誤芽腫(症候群)　**RALPH**
腎(臓)・尿管・膀胱　**KUB**
腎(臓)・尿管および脾臓　**KUS**
塵肺症　**pneumoultra**
滲出液　**eff, exud, WOFL**
滲出性中耳炎　**EOM, OME, SOM**
滲出線　**EL**
震純音　**WPT**
蕁麻疹　**UT**
親近感・包容力・協調力・持続力・責任能力　**ACCCA**
親水性・親油性数　**HL number**
親水性・親油性バランス　**HLB**
親水性/親油性(数)　**HL**
親水性/親油性(比)　**H/L**
親水性相互作用クロマトグラフィ　**HILIC**
親水軟膏　**HO**
親密　**rap**
親密な　**Int**
親和性定数　**pA_2**

し

す

スイカ状の胃　**WS**
スイス救急飛行隊　**SAR**
スイス(型)無γグロブリン血症　**SAG**
スウェーデン老年者高血圧降圧薬有用性調査　**STOP**
スカベンジャー受容体　**SR**
スカンジウム　**Sc**
スカンジナビアシンバスタチン臨床試験　**4S**
スカンジナビアの　**Scand**
スカンジナビア薬局方　**CMS**
スギ花粉抗原　**SBP**
スギ花粉症　**CP**
スギ花粉症抗原　**CPAg**
スクアレン　**SQ**
スクシニル(基)　**suc**
スクシニルコリン　**SCC, SCH, sch, SUX**
スクシニルジコリン　**SDC**
スクシニル補酵素A　**succinyl CoA**
スクシノデヒドロゲナーゼ　**SUDH**
スクラルフェート(＝ショ糖硫酸エステルアルミニウム塩)　**SCR**
スクリーニング細菌尿　**ScBU**
スクリーン濾過圧　**SFP**
スクループル　**S, s, scp, SCR, scr, scrup**
スケジュール　**sched, sked**
スケジュール変更　**SC**
スコポラミン　**SCOP, scop**
スズ　**Sn**
スズメバチ毒　**YJV**
スター・エドワーズ弁　**SE valve**
スタイン・レベンタール(症候群)　**SL**
スタイン・レベンタール症候群　**SLS**
スタージ・ウェーバー(症候群)　**SW**
スタージ・ウェーバー症候群　**SWS**
スタッフ能力開発　**SD**
スタヒロコッカス(属)　**S, STAPH, staph, Staph.**
スタントン数　**St**
スタンフォード・ビネー(知能試験)　**SB, S-B**
スタンフォード・ビネー知能尺度　**SBIS**
スタンフォード催眠感受性尺度　**SHSS**
スタンフォード知能テスト　**SIT**
ズダンブラックB染色　**SBB**
スチュアート・プラウアー因子　**SPF**
スチルブ　**sb**
スチール様毛髪症候群　**SHS**
スチレンリンゴ酸ネオカルチノスタチン　**SMANCS**
ステアリン酸　$\mathbf{C_{18=0}}$
ステアリン酸アルミニウムの油性結晶ペニシリン　**PAM**
スティックラー症候群　**SS**
スティッフマン症候群　**SMS**
スティーブンス・ジョンソン(症候群)　**SJ, S-J**
スティーブンス・ジョンソン症候群　**SJS**
ステージ特異的胎児抗原　**SSEA**
ステラジアン　**sr, sterad**
ステルンベルグ・リード(細胞)(＝多核巨細胞)　**SR**
ステロイド依存性喘息　**SDA**
ステロイド過敏ネフローゼ症候群　**SSNS**
ステロイド結合血漿(蛋白)　**SBP**
ステロイド受容体　**SR**
ステロイドスルファターゼ　**STS**
ステロイド抵抗性拒絶(反応)　**SSR**
ステロイド抵抗性喘息　**SRA**
ステロイド反応性ネフローゼ症候群　**SRNS**
ステロイドホルモン　**SH, STH**
ステロイド離脱症候群　**CWS**
ステンセン管　**SD**
ステンレス鋼歯冠　**SSCr**
ストーク　**St**
ストークス・アダムス(症候群)　**SA**
ストークス・アダムス発作　**SAA**
ストップ　**STOP**
ストマイ　**SM**
ストーマ療法(士)　**ET**
ストラチャン・スコット(症候群)　**SS**
ストリキニン　**STC**
ストレージプール病　**SPD**

ストレス後エタノール消費 **PSEC**
ストレス心電図検査法 **SECG**
ストレス(性)(尿)失禁 **SI, SUI, USI**
ストレスによる無痛覚症 **SIA**
ストレス方式 **SF**
ストレス誘発感覚脱出 **SIA**
ストレッチングあくび症候群 **SYS**
ストレートバック症候群 **SBS**
ストレプトアビジン **SA**
ストレプトキナーゼ **SK, STK**
ストレプトキナーゼ・ストレプトドルナーゼ **SKSD, SK/SD**
ストレプトキナーゼ活性化 **SAK, SKA**
ストレプトコッカス(属) **S, SC, STR, str., STREP, Strep, strep., strept., streptoc.**
ストレプトゾ(ト)シン糖尿病 **SZD**
ストレプトゾシンの頻回投与による真性糖尿病 **MDSDM**
ストレプトゾ(ト)シン **STZ, SZ**
ストレプトゾ(ト)シン,マイトマイシン,フルオロウラシル **SMF**
ストレプトドルナーゼ **SD**
ストレプトドルナーゼストレプトキナーゼ **SD-SK**
ストレプトニグリン **SM**
ストレプトバシラス(属) **S**
ストレプトマイシン **S, SM, STM, strep**
ストレプトマイシンとイソニコチン酸ヒドラジド **SH**
ストレプトミセススブチリシンインヒビター **SSI**
ストレプトリジン **SL**
ストレプトリジンO **SLO**
ストレプトリジンS **SLS**
ストレプトリジンS血清抑制因子 **SISS**
ストロボスコープ **strobo**
ストロボスコープで計測された **strobed**
ストロボスコープで照明された **strobed**
ストローマ吸着防御抗原 **SAPA**
ストロンギロイデス(属) **S**
ストロンチウム **Sr**
ストロンチウム単位 **SU**
スネレン表 **SC**
スーパーオキシドジスムターゼ **SD, SOD**
スーパーファミリー **SF**
スパルフロキサシン **SPFX**
(最大拡張時の手親指小指間の)スパン **DS**
スピーカー **SP, spkr**
スピラマイシン **SPM**
スピリルム(属) **S, Sp**
スピロノラクトン **SC8109**
スピロヘータ(属) **Spir.**
スピロメトラ(属) **S**
スピンエコー法 **SE**
スピン免疫(測定)法 **SI, SIA**
スフィンゴミエリン **SM, SPH**
スプレーグ・ドーリー(ラット) **SD**
スプーン半分 **c.medium**
スプーンとフォーク **spork**
スペイン系アメリカ人 **SA**
スペイン語(の) **Span**
スペイン国際放射線医学センター **CIRM**
スペイン人(の) **Span**
スペクチノマイシン **SPCM**
スペクト **SPECT**
スペクトル心電図 **SPCG**
スベドベリ浮上定数 **SF units**
スペルミジン **SPD, Spd**
スペルミン **Sp, Spm**
スポーツ医学 **SM**
スポット形成細胞 **SFC**
スポロトリクム(属) **S**
スポロトリクム症 **SPORO**
スポロトリックス(属) **S**
スマック **SMAC**
スミス・ピーターセン(釘) **SP, S-P**
スミス・レムリ・オピッツ症候群 **SLOS**
スミス表面抗原 **SSA**
ズーム **zm**
スムーズ型 **S form**
スムースラフミューテイション **SRM**
スモールアウトラインパッケージ **SOP**
スモン(病) **SMON**
スライク **sl**
スライス **sl**
スライドラテックス凝集試

験 **SLAT**
スリット脳室症候群
SVS
ズルジャー・オグデン(症候群) **ZO**
スルタミシリン **SBTPC**
スルバクタム **SBT**
スルバクタム・セフォペラゾン **SBT/CPZ**
スルファ剤 **SF**
スルファサラジン **SSA**
スルファジメトキシン
SDM
スルファチアゾール **ST**
スルファニルアミド(=スルホンアミド)
SNM, sulfa
スルファメトキサゾール
SMX, SMZ, STX
スルファメトキサゾールトリメトプリム
SMX/TMP, ST
スルファメトキシピラジン
SMP
スルファルスフェナミン
Sar
スルフイソキサゾール
SI, SIX, SSX
スルフイソミジン **SID**
スルフィンピラゾン
SPZ
スルフヒドリル **SH**
スルフヒドリル基 **SH**
スルフヘモグロビン
SHB, S Hb
スルホコハク酸ジオクチルナトリウム **DOSS, DSS**
スルホサリチル酸 **SSA**
スルホニル尿素 **SU**
スルホプロピル **SP**
スルホベンジルペニシリン(=スルベニシリン)
SBPC
スルホリシノレイン酸
SRA
スルホンアミド(=スルファニルアミド) **SA**
スルホンアミド抵抗(性)の
SR
スルホン酸ポリエチレン
PES
スレオニン **T**
スローン・ケタリング研究所 **SKI**
スローン・ケタリング記念癌センター **MSKCC**
スワイヤー・ジェームス症候群 **SJS**
スワン・ガンツカテーテル
SG, SGC, SG cath
すぐさま **stat., Stat**
すたれた **obs, obs., OBS, Obs**
すなわち **ie, i.e., sc., viz, viz.**
すべての **q.q.**
ずり応力応答成分
SSRE
ずり(応力)惹起血小板凝集
SIPA
すりつぶす **conter**
吸わせよ **sug.**
吸わせるべき **sugend.**
好きなだけ **q.l., q.pl.**
図 **Abb., Abbild, diag, fig, IL, Il, il, ill, illus**
図解 **IL, Il, il, ill, illus**
図解された **il**
図解した **illus**
図解する **il**
図示された **il**
図示する **il**
図式的投影法 **SPT**
図表 **dia**
図表生物医学文献システム
ABLS
据え置きにした **def**
酢 **A, acet.**
澄んだ **cl, clr**
頭上 **OVH**
頭痛 **HA**
頭痛・不眠・うつ(症候群)
HID
頭痛単位係数 **HUI**
水温 **WT**
水化 **Hyd.**
水解小体 **L**
水解輸送 **HRT**
水銀 **Hg, Hydrarg, Hydrarg.**
水銀-2-水酸化プロパン
MHP
水銀柱 **Hg**
水銀の還元・気化原子吸光分析 **CVAAS**
水剤をつくれ **ft.m.**
水酸化イオン **OH-**
水酸化エチルメタクリレイト **HEMA**
水酸化カリウム **KOH**
水酸化酵素 **OHlase**
水酸化肪脂酸 **HFA**
水酸化ステロイド脱水素酵素 **HSD**
水酸化ナトリウム
NaOH
水酸化物 **OH**
水酸化プロゲステロン
OHP
水酸化リチウム **LiOH**
水酸化リン灰石 **HAP**
水酸基 **OH**
水晶 **Xtal**
水晶体 **L**
水晶体基底膜 **LBM**
水晶体後部線維増殖症
RLF
水晶体超音波乳化吸引術
PEA
水晶体(核)摘出(術) **LE**
水晶体乳化 **PE**
水晶体囊外摘出術 **ECCE**

水晶体嚢内摘出術　**ICCE**
水晶微量天秤法　**QCM**
水腫　**E，ed**
水腫肺症候群　**WLS**
水蒸気飽和状態　**ATPS**
水蒸気飽和状態の体温と大気圧　**BTPS**
水質汚染管理　**WPC**
水質汚染管理活動　**WPCA**
水生生物研究室　**ABL**
水性懸濁液　**AS**
水性の　**A，a，AQ，aq，aq.，aqu**
水製エキス　**extr.aq.**
水素　**H**
水素1(＝プロチウム)　**^{1}H**
水素2　**^{2}H**
水素3　**^{3}H**
水素イオン　**H^{+}**
水素イオン指数　**pH，P_{H}**
水素イオン濃度　**cH^{+}，[H^{+}]**
水素炎イオン化検出器　**FID**
水素発生原子吸光分析　**HGAAS**
水中油型　**O/W**
水中油中水型乳剤アジュバント　**WOW**
水柱センチメートル　**cmAq，cmH_2O**
水(分)貯留　**WR**
水痘　**Chix，chpx.，ch.px，Cp，V**
水痘帯状疱疹　**VZ**
水痘帯状疱疹ウイルス　**VZV**
水痘帯状疱疹免疫グロブリン　**VZIG，VZIg**
水痘生ワクチン　**LVV**
水筒　**WB**
水道水　**aq.font.**
水頭症・無脳回(症)・網膜形成異常〔異形成〕　**HARD**
水熱分解同時誘導体化法　**SHD**
水分出納　**IN.OUT**
水分制限　**FR**
水分貯留　**FR**
水分貯留係数　**WRC**
水分補給　**Hyd.**
水平(の)　**hor**
水平外転/内転　**HAb/HAd**
水平可視光彩径　**HVID**
水平(性)眼振　**ny.hor**
水平軸　**x-axis**
水平の　**H，horiz**
水平面　**H，hor**
水疱　**mal.**
水疱形式で　**mal.**
水疱性口峡炎　**HA**
水疱性口内炎　**VS**
水疱性口内炎ウイルス　**VSV**
水疱性類天疱瘡　**BP**
水薬の1服量　**h.**
水溶液　**AS**
水溶性アジュバント　**WSA**
水溶性抗生物質　**WSA**
水溶性食物繊維　**SDF**
水溶性の　**WS**
水溶性プロカインペニシリンG　**APPG**
水様下痢・低塩酸・低カリウム血・アルカローシス　**WDHHA**
水様下痢・低カリウム血症・無胃酸(症候群)　**WDHA**
水様下痢・低カリウム血症・無塩酸(症候群)　**WDHH**
水様下痢症候群　**WDS**
水様の　**A，a**
水力学的な　**Hydr，Hydr.**
水力学的平衡カプセル　**HBC**
水力学的平衡系　**HBS**
水力振盪症　**HC**
水力の　**Hydr，Hydr.**
吸取紙　**chart bib.**
垂直　**perp，V**
垂直(性)圧迫　**vert.comp.，vert.compr.**
垂直型アクリルアミドゲル電気泳動　**V-PAGE**
垂直(性)眼振　**ny.vert**
垂直照射断層撮影(法)　**VRT**
垂直性亜脱臼　**VS**
垂直選択的な　**VS**
垂直帯胃形成術　**VBG**
垂直の　**perp，V，vert**
垂直輪異形成(術)　**VRG**
衰弱　**AT，debil.，MAR**
衰弱した　**debil.**
衰弱性壊疽　**decub.**
(膵)島細胞　**IC**
推奨1日摂取量　**RDI**
推薦　**rec，recomm，Recomm**
推薦する　**rec，recomm，Recomm**
推測　**calc，caln**
推測する　**calc**
推定運動単位　**MUE**
推定学習能力　**ELP**
推定肝血流量　**EHBF**
推定乾燥重量　**EDW**
推定クレアチニンクリアランス　**ECC**
推定在胎月齢　**EGA**
推定された　**est**
推定糸球体濾過量　**eGFR**
推定重量　**est wt**
推定受胎日　**EDC**
推定出血量　**EBL**

す

推定出産日　**EDOC**
推定胎児体重　**EFW**
推定入院期間　**ELOS**
推定分娩日　**EDL**
推定平均値　**GA**
随意的可動範囲　**VROM**
随意的努力　**VE**
随意的な　**vol**
随意の　**Opt，opt，opt.，voly**
随意不妊協会　**AVS**
随時読出し可能メモリ　**RAM**
随伴陰性変動　**CNV**
随伴染色体　**SAT chromosome**
睡眠　**Sl**
睡眠開始 REM（＝レム）期　**SOREMP**
睡眠開始後覚醒　**WASO**
睡眠覚醒リズム・見当識・体動〔言動〕・要求〔訴え〕　**SOAD**
睡眠過剰・睡眠時無呼吸（症候群）　**HSA**
睡眠関連呼吸障害　**SRBD**
睡眠時間　**HS，SPT**
睡眠時周期性運動　**PMS**
睡眠時代謝率　**SMR**
睡眠時電気的てんかん重延状態　**ESES**
睡眠時無呼吸　**SA**
睡眠時無呼吸過眠症候群　**SAHS**
睡眠時無呼吸症候群　**SAS**
睡眠時無呼吸不眠症候群　**SAIS**
睡眠障害国際分類　**ICSD**
睡眠障害性呼吸　**SDB**
睡眠障害センター連合　**ASDC**
睡眠精神生理研究協会　**APSS**
睡眠潜時反復検査　**MSLT**
睡眠相後退　**DSP**
睡眠相遅延不眠症　**DSPS**
睡眠促進物質　**SPS**
睡眠段階変化頻度　**SSCF**
睡眠の開始と持続障害　**DIMS**
睡眠発現レム期　**SOREMP**
睡眠ポリグラフ検査　**PSG**
睡眠ポリグラム　**PSG**
睡眠薬　**SM**
膵アミラーゼ　**PA**
膵胃吻合　**PG**
膵炎関連蛋白質　**PAP**
膵液　**PJ**
膵液蛋白　**PJP**
膵からのインスリン分泌量　**AIEP**
膵管　**PD**
膵管充填　**DI**
膵管胆道合流異常　**AAPABIDS**
膵管内超音波検査（法）　**IDUS**
膵癌　**PC，PCA，PK**
膵癌関連抗原　**PCAA**
膵癌胎児抗原　**POA**
膵機能検査　**PFT**
膵機能診断〔テスト〕　**PFD**
膵空腸吻合　**PJ**
膵腎同時移植　**SPK**
膵静脈　**PV**
膵切除された　**PX**
膵石蛋白　**PSP**
膵全摘（出）術　**TP**
膵臓　**PANC**
膵臓機能不全　**PI**
膵臓の　**pancreat**
膵臓抑制試験　**PST**
膵単独移植　**PTA**
膵胆管の　**PB**
膵抽出物　**PE**
膵トリプシン抑制因子　**PTI**
膵島活性化蛋白　**IAP**
膵島細胞移植術　**PICT**
膵島細胞癌　**ICC**
膵島細胞抗体　**ICA，ICAb**
膵島細胞腫瘍　**ITP**
膵島細胞膜抗体　**ICSA**
膵島腺腫アミロイドポリペプチド　**IAPP**
膵頭十二指腸切除　**PD**
膵頭部癌　**PKK**
膵（臓）嚢性線維症　**CFP**
膵尾部切除術　**DP**
膵分泌性トリプシン抑制因子　**PSTI**
膵ペプチド　**PP**
膵ポリペプチド　**PP**
膵由来ヒトインスリン　**PHI**
膵ランゲルハンス島細胞質抗体　**ICCA**
膵リパーゼ　**PL**
膵攣縮寛解ポリペプチド　**PSP**
錐体　**PYR**
錐体外路系　**EPS**
錐体外路症候（学）　**EPS**
錐体外路症候群　**EPS**
錐体外路症状　**EPS**
錐体外路チロキシン　**ETT**
錐体外路副作用　**EPSE**
錐体隆起　**PE**
錐体路　**PT**
錐体路ニューロン　**PTN**
錐内線維筋　**IFM**
（脳脊）髄液　**C，CSF，LCR，LCS**
髄液　**SF，Syn FI**
（脳脊）髄液圧　**CSFP，CSP**

髄液細胞数算定　**SFC**
髄液の　**syn，synov**
(脳脊)髄液ワッセルマン反応　**CSF-WR**
髄外動静脈奇形　**EAVM**
髄芽腫　**MB**
髄核ヘルニア　**HNP，NPH**
髄腔内注射　**IT**
髄腔内注入　**EL**
髄腔内の　**ITh**
髄索性組織球性細網症　**HMR**
髄条　**SM**
髄軸の　**PA**
髄質外層集合管　**OMCD**
髄質集合尿細管　**MCT**
髄質性海綿腎　**MSK**
髄質内層集合管　**IMCD**
髄鞘　**myel**
髄鞘(＝ミエリン)関連糖蛋白　**MAG**
髄線　**med ray**
髄線実質　**med ray par**
髄内釘固定法　**IMN**
髄内動静脈奇形　**IAVM**
髄内の　**IM**
髄膜　**men，mening**
(脳脊)髄膜炎　**CSM**
髄膜炎　**men，mening，mgtis，syn，synov**
髄膜炎菌　**Nm**
髄膜癌腫症　**MC**
髄膜菌性(脳脊)髄膜炎　**MM**
髄膜血管の　**MV**
髄膜腫　**M，Men**
(脳脊)髄膜の　**men，mening**
髄膜脳炎　**ME**
髄膜白血病　**ML**
髄膜脈管の　**MV**
髄様癌　**MC**
数学　**math，math**
数学的な　**math，math**
数学(上)の　**math，math**
数滴ずつ　**gutt.quibusd.**
皺襞　**P**
皺襞細胞指数　**FI**
趨化力　**CA**
優れた　**exc**
鈴木万能微細印象法＝スンプ法　**SUMP**
砂袋　**SB**
鋭い　**SH**
鋭い/鈍い　**S/D**
座っている　**sitg，sttg**
寸法　**dim，dim.**

す

せ

ゼアチン **Zea**
セクレチン **SEC**
セクレチンテスト **S test**
セクレチンパンクレオザイミン検査 **SPT**
セクレチン様免疫反応性 **SLI**
セコナール **Sec**
セザリー症候群 **SS**
セシウム **Cs**
セシウム 129 ^{129}**Cs**
セシウム 131 ^{131}**Cs**
セ氏 **C, CEL, Cel, Cels**
セスタン・シュネ(症候群) **CC**
ゼータ赤血球沈降速度 **Z-ESR**
ゼータ沈降速度率〔比〕 **ZSR**
セチルトリメチル塩化アンモニウム **CTAC**
セチルトリメチル臭化アンモニウム **CTAB**
セービン・フェルドマン(色素試験) **SF**
セービン・フェルドマン(色素)試験 **SFT**
セファクロル **CCL**
セファセトリル **CEC**
セファゾリン **CEZ, CZ**
セファタメトピボキシル **CEMT-PI**
セファトリジン **CFT**
セファドロキシル **CDX**
セファピリン **CEP, CEPR**
セファマンドール **CMD**
セファマンドル **CMO**
セファランチン **Ceph**
セファリンコレステロール架状〔綿状〕試験 **CCF test**
セファリンコレステロール架状〔綿状〕反応 **CCF**
セファリンコレテロールレシチン架〔綿〕状反応 **CCLF**
セファリン架状〔綿状〕検査 **ceph floct**
セファレキシン **CEX**
セファログリシン **CEG**
セファロスポリン **CEP**
セファロスポリン系抗生物質 **CEPs**
セファロチン **CET, CF, CR**
セファロリジン **CER**
セフィキシム **CFIX**
セフェム系抗生物質 **CEP**
セフォジジム **CDZM**
セフォチン **CET**
セフォペラゾン **CPZ**
セフジニル **CFDN**
セフスロジン **CFS**
セフゾナム **CZON**
セフタジジム **CAZ**
セフチゾキシム **CZX**
セフチブテン **CETB**
セフテゾール **CTZ**
セフテラムピボキシル **CFTM-PI**
セーブトライアル **SAVE**
セフトリアキソン **CTRX**
セフピミゾール **CPIZ**
セフピラミド **CPM**
セフピラミドナトリウム **CPM**
セフピロム **CPR**
セフブペラゾン **CBPZ**
セフポドキシムプロキシチル **CPDX-PR**
セフミノクス **CMNX**
セフメタゾール **CMZ**
セフメノキシム **CMX**
ゼブラ小体 **ZB**
セフラジン **CED, CER**
セフロキサジン **CXD**
セフロキシム **CXM**
セフロキシムアキセチル **CXM-AX**
セブンスデイ教派 **SDA**
セホキシチン **CFX**
セホタキシム **CTX**
セホチアム **CTM**
セホチアムヘキセチル **CTM-HE**
セホテタン **CTT**
セボフルラン **S**
セミコロン **sem**
セムリキ森林ウイルス **SFV**
セメント質エナメル質境界(線) **CEJ, cej, c.e.j.**
セメント質骨化線維腫 **COF**
セラチア(属) **S**
ゼラチン **gel**
ゼラチン・亜テルル酸塩・タウロコール酸塩 **GTT**
ゼラチン凝集試験 **GAT**
ゼラチンの **gel**
ゼラチンベロナール緩衝液 **GVB**
ゼラチン粒子凝集(法) **PA**
セラミック製人工耳小骨 **CORP**
セラミド **CER, Cer**
セラミドジヘキソシド **CDH**
セラミドトリヘキソシド **CTH**
セリアックスプルー **CS**
セリウム **Ce**
ゼリーに混入して

gel.quav.
セリル　Ser
セリン　S, Ser, ser
セリングリセロホスファチド　SGP
セリン蛋白質分解酵素阻害因子　Serpins
セリンデヒドラーゼ　SDH
セリンヒドロキシメチルトランスフェラーゼ　SHMT
セル・プロセッシング・センター　CPC
セルレイン・セクレチン試験　CS-T
セルロース　cell
セルロースアセテート　CA
セルロースアセテート電気泳動法　CAEP
セルロースアセテート膜上のコロニー形成単位　CFU-ML
セルロースアセテート膜(免疫)電気泳動法　CAM
セルロースアセトプロピオン酸　CAP
セルロースイオン交換体　CIDS
セルローストリアセテート　CTA
セルロプラスミン　Cp, CP, CRPL
セレニウム75　^{75}Se
セレン　Se
セレン含有蛋白糖(類)　SEPS
ゼロ　nil., Z
セロイド・リポフスチン症　CLF
ゼロックス放射線図　XR
ゼロ低価　0-L
セロトニン・ノルアドレナリン再取込み阻害薬　SNRI
セロトニン運搬蛋白　SERT
セロトニン結合蛋白　SBP
セロトニン作働性神経　SN
セロトニンド(ー)パミン拮抗薬　SDA
セロトニンのベンジル同族体　BAS
ゼロ発射　ZD
ゼロ頻度　ZF
ゼロラジオグラフィ　XR
ゼロラジオグラフィ装置　XR
セングスターテン・ブレークモア管　S-B tube, SB Tube
セングステークン・ブレークモア管　SBT, S-B T
センチ(=10−2)　c
センチグラム　Cg, cg, cg., cgm, cgm., cnt, ct gr
センチストーク　cSt
センチポアズ(=1/100ポアズ)　cP, cp.
センチメートル　cent, cent., CM, cm
センチメートル/秒　cmps, cm/s, cm/sec
センチメートルグラム秒　CGS, cgs, c.g.s.
センチモルガン　cM, cmo
センチリットル　cl
セントルイス脳炎　SLE
セントルイス脳炎ウイルス　SLEV
セイント・ジュード医学弁　SJM
セカンドオピニオン　SO
センター　ctr
センダイウイルス　HVJ
せき　tus.
せきの発作時　tuss.urg.
せん(譫)妄による行動学的異常を評価する基準　DRS
世界医師会　AMM, WMA
世界医事法学会　WMLA
世界医療援助　WMR
世界エイズ・結核・マラリア対策基金　GFATM
(WHO)世界エイズ対策計画　GPA
世界解剖・臨床病理学会　WASP
世界核医学連盟　WFNMB
世界家庭医学会議　WONCA
世界環境開発委員会　WCED
世界環境問題情報局　OMIPE, WOIEP
世界気候観測計画　WCRP
世界気象機関　WMO
世界血友病学会　WFH
世界健康財団連合　FWHF
世界健康統計年報　WSA
世界公衆衛生協会連盟　WFPHA
世界作業療法学連盟　WFOT
世界獣医解剖学協会　AMAV, WAVA
世界獣医家禽学協会　WVPA
世界獣医師会　WVA
世界獣医学史協会　WAHVM
世界獣医寄生虫学協会　WAAVP

世界獣医食品衛生学協会　**WAVFH**
世界獣医生理学・薬理学・生化学協会　**WAVPPB**
世界獣医微生物学・免疫学・伝染病学協会　**WAVMI**
世界獣医病理学協会　**WAVP**
世界集中治療医学会　**WCICCM**
世界集中治療医学会連合　**WFSICCM**
世界消化器内視鏡学会　**OMED**
世界消化器内視鏡学会アジア太平洋分科会　**OMED AP**
世界消化器病学会　**OMGE**
世界小動物獣医学協会　**WSAVA**
世界小児外科学会連盟　**WFAPS**
世界食糧計画　**WFP**
世界神経学連合　**FMN**
世界神経学連盟　**WFN**
世界神経放射線学会連合　**WFNRS**
世界身体障害者機構　**WOIH**
世界性科学学会　**WAS**
世界精神医学連合　**WPA**
世界精神衛生連盟　**WFMH**
世界精神健康連合　**FMSM**
世界対癌連合　**IUAC**
世界大衆薬製造協会　**WFPMM**
世界超音波医学学術連合　**WFUMB**
世界知的所有権機関　**WIPO**
世界治療連盟　**WFH**
世界的な　**univ**
世界的に　**univ**
世界標準委員会　**COWS**
世界物理療法学会　**WCPT**
世界貿易機関　**WTO**
世界保健機関　**OMS, WGO, WHO**
世界保健総会　**WHA**
世界麻酔学会連合　**WFSA**
世界薬学史学会機構　**UMHP**
世界予防接種助言者会議　**GAG**
世界リハビリテーション基金　**WRF**
世代　**GEN, gen**
背(中)　**bk**
脊椎奇形・鎖肛・気道食道瘻・橈骨欠損　**VATER**
精神発達遅滞児全国協会　**NSMHC**
世紀　**cent, cent.**
正円窓　**RW**
正円窓膜　**RWM**
正栄養士　**RD**
(米国の)正看護師　**RN**
正眼視　**E**
正確に　**No, No., no., xact**
正規テスト希釈度　**RTD**
正弦〔サイン〕波ジアテルミー　**SW dia.**
正式な訓練　**FT**
正色(素)性正(赤血)球性貧血　**NNA**
正色(素)性正赤血球性貧血　**NCNCA**
正色素性赤血球　**NCE**
正視　**EM, Em, em**
正常　**n, N, n, NP**
正常,自然腟分娩　**NSVD**
正常・満期・自然分娩　**NFTSD**
正常圧　**NP**
正常圧水頭症　**NPH**
正常以下の　**SM**
正常位肝移植　**OLT**
正常イヌ血清　**NDS**
正常ウサギ血清　**NRS**
正常ウサギ免疫グロブリン　**NRIg**
正常ウマ血清　**NHS**
正常栄養の　**NN**
正常下限　**LLN, LNL**
正常型プリオン蛋白　**PrP^{C}**
正常可動域　**NR(O)M, NROM**
正常眼圧　**TN, Tn**
正常眼圧緑内障　**NTG**
正常緩衝塩基　**NBB**
正常気圧　**An**
正常気圧・温度　**NPT**
正常血圧・体温　**NPT**
正常血圧ウィスターラット　**NWR**
正常血圧者　**NT**
正常血圧(性)の　**NT**
正常血圧ラット　**NR, NTR**
正常月経周期　**NMP**
正常血清　**NBS, NS**
正常血清アルブミン　**NSA**
正常血清チ〔サイ〕ロキシン　**T_4N**
正常限界　**NL**
正常骨髄　**NBM**
正常骨髄抽出物　**NBME**
正常(電気)軸偏位　**NAC**
正常自然分娩　**NSD**
正常自然満期産　**NSFTD**
正常出産時体重　**NBW**
正常小児期疾患　**NCD**
正常上皮細胞　**NE**

正常食塩液　**NS sol**
正常女性外性器〔外陰部〕　**NEFG**
正常女性染色体型　**XX**
正常女性の染色体　**46 XX**
正常腎機能　**NRF**
正常心室中隔肺動脈閉鎖　**PAIVS**
正常性欲(・性交・絶頂期)　**NL**
正常赤血球　**NRBC**
正常組織　**NT**
正常帯　**NZ**
正常体温　**NT**
正常体温・正常脈拍　**STP**
正常対照　**NC**
正常耐糖能　**NGT**
正常男児　**NMI**
正常男性(性)染色体型　**XY**
正常男性染色体型　**XY**
正常腟鏡検査所見　**NCF**
正常値の上限　**ULN**
正常抽出ホルモン　**NH**
正常中性脂肪血　**NTG**
正常腸音　**BSN, NBS**
正常低比重リポ蛋白　**NLDL**
正常頭蓋の　**NC, normoceph**
正常洞調律　**NSR**
正常な　**nor, norm**
正常な外眼運動　**NOM**
正常ナトリウム(食)　**NS**
正常に開いた　**NO**
正常に閉鎖した　**NC**
正常乳腺組織　**NBT**
正常の　**NL, NR**
正常脳幹　**NBS**
正常の大きさ,形,位置　**NSSL**
正常の大きさと形　**NSS**
正常の温度と気圧　**NT & P**
正常排尿筋反射　**NDR**
正常範囲　**NR, NZ**
正常範囲内　**cin NL, WLN, WNL**
正常反応　**NR**
正常ヒトグロブリン　**NHG**
正常ヒト(保存)血漿　**NHP**
正常ヒト血清　**NHS**
正常ヒト腎臓　**NHK**
正常ヒト蛋白　**NHWM**
正常ヒト保存血漿　**NHPP**
正常沸点　**NBP**
正常分子量レニン　**NMS**
正常分娩　**ND**
正常糞便抗原　**NFA**
正常分娩後の　**NPP**
正常マウス血清　**NMS**
正常満期分娩　**NFTD**
正常ヤギ血清　**NGS**
正常ラクターゼ活性　**NLA**
正常ラット腎　**NKR, NRK**
正常ラット腎(細胞)におけるキリステン肉腫ウイルス　**KNRK**
正常リズムと心拍数　**RRR**
正常流(量)　**NF**
正常量　**ND**
正常リンパ球移入試験　**NLT**
正常レニン本態性高血圧(症)　**NREH**
正睡眠　**OS**
正赤芽球　**NB, nbl**
正染性正赤芽球　**N・Ebl-o**
正染性赤芽球　**OEb**
正染性の　**Ortho, ortho**
正染性白質萎縮(症)　**OLD**
正中縦断(面)　**MLS**
正中仙骨動脈　**MS**
正中前頭部　**MF**
正中中心部　**MC**
正中頭頂部　**MP**
正中の　**md, md., mdn, MED, Med, med., ML**
正中背側の　**MD**
正中隆起　**ME**
正の　**P**
正のフィードバック　**PFB**
正方形の　**qua**
正または誤　**T/F**
生化学　**Biochem, biochem, biochem.**
生化学士　**M.Bi.Chem**
生化学者　**Biochem, biochem, biochem.**
生化学の　**Biochem, biochem, biochem.**
生化学博士　**D.Bi.Chem, Dr.Bi.Chem.**
生活関連動作　**APDL**
生活支持と環境管理組織　**LSECS**
生活と健康の質　**QLH**
生活年齢　**CA**
生活の　**vit**
生活の質　**QOL**
生活の神聖さ　**SOL**
生活費　**COL**
生活満足指数　**LSI**
生活歴　**CV**
生検　**Bx**
生検掻爬　**B & C**
生合成ヒト成長因子　**B-HGH**
生後感染　**PNI**
生後日数　**DAB**
生産　**LB**
生児出産　**LB**

生歯　**Dent, dent.**
生殖・泌尿器(の)　**GU**
生殖遺伝子副体　**Fepisome**
生殖器　**GEN, gen, genit**
生殖(器)の　**GEN, gen**
生殖(器)の腹腔鏡手術　**RLS**
生殖泌尿器系　**GUS**
生殖不能の　**st, ster**
生殖補助技術　**ART**
生殖力　**fert**
生成物　**P, prod**
生存因子　**SF**
生存可能出生　**VB**
生存可能損失年　**YPLL**
生存期間の延長　**ILS**
生存時間　**ST**
生存している運動神経　**SMN**
生存しており健康である　**L & W**
生存数　l_x
生存性・脆弱性比　**S/V**
生存胚　**LE**
生存未熟女児　**ILFC**
生存率　**px**
生存率・疫学・最終結果　**SEER**
生息場所　**habit**
生体解剖　**vivi**
生体解剖反対同盟　**AVS**
生体現象記録装置システム　**CWG**
生体工学　**bioeng**
生体工具　**BE**
生体自己制御　**BF, BFB**
生体実験　**vivi**
生体腎移植ドナー　**LRC**
生体超音波顕微鏡　**UBM**
生体内画像選択分光器　**ISIS**
生体内で　**in viv., IV, i.v.**
生体の　**vit**
生体防衛指数　**HDI**
生体免疫検定　**BIA**
生態学・疫学研究室　**EEL**
生長　**V, Veg, veg**
生年　**YOB**
生年月日　**BD, DB, D/B, DOB**
生合成ヒトインスリン　**BHI**
生物　**org**
生物医科学協会　**BSC**
生物医科学研究所　**BRI**
生物医科学支持基会　**BSSG**
生物医学　**biomed**
生物医学工学研究協同体　**BERC**
生物医学の　**biomed**
生物汚染　**biocon**
生物科学　**biosci**
生物科学士　**M.Bi.S**
生物科学者　**biosci**
生物科学情報委員会　**COBSI**
生物化学戦　**BCW**
生物化学的酸素要求量　**BOD**
生物科学の　**biosci**
生物科学博士　**D.Bi.Sc**
生物学　**bio, Biol, biol**
生物学・医学部　**DBM**
(英国)生物学研究所　**IB**
生物学研究所　**BRI**
生物学者　**Biol, biol**
生物学周辺科学　**BIOS**
生物学的　**Biol, biol**
生物学的応答調節物質　**BRM**
生物学的汚染指数　**BIP**
生物学的活性　**BA, F**
生物学的活性単位　**UBA**
生物学的偽反応体　**BFR**
生物学的偽陽性(反応)　**BFP**
生物学的許容限界　**BTL**
生物学的許容値　**BLV**
生物学的検定　**BA**
生物学的効果比　**RBE**
生物学的実験　**bioex**
生物学的水質汚染指数　**BIP**
生物学的製剤製造の施設許可申請　**ELA**
生物学的精神医学　**BP**
生物学的戦争　**BW**
生物学的単位　**BU**
生物学的低下　**biodet**
生物医学的な　**BM**
生物学的に清浄な　**bioclean**
生物学的に退化可能な　**biodeg**
生物学的に破壊可能な　**biodes**
生物学的妊娠反応　**BPT**
生物学的曝露指数　**BEI**
生物学的半減期　**BHL, BHT, Tb**
生物学的反応　**BR**
生物学的防御　**biodef**
生物学的連続記録センター　**BSRC**
生物学と電子工学　**bionics**
生物学の　**bio**
生物学標準局　**DBS**
生物工学　**BE, bioeng**
生物工学会　**BES**
生物工学士　**M.Bi.Eng**
生物工学と人間研究　**BHR**
生物工学博士　**D.Bi.Eng**
生物サイバネティクス　**biocyb**
生物時間測定　**biochron**
(FDA の)生物製剤評価・研究センター　**CBER**

生物性電位　**BP**
生物(学)的価値　**BV**
生物電気修復成長学会
BRAGS
生物電子工学　**BE**
生物反応修飾〔変換〕物質
BRM
生物物理学　**Biophys**
生物物理学士
M.Bi.Phy
生物物理学者　**biophys**
生物物理学の　**biophys**
生物物理学博士
D.Bi.Phy
生物物理プロフィール評価
BPS
生物分類(番号)　**OID**
生命維持装置　**LSS**
生命延長　**ILS**
生命科学医学情報コンピュータ　**LSMOC**
生命科学研究室　**ABL**
生命期間の限られた細胞
CLLS
生命救助サービス　**LSS**
生命救助本部　**LSS**
生命記録　**vit rec**
生命徴候　**VS**
生命徴候安定　**VSS**
生命徴候正常　**VSN**
生命の　**vit**
生命の快適さ　**AOL**
生命の尊厳　**SOL**
生命を脅かす　**TL**
生来性精神疾患状態　**cps**
生来の　**N, n.**
生理学　**P**
生理学的完全弁　**PFV**
生理学的死腔　**Vd p**
生理学的薬力学的モデル
PBPK
生理学的容積　**VP**
生理学的老化率　**PAR**
生理学の　**PHYS, physio, physio., Physiol, physiol**
生理食塩液浣腸　**SE**
生理食塩水　**NS, NSS, NS sol, PhyS, SS**
生理食塩水浣腸　**NSE**
生理食塩水抽出リステリア属　**SEL**
生理的許容量・上下肢・聴力・視力・感情的許容量・心的安定性
PULHEEMS
生理的作業負荷指数
PWI
生理的食塩　**PhyS**
生理的食塩水　**PSS**
生理的評価委員会　**PEB**
成功　**suc**
成功した　**S**
成功者　**suc**
成功する　**suc**
成人　**A**
成人T細胞性白血病ウイルス　**ATLV**
成人T細胞性白血病誘導因子　**ADF**
成人T細胞性白血病リンパ腫　**ATL-L**
成人T細胞(性)白血病
ATL
成人T細胞(性)白血病(関連)抗原　**ATLA**
成人T細胞(性)リンパ腫
ATL
成人型結節性動脈周囲炎
APN
成人型呼吸窮迫症候群
ARDS
成人型多囊胞症
APCD, APD
成人型糖尿病　**MOD**
成人型ヘモグロビン
Hb A
成人胸腺摘出(術)　**ATx**
成人呼吸器疾患　**ARD**
成人女性　**AF**
成人多囊胞性腎疾患
APKD
成人男性　**AM, A/M**
成人T細胞性白血病ウイルスI(II, III…)型
ATLV-I, II, III…
成人T細胞(性)白血病ウイルス性抗原　**ATLA**
成人突然死症候群
SMDS
成人(型)の　**A**
成人の去勢　**AC**
成人の特異感情障害
SEHA
成人発症型糖尿病
MODM
成人発症(型)糖尿病
AOD, AODM
成人病　**AD**
成人ファンコニ症候群
AFS
成人毎日必要最小量
MADR
成熟　**MAT**
成熟T細胞特異抗原
RTSA
成熟Tリンパ球特異抗原
PTSA
成熟胸腺細胞　**M-Thy**
成熟指数　**MI, MQ**
成熟した　**M, m, MAT**
成熟する　**MAT**
成獣胸腺摘除　**ATx**
成層圏変化検出のためのネットワーク　**NDSC**
成長　**V, Veg, veg**
成長監視ユニット　**GCU**
成長関連蛋白　**GAP**
成長調節遺伝子　**GRO**
成長と発育　**G and D, GD, G/D**
成長と分化ホルモン
GDH
成長不全　**GF**
成長ホルモン　**GDH,**

GH, SH
成長ホルモン(＝ソマトトロピン) STH
成長ホルモン結合蛋白 GHBP
成長ホルモン欠乏症 GHD
成長ホルモン神経分泌異常症 GH-NSD
成長ホルモン調節神経分泌系異常 GHND
成長ホルモン分泌抑制因子 GIF
成長ホルモン分泌抑制ホルモン GHIH
成長ホルモン放出因子 GHRF, GRF
成長ホルモン放出因子ニューロン GRF
成長ホルモン放出ペプチド GHRP
成長ホルモン放出ホルモン GHRH, GRH
成長ホルモン放出抑制因子 GHRIF, GRIF
成長ホルモン放出抑制ホルモン GIH
成長抑制の GI
成分 C, cmpt, compo, constit, elem
成分栄養(チューブ) ED
成分栄養・味の素・千葉大学 ED-AC
成分栄養チューブ ED tube
成分経腸栄養法 EEH
成分の elem
西部ウマ脳炎 WEE
西部ウマ脳炎ウイルス WEEV
西部の W
西部脳炎 WE
西部脳脊髄炎 WE
西部薬局・化学協会 WPCC
西北蒼朮 AC
西洋ワサビペルオキシダーゼ HRP, HRPO
西暦 AD
西暦紀元前 B.C.
声音振盪 VF, V.F.
声質 VQ
声帯 SB, TC, VC, v.c.
声帯機能異常 VCD
声帯共鳴 VR, V.R.
声帯溝症 SV
声帯速度指数 VVI
声門上喉頭部分摘出 SSL
制癌剤動注兼塞栓療法 TCE
制御できない OOC
制限 def, lim, rest
制限酵素切断片長多型性 RFLP
制限された lmtd., ltd., R, rest, rstr
制限する lim, rest
制限目標遺伝子解析法 RLGS
制度 Inst, inst, Instn
制度(上)の Inst, inst
制尿法 ADP
姓不明 LNU
姓名症候群 NAME syndrome
姓名不明 NU
性 G, g, GEN, gen
性科学研究所 ISR
性格異常 CD
性格疾患 CD
性(行為)感染症 STD
性器 GEN, gen, genit
性器の GEN, gen
性器発育異常 GD
性器発育不全 GD
性機能指数 SFI
性クロマチン SC
性クロマチン検査 SCT
性決定染色体 X-chrome
性交 SI
性交後試験 PCT
性交後の PC, PIC
性行為獲得性〔後天性〕免疫不全(症候群) SAID
性行為感染状態 STC
性行為感染反応性関節炎 SARA
性行動中枢 SBC
性項目表 SI
性細胞輸卵管内注入法 GIFT
性質 char
性ステロイド結合グロブリン GBG, SSBG
性制限蛋白 Slp
性染色体が1つだけ存在 XO
性腺刺激ホルモン GDH, GTH, GTP
性腺刺激ホルモン(＝ゴナドトロピン) SGTH
性腺刺激ホルモン増強因子 GEF
性腺刺激ホルモン放出因子 GnRF, GRF
性腺刺激ホルモン放出ホルモン GnRH, GRA, GRH
性腺刺激ホルモン抑制因子 GIF
性腺刺激ホルモン抑制物質 GIM
性腺ステロイド結合グロブリン GSBG
性対象者 sex
性知識および態度テスト SKAT
性的嫌がらせ SH
性的個性指数 SPI
性的な sex

性的二系核　**SDN**
性的不能(症)　**IMP, Impo**
性転換(者)　**TS**
性の　**sex**
性能　**p**
性犯罪者　**so**
性比　**SR**
性病　**VD, vee dee, VL**
性病・梅毒　**VDS**
性病医認定書　**DV**
性病クリニック(外来)　**VDC**
性病研究医学協会　**MSSVD**
性病研究所梅毒検査法　**VDRL**
性病実験研究所〔検査室〕　**VDEL**
性病症例　**VC**
性病性リンパ(節)疾患　**LPV**
性病性リンパ肉芽腫　**LGV, LVG**
性病性リンパ肉芽腫性結膜炎　**LGV conjunctivitis**
性病注意　**VDA**
性病と皮膚科認定書　**DV & D**
性病なし　**NVD**
性病の　**ven**
性病分局　**VDB**
性病予防協会　**SPVD**
性病予防全国連合　**NAPVD**
性分化スケール　**SDS**
性ホルモン　**SH**
性ホルモン結合グロブリン　**SHBG**
性ホルモン結合血漿蛋白　**SBP**
性ホルモン結合蛋白　**SHBP**
性欲阻害　**ISD**
性・薬物全国フォーラム　**NSDF**
青酸　**HCN**
青少年麻薬取締局　**JND**
青色ゴムまり様母斑(症候群)　**BRBN**
青色光網膜傷害　**BLH**
青色熱ルミネセンス　**BTL**
青色の　**B, Bl, bl, caerul.**
青錐(状)体色素　**SWS cone pigment**
青年期人口　**AP**
青年(期)自殺　**AS**
青斑核　**LC**
青緑色　**bG**
政府　**govt**
政府の　**Gov**
星細胞腫　**AST**
星状X線スペクトル　**SXS**
星状神経節ブロック　**SB, SGB**
脆弱X症候群　**FXS**
(Down syndromeに伴う)脆弱X染色体による精神発達遅滞　**FMR-1**
脆弱性　**frag**
脆弱性・硬度比　**v/h**
脆弱性試験　**frag. test**
脆弱部　**fra, FS**
清潔間欠導尿　**CIC**
清潔看護師　**SN**
清掃　**hskpg.**
清掃された　**cld**
晴朗・静穏・平和　**STP**
聖路加病院　**SLHC**
精液　**sem., Semf, SF**
精液検査　**SFA**
精液酸ホスファターゼ　**SAP**
精液の　**sem**
精液ヒアルロニダーゼ単位　**HUS**
精液分析　**SA**
精管摘出マイクロサージェリー〔顕微(鏡)手術〕　**MEDS**
精研式自閉症用行動評定表　**CLAC**
精索水瘤　**HFS**
精子・頸管粘液接触試験　**SCMC**
精子異常　**SA**
精子核膨化因子　**SNDF**
精子形成活動試験　**SAT**
精子進入部位　**SEP**
精子頭部　**SH**
精子特異性抗原　**SSA**
精子被覆抗原　**SCA**
精神・臓器症候群　**POS**
精神(科)医　**P**
精神医学　**P, Psy, psy, PSYCH, Psych, psych, psychiat**
精神科　**Psy, psy**
精神医学抄録探索・修正　**PASA**
精神医学的疫学研究のための面接基準　**PERI, PERT**
精神医学的戦略委員会　**PSB**
精神医学的飛行逃避　**PFA**
精神医学と神経(病)学　**PN, P & N**
精神医学の　**PS, psychiat**
精神異常(性)性(的)攻撃者　**MDSO**
精神運動　**PK**
精神運動の　**PK**
精神運動発達指数　**PDI**
精神運動発作　**PS**
精神運動領域　**P**
精神衛生　**MH**

せ

精神衛生管理　**MHA**
精神衛生教育全国情報センター　**NCMHE**
精神衛生協会　**MHA**
精神衛生全国委員会　**NCMH**
精神衛生全国連合　**NAMH**
精神科医療ソーシャルワーカー　**PSW**
精神科医療ソーシャルワーク　**PSW**
精神化学　**PSYCHEM**
精神科救急サービス　**PES**
精神科資格認定書　**D.Psy.**
精神科社会学士　**MPSW**
精神科集中治療室　**PICU**
精神科専門医資格　**DPM**
精神科ソーシャルワーカー協会連合　**AAPSW**
精神科的家庭治療サービス　**PHTS**
精神科評価用紙　**PEF**
精神機能作用　**ment**
精神研究施設　**MRI**
精神健康クリニック　**MHC**
精神疾患診断と統計マニュアル　**DSM**
精神疾患なし　**NMI**
精神社会的問題の臨床鑑定　**CAPP**
精神障害者のため正看護師　**RNMS**
精神障害の　**MI, psychopath, Psy-path, psy-path**
精神障害の診断と統計の手引き　**DMS**
(米国精神医学会による)精神障害分類基準　**DSM**
精神状態　**MS**
精神状態検査　**MSE**
精神状態検査記録　**MSER**
精神状態質問表　**MSQ**
精神情動疾患　**PAD**
精神神経科医　**PN**
精神神経学　**PN**
精神神経症の　**PN**
精神神経的個性　**psycho**
精神神経免疫学　**PNI**
精神身体医学　**PsychosMed**
精神身体調査　**PSI**
精神身体の　**psychosom, psy-som**
精神衰弱　**Pt**
精神生理学　**Psychophysiol, psychophysiol.**
精神生理学の　**Psychophysiol, psychophysiol.**
精神測定学　**psychomet**
精神測定年鑑　**MMY**
精神(発達)遅滞　**MR**
精神遅滞　**MD**
精神(発達)遅滞児　**MR**
精神(発達)遅滞の　**feeb, MR**
精神遅滞の　**MD**
精神的無精子症　**PA**
精神電流現象　**PGP**
精神電流反射　**PGR**
精神年齢　**IA, MA, PA**
精神(的)の　**ment**
精神の　**spir**
精神発達遅延　**Schwach**
精神発達遅滞児　**CRMD**
精神皮膚電流抵抗　**PGSR**
精神皮膚電流反射　**PGSR**
精神皮膚電流反応　**PGSR**
精神病　**MI, P**
精神病・間欠性低ナトリウム血・多渇(症候群)　**PIP**
精神病院　**MI, psycho**
精神病院医療管理者協会　**AMSMH**
精神病質　**Psy-path, psy-path**
精神病正看護師　**RMN**
精神病性痴呆　**PD**
精神病的うつ病　**PD**
精神病棟　**psycho**
精神病の全身麻痺　**GPI**
精神病理学　**psychopathol**
精神病理の　**psychopath, psychopathol**
精神物理学　**psychophys**
精神分析　**PA, ps.an., PSAn, PsAn, psychoan**
精神分析者　**PA, ps.an., PSAn, PsAn**
精神分析する　**ps.an., PSAn, PsAn**
精神分析専門医　**ps.an., PSAn, PsAn**
精神分析の　**ps.an., PSAn, PsAn**
精神変換薬　**MADs**
精神変調指数　**MDI**
精神保健センター　**MHC**
精神療法　**psychother**
精製した　**dep.**
精製ジフテリアトキソイド　**PTAP**
精製水　**Aq.puri.**
精製胎盤蛋白　**PPP**
精製ツベルクリン蛋白　**PPD**
精製ツベルクリン蛋白一般用　**PPDS, PPPD-S**
精製痘苗　**PVL**

精製ブタインスリン **PPI**
精巣〔睾丸〕炎 **orch**
精巣自己検査 **TSE**
精巣挙筋の **crem, cremas**
精巣挙筋反射 **CR**
精巣決定因子 **TDF**
精巣鞘膜 **TVT**
精巣性女性化症候群 **TFS**
精巣〔睾丸〕摘除(術) **ORCH**
精巣内精子回収 **TESE**
精嚢 **sem.ves., SV**
精嚢ミクロソーム **SVM**
精留した **rct.**
製作者 **mfr**
製剤した **PP**
製造(する) **manu, manuf**
製造許可申請 **PLA**
製造された **mfd**
製造(業)者 **mfr**
製造物責任 **PL**
製造物責任予防 **PLP**
製品 **manu, manuf, mfr**
製品概要 **SPC**
製品保証 **PL**
製薬協会員 **MPS**
製薬協会財団 **PMAF**
静穏睡眠 **QS**
静止圧 **SP**
静止する **R**
静止電位 **RP**
静水圧 **HP**
静水性肺水腫 **HPE**
静水柱圧利用排液 **WSD**
静水の **Hyd.**
静電単位 **ESU**
静電の **es**
静電容量 **K**
静(的)肺コンプライアンス **CST**
整形外科 **ORS, orth, Ortho, ortho**
整形外科(学) **OS**
整形外科医 **D.Sc.Os., OR, orthop, OS**
整形外科学士 **M.S.Ortho**
整形外科学修士 **M.Ch.Orth.**
整形外科看護師全国協会 **NAON**
整形外科技術者全国委員会 **NBOT**
整形外科技術者全国協会 **NAOT**
整形外科基礎研究会 **ORS**
整形外科矯正器と義肢製造協会 **OALMA**
整形外科検査 **OE, OX, Ox, O_x**
整形外科検査・特殊 **OCSP**
整形外科資格認定書 **DOrth**
整形外科疾患 **Ortho, ortho**
整形外科における研究と教育のための基金 **OREF**
整形外科の **O, OR, Ortho, ortho**
整骨医 **OD, Osteo**
整骨医学 **Osteo, osteo**
整骨医学博士 **D.O.**
整復 **red**
整復する **red**
臍下1指幅 **U/1**
臍上1指幅 **1/U**
石炭酸係数 **PC, Pc**
石炭酸フクシン **CF**
石炭酸メチルブルー **CMB**
石油 **petr**
赤外吸収,放電発光陰極光 **GDOS**
赤外線(照射) **IR ray**
赤外線肝スキャナー **ILS**
赤外線吸収分光計測 **IR**
赤外線凝固薬 **IRC**
赤外線金属反射吸収スペクトル法 **IRAS**
赤外線の **IR**
赤外線光凝固 **IRC**
赤外(線)の **IF, IFR, infra**
赤外部の **IF**
赤芽球 **Ebl**
赤芽球系・骨髄球系比 **E/M ratio**
赤芽球コロニー群形成細胞 **BFU-E**
赤芽球コロニー群刺激細胞 **BPA**
赤芽球コロニー形成単位 **CFU-E**
赤芽球性白血球 **EBL**
赤芽球性白血病ウイルス **SFFV**
赤芽球性不応性貧血 **RAEB**
赤芽球増加型不応性貧血 **RAEM**
赤芽球増殖性プロトポルフィリン症 **EPP**
赤芽球バースト形成単位 **BFU-E**
赤芽球分裂 **Em**
赤芽球癆 **PRCA**
赤核 **RN**
赤核脊髄路 **RST**
赤褐色 **rBr**
赤十字 **RC**
赤十字国際委員会 **CIRC, ICRC**
赤色骨髄 **RM**
赤色コロイド試験 **RCT**
赤色静脈血 **RVB**
赤色軟化 **RS**
赤色熱発光 **RTL**
赤色の **E**

せ

赤色斑　**P**
赤錐体色素
LWS cone pigment
赤沈　**BSR，SR，S.R.，VES**
赤橙色　**RO**
赤白血病　**EL**
赤白血病ウイルス　**ELV**
赤脾髄　**RP**
赤痢　**dysen**
赤痢菌(属)　**S，Sh，Shig**
赤痢菌サルモネラ(寒天培地)　**SS**
赤痢菌サルモネラ菌寒天(培地)　**SS agar**
赤痢菌様毒素　**SLT**
咳とくしゃみ　**C & S**
脊髄　**RM，SC，sp.cd**
脊髄・小脳路黒核変性
SCND
脊髄圧　**SFP**
脊髄圧波　**SPW**
脊髄圧迫　**CC**
脊髄液　**sp fl**
脊髄腔造影(法)　**Myelo**
脊髄腔内　**IT**
脊髄腔内注入　**EI**
脊髄血流量　**SCBF**
脊髄後角　**SDH**
脊髄後頭痛　**PSH**
脊髄コンピュータ断層撮影(法)　**CTM，SCT**
脊髄刺激　**SCS**
脊髄視床路　**STT**
脊髄集中治療部(病棟)
SICU
脊髄小脳変性症　**SCD**
脊髄性筋萎縮症　**SMA**
脊髄性進行性筋萎縮症
SPA，SPMA
脊髄造影　**MLG**
脊髄造影図　**myel**
脊髄造影図予約済み
myel.sched.
脊髄損傷　**SCI**
脊髄損傷サービス(科)
SCIS
脊髄損傷ユニット(病棟)
SCIU
脊髄電図検査　**EMG**
脊髄内の　**IR，isp**
脊髄傍の　**PS，PV**
脊髄麻酔　**Sp**
脊髄誘発電位　**ESCP，SEP，SpEP**
脊柱　**SP，Sp，sp，WS**
脊柱角　**CVA**
脊柱管　**VC**
脊椎　**SP，Sp，sp**
脊椎圧迫　**vert.comp.，vert.compr.**
脊椎間の　**IV**
脊椎骨端異形成症　**SED**
脊椎指圧療法　**Chiro**
脊椎指圧療法士　**Chiro**
脊椎性尾神経根症　**SCR**
脊椎性尾髄症　**SCM**
脊椎穿刺　**SPT**
脊椎穿刺針　**SN**
脊椎前方固定術　**ASF**
脊椎破裂　**SB**
脊椎分裂・水頭症協会
ASBAH
脊椎傍の　**paravert**
脊椎傍ブロック　**PVB**
脊椎麻酔　**sp.an.**
脊椎麻酔・硬膜外麻酔併用法　**CSE**
脊麻　**sp.an.**
責任のある　**RESP，Resp，resp，resp.**
積　**P**
積算筋電図　**IEMG**
積分視覚濃度　**IOD**
切開　**Inzi，S，s，sec，sect，sect.**
切開(術)　**INC，inc，inc.**
切開した　**sec，sect，sect.**
切開する　**I，incid.**
切開の　**INC，inc，inc.**
切開排膿　**I & D**
切腱術　**tenot**
切除　**Ex，ex，exc，excis，rem**
切除(術)　**Res，res**
切除する　**excis，rem，Res，res**
切除生検　**exc.bx**
切除断端　**SM**
切除度　**R**
(乳歯の)切歯　**I，i**
切歯・犬歯・小臼歯・大臼歯　**ICPM，ICPMM**
切歯下顎面角　**IMPA**
切歯近位の　**IP**
切歯髄の　**IP**
切断　**Amp，S，s，sec，sect，sect.**
切断(する)　**X**
(肢)切断患者　**ampt**
切断した　**amp，sec，sect，sect.**
切断術〔法〕　**AMP，amp，ampt**
切断する　**amp，sev**
切端唇側壁の　**ILa**
切迫心筋梗塞(症)　**IMI**
切片　**S，s，sec，sl**
石灰　**L**
石灰化歯牙嚢胞　**COC**
石灰塵肺　**CWP**
石鹼浣腸　**ES，SE，SSE**
石鹼水　**SS**
石鹼水浣腸　**SSE，S & W enema**
石鹼清拭　**SB**
石鹼溶液　**SS**
舌　**TNG**
舌咽呼吸　**GPB**
舌咽神経痛　**GPN**
舌縁　**ML**

舌下顎反射　**LMR**
舌下頸動脈絞扼　**HCE**
舌下の　**SL, sl, subl, subling**
舌癌　**ZK**
舌骨下筋　**IS**
舌骨体　**HB**
舌喉頭蓋ひだ　**GEF**
舌側歯肉の　**LG**
舌側遠心の　**LD**
舌側の　**ling**
舌と歯溝　**T & G**
舌(側)の　**L**
舌の　**ling**
舌の・歯溝の・数珠状の　**TGB**
舌扁桃　**LT**
舌扁桃肥大　**ZMH**
舌偏位　**glos.dev**
舌保持器　**TRD**
(ヒツジ)赤血球　**E**
赤血球　**Er, er, ERY, Ery, eryth, GR, RBC, rbc, RC**
赤血球・抗赤血球複合体　**EA**
赤血球・抗赤血球補体複合体　**EAC**
赤血球/血漿比　**RBC/P**
赤血球 MAP　**MAP**
赤血球アデノシンデアミナーゼ　**RBC-ADA**
赤血球円柱　**RC**
赤血球吸着ウイルス　**HAV, HA virus**
赤血球吸着現象　**HAD**
赤血球吸着反応試験　**HA test**
赤血球凝集　**RCA**
赤血球凝集価　**HAT, HT**
赤血球凝集活性　**HA**
赤血球凝集抗体　**HA**
赤血球凝集試験　**HA**
赤血球凝集植物性血球凝集素　**EPHA**
赤血球凝集性抗ペニシリン抗体　**HAPA**
赤血球凝集性脳脊髄炎　**HE**
赤血球凝集性ペニシリン抗体　**HPA**
赤血球凝集素　**HA**
赤血球凝集素単位　**HU**
赤血球凝集素ノイラミニダーゼ　**HN, HANA**
赤血球凝集素抑制　**HAI**
赤血球凝集単位　**HAU, HU**
赤血球凝集脳脊髄炎ウイルス　**HEV**
赤血球凝集反応　**HAR**
赤血球凝集抑制(滴定濃度)　**HAI**
赤血球凝集抑制試験　**HAIT, HIT, HI test**
赤血球凝集抑制反応　**HAIR**
赤血球グルタチオン還元酵素　**EGR**
赤血球係数　**VG**
赤血球結合抗原抗グロブリン試験　**RCLAAT**
赤血球抗血清　**EA**
赤血球抗体複合体　**EA**
(ヒツジ)赤血球抗体補体複合体　**EAC**
(ヒツジ)赤血球抗体ロゼット形成細胞　**EA-RFC**
赤血球コプロポルフィリン　**ECP**
赤血球産生微小環境　**HIM**
赤血球酸ホスファターゼ　**EAP**
赤血球受容体　**ER**
赤血球新生促進刺激因子　**ESF**
赤血球数算定　**RBC, rbc**
赤血球成熟因子　**EMF**
赤血球沈降速度　**BSR, ESG, ESR, VES**
赤血球沈降反応　**BSR**
赤血球鉄交換率　**RIT**
赤血球鉄交代　**RCIR, RCIT**
赤血球鉄交替率　**EITR, RITR**
赤血球鉄交代率　**RCIRR**
赤血球鉄利用(率)　**RCI-Ut**
赤血球鉄利用率　**RCU**
赤血球トランスケトラーゼ　**ETK**
赤血球トリヨードチ〔サイ〕ロニン　**T-e**
赤血球の　**E**
赤血球の平均の厚さ　**MCAT**
赤血球パック　**PRC**
赤血球付着　**RCA**
赤血球(大小)不同(症)　**aniso**
赤血球浮遊　**RCS**
赤血球プロトポルフィリン　**EP**
赤血球分布幅　**RDW**
赤血球免疫付着　**RCIA**
赤血球容積　**CV, RBCV, RCV, VRBC**
赤血球両受体　**EA**
赤血球両受体補体　**EAC**
赤血球利用率　**RIU**
赤血球ロゼット形成細胞　**ERFC, E-RFC**
浙江白朮　**ACO, AO**
接眼ミクロメータ単位　**OMU**
接近速度　**SOA**
接合　**conjug.**
接合(部)型表皮水疱症　**JEB**
接合部　**jct**

接合部異所性頻拍　**JET**
接合部(性)頻拍(症)　**JT**
接耳　**a.c.**
接触　**cont, cont.**
接触・保菌容疑者　**C, c**
接触過敏症　**CHS**
接触感染症　**CD**
接触感度　**CS**
接触蕁麻疹　**CU**
接触蕁麻疹症候群　**CUS**
接触性膿疱性皮膚炎　**CPD**
接触性皮膚炎　**CD**
接触電位差　**CPD**
接触伝染病　**CD**
接触複合走査　**CCS**
接種(法)　**inoc, inoc.**
接種後の　**PI, Postinoc**
接種した　**inoc, inoc.**
接種する　**INOC, inoc**
接種前の　**Preinoc**
接地　**E, grd**
接地線　**gnd**
絶縁抵抗　**IR**
絶食　**NBM, NPM, NPO**
絶食で　**esur.**
絶対安静　**ABR, SBR, SCB**
絶対アンペア　**abamp**
絶対温度　**°A, A, T, *T***
絶対大気圧　**ATA, ata**
絶対構造　**US**
絶対心濁音界　**ACD**
絶対性不整脈　**AA, Aa**
絶対潜時　**AL**
絶対大気圧　**ATA, ata**
絶対抵抗単位　**ARU**
絶対的就床安静　**CBR**
絶対の　**A, abs**
絶対標高　**abs alt**
絶対不応期　**ARP**
絶対不整脈　**AA**
絶対リスク減少率　**ARR**
絶対零度　**K**
絶望スケール　**HS**
摂氏　**C, CEL, Cel, Cels**
摂氏(温度)　℃
摂氏(=℃)　**CENT, Cent, cent, centi**
摂氏温度単位　**CTU**
摂氏度　℃
(経口)摂取　**ingest**
摂取　**I**
摂取せよ　**su, su.**
摂取(量)と排出(量)　**I & O**
摂取率　**upt**
摂取量と排泄量を測定・記録(せよ)　**M & R I & O**
摂食態度検査　**EAT**
(分)節　**sec, sect, sect.**
節前の　**pregang**
節点　**NP**
説明する　**expl**
説明できる　**A**
説明と同意　**IC**
積極的診断法　**VDA**
積極的心理的態度　**PMA**
積極的な　**A, a**
積極的な特異的免疫療法　**ASI**
狭い　**lmtd., ltd.**
千　**M, m.**
千分の　**vT, v.T.**
千分率　**vT, v.T.**
仙骨　**S, sac**
仙骨横位　**SLT**
仙骨岬角　**SP**
仙骨神経　**S**
仙骨恥骨間の　**SP**
仙骨恥骨の　**Sp, sp**
仙骨の　**S, sac**
仙骨左後位　**SLP**
仙骨左前位　**SLA**
仙坐骨切痕　**ss notch**
仙(骨)坐骨の　**s.s.**
仙髄排尿反射中枢　**SMC**
仙台ウイルス　**SV**
仙腸関節　**SIJ, SI jt**
仙腸骨の　**SI**
仙腸装具　**SIO**
仙(骨)腸(骨)の　**sac-il**
仙椎(S 1のように使う)　**S**
仙椎の　**S**
仙尾下恥骨点　**SCIPP**
仙尾骨の　**SC**
占拠している　**Occup, occup**
占拠する　**Occup, occup**
先進部　**Pr**
先祖　**prog**
先体反応　**AR**
先端　**X, x**
先端(肢端)骨溶解(症)　**AOL**
先端衝撃　**AI**
先端肥大性心筋症　**AHCM**
先端放射性の　**AR**
先天異常　**PAVM**
先天(性)奇形　**CM**
先天性異常造血性貧血　**CDA**
先天性横隔膜ヘルニア　**CDH**
先天性外転欠損　**CAD**
先天性角化異常症　**DKC**
先天性角膜上皮異栄養症　**CECD**
先天性片側性形成異常・魚鱗癬様紅皮症・肢欠損症候群　**CHILD**
先天性眼振　**CN**
先天性肝線維化症　**CHF**
先天性胸腺異形成(症)　**CTD**
先天性巨大結腸症　**HSCR**
先天性魚鱗癬様紅皮症

CIE
先天性筋ジストロフィ **CMD**
先天性クロール下痢症 **CCD**
先天性形成不良性貧血 **CHA**
先天性限局皮膚欠損 **CLAS**
先天性甲状腺機能低下症 **CH**
先天性股関節疾患 **CHD**
先天性股関節脱臼 **CDH, CHD, DDH, LCC**
先天性骨形成不全 **OI congenita**
先天性骨髄性ポルフィリン症 **CEP**
先天性重症筋無力症 **CMG**
先天性心(臓)疾患 **CHD**
先天性心疾患 **CC**
先天性心臓弁膜症 **CVD**
先天性心不全 **CHF**
先天性脊椎骨端骨異形成症 **SED congen**
先天性全身脂肪萎縮 **CGL**
先天性代謝異常 **IEM**
先天性多嚢胞疾患〔病〕 **CPD**
先天性多発性関節拘縮症 **AMC**
先天性多弁膜症 **CPVD**
先天性男性化副腎過形成(症) **CVAH**
先天性胆道運動障害 **CBD**
先天性胆道拡張症 **CBD**
先天性胆道閉鎖症 **CBA**
先天性腟欠損 **CAV**
先天性中枢性過呼吸症候群 **CCHS**
先天性腸無神経節症 **CIA**
先天性殿部過形成 **CDH**
先天性内因子欠損症 **CIFD**
先天性内反足 **CCF**
先天性尿路奇形 **CUD**
先天性尿路変形 **CUD**
先天性ネフローゼ **CN**
先天性の **B**
先天性嚢胞性腺腫様奇形 **CCAM**
先天性梅毒 **LC**
先天性肺胞異形成 **CAD**
先天性肺リンパ管拡張症 **CPL**
先天性ハインツ(小)体(性)貧血 **CHBA**
先天性非球状赤血球(性)溶血(性疾患) **CNHD**
先天性非球状赤血球(性)溶血性貧血 **CNSHA**
先天性非進行性ミオパシー **CNM**
先天性皮膚カンジダ症 **CCC**
先天性風疹症候群 **CRS**
先天性封入体溶血性貧血 **CIBHA**
先天性不応性鉄芽球性貧血 **CRSA**
先天性副腎過形成 **CAH**
先天性副腎性男性化 **CAV**
先天性副腎皮質過形成 **CAH**
先天性変形なし **NCD**
先天性無力性硬化性筋ジストロフィ **CASMD**
先天性翼状片関節異形成症 **PAMC**
先天性リパーゼ欠損症 **CPLD**
先天的四肢欠損(症) **CLD**
先天的な **inher, N, n.**
先天(性)の **CONG, cong., congen**
先天(性)梅毒 **CS**
先天放出機構 **IRM**
先発医薬品 **BND**
尖圭コンジローマ **CA**
尖頭合指(症) **ACS**
尖頭症 **oxycephs**
尖頭多合指(症) **ACPS**
全 **T, tot**
全(反応) **W**
全アデニンヌクレオチド **TAN**
全アンモニア窒素 **TAN**
全胃温存膵頭十二指腸切除術 **SSPPD**
全インド医科学研究所 **AIMS**
全遠視 **HT**
全オゾン分布分光器 **TOMS**
全カリウム量 **TBK**
全〔総〕カルシウム量 **TBC**
全か無(か)の法則 **ANG, ANL, AON**
全冠(状動脈)血流量 **TCF**
全荷重 **FWB**
全〔総〕換気 **VT, V_T**
全関節置換関節形成(術) **TARA**
全関節置換術 **TJR**
全顎X線写真 **FMX**
全顎X線写真撮影法 **FMX**
全〔総〕クリアランス **TBC**
全血 **B, QB, WB**
全血液量 **TBV**
全血活性化凝固時間 **WBACT**
全血活性化部分トロンボプラスチン時間 **WBAPTT**

せ

全血顆粒球数　**TBGP**
全血カルシウム再沈着時間　**WBRT**
全血管抵抗　**TVR**
全血球計算　**CBC**
全血凝固時間　**WBCT**
全血漿カテコールアミン　**TPC**
全血漿コレステロール　**TPC**
全血漿量　**TPV**
全血単位　**U/WB**
全血窒素　**WBN**
全血の比重　**Gb**
全血部分トロンボプラスチン時間　**WBPTT**
全血ヘマトクリット　**WBH**
全血葉酸　**WBF**
全血(液)量　**QBV**
全血量　**WBV**
全結腸鏡検査(法)　**TC**
全結腸切除(術)　**TC**
全交連　**ALC**
全固形物　**TS**
全国イヤモールド研究所協会　**NAEL**
全国ウィルムス腫瘍研究(グループ)　**NWTS**
全国家族計画　**NFP**
全国環境政策法　**NEPA**
全国看護学生連合　**NSNA**
全国看護師教育連合会　**NLNE**
全国救急ヘリコプターパイロット協会　**NEMSPA**
全国協同胆石研究国内協力　**NCGS**
全国結核協会　**NTA**
全国公衆衛生看護協会　**NOPHN**
全国骨髄ドナー登録制度　**NMDP**
全国疾病治療指標　**NDTI**
全国出生調査　**NFS**
全国身障児学会　**NSCC**
全国専門医学研修計画　**NRMP**
全国的な　**Nat**
全国糖尿病記録グループ　**NDDG**
全国病院退院調査　**NHDS**
全国ホスピス協会　**NHO**
全高調波ひずみ(率)　**THD**
全左(心)室拍出仕事量　**TLVSW**
全細胞溶解産物　**WCL**
全人工膝関節　**TKP**
全〔総〕上皮小体ホルモン分泌(率)　**TPTHS**
全収縮期雑音　**HSM**
全心血管管理部(室)　**CCCU**
全心臓容積　**TCD**
全心電図　**OCG**
全死亡率中の割合　**PMI**
全自動血液塗抹装置　**ABSP**
全身　**GK, WB**
全身アナフィラキシー陽性　**ASA**
全身ガス拡散能力　**D**
全身活動　**WBA**
全身カンジダ症　**SC**
全身菌毒性臓器不全　**STOF**
全身クリアランス　**Q_B**
全身血圧　**SAP**
全身血管抵抗　**SVR, TSPR**
全身(体循環)血管抵抗指数　**SVRI**
全身血流量　**SBF**
全身高熱　**WBH**
全身高熱療法　**TBH**
全身骨塩密度　**TBBMD**
全身骨塩量　**TBBMC**
全身骨ミネラル　**TBBM**
全身酸素輸送　**SOT**
全身シャワー　**WBS**
全身シュワルツマン反応　**GSR**
全身照射　**TBI, TBX, WBR**
全身症状　**GA**
全身状態　**AZ, GC, PS**
全身静脈内血栓溶解療法　**IVCT**
全身進展型　**ED**
全身水分　**TW**
全身水分量　**TBW, TBWA**
全身スキャン　**WBS**
全身性アスペルギルス症　**SA**
全身性ウェゲナー肉芽腫症　**GWG**
全身性エリテマトーデス　**LES, SLE**
全身性炎症性疾患　**SID**
全身性炎症反応症候群＝サーズ　**SIRS**
全身性カルニチン欠乏症　**SCD**
全身性乾燥症候群　**SSS**
全身性強直性間代性発作　**GTCS**
全身性硬化症　**SSc**
全身性高体温　**SH**
全身性高熱　**SH**
全身性紅斑性狼瘡(＝SLE)　**LES**
全身性骨化多発性筋炎　**POG**
全身性細菌感染　**SBI**
全身清拭　**BB**
全身性腺腫脹　**GGE**
全身性胎生毛性多毛(症)　**UHL**
全身性動脈硬化症　**GAS**

全身性動脈性高血圧　**SAH**
全身性の　**sys, syst**
全身性能動性免疫療法　**SAI**
全身性麻痺　**GP**
全身性毛細管漏出症候群　**SCLS**
全身窒素　**TBN**
全身抽出物　**WBE**
全身貯留　**WBR**
全身デジタルスキャナー　**WBDS**
全身電気伝導度測定法　**TOBEC**
全身電子線照射療法　**TSEB**
全身ニュートロン活性化　**TBNA**
全身ニュートロン活性化分析　**TBNAA**
全身熱量計　**BDC**
全身反応　**SR**
全身表面(積)　**TBS**
全身表面積　**TBSA**
全身ヘマトクリット　**TBH**
全身放射線照射　**WBI**
全身発疹　**GR**
全身麻酔　**GA**
全身麻酔(法)下で　**UGA**
全身麻痺　**PG, TP**
全身リンパ節放射線照射　**TLI**
全(総)重量　**nt**
全食事カロリー　**TDC**
全神経活動電位　**WNAP**
全脂質　**TL**
全脂質抽出物　**TLE**
全時間　**TT**
全消化(可能)栄養分　**TDN**
全消化(可能)カロリー　**TDE**
全循環蛋白　**TCP**
全循環ヘモグロビン　**TCH**
全腎血管抵抗　**TRR**
全腎血漿流量　**TRPF**
全腎血流量　**TRBF**
全障害者医療補助金　**TDB**
全膝関節置換術　**TKA**
全世界情報網(＝インターネット通信網の1つ)　**WWW**
全赤血球鉄　**TRI**
全赤血球容積　**TRCV**
全脊椎麻酔　**TSB**
全相関分光法　**TOCST**
全組織標本　**wm**
全層角膜移植(術)　**PK, PKP**
全層植皮　**FTG, FTSG**
全層皮膚移植片　**FTG**
全大腸内視鏡検診　**TCF**
全体液(量)　**TBF**
全体血管抵抗　**TSVR**
全体脂肪(量)　**TBF**
全体循環抵抗　**TSR**
全体の　**GEN, gen, gen'l**
全体平均　**GA**
全〔総〕蛋白(量)　**tot.prot., TP**
全蛋白ツベルクリン　**TPT**
全抵抗　**Rt, TR**
全トレポネマ・パリズム補体結合試験　**WTPCF**
全〔総〕尿(中)性腺刺激ホルモン　**TUG**
全尿道長　**TPL**
全〔総〕尿量　**TVU**
全尿量　**TUV**
全乳　**WM**
全乳房切断術　**TM**
全脳放射線治療　**WBRT**
全反射吸収　**ATR**
全反射螢光X線分析法　**TRXF, TXRF**
全反応　**TR, WR, W-response**
全反応指数　**TRI**
全白血球　**TWBC**
全肺(活量)　**TL**
全肺胸部コンプライアンス　**CT**
全肺気量　**TLC**
全肺血管抵抗　**TPR, TPVR**
全肺血流量　**TPBF**
全肺断層撮影(法)　**WLT**
全肺抵抗　**RL**
全肺容積　**TLV**
全発達遅滞　**PDR**
全般安全度　**OSR**
全般改善評点　**GIR**
全般的生産コード　**UPC**
全般てんかん　**GE**
全般閉塞性肺疾患　**GOLD**
全般有効度　**GUR**
全非経口的栄養法　**TPA**
全ブタクサ抽出物　**WRE**
全米眼科学協会　**PAAO**
全米歯科学協会　**PAOA**
全米心理学会　**ISP**
全ホモジネート　**WH**
全補体　**WC, WC'**
全末梢血管抵抗　**TPR, TPVR**
全埋没人工心臓　**TIAH**
全免疫反応性血清ペプシノゲン　**TISP**
全溶解固形物　**TDS**
全リンパ球分画　**WLF**
全リンパ節照射　**TNI**
全流量　**TF**
(完)全理学的検査　**CPX, C Px**
全量　**ad, TD, t.m.**
全量注入　**TDI**
全量まで　**ad pond.om.**
専門医　**SP, sp, spec**

専門医助言委員会　**SAC**
専門医団体　**MS, MSpC**
専門化　**spec, specif**
専門家　**SP, sp**
専門化されていない　**NS**
専門看護師　**CNS**
専門標準検閲機構　**PSSO**
専門別集中治療病棟　**SCU**
専用手術室　**XOR**
泉門　**F**
浅後頭動脈・中大脳動脈　**SOA-MCA**
浅指屈筋　**FDS**
浅側頭動脈　**STA**
浅側頭動脈・後大脳動脈　**STA-PCA**
浅側頭動脈・上小脳動脈　**STA-SCA**
浅側頭動脈・中大脳動脈（吻合術）（＝ST-MC）　**STA-MCA**
浅側頭動脈・中大脳動脈（吻合術）（＝STA-MCA）　**ST-MC**
浅側頭動脈・中大脳動脈（吻合術）　**STA-MCA**
浅大腿静脈　**SFV**
浅達性II度熱傷　**SDB**
浅腸骨回旋動脈　**SCIA**
浅葉耳下腺摘出術　**SP**
洗眼剤　**collyr.**
洗浄　**IRRG, irrg, irrig**
洗浄液　**LF, lot.**
洗浄可能基剤　**WB**
洗浄剤　**lot.**
洗浄された膀胱　**WB**
洗浄赤血球　**WRBC, WRC**
洗髪　**HB, Hs, Sp**
洗鼻剤　**collun.**
染色体　**chromo, cs**
染色体均質染色領域　**HSR**
染色体（間）交叉〔差〕　**ICC**
染色体交叉〔差〕　**Xta**
染色体短腕　**P**
染色体長腕　**q**
染色体長腕の螢光斑　**Y body**
染色体動原体蛋白　**CENP-B**
染色体の座　**l**
染色体不安定部　**FS**
染色体リボ核酸　**chRNA, cRNA**
染色（済み）尿沈渣　**SUS**
染色分体　**ct**
前　**A, a**
前アブミ骨ひだ　**ASF**
前意識の　**Pcs**
前腋窩　**ant.ax.**
前腋窩線　**AAL**
前下行枝　**AD**
前下交通動脈　**AICA**
前下行動脈　**ADA**
前下象限　**AIQ**
前下小脳動脈　**AICA**
前下垂体甲状腺刺激　**TSP**
前下腸骨棘　**AIIS**
前外シルヴィウス脳回　**AES**
前外側（壁）心筋梗塞　**ALMI**
前外方回旋不安定性　**ALRI**
前冠（状）動脈洞　**ACS**
前額面　**F**
前臼歯形成不全・多汗症・（壮年性）白毛症　**PHC**
前臼歯無歯（症）・多汗症・壮年性白毛症（＝ボエーク症候群）　**PHC**
前胸腺細胞　**Pro-thy**
前胸腺刺激ホルモン　**PTTH**
前胸部　**PC**
前胸部横径　**ACD**
前胸部加速度追跡　**PACT**
前胸部聴診器　**PCS, Prec steth**
前胸部の　**precord**
前胸壁　**ACW**
前胸壁有茎皮弁　**DP flap**
前胸膜外線　**AEPL**
前期破水　**PROM**
前距腓靱帯　**ATF**
前嗅神経核　**AON**
前屈　**AF, FF, ff**
前屈小発作　**PPM**
前駆出期　**PEP**
前駆出期時間　**PET**
前駆の　**prec**
前月経期　**PMP**
前脛骨の　**ant.tib.**
前脛骨部色素斑　**PPP**
前傾　**AV**
前傾・前屈　**AV-AF, AV/AF**
前傾の　**AV**
前口蓋弓　**AFP**
前交通動脈　**ACA**
前交通動脈（瘤）　**Acom, A-com**
前交連　**AC, CA**
前後位と側位　**ap/lat**
（頭部）前後径　**OFD**
前後径　**APD, A-PD, FOD, OF**
前後（方向）の　**A & P, AP, A-P**
前後（方向）の（像）　**AP, A-P**
前後方向第一斜位　**LPO**
前後方向第二斜位　**RPO**
前骨髄細胞白血病　**PML**
（脊髄神経）前根　**VR, vr, v.r.**
前（神経）根　**VNR**
前（神経）根・胸髄　**VRT**

前(神経)根・頸髄　**VRC**
前根応答　**VRR**
前根反射　**VRR**
前鼓室狭部　**ATI**
前十字靱帯　**ACL**
前上顔面静脈の　**ASV**
前上棘　**ant.sup.sp., ASS**
前上象限　**ASQ**
前上腸骨棘　**ASIS**
前初期抗原　**PENA**
前視床下核　**NHA**
前視床穿通動脈　**ATPA**
前斜　**Ao**
前斜角(筋)　**SA**
前斜角筋症候群　**SAS**
前進の　**FWD**
前縦靱帯　**ALL, ant.long.ligs.**
前縦靱帯骨化症　**OALL**
前赤芽球　**PEb, ProEbl**
前脊髄視床路　**AST**
前脊髄動脈症候群　**ASAS**
前側乳頭筋　**ALPM**
前大脳動脈　**ACA**
前柱　**AC**
前置胎盤　**plac.prev., PP**
前ツチ骨靱帯　**AML**
前ツチ骨ひだ　**AMF**
前庭　**vest**
前庭温熱刺激反応　**CVR**
前庭核　**VN**
前庭眼反射　**VOR**
前庭機能　**VF**
前庭左右不均衡　**VA**
前庭神経核の外側核　**LVN**
前庭神経核の内側核　**MVN**
前庭脊髄反射　**VSR**
前庭漸増現象　**VR**
前庭動眼反応　**VOR**
前庭の　**V, vest**
(胃癌の)前庭部(領域)　**A**
前庭膜　**VM**
前頭右側横位　**FDT**
前頭骨・腸骨　**fi**
前頭左側横位　**FLT**
前頭左側後位　**FLP**
前頭左側前位　**FLA**
前頭頭頂の　**FP**
前頭(部)の　**F**
前頭(葉)皮質　**FCX**
前頭皮質　**FC**
前頭部間欠律動的デルタ波　**FIRDA**
前頭弁　**FF**
前頭葉　**FL**
前頭葉眼球運動野　**FEF**
前頭葉超音波療法　**PST**
前内側脊椎静脈　**AIVV**
前内方回旋不安定性　**AMRI**
前乳頭筋　**APM**
前脳底動脈症候群　**RBAS**
前白血球性症候群　**PLS**
前白血病　**PL**
前鼻棘　**ANS**
前吻側腹側核　**V.o.a.**
前負荷係数　**PI**
前部虚血性視神経症　**AION**
前腹側(核)　**VA**
前賦活体　**PA**
前壁　**AW**
前壁梗塞　**AWI**
前壁心筋梗塞　**AMI, AWMI**
前壁中隔梗塞　**ASMI**
(寄生虫の)前鞭毛期　**PM**
前方後頭位　**OA**
前方固定　**AIF**
前方切除術　**AR**
前方の　**A, a, AN, ANT, ant**
前(眼)房　**AC, A/C, a.c.**
前房の　**V**
前房分化症候群　**ACCS**
前房レンズ　**AC-IOL**
(眼の)前脈絡膜動脈　**AChA**
前葉ホルモン　**ALH**
前リンパ芽球　**pLb**
前リンパ球　**pLc**
前リンパ球性白血病　**PL, PLL**
前リンパ節　**ALN**
前立腺　**pros, prost**
前立腺圧係数　**PPC**
前立腺圧出液　**EPS**
前立腺癌　**Cap, PC, PCA, pCa**
前立腺間質液　**PIF**
前立腺(特異)抗原　**PA**
前立腺抗細菌性因子　**PAF**
前立腺上皮内腫瘍　**PIN**
前立腺性血清酸性ホスファターゼ　**PSAP**
前立腺性酸性ホスファターゼ　**PAcP, PAP**
前立腺生体組織内深部レーザー凝固術　**ILCP**
前立腺精嚢腺液　**PVF**
前立腺摘出後感染　**PPI**
前立腺特異抗原　**PSA**
前立腺特異酸性ホスファターゼ　**PSAP**
前立腺の　**prostat**
前立腺針生検　**NBP**
前立腺肥大　**BHP, PH**
前立腺部尿道長　**PPL**
前立腺分泌　**PS**
前立腺マッサージ　**PM**
前立腺未分化小細胞癌　**SCUCP**
前腕　**BE, FA, UA**
前腕回外　**FS**
前腕回外した　**FS**
前腕回内した　**FP, f.p.**
前腕血管抵抗　**FVR**

せ

前腕血流量　**FBF**
前腕切断　**BEAMP**
前腕阻血運動試験　**FIET**
(脊柱)前彎(症)　**lord**
栓　**epistom.**
栓球　**TBC**
穿開術　**paracent**
穿孔　**P, p, pent, perf**
穿孔した　**perf**
穿孔する　**P, p, pent**
穿孔性消化性潰瘍　**PPU**
穿孔性の　**perf**
穿刺　**punct**
穿刺(術)　**paracent**
穿刺吸引(生検)　**FNA**
穿刺吸引細胞診　**ABC, FNAC**
穿刺吸引生検　**FNB**
穿刺する　**punct**
穿通枝領域アテローム硬化性疾患　**BAD**
閃光写真脾門脈造影法　**SSP**
閃光融合域(検査)　**FFT**
旋光分散　**ORD**
喘息　**asth**
喘息症状　**SOA**
喘息性気管支炎　**AB**
喘息の診断と治療の国際報告　**ICR**
喘息のためのガイド　**GINA**
喘息を伴う慢性気管支炎　**CBA**
戦時緊急処方　**WEF**
戦場輸血班　**FTT**
戦争捕虜　**POW**
戦争捕虜症候群　**POM**
戦略情報システム　**SIS**
煎剤　**dec., decoct., det., Dt**
腺　**GL, Gl, gl, gl., gland., Gll**
腺癌　**AC, ACA, ad-ca, Ad-Ca, adenoca**
腺結膜咽頭ウイルス　**ACP-virus**
腺上皮　**GE**
腺腫　**A**
腺腫様過形成　**AH**
腺の　**GL, Gl, gl, gl., gland.**
腺平上皮癌　**as**
腺様増殖症　**AV**
腺様嚢胞(性)癌　**ACC, Acc**
漸増シャトルウォーキングテスト　**ISWT**
漸増抵抗　**PR**
漸増抵抗運動　**PRE**
潜(熱)　**L**
潜函病　**DCS**
潜(刺激)期　**LP**
潜血　**OB**
潜血・陰性　**OBN**
潜血・陽性　**OBP**
潜行性の　**insid**
潜在悪性度不明基質腫瘍　**STUMP**
潜在(性)心筋障害　**LCM**
潜在〔潜伏〕性遠視　**HL, Hl, H/L**
潜在性原発性悪性腫瘍　**OPM**
潜在性線維性肺胞炎　**CFA**
潜在性の　**pot, poten**
潜在的致死障害　**PLD**
潜在的致死障害回復　**PLDR**
潜在的に自己支持のできる視力障害者への援助　**APSB**
潜在的に致命的な不整脈　**PLA**
潜在的余命損失年数　**PYLL**
潜在(性)二分脊椎　**SBO**
潜水病　**CAD**
潜伏期　**ICP, IP, LP**
潜伏期(間)　**LP**
潜伏時弛緩　**LR**
潜伏(性)の　**LAT**
潜伏梅毒　**LL**
線　**l, LL**
線維　**fib**
線維芽細胞　**FIB, Fibro**
線維芽細胞インターフェロン　**FIF, FIFN**
線維芽細胞化学走性因子　**FCF**
線維芽細胞活性化因子　**FAF**
線維芽細胞コロニー形成細胞　**FCFC**
線維芽細胞成長因子　**FGF**
線維芽細胞増殖因子　**FBPF**
線維芽細胞由来成長因子　**FDGF**
線維芽細胞様の　**FL**
線維筋性異形成　**FMD**
線維筋性過形成　**FMH**
線維性過形成　**FH**
線維筋痛症候群　**FS**
線維筋(性)の　**FM**
線維細胞　**FC**
線維性滑膜　**FS**
線維性骨炎　**OF**
線維性骨皮質欠損　**FCD**
線維性蛋白質　**F protein**
線維性肺疾患　**FLD**
線維石灰化膵性糖尿病　**FCPD**
線維腺腫　**FA**
線維素　**cell**
線維層　**FL**
線維束性攣縮　**fasc, fasci**
線維素原　**FBG, FG, FI, Fib, fib, fibrin**

線維組織　**FT**
線維素性有孔ガラス玉　**CPB**
線維素様壊死　**FN**
線維素溶解活性　**FA**
線維(性)の　**F, fib**
線維(性)嚢胞の　**FC**
線維斑　**FP**
線維(性)攣縮　**fibr, fibrill**
線維攣縮　**Fib, fib**
線エネルギー付与　**LET**
線形計画法　**LP**
線形の　**lin, lin.**
線形濃度勾配アクリルアミドゲル　**LPG**
線源・腫瘍間距離　**STD**
線源・皮膚間距離　**SSD**
線源・表面間距離　**SSD**
線源アイソセンター間距離　**SID**
線源皮膚間距離　**FSD**
線源皮膚距離　**FHA, FHD**
線源表面間距離　**FSD**
線源フィルム間距離　**SFD**
線源プレート間距離　**FPD**
線条(体)　**ST, Str**
線条外　**ES**
線条角膜症　**SK**
線条体　**CS**
線条体黒質変性症　**SND**
線状炎症性イボ状表皮性母斑　**LIVEN**
線状骨折　**L fx**
線状赤血球凝集素　**FHA**
(放射線の)線質係数　***Q***
線像強度分布　**LSF**
線虫　**nema**
線虫学　**nemat**
線虫の　**nema**
線虫類　**nema**
線(状)の　**lin, lin.**
線幅因子　**LW**
線毛運動周波数　**CBF**
線毛細胞　**CC**
線毛上皮　**CE**
線毛上皮細胞　**CEC**
線毛不動症候群　**ICS**
線量　**D, d., D, d., dos.**
線量強度　**DI**
線量当量　**DE**
線量率計　**r meter, r-meter**
選択視　**PL**
選択すべき緩下剤　**LOC**
選択性イオンモニタリング　**SIM**
選択性指数　**SI**
選択的胃迷走神経切断　**SGV**
選択的胃迷走神経切離術　**SV**
選択的エストロゲン受容体調整　**SERM**
選択的カルシウム動注負荷後肝静脈採血法　**ASVS**
選択的気管支動脈造影法　**SBAG**
選択的近位迷走神経切離術　**SPV**
選択的頸部照射　**ENI**
選択的外科手術　**elect.surg**
選択的消化管内殺菌(法)　**SDD**
選択的情報サービス　**SDI**
選択的セロトニン再取込み阻害薬　**SSRI, SSRIs**
選択的臓器動脈造影　**SVA**
選択的単一胚移植法　**eSET**
選択的低アルドステロン症　**SHA**
選択的な　**elect**
選択的肺胞気管支造影法　**SAB**
選択的光温度解除　**SP**
選択的美容手術　**ECS**
選択的腹腔動脈造影　**SCA, SCAG**
選択的迷走神経切離術　**SV**
選択的流産　**EAB**
選択的領域リンパ節郭清　**ELND**
選択反応　**CR**
選別・応急処置・後方搬送　**3T**
遷延性(持続性)ウイルス症候群　**PVS**
遷延性可逆性虚血性神経症候　**PRIND**
遷延性局所反応　**LLR**
遷延性睡眠時無呼吸　**PSA**
鮮明な　**brt**
蠕動波　**PW**

そ

ソジウム（＝ナトリウム） **Na**
ソーシャルワーカー **SW**
ソーセージ様膣クリーム **AVC**
ソーダ **sod**
ソックス **SOx**
ソドミー **Sod**
ソナー **sonar**
ゾニサミド **ZNS, ZSM**
ゾピクロン **ZPC**
ソフトコンタクトレンズ **SCL**
ソプラノ **sop**
ソマトスタチン **GIF, Smst, SOM**
ソマトスタチン（＝GIF） **SS**
ソマトスタチン受容体 **SSTR**
ソマトスタチンニューロン **SSN**
ソマトスタチン様免疫反応性 **SLI**
ソマトトロピン **SH**
ソマトトロピン〔成長ホルモン〕阻止因子 **SIF**
ソマトトロピン〔成長ホルモン〕放出因子 **SRF**
ソマトトロピン〔成長ホルモン〕放出因子ホルモン **SRFH**
ソマトトロピン〔成長ホルモン〕放出ホルモン **SRH**
ソマトトロピン〔成長ホルモン〕放出抑制因子（＝ソマトスタチン） **SRIF**
ソマトトロピン〔成長ホルモン〕放出抑制ホルモン **SRIH**
ソマトメジン **SM**
ソマトメジンA **SMA, SM-A**
ソマトメジンC **SM-C**
ソラマメ斑紋状ウイルス **BBMV**
ソラレン **PSOR**
ソラレン長波長紫外線 **PUVA**
ゾリンジャー・エリソン（症候群） **ZE, Z-E**
ゾリンジャー・エリソン症候群 **ZES**
ソルビトール **Sorb**
ソルビトール脱水素酵素 **SDH, SODH**
ソルビトール脱水素酵素〔デヒドロゲナーゼ〕 **SD, Sorb D, SORD**
ソルブド **SOLVD**
ゾーン **Z**
ソンディテスト **ST**
ソンネ赤痢菌 **SS**
その後変化なし **SP, S/P**
その側に貼付せよ **lat admov**
その他 **ms, usw.**
その他の **misc**
その他の報告 **MR**
その名前を表示せよ **s.sn., s.s.n**
その日のうちに **i.d.**
その他 **O, o**
それから **T/**
それぞれ **RESP, Resp, resp, resp., sing.**
それの **qour.**
そんなに熱くない **NSH**
狙撃X線撮影 **spot**
阻害 **I**
阻害の **inhib**
阻害物質定数 **K_i**
阻止 **I, inhib**
阻止因子 **IF**
（細菌発育）阻止抗生物質量 **IAD**
阻止する **inhib**
咀嚼・吸入〔吸引〕・嚥下 **CSS**
咀嚼する **trit.**
祖父 **GF, GR-FR**
祖父と祖母 **gaffer & gammer**
祖母 **GM, GR-MO**
素因 **Disp., disp.**
素質 **constit**
素質的に劣性な精神病質 **CPI**
素質（性）の **constit**
粗性炭酸カリ **pot.**
粗造型コロニー **R**
粗造性 **R**
粗造な **R**
粗大運動活性 **GMA**
粗大かつ喘鳴性の（呼吸） **C & H**
粗大水泡性ラ音 **RL**
粗大な **C**
粗大粉末にせよ **grmp**
粗動 **fl**
粗マリファナ抽出物 **CME**
粗面小胞体 **GER, rER, RER, RM**
粗面の **rs**
組織 **T**
組織圧 **TP**
組織因子 **TF**
組織化学 **HC**
組織学 **Hist., Histol**
組織学者 **Hist., Histol**
組織学的外膜癌浸潤程度 **a0-3**
組織学的癌肛門側断端 **aw**
組織学的骨置換率 **HIR**
組織学的漿膜下癌浸潤度 **ss**
組織学的漿膜癌滲出度 **si**

組織学的漿膜面癌露出および浸潤度　**sei**
組織学的漿膜面癌露出度　**se**
組織学的剝離面癌露出　**ew**
組織活動性指標　**HAI**
組織灌流係数　**TPI**
(病理)組織技士　**HTL**
組織球性悪性リンパ腫　**ML-H**
組織(腫瘍)空中線量比　**TAR**
組織コロイド浸透圧　**TOP**
組織再生誘導法　**GTR**
組織最大線量比　**TMR**
組織細胞様血管腫様病変　**HHLL**
組織修復細胞　**TRC**
組織障害因子　**TDF**
組織静水圧　**THP**
組織浸潤性　**TI**
組織性プラスミノゲンアクチベータ　**tPA, t-PA**
組織増殖　**Veg, veg**
組織増大術　**CAL**
組織耐量　**TTD**
組織抵抗　**Rti**
組織適合遺伝子座　**HL**
組織適合抗原　**HA, HLA**
組織適合性Y抗原　**H-Y antigen**
組織当量　**TE**
組織培養　**TC**
組織培養ウロキナーゼ　**TCUK**
組織培養感染量　**TCID**
組織培養培地　**TCM**
組織培養量　**TCD**
組織ピーク線量比　**TPR**
組織ポリペプチド抗原　**TPA**
組織ポリペプチド抗原反応推進要素　**TRE**
組織脈管形成因子　**TAF**
組織ラクターゼ活性　**TLA**
組成　**Comp., comp., compn, constit, cp, cp.**
疎水性クロマトグラフィ　**HIC**
疎水性蛋白　**HP**
遡及抑制　**RIC**
鼠径下　**SI**
鼠径(部)の　**Ing., ing**
鼠径部肉芽腫　**GI**
鼠径ヘルニア　**IH**
(救急)蘇生(法)　**resus**
蘇生後死亡　**DAR**
蘇生させない指示　**ONTR**
蘇生されない　**NTBR**
蘇生術適応除外　**DNR**
蘇生不可〔不要〕　**DNR**
(救急)蘇生法　**RESC, resc**
蘇生法を行わないという指示書　**DNR-Order**
双球菌(属)　**D**
双極細胞　**BC**
双極性感情障害　**BP**
双極(性)電気凝固(法)　**BPEC**
双極導出　**BP**
双極(性)の　**BP**
双子菌　**G**
双胎間輸血症候群　**TTTS**
爪床　**NB**
早期胃癌　**EGC**
早期冠(状)動脈(疾患)治療　**PCC**
早期記憶　**EM**
早期検体　**EMS**
早期抗原拡散型　**EA-D**
早期後発射　**EAD**
早期興奮症候群　**PES**
早期後脱分極　**EAD**
早期視細胞電位　**ERP**
早期転移因子　**ETn**
早期頭頂部反応　**EVR**
早期妊娠試験　**EPT**
早期の　**E, e**
早期標識ピーク　**ELP**
早期標識ビリルビン　**ELB**
早期幼児自閉症　**EIA**
早産児　**PI, prem**
早熟指数　**PI**
早熟の　**prem**
早朝　**dilne.**
早朝こわばり　**EMS**
早朝に　**p.m., prim.luc.**
早朝尿　**EMU**
早発黄疸　**IP**
早発急速進行性肺成熟　**PALM**
早発性痴呆　**DP**
早発(性)痴呆　**Demen Prae**
早発卵巣不全(症)　**POF**
走化力　**CA**
走査イオンコンダクタンス顕微鏡　**SICM**
走査型オージェ電子顕微鏡　**SAM**
走査型キャパシタンス顕微鏡　**SCaM**
走査型近接場光顕微鏡　**SNOM**
走査型探査顕微鏡　**SXM**
走査型電位顕微鏡　**SPoM**
走査型電子顕微鏡　**SEM**
走査型電気化学顕微鏡　**SECM**
走査型トンネル顕微鏡　**STM**
走査型熱顕微鏡　**SThM**
走査型光音波顕微鏡　**SPAM**

走査型レーザー音響顕微鏡　**SLAM**
走査型レーザー断層撮影法　**SLT**
走査近視野光学顕微鏡　**NFOSM**
走査螢光顕微鏡　**OSFM**
走査磁力顕微鏡　**SMFM**
走査電顕像のコンピュータによる評価　**CESEMI**
走査透過型電子顕微鏡　**STEM**
走査トンネル電位計　**STP**
走査トンネル分光法　**STS**
走査プローブ顕微鏡　**SPM**
相　**ph**
相加　**addn**
相関関係　**r**
相関係数　**CC**
相関二次元　**COSY**
相関法　**COSY**
相互意識のひずみ　**IM**
相互連結樹状細胞　**IDC**
相似係数　**SC**
相似している　**analog**
相似度指数　**SI**
相線　**PL**
相対運動速度　**SRM**
相対塩濃度　**RSC**
相対危険度　**ERP**
相対湿度　**rel hum, RH**
相対消費率　**RCR**
相対的　**rltv**
相対的緩徐洞調律　**RSSR**
相対的肝濁音界　**RHD**
相対的結合活性　**RBA**
相対的結合能　**RBA**
相対的腎機能　**RF**
相対的心濁音界　**RCD**
相対的生物学的効果　**RBW**
相対的生物学的効果直線エネルギー移送　**RBELET**
相対的生物学的効果比　**REB**
相対的脊髄灌流圧　**RSPP**
相対的な　**rel**
相対的反応　**RR**
相対的リスク　**RR**
相対比放射能　**RSA**
相対標準偏差　**RSD**
相対不応期　**RRP**
相対リスク減少率　**RRR**
相談　**cons**
相談サービス　**CS**
相当する　**cntn**
相当体重　**AGA**
相当体重(児)　**AFD**
相当体重児　**AFD infant, AGA infant**
相同染色分体間交換　**HCI**
相反の　**Recip, recip.**
相補DNA　**cDNA**
相補性決定領域　**CDR**
相補性リボ核酸　**cRNA**
相補デオキシリボ核酸　**cDNA**
捜索・救助・医療　**SRM**
挿管　**tub**
挿管連続陽圧　**ICPP**
挿入　**ins**
挿入・欠失　**ID**
挿入配列　**IS**
挿話的な　**epis**
造影CT　**CECT, CE-CT**
造影剤　**CM**
造影剤心筋出現図　**CMAP**
造影剤増強コンピュータ断層撮影(法)　**CECT**
造影剤腎症　**CIN**
造影増強効果　**CE**
造血異形成　**HPD**
造血幹細胞　**HSC**
造血幹細胞の可逆的抑制因子　**SCI**
造血性細胞増殖因子　**HCGF**
造血性プロトポルフィリン症　**EP**
造血臓器　**BFO**
造血増殖因子　**HPGF**
造袋(術)　**marsup**
造鼻術　**rhino**
(女の)曽孫　**GGD**
曽孫(男)　**GGS**
掻爬除去　**Aus**
巣状壊死　**FN**
巣状型肺気腫　**FE**
巣状血管性頭痛　**FVH**
巣状硬化性糸球体腎炎　**FSG, FSGN**
巣状硬化性変化　**FSS**
巣状糸球体硬化症　**FGS**
巣状糸球体腎炎　**FGN**
巣状増殖型ループス腎炎　**FPLN**
巣状増殖性糸球体腎炎　**FPG**
巣状皮膚形成不全　**FDH**
巣状分節状糸球体硬化症　**FSGS**
巣状分節状糸球体硬化症(マウス)　**FGS**
象牙質エナメル質境界　**DEJ**
象牙質形成不全(症)　**DI**
創液　**WOFL**
創開離強度　**WBS**
創傷　**W, w, WD, wd, wds, WND, wnd**
創傷清拭〔清浄化〕　**deb**
創傷チェック　**WC, w.c.**
創傷治癒　**WH**

創傷と皮膚　**W & S**
創傷による死亡　**DOW**
創傷ホルモン　**WH**
創造科学技術推進事業　**ERATO**
創面切除(術)　**deb**
痩身値　**S/V**
装着　**ins**
装着器皮膚間隔　**ASD**
装置　**app, appar, eqpt, equip**
装備　**eqpt, equip**
僧帽(筋)　**trap**
僧帽筋皮弁　**TRMC**
僧帽雑音　**MS**
僧帽の　**mi**
僧帽弁　**MV**
僧帽弁・心室中隔間距離　**EPSS**
僧帽弁・半月弁　**MV-SV**
僧帽弁逸脱症候群　**MVP, MVPS**
僧帽弁開大術　**MV**
僧帽弁開放　**Mo**
僧帽弁開放音　**MO, MOS, OS**
僧帽弁可動域　**MVE**
僧帽弁機能不全　**MI**
僧帽弁逆流　**MR**
僧帽弁逆流指数　**MRI**
僧帽弁逆流症　**MI**
僧帽弁逆流面積　**MRA**
僧帽弁逆流量　**MRF**
僧帽弁狭窄指数　**MSI**
僧帽弁狭窄症　**MS, MVS**
僧帽弁狭窄閉鎖不全(症)　**MSI, MSR**
僧帽弁形成術　**MAP**
僧帽弁口　**MVO**
僧帽弁口圧勾配　**MVG, MV gard**
僧帽弁後尖　**PML**
僧帽弁(拡張期)後退速度　**MVDDR**
僧帽弁口閉鎖症　**MA**
僧帽弁口野(部)　**MVOA**
僧帽弁交連切開(術)　**MC**
僧帽弁疾患　**MD, MVD**
僧帽弁前尖　**AML**
僧帽弁大動脈弁置換(術)　**MAVR**
僧帽弁置換術　**MVR**
僧帽弁バルーン切開(術)　**MBV**
僧帽弁不全　**mit insuf**
僧帽弁閉鎖　**Mc**
僧帽弁閉鎖音　**MC**
僧帽弁閉鎖不全　**IMLC**
僧帽弁閉鎖不全(症)　**IM**
僧帽弁閉鎖不全症　**MR**
僧帽弁弁口面積　**MVA**
僧帽弁輪　**MVR**
層空気流　**LAF**
層空気流室　**LAFR**
層状〔葉状〕魚鱗癬　**LI**
層を重ねて　**sss**
総　**T, tot**
総医学評議会　**GMC**
総〔全〕胃容量　**TSV**
総エストロゲン(排出)　**TE**
総塩基　**TB**
総L鎖濃度　**TLC**
総カルシウム量　**TC**
総肝管　**CHD**
総肝血流量　**THBF**
総肝動脈　**AHC, CHA**
総海綿骨量　**TTBV**
総〔全〕還元糖　**TRS**
総胸腺リンパ球　**TTL**
総駆出時間　**TET**
総血清前立腺性酸ホスファターゼ　**TSPAP**
総血清胆汁酸　**TSBA**
総血清蛋白　**TSP**
総血清ビリルビン　**TSB**
総計　**Σ**
総計で　**Z, Z-**
総頸動脈　**CCA**
総ゴナドトロピン活性　**TGA**
総コリンエステラーゼ　**TChE**
総コレステロール　**T.CH, T-CHO**
総コレステロール血清中　**CT**
総コレステロール量　**TC**
総交換可能チ〔サイ〕ロキシン　**TET**
総交換能力　**TEC**
総交替アルブミン　**TEA**
総(血中)好酸球数　**TEC**
総合活動　**A**
総合環境対策補償責任法　**CERCLA**
総合健康推進計画　**THP**
総合識別　**TD**
総合喘息性格テスト　**CAI**
総合的精神症状評価尺度　**CPRS**
総合的な評価　**OA**
総合的品質管理　**TQC**
総合病院　**Gen Hosp, GH**
総合病院運営と医学情報システム　**THOMIS**
総呼吸コンダクタンス　**TRC**
総再生産率　**GRR**
総酸性リン酸分解酵素　**TAP**
総酸素含量　**OT**
総酸素要求量　**TOD**
(胃液の)総酸度　**A, a**
総酸排泄(量)　**NAE**
総ジギタリス飽和量　**TDD**
総子宮内容積　**TIUV**
総指伸(筋)　**EDC**
総重量　**grwt**
総〔全〕食事性蛋白　**NDP**

総食物繊維量　**TDF**
総脂肪酸　**TFA**
総時間　**TT**
総時間等量　**WTE**
総循環アルブミン　**TCA**
総静脈栄養　**TPN**
総睡眠時間　**TST**
総生存　**OS**
総〔全〕静的コンプライアンス　**TSC**
総説　**REV, rev.**
総組織適合性割合　**NHR**
総代謝可能エネルギー　**TME**
総体重　**TBW**
総体循環抵抗　**TSR**
総体積　**TV**
総胆管　**CBD**
総胆汁酸　**TBA**
総チ〔サイ〕ロキシン　**TT, TT_4**
総窒素　**TN**
総腸骨静脈　**CIV**
総腸骨動脈　**CIA**
総鉄結合能　**TIBC**
総電子数　**TEC**
総トリハロメタン　**TTHM**
総トリヨードチ〔サイ〕ロニン　**TT_3**
総投与量　**TD**
総特殊出生率　**TFR**
総動脈幹　**TA, TAC, TRNG**
総動脈管開存　**PTA**
総内腸骨動脈　**CIIA**
総〔全〕二酸化炭素　**Tco_2**
総白血球　**TWBC**
総肺活量　**CPT**
総肺コンプライアンス　**TLC**
総肺静脈灌流異常症　**TAPVC, TAPVD, TAPVR**
総発情ホルモン　**TO**
総排泄窒素　**TEN**
総ヒドロキシアパタイト　**THA**
総ヒドロキシプロリン　**THP**
(血清)総ビリルビン　**TBI**
総ビリルビン(定量法)　**T bili**
総ビリルビン(量)　**TB, TBIL**
総分岐鎖アミノ酸とチロシンの比　**BTR**
総腹骨盤照射　**WAP**
総ヘモグロビン量　**THb**
総便中窒素　**TFN**
総免疫反応性(インスリン)　**TIR**
総有機炭素　**TOC**
総〔全〕容量　**TV**
総リン　**TP**
総リン脂質　**TPL**
総リンパ球数　**TLC**
総リンパ節軸照射　**TANI**
総流産率　**TAR**
総レニン基質　**TRS**
総〔全〕ロゼット形成細胞　**TRFC**
総和　**sum**
総〔全〕B_{12}結合能　**TBBC**
聡明因子　**C-factor**
増悪　**aggrav, Ex, ex, exac**
増悪した　**AGG, agg.**
増悪する　**Ex, ex, exac**
増加(する)　**INC, inc, inc., INCR, Incr, incr.**
増加した　**INC, inc, inc.**
増加する　**aug., icr**
増加率　**MR**
増刊　**supps**
増感効果比　**ER**
増強　**INC, inc, inc., INCR, Incr, incr.**
増強性インスリン耐性試験　**AITT**
増強ヒスタミン試験　**AHT**
増殖　**H, mult**
増殖(症)　**V, Veg, veg**
増殖因子　**GF**
増殖鎌状網膜症　**PSR**
増殖刺激活性体　**MSA**
増殖性肝(臓)小結節　**HLN**
増殖性細胞核抗原　**PCNA**
増殖性糸球体腎炎　**PGN**
増殖性出血(性)腸疾患　**PHE**
増殖性硝子体網膜症　**PVR**
増殖性腎疾患　**PKD**
増殖性天疱瘡　**PVeg.**
増殖性糖尿病性網膜症　**PDR**
増殖性乳房疾患　**PBD**
増殖性ヘルパー細胞　**PHC**
増殖性網膜炎　**RP, RPr**
増殖前糖尿病(性)網膜症　**PPDR**
増殖帯　**PZ**
増殖能　**PC**
増殖分層　**GF**
増殖網膜症光凝固(術)　**PRP**
増殖抑制因子　**PIF**
増殖率　**MR**
増大(する)　**INC, inc, inc., INCR, Incr, incr.**
増大した　**INC, inc, inc.**
増大している　**INCR, Incr, incr.**
増分　**INC, inc, inc.,**

INCR, Incr, incr.
増幅 **amp**
槽内の **IC**
操作 **Man, MANIP, manip**
操作する **man**
叢 **pl, Pll, plx**
騒音汚染レベル L_{np}
騒音起因の聴力不良 **NIHL**
騒音計 **SLM**
騒音計のA特性デシベル **dBA**
騒音による永久的閾値変動 **NIPTS**
騒音分析器 **son an**
騒音防止協会 **NAS**
騒音防止全国協議会 **NCNA**
臓器獲得計画 **OPPs**
臓器許容量 **OTD**
臓器血流 **OBF**
臓器組織共同センター **OSCC**
臓器転移 **M**
(癌の)臓器転移の有無程度 M_{0-1}
躁うつ(病)の **MD**
躁うつ病 **MDI, MDP**
躁うつ病患者 **MD**
躁(病)エピソード **ME**
躁状態評価尺度 **MS Scale**
躁病 **M**
即時型アレルギー(反応) **IAR**
即時型過敏症 **ITH**
即時型過敏反応 **IHR**
即時型黒化 **IT**
即時型色素黒化 **IPD**
即時型喘息反応 **IAR**
即時(型)過敏症 **IH**
即時全身反応 **IGR**
即時早期抗原 **IEA**
即時乳房再建 **IBR**
即発γ線分析 **PGA**
束 **BD, BDL, fasc, fasc.**
(副腎皮質の)束状帯 **ZF**
足学士 **M.Pd**
足関節血圧指数 **API**
足関節血流量 **AF**
足関節収縮期圧 **AP**
足関節-上腕血圧比 **ABI**
足顆圧指標 **API**
足根管症候群 **TTS**
足根中足(関節) **TMT**
足根中足関節 **TM**
足根中足骨の **TM**
足指血圧と上腕動脈収縮期圧との比 **TPI**
(マウスやモルモットの)足蹠反応 **FPR**
足治療科協会員 **MChS**
足底疣 **PW**
足底の **pl, PL, P.L.**
足底板 **F.B.**
足背動脈 **DP**
足背動脈皮弁 **DP flap**
足部白癬(水虫) **t.pedis**
足浴 **FB**
促進 **AC, ac, Acc, acc, accel, facil**
促進凝固時間 **ACT**
促進グロブリン **AC-G, AcG**
促進剤 **prom**
促進する **facil**
促進反応 **AR**
促進物質 **AC**
促迫状心室調律 **AVR**
速中性子 **FN**
速度 **R, S, vel, vel., veloc, veloc.**
速度(=m/s) **V, v**
速度定数 **k**
速度波形 **VWF**
速反応 **QR**
側咽頭間隙 **PPS**
側キヌタ骨ひだ **LIF**
側嗅神経路 **LOT**
側屈 **lat.bend.**
側屈(の) **LB**
側後眼窩前頭皮質 **LPOF**
側後天蓋核 **LDT**
側坐核 **NA**
側索 **LB**
側鎖 **R**
側鎖ケト酸 **BCKA**
側視空輸レーダー **SLAR**
側視床下部領域 **LHA**
側側(=吻合法の1つ) **SS**
側側門脈大静脈シャント **SSPS**
側中隔核 **LSN**
側中脳静脈 **LMV**
側頭・後頭・頭頂の **TOP**
側頭下顎骨の **TM**
側頭筋 **TM**
側頭頭頂の **TP, T−P**
側頭動脈炎 **TA**
側頭の **temp**
側頭部の **T**
側頭平面 **PT**
側頭葉 **TL**
側頭葉てんかん **TLE**
側脳室 **LV**
側脳室神経 **LVN**
側脳室幅 **LVW**
側脳室幅/大脳半球幅比 **LVW/HW**
側副血行 **collat.circ.**
側副の **col, collat**
側副路 **BP**
側腹部 **fl**
側壁 **LW**
側壁圧 **LWP**
側方眼球運動 **LEM**
側方二倍線量X線撮影(法) **LDER**
側方の **L, lat, lat.**

そ

側方発育型腫瘍　**LST**
側方捕獲制御　**LGC**
側傍巨大細胞　**PGL**
粟粒結核(症)　**mil.TB**
測定　**determin, detn, meas, mst**
測定(する)　**meas**
測定誤差　**E of M**
測定最小限界　**MDL**
測定した　**meas**
測定する　**meas**
測定できる　**M**
測定と記録　**M & R**
測定不可の　**NM**
測定不能　**NTS**
測定方法論的薬剤干渉　**MDI**
属　**GEN, gen**
塞栓　**emb**
塞栓症　**E**
塞栓の　**E**
塞栓療法に用いるデンプン製剤　**DSM**
続発症　**seq.**
続発症なし　**NS**
続発症なしに　**Ṡ seq.**
続発性トルコ鞍空虚症候群　**SESS**
続発性の　**sqq, sqq.**
続発性肺血鉄症　**SPH**
続発性貧血　**SA**
続発性無月経　**SA**
続発性緑内障　**SG**
底　**F, Fd, FU**
注ぐ　**inf.**
即効の　**QA**
卒業後の　**postgrad**
卒業証書　**dpl.**
卒後医学教育　**GME**
卒後医療教育協議会　**COGME**
卒後年　**PGY**
卒後の　**PG**
外上右 1/4(区)　**OURQ**
外からの眼検査　**EEE**
外くるぶし　**LM**
外の　**ext, ext.**
空色の　**caerul.**
損失の百分率増加　**PIL**
損傷　**inj**
損傷(部位)　**les**
損傷後の　**PI, P/I**
損傷された　**inj**

そ

た

タイ・サックス病　**TSD**
ダイアナモンキー　**CDI**
ダイアモンド・ブラックファン(症候群)　**DB**
ダイオドラスト・クリアランス　**Cd**
ダイオドラスト除去率　**ED**
ダイオドラスト尿細管排泄最大量　**TmD**
ダイコム(＝医用画像規格)　**DICOM**
ダイテルス核　**DN**
タイトレンズ症候群　**TLS**
ダイナミックレンジ　**DR**
ダイノルフィン　**DYN**
タイプａ行動型　**TABP**
タイミング　**T**
ダイン　**d, dyn**
タウ　**T**
タウシヒ・ビング(症候群)　**TB**
タウ蛋白キナーゼ　**TPK**
ダウノマイシン　**DM**
ダウノマイシン,ビンクリスチン,プレドニゾロン　**DVP**
ダウノルビシン　**DAUNO, DNR, DRB, DRC**
ダウノルビシン,アザシチジン,アラビノシルシトシン,プレドニゾン,ビンクリスチン(＝オンコビン)　**DZAPO**
ダウノルビシン,アラビノシルシトシン,エトポシド　**DAV**
ダウノルビシン,アラビノシルシトシン,チオグアニン　**DAT**
ダウノルビシン,アラビノシルシトシン,チオグアニン,ビンクリスチン,プレドニゾン　**DATVP**
ダウノルビシン,アラビノシルシトシン,ビンクリスチン　**DAV**
ダウノルビシン,シクロシチジン,6-メルカプトプリン,プレドニゾロン　**DCCMP**
ダウノルビシン,シクロヘキシルクロロエチルニトロソ尿素,ビンクリスチン　**DCV**
ダウノルビシン,シクロホスファミド,6-メルカプトプリン,プレドニゾン　**DCMP**
ダウノルビシン,シタラビン,6-メルカプトプリン,プレドニゾロン　**DCMP**
ダウノルビシン,シタラビン,チオグアニン　**DCT**
ダウノルビシン,シタラビン,プレドニゾロン　**DCP**
ダウノルビシン,シタラビン,プレドニゾロン,6-メルカプトプリン　**DCPM**
ダウノルビシン,ビンクリスチン,L-アスパラギナーゼ,プレドニゾン　**DVLP**
ダウノルビシン,ビンクリスチン(＝オンコビン),アラビノシルシトシン,プレドニゾン　**DOAP**
ダウノルビシン,ビンクリスチン,プレドニゾロン　**DVP**
ダウノルビシン,ビンクリスチン,プレドニゾン,L-アスパラギナーゼ　**DVPA, DVPL-ASP**
ダウリング・デゴス病　**DDD**
タウロコール酸　**TCA**
タウロリトコール酸　**TLCA**
ダウン症　**Mongo**
ダウン症候群　**DS**
ダウン症児　**DSC**
ダカルバジン　**DTIC**
ダカルバジン,アミノメチルニトロソウレア,ビンクリスチン　**DAV**
ダカルバジン,アミノメチルニトロソウレア,ビンクリスチン,ペプロマイシン　**DAVP**
タキキニン　**TK**
ダクチノマイシン　**DACT**
ダクチノマイシン,メトトレキサート,シクロホスファミド　**DMC**
ダース　**dz, dz.**
タタソール症候群　**MODY**
ダ(ッ)フィＡ＋(血液型)　**FYA**
ダ(ッ)フィＡ－(血液型)　**FYAN**
ダ(ッ)フィＢ＋(血液型)　**FYB**
ダ(ッ)フィＢ－(血液型)　**FYBN**
ターナー型性器発育異常　**XO**
ターナー型生殖器発育不全　**XO**
ターナー症候群　**45X syndrome, 45XO syndrome, TS**
ダニ　**DF**
ダニ抗原　**MTAg**

ダニ媒介ウイルス　**TV**
ダニ媒介脳炎　**TBE**
タバコ　**tob**
タバコ壊死ウイルス　**TNV**
タバコ壊死サテライトウイルス　**TNSV**
タバコ煙(溶液)　**CS**
タバコ環状斑ウイルス　**TRSV**
タバコごろごろウイルス　**TRV**
タバコ糖蛋白　**TGP**
タバコと健康研究所　**TAHRI**
タバコモザイクウイルス　**TMV**
ダフィ血液型抗原　**DARC**
ダブコ　**DABCO**
ダブルプロダクト　**PRP**
ターミナルケア　**TC**
タム・ホースフォルムコ蛋白(質)　**THP**
タモキシフェン　**T, TAM**
タラ肝油　**CLO**
タランピシリン　**TAPC**
タリー・ニーベルク症候群　**TNS**
タリウム　**Tl**
タリウム 201　**^{201}Tl**
タリウム心筋シンチグラフィ　**TMS**
ダルクシェーヴィチ核　**ND**
ダルシトールリジン乳糖鉄　**DLLI**
ダール食塩感受性ラット　**DSR**
ダール食塩抵抗性ラット　**DR**
タールとニコチン　**T/N**
ダルトン　**Da**
タロース　**Tal**
タングステン　**W**
タンジェント　**tan**
ダンシル　**DNS, Dns**
タンタル　**Ta**
タンタルムガーゼ　**TaG**
タンニン酸処理感作赤血球凝集反応　**TRC**
タンニン酸処理血球凝集反応　**BDBR**
タンニン酸処理赤血球　**TRC**
タンニン酸処理赤血球凝集(反応)　**TCH, TRCA**
タンニン酸処理赤血球凝集反応　**TEA, TRCH**
タンニン酸処理赤血球凝集抑制免疫学的検定(法)　**TRCHII**
ダンピング症候群　**DS**
タンポン　**Tp**
たくさんの　**amp., ampl.**
ただちに　**extempl, immed, stat., Stat**
ただちにビンを閉め(させ)よ　**illic.lag.obturat.**
たとえば　**e.g., p.e., pex, p.ex., v.g., z.B., zE**
たぶん　**prob**
互いに向きあって　**F & F**
手綱　**HB**
他科依頼　**C, cons, consult**
他眼固視平面視野　**SC**
他原因による死亡　**DOC**
他側送信補聴器　**CROS**
他の線維血管組織　**FVE**
他の場所に　**ew**
他の部位　**OL**
他病棟へ　**t.o.w.**
他部位では認められない　**NEM**
他部位に適応されない　**NEI**
他部位に含まれない　**NIE**
他法をとるべからず　**na, n.a.**
打診　**P, percus**
打診・聴診・振とう音　**PA & F**
打診音　**PN, PT**
打診時振動　**DTP**
打診と聴診　**P/A, P & A**
打診法　**Percuss & ausc**
田中・ビネー式知能検査　**TBSI**
立ち会い診察　**C**
立ち寄る　**DI**
立会い医　**cons**
立っている　**stdg**
立てよ　**St, st.**
多因子解析　**MFA**
多因子(性)の　**MF**
多価肺炎球菌多糖類　**PPS**
多価肺炎球菌多糖ワクチン　**PPV**
多価不飽和脂肪酸/飽和脂肪酸比　**P/S**
多核巨大細胞　**MGC**
多核好酸球　**PE**
多核好中球　**PN**
多核芳香性水酸化炭素　**PAH**
多環芳香族炭化水素　**PAH**
多顆粒性好塩基球　**FGB**
多菌型　**MB**
多極性(神経細胞)　**mp**
多義の　**amb**
多グリコール酸　**PGA**
多クローン骨髄形質細胞増加　**POMP**
多クローン性 B 細胞活性　**PBA**
多クローン性 B 細胞活性化物質　**PBA**

多クローン性B細胞活性 PBA
多クローン性Bリンパ球マイトゲン PBM
多クローン性プラーク形成細胞 PC-PFC
多元酵素免疫測定法 EMIT
多元的誘発電位 MEP
多血小板血漿 PRP
多血の plteh
多形核(白血球) POLY, poly, polys
多形核顆粒球 PMNG
多形核球 PM, PMNs
多形核好塩基球 PMB, P.M.B.
多形核好塩基性白血球 PMB
多形核好酸性(白血病) PME, P.M.E.
多形核好中球 PMN, PMNN, PNL
多形核の PM, PMN
多形核白血球 PML, PMNL
多形球性白血病 PL
多形(性)後角膜ジストロフィ PPCD
多形紅斑 EM
多形後部ジストロフィ PPD
多形滲出性紅斑 EEM
多形性δ波 PDA
多形性黄色星状膠細胞腫 PXA
多形性膠芽腫 GBMF
多形性の polymorph
多形(性)低分化腺癌 PLGA
多形日光疹 PLE
多系統萎縮症 MSA
多言語失語症 MLA
多結節性の MN
多源性心房性調律 MAR
多源性心房頻拍 MAT, MAT
多孔性人工関節 PCA
多抗原ワクチン MAV
多骨性線維性骨形成異常 PFD
多剤抗生物質抵抗型 MAR
多剤耐性(癌化学療法) MDR
多剤耐性(癌化学療法の1つ) MDR
多剤耐性結核菌 MDR-TB
多剤耐性緑膿菌 MDRP
多剤併用療法 MDT
多剤(化学)療法 MAT
多産 fert
多小水疱体 MVB
多小水疱(性)の MV
多小胞体 MVB
多小胞(性)の MV
多次元尺度法 MDS
多刺創 MSW
多肢選択問題 MCQ
多指(趾)・無孔肛門・脊椎骨奇形(症候群) PIV
多指(趾)(症)・無孔肛門・脊椎骨奇形(症候群) PIAVA
多重圧縮錠剤 MCT
多重欠損症 MD
多重欠損症候群 MDS
多重欠乏症 MD
多重人格障害 MPD
多重乳剤アジュバント WOW
多焦点性心房頻拍 MFAT, MFT
多種因子介入的研究(=高血圧治療に関する大規模試験) MRFIT
多種下垂体ホルモン欠損症 MPHD
多種スルファターゼ欠損症 MSD
多数回手術腰部 MOB
多数の粗(大)水泡性ラ音 RL_3
多染性正赤芽球 N・Ebl-p
多染性赤芽球 Ebl-p
多腺性自己免疫症候群 PGA
多腺性自己免疫性症候群 PGAS
多相 pyph
多相遺伝性薬剤耐性 PDR
多相スクリーニング MHS
多相性格表 MPI
多相的健康診断システム MHTS
多層性小胞 MLV
多臓器異常回転症候群 MOMS
多臓器機能障害症候群 MODS
多臓器不全 MOF
多断面再構成 MPR
多中心性細網組織球症 MR
多中心の PC
多動行動症候群 HBS
多動児 HAC
多動症候群 HKS
多糖類 PS
多内分泌欠乏性自己免疫性糸状菌症 MEDAC
多人数用透析液供給装置 HD
多能性幹細胞 PSC
多嚢胞性肝疾患 PCLD, PLD, PDL
多嚢胞性疾患 PCD
多嚢胞性腎(病) MCK, MCKD
多嚢胞性脳症 MCE
多嚢胞性卵巣 PCO

多囊胞性卵巣疾患 **PCOD**
多囊胞性卵巣症候群 **PCOS, POS**
多囊胞卵巣症候群 **POP**
多囊胞卵巣病 **POD**
多発異栄養症 **DP**
多発(性)筋炎と皮膚筋炎 **PDM**
多発血管炎性肉芽腫症 **GPA**
多発根神経障害 **PRN**
多発(性)腎炎 **PN**
多発神経炎 **PN**
多発神経症 **PNP**
多発性一過性白色斑点症候群 **MEWDS**
多発性外骨(腫)症・精神遅滞(症候群) **MEMR**
多発性外傷〔損傷〕 **mul.inj**
多発性眼コロボーマ **MOC**
多発性筋炎 **PM**
多発性筋炎/皮膚筋炎 **PM/DM**
多発性結節性黄色腫 **XTM**
多発性原発性悪性腫瘍 **MPM**
多発性硬化症 **MS**
多発性硬化症感受性 **MSS**
多発性硬化症感受性遺伝子 **MSSG**
多発性硬化症関連因子 **MSAA**
多発性骨髄腫 **MM**
多発性骨髄腫グロブリン **M.gl**
多発性骨端異形成症 **MED**
多発性コレステロール塞栓症候群 **MCES**
多発性自己癒合性扁平上皮癌 **MSHSC**
多発性神経炎・臓器肥大症・内分泌異常症・M蛋白・皮膚病変(症候群) **POEMS**
多発性神経根炎 **PRN**
多発性神経障害・眼筋麻痺・白質脳症・仮性腸閉塞症 **POLIP**
多発性先天(性)異常 **MCA**
多発性先天(性)奇形 **MCA**
多発性対称性脂肪腫症 **MSL**
多発性チック疾患 **MTD**
多発性内分泌欠乏症・アジソン病・カンジダ症(症候群) **MEDAC**
多発性内分泌腺腫症 **MEA**
多発性内分泌腺腫瘍 **MEN**
多発性内分泌腺腫瘍症 **MEN**
多発性内分泌性腺腫 **MEA**
多発性軟骨性外骨腫 **MCE**
多発性軟部組織損傷 **MSTI**
多発性粘膜神経腫 **MMN**
多発性脳梗塞性痴呆 **MID**
多発性囊胞腎 **PCKD**
多発性皮脂囊腫(症) **SCM**
多発性母斑性基底細胞腫 **NBCE**
多発性リンパ腫性ポリポーシス **MLP**
多発(性)動脈炎 **PA, PAr**
多発(性)の **mult**
多発囊胞脂肪膜性骨形成異常 **PLO**
多発囊胞性肝疾患 **PCHD**
多発発育異常 **DP**
多病巣性好酸球性肉芽腫 **MEG**
多不飽和脂肪酸 **PUFA**
多分割照射 **MFD**
多(数)弁置換(術) **MVR**
多併用予防処置 **MPM**
多房性胸腺囊胞 **MTC**
多房性腎囊胞 **MLCN**
多房性囊胞状腎癌 **MCRCC**
多面人格尺度 **MSRPP**
多毛症の家族歴 **FHH**
多目的カプセル **APC**
多目的食品 **MPF**
多様活動性 **MUA**
多様な **mpx, MPX, mux**
多量 **HD**
耐える **tol**
蛇行性穿孔性弾性線維症 **EPS**
唾液 **sal**
唾液(腺型)アミラーゼ **SA**
唾液試料 **SS**
唾液腺ウイルス **SGV**
唾液腺管癌腫 **SDC**
唾液涙腺炎(ウイルス) **SDA**
堕胎法律廃止全国連合 **NARAL**
堕胎薬 **A-pill**
楕円形標的細胞 **OTC**
楕円赤血球症 **El**
楕円体 **sphr**
大うつ病 **MD**
大運動細胞 **LMC**
大円(筋) **TM**
大カロリー **C, Cal**
大カロリー(=kcal) **Cal**

大会　**cong，cong.**
大学　**coll，U，Univ，univ**
大学医療情報ネットワーク　**UMIN**
大学開発　**AD**
大学間教育交流プログラム　**CUPP**
大学病院センター　**CHu**
大学臨床教員協会　**AUCAS**
大感情障害　**MAD**
大(血)管ヘマトクリット　**LVH**
大環状化合物国際シンポジウム　**ISMC**
大顆粒小胞　**LGV**
大顆粒白血球　**LGL**
大顆粒リンパ球　**LGL**
大臼歯　**M**
大気　**AT**
大気圧　**ATPS，B**
大気圧,乾燥状態　**ATPD**
大気圧イオン化法　**ACI**
大気圧化学イオン化法　**APCI**
大気圧下の酸素　**OAP**
大気圧スプレー法　**APS**
大気管理支援センター　**SCRAM**
大気質計画標準課　**OAQPS**
大気測定情報修正組織　**AIRS**
大気中の有害化学物質　**HAPs**
大気浮遊物質　**SPM**
大気放射線局　**OAR**
大胸筋皮弁　**PM-MC flap，PMMF**
大規模集積回路　**LSI**
大凝集アルブミン　**MAA**
大血管転位症　**TGA，TGV**
大結節　**GT**
大後頭孔　**FM**
大後頭三叉〔差〕神経症候群　**GOTS**
大後頭動脈・中大脳動脈バイパス　**OA-MC bypass**
大再生結節　**MRN**
大細胞石灰化セルトリ細胞腫　**LCCSCT**
大心臓静脈血流量　**GCVF**
大食細胞成長因子　**MGF**
大食症　**Bul**
大〔高〕振幅徐波活動　**LSWA**
大斜径　**OM**
大衆薬　**OTCD**
大学教員の教育能力開発　**FD**
大静脈　**VC**
大静脈膜性閉塞(症)　**MOVC**
大豆　**SB**
大豆凝集素　**SBA**
大豆トリプシン抑制因子　**SBTI，STI**
大豆油食　**SBOM**
大豆(トリプシン)抑制因子　**SBI**
大豆レクチン　**SBL**
大切な　**impt**
大泉門　**AF，A-F**
大槽　**CM**
大多数　**maj**
大腿　**AK，a.k.，OS，Th，UPL**
大腿(骨)　**fem，fem.**
大腿・下腿動脈バイパス　**F-C**
大腿・大腿動脈(バイパス)　**F-F**
大腿-膝窩静脈バイパス　**FPVB**
大腿外側　**fem.ext.**
大腿義肢　**AKP**
大腿ギプス　**OSG**
大腿脛骨角　**FA，FTA**
大腿(骨)頸部骨折　**FNF**
大腿血圧　**FBP**
大腿広筋膜　**FL**
大腿骨・腓骨・尺骨症候群　**FFU**
大腿骨骨頭端線離開　**SCFE**
大腿骨中心臼蓋角　**CEW**
大腿骨頭壊死　**ONFH**
大腿骨頭虚血性壊死　**INFH**
大腿骨頭無腐性壊死　**ANF**
大腿四頭筋　**quad**
大腿四頭筋伸展運動　**QEE**
大腿周長　**OSU**
大腿静脈　**FV**
大腿静脈結紮術　**FVL**
大腿神経伸展テスト　**FNST**
大腿動脈　**FA**
大腿動脈圧　**FAP**
大腿動脈血流量　**FABF**
大腿動脈ライン　**FAL**
大腿内側　**fem.int.**
大腿の　**FEM，fem.**
大腿部の　**fem**
大腸閉塞　**LBO**
大腸　**LB，LI**
大腸 X 線検査　**DDL**
大腸癌および直腸癌　**CRC**
大腸癌で発見された　**DCC**
大腸菌　**E，EC，E coli，E.coli**
大腸菌人工染色体　**BAC**
大腸菌ポリペプチド　**ECP**
大腸菌マルトース結合蛋白　**MalE**

大腸菌由来蛋白　**ECP**
大腸性消化不良　**CD, DC**
大腸腺腫症　**AC**
大腸腺腫性ポリポーシス　**APC**
大腸腺腫様ポリープ　**APC**
大腸直腸外科　**CRS**
大腸停滞　**CR**
大腸内視鏡　**CF, CFS**
大腸内視鏡術　**CF**
大腸ファイバースコープ　**FCS**
大腸ポリポーシス　**PC**
大転子　**GT**
大転子間　**BIT**
大動脈　**A, Ao, AO, Ao**
大動脈(弁)　**A**
大動脈・冠(状)動脈バイパス(術)　**A-C bypass**
大動脈・冠(状)動脈バイパス移植(術)　**ACBG**
大動脈・大腿(動脈)バイパス　**AFB**
大動脈・肺動脈中隔欠損症　**APSD**
大動脈・冠(状)動脈吻合バイパス　**ACBG**
大動脈圧　**AOP, AP**
大動脈圧脈波　**AOP**
大動脈開放　**Ao**
大動脈冠(状)動脈の　**AC**
大動脈弓　**AA**
大動脈球　**AK**
大動脈弓症候群　**AAS, ABS**
大動脈弓離断(症)　**IAA**
大動脈(弁)狭窄　**aort.sten**
大動脈駆出音　**AES**
大動脈径　**AOD, ARD**
大動脈口　**AO**
大動脈後壁　**AoPW**
大動脈収縮期血圧　**ASP**
大動脈縮窄　**Coarc**
大動脈縮窄(症)　**C of A**
大動脈縮窄症　**COA, CoA**
大動脈縮窄複合　**COAC**
大動脈前壁　**AoAW**
大動脈窓　**AW**
大動脈造影法　**AOG**
大動脈中隔欠損　**APW, ASD**
大動脈中隔欠損(症)　**Ap window**
大動脈中隔欠損症　**AP Fistel, AP fistula**
大動脈転位(症)　**T of A**
大動脈内カウンターパルセイション　**IACP**
大動脈内カウンターパルセイションバルーン　**IACB**
大動脈内血管内超音波検査(法)　**ICEUS**
大動脈内の　**IA, i.a.**
大動脈内バルーン　**IAB**
大動脈内バルーンカウンターパルセイション　**IABC, IABCP**
大動脈内バルーンパンピング法　**IABP**
大動脈内バルーン補助　**IABA**
大動脈内バルーンポンプ　**IABP, IBP**
大動脈の解離性動脈瘤　**DAA**
大動脈肺動脈窓　**AP Fistel**
大動脈不全　**AINSUF**
大動脈平均圧　**AoMP**
大動脈閉鎖不全症　**AR**
大動脈弁　**AoV, AV, AV**
大動脈弁逸脱　**AVD**
大動脈弁下狭窄症　**Sub.AS**
大動脈弁下部狭窄　**SAS**
大動脈弁下部狭窄(症)　**SS**
大動脈弁逆流　**aort.regurg.**
大動脈弁狭窄(症)　**Asten, A sten., AVS**
大動脈弁狭窄兼閉鎖不全　**ASR**
大動脈弁狭窄症　**AS**
大動脈弁駆出量　**AVSV**
大動脈弁形成術　**AVP**
大動脈弁口径　**AVO**
大動脈弁疾患　**AVD**
大動脈弁上部狭窄　**SVAS**
大動脈弁上部狭窄症　**SAS**
大動脈弁上部狭窄症候群　**SASS**
大動脈弁置換術　**AVR**
大動脈弁超音波心臓検査図　**AVE**
大動脈弁閉鎖　**AC, AVA**
大動脈弁閉鎖不全(症)　**AI, Alnsuf, A insuf.**
大動脈弁膜下狭窄　**SVAS**
大動脈弁無冠尖　**NCC**
大動脈弁領域　**AVA**
大動脈弁輪拡張症　**AAE**
大動脈弁輪形成術　**AAP**
大動脈流量　**AF**
大頭の　**macrocephs**
大脳脚　**CC, CP, PEC, PED**
大脳の損傷範囲　**ECL**
大脳半球の側頭・後頭・頭頂葉の連合野　**TOP**
大脳皮質　**CX**

大脳誘発電位　**CEP**
大白色腎　**LWK**
大発色団　**LC**
大便連鎖球菌　**SF**
大発作　**GM, GM seizzure**
大発作痙攣疾患　**GMCD**
大縫線核　**NRM**
大麻　**GB**
大容量記憶装置　**MSS**
大容量穿刺(術)　**LVP**
大リンパ球　**LL**
大量　**HD, M, m, mas., mass, mass.**
大量(の)　**LA**
大量吸引症候群　**MAS**
大量硝子体出血　**MVH**
大量静脈内メチルプレドニゾロン投与　**HIMP**
大量静脈瘤出血　**MVH**
大量の　**mass, mass.**
大量非経口投与(注射)　**LVP**
大量メチルプレドニゾロン　**HDMP**
大量メトトレキサート　**HDMTX**
太陽に反応する皮膚の型　**ST**
代謝　**met, metab**
代謝回転数　**TO number**
代謝可能エネルギー　**ME**
代謝監視機構　**MMS**
代謝拮抗物質　**AM**
代謝クリアランス率　**MCR**
代謝産物　**M, met, metab**
代謝指数　**MI**
代謝性冠(状動脈)拡張　**MCD**
代謝当量　**MET, METS**
代謝の　**MET, met, metab**
代謝抑制検査　**MIT**
代謝率　**MR**
代償　**comp, compen, compo, cpe**
代償塩基　**CB**
代償作用　**CA**
代償障害　**decompn**
代償する　**compen**
代償性(心疾患)　**comp**
代償性心(臓)疾患　**CHD**
代償なしで　**WOC**
代償の　**compen**
代償不全　**decompn**
代数的な　**alg**
代数の　**alg**
(米国)代替医療局　**OAM**
代表的な　**repr, typ, typ.**
代用L鎖　**SLC**
代理(人)　**SUB, sub, subst**
代理的試行錯誤　**VTE**
代理ミュンヒハウゼン症候群　**MSBP, MSP**
台湾急性呼吸　**TWAR**
体　**COR**
体位　**P, Pos, pos**
(異常)体位眼振　**PN**
体位性アルコール性眼振　**PAN**
体位性縮瞳反応　**PMR**
体位ドレナージ　**PD**
体育　**PED**
体液　**F, FL, Fl, fl, fld, fluid.**
体液性抗体産生　**HAP**
体液性免疫　**HI**
体液(性)免疫能プロフィール　**HIP**
体温　**BT, KT, T, t, T_b, Temp, temp, temp.**
体温・脈拍・呼吸　**TPR, T.P.R.**
体温計　**ther**
体温正常　**TN**
体温と乾燥状態の大気圧　**BTPD**
体温と血圧　**BTP**
体温と脈拍　**T & P, T＋P**
体外液体喪失　**EFL**
体外希釈値　**EDV**
体外式肝灌流　**ECLP**
体外式心肺補助法　**ECLHA**
体外式生命維持装置　**ECLS, ELS**
体外受精　**IVF**
体外受精と胚移植　**IVF & ER**
体外受精と胚移植(法)　**IVF-ET**
体外受精卵卵管内移植法　**ZIFT**
体外循環　**CEC, ECC**
体外循環後症候群　**PPS**
体外循環左(心)室補助装置　**PLVS**
体外循環容量　**ECV**
体外衝撃波結石破砕装置　**ESWL**
体外衝撃波砕石術　**ESWL**
体外照射　**ECI**
体外人工肺炭酸ガス〔二酸化炭素〕除去装置　**$ECCO_2R$**
体外腎砕石術　**ECSWL**
体外心マッサージ　**ECM**
体外成熟　**IVM**
体外成熟-体外受精-胚移植法　**IVM-IVF**
体格がよく栄養良好な　**WDWN**
体格がよく栄養良好な黒人男性　**WDWNBM**
体格がよく栄養良好な白人

女性 **WDWNWF**
体格がよく栄養良好な白人男性 **WDWNWM**
体格指数 **BMI**
体格の良い **WD**
体格不良の **UD**
体幹絶縁 **BF**
体幹の **som, somat**
体血管抵抗 **SVR**
体形 **fm**
体系体系工学 **SSE**
体型指数 **IB**
体験 **exp, exper**
体験外の **OOBE**
体験型 **EB**
体細胞 **SCE**
体細胞超変異 **SHM**
体細胞由来胚性幹細胞 **ntES**
体臭 **BO**
体重 **av, BM, BW, KG, WT, Wt, wt.**
体重・身長・外貌・知性・性発育 **WHAMES**
体重・身長・体温 **WAT**
体重・身長指数 **WLI**
体重移動頻度 **WTF**
体重管理プログラム **WMP**
体重減少 **WL**
体重負荷によるロッキング膝 **WALK**
体重を気にする人 **WW**
体重をマッチさせたコントロール **WMC**
体脂 **BF**
体静脈還流異常 **ASVR**
体質 **constit**
体質性早熟 **IPP**
体質性の再生不良性貧血 **CAA**
体質(性)の **constit**
体水分 **BW**
体性感覚視床 **SST**
体性感覚誘発電位 **SEP**
体性感覚誘発反応 **SER, SERS**
体性神経系 **SNS**
体性知覚誘発電位 **SSEP**
体積 **V, v, VOL, vol, vol.**
体積駆出 **VE**
体積百分率 **vol%**
体知覚誘発電位 **SPEs**
体動 **BM**
体内受精 **IVF**
体内レーザー砕石術 **ICL**
体肺抵抗比 **Pp/Ps, Rp/Rs**
体表1 m^2あたりの量 **M_2**
体表面火傷 **BSB**
体表面積 **BSA, SA**
体表面電位分布図 **BSPM**
体プレスチモグラフィ **BP**
体力指数 **PFI**
対応 **corr, corresp**
対応する **corr, corresp**
対角結合線(=CD) **DC**
対角線(の) **diag, diag.**
対光調節 **L & A**
対光反射 **LR**
対向電気泳動 **CEP**
対向免疫電気泳動(法) **CIE**
対向流遠心洗浄法 **CE**
対向流電気泳動法 **CEP**
対向流分配 **CCD**
対抗して **adv.**
対人依存特性尺度 **IDI**
対人関係精神療法 **IPT**
対称 **Sym, sym**
対称性 **Sym, sym**
対称性緊張性首反射 **STNR**
対称性の **S, s, Sym, sym**
対称的な **s**
対称点 **PS**
対象 **Obj, obj**
対象分類検査 **OCT**
対照 **C, con, cont, cont.**
対照群 **CG**
対照血清 **CS**
対照する **comp**
対数 **log**
対側閾値移動 **CTS**
(反)対側(性)の **contralat, contralat.**
対比浴 **CB**
対らせんフィラメント **PHF**
対立遺伝子特異的オリゴヌクレオシド **ASO**
対立した **opp**
対立する **opp**
苔状線維 **MF**
耐荷重 **WBAT, WBTT**
耐久因子 **EF**
耐性 **R, Res, res, resis, resist, tol**
耐性因子 **RF, R factor**
耐性伝達因子 **RTF**
耐性のあるような **AS TOL**
耐性フレンド白血病細胞 **RFLC**
耐性率 **RR**
耐糖曲線 **GTC**
耐糖能障害 **IGT**
耐熱性アルカリホスファターゼ **HSAP**
耐熱性直接溶血毒 **TDH**
耐熱性内毒素 **ST**
耐熱性乳酸脱水素酵素 **HIDH**
耐熱性乳酸デビドロゲナーゼ〔脱水素酵素〕 **HLDH**

た

耐熱性無細胞性の百日咳・ジフテリア・テタヌス・ワクチン **HSAPDT**
耐容量 **TD**
待機して **OC**
胎芽 **emb**
胎芽性プレアルブミン **EPA**
胎向 **P**
胎児 **emb, fet**
胎児アルコール症候群 **FAS**
胎児エコー **FE**
胎児学 **fetol**
胎児学者 **fetol**
胎児学の **fetol**
胎児肝移植 **FLT**
胎児肝細胞 **FLC**
胎児肝臓 **FL**
胎児危険 **FD**
胎児鏡 **FS**
胎児胸腺 **FT**
胎児胸腺臓器官培養 **FTOC**
胎児抗原 **EA**
胎児呼吸運動 **FBM**
胎児後月齢 **PnM**
胎児採血 **FBS**
胎児時間尿産生率 **HFUPR**
胎児子宮内モニター **IFM**
胎児集中治療室 **FICU**
胎児循環遺残症 **PFC**
胎児心音 **FHS, FHT, KHT**
胎児心音図 **FPCG**
胎児心電図 **FECG, FEKG**
胎児心拍 **FHB**
胎児心拍陣痛図 **fetal CTG**
胎児心拍数 **FHR**
胎児心拍数一過性徐脈 **FHR deceleration**
胎児心拍数一過性頻脈 **FHR acceleration**
胎児心拍数基線 **FHR baseline**
胎児心拍数基線細変動 **FHR baseline variability**
胎児心迫数基線細変動 **STV**
胎児心拍数陣痛計 **CTG**
胎児心拍数陣痛図 **CTG**
胎児水痘症症候群 **FVS**
胎児性アルコール効果(＝妊婦の飲酒による影響) **FAE**
胎児性癌抗原 **NEA**
胎児性タバコ症候群 **FTS**
胎児性ヘモグロビン **HbF**
胎児赤芽球症 **EBF, EF, FE**
胎児先進部 **PP**
胎児胎盤系 **FPU**
胎児胎盤不均衡 **FPD**
胎児頭皮血液 **FSB**
胎児頭部 **HF**
胎児軟骨形成異常(症) **CDF**
胎児の **F**
胎児脳波 **FEEG**
胎児ヒダントイン症候群 **FHS**
胎児ヘモグロビン **fetal h., HbF, Hb P, HgF**
胎児扁桃 **FT**
胎児硫酸グリコ蛋白抗原 **FSA**
胎生学 **EMB, Emb, emb, embry, embryol**
胎動 **FM**
胎嚢 **GS**
胎盤・卵巣・子宮 **POU**
胎盤アルカリ性ホスファターゼ **PAP**
胎盤アルカリホスファターゼ **PLAP**
胎盤エキス **EE**
胎盤機能不全症候群 **PDS**
胎盤血流量 **PBF**
胎盤性スルファターゼ欠損症 **PSD**
胎盤性ロイシンアミノペプチダーゼ **PLAP**
胎盤蛋白 **PP**
胎盤蛋白 5 **PP5**
胎盤乳腺刺激ホルモン **PLH**
胎盤性ラクトゲン **PL**
胎便 **mec**
胎便吸引 **Mec Asp**
胎便吸引〔嚥下〕症候群 **MAS**
胎便抗原 **MA**
退院 **DC, D/C, dc, Dis, disch, Ent**
退院(させる) **disc**
退院後計画協会 **HDPA**
退院後心配なし **NRAD**
退院後のケア **PHC**
退院時健康状態 **COD**
退院時診断 **DD**
退院した **DC, disch**
退院する **disch**
退院調査 **HDS**
退院の **OH**
退院要約 **DS**
退役軍人 **Vet**
退役軍人管理〔運営〕 **VA**
退役軍人局 **V Adm, Vet Adm, Vet Admin**
退役軍人でない **NV**
退化 **deg, Deg, deg., degen**
退化アミロイド **DAM**
退化する **deg**

退行性反応　**DeR**
退縮　**retr, retr.**
退縮の　**R, rec**
退職後生活扶助法
ERISA
帯　**bd, bd., Cd, Z**
(脳の)帯核　**DB**
帯下　**meno**
帯状回　**CG**
帯状束回　**CG**
帯状ヘルペス　**HZ**
帯状ヘルペスウイルス
HZV
帯状疱疹　**zos**
帯状疱疹後神経痛　**PHN**
帯状疱疹状の　**zos**
帯状疱疹免疫グロブリン
Z/G, ZIG, ZIg
帯状疱疹免疫血漿　**ZIP**
帯状疱疹免疫プラズマ
ZIP
第一頭位第一分類　**LOA**
第一横位第一分類(＝LAA)　**LScA**
第一横位第一分類(＝LScA)　**LAA**
第一横位第二分類(＝LAP)　**LScP**
第一横位第二分類(＝LScP)　**LAP**
第一額位(＝LBA)　**LFA**
第一額位(＝LBP)　**LFP**
第一額位(＝LBT)　**LFT**
第一額位(＝LFA)　**LBA**
第一額位(＝LFT)　**LBT**
第一顔位　**RMA, RMT**
第一顔位(＝頤部後方)
RMP
第一胸椎・第二胸椎…など
T_1〔T_2…〕, T1〔T2…〕
第一骨盤位第一分類
LSA
第一骨盤位第二分類
LSP, LST
第一次硝子体過形成遺残
PHPV
第一斜位　**ROP**
第一診断　**prim.diag**
第一世代　**F_1**
第一鉄の　**Fe^{2+}**
第一頭位　**OLT**
第一頭位第二分類
LOP, LOT
第一の　**P**
第五腰椎・第一仙椎
L5-S1
第三の　**T, t, T, t, ter, tert**
第三脳室前腹壁にある終末器官　**OVLT**
第三脳室嚢胞　**TVC**
第三脳室腹側前方
AV3V
第二横位第一分類(＝RScA)　**RAA**
第二横位第一分類(＝RAA)　**RScA**
第二横位第二分類(＝RScA)　**RAP**
第二横位第二分類(＝RAP)　**RScP**
第二額位　**RBA, RBP, RBT**
第二額位(＝LFP)　**LBP**
第二顔位　**LMA, LMT**
第二顔位(オトガイ部後方)
LMP
第二骨盤位第一分類
RSA, SRA
第二骨盤位第二分類
RSP, RST
第二斜位　**LOP**
第二斜位(の)　**LAO**
第二世代　**F_2**
第二大動脈音　**A_2, II A**
第二大動脈音が第二肺動脈音より大　**A_2P_2**
第二鉄の　**Fe^{3+}**
第二頭位　**ODT**
第二頭位第一分類　**ROA**
第二頭位第二分類
ROP, ROT
第二の　**sec, sec.**
第二の意見　**SO**
第六感　**ESP**
第Ⅰ因子　**F Ⅰ**
第Ⅰ〔Ⅱ,Ⅲ〕期梅毒
L Ⅰ〔L Ⅱ, L Ⅲ〕
第Ⅰ期癒合　**PP, P.P.**
第Ⅱ因子　**F Ⅱ**
第Ⅱ期癒合　**ps**
第Ⅲ因子　**F Ⅲ**
第Ⅳ因子　**F Ⅳ**
第Ⅴ因子　**F Ⅴ**
第Ⅶ因子　**F Ⅶ**
第Ⅷ因子　**F Ⅷ**
第Ⅷ因子関連抗原
Ⅷ R：AG, Ⅷ RAg, Ⅷ RAG
第Ⅷ因子関連フォンヴィレブランド因子
Ⅷ R：WF, Ⅷ WF
第Ⅷ因子凝固活性　**Ⅷ：C**
第Ⅷ因子凝固抗原
Ⅷ CAG
第Ⅷ因子フォンヴィレブランド因子　**Ⅷ R：WF**
第Ⅸ因子　**F Ⅸ**
第Ⅹ因子　**F Ⅹ**
第Ⅹ因子抗原　**X：Ag**
第Ⅻ因子　**F Ⅻ**
第XIII因子　**F XIII**
第1,2,3…術後日
PO Ⅰ, Ⅱ, Ⅲ…etc.
第1～3度心(臓)ブロック
HB1°〔2°, 3°〕
(腰神経の)第1～第5腰椎
L1-L5, L_{1-5}
第1期　**f/s**
第1〔2,3…〕胸髄前根
VRT_1〔VRT_2, VRT_3…etc.〕
第1〔2,3…〕胸椎など
D_1〔D_2, D_3…〕
第1〔2,3…〕頸髄前根

た

VRC$_1$〔VRC$_2$, VRC$_3$, etc.〕
第1頸椎～第7頸椎 **C1-7**
第1斜位 **RAO**
第1心音 **S1**
第1親世代 **P$_1$**
第1背側骨間(筋) **FDI**
第1〔2,3…〕腰髄前(神経)根 **VRL$_1$〔VRL$_2$, VRL$_3$, etc.〕**
第1〔2〕腰椎腹側(神経)根 **L$_1$〔L$_2$〕VR**
第2心音 **S2**
第3学年医学生 **MS Ⅳ**
第3期 **t/s**
第3心音 **S3**
第4学年医学生 **MS Ⅲ**
第4級アンモニウム化合物 **QAC**
第4心音 **S4**
第4の **Q**
第5の **quint.**
第5脳神経下顎枝 **V$_3$**
第5脳神経眼枝 **V$_1$**
第5脳神経上顎枝 **V$_2$**
滞在期間 **LOS, LS**
滞留 **detn**
滞留時間 **det.time**
態度 **beh**
平らな **f**
多汗(症) **HH**
高い疑惑指数 **HIOS**
高さ **ALT, alt, H, h, Hgt, Ht**
高田・荒反応 **TAR, TR**
高田反応 **TR**
高める **elev**
卓上分析器 **DAT**
託児所 **DCC/N, Nsy**
濁音 **M, m.**
足し算 **add.**
助け **assist**
助ける **Asst, asst**
正しい **C, OK**
正しい定量 **Q.R., q.r.**
正しく沸騰させよ **coq.s.a.**
立会診察 **cons, consult**
脱感作テスト **DST**
脱臼 **acetab, dis, DISL, Disl, disloc, Lx, LX**
脱臼骨折 **Fx-dis.fx-dis**
脱臼した **DISL, Disl, disloc**
脱臼する **DISL, Disl, disloc**
脱シアル化オロソムコイド **ASOM**
脱出 **H, her., hern**
脱脂肪乾燥肝 **FEDL**
脱脂乳 **SM**
脱脂乳を飲む **DSM**
脱水(症) **dehyd**
脱水した **dehyd**
脱水素酵素 **DH**
脱水になった **dehyd**
脱線維素症候群 **DFS**
脱炭酸酵素 **DC**
脱炭酸酵素阻害薬 **DCI, DCL**
脱着電離 **DI**
脱同期性睡眠 **DS**
脱分極性後電位 **DAP**
脱飽和 **desat**
脱飽和した **desat**
脱落(性)の **D, d., dec**
脱力 **W**
脱力・萎縮・線維束攣縮 **WAF**
脱力又は萎縮 **W/A**
達成比 **AR**
縦切 **l sect**
縦軸 **y**
縦軸の **l, L**
縦線 **Ord, ord, ord.**
縦の **long**
縦の(断面) **l, L**
玉軸受け **bb**
卵アルブミン **EA, OVA**
丹毒 **ERY**
団体 **cong, cong.**
男性 **M, m**
男性(の) **M, m, mas., masc**
男性/女性(比) **M/F, M：F**
男性インポテンス検査 **MIT**
男性型はげ **MPB**
男性化副腎過形成 **VAH**
男性偽半陰陽 **MPH**
男性(性)染色体 **Y**
男性染色体 **Y chrom**
男性同性愛者 **HM, Homo, homo.**
男性同性愛の **Homo, homo.**
男性〔雄〕特異的抗原 **MSA**
男性と女性 **M-W**
男性乳癌 **MBC**
男性ホルモン結合蛋白 **ABP**
担架患者 **LP**
担癌動物 **CBA, TBA**
担体結合鉄 **Cf-Fe**
担鉄赤芽球 **SB**
担鉄赤血球 **S**
単一 **Mo**
単一型 **unif**
単一型の **unif**
単一形 **mono**
単一光子計測 **SPC**
単一光子放射型コンピュータ断層撮影法 **SPECT**
単一臍動脈 **SUA**
単一振動 **vs, vs.**
単一性の **unis**
単一相 **SP**
単一提携の **unicorp**

単一ネフロン糸球体血漿流量　**SNGPF**
単一ネフロン糸球体血流量　**SNGBF**
単一ネフロン糸球体濾過率　**SGFR, SNGFR**
単一の　**sgl, sing., spl, spl.**
単一胚移植法　**SET**
単一律動性前頭部Δ〔デルタ〕波　**MFD**
単位　**E, U**
単位時間あたりのガス量〔気流〕(速度)　$\dot{V}$
単位時間あたりの気流容積〔容量〕　V_E
単位時間血(液)流量　$\dot{Q}$
単位時間の呼吸数　**f**
単位進化時間　**UEP**
単位量　**UD**
単エネルギーX線吸収測定装置　**SXA**
単凹面の　**SCV**
単音　**monot**
単核球　**M**
単核球(細胞)因子　**MCF**
(伝染性)単核細胞(症)　**Mono**
単核細胞　**MC, MNC, mon, mono, Monos**
単核細胞組織因子　**MCTF**
単核性(貪)食細胞　**MNP**
単核性食細胞系　**MPS**
単核性白血球　**MNL**
単核(性)の　**MN**
単眼の　**mono**
単眼妨害　**MD**
単関節(性)関節炎　**MAA**
単球　**Mo, mon, mono, Monos**
単球/リンパ球比　**M : L, M/L**
単球コロニー刺激因子　**M-CSF**
単球コンディション培養液　**MOCM**
単球性白血病　**MoL**
(伝染性)単球増加(症)　**Mono**
単球特異抗原　**MoA**
単球遊走性蛋白　**MCP**
単極胸部導出〔誘導〕　**V**
単極性うつ病　**UD**
単極電気凝固　**MPED**
単極の　**UP**
単極誘導　**MP**
単クローンBリンパ球　**MBL**
単クローン抗膵島細胞自己抗体　**MICA**
単クローン成分　**M component**
単クローン性免疫グロブリン血症　**MG**
単型　**monot**
単型の　**monot**
単光子吸収法　**SPA**
単語理解　**WU**
単細胞蛋白質　**SCP**
単鎖〔一本鎖〕DNA高次構造多型解析(法)　**SSCP**
単シナプス反射　**MSR**
単シロップ　**ss., SS**
単収縮　**Z**
単心室　**SV, UVH**
単心室房室結合　**UAVC**
単心房　**SA**
単耳大きさ平衡テスト　**MLBT**
単色視　**MV**
単純化　**spif**
単純化口腔衛生指数　**OHI-S**
単純型糖尿病性網膜症　**SDR**
単純酵素拡散　**SRED**
単純骨折　**FS**
単純じん肺　**SP**
単純性鼻炎　**Rh.s.**
単純性表皮水疱症　**EBS**
単純性ヘルペスチミジンキナーゼ遺伝子　**HSTK**
単純低カルシウム血性テタニー　**SHT**
単純頭蓋撮影　**PCG**
単純な　**simp., spl, spl.**
単純乳房切除(術)　**SM**
単純反応　**SR**
単純反応時間　**SRT**
単純部分発作　**SPS**
単純ヘルペス　**HS**
単純ヘルペスウイルス　**HSV, HXV**
単純ヘルペスウイルスチミジンキナーゼ　**HSVtk**
単純ヘルペスウイルス脳炎　**HSVE**
単純ヘルペス角膜炎　**HKS, HSK**
単純ヘルペス脳炎　**HSE**
単純放射状酵素拡散法　**SRED**
単純放射状免疫拡散法　**SRID**
単純疱疹　**HS**
単振動　**SV**
単数の　**S, s, sing.**
単旋律の　**mono**
単線維筋電図検査(法)　**SFEMG**
単相性活動電位　**MAP**
単相性反応・時間装置　**SCRAP**
単側波帯　**SSB**
単調洞性デルタ波　**MSDA**
単調な　**monot**
単凸面の　**SCX**
単独甲状腺刺激ホルモン欠乏(症)　**ITSHD**
単独ゴナドトロピン欠損症　**IGD**
単独心血管奇形　**ICM**

た

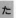

単独成長ホルモン欠損症 **IGHD**
単独注射 **SI**
単独非対称中隔肥大 **IASH**
単独ラクターゼ欠損症 **ILD**
単発性線維性腫瘍 **SFT**
単病巣好酸球(性)肉芽腫 **UEG**
炭化水素 **HC**
炭化水素グリコール効果 **H-G effect**
炭酸・重炭酸緩衝液 **CB, CBB**
炭酸飲料 **CB**
炭酸塩 **carb, carb.**
炭酸ガス含有量 **CO_2**
(血中)炭酸ガス含量 **CO_2 content**
炭酸ガスナルコーシス **CO_2 narcosis**
炭酸ガス濃度単位 **CDCM**
炭酸ガス(吸入)法 **CDT**
炭酸クロロフォルム抽出物 **CCE**
炭酸シクロヘキシルアミン **CHC**
炭酸水 **aq.aerat.**
炭酸水素イオン **HCO_3^-**
炭酸水素ナトリウム **$NaHCO_3$, sod.bicar**
炭酸脱水酵素 **CA**
炭酸脱水酵素活性 **CAA**
炭酸脱水酵素阻害剤 **CAI**
炭酸脱水素酵素阻害剤 **CAH-I**
炭酸ナトリウム **Na_2CO_3**
炭酸の **carb**
炭酸リチウム **Li_2CO_3**
炭水化物 **C, CARB, carb, carbo, CHO, COH, KH**
炭水化物・脂肪・蛋白質 **CFP**
炭水化物・蛋白・脂質 **CHO P F**
炭水化物結合蛋白(質) **CBP**
炭水化物抗原 **CA**
炭水化物代謝指数 **CMI**
炭水化物由来高血糖 **CIH**
炭素 **C**
炭素・コバルト・タングステン合金 **carboloy**
炭素・酸素・窒素・硫黄のアイソトープ **ICONS**
炭素・水素・窒素 **CHN**
炭素/窒素(比) **C/N**
炭素 11 **^{11}C**
炭素 12 **^{12}C**
炭素 13 **^{13}C**
炭素 14 **^{14}C**
炭素質の **carb**
炭素繊維強化プラスチック **CFRP**
炭疽抗血清 **AAS**
胆管 **BD**
胆管癌 **GGK**
胆管検査 **BDE**
胆管細胞癌 **CCC**
胆管消失症候群 **VBDS**
胆管腺症 **BDA**
胆管探査 **BDE**
胆管胆汁 **A bile, A-bile**
胆管閉鎖(症) **BA**
胆汁コレステロール濃度 **BCC**
胆汁酸 **BA**
胆汁酸喪失症候群 **BALS**
胆汁糖蛋白質 **BGP**
胆汁リン脂質濃度 **BPC**
胆膵管鏡 **CPS**
胆石 **C, GS**
胆石症 **cholelith, CL**
胆(道)疝痛 **BC**
胆道鏡的乳頭切開術 **CPT**
胆道造影法 **CAG**
胆道痛 **BTP**
胆嚢 **GB, GB, G.B., VES, ves.**
胆嚢炎 **chole**
胆嚢癌 **GBK**
胆嚢系 **GBS**
胆嚢色素結石 **GBPS**
胆嚢疾患 **GBD**
胆嚢切除(術) **chole, cholecyst**
胆嚢造影検査 **GB, GB exam**
胆嚢造影図 **CCG**
胆嚢胆汁 **B bile, B-bile**
胆嚢摘出後症候群 **PCS**
胆嚢摘出(術) **chole, cholecyst**
胆嚢動脈 **CA**
段階 **ph, stg**
段階冠(状)動脈治療室 **PCCU**
段階的運動テスト **GXT**
段階的患者管理 **PPC**
段階的患者管理棟 **PPCU**
段階的患者管理部門 **PCU**
段階的患者管理問題 **SMP**
段階的集団ケア **PPC**
段階的治療 **SC**
淡蒼球 **GP, Gpm**
蛋白 **PR, Pr, PRO, PROT, prot**
蛋白(質) **P**
蛋白・ビタミン・ミネラル **PVM**
蛋白・ビタミン・無機質 **PROVIMI**
蛋白エネルギー低栄養

PEM
蛋白カルボキシルメチラーゼ **PCM**
蛋白カロリー諮問グループ **PAG**
蛋白カロリー低栄養 **PCU**
蛋白結合 **PB**
蛋白結合チロキシン **PBT_4**
蛋白結合鉄 **PB-Fe**
蛋白結合の **PB**
蛋白結合ヨウ素 **PBI**
蛋白欠乏性膵性糖尿病 **PDPD**
蛋白合成 **PS**
蛋白効率比 **PER**
蛋白脂質複合体 **PLC**
蛋白質脱リン酸酵素 **PPTS**
蛋白質中のセリンリン酸化酵素 **SerK**
蛋白質の最終糖化物 **AGE**
蛋白質分解酵素阻害薬 **Pi, PI**
蛋白食 **PD**
蛋白操作 **PMN**
蛋白喪失性胃腸症 **PLGE**
蛋白喪失性腸症 **PLE**
蛋白(質)チロシンキナーゼ **PTK**
蛋白同化ステロイド **AS**
蛋白透過性血液濾過 **PPHDF**
蛋白物質 **P subst**
蛋白分解酵素 **PCR**
蛋白分画 **PF**
蛋白メチルエステラーゼ **PM**
断指趾型先天性掌蹠角化症 **KHM**
断食の **imprans**
断節 **mut**
断節された **mut**
断続性眼球運動 **SM**
断層撮影 **tomo., Tomo**
断層撮影図 **tomo., Tomo**
断層撮影法 **TG**
断層心エコー図 **2DE, 2-DE**
断層心エコー図法 **2DE, 2-DE**
断熱高速通過 **AFP**
断片 **frag**
断面 **XS, X-sect, x sect.**
断面積 **XSA**
断裂性心房活動 **FAA**
短胃動脈 **AGB, SGA**
短下肢装具 **SLC, SLS**
短下肢副子 **SLS**
短期化学療法 **SCC, SOC**
短期感作 IgG 抗体 **IgG S-T S**
短期記憶 **STM**
短期刺激療法 **BST**
短期滞在 **SS**
短期貯蔵 **STS**
短期入院 **SS**
短期曝露限界 **STEL**
短期目標 **STG**
短棘分節運動 **SSB**
短弧キセノン燈 **SXL**
短後毛様動脈 **SPCA**
短鎖脂肪酸 **SCFA**
短小活動電位 **BSAP**
短小指屈筋 **FDM, FDQB**
短肢性小人症 **CHH**
短指伸筋 **EDB**
短時間増強感覚指数 **SISI test**
短掌筋 **PB**
短潜時体性知覚誘発電位 **SLSEP, SSEP**
短腸症候群 **SBS**
短橈側手根伸筋 **ECRB**
短反転時間回復 **STIR**
短波 **SW**
短波ジアテルミー **SWD, SW dia.**
短波長紫外線 **UVC**
短波長赤外線 **IRA**
短波透熱療法 **dia sw**
短波透熱量法 **SWD**
短腓骨 **PB**
短母指外回転(筋) **APB**
短母指屈筋 **FPB**
短母指伸筋 **EPB**
短絡 **B**
短絡電流 **SCC**
短腕 **SA, S/A**
弾性 **E**
弾性原線維 **EF**
弾性線維偽黄色腫 **PXE**
弾性反跳粒子検出法 **ERDA**
暖房加湿空気 **WHA**
痰 **spt**
端 **ext, ext., extr, extrem**
端側 **ES**
端側(吻合) **ETS**
端々(吻合術) **EE**
端々吻合 **EEA**
端末 **TRML**
端末中間処理 **TIP**
誕生年 **YOB**

ち

サクランボ赤色斑(点)筋ミオクローヌス(症候群) **CRSM**
チアゾリドマイシン **THZ**
チアノーゼ **C, cy, cyan**
チアノーゼ性心(臓)疾患 **CHD**
チアノーゼ性先天性心疾患 **CCHD**
チアノーゼの **cy, cyan**
チアベンダゾール **TBZ**
チアミン **THI, Thi**
チアミン-8-(メチル-6-アセチル・ジヒドロチオクテート)-ジスルフィド **TATD**
チアミンアリルジスルフィド **TAD**
チアミン一リン酸 **TMP**
チアミンジスルフィド **TDS**
チアミン二リン酸 **TDP**
チアミンピロホスファターゼ **TPP**
チアミンピロリン酸 **THPP, ThPP, TPP**
チアンフェニコール **TP**
チミジン一リン酸 **TMP**
チェス疫学調査 **CHESS**
チェック **Ch**
チェックした **ckd**
チェックする **CK, ck**
チェディアック・東病 **CHD**
チェディアック・東(症候群) **CH**
チェディアック・東症候群 **CHS**
チェーン・ストークス呼吸 **CSB, CSR**
チーエン試験 **ZT**
チオ **s**
チオアセタゾン **TBA**
チオアセタミド **TAA**
チオイノシン **Sno**
チオウラシル **TU**
チオウリジン **Srd, sU**
チオウリジン(=sU, Srd) **S**
チオカルバニジン **THC**
チオカルバニリジン **TC**
チオグアニン **TG**
チオグアニン,ビンクリスチン(=オンコビン),アラビノシルシトシン,プレドニゾン **TOAP**
チオグアノシン **TGR**
チオグリコール酸 **TG**
チオグリコール酸塩培地 **TGC medium**
チオグリコール酸 **TGC**
チオシアン酸カリウム **KCNS**
チオセミカルバジド **TSC**
チオセミカルバゾン **TSC**
チオトリエチレンホスホルアミド **Thio-TEPA, thio-TEPA, Thiotepa, thiotepa**
チオドロール **TD**
チオバルビツール酸 **TBA**
チオバルビツール酸反応 **TBA reaction**
チオバルビツール酸反応物質 **TBARS**
チオヒポキサンチン **Shy**
チオプロニン **TP**
チオプロペラジン **TPZ**
チオペンタールナトリウム **STP**
チオホスホルアミド(=チオテパ) **TSPA**
チオ硫酸・クエン酸・胆汁酸・ショ糖培地 **TCBS**
チオ硫酸塩 **Thio**
チオ硫酸ナトリウム **hypo**
チオ硫酸ナトリウムクリアランス **Cthio**
チオ硫酸ナトリウム除去率 **ETHIO**
チカルシリン **TIC, TIPC**
チクロピジン **TC, TP**
チタン **Ti**
チトクローム **C, CYT**
チトクロ(ー)ム P 450 **P-450**
チトクローム P 450 **CYP**
チトクローム系 **cyt.sys.**
チトクローム酸化酵素 **COX**
チニダゾール **TDZ**
(腸)チフス菌 **S.typhi**
チフス菌 **ST, S.typhi.**
チフス様赤痢 **TD**
チーフレジデント **CR**
チマダニ(属) **H**
チミジン **T, TdR**
チミジン(5′-)三リン酸 **TTP**
チミジン因子 **TF**
チミジンキナーゼ **TK**
チミジンキナーゼ欠乏の **TKD**
チミジン合成酵素 **TS**
チミジン二リン酸 **TDP**
チミジンホスホリラーゼ **TP**
チミン **T, Thy**
チミン・アデニン・グアニン **TAG**
チミンデオキシリボシド

Tdr
チーム看護の　**TN**
チームリーダー　**TL**
チモール混濁
thym.turb., TT
チモール混濁試験　**TTT**
チモールブルー　**TB**
チモール綿状反応　**TFT**
チャイニーズハムスター
CH
チャイニーズハムスター卵巣　**CHO**
チャーグ・ストラウス症候群　**CSS**
チャコール・イースト抽出物　**CYE**
チャコールウイルス移送培養液　**CVTR**
チャンス蛋白尿・血尿
CPH
チョコレート血液(寒天培地)　**CB**
チョコレート血液寒天培地
CB agar
チョコレート被覆錠
CCT
チラミン　**Ty**
チール・ネールゼン(法/染色)　**ZN**
チール・ネールゼン染色(法)　**ZNS**
チ〔サイ〕ロカルシトニン
TC, TCA, TCT
チ〔サイ〕ロキシン　**T, Ty**
チ〔サイ〕ロキシン(＝テトラヨードチ〔サイ〕ロニン)　**T_4**
チ〔サイ〕ロキシン結合アルブミン　**TBA**
チ〔サイ〕ロキシン結合凝固素　**TBC**
チ〔サイ〕ロキシン結合グロブリン　**TBG**
チ〔サイ〕ロキシン結合グロブリン指数　**TBGI**
チ〔サイ〕ロキシン結合指数試験　**TBI-test**
チ〔サイ〕ロキシン結合蛋白
TBP
チ〔サイ〕ロキシン結合能
TBC, TBG cap
チ〔サイ〕ロキシン結合プレアルブミン　**TBPA**
チ〔サイ〕ロキシン特異的活性　**T_4SA**
チ〔サイ〕ログロブリン
TG, Tg, Thg, THGL
チ〔サイ〕ログロブリン凝集
TA
チ〔サイ〕ログロブリン凝集試験　**TA test**
チ〔サイ〕ログロブリン血液凝集反応　**TGHA**
(抗)チ〔サイ〕ログロブリン抗体　**TgAb**
チ〔サイ〕ログロブリン抗体
TA, TGA
チロシン　**Tyr, Y**
チ〔サイ〕ロシンアミノトランスフェラーゼ　**TAT**
チロシンエチルエステル
TEE
チ〔サイ〕ロシン水酸化酵素
TH
チロシン水酸化酵素
THO
チロシン脱リン酸化酵素
PTP
チロシンヒドロキシラーゼ
TOH
チ〔サイ〕ロトロピン受容体抗体　**TRAb**
チンキ　**Tct.**
チンキ(剤)　**T, tinc, tinct.**
チンパノグラム　**TG**
チンパンジー　**PTR**
チンパンジー白血球抗原
Chl-A
チンパンジー(の)鼻かぜウイルス　**CCA**
チンメルマン(発色)反応
ZM
ちらつき視野　**FFF**
血・汗・涙　**BS & T**
地域　**dist**
地域医師　**LMD**
地域医療官　**RMO**
地域医療事務官　**DMO**
地域看護のための中央審議会　**CCDN**
地域教育者訓練センター
RTTC
地域共同体を基にした健康開発計画　**CBHDP**
地域緊急医療システム
SAMU
地域獣医事務所　**DVO**
地域中毒治療センター
RPTC
地域病院委員会　**RHB**
地域病院顧問・専門医協会
RHCSA
地域病院事務局　**RHO**
地域薬剤搬送システム
LDDS
地域を統合した非伝染病の調査計画　**CINDI**
地球衛生学　**geohy**
地球オゾン観測組織
GO_3OS
地球環境モニタリング計画
GEMS
地球圏・生物圏国際協同計画　**IGBP**
地区医師　**LMD**
地区看護行政官　**DNO**
地区検疫官　**RMO**
地中海カポジ肉腫
MEKS
地中海性貧血　**thal, Thal**
地中海斑点熱　**MSF**

ち

治験(新)薬 **IND**
治験施設支援機関 **SMO**
治験事務局担当者 **SMA**
治験責任医師 **PI**
治験総括報告書 **CTR**
治験モニタリング担当者 **CRA**
治験薬概要書 **IB**
治験薬管理 **IP**
治験薬申請 **IND**
治効中間投与量 **CD50**
治効量 **DC**
治癒過程期 **Stage H**
治癒した心筋梗塞 **HMI**
治癒の証明 **v**
治癒(線)量 **CD**
治癒良好 **HW**
治癒良好・後遺症なし **WHNS**
治癒良好・残遺なし **WHNR**
治癒良好で無症状の **WHNS**
治癒良好な **WH**
治療 **RX, Rx., Th, THER, ther, Tmt, tmt., tr, treat, trmt, TRT, trt, TX, Tx, tx**
治療医師 **Rx Phys**
(照射)治療可能比 **TGF**
治療可能比 **TR**
治療群 **TG**
治療計画 **T, tr pl, TrPl**
治療計画カンファレンス **TPC**
治療された **Rxd**
治療指数 **TI**
治療社会クラブ **TSC**
治療情報システム **MIS**
治療食調理室 **DK**
治療中止 **TD, T/D**
治療中止(された) **TD**
治療的運動 **ther.ex, th.ex**
治療的演劇グループ **TPG**
治療的角膜表層除去術 **PTK**
治療的血漿交換 **TPE**
治療的放射線医学 **TR**
治療的流産 **TA, TAB**
治療の **cur, ther, THERAP**
治療反応性尺度 **TRS**
治療反応評価法 **TRAM**
治療日 **D/T**
治療方式 **R**
治療目標 **GOT**
治療薬物効果 **TSA**
知覚 **pcpt**
知覚活動電位 **SAP**
知覚しうる **S**
知覚消失〔脱失〕の **anesth**
知覚神経伝導速度 **SAP, SNCV**
知覚騒音レベル **PNL**
知覚速度 **PS**
知覚脱失〔消失〕 **ANA, Anaes, Anaesth, Anes, anes, anesth**
知覚脱失〔消失〕の **ANA, Anaes, Anaesth, Anes, anes**
知覚低下 **↓sen**
知覚低下した **sense.decr.**
知覚(神経)伝導速度 **SCV**
知覚度 **RPE**
知覚ニューロン **SN**
知覚認識運動機能 **PCMF**
知覚の **sens**
知覚の低下 **DSP**
知覚誘発反応 **SER**
知識・技能および能力 **KSA**
知識・態度・実技 **KAP**
知識・能力・技術および習慣 **KASH**
知性 **intell**
知能 **intell**
知能係数 **CI**
知能指数 **IQ**
知能状態小検査 **MMSE**
知能の高い **intell**
知能偏差値 **SS**
恥骨後前立腺摘出術 **RPP**
恥骨後尿道固定術 **RPU**
恥骨上結合 **SP**
恥骨上穿刺 **SP**
恥骨上前立腺切除術 **SPP**
恥骨上の **SP**
恥骨上膀胱穿刺 **SPA**
恥骨の **pub**
恥骨尾骨(筋) **PCG**
恥毛 **PH**
致死抗原 **AL**
致死時間 **LT**
致死性家族性不眠症 **FFI**
致死性正中(部)肉芽腫 **LMG**
致死の **l, L**
致死濃度 **LC**
致死量 **DL, FD, F.D., LD**
致命的な **l, L**
智歯 **WT**
遅延 **dly**
遅延一次縫合 **DPS**
遅延型アレルギー反応 **DeAR**
遅延型過敏症反応 **DTHR**
遅延型過敏反応のエフェクターT細胞 **TDTH**
遅延型感受性 **DS**
遅延型黒化 **DT**
遅延型の **dlyd**

遅延型反応　**LPR**
遅延型皮膚過敏症　**DCH**
遅延(型)過敏症　**DH, DHS, DTH**
遅延(型)過敏(症)反応　**DHR**
遅延(性)紅斑(線)量　**DED**
遅延後脱分極　**DAD**
遅延作用　**DA, PA**
遅延作用錠(剤)　**DAT**
遅延した　**RET, ret, retard**
遅延性非定型的眩暈症　**PAV**
遅延聴力フィードバック　**DAF**
遅延電位　**LP**
遅延なし　**ND**
遅延(型)皮膚過敏(症)　**DCN**
遅延(型)皮膚過敏反応　**DSHR**
遅延不活性因子　**S**
遅延分娩　**DD**
遅作用酸性蛋白酵素　**SMP**
遅滞　**retard**
遅滞した　**r, RET, ret, retard**
遅滞する　**r**
遅発型アレルギー反応　**LAR**
遅発型呼吸性全身症候群　**LRSS**
遅発型喘息反応　**LAR**
遅発性異種移植　**DXR**
遅発性ウイルス感染症　**SVI**
遅発性外傷性脳内血腫　**DTICH**
遅発性肝不全　**LOHF**
遅発性虚血性神経脱落症状　**DIND**
遅発性骨形成不全　**OI tarda**
遅発性ジスキネジア　**TD**
遅発性脊椎骨端骨異形成症　**SED tarda**
遅発性ネフローゼ(症候群)　**LN**
遅発性分娩後出血　**LPPH**
遅発性免疫グロブリン欠乏(症)　**LID**
遅発脊髄圧迫症候群　**SSCCS**
遅発聴覚誘発反応　**LAER**
遅発皮膚反応　**LCR**
遅攣縮酸化物　**so**
痴呆指数　**DI**
置換　**displ**
置換・省略・歪み・付加　**SODA**
置換因子　**RF**
置換する　**displ**
緻密層　**ZC**
小さい　**lit, lit., mi, min, pv., sm, sml**
小さくて強い螢光を発する細胞　**SIF cells**
小さな痛み　**PC**
近い　**JUXT, juxt, nr, P**
力　**F, P, V, V**
力と調律　**F & R**
力分野の分析　**FFA**
力・速度・長さ　**FVL**
蓄積　**accum**
蓄積外傷疾患　**CTD**
蓄積した　**accum**
蓄積的疲労徴候調査　**CFSI**
蓄積の　**cum**
蓄電器　**cond**
蓄尿器　**UR**
蓄尿ビン　**UR**
父(親)　**P**
父親　**F, FR**
父方の叔父　**PU**
父方のおば(＝伯母,叔母)　**PA**
父方の祖父　**pat.gf, PGF**
父方の祖母　**pat.gm, PGM**
父と娘　**f/d**
縮れ毛症候群　**KHS**
縮れ毛病　**KHD**
窒素　**Az, N**
窒素1回呼吸法　**SBN**
窒素13　**^{13}N**
窒素固定遺伝子　**nif genes**
窒素コントロール単位　**NCU**
窒素酸化物　**NO_x**
窒素酸化物合成酵素　**NOS**
窒素測定　**AZM**
窒素分圧　**P_{N2}**
窒素リン　**NP**
窒素リン検出装置〔剤〕　**NPD, NP detector**
窒息ガス　**CG**
窒息を伴う胸郭形成不全　**ATD**
腟　**An, V, VAG, Vag, vag.**
腟炎　**vag.**
腟検　**VE**
腟後隙　**RVS**
腟後壁　**PVW**
腟酸ホスファターゼ　**VAP**
腟上皮内異形成(症)　**VID**
腟上皮内癌　**VIN**
腟上皮内新生物　**VAIN**
腟式子宮切除(術)　**VAG HYST, Vag hyst, vag.hyst.**
腟式子宮全摘出術　**VTH**
腟式子宮摘出(術)

ち

VAG HYST, Vag hyst, vag.hyst.
膣式全子宮摘出(術) **TVH**
膣スミア **VS**
膣スメア指数 **SI**
膣洗浄スメア **VIS**
膣洗浄塗抹(標本) **VIS**
膣電図 **EVG**
膣トリコモナス **TV**
膣トリコモナス症 **TV**
膣と外陰部 **VV**
膣内洗浄 **VI**
膣内避妊用フィルム **VCF**
膣内リング **IVR**
膣に **pro vagin.**
膣の **VAG, Vag, vag.**
膣・子宮膣部・子宮頸内膜 **VCE**
茶色(の) **Br, Br., brn**
茶さじ **t, tsp**
茶さじ1杯 **cochl.infant., coch.parv.**
茶さじ1杯の **t, teasp, tsp**
茶剤 **SP, Sp.**
着色された **cld**
着色せよ **color.**
着床 **I**
着床前遺伝子診断 **PGD**
着用式人工糸球体 **WAG**
中(間部) **MS**
中位鉗子分娩 **MFD**
中位指皺襞 **MFC**
中位手掌皮膚溝 **MPC**
中位の **med, med., mm**
中咽頭 **OP**
中央 **cen, cen.**
中央(線) **ML, m.l.**
中央エコー **ME**
中央演算処理装置 **CPU**
中央器材室 **CS**
中央検査室 **CPHL**
中央材料室 **CRS, CSR**
中央雑誌索引 **IDX**
中央食料技術研究所 **CFTRI**
中央前小脳静脈 **PCV**
中央帯壊死 **CZN**
中央値 **M, m, md, md., mdn, MED, Med, med.**
中央の **cen, cen., mid**
中央部の左 **m/l**
中央部の右 **m/r**
中央縫合 **MR**
中央膨張因子 **CEF**
中央麻薬捜査局 **CNB**
中央薬物研究所[インド] **CDRI**
中央ヨーロッパダニ媒介脳炎 **CETE**
中央ヨーロッパ脳炎 **CEE**
中央ヨーロッパ脳炎ウイルス **CEev**
中外シルビウス脳回 **MES**
中肝臓静脈 **MHV**
中肝動脈 **MHA**
中華レストラン(性)症候群 **CRS**
中華レストラン(性)喘息 **CRA**
中間 **M, m**
中間(期) **int, int.**
中間位 **IM**
中間外側路 **ILC**
中間会話声域 **MSL**
中間型低比重リポ蛋白 **ILDL**
中間冠(状動脈)疾患治療部門 **ICCU**
中間冠(状動脈)症候群 **ICS**
中間冠(状)動脈症候群 **ICAS**
中間ケア施設 **ICF**
中間呼気流量 **MEF**
中間糸状体 **IF**
中間質 **MI**
中間時に **hor.interm.**
中間周波数 **IF**
中間層植皮 **STSG**
中間治療保育室 **ICN**
中間的不活性物 **I**
中間点 **mpt**
中間内部放射線量 **MIRD**
中間に **ad int.**
中間尿検体 **MSU**
中間尿試料 **MSU**
中間の **I, inter.**
中間の初期 **MI**
中間の方法で **v.i.**
中間板 **Z-disk**
中間版(=Z線/Z板) **Z**
中間比重リポ蛋白 **IDL**
中間層皮弁 **STG**
中間頻度 **IF**
中間フィラメント **IF**
中間フィラメント蛋白 **IFP**
中間物 **intermed**
中間変動 **IM**
中間量 **ID**
中間量群 **IDG**
中間彎曲動脈 **ICXA**
中隔 **S, sept, sept.**
中隔・視束前野・視床下部系 **SPH-system**
中隔核 **SEPT**
(鼻)中隔形成(術) **septo**
中隔欠損(症) **SD**
中隔壁厚 **SWT**
中隔彎曲 **SD**
中規模集積回路 **MSI**
中ぐらいの大きさの **mg**
中空型人工腎臓 **HFK**
中結腸静脈 **VCM**
中結腸動脈 **MCA**
中抗原腫瘍 **MAT**

中後眼窩前頭皮質　**CPOF**
中硬膜動脈　**MMA**
中鎖脂肪　**MCT**
中鎖脂肪酸　**MCFA**
中鎖脂肪酸ミルク　**MCT**
中鎖トリアシルグリセロール　**MCT**
中鎖トリグリセリド油　**MCT oil**
中子宮動脈　**MUA**
中止　**DC, D/C, D/c, Dc, dc, d/c**
中止した　**Dc′d, dc′d, DXD, dxd**
中止する　**DC, D/C, D/c, Dc, dc, d/c, DISC, disc, disc.**
中手網部　**MH**
中手骨手根骨(関節)　**CM**
中手骨の骨皮質幅測定　**MCI**
中手根の　**MC**
中手指節関節　**MCPJ, MP, MPJ**
中手指節関節の　**MCP, MCPH, MP**
中手(骨)の　**MC**
中心　**cen, cen., ctr**
中心(線)　**ML, m.l.**
中心(顎)位　**CJR**
中心灰白質　**CGM**
中心核　**CM**
中心核病　**CCD**
中心窩同時視　**SFP**
中心血液量　**CBV**
中心咬合　**CO**
中心サービス　**CS**
中心視野　**CVF**
中心周囲域　**PC**
中心出血性壊死　**CHN**
中心循環血液量　**CCBV**
中心鞘　**CS**
中心静脈　**CV**
中心静脈圧　**CVP, ZVD**
中心静脈栄養　**TPN**
中心静脈カテーテル　**CVC, CV cath**
中心静脈注射　**CV**
中心静脈の　**CV**
中心静脈閉塞(症)　**CVO**
中心線　**CL**
中心側頭部に棘波をもつ良性小児てんかん　**BCECT**
中心側頭部脳波焦点を伴う小児良性てんかん　**BECCT**
中心点　**mpt**
(網膜)中心動脈圧　**CAP**
中心乳管　**LD**
中心の　**cen, cen., ctl**
中心被蓋路　**CTT**
中心微小管　**CMT**
中心肥満指数　**COI**
中心部　**C, c, cs**
中心臨界融合頻度　**central CFF**
中耳　**ME**
中耳液　**MEF**
中耳炎　**OM**
中耳炎,急性カタル性　**OMAC**
中耳炎,急性化膿性　**OMAS**
中耳炎・急性カタル性　**OMCA**
中耳炎・慢性カタル性　**OMCC**
中耳炎・慢性化膿性　**OMChS**
中耳管　**MEC**
中耳滲出液　**MEE**
中旬　**mom**
中(間)周波数　**MF**
中指　**M**
中指(趾)節骨　**MP**
中水泡性ラ音　**Rl**
中枢　**cen, cen.**
中枢興奮機構　**CEM**
中枢興奮状態　**CES**
中枢神経　**CN**
中枢神経系　**CNS, SNC, ZNS**
中枢神経系損傷　**CNS injury**
中枢神経系の情報伝達　**INPRCNS**
中枢神経系白血病　**CNS-L**
中枢神経系容積〔体積〕　$\mathbf{V}_{\mathrm{CNS}}$
中枢神経系抑制薬　**CNS depressant**
中枢神経心肺蘇生術　**CCPR**
中枢(性)神経(原)性過呼吸　**CNH**
中枢性協調障害　**ZKS**
中枢性抗コリン症候群　**CAS**
中枢性睡眠時無呼吸　**CSA**
中枢性尿崩症　**CDI**
中枢性肺胞低換気　**CAH**
中枢性肺胞低換気症候群　**CAH**
中枢聴神経系　**CANS**
中枢伝導時間　**CCT, CTT**
中枢(性)の　**cen, cen.**
中枢優先治療　**PPT**
中枢抑制状態　**CIS**
中性アミノ酸　**NAA**
中性およびイオン衝撃発光分光　**SCANIIR**
中性化　**net**
中性好細胞　**Neutro**
中性子　**n**
中性脂質　**NL**
中性子線量の単位　**n**
中性脂肪　**NF**
中性子放射化学分析法　**RNAA**
中性子保護療法　**NCT**

ち

中性赤(指示薬)　**NR**
中性デタージェント線維　**NDF**
中性の　**N, net, neut**
中性濃度　**ND**
中性〔中間型〕プロタミンハーゲドルン(インスリン)　**NPH**
中性分画　**NF**
中潜時反応　**MLR**
中足骨バー　**MT bar**
中足指節関節　**MPJ, MTP**
中足指節の　**MP, MTP**
中足(骨)の　**meta, MT**
中速イオン散乱分光法　**MEIS**
中大脳動脈　**MCA**
中大脳動脈血栓症　**MCAT**
中大脳動脈症候群　**MCAS**
中断する　**DISC, disc, disc.**
中直腸動脈　**MRA**
中東呼吸症候群　**MERS**
中毒　**intox**
中毒学　**tox, Tox, tox.**
中毒させる　**intox**
中毒性結節性甲状腺腫　**TNG**
中毒性甲状腺腫　**TG**
中毒性ショック症候群　**TSS**
中毒性ショック症候群1型　**TSST-1**
中毒性ショック症候群外毒素　**TSSE**
中毒性ショック症候群毒素　**TSST**
中毒性多結節性甲状腺腫　**TMNG**
中毒性表皮融解壊死型薬疹　**TEN**
中毒性表皮融解症　**TEN**
中毒性物質　**TS**
中毒性めまい　**TV**
中毒単位　**TU, T.U.**
中毒(性)の　**tox, Tox, tox.**
中毒量　**Dtox, TD**
中等大に　**mod, mod.**
中等大の　**mg**
中等度異形成　**MD**
中等度高血圧治療研究　**TOMHS**
中等度腎不全　**MRF, MRI**
中等度膵炎　**MOP**
中等度に　**mod, mod.**
中等度の　**MOD, mod**
中等の　**mm**
中等量の中水泡性ラ音　**RL_2**
中等量メトトレキサート　**IMD**
中内側傍索状視床切除　**CM-Pf**
中脳　**Mes**
中脳中心灰白質　**PAG**
中脳の　**Mes**
中脳縫合　**MR**
中脳網様体　**MRF**
中波長紫外線　**UVB**
中波長赤外線　**IRB**
中背側視床核　**MD**
中肺葉　**ML**
中胚葉混合肉腫　**MMS**
中(間)頻度　**MF**
中分子　**MM**
中分子物質　**MMS**
中部標準物質　**IS**
(肺)中葉症候群　**MLS**
中和価　**NV**
中和抗体　**NA**
中和手技　**NT**
中和する　**neut, NT**
中和するまで　**ad neut.**
中和反応　**NT**
中(部)1/3(区)　**middle/3**
虫垂　**AP, APP, app, app., Appx, V**
虫垂炎　**App, app, Appe, appe.**
虫垂切除　**Appe, appe.**
虫垂切除(術)　**APPY, Appy, appy**
虫垂切除術　**AP, App**
(指の)虫様筋　**LBM**
虫卵・潜血・寄生虫　**OBP**
虫卵・嚢胞・寄生虫　**OCP**
虫卵周囲沈降試験　**COP test**
虫卵周囲沈降反応　**COP**
虫卵と寄生虫　**O & P**
肘下　**BE**
肘下の副木　**SAS**
肘外反角度　**CA**
肘管症候群　**CUTS**
肘上　**AE**
肘上切断　**AE AMP**
肘静脈からの瀉血　**V.s.B.**
肘前の　**ac**
抽出液　**ext fl**
抽出可能な核酸　**ENA**
抽出された　**ext, ext., extd**
抽出水硫化　**DHD**
抽出物　**abstr., Ex., Ex, ex, Ext., ext, ext., Extr.**
注意　**rem**
注意欠陥障害　**ADD**
注意欠陥多動障害　**ADDH, ADHD, AD/HD**
注意(力)欠乏疾患　**ADD**
注意深く　**caut**
注意深く混和せよ　**m.caute**

注射　**Inj, inj, Inj., inject**
注射剤　**Inj, inj, Inj., inject**
注射剤をつくれ　**ft.injec.**
注射する　**inj**
注射電極カテーテル　**IEC**
注射薬物乱用者　**IDU**
注射用蒸留水　**WFI**
注射用滅菌水　**SWI**
注射用滅菌水〔無菌水〕　**SWFI**
注射量　**ID**
注視眼振　**GN**
注釈　**annot**
注腸　**EN, en, en.**
注入　**INF, Inf, inf**
(造影剤)注入肝動脈血管造影　**IHA**
注入硬化療法　**IST**
注入尿路造影像　**IUG**
昼間の居室　**DR**
昼夜騒音レベル　**L_{dn}**
柱　**col, pir**
鋳造(物)　**C**
著効　**CR**
著作　**compo**
著者　**A**
著者の　**auct.**
張力時間係数　**TTI**
貯蔵　**S**
貯蔵ヒト血清　**PHS**
貯蔵プール欠乏症　**SPD**
貯留　**ret**
長下肢装具　**LLB, LLS, SKA orthosis**
長脚　**LL**
長脚円柱(状)ギプス包帯　**LLCC**
長脚ギプス包帯　**LL cast**
長脚歩行ギプス帯　**LLWC**
長期(間)　**LT**
長期外来透析　**CAPD**
長期記憶　**LTM**
長期記録心電図　**LTEC**
長期ケア　**LTC**
長期ケア施設　**LTCF**
長期骨髄培養　**LTBMC**
長期酸素療法　**LTOT**
長期持続性菌血症　**BLD**
長期就床安静　**CBS**
長期生存の　**LTS**
長期貯蔵　**LTS**
長期廃疾　**LTD**
(HIV の)長期非進行者　**LTNP**
(HIV 抗体の)長期非変換者　**LTNS**
長期抑圧(脳)　**LTD**
長期療養　**LTC**
長距離ゼログラフィ　**LDX**
長経路(遮断)徴候　**LTS**
長後毛様動脈　**LPCA**
長鎖　**LC**
長鎖脂肪酸　**LCFA**
長鎖脂肪酸酸化　**LCFAO**
長鎖中性脂肪　**LCT**
長鎖末端反復　**LTR**
長上肢ギプス包帯　**LAC**
長上肢舟状骨ギプス包帯　**LANC**
長寿の　**MB**
長周期原線維　**LSF**
長指屈筋　**FDL**
長(時間)持続(性)増強作用　**LLP**
長(時間)持続(性)脱分極　**LLD**
長時間作用(性)神経弛緩薬　**LAN**
長時間作用(性)の(薬)　**LA**
長時間相乗作用　**LTP**
長趾伸筋　**EDL**
長掌(筋)　**PL**
長肘下(ギプス包帯)　**LBE**
長頭人種　**dolichocephs**
長橈側手根伸筋　**ECRL**
長波長紫外線　**UVA**
長波長赤外線　**IRC**
長波透熱療法　**dia lw**
長腓骨筋　**PL**
長母指外転(筋)　**APL**
長母指屈筋　**FHL, FPL**
長母指伸筋　**EHL, EPL**
長腕副子　**LAS**
重複　**dup**
重複時間　**DT**
張力　**ten, tens, tns, tnsn**
頂　**VTX, vtx, Vx, vx, V, v**
鳥距溝　**CAS**
鳥様顔貌　**VG**
鳥類から感染する気管支炎　**AIB**
朝食　**B, bkf, bkfst, bkft, brek, Brkf, brkf, brkt, jentac.**
朝食後　**post jentac**
朝食前　**a.j.**
朝食前に　**ant.jentac.**
朝鮮出血熱　**KHF**
朝昼兼用食　**brunch**
超易溶性　**vs, vs.**
超遠心(分離)の　**UC**
超遠心分析　**UCA**
超遠心分離　**UCF**
超音波　**HIFU, US, USW, UTS, UTZ**
超音波画像　**UI**
超音波カルジオグラム　**UCG**
超音波気管支鏡　**EBUS**
超音波検査　**echo, US**
超音波検査(法)　**US**
超音波検査(法)　**USE**
超音波検査図　**USG**
超音波検査での(妊娠)週　**WBUS**

超音波周波数　**UF**
超音波手術吸引装置　**CUSA**
超音波心臓検査法　**UCG**
超音波診断(法)　**USG**
超音波心断層図　**UCT**
超音波診断法　**US**
超音波スキャニング　**USS**
超音波チップ　**US tip**
超音波動脈撮影図　**UA**
超音波ド(ッ)プラー法　**UDS**
超音波内視鏡　**UE**
超音波内視鏡下カラード(ッ)プラー法　**CDEUS**
超音波内視鏡検査　**EUS**
超音波ネブライザー　**USN**
超音波の　**US**
超音波脳造影　**UEG**
超音波の強度　**I**
超音波腹腔鏡　**ULS**
超可変領域　**HVR**
超過時間　**OT**
超急性拒絶反応　**HAR**
超急速死要因　**VFDF**
超小型演算処理装置　**MPU**
超抗原　**SAG**
超高圧　**EHT**
超高圧高分解能透過型電子顕微鏡　**HV-HR-TEM**
超高電圧電子顕微鏡　**HVEM**
超高温　**UHT, ULT**
超高周波　**UHF**
超高周波(数)　**SHF, shf**
超高純度　**UP**
超高(度)真空　**UHF, UHV**
超高速　**SHS**
超高速コンピュータ断層撮影(法)　**UFCT**
超高電圧　**UHV, uhv**
超高度の　**XH**
超高濃度陰影部分　**VHDA**
超高比重リポ蛋白　**VHDL**
超高頻度　**VHF**
超高頻度人工換気法　**UHFV**
超高分子ポリエチレン　**UHMWPE**
超高分子量　**UHMW**
超硬度の　**XH**
超酸化物不均化酵素　**SOD**
超心理学　**Parapsych**
超重量の　**XH**
超紫外線　**EUV**
超視,視察,偶聴　**SIOH**
超清浄空気　**UCA**
超大規模集積回路　**VLSI**
超短波　**UKW, USW**
超張力　**UTS**
超伝導量子干渉(計)　**SQID**
超伝導量子干渉計　**SQUID**
超低域　**VLR**
超低カロリー食　**VLCD, VLED**
超低高度　**VLA**
超低周波　**UIF**
超低周波(数)　**VLF**
超低出生(時)体重　**VLBW**
超低体温体外循環　**DHCPB**
超低窒素　**VLN**
超低比重　**VLD**
超低比重リポ蛋白　**VLDL, VLDLP**
超低比重リポ蛋白コレステロール　**VLDLC**
超低比重リポ蛋白トリグリセリド　**VLDTG, VLD-TG**
超微細の　**XF**
超微量(散布)　**ULV**
超免疫反応　**HR**
超粒子放射線撮影(法)　**MR**
超臨界流体クロマトグラフィ　**SFC**
超臨界流体抽出　**SCFE, SFE**
腸　**B, BO, bo., intest**
腸炎ビブリオ　**VP**
腸音正常活発　**BSNA**
腸カルシウム結合蛋白　**ICBP**
腸肝クリアランス　**EHC**
腸肝循環　**EHC**
腸型　**IT**
腸間膜血流　**MBF**
腸間膜静脈下大静脈シャント(術)　**MCS**
腸間膜節　**MN**
腸間膜組織炎　**MP**
腸管仮性閉塞症　**IP**
腸管型グルカゴン　**GTG**
腸管凝集性大腸菌　**EAggE**
腸管グルカゴン　**EG**
腸管結節性リンパ過形成　**INLH**
腸管出血性大腸菌　**EHEC**
腸管組織侵入性大腸菌　**EIEC**
腸管ドレナージ　**ED**
腸管病原性大腸菌　**EPEC**
腸管付着性大腸菌　**EAEC**
腸管ベーチェット病　**IB**
腸管膜血管閉塞症　**MAO**
腸球菌　**E**
腸クロム親和細胞　**EC cell**

腸クロム親和様(型)　ECL
腸脛靱帯摩擦症候群　ITFS
腸骨移植片　IBG
腸骨下腹神経ブロック　IINB
腸骨棘突起間距離　ISP
腸骨前上棘・顆部間距離　SMD
腸骨鼠径神経ブロック　IINB
腸骨大腿骨帯　Y band
腸骨稜骨移植(片)　ICBG
腸刷子縁　IBB
腸細胞病原性サルウイルス　ECMO virus
腸雑音　BS, BT
腸雑音正常　BSR
腸重積症　invagi
腸症に関連したT細胞リンパ腫　EATL
腸性先端〔肢端〕皮膚炎　AE
腸腺縫合　CGS
腸線による縫合　CS
腸チフス　TA, TD
腸チフス・パラチフス(ワクチン)　TPT
腸チフス・パラチフスA・パラチフスB(混合ワクチン)　TAB
腸チフス・パラチフスABC(ワクチン)　TABC
腸チフス・パラチフス腸炎　TPE
腸毒素　Ent
腸糖蛋白　IGP
腸内クロマフィン様細胞　ECL cell
腸内細菌性共通抗原　ECA
腸内細胞傷害性仔ウシウイルス　ECBO
腸内細胞傷害性仔トリウイルス　ECAOV
腸内細胞傷害性仔ヒツジウイルス　ECSO virus
腸内細胞性仔ネコウイルス　ECCO
腸内細胞性仔ブタウイルス　ECPO virus
腸内病原性大腸菌付着因子　EAF
腸内膜リンパ節　MLN
腸粘液抗原　IMA
腸粘膜リンパ球　GML
腸(管)の　int, int.
腸の　intest
腸排泄物　alv.deject.
腸(粘膜)肥満細胞　IMC
腸病原性大腸菌　EEC
腸吻合術　EA
腸ペプチダーゼ　EP
腸平滑筋推進運動　MLSB
腸平骨筋の推進性運動　LBS
腸閉塞　BO, Obst, obst
腸壁気腫　PI
腸埋伏　BI
腸溶(錠)　EC
腸溶剤　ECT
(錠剤の)腸溶皮　EC
腸溶被ビオホルム　ent-vio
腸リンパ球　IL
徴候　S, s, SG, sgs, Sx, sx
徴候と症状　SS, S & S, sx & sx
徴候または症状　S or S
澄明細胞癌　CCE
潮解して　PD
潮解の　deliq
蝶形骨洞　SpS
蝶形骨洞の　sph, sph.
蝶篩骨縫合　SE
調合　Comp., comp., cp, cp.
調査　invest, Res, res, rsch, survill
調査→疑問→読書→評論→叙述　SQ3R
調査質問　SQ
調査指導　SI
調査者　surv
調査者の報告　IR
調査する　surv, sv
調査データ分析プログラム　SDA
調査表　sched
調剤過誤　AD
調剤室　Disp., disp.
調剤錠　DT
調剤情報　DI
調剤する　Disp., disp.
調剤せよ　D, Disp., disp.
調剤部　PHAR, Phar, phar
調節　A, a, a., Acc, ACC, acc, accom, mod, mod., regs
調節肝臓外胆汁ドレナージ　CEBD
調節近点　NPA
調節呼吸(法)　CR
調節された　adj
調節式圧開放弁　APL valve
調節式機械的換気(法)　CMV
調節する　adj
調節〔調整〕性輻輳対調節(比)　AC/A
調節部分再呼吸式麻酔法　CPRAM
調節ホルモン　RH
調節卵巣刺激法　COS
調製した　Ppt, ppt., praep.
調製食品　deli

ち

調整標準化偏差値 **Z**
調和 **harm**
聴音の **acous, acous.**
聴覚閾値 **HT**
聴覚および生物聴覚委員会 **CHBA**
聴覚学 **audio, audiol**
聴覚訓練 **au tr**
聴覚言語局全国連合 **NAHSA**
聴覚原性の **audio**
聴覚性電気眼球運動図 **AOG**
聴覚と理解 **auding**
聴覚の **a, acous, acous., acst, aud**
聴覚脳幹反応 **ABR**
聴覚の記憶幅 **AMS**
聴覚誘発電位 **AEP**
聴覚誘発反応 **AER**
聴解 **auding**
聴骨筋反射 **AMR**
聴取距離 **HD**
聴神経腫(瘍) **AN**
聴神経腫瘍 **AT**
聴診(法) **A, aus., AUSC, ausc, auscul**
聴診器 **Stetho**
聴診と触診 **A & P, A+P**
聴診(法)と打診(法) **Aus & Perc**
聴診と打診 **A & P, A+P**
聴性脳幹反応 **ABER, ABR, BEAR, BERA**
聴力曲線 **AC**
聴力計 **audio**
聴力検査 **HT**
聴力障害された **HI**
聴力図 **audio**
聴力測定 **audio**
聴力損失 **HL**
聴力損失・難聴 **HL, h.l.**
聴力の社会適応指数 **SAI**
聴力疲労試験 **TDT, TdT**
聴力レベル **HL, HTL**
直筋 **rect, rect.**
直後に **subind.**
直鎖型アルキルベンゼンスルホン酸塩(=linear ABS) **LAS**
直鎖脂肪酸 **NFA**
直視下僧帽弁交連切開術 **OMC, OMVC**
直視下レーザー(補助)前立腺切除術 **VLAP**
直接遠心浮遊法 **DCF**
直接閲覧 **DA**
直接型ビリルビン **DB, DBil**
直接観察評価 **DOE**
直接冠(状)動脈拡張術 **DCA**
直接監視下短期化学療法 **DOTS**
直接凝集試験〔検査〕 **DAT**
直接凝集妊娠検査 **DAPT, Dapt**
直接クームス(試験) **DC**
直接クームス試験〔検査〕 **DCT**
直接経口抗凝固薬 **DOAC**
直接抗グロブリン試験〔検査〕 **DAGT, DAT**
直接抗グロブリンロゼット形成の **DARF**
直接喉頭鏡検査(法) **DL**
直接質問で **ODQ**
直接シリコンチューブ挿入 **DSI**
直接視力 **DV**
直接に **stat., Stat**
直接の **dir**
直接皮質反応 **DCR**
直接(型)ビリルビン **DB, D-Bil**
直接メモリ転送 **DMA**
直接免疫蛍光(検査) **DIF**
直接免疫蛍光抗体法 **DFA**
直接遊走抑制 **DMI**
直接落射蛍光フィルター法 **DEFT**
直接卵胞内受精 **DIFI**
直線加速 **A**
直線加速器 **linac, LINAC**
直線の **lin, lin.**
直腸 **R, rect, rect.**
直腸S状結腸X線像 **PSG**
直腸S状結腸鏡 **RSS**
直腸S状(結腸)部(の) **Rs, RS**
直腸S状部 **S**
直腸温 **RT, TR, T(R)**
直腸カテーテル **RT**
直腸から **PR, pr, p.r., p rec, p.rec.**
直腸癌 **RC, Rca, RCa, RK**
直腸灌注 **procto**
直腸鏡検査 **PROCTO, procto**
直腸鏡検査の **PROCTO, procto**
直腸検査 **RE, R/E**
直腸後隙 **RRS**
直腸肛門S状結腸鏡検査 **proct**
直腸肛門S状結腸摘出手術 **proct**
直腸肛門医 **PROCT, Proct, proct.**
直腸肛門炎 **proct**

直腸肛門大腸鏡検査　**proct**
直腸肛門麻痺　**proct**
直腸坐剤　**RS**
直腸指診　**DER, DRE**
直腸上部癌　**Ra**
直腸側腔　**PaRS**
直腸脱　**RP**
直腸腟の　**RV**
直腸腟瘻　**RV fist**
直腸で　**pro rect.**
直腸動脈神経叢　**PRI**
直腸内視鏡的超音波検査　**REUS**
直腸内の　**IR　, I.r.**
直腸に　**pro rect.**
直腸の　**(R), R, rect, rect., rtl**
直腸病学　**PR, Pr, PROCT, Proct, proct., PROCTO, procto**
直腸病専門医　**PR, Pr, PROCT, Proct, proct.**
直腸由来の鮮血　**BRBPR**
直部　**PR**
直立姿勢(をとる)　**STA**
直流　**DC, D.C., dc, d.c.**
直流除細動　**DC shock**
直流電位　**DC potential**
直流電気除細動　**DC**
直流電気の　**glv**
直流電流の　**Galv, galv**
直列　**S, s, ser**
直列弾性要素　**SE**
直角　**RA**
直角の　**perp**
直径　**di, Dia, dia., diam, diam.**
直径指数〔係数〕安全方式　**DISS**
直径の　**di**
著作権　©
沈うつ　**hyp, hypo**
沈下性潰瘍　**GU**
沈降　**SED, Sed, sed, sed.**
沈降係数　**S**
沈降時間　**sed.time, ST**
沈降した　**pptd**
沈降赤血球　**SRC**
(赤血球)沈降速度　**SR, S.R.**
沈降速度　**sed.rt**
(赤血球)沈降速度検査　**SRT**
沈降定数　**s**
沈降定数のスベドベルグ単位　**S**
沈降薄層クロマトグラフィ　**PTLC**
沈降反応　**PT**
沈渣　**SED, Sed, sed, sed.**
沈積〔沈着〕物　**dep.**
沈殿　**SED, Sed, sed, sed.**
沈殿時間　**sed.time**
沈殿した　**pp, PP, pp., pptd, praec.**
沈殿する　**pcpt, PPT, Ppt, ppt, precip**
沈殿速度　**sed.rt**
沈殿反応　**pcpn., pcpt, PPT, Ppt, ppt, ppta, pptn, precip**
沈殿率　**sed.rt**
沈黙療法　**sitr, ST**
陳旧性結核　**OT**
陳旧性心筋梗塞(症)　**OMI**
陳旧性治癒骨折　**OHF**
鎮静させる　**sed, sed.**
鎮静の　**sed, sed.**
鎮静薬　**sed, sed.**
鎮痛性の　**anal**
鎮痛薬　**anal**

つ

ツィンマーマン・レーバンド症候群　**ZLS**
ツィンマーマン就学前言語スケール　**ZPLS**
ツェツェバエ　**G**
ツェルヴェガー症候群　**ZS**
ツォンデック・アッシュハイム反応　**ZA Ra**
ツベルクリン　**T, tbcn., TC**
ツベルクリン・アルブミン陰性　**TAf**
ツベルクリン検査された　**TT**
ツベルクリン単位　**TE, TU, T.U.**
ツベルクリン沈殿　**TP**
ツベルクリン反応　**TR, Tu.R.**
ツベルクリンボルチン　**TV**
ツベルクリン濾液　**TF**
ツベルシジン　**TBC**
ツボ圧迫低周波療法　**SSP**
ツボクラリン　**TC**
ツリウム　**Tm**
ツルゴール　**tur, turg**
ツボ　**lag.**
つがい飼育した　**PF**
つき砕いた　**c**
つくらせよ　**F, F., f, f.**
つくる　**fac., ft.**
(それらを)つくれ　**ft.**
(それを)つくれ　**ft.**
つくれ　**F, F., f, f.**
つわり指数　**EI**
釣り合い　**equilib**
椎間板　**Z**
対　**pr, prs, vs, vs.**
対の　**gem-**
対麻痺　**para, Para, para.**
対麻痺の　**para, Para, para.**
追加　**add., addend., Nachtr, suppl**
追加試薬なしに　**WAR, w.a.r.**
追加診断なし　**NAD**
追加的適格症状　**AQS**
追加の　**add., addnl**
追求　**FT**
追記　**p.s.**
追跡　**fl**
追跡する　**fol**
追跡調査　**FL up, fl up, FU, F/U, f/u**
追跡治療　**RC**
椎　**vert**
椎間関節症候群　**LFS**
椎間関節複合　**IVJC**
椎間板線維血管組織　**FVD**
椎間板造影法　**Disco**
椎間板ヘルニア　**HD, HID, HIVD, IDP, PID, PIVD, RIVD**
椎弓切開(術)　**lami**
椎弓切除(術)　**LAM, Lam, lam**
椎骨　**vert**
椎骨強直性骨増殖症　**VAH**
椎骨後下小脳動脈分岐部動脈瘤　**VA-PICA**
椎骨刺激症候群　**VIS**
椎骨動脈　**VA**
(脊)椎骨の　**vert**
椎骨の　**V**
椎骨脳底(動脈)　**VB**
椎骨脳底(動脈)系　**VBS**
椎骨脳底動脈　**VBG**
椎骨脳底動脈虚血　**VBI**
椎骨脳底動脈循環不全　**VBI**
椎骨脳底動脈(循環)不全(症)　**VBAI**
椎骨脳底動脈(循環)不全(性)眼振　**VBAIN**
椎体間の　**I-B**
槌状趾　**HT**
通院　**OV**
通過　**pas**
通過時間　**PT**
通過者　**pas**
通気　**insuf, insuf.**
通気口選択　**SAV**
通勤医　**ext, ext.**
通常会話声　**OCV**
(リーボウの)通常型間質性肺炎　**UIP**
通常型間質性肺炎　**UIP**
通常(型)間質性肺炎　**UIP**
通常居住地　**UPOR**
通常水　**aq.com.**
通常治療　**uc**
通常投与メトトレキサート,ブレオマイシン,アドリアマイシン,シクロホスファミド,ビンクリスチン(=オンコビン),デキサメタゾン　**m-BACOD**
通常の　**conv, Ord, ord, ord.**
通常の健康状態　**USH, USOH**
通常の健康良好状態　**USOGH**
通常の透過型電子顕微鏡　**CEM, CTEM**
通常の方法で　**mor.sol.**
通常ヘパリン　**RH**
通常方法で使用せよ　**utend.mor.sol.**
通達　**Inst, inst**
通知　**info, infor**
通知する　**ntfy**
通年性アレルギー性鼻炎

PAR
通年性アレルギー性鼻結膜炎　**PARC**
通用年　**CY**
痛覚・触覚・振動覚・位置覚　**PPT vip.pos**
痛覚脱失(症)　**anal**
痛覚鈍麻　**hyp**
杖の助けを借りて歩く　**WWAC**
月　**M, m, MO, mo, mon, mos, mth**
月の仕事水準　**WLM**
月・日・年　**MDY**
次の　**f, ff, fl, fol, sq., subq**
次のもの　**seq.**
次のように　**udf**
作られるように　**ut ft**
続き番号　**sno**
続ける　**KO, K/o, pro**
包　**cap, cap., caps., capsul.**
常に　**sem.**
角　**A, Ang, ang.**
壺　**oll**
妻　**F, ux., W, w, w.**
爪・膝蓋骨症候群　**NPS**
爪・膝蓋骨症候群1型　**NPS1**
爪・膝蓋(症候群)　**NPa**
冷たい　**c, frig.**
冷たい飲料水　**CDW**
強い　**fort., str**
強い衝動・軽度の不安　**HILA**
強さ　**st, str**
強さ・時間　**S-D**
強さ・持続曲線　**I-D curve**
(音の)強さの弁別域　**ADL**
強さの弁別域　**DLI, IDL**
(音の)強さのレベル　**IL**

て

デアミノ・アルギニン・バソプレシン **dAVP**
デアミノ-8-D-アルギニンバソプレシン(＝酢酸デスモプレシン) **DDAVP**
デアメリンS **DS**
デオキシコール酸寒天培地 **DCA**
テイ・サックス(病) **TS**
ディエゴ血液型 **DI**
ディオプター **dptr**
デイケア麻酔に関する学会 **SAMBA**
テイコプラニン **TEIC**
ティーシーピーアイピー **TCP/IP**
ディーゼル排気ガス微粒子 **DEP**
ディー・ブイ・ディー **DVD**
デイホスピタル **DH**
ディルドリン **HEOD**
ディレクター **Dir**
デオキシ-D-グルコース **DDG**
デオキシアデニル酸 **A**
デオキシアデノシン **DA，dAdo**
デオキシアデノシン一リン酸 **dAMP**
デオキシアデノシン二リン酸 **DADP**
デオキシアデノシン三リン酸 **DATP**
デオキシイノシン **DI**
デオキシウリジン **DU**
デオキシウリジン-5′-リン酸 **DUMP，dUMP**
デオキシウリジン一リン酸 **dUMP**
デオキシウリジン二リン酸 **dUDP**
デオキシグアニル酸 **dGp，G**
デオキシグアニレート **dG**
デオキシグアノシン **DG**
デオキシグアノシン-5′-リン酸 **dGMP**
デオキシグアノシン一リン酸 **dGMP**
デオキシグアノシン二リン酸 **DGDP**
デオキシグルコース **DG**
デオキシコホルマイシン **DCF**
デオキシコール酸 **DC，DCA**
デオキシコール酸塩 **DC**
デオキシコール酸ソーダ **NaDOC**
デオキシコール酸ナトリウム **DOC，NaDOC，SDC**
デオキシコルチコイド **DOCS**
デオキシコルチコステロン **DOC**
デオキシコルチコステロングルコシド **DCG，DOCG**
デオキシコルチゾール **Compound S**
デオキシコレート・クエン酸・乳糖・サッカロース寒天 **DCLS**
デオキシサイクリン(＝DOXY,DMCT) **DOTC**
デオキシシチジル酸 **dCp**
デオキシシチジン一リン酸 **dCMP**
デオキシシチジンキナーゼ **DCK**
デオキシシチジン三リン酸 **DCTP，dCTP**
デオキシスパーガリン **DSP**
デオキシチミジン **CdR，dT，dThd**
デオキシチミジン一リン酸 **DTMP，dTMP**
デオキシチミジン三リン酸 **dTTP**
デオキシチミジン二リン酸 **dTDP**
デオキシヌクレオシド一リン酸 **DNMP**
デオキシヒドロコルチコステロン **Compound A**
デオキシフルオロウリジン **5′-DFUR**
デオキシリボ核酸 **ADN，DMS，DNA，DNS**
デオキシリボ核酸・ヒストン **hDNA**
デオキシリボ核酸指数 **DI**
デオキシリボ核酸ポリメラーゼ **DNA-P**
デオキシリボ核酸リン **DNA-P**
デオキシリボ核蛋白 **DNP，Dnp**
デオキシリボース **DR，dRib**
デオキシリボヌクレアーゼ **DNase**
デオキシリボヌクレオチド三リン酸 **dNTP**
テオフィリン **T，TH**
デカ(＝×10) **da，deca**
デカグラム **dag，decag，dkg**
デカメートル **dam，dkm**
デカリットル **dal，dkl**
デカルバモイルマイトマイ

シンC **DCMMC**
デカン酸ハロペリドール **HD, HLD, HL-D**
デカン酸フルフェナジン **FPZ-D**
テキサスレッド **TR**
テキサスレッド標識ストレプトアビシン **TRA**
デキサメタゾン **DEX, DXM**
デキサメタゾン,アラビノシルシトシン,カルボプラチン,エトポシド **DACE**
デキサメタゾン抑制試験 **DST**
デキサメタゾンリン酸ナトリウム **DSP**
テキスト **Schr.**
デキストラン **DX**
デキストラン結合チャコール **DCC**
デキストラン反応(性)抗体 **DRA**
デキストランブルー **DB**
デキストラン硫酸 **Dxs**
デキストロメトルファン **DM**
デキセドリン錠 **dexies**
テクネシウムエチルシステイン二量体 **ECD**
テクネチウム **Tc**
テクネチウム・ヘキサメチル・プロピレナミン・オキシム **HMPAO**
テクネチウム 99 m **^{99m}Tc, Tc^{99m}**
テクネチウム 99 m ピロリン酸塩 **PYP**
テクネチウムイオウコロイド **TSC**
デシ(=10^{-1},1/10) **d**
デジェリーヌ・クルンプケ(症候群) **DK**
デシグラム **dg, dgm**
デジコム **digi-com**
デジタル・アナログ(変換) **DA, d-to-a**
デジタル・アナログ変換器 **DAC**
デジタルラジオグラフィ **DR**
デジタル/アナログ(比) **D/A**
デジタル X 線映像法 **DXI**
デジタル画像伝送システム操作 **MPACS**
デジタル〔電子〕計算機 **digi-com**
デジタル減算静脈血管造影(法) **DVSA**
デジタル減算静脈造影(法) **DSP**
デジタル減算処理 X 線像 **DSR**
デジタル減算処理血管像 **DSR**
デジタル減算処理血管造影法 **DSA**
デジタル減算処理血管断層撮影 **DSAT**
デジタル減算処理間接撮影 **DSF**
デジタルコーンビーム映像法 **DCI**
デジタル式自動周期調節 **DAFC**
デジタル自動類型認知 **DAPR**
デジタル信号処理技術を応用した補聴システム **CLAIDHA**
デジタルスキャンコンバーター **DSC**
デジタルファンビーム走査法 **DFS**
デジタル走査撮影法 **DS**
デジタル操作システム **DOS**
デジタルディスプレイ **DD**
デジタルペンシルビーム走査法 **DPS**
デジタル透視血管造影法 **DFA**
デジタル透視法 **DF**
デジタル動的シミュレーター **DDS**
デシネム **dn**
デシベル **dB, db**
デシベル SPL **dB SPL**
デシベル音圧レベル **dB SPL**
デシメートル **dec, dec., decim, dm**
デシモルガン **dM, dmo**
デジェリーヌ・ソッタ(症候群) **DS**
デシリットル **dl**
デスオキシエフェドリン **DOE**
デスオキシコルチコステロングルコシド **DOCG**
デスオキシコルチコステロントリメチル酢酸塩 **DTMA**
デスオキシピリドキシン **DOP**
デスオキシリボ核酸 **DRNA**
デスオキシリボース **DR**
デスグリシナミド・アルギニン・バソプレシン **DGAVP**
デスクロロベンゾイルインドメタシン **DBI**
テストステロン **T**
テストステロン・エストラジオール結合グロブリン **TEBG, TeBG**
テストステロン・フェニルプロピオネート **TPP**
テストステロングルクロニ

ド　**TG**
テストステロン結合グロブリン　**TBG，TeBG**
テストステロン結合親和性　**TBA**
テストステロン結合蛋白　**TBP**
テストステロン産生率　**TPR**
テストステロン不妊(雌)ラット　**TSR**
テストなし　**NT**
テスパミン　**TEPA**
デスフェリオキサミン　**DF，DFX**
デスベンゾイルアセメタシン　**DBA**
デスベンゾイルデスメチルアセメタシン　**DBMA**
デスベンゾイルデスメチルインドメタシン　**DBMI**
デスメチルアセメタシン　**DMA**
デスメチルイミプラミン　**DMI**
デスメチルインドメタシン　**DMI**
デスメチルジアゼパム　**DMDZ**
デスメチルデスクロロベンゾイルアセメタシン　**DMBA**
デスメチルデスクロロベンゾイルインドメタシン　**DMBI**
デスメ膜　**DM**
テスラ　**T**
データ援助と管理　**DAC**
データ計算流動評価　**DAFA**
データ収集　**dacor**
データ修正　**datacor**
データ修正者　**datacor**
データ取得監視器具　**DAME**
データ操作器具　**DPE**
データ伝達　**datacom**
データ取り込み時間　**ACQST**
データなし　**ND**
テタニー型　**T-type**
テタニー持続時間　**Dt**
テタニー性(攣縮)　**Te**
テタニー性攣縮　**ADTe**
テタヌス後促進　**PTF**
データバンク　**DB**
データ分析・換算システム　**DARES**
データベース　**DB**
データベース管理システム　**DBMS**
データベースロック　**DBT**
データマネジメント　**DM**
テトライソプロピルチタン　**TPT**
テトラエチルアンモニウム　**TEA**
テトラエチル鉛　**TEL**
テトラエチルピロリン酸　**TEEP，TEP，TEPP**
テトラカイン・エピネフリン・コカイン　**TAC**
テトラグリシン　**TG**
テトラクロロエチレン　**TCE**
テトラクロロサリチルアニリド　**TCSA**
テトラクロロジフェニルエタン　**TCE，TDE**
テトラサイクリン　**T，TC，TCN，TE**
テトラサイクリン蛍光試験　**TFT**
テトラサイクリン耐性淋菌　**TRNG**
テトラサイクリンメチレンリジン　**MLTC**
テトラシアノエチレン　**TCNE**
テトラヨウ素サイロ酢酸　**tetrac**
テトラゾリウム還元　**TR**
テトラゾリウム還元阻止(試験)　**TRI test**
テトラゾリウム紫　**TV，VT**
テトラゾール　**TT**
テトラデシル硫酸ナトリウム　**STD，TSS**
テトラニトロブルーテトラゾリウム　**TNT**
テトラニトロメタン　**TNM**
テトラヒドロ-11-デスオキシコルチゾル　**THS**
テトラヒドロウリジン　**THU**
テトラヒドロキシキノン　**THQ**
テトラヒドロコルチゾール　**TH，THC，THF**
テトラヒドロコルチゾン　**THC，THE**
テトラヒドロステロイド　**THS**
テトラヒドロデオキシコルチコステロン　**THDOC**
テトラヒドロデオキシコルチゾール　**THS**
テトラヒドロパパベロリン　**THP**
テトラヒドロピラニルアドリアマイシン　**THP-ADM**
テトラヒドロフラン　**THF**
テトラヒドロフルオレノン　**THF**
テトラヒドロフルフリルアルコール　**THFA**
テトラヒドロ葉酸

TH_4, THF, THFA
テトラヒメナ(属) T
テトラヒメナカルシウム結合蛋白 TCBP
テトラフェニルテトラゾリウム TPT
テトラフェニルホウ酸 TPB
テトラフルオロエチレン teflon, TFE
テトラブロムフェノールフタレインエチルエステル TBPE
テトラベナジン TBZ
テトラメチル-p-フェニレンジアミン TMPD
テトラメチルアンモニウム TMA
テトラメチルウレア TMU
テトラメチルシクロブタンジオール TMCD
テトラメチルシラン TMS
テトラメチル鉛 TML
テトラメチルピペリジン-N-オキシド TEMPO
テトラメチルベンジジン TMB
テトラメチルローダミンイソチオシアネイト TRITC
テトラメチルロダミンイソチオシアネート TMRITC
テトラヨウ素〔サイ〕ロニンレジンスポンジ取り込み試験 T_4-test
テトラヨードフェノールフタレインナトリウム TIPPS
テトロドトキシン TTX
テナガザル白血病ウイルス GALV
テナガザルリンパ肉腫ウイルス GaLV
デナリウス重量 dwt
テニア(属) T
デニス・ブラウン副子 DBS
デニス小児発育検査〔試験〕 DCD
テニス肘 TE
テネイシン TN
テノイルトリフルオロアセトン TTA
テノール・バリトン・バス TBB
デビック症候群 DS
デヒドロアスコルビン酸 DHA
デヒドロイソアンドロステロール DHIA
デヒドロイソアンドロステロン DHIA
デヒドロエピアンドロステロン DEA, DEAS, DHEA
デヒドロキシフェニルグリコール DHPG
デヒドロキシマンデル酸 DHMA
デヒドロゲナーゼ DH
デヒドロコール酸 DH
デヒドロ酢酸 DHA
デヒドロテストステロン DHT
デフェロキサミン DF, DFO, DFOM
デホスホホスホリラーゼキナーゼ DPPK
デメクロサイクリン DMC
デメチルクロルテトラサイクリン DMCTC
デメロール DEM, Dem
デモステロール・コレステロール変換酵素 DCE
デュアルスクリーン DS
デュークス分類(＝大腸・直腸癌の分類) Dukes A,B,C
デュシェーヌ(型)筋ジストロフィ DMD
デュシェーヌ(型)ジストロフィ DD
デュピュイトラン病 DD
デュビン・ジョンソン(症候群) DJ
デュビン・ジョンソン症候群 DJS
デュボイスオレイン酸アルブミン複合体 DOAC
デュルベックリン酸塩緩衝塩 DPBS
テラ(＝10^{12}) T
テラジュール TJ
テラヘルツ THz
テラマイシン TM
デルタアミノレブリン酸 DALA, D-ALA
デルタ型の Delt
デルタ睡眠誘発ペプチド DSIP
デルタ波 D/W
テルビウム Tb
デルフィアシステム DELFIA
テルブタリン TRB
デルフラー・スチュアート(試験) D/S
デルフラー・スチュアート試験 D-S test
テルペンチン turp
デルマタン硫酸 DS
テルル Te
テレタイプライター TTY
テレビ TV
テレビてんかん TV epilepsy
テレフタル酸ポリエチレン PET
テレメトリ TELE,

Tele, tele
テロ対策委員会 CTC
テロメア結合蛋白 TRF
デング出血(性)熱 DHF
デング出血(性)熱ショック(症候群) DHFS
デング(熱)ショック症候群 DSS
デンバー透析病 DDD
デンバー発育スクリーニング検査〔試験〕 DDST
デンプン様小体 CA
デンマークでの抗不整脈III群薬の大規模試験 DIAMOND
テンジクネズミ GP
できるだけ多く AMAP
できるだけ早く ASAP, asap
てんかん Ep, Epi, Epil
てんかん患者 Epil
てんかん患者の突然死 SUDEP
てんかん重積状態 SE
てんかんの Epil
大さじ1杯の T
手足 mem
手足口病 HFMD
手足治療士協会員 FChS
手足の治療 chir
手洗看護師 SN
手紙 corr, corresp
手鏡細胞 HMC
手首 WR, Wr, wr, wr.
手血流量 HBF
手先の器用さ dex, dext, dext.
手近に OH
手の舟状骨骨折用の肘下ギプス SANC
手のひらの vol
手引き man
手膝(試験) H-K
出口 out
出口創 WOX, WX, W/X
電気メッキした Galv, galv
低圧 LP
低圧化学的気相成長法 LPCVD
低イオン強度溶液 LISS
低位右(心)房 LRA
低位(子宮)頸部横帝王切開 LCTCS
低位前腋窩線 LAAL
低位前方切除術 LAR
低位出口鉗子 LOF
低位出口鉗子分娩 LOFD
低エネルギーイオン散乱分光法 LEIS
低エネルギー荷電粒子 LECP
低エネルギー電子顕微鏡 LEEM
低栄養の UN
低塩(分) lo.salt
低塩(分)食 LSD
低温 LT
低温科学 CS
低温視覚施設 LTOF
低温滅菌血漿蛋白溶液 PPL, PPPL
低カリウム LoK, LoKa
低カリウムイオン LK^+
低カリウムデキストラン LPD
低カルシウム LoCa
低カルシウム(食) lo.calc
低カロリー LC
低カロリー(食) lo.cal
低カロリー炭水化物栄養補給 HCF
低カロリー蛋白食 HPF
低拡大(顕微鏡) LP
(顕微鏡の)低拡大野 LPF, lpf, l.p.f.
低眼圧緑内障 LTG
低開発国 UDC
低灌流充血 LPH
低(大)気圧 LAP
低吸収域 LDA
低強度X線顕微鏡 LIXIscope
低緊張性十二指腸造影 HDG
低血圧 Hpo-T, LBP
低血清結合鉄 LBI
低血糖(症) HG
低血糖指数 HI
低血糖性昏睡 HGC
低形成性白血病 HL
低減率 LRR
低ゴナドトロピン性性(腺)機能低下〔不全〕症 HH
低コレステロール lo.chol
低抗原腫瘍 LAT
低酸性・虚血性ニューロン損傷 HINI
低酸素換気刺激 HVD
低酸素換気反応 HVR
低酸素後企図性ミオクローヌス PHIM
低酸素性・虚血性損傷 HIL
低酸素性・虚血性脳障害 HIE
低酸素(症)性応答 HR
低酸素性肺血管攣縮 HPV
低心拍出量(症候群) LCO(S)
低心拍出量症候群 LOS
低出生体重 LBW
低出生体重児 LBWI, LOWBI
低色素血症 hypo
低周波数 LF, lf
低周波数型疲労 LFF

低周波置鍼〔針〕(療法) LFEA
低周波中周波 LFMF
低侵襲冠(状)動脈バイパス手術 MIDCAB
低侵襲手術法 MIST
低侵襲心臓外科手術 MICS
低脂肪 lo.fat
低脂肪(食) LF
低脂肪・(低)コレステロール(食) LFC
低脂肪食 LFD
低浸透圧ショック治療 HOST
低親和性血小板因子 LAPF
低繊維食 LFD
低速電子線回折 LEED
低速陽電子線回折 LEPD
低代謝患者 PM
低体温性虚血 HI
低体温(症)用酸素加温器 HOW
低体重出生矮小症 LBWD
低体積 LV
低炭水化物 LC, Lo CHO
低蛋白 LP
低蛋白食 LPD
低張力 LT
低点 LP
低鉄ジアミノアルシアンブルー LID-AB
低電圧焦点 LVF
低電圧徐波 LVS
低電圧速(波) LVF
低電位速波脳波 LVF-EEG
低トロンボプラスチン血症 HTP
低度異形成 LGD
低ナチュラルキラー症候群 LNKS
低ナトリウム LoNa, LS
低ナトリウム食 LSD
低尿酸血症 HUC
低粘稠度係数 LVI
低濃度 lo-d
低濃度域 LDA
低パーセント白血病 LPL
低反応率補充誤差 DRL
低反応レベルレーザー治療 LLLT
低比重 LD, lo-d
低比重リポ蛋白 LDL
低比重リポ蛋白関連蛋白 LRP
低比重リポ蛋白分布指数 LDI
低比重リンパ球 LDL
低皮切位帝王切開 LFCS
低頻度 LF, lf
低頻度換気 LFV
低頻度(形質)導入 LFT
低フィブリノゲン血漿 HFP
低分化型腺癌 por
低分化リンパ球性悪性リンパ腫 ML-PDL
低分化リンパ球性リンパ腫 PDLC
低分子(量)デキストラン LMD, LMDX
低分子ヘパリン LMH
低分子量 LMW
低分子量キニノゲン LMWK
低分子量デキストラン LMWD
低ヘモグロビン血症 HHB, HHb
低補体血症性血管炎・蕁麻疹様症候群 HVUS
低補体血症性糸球体腎炎 HCGN
低摩擦関節形成術 LFA
低密度 LD, lo-d
低密度ポリエチレン LDPE
低有用周波数 LUF
低ヨード症 HIO
低容量〔容積〕 LV
低リン酸血症性ビタミンD抵抗性くる病 HVDRR
低リン酸血(症)性骨疾患 HBD
低レニン・正常アルドステロン LRNA
低レニン血症性低アルドステロン血症 HH
低レニン血症性低アルドステロン症 SHH
低レニン本態性高血圧(症) LREH
低レベル廃棄物 LLW
定位深部脳波 SDEEG
定位穿刺生検 SFNB
定位脳手術装置 Stereo, stereo
定期安全性最新報告 PSUR
定期健康診断 PHE
定期的測定不要 NPCR
定義 def
定義を下す def
定型うつ病 MDD
定刻に OT
定時崩壊 TD
定常誤差 CE
定常状態 SS
定常状態血漿インスリン SSPI
定常状態血漿ブドウ糖 SSPG
定常人口 L_x
定数 C, const, k
定数・常数を示す記号 K
定数の def
定性〔質的〕分析

qual.anal
定着時定数 **FTC**
定容量における比熱 **CV**
定量 **determin, detn**
定量液 **VS**
定量構造・抗腫瘍活性関係 **QSAR**
定量沈降分析 **QPA**
定量的冠動脈造影(法) **QCA**
定量的構造物性相関 **QSPR**
定量的コンピュータ断層撮影(法) **QCT**
定量的仙腸骨シンチグラフィ **QSS**
定量的超音波法 **QUS**
定量的デジタルX線撮影(法) **QDR**
定量的な **qt, qual**
定量的バフィコート分析 **QBCA**
定量的ピルケー皮内反応 **QP**
定量的漏れ試験 **QLT**
定量噴霧式吸入器 **MDI**
底エコー **BE**
底屈 **PF, plant-flex**
底質 **dep.**
抵抗 **R**
抵抗(性) **Res, res, resis, resist**
抵抗運動 **RM**
抵抗する **Res, res**
抵抗静電容量 **RC**
抵抗のない **non obs.**
抵抗誘発因子 **RIF**
泥膏 **past.**
帝王切開(術) **C, CS, C.S., C/S, c/s, C/sec**
帝王切開後の経腟出産 **VBAC**
帝王切開術 **CS**
帝王切開出産 **CB**
帝王切開分娩 **CD**
帝王切開率 **CSR**
(英国)帝国癌研究基金 **ICRF**
訂正した **cor, cor., corr**
訂正する **C, cor, cor.**
訂正なしで **SC, s.c.**
停止 **ins**
停止した **arr**
停滞時間 **RT**
停留精巣〔睾丸〕 **UDT**
停留肺液 **RLF**
提供者 **D**
提供者協力委員会 **CODE**
提携医師 **AfP, AfPh**
提携した **affil**
提出 **exh**
提出する **exh**
程度 **Deg, deg.**
程度・粗造性・気息性・無力性・努力性 **GRBAS**
溺死 **DIW**
摘出 **av, Ex, ex, Ext, ext, rem**
摘出する **Del, del., rem**
滴 **gt., gtt., gtts.**
滴下で **stillat**
滴状類乾癬 **PG**
滴注 **instill**
滴定酸 **TA**
滴定する **titr**
滴を **gtts.**
適応 **A, a, a.**
適応(症) **ind, ind., indic**
適応がある **indic**
適応最小二乗法 **ALS**
適応した **adj**
適応障害の **malad**
適応水準 **AL**
適応できない **NA**
適応のある **I**
適格な **elig**
適合・上司・創造・外交 **ABCD**
適した **adeq, adq**
適時 **JIT**
適切でない **NA, OOO**
適切な **app, pert**
適切な補助呼吸 **AAV**
適正人口と環境に関する学会 **COPE**
適性体重児 **AGA infant**
適性発育 **AGA**
適性発育(児) **AFD**
適性発育児 **AFD infant**
適当な硬さの **deb.spis.**
適当な基剤に入れて **idon.vehic.**
適当な用法に従って **dir.prop.**
適当な指示のもとに **d.p.**
適当な賦形剤に **indo.vehic.**
適当量 **q.p.**
適用 **appl, applic, ind, ind., indic**
適量 **OD, q.s., q.suff., q.v.**
適量に **q.s.ad**
適齢期の **nube**
敵意と敵意傾向 **HDH**
敵意と敵意傾向のための質問票 **HDHQ**
哲学士 **Ph.B.**
鉄 **Fe, Fer.**
鉄芽球性貧血 **SA**
鉄欠乏 **FeD**
鉄欠乏性貧血 **Fe def, IDA**
鉄結合グロブリン **IBG**
鉄結合蛋白 **IBP**
鉄結合能 **IBC**
鉄の **Fe^{2+}, Fe^{3+}**

鉄(＝^{59}Fe)の赤血球利用率 **%^{59}Fe util**
鉄ヘマトキシリン **IH**
鉄・キニシン・ストリキニン **IQ & S**
徹夜 **ON**
天蓋網状系 **TR**
天然〔未変性〕DNA **nDNA**
天然痘 **smpx**
天疱瘡 **P**
(接触)伝染 **contag**
伝染 **INF, inf, inf., infect**
伝染(病) **commun**
伝染性胃腸炎 **TGE**
伝染性気管支ウイルス **IBV**
伝染性気管支炎ワクチン **IBV**
伝染性疾患管理局 **DCDC**
伝染性単核球症 **IM**
伝染性単核細胞症 **MI**
伝染性単核症受容体 **IMR**
伝染性軟属腫 **MC**
伝染性軟属腫ウイルス **MCV**
伝染性の **contag**
伝染性膿疱性口内炎 **CPS**
伝染(性)の **com, comm**
伝染病 **CD, C.D., commun.dis**
伝染病監視センター〔米国〕 **CDSC**
伝達 **comm, Tr, tr, transm**
伝達因子 **TA, TF**
伝達可能ウイルス性痴呆 **TVD**
伝達可能ミンク脳症 **TME**
伝達関数 **TF**
伝達された **t**
伝達障害 **comm dis**
伝達できる **comm**
伝達不応期 **RPT**
伝達抑制 **DT**
伝統的産婆 **TBA**
伝導 **cond**
伝導時間 **CT**
伝導静脈 **CV**
伝導速度 **CV**
伝導率 **cond, conduct**
典型的な **repr, typ, typ.**
点 **P, pnt, pt, pt.**
点眼液をつくれ **ft.collyr.**
点眼剤 **coll.**
点検し,必要なら修正する **ITCAN**
点耳薬 **aurist.**
点状角膜炎 **KP**
点状出血 **petech, PH**
点状上皮角膜症 **PEK**
点滴 **DI**
点滴静(脈内)注(射) **IVD**
点滴静注腎盂撮影(法) **DIP**
点滴静注胆道撮影法 **DIC**
点滴静脈注射 **DIV**
点滴注入 **instill**
(薬剤)点滴注入流産時間 **IAT**
点広がり関数 **PSF**
点鼻 **NB**
点鼻剤 **collun.**
点鼻薬 **narist.**
展示 **exh**
展示する **exh**
展布硬膏 **emp.ext.**
添加 **addn**
転位 **dis, DISL, Disl, disloc, inv**
転位した **DISL, Disl, disloc, iv**
転位する **DISL, Disl, disloc**
転移 **M, MET, met, metas, Mets**
転移RNA **tRNA, t-RNA**
(癌の)転移あり **M_1**
転移因子 **TF**
転移する **metas, trs**
転移性栄養膜疾患 **MTD**
転移性黒色腫 **MM**
転移性腎細胞癌 **MRCC**
転移性脊髄圧迫 **MCC**
転移性乳癌 **MBC**
転移デオキシリボ核酸 **t-DNA**
(癌の)転移なし **M_0**
転移(性)の **met, metas**
転移リボ核酸 **tRNA, t-RNA**
転換性非ウイルス産出細胞 **CNVP cell**
転換帯 **TMZ**
転換電子メスバウアー分光法 **CEMS**
転形〔変調〕率 **MR**
転座 **t**
転子 **troch.**
転写因子 **NF, TF**
殿部の **Glut**
電圧 **V**
電圧・電流反応性 **VAR**
電圧依存性陰イオン(選択性)チャンネル **VDAC**
電圧計 **Vm**
電圧上昇比率 **RRV**
電位 **pot, vltge**
電位開放カルシウムチャンネル **VGCC**
電位差 **PD**
電位差計 **pots**
電位図 **EGM**

電界　EF
電界効果型トランジスタ　FET
電界ベクトル　E
電界放射型電子銃　FEG
電界放射顕微鏡　FEM
電界放射電子分光法　FEES
電荷　E, e
電荷/電子質量比　E/M, e/m
電荷結合素子　CCD
電荷注入装置　CID
電荷の零〔ゼロ〕点　ZPC
電解イオン顕微鏡検査　FIM
電解イオン脱離　FD
電解質　LYTES, lytes
電解質平衡異常　EI
電気　elec
電気胃図　EGG
電気エアロゾール療法　EAT
電気泳動　ELP, EP
電気泳動度移動アッセイ　EMSA
電気泳動分析　GMSA
電気化学検出器　ECD
電気化学石英結晶マイクロバランス　EQCM
電気化学的電位勾配　ECPOG
電気化学の　EC
電気加熱気化法　ETV
電気感覚計器板　ESP
電気眼球運動図　EOG
電気眼球図記録法　EOG
電気眼振計　ENG, EOG, Nysta
電気眼振図　ENG
電気乾燥術　ED
電気乾燥法　EDN
電気起因性化学発光　ECL
電気技師　EE
電気キモグラフ　EKY
電気キモグラム　EKY
電気経頭蓋刺激　ETS
電気痙攣治療　Es
電気痙攣療法　ECT
電気勾配検出器　PGD
電気交流　VA
電気呼吸記録計　EPG
電気呼吸記録図　EPG
電気式胎児監視　EFM
電気刺激　ES
電気刺針術　EAC
電気(的)射精　EEJ
電気ショック　ES
電気ショック〔痙攣/衝撃〕療法　EST
電気ショック治療　ET
電気ショック療法　EKT, ET
電気神経検査　ENoG
電気診断　ED, EDX, EDx
電気診断法　El Dx
電気浸透流　EOF
電気親和性　EA
電気親和力　E, E_0
電気水圧衝撃波砕石術　ESWL
電気水圧砕石術　EHL
電気生理学的異常　EA
電気生理学的検査　EPS
電気生理学的行動修正　EBM
電気生理学的な　EP
電気穿孔用緩衝液　EB
電気沈降素　EP
電気的筋刺激　EMS
電気的差動治療　Edit
電気的刺激による鎮痛　ESPA
電気的零点　EZ
電気的全写法　EPG
電気的全心収縮期　EMS
電気的に安定な　stat
電気瞳孔計　EPG
電気透析　ED
電気に関する　elec
電気の　elec, elect
電気脳刺激装置　EBS
電気鍼療法　EA, EAP
電気火花びらん　ELOX
電気皮膚電位　GSP
電気皮膚反応　EDR, ESR
電気分解　electrol
電気変性反応　EaR, Ea.R.
電気麻酔　EA, EN
電気免疫拡散　EID
電気免疫定量法　EIA
電気量　Q
電気療法師　TET
電極電位　E
電極の　term
電撃痙攣閾値　MET
電撃ショック　ECS
電撃性紫斑病　PF
電撃療法　ECT
電子　E, E, e
電子化診療記録統合管理　DACS
電子凝固術　EC
電子キロボルト　ekV
電子計算機　cmptr, compu
電子計算機処理　compu
電子計算機で処理する　compu
電子顕微鏡　EM
電子顕微鏡検査　EM, EMC
電子顕微鏡検査と微細分析　EMMA
電子顕微鏡所見　EM
電子工学　electro
電子磁気放射制御　conelrad
電子衝撃イオン化　EI
電子衝撃イオン化法　EI mass spectrometry

電子常磁性共鳴　**EPR**
電子数値積算機つきコンピュータ　**ENIAC**
電子スピン共鳴　**ESR**
電子線エネルギー損失分光法　**EELS**
電子線記録装置　**EBR**
電子線超音波顕微鏡による観察　**EAM**
電子損失分光検査法　**ELS**
電子的症例報告書　**eCRF**
電子的情報処理　**EDP**
電子データ収集(システム)　**EDC**
電子データ処理システム　**EDPS**
電子伝達フラビン蛋白　**ETF**
電子伝達粒子　**ETP**
電子微量分析器　**EMA**
電子プローブ微細X線分析　**EPMA**
電子プローブ微細X線分析器　**EPMA**
電子捕獲　**K**
電子捕獲型検出器　**ECD**
電子捕捉検出器　**EC detector**
電子ボルト　**eV**
電磁気共鳴　**EMR**
電磁血流計　**EMF**
電磁障害　**EMI**
電磁単位　**EMU, emu**
電磁の　**EM, em**
電磁場　**EMF**
電磁パルス　**EMP**
電磁放射　**EMR**
電気　**batt**
電導収縮解離　**EMD**
電場　**EF**
電場刺激　**EFS**
電流　**c, cur**
電流強度　**CS**
電流計　**AM, Am, am**
電流脳写法　**REG**
電流密度　**J**
電量フローインジェクション滴定法　**CFIT**
電話健康相談　**MIL**
電話指示　**PO, P/O, TO, T.O., T/O, t.o.**
電話による医学情報サービス　**MIST**
電話のない　**NP**
電話連絡　**PC, TC, T/C, Tc, t.c.**

と

デブレ・セミレーニュ(症候群) **DS**
ドイツ医学週刊誌 **DMW**
ドイツ眼科学会 **DOG**
ドイツ癌研究センター **DKFZ**
ドイツ救難飛行隊 **DRF**
ドイツ語 **Ger**
ドイツ工業規格 **DIN**
ドイツ人 **Ger**
ドイツ赤十字 **DRK**
ドイツの環境保護庁 **UBA**
ドイツの生殖医療に関する基本法 **ESchG**
ドイツ平面 **DH, DHE**
ドイツ薬局方 **DAB, P.G., Ph.G.**
ドイツ臨床化学会 **GSCC**
トイレットペーパー **TP**
ドゥブレ・ドゥ・トニ・ファンコニ(症候群) **DTF**
トウモロコシ湯煎液 **CSL**
ドゥルベコ変法イーグル培地 **DMEM**
トゥーレット症候群 **TS**
トカイニド **Tc**
ドキシサイクリン(=DOXY,DOTC) **DMCT**
ドキシサイクリン(=DMCT,DOTC) **DOXY**
トキシン **tox, Tox, tox.**
トキソイド・抗毒素合剤 **TAM**
トキソイド・抗毒素沈降物 **TAF**
トキソピリミジン **TXP**
トキソプラズマ **Tp**
トキソプラズマ(属) **T**
トキソプラズマ・風疹・サイトメガロ・ヘルペス・ウイルス(症候群) **TORCH**
トキソプラズマ症 **TOXO, Toxo**
トキソプラズマ皮膚試験抗原 **TSTA**
トキソプラズマ病 **Tp**
ドキソルビシン(=アドリアマイシン) **DOX, DXR**
ドクター中心システム **DOS**
トコキノン10 **E_{10}**
ドコサヘキサエン酸 **DHA**
トコフェロール **T**
トコフェロールキノン **TQ**
トコフェロール欠乏の **TD**
トコフェロールを補充(添加)した **TS**
ドサンクティス・カッキオーネ〔症候群〕 **DSC**
トシル(基) **Tos, tos, Ts**
トシルアルギニンメチルエステル **TAME**
トスフロキサシン **TFLX**
トッド殺虫ガス発生器 **TIFA**
トッド単位 **TU**
ドップラーカルジオグラフィ **DCG**
ドデカニル無水コハク酸 **DDSA**
ドデシルジアミノエチル塩酸グリシン **DAG**
ドデシル硫酸ナトリウム **SDS**
ドデシル硫酸ナトリウムポリアクリルアミドゲル電気泳動 **SDS-PAGE**
ドナー限定輸液 **DST**
ドナー限定輸血 **DST**
ドーナト・ラントシュタイナー抗体 **D-L Ab**
ドーナト・ラントシュタイナー(抗体) **DL**
ドーナト・ラントシュタイナー検査 **DLT**
ドーナト・ラントシュタイナー現象 **DL**
トノグラフィ **Tng**
ド(ー)パ **DOPA, Dopa**
ド(ー)パ酸化酵素 **dopase**
ド(ー)パ反応 **DOPA reaction**
ド(ー)パ反応性筋緊張異常症 **DRD**
ド(ー)パミン **DA, Da, DM, DOA, DOPAmine, DOPAMINE**
ド(ー)パミン-β-ヒドロキシラーゼ **DBH**
ド(ー)パミン作動性神経 **DN**
ド(ー)パミン作用(性) **DA**
ド(ー)パミン受容体 **DA-R**
ド(ー)パ誘発運動障害 **DID**
ドブタミン **DOB**
ドブタミン(負荷)心エコー法 **DSC**
ドブニウム **Db**
ド(ッ)プラー超音波診断法 **DS**
ド(ッ)プラー超音波流量計 **DUF**

トブラマイシン **TM, TOB**
トブラマイシン定量(法) **STA**
トムソン徴候 **T-sign**
トヨマイシン **TY**
トヨマイシンA3 **A3**
ドライシロップ **DS**
トリ〔ライ〕トンX **Tx**
ドラクンクルス(属) **D**
トラコーマ **TR, Tr, trach, trch**
トラコーマクラミジア **CT**
トラコーマ封入体(性)結膜炎(因子) **TRIC**
ドラッグマスターファイル **DMF**
トラネキサム酸 **t-AMCHA, TAMCHA**
(常用/薬用)ドラム **dr, dr.**
ドラム液量 **fl dr**
ドラム薬用度量衡法 **dr ap, dr.ap.**
トラリ **TRALI**
トランス **trans, Xfmr**
トランスアルドラーゼ **TA, TRA**
トランスケトラーゼ **TK, TRK**
トランスケトラーゼ活性 **TKA**
トランスコバラミン **TC**
トランスコルチン **TC**
トランスサイレチン **TTR**
トランスデューサー **XDR**
トランスフェリン **TF, Tf, TFN, Tr**
トランスフェリン結合フェリチン **Tf-Fe**
トランスフェリン受容体 **TFR**
トランスフォーミング増殖因子 **TGF**
トランスポゾン **MGE, Tn**
トランスミッターオフ **X-off**
トランスミッターオン **X-on**
トランスレチノイン酸 **TRA**
ドーランド図解医学辞典 **DIMD**
トリアシルグリセロール **TG**
トリアセチルオレアンドマイシン **TAO, TOM**
トリアセチルジフェノールイサチン **TDI**
トリアトーマ(属) **T**
トリアニンジル塩化エチレン **TACE**
トリアムシノロン **Tr, Triam**
トリアリルシアヌール酸 **TAC**
トリウム **Th**
トリエタノールアミン **TEA, TEM**
トリエチルアミノエチル **TEAE**
トリエチレン・チオホスホラミド **TESPA**
トリエチレングリコール **TE**
トリエチレンチオリン酸アミド **TSPA**
トリエチレンテトラミン **TETA**
トリエチレンホスホラミド **TEPA**
トリエチレンメラミン **TEM**
トリオーズホスフェイトイソメラーゼ **TPI**
トリオースリン酸 **TP**
トリガー **trig**
トリカルボン酸(回路) **TCA**
トリキネラ(属) **T**
トリグリセリド **TG, TGL, TRIG, Trig, trig.**
トリグリセリド脂肪酸 **TGFA**
トリグリセリド豊富リポ蛋白 **TRL**
トリグリセリドリパーゼ **TGL**
トリクロル酢酸 **TCA**
トリクロル酢酸塩 **TCA**
トリクロル酢酸法 **TCA method**
トリクロロエタノール **TCA**
トリクロロエチレン **TCE, TRI**
トリクロロカルバニリド **TCC**
トリクロロフェノール **TCP**
トリクロロフルオロメタン **TCFU**
トリコスタチンA **TSA**
トリ骨髄芽球性ウイルス **AMV**
トリコマイシン **TRM**
トリコモナス **T**
トリコモナス(属) **Trich, trich.**
トリコモナス症 **Tricho**
トリコモナス性腟炎 **TV**
トリサイロニン **TRIT**
トリス・酢酸・エチレンジアミンテトラ酢酸(緩衝液) **TAE**
トリス・ヒドロキシメチル・アミノメタン **TRIS, Tris, tris**
トリス・ヒドロキシメチ

ル・メチルアミン　**TRIS, Tris, tris**
トリス・ホウ酸・エチレンジアミンテトラ酢酸(緩衝液)　**TBE**
トリ膵臓性ポリペプチド　**APP**
トリ膵ペプチダーゼ　**APP**
トリス緩衝食塩水浮遊液　**STBS**
トリ赤芽球症ウイルス　**AEV**
トリ胎仔腎　**ECK**
トリチウム　**T, *t***
トリチウム核磁気共鳴　**TNMR**
トリチウム化チミジン　**^{3}H-TdR**
トリチウムチミジン　**TTh**
トリチオパラメトキシフェニルプロペン　**TMPP**
トリチル(基)　**tr**
トリニトログリセロール　**TNG**
トリニトロトルエン　**TNT**
トリニトロフェニル基　**TNP**
トリニトロフロログルシノール　**TNPG**
トリニトロベンゼンスルホン酸　**TNBS**
トリニトロール塩化ベンゼン　**TNCB**
トリ白血病ウイルス　**ALV**
トリ白血病複合体　**ALC**
トリパノソーマ(属)　**T**
トリハロメタン　**THM**
トリヒドロキシインドール　**THI**
トリヒドロキシメチルアミノメタン　**THAM**
トリピリジルトリアジン　**TPTZ**
トリフェニル酢酸デスオキシコルチコステロン　**DCTPA**
トリフェニルスズ　**TPT**
トリフェニルメタン　**TPM**
トリフェニルメチル　**trityl-**
トリフェニルメチルホスホニウム　**TPMP**
トリプシン　**TPS, Tr**
トリプシン・アルデヒド・フクシン　**TAF**
トリプシン活性化蛋白　**TAP**
トリプシン結合活性　**TBA**
トリプシン不溶セグメント　**TIS**
トリプシン様免疫活性　**TLI**
トリプシン抑制能(検定法)　**TIC**
トリプチケースソイブロス　**TSB**
トリプトファニル転移リボ核酸合成酵素　**TRPRS**
トリプトファン　**TP, Trp, TRY, Try, Tryp, W**
トリプトファン・ペプトン・ブドウ糖(ブロス)　**TPG**
トリプトファンオペロン　**trp operon**
トリプトファン過塩素酸(試験)　**TA**
トリプトファン過塩素酸(反応)　**TA**
トリプトファン合成酵素　**T'ase**
トリプトファン水酸化酵素　**Try H**
トリプトファン負荷試験　**TLT**
トリプトファンペルオキシダーゼ　**TPO**
トリプトファン豊富プレアルブミン　**TRPA**
トリプトン・ブドウ糖・酵母(寒天培地)　**TGY**
トリプトングルコースエキスミルク寒天　**TGE-AGAR**
トリプルX症候群　**XXX**
トリフルオペラジン　**TFPZ**
トリフルオロエタノール　**TFE**
トリフルオロ酢酸　**TFA**
トリフルオロチミジン　**F3T, F3TDR, TFT**
トリフルオロテノイルアセトン　**TTA**
トリブロモエタノール　**E107**
トリブロモサリチルアニリド　**TBS**
トリヘキシフェニジル　**THP**
トリホスホイノシチド　**TPI**
トリホスホピリジンヌクレオチド　**TPN**
トリポックスウイルス　**FPV**
トリマイコバクテリウム複合体　**MAC**
トリメタジオン　**TMO**
トリメタファン　**TMP**
トリメチルアミノオキシド　**TMA**
トリメチルアミン　**TMA**
トリメチルコルヒチン酸　**TMCA**
トリメチル酢酸デスオキシコルチコステロン

DCTMA
トリメチルシリル(基) **TMS**
トリメチルヒ素化合物 **TMA**
トリメチルベンズアントラセン **TMBA**
トリメチルリン酸 **TMP**
トリメトキシアンフェタミン **TMA**
トリメトキシフェニルアミノプロパン **TMA**
トリメドキシム **TMB-4**
トリメトプリム **TMP**
トリメトプリム・サルファメトキサゾール **TMP-SMX**
トリヨウ化チロ酢酸 **TRIAC**
トリヨード・チ〔サイ〕ロニン結合能指数 **TBCI**
トリヨードチ〔サイ〕ロニン **T_3, TIT, TITH, TITh, TRIT**
トリヨードチ〔サイ〕ロニン指数 **T_3 Index**
トリヨードチ〔サイ〕ロニン摂取(検査) **T_3RU, T_3U**
トリヨードチ〔サイ〕ロニン摂取率 **T_3U**
トリヨードチ〔サイ〕ロニン放射(標識)免疫検定(法) **T_3 RIA**
トリレンジイソシアネート **TDI**
トール **Torr, torr**
トルイジンブルー **TB**
トルイジンブルー異染色 **TBM**
トルイジンブルーエオジン **TB-E**
トルエン-2,4-ジイソシアネイト **TC**
トルエンジイソシアネート **TDI**
トルエンスルホニルアルギニンメチルエステル **TANe**
トルコ鞍内クモ膜下腔嵌入 **ISH**
トルゴール **turg**
トルブタマイド **D860**
トルブタミド **tolb**
トルブタミド・グルカゴン試験 **TGT**
トルブタミド試験 **TBT**
トルブタミド負荷試験 **TTT**
トレオニン **Thr**
トレッドミル運動 **TE**
トレッドミル運動試験 **TET**
トレッドミル試験 **TMT, TM test**
トレッドミルスコア **TS**
トレッドミルストレス検査 **TST**
トレッドミルストレス試験 **TMST**
トレッドミルテスト **ETT**
トレードマーク **TM**
ドレナージ **dge, drain, drg, drng**
トレハロースジミコレート **TDM**
トレポネーマ(属) **T, Trep**
トレポネーマ偽陽性 **TFP**
ドレーン **dr**
トレンデレンブルク(体位) **Trend**
トロエル・ジェネー(症候群) **TJ**
トロサ・ハント症候群 **THS**
トローチ **troch., troch.**
トローチ剤をつくれ **ft.troch.**
ドロフィン **dolo**
ドロフィン錠 **dollies**
トロポニンC **TNC**
トロポニンI **TNI**
トロポニンT **TNT**
トロポミオシン **TM**
トロメタミン **THAM**
トロン **Tn**
トロンビン **Th**
トロンビンアンチトロンビン(Ⅲ複合体) **TAT**
トロンビン感受性蛋白 **TSP**
トロンビン凝固時間 **TCT**
トロンビン時間 **TT**
トロンビン増加性フィブリノペプチドB **TIFPB**
トロンビンヒルジン複合体 **THC**
トロンビンレセプター **Part**
トロンボエラストグラフ **TEG**
トロンボエラストグラフィ **TEG**
トロンボエラストグラム **TEG**
トロンボキサン **Thx, Tx, TX**
トロンボキサンA **TxA, TXA**
トロンボキサンA_2 **TxA_2**
トロンボキサンB **TB, TXB**
トロンボキサンB_2 **TxB_2**
トロンボスポンジン **TS**
トロンボスポンジン1 **Thbs**
トロンボテスト **TT**
トロンボプラスチン

TPL
トロンボプラスチン活性化(試験) TAT
トロンボプラスチンスクリーニング試験 TST
トロンボプラスチン生成試験 TGT
トロンボポエチン Tp, TPO
トロンボモジュリン TM
トワイニングの鞍結節と内後頭隆起を結ぶ線 TTT line
ドワイヤー法 DI
トンネル音響顕微鏡 TAM
リーシュマニア・ドノヴァン LD
どうぞ pls
ときどき Occ, occ, occas
ときどきの Occ, occ, occas
とくに bsd
どこでも健康な機会に恵まれた人々 HOPE
とても高い vh
とても良い VG, V/G
とても古い VSO
どのような様式で q.m.
ともに sim., tog
ともに研和せよ ter.sim.
ともに生じたある物 UAF
とらせよ su, su.
とくに esp, espec
土壌 S
土製の fict.
土着集積データ法 NPD
土着の Nat
吐血 hematem
吐心〔悪心〕・嘔吐・下痢・便秘 NVDC
吐出物 eruct
吐物 emet
図書館目録 lib cat
図書検索 LS
努力呼気曲線 FES
努力呼気肺活量 FEV
努力性 S
努力性吸気曲線 FIS
努力性吸気肺活量 FIV, FIVC
努力性吸気流量 FIF
努力性呼気時間 FET
努力性呼気肺活量 FEC
努力性呼気量 FVE
努力性肺活量 FVC
努力性肺活量分析 FVCA
努力性無呼吸持続試験 DVA test
取らせよ,服用させよ CAP, cap, cap.
取る sum.
取れ R, r., rc.
兎唇 CL, HL
兎唇・口唇裂 CL/CP
度 D, d, Deg, deg.
度数 F, freq
時計音による右耳聴能距離 HDRW
時計音による左耳聴能距離 HDLW
時計回りの CKW, ckw, CW, cw, cws
徒手筋力検査 MMT
徒手抵抗運動 MRE
徒手の M
留め針 P
閉ざされた cl, cld
閉じた cl, cld
閉じる cl
閉込め症候群 LIS
登上線維 CF
塗布剤 lin, lin., linim
塗布剤をつくれ ft.linim.
塗布させる ft.ung.
塗布せよ applicand.
塗抹した unct.
溶かした sol.
溶かせ SOLV, solv.
当価重量 Z
当該疾患による死亡 DCD
当直〔待機〕レジデント ROC
当分 pro tem.
当量の Eq, eq, EQU, equiv
同一例 SC
同位元素 I
同位元素希釈質量分光法 ID-MS
同位元素脳槽造影(法) ICG
同位元素標識免疫沈降反応 RIP
同位体 I
同意語 syn
同意説明文書 ICF
同化する〔した〕 assim
同価の Eq, eq, EQU, equiv
同期式間欠的強制換気 SIMV
同期性の sync, synch
同期的間欠的強制換気(＝SIMV) synchronized IMV
同心(性)針筋電図検査(法) CNEMG
同心(性)針電極 CNE
同心半球型エネルギー分析器 HSA
同心半球型分光器 CHA
同所性肝移植 OLT, Olt
同所性心臓移植 OHT
同時黄斑知覚 SMP
同時視 SP
同時スキャン RTS
同時性尿道膀胱内圧測定 SUCM

同時代の　**contemp**
同時多項目アレルゲン特異的 IgE 抗体検査　**MAST**
同時多重チャンネル自動分析器　**SMA**
同時〔即時〕超音波検査(法)　**RTU, RTUS**
同時聴覚フィードバック　**SAF**
同時の　**Sim**
同時分析装置　**SMAC**
同軸の　**coax**
同種移植人工キヌタ骨　**HIP**
同種移植による活性化マクロファージ　**AIM**
同種骨髄移植　**ABMT**
同種混合リンパ球培養反応　**allogenic MLCR**
同種細胞向抗体　**HCTA**
同種細胞親和性の　**HCT**
同種属イヌジステンパー抗血清　**HCD**
同種の　**i**
同種培養癌細胞刺激誘導キラー細胞　**allo-TLAK**
同種破傷風免疫グロブリン　**HTIG**
同種白血球抗体　**HLA**
同種免疫リンパ球細胞傷害性　**ALC**
同性愛(者)の　**H**
同相弁別比　**CMR, CMRR, DF**
同側視蓋　**IOT**
同側乳腺腫瘍再発　**IBTR**
同側の　**homolat**
同調　**SYN**
同調の　**sync, synch**
同定　**ID, iden**
同定する　**iden**
同毒療法　**homo**
同毒療法の　**homo**
同等部　**part.aeq.**
同年齢の　**contemp**
同(等の)部分　**p.ae.**
同部分　**p.aeq.**
同腹子　**LM**
同胞　**sib, sibs, SS**
同名半盲　**HH**
同様に　**ejusd.**
同量　**tal.dos., t.d.**
同量 4 個が与えられるべし　**d.t.d.no Ⅳ**
同量 6 個を送れ　**mitt.tal.vi**
同量投与せよ　**dent.tal.dos.**
同量に分割せよ　**div.in p.aeq.**
同量の　**t**
同量を送れ　**mitt.tal., mtd, m.t.d.**
同量を服用　**sum tal**
同僚審査機構　**PRO**
同類の　**i**
同腕染色体　**i**
投薬　**adm, Adm, med, med., meds, MEDS, PS, Rp, RX, Rx.**
投薬される　**ad hib.**
投薬する　**D**
投薬停止後再発　**PDR**
投与　**adm, Adm**
投与する　**Disp., disp., adhib.**
投与せよ　**DD, Disp., disp.**
投与量規制因子　**DLF**
投与量規制毒性　**DLT**
豆莢斑紋状ウイルス　**BPMV**
東大式人格表　**TPI**
東南アジア医学情報センター　**SEAMIC**
東南アジア小児科学会　**APSSEAR**
東南アジアリウマチ連合　**SEAPAL**
東部ウマ脳炎　**EEE**
東部ウマ脳脊髄炎ウイルス　**EEE virus**
東部腫瘍学共同体　**ECOG**
東部精神病研究会　**EPRA**
東洋系米国人による骨髄ドナー登録組織　**AADP**
東洋人　**O**
東洋人の女性　**f/o**
東洋人夜間死亡症候群　**ONDS**
東洋と西洋　**OW, ow**
到達可能な　**A**
到達して　**on approv**
到着時間　**PXin**
到着時出産〔出生〕　**BOA**
到着日　**DOA**
到着前に　**PTA**
洞　**An, S, s, sin, sin.**
洞結節　**SN**
洞結節回復時間　**SNRT, SRT**
洞結節機能不全　**SND**
洞結節有効不応期　**SNERP**
洞室頻拍症　**SVT**
洞性徐脈　**SB**
洞性早期収縮　**SPS**
洞性不整脈　**SA**
洞組織反応　**SH**
洞大動脈除神経　**SAD**
洞調律　**SR**
洞停止　**SA**
(鼓室)洞摘出(術)　**A**
洞頻脈　**ST**
洞(機能)不全症候群　**SSS**
洞房回復時間　**SART**
洞房結節　**SAN, SAN**
洞房結節動脈　**SANA**
洞房伝導時間　**SACT**

と

洞房の　**SA, S-A**
洞房ブロック　**SAB**
凍結乾燥(法)　**LY, ly, ly.**
凍結乾燥下下垂体前葉(組織)　**LAP**
凍結乾燥した　**lyo**
凍結乾燥豚皮　**LPS**
凍結血漿　**FP**
凍結水　**aq.aster., aq.astr.**
凍結赤血球　**FRC**
凍結切片　**FS, f.s., FX, FZ**
凍結切片赤血球　**FZRC**
凍結切片用免疫組織化学　**IHC-F(r)**
凍結による破裂膀胱　**CEB**
凍結保存受精卵　**FP**
討議室　**CR**
討論の統率者　**DL**
透過性　**P**
透過性因子　**PF**
透過性係数　**PQ**
透過性指数　**PI**
透過性増強因子　**PIF**
透過損失　**TL**
透過(型)電(子)顕(微鏡)　**TEM**
透過(型)電(子)顕(微鏡)法　**TEM**
透過率　**T**
透光率　**Tr**
(X線)透視(検査)　**fluor, fluoro, FX**
(X線)透視(法)　**DL**
透視診断法　**Fl**
透析後白血球抽出物　**DLE**
透析従来法　**CD**
透析前ヒト血清　**PDA, PDS**
透析中非経口栄養法　**IDPN**
透析(性)平衡異常症候群　**DDS**
透析前体重量　**WW**
透熱療法　**Dia, dia., diath**
透明帯　**ZP**
透明帯開窓法　**PZD**
透明帯下注入法　**SUZI**
透明帯下(精子)注入法　**SUZI**
透明帯除去ハムスター卵子を用いる精子侵入〔貫通〕試験　**ZSPT**
透明中隔　**SEP, SP**
透明度　**trany**
透明な　**crys, cryst, vitr, vitr.**
透明領域　**TR**
(拘束)胴ベルト　**WB**
疼痛　**dol.**
疼痛・感覚異常・蒼白・無脈・麻痺・疲労・冷感　**6P1C**
疼痛・麻痺・感覚異常・脈拍喪失の4症状　**4P symptom**
疼痛機能不全症候群　**PDS**
疼痛強度差　**PID**
疼痛時　**dol urg**
疼痛側に　**lat.dol.**
疼痛と灼熱痛　**P & B**
疼痛部　**part.dolent.**
疼痛部位に　**part.dolent.**
疼痛部に　**ad part.dolent.**
淘汰係数　**s**
陶材　**P**
動因　**agt, agt., D**
動員　**mob**
動眼神経(核)　**OMN**
動眼神経核　**OCN**
動眼神経の　**OM**
動悸　**pal, palp, palpi, palpit**
動機分析検査　**MAT**
動原体　**cen, cen.**
動作　**p**
動作解析　**PA**
動作中の受傷　**WIA**
動作誘発気管支収縮　**EIB**
動静脈奇形　**AVM**
動静脈酸素較差　**AVO_2**
動静脈酸素分圧較差　**$AVD\text{-}O_2$**
動静脈シャント　**AVS, A-V S**
動静脈の　**AtV, AV, A-V**
動静脈(口径)比　**AVR, A-V R**
動静脈吻合　**AVA**
動静脈利用比　**DAV**
動静脈瘻　**AVF**
動静脈フィステル　**AVF**
動的〔動態〕家族描画法　**KFD**
動的空間再構築装置　**DSR**
動的心電図検査　**DCG**
動的精神医学　**DP**
動電クロマトグラフィ　**EKC**
動(的)肺コンプライアンス　**Cdyn**
動物　**anim**
動物医学センター　**AMC**
動物学　**Zool**
動物学の　**Zool**
動物行動学会員　**FES**
動物産科学　**OB**
動物飼育条件　**GB**
動物疾病研究協会　**ADRA**
動物蛋白因子　**APF**
動物の疾病と寄生虫　**ADP**
動物命名規約　**Zoo C**
動物薬センター　**CVM**

動物流行性出血性疾患 **EHD**
動脈 **A, a, a., Aa, AA, aa., ART, Art, art.**
動脈・終末呼気炭酸ガス分圧較差 **α-ETCO$_2$**
動脈・静脈 **AV, A-V**
動脈・静脈の **A/V**
動脈・深部静脈(注射) **a/dv**
動脈・肺胞酸素分圧比 **a/A**
動脈/静脈比 **A/V**
動脈圧 **AP, TA, TA, T.A.**
動脈ガス塞栓症 **AGE**
動脈管 **DA**
動脈間圧勾配 **IAPG**
動脈管開存症 **PDA**
動脈管切断術 **PDA-division**
動脈血 **a, a.**
動脈血・肺胞気炭酸ガス分圧較差 **a-ADCO$_2$, a-APCO$_2$**
動脈血・肺胞気窒素分圧較差 **a(-)ADN$_2$**
動脈血圧 **ABP**
動脈血ガス **ABG, ABGs**
動脈血ガス分析 **BGA**
動脈血ガス量 **Va**
動脈血酸素含量 **Cao$_2$**
動脈血酸素分圧 **PaO$_2$**
動脈血酸素飽和度 **SaO$_2$**
動脈血栓症 **AT**
動脈血中ケトン体比 **AKBR**
動脈血中炭酸ガス含量 **Ca$_{Co2}$**
動脈血二酸化炭素〔炭酸ガス〕分圧 **PCO$_2$ art**
動脈血二酸化炭素分圧 **PaCO$_2$**
動脈硬化(症) **AS, A-S, ASC, asc, asc., ATS**
動脈硬化回復の監視研究 **MARS**
動脈硬化指数 **AI**
動脈硬化集積指数 **AIA**
動脈硬化性冠(状)動脈疾患 **ASCAD, ASCVD**
動脈硬化性高血圧性心血管疾患 **ASHCVD**
動脈硬化性腎炎 **ASN**
動脈硬化性心血管病 **ASCVD**
動脈硬化性心(臓)疾患 **AHD**
動脈硬化性心疾患 **ASHD**
動脈硬化性閉塞性疾患 **AOD**
動脈硬化性末梢血管疾患 **ASPVD**
動脈硬化(性)の **ASC, asc, asc.**
動脈撮影 **AG**
動脈周囲炎 **PA**
動脈性オキシヘモグロビン **SpO$_2$**
動脈性高血圧 **AH**
動脈性毛細(血)管の **AC**
動脈塞栓症 **AE**
動脈内化学療法,化学療法動注法 **IAC**
動脈内心電図 **IAE**
動脈内デジタル減算血管造影法 **IADSA**
動脈内の **IA, i.a., i arter.**
動脈内分圧 **Pa**
動脈内リエントリー性頻拍 **IART**
動脈(性)の **a., ART, Art, art.**
動脈ピーエイチ **pHa, PH art**
動脈平滑筋細胞 **ASMC**
動脈閉塞性疾患 **AOD**
動脈弁狭窄兼閉鎖不全 **ASI**
動脈門脈シャント **AP shunt**
動脈瘤 **An, AN**
動脈瘤様骨嚢腫 **ABC**
動揺病感受性 **MSS**
(人工呼吸器の)動力圧 **DP**
登校拒否症 **SP**
登録 **Reg, reg, reg.**
登録看護学生計画 **RSNP**
登録作業療法士 **OTR**
登録された **Reg, reg, reg.**
登録されていない **NL**
登録した **Reg, reg, reg.**
登録商標 **®, RTM**
登録簿 **Reg, reg, reg.**
登録臨床看護教師 **RCNT**
痘瘡形成単位 **PFU**
等圧点 **EPP**
等価温感 **EW**
等価焦点 **EF**
等価線量 **H$_T$**
等価騒音レベル(=Leq) **LAeq**
等価騒音レベル(=LAeq) **Leq**
等価入力雑音レベル **L$_n$**
等差級数 **AP**
等尺性収縮期 **ICP**
等尺性収縮時間 **ITG**
等尺性収縮張力 **IST**
等時性の **isochr**
等速(度)電気泳動 **ITP**
等電点 **IEP, ip, I.p., pH$_I$, PI**
等電点電気泳動 **IEF**
等濃度トレーサー **IDT**

と

等比級数 **GP**
等比重液 **IBS**
等分に **pt.aequ.**
等方向性の **iso, isot**
等方帯 **I band, I disk**
等容圧流量 **IVPF**
等容拡張時間 **IRT**
等容収縮期 **iCT, ICT**
等容性弛緩 **Ir**
等容性収縮 **IC**
等量 **p.ae., p.aeq.**
等量減張期 **IVRT**
等量に分割せよ **D.in P.aeq.**
統一原子質量単位 **u**
統一臓器提供運動 **UAGA**
統計(学) **stat, statist, stats**
統計学的に有意な **SS**
統計学的分析システム **SAS**
統計学的有意差なし **NSS**
統計的相関係数 **r**
統計的品質管理 **SQC**
統計的品質管理手技 **SQCP**
統計データ分析プログラム **SDA**
統計(学)の **statist**
統合型の医学用語システム **UMLS**
統合失調症 **S, Sc, Sch, schiz, SZ, Sz**
統合失調症家族歴 **SFH**
統合失調症残存状態 **SRS**
統合失調症スペクトル **SS**
統合生命維持システム **ILSS**
道路交通災害 **RTA**
銅 **Cu**
導出する **Del, del.**
導入 **I**
糖 **sug**
糖衣錠 **SCT**
糖衣の **sc**
糖化アルブミン **GA**
糖原病 **GSD**
糖剤 **conf.**
糖鎖抗原 15-3 **CA15-3**
糖鎖抗原 19-9 **CA19-9**
糖鎖抗原 50 **CA50**
糖鎖抗原 125 **CA125**
糖鎖抗原腫瘍マーカー **NCC-ST439**
糖漬菓 **conf.**
糖質 **C, CARB, carb, carbo, CHO, COH, KH**
糖質コルチコイド受容体 **GCR**
糖質コルチコイド併用糖負荷テスト **GGTT**
糖質コルチコイドレセプター **GR**
糖質スフィンゴ脂質 **GSLs**
糖蛋白 **GP, THP**
糖蛋白質糖鎖不全症候群 **CDGS**
糖とアセトン **S & A, S/A**
糖尿病性腎症 **DN**
糖尿病性腎臓病 **DKD**
糖尿病 **Db, Dia, diab, DM, dm.**
糖尿病管理 **DBM**
糖尿病管理合併症試験 **DCCT**
糖尿病傾向 **DP**
糖尿病係数 **ID**
糖尿病(性)ケトアシドーシス **DK, DMKA**
糖尿病(性)糸球体硬化(症) **DGS**
糖尿病(性)神経障害〔ニューロパシー〕 **DN**
糖尿病性筋萎縮症 **DA**
糖尿病性ケトアシドーシス **DKA**
糖尿病性ニューロパシー **DAN**
糖尿病性網膜症 **Ret.diab.**
糖尿病性リポイド類壊死(症) **NLD**
糖尿病性類脂肪性壊死 **NLD**
糖尿病に伴うペプチド **DAP**
糖尿病(性)の **diab**
糖尿病の **DB**
糖尿病の親をもつ子供 **ODP**
糖尿病の家族歴 **FHD**
糖尿病の母 **DM**
糖尿病の母の胎児 **FDM**
糖尿病母体の出生児 **IDM**
糖尿病(性)網膜症 **DR**
糖非生成/糖生成比 **NGGR**
糖蜜 **syr**
糖リポ蛋白 **GLP**
糖・アセトン・重酢酸試験 **SAD test**
頭(部) **he, he.**
頭位 **KL**
頭位眼振 **posit.ny**
頭位変換眼球反射 **OCR**
頭位変換眼振 **PN**
頭囲 **HC, HG, KU**
頭蓋 **Cr, cr**
頭蓋 CT 検査 **CCT**
頭蓋咽頭腫 **CRP**
頭蓋外・頭蓋内 **EC-IC**
頭蓋外・内動脈バイパス **EIAB**
頭蓋外動脈疾患 **EAD**
頭蓋外の **EC**
頭蓋下顎顔面の **CMF**
頭蓋学 **craniol**

頭蓋計測法　craniom
頭蓋経皮電気刺激法　TCES
頭蓋最大横径　BPD
頭蓋脊椎の　CrSp
頭蓋頂　VTX, vtx, Vx, vx
頭蓋頂鋭波　V
頭蓋内・(頭蓋)外バイパス術　EC-IC bypass
頭蓋内圧　ICP
頭蓋内圧カテーテル　ICPC
頭蓋内圧亢進　ICH, IICP
頭蓋内圧測定装置　ICP
頭蓋内陥入　BI
頭蓋内血腫　IH
頭蓋内刺激　ICS
頭蓋内自己刺激　ICSS
頭蓋内出血　ICB, ICH
頭蓋内腫瘍　iCT, ICT
頭蓋内増強　ICR
頭蓋内動脈瘤　ICA
頭蓋内内頸動脈　IICA
頭蓋内の　IC
頭蓋の　cran
頭蓋癆(=ろう)　CT
頭頸部　H and N
頭頸部運動　H & N mot.
頭(部)頸部癌(腫)　HNC
頭頸部外科　HNS
頭頸部扁平上皮癌　SCCHN
頭長筋　LC
頭(蓋)頂　V, v
頭頂　VTX, vtx, Vx, vx
頭頂間溝　IPS
頭頂・後頭の　PO
頭頂・殿部(長)　CR
頭(蓋)頂一過性鋭波　V wave
頭頂踵間距離　CH
頭頂の　pari
頭頂部緩反応　SVR
頭頂部の　P
頭低位　HD
頭殿長　CRL
頭(部)と頸(部)　H & N
頭(部)の　ceph
頭皮静脈　SV
頭皮脳波　scalp EEG, SEEG
頭部・頸部・骨幹部　HNS
頭部・腹部(比)　H/A
頭部圧迫　HC
頭部外傷　HI
頭部外傷後遺症　PTB
頭部外傷後症候群　PHIS
頭部外傷症候群　HTS
頭部外傷処理手順　HIR
頭部外傷ユニット　HIU
頭部水平　HF
頭部低下　HD
頭・腕・体幹部　HAT
橈骨　r, rad, rad.
橈骨・尺骨・短指骨　RUS
橈骨血管造影　VAG
橈骨骨膜反射　RPR
橈骨手根骨の　RC
橈骨先端脈　a-r pulse
橈骨側手根屈筋　FCR
橈骨頭亜脱臼　RHS
橈骨動脈カテーテル　RAC
橈骨動脈偽動脈瘤　RAPA
橈骨動脈造影　VAG
橈骨の　rad, rad.
橈側手根屈筋　FCR
橈側の　Ra, rad, rad.
瞳孔　P
瞳孔間距離　IPD, PD
瞳孔対光反射　PLR
瞳孔直径の増加　IPD
瞳孔の正円形と等大　R.R. & E
瞳孔は円形で左右同じ大きさ・対光反射・輻輳反射も正常　PERRLA
瞳孔は等しく光線と調節に反応する　PERLA
瞳孔膜遺残症　PPM
同毒療法の　Homeo
遠い　R, r.
時　Z, Zt
毒　pois
毒(物)　P
毒血症　tox, Tox, tox.
毒蒸気検出器　TVD
毒蒸気減衰器　TVD
毒性　T, tox, Tox, tox.
毒性骨化骨膜炎　POT
毒性の　V, Vi, vir.
毒性物質管理法　TOSCA
毒性容器防止法　PPPA
毒素　tox, Tox, tox.
毒素・抗毒素　TA, T.A., TAT, T.A.T.
毒素・抗毒素反応　TAT reaction
毒素原性大腸菌　ETEC
毒素性ショック毒素　TST
毒素免疫療法　VIT
毒(性)の　tox, Tox, tox.
毒の　ven
毒物学　tox, Tox, tox.
毒物学者　tox, Tox, tox.
毒物情報システム　TOXIN
毒物情報センター　PIC
毒物単位　TU, T.U.
毒物データバンク(の一種)　TDB
毒薬標を貼って　s.s.v.
毒力　V, VI
毒力抗原　Vi antigen
独身の　S, sing.

独身の・結婚した・妻(夫)を失った・離婚した・別居した　**SMWDSep**
独立血液疾患症候群　**IHS**
独立研究所　**IL**
独立検査室　**IL**
独立した　**I, ind, ind.**
独立データ監視委員会　**IDMC**
独立倫理委員会　**IEC**
匿名アルコール中毒者　**ALANON**
匿名断酒会　**AA**
特異性可溶性物質　**SSS**
特異性滲出性円板状苔癬状慢性皮膚炎　**Oid-Oid disease**
特異体質薬剤反応　**IDR**
特異聴力感応抵抗　**x**
特異的　**S**
特異的活性　**SA**
特異的視床投射系　**STPS**
特異的遮断因子　**SBF**
特異的赤血球吸着　**SRCA**
特異的な　**sp, sp., spec, specifi**
特異的内毒素　**ES**
特異的に用意されていない　**NSPF**
特異的反応　**SR**
特異的マクロファージ活性化因子　**SMAF**
特異的マクロファージ武装化因子　**SMAF**
特異的免疫反応増強因子　**SIREF**
特殊ウイルス・白血病計画　**SVLP**
特殊ウイルス癌計画　**SVCP**
特殊X線(検査)　**sp.xr**
特殊学習不適合　**SLD**
特殊顆粒欠損症　**SGD**
特殊感覚　**SS**
特殊感覚器　**SSO**
特殊経管栄養　**STF**
特殊専門能力テスト　**CAT, C-A-T**
特殊装置　**SE**
特殊体性求心性の　**SSA**
特殊投射系　**SPS**
特殊動的作用　**SDA**
特殊内臓遠心性(神経)　**SVE**
特殊内臓求心性(神経)　**SVA**
特殊の　**sp, sp.**
特殊平均に属する　**SPA**
特殊平均を含む　**IPA**
特性指数　**PI**
特徴　**char**
特徴的な　**char**
特定行動目標　**SBOs**
特定食物の嫌悪　**LFA**
特定病原体非依存状態　**SPF**
特典　**priv**
特に　**i.b.**
特発性肺高血圧症　**EPH**
特発骨折　**SF**
特発性CD4 T細胞リンパ球減少症　**ICL**
特発性うっ血性心筋症　**ICCM**
特発性炎症性腸疾患　**IBD**
特発性外反膝　**IGV**
特発性潰瘍性大腸炎　**IUC**
特発性拡張型心筋症　**IDC**
特発性下垂体機能低下症　**IHP**
特発性眼瞼痙攣　**IB**
特発性間質性肺炎　**IIP**
特発性間質性肺線維症　**IIPF**
特発性急性細菌性腹膜炎　**SABP**
特発性急速進行性糸球体腎炎　**idiopathic RPGN, IRPGN**
特発性強直性脊椎炎　**IAS**
特発性起立性低血圧　**IHO**
特発性起立性低血圧(症)　**IOH**
特発性起立性低血圧症候群　**IOHS**
特発性血小板減少性紫斑病　**ITP**
特発性高アルドステロン症　**IHA**
特発性高カルシウム尿症　**IHC, XIH**
特発性好酸球増多症候群　**IHES, IHS**
特発性好中球減少症　**INP**
特発性後天性不応性鉄芽球性貧血　**IARSA**
特発性後天(性)溶血性疾患　**IAHD**
特発性呼吸器疾患　**IRD**
特発性呼吸窮迫症候群　**IRDS**
特発性骨髄線維症　**IM, IMF**
特発性骨髄増殖　**IMP**
特発性細菌性腹膜炎　**IBP, SBP**
特発性再発性膵炎　**IRP**
特発性自己免疫(性)溶血性貧血　**IAHA**
特発性視床下部性性機能低下〔不全〕(症)　**IHH**
特発性周期性浮腫　**ICO**
特発性手根管症候群　**ICTS**
特発性出血性壊死　**SHM, SHN**

特発性食事後症候群 **IPS**
特発性食道潰瘍 **IEU**
特発性心運動亢進症 **IHHS**
特発性心拡大 **ICM**
特発性心筋疾患 **IDM**
特発性心筋症 **ICM, IMP**
特発性心筋肥大 **IMH**
特発性新生児呼吸窮迫障害 **IRDNI**
特発性心(筋)肥大 **ICH**
特発性成長ホルモン欠損症 **IGD**
特発性脊椎硬膜外血腫 **SSEH**
特発性線維化肺胞炎 **IFA**
特発性線維増殖症 **IF**
特発性僧帽弁逸脱症 **IMVP**
特発性側彎症 **IS**
特発性大腿骨頭壊死 **INFH**
特発性中心性漿液性脈絡網膜症 **ICSC**
特発性中心線(部分)破壊病 **IMDD**
特発性長期下痢(症) **IPD**
特発性腸偽閉塞(症) **IIP**
特発性聴力損失 **SHL**
特発性低ゴナドトロピン性性機能低下〔不全〕症 **IHH**
特発性乳児高カルシウム血症 **IIH**
特発性乳腺腫瘍 **SMT**
特発性ネフローゼ症候群 **INS**
特発性捻転ジストニー **ITD**
特発性の **spon, spon., spont**
特発性肺血鉄症 **IDPH**
特発性肺線維症 **IPF**
特発性肺ヘモジデリン沈着症 **IDPH, IPH**
特発性破壊性関節炎 **IDA**
特発性パーキンソン病 **IPD**
特発性皮質性骨化過剰症 **ICH**
特発性微小病変型ネフローゼ症候群 **IMLNS**
特発性微小変化ネフローゼ症候群 **MCINS**
特発性肥大性骨関節症 **IHO**
特発性肥大性大動脈狭窄(症) **IHAS**
特発性肥大性大動脈弁下狭窄症 **IHSS**
特発性不応性鉄芽球性貧血 **IRSA**
特発性副甲状腺機能低下症 **IHP**
特発性副腎過形成 **IAH**
特発性腹膜後線維症 **IRF**
特発性プラズマ細胞リンパ節腫脹 **IPL**
特発性ヘモクロマトーシス **IHC**
特発性無菌壊死 **IAN**
特発性無効赤血球産生 **IIE**
特発性モノクローナル免疫グロブリン異常症 **IMG**
特発性門脈圧亢進症 **IPH**
特発性リンパ節疾患症候群 **ILS**
特発的に起こった **spon, spon.**
特発(性)の **spnt**
特別 **sp**
特別会員 **Fel, fel**
特別ケア病棟 **SCU**
特別研究員 **Fel, fel**
特別サービス **SS**
特別施設 **SF**
特別高い効率 **EHP**
特別注文 **so**
特別治療 **SI**
特別な **espec, partic, spec**
特別の **sp, spl, X**
特変なし **n.B, NB**
特有の心電図波形をみる心室性頻拍の特殊型 **TdP**
特有の名で **n.p.**
読字指数 **RdQ**
読字不能 **URED**
読書学年 **RG**
読書年齢 **RdA**
読書療法 **bibliother**
読書療法士 **bibliother**
読書療法の **bibliother**
読書力試験 **RT**
床ずれ **decub., P/sore**
年 **A**
年上の **SR, Sr**
年下の **jr**
年をとった **O**
凸(形)の **CX, Cx, cx.**
凸面の **CX, Cx, cx.**
突起 **Proc, proc, Procc, prom**
突出 **PRO, proj**
突出した **prom**
突出する **proj**
突然冠(状)動脈死 **SCD**
突然死 **SD**
突然死虚血性心疾患 **SDIHD**
突然死症候群 **SDS**
突然死心疾患 **SDHD**
突然心臓死 **SCD**
突然変異(発生)率 **MF**
突発性自己免疫性甲状腺炎 **SAT**

突発性(薬剤)中止下痢(症)
PWD
突発性難聴　**SD**
特記すべきことなし　**NC**
特記すべき疾患なし
NAD
特許　**pat, pat.**
特許医薬品　**pat.med**

特許権補助証明書　**SPC**
乏しい　**po'**
伴わない　**Ō**
取扱いが難しい菌群
GDO
取消　**canc**
取込み点　**Ep**
貪食能をもつ上皮　**FAE**
鈍縁枝　**OM**
頓服　**1 sum.**
頓服水剤をつくれ　**fh., ft.haust.**
頓用　**1 sum.**

な

ナイスタチン　**NYS**
ナイセリア(属)　**N**
ナイトホスピタル　**Ni.Hos**
ナイトロジェンマスタード-*N*-オキシド　**NMO**
ナイハン・レッシュ(症候群)　**NL**
ナイフとフォーク　**knork**
ナイロビヒツジ病　**NSD**
ナイロン繊維　**NF**
ナキガオオマキザル　**CNI**
ナグビブリオ　**NAG vibrios**
ナーシングホーム　**NH**
ナーシングホームケア　**NHC**
ナースステーション　**NS**
ナースプラクティショナー　**NP**
ナチュラルキラー(細胞)　**NK**
ナチュラルキラーT細胞　**NKT**
ナチュラルキラー細胞　**NK cell**
ナチュラルキラー標的構造　**NKTS**
ナックル・ベンダー(副子)　**KB**
ナトリウム　**Na, Natr, sod**
ナトリウム・リチウム対移送　**SLC**
ナトリウム-L-アスコルビン酸　**SA**
ナトリウムカリウム活性化アデノシン三リン酸　**NaK ATPase**
ナトリウム制限食　**SRD**
ナトリウム排泄因子　**SEF**
ナトリウム排泄増加ホルモン　**NH**
ナトリウム分画排泄率　**FENa**
ナトリウム平衡　**SB**
ナトリウム利尿ペプチド　**NP**
ナトリウム利尿ホルモン　**NaH**
ナノ($=10^{-9}$)　**n**
ナノキュリー　**nC, nCi**
ナノグラム　**m**γ
ナノグラム($=10^{-9}$g)　**ng**
ナノグラム/ミリリットル　**ng/ml**
ナノ単位　**nU**
ナノ秒　**ns, nsec**
ナノファラド　**nF**
ナノメートル　**nm**
ナノモル　**nmol**
ナノモル(の)　**nM**
ナノリットル　**nl**
ナフォキシジン　**NAF**
ナフシリン　**NAF, NF, NFPC**
ナフタリン・クレオソート・ヨードホルム末　**NCI powder**
ナフタレンジイソシアネイト　**NDI**
ナフチル　**NAPH**
ナフトール　**naph**
ナリジクス酸　**NA, ND**
ナリジクス酸セトリミド寒天　**NAC**
ナルトレキソン　**NTX**
ナロキソン　**NLX, Nx**
なし　**N**
などなど　**usf**
なまけもの白血球症候群　**LLS**
なめ薬　**elect.**
名古屋運動失調性マウス　**RMN**
名前で個別されない　**NOIBN**
名前で索引されない　**NOIBN**
名前の明らかな　**ony**
名前不明　**FNU**
投げ出されない　**NTO**
無い　**abs**
内(因性)因子　**IF**
内因子抗体　**IFA**
内因性オピオイド系　**EOS**
内因性急死　**SUD**
内因性交感神経刺激作用　**ISA**
内因性ジギタリス様物質　**EDLF**
内因性の　**E**
内因性発熱物質　**EP**
内因性辺縁系電位　**ELP**
内因性モルヒネ様ペプチド　**EOP**
内エナメル上皮　**IEE**
内外側　**ML**
内外側斜位　**MLO**
内果　**MM, mm**
内科(学)　**I, IM, Int.Med.**
内科・外科会員　**FFPS**
内科・外科事務局　**BuM & S**
内科・外科主任　**Ch Bu Med**
内科医　**I, INT, Int**
内科医助手　**PA**
内科医と外科医　**P & S**
内科および外科有資格者　**L.M.S.**
内科学　**M, MED, Med, med.**
内科学・外科学事務局　**BMS**
内科学士　**M.Int.Med.**
内科学と外科学

Med Surg
内科学博士 D.M.
内科グループ IMG
内科研究学会 SPR
内科と外科 M & S
内科認定書
D.Phs.Med.
内科レジデント入院記録
MRAN
内顆 IM
内胸動脈 ITA
内筋麻痺 IP
内境界膜 ILM
内血液・脳関門 IBBB
内径 ID, IW
内原形質 E
内頸(静脈) IJ, I-J
内頸静脈 IJV
内頸静脈圧 IJP
内頸動脈 IC, ICA
内頸動脈・後交通動脈分岐部 ICPC
内頸動脈後交通動脈(瘤)
ICPC
内頸動脈速度 VICA
内頸動脈閉塞(症) ICAO
内頸動脈流 ICAF
内肛門括約筋 IAS
内固定 IF
内骨折面 IFF
内左 IL
内在性脳内鎮痛系
EBAS
内細胞塊 ICM
内耳 IE
内耳炎 OI
内耳道 IAC, IAM
内耳の IA
(左(心)室)内周短縮速度
VCF
内視鏡下胆嚢切除(術)
IC
内視鏡下副鼻腔手術
FES
内視鏡機械的砕石バスケット鉗子 EML
内視鏡的機械的結石破砕術
EML
内視鏡的逆行性括約筋切断
ERS
内視鏡的逆行性膵管カニュレーション ERCP
内視鏡的逆行性膵管造影
ERP
内視鏡的逆行性大腸挿入法
ERBIM
内視鏡的逆行性胆道膵管造影法 ERCP
内視鏡的逆行性胆道造影法
ERC
内視鏡的逆行性胆道ドレナージ ERBD
内視鏡的逆行性胆嚢造影
ERCC
内視鏡的逆行性胆嚢胆管ドレナージ ERGBD
内視鏡的逆行性内胆道ドレナージ ERIBD
内視鏡的経鼻的胆道ドレナージ ENBD
内視鏡的硬化塞栓療法
EIS
内視鏡的(食道静脈瘤)硬化療法 Sclero
内視鏡的硬化療法 EIS
内視鏡的食道静脈瘤結紮術
EVL
内視鏡的食道静脈瘤硬化術
ES
内視鏡的膵管口切開術
EPST
内視鏡的膵管胆管造影法
EPCG
内視鏡的膵生検 EPB
内視鏡的切除術 ER
内視鏡的胆管ドレナージ
ENBD
内視鏡的胆汁ドレナージ
EBD
内視鏡的超短波凝固治療
EMCT
内視鏡的乳頭括約筋切開術
EPT, ES, EST
内視鏡的乳頭切開術
ES, EST
内視鏡的粘膜切除術
EMR
内視鏡的分割的粘膜切除術
EPMR
内視鏡的リンパ管造影法
ELG
内斜位 E, EP, ES
内斜視 ET, ST
内前頭骨過形成 HFI
内旋 IR
内側踵くさび IHW
内側基底視床下部 MBH
内側基底視床下部の
MBH
内側脛骨症候群 MTS
内側脛骨ストレス症候群
MTSS
内側視床 MT
内側視床下部 MH
内側膝状体 MGB
内側膝状体(核) MGN
内側縦束 FLM, MLF
内側縦束症候群 MLFS
内側前脳束 MFB
内側層間核 MIN
内側足底 MP
内側側副靱帯 TCL,
TLC
内側側副靱帯 MCL
内側中隔核 MSN
内側二対体前部 MPO
内側の M, med, med.
内側の長さ IL
内側半月 med.men
内側半月(板)切除(術)
med.men
内側腓腹(筋) MG
内側腹側 VM
内側毛帯 LM, ML
内側翼状突起 MPP

(視床下部)内側隆起 **ME**
内層 **IL**
内蔵の **SPL**
内臓核 **VN**
内臓血流量 **SBF**
内臓転位 **SI**
内臓動脈閉塞 **SAO**
内臓の **visc**
内臓幼虫移行症 **LMV, VLM**
内臓リーシュマニア症 **VL**
内大脳静脈 **ICV**
内直筋 **MR**
内腸骨動脈 **IIA**
内転 **add, ADD**
内転筋 **add.**
内転する **add.**
内転足 **TV**
内転中足(症) **MTA**
内毒素単位 **EU**
内尿道口 **IUM**
内乳(房)動脈 **IMA**
内乳(房)動脈移植 **IMAG, IMAI**
内乳(房)動脈移植片 **IMG**
内乳(房)動脈バイパス(術) **IMAB**
内乳房リンパシンチグラフィ **IML**
内乳房リンパ節 **IMN**
内(の) **int, int.**
内の **int, int.**
内反股 **CV**
内反足 **TEV**
内反中足(症) **MTV**
内反捻転骨切り術 **VRO**
内反ポリープ状直腸過誤腫 **IPHR**
内背側の **MD**
内皮下間隙 **ss**
内皮下腔 **SES**
内皮下の **SE**
内皮型 NOS **eNOS**
内皮型一酸化窒素合成酵素 **eNOS**
内皮細胞 **EC**
内皮細胞増殖因子 **AFGF, ECGF**
(角膜)内皮性・(角膜)上皮性ジストロフィ **EECD**
内皮増殖因子 **EPF**
(血管)内皮肉腫 **VABES**
内皮の **En**
内皮由来一酸化窒素 **EDNO**
内分泌学 **endo, endocrin, Endocrin, endocrin.**
内分泌学者 **endocrin**
内分泌学の **endocrin**
内分泌学会 **Endoc Soc, ES**
内分泌・代謝 **E & M**
内分泌学 **endocr**
内分泌代謝の **E & M**
内分泌の **endo, endocr**
内部 **int, int., intest**
内部(の) **int, int.**
内部エネルギー **E**
内部吸収量 **IAD**
内部径 **ID**
内部精度管理 **IQC**
内部弾性線維 **IE**
内部弾性板 **IEL**
内部抵抗 **Ir**
内部の **W/I**
内閉鎖筋 **OI**
内方プリズム基底 **BI**
(脳の)内包 **CAI**
内包 **IC**
内膜・中膜の壁厚 **IMT**
内面逆相 **ISRP**
内用 **ad us.int., us.int.**
内容 **cont, cont., contag, contg**
内容(物) **C**
内容物 **cont, cont.**
内容〔薬名〕を明記せよ **d.s.n.**
内・外科学の **MC**
中 1/3 **m/3, M/3**
長い **l, Lg, lg., long.**
長い管 **LT**
長さ **dim, dim., l, L**
長さ・幅・高さ **LBH**
長さ/直径比 **L/D ratio**
謎解きテスト **DST**
謎の熱 **QF**
夏時間 **DST**
斜めの **diag, diag., OBL, obl**
何もされない **ND**
生ワクチン **LV**
鉛 **Pb, Pb.**
鉛中毒 **PBI**
鉛・ジルコニウム・チタン **LZT**
涙の **lacr**
涙・耳介・歯・指(症候群) **LADD**
滑らかな粉末 **pulv.subtil.**
何回も手術を受けた腰 **MOP**
何の疾患も見つからず **NDF**
南方振動指数 **SOI**
軟カプセル **cap.moll.**
軟鶏眼 **HM**
軟口蓋 **SP**
軟口蓋咽頭形成術 **UPPP**
軟骨 **C, cart, Cc**
軟骨外胚葉性形成異常〔異形成〕 **CED**
軟骨基質不全 **CMD**
軟骨結合 **Syn**
軟骨石灰化(症) **CC**
軟骨軟化(症) **CM**

な

軟骨肉腫　**ch s**
軟骨粘液線維腫　**CMF**
軟骨誘導因子　**CIF**
軟骨由来増殖因子　**CDGF**
軟膏　**oint, Ug., UNG, ung., ungt.**
軟膏をつくれ　**ft.ung.**
軟膠嚢　**cap gel el.**
軟性 S 状結腸鏡　**FS**
軟性弾性被膜　**SEC**
軟性の　**moll.**
軟性ビデオ腹腔鏡　**FVL**
軟部腫瘍　**SPT**
軟部組織弛緩　**STR**
軟部組織石灰化　**STC**
軟便　**SF**
軟 X 線域　**SXR**
軟(性)2 孔式〔二重式〕カテーテル　**FDLC**
難産指数　**DI**
難治性アトピー性皮膚炎　**IAD**
難治性足底角化症　**IPK**
難治性鉄芽球性貧血　**RSA**
難聴　**HH, h/h, HOH**
難聴児全国協会　**NDCS**
難聴者全国連合　**NAD**
難聴者のためのアレキサンダーグラハムベル協会　**AGBAD**
難聴者のための米国無力協会　**AAAD**
難聴中央研究所　**CID**

に

ニアミス突然乳児死亡症候群　**NMSIDS**
ニオブ　**Nb**
ニコチニル　**Nic**
ニコチン　**N**
ニコチンアミド　**N**
ニコチンアミドアデニンジヌクレオチダーゼ　**NADase**
ニコチンアミドアデニンジヌクレオチド　**NAD, NADH**
ニコチンアミドアデニンジヌクレオチドリン酸　**NADP**
ニコチンアミドヌクレオチド脱水素酵素〔デヒドロゲナーゼ〕　**NND**
ニコチンアミドモノヌクレオチド　**NMN**
ニコチン酸　**NiA, NICA**
ニコチン酸アミド　**NAA**
ニコチン酸脱水素酵素　**NAD**
ニコチン酸デヒドロゲナーゼ　**NAD**
ニコチン酸モノヌクレオチド　**NAMN**
ニコチン刺激性ニューロフィジン　**NSN**
ニコチン性アセチルコリン受容体　**nAChR**
ニコチン置換療法　**NRT**
ニコラ・デュラン・ファーブル(病)　**NDF**
ニコル・ノーヴィ・マックニール(培地)　**NNM**
ニッケル　**Ni**
ニッシェ　**N**
ニッスル小体　**NS**
ニット　**nt**
ニットダクロン　**KD**
ニッポストロンジルスブラジリエンシス(=ブラジル鉤虫)　**Nb**
ニト　**nt**
ニトラゼパム　**NZP**
ニトリロ三酢酸　**NTA**
ニトロアルギニンメチルエステル　**NAME**
ニトログリセリン　**NG, nitro, NTG**
ニトログリセリン軟膏　**NGO, NTGO**
ニトロゲンマスタード-*N*-オキサイド　**NH_2N-Ox**
ニトロゲンマスタード　**mustrgen, NH_2, NM**
ニトロゲンマスタード(=メクロルエタミン)　**HN2, HN_2**
ニトロゲンマスタード,アドリアマイシン,シクロヘキシルクロロエチルニトロソ尿素　**NAC**
ニトロセルロース　**NC, nitro**
ニトロセルロースフィルター　**NF**
ニトロセルロース膜　**NCM**
ニトロソグアニジン　**NG**
ニトロソジエチルアミン　**NDEA**
ニトロソジメチルアニリン　**NDMA**
ニトロテトラゾリウムブルー(染色)　**NTB**
ニトロバクター(属)　**N**
ニトロフェニルスルフェニル　**Nps**
ニトロフラゾン　**NF**
ニトロフラントイン　**NF**
ニトロプルシッド　**SNP**
ニトロプルシド　**NP, NTP**
ニトロブルーテトラゾリウム(試験)　**NBT**
ニトロブルーテトラゾリウム色素　**NTD**
ニトロブルーテトラゾリウム試験　**NBT T, NBT test**
ニトロン　**Nt**
ニバリン　**NV**
ニフェジピン　**NIF**
ニホニウム　**Nh**
ニーマン・ピック(病)　**NP**
ニーマン・ピック病　**NPD**
ニムスチン　**ACNU**
ニューイングランド医学雑誌　**NEJM**
ニューカッスルウイルス病　**NVD**
ニューカッスル病　**ND**
ニューカッスル病ウイルス　**NDV**
ニューカッスル病ウイルスの亢進　**END**
ニュージーランド黒色(マウス)　**NZB**
ニュージーランド白色(マウス)　**NZW**
ニュートリノ　*ν*
ニュートロン放射化分析　**NAA**
ニュートン　**N**
ニュートンメートル　**Nm**
ニューモシスチス・カリニ肺炎　**PCP**
ニューヨーク医学会　**NYAM**
ニューヨーク血液センター　**NYBC**
ニューヨーク心臓協会　**NYHA**
ニューヨーク大学医学セン

ター **NYUMC**
ニューヨーク病院・コーネル医学センター **NYH-CMC**
ニューロキニンA **NKA**
ニューロテンシン **NT**
ニューロパシー **N**
ニューロパシー関連蛋白 **NAP**
ニューロフィジン **NP**
ニューロペプチドY **NPY**
ニューロメジン **NM**
ニール・ムーサー反応 **NMR**
ニワトリ赤血球 **CE, CRBC**
ニワトリ胎起源 **CEO**
ニワトリ胎致死孤児ウイルス **CELO**
ニワトリ肉腫ウイルス **ASV**
ニワトリ胚線維芽細胞 **CEF**
ニワトリ卵白リゾチーム **HEL**
ニワトリリンパ肉腫ウイルス **ALSV**
ニンジンサポニン **GS**
に属する **pert**
二塩化ジアミンシスプラチン **CPDD**
二塩基リン酸ナトリウム **DSP**
二塩酸トリエチレンテトラミン **TETA**
二期の **PSI**
二孔式カテーテル **DLC**
二抗体固相法 **DASP**
二酢酸エチノジオール **EDDA**
二酸化硫黄 **SO_2**
二酸化炭素 **CD, CO_2**
二酸化炭素結合(力) **CO_2 comb**
二酸化炭素結合力テスト **CPT**
二酸化炭素ナルコーシス **CO_2 narcosis**
二酸化炭素排出量 **V_{CO_2}**
二酸化炭素〔炭酸ガス〕分圧 **PCO_2, P_{CO_2}**
二酸化炭素療法 **CO_2T**
二次悪性新生物 **SMN**
二次イオン質量分析法 **SIMS**
二次外傷救命処置 **ATLS**
二次ガス効果 **SGE**
二次救命処置 **ALS**
二次元エコー図 **2DE, 2-DE**
二次元エコー図法 **2DE, 2-DE**
二次交叉〔差〕免疫電気泳動法 **CIE**
二次手術 **SLO**
二次循環救命処置 **ACLS**
二次小児救命処置 **PALS**
二次心臓救命処置 **ACLS**
二次性(続発性)骨髄異形成症候群 **SMDS**
二次性〔続発性〕シェーグレン症候群 **SSS**
二次性上皮小体機能亢進(症) **SHP**
二次性全般てんかん **SGE**
二次性の **sec, sec.**
二次性肥大性骨関節症 **SHO**
二次体性感覚野 **S II**
二次中性粒子質量分析法 **SNMS**
二次的の **sec, sec.**
二次的無効 **SF**
二次の **PSI**
二次発作 **SA**
二次リソソーム **SL**
二次療法 **SC**
二色グアヤック試験 **BCG test**
二重エネルギーX線吸収測定法 **DER, DRA**
二重エネルギーX線吸収法 **DEXA**
二重エネルギーX線骨塩量測定装置 **DXA**
二重凹面 **DCC**
二重管気管内チューブ **DLET**
二重結合 **δ**
二重光子吸収法 **DPA**
二重鎖(=DNA) **DS, ds**
二重鎖DNA〔デオキシリボ核酸〕 **dsDNA**
二重鎖リボ核酸 **dsRNA**
二重振動 **dv**
二重凸面 **DCx**
二重の **D, dbl, gem-**
二重の動静脈瘻 **d-AVF**
二重標識アイソトープ〔同位元素〕誘導体法 **DID**
二重膜 **DM**
二重膜濾過法 **DF**
二重免疫拡散 **DID**
二重免疫拡散法 **IDDT**
二重盲(検) **DBn**
二重盲検比較試験 **DB-CT**
二重盲検法 **DBT**
二重モード・二腔ペーシング・二腔センシング(ペースメーカー) **DDD**
二重濾過血漿交換法 **DFPE**
二重濾過血漿分離交換法 **DFPP**
二相性気道内陽圧 **BIPAP**

二相性喘息反応　**DAR**
二相性陽圧呼吸　**BIPAP**
二段脈　**bid., b.I.d., bigem.**
二段ロケット免疫電気泳動法　**DDRIE**
二点同時刺激　**DSS**
二動原体染色体　**dic**
二頭筋腱反射　**BTR**
二頭筋反射　**BJ**
二頭(筋)の　**Bi, bic**
二ナトリウム化合物　**disod**
二倍強力　**DS**
二分脊椎　**SB**
二腹の　**digas**
二弁置換　**DVR**
二本鎖の　**DS**
二葉円板弁　**SJM**
二卵性(双胎)　**DZ**
二卵(性)双生児　**ZZ**
二リン酸塩　**DP**
二硫化チアミンプロピル　**TPD**
二硫化テトラエチルジザルフィド　**TETD**
二硫化テトラエチルチウラム　**TTD**
二硫化テトラメチルチウラム　**TMTD**
二連脈　**bigem.**
日本 DNA データバンク　**DDBJ**
日本医学会　**JAMS, JMA**
日本医学放射線学会　**JRS**
日本医薬監視研究所　**JIP**
日本医薬情報センター　**JAPIC**
日本医薬品一般名称　**JAN**
日本医用器械工業会　**JAMEI**
日本医療情報学会　**JAMI**
日本インターネット医療協会　**JIMA**
日本エイコサ・ペンタエン酸検証研究　**JELIS**
日本海外健康管理センター　**JOHAC**
日本外傷学会　**JAST**
日本解剖学用語　**NAJ**
日本科学技術情報センター　**JICST**
日本科学技術情報センターオンライン文献検索システム　**JOIS**
日本化学プログラム交換機関　**JCPE**
日本画像医療システム工業会, ジラ　**JIRA**
日本学術会議　**JSC**
日本癌研究資源バンク　**JCRB**
日本看護協会　**JNA**
日本キリスト教海外医療協力会　**JOCS**
日本血液検査器械検定協会規格　**JHS**
日本血球凝集ウイルス　**HVJ**
日本工業規格　**JIS**
日本鉱物科学会　**JAMS**
日本国際医療技術交流財団　**JIMTEF**
日本国際協力事業団　**JICA**
日本昏睡スケール　**JCS**
日本災害・産業医学会雑誌　**JJTOM**
日本財団法人海外邦人医療基金　**JOMF**
日本産業安全協会　**JISA**
日本産業衛生学会　**JAIH**
日本集中治療医学会　**JSICM**
日本消化器病週間　**JDDW**
日本食品添加物協会　**JFAA**
日本人動脈硬化指数　**AIJ**
日本人に適応されるコレステロール指数　**CIJ**
日本人皮膚型　**JST**
日本整形外科学会　**JOA**
日本製薬工業協会　**JPMA**
日本赤十字社　**JRC**
日本セックスカウンセラー・セラピスト協会(現,日本性科学学会)　**JASCT**
日本特別チーム　**JST**
日本人間工学会　**JEA**
日本脳炎　**B-encephalitis, JE**
日本脳炎ウイルス　**JEV**
日本脳卒中スケール　**JSS**
日本脳卒中データバンク　**JSD**
日本脳卒中協会データバンク部門　**JSSRS**
日本農林規格　**JAS**
日本版前選別発達質問　**JPDQ**
日本版デンバー式発達スクリーニング検査　**JDDST**
日本版ミラー幼児発達スクリーニング検査　**JMAP**
日本版レーヴン色彩マトリックス(検査)　**JRCPM**
日本標準商品分類　**JSCC**
日本ボランティアセンター　**JVC**
日本麻酔学会　**JSA**
日本薬局方　**JP**
日本輸液栄養雑誌　**JJPEN**
日本ラジオアイソトープ協

会　JRIA
日本臨床化学会　JSCC
日本臨床検査標準委員会
JCCLS
日本臨床病理学会　JSCP
日本老人高血圧治療効果試験　JATA
匂い　O
肉眼視　Nv, NV
肉眼的外膜癌浸潤程度
A0-3
肉眼的癌肛門側断端
AW
肉眼的癌リンパ節転移有無程度　N(+)0-4,
N(−)0-4
肉眼的癌リンパ節転移の程度　N(+)0-4,
N(−)0-4
肉眼的剝離面癌露出　EW
肉眼(的)の　macro
肉芽腫性過敏反応　GHR
肉芽腫性大腸炎　GC
肉芽腫性腸疾患　GBD
肉芽組織　g/t
肉汁　juscul.
肉腫　SA, sarc
肉腫ウイルス　SV
肉腫成長因子　SGF
肉と野菜　MV
肉の入っていない　MF
肉胞子虫(属)　S
濁った　cldy, turb
西(の)　W
西ナイルウイルス　WNV
西ナイル脳炎　WNE
偽の　SP
日常コミュニケーション能力　CADL
日常コミュニケーション能力検査　CADLT
日常生活動作　ADL,
BADL
日常生活動作テスト
ADL-T
日常的膀胱容量　OBC
日常の習慣　DH
日内の　d
日光蕁麻疹　SoU, SU
日光性角化症　SK
日光皮膚炎　SB
日光保護因子　SPF
日差血糖変動幅　MODD
日周期　circad
日周期で　circad
日周期の　circad
日中　i.d.
日直医　MOD, OD
入院　Ad, adm,
adm., Adm., HA,
hosp, HS
入院患者行動評価スケール〔尺度〕IBRS
入院患者用多次元的精神症状評価尺度〔スケール〕
IMPS
入院期間　DHS, HD
入院期日　HOD
入院記録　HR
入院させる　hosp
入院時診断　AD
入院前検査　PAT
入院前評価チーム　PAT
入院と退院　A & D,
A and D
入院と治療　H & T
入院(年月)日　D/A
入院日　DOA
入院前(に)　PTA
入院前に　PTH
入学前行動質問票　PBQ
入射線量　ED
入退院　A & D,
A and D
入眠時レム段階
SOREMP
入浴　B, BAL, bal.,
TB
入浴可　BRP
入力・出力　in-out
入力・出力操作　IOP
入力/出力　I/O, I & O
入力端子1　G1
入力端子2　G2
乳癌　BC, MMK
乳癌化学療法に対するアンケート　BCQ
乳癌抗原　BCA
乳癌刺激物　MTI
乳癌凍結切片　BCFS
乳剤　Emul.
乳剤をつくれ　ft.emuls.
乳酸　LA, lact
乳酸/ピルビン酸(比)
L/P
乳酸アシドーシス　LA
乳酸アシドーシス閾値
LAT
乳酸エステル　lac, lact
乳酸塩　lac, lact
乳酸塩・ピルビン酸塩比
LPR, L/P ratio
乳酸加リンゲル(液)
lat.Rin., LR
乳酸加リンゲル液　LRS
乳酸カルシウム
Ca.lact.
乳酸桿菌(属)　L
乳酸桿菌維持培地
LMM
乳酸血症・卒中発作を伴うミトコンドリア脳筋症
MELAS
乳酸酸化酵素　LOD
乳酸脱水素酵素　LAD,
LADH, LD, LDH
乳酸脱水素酵素ウイルス
LDV
乳酸デヒドロゲナーゼ
LADH, LD
乳酸ナトリウム　SL
乳酸ポリマー　PLA
乳酸リンゲル液　RL
乳汁中の乳酸桿菌ドナー因子　LLD factor

乳汁分泌　**lact, lac**
乳汁分泌・無月経・高プロラクチン血症症候群　**GAHS**
乳児　**B**
乳児遺伝性無顆粒球症　**IGA**
乳児壊死性脳脊髄症　**INE**
乳児核大脳変性(症)　**INCD**
乳児型結節性多発動脈炎　**IPN**
乳児型結節性動脈周囲炎　**IPN**
乳児環状紅斑　**AEI**
乳児行動記録　**IBR**
乳児広汎〔び漫〕性脳硬化症　**IDBS**
乳児死亡　**ID**
乳児死亡率　**IMR**
乳児出血性疾患　**HDI**
乳児水頭症　**IH**
乳児多囊胞腎病　**IPKD**
乳児ネフローゼ(症候群)　**IN**
乳児両側線条体壊死　**IBSN**
乳児レフスム症候群　**IRD**
乳脂肪　**BF**
(牛)乳脂肪球皮膜　**MFGM**
乳腺刺激ホルモン　**LGH, LTH, MTH**
乳腺刺激ホルモン(=プロラクチン)　**MH**
乳腺腫瘍ウイルス　**Mtv, MTV**
乳濁　**emul, emuls.**
乳濁液　**emul, emuls.**
乳(様)突(起)の　**mast**
乳糖　**LTS, s.l.**
乳糖・サッカロース・尿素寒天培地　**LSU**
乳糖吸収不全　**LM**
乳糖負荷試験　**LTT**
乳糖不耐症　**LI**
乳頭　**NIP, p, pap**
乳頭筋　**PM**
(網膜)乳頭径　**DD**
乳頭径　**pd**
乳頭腫ウイルス　**PV**
乳頭上新生血管　**NVD**
乳頭線　**ML**
乳頭腺癌　**pap**
乳頭体　**M, MB**
乳頭体視床路　**MT, TMT**
乳頭の　**Pap**
乳頭様の　**mast**
乳酸デヒドロゲナーゼ　**LAD**
乳び球　**CM**
乳房　**Br**
乳房温存療法　**BCT**
乳房検査　**BE**
乳房撮影(法)　**MAMMO**
乳房自己検査　**BSE**
乳房腫瘍　**BT, MT**
乳房腫瘍因子　**MTA**
乳房生検　**BB, B Bx, br.bx**
乳房切除(術)　**mast**
乳房切除後疼痛症候群　**PMPS**
乳房切断(術)　**mast**
乳房の高さ　**BH**
乳幼児　**INF, inf, inf.**
乳幼児黒内障性家族性精神遅滞　**IAFI**
乳幼児突然死　**SID**
乳幼児突然死症候群　**SIDS**
乳幼児の　**INF, inf, inf.**
乳幼児発達スケール　**KIDS**
尿　**H, Ha, Hr, UR, Ur, ur**
尿(の)　**U**
尿アルカリホスファターゼ　**UAP**
尿(中)アルドステロン　**UA**
尿(中)ウロビリノゲン　**UU**
尿(中)ウロポルフィリン　**UUP**
尿うっ滞　**UR**
尿遠心分離沈渣の顕微鏡所見　**Mic**
尿(中)カリウム　**UK**
尿(中)カリクレイン　**UKa**
尿(中)カリクレイン　**UK**
尿管　**HL**
尿管口　**UO**
尿管後方圧　**UBP**
尿管骨盤の　**UP**
尿管腎盂の　**UP**
尿管腟瘻　**UV fistula**
尿管内圧検査法　**UMG**
尿管の　**ure**
尿管膀胱移行(結合)部　**UVJ**
尿管膀胱移行(結合)部狭窄　**UVJ-stenosis**
尿管膀胱角　**UVA**
尿管膀胱の　**UV**
尿クレアチニン　**UCRE**
尿検査　**UA, U/A, Ua, ur anal, ur.anal., Ux**
尿検査・通常および顕微鏡法　**UR & M**
尿検査と顕微鏡検査(法)　**UA & M**
尿(中)コプロポルフィリン　**UCP**
尿(中)コプロポルフィリン検査　**UCPT**
尿細管・間質性疾患　**TID**

尿細管間質性腎炎　TIN
尿細管間質性腎障害　TIN
尿細管基底膜　TBM
尿細管再吸収　TR
尿細管最大排泄量　Tm
尿細管最大輸送量　Tm
尿細管糸球体フィードバック　TGF
尿細管水分再吸収　TRW
尿細管排泄率　TRFR
尿細管パラアミノ馬尿酸塩再吸収極量　TmPAH
尿細管ブドウ糖(再吸収能)最大量　Tm, Tm_G, TmG, Tmg
尿細管無機リン再吸収量　TRP
尿細管リン再吸収率　%TRP
尿産生(率)　UPD
尿酸　U, UA, U/A
尿酸/クレアチニン(比)　UA/C
尿酸塩　MSU
尿酸クリアランス　Cua
尿酸窒素　UAN
尿失禁　UI
尿重量オスモル濃度　UOsm
尿(容量)浸透圧　Uosm
尿浸透圧　UOsm
尿(中)絨毛性ゴナドトロピン　UCG
尿水力学検査　UDS
尿生殖隔膜　UGD
尿生殖器萎縮(症)　UGA
(泌)尿生殖器の　UG, uro-gen
尿生殖器の　GU, G-U
尿生殖洞　UGS
尿性器の　UG, uro-gen
尿潜血　UB
尿素　U, u
尿素洗い出し試験　UWT
尿素クリアランス　Cu, Curea, UC
尿素クリアランス(検査)　UCL, U Cl
尿素呼気テスト　UBT
尿素サイクル酵素疾患　UCE
尿素窒素　UN, Urea N
尿蛋白　UP
尿中・血漿中濃度　U/P
尿中17-オキソステロイド　urinary 17-OS
尿中17-ケトステロイド　urinary 17-KS
尿中17-ヒドロキシコルチコステロイド　urinary 17-OHCS
尿中アルブミン排泄量　UAE
尿中グルコース　UG
尿中ゴナドトロピン　UP
尿中ゴナドトロピン分画　UGF
尿中ゴナドトロピンペプチド　UGP
尿中ナトリウム　UNa
尿中ナトリウム濃度　U_{Na}
尿中ナトリウム排泄　FENa
尿中尿素　UU
尿中尿素窒素　UUN
尿中尿素窒素排泄　UUN
(排泄)尿中のブドウ糖と窒素との比　D/Nr
尿中ブドウ糖/窒素(比)　DN, D/N
尿中ブドウ糖濃度　Gu
尿中溶質濃度　UV/P
尿窒素　UN
尿(中)トリプシン抑制〔阻害〕物質　UTI
尿毒症性髄質嚢胞病　UMCD
尿道　U, u, UA, ureth
尿道圧　P ura
尿道および子宮頸の(培養)　U & C
尿道カテーテル　UC
尿道カテーテル挿入　UCI
尿道カテーテル抜去　UCO
尿道カテーテル法　UC
尿道坐薬　Suppos.ureth., supp.ureth.
尿道前立腺部　PU
尿道造影　UG
尿道造影撮影法　UG
尿道操作症候群　UMS
尿道ドレナージ　UD
尿道内圧曲線　UPP
尿道内圧測定　UPP
尿道内カテーテル　IUC
尿道に　pro ureth.
尿道の　ura, ureth
尿道排泄物　UD
尿道閉鎖圧　UCP
尿道閉鎖圧曲線　UCPP
尿道膀胱撮影　UVG
尿道膀胱造影法　UCG
尿糖　HZ, Hz, US
尿妊娠検査　UPT
尿(中)乳酸脱水素酵素　ULDH
尿の　U, UR, Ur, ur
尿濃度　UC
尿排出　UO
尿培養　UC, U/C
尿培養と感受性　UC & S
尿分析　ur anal, ur.anal.
尿部分標本　UA
尿閉症候群　OVS
尿(中)ホルムアルデヒド　UF
尿崩症　DI
尿(中)ムラミダーゼ活性　UMA

尿免疫電気泳動(法)　**UIEP**
尿流曲線　**UFMG**
尿流量(率)　**Q**
尿流量測定　**UFM**
尿量　**UQ, UV**
尿量適量　**U/O adeq**
尿路　**UT**
尿路カテーテル挿入　**UCI**
尿路カテーテル抜去　**UCO**
尿路感染(症)　**UTI**
尿路感染症　**UTIs**
尿路奇形　**UTM**
尿路上皮基底膜　**UBM**
尿路排出　**UO, UOP**
尿路排泄量　**UV**
尿濾過率　**UFR**
尿(中)Cペプチド　**UCP**
尿・血漿比　**U/P**
人気のある　**pop**
人間開発指数　**HDI**
人間工学　**HE**
人間自由度指標　**HFI, hFI**
人間生活の基本的欲求　**BHN**
人間尊重の態度　**PCA**
人間と生物環境計画　**MAB**
人間の　**mort**
人間発達研究所　**IHD**
人・年　**PY**
任意　**arb**
任意単位　**AU**
任意の　**arb**
任意の型　**OF**
任意ポリメラーゼ鎖反応　**AP-PCR**
任意量　**q.l., q.p., q.pl., q.v.**
妊産婦死亡調査委員会　**MMC**
妊産婦・新生児・子どもの健康パートナーシップ　**PMNCH**
妊娠　**GEST, Mat, pg, preg, Sgt, SS**
妊娠1回・出産0回・流産1回　**Gr_1　P_0　AB_1**
妊娠1回・流産1回　**$grav.\dot{T}/Ab.\dot{T}$**
妊娠回数・流産回数・出生児数　**Para**
妊娠関連α糖蛋白　**PAG**
妊娠関連αマクログロブリン　**PAM**
妊娠関連グロブリン　**PAG**
妊娠関連血漿蛋白　**PAPP**
妊娠関連蛋白　**PAP**
妊娠期　**GS**
妊娠血清　**PS**
妊娠高血圧症　**PAH**
妊娠時一過性甲状腺機能亢進症　**GTH**
妊娠した　**Gr, PG, Pg, pg, pg., preg**
妊娠していない　**NPG**
妊娠性急性脂肪肝　**AFLP**
妊娠性絨毛性腫瘍　**GTN**
妊娠性瘙痒性蕁麻疹様丘疹兼局面症　**PUPPP**
妊娠性疱疹因子　**HG factor**
妊娠中絶　**TOP**
妊娠中絶手術　**STOP**
妊娠中絶避妊相談研究協会　**ACCRA**
妊娠中の　**grav.**
妊娠中予後不良徴候　**PBSP**
妊娠糖尿病　**GDM**
妊娠特異(的)β_1糖蛋白質　**SP-1, SP1, SP_1**
妊娠と出産の合併症　**PBC**
妊娠尿　**PU**
妊娠尿中絨毛性ゴナドトロピン　**PU**
妊娠尿ホルモン　**PUH**
妊娠の　**GEST, Gr, PG, Pg, pg, pg.**
妊娠(性)ヘルペス　**HG**
妊娠(性)疱疹　**HG**
妊娠誘発高血圧　**PIH**
妊娠誘発性ブドウ糖不耐(症)　**PIGI**
妊娠率　**PR**
妊馬血清ゴナドトロピン　**PMSG**
妊馬血清性ゴナドトロピン　**PMG**
妊馬血清ホルモン　**PMS**
妊婦　**G, g., gr., Grav, grav., gravid., PW**
妊婦血清　**PS**
妊婦自身の出生時体重　**MBW**
認可された重度視力障害者精神治療士協会　**ABCP**
認可された物理療法　**LPT**
認証標準物質　**CRM**
認識　**recog**
認識(機能試験)　**COG**
認識因子　**RF**
認識行動療法　**CBT**
認知不能(症)　**AGN, agn**
認知領域　**C**
認知療法　**CT**
認定看護師　**CN**
認定記録技士　**ART**
認定された　**C, CERT, Cert, cert, cert.**
認定されていない　**NA**
認定糖尿病教育士　**CDE**

ぬ

ヌクレオカプシド　**NC**
ヌクレオシド　**N，Nuc**
ヌクレオシド 5′-モノホスフェート〔一リン酸〕　**NMP**
ヌクレオシド 5′-ホスフェート（リン酸）　**NDP**
ヌクレオシド三リン酸　**NTP**
ヌクレオシドホスホリラーゼ　**NP**
ぬるま湯浣腸　**TWE**
抜け出された　**TO**

ね

ネオアジュバント化学療法 **NAC**
ネオアルスフェナミン **neo, neoars**
ネオカルチノスタチン **NCS**
ネオジミウム **Nd**
ネオジミウム・イットリウム・アルミニウム・ガーネット **Nd-YAG**
ネオスポリン軟膏 **NSO**
ネオテトラゾリウム(染色) **NT**
ネオトラマイシン **NTM**
ネオプテリン/ビオプテリン(比) **N/B**
ネオマイシン **N, NE, NM**
ネオマイシン卵黄 **NEY**
ネオマイシン卵黄寒天(培地) **NEYA**
ネオン **Ne**
ネカトール(属) **N**
ネグリ(小)体 **NB**
ネコエイズ **FAIDS**
ネコ海綿状脳症 **FSE**
ネコ線維肉腫ウイルス **FSV**
ネコ伝染性腹膜炎ウイルス **FIPV**
ネコ肉腫ウイルス **FeSV**
ネコに腫瘍を発生する細胞膜抗原 **FOCMA**
ネコのウイルス性鼻気管支炎 **FVR**
ネコの目症候群 **CES**
ネコ白血病ウイルス **FeLV, FelV, FLV**
ネコ汎白血球減少症ウイルス **FPV**
ネコひっかき(病) **CS**
ネコひっかき病 **CSD**
ネズミ肝炎 **MH**
ネズミ形質細胞腫 **MPC**
ネズミ後天性免疫不全症候群 **MAIDS**
ネズミサイトメガロウイルス **MCMV**
ネズミ神経芽(細胞)腫 **MNB**
ネズミ赤芽球症ウイルス **MEV**
ネズミ赤白血病 **MEL**
ネズミ赤白血病細胞 **MELC**
ネズミチフス菌 **ST**
ネズミ内因子濃縮物 **RIFC**
ネズミ肉腫ウイルス **MSV**
ネズミ乳腺腫瘍ウイルス **MuMTV**
ネズミノミ(属) **X**
ネズミ(複合)白血病ウイルス **MuLV, MULV**
ネズミ白血病ウイルス **MLV**
ネチルミシン **NTL**
ネットワーク管理センター **NCC**
ネトルシップ伴性眼白子(症) **XOAN**
ネーパー **Np**
ネプツニウム **Np**
ネブラスカウシ下痢ウイルス **NCDV**
ネフローゼ症候群 **NS**
ネム **N**
ネンブタール **Nemb**
ネンブタールカプセル **nemmies**
寝小便 **enur**
(加)熱 **Ht, ht**
熱 **fev**
熱(病) **feb.**
熱安定性の **HS**
熱イオン化検出器 **TID**
熱エネルギー分析器 **TEA**
熱音響測定 **TS**
熱が上昇したときに **ag.feb.**
熱加変性ゼラチン **MFG**
熱希釈法による心拍出量 **COTD**
熱凝固 **HA**
熱凝集グロブリン **HAG**
熱螢光線量計 **TLD**
熱交換器内蔵人工肺 **TDO**
熱殺菌された **HK**
熱殺菌リステリア菌 **HKLM**
熱産生 **HP**
熱ショック蛋白 **HSP**
熱処理血漿分画 **HTPF**
熱死点 **TDP**
熱重量測定 **TG**
熱湿交換器 **HME**
熱傷指数 **BI**
熱傷集中監視室 **BCU**
熱傷深達度指標 **BDI**
熱傷面積 **BSA**
熱傷様口腔(粘膜)症候群 **SMS**
熱傷様皮膚症候群 **SSS**
熱傷予後指数 **PBI**
熱ストレス指数 **HSI**
熱性の **feb.**
熱性痙攣 **FC**
熱接着包装 **HS**
熱単位 **TU**
熱帯医学 **TM, Trop Med**
熱帯医学衛生学認定書 **DTMH**
熱帯医学士 **DTM**
熱帯医学認定書 **DTM**
熱帯環境データ **TREND**
熱帯獣医認定書 **DTVM**
熱帯スプルー **TS**

熱帯性痙性脊髄麻痺　**TSP**
熱帯性好酸球増加症　**THE**
熱帯性脾腫症候群　**TSS**
熱帯熱原虫　**PV**
熱帯熱マラリア原虫　**PF**
熱帯の　**t, trop**
熱帯肺好酸球症　**TPE**
熱帯病研究と訓練特別計画　**TDR**
熱帯病(のための)病院　**HTD**
熱治療技士　**FTT**
熱伝達の係数　**K**
熱伝導性　**TC**
熱伝導性検出器　**TCD**
熱湯　**aq.bul., aq.bull., aq.ferv.**
熱の　**therm**
熱のある　**fev**
熱板試験　**HPT**
熱病　**fev**
熱病の　**fev**
熱不安定因子　**HLF**
熱不安定腸毒素　**LT**
熱不安定の　**TL**
熱不活化ウシ胎仔血清　**HIFBS, HIFCS**
熱不活化された　**HI**
熱不活性化点　**TIP**
熱不耐性　**HL**
熱放出緩和姿勢　**HELP**
熱容量　**C**
熱力関数　**S**
熱量管理システム　**CCS**
熱ルミネッセンス　**TL**
熱レーザー角膜形成　**TLK**
熱レンズ分光法　**TL**
熱〔温湿布〕・超音波・マッサージ　**HUM**
熱・(患部)不使用・発赤・疼痛・膿・腫脹(などの感染症状)　**HARPPS**

年　**Y, yr, yrs**
年月日　**D, d**
年鑑　**yearb, yrb**
年金　**pens**
年ごとに　**PA, p.a.**
年摂取限度　**ALI**
年代　**A**
年に　**p.a.**
年百分率　**apr**
年報　**Ann, ann, Annls, AR, Jahrb, Jber**
年齢　**A, aet., Lj, YO, Y/O, y/o**
年齢〜歳　**Y/A**
年齢相応の　**p.rat.aetat.**
年齢相当の　**aeq**
年齢に応じた　**ae.**
年齢に応じて　**aet., p.rat.aetat., pro rat.aet.**
年4回の　**qr, quart**
捻挫　**spr**
捻出因子　**FF, F factor**
捻転ジストニー　**TD**
捻髪音　**crep, crep.**
捻髪音の　**crep, crep.**
(類)粘液(状の)　**muc**
粘(膜)液　**MF**
粘液　**M, muc**
粘液・均一性・粗糙変異　**MSRM**
粘液顆粒　**MG**
粘液刺激物質　**MSS**
粘液腫　**MYX**
粘液水腫の　**My**
粘液性腺癌　**muc**
粘液糖蛋白　**MGP**
粘液(性)の　**muc**
粘液膿性子宮頸(管)炎　**MPC**
粘液(化)膿(性)の　**muco-pur**
粘液流量率　**MFR**
粘滑薬　**MUC**

粘性　**h, visc**
粘性蛋白質分解酵素　**MPS**
粘着　**adh, adhes**
粘着性　**h, visc**
粘着性の　**adh, adhes, visc**
粘稠度　**h, v**
粘(稠)度　**visc**
粘(稠)度指数　**VI**
粘膜　**M, MM**
粘膜下　**sm, SM**
粘膜外十二指腸筋切開術　**EDN**
粘膜下口蓋裂　**SCP**
粘膜下腫瘍　**SMT**
粘膜下切除術　**SMR**
粘膜下の　**SM**
粘膜関連リンパ組織　**MALT**
粘膜機能検査　**MFT**
粘膜筋板(まで)　**mm**
粘膜系リンパ組織　**MALT**
粘膜上皮内　**ep**
粘膜性潰瘍性大腸炎　**MUC**
粘膜層癌　**mca**
粘膜内　**m**
(光顕でみられる)粘膜内癌　**m**
粘膜皮膚カンジダ症　**MCC**
粘膜皮膚眼症候群　**MCOS**
粘膜皮膚リーシュマニア症　**MCL**
粘膜皮膚リンパ節関節炎　**MCLA**
粘膜皮膚リンパ節症候群　**MLNS**
粘膜肥満細胞　**MMC**
粘膜病ウイルス　**MDV**
粘膜リンパ球抗原　**MLA**

の

ノイキノン　**NEQ**
ノイラミニダーゼ　**N, NA**
ノイラミニダーゼ処理ヒツジ赤血球　**NSRBC**
ノイラミニダーゼ阻害　**NAI, NI**
ノイラミン酸　**Neu**
ノカルジア(属)　**N**
ノカルジア水溶性窒素　**NWSN**
ノカルジアルブラ細胞壁骨格　**N-CWS**
ノースウェスタン大学制定障害度　**NUDS**
ノースウェスタン文章構文テスト　**NSST**
ノックアウトされていない　**XKO**
ノックアウトした〔された〕　**KO, K/O**
ノドジロオマキザル　**CCA**
ノーナン症候群　**NS**
ノバルセノベンゾール　**NAB**
ノベリウム　**No**
ノボビオシン　**NB**
ノーマン・ウッド(症候群)　**NW**
ノーマンズランド　**NML**
ノルアドレナリン　**NA, Nad, NAdr, NOR**
ノルアドレナリン負荷試験　**NA-test**
ノルエチステロン　**NET**
ノルエピネフリン　**NE, NEP**
ノルジヒドログアヤレト酸　**NDGA**
ノールズ研究用音響的人体模型　**KEMAR**
ノルトリプチリン　**NT**
ノルバリン　**Nva**
ノルフロキサシン　**NFLX**
ノルメタ・アドレナリン　**NMA**
ノルメタネフリン　**NM, NMN, normet**
ノルメトアドレナリン　**NM**
ノルロイシン　**Nle, norleu**
ノンストレス試験　**NST**
ノンネ(グロブリン試験)　**N**
ノンネ・アペルト反応　**NA**
ノンネ・フロアン(症候群)　**NF**
ノンネテスト　**N**
ノンレム　**NON-REM**
ノンレム睡眠　**NREM, NREMS**
のんきさと思考的外向　**R.T**
伸ばす　**st, str**
延ばした　**def**
延ばす　**elong**
野　**A, S**
飲ませる　**ad hib.**
(薬を)飲む　**rc.**
飲む　**bib., R, r.**
飲む・飲んだ・飲まれた　**DDD**
能動酸化法　**AOM**
能動性の　**A, a, act**
能動的運動範囲　**AROM**
能動的運動補助範囲　**AAROM**
能弁　**W**
能力　**C, c, c., cap**
脳　**BRA**
脳アミロイド血管症　**CAA**
脳炎　**E**
脳炎後パーキンソン症候群　**PEP**
脳下垂体アルコールブロック　**NALP**
脳回転状萎縮に伴う高オルニチン血症　**HOGA**
脳肝腎(症候群)　**CHR**
脳肝腎症候群　**CHRS**
脳眼顔面・骨格(症候群)　**COFS**
脳眼形成不全・筋ジストロフィ　**COD-MD**
脳幹聴覚誘発電位　**BAEP**
脳幹聴覚誘発反応　**BAER**
脳幹電気反応　**BSER**
脳幹(誘発)反応　**BSER**
脳幹反応　**BSR**
脳幹網様体　**BSRF**
脳幹誘発電位　**BSEP**
脳幹誘発反応聴力検査(法)　**BERA**
脳関連T細胞抗原　**BAT**
脳関連テータ抗原　**BAT**
脳灌流圧　**CPP**
脳弓　**F, FX**
脳機能係数　**BFI**
脳クモ膜下静脈圧　**CSAVP**
脳グルコース酸比　**CGOQ**
脳外科(学)　**NSurg, N.Surg**
脳外科医　**N surg**
脳(神経)外科経過記録　**NSPN**
脳外科検査　**NSX**
脳外科の　**N surg**
脳血液量　**CBV**
脳血管撮影　**CRAG**
脳血管疾患　**CVD**
脳血管障害　**Apo, CVE**
脳血管性痴呆　**VD**
脳血管造影　**AEG**

脳血管造影法　**CAG**
脳血管抵抗　**CVR**
脳血管(性)の　**CV**
脳血管反応性　**CVR**
脳血管不全(症)　**CVI**
脳血管閉塞性疾患　**CVOD**
脳血管発作〔障害〕　**CVA**
脳血栓症　**CT**
脳血流量　**CBF**
脳研究所　**BRI**
脳腱黄色腫症　**CTX**
脳交連　**CC**
脳呼吸比　**CRQ**
脳梗塞　**Apo, CI**
脳硬膜動脈・筋血管癒合術　**EDAMS**
脳硬膜動脈血管癒合術　**EDAS**
脳酸素消費比率　**$CMRO_2$**
脳酸素消費量　**$CMR\text{-}O_2$**
脳酸素代謝予備　**CO_2MR**
脳酸素代謝率　**$CMRO_2$**
脳心筋炎　**ECM, EMC**
脳心筋炎ウイルス　**EMCV, EMC virus**
脳心臓滲出液　**BHI**
脳心臓滲出液緩衝液　**BHIB**
脳心臓滲出液培地　**BHI medium**
脳心肺蘇生術　**CCPR**
脳出血　**Apo, HC**
脳死　**BD**
脳室　**V, v, VENT, vent, ventric**
脳室・脳比　**VBR**
脳室(随)液　**VF**
脳室(髄)液圧　**VFP**
脳室頸静脈(シャント)　**VJ**
脳室頸静脈心臓(シャント)　**VJC**
脳室周囲高信号域　**PVH**
脳室周囲出血　**PVH**
脳室周囲髄液浮腫　**PVE**
脳室周囲性白質軟化症　**PVL**
脳室周囲低吸収域　**PVL**
脳室周囲の超音波輝度が高い所見　**PVE**
脳室上衣下出血　**SEH**
脳室心房シャント　**V-A shunt**
脳室髄液　**VCSF**
脳室造影　**CVG**
脳室造影〔撮影〕　**VG**
脳室造影〔撮影〕図　**VGM**
脳室造影〔撮影〕法　**VEG**
脳室内圧　**IVP**
脳室内血腫　**IVH**
脳室内出血　**IVCG, IVH**
脳室内の　**icv, ICV**
脳室内連絡　**CIV**
脳室の　**V, v, VENT, vent, ventric**
脳室腹腔シャント　**VP shunt, v-p shunt, V-P shunt**
脳室腹腔シャント術　**V-P**
脳室腹腔シャント　**VPS**
脳室腹腔の　**VP, V/P**
脳室(内)へ　**icv, ICV**
脳神経　**CN, Cr ns, cr.ns.**
脳神経外科世界連合　**WFNS**
脳神経徴候　**CN sign**
脳神経伝達物質　**BNT**
脳神経麻痺　**CNP**
脳振とう後症候群　**PCS**
脳深部刺激　**DBS**
脳腫瘍　**BT, CT**
脳腫瘍頭痛　**BTH**
脳磁気図計　**MEG**
脳磁気図検査法　**MEG**
脳磁図　**MEG**
脳障害　**BD**
脳障害なし　**NBD**
脳静脈撮影　**CVG**
脳震盪　**comm.cer.**
脳セクター〔扇形〕スキャン　**CSS**
脳性灰白髄炎　**CP**
脳性小児麻痺　**CP**
脳性早熟　**CPP**
脳性の　**cereb**
脳性麻痺　**CP**
脳性(小児)麻痺診療所　**CPC**
脳脊髄(液)　**CS**
脳摂取指数　**BUI**
脳卒中　**Apo, APO, Apo**
脳卒中易発症高血圧自然発症ラット　**SHRSP, SHRSP, SHR-SP**
脳卒中治療センター　**STC**
脳卒中病院前救護　**PSLS**
脳組織圧　**BTP**
脳組織灌流圧　**CTPP**
脳損傷　**BD**
脳槽圧　**CP**
脳代謝率　**CMR**
脳蛋白溶剤　**BPS**
脳底頭蓋骨折　**BSF**
脳底動脈　**BA**
脳底動脈型片頭痛　**BAM**
脳底動脈頂点動脈瘤　**BA top**
脳底動脈不全(症)　**BAI**
脳電位分布図(法)　**BEAM**
脳動脈硬化(症)　**CAS**
脳動脈硬化症　**HAS**
脳ナトリウム利尿ペプチド　**BNP**
脳内圧亢進(症)　**ICH**
脳内温度増加指数　**CTI**
脳内血腫　**ICH, IH**
脳内出血　**ICH**

(大)脳内の　**IC**
(大)脳の　**cereb**
脳の化学的刺激　**CSB**
脳の障害された　**BI**
脳の電気刺激　**ESB**
脳波　**EECG, EEG**
脳波記録　**EECG**
脳波計　**EEG**
脳波検査　**EECG**
脳波周波数分析装置　**EEG frequency analyzer**
脳波聴力検査　**EEG A**
脳波反応　**EER**
脳波分析　**EEGA**
脳皮質　**CC**
脳皮質灌流速度　**CPR**
脳ブドウ糖代謝率　**CMRG, CMR glu**
脳浮腫　**BE**
脳平均通過時間　**MTT**
脳閉塞性血栓動脈炎　**CTO**
脳膜炎・風疹・流行性耳下腺炎　**3M**
脳誘発電位　**BEP**
脳リピドーシス　**CLIP**
脳梁　**CC**
脳梁膝　**GOC**
脳・筋血管癒合術　**EMS**
脳・ミオシン・血管疾患　**EMS**
農業生物学　**agro**
農業生物学者　**agro**
農業生物学の　**agro**
濃厚な　**conc.**
濃縮　**CONC, conc, conc., concentr, concn**
濃縮血球量　**TPCV**
濃縮された　**CONC, conc, conc., concd, concd., concentr**
濃縮した　**cond**
濃縮性胆汁症候群　**IBS**
濃縮赤血球　**CRC**
濃縮赤血球液　**PC**
濃縮物　**conc, concentr, concn**
濃縮容積　**CV**
濃淡強調CT　**CECT, CE-CT**
濃度　**C, CONC, conc, conc., concentr, concn, dens**
濃度傾斜遠心分離沈降　**DGCS**
(薬物血中)濃度時間曲線下面積　**AUC**
濃度不明　**DU**
濃(厚層)塗抹標本　**DT**
膿胸後リンパ腫　**PAL**
(水晶)嚢外白内障摘出(術)　**XCCE**
嚢外レンズ摘出術　**ECLE**
嚢腫　**Cy**
嚢性中心壊死　**CMM**
嚢内白内障摘出(術)　**ICCE**
嚢内レンズ摘出術　**ICLE**
嚢胞　**Cy**
嚢胞腎　**PCK, PKD, PRD**
嚢胞性線維症　**CF, C.F.**
嚢胞性線維症因子　**CFF**
嚢胞性線維症因子活性　**CFFA**
嚢胞性線維症患者　**CFP**
嚢胞性線維症蛋白　**CFP**
嚢胞性線維性骨炎　**OFC**
嚢胞線維症膜貫通型調節物質　**CFTR**
嚢胞様〔状〕黄斑浮腫　**CME**
残っている　**remg**
残り　**reliq, reliq.**
除いた　**exc**
望まれた　**prefd**
後の　**P**
喉　**Th**
喉に　**gutt.**
飲物　**bev**

は

バイアル **V**
ハイイロキツネザル **HGG**
パイエル板 **PP**
バイオクリーン **BC**
バイオチン **VR**
バイオフィードバック **BF, BFB**
バイオマイシン **Vm, VM**
バイオレット **V, v**
バイカル国際生態学研究センター **BICER**
バイスペシフィック抗体 **BS**
バイタルサイン **V.S., V/S, v.s.**
バイタルサインOK **VSOK**
バイタルサイン安定 **V/S/S**
ハイデンハイム・鉄・ヘマトキシリン **HIH**
バイト **b**
パイナップル **PA**
ハイネ・メイディーン(病) **HM**
バイパス **B, BP**
バイパス移植(片) **BPG**
バイパス血管形成血行再建術調査(＝BART) **BARI**
バイパス血管形成血行再建術比較試験(＝BARI) **BART**
ハイパーテキスト記述言語 **HTML**
パイフェル菌 **Pf**
ハイブリッド顆粒球 **HG**
ハイブリッド血管モデル **HVM**
ハイブリドーマ成長因子(＝IL-6) **HGF**
ハイブリドーマバンク **HB**
ハイブリドーマプラズマ細胞増殖因子 **HPGF**
ハイマン腎炎抗原複合体 **HNAC**
ハイリスク妊娠 **HRP**
パイログロブリン **Pyro**
ハインツ小体 **HB**
パイント **O, P, PT, pt**
ハーヴェーマウス肉腫ウイルス **HaMSV**
ハウエル・ジョリー(小体) **HJ**
ハウエル・ジョリー小体 **HJB**
ハウシップ・ロンベルグ(症候群) **HR**
ハウスダスト **HD**
ハウスダストダニ **HDM**
バウヒニア紫斑凝集素 **BPA**
バウムテスト **TTT**
ハウンスフィールド単位 **H, HU**
バカンピシリン **BAPC**
バーキットリンパ腫 **BL**
パーキンソニズム **Parkin, PKN**
パーキンソン痴呆症候群 **PD, PDC**
パーキンソン病 **PD**
バクテリア **bact**
バクテリウム(属) **BACT, Bact, bact, bact.**
バクテリオクロロフィル **BChL**
バクテリオフェオフィチン **BPheo**
バクテリオロドプシン **BR**
バクテロイデス(属) **B**
バークリウム **Bk**
ハーゲマン因子 **HaF, HF**
パジェット病 **PD**
パジェット(病)様メラニン細胞増加(症) **PM**
バシジオボルス(属) **B**
バシトラシン **B, BC, BTRC**
バシトラシンX **BX**
ハジナ・デーモン(肉汁) **HD**
ハジュ・チェネー症候群 **HCS**
バシラス **B, B., Bac, Bac.**
パス **PAS**
パスカル **Pa**
パスカル(＝プログラミング言語) **PASCAL**
パスツール研究所 **IP**
パスツレラ(属) **P, Past, Past.**
バスキュラーアクセス **VA**
バーゼル解剖学用語 **BNA**
パーセント **pc, pct**
パーセント肺活量 **%VC**
バソトシン **VT**
バソプレシン **VP**
バター **but.**
ハーター・ジー(症候群) **HG**
パータクチン **PRM**
パタスモンキー **EPA**
パターン解析 **PA**
パターンシフト視覚誘発反応 **PSVER**
パターン認識受容体 **PRR**
パターン変換視覚誘発電位 **PRVEP**
パーチ **P**
バチ状指・チアノーゼ・浮

腫　**CCE**
ハッカ水
aq.menth.pip.
パック/日　**p/d**
バックグラウンド　**BG**
バックグラウンド減算法
BG subtraction
(甲状腺)ハッサル小体
HC
ハッサル小体　**HB**
バッセン・コルンツヴァイク(症候群)　**BK**
ハッチンソン・ウェーバー・ポイツ(症候群)
HWP
ハッチンソン・ギルフォード症候群　**HG**
ハッチンソン・ギルフォード早老症候群　**HGPS**
ハッチンソン・ベック(病)
HB
バッテン病　**BD**
バッド・キアリ(症候群)
BC
バッドキアリ症候群
BCS
パップ(剤)　**cat, cat.**
パップ剤をつくれ
ft.catapl., ft.cataplasm.
バップス　**VAPS**
ハーディー・ランド・リッター色覚異常検査表
HRR, HRR plates
バーディック吸引(器)
Burd
ハーディング・パッセー(黒色腫)　**HP**
ハーディング・パッセイ黒色腫　**HPM**
バード・ピック(症候群)
BP
バート型ヘモグロビン
Hb Bart
ハト血清　**PS**
ハードコンタクトレンズ
HCL
ハートナップ(病)　**H**
ハートナップ病
H disease
ハートマン液　**HS**
バーナー・モリソン(症候群)　**VM**
バナジウム　**V**
バーナード・スーリエ症候群　**BSS**
パナマレッド　**PR**
ハーニウム　**Ha**
バニリルマンデル酸
VMA
バニル酢酸　**VLA**
バニル乳酸　**VLA**
ハネ　**HANE**
パネルディスカッション
PD
ハノーバー集中(治療)スコア　**HIS**
ハーバード医科大学
HMS
ハーバードポンプ　**HP**
パパニコロー(検査・分類・染色)　**PAP**
パパニコロー癌研究所
PCRI
パパニコロー染色
Pap sm
パピヨン・ルフェーブル症候群　**PLS**
パピローマ　**Pap**
バビンスキー(反射)
Bab
バビンスキー・ナジェット(症候群)　**BN**
ハープ・ディンマー(症候群)　**HD**
ハブカ　**HABCA**
バブコック知能検査
BTME
ハプトグロビン　**HP, Hp, Hpt**
ハプトグロビン・ヘモグロビン複合体
Hp-Hb complex
ハフニウム　**Hf**
ハプロタイプ頻度　**Hf**
パブロン　**PAV**
ハベカシン　**HBK**
パポバウイルス　**papova**
ハマン・リッチ(症候群)
HR
パミ　**PAMI**
パーミル　**vT, v.T.**
ハミルトンうつ病(尺度)
HAMD
ハミルトンうつ病評価尺度
HDS, HRSD
ハミルトン評点尺度
HRS
ハミルトン不安(尺度)
HAMA
ハミルトン不安評点尺度
HARS
ハムスター胚細胞　**HEC**
ハムスター胚線維芽細胞
HEF
ハムスター白血病ウイルス
HALV
パラ　***p*-**
パラヒドロキシメルクリ安息香酸　**PHMB**
パラアミノ安息香酸
PABA
パラアミノ安息香酸カリウム　**KPAB**
パラアミノサリチル酸
PAS, PASA
パラアミノサリチル酸カルシウム　**PAS**
パラアミノ馬尿酸
PAH, PAHA
パラアミノ馬尿酸塩
PAH
パラアミノ馬尿酸ナトリウム除去率　$\mathbf{E}_{PAH}$
パラアミノプロピオフェノ

ン **PAP, PAPP**
パラアミノメチル安息香酸 **PAMBA**
バラ色粃糠疹 **PR**
パラインフルエンザウイルス **HA virus, PIV**
パラオキシプロピオフェノン **PPP**
パラクアット **PPV**
パラクロロ第二水銀〔メルクリ〕安息香酸塩 **PCMB, *p*CMB**
パラクロロ第二水銀〔メルクリ〕フェニルスルホン酸 **PCMPS**
パラクロロ第二水銀〔メルクリ〕ベンゼンスルホン酸 **PCMBS**
パラクロロニトロベンゼン ***p*-CNB**
パラクロロフェニルアラニン ***p*-CPA, PCPA, *p*CPA**
パラコート中毒の重症度指数 **SIPP**
パラジクロロベンゼン **parad, PDB**
パラジメチルアミノベンズアルデヒド **PDAB**
パラジウム **Pd**
パラチオン **DNTP**
パラチフスA **PA**
パラチフスB **PB**
パラチフスC **PC**
パラトリルイソプロピルカルボニル **PTIC**
パラトリルメチルカルビノール **PTMC**
パラトルモン **PT**
バラニー協会 **B.S.**
パラニトロアニリン **pNA**
パラニトロカテコール **PNC**
パラニトロビフェニル **PNB**
パラニトロフェニルガラクトシド **PNPG**
パラニトロフェニルグリセリン **PNPG**
パラニトロフェニル硫酸 **p-NPS**
パラニトロフェニルリン酸塩 **PNPP**
パラニトロフェノール **PNP, P-NP, p-NP**
パラニトロブルーテトラゾリウム **PNBT**
パラノイア **PA, Pa**
パラヒドロキシフェニル酢酸 ***p*-HPLA, P-HPLA**
パラヒドロキシフェニルサリチルアミド **PHPS**
パラヒドロキシフェニルピルビン酸 ***p*-HPPA**
パラフィン **par**
パラフィン紙 **chart cera.**
パラフィン乳剤のフェノールフタレイン **PPP**
パラフィン浴 **PB**
パラフェニルフェノール ***P*-PHP, P-PHP**
パラフェニレンジアミン **PPD**
ハラーフォルデン・シュパッツ症候群 **HSS**
ハラボーデン・シュパッツ病 **HSD**
パラホルムアルデヒド **PFA**
パラメタゾン **PM**
パラメトキシアンフェタミン **PAM, PMA**
パラメルクリ安息香酸 **PMB**
パラメルクリベンゼンスルホン酸 **PMBS**
バラライム **BL**
バランス式前腕装具 **BFO**
バランス前腕補助具 **BFP**
バランチジウム(属) **B**
バリアント型CJD **vCJD, v-CJD**
バリウム **Ba**
バリウム嚥下 **Ba swallow**
バリウム粥 **BM**
バリウム浣腸 **BaE, BaEn, Ba enem.**
バリウム注腸(検査) **BE**
バリオチン **VT**
パリ解剖学用語 **NAP, PNA**
ハリガネムシ類 **G**
ハリス・クローネ子宮マニピュレーター注射器 **HUMI**
バリストカルジオグラフ **BCG**
バリストカルジオグラム **BCG**
ハリネズミ **Hh**
バリール・矢口・エベランド **BYE**
バリン **V, VAL, Val, val.**
バリン・アルギニン・バソプレシン **VDAVP**
(側彎症に対する)ハリントン法 **HI**
ハリントンロッド装具 **HRI**
バー療法(＝脳腫瘍治療法の1つ) **BAR-therapy**
バル(＝ジメルカプロール) **BAL**
バルサム **BAL, bal., bals.**
バルサルバ試験 **PDV**
パルス・ド(ッ)プラー心エ

コー図　**PDE**
パルス/秒　**PPS, p.p.s.**
パルス位相変調　**PPM**
パルスオキシメーター表示酸素飽和度　**SpO_2**
パルス周波数変調　**PFM**
パルス振幅変調　**PAM**
パルス数変調　**PNM**
パルス遅延時間　**PD**
ハルステッド・ライタン(検査)　**HR**
ハルステッド・ライタン神経心理学的検査　**HRNB**
ハルステッド失語検査　**HAT**
パルスド(ッ)プラー超音波法　**PDU**
パルス幅変調　**PDM, PWM**
パルスフィールド電気泳動法　**PFGE**
バルトネラ(属)　**B**
ハルトマン数　**Ha**
バルトリン・尿道・スキーン腺　**BUS glands**
バルトリン腺とスキーン腺　**B & S glands**
バルビツレート　**Barb, barb**
バルプロ酸　**VPA**
パルミチン酸　**$C_{16=0}$**
パルミチン酸イソプロピル　**IPP**
パルミトオレイン酸　**$C_{16=1}$**
バルーン閉塞下逆行性経静脈的塞栓術　**B-RTO**
バルーン拡張式血管内ステント　**BEIS**
バルーンカテーテル僧帽弁開大術　**CBV**
バルーン心房中隔切開術　**BAS**
バルーン心房中隔裂開術　**BAS**
バルーンチューブ　**BT**
バルーン大動脈弁形成術　**BAV**
バルーン閉鎖式肝動脈造影　**BOHA**
バルーン閉塞動注法　**BOAI**
バレット食道　**BE**
バレル　**BBL, BLS**
ハレルフォルデン・シュパッツ(症候群)　**HS**
ハレルマン・ストレフ症候群　**HSS**
パロキシプロピオン　**POP**
ハロゲン　**Hal, hlg**
ハロゲン化ジメチル(-2-ヒドロキシ-5-ニトロベンジル)スルホニウム　**HNB-DMSH**
ハロセン　**H**
ハロタ〔セ〕ン　**HAL**
ハロタン　**H**
ハロタ〔セ〕ン・酸素・ガス〔亜酸化窒素〕　**HOG**
ハロタ〔セ〕ン・%・時　**HPH**
ハロタ〔セ〕ン肝炎　**HH**
ハロタ〔セ〕ン麻酔　**HA**
ハロペリドール　**HAL, HLP**
パロモマイシン　**PRM**
パワーユニット　**PU**
バーン　**b**
パン・バター心膜炎　**B & B pericarditis**
ハンガヌチウ・ダイヘル　**HD**
パン屑　**mic.pan.**
ハンクス平衡食塩水　**HBSS**
パンクレオザイミン　**PCZ, PZ**
パンクレオザイミン・コレシストキニン　**PZ-CCK**
パンクレオザイミン・セクレチン試験　**PS test**
バンコマイシン　**VA, VCM**
バンコマイシン,コリスチン,アニソマイシン　**VCA**
バンコマイシン耐性黄色ブドウ球菌　**VRSA**
バンコマイシン耐性腸球菌　**VRE**
ハンスフィールド値　**HN**
ハンセン・ストリート釘　**HSN**
ハンセン(らい)病　**L**
ハンセン病　**HD**
ハンセン病救助協会　**LEPRA**
ハンセン病撲滅レオナルド記念館　**LMEL**
ハンター・ドリフィールド(曲線)　**H and D, H & D**
ハンター・フルラー(症候群)　**HH**
ハンタウイルス肺症候群　**HPS**
パンチカード機械　**PCM**
パンチカード方式　**PCS**
パンチ生検　**PB**
ハンチントン(舞踏)病　**HD**
ハンチントン舞踏病　**HC**
ハンディキャップ(のある)　**hcap, HCAP, hcp, HCP**
パンディー反応　**P**
バンデリアマメレクチン1　**BSL1**
ハンド・シューラー・クリスチャン病　**HSC**
ハンド検査　**HT**
パンと水　**b & w**

ハンブルグ抗不整脈薬大規模試験 **CASH**
ハンブルグ式児童用ウェクスラー知能テスト **HAWIK**
ハンブルグ式成人用ウェクスラー知能テスト **HAWIE**
ハンブルグ精神障害評価尺度 **HRPD**
パンフレット **pam.**
バップス **VAPS**
ハト(＝鳩) **pgn**
(太鼓)ばち指形成 **C**
はっきりした異常なし **NAA**
はっきりした所見 **sig.F.**
はっきりした脳障害 **DBD**
吐き気がする **S**
吐き出したもの **V**
吐き出す **expt, expt.**
汎用コンピュータ **GPC**
波高分析器 **PHA**
波状熱の凝集反応試験 **ABR test**
波数 **WN**
波長 **λ, ψ, WL**
波動 **fluc**
波動する **fluc**
波動物 **fluc**
波動変動式終末呼気陽圧呼吸法 **F-PEEP**
派生染色体 **der**
派生的な **deriv, deriv.**
破壊 **dest**
破壊する **dest**
破壊性奇胎 **IM**
破壊性絨毛腺腫 **CA, CAD, CD**
破壊性脊椎症 **DSA**
破壊胞状奇胎 **DM**
破骨細胞 **OCL**
破骨細胞活性化因子 **OAF**
破骨細胞刺激因子 **OSF**
破骨細胞様巨細胞 **OCLG, OLGC**
破砕因子 **CF**
破傷風 **TE, Te, Tet, tet**
破傷風・ジフテリア(トキソイド) **TD, Td**
破傷風・百日咳 **TP**
破傷風・百日咳ワクチン **TPV**
破傷風抗毒素 **TAT**
破傷風抗毒素血清 **TAS**
破傷風抗毒素皮膚試験 **TATST**
破傷風トキソイド **tet.tox., TT**
破傷風トキソイド抗体 **TTA**
破傷風毒素 **TET**
破傷風免疫グロブリン **TIG, TIg**
破水 **ROM, rupt.memb**
破綻 **BTB**
破綻出血 **BB**
破片 **frag**
破膜 **ROM, rupt.memb**
破裂(した) **rupt**
破裂した **RPTD, rupt'd**
馬蹄形裂孔 **HST**
馬尿酸 **HA**
馬尿酸-L-ヒスチジル-L-ロイシン **HHL**
馬尿酸グリシルグリシン **HGG**
馬力 **HP, PS**
歯 **t**
歯の **den, Odont, odont.**
歯磨き指導 **TBI**
場所 **l, pl**
場理論 **S-S**
葉 **fo., fol, h, hb**
葉巻タバコ喫煙本数/日 **c/d**
播種 **dissem**
播種された **dissem**
播種した **dissem**
播種状掌蹠汗孔角化症 **PPPD**
播種状表在性光線性角化症 **DSAK**
播種する **dissem**
播種性エリテマトーデス **LED**
播種性エリテマトーデス〔紅斑性狼瘡〕 **DLE**
播種性黄色腫 **XD**
播種性血管内凝固(症候群) **DIC**
播種性血管内凝固障害 **DIC**
播種性好酸球性膠原病 **DECD**
播種性紅斑性狼瘡 **LED**
播種性特発性骨増殖症 **DISH**
播種性の **dissem**
播種性表在性光線性汗孔角化症 **DSAP**
播種性腹膜平滑筋腫症 **LPD**
灰色 **g**
灰色の **g**
背臥位(仰臥位)拡張期圧 **SDBP**
背臥の **SU, sup, SUP, sup.**
背屈 **DF, dorsi, dorsifl**
背屈小発作 **RPM**
背景 **BG**
背景音楽 **BGM**
背景活動 **BA**
背景の **bkg**
背側運動核 **DMN**
背側延髄網様体 **DMRF**

背側骨間(筋)　**DI**
背側索　**DLF**
背側子宮動脈　**DUA**
背側脊髄小脳路　**DSCT**
(視床下部)背側内側(核)　**MD**
背側の　**D, d., dor**
背側迷走神経核群　**DVC**
背側網様核　**RD**
背腸骨筋　**DI**
背痛　**BA, B/A**
背内側核　**DM**
背内側の　**DM**
背(面)の　**D, d., dor**
背部　**bk**
背部清拭　**BC**
背部痛　**BA, B/A**
背部の　**D**
背腹の方向　**DV**
背面　**vo**
肺　**L, LU, Lu**
肺アンジオテンシンI変換酵素　**PACE**
肺因子　**PF**
肺移植　**LTX**
肺炎　**PN, Pn, pn, pneu, Pneumo, pneumo, PNM**
肺炎球菌　**Pn**
肺炎球菌多糖類ワクチン　**PPS**
肺炎球菌ワクチン　**PV**
肺肝境界　**LLB, LLG**
肺活量　**CV, VC, VIT CAP, vit.cap., VK**
肺活量計　**Sp**
肺活量測定(法)　**SP**
肺開放音　**PO**
肺換気/血流(肺スキャン)　**V/Q**
肺換気血流スキャン　**VPLS**
肺間質水腫　**PIE**
肺間質性気腫　**ITE, PIE**
肺癌　**LC, LK**
肺気腫症　**PE**
肺吸虫(属)　**P**
肺基底膜　**LBM**
肺機能　**PF**
肺機能検査　**PFT**
肺機能スコア　**PFS**
肺ケアチーム　**PCT**
肺血液量　**LBV, PBV**
肺血管外液量　**PEV**
肺血管(性)高血圧(症)　**PVH**
肺血管疾患　**PVD**
肺血管抵抗　**PVR**
肺血管抵抗指数　**PVRI**
肺血管閉塞(性)疾患　**PVOD**
肺血栓症　**PT**
肺血栓塞栓疾患　**PTED**
肺血栓塞栓症　**PTE**
肺血流量　**PBF, Qp**
肺原因不明組織球増殖症　**PHX**
肺結核　**PP, PT, PTB, TP**
肺コンプライアンス　**CL**
肺好酸球症　**PE**
肺好酸球増多症　**PIE**
肺高血圧　**PH**
肺高血圧症　**PHT**
肺高血圧(症)を伴う胎児循環遺残(症)　**PFCPH**
肺梗塞　**PI**
肺細動脈抵抗　**PAR**
肺細胞　**LC**
肺小細胞〔燕麦細胞〕癌　**SCCL**
肺小細胞癌　**SCLC**
肺小動脈抵抗　**PAR**
肺心臓疾患　**PHD**
肺伸展受容器　**PSR**
肺枝狭窄(症)　**PBS**
肺実質　**LP**
肺実質組織量　**Vt**
肺疾患　**PD, PUD, PuD, Pu D, Pul**
肺疾患管理部門　**PCU**
肺疾患の所見なし　**NEPD**
肺疾患(性)貧血　**PDA**
肺集中治療室　**PICU**
肺循環　**PC**
肺硝子膜症　**PHM**
肺磁図　**MPG**
肺静脈　**PV**
肺静脈圧　**PL, PVP**
肺静脈うっ血　**PVC**
肺静脈還流異常症　**APVD**
肺静脈狭窄　**PVS**
肺静脈閉塞(閉鎖)(症)　**PVO**
肺静脈閉塞病　**PVOD**
肺水腫　**PE**
肺水腫液　**PEF**
肺切除　**PNX**
肺生検　**LB**
肺性心　**CP, PHD**
肺性肥大性骨関節症　**PHO**
肺洗浄　**PT**
肺腺癌細胞　**LAC**
肺塞栓　**PE**
肺塞栓症　**PE**
肺大食細胞　**PM**
肺体重比　**LBWR**
肺通過時間　**PTT**
肺抵抗　**Rp**
肺毒性単位　**UPTD**
肺動静脈瘻　**PAF, PA-VF**
肺動脈　**PA, PAVM**
肺動脈圧　**Pa, PAP**
肺動脈圧・肺静脈圧　**Pa-Pv**
肺動脈圧/体血圧(比)　**Pp/Ps**
肺動脈陰影欠損　**PAFD**
肺動脈拡張期圧　**PADP**
肺動脈拡張期の　**PAd**

肺動脈拡張終期圧　PAEDP
肺動脈幹　PAT, PT
肺動静脈奇形　PAVM
肺動脈狭窄　PAS
肺動脈狭窄(症)　PS
肺動脈狭窄兼閉鎖不全　PSI
肺動脈狭窄兼閉鎖不全症　PSI
肺動脈狭窄症　PS
肺動脈血栓塞栓症　PATE
肺動脈血栓動脈内膜剝離　PATE
肺動脈血流量　PAF, Q_{PA}
肺動脈高血圧　PAH
肺動脈絞扼術　PAB
肺動脈疾患の重症度指数　IPVD
肺動脈楔入(＝せつにゅう)圧　PAWP
肺動脈楔入圧　PWP
肺動脈楔入(＝せつにゅう)部　PAW
肺動脈造影　PAG
肺動脈第二音　P2, P_2
肺動脈低血圧　PAH
肺動脈抵抗　PAR
肺動脈平均圧　PAMP
肺動脈閉鎖　OAP
肺動脈閉鎖(症)/肺動脈弁狭窄(症)　PA/PS
肺動脈閉鎖圧　PAOP
肺動脈閉塞(圧)　PAo
肺動脈弁(＝右房)　PV
肺動脈弁開放速度　PVOV
肺動脈弁狭窄　pul sten
肺動脈弁狭窄(症)　PVS, VPS
肺動脈弁置換術　PVR
肺動脈弁不全(症)　PI
肺動脈弁閉鎖(音)　PC
肺動脈弁閉鎖不全　PI, PR
肺動脈弁閉塞症　PA
肺動脈弁輪形成術　PAP
肺内ガス混合指数　PMI
肺内ガス混合比　ER
肺内皮細胞膜　PEM
肺(性)の　P
肺の　PUL, Pul, pul, PULM, pulm
肺の拡散能　DL
肺の気圧性外傷　PBT
肺ヒアリン膜　PHM
肺表面活性物質　PS
肺微細珪肺　pneumoultra
肺微小塞栓術　PME
肺微石症　PML
肺不全　PI, pul ins
肺不全指数　PII
肺幅　LW
肺平均通過時間　PMTT
肺胞　ALV, alv, alv.
肺胞・毛細管　A-C
肺胞・毛細管ブロック　A-C block
肺胞１回換気量　V_TA
肺胞圧　PA
肺胞音　VS
肺胞拡散能　AD capacity
肺胞管　AV
肺胞換気(量)　alv vent, alv.vent.
肺胞間質性肺疾患　AILD
肺胞気　A
肺胞気・動脈血酸素分圧較差　A-aDo_2, A-aDO_2
肺胞気・動脈血炭酸ガス分圧較差　A-aDCO_2, A-aPco_2
肺胞気・動脈血窒素分圧較差　A(-)aDN_2
肺胞気酸素濃度　FAO_2
肺胞気酸素分圧　PaO_2, PAO_2
肺胞気二酸化炭素圧　$PACO_2$, P_ACO_2
肺胞気二酸化炭素〔炭酸ガス〕濃度　$FACO_2$
肺胞気容積〔容量〕　$\dot{V}_A$, V_A
肺胞腔　AS
肺胞細胞癌　ACC
肺胞死腔　Vd alv
肺胞死腔換気量　V_DA
肺胞死腔量　V_DA
肺胞終末毛細管　c′
肺胞硝子膜症　HMD
肺胞上皮増生　AEH
肺胞大食細胞　PAM
肺胞蛋白症　ALP, PAP
肺胞低酸素血管攣縮　PAHVC
肺胞内圧　Palv
肺胞内の　IA, i.a.
肺胞二酸化炭素〔炭酸ガス〕分圧　PCO_2A
肺胞の　ALV, alv, alv.
肺胞嚢　AS
肺胞微石症　MAP, PAM
肺胞壁基底膜　AWBM
肺胞マクロファージ　AM
肺胞マクロファージ由来成長因子　AMDGF
肺胞毛細(血)管膜　ACM
肺胞毛細(血)管膜透過性　ACMP
肺胞容量〔容積〕　VA
肺毛細管　PC
肺毛細(血)管血液量　VC, V_C, Vc
肺毛細管血流　Qc
肺毛細管血流量　PCBF
肺毛細管楔入圧　Po
肺毛細管蛋白漏出　PCPL

肺毛細血管圧　**PCP**
肺毛細血管血流量　**Qpc**
肺毛細血管楔入圧　**PCWP**
肺門部リンパ節　**HN**
肺門リンパ節　**HLN**
肺容積　**LV**
肺容量減少　**LVR**
肺容量減少手術　**VRS**
肺容量減少(手)術　**LVRS**
肺葉外腐骨(分離片)形成　**ELS**
肺葉内肺分画症　**ILS**
肺流量　**PF**
胚　**emb**
胚移植　**ET**
胚移植術　**ET**
胚芽層出血　**GLH**
胚細胞癌　**ECC**
胚細胞腫　**G**
胚成長発育因子　**EGDF**
胚性幹細胞　**ES**
胚中心　**GC**
胚中心Bリンパ球　**GCB**
胚中心細胞　**GCC**
胚盤胞移植　**BT**
胚置換　**ER**
配偶者間人工授精　**AIH**
配偶者や恋人など親密な関係にある，またはあった者から振るわれる暴力　**DV**
配偶子卵管内移植法　**GIFT**
配合禁忌　**contra**
配合禁忌の　**contra, incompat**
配分　**dis**
配列　**AL, al**
配列順(序)　**Seq, seq**
倍加時間　**Td**
倍数　**pl**
倍率　**MF**
梅毒　**Σ, L, lu., SY, syph**
梅毒学　**syph**
梅毒学者　**syph**
梅毒螢光トレポネーマ抗体試験　**FTAT**
梅毒血清反応　**STS**
梅毒検査　**LT**
梅毒性骨軟骨炎　**SOC**
梅毒性心疾患　**LHD, SHD**
梅毒性の　**syph**
梅毒トレポネーマ　**TP**
梅毒トレポネーマ・メチレンブルー試験　**TPMB**
梅毒トレポネーマ感作赤血球凝集試験　**TPHA test**
梅毒トレポネーマ凝集(試験)　**TPA**
梅毒トレポネーマ血球凝集反応　**TPHA**
梅毒トレポネーマ不動化(試験)　**TPI**
梅毒トレポネーマ不動化試験　**TIT, TPI test**
梅毒トレポネーマ不動化付着　**TPIA**
梅毒トレポネーマ補体(結合試験)　**TPC**
梅毒トレポネーマ補体結合試験　**TPCF test**
梅毒トレポネーマ免疫付着(試験)　**TPIA**
梅毒の血清学的検査　**SU**
梅毒標準検査　**STS**
排液　**drain, drg, drng, ext.liq.**
排液(法)　**dge**
排液管　**dr**
排出　**excr**
排出する　**excr**
排出性尿路造影〔撮影〕図　**XU**
排出性膀胱造影〔撮影〕図　**XC**
排出用経皮胃造瘻(術)　**VPG**
排出量　**Vo**
排泄　**excr**
排泄(物)　**DC, D/C, dc**
排泄されるまで使う　**UUE**
排泄指数　**EI**
排泄した　**DC**
排泄する　**evac, excr**
排泄性尿路造影　**EXU**
排泄物　**disc**
排尿筋括約筋協調不全　**DSD**
排尿筋の収縮不全を伴う膀胱過活動　**DHIC**
排尿筋不安定症　**DI**
排尿後膀胱造影図　**PVC**
排尿した　**vd**
排尿していない　**HNV**
排尿時尿路造影図　**MCUG**
排尿時の　**vdg.**
排尿時膀胱造影〔撮影〕(法)　**VCG**
排尿時膀胱造影〔撮影〕図　**VCG**
排尿時膀胱造影法　**MCG**
排尿時膀胱内圧/尿流量図　**P/F chart**
排尿時膀胱尿道造影　**VUG**
排尿時膀胱尿道造影〔撮影〕図　**VCG, VCU, VCUG**
排尿時膀胱尿道造影〔撮影〕法　**VCUG**
排尿時膀胱尿道造影法　**MCUG**
排尿する　**PU, vd**
排尿パック　**HP**
排尿(後)膀胱　**VB**
排尿流速　**VER**
排尿流量　**VER**

排尿量　**VV**
排膿　**drg, drain, drng**
排膿(法)　**dge**
排便　**BM, BO, DEF, def.**
排便訓練　**TT**
排便する　**def**
排膿　**drain**
排卵している　**OV**
排卵法　**OM**
排卵誘発ホルモン　**OIH**
敗血症重症度スコア　**SSS**
敗血症性肺水腫　**SPE**
敗血性皮膚潰瘍性疾患　**SCUD**
培地　**M, m, med, med.**
培地赤血球脆弱性　**MCF**
培養　**cult**
培養T細胞　**CTC**
培養液　**CM**
培養胸腺上皮　**CTE**
培養血管平滑筋細胞　**CVSMC**
培養コロニー形成細胞　**CFC-C**
培養コロニー形成単位　**CFU-C**
培養されていない　**NC**
培養されない　**NG**
培養上皮細胞移植　**CEA**
培養と感受性　**C/S, c/s, C & S, C+S**
廃棄物処理に関する法律　**RCRA**
廃疾　**DB, dis, disab**
廃疾保険　**DI**
廃水処理プラント　**WWTP**
媒介　**transm**
媒介者　**V, *V*, vehic.**
媒介動物　**vect**
媒介物質　**M**
媒質　**M, m, med, med.**
博士　**d**
白衣効果　**WCE**
白衣高血圧(症)　**WCH**
白花朝鮮アサガオ凝集素　**DSA**
白人　**C, Cau, Cauc, wt.**
白人既婚女性　**WMF**
白人既婚男性　**WMM**
白人小児　**CC, WC, W/C, wh ch**
白人女性　**C♀, WF, W/F, wf**
白人成人　**W/A**
白人成人女性　**CAF, WAF**
白人成人男性　**CAM, WAM**
白人男性　**C♂, WM, W/M**
白人の成人　**CA, C/A**
白色脂肪組織　**WAT**
白色上皮　**W**
白質切截　**lobo**
(大脳)白質損傷　**WML**
白質脳炎　**LE**
白癬菌(属)　**T**
白体　**CA**
白内障　**CAT, Cat, cat.**
白内障吸引灌流装置　**AID**
白(色)脾髄　**WP**
白ろう病　**VWF**
麦芽エキス肝油　**DCL**
麦芽ミルクセーキ　**malt**
(心)拍出量記録器　**COR**
拍出力　**O**
拍動/秒　**BPS**
拍動/分　**ppm**
拍動指数　**PI**
拍動性周波発振器　**BFO**
拍動性電磁場　**PEMF**
拍動性補助装置　**PAD**
拍動流　**pc**
(水晶体嚢)剥脱　**CE**
剥奪症候群　**DS**
剥離　**desq**
剥離式包装(薬包)　**SP**
剥離内膜　**IF**
博士号　**PhD, ph.D.**
箔　**F**
薄束　**FFG**
薄層クロマトグラフィ　**TLC**
薄層電気泳動　**TLE**
曝露　**Ex, ex, exp, X, x**
曝露群寄与危険率　**EARP**
曝露時間　**S**
曝露前に　**PE**
爆発的運動行動　**EMB**
爆発的精神行動　**EMB**
爆発的濾胞増殖(過形成)　**EFH**
箱　**scat.**
箱に入れて　**in scat**
箱に入れよ　**dent.ad.scat.**
箱庭療法　**SPT**
初め　**beg**
初めての　**V**
始まり　**beg**
始まる　**beg**
始める　**beg**
端　**ext, ext.**
橋本甲状腺炎　**HT**
橋渡し研究　**TR**
裸での体重　**NW**
裸の包装　**SP**
白金　**plat, Pt**
白血球　**GB, G.B., L, leuko, Lkc, W, WBC, WC**
白血球(数)　**WBC**
白血球アスコルビン酸　**LAA**

白血球アルカリホスファターゼ　**LAP**
白血球アルカリホスファターゼ活性　**LAPA**
白血球アルカリホスファターゼ染色(法)　**LAP stain**
白血球因子抗原 1　**LFA-1**
白血球インターフェロン　**LeIF**
白血球エステラーゼ　**LE**
白血球エラスターゼ　**LE**
白血球円柱　**WC**
白血球活性化因子　**LAF**
白血球関連抑制活性　**LIA**
白血球吸着抑制〔阻止〕因子　**LAIF**
白血球凝血促進活性　**LPCA**
白血球凝集　**LA**
白血球共通抗原　**LC**
白血球結合型ヘルペスウイルス　**LAHV**
白血球減少因子　**LPF**
白血球抗原　**LA**
白血球抗原因子 3　**LAF-3**
白血球抗原感受性テスト　**LAST**
白血球コロニー形成ユニット　**LCFU, L-CFU**
白血球自動測定器　**LARC**
白血球除去赤血球　**LPRC**
白血球浸潤因子　**LIF**
白血球数　**WC, WCC**
白血球数と分画　**WBC diff**
白血球性発熱物質　**LP**
白血球接着　**LA**
白血球接着不全(症)　**LAD**
白血球接着分子　**LAM, leu-CAM**
白血球走性因子活性　**LFA**
白血球増多因子　**LPF**
白血球増多誘発因子　**LIF**
白血球窒素　**WBN**
白血球チロシンキナーゼ　**ltk**
白血球伝達　**LCP**
白血球透析物　**LD**
白血球特異(的)活性　**LSA**
白血球トロンボプラスチン　**LTP**
白血球内因性メディエータ　**LEM**
白血球内皮細胞接着分子 1　**LECAM-1**
白血球粘着阻止(試験)　**LAI**
白血球破壊(破砕)性血管炎　**LCV**
白血球ヒスタミン放出(試験)　**LHR**
白血球百分率数　**DLC**
白血球有糸核分裂因子　**LMF**
白血球遊走因子　**LCF**
白血球遊走技術　**LMT**
白血球遊走試験　**LMT**
白血球遊走増強　**LME**
白血球遊走促進因子　**LMAF**
白血球遊走抑制　**LMI**
白血球遊走阻止因子　**LIF**
白血球遊走阻止検査　**LIT**
白血球遊走抑制試験　**LMIT**
白血球遊走抑制因子　**LMIF**
白血球遊走抑制反応　**LMIR**
白血球由来インターフェロン　**LIF**
白血球抑制因子　**LIF**
白血病ウイルス　**LV**
白血病関連抗原　**LAA**
白血病細胞　**LC**
白血病細胞由来抑制活性　**LIA**
白血病性(細)網内(皮)症　**LRE**
白血病阻止因子　**LIF**
白血病有意線量　**LSD**
抜管　**extub**
抜管した　**extub**
抜管する　**extub**
抜糸　**DSO, SR**
抜歯　**Ex, ex, Ext, ext**
抜歯(された)　**TE**
発育　**dev, devel, dvlp**
発育異常緑内障　**DG**
発育学　**som**
発育指数　**DQ**
発育した　**devd, devel**
発育する　**dev, dvlp**
発育遅延　**GR**
発育年齢　**DA, D.A.**
発育のない　**NG**
発育歴　**DH**
発音持続時間　**PT**
発刊予定　**MBI**
発汗　**persp**
発汗過多(症)　**HH**
発癌剤　**BBN**
発見されたもの　**q.e.i.**
発見されない　**nei**
(症状)発現　**manif, manifest**
発光スペクトル検出器　**ESD**
発光ダイオード　**LED**
発行された　**pub**
発行者　**pub**
発語オーケー　**sp.o.k.**
発酵学　**zymol**
発酵の　**F**

発散 **div, div.**
発射 **Dis, disch**
発射間間隔 **IDI**
(疾患の)発症および経過 **O & C, O+C**
発症後病院到着前心疾患対策 **PHCC**
発症直後(に) **IAO**
発振器 **osc**
発情 **Ht, ht**
発生 **occ**
発生学 **AER, EMB, Emb, emb, embry, embryol**
発生源入力システム **OES**
発生時間 **GT**
発生率 **IN**
発声指数 **PQ**
発達 **dev, devel, dvlp**
発達眼窩研究室 **DORL**
発達させる **dev**
発達指数 **EQ**
発達障害 **DD**
発達スクリーニングテスト **MN**
発達する **dvlp**
発達年齢 **DA**
発達文章段階 **DSS**
発達率技術 **DART**
発痛点 **trig.pnt., trig.pt.**
発痛物質 **PPS**
発展因子分析 **EFA**
発熱 **fev**
発熱が続く間 **feb.dur.**
発熱がないときに **abs.feb.**
発熱している **feb.**
発熱時に **adst.feb.**
発熱性外毒素 **PE**
発熱性ダニ媒介脳炎 **PTBE**
発熱中 **aggred.feb.**
発熱様物質放出因子 **PRF**
発病力 **V**
発疱膏 **emp.vesic.**
発疱剤 **mal.**
発疱で **mal.**
花 **flor.**
放す **mitt, mitt.**
鼻アレルギー **NA**
鼻カニューレ **NC**
鼻からの距離 **DFN**
鼻クリアランス **NC**
鼻と咽喉 **NT, N & T, N & thr**
鼻の **N, n, NAS**
鼻変形 **ND**
鼻ポリープ **NP**
鼻ポリープ切除術 **NP**
鼻マスク人工換気〔呼吸〕法 **NMV**
鼻マスクによる間欠陽圧補助呼吸 **NIPPV**
離れた **R, r.**
母(親) **M**
母親健康プログラム **MHP**
母親態度スケール(尺度) **MAS**
母親と父親 **M & F**
母親乳児ケア **MIC**
母方の叔父 **MU**
母方のおば **MA**
母方の祖父 **mat.gf, MGF**
母方の祖母 **mat.gm, MGM**
幅 **W, w**
幅広い切痕のあるP波 **WNPW**
早い **q**
早く **Ce**
早くわかるX線診断システム **IDX**
速い **f, qk, rap**
速さ **vel, vel., veloc, veloc.**
払いのけ反射 **WR**
腹 **ABD, Abd, abd, abd., abdo, ABDOM, Abdom, abdom**
腹(部)当てガーゼ **ABD (pad)**
腹の **ABD, Abd, abd, abd., abdo, ABDOM, Abdom, abdom, ven, vent, ventr**
針穴視力 **VA_{ph}**
針生検 **CNB**
針による肝生検 **NLB**
(注射)針をオープンに保て **KNO**
万国時間 **UT**
反回神経 **RLN**
反回神経麻痺 **RL, RNP**
反回の **rec, recur**
反響音 **ES**
反屈束 **FR**
反屈の **RF**
反社会的人格 **ASP**
反社会的な **AS**
反時針方向 **ACW**
反射 **ref, refl, refl.**
反射吸収性分光 **RAS**
反射係数 **RC**
反射光電式プレチスモグラフ **RPP**
反射する **refl, refl.**
反射性交感神経性異栄養症 **RSD**
反射性神経血管症候群 **RNS**
反射性寝返り運動 **RU**
反射性排尿収縮 **RMC**
反射抑制肢位 **RIP**
反対 **opp**
反対側衝撃 **CC**
反対側腎血漿流量

は

CRPF
反対側の耳を遮蔽して **OEM**
反対の **con., cont, cont., OP, Op, op, opp**
反転 **inv, REV, rev.**
反転回復法 **IR**
反転時間 **TI**
反時計方向 **CCW**
反応 **R, react, RESP, Resp, resp, resp., Rxn, RXN, rxn, rxns**
反応・刺激比 **RSR**
反応細胞 **RC**
反応時間 **RT**
反応刺激 **RS**
反応状態 **RC**
反応する **R, RESP, Resp, resp, resp.**
反応性気道疾患〔障害〕症候群 **RADS**
反応性好酸球性胸膜炎 **REP**
反応性充血 **RH**
反応性神経性うつ病 **RND**
反応性蛋白 **RP**
反応性電圧・電流 **RVA**
反応性リンパ細網細胞増生 **RLH**
反応漸減 **RD**
反応増加 **RI**
反応速度定数 **k**
反応のある **RESP, Resp, resp, resp.**
反応半減期 **T1/2**
反応物 **R**
反応率 **RR**
反応量と誤差の関係 **RER**
反復 **rec, recur**
反復運動症候群 **RMS**
反復最大負荷 **RM**
反復作用 **RA**
反復作用錠 **RAT**
反復刺激後増強 **PTP**
反復ストレス症候群 **RSS**
反復すべし **inter.**
反復性心房興奮 **RAF**
反復せよ **iter., reit., REP, rep., rept, rept.**
反復配列 **TRA**
半 **S, s, s.**
半円束 **FI**
半円の **SC**
半価層 **hvl, HVT, HWS**
半規管機能低下 **CP**
半規管麻痺 **CP**
半球 **H, Hemi**
半球間伝達時間 **IHTT**
半球血栓性梗塞 **HTI**
半球血流量 **HBF**
半球幅 **HW**
半月神経節ブロック **GGB**
半月弁 **SV**
半月弁閉鎖 **SC**
半径 **r, rad, rad.**
半径の **Ra**
半減期 **HL, HT,** $t_{1/2}$**, t1/2**
半腱様(筋) **ST**
半合成ヒトインスリン **SHI**
半さじ **c.medium**
半身照射 **HBI**
半浸透表面 **SPS**
半水平位 **SH**
半垂直位心電図 **SV**
半数染色体数 **N**
半数〔50%〕致死温度 LT_{50}
半数致死線量 **HWD**
半数致死量 LD_{50}
半数卵感染量 EID_{50}
半側麻痺 **hemi**
半値全幅 **FWHM**
半値半幅 **HWHM**
半致死量 **MDL**
半デスモゾーム **hd**
半導体検出器 **SSD**
半軟食 **SS**
半分 $\overline{SS}$, $\overline{SS}$, $\dot{S}\dot{S}$, **S, s, s., sem, sem., S-S, ss,** $\overline{SS}$, **ss.**
半分の **Dim., dim., HF, hf.**
半分を **FS**
半膜様の **SM**
半量 **ss.**
汎アレルギー状態 **PAS**
汎小葉型肺気腫 **PE**
汎小葉性肺気腫 **PLE**
汎収縮期雑音 **HSM**
汎適応症候群 **AAS, GAS**
汎発性高血圧性細動脈症 **AHD**
汎発性食道痙攣 **DES**
汎発性分化型リンパ球性リンパ腫 **DWDL**
汎網膜光凝固 **PRP**
汎用コリメーター **GP**
汎 T 細胞抗原 **Pan T**
阪大式知能検査 **OISA**
伴性高 IgM 症候群 **XLHM**
伴性若年性網膜分離(症) **XLJR**
伴性精神遅滞 **XLMR**
伴性低リン酸(塩)血(症) **XLH**
伴性無 γ グロブリン血症 **XLA**
伴性免疫不全症 **Xid**
伴性優性 **XD**
伴性劣性魚鱗癬 **XLI**
伴性劣性重症複合免疫不全症 **XSCID**
伴性劣性精神(発達)遅滞

XRMR
伴性劣性鉄芽球性貧血
XLSA
伴性劣性の **XLR, XR**
伴性劣性リンパ増殖症候群
XLP
版 **ed**
斑(紋) **Mac**
斑点関連絨毛 **PAV**
斑点状抗核抗体
FANA, SANA
斑点のある白い(粘膜)
WPN
晩期運動障害 **TD**
晩期全身(性)結核 **LGT**
晩期妊娠代謝性中毒症
MTLP
晩に **v.**
晩発性小脳皮質萎縮症
LCCA
晩発性皮質性小脳変性症
LCCD
晩発性皮膚ポルフィリン症
PCT
番号 **N, n, N, n., No, No., no., No., no., nos, Nr, Nr., num**
番号を付された **num**
範囲 **lim, regs**
瘢痕期 **Stage S**
瘢痕形成 **C**
瘢痕(性)類天疱瘡 **CP**

ひ

ヒアリンの　**HYLO**
ヒアリン膜症候群　**HMS**
ヒアルロン酸　**HA**
ピーエイチ　**pH**，**P_H**
ピエゾ電気の　**PZE**
ピエール・ロバン症候群　**PRS**
ヒオスシン　**H**
ビオチンカルボキシル運搬蛋白質　**BCCP**
ヒオデオキシコール酸　**HDCA**
ビオプテリン　**BP**
ビーカー　**bkr**
ビグアナイド剤　**BG**
ピーク気道圧　**PAP**
ピーク駆出までの時間　**TPE**
ピークフロー　**PFR**
ピグミ・チンパンジー　**PPA**
ピコ(＝10^{-15})　**P**
ピコキュリー　**pC**，**pc**，**pCi**
ピコグラム　**pg**
ピコピコグラム　**ppg**，**ppg.**
ピコ秒　**ps**，**PSEC**
ピコファラド　**pF**
ピコメートル　**pm**
ピコモル　**pM**
ピコリットル　**pl**
ピシバニール　**PIC**
ビジョルク・シャイリー(弁)　**B-S**
ビス　**bis**
ヒス・プルキンエ系　**HPS**
ビスエーテル　**BCME**
ヒスキー・ネブラスカ学習適性検査　**HNTLA**
ビスクロロエチルニトロソウレア，ビンクリスチン，アドリアマイシン，プレドニゾン　**BVAP**
ビスクロロエチルニトロソ尿素(＝カルムスチン)　**BCNU**
ビスクロロエチルニトロソ尿素，アラビノシルシトシン，シクロホスファミド　**BAC**
ビスクロロエチルニトロソ尿素，アラビノシルシトシン，シクロホスファミド，6-チオグアニン　**BACT**
ビスクロロエチルニトロソ尿素，エトポシド，アラビノシルシトシン，シクロホスファミド　**BEAC**
ビスクロロエチルニトロソ尿素，エトポシド，アラビノシルシトシン，メルファラン　**BEAM**
ビスクロロエチルニトロソ尿素，シクロホスファミド，アドリアマイシン，プレドニゾン　**BCAP**
ビスクロロエチルニトロソ尿素，シクロホスファミド，ビンブラスチン，プロカルバジン，プレドニゾン　**BCVPP**
ビスクロロエチルニトロソ尿素，シクロホスファミド，プレドニゾン　**BCP**
ビスクロロエチルニトロソ尿素，シクロホスファミド，プロカルバジン，プレドニゾロン　**BCPP**
ビスクロロエチルニトロソ尿素，ヒドロキシ尿素，ダカルバジン　**BHD**
ビスクロロエチルニトロソ尿素，ヒドロキシ尿素，ダカルバジン，ビンクリスチン　**BHD-V**
ビスクロロエチルニトロソ尿素，ビンクリスチン，ダカルバジン　**BVD**
ビスクロロエチルニトロソ尿素，ビンクリスチン(＝オンコビン)，プレドニゾン　**BOP**
ビスクロロエチルニトロソ尿素，ビンクリスチン(＝オンコビン)，プロカルバジン，プレドニゾン　**BOPP**
ビスクロロエチルニトロソ尿素，メトトレキサート，プロカルバジン　**BMP**
ビスクロロメチルエーテル　**BCME**
ビスジアゾ化ベンチジン　**BDB**
ヒス心室時間　**HV interval**，**HV time**
ヒス束　**BH**，**HB**
ヒス束下ブロック　**HV block**
ヒス束上ブロック　**AH block**
ヒス束電位図　**HBE**
ヒス束内ブロック　**BH block**
ヒスタグロビン　**HG**
ビスタマイシン　**VSM**
ヒスタミン　**HA**，**Hist**，**hist**
ヒスタミン・イオン転換　**HIT**
ヒスタミン2受容体　**H2R**
ヒスタミンウサギ血清アルブミン接合　**HRSA**
ヒスタミン含有ニューロン　**HN**
ヒスタミン吸入試験　**HIT**

ヒスタミン丘斑試験 **HWT**
ヒスタミン固定力 **HPP**
ヒスタミン受容体 **HR**
ヒスタミン増感因子 **HSF**
ヒスタミンチャレンジ試験 **HCT**
ヒスタミン放出活性 **HRA**
ヒスタミンメチルトランスフェラーゼ **HMT**
ヒスタミン誘発試験 **HPT**
ヒスタミン誘発性抑制因子 **HSF**
ヒスタミン遊離因子 **HRF**
ヒスタミン遊離試験 **HRT**
ヒスタミン様物質 **H-subst**
ヒスタミン抑制放出因子 **HIRF**
ヒスチジル **His**
ヒスチジン **H，HI，Hi，His，HIS，Hist，hist**
ヒスチジン血症 **Hist，hist**
ヒスチジンデカルボキシラーゼ **HDC**
ヒスチジンリッチグリコプロテイン **HRG**
ヒスチジン類似 α ヒドラジン **AHH**
ヒステリー **HV，Hy，hy，HYS，hys.**
ヒステリー性変換反応 **HCR**
ヒステリーの **HYS，hys.**
ヒストサイトーシス X **HX**
ヒストプラズマ(属) **H**
ヒストプラズマ症 **histo**
ヒストプラズマ組織抑制因子 **HIF**
ビストリメチルシリトリフルオロアセトアミド **BSTFA**
ビスマス **Bi**
ビスリン酸 **P_2**
ヒ素 **As**
ビタミン **V，Vit，vit**
ビタミンA **VA**
ビタミンA欠乏(症) **VAD**
ビタミンB **VB**
ビタミンB_{12r} **cob II**
ビタミンB_{12s} **cob I**
ビタミンB群 **vit Bcx**
ビタミンB複合体 **B vit.compl**
ビタミンC **VC**
ビタミンD **D，VD**
ビタミンD依存性(くる病) **VDD**
ビタミンD依存性くる病 **DDR，VDDR**
ビタミンD結合蛋白 **DBP**
ビタミンD抵抗性くる病 **VDRR**
ビタミンD不足骨障害 **HVDO**
ビタミンE **E，VE**
ビタミンF **VF**
ビタミンG **VG**
ビタミンH **VH**
ビタミンI **VI**
ビタミンJ **VJ**
ビタミンK **VK**
ビタミンK_1 **K_1**
ビタミンK_2 **K_2**
ビタミンK_3 **K_3**
ビタミンK欠乏誘導蛋白 **PIVKA**
ビタミンL **VL**
ビタミンM **VM**
ビタミンP **vit P，VP**
ビタミンPP **vit PP，VPP**
ビタミンT **V.T**
ビタミンU **VU**
ビタミン化学者協会 **AVC**
ピック病 **PD**
ヒックマンライン **HL**
ヒツジ **Sh**
ヒツジ細胞凝集試験 **SCAT**
ヒツジ膵臓ポリペプチド **OPP**
ヒツジ成長ホルモン **OGH**
ヒツジ精嚢 **SSV**
ヒツジ赤血球 **SE，SRBC，SRC**
ヒツジ赤血球凝集テスト **SEAT**
ヒツジ赤血球凝集反応 **SCAT**
ヒツジ赤血球抗原 **SLEA**
ヒツジ赤血球抗体 **SLEA**
ヒツジ赤血球ロゼット形成能 **SERFC**
ヒツジ胎盤ラクトゲン **OPL**
ヒツジ乳腺刺激ホルモン **OLH**
ヒツジプロラクチン **OP**
ヒツジ(赤血球)ロゼット形成細胞 **SRFC**
ピッチ期間比 **PPQ**
ピッチバランス **PB**
ピッツバーグ肺炎因子 **PP，PPA**
ピーテン **PTEN**
ビット/秒 **bps**
ヒッペル・リンダウ症候群 **HLS**
ビデオ記録装置 **EVRS**

ひ

ビデオコントラスト増強
VEC
ビデオ増幅顕微鏡　**VIM**
ビデオ表示装置　**VDU**
ビデオレコーダー　**VTR**
ヒト　**H, h, HSA, per**
ヒトリンパ芽球(性)インターフェロン　**HLBI**
ヒトαフェトプロテイン
HAFP
ヒトB細胞特異抗原
HBSA
ヒトBリンパ球抗原
HBLA
ヒトNK細胞　**HNK**
ヒトT細胞好性ウイルスIII型　**ARV**
ヒトT細胞特異抗原
hTS
ヒトT細胞白血病ウイルス　**HTLV**
ヒトT細胞白血病ウイルス関連膜抗原
HTLV-MA
ヒトTリンパ球抗原
HTLA
ヒトTリンパ球向性ウイルス　**HTLV**
ヒトTリンパ球向性ウイルスI〔II/III〕型
HTLV-I〔II, III〕
ヒトTリンパ球向性ウイルス関連気管支・肺胞異常症　**HABA**
ヒトTリンパ球向性ウイルス関連膜抗原
HTLV-MA
ヒトアジュバント病
HAD
ヒト遺伝子組換え型腫瘍壊死因子　**RH-TNF**
ヒトインターフェロン
HuIFN
ヒト栄養　**HN**
ヒトエンテロウイルス
HEV
ヒト黄体化ホルモン
hLH
ヒト黄体刺激ホルモン
hPr, hPRL
ヒトオウム病ウイルス
HPV
ヒト下垂性性腺刺激ホルモン　**hHG**
ヒト下垂体性腺刺激ホルモン　**hPG**
ヒト下垂体の　**HP**
ヒト下垂体卵胞刺激ホルモン　**hPFSH, hPPSH**
ヒト顆粒球性エールリヒア症　**HGE**
ヒトカルシトニン　**hCT**
ヒト冠状ウイルス　**HCV**
ヒトガンマグロブリン
HGG, hGG
ヒト旧ツベルクリン
HOT
ヒト狂犬病免疫グロブリン
HRIG, HRIg, RIgH
ヒト胸腺抗血清
HUTHAS
ヒト胸腺細胞抗原　**HTA**
ヒト胸腺白血病　**HTL, HTLA**
ヒト胸腺白血病関連抗原
HThyL
ヒト形質細胞抗原
HPCA
ヒト(型)結核菌　**MTB, M tuberc., M.tuberc**
ヒト血球凝集試験
HCAT
ヒト血小板懸濁液　**HPS**
ヒト血小板抗原　**HPA**
ヒト血小板濃縮物
SD-PC
ヒト血小板由来成長因子
hPDGF
ヒト血清　**HS**
ヒト血清アルブミン
HSA, HuSA
ヒト血清胸腺因子
HSTF
ヒト血清蛋白　**HSP**
ヒト血清プレアルブミン
HSP
ヒト好塩基球脱顆粒試験
HBDT
ヒト甲状腺アデニルシクラーゼ刺激物質
HTACS
ヒト甲状腺刺激因子
hTS
ヒト甲状腺刺激抗体
hTSAb
ヒト甲状腺刺激ホルモン
hTS, hTSH
ヒト好中球エラスターゼ
HNE
ヒト好中球コラゲナーゼ
HNC
ヒト抗マウス抗体
HAMA
ヒト呼吸器コロナウイルス
HRCV
ヒト黒色腫細胞系　**HMV**
ヒト骨格成長因子　**hSGF**
ヒト骨肉腫　**HOS**
ヒトコロナウイルス感受性
HCVS
ヒト臍静脈　**HUV**
ヒト臍帯血清　**HCS**
ヒト臍帯静脈移植片
HUCVG
ヒト臍帯静脈内皮細胞
HUVECs
ヒトサイトメガロウイルス
HCMV, human CMV
ヒト耳下腺リゾチーム
HPL
ヒト絨毛性性腺刺激ホルモン　**hCG**
ヒト絨毛性ソマトトロピン

ひ

HCS
ヒト絨毛性ソマトマンモトロピン(＝ヒト胎盤性ラクトゲン) HCS, hCS, hcs, HCSM, hCSM
ヒト絨毛性卵胞刺激ホルモン hCFSH
ヒト腫瘍幹細胞効力検定 HTSCA
ヒト腫瘍コロニー効力検定 HTCA
ヒト上皮細胞 HEP
ヒト腎(細胞) HK
ピトシン pit
ヒト神経芽(細胞)腫 HNB
ヒト腎細胞 HKC
ヒト心房性ナトリウム利尿ペプチド HANP
ヒト心房性ナトリウム利尿ホルモン hANP
ヒト膵成長ホルモン放出因子 hpGRF
ヒト膵トリプシン抑制因子 HPTIN
ヒト膵ポリペプチド hPP
ヒト性腺刺激ホルモン HG, hG
ヒト成長〔生長〕因子 HG, hG
ヒト成長ホルモン hGH
ヒト成長ホルモン刺激因子 HGRF, hGRF
ヒト赤白血病 HEL
ヒト赤血球 HRBC, HuE, HuRBC
ヒト赤血球凝集試験 HEAT
ヒト赤血球抗原 HEA
ヒト赤血球試験 HEA
ヒト線維芽細胞 HF
ヒト線維芽細胞インターフェロン HFI, hFI, HFIF, hFIF
ヒト胎児線維芽細胞 HEF
ヒト胎児の二次口蓋の間葉組織から樹立された細胞 HEPM
ヒト胎児肺 HFL, hFL
ヒト胎盤(性)甲状腺刺激ホルモン hPT
ヒト胎盤性乳腺刺激ホルモン HCS
ヒト胎盤性ラクトゲン HPL, hPL
ヒト胎盤調整培地 HPCM
ヒト胎盤培養基 HPCM
ヒト大網小動脈由来内皮細胞 HOME
ヒト唾液糖蛋白 HSGP
ヒト多剤耐性蛋白 hMRP
ヒト腸上皮(細胞) HIE
ヒト治療量 HTD
ヒトT細胞白血病 HTL
ヒトT細胞白血病ウイルスI型関連脊髄症 HAM
ヒトT細胞白血病ウイルスI型関連気管支肺病変 HAB
ヒトT細胞白血病ウイルスI〔II/III〕型 HTLV-I〔II, III〕
ヒトT細胞白血病ウイルス脊髄症 HAM
ヒトT細胞リンパ腫 HTL
ヒトTリンパ球向性ウイルスI型関連気管支肺病変 HAB
ヒトTリンパ球向性ウイルスI型関連脊髄症 HAM
ヒト糖尿病性神経障害 HDN
ヒトと動物の結束 HAB
ヒトトロンビン HT
ヒト内因子濃縮 HIFC
ヒト内皮細胞 HEC
ヒト二倍体狂犬病ワクチン HDRV
ヒト二倍体細胞 HDC
ヒト二倍体細胞株(系) HDCS
ヒト乳癌細胞膜プロテイナーゼ HMCCMP
ヒト乳逆転写酵素 HMRTE
ヒト乳腺腫瘍 HBT
ヒト乳頭腫ウイルス HPV
ヒト乳頭腫ウイルス感染 HPV
ヒトニューロフィシン HNP
ヒト尿カリクレイン HUK
ヒトの Hu
ヒトの腸の HE
ヒトの乳癌と卵巣癌 HBOC
ヒトの発育と家庭生活 HDFL
ヒトノミ(属) P
ヒト胚腎(細胞) HEK
ヒト胚肺 HEL
ヒト胚肺線維芽細胞 HELF
ヒト胚脾臓 hES
ヒト胚皮膚 hES
ヒト肺胞マクロファージ HAM
ヒト肺野 HLF
ヒト破傷風抗毒素 HTAT
ヒト破傷風免疫グロブリン hTIg
ヒト白血球 HL
ヒト白血球インターフェロン HLI

ヒト白血球インターフェロン環境 **HUIFM**
ヒト白血球エラスターゼ **HLE**
ヒト白血球抗原 **HLA, HLA antigen**
ヒト白血球抗原 A **HLAA**
ヒト白血球抗原 B **HLAB**
ヒト白血球抗原 D **HLAD**
ヒト白血球抗原 L **HLAL**
ヒト白血球分化抗原 **HLDA**
ヒトパルボウイルス **HPV**
ヒト反応 **H**
ヒト微小血管内皮細胞 **MvEC**
ヒト皮膚血管内皮細胞 **HMVECs**
ヒト表皮性成長因子 **hEGF**
ヒトブドウ糖排出量 **HGO, hGO**
ヒトプロラクチン **hPL, hPr, hPRL**
ヒト閉経期ゴナドトロピン・ヒト絨毛性ゴナドトロピン **hMG-hCG**
ヒト閉経期ゴナドトロピンに関する国際文献機関 **IRP-HMG**
ヒト閉経期尿性性腺刺激ホルモン **hMG**
ヒト閉経期の **HMP**
ヒトヘルペスウイルス **HVH**
ヒトヘルペスウイルス 1〔2,3…7〕型 **HHV1〔2,3…7〕**
ヒト乏塩アルブミン **HSA**
ヒト包皮上皮細胞 **HFEC**
ヒト包皮線維芽細胞 **HFF, hFF**
ヒトマクロファージ走化性および活性化因子 **rhMCAF**
ヒトマクロファージ増殖因子 **hMDGF**
ヒト末梢血単核細胞 **HPMC**
ヒト末梢血白血球 **HPBL**
ヒト末梢血リンパ球 **HPL**
ヒト末梢神経ミエリン抽出物 **HPNME**
ヒト免疫グロブリン **HIg**
ヒト免疫グロブリン A の異種型マーカー **Am**
ヒト免疫グロブリン G の異種型マーカー **Gm**
ヒト免疫血清グロブリン **HISG**
ヒト免疫状態調査 **HISS**
ヒト免疫不全ウイルス **HIV**
ヒト免疫不全ウイルス感染症 **HIV infection**
ヒト免疫不全ウイルス関連歯周炎 **HIV-P**
ヒト免疫不全ウイルス抗体 **HIV-AB**
ヒトモル甲状腺刺激ホルモン **hMT**
ヒドララジン **HDZ, HYD**
ヒト卵管液 **HOF**
ヒト卵巣癌 **HOC**
ヒト卵胞刺激ホルモン **HFSH, hFSH**
ヒトリンパ球 **HL**
ヒトリンパ球インターフェロン **HLI**
ヒトリンパ球抗原 **HLA**
ヒトリンパ球抗原 B **HLAB**
ヒトリンパ球抗原 C **HLAC**
ヒトリンパ球抗原 D **HLAD**
ヒトリンパ球抗体 **HLA**
ヒト累積卵母細胞複合 **COC**
ヒトレオウイルス様の **HRVL**
ヒトレッシュ・ナイハン（細胞） **HLN**
ヒトレトロウイルス性疾患 **HRD**
ヒドロキシ **OH**
ヒドロキシ・ヘプタデカトリエノン酸 **HHT**
ヒドロキシアシル・コエンザイム A デヒドロゲナーゼ **HADH**
ヒドロキシアパタイト **HA, HAP**
ヒドロキシイソバレリン酸 **Hyv**
ヒドロキシインドール **HI**
ヒドロキシインドール-*O*-メチル転移酵素 **HIOMT**
ヒドロキシインドール酢酸 **OH IAA**
ヒドロキシエイコサテトラエン酸 **HETE**
ヒドロキシエチルセルロース **HEC**
ヒドロキシエチルデンプン **HES**
ヒドロキシエチルメチルセルロース **HEMA**
ヒドロキシエルゴカルシフェロール **HEC**
ヒドロキシコバラミン **OHB_{12}**

ヒドロキシコルチコイド **HC, HOC**
ヒドロキシコルチコステロイド **HCS, OH, OHCS, OHCs**
ヒドロキシコルチゾン **HCT**
ヒドロキシコレカルシフェロール **OHC**
ヒドロキシコレカルシフェロール(=ビタミンD) **HCC**
ヒドロキシ脂肪酸 **OHFA**
ヒドロキシダウノマイシン,ビンクリスチン(=オンコビン),アラビノシルシトシン,プレドニゾン,ブレオマイシン **HOAP-BLEO**
ヒドロキシダウノマイシン,ビンクリスチン(=オンコビン),プレドニゾン **HOP**
ヒドロキシデオキシコルチコステロン **OH-DOC**
ヒドロキシトリプタミン(=セロトニン) **HT, HTA**
ヒドロキシトリプトファン(=セロトニン前駆体) **HTP**
ヒドロキシニトロベンジルブロミド **HNB**
ヒドロキシ尿素 **HU, HUR, HYD**
ヒドロキシの **ho**
ヒドロキシフェニル・シンコニン酸 **HPC**
ヒドロキシフェニル・フェニルヒダントイン **HPPH**
ヒドロキシフェニル酢酸 **HPAA**
ヒドロキシフェニル乳酸 **HPLA**
ヒドロキシフェニルピルビン酸 **HPPA**
ヒドロキシフェニルピルビン酸酸化酵素 **HPPO**
ヒドロキシプロピルセルロース **HPC**
ヒドロキシプロピルメチルセルロース **HPC**
ヒドロキシプロリン **HPR, HYP, Hyp, Hypro, OHP**
ヒドロキシヘキサミド **HH**
ヒドロキシメステロン **HMS**
ヒドロキシメチル **hm**
ヒドロキシメチル・ウラシル **HMU**
ヒドロキシメチルグルタリル **HMG**
ヒドロキシメチルグルタリルコエンザイムA還元酵素 **HMG-CoA reductase**
ヒドロキシメチルシトシン **HMC**
ヒドロキシメチルフルフラル **HMF**
ヒドロキシラーゼ **OHlase**
ヒドロキシリジン **HYL, Hyl**
ヒドロキシリン **Hydrox**
ヒドロキシルメチルセルロース **HMC**
ヒドロキシルラジカル **OH**
ヒドロキソコバラミン **OH-Cbl**
ヒドロクロロチアジド **HCT, HCTZ, Hctz**
ヒドロコルチゾン **F, HC, HCT, Hyd**
ヒドロコルチゾン・インスリン・トランスフェリン・エストラジオール・セレン **HITES**
ヒドロコルチゾン試験 **HT**
ヒトロタウイルス **HRV**
ビトロネクチン **VN**
ビトロネクチン受容体 **VNR**
ヒドロペルオキシ・エイコサ・テトラエノイン酸 **HPETE**
ヒドロペルオキシアラキドン酸 **HPAA**
ピーナッツ凝集 **PNA**
ビニルエーテル **Vin**
ピバンピシリン **PVPC**
ビーピーエムシー **BPMC**
ビフィズス菌 **Lac-B**
ピブメシリナム **PMPC**
ビブリオ(属) **V, *V.***
ピペコリン酸 **PA**
ピペミド酸 **PP, PPA**
ピペラシリン **PIP, PIPC**
ピペラジン-*N*,*N'*-ビス(2-エタンスルホン酸) **PIPES**
ヒポキサンチン **HX**
ヒポキサンチン・アミノプテリン・チミジン培地 **HAT medium**
ヒポキサンチン・チミジン **HT**
ヒポキサンチン(グアニン)ホスホリボシルトランスフェラーゼ **HGPRT**
ヒポキサンチンホスホリボシルトランスフェラーゼ **HPRT**
ヒポキサンチンリボシド **HXR**
ヒポクラテス **HIPP**

ヒポコンドリー(症) **Hs**
ヒマシ油 **CO**
ヒマシ油・温浴・浣腸 **OBE**
ピマリシン **PMR**
ヒュー・パウエルのデジタル表示装置 **HP-D**
ヒューナー試験 **HT**
ビュルガー・グリュッツ(症候群) **BG**
ピューロマイシン **PM**
ヒヨコ感染量 **CID**
ヒヨコ細胞凝集量 **CCA**
ヒヨスチン・モルヒネ・カクタス・皮下注射剤 **HMC hypodermic tablets**
ピラジナミド **PZA**
ヒラメ筋 **GS, SOL**
ピリジル酢酸第二水銀 **PMA**
ピリジン **Pyr, pyr**
ピリジンアルドキシムメチオジド **PAM**
ピリジン酢酸 **PAA**
ビリダンス連鎖球菌(性)心内膜炎 **SVE**
ピリチオン亜鉛 **ZPT**
ピリドキサミン **PM**
ピリドキサミンリン酸 **PMP**
ピリドキサ(ー)ル **PL**
ピリドキサ(ー)ル **Py**
ピリドキサ(ー)ル-5′-リン酸 **P-5′-P**
ピリドキサ(ー)ル-5′-リン酸 **PyrP**
ピリドキサ(ー)ルリン酸 **PLP**
ピリドキサ(ー)ルリン酸 **PALP**
ピリドキサレイテッド・プリペライズド・ヘモグロビン液 **Pr-Pl-Hb**
ピリドキシン **PIN, PN**
ピリドキシン-5′-リン酸 **PNP**
ピリドキシン欠乏食 **PDD**
ピリドンカルボン酸 **PCA**
ピリベンザミン **PBZ**
ピリミジン **Py, Pyr, pyr**
ピリミジン-5′-ヌクレオチダーゼ **P5N**
ピリミジンヌクレオシド **Pyd, Y**
ピリメタミンキニーネ **PQ**
ビリルビン **BIL, bil, bili, bilirub, BR**
ビリルビン/アルブミン(比) **BIL/ALB**
ビリルビングルクロノシドグルクロノシル転移酵素 **BGGT**
ビリルビン最小濃度 **MCBR**
ビリルビン産生 **BRP**
ビリルビンジグルクロナイド **BDG**
ビリルビンモノグルクロナイド **BMG**
ビルギニウム **VI**
ヒルゲンライナー・パーキンス **H-P**
ピル後乳汁分泌無月経 **PPGA**
ヒルシュスプルング関連腸炎 **HAEC**
ヒルシュスプルング病 **HD, HSCR**
ビールショウスキー・ヤンスキー(症候群) **BJ**
ピルビン酸塩 **Pyr, pyr**
ピルビン酸カルボキシラーゼ **PC**
ピルビン酸キナーゼ **PK, PVK**
ピルビン酸酸化因子 **POF**
ピルビン酸酸化酵素 **PO**
ピルビン酸脱水素酵素 **PDH**
ピルビン酸脱水素酵素複合体 **PDHC**
ピルプロフェン **PPF**
ビルレンス抗原 **Vi antigen**
ビルロートⅠ法 **B-Ⅰ, BⅠ**
ビルロートⅡ法 **B-Ⅱ, BⅡ**
ピレンデカン酸 **PDA**
ピロカルピン **PL**
ピログルタミン酸 **pyroglu**
ピロコッカスフリオサス **Pfu**
ビロードクサフジ凝集素 **VVA**
ビロードクサフジレクチン **VVL**
ピロホスファターゼ **PP**
ピロミド酸 **PA**
ピロリジンジチオカルボン酸 **PDTC**
ピロリジンメチルテトラサイクリン **PLM-Tc**
ピロリンカルボキシ酸 **pc**
ピロリン酸塩 **PP, PYP, Pyro**
ピロリン酸関節症 **PA**
ピロルニトリン **PN, PRLN**
ピロロキノリンキノン **PQQ**
ビン **bot, lag., phial, V**
ピン **P**
ビンカロイコブラスチン **VLB**
ピンク **P**

ビンクリスチン **VC, VCR**
ビンクリスチン,6-メルカプトプリン,プレドニゾロン **VMP**
ビンクリスチン,6-メルカプトプリン,プレドニゾン **VMP**
ビンクリスチン,L-アスパラギナーゼ,プレドニゾン **VLP**
ビンクリスチン,アクチノマイシン,プレドニゾン **VAP**
ビンクリスチン,アクチノマイシン,メトトレキサート,プレドニゾン **VAMP**
ビンクリスチン,アクチノマイシンD,シクロホスファミド **VAC**
ビンクリスチン,アクチノマイシンD,シクロホスファミド,アドリアマイシン **VACA**
ビンクリスチン,アクチノマイシンD,ブレオマイシン **VAB**
ビンクリスチン,アドリアマイシン,6-メルカプトプリン,プレドニゾロン **VAMP**
ビンクリスチン,アドリアマイシン,塩酸ニムスチン **VAN**
ビンクリスチン,アドリアマイシン,シクロホスファミド **VAC**
ビンクリスチン,アドリアマイシン,シスプラチン **VAC**
ビンクリスチン,アドリアマイシン,デキサメタゾン **VAD**
ビンクリスチン,アドリアマイシン,デキサメタゾン,アクチノマイシンD **VADA**
ビンクリスチン,アドリアマイシン,フルオロウラシル,メトトレキサート(=アメトプテリン),シクロホスファミド **VAFAC**
ビンクリスチン,アドリアマイシン,プレドニゾン,アラビノシルシトシン **VAPA**
ビンクリスチン,アドリアマイシン,プロカルバジン **VAP**
ビンクリスチン,アドリアマイシン,メチルプレドニゾロン **VAMP**
ビンクリスチン,アメトプテリン,6-メルカプトプリン,プレドニゾロン **VAMP**
ビンクリスチン,アメトプテリン,6-メルカプトプリン,プレドニゾン **VAMP**
ビンクリスチン(=オンコビン),アラビノシルシトシン,プレドニゾン **OAP**
ビンクリスチン,シクロホスファミド(=エンドキサン),6-メルカプトプリン,プレドニゾロン **VEMP**
ビンクリスチン,シクロホスファミド(=エンドキサン),6-メルカプトプリン,プレドニゾン **VEMP**
ビンクリスチン,カルボコン,アドリアマイシン **VCQ**
ビンクリスチン,カルボコン,フルオロウラシル,プレドニゾロン **VQFP**
ビンクリスチン,カルムスチン,シクロホスファミド,メルファラン,プレドニゾン **M2, M-2**
ビンクリスチン(=オンコビン),ジアンヒドロガラクチトール,アドリアマイシン,プラチノール **ODAP**
ビンクリスチン,シクロホスファミド,6-メルカプトプリン,プレドニゾロン **VCMP**
ビンクリスチン,シクロホスファミド,アドリアマイシン,プレドニゾン **VCAP**
ビンクリスチン,シクロホスファミド(=エンドキサン),ナツラン,プレドニゾロン **VENP**
ビンクリスチン,シクロホスファミド(=エンドキサン),ナツラン,プレドニゾン **VENP**
ビンクリスチン,シクロホスファミド,フルオロウラシル **VCF**
ビンクリスチン,シクロホスファミド(=エンドキサン),プレドニゾロン **VEP**
ビンクリスチン,シクロホスファミド(=エンドキサン),プレドニゾロン,アドリアマイシン **VEPA**
ビンクリスチン,シクロホスファミド,プレドニゾン **VCP**
ビンクリスチン,シクロホスファミド(=エンドキサン),マイトマイシンC

VEM
ビンクリスチン,シクロホスファミド(=エンドキサン),メトトレキサート,プレドニゾン **VEMP**
ビンクリスチン,シクロホスファミド,メルファラン,プレドニゾン **VCMP**
ビンクリスチン,ダウノルビシン,プレドニゾン **VDP**
ビンクリスチン,ダクチノマイシン,ブレオマイシン,シスプラチン,シクロホスファミド **VDBCC**
ビンクリスチン,ドキソルビシン,デキサメタゾン **VDD**
ビンクリスチン,ビスクロロエチルニトロソ尿素,アドリアマイシン **VBA**
ビンクリスチン,ビスクロロエチルニトロソ尿素,アドリアマイシン,プレドニゾン **VBAP**
ビンクリスチン,ビスクロロエチルニトロソ尿素,メルファラン,シクロホスファミド,プレドニゾン **VBMCP**
ビンクリスチン,フルオロウラシル,アドリアマイシン,マイトマイシンC **VFAM**
ビンクリスチン,ブレオマイシン,シスプラチン **VBC**
ビンクリスチン,ブレオマイシン,メトトレキサート **VBM**
ビンクリスチン,プレドニゾロン **VP, V-P**
ビンクリスチン,プレドニゾン **VP**
ビンクリスチン(=オンコビン),プレドニゾン,L-アスパラギナーゼ **OPAL**
ビンクリスチン,プレドニゾン,シクロホスファミド,アラビノシルシトシン **VPCA**
ビンクリスチン,プレドニゾン,シクロホスファミド,メトトレキサート,フルオロウラシル **VPCMF**
ビンクリスチン,プレドニゾン,ビンブラスチン,クロラムブシル,プロカルバジン **VPBCPr**
ビンクリスチン(=オンコビン),プロカルバジン,プレドニゾン **OPP**
ビンクリスチン,メトトレキサート,アドリアマイシン,アクチノマイシンD **VMAD**
ビンクリスチン,メトトレキサート,プレドニゾロン **VMetP**
ビンクリスチン,メルファラン,シクロホスファミド,プレドニゾン **VMCP**
ヒンズ・ツー〔スリー〕 **Hind** II〔III〕
ビンスワグナー型血管性痴呆 **VDBT**
ピン痛覚 **PP**
ビンデシン **VDN, VDS**
ビンデシン,エトポシド,プロカルバジン,プレドニゾン,ブレオマイシン **FEPP-B**
ヒントン(梅毒検査) **Hint**
ヒントン試験 **Hint test**
ビンブラスチン **VB, VBL, Vbt, VLB**
ビンブラスチン,アクチノマイシンD,ブレオマイシン **mini-VAB**
ビンブラスチン,アクチノマイシンD,ブレオマイシン,シスプラチン,シクロホスファミド **VAB-6**
ビンブラスチン,アドリアマイシン,チオテパ **VATH**
ビンブラスチン,アドリアマイシン,チオテパ,ハロテスチン **VATH**
ビンブラスチン,アドリアマイシン,ブレオマイシン,シクロヘキシルクロロエチルニトロソ尿素〔ウレア〕,ダカルバジン **VABCD**
ビンブラスチン,アドリアマイシン,マイトマイシンC **VAM**
ビンブラスチン,イホスファミド,(硝酸)ガリウム **VIG**
ビンブラスチン,イホスファミド,シスプラチン(=プラチノール) **VIP**
ビンブラスチン,エトポシド,プレドニゾン,アドリアマイシン **VEPA**
ビンブラスチン,エトポシド,プレドニゾン,アドリアマイシン,ブレオマイシン **VEPA-B**
ビンブラスチン,ダカルバジン,シスプラチン(=プラチノール) **VDP**

ひ

ビンブラスチン,ブレオマイシン　**VB**
ビンブラスチン,ブレオマイシン,シスプラチン(＝プラチノール)　**VBP**
ビンブラスチン,ブレオマイシン,メトトレキサート　**VBM**
ビンロシジン　**VRD**
ビンを振盪した後に　**p.p.a.**
ひきがね点　**trig.pnt.,trig.pt.**
ひずみ　**str**
ひだ　**Lig, lig, lig., Lig, lig, lig., ligg, ligg., ligg, ligg., ligs, P**
ひとつまみの　**pug.**
ひと握り　**m., man., manip., p.**
び漫〔広汎〕性間質性線維化肺炎　**DIFP**
び漫性間質性肺炎　**DIP**
び漫〔広汎〕性細網肉腫　**DHL**
び漫〔広汎〕性糸球体腎炎　**DGN**
び漫〔広汎〕性軸索損傷　**DAI**
び漫〔広汎〕性視床投射　**DTPS**
び漫〔広汎〕性増殖性糸球体腎炎　**DPGN**
び漫〔広汎〕性増殖性ループス腎炎　**DPLN**
び漫〔広汎〕性特発性硬化性骨増殖症　**DISH**
び漫〔広汎〕性特発性骨増殖症　**DISH**
び漫〔広汎〕性内膜肥厚　**DIT**
び漫〔広汎〕性粘着性大腸菌　**DAEC**
び漫性の　**D**
び漫〔広汎〕性脳損傷　**DBI**
び漫〔広汎〕性肺胞障害　**DAD**
び漫〔広汎〕性汎細気管支炎　**DPB**
び漫〔広汎〕性表層角膜炎　**KSD**
び漫〔広汎〕性腹膜炎　**Panperi**
び漫〔広汎〕性未分化リンパ球性リンパ腫　**DPDL**
び漫〔汎発〕性淋菌感染　**DGI**
び漫〔広汎〕性リンパ腫混合型　**DM**
び漫〔広汎〕性リンパ腫小切れ込み核細胞型　**DSC**
び漫〔広汎〕性リンパ腫大細胞型　**DL**
び漫〔広汎〕性レビー小体病　**DLBD**
びらん　**Er**
びらん性骨関節炎　**EOA**
びらん性変形性関節症　**EOA**
引き金　**trig**
引き出す　**deriv**
引き離す　**dissoc**
火花放電イオン化固体質量分析法　**SSMS**
日　**D, d, D, d., da**
日ごとに　**dd.in d.**
日ごとの　**pd, p.d.**
日付　**D, d**
日付なし　**ND**
日内最高体温　**T-max, T_{max}**
日々　**in d.**
日々起こる慢性的頭痛　**CDH**
日焼け　**SB**
日焼けした　**BKD, br**
日焼け防止指数　**SPF**
日和見感染　**OI**
比　**R, r, rat**
比較　**Vergl**
比較医学士　**DCM**
比較遠心力　**RCF**
比較ゲノム交配　**CGH**
比較上の　**comp**
比較する　**comp, CP, cp, cp.**
比較生物学研究所　**ICB**
比較的大きい軽度減速　**FMVD**
比較的気体膨張　**RGE**
比較的停留時間　**RRT**
比較的な　**rel**
比較的に　**rel**
比較的薬剤強度　**RDI**
比較的流量率　**RF**
比較に適した　**comp**
比較(的)の　**comp**
比較の　**compar, vgl.**
比色定量計　**MR**
比色分析　**color.**
比重　**d, g, GD, SG, Sg, s.g, sg, spec.gr., sp.G, Sp.Gew., SP GR, Sp Gr, sp.gr**
(液体)比重測定(法)　**HHM**
比熱　**sp.ht**
比放射能　**S, SA**
比喩的に　**FIG**
比率　**prop**
(脈の)比率とリズム　**r & r**
比率のとれた　**ppn**
比率目盛　**Rs**
比率を保った　**prop**
比例　**ppn**
比例して　**in pro**
比例動作・積分動作・微分動作　**PID**
皮下(の)　**subcut, subcut.**
皮下(注射)　**HRPO**

ひ

皮下気腫　**SCE**
皮下神経刺激　**SCNS**
皮下注射　**H, hypo, IS, SC, sci**
皮下注射器　**H**
皮下注入　**H inf**
皮下に　**hypo, sc, subcu, subcu., subcut, subcut.**
皮下熱傷　**DB**
皮下の　**H, hype, hypo, SC, sc, SQ, sq, subcu, subcu., Sub-Q, subq, sub-q**
皮下ヒスタミン試験　**SHT**
皮下用錠剤　**HT, h.t.**
皮脂厚　**SFT**
皮質　**C, cort, cort.**
皮質遠心性抑制　**CFI**
皮質拡大因子　**CMF**
皮質下の　**SC**
(腎)皮質血流(量)　**CBF**
皮質視覚　**CV**
(腎)皮質集合尿細管　**CCT**
皮質錐体外路系　**COEPS**
皮質(性)体性感覚誘発電位　**CSEP**
皮質(性)体性感覚誘発反応　**CSER**
皮質(性)の　**cort, cort.**
皮質脳波　**ECC, ECoG**
皮質部集合尿細管　**CCD**
皮質味領域　**CTA**
皮質誘発電位　**CEP**
皮質(性)誘発反応　**CER**
皮(膚分)節　**derm**
皮内(の)　**IC, ic**
皮内試験　**IT**
皮内注射　**IC, ic**
皮内テスト　**IDT**
皮(膚)内の　**ID, id, i.d., i derm**
皮内の　**i cut**
皮内反応　**iCT, ICT, IDR**
皮膚　**SK, SKI**
皮膚・頭・目・耳・鼻・咽喉　**SHEENT**
皮膚・視覚認知　**DOP**
皮膚・梅毒学技士　**DST**
皮膚・フィルム(間)距離　**SFD**
皮膚T細胞白血病リンパ腫　**CTCL**
皮膚T細胞リンパ腫　**CTCL, CTLL**
皮膚悪性黒色腫　**CMM**
皮膚悪性リンパ腫　**CML**
皮膚移植(片)　**SG**
皮膚インピーダンス　**Sz**
皮膚壊死毒素　**DNT**
皮膚エリテマトーデス　**CLE**
皮膚炎　**Derm**
皮膚塩基性過敏症　**CBH**
皮膚温記録図　**DTG**
皮膚温度　**ST, Ts**
皮膚温度回復時間　**STRT**
皮膚温度検査　**STT**
皮膚科医　**D, Derm, derm, derm., DM**
皮膚潰瘍　**DU**
皮膚科学　**D, Derm, derm, derm., Derma, DM**
皮膚科学士　**M.S.Derm**
皮膚型結節性動脈周囲炎　**PNC**
皮膚科認定書　**DDM**
皮膚科の　**derm**
皮膚感作抗体　**SSA**
皮膚肝性ポルフィリン症　**CHP**
皮膚関連リンパ組織　**SALT**
皮膚筋炎　**DM, DMS**
皮膚螢光　**SF**
皮膚血管炎　**CV**
皮膚血流(量)　**CBF**
皮膚紅斑(線)量　**HED**
皮膚呼吸因子　**SRF**
皮膚コンダクタンス　**SC**
皮膚コンダクタンス反応　**SCR**
皮膚試験〔反応〕　**ST**
皮膚試験単位　**STU**
皮膚試験(用)量　**STD**
皮膚自己検査　**SSE**
皮膚糸状菌症　**DMT**
皮膚針刺試験　**SPT**
皮膚水分喪失　**CWL**
皮膚線維芽細胞　**SF**
皮膚線量　**SD, S.D.**
皮膚単位　**SU**
皮膚単位量　**HED, SUD**
皮膚抵抗　**SR**
皮膚(電気)抵抗反射　**SRR**
皮膚抵抗反射　**SPR**
皮膚(電気)抵抗反応　**SRR**
皮膚抵抗変化　**SRC**
皮膚電位　**EDA, SP**
皮膚電位活動　**SPA**
皮膚電位反射　**SPR**
皮膚電位反応　**SPR**
皮膚電位レベル　**SPL**
皮膚電気抵抗　**ESR**
皮膚電気抵抗図　**EDG**
皮膚電気抵抗水準　**SRL**
皮膚電気反射　**GSR**
皮膚電気反射(聴力検査)　**GSR**
(急性熱性)皮膚粘膜リンパ節症候群　**MCLS**
皮膚反応〔惹起〕因子　**SRF**
皮膚反応因子　**SFR**
皮膚反応惹起抗原　**SRA**
皮膚病学の　**derm**

皮膚表面脂質　**SSL**
皮膚防御因子　**SPF**
皮膚毛細血管血流量　**PBF**
皮膚用の　**FS**
皮膚良性リンパ節症　**LBC**
皮膚リンパ球腫　**LABC**
否定的態度　**NA**
批判的親　**CP**
尾形の　**C**
尾骨　**cocc**
尾骨の　**CO, COC, Coc, coc., cocc**
尾状核　**CN, NCd**
尾状被殻　**CP**
尾側退行症候群　**CRS**
尾側の　**C, CD, Cd, cd**
尾(側)の　**Caud**
尾部の　**Caud, CD, Cd, cd**
拡がる　**ext, ext.**
披裂　**Fiss, fiss**
披裂喉頭蓋の　**AE**
披裂喉頭蓋ひだ　**AE fold**
披裂部　**ary**
泌尿器科(学)　**U, UR, Ur, Ur., uro, Uro, URO, Urol, urol, urol.**
泌尿器科医　**U, UR, Ur, Ur., Urol, urol, urol.**
泌尿器疾患診断指数　**UDI**
泌尿器治療ユニット　**UCU**
泌尿器(科)の　**uro, Uro, URO**
泌尿器の　**UR, Ur, ur**
泌尿生殖器結核　**UGT**
肥厚　**HYP, Hyp, hyp.**
肥厚性〔肥大性〕ニューロパシー　**HN**
肥厚性瘢痕　**HS**
肥厚性鼻炎　**Rh.hyper.**
肥厚性幽門狭窄(症)　**HPS**
肥厚性リンパ球(性)胃炎　**HLG**
肥大　**HYP, Hyp, hyp.**
肥大型心筋症　**HC, HCM**
肥大型心筋症症候群　**HHCS**
肥大型閉塞性心筋症　**HOCM**
肥大下鼻甲介　**HIT**
肥大性〔肥厚性〕筋性大動脈弁下部狭窄(症)　**HMSAS**
肥大性骨関節炎　**HOA**
肥大性骨関節症　**HO**
肥大性浸潤性腱炎　**HIT**
肥大〔肥厚〕性大動脈弁下部狭窄(症)　**HSAS, HSS**
肥大性肺性骨関節炎　**HPO**
肥大性肺性骨関節症　**HPO**
肥満換気低下症候群　**OHS**
肥満患者治療部　**WPCU**
肥満高血圧　**OHT**
肥満細胞　**MC**
肥満細胞カルボキシペプチダーゼA　**MC-CPA**
肥満細胞成長因子　**MCGF**
肥満細胞脱顆粒ペプチド　**MCDP**
肥満細胞プロテアーゼ1　**MCPT-1**
肥満細胞変性試験　**MDT**
肥満細胞用培養液　**MCM**
肥満指数　**OI**
肥満症　**O**
肥満症研究会　**ASO**
肥満正常血圧(者)　**ONT**
肥満の　**O, OB**
非アトピー性喘息　**NABA**
非アトピー性皮膚炎　**NAD**
非アドレナリン作動性,非コリン作動性(神経)　**NANC**
非アドレナリン作動抑制性神経　**NAIN**
非アドレナリン作動(性)抑制反応　**NAIR**
非アルコール性脂肪肝障害　**NAFLD**
非アルコール性脂肪性肝炎　**NASH**
非アルコール性の　**NA**
非悪性　**NM**
非悪性の(腫瘍)　**N**
非イオン性界面活性剤　**NIS**
非インスリン依存型糖尿病　**NIDD**
非インスリン治療疾患　**NITD**
非運動性の(細菌)　**NM, nm**
非エステル化コレステロール　**NEC, UC**
非エステル化(遊離)脂肪酸　**UFA**
非エステル結合型脂肪酸　**NEFA**
非汚染〔無菌的〕中間尿採取　**CCMSU**
非汚染〔無菌的〕排泄検体　**CVS**
非汚染排泄検体(尿)　**CL void**
非応答者　**NR**

非化膿性中耳炎　**NOM**
非加熱血清レアギン(試験)　**USR**
非外傷性正常頭部の　**ATNC**
非外傷(性)の　**AT**
非角化性癌　**NKC**
非活動性の　**inac**
非活動性肺疾患　**NAPD**
非冠(状)静脈洞　**NCS**
非貫壁性心筋梗塞(症)　**NTMI**
非開胸(式)心(臓)マッサージ　**CCM**
非開業の　**NP**
非塊状の　**UA**
非潰瘍性消化不良　**NUD**
非癌性白ハツカネズミ　**CFW**
非観血的整復　**CR**
非共鳴多光子イオン化　**NRMPI**
非局方の　**unof, unoff**
非均等型左(心)室肥大　**ALVH**
非協力的な　**uncoop**
非急速眼球運動(睡眠)　**NREM**
非急速眼球運動の　**NON-REM**
非急速眼球運動睡眠　**NREMS**
非球形溶血性貧血　**NSHA**
非強調コンピュータ断層撮影法　**NECT**
非揮発性の　**NV**
非揮発性物質　**NVM**
非喫煙者　**NS, NSM**
非器質性発育不良　**NFTT**
非機能的細胞外液　**non-functional ECF**
非凝集(性)の　**NAG**
非凝集の　**UA**
非ケトン性高血糖(性)高浸透圧(性)昏睡　**NKHHC**
非ケトン性高血糖症　**NKHG**
非ケトン性高浸透圧症候群　**NKHS**
非ケトン性高浸透圧性昏睡　**NKHOC**
非ケトン性高浸透圧性糖尿病性昏睡　**NKHDC**
非ケトン性昏睡　**NKC**
非血縁ドナー　**URD**
非経口的栄養補給　**TF**
非経口的に　**parent**
非経口の　**parent**
非経口不活化(ワクチン)　**KP**
非経口薬協会　**PDA**
非経腸栄養法　**TPN**
非結核性マイコバクテリア　**NTM**
非結合　**NC**
非結合 TBG　**UTBG**
非結合チ〔サイ〕ロキシン結合グロブリン　**UTBG**
非結合ビリルビン　**BU**
非コラーゲン蛋白　**NCP**
非コリン作動興奮性神経　**NCEN**
非コレラビブリオ(菌)　**NCV**
非公式の　**unof, unoff**
非甲状腺疾患　**NTI**
非行の研究と治療研究所　**ISTD**
非高比重リポ蛋白　**NHDL**
非骨化性線維腫　**NOF**
非硬変性門脈線維症　**NCPF**
非(肝)硬変の　**NC**
非構造(蛋白)　**NS**
非膠原蛋白　**NCP**
非再呼吸　**NR**
非再燃性の　**unrem, unremit**
非細菌性咽頭炎　**NBP**
非細菌性血栓性心内膜炎　**NBTE**
非細菌性結膜炎　**NBC**
非細菌性前立腺炎　**NBP**
非細胞核蛋白　**NHP**
非菜食主義者　**NV**
非産生細胞　**NP**
非十分量　**NSO**
非小細胞性肺癌　**NSLC**
非小細胞(性)肺癌　**NSCLC**
非手術　**no op**
非手術的生検法　**NOBT**
非心原性肺水腫　**NCPE**
非心(臓)原性浮腫　**NCE**
非心臓性胸痛　**NCCP**
非処方箋薬を扱う薬局の監視者　**OOTCDE**
非刺激　**NS**
非実質(性)細胞　**NPC**
非持続性心室性頻脈　**NSVT**
非持続性心室頻拍　**VT-NS**
非食細胞の　**NP**
非侵襲性頸動脈検査　**NICE**
非侵襲性血流検査　**NIFS**
非侵襲治療学会　**SMIT**
非神経細胞(性)エノラーゼ　**NNE**
非脂肪組織　**FFM**
非修復作用　**NRA**
非商標名　**INN**
非常に　**V, v**
非常に感受性の高い　**VS**
非常に危険な物質　**EHSs**
非常に緊急の　**VU**
非常に正確に混和せよ　**m.accur.**
非常に低い出生率　**VLBR**

非常に良い健康状態 **VGH**
非湿性咳 **NPC**
非新生物症候群 **NNS**
非種痘群の余分発生率 **EIRN**
非ステロイド抗炎症化合物 **NOSAC**
非ステロイド性抗炎症薬 **NSAID(s)**
非ステロイド性抗男性ホルモン **NSAA**
非水銀性非腐蝕性 **NMNC**
非水疱型先天性魚鱗様紅皮症 **NBCIE**
非水溶性食物繊維 **IDF**
非セミノーマ〔非精上皮腫〕性精巣胚細胞腫瘍 **NSGCTT**
非セミノーマ〔非精上皮腫〕胚細胞腫瘍 **NSGCT**
非正視 **Am, am**
非生殖器皮膚線維芽細胞 **NGSF**
非生体内で **IV, i.v.**
非全身反応 **NSR**
非性病の **NV**
非接種の **NV**
非接触型眼圧計 **NCT**
非精上皮腫性精巣〔睾丸〕腫瘍 **NSTT**
非精上皮腫瘍性睾丸〔精巣〕腫瘍 **NSGCT**
非線型混合効果モデル **NONMEM**
非増殖性網膜症 **NPR**
非増殖(性)糖尿病(性)網膜症 **NPDR**
非代償性肝硬変 **DC**
非代償(性)の **decomp, uncomp**
非対称 **A, a, asym**
非対称性緊張性頸反射 **ATNR**
非対称性心肥大 **ASH**
非対称性先端肥大 **AAH**
非対称性中隔肥厚 **ASH**
非対称的な ***uns-*, uns**
非対称(性)の **A, a, asym**
非対称の **unsym**
非脱分極性筋弛緩薬 **CBA**
非蛋白結合の **NPB**
非蛋白(性)呼吸比 **NPRQ**
非蛋白質性窒素 **NPN**
非蛋白スルフヒドリル(基) **NPSH**
非弾性電子トンネリング分光法 **IETS**
非弾性平均自由行程 **IMFP**
非チアノーゼ性心疾患 **NCCHD**
非中毒性甲状腺腫 **NTG**
非中毒性多結節(性)甲状腺腫 **NTMNG**
非治癒サルコイドーシス **NCS**
非直視下僧帽弁交連切開術 **CMC**
非腸管線維芽細胞 **NIF**
非通常型間質性肺炎 **UIP**
非デンプン性多糖 **NSP**
非定型群 **I group**
非定型抗酸菌 **AM**
非定型抗酸菌症 **AM**
非定型的抗酸菌 **AAFB**
非定型的線維黄色腫 **AFX**
非定型的乳房切除術 **MRM**
非定型的有糸核分裂像 **AMF**
非定型母斑症候群 **AMS**
非転移性栄養膜〔絨毛性〕疾患 **NMTD**
非転移性妊娠性栄養膜〔絨毛性〕疾患 **NMGTD**
非同時性の **async**
非特異化ウシ血清 **DBS**
非特異性コリンエステラーゼ **nsCHE**
非特異性腟炎 **NSU, NSV**
非特異性尿道炎 **NSU**
非特異性反応性肝炎 **NSRH**
非特異的 ST-T(波) **NSSTT**
非特異的エステラーゼ **NSE**
非特異的肝細胞異常 **NHA**
非特異的交叉〔差〕反応抗原 **NCA**
非特異的呼吸器疾患 **URD**
非特異的食道運動機能不全 **NEMD**
非特異的性器感染 **NSGI**
非特異的の **NS**
非特異的非びらん性胃炎 **NNG**
非特異的遊離 **NSR**
非特異(的)な **nonspec**
非特異抑制因子 **NSF**
非特殊投射系 **DPS**
非糖還元性物質 **NGRS**
非糖尿病(性)の **ND**
非内因性の **NE**
非内分泌性低身長 **NESS**
非人間の **NH**
非妊娠血清 **NPS**
非白人女性 **NF**
非白人男性 **NM**
非発酵性細菌 **NFB**
非破壊性検査 **NDT**
非配偶者間人工授精 **AID**
非ヒストン染色質 **NHC**

非ヒストン染色体　**NHC**
非ヒストン染色体蛋白(質)　**NHCP**
非ヒストン蛋白　**NHP, NHPP**
非必須アミノ酸　**NEA, NEAA**
非肥満(本態性)高血圧　**NHT**
非肥満性糖尿病　**NOD**
非肥満の　**NO**
非病期　**DFI**
非病生存　**DFS**
非病理的　**NP**
非標準　**non std**
非標準項目　**NSI**
非ブタノール抽出ヨウ素(症候群)　**NBEI**
非ふるえ熱産生：体温調節性　**NST：T, NST(T)**
非ふるえ熱産生：不可避的　**NST：O, NST(O)**
非分化細胞　**NDC**
非分割性の　**i**
非分散型赤外線分析計　**NDIR**
非分葉核(好中球)　**nonsegs**
非付着性白血病　**NAL**
非糞抗原　**NFA**
非ペニシリナーゼ産生淋菌　**NPPNG**
非ヘモグロビン蛋白　**NHP**
非弁〔心臓〕疾患　**NVD**
非弁膜症心房細動　**NVAF**
非変質性細菌性抗原　**UBA**
非閉塞性腸(管)虚血　**NOII**
非閉塞性肥大型心筋症　**HNCM**
非ホジキン悪性リンパ腫　**NHML**
非ホジキン(性)リンパ腫　**NHL**
非抱合型ビリルビン　**UB**
非発作性(房室)接合部頻拍(症)　**NPJT**
非麻痺性ポリオ　**NP polio**
非免疫学的接触蕁麻疹　**NICU**
非免疫グロブリン　**NIg**
非免疫性腎疾患　**NIRD**
非免疫性胎児水腫　**NIHF**
非免疫ヒツジ(血清)　**NIS**
非滅菌管理経腟分娩　**USCVD**
非滅菌自然経腟分娩　**USUCVD**
非羊水の　**NA**
非羊膜の　**NA**
非抑制性インスリン様活性　**NSILA**
非抑制排尿(筋)容量　**UDC**
非流暢な　**NF**
非淋菌性外陰腟炎　**NGV**
非淋菌性尿道炎　**NGU**
非罹患表皮　**UE**
非連続性の　**incoher**
非 A 非 B 型肝炎　**NANB**
非 A 非 B 型肝炎ウイルス　**NANBV**
非 A 非 B 非 C 型肝炎　**NANBNCH**
非 B 型(肝炎)　**NB**
飛行時間　**TOF**
飛行時間型質量分析法　**TOFMS**
飛行適性評価　**FAR**
疲労試検　**FT**
秘書　**sec, sec., sed, sed.**
秘匿式麻酔安全報告　**CAIR**
被移植者　**Recip, recip.**
被殻　**pu, PUT**
被殻出血　**PH**
被蓋網様体核　**NRT**
被虐待児症候群　**BCS**
被虐待婦人症候群　**BWS**
被検者　**S, ss, su, su., subj, Vp.**
被験者　**S, ss, su, su., subj**
被験者の身長　**SHUT**
被覆加工圧縮錠剤　**CCT**
被覆加工錠　**CT**
被覆された　**ctd**
被覆小胞　**CV**
被覆線維　**SF**
被膜　**cap, cap., caps., capsul., oa**
被膜厚　**OAD**
被膜外拡散　**ECS**
被膜高　**OAH**
被膜長　**OAL**
被膜幅　**OAW**
悲観的尺度　**HS**
費用　**chg**
費用対効果分析　**CEA**
費用対効用分析　**CUA**
費用対利益分析　**CBA**
備考　**Misc**
脾　**S**
脾コロニー形成細胞　**CFC-S**
脾指数　**SI**
脾腫　**SP**
脾静脈　**SV, VL**
脾樹状細胞　**SDC**
脾膵分離　**SPD**
脾臓　**S, sp, SP**
脾臓壊死ウイルス　**SNV**
脾臓コロニー形成単位　**CFU-S**
脾臓細胞　**SC, SPC**

脾臓体重比　**SBR**
脾摘重篤後感染(症候群)　**OPSI(syndrome)**
脾摘出術　**SpX**
脾動脈　**SA**
脾動脈塞栓術　**SAE**
脾内圧　**ISP**
脾フィブリン溶解蛋白酵素　**SFP**
脾門脈造影　**SPG**
脾リンパ球　**SL**
脾・腎・肝　**SKL**
腓骨　**FIB**
腓骨筋萎縮症　**PMA**
腓腹筋　**gast, Gastroc, gastroc, GS**
微温湯　**aq.tep.**
微温湯浣腸　**TWE**
微細構造　**FS**
微細振動　**MT, MV**
微細電子工学　**ME**
微細動脈瘤　**MA, Mic**
微細な　**F**
微細脳機能障害　**MBD**
微細脳機能障害症候群　**MBD**
微小管　**MT, MTS**
微小管結合蛋白　**MAP**
微小管蛋白　**MTP**
微小管付属蛋白質　**MAPs**
微小凝集アルブミン　**MIAA**
微小螢光測定(法)　**MFM**
微小血管圧　**MVP**
微小血管減圧術　**MVD**
微小血管研究　**MVR**
微小血管障害性溶血性貧血　**MAHA**
微小残存病変　**MRD**
微小終板電位　**MEPP**
微小絨毛　**MV**
微小絨毛膜　**MVM**
微小循環　**MC**
微小循環による防御機構　**MDS**
微小循環領域の血流を調節する機構　**MFRS**
微小腎疾患　**MRD**
微小染色体　**DM**
微小(大)脳機能不全　**MCD**
微小嚢胞　**MV**
微小プロラクチノーマ　**MIPM**
微小変化型ネフローゼ症候群　**MLNS**
微小変化群　**MC**
微小変化腎障害　**MCN**
微小変化ネフローゼ症候群　**MCNS**
微晶質の　**microcryst**
微晶性の　**microcryst**
微生物回路　**CML**
微生物学　**microbiol., Microbiol**
微生物学研究科　**MRD**
微生物学研究施設　**MRE**
微生物学士　**B.Mic., M.Mic**
微生物学的(検定)　**MB**
微生物学的安全指数　**MSI**
微生物学認定書　**Dip.Micro.**
微生物学(的)の　**microbiol., Microbiol**
微生物と食品基準諮問委員会　**NACMCF**
微分熱重量測定　**DTG**
微量元素　**TE**
微量の　**T**
微量免疫螢光検査法　**MIF**
鼻胃経管栄養　**NG fdgs**
鼻胃の　**NG**
鼻咽頭　**NP**
鼻咽頭エアウェイ　**NPA**
鼻咽頭癌　**NPC, NPCa**
鼻咽頭吸引　**NPA**
鼻咽頭の　**NP**
鼻咽頭培養　**NPcult**
鼻咽頭ファイバースコープ　**NPF**
鼻炎　**rhin**
鼻科医　**Rhin**
鼻科学　**Rhi, rhinol**
鼻科学者　**rhinol**
鼻科学の　**rhinol**
鼻科専門医　**Rhin**
鼻空腸の　**NJ**
鼻腔・上顎洞気流動態図　**RMAG**
鼻腔栄養　**NG fdgs**
鼻腔栄養チューブ　**NG tube**
鼻腔栄養の　**NG**
鼻腔関連リンパ組織　**NALT**
鼻腔抵抗　**NAR**
鼻腔内の　**IN**
鼻形成術　**rhino**
鼻甲介　**turb**
鼻汁塗抹　**NS**
鼻出血　**epis**
鼻洗　**NW**
鼻胆管ドレナージ　**NBD**
鼻中隔矯正術と下鼻介切除術　**Devi-Con**
鼻中隔再建(術)　**NSR**
鼻中隔節　**CSN**
鼻中隔彎曲矯正手術　**Devi**
鼻中隔彎曲症　**Devi, DSN**
鼻内の　**IN**
鼻内領域　**EA**
鼻閉　**NO, NV**
鼻傍癌　**PNC**
鼻翼　**AN**
鼻涙管　**ND, NLD**
鼻涙腺反射　**NLR**

避妊技術　**CT**
避妊手技　**CT**
避妊薬後無月経　**PP**
秀でる　**exc**
東　**E**
東海岸熱　**ECF**
東回りの　**EB**
光　**l, L, Lt, lt., lt**
光アレルゲン　**PA**
光イオン化検出器　**PID**
光音響分光法　**PAS**
光カロリメトリー分光法　**PCS**
光化学治療　**PCT**
光眼瞼反射　**PPR**
光過敏症・魚鱗癬・もろい毛髪・知能障害・生殖能低下・短身長　**PIBIDS**
光開始化学発光　**PICL**
光感受脱落　**PDD**
光恐怖　**PT**
光凝固　**LC, LK, PC, PHC, photocoag**
光駆動　**PD**
光痙攣反応　**PCR**
光散乱指数　**LSI**
光刺激　**PS**
光刺激発光　**PSL**
光受容器膜　**PRL**
光照射治療　**PRT**
光磁気ディスク　**MOD**
光第二高調波発生　**SHG**
光ディスク　**OD**
光投射　**LProj**
光透過性電極　**OTE**
光透過性薄層電極　**OTTLE**
光認知　**LP**
光反応　**LR, PR**
光反応酵素　**PRE**
光反応性　**PHR**
光反応の　**PR**
光ファイバーの　**FO**
光ミオクローヌス反応　**PMR**
光力学的診断　**PDD**
光励起発光　**OSL**
低い　**l, L, LO, niedr**
膝　**K, KN, Kn, kn**
膝(より)上の　**AK, a.k.**
膝折れ防止用プラスチック短下肢装具　**SKAO**
膝・踵装具　**KAO**
膝・踝・足装具　**KAFO**
肘　**C, el, elb**
肘下の　**UE**
肘知覚電位　**ESEP**
肘反射　**EJ**
肘・手関節・手指装具　**EWHO**
菱形の　**rhom**
額　**F**
左　**l**
左(の)　**l, L, laev., sinist.**
左足　**LF**
左足増高単極肢誘導　**aVF**
左胃静脈　**LGV**
左胃静脈下大静脈吻合術　**LGV**
左胃大網膜動脈　**AGES**
左胃動脈　**LG, LGA**
左上(象限)　**LA**
左上の　**LU**
左後斜位　**LPO**
左頤横位　**MLT**
左頤後位　**LMP, MLP**
左頤前位　**MLA**
左下横隔膜動脈　**APIS**
左下眼瞼　**LLL**
左下胸骨縁　**LLSB**
左下肩甲骨縁　**LLSB**
左下肢　**LLE, LLL, LLX**
左下斜(筋)　**LIO**
左下腿　**LLL**
左下大静脈　**LIVC**
左下直(筋)　**LIR**
左下(肺)(野)　**LLL**
左下部　**L & B, LB**
左下腹部　**LLQ**
(肺の)左下葉　**LLL**
左下(肺)葉　**LLLL**
左(肺)下葉ラ音なし　**LLLNR**
左外(側)縁　**LLB**
左外斜視　**LXT**
左外側心室早期興奮　**LLVP**
左外側大腿　**LLT**
左外側大腿の　**LLF**
左外側の　**LL, lt.lat**
左外直(筋)　**LLR**
左回旋動脈　**LCA**
左回転　**LR**
左肩後位　**ScLP**
左肩前位　**ScLA**
左肝静脈　**LHV**
左肝動脈　**LH, LHA**
左冠(状)静脈洞　**LCS**
左冠尖　**LCC**
左冠(状)動脈　**LCA**
左冠(状)動脈主幹部　**LMC, LMCA, LMT**
左冠(状)動脈前下行枝　**LAD, LADCA**
左季肋部　**LHC**
左肩甲骨縁　**LSB**
左結腸動脈　**LCA**
左頸動脈　**LCA**
左頸動脈(血管)内膜切除(術)　**LCE**
左交感神経　**LSN**
左後下束ブロック　**LPIFB**
左後下の　**LPI**
左後心室早期興奮　**LPVP**
左後束ブロック　**LPFB**
左後頭位　**LO**
左後頭横側位　**OLT**
左後頭部　**lo, LO**
左後内頸動脈　**LPICA**

左後方下行動脈　**LPDA**
左黒質　**LSN**
左三角(筋)　**LD**
左鎖骨下静脈　**LSCV, LSV**
左鎖骨下動脈　**LSA, LSCA**
左鎖骨中央線　**LMCL**
左下(象限)　**L & B, LB**
左下象限　**LW**
左下の　**LL**
左上(部)1/4 区　**LUQ**
左上オリーブ(核)　**LSO**
左上外(部)1/4 区　**LUOQ**
左上外殿部　**LUOB**
左上眼瞼　**LUL**
左上胸骨縁　**LUSB**
左上肩甲骨縁　**LUSB**
左上肢　**LA, LUE, LUL**
左上斜(筋)　**LSO**
左上斜位　**LH**
左上斜視　**LH**
左上象限　**ULQ**
左上大静脈　**LSVC**
左上大静脈遺残　**PLSVC**
左上直(筋)　**LSR**
左上肺(野)　**LUL**
左(肺)上葉　**LUL**
左(肺)上葉切除術　**LUL**
左上腕　**LUA**
左示指　**LIF**
左耳介　**LA**
左視覚　**VL, VLE**
左視野　**LVF**
左斜位鼠径ヘルニア　**LOIH**
左腎静脈　**LRV**
左腎動脈　**LRA**
左正中(の)　**LM**
左仙骨　**LS**
左仙骨側方　**LSL**
左仙骨部横位　**LST**
左仙骨部後位　**LSP**
左前三角　**LAT**
左前小開胸　**LAST**
左前上束ブロック　**LASFB**
左前上の　**LAS**
左前上ヘミブロック　**LASH**
左前脊椎動脈　**LASA**
左前頭(部)開頭(術)　**LFC**
左前頭極　**LFp**
左前頭部　**LF**
左前腕　**LF, LFA**
左側臥位　**lar, LLD**
左側頭　**t.s.**
左側頭後部　**LPT**
左側頭前部　**LAT**
左側頭中部　**LMT**
左側頭部　**L-T**
左鼠径ヘルニア　**LIH**
左総頸(動脈)　**LCC**
左総頸動脈　**LCCA**
左大血管転位症　**LTGA**
左大腿　**LT**
左大腿前面　**LAT**
左大腿直(筋)　**LRF**
左大腿動脈　**LFA**
左大腿ヘルニア　**LFH**
左体性感覚誘発電位　**LSEP**
左短脚固定器　**LSLB**
左中・側会陰切開(術)　**LMLE**
左中外側会陰切開(術)　**LME**
左中外側の　**LML**
左中指　**LMF**
左中耳炎　**LOM**
左中耳炎・化膿性・急性　**LOMSA**
左中耳炎・化膿性・慢性　**LOMSC, LOMSCh**
左中心部　**LC**
左中大脳　**LMC**
左中大脳動脈　**LMCA**
左中大脳動脈血栓症　**LMCAT**
左長脚装具　**LLL brace**
左直接鼠径ヘルニア　**LDIH**
左腸骨窩　**LIF**
左腸骨部　**LIR**
左椎骨動脈　**LVA**
左手　**LH, m.s.**
左手増高単極肢誘導　**aVL**
左手側　**LHs**
左手で　**CS**
左殿(筋)　**LG**
左殿(部)の　**LG**
左殿部　**LB**
左と右　**L & R**
左(冠(状)動脈)回旋枝　**LCX**
左動脈圧　**LAP**
左頭頂部　**LP, L-P**
左橈骨動脈　**LRA**
左内胸動脈　**LITA**
左内頸(動脈)　**LIC**
左内頸動脈　**LICA**
左内直(筋)　**LMR**
左尿管口　**LUO**
左の　**G, g, g., Li, S, s, sin, sin.**
左半球　**LH**
左背後位　**LDP**
左背前位　**LDA**
左肺静脈　**LPV**
左肺動脈　**LPA**
左尾状核　**LCN**
左腹側側方殿部　**LVLG**
左方向　**l**
左巻き二重鎖らせん DNA　**Z-DNA**
左耳　**a.l., AL, AS, A.S., a.s., LE**
左無名静脈　**LIV**
左門脈　**LPV**
左腰部　**LLR**
左卵管卵巣摘出(術)　**LSO**

左下肋部　LHC
左肋間縁　LICM
左肋間腔　LICS，LIS
左肋骨縁　LCB，LCM
左＜右　L＜R
左＞右　L＞R
左→右　L→R
必須アミノ酸　EAA
必須脂肪酸　EFA
必須脂肪酸欠乏　EFAD
必須瞬間換気量　MMV
必須蛋白比　NPR
必須蛋白利用　NPU
必須リン脂質　EPL
必要証明書　CON
必要な　nec，req
必要なとき　si op.sit
必要ならば　if nec，si op.sit，S op S，S.op.s，s.op.s.，S OP SIT，s.op.sit，SOS，s.o.s.
必要に応じて　A/N，prn，p.r.n.，quot.op.sit
必要に応じて変え・観察し・修理する　MOD/IRAN
一晩おきに　alt.noc.，alt.noct.
一晩じゅう　ON
人差し指　In，ind，ind.
等しい　aeq.，eq
百　C，c.
百日咳　pert，WC
百日咳・ジフテリア・破傷風　PDT
百日咳・ジフテリア・破傷風の新タイプ3種混合ワクチン　APDT
百日咳凝集反応　BPAG
百日咳毒素　PT
百日咳(菌)ワクチン　HPV
百日咳ワクチン・ジフテリアトキソイド　PVDT
百分位数　P
百分率　pct
百分率階数　PR
百万マウス　megamouse
百万命令毎秒　MIPS
氷点　FP
氷点浸透圧計　FPO
表　Tab，tbl，Tbl
表現　expn
表現型　pheno
表在拡大型黒色腫　SSM
表在性筋腱膜系　SMAS
表在性点状角膜炎　KSP
表在性の　subl.
表在大腿動脈　SFA
表在(性)点状角膜炎　SPK
表在(性)の　sup，SUP，sup.，superf，superfic
表示させよ　Sig，sig.
表示して与えよ　D.S.，d.s.
表示する　descr
表示せよ　Sig，sig.
表情　expn
表層角膜移植術　LK
表層点状角膜炎　KPS
表皮菌(属)　E
表皮細胞　EC
表皮細胞表面蛋白　ECSP
表皮真皮結合部　DEJ
表皮水疱症　EB
表皮熱傷(＝I度熱傷)　EB
表皮剥脱　Abr，abr
表皮剥脱擦過傷　abras
表皮剥脱素　ET
表皮剥離性角質増殖　EH
表面　S，sur
表面X線　SFXR
表面化学分析　SCA
表面活性物質　SAM，SAS，SF
表面活性物質様活性　SLA
表面活性リン脂質　DPL
表面結合(蛋白)　SB
表面抗原　SA
表面上皮　SEP
表面線量　SD
表面増感共鳴ラマン散乱分光法　SERRS
表面増強ラマン散乱　SERS
表面弾性波　SAW
表面張力　σ，ST
表面プラズモン共鳴　SPR
表面膜免疫グロブリン　SMIg
(膜)表面免疫グロブリン　SIg，sIg
秒　S，s，sec，sec.
病因　agt，agt.，etiol，pathogen
病因生成物　DFP
病因論　Path，path.
病院　H，Hosp，hosp.，spital
病院・研究所図書館協会　AHIL
病院医師組織　HPO
病院医薬協会　HPA
病院外来部　HOPD
病院活動分析　HAA
病院管理　HAD
病院管理委員会連合　AHMC
病院管理学士　BSHA，MSHA
病院管理者　HAD
病院管理認定書　Dip.HA.
病院救急管理率　HEAR
病院供給源管理　HRA
病院公的関係協会　AHPR

病院顧問協会　**AHC**
病院産業協会　**HIA**
病院自動化　**HA**
病院情報システム　**HIS**
病院住込医師　**HP**
病院洗濯業者協会　**SHLM**
病院治療　**HT**
病院到着時間　**HAT**
病院到着前出産　**BBA**
病院図書館審議会　**HLC**
病院と福祉の管理者協会　**AHWA**
病院入院患者調査　**HIPE**
病院認定マニュアル　**AMH**
病院認定連合委員会　**JCAH**
病院搬送指示　**HTO**
病院報告　**HR**
病院保険　**HI, hosp ins**
病院補充　**HR**
病院用の国際疾患分類　**H-ICDA**
病院倫理委員会　**HEC**
病気　**D, sk**
病気状態で生存　**AWD**
病気なし　**ND**
病気の　**S**
病気の悪化　**PD**
病気の進行　**PD**
病気の費用　**COI**
病気ヒッピーのための医療援助　**MASH**
病気保険プログラム　**HIP**
病期　**st, stg**
病期分類する　**stg**
病苦　**compl**
病原性の　**Path, path.**
病原体　**Path, path.**
病原体関連分子認識パターン　**PAMP**
病死　**DWD**
病床看護終了　**CBOC**
病状要約　**Rev of Sym**
病巣　**foc**
病巣の　**f, foc**
病巣部　**FZ**
病訴　**COMP, comp, compl, compl., complt**
病訴のない　**no compl**
病的骨折　**Path Fx**
病的習慣疾患　**PHD**
病的状態　**PS**
病的盗癖　**klepto**
病的肥満の　**MO**
病棟　**W, Wd**
病棟行動評点尺度　**WBRS**
病棟事務　**CC**
病棟主任　**WM**
病棟雰囲気尺度　**WAS**
病棟分娩　**WC**
病変内の　**il, i lesion**
病変部　**FZ**
病変部に　**Par.aff.**
病変部に適用　**p.a.a., psa, p.s.a.**
病理解剖　**post**
病理学　**PA, pa, Path, path., Pth**
病理学・細菌学資格認定書　**DMPB**
病理学検査室　**PAL**
病理学者　**Path, path.**
病理学的証拠なし　**NEP**
病理学的病期　**PS**
病理学の　**Path, path.**
病理診断　**Path Dx**
病理組織学的収縮不全度　**HCFI**
病理組織学的リンパ管侵襲の有無と1～3の程度　**ly 0-3**
病理組織学的リンパ節有無程度　**n(+)0-4, n(−)0-4**
病理組織学的リンパ節転移の程度　**n(+)0-4, n(−)0-4**
病理的診断なし　**NPD**
病歴　**An, ANM, CH, Hist, hist, Hx, Hy, MH, M Hx**
病歴課　**MRD**
病歴学士　**B.S.Med.Rec., B.S.Med.Rec.Lib.**
病歴士　**MRL**
病歴室　**MRL**
病歴対照試験　**HCT**
病歴と理学的検査　**HPE**
病歴と理学所見　**H & P**
病歴保管者　**MRL**
病歴用紙　**MHS**
描写する　**descr**
評価　**eval**
評価する　**eval**
評価と計画　**A/P**
評価不能　**NE**
評論　**R**
標準以下の　**substd**
標準塩基　**BS**
標準温度・気圧・飽和　**STPS**
標準温度・標準気圧　**STP, s.t.p.**
標準温度・標準気圧・標準乾燥状態　**STPD**
標準化　**standard, std**
標準化・評価　**S/E**
標準化された　**stand, standard, std**
標準化試験　**ST**
標準化死亡比　**SMR**
標準化相対危険　**SRR**
標準家族相互作用試験　**SFIT**
標準型　**SF**
標準クエン酸食塩水　**SSC**
標準経管栄養　**Std TF**

標準検査(用)量　**STD**
標準誤差　**SE**
標準作用温度　**SOT**
標準試験(用)量　**STD**
標準重炭酸塩　**SB**
標準重炭酸塩濃度　**SB concentration**
標準手技　**SP**
標準水素電極　**NHE**
標準精神医学用語集　**Stan Psych**
標準操作手技　**SOP**
標準代謝率　**SMR**
標準耐糖テスト　**SGTT**
標準的カポジ肉腫　**CKS**
標準的治療　**ST**
標準当量偏差　**NED**
標準得点　**SS，Z**
標準なし　**ns**
標準二段階法　**STS**
標準年齢研究　**NAS**
標準の　**stand，std**
標準針金測径器　**SWG**
標準平均温度　**TM**
標準偏差　σ，**SD，SEM，z**
標準毎分立方フィート　**SCF/min**
標準(光学)密度　**DS**
標準模擬患者　**SP**
標準容積(体積)　V_{o}
標準量　**ND**
標識細胞百分率　**%LC**
標識指数　**LI**
標識認識蛋白　**SRP**
標識分裂細胞百分率　**%LM**
標識リンパ芽球　**LBL**
標題　**t**
標題・副題と見出し　**TSAC**
標題ページ索引　**TPI**
標的　**tgt，trgt**
標的域　**TA**
標的器官　**TO**
標的結合能　**TBC**
標的細胞　**TC**
標本　**exx，SPEC，spec**
昼　**M，m.，N**
昼間の　**d**
広い　**ext，ext.，lat，lat.**
広さ　**W**
品質　**Q**
品質確認試験　**QVT**
品質化されていない　**unqual**
品質管理　**QC**
品質管理情報　**QCI**
品質管理水準　**QCL**
品質管理データ　**QCD**
品質向上・納期厳守・原価削減　**QDC**
品質保証　**QA**
品質保証基準　**QAS**
品質保証局　**BQA**
品質保証プログラム　**QAP**
貧血誘発因子　**AIF**
貧者用として　**PP，P.P.，Pp，p.p.**
頻回再発　**FR**
頻回注射療法　**MIT**
頻度　**F，freq**
(心)頻拍　**tach，tachy，tachy.**
頻脈　**tach，tachy，tachy.**

ふ

ファイバーオプティク化学センサー　**FOCS**
ファイバー気管支鏡　**FBS**
ファイバースコープ付胃カメラ　**GTF**
ファイフェレラ属　**Pf**
ファカルティ・ディベロプメント　**FD**
ファーストユース症候群　**FUS**
ファブリチウス嚢　**BF**
ファーブル・ラクショ(病)　**FR**
ファミリーナースプラクティショナー　**FNP**
ファミリープラクティス　**FP**
ファラー現象　**F**
ファラデー定数　**F**
ファラド　**F，f，far**
ファルコナー・ウェッデル(症候群)　**FW**
ファロー五徴症　**P/F**
ファロー四徴(症)　**Tet，TF，T/F，TOF，T of F**
ファンギーソン染色　**VG**
ファンコニ・ヘグリン症候群　**FH**
ファンコニ症候群　**FS**
ファンコニ貧血　**FA**
ファンデンベルグ(試験)　**VdB**
ファンデンベルグ試験　**Vend**
フィコエリトリン　**PE**
フィコシニアン　**PC**
フィステル　**fist**
フィックの垂直軸　***z* axis of Fick**
フィックの縦軸　***y* axis of Fick**
フィックの横軸　***x* axis of Fick**
フィッシャー・レース(表記法)　**FR**
フィッシャー症候群　**FS**
フィッシュバーグ希釈試験　**Fish dill**
フィッシュバーグ濃縮試験　**Fish conc**
フィッシュ法　**FISH**
フィート　**f**
フィート(＝footの複数形)　**Ft，ft**
フィート/秒　**fos，FPS**
フィート輝度　**FTL，ft-L**
フィート燭光　**ft-c**
フィードバック　**FB**
フィードバック機構　**FM**
フィードバックコントロールシステム　**FCS**
フィードバックシステム　**FBS**
フィードバック制御　**FR**
フィブリノゲン　**FBG，FG，FI，Fib，fib，fibrin**
フィブリノゲンガスクロマトグラフィ　**FGC**
フィブリノゲン関連抗原　**FRA**
フィブリノゲン関連(性)の　**FR**
フィブリノゲン摂取試験　**FUT**
フィブリノゲン分解産物　**FgDP**
フィブリノゲン分解物　**FDP**
フィブリノペプチド　**FP**
フィブリノペプチドA　**FPA**
フィブリノペプチドB　**FPB**
フィブリン　**Fbn，FIB**
フィブリン・フィブリノゲン分解産物　**fdp/Fdp，FSP**
フィブリン安定化因子　**FSF**
フィブリン分解産物　**FBP，FDP**
フィブリン分解産物D二量体　**DD**
フィブリンモノマー　**FM**
フィブリンモノマーテスト　**FMT**
フィブリンモノマー溶解複合体　**FMSC**
フィブロネクチン　**FN**
フィブロネクチン受容体　**FNR**
ブイヨン濾液　**BF**
フィラデルフィア染色体　**Ph，Phi**
フィラリア　**F**
フィラリア仔虫　**Mf，mf**
フィールドイオン化質量分析法　**FI-MS**
フィールドデソープション質量分析法　**FD-MS**
フィールドフロー分別　**FFF**
フィルムバッジ　**FB**
フィロキノン　**K_1**
フィンゼン単位　**FU**
フート/分　**fpm**
フェイル・クリペル症候群　**FK**
フェークトリン単位　**VE**
フェナジンメト硫酸　**PMS**
フェナセチン・アスピリン・カフェイン　**PAC**
フェナセチン・アスピリン・デスオキシエフェドリン　**PAD**
フェナントレン　**Ph**

フェニトイン　**PHT, PT, PTN**
フェニル　**PH**
フェニルアラニン　**F, P, PA, PHA, Phe**
フェニルアラニン・リジン・バソプレシン　**PLV**
フェニルアラニン水酸化酵素　**PAH**
フェニルアラニンとメトトレキサート　**PM**
フェニルアラニンマスタード　**L-PAM**
フェニルイソチオシアネート　**PITC**
フェニルイソプロピルヒドラジン　**PIH**
フェニルエタノールアミン-*N*-メチルトランスフェラーゼ　**PNMT**
フェニルエチルアミン　**PEA**
フェニルエチルアラニン　**PEA**
フェニルエチルアルコール　**PEA**
フェニルエチルジグアニド　**PEDG**
フェニルエチルマロンアミド　**PEMA**
フェニルエチルメチルエチルカルボノール　**PEMEC**
フェニル過酢酸　**PPAA**
フェニルグリオキサール　**PGO**
フェニルグリシン　**Phgly**
フェニルケトン尿症　**PKU**
フェニル酢酸　**PAA**
フェニルセファロース　**PS**
フェニルチオカルバミド　**PTC**
フェニルチオカルバモイル　**PTC**
フェニルチオ尿素　**PTU**
フェニルチオヒダントイン　**PTH**
フェニルトリメチルアンモニウム　**PTM, PTMA**
フェニルヒドラジン　**PhH**
フェニルピルビン酸　**PPA**
フェニルピルビン酸陽性の　**PPA pos**
フェニルブタゾン　**PBZ**
フェニルブチルカルビノール　**Ph BC**
フェニルメチルスルホニルフッ化物　**PMSF**
フェニレフリン　**PE**
フェネチシリン　**PEPC**
フェネチシリンカリウム　**PE-K**
フェネチルビグアナイド　**DBI, PEBG**
フェノキシエチルペニシリン(＝フェネチシリン)　**PEPC**
フェノキシプロピルペニシリン　**PPPC**
フェノキシベンザミン　**POB**
フェノキシメチルペニシリン　**PCV**
フェノチアジン　**PTZ**
フェノバルビタール　**PB, phen**
フェノバルビタールとベラドンナ　**P & B**
フェノバルビタールナトリウム　**PBS**
フェノバルビトン　**PB**
フェノール係数　**PC, Pc**
フェノールスルホンフタレイン　**PSP**
フェノールスルホンフタレイン排泄試験　**PSP test**
フェノールフタレイン　**P, phenolp**
フェノールフタレイン二リン酸塩寒天培地　**PPm**
フェノールフタレインモノ-β-グルクロン酸塩　**PMG**
フェノールレッド　**PR**
フェムト(＝10^{-15})　**f**
フェムトグラム(＝10^{-15}g)　**fg**
フェムトメートル(＝10^{-15}メートル)　**fm**
フェムトモル(＝10^{-15}モル)　**fmol**
フェムトリットル(＝10^{-15}リットル)　**fL, fl**
フェリチン　**FER, Ft**
フェリックス・ヴァイル(反応)　**FW**
フェリックス・ヴァイル反応　**FWR**
フェルティ症候群　**FS**
プエルトリコ人　**PR**
フェルミ　**F**
フェルミウム　**Fm**
フェレドキシン　**Fd**
フェロー　**F**
フェンサイクリジン　**PCP**
フェンホルミン　**Phen**
フォーグト・小柳(症候群)　**VK**
フォーグト・小柳・原田(症候群)　**VKH**
フォーグト・シュピールマイヤー(症候群)　**VS**
フォーグトの緑内障斑　**GL**
フォーゲス・プロスカウアー検査〔試験〕

VP test，V-P test
フォーゲス・プロスカウアー反応 **VPR**
フォーゲス・プロスカウエル半固形寒天培地 **VP**
フォーゲス・プロスカウアー(試験/反応) **VP**
フォーゲル・ジョンソン寒天(培地) **VJ**
フォスター・ケネディ症候群 **FK**
フォックス・フォーダイス(病) **FF**
フォト **ph**
フォートラン **FORTRAN**
フォトルミネセンス法 **PL**
フォーリーカテーテル **FC**
フォリン・ウー反応 **FWR**
フォリン・ウー法 **FWM**
フォルスマン抗原 **F-antigen**
フォルノー710 **F 710**
フォレル野 **FF**
フォン **P，ph，v**
フォンヴィレブランド症候群 **vWS，vWs**
フォンヴィレブランド病 **vWD，VWD**
フォンヴィレブランド病因子 **vWF，VWF**
フォンヒッペル・リンダウ病 **HLD，VHL**
フォンレックリングハウゼン病 **VRD**
フコース **Fuc**
フザリウム(属) **F**
ブジー **Buginar**
フシジン酸 **FA，FSD**
フジマメ凝集素 **DBA**
フジラジオグラフィ **FCR**
ブースビー・ラブレス・ブルブリアン(酸素マスク) **BLB**
ブスルファン **BSF，BUS**
フソバクテリウム(属) **F**
フソバクテリウム属 **FB**
ブタ胃ムチン **HGM**
ブタガストリン放出ペプチド **pGRP**
ブタカルシトニン **PCT**
ブタキロシド **PT**
ブタクサ **RAG，RW，Rw**
ブタクサ過敏(性) **RWS**
ブタクサ花粉 **RWP**
ブタクサ抗原 **RA**
ブタ水疱性発疹ウイルス **VESV**
ブタ水疱病 **SVD**
ブタ膵ポリペプチド **PPP**
ブタストレス症候群 **PSS**
ブタ成長ホルモン **PGH**
ブタ腸腺腫症 **PIA**
ブタトリプシン **PTr**
ブタ内因子濃縮物 **HIFC**
ブタノール抽出性ヨード **BEI**
ブタ流行性肺炎 **SEP**
フタル酸ジブチル **DBP**
ブチル **Bu**
ブチル酸ヒドロコルチゾン・クリーム **HB**
ブチルヒドロキシアニソール **BHA**
ブチルフェニルメチルカルバメイト **BPMC**
フッカー・フォーブス法 **HF**
フッ化デカリン **FDC**
フッ化ナトリウム **NaF**
ブッシェル **BUS**
フッ素 **F**
フッ素18 **F-18，^{18}F**
フッ素18標識陽電子放射型断層撮影(法) **PET-FDG**
フッ素と液体酸素 **flox**
フッ素リン酸ジイソプロピル **DPF**
フット **F，f，Ft，ft**
フート・ポンド **ft lb，ft-lb，FT-Lb**
プテロイルグルタミン酸 **PGA，PteGlu**
プテロイルジグルタミン酸 **PDGA**
プテロイルトリグルタミン酸 **PTGA**
プテロイルヘプタグルタミン酸 **PHGA，PteGlu7**
フート **F，f，Ft，ft**
フート・ランベルト **FL**
ブドウ球菌(属) **S，STAPH，staph，Staph.**
ブドウ球菌エキス **SE**
ブドウ球菌(赤)血球凝集抗体 **SHA**
ブドウ球菌食中毒 **SFD**
ブドウ球菌性中毒性ショック症候群 **STSS**
ブドウ球菌性熱傷様皮膚症候群 **SSSS**
ブドウ球菌蛋白A **SP，SpA，SPA**
ブドウ球菌(性)中毒性表皮壊死融解症 **STEN，S-TEN**
ブドウ球菌腸毒素A **SEA**
ブドウ球菌腸毒素B **SEB**
ブドウ球菌腸毒素B抗血清 **SEBA**
ブドウ球菌腸毒素D

ふ

SED
ブドウ球菌腸毒素 F SEF
ブドウ球菌腸内毒素 SE
ブドウ球菌腸内毒素 E SEE
ブドウ球菌(性)の staph
ブドウ球菌バクテリオファージ製剤 SPL
ブドウ球菌プロテアーゼ SP
ブドウ酒 vim
ブドウ酒様血管腫 PWS
(右旋性)ブドウ糖 D
ブドウ糖 DXT, G, g, Glu, GLU, glu., gluc
ブドウ糖・インスリン・カリウム(療法) GIK
ブドウ糖・システイン血液寒天 GCBA
ブドウ糖・ショ糖・デンプン寒天 DSS
ブドウ糖・食塩比 D/S
(尿中の)ブドウ糖/窒素比 D-N ratio, D：N ratio
ブドウ糖-3-リン酸 G3P
ブドウ糖-食塩水 DS
ブドウ糖アミノゲン液 DAS
ブドウ糖依存インスリン放出ペプチド GIP
ブドウ糖依存向インスリンペプチド GIP
ブドウ糖インスリン負荷試験 GITT
ブドウ糖液 G/W
ブドウ糖含有リン酸緩衝食塩水 GPBS
ブドウ糖酵素 GK
ブドウ糖最大移送値 TmG
ブドウ糖酸化酵素 GO, g.o., GOD
ブドウ糖食塩液 D/S
ブドウ糖水溶液 D/W
ブドウ糖(検査)スティック DS
ブドウ糖生理食塩液 D/NS
ブドウ糖摂取 GU
ブドウ糖ゼラチンベロナール(溶液) DGV
ブドウ糖耐性因子 GTF
ブドウ糖脱水素酵素 GDH
ブドウ糖電解質溶液 GES
ブドウ糖と生食水 G/S
ブドウ糖非発酵グラム陰性桿菌 GNF-GNR
ブドウ糖フェノール液 DP fluid
ブドウ糖負荷 gluc.tol, glu.tol
ブドウ糖負荷試験 GTT
ブドウ糖輸送系 GTS
ブドウ糖輸送量 GT
ブドウ糖療法 GT
ブドウ膜炎・緑内障・前房出血(症候群) UGH
ブドウ膜炎・緑内障・前房出血および硝子体出血(症候群) UGH＋
フートキャンドル fc
フートポンド FP, fp
フートポンド/秒 FPS, fps
フトラフール FT207
フトラフール,アドリアマイシン,シクロホスファミド,シスプラチン(＝プラチノール) FACP
フトラフール,アドリアマイシン,マイトマイシンC FURAM
フートランベルト FTL, ft-L
プトレシン Pu
プトレッシン Put
フマラーゼ FUM
フマル酸還元酵素 FRD
フマル酸ヒドラターゼ FH
フマレート FUM
ブライアン高抗体価株・ラウス肉腫ウイルス BH-RSV
ブライアン標準株・ラウス肉腫ウイルス BS-RSV
プライス沈降反応 PPR
プライバシー保守の 3 大条件：教育・法的規制・技術 3E
フライブルグ人格特性尺度 FPI
プライマリケア PC
プライマリケア医師 PCP
プライマリケア国際分類 ICPC
プライマリケアにおける保健問題の国際分類 ICHPPC
プライマリケア網 PCN
プライマリヘルスケア PHC
フライングスポット顕微鏡 FSM
プラウニッツ・キュストナー PK, P-K
プラウニッツ・キュストナー試験 PKT
プラウニッツ・キュストナー反応 PK reaction, PKR
ブラウン・セカール(症候群) BS
ブラウンキツネザル LFF
プラーク形成細胞 PFC
プラーク形成単位 PFU
フラグメント frag

フラジェリン重合体 **POL**
フラジオマイシン **FRM**
ブラジキニン **BK**
ブラジキニン増強因子 **BPF, BPP**
プラシボ **P, PBO, PL, PLBO**
フラスコ **lag.**
プラストキノン **PQ**
プラストキノン9 **PQ-9**
ブラストミセス(属) **B**
プラズマクリットテスト **PCT**
プラズマ細胞疾患 **PCD**
プラズマ細胞腫 **PCT**
プラズマ脱離マス分光 **PDMS**
プラズマトロンボプラスチン因子 **PTF**
プラズマトロンボプラスチン成分 **PTC**
プラズマトロンボプラスチン成分欠損 **PTCD**
プラズマトロンボプラスチン前駆物質 **PTA**
プラズマプロトロンビン転化因子 **PPCF**
プラズマプロトロンビン転化促進因子 **PPCA**
プラスミド **P**
プラスミノゲン **Pg, plg, PLg, PLG**
プラスミノゲンアクチベータ **PA**
プラスミノーゲン活性化因子 **PLA**
プラスミノゲン活性化抑制因子 **PAI**
プラスミン **PL, Pln**
プラスミン・抗プラスミン複合体 **PIC**
プラスミン α_2 抗プラスミン複合体 **PA**
プラスミン α_2 プラスミンインヒビター複合体 **PIC**
プラスモジウム(属) **P**
プラセオジミウム **Pr**
プラセボ **ADT, P, PBO, PL, PLBO**
プラゾシン **PZ**
フラゾリドン **FZ**
プラダー・ウィリ症候群 **PW, P-W, PWS**
プラダー・ラブハート・ウィリ症候群 **PLWS**
フラダンチン **FD**
プラチナ **plat, Pt**
ブラックファン・ダイヤモンド(症候群) **BD**
ブラックモンガベイ **CAL**
ブラックライト **BL**
フラビンアデニンジヌクレオチド **FAD, FADN**
フラビンアデニンジヌクレオチド還元型 **FADH$_2$**
フラビン含有酸素酵素 **FMO**
フラビンモノヌクレオチド **FM, FMN**
フラビンモノヌクレオチド還元型 **FMNH**
フラボバクテリア髄膜炎 **Fl.m**
プラリドキシム **PAM**
ブラロック・タウジヒ **BT**
ブラロック・タウジヒシャント **BT shunt**
プランク定数 **H**
フランクフルト愁訴質問リスト **FBF**
フランクリン **Fr**
フランシウム **Fr**
フランシセラ(属) **F**
フランス国立骨髄ドナーバンク **GMFT**
フランス式(カテーテルサイズ) **Fr**
フランス製鋼ゾンデ **FSS**
フランス臨床生物学会 **FSBC**
ブランチ **brunch**
ブランデー **s.v.g., S.V.gal., s.v.t.**
ブランド・ホワイト・ガーランド症候群 **BWG syndrome**
プランマー・ビンソン症候群 **PV, PVS**
フーリエ級数 **FS**
フーリエ変換 **FT**
フーリエ変換型マイクロ波分光(計) **MWFT**
フーリエ変換質量分析計 **FTMS**
フーリエ変換赤外分光器 **FTIR**
フーリエ変換を利用したデコンボリューション **FSD**
プリオン蛋白 **PrP**
フリージンガースコア **FS**
プリズム **Pr**
プリズムジオプトリー **PD**
プリズムの **prism**
フリッカー周辺視野 **FP**
フリッカー中心視野 **FC**
フリッカー融合頻度 **FFF**
フリーデリックセン・ウォーターハウス(症候群) **FW**
フリードマン妊娠試験法 **FRIED test**
フリードマン反応 **Fr.R**
フリードリ〔ライ〕ヒ失調症 **FA**
ブリネル硬度数 **BHN**
フリーフロー電気泳動法

FFE
フリーマン-シェルドン(症候群) **FS**
プリミドン **PRM**
ブリュイ **B, br**
フリーラジカル **FR**
フリーラジカル検出法 **FRAT**
ブリリアントイエロー **by**
ブリリアントグリーン **BG**
ブリリアントグリーン乳糖胆汁ブイヨン **BGLB**
ブリリアントクレシルブルー **BCB**
プリン **Pur**
プリン-5′-ヌクレオチダーゼ **PNP**
ブリンクマン指数 **BI, B.I.**
プリンツメタル型狭心症 **PMA**
プリンヌクレオシド **Puo, R**
プリンヌクレオシドホスホリラーゼ **PN**
プリンヌクレオチドサイクル **PNC**
プリンヌクレオチドリン酸分解酵素 **PNP**
フルオシノニド **Fc**
フルオライドナンバー **FN**
フルオレ(ス)セイン **FL, Fl**
フルオレ(ス)セイン/蛋白(比) **F/P**
フルオレ(ス)セインイソシアネイト **FIC**
フルオレ(ス)セインイソチオシアネート **FITC**
フルオレ(ス)セイン酢酸水銀 **FMA**
フルオレ(ス)セイン二酢酸 **FDA**
フルオレ(ス)セイン標識抗体 **FA**
フルオロウラシル **5-FU, FU, FUra**
フルオロウラシル,アドリアマイシン,シクロホスファミド **FAC**
フルオロウラシル,アドリアマイシン,シクロホスファミド,ストレプトゾ(ト)シン **FACS**
フルオロウラシル,アドリアマイシン,シクロホスファミド,レバミゾール **FAC-LEV**
フルオロウラシル,アドリアマイシン,マイトマイシン **FAM**
フルオロウラシル,アドリアマイシン,マイトマイシンC,アルキル化剤 **FAMA**
フルオロウラシル,アドリアマイシン,マイトマイシンC,ストレプトゾ(ト)シン **FAM-S**
フルオロウラシル,アドリアマイシン,メチルクロロエチル-シクロヘキシルニトロソ尿素 **FAMe**
フルオロウラシル,イミダゾール,ビンクリスチン,ビスクロロエチルニトロソ尿素 **FIVB**
フルオロウラシル,エトポシド,シスプラチン **FEC**
フルオロウラシル,シクロホスファミド,アドリアマイシン,シスプラチン **FCAC**
フルオロウラシル,シクロホスファミド,プレドニゾン **FCP**
フルオロウラシル,シクロホスファミド,マイトマイシンC,クロモマイシン **FAMA**
フルオロウラシル,シクロホスファミドA,マイトマイシンC,トヨマイシン **FAMT**
フルオロウラシル,ビンクリスチン(=オンコビン),マイトマイシンC **FOMI**
フルオロウラシル,マイトマイシン,ストレプトゾ(ト)シン **FMS**
フルオロウラシル,マイトマイシンC **FMA**
フルオロウラシル,マイトマイシンC,シタラビン **FMC**
フルオロウラシル,マイトマイシンC,放射線照射 **FUMIR**
フルオロウラシル,メチルクロロエチル-シクロヘキシルニトロソ尿素,ビンクリスチン **FMV**
フルオロウラシル,ラゾキサン,メチルクロロエチル-シクロヘキシルニトロソ尿素 **FIME**
フルオロウラシル,ロイコボリン,シスプラチン(=プラチノール) **FLEP**
フルオロウリジン一リン酸 **FUMP**
フルオロウリジン三リン酸 **FUTP**
フルオロカーボン **FC**
フルオロビプロフェン **FP**
フルオロフェニルアラニン **FPA**
フルオロメトロン **FML**

フルオロヨードアラビノシルシトシン　**FIAC**
ブルガリア乳酸菌(属)　**LB**
ブルガリア乳酸菌因子　**LBF**
ブルギア(属)　**B**
プルキンエ細胞　**PC**
プルキンエ線維　**PF**
プルキンエ層　**PL**
フルクトース一リン酸　**FMP**
フルクトース 1,6-ジホスファターゼ　**FDPase**
フルクトース 1,6-二リン酸　**FDP**
フルクトース二リン酸　**FDP**
フルクトース二リン酸アルドラーゼ　**FDPALD**
フルクトース 1,6-ビスホスファターゼ　**FBPase**
フルクトース 1-リン酸　**F-1-P, F1P**
フルクトース 6-リン酸　**F-6-P, F6P**
フルクトース 6-リン酸キナーゼ　**FPK**
ブルークロス　**BC**
フルコナゾール　**FCZ**
フルシトシン　**FC**
ブルーシールド　**BS**
ブルースター　**B**
ブルセラ(属)　**B, B., BR, Br, BRBA, Bruc**
ブルセラアボータス　**BA**
フルダラビン,アラビノシルシトシン,顆粒球コロニー刺激因子,イダルビシン　**FLAG-ida**
ブルータングウイルス　**BTV**
ブルック反応試験　**BRT**
ブルーテトラゾリウム(染色)　**BT**
プルトニウム　**Pu**
ブルトンチロシンキナーゼ　**Btk**
ブルーバイオレット　**BV**
ブルーレイディスク　**BD**
プールヒト血漿　**PHP**
フルフェナジン　**FPZ**
フルラー〔ハーラー〕症候群　**HS**
プルーンベリー奇形　**PBA**
プルーンベリー症候群　**PBS**
プレ-β-リポ蛋白　**pre-β-Lp**
フレア(発赤拡張)細胞　**F+C**
プレアルブミン　**PA**
ブレオマイシン　**BLEO, Bleo, BLM**
ブレオマイシン,アドリアマイシン,シクロヘキシルクロロエチルニトロソ尿素,ビンクリスチン(=オンコビン)　**BACO**
ブレオマイシン,アドリアマイシン,シクロヘキシルクロロエチルニトロソ尿素,ビンクリスチン(=オンコビン),ニトロゲンマスタード　**BACON**
ブレオマイシン,アドリアマイシン,シクロホスファミド,クエン酸タモキシフェン　**BACT**
ブレオマイシン,アドリアマイシン,シクロホスファミド,ビンクリスチン(=オンコビン),デキサメタゾン　**BACOD**
ブレオマイシン,アドリアマイシン,シクロホスファミド,ビンクリスチン(=オンコビン),プレドニゾン　**BACOP**
ブレオマイシン,アドリアマイシン,ビンブラスチン,イミダゾールカルボキサミド,プレドニゾン　**BAVIP**
ブレオマイシン,アドリアマイシン,プレドニゾン　**BAP**
ブレオマイシン,アドリアマイシン,メトトレキサート,ビンクリスチン(=オンコビン),ニトロゲンマスタード　**BAMON**
ブレオマイシン,イホスファミド,シスプラチン(=プラチノール)　**BIP**
ブレオマイシン,エトポシド,シスプラチン(=プラチノール)　**BEP**
ブレオマイシン,エルジシン,ロムスチン,ダカルバジン　**BELD**
ブレオマイシン,シクロヘキシルクロロエチルニトロソ尿素,アドリアマイシン,ベルバン　**B-CAVe**
ブレオマイシン,シクロホスファミド(=エンドキサン),6-メルカプトプリン,プレドニゾロン　**BEMP**
ブレオマイシン,シクロホスファミド,ダクチノマイシン　**BCD**
ブレオマイシン,シクロホスファミド,ビンクリスチン,プロカルバジン,プレドニゾン　**BCVPP**
ブレオマイシン,ダカルバジン,ビンクリスチン(=オンコビン),プレドニゾン,アドリアマイシン

B-DOPA

ブレオマイシン,ビンクリスチン(＝オンコビン),アドリアマイシン,プレドニゾン **BOAP**

ブレオマイシン,ビンクリスチン,シクロホスファミド,プレドニゾロン **BVCP**

ブレオマイシン,ビンクリスチン(＝オンコビン),ストレプトゾトシン,エトポシド **BOSE**

ブレオマイシン,ビンクリスチン(＝オンコビン),ナツラン,プレドニゾロン **BONP**

ブレオマイシン,ビンクリスチン(＝オンコビン),プレドニゾン **BOP**

ブレオマイシン,ビンクリスチン(＝オンコビン),プレドニゾン,アドリアマイシン,メトトレキサート **BOPAM**

ブレオマイシン,ビンクリスチン(＝オンコビン),プロカルバジン,プレドニゾロン **BOPP**

ブレオマイシン,ビンクリスチン(＝オンコビン),ロムスチン,ダカルバジン **BOLD**

ブレオマイシン,マイトマイシンC **BM**

ブレオマイシン,メクロルエタミン,ビンクリスチン(＝オンコビン),プレドニゾン **BLEO-MOP**

ブレオマイシン,メクロルエタミン,ビンクリスチン(＝オンコビン),プロカルバジン,プレドニゾン **B-MOPP**

フレオン **F**

フレオン12 **F-12**

プレカリクレイン **PKK**

プレカリクレイン活性化因子 **PKA**

プレグナンジオール **P_2, PD, P-diol**

プレグナンジオールグルクロン酸化合物 **PG**

プレグナンジオールグルクロン酸ナトリウム **NaPG**

プレグナントリオール **P_3**

プレドニゾロン **PDL, pred, prednis, PSL**

プレドニゾロンブドウ糖負荷試験 **PGTT**

プレドニゾン **P, PDN, PRED, pred, prednis**

プレドニゾン,アラビノシルシトシン,チオグアニン,シクロホスファミド,ビンクリスチン(＝オンコビン) **PATCO**

プレドニゾン,ビンクリスチン(＝オンコビン),アラビノシルシトシン,シクロホスファミド **POACH**

プレドニゾン,ビンクリスチン(＝オンコビン),メトトレキサート,プリネトール **POMP**

プレドニゾン,フルオロウラシル,タモキシフェン **PFT**

フレーム/秒 **fps**

フレームを用いない原子吸光法 **FLAAS**

フレロキサシン **FLRX**

フレンチ(サイズ) **F**

フレンチ(スケール) **FR, Fr**

フレンチゲージ **FG**

フレンチ番号 **F**

フレンド(ウイルス) **FR**

フレンド・モロニー・ラウシャー(抗原) **FMR**

フレンドウイルス **FV**

フレンドウイルス感受性遺伝子4 **Fv-4**

フレンドウイルス赤血球増加症 **FVP**

フレンドウイルス貧血 **FVA**

フレンド白血病ウイルス **FLV**

フレンド白血病細胞 **FLC**

フレンド病ウイルス **FDV**

フローインジェクション分析 **FIA**

フローインジェクション分析器 **FIA**

プロインスリン **PI**

プロインスリン様成分 **PLC**

フロイントアジュバント **FA**

フロインド完全アジュバント **FCA**

プロオピオメラノコルチン **POMC**

プロカインアミド **PA**

ブローカ帯 **DBB**

プロカルバジン **PCB, PCZ**

プロカルバジン,イグロサミド,メトトレキサート **PRIME**

プロカルバジン,ビンクリスチン(＝オンコビン),シクロヘキシルクロロエチルニトロソ尿素 **POC**

プロカルバジン,ビンクリスチン(＝オンコビン),シクロヘキシルクロロエ

チルニトロソ尿素，シクロホスファミド **POCC**
プロカルバジン・アルケラン・硫酸ビンブラスチン **PAVe**
プログラム **prog**
プログラム案内 **PG**
プログラム化された電気生理学的刺激 **PES**
プログラム可能な埋込み式薬物システム **PIMS**
プロゲステロン **P, PG, P_4**
プロゲステロン受容体 **PgR, PGR, PR**
プロゲステロン受容体試験 **PRA**
プロゲストゲンチャレンジ試験 **PCT**
プロコラーゲン **PC**
プロコラーゲンペプチド **P-P**
フローサイトメトリー **FCM**
プロスタグランジン **PG**
プロスタグランジンA **PGA**
プロスタグランジンB **PGB**
プロスタグランジンC **PGC**
プロスタグランジンD **PGD**
プロスタグランジンE **PGE**
プロスタグランジンE代謝産物 **PGEM**
プロスタグランジンF **PGF**
プロスタグランジンG **PGG**
プロスタグランジンH **PGH**
プロスタグランジンI **PGI**
プロスタグランジンI_2(＝プロスタサイクリン) **PGI_2**
プロスタグランジンJ **PGJ**
プロスタグランジンX **PGX**
プロスタグランジン合成酵素 **PGS**
プロスタグランジン合成酵素阻害薬 **PGSI**
プロスタグランジンシクロオキシゲナーゼ **PCO**
プロスタグランジン様物質 **PLS**
プロスタグランジン類 **PGs**
プロスタサイクリン合成刺激血漿因子 **PSPF**
プロスタサイクリン産生刺激因子 **PSF**
プロスチオン **PR**
フロセミド **FRS, FSM**
フローセン・酸素・笑気麻酔 **FOG**
プロタミン亜鉛インスリン **PZI**
プロタミンインスリン **PI**
プロタミン硫酸試験 **PST**
プロチオナミド **PTH**
ブロチゾラム **BZL**
フロッピーディスク **FD**
プロテアーゼトキソイド **PT**
プロテインC **PC**
プロテインCインヒビター **PCI**
プロテインキナーゼ **PK, PKase**
プロテインキナーゼA **PKA**
プロテインキナーゼC **PKC**
プロテインキナーゼ活性化比 **PKAR**
プロテウス(属) **P**
プロテオグリカン **PG**
プロテオース・イースト・ブドウ糖(ブイヨン) **PYG**
プロテオリピドアポ蛋白 **PLP**
プロテオリピド蛋白 **PLP**
プロテスタント(の) **P, PROT, Prot**
プロテーゼ **pros, prosth**
プロテーゼの **pros**
プロトアクチニウム **Pa**
プロトポルフィリン **PP, PROTO**
プロトポルフィリン症 **PP**
プロトロンビン **PRO, prothrom, PTB**
プロトロンビン・プロコンバーチン(・スチュワート因子活性)検査 **P & P test, P+P-test**
プロトロンビン活性 **PA, PTA**
プロトロンビン含量 **prothr.cont**
プロトロンビン交換因子 **PCF**
プロトロンビン時間 **proth.time, pro-time, pro.time, Pro-X, PT**
プロトロンビン時間国際標準比〔値〕 **PT-INR**
プロトロンビン時間コントロール〔対照〕 **PRTH-C**

ふ

プロトロンビン消費時間 **PCT**
プロトロンビン複合体 **PTC**
プロトロンビン複合体濃縮物 **PCC**
プロトロンビン複合体濃度 **PCC**
プロトン画像 **PDI**
プロトンスペクトロスコープ画像 **PSI**
プロトンポンプ阻害薬 **PPI**
プロパジン **P**
プロパフェノン **Pr**
プロピオニルCoAカルボキシラーゼ **PCC**
プロピオニルエリスロマイシンラウリル硫酸塩 **PELS**
プロピオニルチオコリン **PTC**
プロピオン酸 **PA**
プロピオン酸塩 **P**
プロピオン酸クロベタゾール **CP**
プロピオン酸テストステロン **TP**
(気管支喘息治療の)プロピオン酸ベクロメタゾン吸入 **BDI**
フロー微小螢光測定 **FMF**
プロピシリン **PPPC**
プロビデンシア(属) **P**
プロピル **PR, Pr**
プロピルチオウラシル **PT, PTU**
プロフィブリノリジン **PFL**
プロフェッショナル・メカニカル・トゥース・クリーニング **PMTC**
プロブコールの量の違いによる再発試験 **PQRST**
プロプラノロール **PP, prop**
プロベネシド **Pb, Pb.**
プロペルジンB因子 **Bf**
プロホスホリパーゼA **PROPLA**
フローボリューム曲線 **FVC**
プロマイシンアミノヌクレオシド腎症 **PAN**
プロマイシンアミノヌクレオシドネフローシス **PAN**
ブロムグラスモザイクウイルス **BMV**
ブロムクレゾールグリーン **BCG**
ブロムクレゾール紫 **BCP**
ブロムスルファレイン **BSP**
ブロムスルホフタレインクリアランス **CBSP**
ブロムフェノールブルー **BPB**
ブロムペリドール **BPD**
ブロムベンジルシアニド **CA**
ブロムワレリル尿素 **BVU**
プロメチウム **Pm**
ブロモアセトアミド **BAA**
ブロモウラシル **BrU, BU**
フロモキセフ **FMOX**
ブロモクリプチン **BC, CB-154**
ブロモスルホフタレイン **BSP**
プロモーター **p**
ブロモチモールブルー **BTB**
ブロモデオキシウリジン **BDUR, BrdU, BrdUrd**
ブロモナフトール **1-BN(2)**
ブロモビニルデオキシウリジン **BVDU**
ブロモベンジルシアニド **BBC**
プロラクチン **P, PR, Pr, PRL**
プロラクチン結合測定(法) **PBA**
プロラクチン産生下垂体腫瘍 **MAPM**
プロラクチン産生腫瘍 **PM**
プロラクチン阻害薬 **PI**
プロラクチン分泌抑制因子 **PIE**
プロラクチン放出因子 **PRF**
プロラクチン放出ホルモン **PRH**
プロラクチン放出抑制因子 **PIF, PRIF**
プロラクチン放出抑制ホルモン **PIH, PRIH**
プロリルヒドロキシラーゼ **PH**
プロリン **P, Pro, prol**
フロレンチウム **FL**
プロログ **PROLOG**
フロントエンドプロセッサ **FEP**
ブンガロトキシン **Bgt, BGT, BTX, BuTX, BuTx**
フッ化指数 **FN**
ふ化補助術 **AH**
ふたのある容器に入れて **in vas.claus.**
ふちのある空胞 **RV**
ぶどう酒 **vin, vin., w**
ふらふらする **unst**
ふるえ **trem, tremb**
不安 **anx**

不安階層表　SUD
不安緊張状態　ATS
不安指数　AI
(テイラー)不安尺度(検査)　MAS
不安障害面接基準　ADIS
不安障害面接試験　ADIS
不安状態　AS
不安状態調査票　ASI
不安神経症　AN
不安定(性)　instab
不安定因子　LF
不安定凝固刺激物質　LASS
不安定狭心症　UA, UAP, USAP
不安定蛋白　LP
不安定な　unst
不安定波螢光免疫測定法　EV-FIA
不安定ペプチド　LP
不安定ヘモグロビン病　UHD
不安な　anx
不安のない妊娠　PWF
不一致の　I
不運な産科歴　POH
不応期　RP
不応性貧血　RA
不穏下肢症候群　RLS
不可逆性鎌状赤血球　ISC
不可能な　disab, imposs, U, un
不快音量域値　UCL
不快音量レベル　ULL
不快音レベル　UCLL
不快感　dis, disc
不快感閾値　TD
不快軽減指数　DRQ
不快指数　DI
不完全右脚ブロック　IRBBB
不完全解明乳児突然死症候群　pSIDS
不完全干渉　DI
不完全干渉性粒子　DI particle
不完全左脚ブロック　ILBBB
不完全心(臓)ブロック　IHB
不完全精巣性女性化症候群　ITFS
不完全男性偽半陰陽　IMP
不完全治癒　IH
不完全な　Imp, imp, imperf, INC, inc, inc., incompl
不完全フロインドアジュバント　ICFA
不完全フロインドアジュバント　FIA, IFA
不完全両脚ブロック　IBBBB
不活化ポリオ(ウイルス)ワクチン　IPV
不活化量　IAD
不活性　i
不活性・活性(ワクチン)　KL
不活性化血清　IAS
不活性化ペプシン　IP
不活性化ポリオワクチン　IPV
不活性の　inac
不感蒸泄水分　IW
不感知距離　NOA
不確実(性)　uncert
不確実な　U
(神経)不確帯　ZI, z.i.
不確定因子　UF
不確定種　SP indet, SP inquir
不確定な病因　UE
不均一核リボ核酸　hnRNA, HnRNA
不規則　irreg
不規則の　A, AB, ABN, Abn, abn, abnor, abnorm
不許可の　nl., n.l.
不具　dsabl
不具の　dsabl
不顕性血管(先天)奇形　OCVM
不顕性の　subclin
不顕性リンパ節転移　OLNM
不合格となった　F
不十分データ　ID
不十分な　def, defic, insuf, insuf.
不治の　incur, incur.
不随意運動　IVM
不随意の　invol
不正(子宮)出血　DFB
不正療法　malprac
不正療法医　malprac
(機能)不全(症)　insuff
不全　F
不全型胎児タバコ症候群　FTE
不全片麻痺　HP
不全対麻痺　para, Para, para.
不全流産　Inc Ab
不整脈　Arry, CA
不整脈原性右室異形成　ARVD
不整脈原性右室異型性症　ARV
不整脈治療に関する調査　JALT
不整脈モニター部門　CAMU
不足　def, defic
不足している　def, defic
不足の　sc
不確かな　equiv
不定期DNA合成　UDS
不定の　indef, V, var
(妊娠)不適黄体期　ILP
不適合な　incompat

ふ

不適合溶血性輸血　**IHBT**
不適合溶血性輸血病　**IHBTD**
不適合数　**IN**
不適切性ホルモン分泌　**IGS**
不適当な　**indeq**
不同視　**An, Anisometr**
不動にする　**immobi**
不動の　**immob**
不妊研究会　**ASHI**
不妊の　**ster**
不燃性の　**non flam**
不平　**compl**
不変　**id.**
不変H鎖領域　**CH**
不変L鎖領域　**CL**
不変在来治療　**UCT**
不変の　**UC, unchg**
不変部　**C region, C-region**
不変母音・子音　**CVC**
不本意な精神病院収容者解放のための米国連合　**AAAIMH**
不本意な脱落　**UDO**
不法の　**nl., n.l.**
不飽和(ビタミン)B_{12}結合能　**UBBC**
不飽和結合能　**UBC**
不飽和鉄結合能　**UIBC**
不飽和の　**unsat**
不満足状態　**UC**
不満足な　**uns, unsat**
(姓名)不明　**N/K**
不明　**X, x**
不明熱　**FUO**
不明の　**NK, U, UK, undet, UNK, unk, unkn**
不明瞭な　**amb, ambig, obsc**
不溶性骨ゼラチン　**IBG**
不溶(解)性の　**insol**
不溶性の　**I, i, NL**
不慮乳幼児突然死　**SUID**
付加　**addn, appos**
付加価値通信網　**VAN**
付加的喫煙抑制　**SSA**
付加の　**add., addnl**
付加物　**adj**
付近の　**adj**
付随体　**s, SAT**
付随的臨床所見　**ACF**
付随の　**accy**
付属　**apx**
付属器　**Ad**
付属の　**adj**
付属物　**adj, AP, APP, app, app., Appx**
付帯的な　**incid**
付録　**addend., Beibl, Nachtr, suppl**
扶養家族　**Dep, dep.**
扶養小児への援助　**AFDC**
負荷試験　**TT**
負荷量　**DL, LD**
負傷した　**WD, wd**
負傷者カード　**FM card**
負のフィードバック　**NFB**
振子様回転検査　**PRT**
振子様回転試験　**DPP**
振子(様)眼振　**ny.und**
振る　**AGIT, agit.**
浮腫　**Ö, ö, E, ed**
浮腫・紅斑・滲出液　**EEE**
浮腫・蛋白尿・高血圧妊娠中毒症　**EPH-gestosis**
浮腫因子　**EF**
浮腫斑　**ME**
浮遊物質　**SS**
婦人・乳児・小児　**WIC**
婦人科　**OB/GYN, ob-gyn**
婦人科医　**GYN, Gyn, gyn**
婦人科外来　**WOU**
婦人科学　**GYN, Gyn, gyn**
婦人科学の　**GYN, Gyn, gyn**
婦人年　**WY**
符号　**S, s, SG, sgs**
部　**bur, pt, pt., Reg, reg, reg.**
部位　**Reg, reg, reg.**
部分　**P̲, p., pt, pt., ss, S̅S̅, ss.**
部分回腸バイパス術　**PIB**
部分荷重　**PWB**
部分寛解　**PR**
部分機能好中球　**PFN**
部分脂質ジストロフィ　**PLD**
部分人工心臓　**PAH**
部分清拭　**PB**
部分弾性成分　**PEC**
部分的　**part, part.**
部分的肝切除された　**PH**
部分的肝切除　**HPX**
部分的結節変形　**PNT**
部分的骨髄芽球症を伴う不応性貧血　**RAPM**
部分的作用薬活性　**PAA**
部分的小腸閉塞(症)　**PSBO**
部分的全層角膜移植(術)　**PPK**
部分的に　**part, part.**
部分的に可溶な　**P sol**
部分的肺静脈還流異常　**PAPVC, PAPVD, PAPVR**
部分的半月板切除　**PM**
部分的脾動脈塞栓術　**PSE**
部分てんかん　**PE**
部分トロンボプラスチン時間　**PTT**

部分の　**part, part.**
部分非経口栄養　**PPN**
部分プロトロンビン時間　**PPT**
部分変性反応　**PRD**
部門　**Dept, dept, DPT**
普通かつ慣例的な　**U & C**
普通生活条件　**OLC**
普通の　**conv**
普遍的な　**univ**
普遍的に　**univ**
触れることができない　**NP**
腐蝕性の　**corros**
腐敗(する)　**DK**
腐敗した　**dec, dec'd**
腐敗する　**dec**
孵化後日数　**Pn**
賦形剤　**V**
賦形薬(剤)　**vehic.**
舞踏病　**CHO**
舞踏病・有棘赤血球症　**CA**
封筒　**env**
封入　**incln**
封入形成単位　**IFU**
封入された　**encl**
封入する　**encl**
封入(小)体　**IB, IncB**
封入体筋炎　**IBM**
封入体性結膜炎　**IC**
封入体病〔疾患〕　**ID**
封入体　**I**
風疹ウイルス　**RV**
風疹ワクチン　**RV**
風疹ワクチン様ウイルス　**RVV**
深く浸込ませる　**SAT, sat.**
深さ　**d**
伏在(静脈)　**saph**
伏在静脈　**SV**
伏在静脈移植片　**SVG**
含まれた　**contd**
含む　**cntn, incl**
含む(こと)　**TC**
服用　**s., z.n.**
服用させよ　**s., sum.**
服用する　**capiend., sum.**
服用せよ　**RX, Rx.**
服用前に振れ　**agit.ante sum., agit. a.us.**
服用量　**D, d., dos.**
副看護師長　**AHN**
(補体系の)副経路　**AP**
副経路性50%溶血活性　**$APCH_{50}$**
副甲状腺機能亢進(症)　**hyperpara**
副甲状腺機能亢進症　**HP, HPT, HPTH**
副甲状腺機能亢進性ホルモン　**HPTH**
副甲状腺機能低下・アジソン・モニリア症〔カンジダ症〕(症候群)　**HAMS**
副甲状腺機能低下症　**HP**
副甲状腺機能低下症・アジソン病・モニリア症〔カンジダ症〕(症候群)　**HAM**
副甲状腺摘出(術)　**para**
副甲状腺摘出術　**PTX**
副甲状腺ホルモン　**PH, PTH**
副甲状腺ホルモン関連蛋白　**PTHrP**
副甲状腺ホルモン分泌　**PTHS**
副交感指数　**PI**
副交感神経　**PNS**
副交感神経系　**PSNS**
副交感神経の　**PS**
副交感神経分割　**parasym div**
副行循環　**collat.circ.**
副行路　**BP**
副作用　**ADR, NW, SE**
副作用質問用紙　**SEQ**
副作用用語集　**ART**
副索引　**SI**
副雑音　**Ng**
副子　**sp, spl**
副次的な　**accy**
副神経核　**NAC**
副腎エピネフリン　**AE**
副腎球状帯刺激ホルモン　**AGTH**
副腎皮質　**AC**
副腎腫細胞　**HNC**
副腎髄質　**AdM, AM**
副腎髄質刺激ホルモン　**CASH**
副腎髄質切除(術)　**ADMX**
副腎性器症候群　**AGS**
副腎脊髄ニューロパシー　**AMN**
副腎切除　**ADX**
副腎体重因子　**AWF**
副腎摘出アロキサン糖尿病　**AAD**
副腎摘出した　**ADX**
副腎摘出の　**Adrex**
副腎の　**adren**
副腎白質ジストロフィ　**ALD**
副腎発育因子　**AGF**
副腎白血球脊髄神経疾患　**AMN**
副腎皮質　**AdC, NNR**
副腎皮質刺激試験　**ACTH-Z method**
副腎皮質刺激ポリペプチド　**ACTP**
副腎皮質刺激ホルモン　**ACTH**
副腎皮質刺激ホルモン放出因子　**ACTH-RF,**

CRF
副腎皮質刺激ホルモン放出ホルモン **ACTH-RH, CRH**
副腎皮質自己抗体 **AA**
副腎皮質抽出物 **ACE**
副腎皮質内層 **X-zone**
副腎皮質(機能)不全(症) **ACI**
副腎皮質ポリペプチド **ACPP**
副腎皮質ホルモン **ACH**
副組織適合性遺伝子座 **MIH**
副左胃動脈 **AGSA**
副鼻腔 **PNS**
副鼻腔炎 **S, S.Pn.**
副鼻腔気管支炎 **SB**
副鼻腔気管支症候群 **SBS**
副鼻腔蓄膿症 **Emp., Empy**
(タバコの)副流煙 **ss**
福祉 **comm**
福祉発展 **COMDEV**
福山型先天性筋ジストロフィ **FCMD**
腹囲 **AC, AG, BU, LU**
腹囲指標(＝肥満度指標) **ACI**
腹会陰式直腸切断術 **APR**
腹外側(核) **VL**
腹外側核 **VL nucleus**
腹外側(核)の **VL**
腹腔圧 **Pabd**
腹腔液 **PF**
腹腔鏡 **LPS**
腹腔鏡下エタノール注入療法 **LEI**
腹腔鏡下遠位胃部分切除(術) **LADPG**
腹腔鏡下完全閉鎖(術) **LTO**
腹腔鏡下骨盤リンパ節郭清(術) **LPLND**
腹腔鏡下生殖手術 **LRS**
腹腔鏡下精巣〔睾丸〕固定(術) **LOP**
腹腔鏡下経胆嚢総胆管診査 **LTCBDE**
腹腔鏡下多嚢胞卵巣多孔術 **LOD**
腹腔鏡下胆嚢摘出(術) **LC**
腹腔鏡下胆嚢摘出術 **Lapa-Chole, lapcholy, LCE**
腹腔鏡下腟式子宮摘出術 **LAVH**
腹腔鏡下虫垂切除術 **LA**
腹腔鏡下超音波法 **LUS**
腹腔鏡下ニッセン胃底皺襞形成(術) **LNF**
腹腔鏡下ヘルニア修復術のうち腹膜外到達法 **TEP**
腹腔鏡下マイクロ波凝固療法 **LMC**
腹腔鏡下卵管凝固 **LSTC**
腹腔鏡下卵管結紮 **LTL**
腹腔鏡下卵管焼灼 **LSTC**
腹腔鏡下卵管バンド結紮 **LTB**
腹腔鏡下卵管不妊手術 **LTS**
腹腔鏡下両側卵管部分切除(術) **LS BPS**
腹腔鏡下レーザー胆嚢摘出術 **LLC**
腹腔鏡検査 **laparo**
腹腔鏡検査(法) **LAP, lap**
腹腔鏡的交感神経遮断術 **ETS**
腹腔鏡的卵管結紮(法) **LSTL**
腹腔常在細胞 **RPC**
腹腔静脈シャント術 **PV shunt, P-V shunt**
腹腔神経叢ブロック **CPB**
腹腔滲出液大食細胞 **PEM**
腹腔滲出液リンパ球 **PEL**
腹腔滲出好中球 **PEN**
腹腔滲出細胞 **PEC**
腹腔動脈 **CA, CT**
腹腔動脈圧迫症候群 **CACS**
腹腔内(注射) **IP**
腹腔内圧 **IAP**
腹腔内温熱灌流療法 **IPHP**
腹腔内化学療法 **IPC**
腹腔内感染 **IAI**
腹腔内授精 **DIPI**
腹腔内ショック **IPS**
腹腔内に **IP, ip, i.p.**
腹腔内の **IAB, IP, ip, i.p.**
腹式呼吸 **abd resp**
腹式子宮全摘術 **ATH, TAH**
腹式子宮全摘術・両卵管卵巣摘出術 **TAHBSO**
腹式子宮摘出(術) **AH**
腹式子宮摘出術 **ABD HYST, Abd Hyst**
腹水 **AF, Ascit Fl**
腹水/血漿(比) **A/P**
腹側 **ABD, Abd, abd, abd., abdo, ABDOM, Abdom, abdom**
腹側頸椎癒着術 **VDS**
腹側後下(核) **VPI**
腹側後外側(核) **VPL**
腹側後内側(核) **VPM**
腹側後内側視床核 **VPM**
腹側正中 **vm.**

腹側脊髄視床路　**VST**
腹側前部の　**VA**
腹側動脈バイパスポンピング　**VABP**
腹側の　**ABD, Abd, abd, abd., abdo, ABDOM, Abdom, abdom, V, v, ven, vent, ventr**
(神経の)腹側被蓋部(野)　**VTA**
腹側無顆粒島状皮質　**AIV**
腹側網状核　**NRV**
腹側網様核　**RV**
腹内側核　**VM, VMN**
腹内側視床下部(ニューロン/核)　**VMH**
腹内側の　**VM**
腹(側)の　**AB**
腹(部)の　**AB**
腹背側の　**VD**
腹部　**ABD, Abd, abd, abd., abdo, ABDOM, Abdom, abdom**
腹部・会陰の　**AP, A-P**
腹部X線写真　**abd XP**
腹部射創　**GSWA**
腹部銃創　**GSWA**
腹部食道　**Ea**
腹部大動脈　**AO**
腹部大動脈瘤　**AAA**
腹部大動脈瘤切除術　**AAA**
腹部に　**p.a.**
腹部の　**ABD, Abd, abd, abd., abdo, ABDOM, Abdom, abdom, ven, vent, ventr**
腹部パッド　**ABD (pad)**
腹部皮膚反射　**AbSR**
腹壁欠損(症)　**VWD**
腹壁脂肪指数　**AFI**
腹壁嚢胞状気腫　**PCI**
腹壁反射　**BDR**
腹膜　**P**
腹膜外前外側椎間板摘出術　**EPALD**
腹膜外内視鏡骨盤リンパ節切除　**EEPLND**
腹膜偽粘液腫　**PP**
腹膜偽(性)粘膜腫　**PP**
腹膜後気体造影法　**Pneumoret**
腹膜後線維腫症　**RF**
腹膜後線維症　**RPF**
腹膜滲出液　**PE, PEF**
腹膜転移　**P**
腹膜透析　**PD**
腹膜透析液　**PDF**
腹膜透析システム　**PDS**
腹膜播種　**P**
腹膜播種・肝転移・漿膜浸潤・リンパ節転移　**PHSN**
腹膜播種の程度　**P_{0-3}**
腹鳴　**G**
複合　**Z, Z-**
複合化学反応　**CCR**
複合型経口避妊薬　**COC**
複合活動電位　**CAP**
複合筋活動電位　**CMAP**
複合近視合併性乱視　**M+Am**
複合血球計測　**CBC**
複合産物　**CP**
複合信号処理器　**MSP**
複合ストレプトマイシン　**COSM**
複合体　**C, Cx**
複合の　**mux**
複合〔複雑〕反応時間　**CRT**
複合ビタミン輸液　**MVI**
複合病変　**CL**
複合粉砕骨折　**CCF**
複合ヨードグリセリン　**I_2KL**
複合連絡　**JC**
複雑型局部疼痛症候群　**CRPS**
複雑な　**compl**
複雑部分てんかん　**CPE**
複雑部分てんかん重積発作　**CPSE**
複雑部分発作　**CPS**
複視　**DV**
複数感染再活性化　**MR**
複数の　**pl**
複性遠視性乱視　**H+Hm, H-Hm**
複性近視性遠視　**CMA**
複製　**dup, repro**
複製開始遺伝子　**ori**
(ウイルスの)複製型分子　**RF**
複製する　**dup, repro**
複方　**co., Comp., comp., cp, cp.**
輻輳　**C, conv, converg**
輻輳近点　**NPC**
輻輳斜視　**conv.strab**
輻輳不全　**CI**
藤紫色　**L**
蓋付膠嚢　**cap gel op.**
再びチェックする　**re.ch**
縁　**MAR, marg**
仏国際軍事医薬委員会　**CIMPM**
沸点　**BP, bp, b.p., EB**
沸湯で　**in aq.bull.**
沸騰　**Coct, coct., EB**
沸騰(させよ)　**bull, bull.**
沸騰時に　**impet-efferv**
沸騰水　**aq.bul., aq.bull., aq.ferv.**
沸騰の終りに　**sub fin.coct.**
物質　**mat, subst**
物質P　**SP**

ふ

物体・フィルム間距離 **OFD**
物理・職業治療認定書 **Dip.P. & OT.**
物理学的半減期 **Tp**
物理学的ミリレントゲン当量 **MREP**
物理的痙攣 **pj's**
物理療法 **PhysTher, phys.ther, PT**
物理療法科 **PM**
物理療法学外来 **PM clinic**
物理療法学士 **B.S.Phys.Ther.**
物理療法協会員 **MCSP**
物理療法士 **B.Phy.Thy., BPT**
物理療法士全国協会 **NAPT**
物理療法とリハビリテーション **PMR, PM & R, PM+R**
物理療法とリハビリテーション科 **PMRS**
物療医学 **PhysMed, Phys Med**
復帰的分裂終了期 **RP**
(作用)物質〔薬/因子〕 **agt, agt.**
太った・40 歳代・女性 **FFF**
太った・40 代〔50 代〕・女性,生殖力のある **4F**
船積み熱ウイルス **SFV**
古い **O**
古い骨の **OB**
分 **m, mi, MIN, min.**
分圧 **P, PP**
分化 **d**
分化凝集力価 **DAT**
分化(型)甲状腺癌 **DTC**
分化細胞 **DC**
分化的分裂間期 **DI**
分化度 **DR**
分画 **F, f, Fract, fract, Seg, seg**
分画の **F, f**
分画排出 **FE**
分割 **div, div., seg**
分割された **seg**
分割する **Seg, seg**
分割量 **part.bic.**
分解 **decomp**
分解する **dec, decomp**
分解型彎曲消化管吻合器 **PCEEA**
分解産物 **DP**
分解指数 **DI**
分解した **dec, dec'd, decomp**
分岐鎖アミノ酸 **BCAA**
分極 **P**
分極活性ゾーン **ZPA**
分光光度計 **SP**
分差 **MD**
分散解析 **ANOV, ANOVA**
分散多変量解析 **MANOVA**
分散比 **F**
分散分析 **ANOV, ANOVA**
分子 **mol, mole**
分子軌道 **MO**
分子層 **ML, MOL**
分子の **mol, mole**
分子(量)比 **Mr**
分子量 **M, Mg, mol.wgt, MOL WT, Mol wt, mol wt, mol.wt., MW, MWt**
分子量限界 **MWCO**
分子量判別上限 **SE**
分子量分布 **MWD**
分枝血管閉塞 **BVO**
分時回転数 **rpm, RPM**
分時換気量 **MBC,** V_E
分時呼吸数 **RRpm**
分時呼吸量 **RMV**
分時最大呼吸量 **MVV**
分時静脈血酸素消費量 mVO_2
分時心拍出量 **CMO, HMV**
分時心拍出量指数 **HMV**
分時肺換気血流比 $\dot{V}Q$
分時肺胞換気量 $\dot{V}_A$, V_A
分時拍出量 **MO**
分時量 **MV**
分腎機能 **SRF**
分腎機能検査 **SRFS**
分腎機能比 **SFR**
分数 **F, f**
分析 **ANAL., anal, anal.**
分析者 **ANAL., anal, anal.**
分析心理学 **Anal.Psychol.**
分析心理学的精神科医 **A(-)P psychiatrist**
分析する **ANAL., anal, anal.**
分析的知能テスト **AIT**
分析電子顕微鏡 **AEM, ATEM**
分析電子顕微鏡検査 **AEM**
分析の **ANAL., anal, anal., analyt**
分析用試薬 **AR**
分節 **Seg, seg**
分節性脊椎固定術 **SSI**
分配 **dis, distr, distrib**
分配クロマトグラフィ **PC**
分配係数 **Kd, PC**
分配する **dist, distr, distrib**
分配量 **VD**
分泌 **S**

分泌(型)　**Se**
分泌遺伝子　**Se**
分泌型免疫グロブリンA　**sIgA, S-IgA**
分泌小胞　**SV**
分泌成分　**SC**
分泌顆粒　**S, SG**
分泌者　**Se**
分泌小滴　**SD**
分泌性中耳炎　**SOM**
分泌率　**SR**
分泌片　**SP**
分布　**distr, distrib, dstr**
分布係数　**Kd**
分布する　**distr, distrib**
分布点　**DP**
分布表　**TD**
(薬物の血中)分布容量　**Vdss**
分服で　**fract.dos., part.vic.**
分別合成比　**FSR**
分別尿　**Fx**
分娩　**Del, del., dely, dlvr, dy, P, part, part.**
分娩・出産・回復　**LDR**
分娩開始　**OOL**
分娩経過図　**PG**
分娩後(の)　**P, Pp**
分娩後室　**PDR**
分娩後出血　**PPH**
分娩後に　**AP**
分娩させる　**Del, del.**
分娩時死産　**IPSB**
分娩した　**dld**
分娩時胎児仮死　**IPFD**
分娩室　**DR, D.R., LR**
分娩前出血　**APH**
分娩前に　**a.p., PTD**
分娩の　**dd, deld, delvd**
分娩日　**DD**
分娩予定日　**CDC, DED, EDC, EDD**
分母　**denom**
分包散剤　**cap.chart., chart, chart.**
分葉核(好中球)　**seg**
分葉核好中球　**Seg, SEGS, Segs, segs, Sg**
分葉性糸球体腎炎　**LGL, LGN**
分量　**D, d.**
分離　**dissoc, isoln, seg, sep**
分離された　**seg**
分離した　**sep**
分離する　**dissoc, seg, sep, sev**
分離せず　**NI**
分離の　**crit**
分離肺換気　**DLV**
分類　**clas, clasn, class**
分類学　**taxon**
分類された　**classif**
分類されていない　**NC**
分類する　**clas**
分類操作上の単位　**OTU**
分類不能型低免疫グロブリン血症　**CVH**
分類不能の　**u, UC, unclas**
分類不能の間質性肺炎　**NCIP**
分類不能の結合組織疾患　**UCTD**
分裂　**div, div., f**
分裂指数　**MI**
分裂症反応　**SR, S/R**
分裂促進因子　**MF**
分裂病国際試験研究　**IPSS**
分裂片　**seq.**
文化的/民族的多様性　**CED**
(引用)文献　**biblio**
文献　**art, lit, lit., ref**
文書　**doc**
文書型定義　**DTD**
文書提示　**doc**
文章完成検査　**SCT**
文章完成テスト　**SCT**
文章での指示　**WO, W/O**
吻合(術)　**ANAS**
吻合部ポリープ状肥厚性胃炎　**SPHG**
吻側延髄腹外側部　**RVLM**
粉砕された　**com, comm, commin**
粉砕する　**trit.**
粉末　**pdr, plv., powd, PULV, pulv., pwd, talc.**
粉末エキス　**PE**
粉末化する　**pulv**
粉末吸入器　**DPI**
粉末にした　**p., plv., powd, red.in pulv., Red.in pulv., r in pulv, r.in pulv.**
粉末にする　**redig.in pulv.**
粉末にせよ　**red.in pulv., Red.in pulv.**
雰囲気　**ATM, atm, atmos**
雰囲気の　**atmos**
噴霧　**Neb**
噴門痙攣　**ACH**
噴門上部興奮伝播時間差　**ECTD**
噴門上部の　**EP**
噴門部　**C**
噴門部癌　**C-K, CK**
糞(便)　**F**
糞線虫(属)　**S**

糞(便)の　**F**
糞便　**F**
糞便中ウロビリノゲン
　FU
糞便封鎖システム
　FcR-AD
糞便連鎖球菌　**SF**

へ

ベーア・シフリン(病)　**BS**
ペア刺激　**PS**
ヘアリーセル白血病　**HCL**
ベイシック　**BASIC**
ヘキサクロルエタン　**HC**
ヘキサクロロシクロヘキサン　**HCC**
ヘキサクロロフェン　**COMPD G-11, G_6, HCP**
ヘキサクロロフェンフェニル水銀　**PMH**
ヘキサジメスリン　**HDM**
ヘキサメチルホスホラミド　**HMP, HMPA**
ヘキサメチルメラミン　**HMM, HXM**
ヘキサメチルメラミン,アドリアマイシン,*cis*-ジアミンジクロロプラチナム　**HAD**
ヘキサメチルメラミン,アドリアマイシン,シクロホスファミド　**HAC**
ヘキサメチルメラミン,アドリアマイシン,メルファラン　**HAM**
ヘキサメチルメラミン,シクロホスファミド,アドリアマイシン,シスプラチン(=プラチノール)　**H-CAP**
ヘキサメチルメラミン,シクロホスファミド,アンホテリシンB,フルオロウラシル　**Hexa-CAF**
ヘキサメチルメラミン,ビンクリスチン(=オンコビン),メトトレキサート　**HOM**
ヘキサメチルリン酸トリアミド　**HMPT**
ヘキサメチレン・ジイソシアネート　**HDI**
ヘキサメチレンテトラミン　**HMT**
ヘキサメチレンビスアセトアミド　**HMBA**
ヘキソキナーゼ　**HK, Hx**
ヘキソキナーゼ1　**HK1**
ヘキソサミニダーゼA　**HEXA, Hex A**
ヘキソサミニダーゼB　**HEXB, Hex B**
ヘキソース　**Hxs**
ヘキソース一リン酸経路　**HMP, HMPS, HMS**
ヘキソース二リン酸　**HDP**
ヘキソン抽出アセトン　**HEA**
ベクター　**vect**
ヘクト(=10^2)　**h**
ヘクトグラム(=100 g)　**hg**
ヘクトパスカル(=mb)　**hPa**
ヘクトメートル(=100 m)　**hm**
ヘクトリットル(=100 *l*)　**hl**
ベクトル　**V, *V***
ベクトル眼電位図計　**VEOG**
ベクトル心磁図　**VMCG**
ベクトル心電図　**VCG, VECG, VKG**
ベクトル心電図法　**VCG**
ヘグリン症候群　**HS**
ベクレル　**Bq**
ページ(頁)　**P, p**
ページェット病　**PD**
ページング・カルジオバージョン・脱細動　**PCD**
ページング刺激　**PI**
ヘス・エドワード分類　**HE classification**
ペスト予防連合委員会　**FCPC**
ヘストン人格調査表　**HPI**
ベスニエ・ベック(症候群)　**BB**
ベスニエ・ベック・シャウマン(症候群)　**BBS**
ペースメーカー　**PM**
ペースメーカー症候群　**PS**
ペースメーカー除細動器　**PCD**
ペースメーカー線　**PMW**
ペースメーカー(興奮)旋回〔輪回〕運動頻拍(脈)　**PCMT**
ペースメーカー媒介頻脈　**PMT**
ベータ　**B, b.**
ペタ(=10^{15})　**P**
ヘタシリン　**DOPIPC**
ベータ線　**β, β ray**
ベタメタゾン　**BM, BMS**
ベーチェット症候群　**BS**
ベーチェット病　**BD**
ベッカー型筋ジストロフィ　**BMD**
ベックうつ病尺度　**BDI**
ヘッシュル回　**HG**
ベッツ・クリューガー母斑　**B-K mole**
ペット　**PET, PETT**
ヘッドアップディスプレイ　**HUD**
ヘッド・ホームズ(症候群)　**HH**
ベッド外で　**OOB**
ベッドサイド　**BS, bs**

ベッドサイドケア　**BSC**
ベッドサイドで　**ABS**
ベッドサイドドレナージ　**BSD**
ベッドサイドにて　**@bs.**
ベッド上安静　**BR**
(疾病でなく性行為による)ベッドでの死　**DIB**
(疾病ではなく性行為による)ベッドでの死　**D in B**
ベッド頭部　**HOB**
ベッドの頭部を上げる　**EHB**
ベッドの長さ　**FOB**
ベッド肺分画　**PBS**
ヘテロ(ジナス)核リボ核蛋白　**hnRNP**
ヘテロ(ジナス)核リボ核酸　**hnRNA，HnRNA**
ヘテロ接合性オルニチントランスカルバモイラーゼ　**HOTC**
ヘテロ接合性家族性高コレステロール血(症)　**hFH**
ヘテロ接合体　**Ht**
ヘテロ接合の　**HET**
ヘテロファゴゾーム　**HP**
ヘテロリボ核酸　**hRNA**
ペニー重量　**dwt**
ペニシラミン　**PC**
ペニシラミン誘発筋無力症　**PIM**
ペニシリウム(属)　**P**
ペニシリナーゼ産生淋菌　**PPNG**
ペニシリン　**P，PC，PCN，Pen，pen，penic，PNC**
ペニシリン,ストレプトマイシン,テトラサイクリン　**PST**
ペニシリン,バシトラシン,ストレプトマイシン,カプリル酸塩　**PBSC**
ペニシリンG　**PCG，PNG**
ペニシリンG耐性肺炎球菌　**PRSP**
ペニシリンV　**PCV，V-cillin**
ペニシリンVカリウム　**PVP**
ペニシリン感受性酵素　**PSE**
ペニシリン感受性肺炎球菌　**PSSP**
ペニシリン群抗生物質　**PCs**
ペニシリン結合蛋白　**PBP**
ペニシリン除去率　$\mathbf{E_{pc}}$
ペニシリン耐性肺炎球菌　**PRSP**
ペニシリン低感受連鎖球菌性肺炎　**PISP**
ペニシロイルポリリジン　**PPL**
ペニスの血圧と上腕動脈収縮期圧との比　**PBI**
ベネズエラウマ脳脊髄炎(ウイルス)　**VEE**
ベネズエラ脳炎　**VE**
ベノア度盛　**B**
ヘノッホ・シェーンライン(症候群)　**HS**
ヘノッホ・シェーンライン紫斑病　**HPS，HSP**
ヘノッホ・シェーンライン紫斑病性腎炎　**HSPN**
ヘノッホ・シェーンライン症候群　**HSS**
ペーパークロマトグラフィ　**PC，PCG**
ヘパプラスチン試験　**HPT**
ペーパーラジオイムノソルベント試験　**PRIST**
ヘパラン硫酸プロテオグリカン　**HSPG**
ヘパリン　**H，HP**
ヘパリン・ノボ・レンテ　**HNL**
ヘパリン依存性(血)小板関連抗体　**HDPAA**
ヘパリン加血漿肝性リパーゼ　**PHHL**
ヘパリン加血漿リポ蛋白リパーゼ　**PHLPL**
ヘパリン加新鮮血液　**Hp-F**
ヘパリン関連血小板減少(症)　**HAT**
ヘパリン関連血小板減少(症)と血栓症　**HATT**
ヘパリン結合性成長因子　**HBGF**
ヘパリン結合成長因子　**HGF**
ヘパリン結合増殖因子1　**HBGF-1**
ヘパリン後脂肪分解活性　**PHLA**
ヘパリンコファクターII　**HC II**
ヘパリン中和活性　**HNA**
ヘパリン添加血漿　**PHP**
ヘパリン補因子　**HC**
ヘパリン誘因性血栓症・血小板減少症候群　**HITTS**
ヘパリン誘発〔誘因〕性血小板減少症　**HIT**
ヘパリン誘発体外LDL沈殿法　**HELP**
ヘパリン誘発体外低比重リポ蛋白沈殿法　**HELP**
ヘビースモーカー　**HS**
ヘビ毒　**SV**
ベビー用軟食　**BSD**
ベフェニウムヒドロキシナフトエート　**BHN**
ペプシノゲン　**PG**
ペプシン　**peps，PPS**

ペプシンユニット **PU**
ペプチケニオ **PTC**
ペプチダーゼ **Pep, PEP**
ペプチド・ヒスチジン・イソロイシン **PHI**
ペプチド HM **PHM**
ペプチド YY **PYY**
ペプチド結合蛋白 **PBP**
ペプトコッカス(属) **P**
ペプトン・デンプン・ブドウ糖 **PSD**
ペプトン・ブドウ糖・酵母抽出物 **PGYE**
ペプレオマイシン **NK631**
ペプレオマイシン,シスプラチン(=プラチノール),マイトマイシンC **PPM**
ペプロマイシン **PEP**
べへノイルアラビノフルラノシルシトシン,ダウノルビシン,6-メルカプトプリン,プレドニゾロン **BH-AC DMP**
べへノイルアラビノフルラノシルシトシン(=エノシタビン) **BH-AC**
ヘマトキシリン・エオジン(染色法) **H and E staining**
ヘマトキシリン・エオジン染色 **HES**
ヘマトキシリン・フロキシン・サフロン **HPS**
ヘマトキシリンエオジン染色 **HE**
ヘマトキシリンとヴァンギーソン(染色) **HVG**
ヘマトクリット **crit, Crit, crit., Crt, crt, hcrit, hemat, HMT, Ht**
ヘマトクリット(値) **Hct**
ヘマトクリット値 **Ht**
ヘマトポルフィリン **Hp**
ヘマトポルフィリン誘導体 **HpD**
ヘミコリニウム3 **HC-3**
ヘミン **X-factor**
ヘミン調節性インヒビター **HRI**
ヘミン調節性レプレッサー **HCR**
ヘム **X-factor**
ヘム〔血色素〕合成酵素 **HS**
ヘムシンターゼ **HS**
ヘモグロビン **Hb, hem, hemo, Hg, HGB, Hgb, hGB, hgb.**
ヘモグロビン・ハプトグロビン(複合体) **Hb-HP**
ヘモグロビン50%酸素(化)圧 **P-50, P_{50}**
ヘモグロビンA **Hb A**
ヘモグロビンA_1 **Hb A_1**
ヘモグロビンA_{1c} **Hb A_{1c}**
ヘモグロビンA_2 **Hb A_2**
ヘモグロビンAとヘモグロビンS **Hb A-S**
ヘモグロビンC **Hb C**
ヘモグロビンD **HbD**
ヘモグロビンE **Hb E**
ヘモグロビンF **HbF**
ヘモグロビンH **Hb H**
ヘモグロビンM **HbM**
ヘモグロビンP **Hb P**
ヘモグロビンS **Hb S**
ヘモグロビンSのホモ接合型 **HbSS**
ヘモグロビンS病 **HbS disease**
ヘモグロビンSC **HbSC**
ヘモグロビンSC病 **HbSC disease**
ヘモグロビン血漿比 **H/P**
ヘモグロビン酸カリウム **KHb**
ヘモグロビン〔血色素〕とヘマトクリット **Hgb & Hct**
ヘモグロビンとヘマトクリット **H & H**
ヘモグロビン濃度 **CGM**
ヘモグロビン飽和度 **S**
ヘモグロビンレポア **Hb Lepore**
ヘモクロマトーシス **HCH, Hch**
ヘモシアニン **HCY**
ヘモフィルス(属) **H**
ヘモフィルス(属)胸膜肺炎 **HP**
ヘモフィルス属の感受性検査用培地 **HTM**
ヘモペキシン **Hx**
ヘモペキシン **Hpx**
ペヨーテ **P**
ヘラー・ネルソン(症候群) **HN**
ペラグラ予防因子 **PPF, PP factor, P.P.factor, P-P factor**
ペラグラ予防の **PP, P-P**
ペラグラ予防ビタミン **vit PP**
ベラドンナ **BD, bella**
ベラドンナエキス **X-Bell**
ベラドンナと阿片 **BO, B & O**
ヘリウム **He**
ヘリウム希釈 **HD**
ヘリウム平衡時間 **HET**
ペリオジック酸・メテナミン銀 **PAMS**
ヘリコバクターピロリ **HP**

ペリディニムクロロフィル(蛋白) **PerCP**
ペリフラックスレーザード(ッ)プラ流量計 **PLDF**
ベリリウム **Be**
ベリリウム肺疾患 **BLD**
ペリレン **Pe**
ベル **B**
ペルオキシソーマルエタノール酸化システム **PEOS**
ペルオキシダーゼ **Po ase, POX, PX**
ペルオキシダーゼ抗ペルオキシダーゼ **PAP**
ペルオキシダーゼ標識抗体 **PTA**
ベルクロラ音 **Velcro**
ベルチエラ(属) **B**
ヘルツ **Hz**
ベルナール・ホルナー症候群 **BH**
ヘルニア **H, her., hern**
ヘルニア板症候群 **HDS**
ヘルパー/サプレッサー(比) **H/S**
ヘルパーT細胞 **HT cell, TH, Th, Thc**
ヘルパーT細胞/サプレッサーT細胞比 **TH/TS**
ヘルパーT細胞因子 **ThF**
ヘルパー因子 **HF**
ヘルパンギーナ **HA**
ベルビュー知能検査 **BIS**
ヘルプ(症候群) **HELLP**
ペルフェナジン **PZC**
ペルフルオロイソブチレン **PFIB**
ペルフルオロ化合物 **PFC**
ペルフルオロトリプロピルアミン **FTPA**
ヘルペス **zos**
ヘルペスウイルス **HV**
ヘルペスウイルス感受性 **HVS**
ヘルペスウイルスサイミリ **HVS**
ヘルペス型ウイルス **HTV**
ヘルペス性膝神経節炎 **HGG**
ヘルペス様ウイルス **HLV**
ベル麻痺 **BP**
ヘルマンスキー・パドラック症候群 **HPS**
ヘルムホルツ自由エネルギー **F**
ベルンハイム基礎培地 **BBM**
ペレグリーニ・シュティーダ(症候群) **PS**
ヘロイン **big H, H**
ヘロイン・モルヒネ・コカイン **HMC**
ヘロイン緊急救命プロジェクト **HELP**
ヘロイン性腎症 **HAN**
ヘロインとコカイン **H & C**
ベロ毒素 **VT**
ベロ毒素産生大腸菌 **VTEC**
ベロナール緩衝液 **VB**
ベロナール緩衝液賦形 **VBD**
ベロナール緩衝シュウ酸塩加生(理)食(塩)水 **VBOS**
ベロナール緩衝生食水 **VBS**
ベーンケン単位 **R**
ベンザチンペニシリンG **BPG**
ベンジオダロン **BZD**
ベンジル **Bzl**
ベンジル・チオウレア **BTU**
ベンジルオキシカルボニル(基) **Z**
ベンジル酸 3α トロパニルエステル **BTE**
ペンシルベニア大学嗅覚鑑定試験 **UPSIT**
ベンジルペニシリン **BPC, PCG**
ベンジルペニシリン・ベンザチン **BPC-G**
ベンジルペニシロイル **BPO**
ベンジルペニシロイルヒト血清アルブミン **BPO-HSA**
ベンジルペニシロイルポリリジン **BPL**
ベンジン **benz, benz.**
ベンズアルデヒド **BzH**
ベンズキアミド **BZQ**
ベンスジョーンズ(蛋白) **BJ**
ベンスジョーンズ蛋白 **BJP**
ベンゼドリン **benz, benz.**
ベンゼン **benz, benz.**
ベンゼン・トルエン・キシレン **BTX**
ベンゼンスルホヒドラジド **BSH**
ベンゼンスルホン酸 **BSA**
ベンゼン(寒天培地)の **BZ**
ベンゾイル **BZ, Bz**
ベンゾイルアルギニンアミド **BAA**
ベンゾイルアルギニンエチルエステル **BAEe**
ベンゾイルアルギニンメチルエステル **BAME**

ベンゾイル化 4,4′-ジアミノスチルベン-2,2′-ジスルホン酸 **MBAS**
ベンゾイルサイアミン-*o*-一リン酸塩 **BTMP**
ベンゾイルペルオキシド **BPO_2**
ベンゾジアゼパン **BDZ**
ベンゾジアゼピン **BZ**
ベンゾジアゼピン誘導体 **BZD**
ベンゾチアジド **BZD**
ベンゾチアディアジン **BTD**
ベンゾピレン **BP**
ベンゾール **BZL**
ベンダー・ゲシュタルト（検査） **BG**
ベンダー・ゲシュタルト検査 **BGT**
ペンタガストリン **PG**
ペンタクロロニトロベンゼン **PCNB**
ペンタクロロフェノール **PCP**
ベンダー試験 **BGT**
ヘンダーソン・ハッガード（吸入器） **HH**
ヘンダーソン・ヘッガード吸入器 **HHI**
ペンタデシルカテコール **PDC**
ペンタマイシン **PNT, PTM**
ペンタミシン **PNT**
ペンタメチルメラミン **PMM**
ベンチレータ（ー） **V, vent**
ペンチレンテトラゾール **PTZ**
ペンテトラゾール **PTZ**
ペントース核酸 **PNA**
ペントタール **pento**
ペントタールナトリウム **Sod Pent**
ベントナイト絮状反応試験 **BFT**
ベントナイト綿状反応試験 **BFT**
ヘンリー **H**
ヘンレのわな〔係蹄〕 **LOH**
ヘンレ（の）わな **LH**
へこんだ **cv**
ヘラー・ドール（手技） **HD**
ヘリックス・ループ・ヘリックス（の DNA 結合モチーフ） **HLH**
部屋 **rm**
部屋から出て **OOR**
平滑型（細菌集落） **S**
平滑筋 **SM**
平滑筋芽腫 **LB, LMB**
平滑筋活性化因子 **SMAF**
平滑筋細胞 **SMC**
平滑筋細胞由来増殖因子 **SDGF**
平滑筋自己抗体 **SMA**
平滑筋肉腫 **LMS, LS**
平滑筋ミオシン H 鎖 **SMMHC**
平均 **M**
平均（の） **aver, avg**
平均１日窒素平衡 **MDNB**
平均１日量 **ADD, MDD**
平均圧 **MP**
平均右（心）室圧 **MRVP**
平均右（心）房圧 **MRAP**
平均右房圧 **RAm**
平均拡張期圧 **AvDP**
平均加算機 **ARC**
平均加重比 **AWR**
平均ガス圧 **P**
平均気道内圧 **MAP**
平均吸気圧 **MIP**
平均吸収時間 **MAT**
平均球面燭光 **mscp**
平均駆出率 **MER**
平均駆出力 **MSF**
平均グリセリン変動域 **MAGE**
平均経過コンピュータ **CAT**
平均螢光強度 **MFI**
平均血圧 **MBP, Pm**
平均血管内圧 **AIP, MIP**
平均血漿濃度 **MPC**
平均血小板体積 **MPV**
平均血糖 **MBG**
平均効果圧 **MEP**
平均呼吸時間 **MTT**
平均故障時間 **MTBF**
平均最小必要量 **AMR**
平均最大呼気流量 **MEF_{50}**
平均最大流量 **MMF**
平均細胞閾値 **MCT**
平均細胞直径 **MCD**
平均左（心）室収縮期（圧） **LVs**
平均左（心）室房圧 **LA_m**
平均左（心）房圧 **MLAP**
平均二乗誤差 **mse**
平均収縮期駆出速度 **MSER**
平均重量 **MW**
平均腫脹時間 **MST**
平均寿命 **$\dot{M}_0$**
平均循環時間 **MCT**
平均循環時間測定装置 **MT**
平均静脈血酸素量 **MVO_2, $M\bar{V}O_2$**
平均上腕動脈（圧） **BAm**
平均除去率 **MCR**
平均心係数 **MCI**
平均腎血流量 **MRBF**
（放射線の）平均身体照射量 **ABD**

平均水平燭光　**mhcp**
平均数　**n**
平均静止電位　**MRP**
平均生存期間　**MST**
平均生存日数　**MSD**
平均赤血球径　**MED**
平均赤血球血色素濃度　**MCC，MCHC**
平均赤血球血色素量　**MCH**
平均赤血球厚径　**MCT**
平均赤血球恒数　**MCC**
平均赤血球寿命　**MRCLS**
平均赤血球直径　**MCD**
平均赤血球ヘモグロビン濃度　**MCHC**
平均赤血球ヘモグロビン量　**MCH，MCHg，MCHgb**
平均赤血球容積　**MCV**
平均絶対誤差　**MAE**
平均絶対偏差　**MAD**
平均全身動脈圧　**mSAP，MSAP**
平均潜伏期　**MIP**
平均線量　**D**
平均体温　**MBT**
平均対照群死　**MCD**
平均大動脈(血)圧　**MAP**
平均滞留時間　**MRT**
平均値の標準偏差値　**SDM，sdm**
平均値標準誤差　**SEM**
平均中間圧　**AMP**
平均注射率　**AIR**
平均直径/厚さ比　**MDTR**
平均的生存期間　**MLS**
平均的内周短縮率　**MCSR**
平均的変化　**MV**
平均動脈(血)圧　**MAP**
平均動脈圧　**MABP**
平均動脈血圧　**MA**
平均投与量・治療量　**AD**
平均尿流量率　**AFR**
平均の　**AV，Av，av.**
平均肺動脈圧　**mPAP，MPAP**
平均排尿比　**AVR**
平均ピーク音響　**APN**
平均輻射温度　**MRT**
平均分解赤外線　**MRIF**
平均偏倚調整　**ada**
平均偏差　**AD，MD**
平均放電間隔　**MIPI**
平均母体グルコース　**MMG**
平均溶解時間　**MDT**
平均溶血量　**MHD**
平均用量　**D**
平均より良い　**BTA**
平均流量率　**MFR**
平均リンパ球排出量　**ALO**
平均レベル　**ML**
平行線維　**PF**
平行の　**par**
平行棒　**//bars**
平衡　**bal**
平衡異常症候群　**DES**
平衡検査　**BT**
平衡状態　**EQ，equilib**
平衡食塩水　**BSS**
平衡定数　**K，K_{eq}，pK**
平衡電解質溶液　**BES**
平衡透析　**ED**
平坦な　**applan.**
平坦脳波　**flat EEG**
平地を10分間歩行させて最大に歩行できる距離　**10 MWD**
平板・血小板　**pl**
平板効率　**EOP**
平方(の)　**sq**
平方インチ　**qu in，sq.in**
平方センチメートル　**cm^2，qcm，sq.cm**
平方デシメートル　**qdm**
平方フィート　**sq.ft**
平方フート　**ft^2**
平方ミリメートル　**mm^3，qmm，sq.mm**
平方メートル　**m^2，qm，sq.m**
平方ヤード　**yd^2**
平面位表示器　**PPI**
平流・直流　**CC**
米国アレルギー学会員　**FACAI**
米国グループ保健協会　**GHAA**
米国リウマチ学会　**ACR**
米国足看護研究所　**AFCI**
米国足整形外科医専門協会　**ACFO**
米国足の外科専門協会　**ACFS**
米国足の整形外科学会員　**FACFO**
米国足放射線医専門協会　**ACFR**
米国アルコール問題審議会　**ACAP**
米国アルコール薬物乱用精神衛生局　**ADAMHA**
米国アレルギー・喘息・免疫学会　**ACAAI**
米国アレルギー学者専門協会　**ACA**
米国アレルギー学会　**AAA**
米国アレルギー研究会　**ASSA**
米国アレルギー喘息免疫学アカデミー　**AAAAI**
米国医学教育委員会　**FSMB**
米国医学教育学会　**AAPE**
米国医学資格審査方式の1つ　**USMLE**
米国医学書出版協会

AAMBP
米国医学生協会　SAMA
米国医学卒後研修認定委員会　ACGME
米国医学連合教育研究財団
AMAERF
米国医科大学協会
AAMC
米国医師(組織)　Amdoc
米国医師会　AAGP, AMA
米国医師会会員
FACP, FAMA
米国医師会雑誌　JAMA
米国医師会薬品情報データベース　AMADIB
米国医師会薬品評価
AMA-DE
米国医史学協会　AAHM
米国医師学会　ACP
米国医師看護師協会
AADN
米国医師協会　AAP
米国医師免許証　AMQ
米国胃腸専門協会　ACG
米国胃腸内視鏡外科学会
SAGES
米国胃腸病学会員
FACG
米国胃腸病協会　AGA
米国遺伝学会　ASG
米国医薬化学連合
USMC
米国医薬品集　PDR
米国医薬品評価研究センター　CDER
米国医療技士専門協会
ACMT
米国医療技術者協会
ASMT
米国医療機能評価機関
JCAHO
米国医療行政行動委員会
AMPAC
米国医療記録協会
AMRA
米国医療ソーシャルワーカー協会　AAMS
米国医療婦人協力者協会
AMAWA
米国医療補助者協会
AAMA
米国医療用ミルク委員会
AAMMC
米国栄養学会　AAN, ANS
米国栄養研究所　AIN
米国疫学協会　AES
米国応用栄養学会
AAAN
米国汚染管理協会
AACC
米国音響協会　ACSOA
米国外国医科(大学)学生
USFMS
米国外傷外科協会
AAST
米国外人医師卒後教育委員会　ECFMG
米国改正食糧サービス協会
ACFSA
米国海兵隊病院　USMH
米国解剖学者協会　AAA
米国化学協会　ACS
米国化学者研究所　AIC
米国科学振興協会
AAAS
米国化学病理学者協会の医学技術者　MTASCP
米国顎顔面外科医協会
ASMFS
米国学術的医療センター協会　AMCC
米国学校保健協会
ASHA
米国眼科・耳鼻咽喉科学会
AAO & O
米国眼科アカデミー
AAO
米国眼科学委員会　ABO
米国眼科学専門医資格者
DABO
米国眼科学会　AOS
米国癌学会　AACR
米国眼球銀行協会
EBAA
米国癌協会　ACS
米国癌検知センター
CDC
米国看護家庭管理専門協会
ACNHA
米国看護協会　ANF
米国看護師協会　ANA
米国看護助産術専門協会
ACNM
米国看護麻酔士協会
AANA
米国看護師協議会　NCN
米国患者同盟　APA
米国癌審議会　UCC
米国癌制圧協会　ASCC
米国関節炎研究会
ASSArth
米国顔面形成再建外科協会
AAFPRS
米国規格協会　ANSI
米国規格局　USBS, USBuStand
米国規格標準局　NBS
米国寄生虫学者協会
ASP
米国気管食道科学協会
ABEA
米国救急医療委員会
ABEM
米国救急医療医師専門協会
ACEP
米国救急ヘリコプター搬送システム
ASHBEAMS
米国吸入療法士協会
AAIT
米国矯正精神医協会
AACP
米国胸部外科医協会

AATS
米国胸部疾患学会　ACCP，ATS
米国魚鱗癬ヘルペス学者協会　ASI & H
米国空軍病院　USAFH
米国軍医総監室　S.G.O.
米国軍病理研究所　AFIP
米国形成外科・再建外科医協会　ASPRS
米国形成外科・再建外科学会　ASPRS
米国形成外科医協会　AAPS
米国外科医師会員　FACS
米国外科学委員会　ABS
米国外科学専門医資格者　DABS
米国外科学会　ACS
米国外科協会　ASA
米国血液バンク協会　AABB
米国血液病学会　ASH
米国結核病医協会　AATP
米国血管学会員　FACA
米国研究室動物専門協会　ACLAM
米国健康医学委員会　ABHP
米国健康教育福祉局　USDHEW
米国健康協会専門委員会　ACHA
米国健康研究所　AHI，SIA
米国健康体育リクリエーション協会　AAHPER
米国健康保険協会　HIAA
米国言語聴覚学会　ASLHA
米国言語聴覚協会　ASHA
米国検査材料協会　ASTM
米国口蓋裂協会　ACPA
米国口蓋裂リハビリテーション協会　AACPR
米国光学会社　AOC
米国公共福祉協会　APWA
米国口腔・形成外科医協会　AAOPS
米国口腔科学会　AAOM
米国口腔外科委員会　ABOS
米国口腔外科医協会　ASOS
米国口腔病理学会　AAOP
米国口腔放射線医学会　AAOR
米国公衆衛生医師協会　AAPHP
米国公衆衛生協会　APHA，ASHA
米国公衆衛生協会員　FAPHA
米国公衆衛生局　USPHS
米国公衆衛生歯科医師協会　AAPHD
米国甲状腺協会　ATA
米国甲状腺腫協会　AGA
米国喉頭科学協会　ALA
米国公用名　USAN
米国呼吸ケア協会　AARC
米国国際開発庁　USAIDS
米国国民医薬品集　NF
米国国立医師国家試験実施委員会　NBME
米国国立衛生研究所　NIH
米国国立科学アカデミー/国立研究協議会　NAS/NRC
米国国立獣医協会　NVMA
米国国立保健統計センター　NCHS
米国国立薬物濫用研究所　NIDA
米国骨疾患医学試験官協会　AAOME
米国骨疾患協会　AOA
米国骨疾患外科医中の一般医専門協会　ACGPOMS
米国骨疾患整形外科医専門協会　ACOP
米国骨疾患専門医協会　AAOC
米国骨疾患内科医専門協会　ACOI
米国骨疾患病院管理者専門協会　ACOHA
米国骨髄ドナー登録協会　AABMDR
米国顧問薬剤師協会　ASCP
米国在郷軍人病院　USVH
米国細菌学者協会　ASB
米国最新薬剤便覧　ADI
米国才能児協会　AAGC
米国細胞学会　ASC
米国産科婦人科医協会　AAOG
米国産科婦人科医専門協会　ACOG
米国産科婦人科学委員会　ABOG
米国産科婦人科腹部外科医協会　AAOGAS
米国産業医学会　AAOM
米国産業衛生協会　AIHA
米国産業衛生専門家会議　ACGIH
米国産業看護師協会　AAIN

米国産業健康協議会
AIHC
米国産業歯科医協会
AAID
米国産業内科医・外科医協会 AAIPS
米国産業ラジウムX線協会 AIRX
米国産婦人科学会員
FACOG
米国産婦人科学専門医資格者 DABOG
米国歯科医学史協会
AAHD
米国歯科医学会 AAD,
AADM
米国歯科医業経営協会
AADPA
米国歯科医療サービス
ADS
米国歯科衛生士協会
ADHA
米国歯科学会員 FACD
米国歯科学生クラブ間評議会 ADIC
米国耳科学会 AOS
米国歯科教育基金
AFDE
米国歯科協会 ADA,
Am Dent
米国歯科矯正委員会
ABO
米国歯科矯正学会 AAO
米国歯牙矯正学校 ASO
米国資格試験認定機関連合
FLEX
米国歯科検査室研究所
DLIA
米国歯科公衆衛生委員会
ABDPH
米国歯科試験協会
AADE
米国歯科助手協会
ADAA
米国歯科大学協会
AADS
米国歯科同業組合
ADTA
米国歯科放射線写真技士協会 ASDR
米国歯科麻酔協会
ADSA
米国式手話 ASL
米国歯周医学会 AAP
米国歯周学委員会 ABP
米国実験生物学会連合
FASEB
米国実験病理学会
ASEP
米国疾病管理予防センター
CDC
米国失明者指導者協会
AAIB
米国耳鼻咽喉科学委員会
ABO
米国耳鼻咽喉科学専門医資格者 DABOt
米国耳鼻咽喉科学会
ALROS
米国耳鳴研究会 ATA
米国社会精神医学協会
AASP
米国社会保健協会
ASHA
米国獣医栄養士協会
AAVN
米国獣医学試験官協会
AABEVM
米国獣医科大学協会
AAVMC
米国獣医学会 AVMA
米国獣医細菌学協会
AAVB
米国獣医病理学者協会
AAVP
米国獣医病理学者専門協会
ACVP
米国集団精神医療協会
AGPA
米国修復歯科学会
AARD
米国手術室看護師協会
AORN
米国女医会 AMWA
米国消化器内視鏡学会
ASGE
米国上顎顔面装具学会
AAMP
米国小児科学委員会
ABP
米国小児皮膚科学委員会
ABPD
米国小児科学専門医資格者
DABP
米国小児科学会 AAP,
APdS, APS
米国小児精神医学会
AACP
米国小児精神医療協会
AAPCC
米国承認名 USAN
米国消費者健康情報調査研究所 CHIRI
米国生薬学会 ASP
米国職業心理学試験委員会
ABEPP
米国食品・薬品公務員協会
AFDOUS
米国食品安全検査局
FSIS
米国食品医薬品局 FDA
米国飼料顕微鏡検者協会
AAFM
米国視力矯正審議会
AOC
米国視力障害者財団
AFB
米国視力障害者のために働く者の協会 AAWB
米国視力測定学会 AAO
米国視力測定協会 AOA
米国視力測定士専門協会
ACO
米国神経科学会 NSA
米国神経学協会 ANA

米国神経学会　AAN
米国神経外科委員会
ABNS
米国神経外科学専門医資格者　DABNS
米国神経外科学会　NSA
米国神経精神科医専門協会
ACN
米国神経病理学者協会
AAN
米国人工臓器協会
ASAIO
米国人口動態統計局
NOVS
米国心身学会　APS
米国新生物疾患研究協会
AASND
米国心臓移植調査
NHTS
米国心臓協会　AHA, Am Heart
米国心臓病学会員
FACC
米国心臓病学専門協会
ACC
米国身体障害者法　ADA
米国身体障害者連合
AFPH
米国人道的心理学協会
AAHP
米国心理学協会　APA
米国心理分析研究所
AIP
米国心理療法協会　APA
米国睡眠障害学会
ASDA
米国頭痛研究協会
AASH
米国生化学者協会
ASBC
米国整形外科委員会
ABOS
米国整形外科学専門医資格者　DABOS
米国整形外科学会
AAOS
米国整形外科協会　AOA
米国整骨外科医学会
ACOS
米国性情報教育協議会
SIECUS
米国生殖泌尿器外科医協会
AAGU
米国精神医学会　SIP
米国精神医学協会　APA
米国精神医学神経学委員会
ABPN
米国精神矯正学協会
AOrPA
米国精神欠陥者のための協会　AAMD
米国精神神経科学専門医資格者　DABPN
米国精神神経認定医
Dip.Amer.Bd.P. & N.
米国精神発達遅滞学会
AAMR
米国精神問題研究会
ASRPP
米国性病学会　AVDA
米国性病研究所　VDRL
米国生物科学研究所
AIBS
米国生物分析委員会
ABBA
米国政府発行の公文書
FR
米国生命記録・公衆衛生統計協会　AAVRP
米国製薬会社協会　PMA
米国製薬協会　ADMA, APA, APhA
米国製薬工業協会
PhRMA
米国生理歯科学会
AAPD
米国赤十字　ARC
米国赤十字看護師サービス
ARCNS
米国専門医制度調整機関
ABMS
米国前立腺癌研究計画
NPCP
米国臓器移植ネットワーク
UNOS
米国総合臨床〔家庭〕医学会
AAFP
米国総合臨床医学認定学会
ABFP
米国大学放射線科医
AUR
米国代償医学会　AACM
米国大腸直腸外科委員会
ABCRS
米国大腸直腸外科医協会
ASCRS
米国代理母斡旋センター
ICA
米国聴覚学会員　FASA
米国聴覚学会誌　JASA
米国聴覚障害者教育のための組織　AOEHI
米国調剤教育財団
AFPE
米国調剤教育審議会
ACPE
米国聴力協会　AHS
米国直腸肛門学会
APrS, APS
米国治療学会　ATS
米国で使用される国際疾病分類　ICDA
米国手の外科学会
ASSH
米国てんかん協会　AES
米国電子顕微鏡学会
EMSA
米国伝染病センター
CDC
米国統合失調症財団
ASF
米国糖尿病学会食
ADA diet
米国糖尿病協会　ADA
米国糖尿病協会食事番号

ADA
米国動物の健康と薬物の協会 AAHPhA
米国東洋医学校
ACTCM
米国毒物管理センター協会
AAPCC
米国特許 US pat
米国内科医外科医協会
AAPS
米国内科学委員会
ABIM
米国内科学会員 FAPS
米国内科学専門医資格者
DABIM
米国内科学リハビリテーション学会議
ACPMR
米国内科学会 ASIM
米国内科外科学有資格者
LCP & SA
米国内科外科学会員
MCPS
米国難聴学会 ASHH
米国難聴指導者 AID
米国人間遺伝学会
ASHG
米国熱帯医学衛生学会
ASTMH
米国熱帯医学協会
AATM
米国熱帯医学財団
AFTM
米国熱帯医学会 ASTM
米国脳神経外科医協会
AANS
米国脳性麻痺学会
AACP
米国脳性麻痺協会
UCPA
米国の生涯教育用の教本と問題集シリーズ
MKSAP
米国の病院で働くリスクマネージャー支援協会
ASHRM
米国の母子家庭生活保護制度の１つ AFDC
米国発語矯正協会
ASCA
米国母親・乳児健康協会
AAMIH
米国微生物学協会 AAM
米国微生物学会 ASM
米国泌尿器科学専門医資格者 DABU
米国泌尿器科学会 AUA
米国皮膚科学専門医資格者
DABD
米国皮膚科学梅毒学協会
AADS
米国皮膚科学会 AAD
米国皮膚科協会 ADA
米国病院管理学会
AAMA
米国病院管理専門協会
ACHA
米国病院協会 AHA
米国病院供給会社
AHSC
米国病院供給(会社)
AHS
米国病院計画協会
AAHP
米国病院計理士協会
AAHA
米国病院工学技術協会
ASHE
米国病院購入代理店協会
AAHPA
米国病院顧問協会
AAHC
米国病院財団 AHF
米国病院歯科主任協会
AAHDC
米国病院足病学者協会
AAHP
米国病院薬剤師会発行の病院医薬品集 AHF, AHFS
米国病院薬剤師協会
ASHP
米国標準協会 ASA
米国病理学委員会 ABP
米国病理学会員 FCAP
米国病理学者登録 ARP
米国病理学者微生物学者協会 AAPB
米国病理学専門医資格者
DABPath
米国病理同学院 CAP
米国病歴士学会
AAMRL
米国腹部外科委員会
ABAS
米国婦人科学協会 AGS
米国物理療法協会
APTA
米国物理療法士登録
ARPT
米国不妊研究会 ASSS
米国法医学委員会
ABLM
米国法医学専門協会
ACLM
米国法医学会 AAFS
米国防火協議会 NFPA
米国膀胱鏡製作会社
ACMI
米国放射線医学委員会
ABR
米国放射線医学専門医資格者 DABR
米国放射線科学会員
FACR
米国放射線学会/国立電機器製造協会
ACR/NEMA
米国放射線技師協会
ASRT
米国放射線技士登録
ARRT
米国放射線協会 ARRS
米国放射線専門協会
ACR

米国保健福祉省　**DHHS**
米国母子健康協会
AAMCH
米国補綴歯科学委員会
ABP
米国ホメオパシー研究所
AIH
米国麻酔医専門協会
ACA，ACAnes
米国麻酔科学会員
FACA
米国麻酔学専門医資格者
DABA
米国麻酔学会　**ASA**
米国免疫学者協会　**AAI**
米国盲人のための印刷所
APHB
米国薬剤コード　**NDC**
米国薬剤コード集
NDCD
米国薬剤師専門協会
ACP
米国薬理学実験治療学会
ASPET
米国薬局方　**USP，USPhar，US phar**
米国薬局方単位　**USPU**
米国薬局方注解　**USD**
米国薬局方薬品情報
USPDI
米国薬効局　**USDEA**
米国輸液栄養学会
ASPEN
米国輸血サービス
NBTS
米国予防医学委員会
ABPM
米国予防医学会員
FACPM
米国予防医学会議
ACPM
米国予防医学専門協会
ACPP
米国リウマチ協会　**ARA**
米国理学療法協会　**APA**
米国理学療法リハビリテーション医学委員会
ABPMR
米国理学療法リハビリテーション学会　**AAPMR**
米国陸軍医療サービス
USAMEDS
米国陸軍歯科研究所
USAIDR
米国陸軍診療所
USAHC
米国陸軍病院　**USAH**
米国リハビリテーション財団　**ARF**
米国リハビリテーション治療協会　**AART**
米国留学のための英語力試験　**TOEFL**
米国臨床医協会　**AAMC**
米国臨床栄養学会
ASCN
米国臨床化学協会
AACC
米国臨床観察学会　**ASCI**
米国臨床管理者専門協会
ACCA，ACCM
米国臨床研究連合
AFCR
米国臨床検査標準委員会
NCCLS
米国臨床腫瘍学会
ASCO
米国臨床病理学会
ASCP
米国臨床薬学・治療学会
ASCPT
米国臨床薬学会　**ACCP**
米国老人協会　**AGS**
米国老人研究財団
AGRF
米国労働省労働安全保健局
OSHA
米国老年者収縮期型高血圧研究　**SHEP**
米大陸心臓学会　**ISC**
併合性副鼻腔炎　**KS**
併発筋炎　**OVLP**
併発部　**IF**
併用　**comb**
並行弾圧成分　**PE**
並列型光活性電位センサー
LAPS
閉回路電圧　**CCV**
閉環状 DNA
closed cDNA
閉胸式心蘇生　**CCCR**
閉経期ゴナドトロピン
MG
閉経後出血　**PMB**
閉経後症候群　**PMS**
閉経後触知可能卵巣
PMPO
閉経後の骨粗しょう(鬆)症
PMO
閉鎖　**C，Cl，cl，clsg，clsr**
閉鎖運動連鎖　**CKC**
閉鎖オリーブ蝸牛束
COCB
閉鎖オリーブ蝸牛電圧
COCP
閉鎖回路テレビ　**CCTV**
閉鎖骨折　**FS**
閉鎖式開胸術　**CT**
閉鎖した　**imperf**
閉鎖時弁音　**CVS**
閉鎖生態系生命維持システム　**CELSS**
閉鎖性頭部外傷　**CHI**
閉鎖帯　**Tj**
閉鎖堤　**TB**
閉鎖導尿　**CBD**
閉鎖容積　**CV**
閉塞　**Obst，obst，Obstruct，Occ，ocl**
閉塞型睡眠無呼吸症候群
OSAS
閉塞後反応性充血
PORH
閉塞する　**Obst，obst**

閉塞性乾燥性亀頭炎　**BXO**
閉塞性気管支細気管支炎　**BBO**
閉塞性気道疾患　**OAD**
閉塞性凝血性大動脈症　**OTAP**
閉塞性頸動脈疾患　**OCAD**
閉塞性血栓血管炎　**TO**
閉塞性血栓性血管炎　**TAO, TSO**
閉塞性呼吸低下　**OH**
閉塞性細気管支炎　**BO, OB**
閉塞性細気管支炎・間質性肺炎　**BIP**
閉塞性細気管支炎性間質性肺炎　**BIP**
閉塞性睡眠無呼吸　**OSA**
閉塞性動脈硬化症　**ASO**
閉塞性動脈疾患　**OAD**
閉塞性肺疾患　**OLD**
閉塞性肺低血圧症　**OPH, Oph**
閉塞性無呼吸　**OA**
閉塞の　**Obst, obst, Obstruct**
壁在性増殖型アスペルギローマ　**PAIC**
壁細胞抗体　**PCA**
壁細胞迷走神経切断　**PCV**
壁側胸膜組織　**PPT**
壁内糸球体硬化症　**IGS**
壁内心筋梗塞　**TMI**
壁反響性陰影　**WES**
壁被覆開口管の　**WCOT**
頁　**pp, PP, pp.**
頁(＝ページ)　**pg**
臍　**U, umb**
臍の　**reg umbilic**
別刷　**repr**
別々に　**sep, separ.**
片腎切除(術)　**UNX**
片側横隔膜　**HD**
片側下肢切除術　**HP**
片側〔半側〕顔面痙攣　**HFS**
片側〔半側〕顔面小人症　**HFM, HM**
片側〔半側〕顔面の過形成　**HFH**
片側(性)緊張(性)気胸　**UTP**
片側痙攣・片麻痺・てんかん(症候群)　**HHE**
片側後方腰椎椎体固定(術)　**UPLIF**
片側骨盤切除術　**HP**
片側人工膝関節置換術　**UKA**
片側性腎血管疾患　**URVD**
片側性母斑性毛細血管拡張症候群　**UNTS**
片側(性)脱力　**UW**
片側尿管閉塞(症)　**UUO**
片側(性)の　**unilat**
片側〔半側〕肥大・腸ウェブ・耳介前方糸状線維腫・先天性角膜混濁(症候群)　**HIPO**
片側卵管卵巣摘出　**USO**
片麻痺　**hemi, Hp**
片麻痺性片頭痛　**HM**
辺縁　**MG, mrg**
辺縁系・視床下部・下垂体・副腎系　**LHPA**
辺縁系中脳部　**LMA**
辺縁組織膜関連蛋白　**LAMP**
辺縁の　**mg, mrg**
辺縁領域リンパ球　**MZL**
弁　**V, v, val, vlv**
弁口面積　**VA**
弁置換　**VR**
弁置換術　**VR**
弁の　**vlv**
弁別閾検査　**DL test**
弁別閾値　**DL**
弁別能　**DS**
弁膜性心疾患　**VDH**
弁膜性心臓疾患　**VHD**
弁輪上僧帽弁置換術　**SMVR**
変圧器　**trans, Xfmr**
変異　**V, v, var**
変異型クロイツフェルト・ヤコブ病　**vCJD, v-CJD**
変異株　**var**
変異体　**var**
変異多数斑紋(マウス)　**W_v**
変域外の　**OR**
変化　**chg, chg's, chng**
変化した　**chg'd**
変化する　**var**
変化なし　**NC**
変化のない　**sta**
変化のない短身　**NVSS**
変化量　**INCR, Incr, incr.**
変株特異的表面抗原　**VSA**
変株表面糖蛋白　**VSG**
変換器　**XDR**
変換酵素　**CE**
変換酵素抑制剤　**CEI**
変形　**deform**
変形性関節炎　**AD, DA**
変形性関節症　**OA, Osteo, osteo, osteoarth**
変形性脊髄症　**SD**
変形性梅毒性関節炎　**ASD**
変形〔奇形〕赤血球　**POIK, poik**
変形〔奇形〕赤血球症　**POIK, poik**
変種　**V, v, var**
変質　**Deg, deg.,**

degen
変質した **denat**
変性 **deg, Deg, deg., degen**
変性円板疾患 **DDD**
変性剤濃度勾配ゲル電気泳動法 **DGGE**
変性細胞 **DC**
変性疾患 **DD**
変性する **deg**
変性性関節疾患 **DJD**
変性の **degen**
変性反応 **DER, DeR, DR**
変動 **fluc, V, v, var**
変動〔変異〕係数 **V**
変動係数 **CV**
変復調装置 **MODEM**
変法 **mod, mod.**
便 **sed.**
便ウロビリノゲン **FU**
便器 **BP, bp.**
便所 **RR, WC**
(糞)便脂肪排泄 **FFE**
便潜血 **FOB**
(糞)便胆汁酸 **FBA**
便通 **BM**
便通正常 **BOR**
便通のあるまで **donec alv.sol.**
便秘 **BNO, Obst, obst**
便秘中 **alv.adstrict.**
便薬 **vehic.**
便利性・親切・信頼 **3C**
便１グラム中の虫卵数 **EPG**
扁挑 **AMG**
(脳の)扁桃 **AM**
扁桃核 **AM**
扁桃周囲炎 **periton**
扁桃周囲膿瘍 **periton, PTA**
扁桃切除(された) **TE**
扁桃切除術 **loto**
扁桃単核細胞 **TMC**
扁桃摘出(術) **TE**
扁桃摘出手術 **lec**
扁桃摘出(術)とアデノイド摘出(術) **T & A**
扁桃とアデノイド **T & A**
扁桃の過形成およびアデノイド **hyper T & A**
扁平円柱上皮接合部 **SCJ**
扁平巨細胞 **fR**
扁平紅色苔癬 **LRP**
扁平上皮 **SE, sq.epithl**
扁平上皮癌 **SC, SCC, SCCA, sq, SQ cell ca, sq.cell ca.**
扁平上皮癌抗原 **SCCA**
扁平上皮乳頭腫 **SCP**
扁平足 **FF**
扁平苔癬 **LP**
扁平苔癬様角化症 **LPLK**
扁平苔癬様病変 **LPL**
扁平頭 **fl hd**
扁平な **f, sq**
扁平板 **FP**
偏位 **D, dev, displ**
偏位(性)鼻中隔 **DNS**
偏移 **dev**
偏差 **D, dev**
偏視 **D, dev**
偏菱形 **rhom**
娩出時間 **ATZ**
編集された **ed**
編集者 **ed**
編集者の **ed, edit.**
編集する **ed**
鞭毛 **GX**

ほ

ポアズ　**P**
ポイツ・ジェガース（症候群）　**PJ**
ホィットニー・デーモン（デキストロース）　**WD**
ボイド・スターンズ（症候群）　**BS**
ホウ酸　**BA，B/A**
ホウ酸亜鉛華軟膏　**BZS**
ホウ酸緩衝食塩水　**BBS**
ホウ素　**B**
ホウ素中性子捕捉療法　**BNCT**
ホウメディカ基準切除　**HMRS**
ホー川症候群　**HRS**
ポケット線量計　**PD**
ホジェン・ピアーソン（懸吊牽引）　**HP，H＆P**
ホジキン病　**HD**
ホジキンリンパ腫　**HL**
ポジトロンエミッションCT　**PECT，PET-CT**
ポジトロンエミッションマンモグラフィ　**PEM**
ホスト細胞因子　**HCF**
ボストン合同薬監視計画　**BCDSP**
ボストン診断学的失語症検査法　**BDAE**
ホスファターゼ　**phos，p tase，PTASE**
ホスファチジル　**Ptd**
ホスファチジルイノシトール　**PI，PtdIns**
ホスファチジルイノシトールーリン酸　**PIP**
ホスファチジルイノシトールグリカン　**PIG**
ホスファチジルイノシトール二リン酸　**PIP**
ホスファチジルエタノールアミン　**PE，PtdEth**
ホスファチジルグリセロール　**PG**
ホスファチジルコリン　**PC，PtdCho**
ホスファチジルセリン　**PS，PtdSer**
ホスファチジン酸　**PA，PtOH**
ホスフィン　**PH_3**
ホスホヘキソースイソメラーゼ　**PHI**
ホスホエタノールアミン　**PEA**
ホスホエノールピルビン酸　**PEP**
ホスホエノールピルベートカルボキシキナーゼ　**PEPCK**
ホスホガラクトースウリジルトランスフェラーゼ　**PGUT**
ホスホグリセリン酸　**PG，PGA**
ホスホグリセリン酸キナーゼ　**PGK**
ホスホグリセルアルデヒド脱水素酵素　**PGD**
ホスホグリセロムターゼ　**PGM**
ホスホグルコネート　**PG**
ホスホグルコムターゼ　**PGM**
ホスホグルコン酸脱水素酵素　**PDG，PGD，PGDH**
ホスホクレアチン　**PC，PCR**
ホスホジエステラーゼ　**PDase，PDE**
ホスホトランスアセチラーゼ　**PTA**
ホスホトランスフェラーゼ系　**PTS**
ホスホピリジンヌクレオチド　**PN**
ホスホフルクトキナーゼ　**PFK**
ホスホペントムターゼ　**PPM**
ホスホマイシン　**FOM**
ホスホマンノースイソメラーゼ　**PMI**
ホスホモノエステラーゼ　**PMase**
ホスホリパーゼ　**PLP**
ホスホリパーゼA　**PLA**
ホスホリパーゼA_2　**PLA2，PL-A_2，PLase A_2**
ホスホリパーゼB　**PLB**
ホスホリパーゼC　**PLC**
ホスホリパーゼD　**PLD**
ホスホリボシルグリシンアミド合成酵素　**GAPS，PRGS**
ホスホリボシルトランスフェラーゼ　**PRT，PRTase**
ホスホリボシルピロリン酸　**PPRibP，PRPP**
ホスホリボシルピロリン酸合成酵素　**PRPS**
ホスホリボースイソメラーゼ　**PRI**
ホスホリラーゼbキナーゼ　**PBK**
ホスホリルコリン　**PC**
ホスホリルコリン結合骨髄腫蛋白　**PC-BMP**
ホスホリルジメチルエタノールアミン　**P-DMEA**
ホスホリンアイオダイド　**PI**
ポーセレン　**P**
ポーター・シルバー（色素原）　**PS，P-S**
ポーター・シルバー色素原

PSC
ボダンスキー単位
BOD Unit, BU
ポイツ・ジェガース症候群
PJS
ホッグズヘッド **HHD**
ホットパック **HP, H.P.**
ホッファー・カスタート（症候群） **HK**
ボドロック（直）径 **BD**
ホートン動脈炎 **HA**
ホパテン酸カルシウム
HOPA
ポビドンヨード **PVP-I**
ホプキンズ症状チェックリスト **HSCL**
ホフマン（反射） **Hoff**
ホフマン反射
Hoff refl, H reflex
ホフマン反応
Hoff resp, H response
ボヘミウム **BO**
ホマトロピン
homatrop
ボーマン嚢 **BC**
ホーミング受容体 **HR**
ホムアトロピン
homatrop
ポムス **POMS**
ホメオパシー **Homeo**
ホメオパシー学修了証書
XDFHom
ホメオパシー **homo**
ホメオパシーの **homo**
ボーメ尺度〔スケール〕
B, B.
ボーメ度 **Be**
ボーメ比重計 **BE**
ホモアルギニン **Har**
ホモゲンチシン酸 **HGA**
ホモゲンチジン酸 **HA**
ホモシスチン尿（症）
HCU
ホモシスチン尿〔症〕 **HC**
ホモシステイン **Hcy**
ホモ接合型タイピング細胞
HTC
ホモバニリン酸 **HVA**
ホモリノレン酸 **$C_{20=3}$**
ポラク・デュラント（症候群） **PD**
ポーラログラフ心筋酸素量
PMCO
ボランティア **vol**
ポリ-β-ヒドロキシ酪酸
PHB
ポリ-2-水酸化メタクリル酸 **PHMA**
ポリ-L-グルタミン酸
PLGA
ポリ-L-リジン **PLL**
ポリ-*N*-*p*-ビニルラクトンアミド **PVLA**
ポリアクリルアミド
PAA
ポリアクリルアミドゲル電気泳動 **PAGE**
ポリアクリル酸 **PAA**
ポリアデニル酸 **Poly A**
ポリアデニレート
polyA, poly-A
ポリアミンアセチルトランスフェラーゼ **PAT**
ポリイソブチルメタクリレート **PIBM**
ポリウリジル酸 **Poly U**
ポリウレタン **PU, PUR**
ポリウレタンエラストマー
PUE
ポリエタノール硫酸ナトリウム **SPS**
ポリエチレン **PE**
ポリエチレンイミン **PEI**
ポリエチレン管 **PET, PE tube**
ポリエチレン基質 **PEM**
ポリエチレングリコール
PEG
ポリエチレングリコール電解質液 **PEG-ELS**
ポリ塩化三フッ化エチレン
PCTFE
ポリ塩化ジベンゾパラジオキシン **PCDD**
ポリ塩化ジベンゾフラン
PCDF
ポリ塩化ビニル **PVC**
ポリ塩化ビフェニル
PCB
ポリオ **PM, Polio**
ポリオウイルス **PV**
ポリオウイルス感受性
PVS
ポリオキシエチレン
POE
ポリオ後萎縮症候群
PPAS
ポリオ（灰白髄炎）後症候群
PPS
ポリオ脊髄神経根炎
PMR
ポリオ生ワクチン **PLV**
ポリオーマ **Py**
ポリオーマウイルス **PV**
ポリオーマウイルス受容体
PVR
ポリグアニル酸 **Poly G**
ポリグルタミン酸
poly, poly Glu
ポリクローナルγグロブリン **PGG**
ポリクローナルリウマチ因子 **pRF**
ポリ酢酸ビニル **PVA**
ポリサッカライドK
PSK
ポリサッカライドクレハ
PSK
ポリシチジル酸 **Poly C**
ポリ臭化ビフェニル
PBB
ポリスチレン **PS**
ポリスチレンラテックス粒

子 **PLP**
ポリチミジル酸 **Poly T**
ポリテトラフルオロエチレン **PTFE**
ポリテトラメチレングリコール **PTMG**
ポリ二塩化ビニル **PVDc**
ポリ二フッ化ビニリデン **PVDF**
ポリ乳酸 **PLA**
ポリヌクレオチドキナーゼ **PNK**
ボリビア出血性熱 **BHF**
ボリビア(出血性)熱 **BF**
ポリビニル **PV**
ポリビニルアルコール **PVA**
ポリビニルスポンジ **PVS**
ポリビニルピリジン-*N*-オキシド **PVPNO**
ポリビニルピロリドン **PVP**
ポリビニルホルマールスポンジ **PTF**
ポリビニルメチルエーテル **PVM**
ポリープ **Po**
ポリープ状嚢胞性胃炎 **GCP**
ポリプロピレン **PP**
ポリプロピレングリコール **PPG**
ポリホスフェイト **pp**
ポリミキシン **P**
ポリミキシン,ネオマイシン,バシトラシン **PNB**
ポリミキシンネオマイシンバシトラシン **PNC**
ポリミキシンＢ **PB, PL, PL-B, PM-B, PMX-B**
ポリミキシンノナペプチド **PMBN**
ポリメタアクリル酸 **PMAA**
ポリメチルメタクリレート **PMMA**
ポリメラーゼ **p**
ポリメラーゼ連鎖反応 **PCR**
ポリリボソーム **PR**
ホール・カスター **HK**
ポール・バンネル試験 **PB, PBT**
ホールインワン技法 **HIO**
ボールソケット関節 **BSJ**
ホルターモニター **HM**
ホルツクネヒト腔 **H, HK Raum**
ホルツクネヒト単位 **H, H unit**
ホルツマンインクブロット手法 **HIT**
ボルツマン定数 **k**
ボルデー・ジャング(桿菌) **BG, B-G**
ボルデ・ジャング培地 **BG medium**
ボルデー・ワッセルマン反応 **BW**
ボルデテラ(属) **B**
ボルデテラ百日咳ワクチン **BPV**
ボルト **V**
ボルトアンペア **VA, va**
ボルト・オーム・ミリアンペア計 **VOM**
ホールト・オーラム(症候群) **HO**
ホールト・オーラム症候群 **HOS**
ボルト・秒 **V・s**
ボルト/分 **V/m**
ボルトン **BO**
ホルナー〔ホルネル〕症候群 **HS**
ポルフィリン **P**
ポルフィリン生合成経路 **PBP**
ポルホビリノゲン **PBG**
ボールベアリング **bb**
ポルホビリノゲンデアミナーゼ **PD**
ホルマリン **formal**
ホルマリン固定パラフィン包埋組織 **FFPE tissues**
ホルマリン酢酸固定液 **FAA fixative**
ホルマリンとエタノール **FE**
ホルマリントリクレゾール **FC**
ホルマリン類毒素 **FT**
ボルマン **B**
ボールマン 1〜4 型 **Borr 1-4**
ボールマン胃癌分類Ⅰ〜Ⅳ型 **Borr 1-4**
ホルミウム **Ho**
ホルミウム・イットリウム・アルミニウム・ガーネット **Ho：YAG**
ホルミル **f**
ホルミルグリシンアミドリボ核酸 **FGAR**
ホルミルメチオニル転移リボ核酸 **f-Met-tRNA**
ホルミルメチオニルメチルリン酸 **FMMP**
ホルミルメチオニン **FMET**
ホルムアミド **FA**
ホルムアルデヒド **formal**
ホルムアルデヒド形成性ステロイド **FGS**
ホルムアルデヒド蒸気 **FV**
ホルムアルデヒド尿素

UF
ホルムアルデヒド誘発螢光 FIF
ホルムイミノグルタミン酸 FIGLU
ホルモン H
ホルモン依存性の HD
ホルモン感受性リパーゼ HSL
ホルモン産生量 HP
ホルモン受容体酵素 HRE
ホルモン受容体部位 HRS
ホルモン反応性の HR
ホルモン非依存性 HI
ホルモン非依存性前立腺癌(腫) HIPC
ホルモン非感受性の HI
ホルモン放出因子 RF
ホルモン放出ホルモン RH
ホルモン補充療法 HRT
ボレリア(属) B
ポレンスケ価 PN, PV
ホロカルボキシラーゼ合成酵素 HCS
ポロニウム Po
ボロメーター〔放射エネルギー測定装置〕の電圧と電流 bolovac
ポワッサン(脳炎) POW
ポンダル pdl
ポンド l, L, lb, lb., lbs., lib., pd, pnd
ポンドフィート lb-ft
ポンド/平方インチ(=ψ, プサイ) psi, p.s.i.
ポンド/平方フィート p.s.f.
ボンベシン様免疫反応 BLI
ほかに摘出されない NOE
ほかに分類されない NOC
(幼児語で)ぽんぽん tum
母音・子音 VC
母音・子音・母音 VCV
母子衛生 MCH
母子関係 MCR
母子健康計画 MCHP
母子健康サービス MCHS
母子保健 MCH
母指 POLL, pull.
母指外転(筋) abd.poll.
母指球の Th
母指屈筋 f.p.
母指対立筋 OP
母指内転(筋) add.poll
母指内転筋 AdP
母趾外反症 HV
母趾徴候 TS
母集団 P, Pop, pop
母質 M, MX
母赤血球 MRBC
母性 Mat
母性健康全国委員会 NCMH
母性(愛)妨害 MD
母乳 BM, FM, HM, MM, WM
母乳栄養でない NBF
母乳化ミルク SMA
母乳単核球 BMMC
母乳で育てる BF
母乳で育てること BF
母乳を飲ませること BF
母斑 BM, BMK, bmk
母斑・心房粘液腫・粘液性神経線維腫・そばかす症候群 NAME syndrome
母斑(様)基底 NBS
母斑(様)基底細胞癌(症候群) NBCC
母斑(様)基底細胞癌症候群 NBCCS
包剤 DRSG, drsg
包帯 DRSG, drsg
歩行 Amb, amb., ambul
歩行訓練 GT
歩行時肺換気量 WV
歩行時肺換気量・分時最大換気〔呼吸〕量(比) WV-MBC
歩行者 ped
歩行想定除痛〔麻酔〕 WIA
歩行(可能)の Amb, amb.
歩行用踵(ギプス) WH
歩行用ボンベ WT
保育 nsg
保菌者 C
保健 hlth.
保健と開発に関するイニシアティブ HDI
保健・社会保障局 DHSS
保健安全法 HSC
保健維持機構 HMO
保健医療研究部 HCSD
保健医療サポート HCS
保健医療資金局 HCFA
保健医療分野支援プロジェクト HSSP
保健科学士 DHS
保健科学推進補助金 HSAA
保健関連職教員援助法 HPEASA
保健サービス管理 HSA
保健産業製造業者協会 HIMA
保健師 HV, Hyg, hyg, PHN
保健師協会 HVA
(米国)保健質的改善法 HCIA
保健従事者 HCW

保健所　**HC**
保健情報財団　**HIF**
保健体育協会　**HPS**
保健ネットワーク組織　**HCNS**
保健の　**sanit**
保健福祉サービス計画合理化研究所　**SPRI**
保健福祉省　**HHS**
保険　**INS, Ins**
保険証書　**C/I**
保護　**PRESS**
保護者　**gdn**
保証された　**C**
保証付きの　**UP**
保障　**scty**
保存　**preserv, PRESS**
保存(する)　**Res, res**
保存修復学　**OpDent**
保存する　**consv, preserv**
保存せよ　**cons., serv, serv.**
保存的な　**con, cons**
保存(的)の　**conserv**
保存ヒト赤血球　**PHE**
保有者　**C**
捕獲 γ 線　**CGR**
捕獲空気泡　**CAB**
哺乳動物学　**mammal**
補遺　**Beibl**
補完的活動パッケージ　**CPA**
補強クロストリジウム培地　**RCM**
補強刺激　**RS**
補欠分子族転移酵素　**PR enzyme**
補酵素　**CO, Co**
補酵素 A　**CoA**
補酵素 A〔コエンザイム A〕合成蛋白複合体　**CoA-SPC**
補酵素 F　**Co-F**
補酵素〔コエンザイム〕Q　**CEQ**
補酵素 R　**CoR**
補酵素型ビタミン B_{12}　**DBCC**
補充現象　**R**
補充的な　**compl**
補充の　**suppl**
補助・調節機械的換気　**ACMV**
補助換気(法)　**AV**
補助機械的換気　**AMV**
補助呼吸　**AR**
補助人工心臓　**VAD**
補助的　**AX**
補助的腸管外栄養　**SPN**
補助的の　**aux**
補助的腹腔鏡下外科手術　**LAS**
補助の　**addnl**
補助(的)療法　**AT**
補償作用　**comp, compen, compo**
補正 QT 時間　**QTc**
補正血液量　**CBV**
補正〔矯正〕していない　**UNCOR, uncor, uncorr**
補正生存率　**CSR**
補正赤血球沈降速度　**CSR**
補足　**Beibl, supps**
補足運動野　**SMA**
補足的な　**compl**
補足の　**suppl**
補体　**C, com**
補体 50%溶血単位　**CH_{50}**
補体依存抗体　**CDA**
補体依存(性)抗体媒介細胞傷害　**CDAMC**
補体依存(性)細胞傷害性　**CDC, CDCC**
補体寒冷活性化現象　**CCA**
補体結合　**CF**
補体結合(力)価　**CFT**
補体結合活性　**CFA**
補体結合抗体　**CBAB, CFA**
補体結合試験　**C'Fix**
補体結合試験〔反応〕　**CFT**
補体結合性膵島細胞質抗体　**CF-ICA**
補体結合阻止試験　**CFIT**
補体結合単位　**CF unit**
補体結合(性)の　**CF, C'F**
補体結合反応　**CBR, CFR, KBR**
補体結合抑制(試験)　**CFI**
補体最終活性化分子　**TCC**
補体制御系　**RCA**
補体制御蛋白遺伝子家系　**CCP-SF**
補体成分　**C**
補体第 1〔〜9〕成分　**C1〔-9〕**
補体第 1 成分のサブユニットの 1 つ　**C1q**
補体第 3 成分受容体　**C3-R**
補体第 3 成分プロアクチベーター　**C3PA**
補体第 3 レセプター　**C3-R**
補体に誘導された好酸球遊走因子　**ECF-C**
補体の 50%溶血量　**HD_{50}**
補体反応副経路　**ACP**
補体非依存性細胞傷害(測定法)　**CICC**
補体別経路　**ACP**
補体要求性中和抗体試験　**CRN**
補体レセプター〔補体受容体〕　**CR**
補体レセプター〔受容(体)〕リンパ球　**CRL**
補聴器　**audio, HA**

ほ

補聴器製作会社協会 **HAIA**
補聴器増幅器 **HAA**
補聴器評価 **HAE**
補聴器補助装置 **ALD**
補聴器マイクロフォン **HAM**
方形回内(筋) **PQ**
方向 **R**
方向優位性 **DP**
方程式 **EQ, eq, eqn**
方法 **meth, pro, proc**
方法論 **metho**
乏血小板血漿 **PPP**
乏突起膠腫 **OLG**
包括 **incln**
包括的医療プラン **CMP**
包括的医療保険プラン **CHIP**
包括的健康計画 **CHP**
包括的病院感染対策 **CHIP**
包帯 **curat.**
包帯(剤) **dr, Dsg, dsg**
包帯交換 **DC**
包虫(属) **E**
包虫症 **HD**
(ヒト)包皮(細胞) **FS**
包埋された **Bur**
芳香 **odoram.**
芳香(族)アミノ酸 **AAA**
芳香(族)アミノ酸脱炭酸酵素 **AAAD, AAD**
芳香性の **ar, arom**
芳香族炭化水素水酸化酵素 **AHH**
芳香の **odorat.**
防御 **def**
防御因子 **PF**
防御と保護 **P & I**
防御の **def**
防腐剤 **AS**
抱合 **conjug.**
抱合胆汁塩 **CBS**
抱水クロラール **CH**
放出因子 **RF**
放出開始時間制御型経口投与システム **TES**
放出光分光検査法 **OES**
放出ホルモン **RH**
放射アレルゲン吸着試験 **RAST**
放射型コンピュータ断層撮影法 **ECT**
放射活性・検出・適応・コンピュータ化 **radiac**
放射活性域 **R**
放射状遠心力 **RCF**
放射状角膜切開 **RK**
放射状乳頭周囲毛細血管 **RPC**
放射状免疫拡散(法) **RID**
放射する **rad, rad.**
放射性アイソトープの半減期記号 **T1/2**
放射性核種 **RN**
放射性核種血管造影 **RNA**
放射性核種血管造影〔撮影〕法 **RA**
放射性核種心室造影図 **RVG**
放射性核種心室造影法 **RVG**
放射性核種脳血管造影図 **RCA**
放射性カドミウム **Cd**
放射性気脳写図 **REG**
放射性健康データ **RHD**
放射性骨髄性白血病 **RML**
放射核シンチグラフィ **RNS**
放射性塞栓粒子 **^{125}I**
放射性鉄 **^{59}FE**
放射性同位元素 **RI**
放射性同位元素療法 **RI therapy**
放射性ニオブ **^{95}Nb**
放射性の **RA, RADA**
放射性脳写法 **REG**
放射性廃棄物 **RADWASTE**
放射性ヒト血清アルブミン **RAHSA**
放射性無機物 **R**
放射性免疫吸着分析 **RISA**
放射性免疫グロブリンシンチグラフィ **RIS**
放射性免疫グロブリン療法 **RIT**
放射性免疫不全 **RID**
放射性ヨウ素 **^{131}I**
放射性ヨウ素123標識ヒト血清アルブミン **^{123}I-HSA**
放射性ヨウ素131標識ヒト血清アルブミン **^{131}I-HSA**
放射性ヨウ素摂取 **RAU**
放射性ヨウ素(甲状腺)摂取率 **RIU**
放射性ヨウ素標識脂肪酸 **RIFA**
放射性ヨウ素標識成長ホルモン **IHGH**
放射性ヨウ素標識トリオレイン **RIT**
放射性ヨウ素標識ヒト血清アルブミン **IHSA, RISA**
放射性ヨウ素標識ヒト血清アルブミン(＝RISA) **RIHSA**
放射性ヨード **RAI**
放射性ヨード摂取率 **RAIU**
放射性リン **^{32}P**
放射線医学 **R, Rad, Radiol, Rnt**
放射線影響研究所 **RERF**

放射線科医　**Rad**
放射線科(分科)会員　**FFR**
放射線科学士　**M.S.Rd**
放射線学者　**R, Rnt, Roent**
放射線学者・麻酔学者・病理学者・精神医学者　**RAPP**
放射線学修士　**M.Rad**
放射線学的安全　**radsafe**
放射線学的視診　**radi**
放射線学的障害　**radhaz**
放射線学的診断　**Rad Dx**
放射線学的半減期　t_r
放射線学的病理学的討論会　**RPC**
放射線学的防御　**raddef**
放射線学的防御管理室〔管理者〕　**RDO**
放射線学の　**radl**
放射線ガスクロマトグラフィ　**RGC**
放射線科専門医資格　**D.R.**
放射線画像システム　**RIS**
放射線学会　**SR**
放射線活性干渉　**RAI**
放射線監視　**ramont**
放射線監視装置　**radmon**
放射線感受性試験　**RST**
放射線管理センター　**RCC**
放射線研究協力者　**RRA**
放射線健康研究室　**RHL**
放射線健康公報　**RHB**
放射線効果　**RR**
放射線(照射)後形成異常(症)　**PRD, PRDX**
放射線コントラスト(造影剤)誘発性腎不全　**PCIRF**
放射線撮影　**radiog**
放射線事故母体医療プログラム　**MMPNC**
放射線写真(の)　**X-ray**
放射線周波数　**RF, rf**
放射線照射野　**fld**
放射線診断学　**DR**
放射線診断認定書　**DDR**
放射線心電図　**recg**
放射線性の　**R**
放射線全国諮問委員会　**NACOR**
放射線専門医　**R, Radiol**
放射線組織連合　**ARO**
放射線蓄積効果　**CRE**
放射線調査管理者　**RadSO**
放射線治療　**Rad, rad ther**
放射線治療計画　**RTP**
放射線治療認定書　**DTR**
放射線同位元素大脳画像法　**RCI**
放射線によるインポテンツ　**RAI**
放射線脳波　**reeg**
放射線の検知と照準　**RADAS**
放射線白血病ウイルス　**RadLV**
放射線被刺激放出による微小波増幅器　**MASER**
放射線標準情報センター　**RSIC**
放射線物理学研究室　**RPL**
放射線防護・線量測定全国委員会　**NCRP**
放射線防護基準　**RPG**
放射線防護全国委員会　**NCRP**
放射線防護(測定)全国協議会　**NCRP**
放射線免疫測定法　**RIA**
放射線予防国際会議　**CIPR**
放射線量測定器　**r meter, r-meter**
放射線療法　**RADIO, RATx, RT**
放射能　**A, a, RA**
放射能の　**R, RA, RADA**
放射反応細胞　**RR cells**
放射標識ジイソプロピルフルオロリン酸　**DF^{32}P**
放射標識免疫沈降(試験)　**RIP**
放射免疫拡散　**RID**
放射免疫吸着試験　**RIST**
放射免疫シンチグラム　**RIS**
放射免疫治療　**RIT**
放射免疫電気泳動　**RIEP**
放射免疫電気泳動法　**RIE**
放射レセプター活性　**RRA**
放射レセプター測定(法)　**RRA**
放線冠　**CR**
放線菌(属)　**A, A.**
放電　**DC, D/C, dc, Dis, disc, disch**
放電した　**disch**
放電する　**disch**
法医学　**FM, foren, for med, LM**
法医毒物学　**for tox**
法医病理学　**FOR**
法則　**r**
法(律)的に別居した　**LS**
法律(の)　**leg**
法律的に　**leg**
法律に関する　**leg**
法律(上)の　**leg**
泡沫安定試験　**FST**
房室・動脈バイパス　**AAB**

房室回帰性頻拍　**AVRT**
房室解離　**AVD, AV Dis, A-V dis**
房室管　**AVC, AV canal, A-V canal**
房室間孔　**AVC, AV canal, A-V canal, AV communis, A-V communis**
房室奇形　**AVM**
房室結節　**AVN, A-VN**
房室結節リエントリー性頻拍　**AVNRT**
房室骨形成異常　**AOD**
房室順次ペーシング　**AVSP, DVI**
房室(接合部)性期外収縮　**JPB**
房室接合部　**AVJ**
房室接合部性期外収縮　**JPBC, JPC**
房室中隔欠損　**AVSD**
房室伝導系　**AVCS**
房室伝導時間　**PQ**
房室の　**AtV, AV, A-V**
房室不応期　**AVRP**
房室ブロック　**AVB**
房室弁開口　**AO**
房室無反応　**AVR**
房水産生率　**F**
房水流出係数　**C**
房水流出率　**C-value**
房水流出量　**C**
胞子　**G**
胞子型コロニー　**G**
胞子の　**G**
胞状奇胎　**HM, Mole**
胞状の　**ALV, alv, alv.**
剖検　**autop**
剖検膵管像　**PMP**
紡錘菌(属)　**F**
紡錘状の　**F**
紡錘状皮膚再建　**FSR**
疱疹　**mal.**
疱疹状皮膚炎　**DH**
(放射性)崩壊(する)　**DK**
崩壊指数　**DQ**
崩壊定数　**λ**
崩壊ミリキュリー　**MCD**
訪問　**V**
訪問看護師協会　**VNA**
訪問した　**vs, v/s**
訪問者　**V, vis, vs, v/s**
訪問の　**vis**
報告　**Nachr**
報告(する)　**rept**
報告した　**reptd, rptd**
報告者　**RP**
報告書　**Rpt**
報告する　**REP, rep.**
報告とメモ　**r & m**
報告なし　**NR**
傍黄斑同時視　**SPMP**
傍気管支リンパ組織　**BALT**
傍骨骨肉腫　**POS**
傍糸球体細胞(数)　**JGC**
傍糸球体細胞腫瘍　**JCT, JGCT**
傍糸球体指数　**JGI**
傍糸球体装置　**JGA**
傍糸球体肉芽(顆粒)形成指数　**JGI**
傍糸球体の　**JG**
傍糸球体複合体　**j-g complex**
傍腫瘍浮腫　**PTE**
傍髄質糸球体　**JMG**
傍正中橋網様体　**PPRF**
傍精巣(睾丸)横紋筋肉腫　**PTR**
傍肺毛細血管(受容体)　**J**
傍皮質域　**pc**
傍濾胞B細胞リンパ腫　**PBCL**
帽状腱膜下血腫　**SGH**
飽和　**S, Sa**
飽和(度)　**SAT, sat., satn**
飽和液　**SS**
飽和回復法　**SR**
飽和させる　**SAT, sat.**
飽和指数　**SI**
飽和した　**S, SAT, sat., sat'd, std**
飽和脂肪酸　**SFA**
飽和水蒸気　**ATPS**
飽和するまで　**ad sat., ad satur.**
飽和分析(法)　**SA**
飽和溶液　**sat.sol., sol.sat.**
飽和硫酸アンモニウム　**SAS**
硼酸水　**BAs**
膀胱　**UB, VES, ves., ves.ur.**
膀胱観察　**BLOBS, bl.obs**
膀胱鏡　**Cysto, cysto.**
膀胱鏡・内視鏡拡張術　**CED**
膀胱鏡兼拡張術　**C & D**
膀胱鏡検査　**CS, CYS, Cysto, cysto.**
膀胱鏡検査と腎盂造影　**C & P**
膀胱鏡の　**Cysto, cysto.**
膀胱頸(部)　**VN**
膀胱頸部　**B.N.**
膀胱頸部狭窄　**VNC**
膀胱頸部狭窄症　**BNC**
膀胱頸(部)閉塞　**BNO**
膀胱子宮頸腔　**VCS**
膀胱充満時排尿速度　**FVC, FVFR**
膀胱腫瘍　**BT**
膀胱造影撮影法　**CG**
膀胱造影〔撮影〕図

Cysto, cysto.
膀胱腟腔　**VVS**
膀胱腟瘻　**VV fistula**
膀胱腟瘻再建　**VVFR**
膀胱ドレナージ　**BD**
膀胱内圧　**Pves**
膀胱内圧測定　**CM**
膀胱内圧測定(法)　**CMG**
膀胱内圧測定図　**CMG**
膀胱尿管逆流(現象)　**VUR**
膀胱尿管接合〔分岐〕部　**VUJ**
膀胱尿管造影〔撮影〕図　**VCUG**
膀胱尿道造影〔撮影〕図　**CUG**
膀胱利尿筋(内)圧　**Pdet**
膀胱留置カテーテル　**BT**
縫合　**N, S**
縫合(術)　**sut**
縫合線　**sut**
膨疹・潮紅反応　**WFR**
膨疹吸収時間　**QRZ**
膨疹紅斑反応　**WER**
膨疹反応時間　**QRZ**
膨張　**exp**
他に特記事項がなければ　**NOS**
他に分類できない　**NEC**
他の　**fgn, O, o, OTH**
他の言葉で言えば　**iow**
他の神経疾患　**OND**
北鮮白朮　**AJ**
北米看護診断協会　**NANDA**
北米放射線医学会　**RSNA**
北極航空医学研究室　**AAL**
発作　**A, atk, Sz, sz**
発作性飲酒狂患者　**dipso**
発作性運動誘発〔誘因〕性ジスキネジー　**PED**
発作性運動誘発性舞踏アテトーゼ　**PKC**
発作性寒冷血色素尿症　**PCH**
発作性催眠ジスキネジー　**PHD**
発作性上室性頻拍　**PST**
発作性上室性頻拍(症)　**PSVT**
発作性心室性頻拍(症)　**PVT**
発作性心房細動　**PAf, PAFIB**
発作性心房性頻拍　**PAT**
発作性心房粗動　**PAF**
発作性脱分極性シフト　**PDS**
発作性の　**parox**
発作性脳律動異常　**PCD**
発作性発射　**PD**
発作性頻拍　**PT**
発作性房室結節回帰(性)頻拍　**PAVNRT**
発作性夜間血色素尿症　**PHN, PNH**
発作性夜間呼吸困難　**PND**
発作性労作性呼吸困難　**PDE**
発作頻度　**SF**
発疹チフスワクチン　**TV**
発赤徴候　**RC sign**
勃起維持(静脈)流出量　**OME**
勃起獲得(静脈)流出量　**OOE**
勃起不全　**ED**
欲するだけ服用せしめよ　**cap quant.**
本　**L, lib.**
本質的な異常なし　**no ess.abn**
本質的な変化なし　**NEC**
本態性血小板血症　**ET**
本態性血小板減少症　**Et**
本態性高血圧　**EH**
本態性高血圧症　**EHT**
本態性高コレステロール血症　**EHC**
本態性高脂血症　**EHL**
本態性混合性クリオグロブリン血症　**EMC**
本態性腎出血　**ERB**
本態性振戦　**ET**
本能的行動またはそれを引き起こさせる状態　**D**
本能的衝動を惹起させる刺激　**Sd**
奔馬調律　**G, g**
奔流状態　**EL, ES**
香港型インフルエンザウイルス　**HK virus**
翻訳阻止蛋白　**TIP**

ま

マイエンブルク・アルテル・ユーリンガー(症候群) **MAU**
マイオジール脳室撮影 **MVG**
マイクロ(＝10^{-6}) μ
マイクロアンペア **μA**
マイクロウェーブジアテルミー **MWD**
マイクロオクタロニー法 **MO**
マイクロオーム **μΩ**
マイクロガンマ(＝ピコグラム)(＝10^{-12}g) **μγ**
マイクロキュリー **μCi**
マイクロキュリー時間 **μC hr., μc.h., μCi-hr**
マイクログラム **γ, μg, mcg, mcgm**
マイクログレイン **mgn**
マイクロクーロン **μC, μcoul**
マイクロ〔μ〕国際単位 **μIU**
マイクロサテライトインスタビリティアッセイ **MIA**
マイクロソフト社のOS **MSDOS, MS-DOS**
マイクロソームエタノール酸化系 **MEOS**
マイクロ単位 **mcU, μU**
マイクロ波 **MW**
マイクロ波合成開口映像システム **SAR**
マイクロ波による組織凝血 **MTC**
マイクロ波プラズマ微量元素質量分析装置 **MIP-MS**
マイクロ波誘導プラズマ **MIP**
マイクロバール **μb, μbar, μ-bar**
マイクロ秒 **μs, μsec**
マイクロファラッド **μF, μf**
マイクロプレート螢光抗体法 **MFA**
マイクロヘンリー **μH**
マイクロボルト **μV**
マイクロホン **mike**
マイクロマイクロ(＝10^{-6}) **μμ**
マイクロマイクロキュリー **μμc**
マイクロマイクログラム **μμg**
マイクロマイクロファラッド **μμF**
マイクロミクロン **μμ**
マイクロミリグラム **μmg**
マイクロミリメートル **μmm**
マイクロメートル **μ, μm**
マイクロモル **μmol**
マイクロラジオグラフィ **MR**
マイクロラジオグラム **MR**
マイクロリットル **λ, μl**
マイクロレントゲン **μR**
マイクロワット **μW**
マイコバクテリウム(属) **M, Myco**
マイコプラズマ **MP**
マイコプラズマ(属) **M**
マイコプラズマによる補体結合反応 **MCF**
マイコプラズマ肺炎 **MP, MPn, MPP**
マイシリン **MC**
マイトゲン活性化蛋白 **MAP**
マイトゲン活性化蛋白キナーゼ **MAPK**
マイトマイシン **Mi**
マイトマイシン,ビンブラスチン,シスプラチン(＝プラチノール) **MVP**
マイトマイシンC **MC, MMC, MTC, MTO C**
マイトマイシンC,アドリアマイシン,シスプラチン(＝プラチノール) **MAP**
マイトマイシンC,エトポシド,シスプラチン(＝プラチノール) **MEP**
マイトマイシンC,ビンクリスチン(＝オンコビン),ブレオマイシン,シスプラチン(＝プラチノール) **MOB-PT**
マイトマイシンC,フルオロウラシル **MF**
マイトマイシンC,フルオロウラシル,アドリアマイシン **MIFA**
マイトマイシンC,フルオロウラシル,シタラビン **MFC**
マイトマイシンC,フルオロウラシル,トヨマイシン,シクロホスファミド(＝エンドキサン) **MFTE**
マイナー・トゥース・ムーブメント **MTM**
マイニッケ混濁反応 **MTR**
マイニッケ清澄反応 **MKR**
マイボーム腺障害 **MGD**
マイヤー **MY, My**
マイヤー・ブリックス(型)性格検査 **MBTI**

マイル　**mil, ml**
マイル/時　**mph**
マイレラン　**GT-41**
マウスγグロブリン　**MGG**
マウスＴリンパ球表面抗原系列　**Lyt**
マウスインターフェロン　**MIF**
マウス肝炎　**MVH**
マウス肝炎ウイルス　**MHV**
マウス肝癌　**MH**
マウス幹細胞様細胞　**MSCLC**
マウス血清アルブミン　**MSA**
マウス抗体産生(試験)　**MAP**
マウス抗ラット血清　**MARS**
マウス骨髄リンパ球抗原　**MBLA**
マウスサイトメガロウイルス　**MCMV**
マウス子宮重量　**MUW, NUW**
マウス子宮重量単位　**MUWU**
マウス子宮単位　**MUU, NUU**
マウス主要組織適合遺伝子複合体　**H-2**
マウス上皮(細胞)　**ME**
マウス精管　**MVD**
マウス赤白血病　**MEL**
マウス赤血球　**MRBC**
マウス単位　**ME, MU**
マウスチ〔サイ〕ログロブリン　**MTg**
マウス特異的Ｂリンパ球抗原　**MSBLA**
マウス特異的リンパ球抗原　**MSLA**
マウス肉腫ウイルス　**MSV**
マウス乳房腫瘍　**MMT**
マウス乳房腫瘍ウイルス　**MMTV**
マウス乳房上皮　**MME**
マウス肺炎ウイルス　**PVM**
マウス胚線維芽細胞　**MEF**
マウス培養肥満細胞　**CMC**
マウス白血病ウイルス　**MLS, MLV**
マウス肥満細胞プロテアーゼ　**MMCP**
マウス表皮成長因子　**mEGF**
マウス羊水　**MAF**
マウス卵巣腫瘍　**MOT**
マウスロゼット形成細胞　**MRFC**
マーカー　**mrkr**
マーカス・ガン(瞳孔)　**MG**
マギル痛み性状評価法　**MPQ**
マクスウェル　**Mx**
マグネシア　**Mag.ust**
マグネシウム　**Mag, mag, Mg**
マグネシウム欠乏(症)　**MD**
マグネシウム乳(剤)　**MOM**
マクバーニー(圧痛)点　**McB, McB pt, Mcp**
マクログロブリン　**M, MG**
マクログロブリン・トリプシン(複合体)　**M-T**
マクロファージ　**MP, Mφ**
マクロファージ化学走化性因子　**MCF**
マクロファージ化学誘導蛋白１　**MCP-1**
マクロファージ拡散因子　**MSF**
マクロファージ活性化　**MA**
マクロファージ活性化因子　**MAF**
マクロファージ凝集因子　**MAF**
マクロファージ凝集反応因子　**MAggF**
マクロファージコロニー形成単位　**CFU-M**
マクロファージコロニー刺激因子　**M-CSF**
マクロファージ消失因子　**MDF**
マクロファージ消失反応　**MDR**
マクロファージ分化因子　**MDF**
マクロファージ遊走阻止因子　**MIF**
マクロファージ遊走阻止試験　**MIT**
マクロファージ由来炎症性蛋白　**MIP**
マクロファージ由来成長因子　**MDGF**
マクロファージ抑制因子　**MIF**
マクロライド類　**MLs**
マサチューセッツ眼科耳鼻咽喉科病院　**MEEI**
マサチューセッツ総合病院　**MGH**
マーシャル・スミス症候群　**MSS**
マーシャル・マーケッティ(手技)　**MM**
マーシュ・ベンダー因子　**MB**
マージン　**MAR**
マース(＝アテローマ疾患に対する高脂血症治療薬

の効果を調査した大規模臨床試験） **MAAS**
マーズコロナウイルス **MERS-CoV**
マスリウム **Ma**
マダニ **I**
マダニ(属) **A**
マチス・スカーレットブルー **MSB**
マチャド・ジョセフ・アゾレア病 **MJAD**
マチャド・ジョセフ病 **MJD**
マッカーシー小児能力尺度 **MSCA**
マッサージ **M, m, mass, mass., MSS**
マッサージと医学体育学の認可団体 **CSMMG**
マッサージと医学体操の指導員 **TMMG**
マッドクス桿(状)体 **MR**
マッハ **M**
マッハ数 **Ma**
マッヘ単位 **ME, MU, UM**
マツヤニ由来精油 **turp**
マーティン・オルブライト(症候群) **MA**
マーティン・ベル症候群 **MBS**
マーティン自殺うつ病調査票 **MSDI**
マーデン・ウォーカー症候群 **MWS**
マトリックス **M, MX**
マトリックス固相分散(法) **MSPD**
マトリックス支援レーザー破壊 **MALDI**
マトリックスメタロプロテイナーゼ **MMP**
マニトール除去率 **E_M**
マネージャー **mgr**
マポ(＝水溶性アルキル化剤の１つ) **MAPO**
マラリア根絶計画 **MEP**
マラリア免疫グロブリン **MIg**
マラリア療法 **MT**
マリー・シュトリュンペル(病) **MS**
マリー・バレー脳炎 **MVE**
マリネスコ・シェーグレン症候群 **MSS**
マリファナ **MJ**
マルタ熱菌のウシおよびブタ株から製造した抗原 **MBP**
マルタ熱抗原 **MBA**
マルチアファバ・ビグナミ病 **MBD**
マルトース結合蛋白 **MBP**
マールブルグウイルス病 **MVD**
マールブルグ病 **MD**
マレイン酸エルゴノビン **EM**
マレイン酸クロルフェニラミン **CPM**
マレク病ウイルス **MDV, vMDV**
マレク病ヘルペスウイルス **MDHV**
マロリー・ワイス(症候群) **MW**
マロリー・ワイス症候群 **MWS**
マロリー(小)体 **MB**
マロンアルデヒド **MA**
マロンジアルデヒド **MDA**
マンガン **Mn**
マンガンスーパーオキシドジスムターゼ **MnSOD**
マン筋力テスト **MMT**
マングースキツネザル **LMO**
マンデル酸 **MA**
マンニットクリアランス **C_{man}**
マンニトール・リジン結晶バイオレット・ブリリアントグリーン(培地) **MLCB**
マンニトールアデニンホスフェート **MAP**
マンノサミン **ManN**
マンノース **Man, MAN**
マンノース-6-リン酸 **MAN-6-P**
マンノース感受性(赤)血球凝集(反応) **MSHA**
マンノース結合蛋白 **MBP**
マンノース抵抗性(赤)血球凝集(反応) **MRHA**
マンノース抵抗性〔耐性〕の **MR**
マンノースリン酸イソメラーゼ **MPI**
マンプス(＝マサチューセッツ総合病院式医療コンピュータ言語) **MUMPS**
マンモグラフィー **MMG**
または **od**
または近似値で **ONO**
まっすぐな **st, str**
まとめ **S, Zus**
まぶしがり **phot, PT**
巻いてある細いガーゼ **NGR**
真っすぐな ***o*-**
真夜中 **MN, M/N, mn**
混ぜよ **M, m, m.**
混ぜる **M, m, m.**
麻疹・風疹・流行性耳下腺炎 **MRM**
麻疹・風疹 **MR**

麻疹ウイルス　**MV**
麻疹脳炎　**ME**
麻疹免疫グロブリン　**MIg**
麻酔　**ANA, Anaes, Anaesth, ansth**
麻酔(法)　**Anes, anes, anesth**
麻酔開始　**X**
麻酔回路　**AC**
麻酔学　**Anes, anes, anesth**
麻酔学士　**Maanes**
麻酔下骨盤検査　**PEUA**
麻酔下診察　**EUA**
麻酔後回復　**PAR**
麻酔後回復室　**PARR**
麻酔後回復部　**PARU**
麻酔剤　**BTM**
麻酔資格認定書　**D.A.**
麻酔と脳神経活動モニター　**ABM**
麻酔の　**A, ANA, Anaes, Anaesth, Anes, anes**
麻酔薬　**anesth, BTM**
麻痺性貝毒　**PSP**
麻痺性小児麻痺　**PIP**
麻痺性腕神経叢炎　**PBN**
麻痺量　**PD**
麻薬　**cotics, intox, NARC, narco**
麻薬・危険薬物管理局　**BNDD**
麻薬永久管理局　**PCNB**
麻薬および危険薬品情報ファイル　**NADDIF**
麻薬監視　**Nar Inv**
麻薬管理局　**NDSB**
麻薬管理者　**NARC**
麻薬協議会国際連合　**UNARCO**
(米国)麻薬局　**DND**
麻薬局　**BN**
麻薬常習者のためのサービス・教育・リハビリテーション　**SERA**
麻薬常用者　**ad**
麻薬捜査官　**NO**
麻薬中毒者回復局　**NRO**
麻薬中毒予防全国連合　**NAPAN**
麻薬取締官　**D-men, NARC**
麻薬に対する代理教育者　**DEAN**
麻薬反対の両親　**PAN**
麻薬連合事務局　**FBN**
増す　**icr**
摩擦　**fric, frict, fx, R**
摩擦音　**FR r, Fr r, fr.r.**
摩擦係数　**f**
摩擦法　**fx**
摩擦力顕微鏡　**FFM**
摩耗故障率　**IFR**
毎朝　**o.m., omn.man., q.a.m., Qm, q.m., sing.auror.**
毎朝または毎夜　**om.mane vel noc.**
毎午後　**Qpm, q.p.m.**
毎時　**QH, qh, q.h.**
毎時間　**o.s.h.**
毎時ミリグラム要素　**mgeh**
毎週　**Qw, q.w., wkly**
毎就寝時に　**QHS, q.h.s.**
毎月　**mtl**
毎年の　**Ann, ann**
毎軟便後に　**post sing.sed.liq.**
毎日　**dd, d.d., de d.in d., in d., o.d., pd, p.d., Qd, q.d., tägl, tgl**
毎日(の)　**quot.**
毎日１回　**u.i.d.**
毎日の　**/d, quotid.**
毎日の観察　**DI**
毎日平均患者負荷　**adpl**
毎秒　**PS, ps, p.s.**
毎秒インチ　**ips**
毎秒回転数　**RPS, rps, r.p.s.**
毎秒心拍出量　**CSO**
毎秒崩壊数　**dps**
毎秒メートルキログラム　**MKS, M.K.S., mks**
毎分～語　**WPM, w.p.m.**
毎分換気量　**AMV, MV**
毎分呼吸量　**MRV,** V_E
毎分心拍出量　**HMO, HMV**
毎分崩壊数　**dpm, DPM**
毎分崩壊量　**dis/min**
毎夕　**Qpm, q.p.m.**
毎夜　**omn.noct., ON, On, o.n., Qn, q.n.**
埋葬された　**Bur**
埋葬した　**SEP**
(歯牙)埋伏(症)　**Impx**
埋伏した　**Imp, imp**
前と同じ　**do., u.s.**
前に　**fore**
前に引用された位置に　**l.s.c.**
前の　**A, a, ANT, ant**
前払い健康保険　**PHP**
巻戻し　**REW**
膜　**M, m., memb**
膜安定化活性　**MSA**
膜安定化作用　**MSA**
膜可溶化抗原　**MS-Ag**
膜拡散能　**DM**
膜型人工肺　**ECMO**
膜型人工肺体外循環　**ECMO**
膜型人工肺と部分体外循環による体外式肺補助　**ECLA**
膜型ループス腎炎　**MLN**

膜螢光抗体法 **MIF**
膜抗原 **MA**
膜自発早期破裂 **SPROM**
膜侵襲複合体 **MAC**
膜性細胞質内封入体 **MCB**
膜性糸球体症 **MGP**
膜性糸球体腎炎 **HGN, MG, MGN**
膜性腎症 **MN**
膜性増殖性糸球体腎炎 I 型 **MPGN-I**
膜性増殖性糸球体腎炎 II 型 **MPGN-II**
膜性中隔動脈瘤 **MSA**
膜(性)増殖性糸球体腎炎 **MPGN**
膜電位 **MP**
膜電位依存性カルシウムチャンネル **VDCCs**
膜電位依存性抑制 **VDB**
膜電位の不安定分屑 **L fraction**
膜内外静水圧(差) **TMP**
膜内外電位差 **TMP**
膜内外電位差勾配 **TPG**
膜内粒子 **IMP**
膜被覆顆粒 **MCG**
膜免疫グロブリン **AgR, MIg**
膜様条虫(属) **H**
膜濾過法血漿交換 **MFPE**
孫息子 **GS**
孫娘 **GD**
優る **exc**
貧しい **P, sc**
待ちリスト **WL**
(終)末期医療 **TC**
末期癌 **TCA**
末期腎不全 **WSRF**
末梢 **periph**
末梢 T 細胞型リンパ腫 **PTCL**
末梢気道 **PAW**
末梢血 **PB**
末梢血管 **PV**
末梢血管血漿量 **PV**
末梢血幹細胞 **PBSC**
末梢血幹細胞移植療法 **PBSCT**
末梢血管疾患 **PVD**
末梢血管抵抗 **PVR**
末梢血管の **PV**
末梢血管不全 **PVI**
末梢血管閉塞性疾患 **PVOD**
末梢血好中球 **PBN**
末梢血赤血球 **PBC**
末梢血単核(細胞) **PBM**
末梢血単核球 **PBM, PMBC**
末梢血単核細胞 **PBMC**
末梢血単核白血球 **PBL**
末梢血白血球 **PBL**
末梢血流量 **PBF**
末梢血リンパ球 **PBL**
末梢血リンパ球インターフェロン誘発試験 **PII**
末梢血リンパ球数 **LS**
末梢高栄養(液) **PHA**
末梢骨定量的 CT **PQCT**
末梢循環障害 **PCI**
末梢循環不全 **PCF**
末梢静脈 **PeV, PV**
末梢静脈圧 **PVP**
末梢静脈血漿 **PVP**
末梢静脈内過栄養 **PIVH**
末梢静脈の **PV**
末梢静脈レニン活性 **PRVA**
末梢神経 **PN**
末梢神経外胚葉腫瘍 **PNET**
末梢神経系 **PNS**
末梢神経刺激装置 **PNS**
末梢神経障害 **PN, PNI, PNP**
末梢神経症状・浮腫・色素沈着 **PEP**
末梢神経病変 **PNL**
末梢スメア **PS**
末梢性気道閉塞症 **PAO**
末梢性胆管癌 **PCC**
末梢性糖尿病網膜症 **PDR**
末梢性動脈疾患 **PAD**
末梢性の **periph**
末梢性肺動脈狭窄 **PPS**
末梢性肺動脈狭窄(症) **PPAS**
末梢性良性腫瘍 **PBN**
末梢全抵抗 **PTR**
末梢抵抗 **PR**
末梢抵抗単位 **PRU**
末梢動脈硬化性閉塞性疾患 **PAOD**
末梢動脈閉塞疾患 **PAOD**
末梢の **dist**
末梢白血球 **PWBC**
末梢非経口的栄養 **PPN**
末梢ブドウ糖取り込み **PGU**
末梢有核細胞 **PNC**
末梢リンパ節 **PLN**
末梢レーザー血管形成(術) **PLA**
末節骨 **TP**
末端 **TRML**
末端型黒色腫 **AM**
末端感覚 **TS**
末端の **t, term**
全く **lit, lit.**
松原皮内反応 **MCR**
松葉杖歩行 **CW**
丸い **r, rd**
丸い頭 **rd hd**
丸く等しい **R+E**
稀な **R, r**
満期 **FT**
満期産生存小児 **TBLC**
満期産生存乳幼児 **TBLI**

満期死産　**FTBD**
満期出産　**FTLB**
満期正常経腟分娩 **FTNVD**
満期正常産　**FTND**
満期正常自然分娩 **FTNSD**
満期正常分娩　**TND**
満期と同等の　**FTE**
満足状態　**sat.cond**
満足度面接調査　**MISS**
満足な　**sat, satis**
(食餌に)満腹した　**F**
慢性T細胞リンパ性白血病　**TCLL**
慢性アルコール性膵炎 **CAP**
慢性萎縮性胃炎　**CAG**
慢性咽頭炎　**PC**
慢性咽頭喉頭炎　**PLC**
慢性エプスタイン・バーウイルス　**CEBV**
慢性炎症性脱髄性神経根ニューロパシー　**CIDR**
慢性炎症性脱髄性多発神経根ニューロパシー **CIDP**
慢性炎症性脱髄性多発ニューロパシー　**CIDP**
慢性炎症性多発ニューロパシー　**CIP**
慢性炎症性腸疾患　**CIBD**
慢性円板状エリテマトーデス〔紅斑性狼瘡〕 **CDLE**
慢性開放(隅)角緑内障 **COAG**
慢性潰瘍性大腸炎　**CUC**
慢性カタル性結膜炎 **CCC**
慢性活動性EBウイルス感染症　**CAEBV**
慢性活動性ウイルス肝炎 **CAVH**
慢性活動性肝炎　**CAH**
慢性活動性肝(臓)障害 **CALD**
慢性化膿性中耳炎 **CSOM, OMPC, OMSC**
慢性化膿性右中耳炎 **ROMSC**
慢性過敏症　**CHS**
慢性顆粒球性白血病 **CGL**
慢性肝炎　**CH**
慢性間欠的腹膜透析 **CIPD**
慢性肝(臓)疾患　**CLD**
慢性間質性腎炎　**CIN**
慢性間質性肺炎　**CIP**
慢性肝性脳症　**CHE**
慢性関節リウマチ **CAR, CRA**
慢性感染性神経障害性(神経向性)物質　**CHINA**
慢性冠(状動脈)不全　**CCI**
慢性寒冷赤血球凝集素病 **CHAD**
慢性(細)気管支炎　**CB**
慢性気管支炎　**BC, CB**
慢性器質性脳症候群 **COBS**
慢性気道閉塞　**CAO**
慢性狭隅角緑内障 **CANAG, CNAG**
慢性偽陽性　**CFP**
慢性虚血性心疾患 **CIHD**
慢性血液透析　**HDC**
慢性高血圧　**CH**
慢性光線性皮膚炎　**CAD**
慢性拘束性肺疾患 **CRPD**
慢性喉頭炎　**LC**
慢性硬膜下血腫 **CSDH, CSH**
慢性呼吸器疾患　**CRD**
慢性呼吸器疾患質問表 **CRQ**
慢性呼吸不全　**CRF, CRI**
慢性骨髄芽球性白血病 **CML**
慢性骨髄性白血病　**CML**
慢性骨髄線維形成　**CMF**
慢性骨髄増殖性疾患 **CMPD**
慢性骨髄単球性白血病 **CMML, CMMoL, MLC**
慢性再発性炎症性多発根ニューロパシー　**CRIP**
慢性再発性膵(臓)炎 **CRP**
慢性糸球体腎炎　**CG, CGN**
慢性持続性肝炎　**CPH**
慢性疾患収容病院　**CDH**
慢性疾患に伴う貧血 **ACD**
慢性受動的うっ血　**CPC**
慢性漿液性中耳炎 **CSOM**
慢性腎盂腎炎　**CP, CPN**
慢性腎炎　**CN**
慢性神経刺激　**CNI**
慢性神経疲労　**CNE**
慢性進行性外眼筋麻痺 **CPEO**
慢性進行性多発関節炎 **PCE**
慢性進行性多発性関節炎 **PCP**
慢性進行性多発性硬化症 **CPMS**
慢性進行性ミエロパシー **CPM**
慢性腎疾患　**CRD**
慢性腎臓病　**CKD**
慢性心不全　**CCF**
慢性腎不全　**CRF, CRI**
慢性膵炎　**CP**
慢性生物学的擬陽性の **CBFP**

慢性石灰化膵炎　**CCP**
慢性潜伏性壊血病　**CSS**
慢性増殖性糸球体腎炎　**CPGN**
慢性代謝性アシドーシス　**CMA**
慢性多発(性)関節炎　**cP，CP**
慢性多発ニューロパシー　**CPN**
慢性胆汁性肝炎　**CCH**
慢性単純苔癬　**LSC**
慢性胆道閉塞　**COBT**
慢性中耳炎　**COM，OMC**
慢性腸管膜虚血　**CMI**
慢性 T 細胞リンパ球性白血病　**TCLL**
慢性低酸素性肺疾患　**CHLD**
慢性的就床安静　**CBR**
慢性的透析　**CHD**
慢性統合失調症　**CS**
慢性動脈閉塞　**CAO**
慢性特発性好中球減少症候群　**CINS**
慢性特発性再発性多発ニューロパシー　**CIRPN**
慢性特発性腸性偽閉塞症候群　**CIIPS**
慢性特発性白血球減少症　**CIN**
慢性特発性腸性偽閉塞症　**CIIP**
慢性肉芽腫(性)炎(症)　**CGI**
慢性肉芽腫症　**CGD**
慢性尿崩症　**CDI**
慢性熱中障害　**CDE，CED**
慢性粘着性中耳炎　**CAOM**
慢性粘膜皮膚カンジダ症　**CMC**
慢性の　**ch，CHR，chr，chron**
慢性脳血管疾患　**CCVD**
慢性脳症候群　**CBS，ChrBrSyn，Chr Br Syn，Chr B Synd**
慢性肺気腫　**CPE**
慢性肺疾患　**CLD**
慢性肺性心　**CPC**
慢性破壊性歯周病　**CDP**
慢性白血病　**CL**
慢性非活動性肝炎　**CIH**
慢性非化膿性破壊性胆管炎　**CNSDC**
慢性非特異性肺疾患　**CNSLD**
慢性皮膚エリテマトーデス　**CCLE**
慢性皮膚粘膜カンジダ症　**CMCC**
慢性び漫性間質性肺疾患　**CDILD**
慢性びらん性胃炎　**CEG**
慢性疲労症候群　**CFS**
慢性ピロリン酸塩関節症　**CPA**
慢性複雑腎盂腎炎　**CCP**
慢性複雑性尿路感染症　**CCU**
慢性複雑膀胱炎　**CCC**
慢性副鼻腔炎　**CS**
慢性腹膜透析　**CPD**
慢性閉塞隅角緑内障　**CCAG**
慢性閉塞性気管支炎　**COB**
慢性閉塞性気管支疾患　**COBD**
慢性閉塞性気道疾患　**COAD**
慢性閉塞性呼吸器疾患　**CORD**
慢性閉塞性動脈疾患　**COAD**
慢性閉塞性嚢胞性肺気腫　**COBE**
慢性閉塞性肺気腫　**COPE**
慢性閉塞性肺疾患　**COLD，COPD**
慢性ベリリウム中毒肺　**CPB**
慢性変性疾患　**CDD**
慢性弁膜性心疾患　**CVHD**
慢性膜性糸球体腎炎　**CMGN**
慢性膜性増殖性糸球体腎炎　**CMPGN**
慢性未分化型(統合失調症)　**CUT**
慢性遊走性紅斑　**ECM**
慢性溶血性貧血　**CHA**
慢性葉性肝炎　**CLH**
慢性リウマチ様骨盤脊椎関節強直症　**PSR**
慢性良性肝炎　**CBH**
慢性リンパ球性甲状腺炎　**CLT**
慢性リンパ球性白血病　**LLC**
慢性リンパ性白血病　**CLL**
慢性リンパ肉腫細胞白血病　**CLSCL**
慢性リンパ肉腫性白血病　**CLSL**
慢性ループス腎症　**MLN**
慢性濾胞性結膜炎　**CFC**

み

ミエリン　**myel**
ミエリン塩基性蛋白　**MBP**
ミエリンオリゴデンドロサイトグリコプロテイン　**MOG**
ミエリン形態　**MF**
ミエロペルオキシダーゼ　**MOP, MPO, PMO**
ミエロペルオキシダーゼ欠乏(症)　**MPOD**
ミエローマ蛋白　**M protein**
ミオカマイシン　**MOM**
ミオキナーゼ　**MK**
ミオクローヌスてんかん　**ME**
ミオグロビン　**Mb, MG, MOY**
ミオシン　**M**
ミオシンＨ鎖　**HC**
ミオシン軽鎖　**MLC**
ミオシン軽鎖キナーゼ　**MLCK**
ミオシン重鎖　**MYH11**
ミオヘモグロビン　**MHb**
ミカエリス・メンテン解離定数　**Km, K_m**
ミカエリス・メンテン(解離)定数　K_m
ミカエリス定数　**Km, K_m**
ミカマイシン　**MKM**
ミクリッツ症候群　**MS**
ミクログロブリン　**M**
ミクロコッカス(属)　**M**
ミクロソーム感作血球凝集反応　**MCHA**
ミクロソーム赤血球凝集テスト〔試験〕　**MHA**
ミクロソーム分画補体結合反応　**MCF**
ミクロソームヘムオキシゲナーゼ　**MHO**
ミクロソームリポ蛋白　**MLP**
ミ〔マイ〕クロトーム　**MT**
ミクロトーム　**microt**
ミクロノマイシン　**MCR**
ミクロフィルトレーション　**MF**
ミクロン　**μ, mu**
ミケティ・ウィルソン症候群　**MWS**
ミコナゾール　**MCZ**
ミコフェノール酸　**MPA**
ミセル安定化室温リン光　**MS-RTP**
ミセル電動クロマトグラフィ　**MEKC**
ミセル電動毛細管クロマトグラフィ　**ME**
ミゾリビン　**MZR**
ミデカマイシン　**MDM**
ミドカイン　**MK**
ミトコンドリア　**M, mit., mt, MT**
ミトコンドリアGOT　**M-GOT**
ミトコンドリアアスパラギン酸アミノトランスフェラーゼ　**mAST**
ミトコンドリア転移RNA　**mt tRNA**
ミトコンドリア外膜　**OMM**
ミトコンドリア抗体　**MA**
ミトコンドリア性チミジンキナーゼ　**TK2, TKm, TKM**
ミトコンドリア性リンゴ酸脱水素酵素　**MDH2, MDHM**
ミトコンドリアデオキシリボ核酸　**mtDNA**
ミトコンドリアメッセンジャーRNA　**mt mRNA**
ミトコンドリア脳筋症　**MELA**
ミトコンドリアのクエン酸合成酵素　**Cs**
ミトコンドリア分画　**MF**
ミトコンドリアリボソームRNA　**mt rRNA**
ミトラマイシン　**MTH, MTM**
ミドルネームなしの　**NMN**
ミドルネームのイニシャルなし　**NMI**
ミドルブルック・デュボス試験　**MD**
ミニガストリン　**MG**
ミニ対象試験　**MOT**
ミニム　**M, m**
ミネソタ教師態度調査票　**MTAI**
ミネソタ失語鑑別診断　**MDDA**
ミネソタ失語鑑別診断検査〔試験〕　**MTDDA**
ミネソタ小児発達〔発育〕調査表　**MCDI**
ミネソタ職業興味調査票　**MVII**
ミネソタ多面的人格目録検査　**MMPI**
ミネソタ満足度質問表　**MSQ**
ミネソタ満足度尺度　**MSS**
ミネラル油　**MO**
ミノキシジル　**Mx**
ミノサイクリン　**MiC, MINO**
ミハエリス・グートマン(小体)　**MG**
ミハエリス・グートマン小体　**M-G body**
ミハエリス・メンテン

M-M
ミプス　**MIPS**
ミベリ汗孔角化(症)　**PM**
ミ〔マイ〕レラン　**GT-41**
ミヤール・ギュブレ(症候群)　**MG**
ミュア・トール(症候群)　**MT**
ミュラー管　**Md**
ミュラー管開存症候群　**PMDS**
ミュラー管阻害〔抑制〕因子　**MIF**
ミュラー管抑制物質　**MIS**
ミュラー細胞活動　**m wave**
ミュラー(管)退行因子　**MRF**
ミュンスター式顆部下腿義足　**KBM**
ミュンヘンアルコール症テスト　**MALT**
ミョウバン・血液・木炭法　**ABC**
ミョウバン沈降物　**AP**
ミョウバン沈殿ジフテリアトキソイド　**diph-tox AP**
ミョウバン沈殿毒素　**APT**
ミラー・アボット(管)　**MA**
ミラー・アボット管　**MA tube**
ミラー・フィッシャー(症候群)　**MF**
ミラー・フィッシャー症候群　**MFS**
ミラノ高血圧ラット　**MHR**
ミラノ正常血圧ラット　**MNS**
ミリ(＝10^{-3})　**m, M, m**
ミリアンペア　**MA, mA, ma.**
ミリアンペア秒　**mas, mAS, MAS**
ミリアンペア分　**mam, mAm, MAM, MaM**
ミリオスモル　**mOs, m osmole**
ミリオスモルの　**MOsm, mOsm, mosm**
ミリオンガロン/日　**mg/d**
ミリオングストローム　**MÅ**
ミリガンマ　**mγ**
ミリ規定(溶液)の　**mN**
ミリキュリー　**mc, mc., mCi, MCU**
ミリキュリー時間　**mch, mc h, mc-h, mc.h., mchr, mc-hr, mCi-hr**
ミリグラム　**mg, mgm**
ミリグラム/キログラム　**mg/kg**
ミリグラム/時　**mg/hr**
ミリグラム時　**MGH, mgh, mg h, mg-hr**
ミリグラム当量　**MEq, mEq, meq**
ミリグラム等量　**ME**
ミリグラム当量/リットル　**mEq/l**
ミリグラムパーセント　**mg%**
ミリグラム要素　**mg-el**
ミリクーロン　**mC, mcoul**
ミリ国際単位　**mIU**
ミリ重量モル浸透圧の　**mOs**
ミリス・スタディ(＝心理的ストレスと冠動脈疾患との強い関連性を示した大規模試験)　**MILIS**
ミリスチン酸　**$C_{14=0}$**
ミリスチン酸イソプロピル　**IPM**
ミリスチン酸酢酸ホルボール　**PMA**
ミリ単位　**mU**
ミリバール　**mb, mbar**
ミリ秒　**millisec, ms, msec**
ミリファラド　**mF, mf**
ミリヘンリー　**mH, mh**
ミリポアフィルター　**MF**
ミリポアフィルター法　**MFM**
ミリボルト　**mV, MV**
ミリマイクロキュリー　**mμc**
ミリマイクログラム　**mμg.**
ミリミクロン　**mμ**
ミリメートル　**mm**
ミリメートル/秒　**mm/sec**
ミリメートル水銀柱(圧)　**millihg**
ミリメートル水銀柱圧　**mmHg**
ミリメートル水柱圧　**mmH_2O**
ミリメートル分圧　**mmpp, mm.p.p.**
ミリモル　**mM, mmol, mmole**
ミリモル/リットル　**mM/L, mM/l**
ミリモルの　**mM**
ミリ容積モル浸透圧の　**MOsm, mOsm, mosm**
ミリラザーフォード　**mrd**
ミリラド　**mrad**
ミリランベルト　**mL**
ミリリットル　**mil, mil., ml, ml.**

ミリリットル/分/平方メートル　**ml/min/m²**
ミリレム　**mrem**
ミリレントゲン　**mR**
ミリレントゲン/時　**mr/hr**
ミリレントゲン/時/メートル　**mrhm**
ミリレントゲン当量　**MREM**
ミリワット　**mW**
ミルウォーキーブレース　**MB**
ミルクアルカリ症候群　**MAS**
ミルクと糖蜜　**M & M**
ミルクの入っていない食事　**MFD**
ミルクリング(検査)　**MR**
ミルクリング検査　**MRT**
ミルクリング検査〔試験〕　**MR test**
ミロキサシン　**MLX**
ミンク細胞病巣誘導ウイルス　**MCF**
みかけの分布容積　**Vd**
未刊行の　**NYP**
未完の　**unfin**
未確定原因　**UDO**
未確定の　**P**
未確認診断の関節炎　**AUD**
未確認成長因子　**UGF**
未確認放射性核種の最大許容濃度　**MPCUR**
未既知アレルギー　**NKA**
未決定原因による出血　**BUO**
未検査　**NE**
未検査の　**UT**
未婚死亡　**DU**
未婚の　**UM**
未婚の母　**UWM**
未(経)産の　**nullip**
未出版の　**NYP**
未処置の出血性ショック　**UCHS**
未証明　**up**
未証明の　**up**
未診断　**NYD**
未診断の　**NYD**
未熟クロマチン凝縮　**PCC**
未熟児　**PI, preemies, preemy**
未熟児出生率　**PBR**
未熟児網膜症　**ROP**
未熟赤血球　**IRBC, iRBC**
未熟染色体濃縮　**PCC**
未熟な　**im**
未熟の　**immat, Pr**
未成熟茶色脂肪(細胞)　**IBF**
未治療の　**UT**
未知　**X, x**
未知因子　**UF**
未知外傷　**INK**
未知の　**U, UK**
未知のアミノ酸　**Xaa**
未知の原因による心筋症　**MUO**
未提示の　**unrep**
未評価　**NE**
未分化B細胞リンパ腫　**UBL**
未分化悪性奇形腫　**MTA**
未分化型(癌)　**ud**
未分化癌　**PDC, UC**
未分化結合組織疾患　**UCTD**
未分化結合組織症候群　**UCTS**
未分化神経外胚葉性腫瘍　**PNET**
未分化腺癌　**PDA**
未分化大細胞性リンパ腫　**ALCL**
未分化大細胞リンパ腫　**LCAL**
未分化の　**im, UD**
未分化の胎芽肉腫　**UES**
未分化リンパ球性リンパ腫　**PDLL**
未分化リンパ腫　**UL**
未亡人　**wid., Wid.**
未亡人(になった)　**W, w**
未亡人〔男やもめ〕になった　**wid., Wid.**
未〔非〕抱合ビリルビン　**UCB, UCBR**
未報告の　**unrep**
未来　**fut**
見かけ上の拡散係数　**ADC**
見かけ上の拡散定数　**ADC**
見かけの　**app, appar, SH**
見かけの経皮的神経刺激　**STNS**
見かけの手術をした　**SO**
見つからない　**NF**
見本　**Ex, ex**
見よ　**S, s, v., vd., vid.**
見られない　**NS**
身分証明　**ID**
身振り認知テスト　**GRT**
眉間・オピスチン線　**GOL**
右　**(R), dext.**
右(の)　**R, R, r**
右胃大網動脈　**RGE, RGEA**
右胃大網膜動脈　**AGED**
右胃動脈　**RG, RGA**
右上の　**r & a, RU**
右頤横位　**MDT**
右頤前位　**MDA**
右から左へ　**R-L, R → L**
右下肩甲骨縁　**RLSB**

右下肢　**RLE，RLL，RLX**
右下斜(筋)　**RIO**
右下大動脈　**RIVC**
右下直(筋)　**RIR**
右下部 1/4 区　**RLQ**
右下腹部　**RLQ**
右下葉　**RLL**
右外頸動脈　**RECA**
右外斜視　**RXT**
右外側大腿　**RLT**
右外側大腿の　**RLF**
右外側の　**RL，rt.lat**
右外直(筋)　**RLR**
右回旋　**RR**
右回転　**RR**
右隔壁　**RS**
右隔壁の　**RS**
右肩後位　**ScRP**
右肝静脈　**RHV**
右肝動脈　**RH，RHA**
右肝葉　**RLL**
右冠状静脈洞　**RCS**
右冠尖　**RCC**
右冠(状)動脈　**RCA**
右利き　**dex，dext，dext.，RH**
右胸骨縁　**RSB**
右頸動脈　**RCA**
右結腸静脈　**VCD**
右結腸動脈　**RCA**
右肩甲骨縁　**rt.scap.bord**
右肩甲前位　**ScDA，ScRA**
右後斜位　**RPO**
右後心室早期興奮症　**RPVP**
右後頭横側位　**ODT**
右後頭側面　**ROL**
右後頭背側位　**ODP**
右後頭部　**RO，R-O**
右後頭腹側位　**ODA**
右黒質　**RSN**
右三角筋　**RD**
右鎖骨下静脈　**RSV**
右鎖骨下動脈　**RSA**
右鎖骨下の　**RS**
右下　**l/r**
右下の　**RL**
右上外側の　**RUL**
右上眼瞼　**RUL**
右上胸骨縁　**RUSB**
右上極　**RUP**
右上肩甲骨縁　**RUSB**
右上肢　**RUE，RUL，RUX**
右上斜位　**RH**
右上斜筋　**RSO**
右上直(筋)　**RSR**
右上内側の　**RUM**
右上肺野　**RUL**
右上部 1/4 区　**RUQ**
右上腹部　**RUQ**
右(肺)上葉　**RUL，R.U.L.**
右上葉気管支　**RUB**
右上腕動脈　**RBA**
右示指　**RIF**
右主気管支　**RMB**
右視野　**RVF**
右斜鼡径ヘルニア　**ROIH**
右縦胸静脈　**VAZ**
右正中(神経)　**RM**
右仙骨横位　**RST，SDT**
右仙骨後位　**SDP**
右仙骨前位　**RSA，SDA**
右仙骨側位　**RSL**
右仙骨部後位　**SRP**
右仙骨部前位　**SRA**
右前横方向　**RFT**
右前下行冠(状)動脈　**RADCA**
右前下腿　**RAT**
右前後方　**RFP**
右前斜位　**RAO**
右前側面　**RFL**
右前頭開頭(術)　**RFC**
右前頭前位　**RFA**
右前頭柱　**RFp**
右前頭部　**RF，R-F**
右側臥位　**rar，rt**
右側頭後部　**RPT**
右側頭中部　**RMT**
右側頭に　**t.d.**
右側頭部　**R-T**
右側頭へ　**temp dext.**
右側頭葉前部　**RAT**
右鼠径ヘルニア　**RIH**
右総頸(動脈)　**RCC**
右総頸動脈　**RCA，RCCA**
右大腿　**RT**
右大腿静脈　**RFV**
右大腿動脈　**RFA**
右大動脈弓　**RAA**
右体性感覚誘発電位　**RSEP**
右濁音界　**RBD**
右中隔　**RS**
右中隔の　**RS**
右中間気管支幹(中幹)　**RIB**
右中指　**RMF**
右中耳炎　**ROM**
右中側方　**RML**
右中大脳(動脈)　**RMC**
右中大脳動脈　**RMCA**
右中大脳動脈血栓症　**RMCAT**
右中葉　**RML**
右中葉気管支　**RMLB**
(肺の)右中葉症候群　**RMLS**
右長脚副木　**RLLB**
右腸骨窩　**RIF**
右椎骨動脈　**RVA**
右手　**m.d.，RH**
右手増高単極肢誘導　**aVR**
右手側　**RHS**
右殿筋　**RG**
右殿筋の　**RG**
右殿部　**RB**

右殿部の　RG
右と左の　R & L
右頭頂部　RP, R-P
右内胸動脈　RIMA, RITA
右内頸(動脈)　RIC
右内頸動脈　RICA
右内直(筋)　RMR
右内直筋　RMR muscle
右乳房生検検査　RBBX
右尿管口　RUO
右(の)　RT, Rt, rt.
右(側)の　dex., dext.
右の　R
右脳底動脈　RBA
右半球　RH
右背後位　RDP
右背前位　RDA
右肺　RL
右肺静脈　RPV
右肺動脈　RPA
右左シャント　rl-sh
右尾状核　RCN
右回りの　CKW, ckw, CW, cw, cws
右耳　AD, Ad, a.d., RE
右門脈　RPV
右薬指　RRf
右卵管卵巣摘出術　RSO
右肋下部　RHC
右肋間腔　RICS
右肋骨縁　RCM
右肋骨縁下(方)に　BRCM
右肋骨間縁　RICM
右/左　R/L
短い　parv., Sh, sh
水　AQ, aq, aq., H_2O, W, w
水嚥下　WS
水ゲージ　EG, WG
水摂取　WI
水治療指導員　THT
水治療法　HT
水治療法〔学〕　Hydro
水と一緒の嚥下　WS
水に入れて　ex aq., in aq.
水の　A, a
水のない　sine aq.
水負荷(試験)　WL
水負荷試験　WLT, WPT
水無脳症　HC
水誘発温熱療法　WIT
水を入れた　WP
水・エチレングリコール　WEG
水/粉(比)　W/P
溝　S
乱れている　OOO
道　M
密集斑　MD
密着帯　Tj
密度　D, d.
密度/湿度比　d/m
密封療法　ODT
緑(の)　g, grn
水俣病　MD
南(の)　so
南カリフォルニア感覚統合検査　SCSIT
南カリフォルニアブルークロス　BCSC
耳　a., aur.
耳音響放射　OAE
耳かけ式補聴器　BTE
耳鳴　OS
耳の　aur., auric
耳の後　p.aur.
脈(拍)　P
脈圧　PP
脈管外の　EV
(癌細胞の)脈管浸潤の有無と程度　V_{0-3}
脈管膜増殖性ループス腎炎　MLN
脈再発頻度　PRF
脈増幅調節　PAM
脈と心音　T & T
脈波伝播速度　PWV
脈拍コード変調　PCM
脈拍数　PR
脈拍と呼吸　P & R
脈頻度　PF
脈変調　PM
脈容積と脈圧　V & T
脈絡叢液　CPF
脈絡網膜変性(症)　CRD
脈管内　IV
明晩　cr.vesp., CV, c.v.
明晩服用せよ　c.n.s.
民間公益団体　NGO
民間診断クリニック　PDC

む

ムコイド(の) **muc**
ムコイドコロニー **M colony**
ムコイド中耳炎 **MOM**
ムコ多糖(体) **MP**
ムコ多糖体症 **MPS**
ムコ多糖類 **MPS**
ムコ蛋白 **MP**
ムコ蛋白結合多糖体 **MBP**
ムコリピドーシス **MC, ML, MLS**
ムコール(属) **M**
ムスカリン様アセチルコリン受容体 **mAChR**
ムスチン,ビンブラスチン,プロカルバジン,プレドニゾン **MVPP**
ムチン・血餅・予防試験 **MCP-test**
ムチン糖蛋白 **MGP**
ムーブメント教育プログラムアセスメント **MEPA**
ムラミルジペプチド **MDP**
ムラミルペプチド **MTP**
ムラミン酸 **Mur**
ムリコール酸 **MCA**
ムンテラ **MT**
向かって **adv.**
無 **N, nil.**
無アルブミンラット **NAR**
無意識の **invol, UC, UCS, Ucs, unc, uncon**
無エコー域 **EFS**
無栄養症 **A**
無煙の **smkls**
無塩 **NAS**
無塩(の) **SF**
無塩の **NSA**
無塩無脂肪(食) **SFFF**
無影響量 **NOAEL**
無汗性先天性外胚葉性形成不全 **ACED**
無柄の **Sess**
無害性雑音 **IM**
無核突然変異 **0-mu**
無開口の **imperf**
無感覚の **D, d.**
無関係な原因による死亡 **DUC**
無関係の **UR**
無顆粒小胞体 **AER**
無顆粒島状皮質 **AI**
無牛乳食 **MFD**
無記録の **NR**
無許可休暇 **UL**
無菌(の) **GF**
無菌室 **BCR, BPR**
無菌水性懸濁液 **SAS**
無菌性壊死 **AN**
無菌性骨壊死症 **ONA**
無菌性骨端壊死 **AEN, AN**
無菌性の塩づけ **SSS**
無菌接続装置 **SCD**
無菌で注射のできる懸濁液 **SIS**
無菌動物 **GFA, GfA**
無期限の **indef**
無機質 **min**
無機質脱落 **demin**
無機炭素 **IC**
無機の **inor, inorg**
無機ピロリン酸塩 **PPi**
無機物挿入関連関節炎 **ERA**
無機リン **Pi**
無機リン酸 **IP**
無グルカゴンインスリン **GFI**
無グルテン食 **GFD**
無グルテンの **GF**
無欠陥 **ZD, Z/D**
無欠点 **ZD, Z/D**
無月経 **Am**
無月経・多毛症 **AH**
無血管帯 **AVZ**
無血小板血漿 **PFP**
無形成発作 **AC**
無茎の **Sess**
無口述の **NM**
無孔の **imperf**
無行為 **ND**
無言(症) **M, m.**
無呼吸 **A, As, NR**
無呼吸,遅脈,チアノーゼ **ABC**
無呼吸指数 **AI**
無効気道クリアランス **IAC**
無効な **vd**
無効になっていない **HNV**
無虹彩(症) **An**
無虹彩ウィルムス腫瘍(症候群) **AWTA**
無作為(比較対照)試験 **RCT**
無作為増幅多形デオキシリボ核酸 **RAPD**
無作為の **ran**
無作為標本 **RS**
無作用 **nato**
無酸素性作業閾値 **AT**
無酸素(性)脳症 **AE**
無色糸菌症 **HHM**
無色の,被嚢のある,毒性のある **SCV**
無条件構造 **US**
無条件刺激 **UCS, UDS, UnCS, unCS, UnS, un.s., US**
無条件の **uncond**
無条件反射 **UCR, UCS, uncond.ref, UR**
無条件反応 **UCR,**

uncond.resp, UR
無実施 NP
無臭の odorl
無脂肪(食) FF
無脂肪乾燥ミルク NFD
無脂肪固体 FFS
無症候性キャリア AC
無症候性原発性胆汁性肝硬変 a-PBC
無症候性甲状腺炎 ST
無症候性細菌尿 ABU, ASB
無症候性自己免疫性甲状腺炎 AAT
無症候性心筋虚血 SMI
無症候性動脈硬化症研究 ACAS
無症候性の NS
無症候性保因者 AsC
無症候性保菌者 AsC
無症候(性)の asx
無症状の subclin
無視する NEG
無歯の edent
無晶形物質 A-mat
無傷羊膜 IBOW
無照射 NR
無塵室 ICR
無識別 NI
無水アルコール AA
無水の A, abs, anh, anhyd
無生物の inor, inorg
無制限に adlib., ad lib., Ad lib.
無性の asex
無線遠隔測定装置 RT
無線心電図 RCG
無測定の NM
無断欠勤 LWC
無痛(症,法) anal
無痛分娩 ASD, CWOP, CWP
無痛分娩教育協会 CWPEA
無痛分娩連盟 CWPL
無定形の amo, amor, amorph
無毒界 L
無毒性量 NOAEL
無透析液限外濾過 DFUF
無動小発作 IPM
無動の A
無乳糖食 LFD
無熱で abs.feb.
無熱(性)の AF, afeb
無能 dsabl
無能にする dsabl
無能の dsabl
無反応 NR
無反応(の) NR
無排卵月経 AM
無ブドウ糖ハンクス溶液 GFH
無プリン/無ピリミジンエンドヌクレアーゼ AP-endonuclease
無補助拡張期圧 UDP
無名神経病学者国際連絡 NAIL
無名神経病者 NA
無名の innom
無名麻薬中毒者 NA
無免疫ウサギ血清 NRS
(膀胱の)無抑制性収縮 UIC
無力(症) asth
無力化する neut
無力性 A
無力性体質 HA
無料 NC
無βリポ蛋白血症 ABL
無γグロブリン血症 AGG
蒸し鍋 BM
鞭打ちに伴う疾患 WAS
麦ダイズ混合 WSB
虫くい現象 MEP
息子 S, s
結び Lig, lig, lig., ligg, ligg.
娘 D, d, Da, da, da., dau, dgtr, dtr.
紫 Pu, V, v
室 rm

め

メイ・グリュンワルド(染色) **MG**
メイ・グリュンワルト・ギムザ(染色) **MGG**
メイ・ヘグリン異常 **MHA**
メガ(＝10^6) **M**
メガオーム **MΩ**
メガキュリー **MC, Mc, mc, MCi**
メガサイクル **MC, Mc, mc, MEG, meg**
メガサイクル/秒 **Mcps, mc p s, mcps, Mc.p.s., mc/s**
メガジュール **MJ**
メガ電子ボルト **MeV, MEV, mev**
メガドリコ脳底動脈 **MBA**
メガバイト **MB**
メガパスカル **MPa**
メガファラド **MF**
メガヘルツ **MHz**
メガボルト **Mev, MV**
メガ〔巨大〕ミトコンドリア **MM**
メキシコ系アメリカ人 **MA**
メキシレチン **MX**
メクロルエタミン,アドリアマイシン,ダカルバジン,シスジアミンジクロロプラチナム,ビンクリスチン(＝オンコビン),シクロホスファミド **MADDOC**
メクロルエタミン,ビンクリスチン,ビンブラスチン,プロカルバジン,プレドニゾン **MVVPP**
メクロルエタミン,ビンクリスチン(＝オンコビン),プレドニゾン,ブレオマイシン,アドリアマイシン,プロカルバジン **MOP-BAP**
メクロルエタミン,ビンクリスチン(＝オンコビン),プロカルバジン,プレドニゾン **MOPP**
メクロルエタミン,ビンクリスチン(＝オンコビン),プロカルバジン,プレドニゾン,アドリアマイシン,ブレオマイシン,ビンブラスチン **MOPP/ABV**
メクロルエタミン,ビンクリスチン(オンコビン),メトトレキサート,プレドニゾン **MOMP**
メクロルエタミン,ビンブラスチン,プロカルバジン,プレドニゾン **MVPP**
メクロレタミン,アドリアマイシン,ブレオマイシン,ビンクリスチン(＝オンコビン),プレドニゾン **MABOP**
メクロレタミン,ビンクリスチン(＝オンコビン),ブレオマイシン **MOB**
メゲストロール,シクロホスファミド,アドリアマイシン **MCA**
メサドン維持(療法) **MM**
メサドン維持治療プログラム **MMTP**
メサンギウム性増殖性糸球体腎炎 **MPN**
メサンギウム増殖性糸球体腎炎 **MesPGN, MPGN, MSPGN**
メサンギウム肥厚 **MT**
メサンギウム毛細管性糸球体腎炎 **MCGN**
メサンギウム細胞 **MC**
メシリナム **MPC**
メシル酸ガベキサート **FOY**
メシル酸ナファモスタット **NM**
メスカリン **Mesc**
メスナ,アドリアマイシン,イホスファミド,ダカルバジン **MAID**
メスナ,アドリアマイシン,インターロイキン-3,ダカルバジン **MAID**
メスナによる尿道保護,イホスファミド,ミトキサントロン,エトポシド **MINE**
メズロシリン **MZ, MZPC**
メドゥサ(の)頭 **caput med**
メセドリン **Meth**
メセナミン **hexa**
メゾ型 **MS**
メゾトリウム **MSTh**
メタ **m**
メタアクリル酸 **MAA**
メタアドレナリン **MA**
メタクリン酸グリコール **GMA**
メタサイクリン **MTC**
メタゾールアミド **ME**
メタネフリン **M, MN**
メタノール抽出残渣 **MER**
メタヒ酸亜鉛 **ZMA**
メタヒドリン **MHD**
メタボリックシンドローム **MS**
メタロチオネイン **MT**
メタロプロテナーゼインヒ

ビター　**TIMP**
メタンスルホニルフルオリド　**MSF**
メタンスルホン酸ナトリウム　**IHMS**
メチオニン　**M, Met, MET, met**
メチオニン・エンケファリン　**met-EK**
メチオニン・スルホキシミン　**MS**
メチオニン転移リボ核酸　**Met-tRNA**
メチシリン　**DMPC, DMPPC, MCI, METH**
メチシリン感受性黄色ブドウ球菌　**MSSA**
メチシリン耐性黄色ブドウ球菌　**MRS, MRSA**
メチシリン耐性コアグラーゼ陰性ブドウ球菌　**MRCNS**
メチシリン耐性表皮ブドウ球菌　**MRSE**
メチマゾール　**MMI**
メチル　**Me, ME-, meth**
メチレン二ホスホン酸　**MDP**
メチレン二リン酸　**MDP**
メチル-6-クロロエチルニトロソウレア　**MCNU**
メチルアゾメタノール　**MAM**
メチルアルコール　**Me, MeOH, metho**
メチルアルソン酸　**MAA**
メチルアンドロステンジオール　**MAD**
メチルイソブチルケトン　**MIBK**
メチルエチルエーテル　**MEE**
メチルエチルケトン　**MEK**
メチル化ウシ血清アルブミン　**MBSA**
メチルキサンチン(免疫抑制)　**PTX**
メチル基受容化学走性蛋白　**MCP**
メチル基転移酵素　**MTFase**
メチルグアニジン　**MG**
メチルグリオキサル　**MG**
メチルグリオキサルビスグアニルヒドラゾン　**MGBG, MGBH**
メチルグリオキサルビスグアミルヒドラーゼ　**MGBG**
メチルグリオキシルビスグアニルヒドラゾン　**methyl-GAG**
メチルグリーンピロニン　**MGP**
メチルグルコシド　**MG**
メチルクロトニル補酵素Aカルボキシラーゼ　**MCC**
メチルクロロエチル-シクロヘキシルニトロソ尿素,シクロホスファミド,プレドニゾン　**MeCP**
メチルクロロエチル-シクロヘキシルニトロソ尿素,フルオロウラシル,アドリアマイシン　**MEFA**
メチルクロロエチルシクロヘキシルニトロソ尿素(＝セムスチン)　**MCCNU**
メチルクロロフェニルイソキサゾリルペニシリン(＝フルクロキサシリン)　**MFIPC**
メチルクロロフェニルイソキサゾールペニシリン(＝クロキサシリン)　**MCIPC**
メチルコバラミン　**MeB$_{12}$, MeCbl**
メチルコラントレン　**MC, MCA**
メチルコラントレン(誘発)肉腫　**MCS**
メチルジクロルフェニルイソキサゾリルペニシリン(＝ジクロキサシリン)　**MDIPC**
メチルジゴキシン　**β-MD**
メチルシトシン　**MeCyt**
メチル臭化ホマトロピン　**HMB**
メチルセルロース　**MC**
メチルチアジアゾールチオール　**MTDT**
メチルチオウラシル　**MTU**
メチルチオレートヨードホルムアルデヒド(染色)　**MIF**
メチルチモールブルー　**MBT**
メチルチロシン　**MT**
メチルテトラヒドロ葉酸　**MeFH$_4$**
メチルド(ー)パ　**MDOPA**
メチルニトロソウレア　**ACNU**
メチルニトロソ尿素　**MNU**
メチルヒスチジン　**MH**
メチルフェニデート　**MPH**
メチルフェニルイソキサゾリルペニシリン　**MPIPC**
メチルフェニルエチルヒダントイン　**MPEH**
メチルブチルケトン

MBK
メチルプレドニゾロン **MePr, MP**
メチルプレドニゾロンパルス療法 **MPPT**
メチルベンジルアミン **MBeA**
メチルベンジルアルコール **MBA**
メチルベンジルニトロソアミン **MBN**
メチルマロニル **mm**
メチルマロニル・コエンザイム〔Co〕A ムターゼ **MMM**
メチルマロニルコエンザイム A **MMCoA**
メチルマロン酸 **MMA**
メチルメタクリル酸 **MMA**
メチルメタンスルホン酸 **MMS**
メチルメチオニンスルホニウムクロリド **MMSC**
メチルメルカプトイミダゾール **MMI**
メチルレッド **MR**
メチルレッド・フォーゲス・プロスカウエル反応用ブイヨン **MR-VP**
メチルロムスチン **Me-CCNU**
メチレンジイソシアネート **MDI**
メチレンジフェニルジイソシアネート **MDI**
メチレンブルー **MB, MEB**
メチレンブルー活性物質 **MBAS**
メチレンブルー還元時間 **MBRT**
メチレンブルー色素 **MBD**
メチレンブルー点滴注入 **MBI**
メチレンブルー複合体 **MBC**
メディエーター **M**
メッケル憩室 **MD**
メッシュ **MeSH**
メッセンジャーRNA **mRNA**
メテノロンエナンテート **MAE, ME**
メトアンフェタミン **MAP**
メトエンケファリン受容体結合性の **MERB**
メトエンケファリン様免疫反応性 **MELI**
メトキシトリプタミン **MT**
メトキシヒドロキシマンデル酸 **MOMA**
メトキシフルラン **MOF**
メトクロプラミド **MCP**
メトクロプラミド,デキサメタゾン,ロラゼパム,オンダンセトロン **MDLO**
メトトレキサート **M, MTX**
メトトレキサート,アクチノマイシン D,クロラムブシル **MAC**
メトトレキサート,アクチノマイシン D,シクロホスファミド **MAC, MAC Ⅲ**
メトトレキサート,アドリアマイシン,シクロホスファミド,シクロヘキシルクロロエチルニトロソ尿素 **MACC**
メトトレキサート,アドリアマイシン,シクロホスファミド,ビンクリスチン(=オンコビン),ブレオマイシン **MACOB**
メトトレキサート,アドリアマイシン,フトラフール **MAF**
メトトレキサート,アラビノシルシトシン,シクロホスファミド,シクロヘキシルクロロエチルニトロソ尿素 **MACC**
メトトレキサート,エトポシド,ヘキサメチロネラミン **MVH**
メトトレキサート,シクロホスファミド(=エンドキサン),ビンクリスチン **MEV**
メトトレキサート,シクロホスファミド(=エンドキサン),ビンクリスチン,プレドニゾン **MEVP**
メトトレキサート,シクロホスファミド **MECY**
メトトレキサート,ビンクリスチン(=オンコビン),L-アスパラギナーゼ,デキサメタゾン **MOAD**
メトトレキサート,ビンクリスチン(=オンコビン),シクロホスファミド,アドリアマイシン **MOCA**
メトトレキサート,ビンクリスチン(=オンコビン),フルオロウラシル **MOF**
メトトレキサート,ビンクリスチン(=オンコビン),プレドニゾン **MOP**
メトトレキサート,ビンブラスチン,アドリアマイシン,シスプラチン **MVAC, M-VAC**
メトトレキサート,ブレオ

マイシン,アドリアマイシン,シクロホスファミド,ビンクリスチン(=オンコビン),ソル・メドロール **M-BACOS**
メトトレキサート,ブレオマイシン,アドリアマイシン,シクロホスファミド,ビンクリスチン(=オンコビン),デキサメタゾン **M-BACOD**
メトトレキサート,ブレオマイシン,ジアミンジクロロプラチン **MBD**
メトトレキサート,ブレオマイシン,シスプラチン **MBC**
メトトレキサート・プレドニゾン **MXP**
メトトレキサート-ロイコボリン,アドリアマイシン,シクロホスファミド,ビンクリスチン(=オンコビン),プレドニゾン,ブレオマイシン **MACOP-B**
メトピロン **SU 4885**
メトプロロール拡張型心筋症 **MDC**
メトヘムアルブミン **MHA**
メトヘモグロビン **metHb, MHb**
メトヘモグロビン還元酵素 **Hb R, MHR, MR, MR-E**
メトミオグロビン **metMb**
メドライン **MEDLINE**
メトリザミドコンピュータ断層撮影大槽造影法 **MCTC**
メートル **M, m**
メートル・キログラム・秒・アンペア **MKSA**
メートルキログラム **MKG, mkg**
メートル・グラム・秒 **MGS**
メートル/秒 **M/S**
メートル角 **Am, am, MA, ma, mW, M.W**
メトルキゾロン **MTQ**
メートルレンズ **ML**
メトロイリーゼ **Metr**
メトロイリンテル **Metr**
メドロキシプロゲステロン **MP**
メトロニダゾール **Met, MTZ**
メナキノン **K_2, MK**
メナキノン6 **MK-6**
メナジオン **K_3**
メナジオン結合 α-グリセロリン酸脱水素酵素 **MAG**
メニエール症候群 **MS**
メニエール病 **MD**
メネトリエ病 **MD**
メバロン酸 **MVA**
メフェナム酸 **ME**
メープルシロップ尿 **MSU**
メープルシロップ尿病 **MSUD**
メプロバメート **MPB**
メペリジン **MEP, mep**
メペリジン・プロメタジン・クロルプロマジン **MPC**
メラニン細胞凝集因子 **MCF**
メラニン細胞刺激因子 **MSF**
メラニン細胞刺激ホルモン **MEH, MSH**
メラニン細胞刺激ホルモン放出因子 **MRF, MSHRF**
メラニン細胞刺激ホルモン放出ホルモン **MRH**
メラニン細胞刺激ホルモン放出抑制因子 **MIF, MRIF, MSH-RIF**
メラニン細胞刺激ホルモン放出抑制ホルモン **MRIH**
メラニン(保有)細胞指数 **MI**
メラニン細胞放出因子 **MRF**
メラニン細胞ホルモン **MH**
メラニン細胞抑制因子 **MIF**
メラノサイト抑制ホルモン **MIH**
メラノーマ抗原 **MEL**
メラノーマ抗原遺伝子1 **MAGE-1**
メラノーマ細胞 **MC**
メラノーマ成長刺激活性 **MGSA**
メラミンホルムアルデヒド **MF**
メラルソプロール **Mel**
メリーランド救急医療サービス研究所 **MIEMSS**
メルカーソン・ローゼンタール(症候群) **MR**
メルカーソン・ローゼンタール症候群 **MRS**
メルカプト **s**
メルカプトアルキルアミン **MAA**
メルカプトイミダゾール **MI**
メルカプトエチルアミン **MEA**
メルカプトプリン **MP**
メルカプトメリン **MT-6**
メルク分子モデルシステム **MMMS**

メルシュ・ヴォルトマン症候群 **MWS**
メルチオレイトホルムアルデヒド溶液 **MF solution**
メルファラン **MPL**
メルファラン,シクロホスファミド(=エンドキサン),ビンクリスチン,プレドニゾン **MEVP**
メルファラン,シクロホスファミド(=エンドキサン),ビンクリスチン,メチルニトロソウレア,プレドニゾン **MEVAP**
メルファラン,シクロホスファミド,ビスクロロエチルニトロソ尿素,プレドニゾン **MCBP**
メルファラン,シクロホスファミド,プレドニゾン **MCP**
メルファラン,プレドニゾン **MP**
メレナ **mel**
メロディー・リズム・アクセント **MRA**
メンキー縮れ毛 **MKH**
メンキー縮れ毛症候群 **MKHS**
メンデレビウム **Md, Mv**
メンバー **mem**
メンブランフィルター法 **HGMF**
メラス **MELAS**
めまい **vert**
めまい〔眩暈〕(感) **DZ**
目方で **pond.**
目盛りをつけた **grad**
眼鏡商組合員 **FADO**
眼と耳 **EE**
眼に **ocul.**
眼ぬぐい液 **Es**
眼の高さ **HE**
眼・歯・指(症候群) **ODD**
名義上の **nom**
名簿 **Reg, reg, reg.**
命日 **D, d.**
命名者 **denom**
命名法 **nm, nomen**
命令 **dir, dir.**
命令書 **WO, W/O**
命令する **Pr**
明暗識別 **LDD**
明確な **d, def**
明示する **def**
明度差閾値 **LD**
明度識別周辺視野測定 **LP**
明度識別中心視野測定 **LC**
明白な **evid**
明白な診断 **ad diag**
明瞭でない **n.l.**
明瞭な効果 **APE**
明瞭な生命険悪状態 **ALTe**
明/暗(比) **LD, L/D**
迷走神経 **X**
迷走神経刺激 **VS**
迷走神経切断および胃腸切開(術) **V & G**
迷走神経切断兼幽門形成術 **V & P**
迷走神経切断後下痢 **PVD**
迷走神経切断とビルロート胃腸吻合(術) **VBG**
迷走神経背側核 **DNV**
迷走神経傍神経節腫 **VBP**
迷入(性)の **aber**
迷路立ち直り反射 **LRR**
瞑想方法 **TM**
雌 **F, Fe, fe**
雌(性)の **fem**
雌の **F, G**
滅菌 **ster**
滅菌器 **ster**
滅菌水 **SW**
滅菌する **ster**
滅菌の **st, ster**
滅菌溶液 **SS**
免疫 **Immun, immun, immun.**
免疫(法,処置) **Immun, immun, immun.**
免疫インターフェロン **IIF**
免疫応答 **Ir**
免疫応答遺伝子 **Ir gene**
免疫芽球性肉腫 **IBS**
免疫芽球性リンパ節症 **IBL**
免疫芽球プラズマ〔血漿〕 **IP**
免疫学 **Immun, immun, immun., Immunol, immunol**
免疫拡散手技 **IDP**
免疫拡散法 **Id, IDT**
免疫拡散補体結合 **IDCF**
免疫学的検査 **IT**
免疫化する **Immun, immun, immun.**
免疫関与疾患 **IMD**
免疫関連抗原 **Ia**
免疫吸着 **IA**
免疫吸着療法 **IAT**
免疫グロブリン **γ, Ig, IG**
免疫グロブリンA **γA, IgA**
免疫グロブリンA分泌細胞 **IgA-SC**
免疫グロブリンD **γD, IgD**
免疫グロブリンE **γE, IgE**
免疫グロブリンF **IgF**
免疫グロブリンG **γG, G, IgG**

免疫グロブリンＧリウマチ因子 **IgG RF**
免疫グロブリンＨ鎖 **IgH**
免疫グロブリンＬ鎖 **IgL**
免疫グロブリンＭ **γM，IgM**
免疫グロブリンＭ分泌細胞 **IgM-SC**
免疫グロブリンＭリウマチ因子 **IgM RF**
免疫グロブリン遺伝子スーパーファミリー **IgGSF**
免疫グロブリン型 **GM**
免疫グロブリン結合因子 **IBF**
免疫グロブリン欠損(症) **ID**
免疫グロブリン消費試験 **iCT，ICT**
免疫グロブリン定量 **IgQ**
免疫グロブリン分泌細胞 **IgSC，ISC**
免疫螢光検査 **IFT**
免疫螢光検査(法) **IFL**
免疫螢光抗体 **IFA**
免疫螢光抗体法 **IF**
免疫螢光測定法 **IFA**
免疫螢光法 **IFT**
免疫血清 **IS**
免疫血清グロブリン **ISG**
免疫欠乏状態 **IDS**
免疫検査 **IT**
免疫抗原認識部位 **IGR**
免疫固定電気泳動法 **IFE**
免疫細胞化学 **IC，ICC**
免疫細胞化学的測定法 **ICA**
免疫細胞毒性 **IC**
免疫サプレッサー **IS**
免疫刺激複合体 **ISCOMS**
免疫食作用 **Ip**
免疫シンチグラム **RAID**
免疫性金銀染色(法) **IGSS**
免疫性腎疾患 **IRD**
免疫生物(学的)活性 **IA**
免疫性溶血性貧血 **IHA**
免疫接触性糸球体症 **ITGP**
免疫接触性蕁麻疹 **ICU**
免疫組織化学 **IHC**
免疫増強療法 **IAT**
免疫増殖性小腸疾患 **IPSID**
免疫測定法 **IA**
免疫体 **IB，IK，I.K.**
免疫妥協宿主 **ICH**
免疫単位 **IE，IU**
免疫調節(性)αグロブリン **IRA**
免疫調節適量 **OID**
免疫(学的)適格細胞 **ICC**
免疫電気泳動(法) **IE**
免疫電気泳動法 **IEA，IEP**
免疫電気向流法 **CIE(P)**
免疫電気浸透法 **IES**
免疫電子顕微鏡法 **IEM**
免疫粘着(反応) **IA**
免疫粘着(赤)血球凝集(反応) **IAHA**
免疫(性)の **Immun，immun，immun.**
免疫バランス **IB**
免疫(学的)反応 **IR**
免疫反応系 **IRS**
免疫反応性インスリン **IRI**
免疫反応性ウシ血清アルブミン **IBSA**
免疫反応性エラスターゼ **IRE**
免疫反応性ガストリン **IRG**
免疫反応性カルシトニン **iCT，ICT**
免疫反応性グルカゴン **IRG，IRGI**
免疫反応性グルコース **IRG**
免疫反応性血漿 **IRP**
免疫反応性上皮小体ホルモン **iPTH，IRPTH**
免疫反応性成長ホルモン **ICH，IGH，IRGH**
免疫反応性ソマトスタチン **IRS**
免疫反応性多発脊髄炎ワクチン **IPV**
免疫反応性トリオシノゲン **IRT**
免疫反応性トリプシン **IRT**
免疫反応性ヒトガストリン **iG**
免疫反応性ヒト絨毛性ゴナドトロピン **IRhCG**
免疫反応性ヒト絨毛性体乳腺成長ホルモン **IRhCS**
免疫反応性ヒト成長ホルモン **IRhGH**
免疫反応性ヒト胎盤性ラクトゲン **IRhPL**
免疫反応性ヒト皮膚コラゲナーゼ **IHSC**
免疫反応性フィブロネクチン **IFN**
免疫反応性副腎皮質刺激ホルモン放出因子 **I-CRF**
免疫反応性プロインスリン **IRP**
免疫反応性プロスタグランジンＥ **iPGE**
免疫反応性プロラクチン **IRP**
免疫反応性モチリン **IRM**
免疫反応物質Ｐ **ISP**

免疫反応(性)ベータエンドルフィン **IB-EP**
免疫比濁法 **TIA**
免疫複合体 **IC, ICX**
免疫複合体糸球体腎炎 **ICGN**
免疫複合体病 **ICD**
免疫不全 **ID**
免疫不全関連ウイルス **IDAV**
免疫不全症候群 **IDS**
免疫付着(粘着)免疫吸着検定 **IAHIA**
免疫付着〔粘着〕免疫吸着検定 **IAIA**
免疫ペルオキシダーゼ **IMPO, IP**
免疫ペルオキシダーゼ法 **IPT**
免疫便潜血検査 **IFOBT**
免疫防御機構 **IDM**
免疫放射定量法 **IRMA**
免疫放射標識定量法 **IRA**
免疫優位エピトープ **IDE**
免疫抑制 **IS**
免疫抑制遺伝子 **Is gene**
免疫抑制酸性蛋白 **IAP**
免疫抑制(性)酸性物質 **IAS**
免疫抑制法 **IM**
免疫抑制薬 **ISD**
免疫リボ核酸 **iRNA**
免疫量 **IMD**
免疫療法 **IT**
免荷 **NWB**
免許を受けた **l, L**
面接 **intvw**
面接する **intvw**
面倒なクロストリジウム関連の下痢 **CDAD**
綿花状白斑 **CWP**
綿状反応 **flocc, FR**
綿弾性包帯 **CEB**

も

モキサラクタム　**LMOX，MOX**
モザイク　**M，mos**
モーズレイ健康調査表　**MMQ**
モーズレイ性格〔人格〕検査　**MPI**
モダリティ・ワークリスト管理　**MWM**
モード　**M，Mo**
モニエール・クーン(症候群)　**MK**
モニリア(＝カンジダ)とトリコモナス　**M & T**
モノアシルグリセロール　**MG**
モノアミン　**MA**
モノアミン酸化酵素　**MAO**
モノアミン酸化酵素 A　**MAOA**
モノアミン酸化酵素 B　**MAOB**
モノアミン酸化酵素阻害薬　**MAOI，RIMA**
モノアミン酸化酵素抑制薬　**IMAO**
モノイソニトロソアセトン　**MINA**
モノエタノールアミン　**MEA**
モノエチルグリシンキシリジド　**MEGX**
モノエチルリン酸　**MEP**
モノエチレングリコール　**MEG**
モノカイン　**MK**
モノグリセリド　**MG**
モノグリセリド加水分解酵素　**MGH**
モノクロタリン　**MC**
(ネズミ)モノクローナル抗体　**MOAB**
モノクローナル抗体　**MA，mAb，MCA，MCAb，MCAB，MOAb**
モノクローナルバンド　**M band**
モノクローナル非特異的抑制因子　**MNSF**
モノクローナルリウマチ因子　**MRF**
モノクロロ酢酸　**MCA**
モノシアロガングリオシド　**GM**
モノのインターネット　**IoT**
モノフルオロアセトアミド　**MFA**
モノフルオロホスフェート　**MFP**
モノブロモ酢酸　**MBA**
モノメチルヒドラジン　**MMH**
モノメチロールジメチルヒダントイン　**MDMH**
モノメトキシトリチル　**mmt**
モノヨード酢酸　**MIA，MIAA**
モノヨードチロシン　**MIT**
モノヨードチ〔サイ〕ロニン　$\mathbf{T_1}$
モラー・アクセンフェルト菌　**MA**
モリブデン　**Mo，moly**
モリブデン 99　^{99}**Mo**
モル　**M，mol**
モル/リットル　**mol/l**
モル液　**MS**
モルガニー・アダムス・ストークス(症候群)　**MAS**
モルガン単位　**mo**
モル吸収係数　**e**
モル消衰係数　**e**
モル旋光度　**MD**
モル濃度　**c，molc**
モルヒネ　**M，m，MOR，morph**
モルヒネ中毒　**ISMUS**
モルヒネとコカイン　**M & C，M+C**
モルヒネ様因子　**MLF**
モルヒネ様化合物　**MLC**
モル分率　**x**
モルモット　**GP**
モルモット γ グロブリン　**GPGG**
モルモットアルブミン　**GPA**
モルモット回腸　**GPI**
モルモット気管　**GPT**
モルモット気管平滑筋　**GPTSM**
モルモット血清　**GPS**
モルモット結腸紐筋　**TCGP**
モルモット抗インスリン血清　**GPAIS**
モルモット腎吸収試験　**GPKA**
モルモット腎抗原　**GPK**
モルモット赤血球　**GPRBC**
モルモット単位　**GPU，MSE**
モルモット腸粘膜ホモジネート　**GPIMH**
モルモット胚　**GPE**
モルモット白血球抗原　**GPLA**
モルモット白血病ウイルス　**GPLV**
モルモット脾　**GPS**
モルモットヘルペスウイルス　**GPHV**
モルモット補体　**GPC**
モルモットミエリン塩基性蛋白　**GPBP**

モレイングラハト黄疸指数　**MG**
モレイングラハト(黄疸)指数　**MG**
モロニー(株)　**Mo**
モロニー・ネズミ白血病　**MLVM**
モロニー肉腫ウイルス　**MSV**
モロニーネズミ肉腫ウイルス　**MSVM**
モロニーネズミ白血病ウイルス　**MMLV, MMuLv**
モロニー白血病ウイルス　**MLV**
モロニーマウス肉腫ウイルス　**MoMSV**
モロニーマウス白血病ウイルス　**Mo-MuLV**
モンゴメリ・アスベルグうつ病係数　**MADS**
モンテカルロ法　**MCM**
モントリオール血小板症候群　**MPS**
モントリオール神経学研究所　**MNI**
モンロー還流排液法　**MTD**
もう一度繰り返せ　**rep.sem.**
もし強度が許せば　**si vir.perm.**
もっと　**mo′**
もどし交配　**BC**
ものすごい体臭　**DBO**
もはや入院の必要なし　**HNLN**
もはや必要なし　**NLN**
文字どおりに　**lit, lit.**
文字どおりの　**lit, lit.**
持ち出す(ために)　**TTO**
模倣　**imit, sml**
模倣者　**sml**
模倣する　**sml**
模倣の　**imit**
毛孔性紅色粃糠疹　**PRP**
毛細管　**Cap**
毛細管拡散能　**CDC**
毛細(血)管血液ガス　**CPG**
毛細(血)管血流　**CBF**
毛細管ゲル電気泳動　**CGE**
毛細管浸透圧　**COP**
毛細(血)管静水圧　**CHP**
毛細管電気クロマトグラフィ　**CEC**
毛細(血)管内腔　**CL**
毛細管領域電気泳動　**CEZ**
毛細管領域電気泳動法　**CZE, CZP**
毛細管濾過係数　**CFC**
毛細血管　**c**
毛細血管圧　**CP**
毛細血管外病変　**ECL**
毛細血管拡張性運動失調(症)　**AT, A-T**
毛細血管拡張性失調症　**AT**
毛細血管基底板　**CBL**
毛細血管基底膜　**CBM**
毛細血管血流速度　**CBV**
毛細血管後小静脈　**PCV**
毛細血管全血の真性血糖　**CWBTS**
毛細血管と線維の比率　**C/F**
毛細血管内血液ガス　**CBG**
毛髪・鼻・指(症候群)　**TRP**
毛様体　**CB**
毛様体機能障害因子　**CDF**
毛様体向神経性因子　**CNTF**
毛様体神経栄養因子　**CNTF**
毛様体動脈圧　**CAP**
妄想　**del**
妄想型統合失調症　**PS**
妄想疾患　**DD**
盲係蹄症候群　**BLS**
盲人教師協会会員　**FCTB**
盲人全国連合　**NFB**
盲人奉仕協会　**BSA**
盲腸　**C**
盲腸通過時間　**OCTT**
盲目的接近　**BA**
盲目の　**bd, bd.**
蒙古症　**Mongo**
蒙古斑　**MS**
網状紅斑性ムチン沈着症候群　**REM syndrome**
網状赤血球産生指数　**RPI**
(副腎皮質)網状体　**ZR**
網(状)赤血球　**Ret, retic, retics**
網赤血球　**R**
網(状)赤血球算定　**retic count**
網(状)赤血球数　**retic.ct**
(細)網内(皮)系　**SRE**
網(状)内(皮)系　**RES**
網膜　**ret**
網膜異常形成　**RD**
網膜黄斑　**ML**
網膜外眼位情報　**EEPI**
網膜下液　**SRF**
網膜芽細胞腫　**RB**
網膜芽腫関連蛋白　**RBAP**
網膜下新生血管　**SRN**
網膜間結合蛋白　**IRBP**
網膜肝内分泌(症候群)　**RHE**
網膜血管炎　**RV**
網膜色素上皮　**RPE**
網膜色素変性症　**Deg.pig., Pig.deg., RPD**

網膜出血　**RH**
網膜上膜　**ERM**
網膜静脈分岐閉鎖症　**BRVO**
網膜神経感覚上皮　**NSR**
網膜神経膠腫性過誤腫　**RAH**
網膜神経節細胞　**RGC**
網膜正常対応　**NRC**
網膜前出血　**PRH**
網膜対応異常　**ARC**
網膜対応欠如　**LRC**
網膜断層解析装置　**OCT**
網膜中心静脈　**CRV**
網膜中心静脈閉塞(症)　**CRO**
網膜中心静脈閉塞症　**CRVO**
網膜中心動脈　**CRA**
網膜中心動脈閉塞(症)　**CRAO**
網膜電位計測　**ERG**
網膜電計　**ERG, erg**
網膜電図　**ERG**
網膜動脈圧　**RAP**
網膜動脈枝閉塞(症)　**BRAO**
網膜内出血　**IRH**
網膜内電図　**EIRG**
網膜内微小血管異常　**IRMA**
網膜内微小血管症　**IRMA**
網膜二重対応　**DRC**
網膜剝離　**RD**
網膜反射　**RR**
網膜微細動脈瘤　**RCM**
網膜分枝静脈閉塞症　**CMD**
網膜由来成長因子　**RDGF**
網脈絡膜欠損・心疾患・後鼻孔閉鎖症・成長障害・知能発育障害(ないし中枢神経系奇形)・外性器低形成(ないし耳介奇形,ないし聾)　**CHARGE**
網様上行賦活系　**RAAS**
網様体　**FR, RB, RF**
網様体脊髄路　**REST**
網様体賦活系　**RAS**
網様の　**RET, ret**
毛様細胞性白血病　**HCL**
木材　**Lig, lig, lig.**
目次　**TOC**
目的　**Obj, obj**
目標　**t**
目標症候評価基準　**TSES**
目標心拍数　**THR**
目標調節式注入法　**TCI**
目標とフィルム間の距離　**TFD**
沐浴　**B, B, b.**
用いよ　**admov., us**
用いられる　**U, utend.**
没食子酸プロピル　**PG**
最も優秀な　**ME**
最もよく純化した　**rctss.**
最もよく精製した　**recfss**
本明・ギルフォード性格検査　**MG**
戻ってくる　**rtn**
戻る　**ret**
桃色　**P**
脆い　**frag**
文部省[米国]　**MOE**
門大静脈吻合　**PCA**
門脈　**PoV, PV**
門脈圧亢進性胃疾患　**PHG**
門脈圧亢進(症)腸血管症　**PHIV**
門脈拡張　**PVD**
門脈肝炎　**PH**
門脈灌流圧　**PPP**
門脈血栓症　**PVT**
門脈血流量　**PVF**
門脈高血圧(症)　**PHTN**
門脈高血圧症　**PHT**
門脈周囲域　**PP**
門脈周囲帯壊死　**PZN**
門脈性肝硬変　**PC**
門脈造影下 CT　**CTAP**
門脈体循環性脳障害　**PSE**
門脈体循環抵抗　**PSR**
門脈大静脈(シャント)　**PC**
門脈大静脈シャント　**PCS**
門脈大静脈吻合術　**PCS**
紋切り型行動　**SB**
問題　**prob**
問題解決情報　**PSI**
問題志向医学情報システム　**PROMIS**
問題志向型看護記録　**PONR**
問題志向型診断記録　**POMR**
問題志向型診療　**POS**
問題志向型診療システム　**POMS**
問題志向病歴　**POR**

や

ヤギ **G**
ヤギ血清 **GS**
ヤギ抗ウサギγグロブリン **GAR, GARGG**
ヤギ抗マウス免疫グロブリンG **GAMG**
ヤグ(レーザー) **YAG**
ヤークス・ブリッジズ検査 **YBT**
ヤケヒョウヒダニ(抗原) **Dp**
ヤコブ・クロイツフェルト(症候群) **JC**
ヤーダッソーン・レーヴァンドヴスキー(症候群) **JL**
ヤッピー感冒 **Yuppie flu**
ヤッフェ・リヒテンシュタイン(症候群) **JL**
ヤード(=約0.9m) **yd**
ヤーヌスキナーゼ1 **Jak-1**
ヤバサル腫瘍 **YMT**
ヤブカ(属) **A**
ヤーリッシュ・ヘルクスハイマー反応 **JHR**
ヤング・ヘルムホルツ説 **YHT**
ヤンスキースクリーニング指数 **JSI**
矢田部・ギルフォード性格検査 **YG test, Y-G test**
夜間3回 **t.i.n.**
夜間(レム睡眠期に一致してみられる)陰茎勃起 **NPT**
夜間間欠的腹膜透析 **NPD**
夜間脚筋(肉)痙攣 **NLMC**
夜間酸素療法 **NOT**
夜間酸素療法試行 **NOTT**
夜間睡眠遮断 **NSD**
夜間多尿(症) **noc., noct.**
夜間に **int.noct.**
夜間膀胱容量 **NBC**
夜尿〔症〕 **enur**
夜尿時膀胱容量 **EBC**
夜盲(症) **XN**
野菜 **veg**
野生型 **WT**
野戦救急車 **FA**
焼けた **br**
焼かれた **ust.**
役に立たない結合の **NSC**
約 **ab., abt, c, c., ca, etw, f, za**
薬(物) **M, med, med., meds, MEDS**
薬援助によるリハビリテーションと教育 **DARE**
薬化学 **phar c**
薬学 **Ph, PHAR, Phar, phar**
薬学会 **PS**
薬学会員 **FPS**
薬学士 **BP, DeePee, M.Phr., M.S.P, Ph.G., Phm.B.**
薬学進歩のためのカナダ財団 **CFAP**
薬学認定書 **Dip.Phar.**
薬学の **phar**
薬学博士 **D.P., D.Pharm.**
薬学部卒業者 **Phm.G.**
薬剤 **M, MED, Med, med., med, med., meds, MEDS**
薬剤疫学 **PE**
薬剤学士 **BSP, B.S.Phar.**
薬剤過敏性腎障害 **DIHN**
薬剤関連ループス **DRL**
薬剤血中濃度モニタリング **TDM**
薬剤師 **AP, Ap, ap, Apoth, apoth., Phar, phar, PHARM, pharm**
薬剤使用評価 **DUE**
薬剤情報センター **DIC**
薬剤職能系正会員 **PPOM**
薬剤性過敏症症候群 **DIHS**
薬剤性錯乱症候群 **PCS**
薬剤相互作用 **DI**
薬剤耐性プラスミド **R**
薬剤中毒者 **ad**
薬剤投与記録 **MAR**
薬剤投与チーム **MAT**
薬剤評価 **DE**
薬剤誘発性腎疾患 **DIRD**
薬剤誘発ループス **DIL**
薬剤溶出性ステント **DES**
薬剤用量・乱用管理情報統合システム **IDAMIS**
薬剤利得計画 **PBS**
薬剤リンパ球刺激試験 **DLST**
薬事委員会 **CPMP, P&TC**
薬ビン **ph**
薬品店 **DS**
薬品取引ニュース **DTN**
薬品の副作用 **SED**
薬物 **meds, MEDS**
薬物・化学および準技術連合 **DCAT**
薬物悪用管理局 **BDAC**
薬物安全委員会 **CSM**
薬物および治療法の研究に使用される動物の福祉

WARDS
薬物化学者 **Ph.C.**
薬物管理局 **DCA**
薬物痙攣療法 **PCT**
薬物血中濃度時間曲線下面積 **AUC**
薬物嗜癖 **AD, DA**
薬物受容体 **DR**
薬物使用調査,医薬品使用評価 **DUR**
薬物代謝酵素 **DME**
薬物治療審査システム **DTSS**
薬物動態の **PK**
薬物〔麻薬〕取締局 **DEA**
薬物の放出・吸収・分布・代謝・排泄 **LADME**
薬物媒介性腫瘍抗原 **DMTA**
薬物反応 **MR**
薬物有害反応 **ADR**
薬物輸送システム **DDS**
薬物乱用規制国際連合基金 **UNFDAC**
薬物乱用研究と教育 **DARE**
薬物乱用に対する法の施行 **DALE**
薬物乱用リハビリテーション **DAR**
薬物乱用リハビリテーションプログラム **DARP**
薬包紙 **chart, chart.**
薬名 **n.p.**
薬名を記して **s.n., s.nom., S.nom., s.sn., s.s.n**
薬名を記して与えよ **dtr.s.n.**
薬用式ポンド **lb ap.**
薬用シロップ **OX, Ox, O_x**
薬用ドラム **dr ap, dr.ap., du**
薬用ポンド **PM**
薬用量 **dos.**
薬力学 **PD**
薬理学 **pha, pharmacol, pharmacol**
薬理学的薬剤干渉 **PDI**
薬理学の **pharmacol, pharmacol**
薬量〔線量〕測定 **dos, dosim**
優しく **lenit.**
優しく親切な看護 **TLC**
薬局 **Disp., disp., DS, Ph, PHAR, Phar, phar**
薬局業務基準 **GPP**
薬局参加の医療評価プログラム **PICEP**
薬局の利益管理 **PBM**
薬局方 **P, PH, Ph, ph., Phar, phar**
薬局方検討会議 **PDG**
軟らかい **moll., S**

ゆ

ユーアールエル(＝インターネット上の情報の住所) **URL**
ユーイング肉腫(骨) **EWS**
ユーエスビー(＝PC インターフェイス) **USB**
ユダヤ人(の) **J**
ユニットリスク **UR**
ユネスコ **UNESCO**
ユビキノン **UQ**
ユビキノン-10 **Q10, Q_{10}**
ユビキノン-6 **Q6, Q_6**
ユビクロマノール 9 **Q_9**
ユビクロメノール 9 **Q_9**
ユビヒドロキノン＝ユビキノール **QH_2, $Q-H_2$**
ユーミン **UMIN**
ユーロトランスプラント(＝欧州の移植臓器配分のための非営利団体) **ET**
ユーロピウム **Eu**
ユンクマン・シェーラー単位 **JSU**
ユンクマン・シューラー(単位) **JS**
ゆさぶられっ子症候群 **SBS**
ゆっくりと **sly**
由来する **deriv**
油酸剤 **oleat.**
油脂 **ol.res.**
油浸域 **OIF**
油性停留浣腸 **OR en**
油中水(型) **W/O**
油中水型 **W/O type**
油中水型乳剤アジュバント **WO**
油中水滴(型)(乳剤) **W/O**
油糖 **elaeos., els.**
油脳室撮影 **OVG**
湯 **HW**
輸液 **Tx**
輸液情報コンサルテーションシステム **ADMICS**
輸液注入器 **IP**
輸血 **BT, BTF, Tx**
輸血・関連後天性免疫欠損症候群 **TAAIDS**
輸血改善協会 **BTBA**
輸血感染ウイルス **TTV**
輸血関連(性)エイズ **TRAIDS**
輸血関連急性肺障害 **TRALI**
輸血協会 **BTA**
輸血後移植片対宿主病 **post-transfusion GVHD, PT-GVHD**
輸血後肝炎 **PTH**
輸血後紫斑病 **PTP**
輸血後単核症 **PTM**
輸血後に **PT**
輸血サービス **BTS**
輸血による伝染病 **TTD**
輸血反応 **TR**
輸出血管抵抗 **RE**
輸出の **eff, effer**
輸送機序 **TM**
(細胞内)輸送蛋白 **Tap**
輸入医薬品の品質管理基準 **GIP**
輸入脚症候群 **ALS**
癒合 **fus**
癒合椎間関節 **FAJ**
癒着 **adh, adhes, fxg**
癒着した **f, fxd**
癒着性の **adhes**
癒着製の **adh**
夕方 **vesp.**
夕刻に **vesp.**
夕食後 **post prand**
夕食前に **ant.prand., a.p.**
友人のいない・孤独な・貧しい・不具の **FIND**
有意差なし **NS, NSD**
有意な **Sig, sig**
有害事象 **AE**
有害事象共通用語集 **CTCAE**
(米国)有害物質規制法 **TSCA**
有害物質放出目録 **TRI**
有核細胞数 **NCC**
有核赤血球 **NRBC**
有核の **nuc**
有機陰イオン結合蛋白 **OABP**
有機化合物の基 **R**
有機金属熱分解気層エピタキシャル成長 **MOCVD**
有機酸可溶性リン **OASP**
有機粉塵毒性症候群 **ODTS**
有限(会社) **lmtd., ltd.**
有効 **PR**
有効 1 回拍出量 **ESV**
有効温度 **ET**
有効下顎骨長 **EML**
有効肝血漿血流量 **EHPBF**
有効肝血漿流量 **EHPF**
有効肝血流量 **EHBF, ELBF**
有効(性)期待係数 **EEI**
有効血(液)量 **EBV**
有効甲状腺率 **ETR**
有効左(心)室拍出仕事量 **ELVSW**
有効酸素運搬 **EOT**
有効収縮期圧 **ESP**
有効循環血液量 **ECBV**
有効焦点距離 **EFL**
有効腎血漿流量 **ERPF**
有効腎血流量 **ERBF**
有効性期待係数 **EEI**

有効生物学的量　**EBD**
有効選択的注視　**OPL**
有効直接照射　**EDR**
有効チロキシン比　**ETR**
有効動脈血(液)量　**EABV**
有効な　**eff, effect**
有効濃度　**EC**
有効濃度試験　**CPT**
有効肺血流量　**EPF**
有効肺血(流)量　**EPBF**
有効馬力　**EHP**
有効半減期　**EFL, EHL, T_e, Teff**
有効不応期　**ERP**
有効毛細血(管)流(量)　**ECF**
有効量　**DE, d.e., deff, E, ED**
有効濾過圧　**EFP, Pf**
有効濾過率　**EFR**
有糸核分裂期　**M**
有糸核分裂蛋白　**MP**
有糸分裂　**M**
有糸分裂期間〔周期〕　**M period**
有糸分裂時間　**MT**
有糸分裂制御蛋白　**MCP**
有糸(核)分裂像　**MF**
有色(人種)の　**C, cld, col**
有資格看護師全国連合　**NFLPN**
有資格歯科技工士　**CDT**
有髄軸索　**MA**
有髄性機械温熱受容器　**MMTN**
有髄の　**myel**
有線テレビジョン　**CATV**
有痛性強直性痙攣発作　**PTS**
有痛性肩症候群　**PSS**
有痛性の　**pnfl**
有痛部に　**loc.dol.**
有毒の　**pois, V, Vi, vir.**
有熱時に　**ad.feb.**
有望な　**P**
有毛細胞　**HC**
幽門狭窄(症)　**PS**
幽門形成(術)　**P**
幽門形成術と迷走神経切断術　**P & V**
幽門側断端組織学的癌浸潤の有無　**aw(+), (−)**
幽門側断端肉眼的癌浸潤の有無　**AW(+), (−)**
幽門洞ガストリン細胞過形成症　**AGH**
幽門洞停留症候群　**RGAS**
幽門保存胃切除術　**PPG**
幽門輪温存膵頭十二指腸切除術　**PPPD**
疣(＝ゆう)腫　**Veg, veg**
疣贅(＝ゆうぜい)状表皮異常症　**EV**
(白血球)遊走因子　**CF**
(白血球)遊走因子不活化物質　**CFI**
遊走刺激因子　**MSF, MStF**
遊走指数　**MI**
遊走性血栓性静脈炎　**TPM**
遊走性心房ペースメーカー　**WAP**
遊走増強因子　**MEF**
遊走阻止因子　**MIF**
遊走阻止因子関連蛋白　**MRP**
遊走抑制〔阻止〕　**MI**
遊離 T_3　**FT_3, fT_3**
遊離 T_4　**FT_4, fT_4**
遊離アミノ酸　**FAA**
遊離基　**FR**
遊離コレステロール　**FC**
遊離酸　**FA**
遊離した　**F**
遊離脂肪酸　**FFA**
遊離脂肪酸相　**FFAP**
遊離赤血球プロトポルフィリン　**FEP**
遊離赤血球ポルフィリン　**FEP**
遊離体　**LB**
遊離チ〔サイ〕ロキシン　**FT**
遊離チ〔サイ〕ロキシン指数　**FTI, FT_4I, FT_3 index**
遊離チ〔サイ〕ロニン 4　**FT_4, fT_4**
遊離鉄結合能　**UIBC**
遊離トリヨードチ〔サイ〕ロニン指数　**FT_4 index**
遊離トリヨードチ〔サイ〕ロニン 3　**FT_3, fT_3**
遊離トリヨードチ〔サイ〕ロニン指数　**FT_3I**
遊離ビリルビン　**FB**
雄性(の)　**M, m, mas., masc**
雄性前核成長因子　**MPGF**
誘導　**guid., I, ind, ind., induc**
誘導型 NOS　**iNOS**
誘導型一酸化窒素合成酵素　**iNOS**
誘導結合プラズマ　**ICP**
誘導結合プラズマ質量分析法　**ICP-MS**
誘導結合プラズマ発光分析　**ICP-AES**
誘導された　**deriv, deriv.**
誘導体化反応超臨界流体抽出　**SFDE**
誘導抵抗　**X**
誘導的な　**deriv, deriv.**
誘導電流の　**far**
誘導物　**deriv, deriv.**
誘発　**I, ind, ind.,**

induct
誘発および寛解因子・性質・部位・重症度・一時的な特徴 **PQRST**
誘発加算脳波嗅覚検査 **ERO**
誘発活動 **TA**
誘発活動電位 **EAP**
誘発筋緊張 **IMT**
誘発筋電図 **EEMG**
誘発月経〔生理〕 **IP**
誘発耳音響放射 **EAE, EOAE**
誘発視覚反応 **EVP**
誘発脊髄電位 **SCEP**
誘発脊髄電図 **EESG**
誘発電位 **EP**
誘発電位検出器 **ERD**
誘発白血病ウイルス **ILV**
誘発反応 **ER, EV**
誘発反応聴力検査(法) **ERA**
誘発分娩感覚 **IDI**
誘発補体結合抗原 **ICFA**
誘発迷路性偏倚 **ILD**
(生体高分子の)融解温度 **Tm**
融解性の **dis**
融解点 **fp**
融合 **F, fus**
融合蛋白 **F protein**
融合蛋白質 **F protein**
融合点 **FUP**
融点 **mp, MPT**
優秀科学者の正規会員 **PSOM**
優秀な **exc**
優先権 **prior**
優性栄養傷害性表皮水疱症 **DDEB**
優性視神経萎縮 **DOA**
優性の **D**
優良医薬品供給基準 **GSP**
優良臨床試験基準 **GCP**
指 **F**
指運動機能指数 **FFQ**
指関節のひび **KC**
指屈曲 **FF**
指先 **FT, FTS**
指先血液 **FTB**
指穿刺 **FS**
指によるタッピング **FT**
指鼻(試験) **FN, F-N**
指鼻試験 **FNV, FTN, F to N test**
指鼻指(試験) **FNF**
指指(試験) **FF**
指指試験 **FTF**
指指鼻試験 **FTFTN**
夢研究所 **IDR**
夢時間 **D time**
許されていない **nl., n.l.**

よ

ヨウ化カリウム　**KI**
ヨウ化カリウム飽和液　**SSKI**
ヨウ化水素酸　**HI**
ヨウ化セシウム　**CsI**
ヨウ化蒼鉛エメチン　**EBI**
ヨウ化テトラメチルアンモニウム　**TMAI**
ヨウ化ナトリウム　**NaI**
ヨウ化物　**iodid.**
ヨウ素　**I**
ヨウ素・アジ化合物反応　**IAR**
ヨウ素123　**^{123}I**
ヨウ素125　**^{125}I**
ヨウ素125トリヨードチ〔サイ〕ロニンレジン摂取率　**$^{125}IT_3RSU$**
ヨウ素131　**^{131}I**
ヨウ素$^{131}T_3$レジンスポンジ摂取率試験　**RT_3U**
ヨウ素$^{131}T_3$レジン摂取率　**RT_3U**
ヨウ素131アドステロール　**^{131}I-adosterol**
ヨウ素131トリヨードチ〔サイ〕ロニンレジン摂取率　**$^{131}IT_3RSU$**
ヨウ素131標識凝集アルブミン　**^{131}I-AA**
ヨウ素131標識大凝集アルブミン　**^{131}I-MAA**
ヨウ素131ポリビニルピロリドン　**^{131}I-PVP**
ヨウ素131ポリビニルピロリドン試験　**^{131}I-PVP test**
ヨウ素131メタヨウ化ベンジルグアニジン　**^{131}I-MIBG**
ヨウ素131ローズベンガル　**^{131}I-RB**
ヨウ素アジ化合物試験　**IAT**
ヨウ素入り溶液　**ILo**
ヨウ素酸　**HIO_3**
(甲状腺)ヨウ素摂取絶対量　**AIU**
ヨウ素標識血清アルブミン　**ISA**
ヨウ素標識大凝集アルブミン　**IMAA**
ヨウ素誘発性甲状腺機能亢進症　**IIH**
ヨーク(抗体)　**Yk**
ヨザル　**ATR**
ヨード・ニトロ・テトラゾリウム　**INT**
ヨード131甲状腺結合指数　**TBI**
ヨードアセトアミド　**IAA，IAM**
ヨードアメーバ　**I**
ヨードアンフェタミン　**[^{123}I]IMP，IMP**
ヨード結合能　**IBC**
ヨード酢酸(＝モノヨード酢酸)　**IAA**
ヨードデオキシウリジン　**IDU**
ヨードホルム蒼鉛パラフィン　**BIP**
ヨードホルム蒼鉛パラフィン泥膏　**BIPP**
ヨードホルム蒼鉛パラフィン軟膏　**BIPP**
ヨハネ協会救急救援助隊　**JUH**
ヨブ症候群　**JS**
ヨリー反応　**JR**
ヨーロッパ――　→欧州も参照
ヨーロッパ産ハリエニシダ凝集素Ⅰ　**UEA-1**
ヨーロッパ人　**Eu**
ヨーロッパの　**Eu**
よく　**ben.**
よく混和せよ　**mb，m.b.**
よく知られた　**wk**
よく知られた事実　**WKF**
よく注意せよ　**NB，N.B.**
よく発達した側副循環　**WDCC**
よく振れ　**agit.bene**
よく分化した　**WD**
よく分化したリンパ球　**WDL**
よく分化したリンパ球性リンパ腫　**WDLL**
よく分化したリンパ性リンパ腫　**WDLL**
よし　**OK**
より詳しくは例をみよ　**FES**
より低い　**l，L**
より若い　**Yr**
よろしい　**OK**
与圧　**compr，comprn**
予期している　**exp**
予見定額払い方式　**PPS**
予後　**prog，progn，PX，Px，px**
予後からみた栄養指数　**PNI**
予測環境濃度　**PEC**
予測基礎代謝量　**PEE**
予測不能突然死　**SUD**
予測無作用濃度　**PNEC**
予想されている　**exp，expt，expt.**
予想している　**exp**
予知　**A**
予知する　**p**
予定　**sked**
予備　**PRESS，Res，res**
予備アルカリ　**Rph**
予備吸気量　**IRV**
予備教育の　**pre-voc**
予備軍医団　**MRC**
予備の　**Pre，pre，prelim，suppl**

よ

予備量　**Rve-vol**
予防　**PR, prevent, pro**
予防医学　**PrevMed, PRM, PVMed**
予防する　**prev**
予防接種　**vacc**
(WHO の)予防接種拡大計画　**EPI**
予防接種後に　**PV**
予防接種痕　**VS**
予防接種痕・左上腕　**VSULA**
予防接種諮問委員会　**ACIP**
予防接種の追加免疫　**booster**
予防接種を受けた　**V**
予防接種をしていない　**NV**
予防的抗生物質　**PA**
予防的抗生物質治療　**PAT**
予防的全脳照射療法　**PWBRT**
予防的頭蓋照射　**PCI**
予防の　**prev, pro, proph, pvnt**
予約　**app, appoint, Appt, appt.**
予約なしの来院(患者)　**WI**
予約を守れなかった　**FTKA**
余暇活動　**LTA**
余暇〔レジャー〕興味調査表　**LII**
余弦　**cos**
余分の　**X**
良い　**F, G, gd**
良い印象　**Gi**
良い状態　**GC**
良くない　**NG**
良さそうな　**F**
夜明けに　**diluc., lucp., luc.prim.**
読み取り枠　**ORF**
読むこと　**R, Rd**
幼仔虫運動停止試験　**MIT**
幼児型多嚢胞症　**IPCD**
幼若細胞凝集反応単位　**CCA unit**
幼稚園児聴力スクリーニングテスト　**KAST**
用語　**T**
用手牽引　**MT**
用手の　**M**
用心して　**caut**
用法　**S., u.**
用法：1 日 3 回 1 包ずつ服用　**Sig. 1 powder t.i.d.s.**
用法：1 日 3 回食後 1/3 ずつ服用　**Sig.1/3 t.i.d. p.c.Sum.**
用法既知に　**dun, d.u.n.**
用法指示　**S, s, /S/, /s/, Sig, sig**
(適)用量　**dos.**
用量強度　**DI**
用量を漸増する　**dpc**
羊水　**AF**
羊水指数　**AFI**
羊水ブドウ糖　**AFG**
羊水量　**AFV**
羊膜嚢　**BOW**
羊膜破水　**RBOW**
羊膜破裂　**RBOW**
要因　**Fac**
要求　**rqmt, rqr**
要求(する)　**req, rqr**
要求されない　**n/r**
要素　**Fac**
要約　**abst, abstr., sum**
要約しない　**unab**
容易な　**ez**
容器を振盪せよ　**agit.vas.**
容積　**cy, V, v, VOL, vol, vol.**
容積/重量　**V/W, v/w**
容積あたり重量　**W/V**
容積圧　**VP**
容積厚さ指数　**VTI**
容積圧反応　**VPR**
(心室)容積過負荷　**VO**
容積胸腔ガス　**VTG**
容積指数　**VI**
容積(中)重量パーセンテージ　**w/v**
容積百分率　**vol%, VPC**
容積補償法　**VCM**
容態　**cond, condn**
容量　**C, c, c., cap, V, v, VOL, vol, vol.**
容量/容量　**V/V**
容量指数　**VG**
容量の　**vol**
揚子江病　**YRD**
葉　**fo., fol, h, hb**
葉酸　**FA**
葉酸カルシウム　**CF**
葉酸拮抗物質　**FAA**
葉酸拮抗薬　**FAA**
葉酸結合蛋白　**FABP**
葉緑素　**chloro**
陽圧　**pos.pr, pos.press**
陽圧換気　**PPV**
陽圧呼吸(法)　**PPB**
陽陰圧呼吸　**PNPB, PNPR, PNPV**
陽極　**A, A, a, a., An**
陽極開放　**AO**
陽極開放強縮　**AOT**
陽極開放クローヌス　**AOC**
陽極開放時音　**AOS**
陽極開放時臭　**AOO**
陽極開放収縮　**AOC,**

AOZ
陽極開放像　AOP
陽極(性)興奮　AnEx, an ex, an.ex., anex.
陽極持続　AD
陽極持続強縮　AnDT
陽極持続強直　ADTe
陽極持続収縮　ADC
陽極の　An
陽極閉鎖　AC
陽極閉鎖音　ACS
陽極閉鎖クローヌス　ACCl
陽極閉鎖臭　ACO
陽極閉鎖収縮　ACC, ANCC, AnCC, AnSZ, ASZ
陽極閉鎖図　ACP
陽極閉鎖性強直性痙攣　ACTe
陽子　P
陽子磁気共鳴　PMR
陽子数　Z
陽性・陰性　p-n
陽性/陰性(比)　P/N
陽性イオンフェリチン　CF
陽性開放収縮　ANOC, AnOC, AnOc
陽性棘波　PSW
陽性棘波パターン　PSP
陽性後電位　PAP
陽性垂直性開散　＋VD
陽性の　POS, Pos, pos
陽性反応適中度　PVP
陽電子　e^+, positron
陽電子再放出顕微鏡　PRM
陽電子消滅 γ 線同時検出　ACD
陽電子断層法　PCT
陽電子放射型横断断層撮影法　PETT
陽電子放射型コンピュータ断層撮影法　PECT
陽電子放射型断層撮影法　PET
陽電子励起オージェ電子分光法　PAES
陽(性)の　P
腰(神経)根症候群　LRS
腰髄の前(神経)根　VRL
腰仙骨の　L-S
腰仙の　LS
腰腸の　IL
腰椎　L, LS, L sp., L-sp, LV, LW, LWS
腰椎・仙腸装具　LSIO
腰椎間板ヘルニア　RLD
腰椎クモ膜下腔腹腔シャント術　LP shunt
腰椎手術不成功症候群　FBSS
腰椎症候群　FBS
腰椎穿刺　LMP, LP, Lumbal, PL
腰椎椎間板ヘルニア　LDH
腰椎椎弓切除(術)　L lam
腰椎内の　IL
腰椎の　L, Lumb, lumb
腰椎腹腔シャント術　LP shunt
腰痛　lum
腰痛(症)　LBP
腰動脈　LA
腰(部)の　L, Lumb, lumb
腰背部痛　LDP
腰部(症)　LB
腰部(下背部)圧痛　LBT
腰部屈曲　LBB
腰部硬膜外麻酔　LEA
腰部(下背部)症候群　LBS
腰部脊柱管狭窄症　LSCS, LSS
腰部椎間板ヘルニア　HLD
腰方形筋　qua
腰傍の　para L
腰・仙椎装具　LSO
溶液　SOL, Sol, sd, sol., soln, Solut, solut, solut.
溶液のアルカリ度を示す記号　POH
溶液をつくれ　ft.sol., ft.solut.
溶解固体　DS
溶解した　dissd, dslv
溶解腫瘍細胞　LTC
溶解する　deliq
溶解性腎炎因子　LyNeF
溶血　Hem, hem., HL
溶血(現象)　haem
溶血・肝酵素上昇・血小板減少(症候群)　HELLP
溶血開始点　HSP
溶血終了点　HEP
溶血性疾患　HD
溶血性尿毒症症候群　HUS
溶血性の　Hem, hem.
溶血性貧血　HA
溶血性貧血抗原　HAA
溶血性免疫体　HIB
溶血素　HL
溶血単位　HU
溶血(反応)抑制　HLI
溶材　solv, solv.
溶質　S, solu
溶存酸素　DO
溶存全有機物　DOC
溶媒　solv, solv.
溶媒添加後　PM
溶連菌感染後糸球体腎炎　PSGN
様式　fm, meth
様相感受性　MS
養子免疫療法　AI
養父　FF

養母　**FM**
抑圧遺伝子感受性変異体　**sus, SUS**
抑うつ　**depr**
抑うつ感情のないうつ病　**DSD**
抑うつ度自己採点の質問　**SRQ-D**
抑制　**I, inhib**
抑制因子　**I, IF, inhib, R, SF**
抑制可能インスリン様活性　**SILA**
抑制肛内反射　**IAR**
抑制細胞　**SC**
抑制細胞活性　**SCA**
抑制された性的興奮　**ISE**
抑制指数　**SI**
抑制する　**inhib**
抑制性T細胞　**Ts**
抑制性T細胞因子　**TsF**
抑制性シナプス後電位　**IPSP**
抑制性接合部電位　**IJP**
抑制定数　$\mathbf{K_i}$
抑制の　**inhib**
抑制〔阻止〕濃度　**IC**
抑制濃度　**CTC**
抑制物質　**I-sub**
抑制物質感受性エステラーゼ　**ISE**
抑制ホルモン　**IH**
抑制薬　**inhib**
抑制量　**ID**
浴室　**BR**
浴槽に　**ad baln.**
翌朝　**c.m., prox.luc.**
翌朝服用　**c.m.s**
翌月　**nM**
翌日　**d.seq., ND, seq.luce.**
翌朝　**cr.mane, m. seq., seq.luce.**
翌夜　**c.n.**
横緩和時間　$\mathbf{T_2}$
横径の　**X, xvse**
横牽引装置　**DTT**
横軸　**x**
横軸の　**X, xvse**
横の　**T, trans**
横向きの　**lat, lat.**
汚れのない　**cl**
吉田肉腫　**YS**
四日熱(マラリア)原虫　**pm**
欲求　**D**
読出し専用メモリ　**ROM**
夜　**n, noct., Noct.**
夜と朝　**n.et m., NM, nm, n & m, n mque, n.mque., noct.maneq.**
夜の　**noc., noct.**
弱い　**feeb, W, w, WK, wk**
弱い・著しい・絶対的濁音　$\mathbf{M_1, M_2, M_3}$
四リン酸ヘキサエチル　**HETP**
四連反応(比)　**TOF**
Ⅳ型コラーゲン　**Type Ⅳ-C**

ら

ライ菌 **ML**
ライ腫(型)ハンセン(病) **LL**
ライ症候群 **RS**
ライター(株蛋白補体結合)試験 **RPCF test**
ライター症候群 **RS**
ライター蛋白(抗原)を用いるコルマー(法) **KRP**
ライター蛋白を用いるコルマー法 **KRP**
ライター病 **RD**
ライト・ギムザ(染色) **WG**
ライトウッド・オールブライト(症候群) **LA**
ライト抗原 **Wr_a**
ライト最大流量計 **WPFM**
ライトマン・フランケル法 **RF**
ライナックでの三次元集光照射システム **SMART**
ライノウイルス **RV**
ライ病 **RD**
ライヘルト・マイスル価 **RMV**
ライム **L**
ライラック(色) **L**
ライリー・デイ(症候群) **RD**
ラウシャー・ネズミ白血病 **MLVR**
ラウス関連ウイルス **RAV**
ラウス肉腫ウイルス **RSV**
ラウス肉腫オンコジーン **src**
ラウリル硫酸ナトリウム **SLS**
ラウンド・ザ・クロック(療法) **RTC**
ラエネック肝硬変 **LC**
ラ音 **rh, rh.**
ラクツロース浣腸 **LE**
ラクトグロブリン **LG**
ラクトバチルス・ガッセリ(菌)(属) **LG, Lg**
ラクトフェリン **LFN**
ラクトペルオキシダーゼ **LP**
ラザフォード **rd**
ラザフォード後方散乱分光法 **RBS**
ラザホージウム **Rf**
ラジアン **rad, rad.**
ラジアン/秒 **rad/s**
ラジウム **Ra**
ラジウムエマナチオン **RE, R.E.**
ラジウム埋没 **rad.imp**
ラジウム療法 **RT**
ラジオアイソトープ **RI**
ラジオアイソトープ血管造影法 **RAG**
ラジオアイソトープジェネレータ **RI generator**
ラジオアイソトープ静脈造影法 **RI venography**
ラジオアイソトープ脳室造影法 **RI ventriculography**
ラジオアイソトープ脳槽〔クモ膜下槽〕造影(法) **RI-cisternography**
ラジオアイソトープミエログラフィ **RI myelography**
ラジオアイソトープリンパ造影シンチグラフィ **RI lymphography**
ラジオアイソトープレノグラム **RI renogram**
ラジオイムノアッセイヒト絨毛性体乳腺成長ホルモン **IRHCS**
ラジオオートグラム **RAG**
ラジオヌクライドコンピュータトモグラフィ **RCT**
ラジオ波焼灼療法 **RFA**
ラジオ免疫沈降法 **RIPA**
ラジオ免疫法 **IRA**
ラセミ化の **DL**
ラセミ体エピネフリン **RE**
ラセミ体の **R, r, rac**
ラーセン・ヨハンセン(症候群) **LJ**
ラタモキセフ **LMOX**
ラッグドレッド繊維 **RRF**
ラッサ熱 **LF**
ラッサ熱ウイルス **LFV**
ラッセル・シルヴァー症候群 **RSS**
ラッセルヘビ毒液 **RVV**
ラッセルヘビ毒時間 **RVVT**
ラット肝ミトコンドリア **RLMD**
ラット血清アルブミン **RSA**
ラット好塩基球性白血病 **RBL**
ラットシナプス終末 **RSE**
ラット出血性脳症ウイルス **HER**
ラット心房性ナトリウム利尿ペプチド **R-ANP**
ラット成長ホルモン **RGH**
ラット脊髄ホモジネート **RSCH**
ラット単位 **RU, R.U.**
ラットの胃の線条 **RSS**
ラット白血病ウイルス

RALV
ラット脾臓細胞 **RSC**
ラットフレンド腫瘍 **RFT**
ラット卵巣重量法 **ROW**
ラット卵巣単位 **rou**
ラテックス **L，Lx，LX**
ラテックス・レゾルシノール・ホルムアルデヒド **LRF**
ラテックス吸着 **LF**
ラテックス吸着試験 **LFT**
ラテックス凝集試験 **LAT，LFT**
ラテックス凝集阻止反応 **LAIR**
ラテックス凝集反応 **LA，LAR**
ラテックス凝集比濁法 **LAPA**
ラテックス(粒子)凝集抑制 **LAI**
ラテックス凝集抑制試験〔検査〕 **LAIT**
ラテックス光学的免疫測定法 **LPIA**
ラテックス直接凝集反応 **LDAR**
ラテックス粒子 **LP**
ラテックス粒子凝集(反応) **LPA**
ラテックス粒子凝集テスト **LPAT**
ラテンアメリカ医学アカデミー協会 **LAANAM**
ラテンアメリカ(人)女性 **LAF**
ラテンアメリカ人 **LA**
ラテンアメリカ(人)男性 **LAM**
ラテン語(の) **L**
ラド **rad，rad.**
ラトケ囊 **RCC**
ラドン **Rn**
ラバーダム **RD**
ラバーベース印象 **Rb Imp**
ラパマイシン **RAPA，RPM**
ラフォラ型ミオクローヌスてんかん **LME**
ラフ型 **R form**
ラマン散乱光の円偏光二色性 **ROA**
ラミニン **LA，LM**
ラミネクトミー **LAM，Lam，lam**
ラム **rhm，Rhm**
ラム症候群 **LAMB syndrome**
ラムゼイ・ハント症候群 **RH syndrome**
ラムノース **Rha**
ラリンゲアルマスク **LM**
ラリンゴマイクロサージェリー **LMS**
ラロン型小人症 **LTD**
ランガット脳炎 **LGE，LGT**
ランキン目盛 **°R**
ラングレイ **LY，ly，ly.**
ランゲルハンス細胞 **LC，L cell**
ランゲルハンス細胞顆粒 **LCG**
ランゲルハンス細胞組織球症 **LCH**
ランゲルハンス細胞組織球増殖(症) **LHC**
ランゲルハンス島 **isl of Lang**
ランダムアクセス記憶装置 **CRAM**
ランタン **La**
ランツ・ランダール法 **RR method**
ランデュ・オースラー・ウェーバー(症候群) **ROW**
ランドー・クレッフナー症候群 **LKS**
ランドリー・ギラン・バレー(症候群) **LGB，LGBS**
ランドリー・クスマウル(症候群) **LK**
ランバ **RUMBA**
ランバート **Lm**
ランベルト **L**
ランバート・イートン筋無力症候群 **LEMS**
ランバート・イートン症候群 **LES**
ランプ付鉗子 **CL**
ランブリア鞭毛虫 **GL**
らせん型の **spir**
らせん上の **spir**
裸眼視 **Nv，NV**
裸眼視力 **VAsc，VA_{sc}**
来院 **V**
来院時(既)死亡 **DOA**
癩性結節性紅斑 **ENL**
落差単位 **HDU**
落屑 **desq**
落屑〔剝離〕性間質性肺炎 **DIP**
落葉状天疱瘡 **PF**
落葉の **D，d.**
酪酸ヒドロキシトルエン **BHT**
酪酸プロピオン酸ヒドロコルチゾン **HBP**
落下する **desc**
乱視 **AS，As，as.，AST，Ast，ast，Astg，astig，Astigm**
乱視矯正角膜切開術 **AK**
乱視計 **astig**
乱視者 **astig**
乱視の **astig**
卵 **Ov，ov.**
卵移植 **e**
卵円孔 **FO**
卵円孔開存 **PFO**

卵円窓　**OW，ow**
卵黄　**EY，vit.，vitel.，vit.ov.**
卵黄寒天　**EYA**
卵黄に溶解した　**vit.ov.sol.，vos.**
卵黄嚢　**YS，y.s.**
卵黄包　**YS，y.s.**
卵黄包〔嚢〕癌　**YSC**
卵黄包〔卵黄嚢〕腫瘍　**YST**
卵核胞　**GV**
卵管鏡下卵管形成　**FT**
卵管結紮　**TL，T.L.**
卵管采周囲癒着　**PFA**
卵管子宮(接合部)　**TUB**
卵管周囲癒着　**PTA**
卵管胎芽移植　**TET**
卵管胎芽期移植　**TEST**
卵管内受精　**HIT**
卵管内授精　**ITI**
卵管卵巣摘出(術)　**S＆O，SO，S-O**
卵管卵巣の　**TO**
卵管卵巣膿瘍　**TOA**
卵管留水症　**Hyd**
卵丘細胞-卵母細胞複合体　**COCs**
卵形の頭　**OVHD**
卵形マラリア原虫　**Po**
卵型頭　**OH**
卵(母)細胞質内精子注入法　**ICSI**
卵細胞成熟抑制因子　**OMI**
卵成熟促進因子　**MPF**
卵成熟誘起因子　**MIS**
卵巣　**Ov，ov.**
卵巣アスコルビン酸減少(法)　**OAAD**
卵巣アンドロゲン性機能亢進　**OAH**
卵巣過剰刺激症候群　**OHSS**
卵巣癌　**OC，Ova Ca，OVC**
卵巣癌研究班　**OCSG**
卵巣機能不全〔機能障害〕　**OvDF**
卵巣楔切除術　**OWR**
卵巣コレステロール消耗　**OCD**
卵巣漿液性境界型腫瘍　**OSBT**
卵巣生殖細胞腫瘍　**OGCT**
卵巣成長因子　**OGF**
卵巣摘出された　**OO**
卵巣摘出術　**OO，OVX**
卵巣摘出術を受けた　**OVX**
卵巣乳頭状漿液性腺癌　**OPSA**
卵巣乳頭腺癌　**OPA**
卵巣未熟奇形腫　**OIT**
卵白アルブミン　**OA**
卵白リゾチーム　**EWL**
卵胞刺激ホルモン　**FSH**
卵胞刺激ホルモン放出因子　**FRF，FSH-RF，RFFSH**
卵胞刺激ホルモン放出因子ホルモン　**FSH-RFH**
卵胞刺激ホルモン放出ホルモン　**FRH，FSH-RH**
卵胞刺激ホルモンレセプター結合抑制因子　**FSHRBI**
卵胞内受精　**IFI**
卵捕獲抑制因子　**OCI**

り

リアクタンス　**Re, react, Xc**
リウマチ熱　**RF**
リウマチ　**rheum**
リウマチ因子　**RF**
リウマチ様因子活性　**RFLA**
リウマチ因子様物質　**RFLS**
リウマチ学　**Rhu**
リウマチ性血管炎　**RV**
リウマチ性疾患　**RD**
リウマチ性心疾患　**RHD, Rh.DH**
リウマチ性僧帽弁狭窄症　**RMS**
リウマチ性多発筋痛症　**PMR, PR**
リウマチ性の　**rh, rheum**
リウマチ性弁膜性心疾患　**RVHD**
リウマチ熱　**rheu fev**
リウマチ様多発(性)関節炎　**RP**
リウマチ様の　**rheum**
リエントリー心室性不整脈　**RVA**
リガンド　**L**
リキソース　**Lyx**
リクリエイション　**rec, Rec**
リクリエイション療法　**RT**
リクリエイション療法士　**RT**
リクルートメント　**R**
リケッチア(属)　**R, R.**
リサミンローダミンB　**LRB**
リーシュマニア(属)　**L**
リーシュマン・ドノバン(小体)　**LD, L-D**
リーシュマン・ドノバン(小)体　**L-D bodies**
リシン　**LYS, Lys**
リジン　**K, LYS, Lys**
リジン・インドール運動性培地　**LIM**
リジン/アルギニン比　**L/A**
リジン-8-バソプレシン　**L-8-V**
リジン血管緊張物質　**LVT**
リジン蛋白不耐症　**LPI**
リジン鉄寒天(培地)　**LIA**
リジンバソプレシン　**LVP**
リス肝炎ウイルス　**GSHV**
リス線維腫ウイルス　**SFV**
リスター型　**L form**
リステリア(属)　**L**
リステリア・モノサイトゲネス　**LM**
リストセチン　**RC, RCT**
リストセチン依存性血小板凝集因子　**RAF**
リストセチン補助因子　**RCOF**
リスト内再認　**WLR**
リスホルム格子　**Lys**
リズム　**R**
リゼルグ酸エチルアミド　**LAE**
リセルグ酸ジエチルアミド　**LSD**
リゼルグ酸モルヒネ　**LSM**
リソソーム　**L, LYS, Lys**
リソソーム関連膜糖蛋白　**LAMP-1**
リソソーム酵素　**LE**
リソソーム酵素放出　**LER**
リソソーム酸リパーゼA　**LIPA**
リソソーム酸リパーゼB　**LIPB**
リゾチーム　**LZM, Lzm, lzm**
リソピン脱水素酵素　**LpOH**
リソピンデヒドロゲナーゼ　**LpOH**
リゾホスファチジルエタノールアミン　**LPE**
リゾホスファチジルコリン　**LPC**
リゾホスファチジン酸　**LPA**
リソレシチン　**LLT**
リゾレシチン　**LL**
リタ(＝急性心筋梗塞に関する大規模試験報告書)　**RITA**
リダクターゼ　**R**
リチウム　**Li**
リチウム誘発多飲(症)　**LIP**
リチャーズ・ランデル症候群　**RRS**
リッチナー・ハンハート(症候群)　**RH**
リットル　**l, L, lit, lit.**
リットル/秒　**lps**
リットル/分　**L/M, L/min, LPM, lpm**
リットル/分/平方メートル　**L/min/m²**
リデール・ウォーカー石炭酸係数試験　**RW, R-W**
リード・スターンバーグ(細胞)　**RS**
リード・スタンバーグ細胞　**R-S cell**

リドカイン **L, LIDO, lidoc**
リドカイン血中濃度 **LBC**
リドカイン組織(中)濃度 **LTC**
リトコール(酸) **LC**
リトル野 **LA**
リニアアクセルレータ(=LINAC) **LA**
リニアック **linac, LINAC**
リニメント(剤) **lin, lin., linim**
リノール酸 **$C_{18=2}$, LA**
リノレン酸 **$C_{18=3}$**
リバ・ロッチ血圧計 **RR, RRS**
リハーサルなし **NR**
リバーストリヨードチ〔サイ〕ロニン **rT3, r-T3**
リバースバンド **R-band**
リパーゼ **LPS**
リハビリテーション **Reha, Rehab, rehab, rehab., rehabil, Rehabili**
リハビリテーション学士 **BSR**
リハビリテーション活動側面 **RAP**
リハビリテーションセンター連合 **ARC**
リーバーミード行動記憶検査 **RBMT**
リピオドール **LP, LPD**
リピオドール注入塞栓術 **LPD**
リビット脱水素酵素 **RDH**
リビドマイシン **LVDM**
リビーン〔レヴィーン〕弁 **LVV**
リファンピシン **REP, Rfm, RFM, RFP, RIF**
リファンピシン,エタンブトール,イソニアジド **REI**
リファンピシン,エタンブトール,イソニアジド,シクロセリン,カナマイシン **REICK**
リファンピン **Rfm, RFM, RFP, RMP**
リフト渓谷熱 **RVF**
リフト渓谷熱ウイルス **RVFV**
リブマン・サックス(病) **LS**
リブロース-5-リン酸〔五炭糖〕 **R5P**
リブロース-5-リン酸塩 **Ru-5-P**
リポアミド脱水素酵素 **LAD**
リポアミドデヒドロゲナーゼ **LAD**
リポイド〔変性〕ネフローゼ **LN**
リポエートトランスアセチラーゼ **LTA**
リボ核酸 **RNA**
リボ核蛋白 **RNP**
リポ核蛋白 **LNP**
リボ核蛋白質 **RNP**
リポキシゲナーゼ **LOX**
リポキシン **Lx, LX**
リポ酸(塩) **Lip**
リポジストロフィ **LD**
リボシルチミジン **T**
リボシルチミン **T, THO**
リボース **R, r, rib**
リボース-5-リン酸 **R5P**
リボスタマイシン **RSM**
リボゾーム **RI**
リボソームRNA **rRNA**
リボゾームデオキシリボ核酸 **rDNA**
リボゾームの **r**
リポソーム免疫溶解試験 **LILA**
リボゾーム様粒子 **RLP**
リボソームリボ核酸 **rRNA**
リポ多糖因子 **LPF**
リポ多糖体症 **LPS**
リポ多糖類 **LPS**
リポ多糖類受容体 **LPSR**
リポ蛋白 **LP**
リポ蛋白(a) **Lp(a)**
リポ蛋白B **LPB**
リポ蛋白X **LpX, LPX**
リポ蛋白結合凝固阻害物質 **LACI**
リポ蛋白欠乏血清 **LPDS**
リポ蛋白電気泳動(法) **LEP, LPE**
リポ蛋白と冠(状)動脈硬化に関する研究 **LCAS**
リポ蛋白リパーゼ **LL, LPL**
リポ蛋白リパーゼ活性 **LPLA**
リポチアミドピロリン酸 **LTPP**
リボチミジン **Thd**
リボチミジン5′リン酸 **TMP**
リボチミジン5′-二リン酸 **TDP**
リボチミジン5′-三リン酸 **TTP**
リポテート **LPT**
リポトロピン **LPH**
リボフラビン **RF, RIB**
リボフラビン5′-モノサルフェート **FMS**
リボフラビン担体蛋白 **RCP**
リポペプチド **LPP**

リポポリサッカライド結合蛋白　**LBP**
リボホリン1　**RPN1**
リマ豆〔アオイ豆〕アグルチニン　**LBA**
リマ豆〔アオイ豆〕トリプシン抑制物質　**LBTI**
リムルス・アメーバ様細胞溶解質　**LAL**
リーメンビューゲル　**RB**
リウマチ熱　**Rh.F**
リュッケ腫瘍ウイルス　**LTV**
リュテラン血液型　**Lu**
リヨン高血圧ラット　**LHR**
リヨン正常血圧系統　**LN**
リヨン低血圧系統　**LL**
リン　**P, ph, phos**
リン・タングステン・モリブデン酸　**PTMA**
リン/酸素比　**P/O ratio**
リンゲル液　**RS**
リン光　**phos**
リンゴ酵素　**ME**
リンゴ酸脱水素酵素　**MD, MDH**
リンゴ線維　**AF**
リンコマイシン　**L, LCM, LM**
リン酢酸　**PAA**
リン酸アルギニン　**PA**
リン酸エステル　**P, Ph, ph, phos**
リン酸塩　**P, Ph, ph, phos**
リン酸オクタカルシウム　**OCP**
リン酸化チロシン　**PY**
リン酸緩衝食塩水　**PBS**
リン酸グリコムターゼ　**GP**
リン酸グリセルアルデヒド　**GAP**
リン酸グリセルアルデヒド脱水素酵素　**GAPD**
リン酸グルコムターゼ　**Gpm**
リン酸クレアチン　**CrP, Crp**
リン酸クロロキン　**CP**
リン酸コデイン　**cod.phos., cp**
リン酸サイクル　**PC**
リン酸三ナトリウム　**TSP**
リン酸ジカルシウム　**DCP**
リン酸ジヒドロアセトン　**DAP**
リン酸ジヒドロキシアセトン　**DHAP**
リン酸ジメチルジクロロビニル　**DDVP**
リン酸脱水素酵素　**PDH**
リン酸トリオルトクレジル　**TOCP**
リン酸トリカルシウム　**tricaphos**
リン酸トリクレシル　**TCP**
リン酸トリフェニル　**TPP**
リン酸トリプトンブロス　**TPB**
リン酸排泄係数　**PEI**
リン酸ピリドキシン　**PNP**
リン酸不使用緩衝液　**PFB**
リン酸フラビン　**FP**
リン酸ポリエストラジオール　**PEP**
リン酸マグネシウムアンモニウム結石　**MAP**
リン酸輸送体化合物　**PCC**
リン酸リボシルとリン酸リビトールの重合体　**PRP**
リン酸六炭糖イソメラーゼ　**HIM**
リン脂質　**PHL, PL, PPL**
リン脂質輸送蛋白　**PTP**
リンタングステン酸　**PTA**
リンタングステン酸ヘマトキシリン　**PTAH**
リンド　**RIND**
リンネ　**Linn**
リンネ式の　**Linn**
リンネ試験　**R, R.**
リンパ　**L, LYM**
リンパ/血漿(比)　**L/P**
リンパ栄養パポバウイルス　**LPV**
リンパ外臓器部位　**ELOS**
リンパ外の　**E**
リンパ芽球化転換試験　**LTT**
リンパ芽球化変換　**LBT**
リンパ芽球性悪性リンパ腫　**MLL**
リンパ芽球性リンパ腫　**LBL, LL**
リンパ芽球様細胞株　**LCL**
リンパ管撮影図　**LAG**
リンパ管侵襲　**v**
リンパ管浸潤度　**LY, ly, ly.**
リンパ管造影像　**LAG**
リンパ管造影〔撮影〕法　**LAG**
リンパ管平滑筋腫症　**LAM**
リンパ球　**L, LY, ly, ly., lymphos, lymphs**
リンパ球(性の)　**lym, lymph**
リンパ球/多形核球(比)　**L/P**
リンパ球b抗原　**Lyb**

リンパ球 t 抗原 **Lyt**
リンパ球移行の **LT**
リンパ球依存抗体 **LDA**
リンパ球化学誘導物質活性 **LCA**
リンパ球活性化因子 **LAF**
リンパ球活性化(抗原)決定基 **LAD**
リンパ球関連ウイルス **LAV**
リンパ球〔白血球〕関連抗原 **LFA**
リンパ球機能関連抗原 **LFA**
リンパ球機能抗原 1 **LFA-1**
リンパ球系/組織球系(細胞) **L/H**
リンパ球欠乏 **LD**
リンパ球検出膜抗原 **LYDMA**
リンパ球抗体リンパ球溶解相互作用 **LALI**
リンパ球コロニー形成単位 **CFU-L**
リンパ球混合培養反応 **MLCR**
リンパ球細胞傷害試験 **LCT**
リンパ球識別混合培養(抗原) **LD**
リンパ球刺激因子 **LSF**
リンパ球刺激試験 **LST**
リンパ球刺激ホルモン(因子) **LSH**
リンパ球指数 **LI**
リンパ球浸潤(性)疾患 **LID**
リンパ球数 **LC**
リンパ球性胃炎 **LG**
リンパ球性間質性肺炎 **LIP**
リンパ球性甲状腺炎 **LT**
リンパ球性抗体 **LA**
リンパ球性脈絡髄膜炎 **LCM**
リンパ球性脈絡髄膜炎(ウイルス) **LCL**
リンパ球性脈絡髄膜炎ウイルス **LCMV**
リンパ球性リンパ腫 **LL**
リンパ球性リンパ肉腫 **LCL**
リンパ球走化因子 **LCF**
リンパ球増殖 **LP**
リンパ球増殖疾患 **LPD**
リンパ球増殖阻害因子 **LGIF**
リンパ球増殖反応 **LPR**
リンパ球増多因子 **LPF**
リンパ球転換 **LT**
リンパ球転換因子 **LTF**
リンパ球転換活性 **LTA**
リンパ球転換試験 **LTT**
リンパ球転換反応 **LTR**
リンパ球伝達 **LCP**
リンパ球糖蛋白 **Lgp**
リンパ球毒性抗体 **LCA, LCTA**
リンパ球毒性試験 **LCT**
リンパ球毒素 **LC, LCT, LT**
リンパ球毒素検定 **CTA**
リンパ球の割合 **LYMPH%**
リンパ球媒介細胞毒性 **LMC**
リンパ球媒介細胞溶解 **LMC**
リンパ球培養液 **LCF**
リンパ球反応性指数 **LRI**
リンパ球プラズマ伝達 **LPP**
リンパ球分離液 **LSM**
リンパ球免疫螢光試験 **LIFT**
リンパ球優位の **LP**
リンパ球優勢型ホジキン病 **LPHD**
リンパ球由来血管新生因子 **LIAH**
リンパ球由来好酸球遊走因子 **ECF-L**
リンパ球由来白血球遊走因子 **LDCF**
リンパ球幼若転換試験 **LTT**
リンパ球様樹状細胞 **LDC**
リンパ球濾胞性細網症 **LFR**
リンパ血管併発 **LVSI**
リンパ骨髄系複合体 **LMC**
リンパ腫 **LY, ly, ly.**
(悪性)リンパ腫研究グループ **LSG**
リンパ腫症候群 **LySLK**
リンパ腫培養 **LC**
リンパ腫ポリープ症 **LOP**
リンパ腫様丘疹症 **LOP**
リンパ腫様肉芽腫 **LYG**
リンパ浸透圧 **OPL**
リンパ(球)性白血病 **LCL**
リンパ性白血病 **LL**
リンパ性白血病ウイルス **LLV**
リンパ性白血病ウイルス・(ウイルス関連)フレンド **LLV-F**
リンパ節 **LG, LN, LYN**
リンパ節 T 細胞 **LNT**
リンパ節細胞 **LNC**
リンパ節疾患症候群 **LAS**
リンパ節症関連ウイルス(＝HIV) **LAV**
リンパ節転移 **LNM, N**
リンパ節転移を伴う腫瘍 **TcNM**

リンパ節透過(性)因子 **LNPF**
リンパ節肥大を伴う洞組織球症 **SHML**
リンパ増殖性悪性病変 **LPM**
リンパ肉芽腫 **L**
リンパ肉芽腫症X **Lg X**
リンパ肉腫 **LS, LSA, Lyp**
リンパ肉腫/細網肉腫 **LSA/RCS**
リンパ肉腫細胞(性)白血病 **LSCL**
リンパ肉腫(細胞性)白血病 **LSL**
リンパ毛細管 **LC**
リンパ網内系 **LR system**
リンパ(細)網内(皮)の **LRE**
リンホカイン活性(化)キラー(細胞) **LAK**
リンホカイン **LK**
リンホトキシン **LT**
リー・フラウメニ症候群 **LFS**
リー・ホワイト **LW**
リー・ホワイト凝固時間 **LWCT**
利子 **int, int.**
利尿筋 **det**
利尿筋内尿道括約筋不〔非〕協調 **DISD**
利尿筋尿道(筋)不〔非〕協調 **DUD**
利尿筋反射亢進 **DH**
利尿時間 **dh**
利用可能なデータなし **NDA**
利用できない **NA**
利用できる情報なし **NIA**
梨状(筋) **PIR**
梨状陥凹 **PS**
梨状陥凹癌 **PSC**
梨状葉 **pc**
理学士 **B.S., B.Sc.**
理学的検査 **PE, PEx, PX, Px**
理学的な **PHY**
理学的評価 **PE**
理学博士 **DS, D.S., D.Sc., Sc.D., SciD**
理学療法 **PhysTher, phys.ther, PT**
理学療法士 **physio, physio., PT**
理解できる **U**
理事 **adm., ADM, commn**
理性感情療法 **RET**
理想(的)体重 **DBW, IBW**
理論的腎臓リン閾値 **TRPT**
理論的成長評価 **TGE**
理論的な **theor**
理論的な高さ **HETP**
理論の **theor**
履歴(書) **CV**
罹患腎 **DK**
罹病率・死亡率 **MM, M & M**
離婚した **D, d, div, div., DV**
離散フーリエ変換 **DFT**
離脱症状・退薬症状・禁断症状 **W/D**
離断 **dissec**
離断性骨軟骨炎 **OCD**
力価決定 **standard**
力学 **dyn**
力学的な **mech**
力動(論) **dyn**
力量型 **dyn**
陸軍医療サービス[米国] **AMS**
陸軍軍医学校Ⅲ法[米国] **AMS Ⅲ method**
陸軍軍医学校[米国] **AMS**
立位 **UP**
立位拡張期血圧 **SDBP**
立位の **st, stdg**
立位末梢血漿レニン活性 **UPPRA**
立方センチメートル **cc, c.c., c.cm.**
立方フット〔フィート〕 **cu ft, cuft**
立体4音声の **SQ**
立体撮影 **Stereo, stereo**
立体視 **STEREO**
立体写真 **Stereo, stereo**
立体的水流吸引器 **SASA**
立体(的)脳波(法) **SEEG, s-EEG**
立体ベクトル心電図 **SV(E)C, SVC, SVECG**
立方 **C**
立方インチ **cu in, in^3**
立方センチメートル **cm^3, cu cm**
立方体の **cu, cu.**
立方(体)の **C, c**
立方の **C, cu, cu.**
立方マイクロメートル **cu μm**
立方ミリメートル **cmm, c mm, cu mm**
立方メートル **cu m, m^3**
立方ヤード **cu yd**
立法 **leg**
立法フート **ft^3**
立法フィート/秒 **cfs**
立法フィート/分 **cfm, cf/m**

り

立法ミリメートル　mm^2
律動　**R**
律動的感覚衝撃療法　**RSBT**
率　**C, c, coef, coeff**
略語　**ABB, abbr**
略語にした　**abbr**
略字　**ABB, abbr**
(傷からの)流血　**go**
流行性角結膜炎　**CCE, EKC**
流行性肝炎関連抗原　**EHAA**
流行性感冒財団　**CCF**
流行性耳下腺炎・ニューカッスル病・インフルエンザウイルス　**MNI virus**
流行性耳下腺炎免疫グロブリン　**MIG**
流行性出血熱　**EHF**
流行性神経筋無力症(＝アイスランド病)　**ENM**
流行性腎症　**NE**
流行の　**epid**
流産　**AB, ab, ab., ABO, Abor, abor, misc**
流出　**F**
流出率　**OR**
流出量　**OV**
流体(の)　**FL, Fl, fl, fld, fluid.**
流体静力学　**Hyd**
流体静力学的中性点　**HIP**
流体静力学の　**Hyd.**
流動　**cur**
流動エキス　**extr.fl., fld.xt.**
流動エキス剤　**ext.fd, fld.ext., fl.ext.**
流動学　**rheol**
流動学の　**rheol**
流入　**infl**
流量　**F, FV**
流量計　**FM**
(尿)流量率　**FR**
留置　**detn**
留置カテーテル　**RC, ret.cath**
留置静脈カテーテル　**IDVC**
粒子計測免疫測定　**PCIA**
粒子サイズ決定　**PS detn**
粒子状有機炭素　**POC**
粒子輸送時間　**PTT**
粒子励起X線分析法　**PIXE**
隆起　**elev**
隆起性皮膚線維肉腫　**DFSP**
硫化水素・インドール・運動性試験培地　**SIM medium**
硫化鉛　**PbS**
硫酸亜鉛混濁試験　**ZnTT, ZST, ZTT**
硫酸アトロピン　**AS**
硫酸アンモニウム結晶　**CAS**
硫酸エステル　**SO_4, sulf, sulf.**
硫酸塩　**sulf, sulf., sulph**
硫酸化因子　**SF**
硫酸化水素添加ヒマシ油〔トウゴマ油〕　**SHCO**
硫酸カドミウム反応　**CdR**
硫酸グリコペプチド抗原　**SGA**
硫酸コレステロール　**cs**
硫酸ジヒドロエピアンドロステロン　**DHEAS, DHEA-S**
硫酸蒼鉛寒天　**BSA**
硫酸デキストラン　**DS**
硫酸デキストロアンフェタミン　**DAS**
硫酸デヒドロエピアンドロステロン　**DHAS, DHA-S, DS**
硫酸鉛　**SO_4**
硫酸(塩)の　**sulf**
硫酸ビンクリスチン　**VCR**
硫酸ビンブラスチン,アクチノマイシンD,ブレオマイシン　**VAB**
硫酸ビンブラスチン,アクチノマイシンD,ブレオマイシン,プラチナム　**VAB-II**
硫酸プロタミン連続希釈試験　**SDPS**
硫酸ヘパリン　**HS**
硫酸ポリミキシンB,バシトラシン,ネオマイシン　**PBN**
硫酸マグネシウム　**Mag.sul, $MgSO_4$**
硫酸マグネシウム・グリセリン・水(浣腸)　**MGW**
硫酸マグネシウム(＝$MgSO_4$)飽和溶液　**SSMS**
硫酸モルヒネ　**MS**
旅行者下痢症　**TD**
両凹の　**bicv**
両下肢　**BLE**
両眼　**BE, binocs**
両眼一緒に　**OU, O.U., o.u.**
両眼視機能検査鏡　**synopt**
両眼視視力　**BVA**
両眼視能　**BVE**
両眼視力　**BV**
両眼単一視　**BSV**
両眼に　**ocul. utro.**
両眼の視覚　**VOU**
両眼離反眼運動　**VEM**

両脚ブロック **BBBB**
両上肢 **BUE**
両心室図 **BVG**
両心室肥大 **BVH**
両心補助装置 **BVAD**
両耳 **AU，A.U.，a.u.**
両耳音の大きさバランス検査 **ABLB test**
両耳間移行減衰 **IA**
両耳間潜時差 **ILD**
両耳鼓膜 **MTAU**
両耳垂プレチスモグラフィ **BAPG**
両耳同時音の大きさ平衡検査 **BSLB**
両受体 **M**
両室肥大 **CVH**
両生類 **amph.**
両性の **bisex**
両性能力 **BP**
両染性細胞 **A**
両染性の **A**
両側 **BS**
両側(性)横隔膜麻痺 **BDP**
両側下部 1/4 区 **BLQ**
両側(性)(卵)管結紮(法) **BTL**
両側頸動脈閉鎖 **BCO**
両側睾丸下降した **T↓↓**
両側上部 1/4 区 **BUQ**
両側精管結紮(法) **BVL**
両側性急性網膜壊死 **BARN**
両側短下肢例 **bilat SLC**
両側中耳炎 **BOM**
両側頭部 **BT**
両側尿管閉塞症 **BUO**
両側(性)の **BIL，Bil，bil.，bilat**
両側の **bds，dplx，dpx**
両側肺門部リンパ節腫大 **BHL**
両側(性)肺門リンパ節腫脹 **BHL，BHLE**
両側(性)肺門リンパ節症 **BHA，BHL**
両側波帯 **DSB**
両側鼻腔咽頭気道 **BNPA**
両側部分卵管摘出(術) **BPS**
両側(性)卵管卵巣摘出(術) **BILAT S＆O，BILAT S×O，BSO**
両大血管右室起始症 **BVRV，DORV**
両大血管左(心)室起始症 **DOLV**
両大転子の **bitroch，BT**
両凸の **bicx**
両頭頂部 **BP**
両乳様突起間線 **BML**
両方の骨 **BB**
両耳とも **AU，A.U.，a.u.**
両レベル設定陽圧呼吸 **BiPAP**
良好な **G，gd**
良性潰瘍 **BU**
良性間葉(性)腫瘍 **BMT**
良性再発性肝内胆汁うっ滞 **BRIC**
良性再発性血尿 **BRH**
良性再発性眩暈症 **BRV**
良性自然気胸 **BSP**
良性上皮(性)腫瘍 **BET**
良性腎硬化症 **BNS**
良性線維性組織球腫 **BFH**
良性前立腺過形成(症) **BPH**
良性前立腺肥大(症) **BPH**
良性増殖性病変 **BPL**
良性単クローン性 γ グロブリン血症 **BMG**
良性単クローン性免疫グロブリン血症 **BMG**
良性中胚葉性腫瘍 **BMT**
良性頭位変換眩暈 **BPV**
良性頭蓋内圧亢進(症) **BIH**
良性軟骨芽細胞腫 **BC**
良性熱性痙攣 **BFC**
良性粘膜天疱瘡 **BMPP**
良性粘膜類天疱瘡 **BMMP**
良性の(腫瘍) **N**
良性肥大性前立腺炎 **BHP**
良性皮膚リンパ腫症 **LCB**
良性発作性頭位眼振 **BPPN**
良性発作性頭位変換眩暈 **BPPV**
良性発作性眩暈 **BPV**
良性三日熱マラリア **BTM**
良性流行性腎症 **BEN**
良性リンパ上皮病変 **BLL**
良性ローランドてんかん **BRE**
(投与)量 **dos.**
量 **amt，am't，Q，qt，R**
量子計数型 X 線撮影 **QR**
量子検出効率 **DQE**
量支持換気 **VSV**
量的に不十分 **QNS**
量不足 **QNS**
領域 **A，Br，regs**
療法 **RX，Rx.，Th，THER，ther，TRT，trt，Tx**
療法士 **T**
緑色螢光蛋白質 **GFT**
緑色の **vir.**
緑色のビン **Vv.**
緑内障 **glau，glauc，**

GLC, Glc
緑膿菌　PA
緑膿菌 K　PAK
(移植の)倫理的・法的・社会的問題　ELSI
淋菌　GC, GC, gc, gono
淋菌性関節炎・皮膚炎症候群　GADS
淋菌性新生児眼炎　GON
淋菌性尿道炎　GCU, GU
淋菌性の　gono
淋菌の　GC, GC, gc
淋菌補体結合試験　GCFT
淋疾　GC, Gc, Gca, gca, GO, Gono, gono
淋疾後尿道炎　PGU
淋病　GC, Gc, Gca, gca, GO, Gono, gono, VDG
輪筋　orbic
輪空胞ミオパシー　RVM
輪状筋　CM
輪状甲状筋　CTM
輪状甲状軟骨間膜　CTM
輪状軟骨後面　PC
輪状軟骨後面癌　PCC
輪状の　cir, cir., Circ, circ, orbic
輪状弁　SAV
隣接した　adj
隣接する　adj
隣接の　P, v, vic
臨界温度　crit.temp.
臨界帯　CB
臨界テスト希釈度　CTD
臨界点　CP
臨界の　crit
臨界比　CR
臨界表　CL
臨界フリッカー融合頻度　CFF
臨界閉鎖圧　CCP
臨界ミセル(形成)濃度　CMC, cmc
臨界ミセル濃度　CMC
臨界融合頻度　CFF
臨死体験　NDE
臨床医学　CM
臨床開発担当者　CRA
臨床科学士　D.Cl.Sci, M.Cl.Sc
臨床(検査)科学者　CS
臨床科学者協会　ACS
臨床学習　BSL
臨床過程　CC
臨床看護　CN
臨床基準時間　CFT
臨床教育　BST
臨床記録　CR
臨床研究　CR
臨床研究〔試験〕コーディネーター　CRC
臨床研究者　CI
臨床研究センター　CRC
臨床研究単位　CRU
臨床検査技師　CT, Med Tech, MT
臨床検査技師資格認定書　DMLT
臨床検査室　Cl Lab
臨床検査室改良事業　CLIA
臨床検査室自動化設計概念　CLAA
臨床検査室情報システム　LIS
臨床検査データ取得システム　CLDAS
臨床検査法　Med Tech
臨床検査モニターシステム　CLMS
臨床検討会　CC
臨床工学技術者　BMET
臨床(的)産婦人科(学)　COG
臨床試験受託機関　CRO, CSR
臨床実習　BST
臨床実地の質　QOCP
臨床手技　Clin proc
臨床診断　Clinical Dx
臨床心理学士　M.Clin.Psychol
臨床心理学者　CP
臨床生化学者協会　Assn Clin Biochem
臨床生殖泌尿器外科医協会　CSGUS
臨床精神薬理研究会　CPRG
臨床生理学的検査 vs 心電図モニタリング　ESVEM
臨床単位　CU, KE
臨床知能検査　KIP
臨床的印象　CI
臨床的自己評価尺度　KSbS
臨床的診断未確定の活動性結核　CUDAT
臨床的精神症状評価尺度　CPRS
臨床的な　Cl, cl, Clin, CLIN, Clin, clin.
臨床的ヒアリン膜疾患　CHMD
臨床的分類　CS
臨床データの相互交換基準　CDI
臨床にて　@bs.
臨床の　Clin, CLIN, Clin, clin.
臨床病理(学)　Clin Path, Clin path., CLP, CP
臨床病理学者協会　ACP
臨床病理検討会　CPC
臨床病理資格〔免状〕　D.C.P.

臨床薬学的業務　**CPP**
臨床薬理学と治療学　**CP & T**
臨終　**EOL**
臨終に　**in extrem.**
臨終の　**mort**

る

ルイサイト　**L**
ルイス数　**Le**
ルクス　**lx**
ルゴール液　**I_2KL**
ルーザー・ミルクマン(症候群)　**LM**
ルーシー・コーニル(症候群)　**RC**
ルシー・レヴィ(症候群)　**RL**
ルシー・レヴィ症候群　**RLS**
ルシフェラーゼ　**Luc**
ルーチン　**R, rout, rt**
ルーチン胆嚢摘出術　**RC**
ルーチン入院時検査　**RALT**
ルーチン尿検査　**RU**
ルテチウム　**Lu**
ルテニウム　**Ru**
ルテニウムレッド　**RR**
ルードウィッヒのアンギナ　**LA**
ルビジウム　**Rb**
ルビンスタイン・テイビ(症候群)　**RT**
ルビンスタイン・テイビ症候群　**RTS**
ループス抗凝固物質　**LA**
ループス腎炎　**LN**
ループス帯試験　**LBT**
ループ電気メス外科切除法　**LEEP**
ループ電気メス焼灼切除法　**LEEP**
ループ電気メス切除法　**LEEP**
ルミクロム　**Lc**
ルミフラビン　**Lf**
ルーメン　**lm**
ルーメン/ワット　**lpw**
ルーメン時　**l hr**
ルーワイ吻合術　**R-Y**
涙液層破壊時間　**BUT**
涙液の　**lacr**
涙嚢鼻腔吻合(術)　**DCR**
累加電位　**SP**
累積の　**cum**
累積分布関数　**CDF**
類骨表面　**OS**
類語　**syn**
類上皮の　**EP**
類似点のある　**comp**
類洞内皮細胞(肝)　**SEC**
類鼻疽　**MELDOS**
類扁桃核　**AMYG**

れ

レイノー(現象) **RA**
レイノー(現象)・食道(運動機能障害)・手指〔足指〕硬化・毛細血管拡張(症候群) **REST**
レイノー現象 **RP**
レイノー症候群 **RS**
レイノー病 **RD**
レイノルズ数 **NR**
レイモン・セスタン(症候群) **RC**
レヴィ(小)体痴呆 **LBD**
レヴィン管 **LT**
レオウイルス **REO virus, RV**
レオウイルス様因子(=ロタウイルス) **HRLA**
レオウイルス様病原体 **RVLA**
レオカルジオグラム **RCG**
レオナルド **Le**
レオパード症候群 **LEOPARD syndrome**
レオミュール(温度目盛) **°R**
レオミュール温度計 **R**
レーキ・ローランド因子 **LLF, L-F f.**
レギュラーインスリン **RI**
レクチン依存性細胞傷害 **LDCC**
レクチン介在によるマクロファージの殺腫瘍細胞作用 **LDMC**
レクチン活性化キラー細胞 **LAK**
レクチン誘導細胞介在細胞傷害 **LICC**
レクチン誘導細胞傷害 **LICC**
レグヘモグロビン **Lb**
レーザー **LASER, laser**
レーザー角膜内切削形成(術) **LASK**
レーザー気化法 **LA**
レーザー隅角形成術 **LGP**
レーザー虹彩切開術 **LI**
レーザー周辺虹彩切除(術) **LPI**
レーザー視力矯正 **LVC**
レーザー心臓血管新生術 **TMR**
レサズリン **R**
レーザー線維柱帯形成術 **LTP**
レーザー走査型検眼鏡 **SLO**
レーザー脱離 **LD**
レーザー脱離質量分析法 **LDMS**
レーザー椎間板減圧術 **LDD**
レーザード(ッ)プラー流速計 **LDV**
レーザード(ッ)プラー流速計測法 **LDV**
レーザード(ッ)プラー流量計測(法) **LDF**
レーザー内視鏡 **LES**
レーザーによる経皮的椎間板減圧術 **PLDD**
レーザーによる口蓋垂軟口蓋形成術 **LAUP**
レーザー熱角膜移植(術) **LTK**
レーザーネフェロメトリー **LN**
レーザーバルーン血管形成(術) **LBA**
レーザー光凝固術 **LPC**
レーザー微小プローブ質量分析器 **LAMMA**
レーザー補助下脊椎内視鏡検査(法) **LASE**
レーザー補助下バルーン血管形成術 **LABA**
レーザー補助下微小吻合(術) **LAMA**
レーザー免疫測定法 **LIA**
レーザー誘起イオン化分光法 **LEIS**
レーザー誘発螢光 **LIF**
レーザー誘発体内衝撃波砕石術 **LISL**
レーザー力顕微鏡 **LFM**
レーザー励起原子螢光分析 **LEAFS**
レジオネラ(属) **L**
レジオネラ症 **LD**
レシチン **L**
レシチン・コレステロール・アシルトランスフェラーゼ **LCAT**
レシチン・スフィンゴミエリン比 **L/S, L/S ratio**
レーシック手術 **LASK**
レジデント **Res, res**
レジデント入会記録 **RAN**
レジデント評価調書 **RAPs**
レジンスポンジ摂取率 **RSU**
レジン摂取率 **RUR**
レジン摂取量 **RU**
レ氏(温度目盛) **°R**
レスタミン反応テスト **RRT**
レスビアニズム **Les**
レセルピン **R, ReS, Res, res, RP**
レーダー運動 **RADAR**
レチノイン酸 **ATRA, RA**
レチノイン酸受容体

RAR
レチノール結合蛋白 **RBP**
レッグ・カルベ・ペルテス（病） **LCP**
レッグ・カルベ・ペルテス病 **LCPD**
レッシュ・ナイハン症候群 **LNS**
レッシュ・ナイハン病 **LND**
レッツ蛋白 **LETS protein**
レッテラー・シーベ（病） **LS**
レット **ret**
レッド **R**
レット症候群 **RS**
レデラー・ブリル（症候群） **LB**
レトロウイルス **RETRO.，RV**
レナンピシリン **LAPC**
レニウム **Re**
レニン・アンジオテンシン **RA**
レニン・アンジオテンシン・アルドステロン **RAA，R-A-A**
レニン・アンジオテンシン・アルドステロン系 **RAAS**
レニン・アンジオテンシン系 **RAS**
レニン活性 **RA**
レニン阻害ペプチド **RIP**
レニン放出 **RR**
レニン放出率 **RRR**
レニン本態性高血圧（症） **REH**
レノグラム **RIR**
レノックス・ガストー症候群 **LGS**
レノン・デリリュ（症候群） **RD**
レーバー遺伝性視神経萎縮症 **LHON**
レバイン心雑音強度分類1～6 **Levine1-6**
レーバー視神経萎縮（症） **LOA**
レーバー先天性黒内障 **LCA**
レバミゾール **LMS，LVM**
レビー小体型老人性痴呆 **SDLT**
レビュー **R**
レビンサール・コールズ・リリー（小体） **LCL**
レプ **REP，rep**
レプトスピラ（属） **L，Lept**
レプトスピラ症凝集素 **LEPTOS**
レプトトリキア（属） **L**
レボ **l**
レボチロキシン **LT**
レポート **Rpt**
レボドパ **LD，L-DOPA，L-dopa，l-dapa，L-dapa**
レボフロキサシン **LVFX**
レボメプロマジン **LP，LPZ，LPz**
レム **REM，REM，rem**
レム期 **REMP**
レム睡眠 **AS，REMS，SREM**
レム睡眠欠損 **REMD**
レム睡眠時行動障害 **RBD**
レムナント様リポ蛋白 **RLP**
レムナント様リポ蛋白コレステロール **RLP-C**
レリー・ワイル（症候群） **LW**
レール・キントベルク（症候群） **LK**
レワンドウスキー・ルッツ（症候群） **LL**
レントゲン **R，ROE，Roent，roent，rtg**
レントゲン/時間 **r/h，r/hr**
レントゲン単位 **RU，R unit**
レントゲン同位元素螢光解析法 **RIFMA**
レントゲン当量 **ER**
レントゲンメーター **R-meter**
冷温水 **CHW**
冷却による血管拡張 **CIVD**
冷却濾過法 **CF**
冷所に **in loc frig**
冷浸（法） **mac.**
冷浸せよ **mac.**
冷水 **aq.fig.，aq.frig.，chw**
冷水治療 **CWT**
冷水溶性の **CWS**
冷阻血時間 **CIT**
冷蔵 **refrig**
冷蔵庫 **refr**
冷凍学 **CS**
励起波長 **Ex，ex**
励起誘導放射による光増幅 **LASER，laser**
例 **exx**
例外 **'cept**
例外的誤差 **EE**
例題 **zE**
霊菌 **SM**
霊長動物実験内科・外科研究室 **LEMSIP**
暦年 **CY**
劣性遺伝性ジストニー **RD**
劣性栄養障害性表皮水疱症

RDEB
劣性の **R, rec**
裂 **G, g**
裂孔原性網膜剝離 **RRD**
裂孔ヘルニア **HH**
裂溝 **Fiss, fiss**
裂傷 **lac**
裂創 **LW**
裂頭条虫(属) **D**
裂毛・知能低下・生殖能低下・短軀症候群 **BIDS syndrome**
裂離骨折 **av.fx.**
連結 **jct, JT, jt, junct**
連合 **Fed**
連合する〔した〕 **assoc, assoc.**
連合弁膜症 **CVD**
連鎖 **Seq, seq**
連鎖桿菌(属) **S**
連鎖球菌(属) **S, STR, str., STREP, Strep, strep., strept., streptoc.**
連鎖球菌感染症に関連する小児自己免疫神経障害 **PANDAS**
連鎖球菌後急性糸球体腎炎 **PSAGN**
連鎖球菌細胞壁 **SCW**
連鎖球菌細胞膜 **SCM**
連鎖球菌スーパー抗原 **SSA**
連鎖球菌性蛋白 **Su-Pr**
連鎖球菌増殖因子 **SPF**
連鎖球菌蛋白 G **SPG**
連鎖球菌毒ショック症候群 **STSS**
連鎖球菌発熱性内毒素 **SPE**
連鎖球菌ポリサッカリド **Su-Ps, SU-PS**
連続 **Seq, seq**
連続した **cont'd, ser**
連続循環型腹膜透析 **CCPD**
連続性雑音 **CM**
連続切片 **ser.sect**
連続装用可能なソフトコンタクトレンズ **EWSCL**
連続体膝システム(インプラント) **CKS**
連続多項目分析装置 **SMAC**
連続多重チャンネル自動分析器 **SMA**
連続多数分析 6 種血清検査 **SMA-6**
連続多数分析 60 分 12 種血清検査 **SMA-12/60**
連続多数〔多種目〕分析器 **SMA**
連続弾性成分 **SE**
連続的アルブテロール噴霧療法 **CAN**
連続的血糖測定装置 **CGM**
連続的に **cont, cont., ser**
連続的(静脈)抜去術 **CS**
連続トロンビン時間 **STT**
連続(性)の **cont, cont.**
連続波 **CW**
連続波ド(ッ)プラー法 **CWD**
連続不透明度監視システム **COMS**
連続流動分析器 **CFA**
連続流量調整器 **CFA**
連邦政府の **Fed**
連邦微生物研究所 **CMI**
連盟 **Fed**
連絡 **comm**
煉薬 **elect.**
練習 **E, Ex, ex, exer**
練乳 **cond.milk**
練乳組成 **EMF**
攣縮 **S, Z, Zuck**

ろ

ロイケラン,メトトレキサート,フルオロウラシル **LMF**
ロイコトリエン **LT, LTs**
ロイコトリエンA 4 **LTA4**
ロイコノストック(属) **L**
ロイコボリン **LEU, LV, LVR**
ロイコボリン,ビンクリスチン(＝オンコビン),メトトレキサート,アドリアマイシン,シクロホスファミド **LOMAC**
ロイコマイシン(＝キタサマイシン) **LM**
ロイシルグリシン **LG**
ロイシン **L, LEU, Leu**
ロイシン・イソロイシン・バリン結合蛋白 **LIV-BP**
ロイシン・エンケファリン **Leu-EK**
ロイシンアミノペプチダーゼ **LA, LAP**
ロイシン反応試験 **LRT**
ロイシン負荷試験 **LTT**
ロイトコリエンB_4 **LTB_4**
ロイトコリエンC_4 **LTC_4**
ロイトコリエンD_4 **LTD_4**
ロイトコリエンE_4 **LTE_4**
ロイトコリエンF_4 **LTF_4**
ロイヤル―― →王立を参照
ロイヤル薬剤師会 **RPSGR**
ロイロクリスチン **LCR**
ローウォルフィア・セルペンチーナ **RS**
ロキシスロマイシン **RXM**
ロキタマイシン **RKM**
ロキタンスキー・アショフ(洞) **RA, RAS**
ロキタンスキー・キュスター・ハウザー(症候群) **RKH**
ロケット免疫電気泳動法 **RIEP**
ロシア春夏脳炎 **RSSE**
ロジウム **Rh**
ローシャーウイルス **RV**
ローション(剤) **lot.**
ローズベンガル抗原 **RBA**
ロスマン・マケイ(症候群) **RM**
ロゼット形成細胞 **RFC**
ロゼット形成試験 **RFT**
ロゼット形成阻止遺伝子 **RIF**
ロゼット形成の **RF**
ローゼンタール・メルカーソン(症候群) **RM**
ローゼンツバイク絵画フラストレーションテスト **Rosenzweig-PF-Test**
ロタウイルス **RV**
ローター症候群 **RS**
ローダミンイソチオシアネート **RITC**
ロッキー山紅斑熱 **RMSF**
ロッテルダム症状チェックリスト **RSCL**
ロートエキス **X-copool, X scopol**
ロバートソン転座 **rob**
ロホトキシン **LTX**
ロボトミー **lobo**
ロマノ・ウォード(症候群) **RW**
ロムスチン **CCNU**
ロメフロキサシン **LFLX**
ロラゼパム **LOR, LRZ**
ロランド膠様質 **SGR**
ロリテトラサイクリン **PRMTC, RTC**
ロールシャッハ(検査) **Ror**
ロールシャッハ試験 **RIT**
ロールシャッハテスト **RPP**
ロールシャッハ内容試験 **RCT**
ロールシャッハ予後評価尺度 **RPRS**
ローレル指数 **RI**
ローレンシウム **Lr, Lw**
ローレンス・バークレー研究所 **LBL**
ローレンス・ムーン・バルデー・ビードル(症候群) **LMBB**
ローレンス・ムーン・ビードル(症候群) **LMB**
ローレンス・ムーン・ビードル症候群 **LMBS**
ローン・ガノン・レバイン(症候群) **LGL**
ローン・ガノン・レバイン症候群 **LGL syndrome**
ロング・エバンスラット **LE**
ロングタームバリアビリティ **LTV**
ロンベルグ(徴候) **Rom, Romb**
ろうエステル **WE**
ろう膏〔膏薬〕をつくれ **ft.cerat.**

ろうそく　**C, c, ca**
濾過　**filt, filt.**
濾過圧　**FP**
濾過器　**filt, filt., flt**
濾過剤　**FA**
濾過されない　**NF**
濾過した　**colat, filt, filt.**
濾過する　**filt, filt., flt**
濾過性溶血性貧血　**FHA**
濾過せよ　**col, col., colet, filt, filt.**
濾過率　**FF, FR**
濾紙　**FP**
濾紙顕微鏡試験　**FPM**
濾紙電気泳動　**PE**
濾紙電気泳動法　**PCE**
濾紙放射免疫吸収試験　**PRIST**
濾胞　**F**
濾胞樹状細胞　**FDC**
濾胞性大小細胞混合型　**FMX**
濾胞性リンパ腫混合型　**FM**
濾胞性リンパ腫小切れ込み核細胞型　**FSC**
濾胞性リンパ腫大細胞型　**FL**
濾胞性リンパ肉腫　**FLSA**
濾胞前期　**PF, prF**
濾胞中心細胞　**FCC**
露出　**Ex, ex, exp**
露出する　**exp**
露髄　**X, x**
露呈　**X, x**
老化促進モデルマウス　**SAM**
老眼　**P, Pb, Pb., PR, Pr**
老犬脳炎　**ODE**
老人　**OM**
老人・生存者・身障者の健康保険社会保障　**OASDHI**
老人医療計画　**eldelcare**
老人神経学　**N-Ger**
老人性うつ病尺度〔スケール〕　**GDS**
老人性角化症　**SK**
老人〔老年〕性痴呆　**SD**
老人性の　**S**
老人性〔老年性〕脳疾患　**SBD**
老人性パーキンソニズム　**sP**
老人と生存者保険　**OASI**
老人の顔　**OF**
老人の聴力障害度調査［米国］　**HHIE**
老人斑　**SP**
老人用統覚検査　**GAT**
老視　**PR, Pr, presby**
老視の　**presby**
老衰　**Cad**
老年医学　**Ger, ger, geriat, Gerontol**
老年性萎縮　**SA**
老年性〔老人性〕黄斑変性（症）　**SMD**
老年性〔老人性〕脈絡網膜黄斑変性症　**SMCD**
老年肉芽腫症　**OGD**
老年の　**S**
老年病学　**Ger, ger, geriat, Gerontol**
老年病学者　**Gerontol**
老婦人　**OW, ow**
老練でない　**NV**
老齢　**OA**
老齢保障　**OAS**
労作後呼吸困難　**PED**
労作時息切れ　**SBE**
労作性狭心症　**EA**
労作性呼吸困難　**DOE**
労働　**A**
労働者救護団　**ASB**
労務　**A**
漏電遮断機　**GFCI**
漏斗　**INF**
漏斗状肺動脈弁狭窄(症)　**IPS**
漏斗部肺動脈狭窄　**Inf.PS**
蠟紙に包んで　**ad chart.cer.**
瘻孔　**fist**
瘻孔症状　**FS**
聾唖　**DD, dee-dee**
聾唖クリニック　**HSC**
六塩化ベンゼン　**BHC**
六炭糖　**Hex, Hxs**
六フッ化硫黄(ガス)　**SF**
肋横角　**CPA**
肋椎の　**CV**
肋軟骨の　**CC**
録音図　**phono**
六角　**hex**
六角の　**hex**
肋間(辺)縁　**ICM**
肋間縁　**IC**
肋間気管(状動脈)幹　**ICBT**
肋間胸骨右縁　**RSB**
肋間腔　**ICS, IKR, IS**
肋間の　**IC, intcl**
肋骨　**C, R, R, R.**
肋骨縁　**CM, c.m.**
肋骨脊柱角　**CVA, cva**
肋骨脊柱角叩打痛　**CVA tend., CVAT**
肋骨脊柱の　**CV**
肋骨中線　**MCL**
肋骨椎体角　**RVA, RV-angle**
肋骨の　**C**
肋骨隆起　**RH**
論証する　**dem**
論説　**edit.**
論文　**MS, Mss, MSS, pa**

わ

ワイデル・イエス/ノー信頼度検査　**WY/NRT**
ワイデル聴覚処理検査　**WAPT**
ワイブチン　**Y-Wye**
ワイヤーガイド　**WG**
ワイヤーによる圧迫固定　**Zugg**
ワイル・フェリックス反応　**WFR**
ワイルダー銀(染色)　**WS**
ワイン　**vim, vin, vin., w**
ワイングラス１杯　**cyath.vin., cyath.vinos.**
ワオキツネザル　**LCA**
ワクシニア免疫グロブリン　**VIG**
ワークショップ　**WS**
ワクチニアウイルス　**VV**
ワクチン　**V, vac, vacc**
ワクチン接種協力機構　**VAA**
ワクチンと予防接種のための世界同盟　**GAVI**
ワクチンの血清型　**VS**
ワシントン会話音鑑別検査　**WSSDT**
ワシントン大学文章完成試験〔検査〕　**WUSCT**
ワセリン　**pet, v**
ワタウサギパピローマウイルス　**CRPV**
ワックス型　**WxP**
ワックスバイト　**WxB**
ワックスビーン凝集原　**WBA**
ワッセルマン検査　**Wass**
ワッセルマン反応　**RW, WaR, WR, Wr**
ワット　**W**
ワット/cm²　**W/cm²**
ワット時　**Whr**
ワット秒　**W-s, W-sec**
ワーデンブルグ症候群　**WS**
ワーラー・ローズ試験〔反応〕　**W-R**
ワーラー自己記述調査票　**WSDI**
ワルタルド細胞遺残　**WCR**
ワルデンシュトレームマクログロブリン血(症)　**WM**
ワルデンストレームマクログロブリン血症　**MGW**
ワルファリン　**WARF, Warf**
ワルファリン用量指数　**WDI**
ワーレンベルグ症候群　**WS**
わきの下　**A**
わずかに　**SL, sl, slt**
わずかに溶ける　**SS**
われわれの臨床で　**IOC**
分ける　**div, div., divid.**
割り当てる　**dist**
話声域　**SR**
話題　**CH, Ch, ch, chap**
輪　**r**
矮小型コロニー　**D**
若い　**Y**
若い回教婦人協会　**YMWA**
若者のための薬物教育　**DEFY**
(学生興味調査票の)私がしたい事　**WILD**
割合　**Fract, fract, R, r**
悪い　**B**
我々に　**nob.**
腕囲・胸の厚さ・腰幅指数　**ACH index**
腕周長　**AC**
腕神経叢ニューロパシー　**BPN**
腕神経叢ブロック　**BB**
腕頭動脈　**BCA**
腕頭の　**BC**
腕偏位試験　**ADT**
彎曲肢症候群　**CS**
彎曲した　**CVD, cvd**
彎曲度　**D**

A

A(弁) **A**
A(領域) **A**
Aノルプロゲステロン **ANP**
(ABO式血液型の)A型 **A**
A型肝炎 **HA**
A型肝炎ウイルス **HAV**
A型肝炎抗原 **HA Ag, HA-Ag**
A型肝炎抗体 **HA**
A型スコットランドインフルエンザウイルス **A Scot**
A群β溶血性連鎖球菌 **GABHS**
A群連鎖球菌 **GAS**
A胆汁 **A bile, A-bile**
A帯 **Ab, A band, Ad**
a波 **a**
(ABO式血液型の)AB型 **AB**
ABC症候群 **ABC syndrome**
ABC法 **ABC method**
ABLB検査 **ABLB test**
ABO式血液型 **ABO**
ABO式血液型(のA,AB,B,O) **ABO**
ACブロック **A-C block**
AC/A比(=調整〔調節〕性輻輳対調節比) **AC/A ratio**
ACD液 **ACDS**
ACE阻害薬の脳卒中再発予防効果における大規模試験 **PROGRES**
ACTH-Z法 **ACTH-Z method**
ADPグルコース **ADP-Glc**
ADPリボシル化 **ADP ribosylation**
AFD児(=AGA児) **AFD infant**
AGA児(=AFD児) **AGA infant**
AGEレセプター **RAGE**
AL(吻合)(=消化管2層吻合) **A-L**
APUD系腫瘍 **APUDoma**
AVシャント **AVS, A-V S**

B

Bリンパ球コロニー形成細胞 **BLCFC, BLCFU**
Bリンパ球活性化因子 **BAF**
Bリンパ球系幹細胞コロニー形成単位 **CFU-BL**
Bリンパ球系細胞株 **BLCL**
Bリンパ球刺激因子 **BSF**
Bリンホトキシン **B-Lt, B-LT**
B型 **B type**
B型肝炎 **HB**
B型肝炎ウイルス **HBV**
B型肝炎コア(抗原) **HBc, HBC, HBcAg**
B型肝炎コア抗体 **HBcAb**
B型肝炎血清免疫グロブリン **HBISG**
B型肝炎抗原 **HB Ag, HB antigen, HBg**
B型肝炎抗体 **HB Ab**
B型肝炎表面 **HBs, HBS**
B型肝炎免疫グロブリン **HBIG, HBIg**
B型肝炎s抗体 **HBsAb, HBsAg, HBs-Ag**
B型日本脳炎 **JBE**
B群連鎖球菌 **GBS**
B群連鎖球菌感染症 **GBS**
B細胞 **B cell**
B細胞クローン過多 **BCE**
B細胞活性化因子 **BAF**
B細胞急性リンパ芽球性白血病 **BALL, B-ALL**
B細胞刺激因子 **BSF**
B細胞性悪性リンパ腫 **B-ML**
B細胞成熟因子 **BMF**
B細胞増殖因子 **BCGF**
B細胞増殖と分化因子 **BGDF**
B細胞特異転写因子(=CD 19) **BSAP**
B細胞白血病・リンパ腫 **B-lym**
B細胞反応性 **BCR**
B細胞分化因子 **BCDF, BDF**
B細胞慢性リンパ(球)性白血病 **B-CLL**
(ビタミン)B複合体 **B comp.**
BB抗原 **BB-Ag**
BCG細胞壁骨格 **BCG-CWS**
BCYE寒天 **BCYE**
BG・抗BG複合体 **BGABG**
BIDS症候群 **BIDS syndrome**
BK母斑 **B-K mole**
BLBマスク **BLB**

C

Cペプチド **CP, C-peptide**
Cペプチド免疫測定値 **CPR**
C型肝炎 **HC**
C型肝炎ウイルス **HCV**
C細胞過形成 **CCH**
C多形式非受容器 **CPN**
C多糖類 **CPS**
c波 **c**
C反応性蛋白(試験) **CRP**
C反応性蛋白検査 **CR-test**
C反応性蛋白抗血清 **CRPA**
C末端 **CT, C-terminal**
C末端副甲状腺ホルモン **PTH-C**
C末端ペプチド **CTP**
C領域 **C region, C-region**
cAMP依存性プロテインキナーゼ **PKA**
CCU症候群 **CCU syndrome**
CCU精神病 **CCU psychosis**
CD分類 **CD**
CD40リガンド **CD40L**
CE弁 **CE valve**
cis-ジクロロ-*trans*-ジヒドロキシ-*bis*-イソプロピラミンプラチナム **CHIP**
CO拡散能 C_{CO}
CPD加新鮮血液 **WB-F**
CPD加保存血液 **WB**
CPL分類(癌の型分類) **CPL**
CRST(皮下石灰沈着症,レイノー症状,手指硬化,多発性毛細血管拡張症)(症候群) **CRST**
CTディスコグラフィ **CT-D**
CTペリドログラフィ **CT-P**
CT断層撮影による血管造影法 **CTA**
C1インヒビター **C1 INH**
C1エステラーゼインヒビター **C1 INH**
C1不活性化因子 **C1 INA**
C1q結合測定法 **C1q BA**
C3活性化因子 **C3 A**
C3活性化因子前駆体 **C3 PA**
C3腎炎因子 **C3 NeF**
C3不活性化因子 **C3 in**
C3不活性物質 **C3 INA**
C4結合蛋白(質) **C4-bp**
C4腎炎因子 **C4 NeF**
C9関連蛋白 **C9 RP**

D

D-アミノ酸酸化酵素 **DAAO**
D-グリセルアルデヒド三リン酸 **D-GAP**
D-グリセロリン酸 **GP**
D-グルコース(=右旋性ブドウ糖) **Glc**
D-ツボクラリン **DTC, d-TC**
D-デオキシエフェドリン **D-O-E**
D-ペニシラミン **D-Pc**
D-リボース **rib**
D型肝炎 **HD**
D型肝炎ウイルス **HDV**
D関連抗原 **DR**
D群連鎖球菌 **GDS**
DDS症候群 **DDS syndrome**
def指数 **def index**
DHL寒天培地 **DHL agar**
DK値 **DK**
DMF指数 **dmf index, DMF Index**
DMF比率 **DMF rate**
DNAポリメラーゼI **pol** I
DNAポリメラーゼII **pol** II
DNAポリメラーゼIII **pol** III
DNA結合蛋白質 **DBP**
DNA合成阻害薬 **IDS**
DNA合成抑制因子 **IDS**
DNA複製エラー **RER**
DNA複製ライセンス因子 **RLF**
DNCB感作試験 **DNCB test**
DOP試験 **DOP test**
DP皮弁 **DP flap**
DSM(=精神障害分類診断基準)診断を下すための面接法 **SCID**
D-2-アミノ-5-ホスホノ吉草酸塩 **AP5**

E

Eセレクチンリガンド(=シアリルルイスX) **ESL-1**
E型肝炎 **HE**
E型肝炎ウイルス **HEV**
EAE蛋白(=MBP) **EAE protein**
EBウイルス **EBV, EB virus**
EBウイルス核抗原

EBNA
EB ウイルス関連特異核抗原 **EBNA**
EC 細胞 **EC cell**
EDTA 含有ベロナール緩衝液 **VBE**
EMG 症候群 **EMG syndrome**
EMO 吸入器 **EMO inhaler**
EMO(＝眼球突出・限局性粘液水腫・変形関節)症候群 **EMO syndrome**
EPR システム **EPR system**
ES 細胞 **ES cell**

F

F プライム **F′**
F プライム菌 **F′bacterium**
F^+菌 **F^+ bacterium**
F^-菌 **F^- bacterium**
FAB(分類)(＝白血病分類方式の１つ) **FAB**
Fc レセプター **FcR, Fc-R**
Fc レセプターによる抗体依存的増強作用(＝ADCC) **FcR-AD**
F-18-デオキシグルコース **FDG**
F II(＝ガンマグロブリン)赤血球凝集試験 **F II-HA**

G

G 型肝炎ウイルス **HGV**
G 骨髄腫蛋白 **GM-P**
(ギムザ染色の)G バンド **G-band**
GAM 寒天 **GAM agar**
GC 寒天培地 **GC agar**

H

H 型物質 **H**
H 抗原 **HA, H antigens**
H 鎖 **HC, H chain**
H 鎖可変領域 **V_H**
H 鎖伝令リボ核酸 **H-mRNA**
H 鎖病 **HCD**
H 鎖不変部 **CH**
H 帯 **H band**
H 弁 **HV**
HAM 症候群 **HAMS**
HAT 培養液 **HAT medium**
HBe 抗原 **HBe Ag, HBe-Ag**
HBs 抗原 **HBsAg, HBs-Ag**
HBs 抗体 **HBsAb**
hCG 試験 **HCG test, hCG test**
HDL コレステロール **HDL cholesterol**
HEPES 緩衝食塩水 **HBS**
HIV 感染症 **HIV infection**
HIV 関連腎症 **HIVAN**
HIV 関連唾液腺病 **HIV-SGD**
HIV 抗体 **HIV-AB**
HIV 免疫グロブリン **HIVIG**
HMG・HCG 療法 **HMG-HCG therapy**
HMG 試験 **HMG test**
HMP 側路 **HMPS**
HPV ワクチン **HPVV**
HTL 関連呼吸器障害 **HAB**
HTLV-I 関連細気管支肺胞異常症 **HABA**
HTP テスト **HTP**
H-Y 抗原 **H-Y antigen**

I

I 帯 **I band, I disk**
I〔封入体〕細胞 **I cell**
I〔封入体〕細胞病 **ICD, I cell disease**
I 領域(遺伝子)関連抗原 **Ia-A, Ia antigen**
Ia 抗原 **Ia antigen**
IBL 様 T 細胞リンパ腫 **IBL-T**
ICU 患者の急性生理学的異常・慢性度による重症度評価システム **APACHE**
ICU 精神病 **ICU psychosis**
Ig 受容体 α・β 鎖 **BCR**
IgA 腎症 **IgA GN**
IgE 特異的 Fc レセプター **FcεR**
IgG レセプター **IgG-R**
IgG 特異的 Fc レセプター **FcγR**
IgG 分泌細胞 **IgG-SC**
IgM-抗 A 型肝炎抗体 **IgM-anti HA**
IgM-抗 B 型肝炎コア抗体 **IgM-anti HBc**
IgM 特異的 Fc レセプター **FcμR**
in situ ハイブリダイゼーション法 **ISH**
IQ の満点 **FS**
IS スパイク **IS spike**
IVIM 法(＝MRI 撮影法の１つ) **IVIM**

J

Jマップ **JMAP**
J鎖 **J chain**

K

K-免疫グロブリン(軽鎖) **KM**
Kaup指数 **BMI**
KBM下腿義足 **KBM Prothese**
KBMソケット **KBM**
KT 50 **KT_{50}**
KW分類 **KW classification**

L

L-アスパラギナーゼ **L-ASP**
L-アスパラギナーゼ,プレドニゾン,ビンクリスチン(=オンコビン),シタラビン,アドリアマイシン **LAPOCA**
L-アミノ酸酸化酵素 **LAAO**
L-アラニン **L-Ala**
L-アラニンアミノペプチダーゼ **AAP**
L-エチル-L-フェニルチオウレア **EPTU**
L-グルタミン酸-L-アラニン-L-チロシンポリマー(合成抗原) **GAT**
L-スレオ-ジヒドロキシフェニルセリン **L-threo DOPS**
L-ド(ー)パ **LD, L-DOPA, L-dopa, l-dapa, L-dapa**
L-トリプトファン **LTP, L-Trp**
L-フェニルアラニンマスタード・ビンブラスチン **PAVe**
L鎖 **LC**
L鎖沈着病 **LCDD**
L鎖の可変領域〔部〕 **V_L**
L鎖(病) **LCD, L-chain**
L鎖不変部 **CL**
*lacZ*遺伝子 ***lacZ***
LAMB症候群 **NAME syndrome**
LB因子 **LBF**
LD抗原 **LD antigen**
LDLコレステロール **LDL-cholesterol**
LDL沈殿法 **HELP**
LE因子 **LEF, LE factor**
LE細胞 **LE cell**
LE試験 **LE test**
LE標本 **LE prep**
LFD児 **LFD infant**
LFG児 **LFG infant**
LGA児 **LGA infant**
LGL症候群 **LGL syndrome**
LPガス **LPG**
LPS結合蛋白 **LBP**
L/S比 **L/S ratio**
L-α-グリセロリン酸 **L-α-GP**
L-3-メトキシ-4-ヒドロキシフェニルアラニン **L-3-MTO**
L-5-ヒドロキシトリプトファン **L-5-HTP**
L(-)-5,6,7,8-テトラヒドロ葉酸 **H_4FA**

M

Mモード心エコー検査 **MME**
m-ヨードベンジルグアニジン **MIBG**
M指数 **MI**
M線 **M line**
M帯 **M line**
M蛋白 **MP, M protein**
m波 **m wave**
M弁 **MV**
MERSコロナウイルス **MERS-CoV**
Mg排泄の分離 **FMg**
MN式血液型 **MN**
MRK症候群 **MRK**
MSH抑制ホルモン **MIH**

N

N-アセチルアスパラギン酸塩 **NAA**
N-アセチル-4-アミノアンチピリン **NAAP**
N-アセチル-*p*-アミノフェノール **APAP, NAPA, NAPAP**
N-アセチルアルギニン **NAA**
N-アセチルガラクトサミン **GalNAc**
N-アセチル-β-D-グルコサミニダーゼ **NAG**
N-アセチルグルコサミン **GlcNAc**
N-アセチル-L-システイン **NAC**
N-アセチル-L-チロシンエチルエステル **ATEE**
N-アセチルトランスフェラーゼ **NAT**
N-アセチルノイラミン酸 **NAcneu, NAN, NANA, NeuAc, NeuNAc**
N-アセチルプロカインア

ミド **NAPA**
N-アセチルマンノサミン **ManNAc**
N-アセチル-ムラミル-L-アラニル-D-イソグルタメート **MDP**
N-アセチルムラミン酸 **MurNAc**
N-(2-アセトアミド)-2-アミノエタンスルホン酸 **ACES**
N-(2-アセトアミド)イミノジ酢酸 **ADA**
N-(1-アニリノナフチル-4)-マレイミド **ANM**
N-アリルノルモルヒネ **NANM**
N-イソプロピル-*p*-ニトロフェニルエタノールアミン **INPEA**
N-エチル-*N*-ニトロソ尿素 **ENU**
N-エチルマレイミド **NEM**
N-カルボキシアミノ酸無水物 **NCA**
N-グリコリルノイラミン酸 **NeuGc, NeuNGc, NGNA**
N-(7-ジメチルアミノ-4-メチルクマリニル)マレイミド **DACM**
N-ターミナルジスルフィドノット **N-DSK**
N-トシル-L-フェニルアラニルクロロメチルケトン **TPCK**
N-トリス(ヒドロキシメチル)メチル-2-アミノエタンスルホン酸 **TES**
N-ニトロソジエタノールアミン **NDELA**
N-ニトロソジエチルアミン **NDEA**
N-ニトロソピペリジン **NPip**
N-ニトロソピロリジン **NO-PYR, NPr, NPYR**
N-ニトロソブチルウレア **NBU**
N-ニトロソブチル-4-ヒドロキシブチルアミン **BBN**
N-ニトロソモルホリン **NMOR, NNM**
N-パルミトイルアラC **PL-AC**
N-ブチル-*N*-ニトロソ尿素 **BNU**
N-ブロモアセトアミド **NBA**
N-ブロモコハク酸イミド **NBS**
N-ヘプチルヒドロキノリン-*N*-オキシド **HOQNO**
N-ベンゾイル-*p*-アミノサリチル酸 **BPAS**
N-ホルミルグリシンアミドリボチド **FGAR**
N-ホルミル-1-メチオニル-1-ロイシル-1-フェニルアラニン **FMLP**
N-メチルテトラゾールチオール **NMTT**
N′-メチルニコチンアミド **MNA**
N-メチル-D-アスパラギン酸 **NMDA**
N-メチル-D-アスパラギン酸塩 **NMDA**
N-メチル-*N*-アミルニトロサミン **MAN**
N-メチル-*N*′-ニトロソ-*N*-ニトログアニジン **MNG**
N末端副甲状腺ホルモン **PTH-N**
Na-トシル-L-アルギニルクロロメチルケトン **TACK**
Nα-トシル-L-リジルクロロメチルケトン **TLCK**
NADアーゼ **NADase**
NADHテトラゾリン還元酵素 **NADH-TR**
NIH脳卒中スケール **NIHSS**
NPHインスリン **NPH insulin**
N-{*p*-(2-ベンズイミダゾリル)フェニル}マレイミド **BIPM**
N,*N*′-ジアセチル-4,4′-ジアミノフェニルスルホン **DADDS**
N,*N*-ジエチル-*m*-トルアミド **DEET**
N,*N*′-ジベンジルメチルアミン **DBMA**
N,*N* ビス(2-ヒドロキシエチル)-2-アミノエタンスルホン酸 **BES**
N,*N*-メチレンビスアクリルアミド **bis**
N,*N*′-2,7-フルオレニルエネビアセトアミド **2,7-FAA**
N-2-ヒドロキシ〔水酸化〕エチルピペラジン-*N*′-2′-エタンスルホン酸 **HEPES**
N-2-ヒドロキシ〔水酸化〕エチルピラペジン-*N*′-2-プロパンスルホン酸 **HEPPS**
N-2-フルオレニルアセトアミド **2-FAA, FAA**

O

o-イソプロピル *N*-フェニ

ルカルバメート **INPC**
o-トルイジンホウ酸試験 **OTB**
o-トルイジン亜砒酸塩試験 **OTAT**
o-トルイジンホウ酸法 **OTB method**
o-ニトロビフェニル **ONB**
o-ニトロフェニル **ONP**
o-ニトロフェニル-*β*-ガラクトシダーゼ **ONPG-GAL**
o-フェニルフェノール **OPP**
o-フタルアルデヒド **OPA，OPT**
O-ベンゾイルチアミンジスルフィド **BTDS**
o-メチルトランスフェラーゼ **OMT**
o-ヨード馬尿酸塩 **OIH**

P

p-アミノ馬尿酸クリアランス **CPAH, CPAH，Cpah，cpah**
p-アミノ馬尿酸ナトリウムクリアランス **CPAH**
p-ジメチルアミノアゾベンゼン **DAB**
p-ジメチルアミノベンズアルデヒド **DMAB(A)**
P セレクチン糖蛋白リガンド **PSGL**
p-テルフェニル **TP**
p-トルエンスルホン酸(試験) **TSA**
p-ニトロフェニルグアニジノベンゾエート **NPGB**
p-ニトロフェニル酢酸 **NPA**
P 糖蛋白 **P-gp**
P 波 **P**
PA(法) **PA**
PAH 除去率 **E_{PAH}**
PE 標識ストレプトアビジン **SA-PE**
P/O 比 **P/O ratio**
POEMS 症候群(＝クロウ・深瀬症候群) **POEMS**
p,*p*′-ジフルオロ *m*,*m*′-ジニトロジフェニルスルホン **FNPS**
PR 間隔 **PR**

Q

(オーストラリア)Q 熱 **Q fever**
Q 波 **Q**
QAP 治療 **QAP (treatment)**
QI 時間 **QI**
QOL 補正生存期間 **QAS**
QOL 補正生存年 **QALY**
QS 間隔 **QS**
QS 幅 **QS**
QT 延長症候群 **LQTS**
QT 時間 **QT**

R

R 波 **R**
RA 因子陰性脊椎関節炎 **SNSA**
RD 現象 **RD**
Rh 因子 **Rh factor, Rh-factor**
Rh 血液型の分類法 **Rh classes**
Rh(溶血性)疾患 **RhD**
Rh 免疫グロブリン **RhIG**
RI 現象 **RI**
RI 静脈造影 **RNV**
RI 脳槽撮影 **IC**
RNA 依存 DNA ポリメラーゼ **RDDP**
RNA 依存性プロテインキナーゼ **PKR**
RNA 合成酵素 **RNAP**
RNA 分解酵素 **RNase**
RPR カードテスト **RPRCT**
R-R 間隔 **RRI**
RS ウイルス **RSV**

S

S-アデノシルメチオニン **SAM，SAMe**
S-アデノシル-L-ホモシステイン **SAH**
S 期 **S period**
S 状結腸 **S**
S 状結腸鏡 **SIG，Sig, sig**
S 状結腸鏡検査(法) **SIG，Sig，sig, sigmo，Sigmoid**
S 状結腸鏡の **SIG, Sig，sig**
S 波 **S**
SARS コロナウイルス **SARS-CoV**
SD 抗原 **SD antigen**
SD スパイク **SD spike**
SF ブイヨン **SF**
SFD 児 **SFD infant**
SH 基 **SH**
SH 抗原 **SH antigen**
SI 単位 **SI**
SIM 培地 **SIM medium**
SISI 検査 **SISI test**
Sm 抗体(＝可溶性核抗体の一種) **Sm Ab**
SR 変異 **SRM**
(心電図の)ST 部分 **ST**

T

t-ブトキシカルボニル **BOC**
T リンパ球クローン **TLC**
T リンパ球コロニー形成細胞 **TL-CFC**
T リンパ球依存幼若化反応 **TDPR**
T リンパ球活性化因子 **TAF**
T リンパ球関連抗原 **TLAA**
T_3レジンスポンジ摂取率 **T_3-RSU**
T 細胞クローン過剰 **TCE**
T 細胞クローン法 **TC**
T 細胞悪性リンパ腫 **T-ML**
T 細胞依存の **TD**
T 細胞活性化因子 **TAF**
T 細胞急性リンパ性白血病 **TALL, T-ALL**
T 細胞抗原受容体(遺伝子) **TCR**
T 細胞抗原の一種 **Thy-1**
T 細胞受容体 **TCR**
T 細胞成人急性白血病 **TALL, T-ALL**
T 細胞性慢性リンパ球性(白血病) **TCCL**
T 細胞増殖因子 **TCGF**
T 細胞増殖因子受容体 **TCGF-R**
T 細胞増殖反応 **TCPR**
T 細胞代替因子 **TRF**
T 細胞特異的チロシンキナーゼ **Tsk**
T 細胞反応性 **TCR**
T 字包帯 **TBA**
T 線維 **T**
T 波 **T**
T 包帯 **T**
TCA 法 **TCA method**
TNF 受容体 **TNFR**
Toll/インターロイキン 1 受容体 **TIR**
Toll 様受容体 **TLR**
tPA・SK 比較大規模治験(=いわゆるガスト治験) **GUSTO**
TSH 結合抑制性免疫グロブリン **TBII**
TTC 還元法 **TTC reduced method**
T 1 強調画像 **T1WI**
T 2 強調画像 **T2WI**

V

V マックス **Vmax**
V 領域のなかの(変化が少ない)骨組み **FR**
VDT 症候群 **VDT syndrome**

X

X-リポ蛋白 **X-Lp**
X 染色体 **X-C**
X 染色体種(または表面)抗原 **SAX**
X 染色体短腕 **Xp**
X 染色体長腕 **Xq**
X 線エネルギー分光学 **XES**
X 線エネルギー分光計 **XES**
X 線コンピュータ断層撮影 **CT scan**
X 線テレビ **XTV**
X 線テレビジョン **RTV**
X 線 **XR, xr**
X 線医学 **Rnt, Roent, roent**
X 線解析試験 **XAT**
X 線回折 **XRD**
X 線回折粉末 **XDP**
X 線管熱容量 **HU**
X 線技術者 **XRT**
X 線吸収広域微細構造 **EXAFS**
X 線吸収端近傍構造法 **XANES**
X 線吸収端微細構造 **NEXAFS**
X 線吸収微細構造法 **XAFS**
X 線螢光 **XRF**
X 線・螢光写真技術者 **XRPT**
X 線螢光撮影法 **PFG**
X 線検査(法) **Xp, X-p, XP**
X 線光電子分光法 **XPS**
X 線撮影をした **x'd**
X 線写真 **'gram, Xp, X-p, XP**
X 線写真オカルト肺癌 **ROLC**
X 線重複撮影 **polyso**
X 線準備 **X prep.**
X 線小角散乱 **SAXS**
X 線上顎粘膜機能試験 **X-MFT**
X 線照射治療 **XRT**
X 線照射量 **RAD**
X 線照度計 **XIM**
X 線処理量 **RAD**
X 線診断学 **DRNT**
X 線専門医 **Rnt**
X 線直接撮影法 **FSM**
X 線的胸腔容量 **RCV**
X 線透視下腰椎穿刺 **FALP**
X 線動態撮影 **kymo**
X 線発光分光学 **XPS**
X 線微小解析器 **XRM**
X 線皮膚紅斑量 **SED**
X 線平面検出器 **FPD**
X 線放射計器 **XEG**

X 線放射顕微鏡　**XRPM**
X 線放出スペクトル　**XES**
X 線〔放射線〕療法　**XRT**
X 線を照射した　**x'd**
X 線 CT　**XCT**
X 谷　**X**
X(線)単位　**X，Xu，XU**
X(染色体)不活化中心　**XIC，Xic**
X(染色体)不活性中心特異転写(物)　**XIST**
X(染色体)連鎖リンパ球増殖性症候群　**XLS**
X(染色体)連鎖魚鱗癬　**XLI**
X(染色体)連鎖高 IgM 血症　**XHIM**
X(染色体)連鎖性痙性対麻痺　**XSPG**
X(染色体)連鎖劣性腎石症　**XRN**
Xg 血液型(抗原)　**Xg antigen**
XXY 症候群　**XXYsyndrome**

Y

Y 染色体　**Y，YC**
Y 染色体性ジンクフィンガー蛋白　**ZFY**
Y 染色体の性決定領域　**SRY**
Y 染色体連鎖男性決定遺伝子座　**SRY**
Y 谷　**Y**
YY 症候群　**YY syndrome**

ギリシャ文字

α アクチン　**ACTN**
α アミノ酸窒素　**AAN**
α イソ酪酸　**αIB, α-IB, AIB**
α エンドルフィン　**aEP, α-EP**
α ガラクトシダーゼ　**Ags, GLA**
α キモトリプシン　**α-chy**
α グリセロホスフェイトデヒドロゲナーゼ　**α-GD**
α ケトグルタレート　**α-KG**
α 抗トリプシン　**αAT, AAT**
α 重鎖病　**αHCD, α-HCD**
α 水酸化酪酸脱水素酵素　**HBD**
α トコフェロール　**α-T**
α ナフタレン酢酸　**NAA**
α ナフチルイソチオシアネート　**ANIT**
α ナフチルチオウレア　**ANTU**
α ナフトフラボン　**ANF**
α ハプトグロビン　**HPA**
α ヒドラジノヒスチジン　**α-HH**
α ヒドロキシブチレートデヒドロゲナーゼ　**HDBH**
α ヒドロキシ酪酸脱水素酵素　**α-HBD**
α フェトプロテイン　**αf, α-f, AFP, aFP**
α フェニル-1-*N*-ブチルニトロン　**PBN**
α フェニルブチル尿素　**PBU**
α フコシダーゼ　**αFUC, α-FUC**
α ブンガロトキシン　**α-Bgt, ABgT, ABTX**
α ヘキサクロロシクロヘキサン　**α-HCH**
α メチル-*m*-チロシン　**α-MMT**
α メチル-*p*-チロシン　**α-MPT**
α メチルジオキシフェニルアラニン　**AMD**
α メチルチロシン　**AMT**
α メチルド(ー)パ　**AMD**
α メチルマンノシド　**αMM, α-MM**
α モザイクウイルス　**AMV**
α リポ蛋白　**α-LP**
α-α′-ジアミノピメリン酸　**DAP**
α-L-フコシダーゼ　**FUCA**
α-*N*-アセチルガラクトサミニダーゼ　**NAGA**
α-ケト-γ-メチルチオ酪酸　**KMTB**
α-ケトグルタル酸　**KG**
α-水酸化酪酸脱水素酵素　**HBDH**
$α_1$アンチキモトリプシン　**$α_1$AC**
$α_1$アンチトリプシン　**$α_1$AT, $α_1$-AT**
$α_1$グロブリン　**A_1**
$α_1$抗トリプシン　**$α_1$AT, $α_1$-AT**
$α_1$酸性糖蛋白　**$α_1$-AG**
$α_1$マイクログロブリン　**$α_1$-MG**
$α_1$ミクログロブリン　**$α_1$-M, $α_1$-MG**
$α_2$プラスミン阻害物質〔インヒビター〕　**alpha-2 PM**
$α_2$アンチトリプシン　**$α_2$AT, $α_2$-AT**
$α_2$グロブリン　**A_2**
$α_2$抗トリプシン　**$α_2$AT, $α_2$-AT**
$α_2$プラスミン阻害物質〔インヒビター〕　**$α_2$-PI, APL**
$α_2$マクログロブリン　**$α_2$-M, alpha-2 M**
β アミノイソ酪酸　**β-AIB**
β アラニン　**β-a, β-Ala**
β エステル分解酵素　**β-Est**
β エンドルフィン　**β-EP**
β エンドルフィン免疫反応性　**BEPI**
β エンドルフィン様免疫反応性　**BELIR**
β ガラクトシダーゼ　**β-gal**
β ガラクトシダーゼ 1　**GLB1**
β ガラクトシダーゼ 2　**GLB2**
(大腸菌の)β ガラクトシダーゼ遺伝子　***lacZ***
β 型トランスフォーミング増殖因子　**TGF-β**
β グルクロニダーゼ　**β-GL, GRD, GRS, GUSB**
β グロブリン　**B**
β 神経成長因子　**BNGF**
β 脂肪刺激放出ホルモン　**β-LPH**
β 遮断薬　**BB**
β 水酸化グルタミン酸　**β-HG, BHG**
β 水酸化酪酸脱水素酵素　**HBD**
β 線　**β ray**
β 超低比重リポ蛋白

β-**VLDL**
βトコトリエノール β-**T-3**
βトコフェロール β-**T**
βトロンボグロブリン β-**TG**
βヒト絨毛性ゴナドトロピン β-**HCG**
βヒドロキシ-βメチルグルタリル・コカルボキシラーゼA **HMG-CoA**
βヒドロキシアシル CoA デヒドロゲナーゼ **HOADH**
βブロッカーによる心発作治験 **B HAT**
βプロピオラクトン **BPL, BPLA**
βブンガロトキシン β-**BuTX**
βメタゾン β-**M**
β溶血性連鎖状球菌 β**HS**, β-**HS**
β(型)溶血連鎖球菌 **BHS**
βラクタマーゼ抵抗性抗菌薬 **BLRA**
βラクトグロブリン **BLG**
βリポ蛋白 β-**LP**, **BL**
βA 4 蛋白 β/**A4**
βリポ蛋白 **BLP**, **BLp**
β-D-ガラクトシダーゼ **beta GAL**
β-フェニル-γ-アミノ酪酸 **PhGABA**
β 2′-デオキシチオグアノシン β-**TGdR**
$β_2$グリコプロテイン 1 **beta2 GP1**
$β_2$ミクログロブリン $β_2$-**MG**, $β_2$-**m**, $β_2$**M**, $β_2$-**M**, B_2**M**, $β_2$**m**, **BMG**
γ **Gm**
γアミノ-β-ヒドロキシ酪酸 **GABOB**
γアミノ酪酸 γ**Abu**, **GABA**
γアミノ酪酸トランスアミナーゼ **GABA-T**
γエンドルフィン γ-**EP**
γオリザノール γ**Oz**
γカルボキシグルタミン酸 **Gla**
γグルタミル-p-ニトロアニリド **GGPNA**
γグルタミルシステイニルグリシン **GSH**
γグルタミルシステイン合成酵素 **GGCS**
γグルタミルトランスフェラーゼ γ-**GT**, **GGT**
γグルタミルトランスペプチダーゼ γ-**GTP**, **GGTP**
γグロブリン **G**, **GG**
γ脂肪刺激放出ホルモン γ-**LPH**
γセミノプロテイン γ-**Sm**, γ-**SM**
γ線 **GR**
γ線検出器 **GARD**
Γトコフェロール Γ-**T**
γヒドロキシ酪酸 **GHB**
γビニル GABA **GVG**
γフェトプロテイン **GFP**
γレントゲン **GR**, **gr**
γ六塩酸ベンゼン γ-**BHC**
γH 鎖病 γ-**HCD**
δアミノレブリン酸 δ-**ALA**
δアミノレブリン酸合成酵素 δ-**ALA-S**
δトコフェロール δ-**T**
δヒドロキシ-γ-オキソ-L-ノルバリン **HON**
δ-9-テトラヒドロ〔四水酸化〕カンナビノール **THC**
Δ′-ピロリン-5-カルボキシル酸 **PC**
εアミノカプロン酸 **EACA**
κ鎖 κ **chain**
μ重鎖病 μ**HCD**
ρ因子 ρ-**factor**

医学略語コンパクト(第2版)
ISBN978-4-263-73186-4

2006年 4月20日　第1版第1刷発行
2018年10月10日　第2版第1刷発行

監修者　富野康日己

発行者　白石泰夫

発行所　医歯薬出版株式会社

〒113-8612　東京都文京区本駒込1-7-10
TEL.(03)5395-7640(編集)・7616(販売)
FAX.(03)5395-7624(編集)・8563(販売)
URL https://www.ishiyaku.co.jp/
郵便振替番号　00190-5-13816

印刷／製本・アイワード

MEMO MEMO MEMO

MEMO MEMO MEMO

MEMO MEMO MEMO

MEMO MEMO MEMO

EMO MEMO MEMO

MEMO MEMO MEM

M